CLINICAL PROCEDURES IN EMERGENCY MEDICINE

ASSOCIATE EDITORS

Catherine B. Custalow, MD, PhD
Associate Professor, Retired
Department of Emergency Medicine
University of Virginia School of Medicine
Charlottesville, Virginia

Arjun S. Chanmugam, MD, MBA
Associate Professor and Director of Education
Department of Emergency Medicine
The Johns Hopkins School of Medicine
Baltimore, Maryland

Carl R. Chudnofsky, MD
Chairman
Department of Emergency Medicine
Albert Einstein Medical Center
Associate Professor
Jefferson Medical College
Philadelphia, Pennsylvania

LTC John McManus, MD, FACEP
Adjunct Assistant Professor
Department of Emergency Medicine
Oregon Health and Science University
Portland, Oregon
Clinical Research Physician
Army Institute of Surgical Research
Brooke Army Medical Center
Fort Sam Houston, Texas

CLINICAL PROCEDURES IN EMERGENCY MEDICINE

FIFTH EDITION

EDITORS

James R. Roberts, MD, FACEP, FAAEM, FACMT
Professor of Emergency Medicine
Vice Chair, Department of Emergency Medicine
Senior Consultant, Division of Toxicology
Drexel University College of Medicine
Hahnemann University Medical Center
Chairman
Department of Emergency Medicine
Director, Division of Toxicology
Mercy Catholic Medical Center
Philadelphia, Pennsylvania

Jerris R. Hedges, MD, MS
Professor and Dean
John A. Burns School of Medicine
University of Hawaii—Manoa
Honolulu, Hawaii
Professor and Vice-Dean, Emeritus
Department of Emergency Medicine
Oregon Health and Science University
School of Medicine
Portland, Oregon

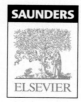

SAUNDERS

ELSEVIER

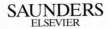

1600 John F. Kennedy Blvd.
Ste 1800
Philadelphia, PA 19103-2899

CLINICAL PROCEDURES IN EMERGENCY MEDICINE   ISBN: 978-1-4160-3623-4
Copyright © 2010 by Saunders, an imprint of Elsevier Inc.

Previous editions copyrighted 2004, 1998, 1991, 1985.

Library of Congress Cataloging-in-Publication Data
 Clinical procedures in emergency medicine / editors, James R. Roberts, Jerris R. Hedges ; associate editors, Catherine B. Custalow ... [et al.].—5th ed.
     p. ; cm.
 Includes bibliographical references and index.
 ISBN 978-1-4160-3623-4
 1. Emergency medicine. I. Roberts, James R., 1946- II. Hedges, Jerris R. III. Title: Emergency medicine.
 [DNLM: 1. Emergency Treatment. 2. Emergencies. WB 105 C641 2010]
 RC86.7.C55 2010
 616.02′5—dc22   2008041760

Acquisitions Editor: Stefanie Jewell-Thomas
Developmental Editor: Dee Simpson
Design Direction: Steven Stave
Illustrations Manager: Kari Wszolek
Marketing Manager: Courtney Ingram

Printed in United States of America

Last digit is the print number: 9 8 7 6 5 4 3 2 1

To Lydia, my eternally supportive wife; to Martha, a newly minted RN with unbridled enthusiasm and passion for emergency medicine; and to Matt, always an inspiration for everything. You all make my life worthwhile.

To Cathy Custalow, MD who picked up the slack everywhere.

To Gary Setnik, MD and Todd Thomsen, MD for their illustrative input.

To Rose Bacher who kept us on target and productive.

To the folks at Elsevier who made this edition a reality: Dee Simpson for gargantuan help with all aspects of this project; to Judy Fletcher, supportive yet again; Berta Steiner who made it all come together.

J.R.R.

As the Fifth edition comes together, I wish to acknowledge the support that Catherine Custalow has brought to this edition by enhancing the overall text and stepping up as I ventured into new areas of responsibility. Without her efforts, this edition would not be possible.

As always, I am appreciative of my family and the years of sacrifice they have made such that this knowledge could be made available to aid future generations of emergency physicians and other practitioners—who themselves seek to alleviate suffering and extend lives.

J.R.H.

To my son, Nick and to the memory of my daughter, Lauren. To James and Doris Bomberger who first were parents and now are friends. To Dr. Harold F. Young for reasons that are obvious to anyone who knows him.

C.B.C.

To my wonderful wife Karen, thank you for your inspiration, support and remarkable partnership; to Sydney, William and Nathan who will always be reminders of what is truly important; to my father who helped to foster the passion of medical education as a public service. Finally to those who practice and teach emergency medicine, may this book serve you well.

A.S.C.

The Fifth edition of the book is dedicated to my past, current, and future residents at Albert Einstein Medical Center… your passion for learning, your devotion to healing, and your zeal for life are truly inspirational.

C.R.C.

My dedication is first in memory of my Grandfather William "Big Daddy" McDonald for his love, wisdom, and guidance. Also, for my family Laura and our two children for their current and future love and support. Finally, for our military personnel who continually sacrifice for our freedom.

J.G.M.

Benjamin S. Abella, MD, MPhil
Assistant Professor, Department of Emergency Medicine
and Associate Director, Center for Resuscitation
Science, University of Pennsylvania, Philadelphia,
Pennsylvania
Artificial Perfusion during Cardiac Arrest

Bruce D. Adams, MD, FACEP
Clinical Professor of Emergency Medicine, Medical
College of Georgia, Augusta, Georgia; Chief,
Department of Clinical Investigation, and Chief,
Department of Emergency Medicine, William
Beaumont Army Medical Center, Fort Bliss, Texas;
Colonel, Medical Corps, United States Army
*Central Venous Catheterization and Central Venous Pressure
Monitoring*

James T. Amsterdam, DMD, MD, MMM, FACEP, FACPE
Professor of Clinical Emergency Medicine, Penn State
University College of Medicine, Hershey; Adjunct
Professor of Emergency Medicine, Drexel University
College of Medicine, Philadelphia; Chair/Service Line
Director, Department of Emergency Medicine, York
Hospital, York, Pennsylvania
Regional Anesthesia of the Head and Neck

Heatherlee Bailey, MD, FAAEM, FCCM
Assistant Professor of Emergency Medicine, Director of
Critical Care Education, and Medical Student Critical
Care Clerkship Director, Department of Emergency
Medicine, Drexel University College of Medicine,
Philadelphia, Pennsylvania
Mechanical Ventilation

J. Dave Barry, MD
Clinical Assistant Adjunct Professor, Department of
Surgery and Emergency Medicine, University of
Texas Health Science Center at San Antonio, San
Antonio, Texas; Adjunct Assistant Professor,
Department of Military and Emergency Medicine,
Uniformed Services University of the Health
Sciences, Bethesda, Maryland; Faculty Emergency
Physician, Department of Emergency Medicine, and
Associate Program Director, San Antonio Uniformed
Services Health Education Consortium (SAUSHEC)
Emergency Medicine Residency Program, Brooke
Army Medical Center, Fort Sam Houston, Texas
Vital Signs Measurement

Steven J. Bauer, MD
Clinical Assistant Professor of Emergency Medicine,
West Virginia University Hospitals-East; Jefferson
Memorial Hospital, Ranson, West Virginia
Alternative Methods of Drug Administration

Lance B. Becker, MD, FAHA
Professor, Department of Emergency Medicine, and
Director, Center for Resuscitation Science,
University of Pennsylvania, Philadelphia,
Pennsylvania
Artificial Perfusion during Cardiac Arrest

Kip Benko, MD, MS
Assistant Clinical Professor of Emergency Medicine,
University of Pittsburgh School of Medicine; Faculty
Staff, Presbyterian University Hospital, Pittsburgh,
Pennsylvania
Emergency Dental Procedures

Edward S. Bessman, MD
Assistant Professor, Department of Emergency
Medicine, The Johns Hopkins University;
Chairman, Department of Emergency Medicine,
Johns Hopkins Bayview Medical Center, Baltimore,
Maryland
Emergency Cardiac Pacing

Courtney A. Bethel, MD
Clinical Assistant Professor of Emergency Medicine,
Drexel University College of Medicine—Medical
College of Pennsylvania and Hahnemann Medical
School; Staff Physician, Mercy Catholic Medical
Center, Philadelphia, Pennsylvania
Burn Care Procedures

Barbara K. Blok, MD
Assistant Professor, Division of Emergency Medicine,
University of Colorado Denver School of Medicine,
Aurora; Assistant Residency Director, Denver Health
Residency in Emergency Medicine, Denver Health
Medical Center, Denver, Colorado
Thoracentesis

Michael E. Boczar, DO
Assistant Clinical Professor, Department of Emergency
Medicine, University of Michigan, Ann Arbor, and
Hurley Hospital, Flint, Michigan
Resuscitative Thoracotomy

Sudip Bose, MD, FACEP, FAAEM
Assistant Clinical Professor, Department of Emergency Medicine, University of Illinois, Chicago; Attending Emergency Physician, Department of Emergency Medicine, Advocate Christ Medical Center, Oak Lawn, Illinois; Former Major, United States Army
Cricothyrotomy and Transtracheal Jet Ventilation

Thomas A. Brabson, DO, MBA, FACOEP, FACEP
Clinical Associate Professor, Department of Emergency Medicine, Philadelphia College of Osteopathic Medicine, Philadelphia, Pennsylvania; Medical Director, Department of Emergency Medicine, City Campus, and Department of Emergency Medical Services, AtlantiCare Regional Medical Center, Atlantic City, New Jersey
Prehospital Immobilization

William J. Brady, MD
Professor of Emergency Medicine and Medicine, University of Virginia; Vice Chair, Department of Emergency Medicine, University of Virginia Hospitals, Charlottesville, Virginia
Basic Electrocardiographic Techniques

G. Richard Braen, MD
Professor and Chairman, Department of Emergency Medicine, and Assistant Dean of Graduate Medical Education, University at Buffalo School of Medicine, Buffalo, New York
Culdocentesis

N. Adam Brown, MD
Clinical Instructor, Robert Wood Johnson, New Brunswick; Attending Physician, Robert Wood Johnson at Rahway, Rahway, New Jersey
Otolaryngologic Procedures

James H. Bryan, MD, PhD
Assistant Professor of Emergency Medicine, Oregon Health and Science University; Assistant Chief, Emergency Medicine, Veterans Affairs Medical Center, Portland, Oregon
Alternative Methods of Drug Administration

Kenneth H. Butler, DO
Associate Professor of Emergency Medicine, Department of Emergency Medicine, University of Maryland School of Medicine; Associate Director, Emergency Medicine Residency, University of Maryland Medical Center, Baltimore, Maryland
Incision and Drainage

Stacie E. Byers, DO, FACEP
Attending Physician, Emergency Medicine, St. Anthony Medical Center, Denver, Colorado
Splinting Techniques

Sharon K. Carney, MD
Clinical Assistant Professor of Emergency Medicine, Department of Emergency Medicine, Drexel University College of Medicine, Philadelphia; Director, Department of Emergency Medicine, Mercy Fitzgerald Hospital, Darby, Pennsylvania
Intravenous Regional Anesthesia

Merle A. Carter, MD, FACEP
Director, Emergency Medicine Residency Program, Albert Einstein Medical Center; Assistant Professor, Jefferson Medical College, Thomas Jefferson University, Philadelphia, Pennsylvania
Compartment Syndrome Evaluation

Theodore C. Chan, MD
Professor of Clinical Medicine, University of California, San Diego; Medical Director, Department of Emergency Medicine, University of California, San Diego, Hospitals, San Diego, California
Basic Electrocardiographic Techniques

Theodore A. Christopher, MD
Professor and Chairman, Department of Emergency Medicine, Thomas Jefferson University, Philadelphia, Pennsylvania
Injection Therapy of Bursitis and Tendinitis

Carl R. Chudnofsky, MD
Chairman, Department of Emergency Medicine, Albert Einstein Medical Center; Associate Professor, Jefferson Medical College, Philadelphia, Pennsylvania
Splinting Techniques

Joseph E. Clinton, MD
Professor and Head, Department of Emergency Medicine, University of Minnesota School of Medicine; Chief, Department of Emergency Medicine, Hennepin County Medical Center, Minneapolis, Minnesota
Basic Airway Management and Decision-Making

Wendy C. Coates, MD
Professor of Medicine, and Chair, Acute Care College, David Geffen School of Medicine at UCLA, Los Angeles; Director, Medical Education, Department of Emergency Medicine, Harbor-UCLA Medical Center, Torrance, California
Anorectal Procedures

Catherine B. Custalow, MD, PhD
Associate Professor, Retired, Department of Emergency Medicine, University of Virginia School of Medicine, Charlottesville, Virginia
Educational Aspects of Emergency Department Procedures

Anthony J. Dean, MD
Assistant Professor of Emergency Medicine and Assistant Professor of Emergency Medicine in Radiology, Director, Division of Emergency Ultrasonography, University of Pennsylvania Medical Center, Philadelphia, Pennsylvania
Bedside Laboratory and Microbiologic Procedures

Paul T. DeFlorio, MD
Adjunct Assistant Professor, Department of Military and Emergency Medicine, Uniformed Services University of the Health Sciences, Bethesda, Maryland; Staff Emergency Physician, Wilford Hall Medical Center, Lackland Air Force Base, Texas
Central Venous Catheterization and Central Venous Pressure Monitoring

Kenneth Deitch, DO
Assistant Professor, Jefferson Medical College, Thomas Jefferson University; Associate Research Director, and Attending Physician, Department of Emergency Medicine, Albert Einstein Medical Center, Philadelphia, Pennsylvania
Intraosseous Infusion

William R. Dennis, MD, MPH
Head of EMS for Navy Medicine East and National Capital Area, Emergency Medicine, Naval Medical Center Portsmouth, Portsmouth, Virginia
Ophthalmologic Procedures

Denis J. Dollard, MD
Clinical Assistant Professor, Department of Emergency Medicine, Drexel University College of Medicine; Director, Emergency Medicine, Mercy Hospital of Philadelphia, Philadelphia, Pennsylvania
Radiation in Pregnancy and Clinical Issues of Radiocontrast Agents

Timothy B. Erickson, MD, FACEP, FAACT, FACMT
Professor, Emergency Medicine and Clinical Toxicology, Associate Head, Department of Emergency Medicine, and Director, Division of Clinical Toxicology, University of Illinois at Chicago, Chicago, Illinois
Procedures Pertaining to Hypothermia and Hyperthermia

Brian D. Euerle, MD
Associate Professor, University of Maryland School of Medicine; Attending Physician, Emergency Department, University of Maryland Medical Center, Baltimore, Maryland
Spinal Puncture and Cerebrospinal Fluid Examination

Charles J. Fasano, DO
Assistant Professor, Department of Emergency Medicine, Jefferson Medical College; Attending Physician, Department of Emergency Medicine, Albert Einstein Medical Center, Philadelphia, Pennsylvania
Physical and Chemical Restraint

Lisa Mackowiak Filippone, MD
Assistant Professor, Emergency Medicine, UMDNJ Robert Wood Johnson Medical School; Attending Physician, Emergency Medicine, Cooper University Hospital, Camden, New Jersey
Ultrasound-Guided Procedures

Michael T. Fitch, MD, PhD
Associate Professor of Emergency Medicine, Wake Forest University School of Medicine, Winston-Salem, North Carolina
Abdominal Hernia Reduction

Brenda A. Foley, MD, FACEP
Clinical Assistant Professor, Department of Emergency Medicine, Thomas Jefferson University, Philadelphia; Attending Physician, Department of Emergency Medicine, Doylestown Hospital, Doylestown, Pennsylvania
Injection Therapy of Bursitis and Tendinitis

Robert T. Gerhardt, MD, MPH, FACEP, FAAEM
Associate Professor, Department of Military and Emergency Medicine, Uniformed Services University of the Health Sciences, Bethesda, Maryland; Staff Physician, San Antonio Uniformed Services Health Education Consortium (SAUSHEC) Emergency Medicine Residency Program, Brooke Army Medical Center, Fort Sam Houston, Texas
Assessment of Implantable Devices

Diane L. Gorgas, MD
Associate Professor and Residency Director, Department of Emergency Medicine, The Ohio State University; The Ohio State University Medical Center, Columbus, Ohio
Vital Signs Measurement; Transfusion Therapy: Blood and Blood Products and Reversal of Warfarin-Induced Coagulopathy

Steven M. Green, MD, FACEP
Professor of Emergency Medicine and Pediatrics, Loma Linda University, Loma Linda, California
Systemic Analgesia and Sedation for Procedures

Brett S. Greenfield, DO, FACOEP/CAQ-EMS
Medical Director, MidAtlantic MedEvac, and Attending Physician, Department of Emergency Medicine, AtlantiCare Regional Medical Center, Atlantic City, New Jersey
Prehospital Immobilization

Maria Halluska-Handy, MD
Assistant Director, Emergency Medicine Residency Program, Albert Einstein Medical Center; Department of Emergency Medicine, Jefferson Medical College, Thomas Jefferson University, Philadelphia, Pennsylvania
Management of Amputations

Richard J. Harper, MS, MD
Associate Professor, Emergency Medicine, Oregon Health and Science University; Chief, Emergency Medicine Service, Portland Veterans Affairs Medical Center, Portland, Oregon
Pericardiocentesis

Richard A. Harrigan, MD
Professor of Emergency Medicine, Temple University; Attending Physician, Department of Emergency Medicine, Temple University Hospitals, Philadelphia, Pennsylvania
Basic Electrocardiographic Techniques

Randy B. Hebert, MD
Attending Physician, Advocate Illinois Masonic Medical Center, Chicago, Illinois
Cricothyrotomy and Transtracheal Jet Ventilation

Jerris R. Hedges, MD, MS
Professor and Dean, John A. Burns School of Medicine, University of Hawaii—Manoa, Honolulu, Hawaii; Professor and Vice-Dean, Emeritus, Department of Emergency Medicine, Oregon Health and Science University School of Medicine, Portland, Oregon
Ophthalmologic Procedures

Christopher P. Holstege, MD
Associate Professor, Departments of Emergency Medicine and Pediatrics, and Chief, Division of Medical Toxicology, University of Virginia School of Medicine; Medical Director, Blue Ridge Poison Center, University of Virginia Health System, Charlottesville, Virginia
Decontamination of the Poisoned Patient

Laura R. Hopson, MD
Assistant Professor, Clinical Track, University of Michigan Health System, Ann Arbor, Michigan
Pharmacologic Adjuncts to Intubation

J. Stephen Huff, MD
Associate Professor of Emergency Medicine and Neurology, University of Virginia Health System, Charlottesville, Virginia
Special Neurologic Tests and Procedures

Charlene Babcock Irvin, MD, FACEP
Research Director, Emergency Medicine Department, St. John Hospital and Medical Center; Associate Clinical Professor, Wayne State University School of Medicine, Detroit, Michigan
Autotransfusion

Tim Janchar, MD
Emergency Physician, Legacy Emmanuel Hospital, Portland, Oregon
Arterial Puncture and Cannulation

Lewis J. Kaplan, MD, FACS
Associate Professor of Surgery, Director, Emergency General Surgery, Yale University School of Medicine, New Haven, Connecticut
Mechanical Ventilation

Eric D. Katz, MD
Program Director and Vice-Chair for Education, Maricopa Medical Center, Phoenix, Arizona
Commonly Used Formulas and Calculations

John J. Kelly, DO, FACEP, FAAEM
Associate Chair, Department of Emergency Medicine, Albert Einstein Medical Center; Associate Professor of Emergency Medicine, Jefferson Medical College, Philadelphia, Pennsylvania
Nerve Blocks of the Thorax and Extremities

Kevin P. Kilgore, MD
Assistant Clinical Professor, University of Minnesota School of Medicine, Minneapolis; Senior Staff Physician, Department of Emergency Medicine, Regions Hospital, St. Paul, Minnesota
Regional Anesthesia of the Head and Neck

Thomas D. Kirsch, MD, MPH
Associate Professor, and Director of Operations, Department of Emergency Medicine, The Johns Hopkins School of Medicine, Baltimore, Maryland
Tube Thoracostomy

Kevin J. Knoop, MD, MS, Capt, MC, USN
Assistant Professor of Military and Emergency Medicine, Department of Military and Emergency Medicine, Uniformed Services University of the Health Sciences, Bethesda, Maryland; Executive Officer, US Naval Hospital, Yokosuka, Japan
Ophthalmologic Procedures

Frederick K. Korley, MD
The Robert E. Meyerhoff Assistant Professor, Department of Emergency Medicine, The Johns Hopkins School of Medicine; Attending Physician, Department of Emergency Medicine, The Johns Hopkins Hospital, Baltimore, Maryland
Management of Increased Intracranial Pressure and Intracranial Shunts

Baruch Krauss, MD, EdM, FAAP, FACEP
Associate Professor of Pediatrics, Harvard Medical School; Senior Associate Physician in Medicine, Division of Emergency Medicine, Children's Hospital Boston, Boston, Massachusetts
Devices for Assessing Oxygenation and Ventilation; Systemic Analgesia and Sedation for Procedures

Diann M. Krywko, MD
Assistant Professor and Emergency Medicine Residency Curriculum Director, Medical University of South Carolina, Charleston, South Carolina; Graduate Lecturer, University of Michigan School of Health Professions, Flint, Michigan
Indwelling Vascular Devices: Emergency Access and Management

Richard L. Lammers, MD
Professor of Emergency Medicine, Michigan State University College of Human Medicine, East Lansing; Research Director, Kalamazoo Center for Medical Studies, Kalamazoo, Michigan
Principles of Wound Management; Methods of Wound Closure

Patricia L. Lanter, MD
Assistant Professor, Emergency Medicine, Dartmouth Medical School, Hanover; Dartmouth Hitchcock Medical Center, Lebanon, New Hampshire
Venous Cutdown

David C. Lee, MD
Clinical Associate Professor, Emergency Medicine, New York School of Medicine, New York; Director of Research, Emergency Medicine, North Shore University Hospital, Manhasset, New York
Bedside Laboratory and Microbiologic Procedures

Matthew R. Levine, MD
Assistant Professor, Department of Emergency Medicine, Northwestern University Feinberg School of Medicine; Attending Physician, Northwestern Memorial Hospital, Chicago, Illinois
Foreign Body Removal

Shan W. Liu, MD, MPH
Instructor, Harvard Medical School; Faculty, Massachusetts General Hospital, Boston, Massachusetts
Peripheral Intravenous Access

Marie M. Lozon, MD
Associate Professor of Emergency Medicine and Pediatrics, University of Michigan Medical School; Director of Children's Emergency Services, University of Michigan Health System, Ann Arbor, Michigan
Pediatric Vascular Access and Blood Sampling Techniques

Matthew L. Lyon, MD
Associate Professor of Emergency Medicine, and Director of Emergency Ultrasound, Department of Emergency Medicine, Medical College of Georgia, Augusta, Georgia
Central Venous Catheterization and Central Venous Pressure Monitoring

Sharon E. Mace, MD, FACEP, FAAP
Professor of Medicine, Department of Medicine, Cleveland Clinic Lerner College of Medicine of Case Western University; Director, Observation Unit, and Director, Pediatric Education/Quality Improvement, Department of Emergency Medicine, Cleveland Clinic; Faculty, Department of Emergency Medicine, Metrohealth Medical Center/Cleveland Clinic Emergency Medicine Residency Program, Cleveland, Ohio
Cricothyrotomy and Transtracheal Jet Ventilation

David E. Manthey, MD
Director, Undergraduate Medical Education, Wake Forest University School of Medicine, Winston-Salem, North Carolina
Abdominal Hernia Reduction

John A. Marx, MD
Adjunct Professor of Emergency Medicine, University of North Carolina, Chapel Hill; Chair, Department of Emergency Medicine, Carolinas Medical Center, Charlotte, North Carolina
Peritoneal Procedures

Phillip E. Mason, MD, Maj, USAF, MC
Faculty Physician, Department of Emergency Medicine, Wilford Hall Medical Center, San Antonio, Texas
Devices for Assessing Oxygenation and Ventilation; Basic Airway Management and Decision-Making

Anthony S. Mazzeo, MD, FACEP, FAAEM
Clinical Assistant Professor, Emergency Medicine, Drexel University College of Medicine, Philadelphia; Attending Physician and Associate Director, Emergency Medicine, Mercy Fitzgerald Hospital, Darby, Pennsylvania
Burn Care Procedures

Douglas L. McGee, DO
Assistant Dean, Jefferson Medical College; Chief Academic Officer, and Emergency Medicine Residency Program Director, Department of Emergency Medicine, Albert Einstein Medical Center, Philadelphia, Pennsylvania
Local and Topical Anesthesia; Podiatric Procedures

John W. McGill, MD
Assistant Professor, University of Minnesota School of Medicine; Senior Associate Faculty, Hennepin County Medical Center, Minneapolis, Minnesota
Tracheal Intubation

Robert M. McNamara, MD
Professor and Chair, Department of Emergency Medicine, Temple University School of Medicine, Philadelphia, Pennsylvania
Management of Common Dislocations

Pauline E. Meekins, MD
Clinical Instructor, Division of Emergency Medicine, Medical University of South Carolina, Charleston, South Carolina
Decontamination of the Poisoned Patient

Dave Milzman, MD, FACEP
Professor of Emergency Medicine and Adjunct Professor of Physiology, Georgetown University School of Medicine; Research Director, and Senior Faculty, Georgetown University/Washington Hospital Center Emergency Medicine Residency, Washington Hospital Center, Washington, DC
Arterial Puncture and Cannulation

Bohdan M. Minczak, MS, MD, PhD
Assistant Professor, and Interim Vice Chairman, Department of Emergency Medicine, Methodist Hospital Division, Thomas Jefferson University Hospital; Associate Professor of Physiology, Philadelphia College of Osteopathic Medicine, Philadelphia, Pennsylvania
Techniques for Supraventricular Tachycardias; Defibrillation and Cardioversion

Daniel S. Morrison, MD, RDMS, FACEP
Assistant Residency Director, Wayne State University/ Sinai-Grace Hospital Emergency Medicine Residency Program, and Assistant Professor of Emergency Medicine, Wayne State University; Director of Emergency Medicine Ultrasound, Detroit Medical Center, Detroit, Michigan
Arthrocentesis

David W. Munter, MD, MBA
Assistant Clinical Professor, Emergency Medicine, Eastern Virginia Medical School, Norfolk; Director, Emergency Medicine Department, Sentara Obici Hospital, Suffolk, Virginia
Esophageal Foreign Bodies

Kathleen A. Neacy, MD
Associate Professor, Loyola University Medical Center, Maywood, Illinois
Tracheostomy Care

Edward A. Panacek, MD, MPH
Professor of Emergency Medicine, University of California, Davis; Director, Office of Clinical Trials, University of California, Davis, Medical Center, Sacramento, California
Balloon Tamponade of Gastroesophageal Varices; Arthrocentesis

Steven J. Parrillo, DO, FACOEP, FACEP
Associate Professor, Philadelphia College of Osteopathic Medicine, and Jefferson Medical College; Attending Physician, Department of Emergency Medicine, Faculty, Emergency Medicine Residency, and Medical Director, Emergency Department, Einstein Elkins Park Hospital, Albert Einstein Medical Center, Philadelphia, Pennsylvania
Arthrocentesis

Margarita E. Pena, MD, FACEP
Associate Residency Director, Emergency Medicine Department, and Medical Director, Clinical Decision Unit, St. John Hospital and Medical Center; Associate Clinical Professor, Wayne State University School of Medicine, Detroit, Michigan
Autotransfusion

James A. Pfaff, MD
Assistant Professor, Department of Military and Emergency Medicine, Uniformed Services University of the Health Sciences, Bethesda, Maryland; Staff Physician, San Antonio Uniformed Services Health Education Consortium (SAUSHEC) Emergency Medicine Residency Program, Brooke Army Medical Center, Fort Sam Houston, Texas
Assessment of Implantable Devices

David Lee Pierce, MD
Assistant Professor of Clinical Emergency Medicine, and Clerkship Director, Emergency Medicine, University at Buffalo School of Medicine, Buffalo, New York
Culdocentesis

Heather M. Prendergast, MD, FACEP
Associate Professor, Emergency Medicine, and Residency Research Director, University of Illinois at Chicago, Chicago, Illinois
Procedures Pertaining to Hypothermia and Hyperthermia

Beatrice D. Probst, MD, FACEP
Associate Professor of Medicine and Surgery, Loyola University Stritch School of Medicine; Assistant Director, Emergency Department, Loyola University Health System, Foster G. McGaw Hospital, Maywood, Illinois
Emergency Childbirth

Robert F. Reardon, MD
Assistant Professor, Department of Emergency, University of Minnesota School of Medicine; Faculty Physician, Department of Emergency Medicine, Hennepin County Medical Center, Minneapolis, Minnesota
Basic Airway Management and Decision-Making; Tracheal Intubation

Emanuel Rivers, MD, MPH
Vice Chairman and Research Director, Department of Emergency Medicine, Henry Ford Hospital, Detroit, Michigan
Resuscitative Thoracotomy

Ralph J. Riviello, MD, MS
Associate Professor, Department of Emergency Medicine, Drexel University College of Medicine; Attending Physician, Hahnemann University Hospital, Philadelphia, Pennsylvania
Otolaryngologic Procedures

James R. Roberts, MD, FACEP, FAAEM, FACMT
Professor of Emergency Medicine, Vice Chair, Department of Emergency Medicine, Drexel University College of Medicine; Chairman, Department of Emergency Medicine, Director, Division of Toxicology, Mercy Catholic Medical Center, Philadelphia, Pennsylvania
Intravenous Regional Anesthesia

Michael S. Runyon, MD
Adjunct Assistant Professor of Emergency Medicine, University of North Carolina, Chapel Hill; Assistant Residency Director, Carolinas Medical Center, Charlotte, North Carolina
Peritoneal Procedures

Brent E. Ruoff, MD
Chief, Emergency Medicine Division, Washington University School of Medicine, St. Louis, Missouri
Commonly Used Formulas and Calculations

Carolyn Sachs, MD, MPH
Associate Clinical Professor, David Geffen School of Medicine at UCLA; Emergency Medicine Center, UCLA Medical Center, Los Angeles, California
Examination of the Sexual Assault Victim

Leonard E. Samuels, MD
Assistant Professor, Emergency Medicine, Drexel University College of Medicine; Hahnemann University Hospital, Philadelphia, Pennsylvania
Nasogastric and Feeding Tube Placement

Gregory Schneider, MD
Attending Physician, Department of Emergency Medicine, Holy Cross Hospital, Fort Lauderdale, Florida
Physical and Chemical Restraint

Robert E. Schneider, MD
Senior Medical Advisor for Workforce Protection, Office of Health Affairs, United States Department of Homeland Security, Washington, DC
Urologic Procedures

Richard B. Schwartz, MD
Chairman, Department of Emergency Medicine, Medical College of Georgia, Augusta, Georgia
Pharmacologic Adjuncts to Intubation

Michael A. Silverman, MD
Instructor of Emergency Medicine, The Johns Hopkins School of Medicine; Chairman, Department of Emergency Medicine, Harbor Hospital, Baltimore, Maryland
Urologic Procedures

Peter Erik Sokolove, MD
Professor, Vice Chair for Education, and Program Director, Department of Emergency Medicine, University of California, Davis, Health System, Sacramento, California
Extensor and Flexor Tendon Injuries in the Hand, Wrist, and Foot; Standard Precautions and Infectious Exposure Management

Cemal B. Sozener, MD
Clinical Lecturer, Department of Emergency Medicine, University of Michigan Medical School, Ann Arbor, Michigan
Indwelling Vascular Devices: Emergency Access and Management

Mark Spektor, DO, MBA
Assistant Professor, SUNY-Downstate; Medical Director, Maimonides Medical Center, Brooklyn, New York
Nerve Blocks of the Thorax and Extremities

Sarah A. Stahmer, MD
Associate Professor of Surgery, and Emergency Medicine Program Director, Division of Emergency Medicine, Department of Surgery, Duke University School of Medicine, Durham, North Carolina
Ultrasound-Guided Procedures

Daniel B. Stone, MD, MBA, FACEP
Assistant Professor, Emergency Medicine, Northwestern University, Chicago, Illinois; Director, Emergency Medicine, Coral Springs Medical Center, Coral Springs, Florida
Foreign Body Removal

Amita Sudhir, MD
Assistant Professor of Emergency Medicine, Department of Emergency Medicine, University of Virginia, Charlottesville, Virginia
Educational Aspects of Emergency Department Procedures

Jacob W. Ufberg, MD
Associate Professor and Residency Director, Department of Emergency Medicine, Temple University School of Medicine, Philadelphia, Pennsylvania
Management of Common Dislocations

Malinda Wheeler, MN, FNP
Director, Forensic Nurse Specialists, Inc., Los Alamitos, California
Examination of the Sexual Assault Victim

Justin Williams, MD
Brooke Army Medical Center, Fort Sam Houston, Texas
Venous Cutdown

Richard Zane, MD
Assistant Professor, Harvard Medical School; Vice Chairman, Brigham and Women's Hospital, Boston, Massachusetts
Peripheral Intravenous Access

HOW THIS MEDICAL TEXTBOOK SHOULD BE VIEWED BY THE PRACTICING CLINICIAN AND THE JUDICIAL SYSTEM

The editors and authors of this textbook strongly believe that the complex practice of medicine, the vagaries of human diseases, the unpredictability of pathologic conditions, and the functions, dysfunctions, and responses of the human body cannot be defined, explained, or rigidly categorized by any written document. *Therefore, it is neither the purpose nor intent of our textbook to serve as an authoritative source on any medical condition, treatment plan, or clinical intervention, nor should our textbook be used to rigorously define a standard of care that should be practiced by all clinicians.*

Our written word provides the physician with a literature-referenced database, and a reasonable clinical guide which is combined with practical suggestions from individual experienced practitioners. We offer a general reference source and clinical roadmap on a variety of conditions and procedures that may confront clinicians who are experienced in emergency medicine practice. This text cannot replace physician judgment, cannot describe every possible aberration, nuance, clinical scenario or presentation, and cannot define rigid standards for clinical actions or procedures. *Every medical encounter must be individualized and every patient must be approached on a case-by-case basis.* No complex medical interaction can possibly be reduced to the written word. The treatments, procedures, and medical conditions described in this textbook do not constitute the total expertise or knowledge base expected to be possessed by all clinicians. Finally, many of the described complications and adverse outcomes associated with implementing or withholding complex medical and surgical interventions may occur, even when every aspect of the intervention has been standard or performed correctly.

The editors and authors of *Clinical Procedures in Emergency Medicine* Fifth Edition

The Fifth edition of *Clinical Procedures in Emergency Medicine* continues the original concept of providing a complete, detailed, and up to date description of many common, and some uncommon, procedures encountered during emergency medical practice. The novice may find the discussions and figures devoted to many procedures somewhat daunting or overwhelming at first; but, hopefully most will eventually appreciate the details and verbiage contained in the text. The goal is to describe an intervention as though it were the nascent clinician's first exposure to the concept, but with a depth that the seasoned operator would also deem helpful. It was difficult to find figures or photographs that convey the details, or elucidate the vagaries, to the extent one might want. The newly added color and additional figures were a much needed update, and morphed into an obvious improvement over previous editions. Many of the photographs were taken by me over 35 years of ED shifts, some were borrowed from other sources, such as the wonderful text by Cathy Custalow. Yet others were originally illustrated by Todd Thomsen with the help of Gary Setnik. No doubt Dr. Thomsen has found his calling, blending amazing art with equally impressive medical expertise. This edition is now available and fully searchable online at expertconsult.com, and MD Consult, with additional figures that will further educate the clinician to the nuances of emergency medicine procedures.

There is, of course, more than one way to approach any patient, or any procedure, so this text is not a dictum. This book does not attempt to define standard of care. It is a compendium of self proclaimed tried and true, but occasionally prospectively tested, techniques, practical hints, and successful tactics gleaned from years of practice, all blended with a modicum of newer modalities (such as ultrasound). As with prior editions, this version also significantly incorporates the personal opinions of the authors and editors. This book is intended to help the clinician and the patients who rely upon them. It's simply a clinical guide, not a legal document. Don't reference this book if you testify in court, for either the defense or the plaintiff. Today's dogma too often becomes tomorrow's heresy, and physician hubris is worse than incompetence. Simply stated, Emergency Medicine, and the human body, too often readily defy the written word, personal opinion, or local custom, and humble even the venerable and universally praised gray haired professor.

Many new authors have been added, as well as a number of new concepts and approaches. My personal thanks are hereby conveyed to those who contributed to previous editions. The updated chapters often merely refine or further manipulate the scholarly work of others who originally assisted us. The current contributors include an enviable blend of friends and colleagues, former students of mine, up and coming stars in their own right, and my prior mentors and role models—all are accomplished physicians, and leaders in their own milieu. Most know more than I know, and most are likely infinitely more capable and facile with procedures. All are capable of writing a text themselves, but are now enlightened and eschew that primal urge since they now know how difficult it is to write even a single chapter. My able and erudite associate editors, Arjun Chanmugam, Cathy Custalow, Carl Chudnofsky, and John McManus provided the bulk of the original editing; but, in the end, my personal bias likely prevailed. If any of our editing changed, altered, or misinterpreted the original thoughts of the contributors, we apologize; but, hard decisions had to be made, and waffling was rarely an option. We attempted to squarely address such omnipresent vague topics as prophylactic antibiotics, and accepted the fact that not all foreign bodies or tendon lacerations will be identified in the heat of the moment. The prescient and sagacious clinician knows that the ability to practice medicine from a book is limited, and one learns best from past experiences; and, for certain, the most instructive past experience is one that was not textbook perfect.

JAMES R. ROBERTS

The emergency physician has the unique responsibility of offering his or her skills at all times to all people (young and old, friendly and hostile, rich and poor). No other health providers are always collectively there at the entrance to the hospital. As emergency physicians, our responsibilities have grown and our horizons have been expanded because of our commitment to people. We have built a system that creates a caring environment from the home to the street and to the hospital, and a system that also integrates firefighters, police officers, paramedics, nurses, clerks, students, pharmacists, and physicians into this caring service. Each new clinical problem and each creative intervention has led to innovations in thought and technical advances. The Fifth Edition of Roberts and Hedges' text, *Clinical Procedures in Emergency Medicine*, takes another step in the pursuit of excellence in the provision of that care.

One of the newest chapters—the use of chemical and physical restraints demonstrates the skill of the authors in integrating the physical (the device) and the chemical (the pharmaceutical). The editors' and the authors' effective integration of the discussion of all the aspects of our care has been the hallmark of this text since the first edition. Each task is described and each goal is defined allowing for a rigorous approach as to how, why, when and with what device and pharmacologic agent each procedure is most safely and effectively performed.

The past 40 years in the history of emergency medicine have seen a remarkably rapid evolution in care. Organized medicine has often been criticized for its inability to change thought patterns and approaches to care, but the ability to change current patterns is the recognized strength of emergency physicians. We have undertaken our responsibilities, created new relationships, and developed new perspectives on clinical medicine in an area where previously no one dared to serve. This text exemplifies and describes the tremendous progress in thought, new techniques, new technology, new pharmaceuticals and their integration for the improved and safer care of the emergency patient. The rapid growth of prehospital care, the ever-increasing roles of emergency care, and the diversity of clinical issues and research dilemmas in emergency medicine have led to the development of a new type of physician in the emergency department. This text defines the breadth of investigative and clinical emergency medicine and the enormous technical skill and intellectual responsibility required of each emergency physician.

These chapters are written by emergency physicians and other physicians working closely with emergency patients who have highly specialized knowledge in particular aspects of emergency medicine. Almost a third of these authors are new contributors to this edition. The further integration of the clinical, investigative and educational roles of the emergency physician has led to the refinement of this Fifth Edition. As the basic science and clinical practice of emergency medicine have further developed, this book has grown to represent a complete view of our specialty. This text offers a balanced analysis of the entirety of the armamentarium at our disposal in the emergency department for the care of those with urgent and emergent problems. The authors attempt to simplify and clarify while focusing on knowledge and process in the environment where we practice. This text permits any practitioner the opportunity to perform his or her first emergency procedures with a foundation that emphasizes evidence and limits bias and ignorance.

This text has filled a void in medical practice. Procedural interventions in the emergency department had previously been largely undefined and certainly inadequately analyzed. The emergency physician who is trained to address the airway, an obstetrical or cardiac emergency for example will be able to utilize this text to review, better understand and develop the requisite cognitive and technical skills. Knowledge of these skills and their indications, as well as the risks and benefits of practice, will permit emergency physicians to achieve the highest level of service and will foster their potential to initiate quality research.

This book is also about motivating physicians to appreciate the clinical norms and expectations in our field. The editors have recognized for years many of the problems defined in the report To Err is Human released by the Institute of Medicine of the National Academy of Sciences in 1999. This text has moved the physician from anecdote to a rigorous analysis. The reader will not only feel more secure while performing an essential procedure with specific technical and pharmaceutical adjuncts but he or she will also become more confident about making the decision not to perform a procedure that entails more risk than benefit to an individual patient. The editors and authors have attempted to enhance education and limit the errors of commission as well as omission while improving the safety and occupational health of the emergency physician.

Recognizing that the emergency department environment is by definition unpredictable and often chaotic, these authors have prepared us to change the human response in an attempt to make errors more difficult to commit. Understanding the remarkable spectrum of responsibility of the emergency physician is our essential task. We shall succeed as health providers if we understand our patients and their needs, the pathophysiology of emergency medicine and its therapeutics, and our procedures and their pitfalls. The Fifth Edition of Roberts and Hedges' *Clinical Procedures in Emergency Medicine* provides enough thought-provoking information about the task, the appropriate technology and the appropriate pharmaceutical at the appropriate dose at the right time to prepare the emergency physician to care for the emergency department patient in a humane and intellectually sound manner. Although few physicians other than emergency physicians will use all the techniques, technology and pharmaceuticals detailed in this text, many other physicians can and will profit immensely from the use of this text. The techniques are well defined, well illustrated, and well referenced by clinicians who obviously use them daily. In this edition, there are many more helpful photographs and graphics with an esthetically pleasing and visually useful commitment to colors. This text remains unique with respect to the depth and breadth with which the editors and authors critically evaluate the tools of

our trade. The two leaders of our field, Roberts and Hedges, are once again assisted by four associate editors in this edition. These respected emergency physicians expand the excellent foundation of editorial contributions and ensure continued successful presentation of this complex material to help guide our clinical care.

The understanding and application of the principles defined in this edition should be considered essential for each emergency physician in his or her attempt to continuously improve the delivery of the best possible health care to our patients.

LEWIS R. GOLDFRANK, MD
Director, Emergency Medicine, Bellevue Hospital Center
New York University Langone Medical Center
Professor and Chair, Emergency Medicine
New York University School of Medicine
Medical Director, New York City Poison Center
New York, New York

VITAL SIGNS AND PATIENT MONITORING TECHNIQUES

CHAPTER 1

Vital Signs Measurement

Diane L. Gorgas and J. Dave Barry

Measuring the temperature, pulse, respiratory rate (RR), blood pressure, and pulse oximetry is generally recommended for all emergency department (ED) patients in addition to an assessment of pain in the appropriate patient population. Vital signs may not only indicate the severity of illness but also dictate the urgency of intervention. Although a single set of values suggests pathology, triage or initial vital signs may be spurious and simply related to stress, anxiety, and fear. Therefore, the *greatest utility of vital signs is their observation over time.* Deteriorating vital signs are an important indicator of a similarly deteriorating physiologic condition, whereas improving values provide reassurance that the patient is responding to therapy. Hence, when a patient undergoes treatment over an extended period of time, remember to repeat the vital signs as appropriate, particularly those that were previously abnormal. In some circumstances, it is advisable to monitor certain vital signs continuously.

Vital signs should be measured and recorded at intervals *dictated by clinical judgment and the scenario and patient's clinical state* or with any significant change in these parameters. Adhering to protocols or disease categories may not be useful or productive. An abnormal vital sign may constitute the patient's entire complaint, as in the febrile infant, or may be the only indication of the potential for serious illness, as in the patient with resting tachycardia.

Emergency medical service (EMS) begins the assessment of the patient's status and vital signs in the prehospital setting. Surges of epinephrine and norepinephrine commonly occur during transport by EMS and these are known to alter the vital signs, leading to increases in heart rates of greater than 10%.[1] *Prehospital vital signs should always be interpreted with the entire clinical scenario in perspective.*

Blood pressure and pulse are frequently evaluated together, as a measure of the blood volume. Although body temperature is usually the last vital sign measured during resuscitation, it has special importance for patients suffering from thermal regulatory failure. With these considerations in mind, the current chapter is organized according to the priorities of patient resuscitation and evaluation.

Additional "vital signs" recently introduced into the practice of emergency medicine are pulse oximetry, capillary refill, and the visual analog or pain scale. Capillary refill is discussed in the blood pressure section of this chapter as an assessment of overall perfusion, circulatory volume, and blood pressure. Assessment of pain as a vital sign is gaining acceptance and is discussed briefly at the end of this chapter. Mental status can be viewed as a summation of measurable vital signs (blood pressure, heart rate, RR, and temperature) with the understanding that significant vital sign abnormalities can cause mental status changes.

 BACKGROUND
CAN BE FOUND ON EXPERT CONSULT

NORMAL VALUES

The range of normal, resting vital signs for specific age groups must be recognized by the clinician to enable identification of abnormal values and their clinical significance. The normal ranges for vital signs are also influenced by gender, race, pregnancy, and residence in an industrialized nation. These ranges have not been validated in ED patients, who have many reasons for vital sign abnormalities, including anxiety, pain, and other forms of distress, in addition to altered physiology from their disease states. *Importantly, ranges of normal vital signs commonly quoted as normal or abnormal in other settings serve only as a guide, and not an absolute criterion, for diagnosis, treatment, further observation, or intervention in the ED.*

Published vital sign norms for children are not as well accepted as for adult patients. Table 1–1 and Table 1–2 report normal vital signs for children by age group as means and standard deviations. In Table 1–1, the values for pulse and blood pressure for 0- to 2-month-olds are adapted from studies of newborn populations (i.e., <7 days).[6–8] During the newborn period, normal arterial blood pressure rises rapidly. Values for pulse and respiration in children older than 3 years reflect an average of male and female values for 0- to 1-, 3-, 9-, and 16-year-old populations. The values for blood pressure reflect an average of male and female values for the

TABLE 1–1 Normal Values for Vital Signs of Infants and Children (Mean ± SD)

Parameter	Age				
	0–2 mo	3–12 mo	1–6 yr	7–12 yr	13–18 yr
Breaths/min	—*	—*	24 ± 3	19 ± 2	17 ± 3
Pulse/min	126 ± 20	131 ± 20	88 ± 9	70 ± 8	64 ± 7
Systolic BP†	72 ± 10	95 ± 15	93 ± 13	100 ± 10	112 ± 12
Diastolic BP	51 ± 9	53 ± 10	55 ± 10	63 ± 10	67 ± 10

*For data on children 0–36 mo, see Table 1–2.
†As an estimate, for children 1–10 yr: 2 × age (in yr) + 90 mm Hg = 50th percentile for systolic BP.
BP, blood pressure; SD, standard deviation.

TABLE 1–2 Normal Respiratory Rates (Breaths/Min) for Children to Age 3 Years (Mean ± SD)

Age (mo)	Awake	Asleep
0–<2	48.0 ± 9.1	39.8 ± 8.7
2–<6	44.1 ± 9.9	33.4 ± 7.0
6–<12	39.1 ± 8.5	29.6 ± 7.0
12–<18	34.5 ± 5.8	27.2 ± 5.6
18–<24	32.0 ± 4.8	25.3 ± 4.6
24–<30	30.0 ± 6.2	23.1 ± 4.6
30–36	27.0 ± 4.1	21.5 ± 3.7

SD, standard deviation.
Adapted from Rusconi F, Castagneto M, Gagliardi L, et al: Reference values for respiratory rate in the first 3 years of life. Pediatrics 94:351, 1994.

TABLE 1–3 Vital Signs During Pregnancy in the Lateral Decubitus Position (Mean ± SD)

Parameter	Trimester		
	1st	2nd	3rd
Pulse rate (beats/min)	77 ± 2	85 ± 2	88 ± 2
Systolic BP (mm Hg)	98 ± 2	91 ± 2	95 ± 2
Diastolic BP (mm Hg)	53 ± 2	49 ± 2	50 ± 2

BP, blood pressure; SD, standard deviation.
Adapted from Katz R, Karliner JS, Resnik R: Effects of a natural volume overload state (pregnancy) on left ventricular performance in normal human subjects. Circulation 58:434, 1978. By permission of the American Heart Association.

1- to 6-month-old and 3-, 9-, and 16-year-old populations.[9] Newer studies have reassessed reference values for RRs in children.[10-14] Table 1–2 reflects the age-related changes and the effect of the state of wakefulness in the RRs of children up to 3 years of age.[11] Hooker and colleagues[10] measured resting RRs in pediatric ED patients up to the age of 18. They noted considerable patient variability and somewhat higher RRs than those shown in Table 1–2.

For the adult population, normal blood pressure values are well established. Although systolic blood pressure increases with age, *normotensive or normal systolic blood pressure* is defined as 90 to 140 mm Hg, and *normotensive or normal diastolic blood pressure* is defined as 60 to 90 mm Hg. Recent discussion in the literature suggests defining an "optimal" blood pressure of 115/75 because blood pressures at or below this level have been associated with minimal vascular mortality.[15] Others suggest expanding the definition of hypertension to integrate a global cardiovascular risk assessment.[16,17] Although most patients have similar blood pressures in both arms, Pesola and coworkers found that 18% of their hypertensive population[13] and 15% of their normotensive population[12] *had a difference of greater than 10 mm Hg in systolic blood pressure between arms.*

In 1928, the New York Heart Association, by consensus, established the normal limits for the resting heart rate of 60 beats/min and 100 beats/min.[18] More recent data indicate that 45 beats/min and 95 beats/min may better define the heart rate limits of normal sinus rhythm in adults of all ages. Spodick[18,19] recommended that the operational definition for the limits of resting heart rate in adults should be 50 beats/min and 90 beats/min. This view is widely supported among cardiologists;[20] however, these ranges may not be applicable to the ED setting. *There is currently no consensus on what con-* stitutes a normal adult RR. Most studies on RR support 16 to 24 breaths/min as the norm for adults.

Pregnancy results in alterations in the normal adult values for pulse and blood pressure. The RR is unchanged, although the physiologic hyperventilation of pregnancy is well recognized. This is a result of the increased tidal volume and decreased residual and expiratory reserve volumes.[21] The resting pulse rate increases throughout pregnancy to 10% to 15% over baseline values. The norms for systolic and diastolic blood pressure are dependent on patient positioning. When the pregnant patient is sitting or standing, the systolic pressures are essentially unchanged. Diastolic pressures decline until approximately 28 weeks' gestation, when they begin to rise to nonpregnant levels. When the pregnant patient is in the lateral decubitus position, both systolic and diastolic pressures decline until the 28th week and then begin to rise to nonpregnant levels (Table 1–3).[22]

RESPIRATION

RR frequency reveals only a glimpse of the entire clinical picture. The pattern, effort, and volume of respiration may be more indicative of altered respiratory physiology. An abnormality in respiration may be a primary complaint or a manifestation of other systemic disease. Increased RRs may be seen in a variety of pulmonary or cardiac diseases, but acidosis, anemia, temperature, stress, and drugs (such as stimulants and salicylates) can significantly alter RR in the absence of cardiopulmonary dysfunction.

Physiology

Breathing is initiated and primarily controlled in the medullary respiratory center of the brainstem. The respiratory center is modulated by the pneumotaxic and apneustic centers in the pons. The pneumotaxic center limits the length of the inspiratory signal and, therefore, can greatly increase or decrease RR. In addition to being modified by other areas of the brainstem, the medullary respiratory center is modified by voluntary centers in the cerebral cortex; pulmonary stretch receptors of the airways; type J or juxtapulmonary capillary receptors of the pulmonary capillaries; arterial baroreceptors of the carotid sinus; and receptors found in skeletal muscle, tendons, and joints. Central and peripheral chemoreceptors also influence RR.[23]

Indications and Contraindications

The only contraindications to careful measurement of RR are the scenarios of respiratory distress, apnea, or upper airway obstruction that require immediate therapeutic intervention. A measurement of RR and effort should be performed as soon as patient care demands allow it in these circumstances.

The respiratory status in both adults and children plays a crucial role in determining the overall assessment of illness. Although it is a sensitive yet nonspecific indicator of respiratory dysfunction, the RR can also predict nonpulmonary morbidity. Several prehospital- and hospital-based illness or injury severity scores feature the RR as a cardinal value. A prehospital RR less than 10 or greater than 29 is associated with a major injury in 73% of children.[24] Other studies link abnormal RRs to in-hospital mortality and the level of care required in the ED.[25,26] Using tachypnea alone as a predictor for pulmonary pathology, infants with a RR of greater than 60 are found to be hypoxic 80% of the time.[27]

Procedure

The RR is the number of inspirations per minute. Measure the RR when the patient is unaware that his or her breathing is being observed, because awareness makes the patient conscious of the breathing pattern, which may alter the rate. One technique is to count respirations while appearing to count the pulse or auscultating the chest. Count for a full minute to most accurately determine the RR. Because the frequency is much less than the pulse, and breathing is less regular, an inaccurate measurement is more likely to occur if the count is taken for only a 15-second interval. Infants, in addition to being principally nasal breathers, are predominantly diaphragmatic breathers, so an infant's RR can easily be determined by observing or palpating the excursion of the chest or the abdominal wall.[28]

Interpretation

RR

A limited number of studies have examined RRs. Older studies found that 91% of healthy males at rest had an RR between 16 and 24 breaths/min.[29] Current texts vary considerably in their definitions of a normal RR and cite published values that range from 8 to 24 breaths/min.

Hooker and associates,[30] in a study that specifically investigated normal RRs in an ED, measured RRs in 110 afebrile ambulatory patients without respiratory complaints (53 females and 57 males). These authors reported a mean rate of 20.1 breaths/min. For patients whose RR was measured again before release from the ED, no significant difference was noted between initial and subsequent RRs. When analyzed by gender, females had a mean RR of 20.9 breaths/

min and males had a mean RR of 19.4 breaths/min, a statistically significant difference. *The researchers concluded that a normal RR in the adult patient population was 16 to 24 breaths/min.*[30] This study also suggested a significant variability in the accurate measurement of RR by different examiners. Rates obtained by nurses versus medical students varied significantly, as did those obtained by medical students versus residents versus attending clinicians.[31] Lim and colleagues[32] found generally good agreement between observers in the RR measurement, but interobserver variability could account for a difference of up to 6 breaths/min. The same observer variability accounted for up to 5 breaths/min.

Other studies have provided additional information on normal resting and sleep state RRs in children younger than 7 years.[10–14] RRs obtained with a stethoscope were higher than those obtained by observation (mean difference, 2.6 breaths/min in awake and 1.8 breaths/min in asleep children). Smoothed percentile curves demonstrated a larger dispersion at birth (5th percentile, 34 breaths/min; 95th percentile, 68 breaths/min), whereas dispersion was less at 36 months of age (5th percentile, 18 breaths/min; 95th percentile, 30 breaths/min).

The RR will generally increase in the presence of fever. It is often difficult to determine whether tachypnea is a primary finding or simply associated with hyperpyrexia. Taylor and coworkers[33] studied 572 children younger than 2 years of age, 42 of whom (7%) were subsequently diagnosed with pneumonia, and found that age-appropriate limits for resting tachypnea in the presence of fever could be defined. A sensitivity and specificity of 74% and 77% for pneumonia was achieved when children 6 months of age had an RR greater than 59 breaths/min, those aged 6 to 11 months had an RR greater than 52 breaths/min and those 1 to 2 years had an RR greater than 42 breaths/min. Therefore, even in the face of physiologic compensation for fever, an interpretation of the RR alone can help predict the presence of pulmonary disease.

Respiratory Pattern and Amplitude

Abnormal respiratory patterns may be characteristic of metabolic or central nervous system pathologic conditions. Hyperventilation and hypoventilation may result from an extensive differential diagnosis including primary pulmonary disorders, such as pneumonia or chest wall pain. Kussmaul respiration describes the hyperventilation pattern seen in diabetics with ketoacidosis. Abnormal respiratory patterns in adults can be used in the differential diagnosis or in determining the location of central nervous system lesions.

The recognition of subtle tachypnea can be difficult in the emergency setting, although this can be the solitary harbinger of disease. Measurement of an accurate RR in this patient population is crucial. Another instance of pathology that can confuse the routine measurement of the RR is diaphragmatic breathing or retractions. The variability in counting respiratory effort versus effective respirations is generally not appreciated in a single recorded value.

Observe the respiratory patterns carefully in children. In infants, distinguish periodic breathing, which may be normal, from apnea. By definition, *periodic breathing* consists of three or more respiratory pauses greater than 3 seconds in duration, with less than 20 seconds between pauses. There is no associated bradycardia or cyanosis. This contrasts with apnea, which is a particular problem in preterm infants. *Apnea* is defined as a respiratory pause of greater than 20 seconds. It may be associated with bradycardia and hypoxia.[28] Periodic breathing and apnea are believed to be disorders on a continuum, both stemming from abnormal physiologic control of respiration. However, periodic breathing is considered a benign disorder, whereas infants with symptomatic apneic episodes resulting in an apparent life-threatening event are thought to be at increased risk for sudden infant death syndrome.[34]

Grunting respiration, produced by expiration against a partly closed glottis, is an infant's attempt to maintain positive airway pressure during expiration for as long as possible. It usually signifies an attempt to maintain alveolar patency during airway obstruction, with parenchymal pathology, or from prematurity of the lung.

PULSE

Examine the pulse to establish the cardiac rate and rhythm. Palpate the peripheral pulses to yield clues about cardiac disease, such as aortic insufficiency, and information about the integrity of the peripheral vascular supply. Doppler ultrasound has utility in the location of a pulse, in the assessment of fetal heart tones beyond the first trimester of pregnancy, for evaluation of peripheral lower extremity vascular insufficiency, and for the evaluation of blood pressure in infants or in patients with low-flow states.

Physiology

Blood flowing into the aorta with each cardiac cycle initiates a pressure wave. Blood flows through the vasculature at approximately 0.5 m/sec; however, pressure waves in the aorta move at 3 to 5 m/sec. Therefore, palpated peripheral pulses represent pressure waves, not blood flow.

Indications and Contraindications

The necessity of repeated pulse evaluations is dictated by the clinical complaint and status of the patient. Continuous monitoring is not routine but may be helpful when the clinical situation may predict significant heart rate variability, as in the setting of sepsis.[35] Although an association between the absence of a radial pulse (or the absence of both radial and femoral pulses) and hypotension has been demonstrated for hypovolemic trauma patients, the variability in individual response prohibits the use of this parameter as an absolute gauge of blood pressure.[36] No contraindications exist to assessment of the pulse rate, but keep in mind a few cautionary notes about the examination of the carotid pulse: Avoid concurrent bilateral carotid artery palpation because this maneuver could endanger cerebral blood flow. In addition, massage of the carotid sinus, found at the bifurcation of the external and internal carotid arteries at the level of mandible angle, may result in reflex slowing of the heart rate. To avoid inadvertent carotid sinus massage, palpate the carotid pulse at or below the level of the thyroid cartilage. In adults with atherosclerotic disease, there is a rare risk of precipitating a cerebrovascular event by vigorous palpation of the carotid artery. Minimize this risk by prior auscultation of the carotid artery. If a bruit is present, gently palpate the carotid pulse, avoiding vigorous palpation.

Procedure

Pulses are palpable at numerous sites, although for convenience the radial pulse at the wrist is routinely used. Use the tips of the first and second fingers to palpate the pulse. The two advantages to this technique are (1) the fingertips are quite sensitive, enabling the pulse to be easily located and counted, and (2) the examiner's own pulse may be erroneously counted if the thumb is used instead of the first and second fingers. Pulses are also easily palpated at the carotid, brachial, femoral, posterior tibial, and dorsalis pedis arteries. Palpate the pulse at the brachial artery to appreciate the pulse contour and amplitude. Locate it at the medial aspect of the elbow and note that it is more easily palpated when the elbow is held slightly flexed.[37] Determine the pulse rate by counting for 1 minute, particularly if any abnormality is present. Common convention in the acute care setting is to count a regular pulse for 15 seconds and multiply the resulting number by 4 to determine the beats per minute.

In newborns, use direct heart auscultation and umbilical palpation as the methods of choice to determine heart rate. Instantaneous changes in the newborn heart rates are best indicated for the resuscitation team by the clinician tapping out each heartbeat.[38] In unstable children, palpate the central arteries, particularly femoral and brachial pulses, instead of the more peripheral arteries. In most circumstances, palpating the heart rate will approximate the actual heart rate within 2%.[39]

Interpretation

Pulse Rate

Consider the individual's physiology when interpreting the pulse. In infants and children, interpret the pulse rate with reference to age. Pulse varies with respiration, increasing with inspiration and slowing with expiration. This is known as a sinus dysrhythmia and is physiologic.

Although *bradycardia* is defined as a heart rate of less than 60 beats/min in adults, a well-conditioned athlete may have a normal resting heart rate of 30 to 40 beats/min.[40] As discussed earlier, a redefinition of bradycardia to less than 50 beats/min and tachycardia to greater than 90 beats/min has been proposed based on a normal healthy population.[20,41,42] These definitions of normal represent 95% of a population and do not speak to any given individual's normal baseline rate.

Consider whether a patient's abnormal pulse rate is a primary or secondary condition. Examine the entire set of vital signs when discerning the cause for the abnormal rate. For example, hyperthermia causes a sinus tachycardia. Drug fever, typhoid fever, and central neurogenic fever are suggested when no corresponding tachycardia is found in a patient with elevated body temperature. Hypothermia, with its reduced metabolic demands, may be associated with bradycardia.

Consider the medications that the patient may be taking or the presence of a mechanical pacemaker. Digitalis compounds, β-blockers, and antidysrhythmics may alter the normal heart rate and the ability of this vital sign to respond to a new physiologic stress. These cardioactive medications may be causing the patient's heart rate abnormality.

Heart Rhythm

In addition to determining the pulse rate, obtain information about the regularity of the pulse by palpation. An irregular pulse suggests atrial fibrillation or flutter with variable block, and accurate assessment of the pulse should be obtained by auscultation of apical cardiac sounds. The apical pulse is frequently greater than the peripheral pulse, reflecting

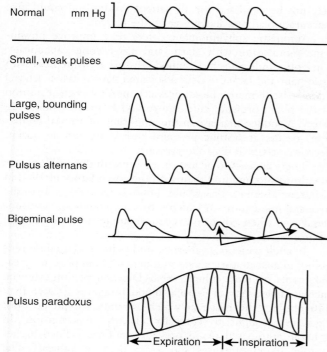

Normal mm Hg

Small, weak pulses

Large, bounding pulses

Pulsus alternans

Bigeminal pulse

Pulsus paradoxus

← Expiration →← Inspiration →

Figure 1–1 Examples of abnormalities of the arterial pulse compared with the normal pulse. The normal pulse pressure is approximately 30 to 40 mm Hg. The pulse contour is smooth and rounded. (The notch on the descending slope of the pulse wave is not palpable.) *(From Bates B: A Guide to Physical Examination and History Taking, 4th ed. Philadelphia, JB Lippincott, 1987.)*

inadequate filling time and stroke volume, with resultant non-transmitted beats. A greater pulse deficit generally reflects more severe disease.

Pulse Amplitude and Contour

Assess the amplitude and contour of the pulse simultaneously. Figure 1–1 compares normal and abnormal pulse amplitudes and contours. Accurate examination and description provide additional clinical information. Superimposition of one patho-physiologic state on another may modify the pulse. For example, sepsis may manifest with variable pulse amplitude, depending on the stage in the development of the disease at which the patient presents. Early in sepsis, cardiac output increases and vascular resistance decreases, causing bounding pulses. In advanced sepsis or septic shock, falling cardiac output and increased vascular resistance are seen, and pulses are diminished.[43]

Definable age-related pulse amplitude and contour changes can be identified. Age-related changes in the arterial pulse are explained by both an increase in arterial stiffness with increased pulse wave velocity and a progressively earlier wave reflection. This leads to increased pulse amplitude in the elderly in all commonly measured sites (carotid, femoral, and radial).[44] In addition to these age-related changes, pulse wave analysis may be useful in determining arterial stiffness and the likelihood of atherosclerotic disease.[45] Although intriguing, the routine measurement of pulse amplitude is not reproducible by simple palpation but instead requires instrumentation not available in EDs.

Pulses during Cardiopulmonary Resuscitation

Palpated "femoral pulses" during chest compression may represent either forward arterial blood flow or "to-and-fro"

movement of blood from the right heart to the venous system. A carotid pulse is preferred when assessing the adequacy of chest compressions during cardiopulmonary resuscitation (see Chapter 17).

ARTERIAL BLOOD PRESSURE

Changes in arterial blood pressure over time may indicate the success of treatment or the worsening of the patient's overall condition. An abrupt reduction in the patient's arterial blood pressure usually indicates the need for immediate intervention or reconsideration of therapy. The current section discusses indirect blood pressure monitoring, rather than intra-arterial techniques, discussed elsewhere. Discussions of the specific use of the Doppler device for pulse and blood pressure measurement and the measurement of orthostatic blood pressure and pulse changes follow this section. As noted earlier, despite an association between the absence of a radial pulse (or the absence of both radial and femoral pulses) and hypotension, in the setting of trauma, the variability in individual response prohibits the use of this parameter as an absolute gauge of blood pressure.[35]

Physiology

Arterial blood pressure indicates the overall state of hemodynamic interaction between cardiac output and peripheral vascular resistance. Arterial blood pressure is the lateral pressure or force exerted by blood on the vessel wall. Arterial blood pressure indirectly measures perfusion, in which blood flow equals the change in pressure divided by resistance.[4] However, because peripheral vascular resistance varies, a normal blood pressure does not confirm adequate perfusion.[46] Mean arterial blood pressure (MAP) can be estimated by adding one third of the pulse pressure (i.e., the difference between the systolic and the diastolic blood pressure) to the diastolic pressure[4,47] or by

$$MAP = \frac{\text{diastolic pressure} \times 2 + \text{systolic pressure}}{3}$$

Indications and Contraindications

Patients with minor ambulatory complaints not related to the cardiovascular system may not receive blood pressure measurements in the ED. Patients with hemodynamic instability need frequent blood pressure monitoring.

In children, there is a significant amount of variability regarding standard situations requiring blood pressure measurement. In general, the younger the patient, the less likely a blood pressure will be obtained.[48] In newborns, infants, and even toddlers, capillary refill is sometimes substituted for a standard blood pressure measurement, although viewing these tests as equivalent can lead to significant errors.

In low-flow states, Doppler measurement of blood pressure may be obtained rapidly. Repeated measurements will provide an evaluation of the adequacy of resuscitation in patients whose blood pressure cannot be auscultated by standard techniques. Placing a catheter for direct intra-arterial measurement of blood pressure has a higher risk of complications, but it may be performed safely in the ED. In particular, direct measurement of arterial pressure during pulseless electrical rhythms may help to discriminate between severe shock and an otherwise non-resuscitatable status.[49–51] Alternative noninvasive devices for continuous blood pressure measurement (CBPM) have been introduced clinically, with varying success. One common method of CBPM utilizes finger cuffs equipped with an infrared photophlethysmograph and sophisticated technology for quantification of finger blood pressure levels. Finapres (Ohmeda, Madison, WI) was the first commercial product employing this technique. Several newer products are on the market today. A number of commercial systems utilize an alternative method of arterial applanation tonometry to measure CBPM. Further study is needed for a solid validation of the devices utilizing these techniques.[52]

Relative contraindications to specific extremity blood pressure measurement include an arteriovenous fistula, ipsilateral mastectomy, axillary lymphadenopathy, lymphedema, and circumferential burns over the intended site of cuff application.

Equipment

The equipment required for indirect blood pressure measurement includes a sphygmomanometer (cuff with inflatable bladder, inflating bulb, controlled exhaust for deflation, and manometer) and a stethoscope or Doppler device (for auscultation) or an oscillometric device.[53-56] A common practice in the prehospital and interhospital transport setting is to forego auscultatory blood pressure measurement with a stethoscope and instead obtain systolic values only via palpation of the first Korotkoff sound. This practice, although sometimes the only feasible method of obtaining any value in a noisy environment, poses significant potential for errors. In a study of critically ill patients transferred between hospitals, palpated systolic blood pressures underestimated manometric values by nearly 30%. According to the American Heart Association Guidelines, to ensure an accurate reading, the sphygmomanometer cuff should be of an appropriate size for the patient. The width of the bladder should be at least 40% of the distance of the limb's midpoint (i.e., from the acromion process to the lateral epicondyle). This published figure of ideal width, when studied in a validation review, may be higher, up to approximately 50%.[57] The length of the bladder should be 80% of the midarm circumference or twice the recommended width.[47] These discrepancies in upper arm size mismatch with cuff size have been demonstrated to produce significant errors in critically ill populations as compared with invasive intraarterial blood pressure measurements.[58] A second study phase from this group showed no marked improvement in agreement of oscillatory and invasive measurements, however, despite correct cuff size.[59]

Manometers in common use are either aneroid, digital, or mercury gravity column. All three types of manometers are convenient for bedside use, although the mercury gravity column must be placed vertically to ensure accurate measurements. An aneroid manometer uses a metal bellows that elongates with the application of pressure. This elongation is mechanically amplified, transmitting the motion to the indicator needle.

Manometers require annual servicing. Mercury columns may require the addition of mercury to bring the edge of the meniscus to the zero mark. The air vent or filter at the top of the mercury column should also be checked for clogging. The aneroid manometer should be calibrated against a mercury column at least yearly. If the aneroid indicator is not at zero at rest, the device should not be used.[60] Digital manometers

may not be validated for all patient groups and could give inaccurate readings depending on the patient.

Automatic sphygmomanometers may improve physiologic monitoring with alarm and self-cycling capabilities. They offer indirect arterial blood pressure measurement with little pain and lack the risks associated with invasive arterial lines.[61] Oscillometric blood pressure monitors detect motion of the blood pressure cuff transmitted from the underlying artery. A sudden increase in the amplitude of arterial oscillations occurs at systolic pressure and MAP, and an abrupt decrease occurs at diastolic pressure.

There appears to be less variability with the oscillometric blood pressure method than with the auscultatory method in children. These results are not, however, generalizable to the neonatal population, in which errors are commonly encountered even when exhaustive measures are taken to control the environment.

In adult patients, numerous studies have focused on reliability of auscultatory versus automated blood pressure measurements. Mercury column versus Dinamap readings showed increased disparity at systolic blood pressures greater than 140 mm Hg, the range at which accuracy should be most rigorously sought to correctly identify hypertension. In general, automated blood pressure readings yielded higher systolic blood pressures and lower diastolic values.[62] The range of error in automated devices was, on average, 4.0 to 8.6 mm Hg.[63] Unfortunately, these studies represent populations without critical illness and do not reflect the accuracy of readings in the extremes of hypertension and hypotension, making generalization to an ED population difficult.

Procedure

Obtain indirect blood pressure measurements at the patient's bedside by palpation, auscultation, Doppler, or oscillometric methods. The technique is straightforward and accurate when well-maintained, calibrated equipment is used by clinicians who follow accepted standards. The patient may be lying or sitting, as long as the site of measurement is at the level of the right atrium and the arm is supported.[47,53] Interestingly, unless the arm is kept perpendicular to the body, measurements will be 9 to 14 mm Hg higher regardless of body position.[54] Hence, allowing the arm to be parallel to the body when supine, but supporting the arm perpendicular to the body when measuring the blood pressure in either the sitting or the standing position, may create a pseudo drop in blood pressure.

To palpate the arterial blood pressure, inflate the cuff to 30 mm Hg above the level at which the palpable pulse disappears. Once properly inflated, palpate directly over the artery and deflate the cuff at 2 to 3 mm Hg/sec. Report the initial appearance of arterial pulsations as the palpable blood pressure. Use the same technique with the Doppler device, with the Doppler auditory signal replacing the palpated pulse. Arterial pressure measurement by palpation and Doppler yields only systolic blood pressure estimates. The Doppler method is preferred when obtaining blood pressures from infants.[64]

When auscultating the blood pressure at the brachial artery, apply the blood pressure cuff about 2.5 cm above the antecubital fossa with the center of the bladder over the artery.[53] Apply the bell of the stethoscope directly over the brachial artery with as little pressure as possible.[65] The *systolic arterial blood pressure* is defined as the first appearance of faint,

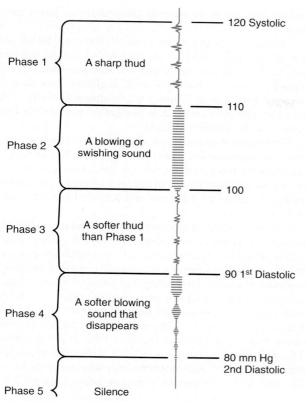

Figure 1–2 **Korotkoff sounds.** Systole—first audible sound. Diastole—sound disappears. *(From Burnside JW, McGlynn TJ: Physical Diagnosis, 17th ed. Baltimore, Williams & Wilkins, 1986.)*

clear, tapping sounds that gradually increase in intensity (Korotkoff phase I). The *diastolic blood pressure* is defined as the point at which sounds disappear (Korotkoff phase V).[53,65] In children, phase IV defines the diastolic blood pressure (Fig. 1–2).[8] Phase IV is marked by a distinct, abrupt muffling of sound when a soft, blowing quality is heard.

It is best to measure by auscultation over the brachial artery because of accepted standardization of the measured values. Alternate sites include the radial, popliteal, posterior tibial, or dorsalis pedis arteries, although any fully compressible extremity artery may be used. Studies correlating direct and indirect blood pressure measurements have demonstrated a good correlation between these methods.[66–68]

Situations exist in which it may not be feasible to obtain upper extremity blood pressure measurements because of patient access issues, particularly those encountered in the prehospital setting. Forearm measurements may be more easily obtained and show fair correlation to standard upper extremity values (within 20 mm Hg in 86% of systolic measurements and 94% of diastolic measurements).[69] Alternatively, noninvasive finger blood pressure measurements have shown promise when compared with standard upper extremity readings. The overall discrepancy in an ED study was 0.1 mm Hg with a standard deviation of ±5.02 mm Hg when comparing finger blood pressures and invasive mean arterial blood pressure via radial artery cannulation.[70]

The accuracy of palpatory, Doppler, and oscillometric methods has also been demonstrated.[71–74] However, when phase I and V Korotkoff sounds are used, indirect methods typically underestimate systolic and diastolic pressure by several millimeters of mercury.[67,75] In addition, during shock,

palpatory and auscultatory methods underestimate simultaneous direct arterial pressure measurements.[76] The flush method, in which return of color after deflation of the cuff is used for estimating blood pressure in infants, may underestimate systolic blood pressure by up to 40 mm Hg.[75] This method is unreliable and is not recommended.

Complications

Complications of indirect blood pressure measurement are minimal when the proper procedure is followed. Inadvertent prolonged application of an inflated blood pressure cuff may result in false elevation of diastolic pressure and in ischemia distal to the site of application, with attendant complications.[4,55] Invasive blood pressure monitoring is associated with a number of potential problems (see Chapter 20).

Interpretation

Normal blood pressure increases with decreasing distance from the aorta. Blood pressure tends to increase with age and is generally higher in males. Individual factors that influence blood pressure include body posture, emotional or painful stimuli, environmental influences, vasoactive foods or medications, and the state of muscular and cerebral activity. Exercise and sustained isometric muscular contraction increase blood pressure in proportion to the strength of the contraction.[4] A normal diurnal pattern of blood pressure consists of an increase throughout the day with a significant, rapid decline during early, deep sleep.[77]

Normal lower limits for systolic blood pressure for infants and children can be estimated by adding 2 times the age (in years) to 70, with the result expressed in millimeters of mercury. The 50th percentile for a child's systolic arterial blood pressure from 1 to 10 years of age can be estimated by adding 2 times the age (in years) to 90 mm Hg. Children older than 2 years are considered hypotensive when systolic blood pressure is less than 80 mm Hg.[78] Children, in particular, are able to maintain MAP until very late during shock.[79] Thus, the finding of a normal blood pressure in a child with signs of poor perfusion should not dissuade the clinician from appropriate treatment. Most adults are considered hypotensive if the systolic blood pressure is less than 90 mm Hg; however, some individuals normally exhibit a systolic pressure in that range. When accompanied by signs of shock, immediate treatment is indicated. In patients with shock, blood flow cannot be reliably inferred from heart rate and blood pressure values.[80,81]

Hypertension

Adults are hypertensive if either the systolic or the diastolic pressure consistently exceeds 140 or 90 mm Hg, respectively.[82,83] Based on a meta-analysis showing strong correlation of blood pressure to vascular and overall mortality down to at least 115/75,[84] some authors[15] have suggested altering the blood pressure definitions to include an "optimal" blood pressure of 115/75 to highlight the vascular risk associated with sustained blood pressures above this level. Other authors[16,17] have suggested incorporating blood pressure into a global cardiovascular risk assessment that includes other associated risk factors. The applicability of population norms for hypertension in a stressful emergency situation is controversial. *One should not make diagnostic or therapeutic decisions based solely on an abnormal initial measurement.* Patients with hypertension require repeat measurement to assess whether ED therapy is required. Because sustained hypertension may be seen in more than a third of initially hypertensive ED patients, careful evaluation and follow-up are required.[85]

The phenomenon of *white coat hypertension* (WCH) is defined as the persistent elevation of blood pressure in the clinical setting only. In order to strictly fit this definition, patients must have a normal ambulatory blood pressure outside of the clinical setting. WCH should not be confused with the *white coat effect* (WCE), a finding of increased blood pressure values in nearly all patients within the clinical setting. The WCE is used to characterize exaggerated hypertension in a normally hypertensive patient, frequently pushing moderately controlled hypertension readings into significantly higher readings while in the clinical setting. The prevalence of WCH is between 20% and 94%, depending on the frequency of clinical setting reassessment.[86-88] Patients in whom WCH or the WCE is most likely to occur are women, nonsmokers, and the elderly.[88,89] It is unclear whether these patients who have isolated clinical setting hypertension (WCH) are at increased risk for developing hypertension and subsequent end-organ damage.[90]

Measurement Errors

Erroneous blood pressure measurements may result from several factors.[83,91] Falsely low blood pressure may be caused by using an overly wide cuff, by placing excessive pressure on the head of the stethoscope, or by rapid cuff deflation.[92,93] Falsely high blood pressure may be caused by the use of an overly narrow cuff, anxiety, pain, tobacco use, exertion, an unsupported arm, or slow inflation of the cuff.

In 470 unselected adults, investigators at Duke University found no spurious effect of cuff size in 350 patients weighing less than 95 kg and with an arm circumference smaller than 35 cm. However, in 120 patients weighing more than 95 kg and with an arm circumference greater than 35 cm, the use of a large cuff reclassified 33% of those with systolic hypertension to borderline, 62% of those with borderline systolic hypertension to normal, and 79% of patients with borderline diastolic hypertension to normal.[94] Of note, 41% of adults observed at the University of Pittsburgh required nonstandard size cuffs, and use of small cuffs was associated with a mean error of 8.5 mm Hg and 4.6 mm Hg in the systolic and diastolic pressures, respectively.[95] Other studies have confirmed relatively high rates of inappropriately diagnosed hypertension among obese patients based on erroneous cuff size.[96]

Hypotensive patients have unreliable Korotkoff sounds. However, Doppler measurements are well correlated with direct arterial systolic pressure in hypotensive patients.[97] An auscultatory gap can be appreciated in hypertensive patients and may mislead the clinician. It is heard during the latter part of phase I and should not be confused with diastolic readings. Auscultation until the manometer reading approaches zero should prevent misinterpretation. In patients with aortic insufficiency or hyperthyroidism, in those who have just finished exercising, and in children younger than 5 years of age, the measurement of diastolic blood pressure should occur at Korotkoff phase IV.

Irregular heart rates also may interfere with accurate blood pressure determination. Take a second or third reading, with 2 minutes of deflation between recordings, and obtain an average when premature contractions or atrial fibrillation are present. Ultrasound methods to measure systolic blood pressure may be more accurate during shock states and in infants.[87,97]

Hemiplegic patients may exhibit different blood pressures in affected and unaffected arms.[98] A flaccid extremity tends to yield lower systolic and diastolic pressures, whereas a spastic extremity tends to yield higher values than the extremity with normal motor tone. Although these differences are generally small, it is preferable to monitor blood pressure in the unaffected limb.

Situational extremes can also lead to misdiagnosis of hypo- or hypertension. The accuracy of a blood pressure measurement aboard an aircraft can have a substantial negative impact on the accuracy of the measurement, with a mean palpation error of 19 ± 22 torr and a mean Doppler error of 8 ± 17 torr.

As noted earlier, numerous errors may occur in the measurement of accurate blood pressure. The only way to combat them is to first be cognizant of practices contributing to them. Unfortunately, few nurses can identify causes of potentially erroneous readings. In a study examining nurses' ability to accurately obtain readings, proper techniques in obtaining systolic blood pressure could be identified 61% of the time, diastolic blood pressure 71%, and an auscultatory gap 54%. Nurses were able to correctly determine faulty equipment 58% of the time, assess cuff size 57%, determine appropriate inflation pressure 29%, determine appropriate deflation rate 62%, and determine correct arm positioning only 14%.[99]

Pulse Pressure

The difference between the systolic and diastolic pressure is termed pulse pressure. Increased pulse pressure (i.e., ≥ 60 mm Hg) is commonly observed in anemia, exercise, hyperthyroidism, arteriovenous fistula, aortic regurgitation, increased intracranial pressure, and patent ductus arteriosus. A narrowed pulse pressure (≤ 20 mm Hg) may be a manifestation of hypovolemia, increased peripheral vascular resistance as seen in early septic shock, or decreased stroke volume.

Differential Brachial Artery Pressures

The presence of systolic blood pressure differences between arms suggests a normal condition if 10–20 mm Hg. If greater, it may indicate advanced focal atherosclerosis, coarctation of the aorta proximal to the left subclavian artery, aortic dissection, other aortic arch syndromes, or other vascular processes preferentially affecting one extremity. The utility of upper extremity bilateral blood pressure measurements has recently come into question. Singer and Hollander[100] found a 10 mm Hg systolic or diastolic difference in 53% of patients in the emergency setting, and a 20 mm Hg or higher difference in 19% of patients. These differences did not appear to be linked to age, gender, race, MAP, cardiovascular risks, or final discharge diagnosis. Smaller interarm differences have been reported by Pesola in the ED setting (18% in hypertensive patients[13] and 15% in normotensive patients[12] when >10 mm Hg cutoff was used).

Pulsus Paradoxus

Normal respiration decreases the systolic blood pressure by approximately 10 mm Hg during inspiration. Pulsus paradoxus occurs when there is a greater than 12 mm Hg decrease in the systolic blood pressure during inspiration. Pulsus paradoxus may occur in patients with chronic obstructive pulmonary disease, pneumothorax, severe asthma, and pericardial tamponade.[101] Other conditions such as an atrial septal defect, aortic insufficiency, and poor left ventricular compliance have been associated with pulsus paradoxus without pericardial fluid.

To measure a paradoxical pulse, place the patient in the supine position lying comfortably, at a 30° to 45° angle, and breathing normally in an unlabored fashion (unusual conditions in a patient suspected of cardiac tamponade, severe asthma, chronic obstructive pulmonary disease, or pneumothorax).[102] Inflate the blood pressure cuff well above systolic pressure and slowly deflate it until first hearing the systolic sounds that are synchronous with expiration (Fig. 1–3). Initially, the arterial pulse will be heard only during expiration, and it will disappear during inspiration. Then deflate the cuff further until arterial sounds are heard throughout the respiratory cycle. A paradoxical pulse can be palpated if it is very large. During palpation, the pulse may completely disappear during inspiration. When present, this technique is a quick bedside confirmation of the possibility of severe tamponade. Palpation for this purpose is best done at peripheral arteries, such as the radial or femoral.

If the difference between these inspiratory and expiratory pressures is greater than 12 mm Hg, the paradoxical pulse is high.[103] Most patients with proven tamponade have a difference of 20 to 30 mm Hg or greater during the respiratory cycle.[104,105] This may not be true of patients with very narrow pulse pressures (typical of advanced tamponade), who have a "deceptively small" paradoxical pulse of 5 to 15 mm Hg. The relative decrease in pulsus paradoxus occurs because the para-

doxical pulse is a function of the actual pulse pressure, and the inspiratory systolic pressure may be below the level at which diastolic sounds disappear.[102] For this reason, the ratio of the paradoxical pulse to the pulse pressure is a more reliable measure. A paradoxical pulse greater than 50% of the pulse pressure is abnormal.[102]

Pulsus paradoxus has been correlated with the amount of impairment of cardiac output by tamponade. In an uninjured patient with pericardial effusion, a pulsus paradoxus greater than 25 mm Hg (in the absence of relative hypotension) is both sensitive and specific for moderate or severe versus mild tamponade.[103] A study of right ventricular diastolic collapse by echocardiography found that an abnormal pulsus paradoxus had a sensitivity of 79%, a specificity of 40%, a positive predictive value of 81%, and a negative predictive value of 40%.[106] The absence of a paradoxical pulse does not rule out tamponade.

In the pediatric population, pulsus paradoxus has been studied to determine the severity of obstructive and restrictive pulmonary disease,[107] most commonly asthma. A value of 15 mm Hg or greater correlates well with clinical score, peak expiratory value, flow rate, oxygen saturation, and the subsequent need for admission.[108]

Despite the disease entities that a widened pulsus paradoxus may suggest, it is a difficult task to perform adequately using only a sphygmomanometer. In a study by Jay and associates,[109] emergency clinicians and critical care specialists were unable to reliably measure pulsus paradoxus in a trained reference subject either by palpation or by sphygmomanometer. The variance of actual versus measured pulsus paradoxus was greater with increasing pulsus paradoxus values into the pathologic range, lowering significantly the positive predictive value of the test.[109] The authors' conclusion was that new aids should be developed and used to reliably predict this important vital sign.

Shock Index

The ratio of the pulse rate over the systolic blood pressure has been suggested as a measure of clinical shock. The shock index (SI) has a normal range of 0.5 to 0.7. A number of clinical scenarios have been studied using the SI as a predictor of severe illness or injury. An SI above 0.85 to 0.90 suggests acute illness in medical patients as well as a marked increase in potential for gross hemodynamic instability in a trauma patient.[110–113] In a study evaluating first-trimester pregnancy, those patients with an SI above 0.83 were 15 times more likely to be diagnosed with an ectopic pregnancy in the ED.[110,114] However, some studies have found that the presenting pulse rate alone had nearly the same predictive power as the SI for severity of illness. Although the SI appears to correlate with left ventricular stroke work index, it has little correlation with systemic oxygen transport in hemorrhagic and septic shock.[111]

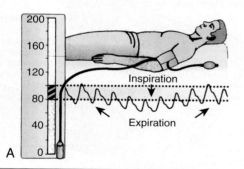

PROCEDURE FOR THE MEASUREMENT OF PULSUS PARADOXUS

Patient should be reclining at a 30° to 45° angle and instructed to breathe normally.

1. Inflate standard blood pressure cuff until Korotkoff sounds over brachial artery disappear.
2. Lower pressure in cuff a few millimeters of mercury per second until first Korotkoff sounds appear during expiration.
3. Maintain pressure at this level and observe disappearance of sounds during inspiration. Record this cuff pressure.
4. Very slowly lower cuff pressure until Korotkoff sounds are heard throughout the respiratory cycle. Record this cuff pressure.
5. The difference between pressures recorded in the two previous steps is then recorded as the measurement (in millimeters of mercury [mm Hg]) of pulsus paradoxus. A pulsus paradoxus >12 mm Hg is abnormal, but nonspecific (see text).

Figure 1–3 *A,* Measurement of pulsus paradoxus. Note that the systolic pressure varies during the respiratory cycle. *B,* Technique for the measurement of pulsus paradoxus. (*A, From Stein L, Shubin H, Weil M: Recognition and management of pericardial tamponade. JAMA 225:504, 1973. Copyright 1973, American Medical Association. Reproduced by permission.*)

DOPPLER ULTRASOUND FOR EVALUATION OF PULSE AND BLOOD PRESSURE

Principles of Doppler Ultrasound

Doppler ultrasound is based on the Doppler phenomenon: The frequency of sound waves varies depending on the speed of the sound transmitter in relation to the sound receiver. Doppler devices transmit a sound wave that is reflected by flowing erythrocytes, and the shift in frequency is detected. Frequency shift can be detected only for blood flow greater than 6 cm/sec.

Indications and Contraindications

Doppler ultrasound is commonly used in the ED for the measurement of blood pressure in low-flow states, evaluation of lower extremity peripheral perfusion, and the assessment of fetal heart sounds after the first trimester of pregnancy. Doppler sensitivity allows the detection of systolic blood pressure down to 30 mm Hg in the evaluation of a patient in shock. In the patient with peripheral vascular disease in whom there is concern about the adequacy of peripheral perfusion, the ankle/brachial index provides a rapid, reproducible, and standardized assessment.[115] Fetal heart sounds provide a baseline assessment of any patient with 12 weeks' gestation or longer in whom there is possible abdominal trauma or fetal distress due to a pregnancy complication. The use of Doppler ultrasound in the evaluation of deep venous thrombosis is a valuable tool; however, it requires specific training and experience to attain proficiency. Discussion of this topic is beyond the scope of this chapter.

Equipment

A nondirectional Doppler device has a probe that houses two piezoelectric crystals. One crystal transmits the signal and the other receives it. Reflected signals are converted to an electrical signal and fed to an output that transforms them to an audible sound. Two commonly used Doppler units are the pocket Doppler stethoscope (model BF4A, Medsonics, Inc., Los Altos, CA) and the ultrasonic Doppler flow detector (model 811, Parks Medical Electronics, Aloha, OR) (Fig. 1–4).

Probes with a frequency of 2 to 5 MHz are best for detecting fetal heart sounds. Frequencies of 5 to 10 MHz are appropriate for limb arteries and veins. The probes should be monitored periodically for electrical damage and integrity of the crystal. Sphygmomanometers used in conjunction with the Doppler device should be calibrated periodically, as described in the section on blood pressure evaluation.

Procedure

Place the Doppler probe against the skin using an acoustic gel as an interface. The gel ensures optimal ultrasound signal transmission and reception and protects the crystals. In an emergency, water-soluble lubricant (e.g., Surgilube or K-Y jelly) may be substituted for commercial acoustic gel. Angle the probe at 45° along the length of the vessel to optimize frequency shifts and signal amplitude.

In the evaluation of peripheral perfusion, place a sphygmomanometer cuff proximal to the arterial pulse and inflate it. Place the probe over the arterial pulse and slowly deflate the cuff. The pressure at which flow is first heard is the systolic pressure *under the cuff.*

In the evaluation of peripheral vascular disease, one may determine the ankle/brachial index. It is standard that this procedure is performed in a formal vascular laboratory. However, an approximation of pressures can be determined in the ED. Usually only the ankle/brachial index is considered for ED purposes. Examine both brachial arteries at the medial

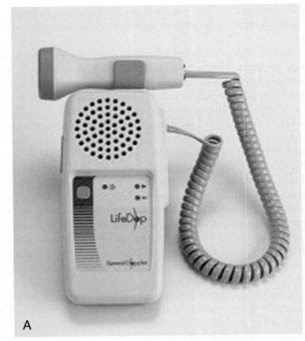

A

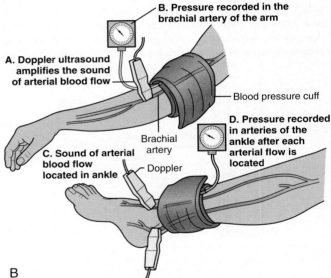

B. Pressure recorded in the brachial artery of the arm

A. Doppler ultrasound amplifies the sound of arterial blood flow

Blood pressure cuff

D. Pressure recorded in arteries of the ankle after each arterial flow is located

Brachial artery

C. Sound of arterial blood flow located in ankle

Doppler

B

Figure 1–4 *A,* Handheld Doppler device with speaker. Devices with an attached stethoscope are also used. *B,* Peripheral vascular testing is performed in a vascular laboratory, but an approximation of the integrity of the peripheral arterial circulation can be gleaned in the ED by calculating the ankle/brachial index, using a Doppler to compare systolic blood pressures in the foot and arm.

aspect of the antecubital fossa. Angle the probe until the most satisfactory signal is obtained. Inflate the cuff and slowly deflate it until the systolic pulse is heard. Repeat the procedure for the posterior tibial and dorsalis pedis arteries of both lower extremities.

In the evaluation of fetal heart tones, because of the variable positioning of the fetus, you may need to examine several locations and angles over the uterus with the probe to search for the optimal signal. It is best to begin in the mid-suprapubic area and then explore the uterus via angulation of the probe. Once tones are located, move the probe along the abdomen to reach a position closer to the origin of the sound.

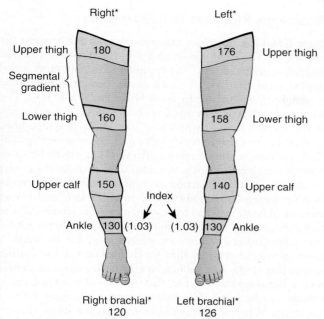

Figure 1–5 Typical pressures in a normal subject. Findings, based on resting pressures, show no evidence of occlusive disease of the large- or medium-sized arteries. Normal findings are as follows: (1) Ankle-to-brachial pressure index ≥1.0. (2) All segmental pressure gradients <30 mm Hg. (3) Upper thigh pressure at least 40 mm Hg above brachial pressure. *Systolic pressure in mm Hg. *(From Doppler Evaluation of Peripheral Arterial Disease: A Clinical Handbook. Fredericksburg, VA, Sonicaid, Inc. Reproduced by permission.)*

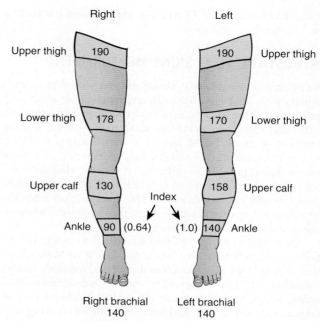

Figure 1–6 Typical pressures in a patient with obstruction of the right popliteal or tibial arteries. Significant findings are as follows: (1) Ankle-to-brachial pressure index <0.9 in right leg. (2) Abnormally high gradient from ankle to below knee and again from below to above knee in right leg. (3) Upper thigh pressures are 50 mm Hg higher than brachial pressures, consistent with normal flow at the aorta-iliac level. Findings are suggestive of a right popliteal occlusion or a right anterior and posterior tibial occlusion, or both. *(From Doppler Evaluation of Peripheral Arterial Disease: A Clinical Handbook. Fredericksburg, VA, Sonicaid, Inc. Reproduced by permission.)*

11

Distinguish fetal heart tones from placental flow by differentiating the quality of the fetal heart tones from the placental flow, which will match the maternal pulse.

Interpretation

As noted earlier, in low-flow states, Doppler ultrasound can detect a blood pressure as low as 30 mm Hg. Calculate the ankle/brachial index of each limb by dividing the higher systolic pressure of the posterior tibial or the dorsalis pedis artery of the limb by the higher of the systolic pressures in the brachial arteries. In normal individuals, the index should be greater than 1.0. Patients with claudication have values between 0.6 and 0.8. Values lower than 0.5 indicate severe impairment and are consistent with rest pain or gangrene.[115] When the lower extremity has been amputated or is injured, brachial/brachial indices can be used (i.e., the systolic blood pressure of the injured or diseased upper extremity compared with the other). Patients with ankle/brachial index values of 0.9 or lower have been found to have increased cardiovascular morbidity and mortality.[116] One study of 323 penetrating extremity wounds found the ankle/brachial index (or the brachial/brachial index) of lower than 0.9 to be 72.5% sensitive and 100% specific for the 29 vascular injuries.[117] Segmental lower extremity pressure measurements may help to identify the level of the obstruction (Figs. 1–5 to 1–7).[118] Obese patients, diabetic patients, or those with calcified vessels that are not compressible may have abnormally high systolic pressures (e.g., 250–300 mm Hg) and indices that do not accurately reflect flow. Normal fetal heart tones should be between

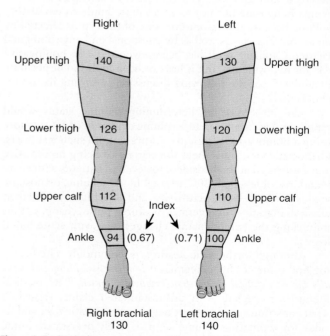

Figure 1–7 Typical pressures in a patient with obstruction of the abdominal aorta or bilateral iliac obstruction. Significant findings are as follows: (1) Ankle-to-brachial pressure index in both legs <0.9. (2) All segmental gradients <30 mm Hg. (3) Both upper thigh pressures are relatively low with respect to brachial pressure. Findings are suggestive of severe aortoiliac occlusive disease. *(From Doppler Evaluation of Peripheral Arterial Disease: A Clinical Handbook. Fredericksburg, VA, Sonicaid, Inc. Reproduced by permission.)*

120 and 140 beats/min. Fetal tones may be heard as early as the 12th week of gestation.

ORTHOSTATIC VITAL SIGNS MEASUREMENT

Orthostatic vital signs have historically been used to evaluate patients with fluid loss, hemorrhage, syncope, or autonomic dysfunction. They are also used to assess the patient's response to therapy. The clinician is often concerned with the accurate detection of acute blood loss or volume depletion. When the clinical syndrome of shock exists, assessment of a blood volume deficit poses little difficulty. It is preferable, however, that volume loss be detected before loss of physiologic compensation and clinical shock occurs. This section addresses the utility of orthostatic vital signs in the detection and monitoring of acute volume depletion.

Many techniques have been advocated to assess volume status. Unfortunately, *most procedures lack a database against which to judge their reliability.* Recommended methods include evaluation of skin color; skin turgor; skin temperature; supine, serial, and orthostatic vital signs; neck vein status; transcutaneous oximetry; and hemodynamic monitoring (e.g., monitoring of central venous pressure). Serial vital sign measurements have been used for assessing blood loss, but they do not reliably detect small degrees of blood loss.[119–121] Up to 15% of the total blood volume can be lost with minimal hemodynamic changes or any alteration of the supine vital signs.[119] A decrease in the pulse pressure occurs with acute blood loss,[121] but the patient's baseline blood pressure values are often unknown. Clinical examination of neck veins adds useful information but is less precise than measurement of central venous pressure. Most clinicians use skin color, temperature, and moisture as a reflection of skin perfusion and sympathetic tone but not as an accurate guide to circulatory volume because the vasomotor tone of the skin is affected by numerous diseases as well as by emotional and environmental factors. Capillary refill has been advocated as a noninvasive test for hypovolemia, but it has not been found to be accurate in adults[122] (see the following discussion regarding its use for children).

The ideal test for determining volume status would rapidly and accurately detect volume depletion of 5% or more using a noninvasive technique. At present, no such test exists. Orthostatic vital signs meet the criteria of being noninvasive and easily used at the bedside. However, in patients with acute blood loss of less than 20% of total blood volume, orthostatic vital signs lack both sensitivity and specificity.[123] Further, ethanol ingestion exaggerates postural pulse changes, thus mimicking the hemodynamic changes seen with acute blood loss.[124]

Although orthostatic testing is commonly cited as a method to detect hypovolemia, *it is often misleading and actually has less clinical value than frequently touted.* The medical literature is replete with unsubstantiated claims regarding what constitutes a positive or negative orthostatic test, and its value for estimating volume status is likely overstated. Some believe that postural hypotension or postural tachycardia occurs with varying degrees of hypovolemia, but they do not define specific criteria for a positive test.[125,126] Other sources (without documentation) perpetuate the notion that relatively small changes in the orthostatic blood pressure or pulse are reliable in detecting hypovolemia, for example, that a decrease of 10 mm Hg or more on assuming the sitting position indicates significant hypovolemia.[127]

Physiologic Response to Hypovolemia

Acute blood loss decreases the pressure gradient between the venules and the right atrium. A fall in this pressure gradient decreases venous return.[128] As a result, cardiac output falls and clinical manifestations of shock ensue. Several homeostatic mechanisms are initiated by acute blood loss (Table 1–4). The dominant compensatory mechanism in shock is a reduction in the carotid sinus baroreceptor inhibition of sympathetic outflow to the cardiovascular system. This increased sympathetic outflow results in several effects: (1) an arteriolar vasoconstriction, which greatly increases total peripheral vascular resistance; (2) a constriction of venous capacitance vessels, thereby increasing venous return to the heart; and (3) an increase of heart rate and force of contraction, which helps to maintain cardiac output despite significant volume loss.[129] These sympathetic reflexes are geared more for the maintenance of arterial pressure than for the maintenance of cardiac output (Fig. 1–8). The value of sympathetic reflex compensation is illustrated by the fact that 30% to 40% of the blood volume can be lost before death occurs while these reflexes are intact. When the sympathetic reflexes are absent, loss of only 15% to 20% of the blood volume may cause death.[129]

Several other reflexes maintain cardiac output in the presence of volume loss. The central nervous system ischemic response stimulates the sympathetic nervous system after the arterial pressure falls below 50 mm Hg and is responsible for

TABLE 1–4 Homeostatic Mechanisms in Hemorrhagic Shock

Sympathetic reflex compensation
  Arteriolar vasoconstriction
  Venous capacitance vasoconstriction
  Increased inotropic and chronotropic cardiac activity
  Central nervous system ischemic response
Selective increase in cerebral and coronary perfusion by means of local autoregulation
Increased oxygen unloading in tissues
Restoration of blood volume
  Renin-angiotensin-aldosterone axis activation
  Antidiuretic hormone secretion
  Transcapillary refill
  Increased thirst resulting in increased fluid intake
  Increased erythropoiesis

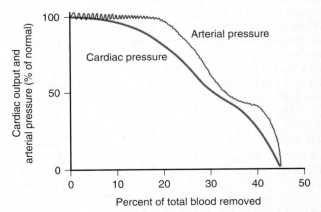

Figure 1–8 The effect of hemorrhage on cardiac output and arterial pressure. *(From Guyton AC: Textbook of Medical Physiology, 6th ed. Philadelphia, WB Saunders, 1981. Reproduced by permission.)*

the second plateau on the arterial pressure curve (see Fig. 1–8).[129] Other compensatory mechanisms that tend to restore the blood volume to a normal level include the release of angiotensin and antidiuretic hormone, which causes arteriolar vasoconstriction and conservation of salt and water by the kidneys.[130] A fluid shift from the interstitium to the intravascular space occurs, helping to restore blood volume over a longer period (1–40 hr).[131,132]

When blood loss results in anemia, part of the loss in oxygen-carrying capacity is countered by an increase in tissue oxygen extraction.[133] Finally, the lost red blood cell mass is slowly replaced by erythropoiesis.

Several investigators[119–121] have examined the changes in blood pressure and pulse that occur in the supine patient with blood loss. Collectively, these studies have shown variable individual hemodynamic responses to acute blood loss of up to 1 L. The frequent inability to detect significant volume loss with supine vital signs and the observation that patients with acute volume loss frequently develop syncope on rising led to the investigation of the use of orthostatic vital signs to detect occult hypovolemia.

Physiologic Response to Postural Changes

When an individual assumes the upright posture, complex homeostatic mechanisms compensate for the effects of gravity on the circulation to maintain cerebral perfusion. These responses include (1) baroreceptor-mediated arteriolar vasoconstriction, (2) venous constriction and increased muscle tone in the legs and the abdomen to augment venous return, (3) sympathetic-mediated inotropic and chronotropic effects on the heart, and (4) activation of the renin-angiotensin-aldosterone system.[134]

These compensatory mechanisms preserve cerebral perfusion in the upright position with minimal changes in vital signs. Currens[135] found that when a normal subject stands, the pulse increases by an average of 13 beats/min, systolic blood pressure falls slightly or does not change, and diastolic pressure rises slightly or does not change. These changes have been confirmed by others.[123–125]

In patients with vasodepressor syncope, the normal compensatory reflexes that preserve cerebral perfusion with postural changes are altered. The normal increased sympathetic tone on standing is paradoxically inhibited, and an exaggerated enhancement of parasympathetic activity (bradycardia) occurs, which can lead to syncope.[136]

Little data exist regarding the true effect of acute blood loss on postural vital signs, and this parameter varies greatly among individuals experiencing hypovolemia. One early study looked at 23 young adult volunteers from whom 500 to 1200 mL of blood was withdrawn.[122] These authors found no reliable change in the postural blood pressure, but a consistent postural increase in the pulse of 35% to 40% was noted after a 500-mL blood loss. In the 6 subjects who were bled approximately 1 L, only 2 were able to tolerate standing; each of them had a postural increase in pulse of greater than 30 beats/min. The other 4 subjects experienced severe symptoms on standing, followed by a marked bradycardia and syncope if they were not allowed to lie down.

Knopp and colleagues[123] phlebotomized 450 to 1000 mL of blood from healthy volunteers. By using the criterion of a pulse increase of 30 beats/min or the presence of severe symptoms (syncope or near-syncope) during a supine-to-standing test, they distinguished accurately between a 1000-mL blood

---

TABLE 1–5 Summary of Orthostatic Tilt Testing*

Test Procedure

1. Blood pressure and pulse are recorded after patient has been supine for 2–3 min
2. Blood pressure, pulse, and symptoms are recorded after patient has been standing for 1 min; the patient should be permitted to resume a supine position immediately should syncope or near-syncope develop

Positive Test

1. Increase in pulse of 30 beats/min or more in adults or
2. Presence of symptoms of cerebral hypoperfusion (e.g., dizziness, syncope)

*The predictive ability of orthostatic vital signs to assess volume status is often overestimated in clinical practice. This suggested guide is based on the ability of the pulse change and patient symptoms to distinguish between no acute blood loss and a 1000-mL acute blood loss in healthy, previously normovolemic volunteers (sensitivity of 98% for detecting 1000-mL acute blood loss).[123] This guide may not be applicable to elderly patients, sick children, medicated patients, and those with autonomic dysfunction.

---

loss and no blood loss. Changes in blood pressure and pulse were not evaluated in the symptomatic subjects. In this study population of 100 normal healthy volunteers with acute blood loss, the sensitivity and specificity using the aforementioned criteria for detecting a 1000-mL blood loss (Table 1–5) were both 98%, giving an accuracy of 96% (2% false-negative results and 2% false-positive results). The investigators were unable to consistently detect a blood loss of 500 mL by using these criteria. In a similar study by Kosowsky and coworkers,[137] the change in heart rate with postural changes after a 500-mL phlebotomy was more discriminatory for the blood loss than blood pressure changes or the change in bioimpedance-based stroke index changes. Of note, these authors found that a heart rate change of 30 beats/min or greater was 13.2% sensitive and 99.5% specific for the 500-mL blood loss versus a heart rate change of 20 beats/min or greater that was 44.7% sensitive and 95.4% specific. Hence, the finding of a significant pulse rise, although insensitive for a 500-mL blood loss, was relatively specific in these healthy adult blood donors.

In the most recent meta-analysis of orthostatic vital signs, the authors concluded that a large postural pulse change (>30 beats/min) or severe postural dizziness precluding the completion of vital sign measurements is required to clinically diagnose hypovolemia secondary to acute blood loss. However, the analysis demonstrates that orthostatic vital signs are often absent after moderate amounts of blood loss, significantly limiting the test's sensitivity (22%) in this scenario.[138]

 TABLE 1–6 Classification of Disorders of Postural Blood Pressure Regulation CAN BE FOUND ON EXPERT CONSULT

Variables Affecting Orthostatic Vital Signs

Many conditions affect the compensatory mechanisms that allow patients to assume the upright posture (Table 1–6).[134] Because of decreased vasomotor tone, limited chronotropic response, and other factors, the elderly have a higher incidence of orthostatic hypotension, which can lead to syncope and fall-related injury,[139] although carotid sinus hypersensitivity may play a greater role in geriatric syncope than orthostasis does.[140] Note that drugs that antagonize the normal autonomic compensatory mechanisms can also produce orthostatic changes. These changes can be severe enough to produce frank syncope, especially in the elderly. However, in one study of euvolemic adult volunteers, orthostatic changes in patients with diabetes or in those using various antihypertensive agents were similar to changes in normal adults.[141] Patients with hypertension may also have abnormal vasomotor responses to tilt testing, demonstrating more instability in small studies.[142]

Even in normal subjects, passive tilting generates a high incidence of orthostatic syncope.[143] Patients with chronic anemia (and a compensated blood volume) seem to have the same postural response as normal subjects.[144] Most of the conditions that affect postural blood pressure regulation involve a pathologic condition that affects the sympathetic nervous system. Orthostatic hypotension caused by autonomic insufficiency is usually not accompanied by tachycardia, whereas the orthostatic hypotension produced by acute volume depletion is commonly accompanied by a pronounced reflex tachycardia.

TABLE 1–7 Commercial Infrared Ear Thermometers
CAN BE FOUND ON EXPERT CONSULT

As noted in Table 1–7, many conditions, diseases, and medications have been implicated as causing abnormal orthostatic vital sign changes. Most variables have been poorly studied. In the elderly, orthostatic vital sign changes in volume-depleted patients have not been studied. In studies of normovolemic nursing home patients, orthostatic hypotension has largely been attributed to autonomic dysfunction and its prevalence has been stated at anywhere from 8% to 40%.[145] In a study of patients 65 years or older, 28% had a drop in systolic blood pressure of greater than 20 mm Hg. The study results showed no increased incidence of orthostatic hypotension among patients with chronic cardiovascular disease, disability, body mass index, or medications, although many of these comorbidities would seem intuitive to increase the risk of orthostasis.[146] Normovolemia orthostatic hypotension in the elderly has been loosely linked to long-term cardiovascular mortality and the risk of subsequent cerebrovascular accidents, but these results have not been consistently observed.[147] Ethanol ingestion exaggerates postural pulse changes up to 8 hours after ingestion,[124] mimicking the hemodynamic changes seen with acute blood loss. However, in the setting of ethanol intoxication and trauma, one must be vigilant for associated occult hemorrhage and not reflexively assign tachycardia to being a result of intoxication alone.

The utility of orthostatic vital signs in children has been questioned. Horam and Roscelli[148] found that healthy adolescents had heart rate changes of 21.5 ± 21.2 beats/min with orthostatic measurements made after 2 minutes of standing. They found similar variation in the systolic blood pressure change (+19 to –17 mm Hg). Bergman and associates[149] found that 25% of clinically normovolemic children had a postural increase in pulse of greater than 20 beats/min and 11% had a postural fall in systolic blood pressure of greater than 20 mm Hg. However, children with fever and diarrhea were included in this "normal" study group. Another study comparing mildly dehydrated children with normal children found a significant difference in the orthostatic rise in pulse between the two groups.[150] Using near-syncope or a change in heart rate of greater than 25 beats/min, orthostatic vital signs have a specificity of 95%, a sensitivity of 75%, and a predictive value of 92% in detecting mild clinical dehydration in children.[150] No difference in orthostatic blood pressure was found between normal and dehydrated children. Considering resting tachycardia as a positive sign of dehydration increased the predictive value of the test.[151] The investigators concluded that in the appropriate clinical setting, an orthostatic increase in pulse greater than 25 beats/min constitutes a positive tilt test, and an orthostatic pulse increase of less than 20 beats/min constitutes a negative test for hypovolemia.[150]

Another complicating factor in interpreting orthostatic vital signs is the development of paradoxical bradycardia in the presence of blood loss. Bradycardia in the face of hemorrhage has generally been considered a preterminal finding of irreversible shock, but bradycardia has been documented in hypovolemic, yet conscious, trauma patients. It has been published that when orthostatic syncope occurred, it was accompanied by hypotension and often bradycardia.[120,121] Many central nervous system factors can contribute to vagal-mediated syncope in ED patients with acute traumatic blood loss. These factors include pain, the sight of blood, stress, and nausea. Several investigators[152,153] described women with hemoperitoneum secondary to ruptured ectopic pregnancy who were hypotensive but did not have tachycardia. Jansen[154] reviewed other cases of this relative bradycardia that occurred in hypotensive patients with acute intraperitoneal bleeding and postulated a parasympathetic mechanism triggered by the presence of free blood in the peritoneal cavity. This bradycardia may be reversed with atropine, but aggressive fluid replacement is the treatment of choice because anecdotal reports mention serious ventricular arrhythmias from atropine used in this setting.[155] Paradoxical bradycardia has also been described in patients with abdominal or thoracic trauma or arterial bleeding from extremity wounds.[155] This paradoxical bradycardia may be more frequently associated with rapid and massive bleeding, whereas patients with a more gradual blood loss tend to have a more typical tachycardiac response. When the patient's clinical presentation is consistent with volume loss or shock, the clinician should not allow the absence of tachycardia to change the assessment.

Indications and Contraindications

When the volume status of a patient is assessed by use of orthostatic vital signs, several points should be remembered. Many factors influence orthostatic blood pressure including age, preexisting medical conditions, the use of medication, and autonomic dysfunction (see Table 1–6). Data relating the effect of blood loss to orthostatic vital signs are limited to phlebotomized healthy volunteers. Great care must be used when extrapolating these data to patients with anemia, dehydration, or painful trauma. The clinician must consider the clinical condition of the patient as well as the orthostatic vital signs in evaluating a patient for volume depletion.

Orthostatic vital signs can be considered as part of the evaluation of any patient with known or suspected volume loss or a history of syncope, except in the presence of these contraindications: The use of orthostatic vital signs is unnecessary and dangerous in a patient with supine hypotension or the clinical syndrome of shock. Orthostatic vital sign evaluation is also contraindicated in patients with a severely altered mental status, in the setting of possible spinal injuries, and in those with lower extremity or pelvic fractures.

The use of medications that block the normal vasomotor and chronotropic response to orthostatic tests also represents a contraindication to use of this test for assessment of volume status. However, when the patient's volume status is believed to be adequate and the clinician seeks to determine whether specific medications may have affected the patient's ability to respond to postural changes, the test may be useful. In the latter situation, the primary finding may be the feeling of near-syncope with little or no change in vital signs.

Orthostatic vital signs are often used to assess a patient's response to therapy. In patients receiving intravenous rehydration therapy, serial orthostatic vital signs are widely used to judge the end point to therapy before release. Johnson and colleagues[156] used this technique to demonstrate that the individual orthostatic vital signs response to saline infusion in women with hyperemesis gravidarum was associated with other measures of rehydration, including weight gain and decreased urine-specific gravity. Although the individual improvement in orthostatic vital signs in response to rehydration was of clinical value, the presenting orthostatic vital signs were considered insufficient as the sole indicator of clinical dehydration in this population.

Technique

Once the decision to obtain orthostatic vital signs has been made, record the blood pressure and pulse after the patient has been in the supine position for 2 to 3 minutes (see Table 1–5). Allow the patient to rest quietly. Do not perform any painful or invasive procedures during the test. Anxiety, fever, and other causes of resting tachycardia may make the test uninterpretable.[149]

Ask the patient to stand, and be prepared to assist the patient if severe symptoms or syncope develop. A supine-to-standing test is more accurate than a supine-to-sitting evaluation. Knopp and colleagues[123] found that the supine-to-sitting test was not reliable for detecting 1000 mL of blood loss (55% false-negative results). If severe symptoms develop (defined as syncope or extreme dizziness requiring the patient to lie down) on standing, the test is considered positive and should be terminated. If the patient is not symptomatic, record the blood pressure and pulse after the patient has been standing for 1 minute. This interval resulted in the greatest difference between the control and the 1000-mL phlebotomy groups in the study by Knopp and colleagues.[123]

A number of studies have been completed on normotensive, normovolemic patients to assess end points for orthostatic vital parameters. These have included sitting-to-standing methods[157] as well as varying rates of postural changes including lying times from 5 to 10 minutes and standing times of 0 to 2 minutes.[158] Complications include syncope with a resulting fall and injury and the possibility of exacerbating an existing fracture or spinal cord injury.

Interpretation

Criteria for positive orthostatic vital sign changes are either tachycardia greater than a specific threshold (see later) or symptoms of cerebral hypoperfusion (e.g., near-syncope).[151] Although blood pressure changes may be seen, they are too variable to be an indicator of blood volume loss. Although specific population-based thresholds for pulse rate and blood pressure changes have some value for identifying patients at high risk for significant volume loss, great individual variability limits the use of this technique as a screening test. That is, a volume loss of 500 mL (and occasionally more) may be associated with a negative orthostatic vital sign assessment (see later).[137,159] However, the use of serial measurements to ascertain the response to therapy of patients considered at risk for volume loss appears to have clinical utility.[156]

In the setting of possible blood loss, if the patient has a pulse rise of 30 beats/min or severe symptoms and if other complicating factors have been excluded, blood loss is highly likely (2% false-positive rate).[123,137] When evaluating the patient with moderate blood loss, there appears to be no advantage to using the SI as a marker of hypovolemia versus previously published tilt test criteria.[160] The presence of a negative test indicates only that an acute blood loss of 1000 mL is unlikely (2% false-negative rate); a blood loss of 500 mL cannot be excluded (43%–87% false-negative rate).[123,137,161]

In children, postural near-syncope or an orthostatic pulse increase of 25 beats/min may be a predictor of mild dehydration. The accuracy of these criteria is increased by the addition of resting tachycardia.[150] However, one cannot quantify the amount of volume depletion with this test in children.

Criteria for significant orthostatic blood pressure changes cannot be definitively set for the following reasons: (1) in the study by Knopp and colleagues,[123] a lack of correlation between blood pressure in the phlebotomy and control groups was seen; (2) a large variability in postural blood pressures has been found in the adult ED population;[162,163] (3) results of studies using passive tilt tables cannot be extrapolated to the bedside use of orthostatic vital signs; (4) studies using healthy patients with acute blood loss may not reflect orthostatic changes that are seen in the elderly or those with chronic bleeding, dehydration, and various other medical problems; and (5) many studies of orthostatic changes never used a criterion standard (measurement of actual volume loss) in their determinations. Because of lack of agreement about the degree of postural blood pressure change that constitutes a positive test result, the most reasonable definition may be any postural fall in blood pressure that results in symptoms of cerebral hypoperfusion.[164]

CAPILLARY REFILL

The capillary refill test is a measurement of the time interval from the release of nailbed or soft tissue pressure (sufficient to blanch the nailbed or superficial soft tissue) until the return to normal coloration. Delayed capillary refill is an indication of reduced skin turgor, often as a result of volume depletion. Measurement of the capillary refill time interval appears to be somewhat accurate in children, but its accuracy in assessing dehydration and reduced perfusion in adults is highly suspect.[122,165] Skin elasticity is the characteristic allowing skin to spring back to its original shape after it has been deformed. The presence of normal skin turgor is a sign of adequate circulatory perfusion, because the speed of refilling the capillary bed after compression is responsible for the return of color to the skin.[38]

Indications and Contraindications

The capillary refill time interval should not be obtained in a dependent extremity, a recently burned or injured extremity, or at the site of an infection or acute injury. Because capillary refill is available without additional equipment and takes only a few seconds to perform, it can be a useful bedside assessment of perfusion and dehydration when used in conjunction with other objective signs of the adequacy of perfusion. It should not be considered accurate as a stand-alone tool. *Capillary refill is not an appropriate alternative to measuring the blood pressure in pediatric patients.*

Procedure

The preferred sites for performing capillary refill are the nailbed, the thenar surface of the palm, and the heel. The current standards are best developed for capillary refill obtained at the nailbed.[165] Regardless of the site chosen, position the extremity at about the level of the right atrium. The minimum pressure necessary to produce blanching yields the most reproducible values. Release the nailbed and begin timing with a stopwatch or simply by counting out "one-thousand-one, one-thousand-two" for an approximation of the interval. Stop the clock when the nailbed becomes pink again. The relative apparent simplicity of the test notwithstanding, significant interobserver reliability has been noted in obtaining measurements.[166] A repeated measurement should be obtained at the same location as the initial test, because alternate sites may have different capillary refill times.

Interpretation

The normal capillary refill interval increases with age, degree of dehydration, and degree of hypoperfusion. Hypothermia, hyponatremia, congestive heart failure, malnutrition, and edema all increase the capillary refill interval. Environmental conditions, which can falsely alter capillary refill, are the ambient temperature[166] and the quality of ambient lighting.[167] Fever alone does not appear to prolong or shorten capillary refill time.[168]

The main difficulty in interpreting the capillary refill interval is that normal values in healthy patients *fall into a wide range*. In 30 normal infants from 2 to 24 months of age, the mean capillary refill interval was 0.8 ± 0.3 seconds. Measurements obtained from the nailbed were more reproducible than those from the heel. Combined results from four studies evaluating capillary refill revealed a pooled sensitivity of 0.60 (95% confidence interval [CI], 0.29–0.91) and a specificity of 0.85 (95% CI, 0.72–0.98) for detecting 5% dehydration in children.[169] The presence of delayed capillary refill greater than 2 seconds when combined with any two or more of absent tears, dry mucous membranes, or ill general appearance predicted clinical dehydration (>5% deficit of body weight) in children (age 1 mo–5 yr) with a 87% sensitivity and 82% specificity.[168]

Frequent monitoring of capillary refill may be useful in assessing responses to rapid fluid resuscitation in children. *The role of serial capillary refill interval measurements for assessing the response to rehydration in adults is unknown but it does not appear to be useful for assessing acute blood volume loss.* In adults, the capillary refill interval was found to be less sensitive and less specific than orthostatic vital signs for detecting a 450-mL blood loss during blood donation.[122]

TEMPERATURE

Detection of abnormal body temperature facilitates proper diagnosis and evaluation of presenting complaints.[170–178]

The inability to maintain normal body temperature is indicative of a vast number of potentially serious disorders, including infections, neoplasms, shock, toxic reactions, and environmental exposures.[170,173] Fever in neutropenic, immunocompromised, and intravenous drug–abusing patients may be more reliable than laboratory tests or clinician assessment in diagnosing serious illness.[173] Infants are particularly sensitive to thermal stress and may demonstrate lower body temperatures during asphyxia or necrotizing enterocolitis.[174–176] Normalization of body temperature after intervention may have important prognostic and therapeutic implications.[173] Some studies report rates as low as 13% in measuring temperature in the critically ill or injured.[179] The pre-triage or home assessment of body temperature is fraught with difficulties and unreliability, whether taken by oral, rectal or tympanic routes, *making the reporting of fever at home very difficult to interpret in the clinical setting.*[180,181]

Physiology

Under normal conditions, the temperature of deep central body tissues (i.e., core temperature) remains at 37°C ± 0.6°C (98.6°F ± 1.08°F).[177,178] Core body temperature can be maintained within a narrow range while environmental temperature varies from as much as 13°C to 60°C (55°F–140°F),[182] whereas surface temperature rises and falls with environmental and other influences. Maintenance of normal body temperature requires a balance of heat production and heat loss. Heat loss occurs by radiation, conduction, and evaporation. Approximately 60%, 18%, and 22% of heat loss, respectively, occurs by these methods. Heat loss is increased by wind, water, and lack of insulation (e.g., clothing). Sweating, vasodilatation, and decreased heat production serve to decrease temperature, whereas piloerection, vasoconstriction, and increased heat production serve to increase body temperature. Heat production is increased by shivering, fat catabolism, and increased thyroid hormone production.

Temperature control occurs by feedback mechanisms operating through the preoptic area of the hypothalamus. Heat-sensitive neurons in this area increase their rate of firing during experimental heating. Receptors in the skin, spinal cord, abdominal viscera, and central veins primarily detect cold and provide feedback to the hypothalamus, which signals an increase in heat production. Stimuli that change the core body temperature result in reflex changes in mechanisms that increase either heat loss or heat production.[182]

Indications and Contraindications

Clinicians generally measure body temperature to determine whether it is outside the normal range and as an indication of pathologic conditions that can affect core body temperature. Because actual core body temperature measurement requires the placement of invasive monitors, such as an esophageal or a pulmonary artery probe, clinicians commonly use estimates of core body temperatures, which conveniently and safely assess abnormalities of core temperature. Unfortunately, all non–core body sites and methods have inherent accuracy limitations, which clinicians have come to accept in assessing most patients.

Oral temperature measurement requires a cooperative adult or child. Patients who are grossly uncooperative, hemodynamically unstable, septic, or in respiratory distress (with an RR > 20) require another method of temperature measurement.[183] This group includes children younger than 5 years and patients who are intubated. Other factors can also influence the reliability of oral temperatures. The recent ingestion of hot or cold beverages can alter oral temperature readings for 5 to 30 minutes and can falsely elevate a normal temperature by up to 2.6° F or mask a fever in the case of cold liquid ingestion.[184]

Special techniques of measuring actual core body temperature may be indicated in certain patients (e.g., those with profound hypothermia, frostbite, or hyperthermia). Measurement of core body temperature is indicated in these individuals because it accurately measures treatment effects. This is the group of patients who will also benefit most from continuous temperature measurements.[185]

Measurement Sites

Core Body Temperature

It has been demonstrated that the following sites accurately reflect core body temperature and its changes: the esophagus (in the distal third), the tympanic membrane (using a direct thermistor in contact at the anterior inferior quadrant of the tympanic membrane),[186,187] and the pulmonary artery.[188]

Other sites may represent core body temperature under certain conditions. For example (1) the rectum, when the temperature is obtained at least 8 cm from the anus using an indwelling thermistor and the body temperature is relatively constant, and (2) the bladder when measured with an indwelling thermistor.[127,189] Data on core temperature in pediatric patients are limited and it is unclear whether bladder, rectal, or oral temperature is a good measurement of core body temperature in children.[190]

Peripheral Body Sites Approximating Core Body Temperature

Digital electronic probes are commonly used for the measurement of oral temperatures in ambulatory patients.[191] Disadvantages include various factors that affect clinical accuracy and sensitivity. The electronic probes must be covered with disposable covers, and even these are not completely effective in preventing contamination of the probe with microorganisms.[192] Disposable single-use oral thermometers are now available and are as reliable as mercury or tympanic membrane (TM) thermometers.[193] In the pediatric population, pacifier thermometers record supralingual readings in infants. The average time needed to record a reading with a pacifier thermometer is 3 minutes and 23 seconds, making their application in emergency medicine limited, although their sensitivity (72%) and specificity (98%) rival alternative methods.[194] Although there are no absolute contraindications for oral temperature assessment, patients with factors shown to produce unreliable results (see later) require temperature measurement at other sites.[183,195,196]

The rectal temperature is often considered the criterion standard of body temperature for ambulatory patients and it is often routine for children younger than 3 years.[197] Its advantages include accuracy, sensitivity, and availability. One intensive care unit study found rectal probe temperatures to demonstrate limited variability or bias when compared with pulmonary artery temperatures.[198] The disadvantages include longer intervals for measurement, safety concerns, and inconvenience. Neutropenia and recent rectal surgery represent relative contraindications to rectal temperature measurement.[199]

Body temperature measurement by infrared radiation (IR) detected from the ear, including the auditory canal and TM, is easy to use, hygienic, convenient, and quick.[200] It can be used as a general screening technique, especially in individuals in whom a very accurate temperature is not clinically sought, such as minor trauma. Although clearly superior to axillary temperature readings,[201] controversy remains regarding the sensitivity and specificity of IR TM readings in the ED. More work is being done in the pediatric population, with an overall sensitivity between 50% and 80% and a specificity of 85%. The lower sensitivities are found in newborns and infants under the age of 3 years.[202,203] Systematic reviews of pediatric studies have pooled data suggesting a 65% sensitivity, which is likely to be unacceptable in the clinical setting.[204] Adult studies, although generally more favorable in recommending IR TM temperatures, have shown gaps in reliability as well.[205] Temporal artery scanning to detect fever is being increasingly examined. In general, these devices show better sensitivity in detecting fever in infants as compared with TM thermistry (66% vs 49% sensitivity)[206] and may be useful in excluding fever as defined as a rectal temperature greater than 38.3° C if the temporal artery readings are less than 37.7° C.[207] The point can be argued that a sensitivity of 60% in any population lacks the required sensitivity to be useful clinically. A theoretical disadvantage of TM temperatures might be a falsely elevated estimate of the core temperature in the presence of otitis media. However, in one study, TMc thermometers accurately reflected oral temperatures in children with otitis media.[208]

Although not a likely ED concern, prehospital providers who might wish to measure IR TM temperature at low ambient temperatures should be aware that below 24.6°C, the TM readings will greatly underestimate core temperatures.[209] EMS personnel should also be aware that in a cohort of exhausted marathon runners, rectal and IR TM temperatures have only moderate correlation.[210] Hence, when hyperthermia or hypothermia is clinically suspected and the IR TM temperature does not confirm an abnormal temperature, a rectal temperature should be obtained.

Axillary and tactile temperature assessments have been demonstrated to be unreliable and insensitive. They should not be used as screening methods for core temperature abnormalities in the ED.[211–213] Similarly, the use of liquid crystal chemophototropic strips applied to the skin of the forehead are not accurate for single measurements or fever screening.[214,215] Single-use Tempa-DOT thermometers, which show increasing temperature dot darkening with increasing temperature, have been adopted by many EDs. The sensitivity of these thermometers for fever identification remains to be determined. The most rudimentary method for temperature measurement, parental assessment by tactile touch, is associated with a measured fever approximately 75% of the time.[216] Clinician estimation of fever is almost identical (70%).[217]

Equipment

Mercury-in-glass thermometers remain popular despite requiring longer equilibration times and having cumbersome cleansing requirements. Electronic methods of temperature measurement are based on the thermocouple principle. Modern electronic thermometers signal once extrapolation of the temperature-time curve occurs.[218] Current in vitro standards call for an accuracy of ±0.1°C (±0.18°F) over the range of 37° to 39°C (98.6°F–102.2°F).[219] Thermistor probes (i.e., small thermocouples with instantaneous readouts) for esophageal and vascular temperature measurement provide continuous temperature readouts when attached to a potentiometer.[5] Thermistor products are available for esophageal, bladder, and rectal probes with appropriate readout monitors.

Noncontact IR ear thermometers were introduced in 1985. These thermometers were initially used only in hospitals, but they are now sold over the counter for home use. The IR ear thermometers work by incorporating an IR sensor in the field of view of the IR emissions from the ear. Ear IR thermometers generally detect naturally occurring IR emissions over a brief time period, generally less than 1 sec. The emissions are converted to an electrical analog signal, which is digitized and analyzed by a microprocessor with resultant digital display.[220] The primary determinant of radiation emission is the temperature of blood perfusing this area, and the warmest spot in the auditory canal is the TM. Thus, current IR ear thermometers are operator-dependent in the same fashion that otoscopy requires proper positioning to enable the examiner to "see" the TM.[221]

Various IR ear thermometers are available commercially with varying operating temperature ranges, features, and reported accuracy. Clinical data assessing relative performance of the many commercial devices are limited. In one study comparing many of these IR thermometers, the Pro-1 and FirstTemp gave significantly higher readings.[221]

Procedure

Begin the temperature measurement by selecting the body site. Consider the accuracy of using a site to reflect core temperature, the site sensitivity to temperature changes, the convenience, the time required, the safety, and the site availability.[199,222] When reusable probes are used, cover the thermometer end with a probe cover. Insert the temperature probe and allow the probe to equilibrate with the temperature of the local body tissues. Proper placement of the temperature probes significantly influences the results for oral, rectal, esophageal, and vascular temperatures.[177,223,224]

Obtain sublingual oral temperatures in either the right or the left posterior sublingual pocket, with the mouth closed.[223] The patient should be sitting upright or lying down, holding the base of the probe with one hand.[191]

A rectal temperature should be obtained with the patient in the left or right lateral decubitus position with clothing removed. Lubricate the probe cover, wear gloves, and insert the probe gently to a depth of 3 to 5 cm to ensure accurate, atraumatic results.[177]

Axillary temperatures are frequently obtained on neonatal patients in incubators because of convenience. The technique is not indicated unless other sites are unavailable.[212,225]

Although not commonly used, temperature measurement of a freshly voided urine specimen can validate temperature measurement at other body sites. A nomogram of expected urinary temperatures has been derived from measurements of oral and urinary temperatures (Fig. 1–9).[226]

An esophageal catheter can be placed for measurement of the core body temperature similar to placement of a nasogastric or orogastric tube (see Chapter 41). The distal tip of the esophageal catheter contains a thermistor to measure the body temperature. In normal adults, insert the catheter approximately 34 cm deep into the esophagus, with the objective of locating the probe tip at the level at which the esophagus is between the aorta and the left atrium. Connect the

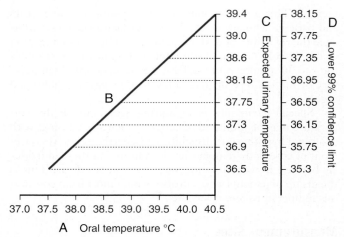

Figure 1–9 Relationship between oral and urinary temperatures constructed as a nomogram. Urinary temperatures are consistently within 1°C to 1.5°C of simultaneously obtained oral temperatures and within 2°C of rectal temperatures. To use the nomogram, locate the oral temperature on the horizontal axis (*A*) and draw a perpendicular line to intersect the diagonal border of the graph (*B*). Follow the dotted horizontal line to the right to determine the expected urinary temperature on the longitudinal axis (*C*). *D,* The far right-hand scale provides a 99% confidence level for the lower range of expected urinary temperatures and finding a value below the 99% confidence level is essentially diagnostic of a factitious fever. (*A–D, From Murray HW, Tuazon CU, Guerrero IC, et al: Urinary temperature: A clue to early diagnosis of factitious fever. N Engl J Med 296:23, 1977. Reproduced by permission of the New England Journal of Medicine.*)

catheter to a potentiometer and allow it to equilibrate briefly before a body temperature reading is taken.

For a pulmonary artery (PA) catheter assessment of core body temperature, place a PA or thermistor-tipped catheter into the PA. A detailed discussion of the placement of PA catheters is beyond the scope of this chapter. Once the PA catheter is in the correct position, obtain the temperature by using the potentiometer attached to the distal thermistor. Because of the risks associated with catheter placement, PA temperatures are generally reserved for patients with another clinical indication for PA pressure monitoring.

Complications

Complications associated with axillary, oral, ear IR, and liquid crystal thermometers are rare or unreported. TM perforation and pain have been reported as complications of thermistor probe placement in the auditory canal. Complications associated with rectal temperature measurements are extremely rare, but include rectal perforation, pneumoperitoneum, bacteremia, dysrhythmias, and syncope.[199,222] Falsely low but supranormal rectal temperature measurements may be seen during shock.[227] Rectal temperatures may also lag behind core temperature changes.

Complications associated with esophageal temperature measurement include those associated with placement of an orogastric or nasogastric tube (see Chapter 41). Confirmation of accurate placement can be verified with a chest radiogram. In addition, spurious temperatures may arise from an improperly calibrated potentiometer, a damaged thermistor, or a proximal esophageal location. Mechanical ventilation or thoracotomy can falsely lower measured esophageal core temperatures. Although anxiety-producing for parents, *biting and breaking a mercury thermometer is generally inconsequential with regard to either glass or mercury ingestion.*

Interpretation

Normal values for body temperature are affected by the following variables: (1) site and methods used for measurement, (2) perfusion, (3) environmental exposure, (4) pregnancy, (5) activity level, and (6) time of day. Clinicians must interpret body temperature with knowledge of the range of normal values at the intended site of measurement. Although the core body temperature remains nearly constant (37.0°C ± 0.6°C or 98.6°F ± 0.18°F), the surface temperature rises and falls with changes in ambient temperature, exercise, and time of day. The definition of *fever* varies by the site of measurement and is defined by a temperature greater than 2 standard deviations (SD) above the mean. *Fever has been defined as an oral temperature of 37.8°C or higher (100.0°F),*[228] *a rectal temperature of 38.0°C or higher (100.4°F),*[229] *or an IR ear temperature of 37.6°C or higher (99.6°F).*[230] Based on the measurement of temperatures in normal, healthy infants, Herzog and Coyne[231] recommend that fever should be defined as rectal temperature of 38°C or higher in infants younger than 30 days old; 38.1°C or higher in infants 30 to 60 days (1–2 mo); and 38.2°C or higher in infants 60 to 90 days old (2–3 mo). *Hypothermia* has been defined as a core body temperature lower than 35°C (<95°F), whereas *hyperthermia* has been defined as a core body temperature higher than 41°C (>105.8°F), with accompanying symptoms and signs.[232] A useful nomogram and formulas for conversion of centigrade to Fahrenheit are provided in Figure 1–10.

Temperature probes that require the transfer of heat energy from local tissues to the temperature probe require a period of equilibration and reliable tissue contact at the intended body site. Acceptable equilibration times for mercury-in-glass thermometers for oral, rectal, and axillary sites are 7, 3, and 10 minutes, respectively. Used in a predictive mode, electronic digital thermometers generally require 30 seconds for oral or rectal temperature equilibration. The predictive mode uses temperature changes versus time to predict an equilibration temperature.

Normal ranges and suggested febrile thresholds for common body sites and methods should be considered in the interpretation of temperature values (Table 1–8). The interpretation of temperature measurements during clinical assessment must consider the use of antipyretics, level of activity, pregnancy, environmental exposure, and patient age. The duration of antipyresis with acetaminophen or aspirin is 3.5 to 4 hours. When both drugs are given together, the duration of action may be extended up to 6 hours.[233] Body temperature is increased during sustained exercise, pregnancy, and the luteal phase of the menstrual cycle. Temperature also increases in later afternoon during diurnal variation. Body temperature is generally reduced with advanced age.

Oral temperature measurements are affected by ingestion of hot or cold liquids,[199] tachypnea,[234] and cold ambient air.[235] Smoking appears to result in little change in oral temperatures.[196,199] Therefore, before taking an oral temperature, the examiner should inquire about these features and possibly delay taking the temperature. Also, Erickson[195] found a 2.7°C (4.9°F) reduction of oral temperature measurement when the probe was placed under the tip of the tongue instead of under the posterior sublingual pocket. When using a mercury-in-glass thermometer, optimum placement time was found to be 7 minutes for oral temperatures in children.[236] Given the extrapolation that occurs with rapid-reading thermocouple devices and IR detectors, it is not surprising that the sensitivity of these devices (whether oral or TM) for fever (as detected by oral mercury thermometers) is only 86% to 88%.[237] Hence, many clinicians have adopted the adage that when a temperature is suspected or crucial in decision making, but not evident with an oral thermocouple probe or IR TM thermometer, measurement with a mercury-in-glass thermometer is indicated.

Axillary temperatures have a low sensitivity but a high specificity for fever; hence, axillary temperatures should not be used to screen for fever.

When rapid changes in body temperature occur, oral and TM temperature measurements appear to be more reliable than rectal temperature. In 20 adults examined during open

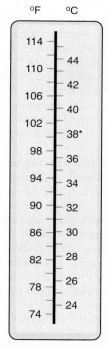

Figure 1–10 Temperature conversion scale. To change Celsius (centigrade) to Fahrenheit, multiply the Celsius temperature by 9/5 and add 32. To change Fahrenheit to Celsius, subtract 32 from the Fahrenheit number and multiply by 5/9. *100.4°F.

TABLE 1–8 Normal Ranges and Suggested Febrile Thresholds for Human Body Temperature (in Healthy Resting Patient)

Body Site	Type of Thermometer	Normal Range (°C)	Fever (°C)
Core*	Electronic	36.4–37.9	38.0
Oral	Mercury-glass, electronic	35.5–37.7	37.8
Rectal	Mercury-glass, electronic	36.6–37.9	38.0
Ear	Infrared emission	35.7–37.5	37.6†

*Temperature obtained with a properly positioned pulmonary artery, esophageal, or tympanic membrane thermistor.
†For unadjusted ear temperature using Thermoscan Pro-1 (Thermoscan, Inc., San Diego, CA).

heart surgery, oral temperatures showed a better correlation with blood temperature during rapid cooling and rewarming.[224] In 12 adults, the average rectal temperature lag during warming was 5.3 minutes during water immersion and 3.8 minutes during exercise.[238] Sublingual (oral) temperature delay (1.3 and 0.9 minutes for the two experiments, respectively) was less than auditory canal delay (1.1 and 4.1 minutes, respectively) in temperature response.

Infrequently, ED patients require constant monitoring of temperature (e.g., in cases of hypothermia or hyperthermia). This can usually be performed using a bladder or esophageal probe attached to a potentiometer. Patients with indwelling central venous or pulmonary arterial catheters may have electronic thermistors inserted into the central circulation to measure core body temperature. As noted earlier, rectal temperature measurements are less desirable for monitoring patients undergoing rapid core temperature changes. Periodic IR TM temperature monitoring may represent one useful option in the hypothermic patient.[239]

The interpretation of ear IR temperatures requires a knowledge of the mode of thermometer operation and ambient temperature. Cerumen occlusion of the ear canal may produce a false low reading.[240] Most IR ear thermometers have different modes that allow users to predict the equivalent temperature at other body sites. IR ear thermometers appear moderately sensitive for fever.[241,242] If these devices are used, the clinician must be aware of the potential for a false low temperature. When in doubt, the measurement should be repeated with a more standard method.

PAIN AS A VITAL SIGN
Background

For centuries, the goal of physicians has been the alleviation of pain. Albert Schweitzer called pain, "the most terrible of all the lords of mankind," and appropriately one of the goals of modern medicine has been to understand and accurately assess pain in hopes of better methods to treat it. A paradigm shift occurred and pain was then being viewed as a mechanism to provide a mechanical warning of actual or potential damage to cells and tissues in a specific body area.

Wheras there is no question that at least temporary pain relief is one thing any clinician can usually accomplish with relative ease, the concept of using pain as "the fifth vital sign" has not met with universal agreement.[243] *Literal interpretation of this concept can be fraught with problems, and because of the subjective nature of pain, measurement and interpretation is, by nature, imprecise.* It is not established that initiatives mandating documentation of pain as the fifth vital sign is associated with improvement of pain management.[244] Pain can cause sympathetically mediated changes in vital signs. However, with regard to the quantitative effect of pain, *it is well established that standard vital signs (pulse, respiration, blood pressure) do not meaningfully correlate with the level of perceived pain, even in patients with substantial pain, regardless of age, gender, or diagnosis.*[245] Adhering to such nonsensical statements as "pain never killed anyone" had engendered such absurd practices as eschewing narcotics for any patient with abdominal pain. Contentions that the judicious use of analgesics will obscure a clinical condition or otherwise adversely affect clinical care are antiquated, unscientific, and inhumane. In short, pain control facilitates the overall ED encounter for both patient and clinician.

Two types of pain are of concern to ED clinicians: *acute pain* defined as the normal predicted physiologic response to a noxious chemical or thermal stimulus. Acute pain is generally time-limited. *Chronic pain* is defined as persistent or episodic pain of a duration or intensity that adversely affects the function or well-being of the patient. Pain of either variety is the most common chief complaint of more than 50% of ED patients, approaching 75% in some studies.[246] In addition to the frequency of this disorder as a chief complaint, special focus should be placed on it based on the Joint Commission on Accreditation of Healthcare Organizations (JCAHO) goals mandating all hospitals develop comprehensive programs for the measurement, treatment, and documentation of pain.[247]

Reliably quantifying pain should be the goal of ED clinicians and is an appropriate step in the triage process. The discrete cognitive process that signals the sensation of pain is inherently influenced by culture, personality, experiences, and the underlying emotional state. The ideal pain measurement in patients continues to depend on methods that can utilize, or control for, subjective experience.

Procedure/Interpretation

Although JCAHO has required organizations to assess the nature and intensity of pain in all patients, there is no perfect measurement tool suitable for the wide variety of patients and clinical settings experienced in EDs. Pain is a complex, subjective, multifaceted, personal experience that is difficult to easily quantify for all individuals. The perfect pain assessment tool for the ED setting would be simple and rapid to administer, while providing a precise, reliable, and valid measure of pain regardless of a patient's age, cultural background, and cognitive or physical impairments. Although numerous instruments to measure acute pain have been proposed, none meets all of the criteria necessary to satisfy this definition. Regardless of the instrument chosen to measure pain, the primary focus should be to allow the patient to personally report her or his pain and to rate it from her or his viewpoint. It is widely accepted that health professionals cannot rate pain intensity as accurately as patients themselves.[248,249] While the patient's reporting of pain intensity can be frustating to the clinician, the patient's self-report of her or his own pain is considered the "gold standard" of initial assessment of pain, and to track or quantitate improvement or worsening of pain. Such reporting is not necessarily a gold standard to mandate specific interventions.[248,250]

Multiple unidimensional acute pain measurement instruments have been published, and many have been independently validated. These tools are limited to quantifying pain severity only and may overlook the other multidimensional aspects of an individual's pain experience. Common unidimensional pain instruments include the verbal rating scale (VRS), numerical rating scale (NRS), visual analog scale (VAS) and graphical rating scales such as the Wong-Baker Faces Pain Scale (WB-FPS) and the Faces Pain Scale—Revised (FPS-R). The VRS is administered by asking the patient to rate the severity of pain using a set of descriptors such as "none," "mild," "moderate," or "severe." These tests are rapid and easy to use, but may be less responsive to changes in pain severity owing to the small number of categories.[251] Language and cultural barriers could limit the effectiveness.

The NRS consists of numbers on a line; patients are asked to score their pain after explanation of the scale.[250] For example, 1 means no pain and 10 means the worse pain ever experienced. The NRS has been validated for verbal administration, but may be difficult to use in patients with cognitive impairment who may have difficulty translating pain into numbers.[248]

Probably the most used pain scale in the ED is the 1 to 10 VAS. The VAS utilizes a 10-cm line bounded on each end by perpendicular stops and descriptors. Zero equates to no pain, and 10 equates to the worst pain ever experienced. The initial score is not as important as a change during treatment. Generally, a change of VAS scales have been shown to be valid and reliable if self-completion is appropriate.[252] However, *there is wide variability in this technique, and at least 13 to 30 mm (1.3–3 cm) change on the scale is required to validate clinically relevant worsening or relief.*[253] Low completion rates may be seen in patients with visual or cognitive impairment. In one ED study, failure rates for the VAS were 15% compared with 0% for the NRS.[254] Graphical rating scales are useful for patients with limited cognitive and expressive abilities, especially children. They may also be helpful to overcome language or cultural differences. In a 2002 Illinois ED survey, the WB-FPS was the most common (81.7% of responding facilities) pain measurement tool used for pediatric pain assessment.[255] The FPS-R was developed to overcome potential cultural differences in how patients perceive tears or the act of smiling.

Multidimensional pain measurement tools attempt to provide more insight by incorporating affective, sensory, and cognitive aspects of the pain experience into the measurement process. In general, multidimensional measurement tools require more time to administer and, thus, are mostly impractical for routine use in the ED. One exception may be the short-form McGill Pain Questionnaire (SF-MPQ), which is reported to take only 2 to 5 minutes to complete.[251] The SF-MPQ has been shown to be reliable and valid,[250] but little study has been performed in the ED setting. These tools may be difficult to administer in patients with hearing or visual difficulties as well as those with limited cognitive abilities such as children or the elderly.

Overview of Visual Analog Pain Scales

It is general knowledge, and a frequent observation, that the patient's use of the commonly applied 1 to 10 VAS, while perhaps helpful to monitor progress of pain control or lack thereof, often overestimates the level of pain from the clinician's standpoint. Conversely, it may underestimate pain in certain stoic individuals or certain cultural groups. A rating of 10 was designed to indicate the "worst pain ever experienced," but this level is commonly chosen by patients with problems clearly of a minor nature. Whereas a rating of 10 may be the patient's understanding of his or her pain level, and used to describe the worst abdominal pain, backache, sprained ankle, arthritis, and so on that *he or she has personally experienced,* such a rating need not mandate a specific pain reduction approach that is always better driven by clinician evaluation and the entire scenario. It is not uncommon, for example, for patients to rate their pain a 12 on a 1–10 scale in an attempt to emphasize their personal experience, anxiety, or fear of receiving inadequate analgesia. It may be a patient's perception that a higher rating will expedite treatment, prompt higher doses of narcotics, or otherwise engender more compassionate care, making this a complex issue indeed. *A common erroneous tactic or subterfuge of litigation proceedings is to incriminate a clinician's diagnosis, treatment, or disposition based on the patient's rendition of the pain scale.* Many benign kidney stones rightly garner a 10 pain rating, but some aortic dissections are totally painless, hardly rendering any pain report equal to the seriousness of the medical condition.

Overall Goal of Pain Relief

The goal of EP pain management is to adequately relieve or control pain without compromising diagnosis, treatment plans, or the safety of the patient. The ideal objective is to totally relieve pain (0 on the pain scale). This goal is difficult, if not impossible to consistently achieve in the complex ED milieu. It is best accomplished by combining clinician experience, real time clinical judgment, repeat evaluation, and discussion with the patient and family. Strict adherence to protocols or relying on a dogmatic approach can be fraught with peril. It is best to treat the patient, not the pain scale.

 REFERENCES CAN BE FOUND ON EXPERT CONSULT

21

CHAPTER 2

Devices for Assessing Oxygenation and Ventilation

Baruch Krauss and Phillip E. Mason

Accurately estimating the severity of airflow obstruction is a critical component of caring for patients with acute exacerbations of asthma and chronic obstructive pulmonary disease (COPD). History and physical examination are the cornerstone of this assessment in emergency medicine practice. However, history and physical alone cannot reliably quantify airflow obstruction in these situations.[1–5] Among patients with obstructive pulmonary disease, wide variation exists in the ability to sense airway obstruction and up to 15% of patients with marked airflow obstruction will not be dyspneic.[6–9] This blunted perception of airway obstruction may be a contributor to fatal and near-fatal asthma attacks.[10] After therapy for acute asthma, patients may have complete resolution of symptoms while severe airflow obstruction is still present.[11] With these difficulties in estimating air flow obstruction, the addition of objective measures provides valuable information in the evaluation of dyspneic patients with obstructive lung disease.

Spirometry is simply the measurement of the volume of air exhaled during a forced expiratory maneuver.[12] This can be interpreted as a function of time to determine the flow rate. Spirometry gives the most complete picture of lung mechanics and is the centerpiece of pulmonary function testing. Whereas many parameters can be derived from a spirogram, the most useful are forced vital capacity (FVC), the total volume exhaled during a forced expiratory maneuver, and forced expiratory volume in 1 second (FEV_1), the average flow rate during the 1st second of the forced expiratory maneuver (Fig. 2–1).

The advent of small handheld devices that can provide standard spirometric parameters has made this technology more amenable to use in the emergency department (ED). However, the most common objective measure of respiratory mechanics used in the ED is the peak expiratory flow rate (PEFR). PEFR is the maximum flow of gas achieved during a forced expiratory maneuver. It correlates well with standard spirometry and has been studied extensively in the ED setting.

INDICATIONS

Evaluation of Acute Asthma Attacks

Currently, no standards exist regarding the measurement of pulmonary function parameters in ED patients, and practice varies widely. However, clinical decisions are rarely made on such parameters, and cannot replace clinical judgment. Whereas most patients with asthma exacerbations can be evaluated, treated and disposition decisions made without formal testing, objective measures of pulmonary mechanics may be used, with PEFR being the most common measure. Several con-

sensus guidelines recommend obtaining an objective measure of airflow obstruction in all patients presenting to the ED with an acute exacerbation of asthma.[13–15] Others have proposed that the decision to measure PEFR in acute asthma should be individualized.[16] If these parameters are to be used, they should be measured at presentation, after initial treatment and periodically thereafter.[13–15]

Evaluation of COPD Exacerbations

PEFR and spirometry testing can yield objective data on airflow obstruction during the ED evaluation of COPD exacerbations and have been used in that role by ED practitioners. However, consensus guidelines do not recommend their use in the acute setting.[17–19]

Differentiating Causes of Dyspnea

PEFR has been studied for its ability to differentiate between COPD and congestive heart failure (CHF).[20] Use of PEFR in this setting has not been studied thoroughly and it is not routinely used for this purpose.

Evaluation of Neuromuscular and Chest Wall Disease

Diseases of the chest wall and neuromuscular system can cause respiratory compromise. Although it is not commonly done in the ED, pulmonary function testing can quantify the degree of impairment and help determine what level of admission is needed.

CONTRAINDICATIONS

Need for Immediate Intervention

Patients with severe respiratory compromise should receive aggressive therapy and no delay should occur for pulmonary function testing.

Conditions that May Be Worsened by Increased Intrathoracic Pressure

Patients performing a forced expiratory maneuver will develop significant elevations of intrathoracic pressure. Pneumothorax or aneurysms of the aorta or cerebral vasculature may be exacerbated by the forced expiratory maneuver. The presence of these conditions should be considered a relative contraindication to pulmonary function testing.

EQUIPMENT

Spirometers can generally be divided into two categories. Volume spirometers measure the amount of gas exhaled and present it as a function of time. Volume spirometers tend to be cumbersome and are not ideally suited to the ED setting. Flow spirometers measure the flow of gas past a certain point and use that information to extrapolate volume and time data. These machines are smaller, simpler to use, and better suited to the ED setting. Flow spirometers determine gas flow by measuring the pressure difference between two points in a tube (pneumotachograph), cooling of a heated wire (hot wire anemometer), or revolutions of a rotating vane. Most handheld spirometers also measure PEFR.

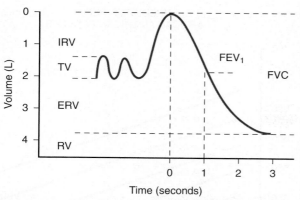

Figure 2–1 Diagrammatic representation of spirometry values. ERV, expiratory reserve volume; FEV_1, forced expiratory volume in 1 second; FVC, forced vital capacity; IRV, inspiratory reserve volume; RV, residual volume; TV, tidal volume.

The most commonly used device to measure PEFR is the "mini-Wright" peak flow meter. These meters provide accurate and reproducible measurements of PEFR.[21] The mini-Wright peak flow meter retains its accuracy over a period of at least 5 years.[22] There is significant variation between types and brands of peak flow meters, and only measurements recorded on the same brand of peak flow meter are useful for comparison with a patient's baseline PEFR.[11,23,24]

PROCEDURE

Calibrate the spirometer in accordance with the manufacturer's directions and examine the peak flow meter to ensure that the measurement bar is resting at the zero line before beginning the procedure. For multipatient devices, attach a sterile mouthpiece to the input orifice.

Prior to initiating the procedure, explain it to the patient and give a few practice runs if the patient is not familiar with it.

Position the patient in the standing position or, if that is not feasible, seated upright in bed. Elevate the chin and hold the neck in a slightly extended position. A nose clip is not required for PEFR measurements but may be useful when performing spirometry.

After a period of normal breathing, ask the patient to take a maximal inspiration and seal her or his lips around the mouthpiece, taking care to keep her or his tongue from partially obstructing it. Initiate a rapid, forceful expiration as soon as possible after reaching maximal inspiration. The PEFR usually occurs during the first 100 msec of expiration, so a prolonged expiration is not necessary for the test. However, when performing spirometry, it is important that a full exhalation occurs. With both tests, it is important to have a forceful and fast exhalation rather than a slow, sustained one. Coach the patient throughout the procedure and remind her or him to continue a forceful and complete exhalation. Three measurements should be obtained for both spirometry and PEFR.[25,26]

PEFR measurements are very sensitive *to patient effort and even a small decrease in patient effort can lead to considerable degradation of the results.*[11,27] Because airflow is greatest when lung volumes are highest and airways are larger, the test is accurate only if performed after a maximal inspiration.

TABLE 2–1 Approximate Values*

	FEV_1 (L)	FVC (L)	FEV_1/FVC ratio (%)
Male	3.0–5.0	3.5–6.0	75–85
Female	2–3.5	2.5–4.0	75–85

*Refer to equations in text for more accurate estimates of normal values. FEV_1, forced expiratory volume in 1 second; FVC, forced vital capacity. Based on Hankinson JL, Odencrantz JR, Fedan KB: Spirometric reference values from a sample of the general U.S. population. Am J Respir Crit Care Med 159:179, 1999.

INTERPRETATION

Obstructive diseases are characterized by a disproportionate decrease in airflow (FEV_1) in relation to the gas exhaled (FVC).[28] A decreased FEV_1/FVC ratio with preservation of FVC indicates the presence of airflow obstruction. Restrictive diseases decrease total lung capacity and therefore decrease FVC to a greater degree than FEV_1. Decreased FVC with a normal or increased FEV_1/FVC ratio is indicative of restriction. It is appropriate to consider the FEV_1/FVC ratio when attempting to determine whether a patient has airflow obstruction. However, in patients with an established diagnosis, FEV_1 is the value that best reflects changes in lung function. Typical values are shown in Table 2–1. These values are dependent on age, gender, ethnicity, and height and can be predicted from mathematical equations.[29]

Isolated measurements of PEFR are not reliable in making the diagnosis of asthma because there are significant variations between individuals. However, it is appropriate to monitor the degree of airflow obstruction in known asthmatics.

Although measures of airflow obstruction are not stand-alone tests, when considered along with other clinical factors, they can guide decisions regarding disposition in acute asthma exacerbations. The highest value of three PEFR or FEV_1 measurements should be used and, whenever possible, compared with the patient's personal best.[13-15] In one study of inner-city patients, only 29% knew their personal best PEFR, and even when known, this number may be unreliable.[30] In these cases, comparison with predicted values is appropriate. Normal PEFR values for adults are shown in Figures 2–2 through 2-4. Values for children are presented in Tables 2–2 and 2–3. The National Asthma Education and Prevention Program has classified the severity of asthma exacerbations based on the results of FEV_1 and PEFR testing (Table 2–4).[13]

 TABLE 2–2 Predicted PEFR for Boys Ages 8–20 Years
CAN BE FOUND ON EXPERT CONSULT

 TABLE 2–3 Predicted PEFR for Girls Ages 8–18 Years
CAN BE FOUND ON EXPERT CONSULT

Multiple guidelines and articles have advocated specific cutoffs for PEFR and FEV_1 values to guide disposition decisions.[13-15] There is variation in these guidelines and there is no consensus that absolute cutoffs exist.[16] When obtained, these values should be viewed as an additional datapoint to be considered, along with other clinical variables, in making dispositions for asthmatics presenting to the ED. Patients with an initial PEFR greater than 70% of personal best or predicted will likely be discharged and those below 35% will

PREDICTED PEFR
CAUCASIAN PATIENTS

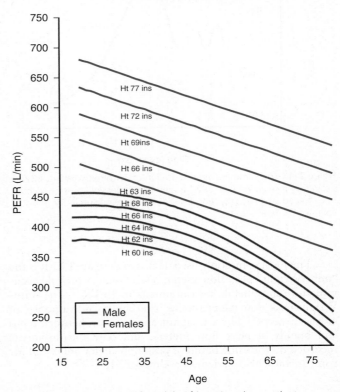

Figure 2–2 Predicted peak expiratory flow rate (PEFR) for adult Caucasian patients. *(Based on equations from Hankinson JL, Odencrantz JR, Fedan KB: Spirometric reference values from a sample of the general U.S. population. Am J Respir Crit Care Med 159:179, 1999.)*

PREDICTED PEFR
AFRICAN AMERICAN PATIENTS

Figure 2–3 Predicted PEFR for adult African American patients. *(Based on equations from Hankinson JL, Odencrantz JR, Fedan KB: Spirometric reference values from a sample of the general U.S. population. Am J Respir Crit Care Med 159:179, 1999.)*

Figure 2–4 Predicted PEFR for adult Mexican American patients. *(Based on equations from Hankinson JL, Odencrantz JR, Fedan KB. Spirometric reference values from a sample of the general U.S. population. Am J Respir Crit Care Med 159:179, 1999.)*

PREDICTED PEFR
MEXICAN AMERICAN PATIENTS

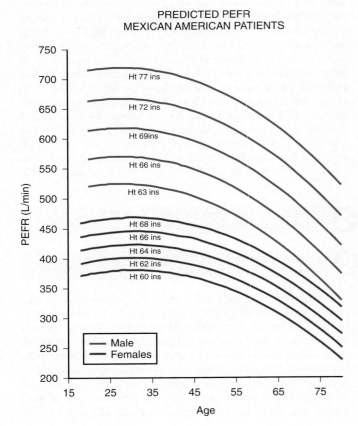

probably need admission. Beyond degree of initial airflow obstruction, response to inhaled bronchodilators is a useful gauge of suitability for outpatient management. A poor response argues in favor of admission, whereas recovery of PEFR or FEV_1 to greater than 70% of personal best is a favorable sign.

NONINVASIVE OXYGENATION MONITORING: PULSE OXIMETRY

Pulse oximetry, the noninvasive measurement of the percentage of hemoglobin bound to oxygen, provides real-time estimates of arterial saturation in the range of 80 to 100% and gives early warning of diminished perfusion while avoiding the discomfort and risks of arterial puncture. As a result, it has become the standard of care in a wide variety of clinical settings.

Technology

Oximetry is based on the Beer-Lambert law, which states that the concentration of an unknown solute dissolved in a solvent

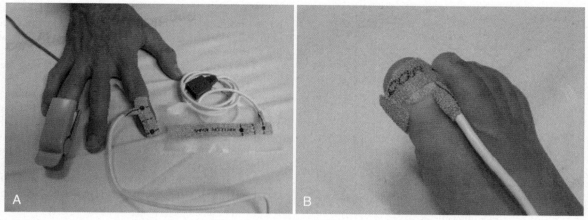

Figure 2–5 *A*, Pulse oximeter sensors attached to the digits. *B*, Pulse oximeter sensors attached to the dorsum of the nose and the earlobe. Only one site is measured at a time.

TABLE 2–4 Severity of Asthma Exacerbations according to Objective Measures of Airflow Obstruction

% Personal Best or Predicted (FEV$_1$ or PEFR)	Severity of Exacerbation
≤30	Life threatening
31–50	Severe
51–80	Moderate
>80	Mild

FEV$_1$, forced expiratory volume in 1 second; PEFR, peak expiratory flow rate.

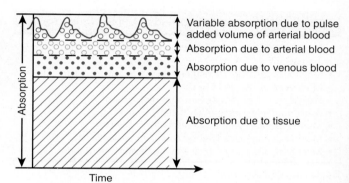

Figure 2–6 Factors influencing light absorption through pulsatile vascular bed. *(From McGough EK, Boysen PG: Benefits and limitations of pulse oximetry in the ICU. J Crit Illness 4:23, 1989.)*

can be determined by light absorption pulse oximetry, combining the principles of optical plethysmography and spectrophotometry. The probe, set into a reusable clip or a disposable patch, is made up of two photodiodes, producing red light at 660 nm and infrared light at 900 to 940 nm, and a photodetector, which is placed across a pulsatile vascular bed such as the finger or ear (Fig. 2–5). These particular wavelengths are used because the absorption characteristics of oxyhemoglobin and reduced hemoglobin are quite different at the two wavelengths. The majority of light is absorbed by connective tissue, skin, bone, and venous blood. The amount of light absorbed by these substances is constant with time and does not vary during the cardiac cycle. A small increase in arterial blood occurs with each heartbeat, which results in an increase in light absorption (Fig. 2–6). By comparing the ratio of pulsatile and baseline absorption at these two wavelengths, the ratio of oxyhemoglobin to reduced hemoglobin is calculated.

Because the pulse oximeter uses only two wavelengths of light, it can distinguish only two substances. As a result, pulse oximeters measure "functional saturation," which is the percentage of oxyhemoglobin compared with the sum of the oxyhemoglobin and reduced hemoglobin. The disadvantage of functional saturation is that the denominator *does not include other hemoglobin species that may be present, such as carboxyhemoglobin and methemoglobin (MetHb)*. The advantage is that the use of only two wavelengths in the oximeter reduces device cost, size, and weight. The CO-oximeter, one example of a commercially available in vitro oximeter and the standard by which pulse oximetry is calibrated, uses four or more wavelengths, measures the "fractional saturation," and is able to measure additional hemoglobin species.

Physiology

The arterial O$_2$ saturation (SaO$_2$) measures the large reservoir of O$_2$ carried by hemoglobin, 20 mL of O$_2$/100 mL of blood, compared with the arterial O$_2$ partial pressure (PaO$_2$), which only measures the relatively small amount of O$_2$, approximately 0.3 mL of O$_2$/100 mL of blood, dissolved in the plasma. The SaO$_2$ correlates well with the PaO$_2$, but the relationship is nonlinear and is described by the oxyhemoglobin dissociation curve (Fig. 2–7). For the hypoxic patient, small changes in SaO$_2$ represent large changes in the PaO$_2$, because these SaO$_2$ values fall on the steep portion of the curve. Conversely, measurements of SaO$_2$ are relatively insensitive at detecting significant changes in PaO$_2$ at high levels of oxygenation because these SaO$_2$ values fall on the plateau portion of the curve.

Currently available pulse oximeters are accurate and precise when saturations range from 70% to 100%. This range is satisfactory because for most patients an O$_2$ saturation of 80% is as much an urgent warning as is one of 67%. Testing of pulse oximeters has shown that at 75% saturation, bias is scattered uniformly with 7% underestimation and 7% overestimation.

Clinical Utility

Pulse oximetry offers a more physiologic means of assessing the adequacy of oxygenation than the arterial blood gas by providing continuous estimated SaO$_2$ measurements. Mea-

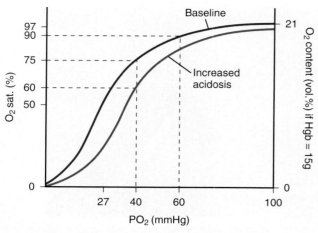

Figure 2–7 Oxyhemoglobin dissociation curve.

TABLE 2–5 Clinical Applications of Pulse Oximetry

- Assess adequacy of preoxygenation before endotracheal intubation
- Monitor oxygenation during emergency airway management
- Monitor ventilator and FI_{O_2} changes
- Provide early indicator of ventilator dysfunction
- Assist routine weaning of O_2 therapy
- Monitor patients with acute respiratory distress
- Monitor during procedural sedation and analgesia
- Monitor during interhospital and intrahospital transport

FI_{O_2}, forced inspiratory oxygen.

surement of SaO_2 is determined from blood gas measurements coupled with knowledge of actual hemoglobin levels in a patient's blood. The SaO_2 measurement is estimated using pulse oximetry (SpO_2). In this chapter, we equate SaO_2 and SpO_2.

Because data on clinical efficacy of routine pulse oximetry monitoring in the ED are limited, clinical value has been extrapolated from anesthesia studies.[31-33] These studies report a decreased incidence and duration of desaturation episodes, fewer adverse events during recovery, and a shortened time to discovery of hypoxia. Therefore, routine monitoring in critically ill patients should result in fewer episodes of severe arterial desaturation and more rapid recognition of the adverse physiologic events that produce arterial desaturation. Patient outcomes should be improved with therapeutic interventions resulting from immediate knowledge of an unfavorable SaO_2.[34]

Indications

Recommended uses of pulse oximetry fall into one of two broad categories: (1) as a real-time indicator of hypoxemia, continuous oximetry monitoring can be used as a warning system, because many adverse patient events are associated with arterial desaturation,[35] and (2) as an end point for titration of therapeutic interventions in order to avoid hypoxia (Table 2–5).

Procedure

The location for the probe is determined by the clinical situation and available probes. A reusable clip-on probe makes the digits easily accessible. Other sites include the earlobe, the nasal bridge or septum, the temporal artery, and the foot or palm of an infant. Tape and splints can be used to secure the digit probe and to minimize motion.

The computer analyzes the incoming data to identify the arteriolar pulsation and displays this in beats per minute; newer devices also display a pulse plethysmograph. Simultaneously, O_2 saturation is displayed on a beat-to-beat basis. Some machines have hard-copy capability and can provide paper documentation of the patient's status. If the oximeter fails to detect pulsatile flow, either the reading will not display or the SaO_2 value will be given with a poor signal quality warning, depending on the machine. It is valuable to evaluate serial measurements and to verify that measurements correlate with other clinical markers.

Interpretation

Patients with good gas exchange have O_2 saturations between 97% and 100%. When the SaO_2 falls below 95%, hypoxia may be present, although patients with obstructive lung disease may live in this range. Oxygen saturations below 90% represent significant hypoxia. In adults and older children with reactive airway disease, as with spirometry, a low isolated early measurement of SaO_2 does not mandate admission because of the wide variability of response to therapy. However, low SaO_2 readings should be heeded as important clinical warning signs. Pulse oximetry may be affected by numerous extrinsic factors, but a decline in oxygen saturation should always prompt an evaluation of respiratory rate (RR) and the adequacy of ventilation and circulation.

Although pulse oximetry represents a significant advance in noninvasive oxygenation monitoring, clinicians must recognize and understand its limitations.[36] Pulse oximetry measures only O_2 saturation. In contrast to arterial blood gas determination or capnography, pulse oximetry provides no direct information on pH or the arterial CO_2 partial pressure (Pa_{CO_2}) levels. Witting and Lueck[37] have empirically demonstrated that a room-air SaO_2 value of 97% or greater strongly rules against hypoxemia and moderate to severe hypercapnia. Their validated study of patients with respiratory complaints receiving arterial blood gas analysis found good discrimination with a room-air SaO_2 value of 96% or less. For hypoxia ($Pa_{O_2} < 70$ mm Hg), this value was 100% sensitive and 54% specific. For hypercapnea ($Pa_{CO_2} > 50$ mm Hg), this value was 100% sensitive and 31% specific. Kelly and colleagues[38] found a cutoff of a room-air SaO_2 value of 92% or less as more accurate for identifying hypoxia in COPD patients.

Pulse oximetry is not a substitute for monitoring ventilation, because there is a variable lag time between the onset of hypoventilation or apnea and a change in oxygen saturation.[39] Therefore, during procedural sedation, monitoring of ventilation is a more desirable goal for prevention of hypoxia than simple pulse oximetry (see "Procedural Sedation and Analgesia," under "Carbon Dioxide Monitoring," later in this chapter). Hypoventilation and resultant hypercapnia may precede a decrease in hemoglobin O_2 saturation by many minutes. Further, supplemental O_2 may mask hypoventilation by delaying the eventual O_2 desaturation that pulse oximetry monitoring is designed to recognize. In preoxygenated animals, airway obstruction was detected within 10 seconds using capnography, but SaO_2 values did not change during the 180-second study periods.[39] Other pulse oximetry limitations are summarized in Table 2–6.

TABLE 2-6 Factors Affecting Pulse Oximetry Readings

- Severe anemia: Satisfactory readings obtained down to hemoglobin level of 5 mg/dL
- Motion-artifact: See text regarding probe sites
- Dyes: Transient effect unless methemoglobinemia results
- Light-artifact: Minimize by covering probe with opaque material
- Hypoperfusion: Inadequate pulse signal will display
- Electrocautery: Minimize by increasing the distance of the sensor from the surgical site
- Deep pigmentation: Use fifth finger, earlobe, or other area of lighter pigmentation
- Dark nail polish: Remove with acetone or place sensor sideways on digit
- Dyshemoglobinemias (e.g., carboxyhemoglobin and methemoglobin): Falsely elevate saturation reading
- Elevated bilirubin: Accurate up to bilirubin level of 20 mg/dL in adults; no problem reported for jaundiced children
- High saturation: Pulse oximetry not useful for monitoring hyperoxemia in neonates
- Fetal hemoglobin: No effect on pulse oximetry; falsely reduced CO-oximetry readings
- Venous pulsations: Artificially lower O_2 saturation; choose probe site above the heart
- Dialysis graft (arteriovenous fistula): No difference from contralateral extremity unless fistula produces distal ischemia

Sources of Interference

Effects of Dyshemoglobinemias

In patients with methemoglobinemia or with elevated carboxyhemoglobin levels, *pulse oximetry does not accurately depict quantitative hemoglobin O_2 saturation changes.*[40,41] Carboxyhemoglobin results in falsely high SaO_2 estimates of hemoglobin O_2 saturation. Low quantities of MetHb will reduce pulse oximetry reading by about half the actual MetHb percentage. However, even large quantities of MetHb (>10%) can result in a stable pulse oximeter reading of 85% regardless of the actual SaO_2. Because pulse oximetry will variably underestimate the percentage of abnormal hemoglobin, a CO-oximeter is required for confirmation of these conditions and quantitative analysis.

Fetal Hemoglobin

Full-term newborns can have up to 75% of total hemoglobin in the form of fetal hemoglobin and up to 5% carboxyhemoglobin. Pulse oximetry remains accurate in the presence of fetal hemoglobin. However, a CO-oximeter will erroneously interpret the carboxyhemoglobin level to be elevated and the oxyhemoglobin level to be artificially reduced. Therefore, when fetal hemoglobin levels are high, CO-oximetry readings should not be used to confirm pulse oximetry readings.

Low Perfusion

To function properly, pulse oximeters require a pulsating vascular bed. Hypotension with vasoconstriction, hypothermia, or the administration of vasoconstricting drugs may reduce the pulsatile component to less than 0.2% of the total signal. At this level, the true signal cannot be distinguished from background noise. Under these conditions, pulse oximeters may display a message indicating an inadequate pulse signal. A change in the location of the sensor to an area with higher perfusion, such as an earlobe, may improve the pulse signal.

Intravenous Dyes

A number of dyes and pigments interfere with the accuracy of pulse oximetry.[42] Methylene blue, the treatment for methemoglobinemia, absorbs light at 660 nm, similar to the absorption of reduced hemoglobin, and can significantly lower pulse oximeter saturation readings to as low as 1%. Low readings also can be seen with other intravenous dyes such as indigo carmine, indocyanine green, and fluorescein, although the rapid clearance of these agents minimizes the phenomenon.

Bilirubin

Hyperbilirubinemia does not affect the accuracy of pulse oximetry. However, hyperbilirubinemia may have an effect on absorption at the lower wavelengths used by CO-oximeters, resulting in a discrepancy between pulse oximeter and CO-oximeter readings.

Skin Pigmentation

Pulse oximeter accuracy is somewhat reduced by deeply pigmented skin. This effect is likely due to a shift in the light-emitting diode's output spectrum as the light output is increased. This effect is small and results in only a slight decrease in accuracy over a large number of samples. Placing the probe on an area of lighter pigmentation, such as the fifth finger or an earlobe, has been suggested as a means to minimize this effect.

Nail Polish

Conflicting data exist about the effect of nail polish on the accuracy of pulse oximetry. Mounting the probe side-to-side on the finger was found to be as accurate as readings on uncovered nails. This technique also circumvents the problem of only partial placement of the probe because of very long fingernails, which may cause a low O_2 saturation reading. An alternative solution to the problem of nail polish is to remove it with acetone. The accuracy of SaO_2 readings in the setting of synthetic nails is unknown. If a poor signal is obtained in the setting of a synthetic nail, either the synthetic nail should be removed or an alternative site for placement used.

High Saturation

Because the O_2 dissociation curve plateaus at saturation levels greater than 90%, a large increase in PaO_2 results in a small increase in saturation. Therefore, an error of a few percentage points could represent a large error in PaO_2. This is inconsequential for most adult patients but is of extreme importance for neonates at risk of retinopathy caused by hyperoxemia.

Venous Pulsations

Increased venous pulsations resulting from right heart failure, tricuspid regurgitation, or placement of a tourniquet or blood pressure cuff above the probe can interfere with accurate readings and lead to artificially lower O_2 saturations, because the pulse oximeter interprets any pulsatile measurement as arterial. Placing the probe on a site above the heart may improve accuracy. Some pulse oximeters have the capability to synchronize pulsations at the probe site to electrocardiographic (ECG) signals, thus enhancing the signal-to-noise ratio.

Anemia

Because pulse oximetry depends on light absorption by hemoglobin, it becomes less accurate and less reliable in conditions of severe anemia when the hemoglobin content falls below 5 mg/dL.[43,44]

Ambient Light

Because the pulse oximeter's photodetector is nonspecific, high-intensity ambient light can produce interference. Surgical, fluorescent, and heating lamps are common sources of this interference. This problem can be corrected by wrapping the probe with a light barrier, such as a dark cloth or other opaque material.

Motion

Motion of the probe can produce considerable artifact and inaccurate readings. Correlating a pulse oximetry signal with an ECG waveform or using alternate probe sites, such as the ear or toe, also may reduce motion artifact. Newer generation pulse oximetry signal processing technology has greatly reduced motion artifact.

Probe Site

The finger is the most common probe site used for adult pulse oximetry. If the finger is inaccessible or unsuitable, other probe sites, such as the earlobe, nose, and forehead (using reflectance instead of transmittance), may be used. It should be noted, however, that the forehead and nasal bridge probes may be less accurate than the finger and ear probes. In infants and small children, an adhesive sensor unit is preferred. Probes also can be secured in place over the heel or lateral foot using a gauze or Coban wrap. Common sites of attachment include the great toe, the heel, and the lateral aspect of the foot.

Electrocautery

Electrical interference from devices such as electrocautery also can impair the accuracy of pulse oximetry. This interference can be reduced by increasing the distance between the surgical site and the probe.

Conclusions

Pulse oximetry is a widely available technology that provides an easy, noninvasive, and generally reliable method to monitor oxygenation. Because measurements are continuous, pulse oximetry allows for earlier detection of clinically unsuspected hypoxic episodes than does intermittent arterial blood gas analysis. Frequent measurements should lead to earlier corrective measures and the prevention of adverse consequences.

CO$_2$ MONITORING

Capnography is the noninvasive measurement of the partial pressure of CO$_2$ in exhaled breath. The CO$_2$ waveform or capnogram represents changes in the CO$_2$ concentration over the time of one respiratory cycle. CO$_2$ measured at the airway can be displayed as a function of time (CO$_2$ concentration over time) or exhaled tidal volume (CO$_2$ concentration over volume). The relationship of CO$_2$ concentration to time is graphically represented by the CO$_2$ waveform or capnogram (Fig. 2–8). Changes in the shape of the capnogram are diagnostic of disease conditions, whereas changes in end-tidal CO$_2$ (E$_T$co$_2$ – the maximum CO$_2$ concentration at the end of each tidal breath) can be used to assess disease severity and response to treatment. This chapter discusses the use of time-

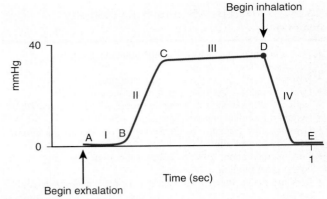

Figure 2–8 Normal capnogram. *(From Krauss B, Hess DR: Capnography for procedural sedation and analgesia in the emergency department. Ann Emerg Med 50:172, 2007.)*

based capnography because this is the only form of CO$_2$ monitoring used in emergency medical service (EMS) and the predominant form used in the ED and because of certain technology characteristics of volume-based capnography that make it not easily adaptable to non-intubated subjects.

Oxygenation and ventilation are distinct physiologic functions that must be assessed in both intubated and spontaneously breathing patients. Pulse oximetry provides real-time feedback about oxygenation whereas capnography provides breath-to-breath information about ventilation (how effectively CO$_2$ is being eliminated by the pulmonary system), perfusion (how effectively CO$_2$ is being transported through the vascular system), and metabolism (how effectively CO$_2$ is being produced by cellular metabolism).

Terminology

The ancient Greeks believed there was a combustion engine inside the body that gave off smoke (*Capnos* in Greek) in the form of the breath. A capnometer is a CO$_2$ monitor that displays a number {i.e., E$_T$co$_2$}. A capnograph is a CO$_2$ monitor that displays a number and a waveform (i.e., the capnogram).

Technology

Capnography became a routine part of anesthesia practice in Europe in the 1970s and in the United States in the 1980s.[45] Capnography was incorporated into the American Heart Association (AHA) guidelines in 2000 and the American College of Emergency Physicians (ACEP) guidelines in 2001 and has become one standard for verification of endotracheal tube placement in the operating room, the ED, and EMS.

Most capnography technology is built on infrared (IR) radiation techniques. These techniques are based on the fact that CO$_2$ molecules absorb IR radiation at a very specific wavelength (4.26 μm), with the amount of radiation absorbed having a close to exponential relation to the CO$_2$ concentration present in the breath sample. Detecting these changes in IR radiation levels, using appropriate photo-detectors sensitive in this spectral region, allows for the calculation of the CO$_2$ concentration in the gas sample.

CO$_2$ monitors measure gas concentration or partial pressure using one of two configurations, depending on the location of the sensor: mainstream or sidestream. Mainstream devices measure CO_2 directly from the airway, with the sensor located on the endotracheal tube. Sidestream devices measure CO_2 by aspirating a small sample from the exhaled breath through tubing to a sensor located inside the monitor. Mainstream systems, because the sensor is located on the endotracheal tube, are configured for intubated patients. Sidestream systems, because the sensor is located inside the monitor, are configured for both intubated and non-intubated patients. The airway interface for intubated patients is an airway adapter placed on the hub of the endotracheal tube; for spontaneously breathing patients, a nasal-oral cannula allows concomitant CO_2 sampling and low-flow oxygen delivery.

Sidestream systems can be high flow (150 cc/min; being the amount of CO_2 in the breath sample required to obtain an accurate reading) or low flow (50 cc/min). Low-flow sidestream systems have a lower occlusion rate (from moisture or patient secretions) and are more accurate in patients with low tidal volumes (neonates, infants, and patients with hypoventilation and low–tidal volume breathing).[46]

CO_2 monitors can be either quantitative or qualitative. Quantitative devices measure the precise E_Tco_2 as either a number (capnometry) or a number and a waveform (capnography). Qualitative devices measure a range in which the E_Tco_2 falls (e.g., 0–10 mm Hg, >35 mm Hg) as opposed to a precise value (e.g., 38 mm Hg). The most commonly used qualitative device is the colorimetric E_Tco_2 detector, consisting of a piece of specially treated litmus paper that turns color when exposed to CO_2. Its primary use is for verification of endotracheal tube placement and position. If the tube is in the trachea, the resultant exhalation of CO_2 will change the color of the litmus paper; if the tube is in the esophagus with no CO_2 in the breath, there will be no color change.

Physiology

The capnogram, corresponding to a single tidal breath, consists of four phases (ascending phase, alveolar plateau, inspiratory limb, dead space ventilation) in which each of these phases has conventionally been approximated as a straight line.[45,47] Phase 1 (dead space ventilation, A–B) represents the beginning of exhalation in which the dead space is cleared from the upper airway. Phase 2 (ascending phase, B–C) represents the rapid rise in CO_2 concentration in the breath stream as the CO_2 from the alveoli reaches the upper airway. Phase 3 (alveolar plateau, C–D) represents the CO_2 concentration reaching a uniform level in the entire breath stream (from alveolus to nose) and concludes with a point of maximum CO_2 concentration (E_Tco_2). This is the number that appears on the monitor display. Phase 4 (D–E) represents the inspiratory cycle in which the CO_2 concentration drops to zero as atmospheric air enters the airway (see Fig. 2–8).

A normal capnogram, for patients of all ages, is characterized by a specific set of elements: It includes four distinct phases, the CO_2 concentration starts at zero and returns to zero (i.e., there is no rebreathing of CO_2), a maximum CO_2 concentration is reached with each breath (i.e., E_Tco_2), the amplitude is dependent on the E_Tco_2 concentration, the width is dependent on the expiratory time, and there is a characteristic shape for all subjects with normal lung function.

Patients with normal lung function, irrespective of age, will have a characteristic rectangular or trapezoidal shaped capnogram and a narrow E_Tco_2-Pco_2 gradient (0–5 mm Hg), with the E_Tco_2 accurately reflecting the Pa_{CO_2}.[48] Patients with

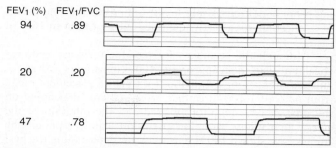

FEV$_1$ (%)	FEV$_1$/FVC
94	.89
20	.20
47	.78

Figure 2–9 Capnogram shape in normal subjects and in patients with obstructive and restrictive lung disease. *(From Krauss B, Deykin A, Lam A, et al: Capnogram shape in obstructive lung disease. Anesth Analg 100:884, 2005.)*

obstructive lung disease will have a more rounded ascending phase and an upward slope in the alveolar plateau (Fig. 2–9).[49] In patients with abnormal lung function from V-Q mismatch, the gradient will widen, depending on the severity of the lung disease, and the E_Tco_2 will be useful only for trending ventilatory status over time and not as a spot check that may or may not correlate with the Pa_{CO_2}.[50,51]

Indications for Intubated Patients

- Verification of endotracheal tube placement
- Continuous monitoring of tube location during transport
- Gauging effectiveness of resuscitation and prognosis during cardiac arrest
- Titrating E_Tco_2 levels in patients with suspected increases in intracranial pressure
- Determining prognosis in trauma
- Determining adequacy of ventilation

Verification of Endotracheal Tube Placement

Unrecognized misplaced intubation (UMI) is the placement of an endotracheal tube in a location other than the trachea, unrecognized by the clinician. This life-threatening condition has been extensively documented in the EMS literature, with early studies reporting a 0.4% to 8% UMI rate. Katz and Falk in 2001[52] were the first to perform a study with the primary outcome of identifying the rate of UMI and noted an alarming rate of 25%. More recent EMS studies have reported UMI rates of 7% to 10%.

After intubation, the presence of a waveform with all four phases indicates that the endotracheal tube is through the vocal cords. A flatline waveform indicates esophageal placement except in selected conditions (obstruction of the endotracheal tube, complete airway obstruction distal to the tube, tracheal placement with inadequate pulmonary blood flow from either poor chest compressions or prolonged cardiac arrest with no circulating CO_2 due to cessation of cellular metabolism).

The accuracy of E_Tco_2 to confirm tracheal location of an endotracheal tube varies based on the type of CO_2 technology utilized. In patients who are not in cardiac arrest, qualitative colorimetric E_Tco_2 and quantitative capnography studies have demonstrated 100% sensitivity and specificity for tracheal placement. In marked contrast, the use of clinical signs for verification has been shown to be unreliable. Fogging or condensation of the tube occurs in 80% of esophageal tubes,[53] chest wall movement can be produced by tracheal or esophageal tubes,[54] and anesthesiologists under ideal operating room conditions, using breath sounds as the sole means of verification, incorrectly identified tube location in 16% of cases.[55]

Although the accuracy of $E_T co_2$ for verifying endotracheal tube placement approaches 100% in patients with spontaneous circulation, sensitivities for tracheal placement range from 62% to 100% in cardiac arrest patients depending on the type of CO_2 monitoring used and the duration of the arrest. In patients with low-perfusion states, capnography studies have shown 100% sensitivity for determining tracheal location of the tube.[56,57] However, the specificity of capnography for esophageal intubation in cardiac arrest is uncertain owing to the small number of esophageal intubations in cardiac arrest studies. When a waveform is present in an intubated patient in cardiac arrest, the endotracheal tube can be assumed to be in the trachea. However, if there is no waveform, the tube may be in the esophagus or in the trachea with no CO_2 reading owing to insufficient pulmonary blood flow.

Colorimetric studies have shown variable sensitivity because the exhaled CO_2 concentration can fall below the detection threshold. Therefore, it is particularly important when evaluating $E_T co_2$ studies to distinguish those involving qualitative colorimetric detection from those using capnography.

Monitoring Tube Position during Transport

Although the presence of UMI (from either initial misplacement of the endotracheal tube or subsequent dislodgment of the tube during transport) has catastrophic consequences, it is preventable. Continuous monitoring of tube position during transport (prehospital to hospital, interhospital, or intrahospital) is essential for patient safety. $E_T co_2$ confirmation of initial endotracheal tube placement and continuous monitoring of tube position has been an accepted standard of care by the American Society of Anesthesiologists and is recommended by other national organizations. In 2005, Silvestri and coworkers[58] studied the impact of continuous $E_T co_2$ monitoring on UMI rate and found a 23% UMI rate in the group that did not use continuous $E_T co_2$ monitoring and a 0% UMI rate in the group that did.

Gauging Effectiveness of Cardiopulmonary Resuscitation

In the 1980s, studies in animal models demonstrated that $E_T co_2$ levels reflect cardiac output during cardiopulmonary resuscitation and can be used as a noninvasive measure of cardiac output. A landmark study in 1988 demonstrated this principle in humans (Fig. 2–10).[59] During cardiac arrest, when alveolar ventilation and metabolism are essentially constant, the $E_T co_2$ reflects the degree of pulmonary blood flow. Therefore, the $E_T co_2$ can be used as a gauge of the effectiveness of cardiac compressions. Because effective cardiac compression leads to a higher cardiac output, the $E_T co_2$ will correspondingly rise from baseline, reflecting an increase in perfusion.

The measurement of $E_T co_2$ varies directly with the cardiac output produced by precordial compression and has been described in both EMS and intensive care unit patients. These studies found $E_T co_2$ levels lower than 3 mm Hg at the onset of cardiac arrest, with higher levels generated during cardiac compressions and a mean peak greater than 7.5 mm Hg just before return of spontaneous circulation (ROSC).[59,60] This peak in $E_T co_2$ level is the earliest sign of ROSC and may occur before palpable hemodynamic signs (pulse or blood pressure).

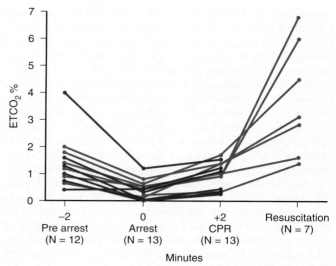

Figure 2–10 End-tidal carbon dioxide concentration ($E_T co_2$) pattern during cardiac arrest. *(From Falk JL, Rackow ED, Weil MH: End-tidal carbon dioxide concentration during cardiopulmonary resuscitation. N Engl J Med 318:607, 1988.)*

Indicator of ROSC

The Falk study[59] also showed that during cardiac arrest, the $E_T co_2$ is the earliest indicator of return of spontaneous circulation. When the heart is restarted, the dramatic increase in cardiac output, and resulting increase in perfusion, leads to a rapid increase in the $E_T co_2$ from baseline as the CO_2 that has built up in the blood during cardiac arrest is effectively transported to the lungs and exhaled.

AHA guidelines emphasize the importance of continuing chest compressions without interruption until a perfusing rhythm is reestablished. Experimental evidence indicates that interruptions in chest compressions are followed by sustained periods during which flow gradually returns to preinterruption levels. Capnographic monitoring virtually eliminates the need to "stop pumping" for the purpose of checking for pulses. Reestablishment of a perfusing rhythm will be immediately accompanied by a dramatic increase in $E_T co_2$, at which point chest compressions can safely be stopped while ECG rhythm and blood pressure are reassessed.[61]

Assessing Prognosis of Cardiac Arrest Resuscitation

$E_T co_2$ can be used as a prognostic indicator of survival in adult cardiac arrest patients. In multiple studies, $E_T co_2$ levels of 10 mm Hg or lower measured 20 minutes after the initiation of advanced cardiac life support accurately predicted death in patients with cardiac arrest. The prognostic value of measuring $E_T co_2$ has been demonstrated in animal and human studies.

Identifying the Etiology of Cardiac Arrest

While not generally used clinically, $E_T co_2$ may be useful in determining the etiology of cardiac arrest. Animal studies reported higher $E_T co_2$ levels at the onset of cardiac arrest caused by primary asphyxia than arrest caused by ventricular fibrillation. A prehospital cardiac arrest study found similar results, reporting higher $E_T co_2$ levels for the asphyxia group (initial rhythm of asystole or pulseless electrical activity associated with conditions such as airway foreign body, aspiration, asthma, or drowning) compared with the ventricular tachycardia/fibrillation group (initial rhythm of ventricular tachycardia/fibrillation associated with acute myocardial infarction).

Titrating E$_T$co$_2$ in Patients with Suspected Increased Intracranial Pressure

E$_T$co$_2$ monitoring has been shown to play a role in avoidance of inadvertent hyperventilation in patients with head injury and suspected increased intracranial pressure. CO$_2$ levels affect blood flow to the brain, with high CO$_2$ levels resulting in cerebral vasodilatation and low CO$_2$ levels resulting in cerebral vasoconstriction. Sustained hypoventilation (E$_T$co$_2$ levels $\geq$ 50 mm Hg) is detrimental to patients with increased intracranial pressure because it results in increased cerebral blood flow and potential worsening of intracranial pressure.

Sustained hyperventilation is also detrimental and is associated with worse neurologic outcome in severely brain-injured patients. Consequently, ventilation with CO$_2$ monitoring to achieve eucapnea is recommended.[62] Prehospital use of E$_T$co$_2$ monitoring reduces the incidence of inadvertent hyperventilation. Severe head-injury patients monitored with continuous E$_T$co$_2$ had a lower incidence of inadvertent hyperventilation than those without E$_T$co$_2$ monitoring.[63] Prehospital blunt trauma victims monitored with continuous capnography were more likely to arrive at the ED appropriately ventilated.[64]

E$_T$co$_2$ monitoring has also demonstrated prognostic value in determining outcome in trauma victims. In a study of blunt trauma patients requiring prehospital intubation, E$_T$co$_2$ levels were able to distinguish the survival from the nonsurvival group.[65]

Indications for Capnography in Spontaneously Breathing Patients

In spontaneously breathing, nonintubated patients capnography can be used for

- Rapid assessment of critically ill or seizing patients.
- Assessment and triage of victims of chemical terrorism.
- Gauging severity and response to treatment in acute respiratory distress.
- Determining adequacy of ventilation in patients with altered mental status.
- Assessment of airway, breathing, and circulation (ABCs) in actively seizing patients.
- Detecting metabolic acidosis in diabetic patients and in children with gastroenteritis.

Assessment of Critically Ill or Seizing Patients

The ABCs of critically ill patients can be rapidly assessed using the waveform and E$_T$co$_2$ values. The presence of a normal waveform denotes a patent airway and spontaneous breathing.[66] Normal E$_T$co$_2$ levels (35–45 mm Hg) signify adequate perfusion.[59,67]

Capnography can be used to assess and triage critically ill patients, victims of chemical terrorism, and actively seizing patients.[68,69] Unlike pulse oximetry, capnography does not misinterpret motion artifact and provides reliable readings in low-perfusion states.

Capnography is the only monitoring modality that is accurate and reliable in actively seizing patients. Capnographic data (RR, E$_T$co$_2$, and capnogram) can be used to distinguish among

- Seizing patients with apnea (flatline waveform, no E$_T$co$_2$ readings, and no chest wall movement).
- Seizing patients with ineffective ventilation (small waveforms, low E$_T$co$_2$ values).
- Seizing patients with effective ventilation (normal waveform, normal E$_T$co$_2$ values).

Assessment and Triage of Victims of Chemical Terrorism

EDs and EMS systems have intensively focused on training to identify and effectively manage mass casualty chemical terrorism events. A noninvasive assessment tool would facilitate the rapid identification of the common life-threatening complications of chemical terrorism.[68] Capnography can rapidly detect the common airway, respiratory, and central nervous system adverse events associated with the nerve agents including apnea, upper airway obstruction, laryngospasm, bronchospasm, respiratory failure, seizures, and coma (Table 2–7).

 TABLE 2–7 Capnographic Identification of Life-Threatening Complications of Nerve Agents CAN BE FOUND ON EXPERT CONSULT

Gauging Severity and Response to Treatment in Acute Respiratory Distress

Capnography provides dynamic monitoring of ventilatory status in patients with acute respiratory distress from any cause including asthma, bronchiolitis, COPD, CHF, croup, and cystic fibrosis. By measuring E$_T$co$_2$ and RR with each breath, capnography provides instantaneous feedback on the clinical status of the patient. RR is measured directly from the airway (nose and mouth), by oral-nasal cannula, providing a more reliable reading than impedance respiratory monitoring. In upper airway obstruction and laryngospasm, impedance monitoring detects chest wall movement, interprets this as a valid breath, and displays an RR, even though the patient is not ventilating. In contrast, capnography will detect no ventilation and shows a flatline waveform.

E$_T$co$_2$ trends can be rapidly assessed, especially in tachypneic patients. A patient with an RR of 30 will generate 150 E$_T$co$_2$ readings in 5 minutes. This provides sufficient information to determine whether the patient's ventilation is worsening despite treatment (increasing E$_T$co$_2$), stabilizing (stable E$_T$co$_2$), or improving (decreasing E$_T$co$_2$) (Fig. 2–11).

Procedural Sedation and Analgesia

Pulse oximetry is the standard technique to monitor procedural sedation in the ED, but capnography can also detect the common adverse airway and respiratory events associated with procedural sedation and analgesia.[70] Capnography is the earliest indicator of airway or respiratory compromise and will manifest an abnormally high or low E$_T$co$_2$ well before pulse oximetry detects a falling oxyhemoglobin saturation, especially in patients receiving supplemental oxygen (Fig. 2–12). Capnography provides a nonimpedance RR directly from the airway (via oral-nasal cannula). This is more accurate than impedance-based respiratory monitoring, especially in patients with obstructive apnea or laryngospasm, in which impedance-based monitoring will interpret chest wall movement without ventilation as a valid breath.

Both central and obstructive apnea can be almost instantaneously detected by capnography (Table 2–8). Loss of the capnogram, in conjunction with no chest wall movement and no breath sounds on auscultation, confirms the diagnosis of central apnea. Obstructive apnea is characterized by loss of the capnogram, chest wall movement, and absent breath sounds. The absence of the capnogram in association with the presence or absence of chest wall movement distinguishes apnea from upper airway obstruction and laryngospasm. Response to airway alignment maneuvers can further distinguish upper airway obstruction from laryngospasm.

Capnography may be more sensitive than clinical assessment of ventilation in detection of apnea. In a recent study, 10/39 of patients (26%) experienced 20-second periods of apnea during procedural sedation and analgesia. All 10 episodes of apnea were detected by capnography but not by the anesthesia providers.[71]

Because the amplitude of the capnogram is determined by $E_T co_2$ and the width is determined by the expiratory time, changes in these parameters affect capnogram shape. Hyperventilation (increased RR, decreased $E_T co_2$) results in a low-amplitude and narrow capnogram, whereas classic hypoventilation (decreased RR, increased $E_T co_2$) results in a high-amplitude and wide capnogram (see Table 2–8). Acute bronchospasm results in a capnogram with a curved ascending phase and upsloping alveolar plateau (see Fig. 2–12). An $E_T co_2$

greater than 70 mm Hg, in patients without chronic hypoventilation, indicates respiratory failure.

Two types of drug-induced hypoventilation occur during procedural sedation and analgesia (see Table 2–8).[70] Bradypneic hypoventilation (type 1), commonly seen with opioids, is characterized by an increased $E_T co_2$ and an increased Pa_{CO_2}. RR is depressed proportionally greater than tidal volume, resulting in bradypnea, an increase in expiratory time, and a rise in $E_T co_2$, graphically represented by a high-amplitude and wide capnogram (see Table 2–8).

Bradypneic hypoventilation follows a predictable course, with $E_T co_2$ increasing progressively until respiratory failure and apnea occur. Although there is no absolute threshold at which apnea occurs, patients without chronic hypoventilation with $E_T co_2$ greater than 80 mm Hg are at significant risk.

Hypopneic hypoventilation (type 2), commonly seen with sedative-hypnotic drugs, is characterized by a normal or decreased $E_T co_2$ and an increased Pa_{CO_2} as airway dead space remains constant (e.g., 150 mL in the normal adult lung) and tidal volume is decreasing. Tidal volume is depressed proportionally greater than RR, resulting in low tidal volume breathing that leads to an increase in airway dead space fraction (dead space volume/tidal volume). As tidal volume decreases, airway dead space fraction increases, which in turn results in an increase in the $Pa_{CO_2} - E_T co_2$ gradient. Even though Pa_{CO_2} is increasing, $E_T co_2$ may remain normal or be decreasing, graphically represented by a low-amplitude capnogram.

The low tidal volume breathing that characterizes hypopneic hypoventilation increases dead space ventilation when normal compensatory mechanisms are inhibited by drug effects. Minute ventilation, which normally increases to compensate for an increase in dead space, does not change or may decrease. As minute ventilation decreases, arterial oxygenation decreases. If minute ventilation decreases further, oxygenation is further impaired. However, $E_T co_2$ may initially be high (bradypneic hypoventilation) or low (hypopneic hypoventilation) without significant changes in oxygenation, particularly if supplemental oxygen is given. Therefore, a drug-induced increase or decrease in $E_T co_2$ does not necessarily lead to oxygen desaturation and may not require intervention.

Hypopneic hypoventilation follows a variable course and may remain stable with low tidal volume breathing resolving over time as central nervous system drug levels decrease and redistribution to the periphery occurs, progress to periodic

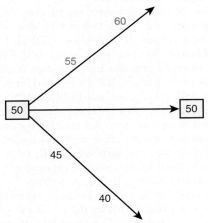

Figure 2–11 $E_T co_2$ trending in acute respiratory distress. Dynamic ventilatory information provided by $E_T co_2$ trends for gauging response to treatment in patients with acute respiratory distress. Trends show worsening despite treatment (increasing $E_T co_2$), stabilized (stable $E_T co_2$), or improving (decreasing $E_T co_2$) ventilatory status.

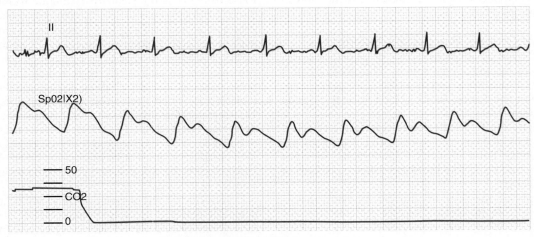

Figure 2–12 Capnographic detection of apnea.

TABLE 2-8 Capnographic Airway Assessment for Procedural Sedation and Analgesia

Diagnosis	Waveform	Features		Intervention
Normal		SpO$_2$ E$_T$CO$_2$ Waveform RR	Normal Normal Normal Normal	No intervention required Continue sedation
Hyperventilation		SpO$_2$ E$_T$CO$_2$ Waveform RR	Normal ↓ Decreased amplitude and width ↑	Reassess patient Continue sedation
Bradypneic hypoventilation (type 1)		SpO$_2$ E$_T$CO$_2$ Waveform RR	Normal ↑ Increased amplitude and width ↓↓↓	Reassess patient Assess for airway obstruction Supplemental oxygen Cease drug administration or reduce dosing
		SpO$_2$ E$_T$CO$_2$ Waveform RR	 ↑ Increased amplitude and width ↓↓↓	
Hypopneic hypoventilation (type 2)		SpO$_2$ E$_T$CO$_2$ Waveform RR	Normal ↓ Decreased amplitude →	Reassess patient Continue sedation
		SpO$_2$ E$_T$CO$_2$ Waveform RR	 → Decreased amplitude →	Reassess patient Assess for airway obstruction Supplemental oxygen Cease drug administration or reduce dosing
Hypopneic hypoventilation with periodic breathing		SpO$_2$ E$_T$CO$_2$ Waveform RR Other	Normal or ↓ ↓ Decreased amplitude → Apneic pauses	

Continued

TABLE 2–8 Capnographic Airway Assessment for Procedural Sedation and Analgesia—cont'd

Diagnosis	Waveform	Features	Intervention
Physiologic variability		SpO$_2$: Normal E$_T$CO$_2$: Normal Waveform: Varying* RR: Normal	No intervention required Continue sedation
Bronchospasm	 50 [CO$_2$] 0 Time	SpO$_2$: Normal or ↓ E$_T$CO$_2$: Normal, ↑, or ↓† Waveform: Curved RR: Normal, ↑, or ↓† Other: Wheezing	Reassess patient Bronchodilator therapy Cease drug administration
Partial airway obstruction	 40 [CO$_2$] 0 Time	SpO$_2$: Normal or ↓ E$_T$CO$_2$: Normal Waveform: Normal RR: Variable Other: Noisy breathing and/or inspiratory stridor	Reassess patient Establish IV access Supplemental O$_2$ (as needed) Cease drug administration Full airway patency restored with airway alignment Noisy breathing and stridor resolve
Partial laryngospasm			Airway not fully patent with airway alignment Noisy breathing and stridor persist
Apnea	 40 [CO$_2$] 0 Time	SpO$_2$: normal or ↓‡ E$_T$CO$_2$: Zero Waveform: Absent RR: Zero Other: No chest wall movement or breath sounds	Reassess patient Stimulation Bag mask ventilation Reversal agents (as appropriate) Cease drug administration
Complete airway obstruction		SpO$_2$: Normal or ↓‡ E$_T$CO$_2$: Zero Waveform: Absent RR: Zero Other: Chest wall movement and breath sounds present	Airway patency restored with airway alignment Waveform present
Complete laryngospasm			Airway not patent with airway alignment No waveform Positive pressure ventilation

E$_T$CO$_2$, end-tidal carbon dioxide concentration; RR, respiratory rate; SpO$_2$, pulse oximetry.
*Varying waveform amplitude and width.
†Depending on duration and severity of bronchospasm.
‡Depending on duration of episode.

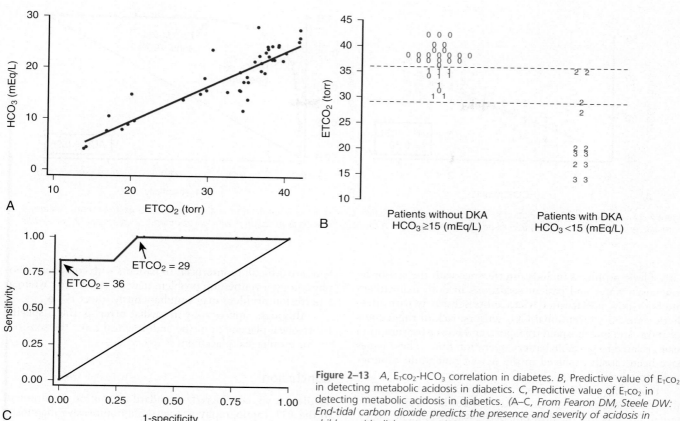

Figure 2–13 *A,* E_Tco_2-HCO_3 correlation in diabetes. *B,* Predictive value of E_Tco_2 in detecting metabolic acidosis in diabetics. *C,* Predictive value of E_Tco_2 in detecting metabolic acidosis in diabetics. *(A–C, From Fearon DM, Steele DW: End-tidal carbon dioxide predicts the presence and severity of acidosis in children with diabetes. Acad Emerg Med 9:1373, 2002.)*

breathing with intermittent apneic pauses (which may resolve spontaneously or progress to central apnea), or progress directly to central apnea.

Determining the Adequacy of Ventilation in Patients with Altered Mental Status

Patients with altered mental status, including those with alcohol intoxication, intentional or unintentional drug overdose, and postictal patients (especially those treated with benzodiazepines), may have impaired ventilatory function. Capnography can differentiate between patients with effective ventilation and those with ineffective ventilation as well as providing continuous monitoring of ventilatory trends over time to identify those patients at risk for respiratory depression.

Detection of Metabolic Acidosis

In addition to its established uses for ventilation and perfusion assessment, capnography is a valuable tool for assessing metabolic status providing information on how effectively CO_2 is being produced by cellular metabolism.

Recent studies have shown that E_Tco_2 and serum bicarbonate (HCO_3) are linearly correlated in diabetes and in gastroenteritis and E_Tco_2 can be used as an indicator of metabolic acidosis in these patients (Figs. 2–13A and 2–14A).[72–74] As the patient becomes acidotic, HCO_3 decreases and a compensatory respiratory alkalosis develops with an increase in minute ventilation and a resultant decrease in E_Tco_2. By increasing minute ventilation, these patients are able to lower arterial CO_2 tension to help correct the underlying acidemia. The more acidotic, the lower the HCO_3, the higher the RR, and the lower the E_Tco_2.

E_Tco_2 can be used to distinguish diabetics in ketoacidosis (metabolic acidosis, compensatory tachypnea, low E_Tco_2) from those who are not (nonacidotic, normal RR, normal E_Tco_2) (see Fig. 2–13B and C). Similarly, E_Tco_2 is correlated with and predicts the HCO_3 in children with gastroenteritis (see Fig. 2–14B). In a study of diabetic children presenting to the ED, E_Tco_2 less than 29 mm Hg identified 95% of the patients with ketoacidosis with 83% sensitivity and 100% specificity. Conversely, no ketoacidosis was detected in patients with E_Tco_2 greater than 36 mm Hg (see Fig. 2–10C).[72] Using these data, nursing triage protocols can be developed to facilitate rapid assessment and treatment of patients in diabetic ketoacidosis.

A similar association between E_Tco_2 and HCO_3 was demonstrated in children with gastroenteritis with maximal sensitivity occurring at E_Tco_2 of 34 mm Hg or less (sensitivity 100%, specificity 60%) and optimal specificity without compromise of sensitivity occurring at E_Tco_2 of 31 mm Hg or less (sensitivity 76%, specificity 96%)[74] (see Fig. 2–14B).

As a potential triage tool for determining the need for oral versus intravenous rehydration, E_Tco_2 could identify patients with a clinically significant acidosis with an E_Tco_2 of 31 mm Hg or less giving a positive likelihood ratio of 20.4 in detecting HCO_3 of 15 mmol/L or less and a ratio of 14.1 for HCO_3 of 13 mmol/L or less. These E_Tco_2 values are 14 or 20 times more likely to occur in an acidotic patient than in a patient with an HCO_3 greater than 13 or 15 mmol/L.

Limitations

Significant technical problems have limited the effective use of capnography and restricted its clinical applications in the

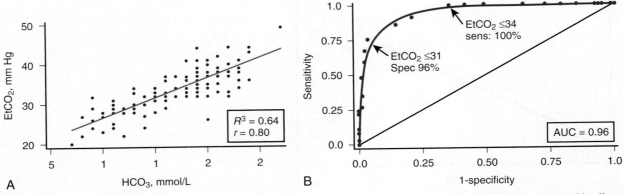

Figure 2–14 *A*, E_TCO_2-HCO_3 correlation in gastroenteritis. *B*, Predictive value of E_TCO_2 in detecting metabolic acidosis in gastroenteritis. *(A and B, From Nagler J, Wright RO, Krauss B: End-tidal carbon dioxide as a measure of acidosis in children with gastroenteritis. Pediatrics;117:260, 2006.)*

past. These problems include interference with the sensor by condensed water and patient secretions in both mainstream and high-flow sidestream devices, cross-sensitivity with anesthetic gases in conventional CO_2 sensors, lack of ruggedness for intra- and interhospital transport, and power consumption issues related to portable battery operation time. These issues have been mostly resolved in the newer generation capnography monitors.

However, problems with accuracy continue to affect high-flow sidestream systems. When the tidal volume of the patient drops below the flow rate of the system (e.g., neonates, infants, hypoventilating patients with low tidal volume breathing), the monitor will entrain room air to compensate, falsely diluting the E_TCO_2 and slurring the ascending phase of the waveform.[75–77]

Early capnography airway interfaces (i.e., nasal cannula) had difficulty providing consistent measurements in mouth-breathing patients and patients who alternated between mouth- and nose-breathing. The newer oral-nasal interface no longer has these problems.

Capnography is most effective when assessing a pure ventilation, perfusion, or metabolism problem. Capnographic findings in mixed ventilation, perfusion, or metabolism problems are difficult to interpret. In patients with complex pathophysiology, a ventilation problem may elevate E_TCO_2, whereas a perfusion problem may simultaneously lower E_TCO_2.

Although capnography in cardiac arrest is 100% specific for tracheal placement of the endotracheal tube, the sensitivity for esophageal placement is uncertain.

Conclusion

While not yet considered a standard or routine requirement in the ED, capnography is a versatile noninvasive diagnostic modality for monitoring ventilatory status in both intubated and nonintubated patients. Clinical applications include verification of endotracheal tube placement and continuous monitoring of tube location, cardiac arrest, head trauma, vital sign assessment in critically ill or injured patients, patients in acute respiratory distress, unconscious or obtunded patients, and metabolic disorders such as diabetes and acute gastroenteritis in children.

 REFERENCES CAN BE FOUND ON EXPERT CONSULT

RESPIRATORY PROCEDURES

CHAPTER **3**

Basic Airway Management and Decision-Making

Robert F. Reardon, Phillip E. Mason, and Joseph E. Clinton

Over the last few decades, several important changes have occurred in emergency airway management. Bag-mask ventilation has been supplemented by intermediate, or backup, ventilation devices like the laryngeal mask airway (LMA), the Combitube, and the laryngeal tube. These have become important devices for the initial resuscitation of apneic patients and for rescue ventilation when intubation fails.[1] Noninvasive positive-pressure ventilation (NPPV) is now used in place of tracheal intubation in some critically ill patients. Despite these advances, basic techniques such as opening the airway, oxygenation, and bag-mask ventilation remain the cornerstones of good emergency airway management.[2,3] Airway maintenance without endotracheal intubation is one of the most important emergency airway management techniques to keep patients alive until a definitive airway can be established.[4]

This chapter describes basic airway skills including opening the airway, O_2 therapy, NPPV, bag-mask ventilation, and intermediate ventilation devices. Because of the complexity of these skills and decisions, providers should develop a simple, organized approach to emergency airway management, being cognizant that when a specific intervention has failed, it is time to move rapidly to a different approach. Developing a simple preconceived algorithm that employs proven techniques and is applicable to a broad range of clinical scenarios will help providers manage difficult, anxiety-provoking emergency airways.

THE CHALLENGE OF EMERGENCY AIRWAY MANAGEMENT

Although other specialists are sometimes available, most emergency airways are managed by emergency clinicians.[5]

Airway management in the emergency department (ED) is much different from airway management in the controlled setting of the operating room. Likewise, conventional airway management tools may be ineffective in the uncontrolled prehospital environment. Major challenges include hypoxia, shock, and the presence of vomit, blood, or excessive secretions in the airway. Many patients are uncooperative and combative, making it impossible to examine their airway prior to choosing an intubation technique. Medical history, allergies, and even the current diagnosis are often unknown before emergency airway management begins. Time constraints, lack of patient cooperation, and the risk of vomiting limit the use of optimal techniques, such as awake intubation. In trauma patients, the risk of cervical spine injury limits optimal head and neck positioning for bag-mask ventilation and laryngoscopy. All of these factors increase the risk of complications due to emergency airway management.[5,6] As many as 1% of all emergency airways require a surgical approach.

BASIC AIRWAY MANAGEMENT TECHNIQUES

Opening the Airway

The first concern in the management of the critically ill patient is *adequacy of the airway*. Upper airway obstruction most commonly occurs when patients are unconscious or sedated. It can also occur with injury to the mandible or muscles that support the hypopharynx. In these situations, the tongue moves posteriorly into the upper airway when the patient is lying supine. Upper airway obstruction caused by the tongue can be relieved by positioning maneuvers of the head, neck, and jaw; nasopharyngeal or oropharyngeal airways; or continuous positive airway pressure (CPAP).

Pulse oximetry (SpO_2) has greatly improved our ability to monitor oxygenation of patients at risk of airway or ventilatory compromise.[7] These monitors are accurate under most conditions,[8] and allow clinically subtle deterioration to be recognized quickly. SpO_2 monitors are standard equipment in all emergency airway settings.

Manual Airway Maneuvers

Airway obstruction in unconscious patients may be due to posterior displacement of the tongue; however, research in obstructive sleep apnea and CPAP shows that the concept of the airway collapsing like a flexible tube may be more accurate[4,9] (Fig. 3–1*A*). Upper airway obstruction may cause snoring or stridor, but an apneic patient or one who is moving

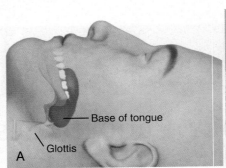 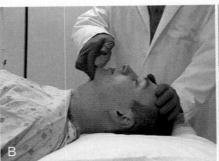 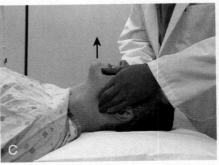

Base of tongue

Glottis

A   B   C

Figure 3–1 *A,* The airway can be obstructed by the tongue and or collapse of the airway. Initial maneuvers for opening the airway include head-tilt/chin-lift *(B)* and jaw thrust *(C)*. *(A–C, From Thomsen Todd, Setnik G [eds]: Procedures Consult—Emergency Medicine Module.Copyright 2008 Elsevier Inc. All rights reserved.)*

minimal air may not exhibit any audible evidence of upper airway obstruction. Therefore, every unconscious patient has a potential upper airway obstruction.

More than 30 years ago, Guildner[10] compared different techniques for opening obstructed upper airways and found that the head-tilt/chin-lift and the jaw-thrust techniques were effective (see Fig. 3–1*B* and *C*). Modern airway textbooks still describe the head-tilt/chin-lift and the jaw-thrust maneuvers, but also describe the "triple airway maneuver," which is a combination of head-tilt, jaw-thrust, and mouth opening.[4,11]

It is widely accepted that the jaw-thrust-only (without head-tilt) maneuver should be performed in patients with suspected cervical spine injury, but this technique is sometimes ineffective and there is no evidence that it is safer than the head-tilt/chin-lift maneuver.[12] In 2005, the American Heart Association (AHA)[13] concluded that airway maneuvers are safe during manual in-line stabilization of the cervical spine, but highlighted evidence that all airway maneuvers cause some spinal movement. Both the chin-lift and the jaw-thrust maneuvers have been shown to cause similar substantial movement of the cervical vertebrae.[14-18] The AHA recommended that "in a victim with a suspected spinal injury and an obstructed airway, the head-tilt/chin-lift or jaw-thrust (with head-tilt) techniques are feasible and may be effective for clearing the airway," while emphasizing that "maintaining an airway and adequate ventilation is the over-riding priority in managing a patient with a suspected spinal injury."[13]

Despite the lack of evidence for the jaw-thrust-only (without head-tilt) technique, many experienced airway providers believe that this technique is effective and valuable.[4,19] It is certainly reasonable to attempt the jaw-thrust-only technique before employing the chin-lift/head-tilt technique in patients with possible cervical spine injury.[11]

Importantly, the addition of CPAP may relieve airway obstruction when simple manual positioning maneuvers fail. Meier and colleagues[9] showed that adding CPAP to the chin-lift and jaw-thrust maneuvers decreased stridor and improved the nasal fiberoptic view of the glottic opening in anesthetized children.

The Head-Tilt/Chin-Lift Maneuver
To perform the head-tilt/chin-lift maneuver, place the tips of the index and middle fingers beneath the patient's chin (see Fig. 3–1*B*). Lift the chin cephalad and toward the ceiling. The upper neck will naturally extend when the head tilts backward during this maneuver. Apply digital pressure on only the bony prominence of the chin and not on the soft tissues of the submandibular region. The final step of this maneuver is to use the thumb to open the patient's mouth while the head is tilted and the neck is extended.

The Jaw-Thrust Maneuver
To perform the jaw-thrust maneuver, place the tips of the middle or index fingers behind the angle of the mandible (see Fig. 3–1*C*). Lift the mandible toward the ceiling until the lower incisors are anterior to the upper incisors. This maneuver can be performed in combination with the head-tilt/chin-lift maneuver or with the neck in the neutral position during in-line stabilization.

The Triple Airway Maneuver
The "triple airway maneuver" is described by many authors as the best manual method for maintaining a patent upper airway.[4,11] The most common description of this maneuver is head-tilt, jaw-thrust, and mouth opening.[4,11] Other authors describe the triple maneuver differently, as a combination of upper cervical extension (head-tilt), lower cervical flexion, and jaw protrusion (jaw-lift).[19] The triple airway maneuver has been described as a technique for providers with advanced airway skills.[11] No studies exist to support the assertion that this technique is more effective than the head-tilt/chin-lift or jaw-thrust maneuvers. However, the triple maneuver is commonly mentioned in the anesthesia literature and is probably very effective.

Patient Positioning

The best way to position a patient's head and neck to open the upper airway is to mimic how patients with upper airway obstruction position themselves, sitting upright while leaning their head and neck forward.[2] This is known as the "sniffing position" and is achieved by flexion of the lower cervical spine and atlanto-occipital extension (tilting the head backward). In the supine adult, this is accomplished by elevating the patient's head 1 to 4 inches (much more in obese patients) while maintaining head-tilt.[2,4] The sniffing position is contraindicated in patients with cervical spine injuries. In young children, this position is often achieved without lifting the head because the occiput of the child is relatively large, so the lower cervical spine is normally flexed when the child is lying supine on a flat surface.

Airway management is usually easiest when patients are in the supine position; however, the lateral position may be best for patients who are actively vomiting and those with excessive upper airway bleeding or secretions. Some evidence suggests that rotating patients to the lateral position may not prevent aspiration.[20] Patients with suspected cervical spine injury should have their head immobilized with in-line stabilization if they need to be rolled to the lateral position. Airway management maneuvers may be limited or difficult when patients are in the lateral position.

Foreign Body Airway Obstruction

Abdominal Thrusts (Heimlich Maneuver), Chest Thrusts, Back Blows/Slaps

The 2005 International Consensus Conference on Cardiopulmonary Resuscitation and Emergency Cardiopulmonary Care[13] evaluated the evidence for different techniques for clearing foreign body airway obstruction. They found good evidence for the use of chest thrusts, abdominal thrusts, and back blows/slaps. However, insufficient evidence exists to determine which technique is the best and which should be used first. Some evidence exists that chest thrusts may generate higher peak airway pressures than the Heimlich maneuver.

The technique of subdiaphragmatic abdominal thrusts to relieve a completely obstructed airway was popularized by Dr. Henry Heimlich and is commonly referred to as the "Heimlich maneuver."[21] The technique is most effective when a solid food bolus obstructs the larynx. In the conscious patient, stand behind the upright patient. Circle the arms around the patient's midsection with the radial side of the clenched fist placed on the abdomen, midway between the umbilicus and the xiphoid. Then grasp the fist with the opposite hand and deliver an inward and upward thrust to the abdomen (Fig. 3–2A). A successful maneuver will cause the obstructing agent

to be expelled from the patient's airway by the force of air exiting the lungs. Abdominal thrusts can also be performed on unconscious, supine patients. For this position, kneel next to the patient's pelvis facing cephalad (see Fig. 3–2B). Place the palmar bases of the hands in an overlapping fashion on the upper abdomen, in the same location as in the upright technique. Deliver inward, upward thrusts with the same objective as the upright method. Abdominal thrusts are relatively contraindicated in pregnant patients and those with protuberant abdomens. Potential risks of subdiaphragmatic thrusts include stomach rupture, esophageal perforation, and mesenteric laceration, compelling the rescuer to weigh the risks and benefits of this maneuver.[22–27] Use a chest position for pregnant patients (see Fig. 3–2C).

Alternatively, manage foreign body airway obstruction with chest compressions (back blows in an inverted infant) identical to those delivered during cardiopulmonary resuscitation (CPR) (see Fig. 3–2D). The theory is the same as for abdominal thrusts, to expel the obstructing agent by forcing air out of the lungs. Some data suggest that chest compressions may create higher peak airway pressures than the Heimlich maneuver.[28] A combined (simultaneous) chest compression and subdiaphragmatic abdominal thrust may produce even higher peak airway pressures and should be considered when the standard techniques fail.

Back blows are often recommended for infants and small children with foreign body airway obstruction. Some authors have argued that back blows may be dangerous and may drive foreign bodies deeper into the airway, but there is no convincing evidence of this phenomenon.[29,30] As for the other techniques, anecdotal evidence suggests that back blows are

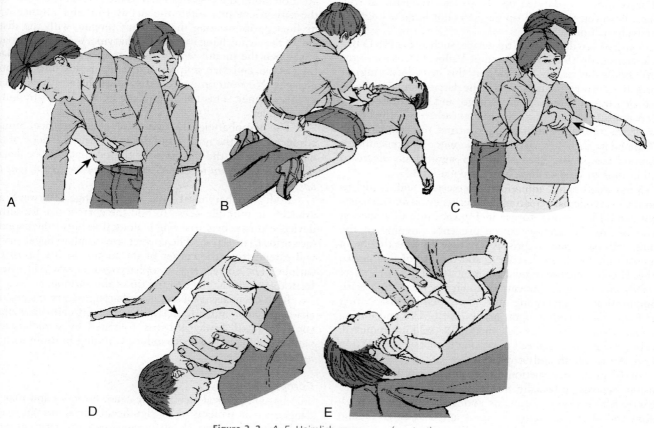

Figure 3–2 *A–E,* Heimlich maneuvers (see text).

effective.[31-33] However, no convincing data indicate that back blows are more or less effective than abdominal or chest thrusts. Back blows may produce a more pronounced increase in airway pressure, but over a shorter period of time than the other techniques. The AHA guidelines suggest back blows in the head-down position (see Fig. 3–2D) and head-down chest thrusts in infants and small children with foreign body airway obstruction.[34] The AHA does not recommend abdominal thrusts in infants, because infants may be at higher risk of iatrogenic injury. From a practical standpoint, back blows should be delivered with the patient in a head-down position, which is easier in infants than in larger children.

Any patient with a complete airway obstruction may benefit from chest compressions, abdominal thrusts, or back blows. Give CPR to all unconscious patients with airway obstruction. It is important to realize that more than one technique is often required to clear foreign body airway obstruction, so multiple techniques should be applied in a rapid sequence until the obstruction is relieved.[13] Perform a finger sweep of the patient's mouth only if a solid object is seen in the airway. It is recommended to suction newborns rather than give them back blows or abdominal thrusts.[34]

Suctioning

Patient positioning and airway opening maneuvers are often inadequate to achieve complete airway patency. Ongoing hemorrhage, vomitus, and particulate debris often require suctioning. Several types of suctioning tips are available. A large-bore dental-type suction tip is the most effective for clearing vomitus from the upper airway because it is less likely to become obstructed by particulate matter. The tonsil tip (Yankauer) suction device can be used to clear hemorrhage and secretions. Its rounded tip is also less traumatic to soft tissues; however, the tonsil tip device is not large enough to effectively suction vomitus.

A large-bore dental-type tip device, such as the HI-D Big Stick suction tip (SSCOR, Inc., Sun Valley, CA; www.sscor.com) should be readily available at the bedside during all emergency airway management. The large-bore tip allows rapid clearing of vomitus, hemorrhage, and secretions.

A limiting feature of many suction catheters is the diameter of the tubing. Vomitus may obstruct the standard $\frac{1}{4}$-inch-diameter catheter.[35] A $\frac{3}{8}$-inch-diameter suction catheter (Conmed Corp.) has been shown to significantly decrease suction time of viscous and particulate material.[36]

Keep suctioning equipment connected and ready to operate; everyone participating in emergency airway management should know how to use it. Interposition of a suction trap close to the suction device prevents clogging of the tubing with particulate debris. A trap that fits directly onto a tracheal tube has been described, and the use of this device allows effective suctioning during intubation.[37]

No specific contraindications to airway suctioning exist. Complications of suctioning may be avoided by anticipating problems and providing appropriate care before and during suctioning maneuvers. Nasal suction is seldom required, except in infants, because most adult airway obstruction occurs in the mouth and oropharynx.

Avoid prolonged suctioning because it may lead to significant hypoxia, especially in children. Do not exceed 15 seconds for suctioning intervals and give supplemental O_2 before and after suctioning. Naigow and Powasner[38] found that suctioning consistently induced hypoxia in dogs and that

it was best avoided by hyperventilation with high-concentration O_2 before and after suctioning.

Perform suctioning under direct vision or with the aid of the laryngoscope. Forcing a suction tip blindly into the posterior pharynx can injure tissue or convert a partial obstruction to a complete obstruction.

Artificial Airways: Oropharyngeal and Nasopharyngeal Airways

Indications and Contraindications

Once the airway has been opened with manual maneuvers and suctioning, artificial airways, such as the nasopharyngeal and oropharyngeal airways, can facilitate both spontaneous breathing and bag-mask ventilation. Semiconscious patients who require a head-tilt/chin-lift or jaw-thrust maneuver to open their airways may develop hypoxia because of recurrent obstruction if these maneuvers are discontinued. O_2 supplementation and a nasopharyngeal airway may be all the support that is necessary.

Patients who are unresponsive or apneic are usually easier to ventilate with a bag-mask device when an oropharyngeal airway is in place. In the ED, patients who tolerate an oropharyngeal airway should probably be intubated.

Artificial Airway Placement

The simplest and most widely available artificial airways are the oropharyngeal and nasopharyngeal airways (Fig. 3–3). Both are intended to prevent the tongue from obstructing the airway by falling back against the posterior pharyngeal wall. The oral airway also may prevent teeth clenching. The oropharyngeal airway may be inserted by either of two procedures. One approach is to insert the airway in an inverted position along the patient's hard palate. When it is well into the patient's mouth, rotate the airway 180° and advance it to its final position along the patient's tongue, with the distal end of the airway lying in the hypopharynx. A second approach is to open the mouth widely, use a tongue blade to displace the tongue, and then simply advance the airway into the oropharynx. No rotation is necessary when the airway is placed in this manner. This technique may be less traumatic but it takes longer.

The nasopharyngeal airway is very easy to place. Simply advance it into the nostril and direct it along the floor of the nasal passage in the direction of the occiput, not cephalad. *Advance it fully until the flared external tip of the airway is at the nasal orifice.*

Both oropharyngeal and nasopharyngeal airways are available in multiple sizes. To find the correct size for either device, estimate by measuring it along the side of the patient's face prior to insertion. The correct size oropharyngeal airway will extend from the corner of the mouth to the tip of the earlobe. The correct size nasopharyngeal airway will extend from the tip of the nose to the tip of the earlobe.

Both oropharyngeal and nasopharyngeal airways provide airway patency similar to that of the head-tilt/chin-lift maneuver. The nasal airway is better tolerated by semiconscious patients and is less likely to induce vomiting in those with an intact gag reflex.

Complications

The nasopharyngeal airway may cause epistaxis and may be dangerous in patients with significant facial fractures and basilar skull fractures. Semiconscious patients with nasopha-

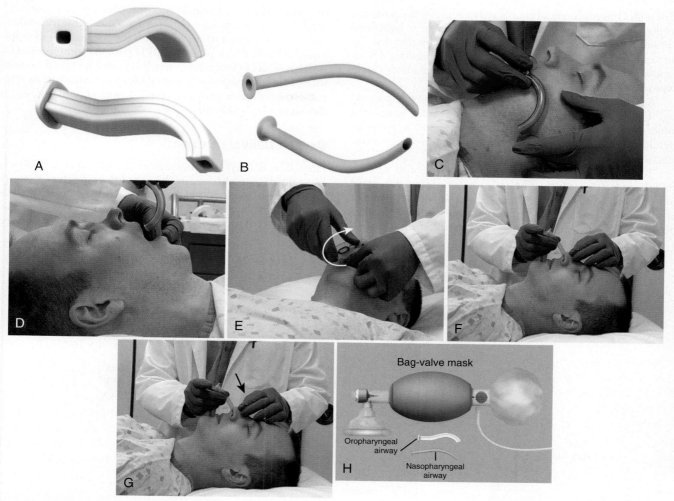

Figure 3–3 Simple artificial airways. Oropharyngeal (*A*) and nasopharyngeal (*B*) airways. To insert the oropharyngeal airway first measure (*C*) then open the mouth with the thumb and index finger (*D*), insert with the *curve upward* and rotate to pass over the base of the tongue (*E*). *It may help to pull the jaw forward during passage.* To insert the nasopharyngeal tube, first measure (*F*), then lubricate and gently pass the entire device through the most patent nostril (*G*) until the flared tip is at the nasal orifice. *H,* A bag-mask is then used to ventilate with either airway in place. *(A–H, From Thomsen T, Setnik G [eds]: Procedures Consult—Emergency Medicine Module.Copyright 2008 Elsevier Inc. All rights reserved.)*

ryngeal airways may deteriorate and require intubation, so they should be monitored closely.

The oropharyngeal airway may induce vomiting when placed in patients with an intact gag reflex. The oropharyngeal airway may also cause airway obstruction if the tongue is pushed against the posterior pharyngeal wall when it is inserted. The oropharyngeal airway should not be used as a definitive airway.

OXYGEN THERAPY

Adequate O_2 delivery depends upon the inspired partial pressure of O_2, alveolar ventilation, pulmonary gas exchange, oxygen-carrying capacity of the blood, and cardiac output. The easiest factor to manipulate is the partial pressure of inspired O_2, accomplished by simply increasing the fraction of inspired oxygen (FI_{O_2}) with supplemental O_2.

Indications and Contraindications

Resuscitate all patients in cardiac arrest or respiratory arrest with 100% O_2. The most certain indication for supplemental

O_2 is the presence of arterial hypoxemia, defined by a PaO_2 <60 mm Hg or arterial oxygen saturation (SaO_2) less than 90%.[39] Normal subjects will begin to experience memory loss at an arterial oxygen partial pressure (Pao_2) of 45 mm Hg and loss of consciousness occurs at a Pao_2 of 30 mm Hg.[40–42] Chronically hypoxemic patients can adapt and function quite well with a Pao_2 of 50 mm Hg or lower.[43]

When tissue hypoxia is present or suspected, give O_2 therapy.[39,44] Shock states resulting from hemorrhage, vasodilatory states, low cardiac output, and obstructive lesions can all lead to tissue hypoxia and should benefit from supplemental O_2. Whatever the cause of the shock state, the administration of O_2 is indicated until the situation can be thoroughly evaluated and cause-specific therapy is instituted.

Respiratory distress without documented arterial hypoxemia is a common indication for O_2 administration, although no evidence exists to support this practice.[45] O_2 therapy for acute myocardial infarction is often recommended, but there is no difference in outcomes between patients receiving O_2 or those receiving room air after myocardial infarction. The AHA gives a class I recommendation for O_2 only in patients with hypoxemia, cyanosis, or respiratory distress.[39,44,46–48]

Although O_2 is routinely administered to acute stroke patients, no convincing evidence exists that this practice is beneficial without documented hypoxia; it is not recommended by current guidelines.[49–51] It is reasonable to administer O_2 to hypotensive patients and those with severe trauma until tissue hypoxia can be definitively excluded.[45]

Administer O_2 to patients with carbon monoxide poisoning. The half-life of carboxyhemoglobin is 4 to 5 hours in a subject breathing room air but can be decreased to approximately 1 hour by the administration of 100% O_2 by nonrebreather face mask at atmospheric pressure.[52]

There are no contraindications to O_2 therapy when a definite indication exists. The risks of hypoxemia are grave and undeniable. O_2 therapy should never be withheld from a hypoxemic patient for fear of complications or clinical deterioration. CO_2 retention is not a contraindication to O_2 therapy. Rather, it demands that the clinician administer O_2 carefully and recognize the potential for respiratory acidosis and clinical deterioration. Although the mechanism of respiratory acidosis developing in COPD patients administered O_2 is debated, its occurrence is not.[53,54] Caution should be used when administering supplemental O_2 to patients with an arterial carbon dioxide pressure (Pa_{CO_2}) over 40 mm Hg, but it should not be withheld.

Oxygen Delivery Devices

High-flow delivery systems provide an FI_{O_2} that is relatively constant despite changes in the patient's respiratory pattern. The Venturi mask is the high-flow delivery device that is widely available (Fig. 3–4A and inset). Room air is entrained into the system through entrainment ports and mixes with the

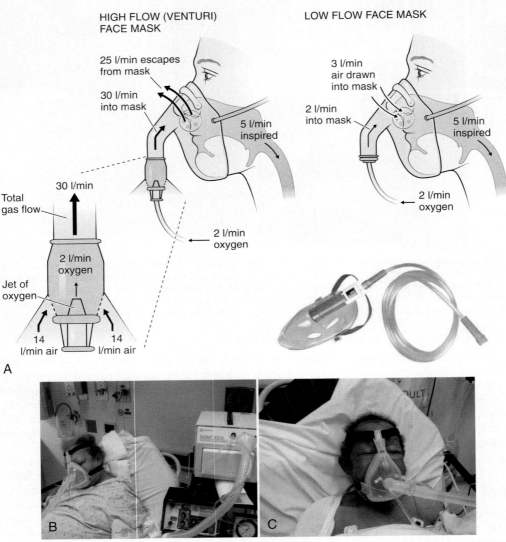

Figure 3–4 *A–C,* Using a wall oxygen source, high-flow oxygen masks provide the entire ventilatory requirement using a Venturi valve. The port size of the valve ensures that the correct proportions of oxygen and entrained (environmental) air *are mixed to obtain a fixed oxygen concentration.* Low-flow oxygen masks do not provide the entire ventilatory requirement. Air is drawn in through the loose-fitting mask to supplement the oxygen flow rate. *A,* A chronic obstructive pulmonary disease (COPD) patient can be accurately given 28% oxygen with this mask. *Inset:* Principle of the venture mask. *B,* Bilevel positive airway pressure (BiPAP) or continuous positive airway pressure (CPAP) has beneficial effects on the physiology of congestive heart failure and COPD and may be used to avoid intubation. The value of CPAP vs. BiPAP is controversial. Note: Severe neck flexion shown here may limit effectiveness of this intervention. Reposition the patient or perform tracheal intubation. *C,* When initiating BiPAP, it is best to let the patient hold the mask on his or her own face for several minutes before securing the mask with the head straps. Patients must be monitored closely for clinical decompensation and mask movement. Extremely anxious or hypoxic patients cannot tolerate the mask and feel smothered, and they are best intubated. Patients with facial hair may have problem with a tight mask fit.

O_2 provided from the O_2 source. The proportion of entrained air, and therefore the FI_{O_2}, is constant and is determined by the velocity of the O_2 jet and size of the entrainment ports. Because the total gas flow (O_2 plus air through entrainment ports) meets or exceeds the patient's inspiratory flow rate, no additional entrainment of air occurs around the mask, thereby minimizing changes in FI_{O_2} as the patient's respiratory pattern changes.[55,56] The mask is continuously flushed by the high flow of gas, preventing the accumulation of exhaled gases in the mask. Venturi masks are packaged with multiple inserts, each with a different size orifice for O_2 inflow. FI_{O_2} is determined by selecting the appropriate colored insert and O_2 flow rate according to the manufacturer's instructions. The inspiratory flow rate for a resting adult is about 30 L/min, a rate matched by the total gas flow provided by the Venturi mask at all settings. However, a patient with respiratory distress may have an inspiratory flow rate of 50 to 100 L/min.[56] If the inspiratory flow rate exceeds the total gas flow delivered by the mask, additional air will be entrained around the mask and the FI_{O_2} will decrease. Masks with higher FI_{O_2} ratings entrain less outside air and, therefore, provide less total flow. Caution should be used with masks rated above 35% in patients with respiratory distress because the FI_{O_2} may be significantly reduced with high inspiratory flow rates.

Low-flow delivery devices provide gas flow that is less than the patient's inspiratory flow rate. The difference between the patient's inspiratory flow and the flow delivered by the device is met by a variable amount of room air being drawn into the system. Patients with normal respiratory rates and tidal volumes will require less outside air than those in respiratory distress and will, therefore, receive a higher FI_{O_2}. As a patient's inspiratory flow changes, so will the FI_{O_2} they receive from a low-flow device.[55,56]

The prongs of a cannula deliver a constant flow of O_2 that accumulates in the nasopharynx and provides a reservoir of oxygen-enriched air for inspiration. The FI_{O_2} delivered by nasal cannulas is determined by many factors including respiratory rate, tidal volume, pharyngeal geometry, and O_2 flow. Most importantly, at a constant O_2 flow rate, the FI_{O_2} varies inversely with the respiratory rate. Despite this limitation, nasal cannulas are very comfortable for patients and are the most common low-flow O_2 delivery device.

Simple masks receive a constant flow of O_2 from the O_2 source and have multiple vent holes. During inspiration, the oxygen-enriched air that has accumulated in the mask, along with room air entrained through the vent holes, is inhaled. During expiration, 200 cc (the approximate volume of the mask) of exhaled gases are deposited in the mask with the rest exiting through the vent holes. The continuous flow of O_2 then partially washes out the mask prior to the next inspiration. The mask itself provides the reservoir of oxygen-rich gas for inhalation. A complex interplay between mask volume, tidal volume, respiratory rate, and O_2 flow determines the FI_{O_2} actually delivered to the patient.

A partial rebreathing mask incorporates a bag-type reservoir to increase the amount of O_2 available during inspiration, thereby requiring less outside air to be entrained. Non-rebreathing masks are similar to partial rebreathing masks but have a series of one-way valves. One valve lies between the mask and the reservoir and prevents exhaled gases from entering the reservoir. Two valves in the side of the mask permit exhalation while preventing the entry of outside air. In practice, one of these valves is often removed to permit inhalation in the event of an interruption of O_2 flow

to the mask. A variable amount of air can still leak around the mask. This outside air and the exhaled gases remaining in the mask dilute the O_2 from the reservoir and prevent the mask from providing 100% O_2. O_2 flow to the mask should be sufficient to prevent collapse of the bag during inspiration. As with all low-flow devices, the FI_{O_2} delivered varies with the patient's respiratory pattern. Many clinicians have the misconception that a non-rebreathing mask can provide an FI_{O_2} near 100%. In practice, a non-rebreathing mask usually delivers an FI_{O_2} of about 70%.

Procedure

In selecting the proper delivery device, consideration should be given to the clinical condition of the patient and the amount of O_2 needed. High-flow systems should generally be used for patients who need precise control of FI_{O_2}, such as COPD patients with chronic respiratory acidosis. Low-flow masks are appropriate for patients who need supplemental O_2 but do not require precise control of FI_{O_2}. Nasal cannulas are best suited to patients who do not require a high FI_{O_2} and will not be harmed by the lack of precise control. In most patients receiving supplemental O_2, an initial FI_{O_2} of 25% to 35% (1–3 L/min) delivered by nasal cannula is appropriate. A higher FI_{O_2}, delivered by mask, may be needed in patients with significant hypoxemia, end-organ dysfunction, or respiratory distress. An initial FI_{O_2} of 24% to 28% delivered by Venturi mask is indicated for patients with hypoxemia and chronic respiratory acidosis.[45,54]

Frequent clinical assessment and SpO_2 are needed in all patients receiving O_2 therapy. Periodic determination of blood gases is imperative for those at risk of developing respiratory acidosis.[57–59] Equilibration of SaO_2 after changes in supplemental O_2 occurs within 5 minutes.[60]

FiO_2 should be titrated to achieve therapeutic goals while minimizing the risk of complications. An SaO_2 of 90% to 95% ($Pao_2 \approx 60$–80 mm Hg) is an appropriate target for most patients receiving supplemental O_2.[45] Increases above these levels do not add appreciably to the O_2 content of blood and are unlikely to confer an additional benefit. One may exceed these parameters in patients with shock and end-organ dysfunction, but the added risk and small potential benefit should be considered on an individual basis. In patients with COPD, SaO_2 of 90% ($Pao_2 \approx 60$ mm Hg) should be the goal of O_2 therapy.[57–59] Mechanical ventilation should be considered when oxygenation goals cannot be achieved without progressive respiratory acidosis.

Preoxygenation for Rapid-Sequence Intubation

Preoxygenation prior to rapid-sequence induction (RSI) and intubation may allow a significantly longer safe apneic period. Providing maximal FI_{O_2} with a non-rebreather mask for 3 to 5 minutes is recommended. Alternatively, a series of eight vital capacity breaths from a high FI_{O_2} system, such as a non-rebreather mask or a bag-valve-mask device, may be used if there is no time for standard preoxygenation.[61]

Preoxygenation, if possible or practical to institute, is one the most important aspects of RSI. It allows much more time for the intubation procedure and significantly increases the chance of successful intubation on the first attempt. Failure to preoxygenate prior to RSI is often a critical factor when a straightforward emergency airway becomes an airway disaster.

Complications of Oxygen Therapy

Worsening of CO_2 retention leading to progressive respiratory acidosis and obtundation in COPD patients is the complication most likely to be seen in the ED. This phenomenon is well documented and was first described by Barach in 1937.[62] It has been attributed to several mechanisms including loss of hypoxic respiratory drive, ventilation-perfusion $(\dot{V}/\dot{Q})$ mismatch and decreased hemoglobin affinity for CO_2 (Haldane effect). This avoidable complication is best prevented by administering O_2 to chronic CO_2 retainers only when there is an indication, administering it at the smallest effective dose, and carefully monitoring clinical and arterial blood gas parameters.

Exposing the lung to excessive concentrations of O_2 can lead to toxicity and, in severe cases, can cause acute respiratory distress syndrome. Injury to the pulmonary parenchyma occurs as a result of the formation of reactive oxygen species. No data describe what concentration or duration of exposure to O_2 leads to toxicity but presumably both of these factors, as well as individual patient characteristics, determine the likelihood of toxicity. The benefits of O_2 therapy in the ED usually outweigh the risks of O_2 toxicity. Fear of toxicity should not prevent the use of O_2 when there is an indication but should encourage the clinician to use the minimum concentration of O_2 necessary to achieve therapeutic goals. High concentrations of O_2 are well tolerated over short periods and may be life saving.

In patients receiving high concentrations of supplemental O_2, nitrogen in the alveoli is largely replaced by O_2. If this O_2 is then absorbed into the blood faster than it can be replaced, the volume of the alveoli will decrease and absorptive atelectasis will occur. Airway obstruction potentiates this problem by preventing the rapid replacement of absorbed gases.

NPPV

NPPV provides patients the benefits of positive-pressure ventilation without endotracheal intubation and its associated risks. Once limited to the treatment of obstructive sleep apnea and chronic respiratory failure, NPPV is now commonly used for acute respiratory failure.

NPPV decreases intubation rates and mortality in the setting of acute pulmonary edema and acute exacerbations of COPD.[63-67] NPPV has fewer infectious complications and is often a good alternative to endotracheal intubation.[68,69]

CPAP describes a constant level of positive airway pressure maintained throughout the respiratory cycle without the provision of greater support during inspiration. The addition of increased pressure during the inspiratory phase is known as pressure support (PS). The combination of CPAP and PS is bilevel positive airway pressure, commonly referred to as BiPAP. The focus of this chapter is the use of BiPAP in the setting of acute respiratory failure (ARF). BiPAP (Respironics, Inc., Murrysville, PA; www.respironics.com) is a trade name for noninvasive ventilators manufactured by Respironics and should not be confused with the term BiPAP as described previously.

CPAP was first used to treat congestive heart failure in 1936 when Poulton[70] described using a vacuum cleaner to generate positive pressure. Neuromuscular disorders were first treated with NPPV in 1987 and it was first used in the setting of ARF in 1989.[71,72] The past decade has seen extensive investigation into noninvasive ventilation and its use in ARF.

Indications and Contraindications

Strong evidence exists for the use of NPPV in acute exacerbations of COPD. Evidence-based guidelines recommend its use in patients who, despite maximal medical therapy, exhibit persistent respiratory distress and respiratory acidosis (pH ≤ 7.35).[57-59] When used in addition to standard medical therapy, NPPV decreases the need for intubation, decreases complications, and improves outcomes in this population.[64,65] NPPV also decreases the need for endotracheal intubation and decreases mortality in patients with respiratory failure secondary to cardiogenic pulmonary edema.[63,64,67] The exact benefits of CPAP versus BiPAP are uncertain, and either is acceptable when NPPV is required. Some studies suggest that CPAP is preferable to BiPAP for acute pulmonary edema; however, no definite consensus has been reached.[67,73-75]

NPPV has been used successfully in the setting of ARF secondary to pneumonia. However, the benefit is not as great in this group as in others and intubation rates are still high.[76-78] Some evidence supports a trial of NPPV in respiratory failure secondary to asthma.[79-82] However, large-scale randomized trials are lacking and it is not certain that the treatment is beneficial in this setting. An attempt to reverse respiratory failure using NPPV is reasonable in selected asthmatics but provisions for more aggressive intervention should be immediately available.

NPPV is especially useful in patients with ARF who have do-not-resuscitate (DNR) status and do not want endotracheal intubation.[83-85] Most patients who refuse intubation will allow NPPV.

Several clinical scenarios exist in which NPPV is likely to fail (Table 3–1). Patients who are in extremis are not candidates for NPPV. When the combination of mental status, respiratory function, and hemodynamics indicate this threshold has been reached, the airway should be managed using traditional endotracheal intubation. Altered mental status is generally considered a contraindication to the use of NPPV. Despite this, there are reports of NPPV success in patients with severely altered mental status.[86-88] In select patients who are able to maintain airway patency, NPPV can be attempted provided the equipment and personnel for endotracheal intubation are immediately available. Patient-ventilator synchrony is crucial to the success of NPPV, and therefore, patients who are agitated or combative are unlikely to be successfully managed with this technique.

In hemodynamically stable patients, NPPV appears to have no significant adverse effects and may actually improve hemodynamics.[76,89-93] However, in decompensated patients or

---

TABLE 3–1 Patient Characteristics Associated with Noninvasive Positive-Pressure Ventilation Failure

Pneumonia, ARDS
Decreased level of consciousness (GCS ≤ 13)
Respiratory rate ≥ 30
Severe disease (Apache II ≥ 29, SAPS II ≥ 35)
pH < 7.25

ARDS, adult respiratory distress syndrome; GCS, Glasgow Coma Score; SAPS, Simplified Acute Physiology Score.

those with a low pulmonary capillary wedge pressure, hemodynamics may be adversely affected by NPPV.[94–96] The adverse hemodynamic effects of NPPV will be no greater than those of conventional mechanical ventilation in the same patient and a trial can be considered for a patient who is otherwise a good candidate.

Patients with facial features or deformities that preclude effective mask fitting are not appropriate candidates for NPPV. The presence of facial hair may also create difficulties with mask fitting but is not a contraindication. Positive pressure applied after recent sinus or upper airway surgery may have adverse results; these conditions are contraindications to its use. Positive pressure alone will not provide a lasting remedy for a fixed obstruction of the upper airway; such patients should be managed with traditional airway techniques. Because significant aerophagia can occur with NPPV, bowel obstruction and recent upper gastrointestinal surgery are relative contraindications. The technique may be employed safely if the mental status is normal and the inspiratory pressures are kept below 20 cm H_2O.

Excessive respiratory secretions predict failure of NPPV and are better managed in the intubated patient. Persistent vomiting is considered a contraindication to NPPV. Suctioning and clearance of vomitus from the airway is difficult during noninvasive ventilation.

Equipment

NPPV can be safely and adequately delivered using standard critical care ventilators or machines specifically designed to deliver BiPAP (i.e., BiPAP Vision, Respironics).

Dedicated BiPAP devices have been extensively studied in the setting of ARF, and this is the strongest argument for using them instead of standard ventilators. These devices are tolerant of the leaks that are inevitable in NPPV and do not sound unnecessary alarms. They are portable, simple to operate, and less expensive than standard ventilators. However, they have fewer monitoring capabilities than standard ventilators and most lack an O_2 blender, which precludes precise determination of FI_{O_2}. Delivery of FI_{O_2} greater than 50% is difficult to achieve with typical BiPAP settings.[97] O_2 blenders and advanced monitoring capabilities are being incorporated into newer devices.

Traditional critical care ventilators can also deliver NPPV. They allow delivery of a precise FI_{O_2} and sophisticated monitoring but do not tolerate leaks as well as machines designed specifically for noninvasive ventilation. Some ventilators now include a dedicated NPPV mode, which may overcome this problem. Regardless of the ventilator chosen, it is critical that it be capable of maintaining airway pressure in the presence of leakage around the mask interface.

Perhaps no piece of equipment is more important to the success of NPPV than the interface between the patient and the ventilator. The oronasal mask eliminates the problem of leakage through the mouth and augments respiratory mechanics more effectively than nasal masks (see Fig. 3–4B).[98–100] It has the disadvantage of being quite claustrophobic and precluding eating, oral suctioning, and effective verbal communication. The volume of the oronasal mask is greater than that of the nasal mask. This increased dead space leads to some degree of CO_2 rebreathing, the effects of which are probably insignificant. Masks containing an exhalation port are optimal for preventing rebreathing and efficiently lowering arterial carbon dioxide pressure (Pa_{CO_2}). The oronasal mask is recommended for patients with ARF and is the most widely used interface in this setting.[101]

Nasal masks are the predominant interface used in chronic respiratory failure but can also be used in the acute setting. They are well tolerated owing the ability to eat and communicate verbally. They do permit significant leakage from the mouth, which can be somewhat uncomfortable. Significant mouth breathing markedly decreases their effectiveness.

Application of NPPV

When using a conventional critical care ventilator, one must decide between pressure- and volume-limited modes of ventilation. Whereas both modes will provide adequate support for most patients, pressure-limited modes tend to be better tolerated and are the most widely used. Pressure-supported ventilation (PSV) is the mode most commonly used for NPPV in ARF. PSV refers only to the provision of ventilatory support during inspiration. CPAP in addition to PSV provides greater support and is preferred.[102] CPAP should initially be set at 4 to 5 cm H_2O. Initial pressure support should be set at 8 to 10 cm H_2O to prevent patient discomfort and intolerance due to high inspiratory pressures. Leakage around the mask is inevitable during NPPV. This can create problems with cycling and is a major cause of patient intolerance of NPPV. For this reason, triggers should be set to their most sensitive levels. If the ventilator has a dedicated NPPV mode, be certain it is selected.

When using a dedicated NPPV machine such as the BiPAP Vision, the spontaneous mode is analogous to PSV and cycles to inspiration only when it is triggered by the patient. This mode is appropriate for most patients. If the respiratory drive is diminished or the inspiratory effort is insufficient to trigger the ventilator, then the spontaneous/time mode should be selected. This mode will function identically to the spontaneous mode unless the patient fails to trigger the ventilator at or above the set respiratory rate, in which case it will cycle automatically to provide the set number of breaths per minute.

Expiratory positive airway pressure (EPAP) is the minimum level of positive pressure supplied during the respiratory cycle and is present during the expiratory phase. It is analogous to CPAP and should be set at 4 to 5 cm H_2O initially. Lower levels may lead to accumulation of expired gases in the circuit and CO_2 rebreathing. Inspiratory positive airway pressure (IPAP) refers to the additional support provided during the inspiratory phase and should be initially set at 8 to 10 cm H_2O initially. An O_2 line should be attached to the designated inlet site in the circuit or a T-piece inserted in the tubing. An initial flow of 4 L/min is reasonable but higher levels (≤ 15 L/min) are appropriate in the presence of significant hypoxemia. If the machine has an O_2 blender, the desired FI_{O_2} should be set.

Before establishing NPPV, consideration should be given to patient criteria associated with failure of NPPV (see Table 3–1). Whereas the technique can be used in a wide variety of patients, selecting patients based on these criteria will ensure a reasonable chance for success. Before starting NPPV, establish standard vital sign monitoring (including SpO_2) and obtain intravenous access. Preparations for endotracheal intubation should be made and a skilled operator immediately available. Although noninvasive ventilation can be done in any position, place the patient in the upright or semi-upright position to optimize respiratory mechanics and lessen the risk of aspiration.

Select a proper-sized mask and attach head straps. Configure the ventilator and turn it on with the initial settings determined as described previously. With the patient properly positioned, hold the mask loosely against the face with constant reassurance and coaching. As the patient becomes accustomed to positive pressure, secure the mask and adjust it to minimize leaks. Do not overtighten the straps because this can lead to patient intolerance and pressure necrosis on the bridge of the nose (see Fig. 3–4C).

Once the patient is tolerating the mask, titrate the pressures to achieve the desired effect of decreasing the respiratory rate and work of breathing. Avoid inspiratory pressures above 20 cm H_2O because they will increase the risk of aerophagia and patient intolerance. Adjust O_2 flow or FI_{O_2} to achieve the desired SpO_2. One should keep in mind that when using a single-limb ventilator circuit and O_2 bleed in (as with the BiPAP Vision), the delivered FI_{O_2} will decrease for a given O_2 flow as the IPAP is increased; therefore, it may be necessary to increase O_2 flow as the IPAP is increased to avoid desaturation.

Monitor the patient minute-to-minute using clinical parameters. A significant deterioration in the patient's condition may indicate the need for endotracheal intubation. Measure arterial blood gases prior to instituting NPPV and again 1 hour later. Further measurement of arterial blood gases is dictated by the response to therapy and clinical situation.

Patient-ventilator synchrony is crucial to the success of NPPV. Patient tolerance may be increased by allowing the patient to hold the mask on her or his own face. This approach allows her or him to get used to the feeling of the NPPV mask while avoiding the sensation of being smothered by the device. The patient should be constantly reassured and coached during the initiation of NPPV. Low-dose neuroleptics or anxiolytics may also be useful in achieving maximal patient compliance and ventilator synchrony.

Cycling from inspiration to expiration is determined differently depending on the mode of ventilation. In PSV, inspiration ends when the flow in the circuit decelerates to a predetermined level. Owing to the inevitable presence of leaks during NPPV, it is possible that the ventilator will not sense a deceleration of flow sufficient to cycle to expiration, leading to persistent inspiratory pressures being delivered to the patient. Achieving a good mask fit with minimal leaks is the best prevention for this complication. Many ventilators also incorporate a backup time-cycling mechanism, which sets a maximum duration of the inspiratory phase.

Patient-ventilator asynchrony may result from failure to sense a spontaneous breath. Once again, minimize leakage around the mask to help remedy this problem. If the ventilator allows manipulation of triggering parameters, flow triggering should be used and set at its most sensitive level.

Although aerosol delivery is less efficient during NPPV than during spontaneous breathing, the efficacy of aerosolized bronchodilators appears to be maintained.[103–105] Deliver aerosols distally in the circuit, ideally between the tubing and the patient interface.[106,107]

Complications

The most common complications of NPPV are typically minor and easily remedied. Discomfort or ulceration over the bridge of the nose can be minimized by avoiding overtightening straps or by using a skin barrier in this location. Sinus and middle ear discomfort may occur in the presence of high inspiratory pressures. This is best managed with a temporary decrease in pressure followed by gradual increase as the patient tolerates. Claustrophobia can occur with the use of the oronasal mask and may lead to patient intolerance of the procedure. If the patient's clinical condition permits, consider loosening the straps and letting the patient hold the mask to his or her face. Low-dose anxiolytics may also be appropriate in some patients.

Major complications of NPPV are rare and include pneumothorax, hypotension, gastric overdistention, and esophageal perforation. Appropriate patient selection and use of proper settings will minimize the occurrence of these conditions. Constant monitoring of the NPPV patient is necessary to immediately detect their occurrence.

BAG-MASK VENTILATION

Bag-mask ventilation is the single most important technique for emergency airway management.[3,19,108] Bag-mask devices are widely available and are standard equipment in all patient care settings. Although the bag-mask method of ventilation appears to be simple, it can be difficult to perform correctly. Having good bag-mask ventilation skills is a prerequisite to more advanced methods of emergency airway management.[3] Manually opening the airway, properly positioning the head and neck, placing an oropharyngeal airway device, and achieving a tight face mask seal are the keys to good bag-mask ventilation.

Indications and Contraindications

Bag-mask ventilation is the most common initial technique for ventilation of apneic patients and for rescue ventilation after failed intubation. Many authors note that bag-mask ventilation is relatively contraindicated in patients with a full stomach, those who are in cardiac arrest, and those who are undergoing RSI.[2,4] These patients have a high risk of stomach inflation and subsequent aspiration. Unfortunately, these are the patients for whom ED providers most commonly use bag-mask ventilation. In ED situations, the need for ventilation and oxygenation always takes priority over potential aspiration.[2]

The only contraindication to attempting bag-mask ventilation is when application of a face mask is impossible. It is often impossible to achieve an effective face mask seal on patients with significant deforming facial trauma and those with thick beards. An intermediate ventilation device, such as a laryngeal mask airway (LMA), is a better choice for initial ventilation in such patients.

Bag-Mask Ventilation Technique

Achieving adequate tidal volumes with bag-mask ventilation requires a tight mask seal and appropriate compression of the bag. However, overaggressive bag-mask ventilation causes stomach inflation and increases the risk of aspiration. The goal is to achieve adequate gas exchange while keeping the peak airway pressures low. Squeezing the bag forcefully and abruptly creates a high peak airway pressure and is more likely to inflate the stomach. Several studies show that increased tidal volume is associated with higher peak airway pressures and increased gastric inflation.[50,108–111] Data also show that decreased inspiratory time increases peak airway pressure and

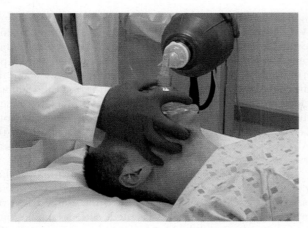

Figure 3–5 One-handed bag-mask ventilation technique can be difficult to perform efficiently. The thumb and index finger control the mask, while the third to fifth fingers lift the mandible up into the mask. It may be possible to place the little finger behind the angle of the mandible to perform a jaw-thrust maneuver. *(From Thomsen T, Setnik G [eds]: Procedures Consult—Emergency Medicine Module. Copyright 2008 Elsevier Inc. All rights reserved.)*

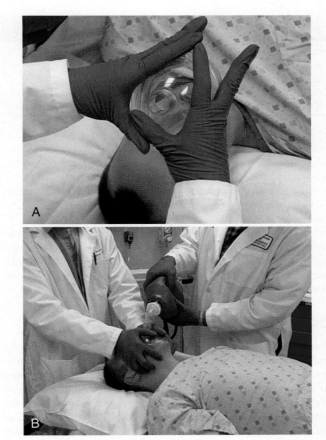

Figure 3–6 With the easier two-handed bag-mask ventilation technique, the mask is controlled by the thenar eminences and thumbs (*A*), while the second through fifth fingers perform a jaw thrust and lift the mandible up into the mask (*B*). One operator controls the mask, the other the bag. *(A and B, From Thomsen T, Setnik G [eds] Procedures Consult—Emergency Medicine Module. Copyright 2008 Elsevier Inc. All rights reserved.)*

increases gastric inflation.[112,113] Therefore, it appears that the best method of bag-mask ventilation is to provide a tidal volume of about 500 mL delivered over 1 to 1.5 seconds.[113] Effective ventilation and oxygenation should be judged by chest rise, breath sounds, SpO_2, and exhaled CO_2 monitoring.

A variety of mask configurations are available to facilitate a tight seal. The most common mask used in ED situations is a transparent disposable plastic mask with a high-volume, low-pressure cuff. This type of mask eliminates the need for an anatomically formed mask and can be used for a wide variety of patients with differing facial features. Various mask sizes are available.

For the single rescuer, only one hand can be used to achieve the seal because the other must squeeze the bag. The rescuer must apply pressure anteriorly while simultaneously lifting the jaw forward. The thumb and index finger provide anterior pressure while the fifth and fourth fingers lift the jaw. The E-C clamp technique is often the most effective: The thumb and index finger form a "C" providing anterior pressure over the mask; while the third, fourth, and fifth fingers form an "E" to lift the jaw (Fig. 3–5). Generally, well-fitting intact dentures should be left in place to help ensure a better seal with the mask.

It has been suggested that effective bag-mask ventilation during CPR requires two hands and, therefore, two rescuers.[114] We suggest using the two-rescuer technique whenever it is practical (Fig. 3–6).

All bag-mask devices should be attached to a supplemental O_2 source (with a flow rate of 15 L/min) to avoid hypoxia. A significant problem with the bag-mask method is the low percentage of O_2 achieved with some reservoirs. The amount of delivered O_2 is dependent on the ventilatory rate, the volumes delivered during each breath, the O_2 flow rate into the ventilating bag, the filling time for reservoir bags, and the type of reservoir used. A 2500-mL bag reservoir and a demand valve are preferred for O_2 supplementation during bag-mask ventilation.[115]

Pediatric bag-mask devices should have a minimum volume of 450 mL. Pediatric and larger bags may be used for ventilation of infants with the proper mask size, but be careful to administer only the volume necessary to effectively ventilate the infant. Avoid pop-off valves because airway pressure under emergency conditions may often exceed the pressure of the valve.[116]

Bag-mask ventilation may be the best method of prehospital airway support in trauma patients and in children. Murray and coworkers[117] performed a large retrospective study suggesting that patients with severe head injury had a higher risk of mortality if they were intubated in the prehospital setting. In the same year, Gausche and associates[118] reported that neurologic outcome and ultimate survival rates of prehospital pediatric resuscitations by emergency medical service (EMS) providers with bag-mask ventilation were as good as with tracheal intubation.

Complications

The main complications of the bag-mask technique are inability to ventilate and gastric inflation. Several factors may lead to difficult bag-mask ventilation. Langeron and colleagues[119] performed a large prospective study of adults undergoing general anesthesia and reported a 5% incidence of difficult mask ventilation. They also identified five independent risk factors for difficult mask ventilation (Table 3–2). When mask ventilation is technically difficult, higher peak airway pressure

TABLE 3–2 Risk Factors for Difficult Mask Ventilation

Presence of a beard
Body mass index > 26 kg/m²
Lack of teeth
Age > 55 yr
History of snoring

From Langeron O, Masso E, Huraux C, et al: Prediction of difficult mask ventilation. Anesthesiology 92:1229, 2000.

is often required in order to provide an adequate tidal volume. In these situations, gastric inflation is more likely and aspiration may occur.

Be vigilant to recognize complications early and take corrective action. Even when bag-mask ventilation is easy and good technique is used, some gastric dilatation will usually occur. Minor gastric distention should not be considered substandard in the setting of prolonged bag-mask ventilation.

Cricoid Pressure (Sellick's Maneuver)

Consider applying cricoid pressure during bag-mask ventilation. Cricoid pressure is often referred to as Sellick's maneuver, because of Sellick's classic article in 1961.[120] The purpose of the technique is to apply external force to the anterior cricoid ring to push the trachea posteriorly, compressing the esophagus against the cervical vertebrae. In theory, cricoid pressure compresses the distensible upper esophagus but not the airway, because the cricoid ring is fairly rigid. Some data suggest that cricoid pressure prevents gastric inflation and subsequent vomiting/regurgitation during bag-mask ventilation and intubation.[120–122] However, there are also conflicting reports and some controversy about whether cricoid pressure is really effective.[121] Nevertheless, cricoid pressure is currently recommended and should be performed when possible during resuscitation and all RSIs.[123,124]

Be aware that excessive or incorrectly applied cricoid pressure can interfere with bag-mask ventilation, direct laryngoscopy, and insertion of the LMAs. When faced with difficult or failed ventilation or intubation, or when using LMAs, consider relaxation of cricoid pressure.[121] Also, be very careful when applying cricoid pressure in infants and young children, whose airways are more pliable and subject to obstruction with excessive cricoid pressure.

The proper technique for applying cricoid pressure (Sellick's maneuver) is to place the thumb and middle finger on either side of the cricoid cartilage with the index finger in the center anteriorly.[120] Apply about 30 N of force to the cricoid cartilage in the posterior direction.[121,124] As a reference, about 40 N of digital force on the bridge of the nose will usually cause pain.[121]

INTERMEDIATE AIRWAY DEVICES

In an emergency airway situation, use these devices for temporary rescue ventilation until tracheal intubation or a surgical airway can be performed.

The LMAs

The laryngeal mask airway (LMA™, LMA North America, Inc., San Diego, CA; www.lmana.com) devices are essential adjuncts for rescue ventilation and difficult intubation.[125,126] LMA devices have been used more than 200 million times worldwide and researched extensively.[127] LMA devices are primary rescue adjuncts in the difficult airway guidelines put forth by the American Society of Anesthesiologists[125] and the Difficult Airway Society.[126] Advanced Cardiac Life Support guidelines suggest that the LMA provides a more secure and reliable means of ventilation than face-mask ventilation.[1] Pediatric Advanced Life Support guidelines acknowledge the LMA as a potential backup device for difficult pediatric airways.[128,129]

All of the LMA devices consist of an airway tube attached to an oval mask, rimmed by an inflatable cuff. The cuffed mask is designed to form a seal around the glottis when the device is properly placed. In fasted patients undergoing general anesthesia, an LMA can often be used instead of a tracheal tube. The LMA-glottic seal allows positive-pressure ventilation and protection of the airway from oral and nasal secretions. LMA devices do not necessarily protect the airway from aspiration of gastric contents. In emergency airway management, LMA devices are used as temporizing airways to allow rescue ventilation and provide a conduit for tracheal intubation.

Several different types of LMA devices are available. For emergency airway management, the original LMA and the intubating laryngeal mask airway (ILMA) are the most practical. Therefore, we describe these devices in detail and do not discuss other LMA devices. Emergency airway providers should be aware that the procedure for placing the ILMA is much different from the procedure for placing the LMA. It is prudent to learn how to use both devices, because many EDs use the ILMA in adults and the LMA in children. Many prehospital providers use the LMA.

The original LMA is now called the LMA Classic. A disposable version of the original LMA, called the LMA Unique, is available. The ILMA is called the LMA Fastrach, and it is specially designed to facilitate tracheal intubation. A disposable version of the intubating LMA, called the LMA Fastrach Single Use, is available.

Both versions of the original LMA (LMA Classic and LMA Unique) have the same design and functional characteristics, so in this chapter both devices are referred to as the *LMA*. Both versions of the ILMA (LMA Fastrach and LMA Fastrach Single Use) have the same design and function characteristics, so they are referred to as the *ILMA* in this chapter. Several other LMA devices are not as practical for emergency airway management and are not discussed in this chapter.

The LMA and the ILMA can be used as rescue devices in cases of failed bag-mask ventilation. Both devices can be inserted in less than 30 seconds and provide effective ventilation in 98% to 99% of patients.[127] The ILMA is more useful in the ED, because it is easier for inexperienced personnel to place and facilitates tracheal intubation.[130–134] Also, when the head is in the neutral position, during in-line stabilization of the cervical spine, the ILMA is more likely to allow successful ventilation and intubation.[135–137]

Patients who are difficult to intubate by direct laryngoscopy are often easy to intubate with the ILMA because many anatomic factors that cause difficult direct laryngoscopy do not affect placement or function of the LMA devices.[138,139] The ILMA is more successful for ventilation and intubation of difficult airways than the LMA, and the failure rate of ILMA intubation of difficult airways is very low (see Chapter 4 for intubation through LMA devices).[127]

The ILMA (ILMA or LMA Fastrach)

The ILMA is an essential rescue ventilation device for the "cannot-intubate/cannot-ventilate" situation. It is also an excellent primary ventilation and intubation device for patients with known difficult airways, especially in cases of severe facial trauma. The ILMA has several advantages over the LMA (see earlier). The ILMA mask is attached to a metal tube and handle. The handle allows one-handed insertion and manipulation. The metal tube has an anatomic curve to fit into the upper airway and is large enough to accept an 8.0-mm cuffed endotracheal tube. The ILMA can be used up to 40 times before being replaced. The disposable ILMA has a hard plastic handle and tube and can be used only once. The ILMA is available only in sizes suitable for adults and children heavier than 30 kg, so the LMA should be used for smaller children and infants.

Indications and Contraindications. The ILMA is indicated as an alternative to bag-mask ventilation or as a conduit for intubation of difficult airways.[140] Its primary use in emergency airway management has been as a rescue device in the cannot-intubate/cannot-ventilate situation. In this situation, adequate ventilation with the ILMA is possible in almost all cases.[127,141,142] Ventilation with the ILMA is probably superior to face mask ventilation with inexperienced providers.[143] The ILMA can also be used as a primary ventilation and intubation device for patients with difficult airways.[140] Tracheal intubation through the ILMA can be accomplished using a blind technique, or with light-wand or fiberoptic guidance (see Chapter 4 for tracheal intubation through the ILMA). Studies of difficult airway management with the ILMA show that almost all patients can be adequately ventilated with the ILMA and 94% to 99% can be intubated through the device.[127,138,140,141,144]

The ILMA is especially useful in patients with difficult face mask ventilation owing to a beard, severe facial trauma, or obesity because none of these factors inhibits ILMA placement. When brisk bleeding above the glottis makes ventilation and intubation difficult, the ILMA can prevent aspiration of blood and facilitate blind or fiberoptic intubation. In patients requiring an urgent cricothyrotomy or percutaneous needle insertion into the trachea, the ILMA can be used to counteract anterior neck pressure. In this capacity, the ILMA provides temporary ventilation and stabilizes the cervical spine during the surgical airway procedure.

The ILMA is contraindicated in patients with less than 2 cm of mouth opening. The ILMA requires 2 cm of space between the upper and the lower incisors in order to be inserted. The ILMA is relatively contraindicated in awake patients, especially those with a full stomach. Insertion of the ILMA in an awake patient will cause coughing, gagging, or vomiting. If the ILMA is inserted when the patient is awake and the stomach is full, there is a high likelihood of vomiting and aspiration. In the ED, the ILMA should be used only if the patient is unconscious or after a paralytic agent has been given. Once the ILMA is inserted and ventilation is established, the patient should not be allowed to wake up or gag. Consider giving a long-acting paralytic agent or multiple doses of succinylcholine after the ILMA is placed and ventilation is adequate.

Although several studies show that the ILMA is safe and effective for ventilation and intubation during in-line cervical spine stabilization, some evidence shows that the ILMA causes posterior pressure on the midportion of the cervical spine.[144-148] The clinical importance of cervical spine

pressure caused by the ILMA is unknown and the device is generally considered safe in patients with an unstable cervical spine injury. Nevertheless, providers should be aware of this concern and make every effort to stabilize the ILMA in these situations. Ventilation with the ILMA may be difficult or impossible in patients with severely distorted upper airway anatomy, especially those with scarring secondary to cervical radiation therapy.

Placement of the ILMA. The first step is to select the appropriate-sized ILMA. The ILMA is available in three sizes: size 3 for children weighing 30 to 50 kg, size 4 for small adults weighing 50 to 70 kg, and size 5 for adults weighing 70 to 100 kg. When there is doubt about which size is appropriate, it is probably better to use the larger size.

After choosing the correct ILMA, completely deflate the cuff while pushing it posteriorly so that it assumes a smooth wedge shape without any wrinkles (Fig. 3–7). Place a small amount of water-based lubricant onto the posterior surface of the ILMA mask just before insertion. Open the patient's mouth and position the posterior mask tip so that it is flat against the hard palate immediately posterior to the upper incisors (Fig. 3–8). Advance the airway straight into the mouth along the hard palate without rotation until the curved part of the airway tube is in contact with the patient's chin. Then rotate the ILMA completely into the hypopharynx by advancing it along its curved axis, keeping the posterior mask firmly applied to the soft palate and posterior pharynx, until firm

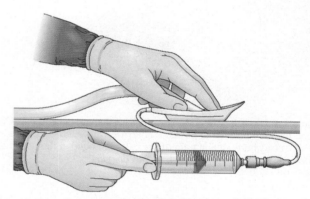

Figure 3–7 Deflation of the laryngeal mask airway (LMA) or intubating laryngeal mask airway (ILMA) cuff using a tabletop. When properly deflated, the cuff should be smooth, wrinkle-free, and concave on its dorsal surface. *(Courtesy of Laryneal Mask Company.)*

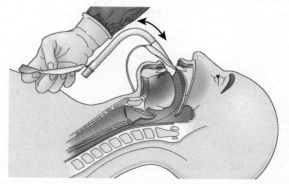

Figure 3–8 **Inserting the ILMA into the mouth.** Lubricate the posterior surface of the ILMA cuff/mask. Open the mouth and place the posterior tip of the ILMA cuff against the anterior hard palate just behind the upper incisors. *(Courtesy of Laryneal Mask Company.)*

resistance is felt (Fig. 3–9). Cricoid pressure impedes proper placement of the ILMA, so consider briefly releasing cricoid pressure while the device is rotated into its final position, wedged into the proximal esophagus.[142,149,150] After insertion, the airway tube should emerge from the mouth directed somewhat caudally. Without holding the tube or handle, inflate the mask cuff (Fig. 3–10). The entire device will normally slide backward a bit when the cuff is inflated. Frequently, only half of the maximum cuff volume is sufficient to obtain a good mask seal. Do not overinflate the cuff; this may make the seal worse. See the instruction manual for maximum cuff volumes. Attach a bag and ventilate the patient, using chest rise, breath sounds, and capnography to confirm adequate gas exchange. If bagging is easy and ventilation is good, the aperture of the ILMA is probably aligned correctly over the vocal cords.

If optimal ILMA placement is not initially accomplished, adjusting maneuvers can be attempted. The purpose of adjusting maneuvers is to align the aperture of the ILMA with the glottic opening. Proper positioning of the ILMA aperture with the glottic opening allows optimal ventilation and facilitates tracheal intubation. Before adjusting the ILMA, consider the patient's position and degree of relaxation; both may affect ILMA function. The ILMA works best in the neutral or sniffing position; cervical extension may interfere with proper placement. The patient should not react to ILMA placement with coughing or gagging because this may interfere with proper placement. Have a single operator perform the adjustment maneuvers by gripping the ILMA handle with one hand, in a "frying pan" grip, and providing bag ventilation with the other hand (Fig. 3–11). After each adjustment maneuver, assess the quality of bag ventilation and mask seal. Easy bag ventilation, good chest rise, and the absence of an audible mask leak are indications of good ILMA alignment with the glottis.

To adjust the position of the ILMA, first gently pull the handle toward you without rotation along the ILMA's curvature. Next, gently push the handle toward the patient's feet without rotating it. Finally, try the "Chandy maneuver," gently rotating the ILMA farther into the hypopharynx and then lifting the handle toward the ceiling above the patient's feet. If these simple maneuvers do not result in adequate ventilation, then consider the "up-down maneuver" (Fig. 3–12). This technique is used to correct down-folding of the epiglottis, which is common with insertion of the ILMA and may interfere with ventilation or intubation. The up-down maneuver is accomplished by rotating the ILMA out of the hypopharynx along its curvature about 5 to 6 cm, while the cuff remains inflated, then sliding it back into position while pressing it against the posterior pharynx. Do not use excessive force when placing or adjusting the ILMA.

If adjusting maneuvers do not result in adequate ventilation, it is likely that the wrong size of ILMA has been used. Incorrect ILMA size is more likely to be a problem if the device is too small, so try a larger ILMA as a reasonable first

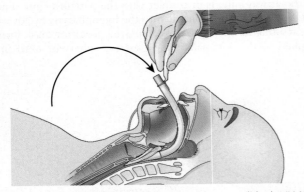

Figure 3–9   Inserting the ILMA into the hypopharynx. Slide the ILMA along the hard palate and posterior pharynx, by rotating the device along its curvature, until the tip of the cuff is wedged in the proximal esophagus. *(Courtesy of Laryneal Mask Company.)*

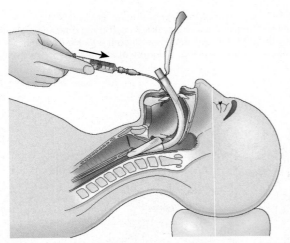

Figure 3–10   ILMA cuff inflation. Let go of the handle while inflating the cuff. The device will normally slide out of the mouth slightly during inflation. Initially inflate the cuff with only half of the maximum cuff volume, then increase inflation as needed. Do not overinflate the cuff. See product manual for maximum cuff volumes. *(Courtesy of Laryneal Mask Company.)*

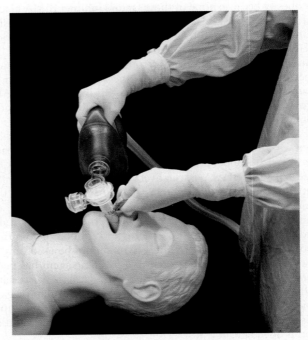

Figure 3–11   ILMA ventilation and adjusting maneuvers. Hold the handle of the ILMA with a "frying pan" grip with one hand and squeeze the ventilation bag with the other hand. Perform adjusting maneuvers while assessing the ease of bag ventilation. Ventilation will be easiest when the distal aperture of the ILMA is optimally aligned with the glottic opening.

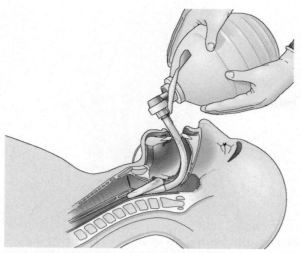

Figure 3–12   The "up-down" maneuver. Rotate the ILMA out of the hypopharynx along its curvature about 5 to 6 cm, while the cuff remains inflated, then slide it back into position while pressing it against the posterior pharynx. This technique is used to correct down-folding of the epiglottis, which may interfere with ventilation or intubation. *(Courtesy of Laryneal Mask Company.)*

approach. If another ILMA size is not available, external anterior neck manipulation/pressure may bring the glottis and ILMA cuff into proper alignment. If the size of the ILMA is not in question, consider completely removing and carefully reinserting the device (see Chapter 4 for intubation through the ILMA and ILMA removal).

Complications. Complications of ventilation and intubation using the ILMA are rare. Episodes of hypoxia are rare after adequate ventilation is established with the ILMA. The risk of aspiration when using the ILMA in the ED is difficult to assess. There are no reports of significant aspiration in descriptive studies of the ILMA. However, most studies have been performed in the controlled environment of the operating room. The risk of aspiration is likely to be much higher in the ED. The ILMA does provide some protection against gastric inflation and passive regurgitation. However, active vomiting while the ILMA is in place would probably lead to aspiration.

Pressure injury to the pharynx may be caused by prolonged use of the ILMA. This complication is very unlikely in the ED. The potential for pressure injury can be prevented by deflating the ILMA as soon as possible after tracheal intubation is achieved.

The LMA (LMA Classic and LMA Unique)

Insertion and tracheal intubation through the LMA are more complicated. The LMA Classic can be used up to 40 times before being replaced. The LMA Unique is a single-use version of the LMA Classic. The LMA Unique has the same dimensions as LMA Classic but is made out of plastic instead of silicone and is very inexpensive. The LMA Classic and LMA Unique are available in all sizes, including pediatric and neonatal sizes. Because the design and functional characteristics of both devices are the same, we use the term *LMA* to refer to both devices.

Indications and Contraindications. The LMA should be considered as a primary rescue device for pediatric emergency airway management, because an ILMA is not available for patients who weigh less than 30 kg. The LMA is also a

good rescue device for adult emergency airway management, when an ILMA is not available. In addition, a very large adult LMA, size 6, is available for patients who weigh more than 100 kg. The largest available ILMA is a size 5. The LMA is a successful rescue device for rescue ventilation in the cannot-intubate/cannot-ventilate situation. The LMA may provide a more secure and reliable means of ventilation than a face mask.[1] The LMA allows adequate ventilation in 98% of adults with known difficult airways and in 90% to 95% of those with unexpectedly difficult airways.[127,151–154] The LMA is useful in patients with brisk bleeding above the glottis or with difficult face mask ventilation owing to a beard, severe facial trauma, or obesity.

Intubation through the LMA is possible, but it requires a smaller endotracheal tube and is more difficult than intubation through the ILMA (see Chapter 4 for intubation through the LMA). Blind intubation through the LMA is not recommended. Most adults with difficult airways can be successfully intubated through the LMA using a flexible fiberoptic scope; however, there is a higher rate of technical problems, hypoxia, and failed intubation compared with the ILMA.[127]

The LMA is particularly useful as a rescue device in difficult pediatric airways.[127] Two descriptive studies and 86 case reports describe the use of the LMA for difficult pediatric airways.[127,155–161] In these reports, ventilation was adequate with the LMA in nearly all pediatric patients.[127,159,161,162] Intubation of pediatric patients through the LMA is usually possible with a small fiberoptic scope.[159,161] Case series and case reports also suggest that the LMA can provide an effective rescue airway in neonatal resuscitation if bag-mask ventilation and endotracheal intubation fail.[163]

The LMA is relatively contraindicated in awake patients, especially those with a full stomach. Insertion of the LMA in an awake patient will cause coughing, gagging, or vomiting. If the LMA is inserted when the patient is awake and the stomach is full, vomiting and aspiration may occur. In the ED, the LMA should be used only if the patient is unconscious or after paralytic agents are given. Once the LMA is inserted and ventilation is established, the patient should not be allowed to wake up or gag. Consider using a long-acting paralytic agent or multiple doses of succinylcholine once adequate ventilation is established.

Decreased mouth opening may make insertion of the LMA difficult or impossible. Insertion of the LMA may also be difficult or impossible in patients with severely distorted upper airway anatomy, especially those with scarring secondary to cervical radiation therapy.

Placement of the LMA. The first step is to select the appropriate-sized LMA. The LMA is available in a wide range of sizes, from size 1 for neonates weighing less than 5 kg to size 6 for adults weighing more than 100 kg. The disposable version is available in sizes 1 through 5, but not size 6. After selecting the proper size, completely deflate the LMA cuff while pushing it posteriorly, so that it forms a smooth wedge shape without any wrinkles (see Fig. 3–7). Place a small amount of water-based lubricant onto the posterior surface of the LMA mask just before insertion. The best patient position for LMA insertion is the sniffing position, with the neck flexed and the head extended. The LMA may be inserted using two different techniques, depending on access to the patient. The most common method is the index finger insertion technique. This is accomplished by holding the LMA like a pen, with the index finger at the junction of the airway tube and the cuff (Fig. 3–13). Have an assistant open the patient's

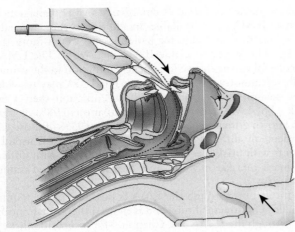

Figure 3–13   LMA insertion. Lubricate the posterior surface of the LMA cuff/mask. Hold the LMA like a pen and place the tip of the index finger at the junction of the airway tube and the cuff. Have an assistant hold the patient's mouth open. Place the posterior tip of cuff against the anterior hard palate just behind the upper incisors.

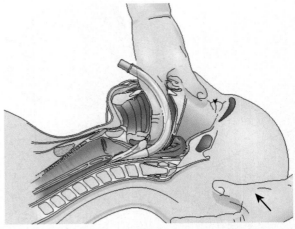

Figure 3–15   LMA insertion. To advance the LMA into its final position, fully extend the index finger and continue to advance the LMA along the posterior hypopharynx until it meets firm resistance. When properly placed, the device may be deeper than expected and the tip of the cuff will be wedged in the proximal esophagus.

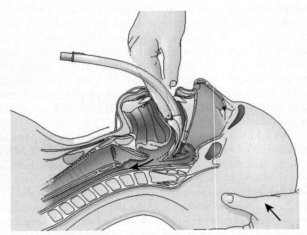

Figure 3–14   LMA insertion. Using the index finger, slide the LMA along the hard palate and posterior pharynx. Use the other hand to apply countertraction on the back of the patient's head.

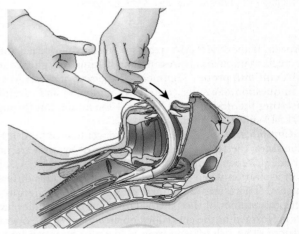

Figure 3–16   LMA insertion. Hold onto the proximal end of the LMA airway tube with the other hand, so that it is not displaced, while carefully removing the inserting hand and index finger from the patient's mouth.

mouth and insert the LMA with the posterior tip pressed against the hard palate just behind the upper incisors. Under direct vision, use the index finger to slide the LMA along the hard palate and into the oropharynx (Fig. 3–14). As the LMA is inserted farther, extend the index finger and push the posterior cuff along the soft palate and the posterior pharynx. Exert counterpressure on the back of the patient's head during insertion. Continue to push the LMA into the hypopharynx until resistance is felt (Fig. 3–15). Use the other hand to hold the proximal end of the LMA airway tube while removing your index finger from the patient's mouth (Fig. 3–16).

An alternative method is the thumb insertion technique. Use this technique when you have limited access to the patient from behind (see www.lmana.com for details). Hold the LMA with your thumb at the junction of the cuff and the airway tube. Place the mask against the hard palate under direct vision as with the index finger technique. Use the thumb to push the LMA into the mouth along the palate and posterior pharynx. Hold the end of the airway tube with the other hand while removing your thumb from the mouth.

After the LMA is fully inserted, let go of the proximal end of the airway tube and inflate the cuff enough to achieve a good seal with the glottis (Fig. 3–17). This may require only half of the maximum cuff volume. Be careful not to overinflate the LMA cuff (see the product packaging for maximal cuff volumes). Attach a bag and ventilate the patient, using chest rise, breath sounds, and capnography to confirm adequate gas exchange. If bagging is easy and ventilation is good, the aperture of the LMA is probably aligned correctly over the glottic opening. Proper positioning of the LMA aperture with the glottic opening allows optimal ventilation.

Several tips or techniques should be considered if LMA ventilation is inadequate. The best way to ensure proper ventilation is to optimize the insertion technique by carefully following the previously discussed directions. Position the patient's head and neck properly and ensure that the patient is deeply anesthetized or paralyzed. Listen for an audible cuff leak to make sure there is a good mask seal. Adjust the cuff volume if necessary to improve the mask seal and ensure optimal ventilation. Simply adding more air to the cuff will

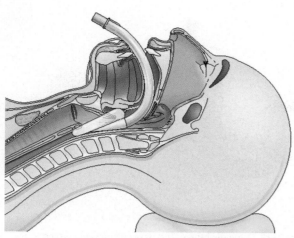

Figure 3–17 LMA cuff inflation. Let go of the LMA while inflating the cuff. The device will normally slide out of the mouth slightly during inflation. Initially inflate the cuff with only half of the maximum cuff volume, and then increase inflation as needed. Do not overinflate the cuff. See product manual for maximum cuff volumes.

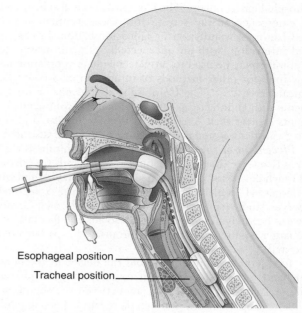

Esophageal position ⎯⎯⎯

Tracheal position ⎯⎯⎯

Figure 3–18 Esophageal-tracheal Combitube. The distal tube and cuff can be placed into either the esophagus (*solid lines*) or the trachea (*dotted lines*). The operator must quickly determine where the tip of the device is located, in order to ventilate the correct airway tube.

not necessarily improve the mask seal with the glottis. Cuff overinflation may cause a leak, whereas deflation and repositioning may improve the seal.

Sometimes adjusting the patient's head and neck position is easier than trying to change the position of the LMA. Move the patient into a better sniffing position or into the chin-to-chest position so see if this improves the LMA cuff seal. If these positions do not help, or are not possible, then try a jaw-thrust or a chin-lift maneuver. Also, apply anterior neck pressure to help push the glottis down into contact with the LMA mask. This technique can be used in combination with any of the maneuvers just discussed.

If mask seal and ventilation are still not optimal after simple repositioning maneuvers, withdraw, advance, or rotate the LMA cuff. Another alternative is to completely remove and reinsert the LMA, with careful attention to the details described earlier. If unsuccessful, change the LMA size. A larger size LMA will usually improve ventilation even if it is more difficult to insert. It is much more common to need to increase LMA size rather than to decrease LMA size. Finally, consider using the ILMA or the Combitube or performing a surgical airway when ventilation with the LMA is not adequate.

Complications. The most important complications associated with using the LMA are aspiration of gastric contents and hypoxia. Remember that the LMA does not protect against aspiration and may actually cause vomiting if the patient gags when the device is placed. In fasted anesthetized patients, the incidence of aspiration is very low, about 2 per 10,000 cases.[127] There are many descriptive studies and case reports of LMA use for difficult airways with no mention of significant aspiration.[127] Although the risk of aspiration is surely higher than 2 per 10,000 when using the LMA in the ED, there is evidence that it provides some protection from passive regurgitation and produces less gastric inflation than bag-mask ventilation.[1]

The cannot-intubate/cannot-ventilate scenarios are the most common reasons for using the LMA in the ED. In this situation, failure to adequately ventilate and oxygenate with the LMA occurs in about 6% of cases. Another 6% of patients with difficult airways suffer episodes of hypoxia during attempts to intubate through the LMA.[127] There is evidence

that the ILMA performs better in the cannot-intubate/cannot-ventilate situation.[127] Failure to ventilate with the ILMA occurs in only about 2% of cases and hypoxia after ILMA placement is very rare. Also, there are more technical difficulties when using the LMA, compared with the ILMA, for difficult airways. This is probably due to the fact that the LMA requires more skill for proper insertion and was not specifically designed to facilitate tracheal intubation.

The Esophageal-Tracheal Combitube

The esophageal-tracheal Combitube (Nellcor, Pleasanton, CA; www.nellcor.com) is an intermediate airway device that can be placed blindly and rapidly.[164] It was designed as a rescue device for difficult and emergency airways. It provides adequate ventilation in up to 95% of patients when it is placed by prehospital providers.[165–167] When the Combitube is placed by physicians, the success rate approaches 100%.[168]

The Combitube has two parallel lumens, a small distal cuff, and a large proximal cuff. When it is placed blindly, the tip will end up in the esophagus in about 90% of cases and in the trachea in about 10% of cases (Fig. 3–18). The longer lumen/tube is used for ventilation when the tip is in the esophagus. It is perforated at the level of the pharynx and occluded at the distal end. The shorter lumen/tube is used for ventilation when the tip is in the trachea. It is open at the distal end, like a standard endotracheal tube. The large proximal cuff/balloon is designed to occlude the pharynx by filling the space between the base of the tongue and the soft palate. The small distal cuff serves as a seal in either the esophagus or the trachea.[165–167,169–171] The Combitube compares favorably with the endotracheal tube with respect to ventilation and oxygenation in cardiac arrest situations.[164,171] In the unconscious patient, the Combitube may provide adequate protection from aspiration.[172]

Indications and Contraindications. The Combitube is a good choice as a primary airway in patients who are unresponsive or in cardiac arrest, especially in the uncontrolled prehospital environment. The Combitube can also be used in any emergency airway setting for rescue ventilation after failed bag-mask ventilation or failed intubation. In cases of failed intubation, with an unexpectedly difficult airway, the Combitube may be used to provide adequate ventilation and allow time for other methods of intubation or a controlled surgical airway.[173,174] The Combitube should not be used in patients with an intact gag reflex and is not recommended in patients shorter than 4 feet tall. It is contraindicated in suspected caustic poisonings or proximal esophageal disorders.

Placement of the Combitube. The Combitube is available in two sizes. The manufacturer recommends the smaller 37 French device for patients 4 feet to 5 feet 6 inches tall, and the larger 41-French device for patients over 5 feet tall. However, studies suggest that the smaller 37-French Combitube can be safely used in patients up to about 6 feet tall.[175,176] The larger 41-French device is appropriate for patients over 6 feet tall.

To insert the Combitube, hold the device in the dominant hand and gently advance it caudally into the pharynx while grasping the tongue and jaw between the thumb and the index finger of the nondominant hand. Pass the tube blindly along the tongue to a depth that places the printed rings on the proximal end of the tube between the patient's teeth and the alveolar ridge.[177] If resistance is met in the hypopharynx, remove the tube and bend it between the balloons for several seconds to facilitate insertion.[177] After insertion, fill the pharyngeal balloon with 100 mL of air, and fill the distal cuff with 10 to 15 mL of air. The large pharyngeal balloon serves to securely seat the Combitube in the oropharynx and to create a closed system in the case of esophageal placement. Because about 90% of placements are esophageal, begin ventilation through the longer (blue) airway tube.[167]

Look for chest rise, good breath sounds, and capnography, without gastric inflation, to confirm proper ventilation. Alternatively, use a Wee-type aspirator device on the shorter (clear) lumen to confirm that the tip is in the esophagus, prior to ventilation through the longer (blue) lumen.[178] The inability to easily aspirate air confirms esophageal placement. Easy aspiration with the Wee-type device indicates a tracheal positioning of the tube and requires changing the ventilation to the shorter (clear) tracheal lumen.

If there is confusion about the location of the Combitube tip, use capnography to ensure that the correct airway tube is being ventilated. However, capnography may be confusing in cases of cardiac arrest.

If the Combitube is in the esophageal position, suction the stomach by passing a catheter through the shorter (clear) lumen into the stomach while the patient is being ventilated via the longer (blue) lumen.[167]

Complications. Inappropriate balloon inflation and incorrect Combitube placement can lead to air leaks during ventilation. The most common placement error is an improper insertion angle. Use a more caudal, longitudinal direction of insertion as opposed to an anteroposterior direction of insertion. The Combitube must also be maintained in the true midline position during insertion to avoid blind pockets in the supraglottic area, which can prevent the passage of the tube.[167] Attention to aligning the ring markings on the tube at the level of the incisors ensures proper positioning of the tube.

The Laryngeal Tube

The laryngeal tube (King LT, King Systems Corporation, Noblesville, IN; www.kingsystems.com) is a relatively new

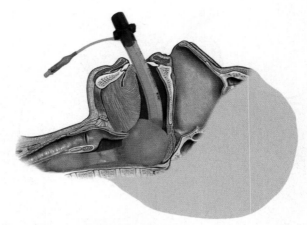

Figure 3–19 Laryngeal tube. The device is properly placed in the hypopharynx. The distal cuff is inflated in the proximal esophagus and the large cuff is inflated at the base of the tongue. The proximal portion of the tube is at the lip line and the distal aperture (between the cuffs) is aligned with the glottic opening. *(Image courtesy of King Systems Corp., Noblesville, IN.)*

supraglottic airway somewhat similar to the Combitube. Like the Combitube, the King LT is designed to isolate the glottic opening between an oropharyngeal cuff and an esophageal cuff (Fig. 3–19). Unlike the Combitube, the King LT has only one airway lumen and a simplified cuff system, so that both cuffs can be inflated with a single airway port. Multiple versions of the King LT have been clinically tested and the latest version is promising.

Like the Combitube, the King LT is designed for blind placement and has a large proximal cuff and small distal cuff. Unlike the Combitube, the tip of the King LT is designed to be placed into the esophagus only. The shape of the King LT and the size of the tip make it unlikely to be placed into the trachea.[179]

When the King LT is properly placed, positive-pressure ventilation is unlikely to cause a gas leak or gastric inflation.[180] Some data show that the King LT may provide a better seal in the oropharynx than the LMA.[181] The King LT-D is a disposable version of the King LT. The King LT-D is designed with the same specifications as the reusable King LT. The King LTS-D is a disposable device exactly like the King LT-D, except for the addition of a distal suction port. There are limited but positive data about the use of the King LT in the emergency and difficult airway settings. The King LT-D is becoming popular in the prehospital setting and is replacing the Combitube in some EMS systems.

Indications and Contraindications. In the ED, indications for using the King LT are the same as those for the Combitube. It appears to be a good rescue ventilation device for failed bag-mask ventilation or failed intubation.[179,182,183] Because the King LT is a supraglottic airway and is designed to be placed blindly, it is relatively contraindicated in patients with foreign body upper airway obstruction.

Placement of the King LT. The first step is to choose the proper size King LT. It is available only in adolescent and adult sizes in the United States. The size 3 is yellow and designed for patients 4 to 5 feet in height, the size 4 is red and designed for patients 5 to 6 feet in height, and the size 5 is purple and designed for patients over 6 feet in height. Several pediatric sizes are available in Europe, but not in the United States.

After determining the appropriate-sized King LT, check the cuffs and then completely deflate them prior to placement. Lubricate the device with a water-based lubricant. The best patient position for insertion of the King LT is the sniffing position, but it can be placed with the head in the neutral position if necessary. Hold the LT at the connector with the dominant hand and hold the mouth open by grasping the chin with the nondominant hand. Introduce the tip of the device into the corner of the mouth while rotating the tube 45° to 90° so that the blue orientation line on the tube is touching the corner of the mouth. Pass the tip of the device into the mouth and under the tongue. As the tip passes under the base of the tongue, rotate the tube back to the midline so that the blue orientation line faces the ceiling. Without exerting force, advance the King LT until the connector is aligned with the teeth. Inflate the cuffs with the minimum volume necessary to create a good seal (see product brochure for maximum cuff volumes). Ventilate with a bag-valve system and confirm placement with chest rise, breath sounds, and capnography.

Complications. Because the King LT is a relatively new device, complications are not extensively documented. The most serious potential complication is tracheal placement. Unlike the Combitube, the tip of the King LT should never go into the trachea. Tracheal placement of the King LT would result in complete airway obstruction and no ventilation of the lungs. Improper placement may result in poor ventilation and injury to the upper airway, especially if the device is not kept in the midline during insertion.

DECISION-MAKING IN EMERGENCY AIRWAY MANAGEMENT

 BOX 3–1 Decision-Making in Emergency Airway Management CAN BE FOUND ON EXPERT CONSULT

The airway provider must have many tools readily available to deal with the acutely compromised airway. It is important to be proficient in a number of different techniques and to tailor their use to the needs of the individual patient. Rescuers should practice potential scenarios before facing patients with a compromised airway. Failure to do so may lead to unnecessarily aggressive management in some situations or to irreversible hypoxic injury as a result of hesitation in others. Deciding who requires a definitive airway and who needs only supportive measures is a formidable task for even the most skilled clinician.

The following parameters should be assessed before the decision is made to establish a definitive airway:

- Adequacy of current ventilation.
- Potential for hypoxia.
- Airway patency.
- Need for neuromuscular blockade (full stomach, teeth clenching).
- Cervical spine stability.
- Safety of the technique and skill of the operator.

Consideration of these factors should guide the clinician in selecting the optimal technique. Choosing the initial approach is often straightforward. Difficulty arises precipitously when the initial approach fails. Time becomes critical as the risk of irreversible hypoxic injury and cardiac arrest

rises. Anxiety then increases and the potential for error increases. Forethought and practice are invaluable when managing these situations.

Rapid Sequence Induction/Intubation (RSI)

Rapid sequence induction of anesthesia has evolved since the introduction of succinylcholine in 1951. The term RSI was initially used as an abbreviation for rapid sequence induction, but is now synonymous with rapid sequence intubation. Initially, the main purpose of RSI was to avoid positive pressure ventilation and prevent gastric inflation in patients at risk of aspiration. RSI has become the most common method of emergency airway management because it provides optimal conditions for direct laryngoscopy.[184-189] Providers using RSI must appreciate the importance of basic skills like preoxygenation, patient positioning and bag-mask ventilation.

Emergency providers should be very careful not to use RSI in a cavalier manner. When giving a paralytic agent, the provider takes complete responsibility for airway maintenance, ventilation, and oxygenation of the patient. Consider awake intubation in patients with known difficult airways. RSI is contraindicated in patients who cannot be orally intubated. RSI should be avoided in patients with laryngotracheal abnormalities caused by tumors, infection, edema or a history of cervical radiation therapy.

One of the most important concepts to understand when using RSI is the concept of optimal laryngoscopy, to maximize first pass success.[190-192] Preparation, preoxygenation, proper patient positioning, anterior neck maneuvers, and good laryngoscopy skills are all important components of optimal laryngoscopy (see Chapter 4). Also, maximizing RSI success requires that providers understand when to avoid RSI. Patient safety during RSI depends on the provider's ability to maintain ventilation and oxygenation if the first attempt at laryngoscopy fails.[192] In this situation, bag-mask ventilation restores oxygenation and allows multiple laryngoscopy attempts. The importance of bag-mask ventilation skills cannot be overstated. Good bag-mask skills allow the emergency airway provider to be less anxious about laryngoscopy and improve the chances of successful RSI.[4]

Difficult Airways and When to Avoid RSI

The term difficult airway is popular, but there is no standard definition of this term. Many use it to describe patients who are difficult to intubate using direct laryngoscopy. Subsequently there is a significant amount of literature dedicated to predicting difficult laryngoscopy. However, even in the best circumstances only 50% of cases of difficult laryngoscopy can be predicted.[193] Many factors such as Mallampati scoring and measurement of thyromental distance have not been found to accurately predict difficult laryngoscopy, especially in the emergency setting.[194,195] Only obvious anatomic and pathologic abnormalities, or a history of difficult intubation are accurate predictors of difficult laryngoscopy (see Chapter 4).[194]

In the emergency setting it is more useful to think of difficult airways as situations where our usual methods of ventilation and intubation fail. Our goal should be to avoid RSI on patients who cannot be ventilated with a bag-mask device and cannot be intubated by direct laryngoscopy. Risk factors for difficult bag-mask ventilation have not been studied as thoroughly, but there is good evidence that the presence

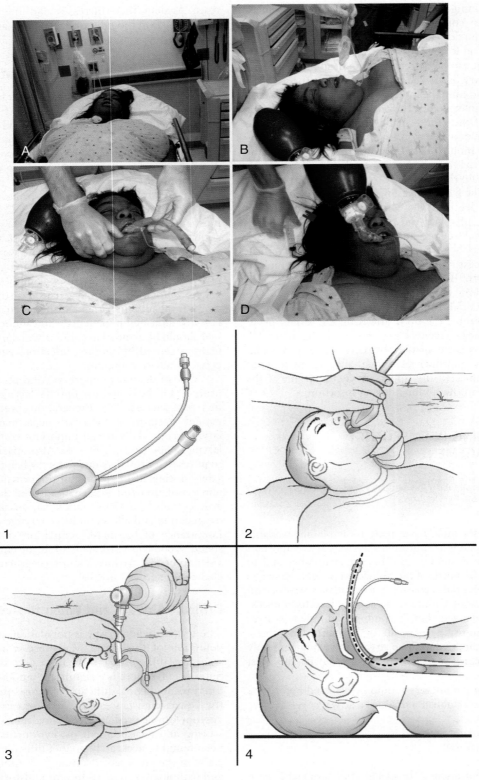

Figure 3–20 *A,* This morbidly obese patient was found asystolic by emergency medical service (EMS). She could not be intubated in the field with multiple attempts and did not survive bag-mask resuscitation. This patient is a candidate for an LMA airway. *B–D,* The LMA is inserted by depressing the jaw, advanced, inflated, and attached to an Ambu bag. Postmortem ventilation was very easy. *E,* Schematic depiction of LMA use. **1,** LMA is an adjunctive airway that consists of a tube with a cuffed mask-like projection at the distal end. **2,** LMA is introduced through the mouth into the pharynx. **3,** Once the LMA is in position, a clear, secure airway is present. **4,** Anatomic detail. During insertion, the LMA is advanced until resistance is felt as the distal portion of tube locates in the hypopharynx. The cuff is then inflated. This seals the larynx and leaves the distal opening of the tube just above the glottis, providing a clear, secure airway (*dotted line*). *(A–E, Redrawn from The American Heart Association in Collaboration with the International Liaison Committee on Resuscitation: Guidelines 2000 for Cardiopulmonary Resuscitation and Emergency Cardiovascular Care. Part 6: Advanced cardiovascular life support. Section 3. Adjuncts for oxygenation, ventilation and airway control. Circulation 102[8 Suppl]:I95, 2000.)*

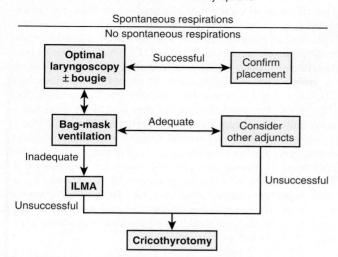

"Awake" intubation—many options

Spontaneous respirations

No spontaneous respirations

Figure 3–21 Emergency airway management algorithm used at Hennepin County Medical Center. The end point of the algorithm is successful tracheal intubation. This algorithm is presented as an example. Individuals and institutions should formulate their own algorithms based on the availability of skills and resources.

Weight (kg)	LMA	Disposable LMA	ILMA
<5	1	—	—
5–10	1.5	—	—
10–20	2	—	—
20–30	2.5	—	—
30–50	3	3	3
50–70	4	4	4
70–100	5	5	5
>100	6	—	—

TABLE 3–3 Laryngeal Mask Airway, Disposable Laryngeal Mask Airway, and Intubating Laryngeal Mask Airway Size Recommendation Based on Weight*

*Note that only standard LMA is available for patients <30 kg.
ILMA, intubating laryngeal mask airway; LMA, laryngeal mask airway.

TABLE 3–4 "Other" Intubation Methods for Emergency Airway Management

Flexible fiberoptics
Rigid/semirigid fiberoptics
Video laryngoscopy
Lighted stylet
Blind nasal
Retrograde
Digital

57

of a beard, obesity, lack of teeth, age over 55 years, and a history of snoring all make bag-mask ventilation more difficult (Table 3–3). The realization that we cannot predict all cases of difficult ventilation and difficult laryngoscopy mandates the need for reliable back-up devices like the ILMA/LMA and the Combitube. There is no doubt that use of the LMA and ILMA has decreased the frequency of failed airways (Fig. 3–20).[138,139,141,196] Finally, if RSI is our usual method of intubation, we must be prepared to perform a surgical airway when laryngoscopy, bag-mask ventilation, and back-up devices fail.[2]

Emergency Airway Management Algorithm

The algorithm presented here summarizes the general approach used in the Department of Emergency Medicine at Hennepin County Medical Center (Fig. 3–21 and Table 3–4). This algorithm is presented as an example. Individual providers and institutions should determine their own algorithms based on the availability of skills and resources. There are many similarities between this algorithm and those put forth by the American Society of Anesthesiologists and the Difficult Airway Society. However, ours is simple and more applicable to emergency airway management. Most published airway algorithms are not ideal for emergency airway management because they do not account for the conditions that we commonly face; patients with full stomachs who are critically ill and often uncooperative, and intubations that cannot be canceled if the airway is too difficult. Also, many algorithms resemble wish lists of equipment and skills that are simply not available to most emergency airway providers. We stress basic airway skills like preparation/preoxygenation, direct laryngos-

copy, and bag-mask ventilation. We also stress the importance of the bougie and the ILMA or LMA as effective basic rescue devices (see Chapter 4 for a discussion of the bougie). Combes and coworkers validated this approach in a large prospective study.[198]

CONCLUSION

Good basic airway management skills, a clear preconceived plan and the availability of proven rescue devices are the keys to dealing with airway emergencies. There are many techniques and devices that can be used to manage emergency airways. However, in difficult situations providers will probably have the best success with techniques and devices with which they are the most familiar.

Acknowledgments

The authors would like to thank Dr. John McGill for his insight and participation in editing this chapter. We would also like to thank Ben Dolan and Ed Peterson for their technical assistance with this chapter.

 REFERENCES CAN BE FOUND ON **EXPERT CONSULT**

CHAPTER 4

Tracheal Intubation

John W. McGill and Robert F. Reardon

Intubation is often the pivotal procedure in the emergency management of a critical patient. If direct visualization of the airway is possible, tracheal intubation is usually straightforward and readily accomplished using direct laryngoscopy. If visualization is difficult or impossible, alternative approaches are usually necessary, and may also prove challenging. This chapter discusses the preparation for intubation and describes the considerations and technical aspects of the various approaches and devices that are used to intubate the trachea. The basic airway management and general decision-making relevant to these techniques are presented in Chapter 3 and should be reviewed before proceeding with this chapter. Chapter 5 discusses the pharmacologic adjuncts for facilitating intubation, and Chapter 6 presents the more invasive approaches to the airway.

GENERAL PREPARATION

Preparation is the key to successful airway management. Two general areas of preparation need addressing before undertaking the first attempt at definitive airway management in the clinical setting. First, prepare mentally and technically. Second, assemble the essential intubation equipment.

Prepare mentally and technically by reading about the procedures, discussing the principles and details with instructors, practicing the techniques on intubation mannequins or in an animal laboratory, and performing the techniques under supervision in a controlled clinical setting. Studies addressing various approaches to tracheal intubation are generally performed under optimal conditions (i.e., with equipment available and with appropriate preparatory training). Also, often hidden within the study findings are individual learning curves. Therefore, do not expect to match the success reported in the literature when first attempting a new intubation technique. Nevertheless, the goal of preparation is to be as high on the learning curve as possible before the clinical application of a new technique. With continued use of the various approaches, one naturally becomes more adept and comfortable with certain devices and techniques than with others. When encountering a difficult airway, it is more important to be skilled in a few approaches at each level of a difficult airway algorithm than to try to master them all. The challenge is to know when to abandon one approach and move on to the next.

Each approach to tracheal intubation has a preferred training format. Orotracheal intubation is well simulated with a mannequin, whereas retrograde intubation is best learned on an animal or cadaver model. Orotracheal intubation is often successful on the first attempt, whereas considerable practice is required to master intubation with a fiberoptic scope. Video instrumentation offers a new dimension to traditional intubation techniques. In preparation for managing critical airway problems, maximal hands-on training is desirable. Ideally, this occurs under the guidance of someone with considerable airway expertise.

The second general area of preparation is making sure that all essential equipment required to perform the airway maneuvers is immediately available and within easy access. This may be accomplished by wall-mounting essential equipment in the emergency department (ED) resuscitation room.[1] Alternatively, place equipment in dedicated adult and pediatric airway carts or tackle boxes in an open, organized, and labeled manner that can be regularly checked and stocked (Fig. 4–1).[2] Essential equipment that is seldom used but is potentially life saving should be clearly identified and placed in an easily accessible location such as a dedicated difficult airway cart. The worst moment to realize that a vital piece of equipment is missing is when someone's life depends on it. The importance of this concept cannot be overstated. Technical expertise cannot substitute for the lack of essential equipment. In airway management, failure has ominous consequences. Mental, physical, and equipment preparation maximizes the chances of success.

AIRWAY ANATOMY

Requisite for a discussion of airway management procedures is a common understanding of airway anatomy and its terminology (Fig. 4–2). The following terms are used frequently in this chapter:

Arytenoid cartilages: the paired cartilages forming the posterior aspect of the laryngeal inlet.

Nasal cavity: from the external nares to the choana.

Nasopharynx: from the end of the nasal cavity (choana) to the level of the soft palate.

Oropharynx: from the soft palate to the upper border of the epiglottis.

Hypopharynx (laryngopharynx): from the epiglottis to the lower border of the cricoid cartilage.

Vallecula: the space at the base of the tongue formed posteriorly by the epiglottis and anteriorly by the anterior pharyngeal wall.

Laryngeal inlet: the opening to the larynx bounded anterosuperiorly by the epiglottis, laterally by the aryepiglottic folds, and posteriorly by the arytenoid cartilages.

Piriform fossae (recesses): the pockets on both sides of the laryngeal inlet separated from the larynx by the aryepiglottic folds.

Corniculate cartilage: the posteromedial portion of the arytenoid cartilage.

Cuneiform cartilage: the anterolateral prominence of the arytenoid cartilage.

Glottis: the vocal apparatus, including the true and false cords and the glottic opening.

Glottic opening (rima glottidis): the opening into the trachea as seen from above through the vocal cords.

PREPARING FOR INTUBATION

Intubation is best performed with two operators, one to perform the intubation, the other to handle equipment, help with positioning, and observe the monitor while keeping track of time. Before intubating, take the following steps in chronological order: (1) attach the necessary monitoring devices and administer oxygen; (2) establish intravenous access; (3) draw up essential medications and *label them if time permits*; (4) confirm that the intubation equipment is available and functioning; (5) reassess oxygenation and maximize preoxygenation; and (6) position

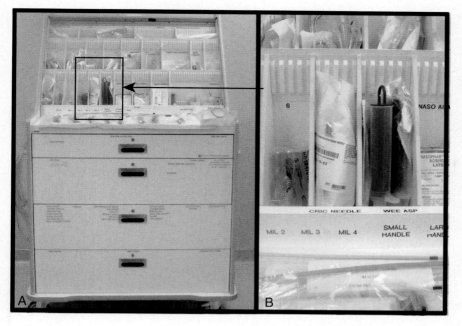

Figure 4–1 *A,* Adult airway cart. Equipment and materials are visible, labeled, and accessible. *B,* Labeling is especially important because it lets you know what is missing. *(Concept of Dr. Ernest Ruiz, Department of Emergency Medicine, Hennepin County Medical Center, Minneapolis, MN.)*

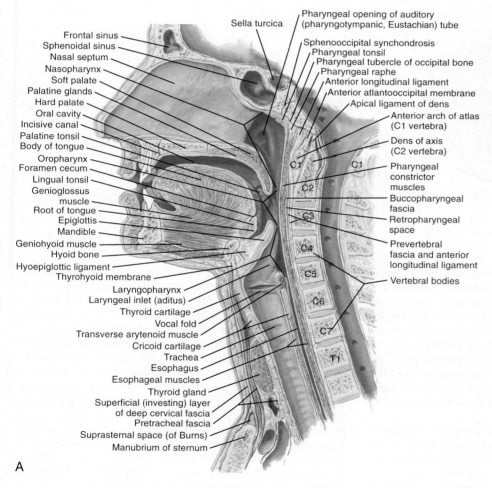

Figure 4–2 *A* and *B,* Anatomy of the upper airway. *C,* View of the larynx, epiglottis, and vocal cords seen with a laryngoscope. *(A, Netter illustrations used with permission of Elsevier Inc. All rights reserved.)*

A

the patient correctly. Assess for a difficult airway, which is not a discrete step but rather a process that may crystallize immediately or progress in an orderly fashion as the clinical situation evolves. In the haste of the moment, it is a common error to forget to preoxygenate or to position the patient optimally. Simple omissions, such as failing to restrain the patient's hands, remove the patient's dentures, or misplace the suction tip, can seriously hamper the success of the procedure. One suggested preintubation checklist is presented in Table 4–1.

In addition to the preparations necessary for optimum patient care, take steps to minimize clinician exposure to potentially infectious materials in patient secretions by wearing gloves, gown, goggles, and mouth protection.

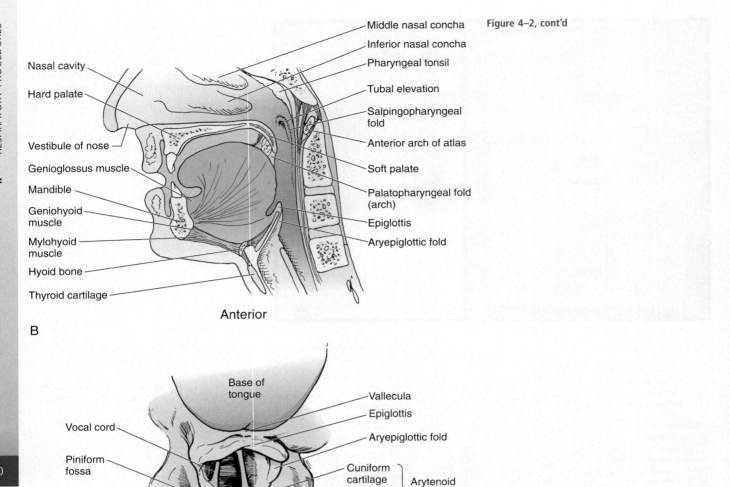

Figure 4–2, cont'd

Middle nasal concha
Inferior nasal concha
Pharyngeal tonsil
Tubal elevation
Salpingopharyngeal fold
Anterior arch of atlas
Soft palate
Palatopharyngeal fold (arch)
Epiglottis
Aryepiglottic fold

Nasal cavity
Hard palate
Vestibule of nose
Genioglossus muscle
Mandible
Geniohyoid muscle
Mylohyoid muscle
Hyoid bone
Thyroid cartilage

Anterior

B

Base of tongue
Vallecula
Epiglottis
Aryepiglottic fold
Vocal cord
Piniform fossa
Cuniform cartilage
Corniculate cartilage
Arytenoid cartilage

Posterior

C

PREOXYGENATION

In cardiac arrest, it is a judgment call as to whether attempts at preoxygenation versus immediate intubation will result in less hypoxic downtime. Impossible to distinctly characterize, real time clinical conditions and available resources allow for variations based on the individual scenario and clinicians approach. Whenever possible, however, preoxygenate all patients in whom tracheal intubation is contemplated. The goal is to maximize alveolar oxygenation in order to limit the risk of hypoxia during intubation attempts. Administer high-flow oxygen, applying it as early as possible with a tight-fitting mask.

Considerable research has been directed toward identifying the optimum method for preoxygenation. Most studies evaluating the efficacy of various preoxygenation approaches have been conducted in the setting of elective intubation. The major focus has been to identify the minimum number of deep breaths that will provide the same degree of oxygenation (denitrogenation) as 3 minutes of a normal volume of breathing of 100% oxygen, the traditional standard. The current recommendation is eight deep breathes over 60 seconds.[3] A reasonable goal is at least eight maximum breaths or 3 minutes of normal tidal volume breathing, both using high oxygen flow rates at 15 L/min. *Such preoxygenation can maintain accept-* *able oxygen saturation for up to 8 minutes in the previously healthy apneic patient.*

The studies addressing the question of how best to preoxygenate patients were conducted under ideal conditions in relatively healthy individuals. It is far more challenging to effectively preoxygenate the critically ill.[4] The principles, nonetheless, are important to keep in mind because not all patients undergoing emergency intubation are in cardiopulmonary extremis and some may be able to follow commands. The groups at greatest risk of rapid desaturation—the obese, the pregnant, and the pediatric patient—will benefit the most. If possible, sit the obese patient up to at least 25° during preoxygenation because significantly higher oxygen tensions can be achieved in this position.[5] In addition to increasing the functional residual volume and decreasing the resistance to inspiration, elevating the head of the bed decreases the chance of aspiration. These advantages can be seen with all patients, although they are most pronounced in the obese.

ASSESSING FOR A DIFFICULT AIRWAY

Difficult airway assessment attempts to predict the patients who will be difficult to ventilate with a bag-valve-mask device or difficult to intubate using direct laryngoscopy. Little data exist on predicting difficult bag-mask ventilation, although

TABLE 4–1 Suggested Preintubation Checklist

1. An assistant should be watching the cardiac monitor, blood pressure, and O_2 saturation while observing the patient for signs of decompensation. The assistant should be instructed to inform the operator if more than 30 sec has elapsed without ventilation.
2. An IV infusion should be running properly. Oxygen should be administered to the patient.
3. Draw the necessary drugs (e.g., atropine, lidocaine, paralyzing agent, induction agent).
4. Attach the bag-valve-mask to an oxygen source (rate of 15 L/min).
5. A stylet should be inserted properly into the tracheal tube.
6. Check the integrity of the balloon and cuff on the tracheal tube.
7. Have tape, twill tape, or a commercial tube stabilizer available.
8. Check the laryngoscope light source. Have a second light source, a selection of blades, and additional endotracheal tubes (ETs) available.
9. Turn on the oral suction device and place it so that it is immediately available near the clinician's right hand. Prepare the catheter suction for postintubation use.
10. Place the syringe to inflate the ET balloon on the stretcher to the right of the patient's head. An option is to attach a syringe to the pilot balloon of the ET tube.
11. If the patient is not pharmacologically paralyzed, restrain the hands.
12. Remove the patient's dentures (delay this action until immediately before intubation if the patient is being bag-mask ventilated).
13. Check the cardiac monitor leads and the rhythm strip immediately before the intubation attempt.
14. Check for optimal head positioning: neck slightly flexed and head extended on the neck (conditions permitting). May be facilitated by placing a towel under the patient's occiput to raise it 10 cm. Obese patients usually require significantly more occiput elevation.
15. Have an aspiration device for esophageal detection (particularly for cardiac arrest) and an end-tidal CO_2 detection device at the bedside.
16. Radiology department should be alerted for the postintubation chest radiograph.

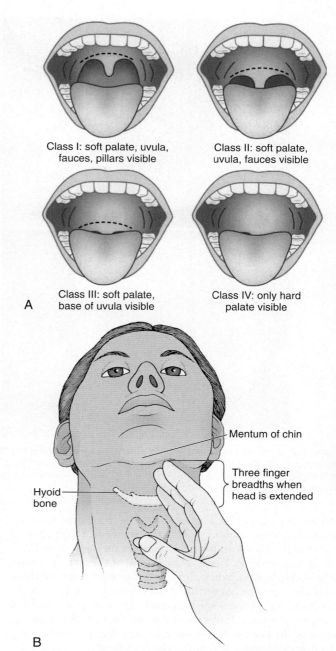

Class I: soft palate, uvula, fauces, pillars visible

Class II: soft palate, uvula, fauces visible

Class III: soft palate, base of uvula visible

Class IV: only hard palate visible

A

Mentum of chin

Three finger breadths when head is extended

Hyoid bone

B

Figure 4–3 *A,* Mallampati classification predicts the difficulty of intubation based on the visibility of the intraoral structures: Intubation difficulty may increase with classes III and IV views. *B,* A difficult intubation also may be encountered if the distance from the mentum of the chin to the hyoid bone in an adult is less than 3 fingerbreadths *when the head is extended.* (*A, From Thomsen T, Setnik G [eds]: Procedures Consult—Emergency Medicine Module. Copyright 2008 Elsevier Inc. All rights reserved.*)

the classic findings of having a beard, being edentulous, being obese, having a history of snoring, or having severe midface trauma have been confirmed (see Chapter 3, Table 3–1).[6] In contrast to the scarcity of studies of difficult ventilation, there is a large body of literature devoted to the airway that is difficult to intubate using direct laryngoscopy. The following discussion addresses clinical conditions and patient anatomy that can contribute to difficult direct laryngoscopy. Bear in mind that there are very few predictors that, in isolation, accurately predict difficult intubation. Rather, the likelihood of a difficult airway increases as the number of positive predictors increases.

Many difficult intubations are predictable if the clinician has adequate time to evaluate the patient before securing the airway. Unfortunately, most intubations in the emergency setting are not elective, nor do they lend themselves to careful evaluation for their degree of difficulty. Unlike the anesthesiologist who usually has the opportunity to evaluate the airway and intubation nuances well before surgery, the emergency clinician must often proceed with an intubation that turns out to be "difficult" only when the patient cannot be readily intubated. Perhaps the most frequently encountered

condition associated with a difficult emergency intubation is the agitated or combative patient. Fortunately, this condition can often be readily eliminated through pharmacologic intervention (see Chapter 5).

The classic predictors of a difficult intubation include a history of previous difficult intubation, prominent upper incisors, limited ability to extend at the atlanto-occipital joint,[7] poor visibility of pharyngeal structures when the patient extends the tongue (Mallampati classification, or the tongue/pharyngeal ratio) (Fig. 4–3A),[8] limited ability to open the

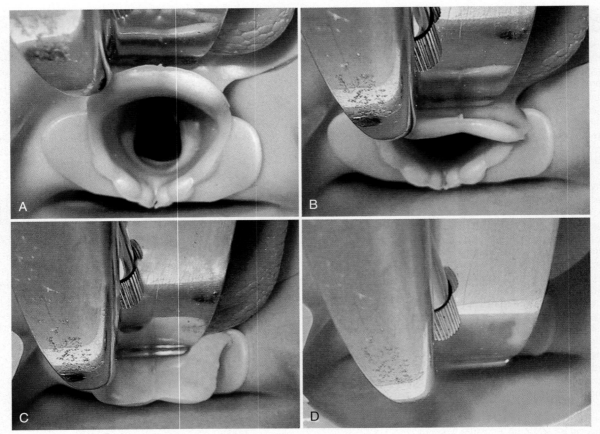

Figure 4–4   Cormack and Lehane grading of laryngeal views during laryngoscopy. *A,* Grade 1: Most of the glottis is visible. *B,* Grade 2: The posterior aspect of the glottis is visible. *C,* Grade 3: Only the epiglottis is seen; no part of the laryngeal inlet is visible. *D,* Grade 4: The epiglottis is not visible. Grades 1 and 2 are usually easily intubated with direct laryngoscopy whereas grades 3 and 4 are often difficult; the ability to see the arytenoid cartilages is the important difference.

mouth (suggested by a space < 3 fingerbreadths between upper and lower incisors),[9] a short distance from the thyroid notch to the chin with the neck in extension (see Fig. 4–3B),[10] and a limited direct laryngoscopic view of the laryngeal inlet (Fig. 4–4).[9] In emergency airway management, many of these predictors are not obtainable.[11] An extensive history is rarely available, the patients are frequently uncooperative, and the presence of trauma limits movement of the neck. Fortunately, some of the key predictors are apparent simply by observing the external appearance of the patient's head and neck.

Patients with neck tumors, thermal or chemical burns, traumatic injuries to the face and anterior neck, angioedema, infection of the pharyngeal and laryngeal soft tissues, or previous operations in or around the airway suggest a difficult intubation because distorted anatomy or secretions may compromise visualization of the vocal cords. Facial or skull fractures may further limit airway options by precluding nasotracheal (NT) intubation. Patients with ankylosing arthritis or developmental abnormalities, such as a hypoplastic mandible or the large tongue of Down syndrome, are difficult to intubate because neck rigidity and problems of tongue displacement can obscure visualization of the glottis.

Besides these obvious congenital and pathologic conditions, the patient with a short, thick neck is one of the more common presentations of a difficult airway. These individuals are easily identifiable by observing the head and neck in profile. Obesity alone may not be an independent predictor of difficult intubation, but obese patients with large circumference necks are likely to be difficult.[12] Facial hair can com-

plicate a difficult airway by rendering bag-mask ventilation ineffective owing to the lack of a good seal. One patient type that does not immediately stand out as a difficult intubation, but can be surprisingly so, is the patient with an unusually long mandibulohyoid distance (the thyroid prominence appearing low in the neck) and a short mandibular ramus.[13] Visualization of the larynx, due to the distance to the larynx and the relative hypopharyngeal location of the tongue, is difficult.

When faced with an anticipated difficult airway, consider all options, including awake intubation and NT intubation. As opposed to elective operating room cases, however, "canceling the case" is rarely an option. Identification of a potentially difficult airway does not necessarily preclude direct laryngoscopy. It does, however, mandate that backup devices be at the bedside if the patient cannot be readily intubated with the laryngoscope.

It should be emphasized that some patients, despite normal-appearing anatomy and the absence of a complicating history, are unexpectedly difficult to intubate. Be prepared for this rare but inevitable occurrence.

DIRECT LARYNGOSCOPY

Despite the proliferation of approaches and devices designed to secure a definitive airway, direct laryngoscopy remains the mainstay of tracheal intubation. The equipment is simple and the approach direct. Visual confirmation of the tube going through the vocal cords is usually possible.

Indications and Contraindications

Any clinical situation in which a definitive airway is necessary, and limited neck motion is permissible, is an indication for direct laryngoscopy. An *unstabilized injured cervical spine* is a relative contraindication to direct laryngoscopy, but should not preclude definitive airway management if a safer means of securing an airway is not available.

Equipment

Laryngoscope

There are two basic blade designs for direct laryngoscopy, curved (Macintosh) and straight (Miller and Wisconsin). Each comes in various adult and pediatric blade sizes. Slight variations in laryngoscopic technique follow from one's choice of blade design, which is often a matter of personal preference. The tip of the straight blade goes under the epiglottis and lifts it directly, whereas the curved blade fits into the vallecula and indirectly lifts the epiglottis via the hyoepiglottic ligament to expose the larynx. Special blades designed for the anterior larynx include the Siker and the Belscope (Avulunga Pty Ltd, New South Wales, Australia).

Each blade type has advantages and disadvantages. The straight blade is often a better choice in pediatric patients, in patients with an anterior larynx or a long floppy epiglottis, and in individuals whose larynx is fixed by scar tissue. It is less effective, however, in patients with prominent upper teeth, and it is more likely to break teeth. Use of the straight blade is also more often associated with laryngospasm owing to its stimulation of the superior laryngeal nerve, which innervates the undersurface of the epiglottis. A straight blade may inadvertently be advanced into the esophagus and initially present one with unfamiliar anatomy until it is withdrawn. The blade has a light bulb at the tip that may slightly hamper vision. The wider, curved blades are helpful in keeping the tongue retracted from the field of vision, allowing for more room in passing the tube in the oropharynx, and they are generally preferred in uncomplicated adult intubations. Aside from patient considerations, some clinicians prefer the curved blade because they find it requires less forearm strength than the straight blade.

The illumination provided by the laryngoscope can make a big difference in the ability to visualize the laryngeal inlet. The importance of these factors is underappreciated, as demonstrated by Levitan and colleagues[14] in their survey of Macintosh blades used in 17 Philadelphia EDs. They found that only 24% of all blades provided the brightness recommended for fine inspection. This finding was largely explained by the fact that the majority of EDs used the A-Mac (American) as opposed to the clearly superior brightness design of the G-Mac (German) or the intermediate brightness of the E-Mac (English).

Tracheal Tubes

The standard adult endotracheal (ET) tube measures approximately 30 cm in length. Tube size is typically printed prominently on the tube and is based on the internal diameter (ID), measured in millimeters. The range is from 2.0 to 10.0 mm, increasing in increments of 0.5 mm. The outer tube diameter is 2 and 4 mm larger than the internal diameter.[15] Tubes are also imprinted with a scale in centimeters that indicates the distance from a tube's distal tip.

Adult men generally accept a 7.5- to 9.0-mm orotracheal tube, whereas women can usually be intubated with a 7.0- to 8.0-mm tube. Larger tubes are theoretically desirable because airway resistance increases as tube size decreases, however, in practice, a 7.5-mm tube is adequate for almost all patients. In emergency intubations, particularly if a difficult intubation is anticipated, many clinicians choose a smaller tube and change to a larger tube later if necessary. Although generally an acceptable practice, this should be avoided in the burn patient because swelling may prohibit subsequent tube placement. For nasal intubation, a slightly smaller (by 0.5 to 1.0 mm) tube is chosen than would be used for orotracheal intubation.

Correct tube size is important in the pediatric population. It is especially important when using an uncuffed tube because a good seal is needed between the ET tube and the upper trachea (Table 4–2). Because tube size is based on the ID, a cuffed tube should generally be one half size (0.5 mm) smaller than an uncuffed tube. The smaller ID of an appropriately sized, small, cuffed tube could theoretically make it more prone to plugging from secretions. Cuffed tubes are available down to a 3-mm ID, although indications for these tubes in neonates and infants are rare. A cuffed tube is used in children with decreased lung compliance who may require prolonged mechanical ventilation. In a child, the smallest airway diameter is at the cricoid ring rather than at the vocal cords, as in adults. Hence, a tube may pass the cords but go no farther. If this should occur, the next smaller sized tube should be passed.

In infants and children, the following formula is a highly accurate method for determining correct uncuffed ET tube size:

$$\text{Tube size} = [4 + \text{age (yr)}]/4$$

For most clinical situations, however, using the width of the nail of the little (fifth) finger as a guide is sufficiently accurate and has been shown to be more precise than finger diameter

TABLE 4–2 Tracheal Tube Sizes for Average Patients*			
Age	Size (Fr)	Internal Diameter (mm)	Equivalent Tracheotomy Tube Size
Premature			
Newborn	12	2.5	00
6 mo	16	3.5	00–0
1 yr	20	4.5	0–1
2 yr	22	5.0	1–2
4 yr	24	5.5	2
6 yr	26	6.0	3
8 yr	28	6.5	4
10 yr	30	7.0	4
12 yr	32	7.5	4
14 yr	34	8.0	5
Adult			
Female	34–36	7.0–8.0	5
Male	36–40	7.5–9.0	6
Special cases			8–10

*A slightly smaller size may be required for nasotracheal intubation.
Modified from Applebaum EL, Bruce DL (eds): Tracheal Intubation. Philadelphia, WB Saunders, 1976.

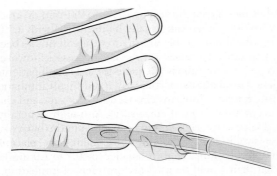

Figure 4–5 Pediatric endotracheal tube size estimation using the fingernail width of the little finger.

(Fig. 4–5).[16] A standard tracheal tube uses a high-volume, low-pressure cuff to avoid pressure necrosis of the tracheal lining. A clinical test for determining correct cuff inflation is to slowly inject air until no air leak is audible while the patient is receiving bag-tube ventilation. This usually occurs with 5 to 8 mL of air if the proper-sized tracheal tube has been selected. Many clinicians use the tension of the pilot balloon as a guide to cuff inflation; slight compressibility with gentle external pressure indicates adequate inflation for most clinical situations. For long-term use, cuff pressure should be measured and maintained at 20 to 25 mm Hg. Capillary blood flow is compromised in the tracheal mucosa when the cuff pressure exceeds 30 mm Hg. In emergency situations, the balloon may simply be inflated with 10 mL of air and adjusted when the patient's condition has stabilized.

Interest in the design of the tracheal tube tip has grown as the Seldinger technique is increasingly applied to intubation. When a tracheal tube is railroaded over a smaller-caliber introducer, whether it is a tracheal tube introducer or a fiber-optic scope, there is a reasonable chance the tube will get hung up on the laryngeal soft tissue.[17] A tracheal tube that has been designed to overcome this problem has a bevel oriented posteriorly and a flexible tip that decreases the distance between the tube and whatever it is being railroaded over (Fig. 4–6).

Check the ET tube cuff for leaks by inflating the pilot balloon before attempting intubation. Prepare the tube for placement by passing a flexible stylet down the tube to increase its stiffness and enhance control of the tip of the tube. Do not extend the stylet beyond the eyelet of the tube. Bend the tube in a gradual curve with a more acute angling in the distal third to more easily access the anterior larynx. Lubricate the tip and cuff of the tube with viscous lidocaine or a water-soluble gel.

Positioning the Patient

Position the patient to optimally align the oral, pharyngeal, and laryngeal axes (Fig. 4–7). The desired position was aptly described by Magill to make the patient appear to be "sniffing the morning air," with the head extended on the neck and the

Figure 4–7 **Head positioning for tracheal intubation.** *A,* Neutral position. *B,* Head elevated. *C,* "Sniffing" position, with flexed neck and extended head. Note that flexing the neck and extending the head lines up the various axes and allows for intubation. This position creates the shortest distance and the straightest line between the teeth and the vocal cords.

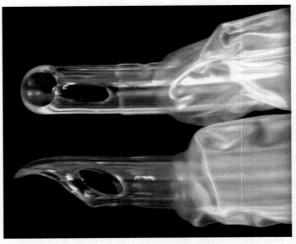

Figure 4–6 Comparison of the standard tracheal tube tip with the Parker Flex-Tip Tracheal Tube. *Note:* When a standard tube is inserted in the normal fashion, the bevel is oriented vertically and toward the patient's left. The Parker tube tip bevel faces posteriorly and may avoid getting caught on laryngeal structures. The flexible tip of the Parker tube also provides a closer fit on an introducer.

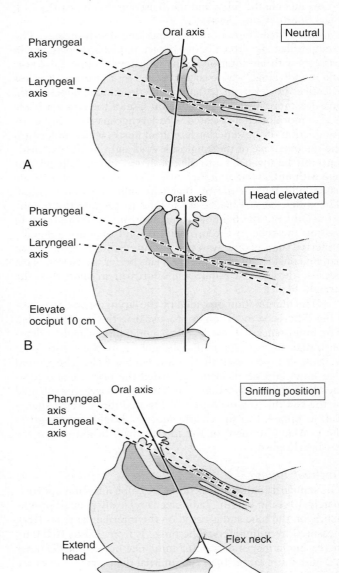

neck slightly flexed relative to the torso. Place a small towel under the occiput (to raise it 7–10 cm) to facilitate positioning in the average adult, but not in a child. Make a slight adjustment to the head position by placing the right hand under the patient's head, during laryngoscopy, and adjusting the extension to optimize glottic visualization (Fig. 4–8). Positioning of the head and neck is a critical step in preparation for intubation; suboptimal head positioning is a common reason for intubation difficulties.

Positioning of the morbidly obese patient is unique because, when the patient is supine, the neck, relative to the torso, is significantly posterior. Hence, achieving the sniffing position in these patients requires more elevation of the head and neck as well as the upper back. One method for achieving the sniffing positioning in the morbidly obese patient is to build a ramp of towels and pillows under the upper torso, head, and neck.[18]

Procedure and Technique

Adults

Stand at the patient's head (see Fig. 4–8). Place the patient in the supine position with the head at the level of the clinician's lower sternum (do not attempt to intubate the patient on a low stretcher). To maintain the best mechanical advantage, keep your back straight and do not hunch over the patient; bend only at the knees. Keep the left elbow relatively close to the body and flex slightly to provide better support. In the severely dyspneic patient who cannot tolerate lying down, perform direct laryngoscopy with the patient seated semierect and the clinician on a step stool behind the patient.[19]

Grasp the laryngoscope in the left hand with the blade directed toward the patient from the hypothenar aspect of your hand. Draw down the patient's lower lip with your right thumb, and introduce the tip of the laryngoscope into the right side of the patient's mouth. Slide the blade along the right side of the tongue, gradually displacing the tongue toward the left as you move the blade to the center of the mouth. If you initially place the blade in the middle of the tongue, it will fold over the lateral edge of the blade and obscure the airway. Placing the blade in the middle of the tongue and failing to move the tongue to the left are two common errors preventing visualization of the vocal cords (Fig. 4–9A–C).

As you move the blade tip toward the base of the tongue, exert a force along the axis of the laryngoscope handle, lifting upward and forward at a 45° angle (see Fig. 4–8). The direction of this force is critical because if the force is too horizon-

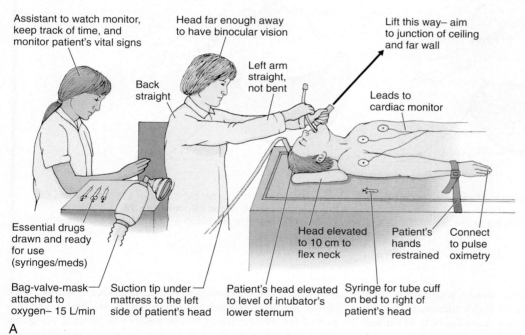

Assistant to watch monitor, keep track of time, and monitor patient's vital signs

Head far enough away to have binocular vision

Lift this way– aim to junction of ceiling and far wall

Back straight

Left arm straight, not bent

Leads to cardiac monitor

Essential drugs drawn and ready for use (syringes/meds)

Head elevated to 10 cm to flex neck

Patient's hands restrained

Connect to pulse oximetry

Bag-valve-mask attached to oxygen– 15 L/min

Suction tip under mattress to the left side of patient's head

Patient's head elevated to level of intubator's lower sternum

Syringe for tube cuff on bed to right of patient's head

A

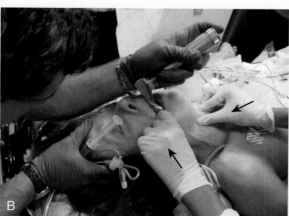

B

Figure 4–8 *A,* Proper positioning of clinician, patient, and assistant for tracheal intubation. The following points are demonstrated: The difficult airway cart is adjacent to the patient; the suction device is at the head of the bed; the patient is in the "sniffing position," with the occiput elevated and the clinician's right hand ready for additional adjustment if necessary; the bed is elevated and the clinician is at the appropriate distance from the patient; the laryngoscope handle is angled at 45°. *B,* Note the assistant manipulating the anterior neck and *retracting the cheek for better views (arrows).*

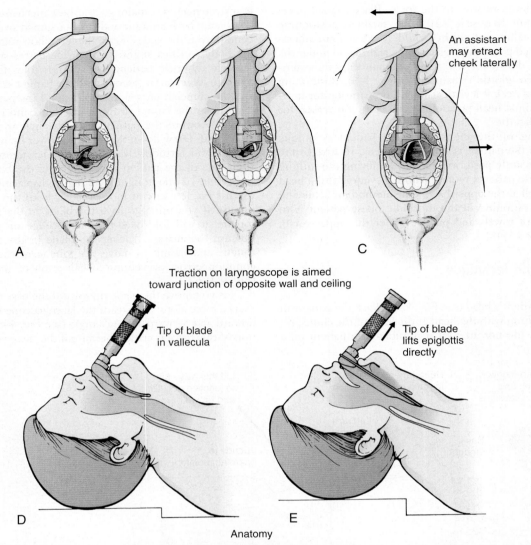

An assistant may retract cheek laterally

A

B

C

Traction on laryngoscope is aimed toward junction of opposite wall and ceiling

Tip of blade in vallecula

Tip of blade lifts epiglottis directly

D

E

Anatomy

Figure 4–9 **Common problems encountered when using the laryngoscope.** *A,* Laryngoscope blade is under the middle of the tongue, with the sides of the tongue hanging down and obscuring the glottis. *B,* Tongue is not pushed far enough to the left, obscuring the glottis. *C,* Correct blade position with the tongue elevated and to the left. *D,* Use of the curved (Macintosh) laryngoscope blade. *E,* Use of the straight (Miller) blade.

tal or too vertical it will result in poor visualization. The epiglottis should come into view with this maneuver. It may help to have an assistant retract the cheek laterally to further expose the laryngeal structures. Avoid bending the wrist because it can result in dental injury if the teeth become a fulcrum for the blade.

The step after visualization of the epiglottis depends on which laryngoscope blade is used. With the curved blade, place the tip into the vallecula, the space between the base of the tongue and the epiglottis. Continued anterior elevation of the base of the tongue and the epiglottis will expose the vocal cords. If the blade tip is inserted too deeply into the vallecula, the epiglottis may be pushed down to obscure the glottis.[8] When using the straight blade, insert the tip under and slightly beyond the epiglottis, directly lifting it up. If the straight blade is placed too deeply, the entire larynx may be elevated anteriorly and out of the field of vision. Gradually withdraw the blade to allow the laryngeal inlet to drop down into view. If the blade is deep and posterior, the lack of recognizable

structures indicates esophageal passage; gradually withdraw to permit the laryngeal inlet to come into view. The use of the curved and straight laryngoscope blades is illustrated in Figure 4–9D and E.

Anterior Neck Maneuvers during Intubation. The larynx can be manipulated from the anterior neck by pressure on the cricoid cartilage, the thyroid cartilage and the hyoid bone. *These are best performed by an assistant.* The technique chosen depends on the purpose of the manipulation. There are two purposes of the anterior neck maneuvers: (1) to prevent gastric regurgitation or gastric insufflation by occlusion of the esophagus and (2) to improve visualization of the larynx during laryngoscopy.

Three techniques are commonly cited:
1. Backward pressure on the *cricoid* of up to 10 to 40 N (1–4 kg) for regurgitation control, called the *Sellick maneuver.*
2. Backward-upward-right-pressure (the *BURP maneuver*) on the *thyroid* cartilage to improve visualization.

3. Pressure over the hyoid, thyroid, and cricoid cartilages termed *optimal-external-laryngeal-manipulation (OELM)*, also called *bimanual laryngoscopy*, for visualization improvement.

Regurgitation Control. A concept first described in 1774 for drowning victims was popularized by Sellick in 1961.[20,21] The theory was that pressure over the cricoid cartilage (the only cartilage that is a complete ring), when directed posteriorly using the thumb and middle finger, compresses the esophagus against the vertebral column and prevents passive regurgitation of gastric contents into the upper airway.[21] This publication led to its widespread standard practice in airway management. Sellick[21] published photos showing an occluded barium column inside a latex sleeve that was placed in the esophagus. The maneuver was performed with the neck in extension as opposed to the common sniffing position currently preferred.

Recent magnetic resonance imaging (MRI) studies have demonstrated that the anatomic concept of the cricoid compressing the esophagus is probably wrong. The esophagus lies lateral to the cricoid 50% of the time. Moreover, it is often displaced laterally when pressure is applied. MRI demonstrates that the most common structure lying posterior to the cricoid is the cricopharyngeus muscle, which forms the inferior portion of the funnel-shaped laryngopharynx and lies cephalad of the esophagus.[22,23] Ample evidence that cricoid pressure prevents regurgitation forces the consideration of a mechanism other than esophageal compression. It may be compression of the laryngopharynx, but that has yet to be demonstrated.

Control of Gastric Insufflation. Cricoid pressure can prevent gastric insufflation from high bag-mask pressures. Paralyzed patients without cricoid pressure tolerate up to 16.5 cm H_2O pressure without experiencing gastric insufflation. An approximate doubling of this pressure to 31.2 cm H_2O causes a 50% increase in the incidence of gastric insufflation. Pediatric studies have demonstrated that cricoid pressures of between 25 and 40 cm H_2O prevent gastric insufflation in children.[24-26]

Cricoid Pressure with a Laryngeal Mask Airway. Cricoid pressure complicates placement of a laryngeal mask airway (LMA). It can make seating of the distal tip of the airway into its proper position more difficult. Once an LMA is in place, cricoid pressure may also hamper efforts to perform tracheal intubation through the LMA. If cricoid pressure interferes with the placement or use of the LMA, then reduce or remove the pressure.[24-26]

Indications and Contraindications. Apply cricoid pressure to prevent passive regurgitation and gastric insufflation that can occur with bag-mask ventilation. The goal is to avoid aspiration. Patients at greatest risk are those who have just eaten or have other conditions such as pregnancy, intestinal obstruction, or simply intoxication, that increase the likelihood of gastric aspiration. It is used routinely in patients undergoing rapid-sequence intubation (RSI) and in patients undergoing bag-valve-mask ventilation. It is contraindicated in patients with suspected cricotracheal injury, active vomiting, sharp foreign bodies in the laryngotracheal region, and unstable cervical spine injury. It should be used with caution in patients with a history of difficult airway.[20]

Procedure for Cricoid Pressure. Identify the cricoid cartilage. Apply backward pressure of 10 to 20 N (1–2 kg) before the patient is fully unconscious and increase the pressure to 30 N (3 kg) with loss of consciousness.[27] A force of 30 N is

approximated by the pressure that causes discomfort when applied to the bridge of the nose. Apply the pressure using the first three fingers. Place the thumb and middle finger on each side of the cricoid and place the index finger in the middle superior portion of the cartilage to help maintain the midline position during application of pressure (Fig. 4–10*A*). Release the cricoid pressure after the patient is successfully intubated and the cuff is inflated or if active vomiting (not regurgitation) occurs. Other indications for release of cricoid pressure are if the laryngoscopic view is inadequate or if, when using an airway device such as the LMA, the device is difficult to place, ventilate, or intubate through.

Complications. The intubating clinician should constantly communicate the help, or lack thereof, of various maneuvers the assistant is performing. The most common complication of cricoid pressure is distortion of the anatomy making intubation more difficult. Fortunately, if recognized, it can be quickly remedied by letting up on the pressure or releasing it entirely. Esophageal rupture can occur in patients who are actively vomiting. Fracture of the cricoid ring can occur with excessive pressure.

Visualization Techniques. Cricoid pressure has also been used to improve visualization of the larynx during laryngoscopy. The "Back" maneuver is used to designate backpressure on the cricoid or thyroid to improve visualization. Two additional visualization techniques exist with better results. They are the BURP technique and the OELM, also called *bimanual laryngoscopy* technique.[28]

BURP Technique for Visualization. Backward pressure on the thyroid cartilage, combined with cephalad pressure and displacement to the right pressure, improves visualization during direct laryngoscopy. The technique was first reported in 1993.[29] A comparison of BURP with simple Back technique in the operating room showed that both maneuvers improved visualization, although the BURP technique was significantly more effective.[30]

PROCEDURE FOR BURP. The technique for BURP can be applied prior to or during laryngoscopy. Place the patient in the sniffing position. This may be done by an assistant as follows: Grasp the lower portion of the thyroid cartilage with the thumb on one side and the index and middle fingers on the other (see Fig. 4–10*B*). Apply pressure in the backward direction and press the larynx against the vertebrae. With continued backward pressure, shift the larynx in an upward direction as far as possible. Exert additional pressure to shift the larynx to the patient's right. The rightward shift in an adult should be no more than 2 cm, because greater displacement has been shown to worsen the laryngoscopic view.[29]

BURP differs from cricoid pressure and cannot be expected to control regurgitation and gastric insufflation in the same way cricoid pressure is intended. The pressure is exerted on the thyroid cartilage. It is a technique for visualization only.

OELM. The technique for OELM also requires an assistant. However, the laryngeal manipulation is first performed by the clinician who is performing laryngoscopy to optimize the glottic visualization. The clinician's hand position is then assumed by the assistant as the clinician removes the right hand to place the tracheal tube.

PROCEDURE FOR OELM. Hold the laryngoscope in the left hand while manipulating the larynx with the right. Hold the larynx by placing the thumb, index, and middle fingers of the right hand on the hyoid bone, thyroid cartilage, and cricoid

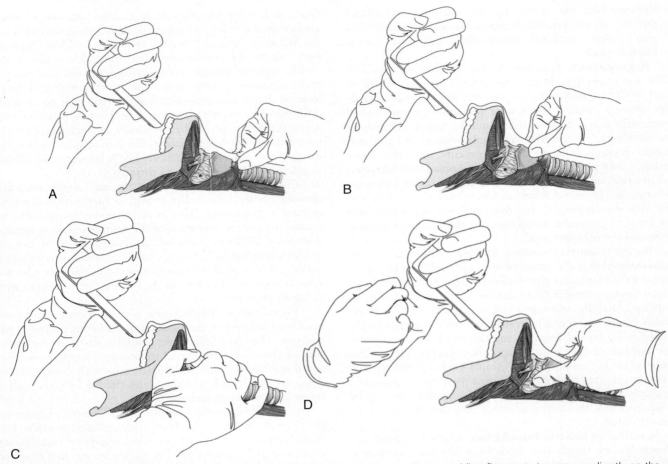

Figure 4–10 **Anterior neck maneuvers during intubation.** *A,* Cricoid pressure, with an assistant providing firm posterior pressure directly on the cricoid cartilage. *B,* Positioning of an assistant's hand, on the inferior portion of the thyroid cartilage, during the BURP maneuver (backward-upward-rightward-pressure). *C,* OELM (optimal external laryngeal manipulation or "bimanual laryngoscopy") step 1: The laryngoscopist optimizes the laryngeal view by reaching around to the patient's neck with the right hand, broadly manipulating the area of the hyoid, thyroid, and cricoid while performing laryngoscopy. *D,* OELM step 2: The assistant's hand replaces the laryngoscopist's hand on the anterior neck, maintaining laryngeal position while the laryngoscopist places the tracheal tube. *(A–D, Courtesy of Department of Emergency Medicine, Hennepin County Medical Center, Minneapolis, MN.)*

cartilage (see Fig. 4–10*C*). Use the pressure of the right hand to displace the larynx posteriorly and to the right until an optimum laryngeal view is obtained with the laryngoscope. Either direction, posterior or to the right, or both, may produce an optimum view. The position of the clinician's right hand is then assumed by an assistant as the clinician intubates the patient (see Fig. 4–10*D*).[31]

Two mechanisms are postulated to explain the improved visualization obtained with OELM. The first is that laryngoscopy displaces the larynx anteriorly and to the left. OELM counters this displacement and improves the view. Second, when the Macintosh blade is used, the maneuver may increase the traction of the laryngoscope blade on the hypoepiglottic ligament, which then lifts the epiglottis out of the line of vision.[31] A similar rationale can be applied to the BURP maneuver. Although the mechanism may be unclear, the improved laryngeal view is not (Fig. 4–11).

Summary. Cricoid pressure remains a common practice in anesthesia and emergency medicine. Objective evidence exists to support its use but the amount of clinical data is meager. Cricoid pressure can interfere with some approaches to intubation. BURP and OELM are similar maneuvers that improve visualization but have no effect on regurgitation.

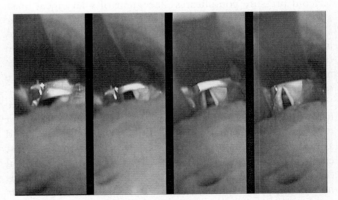

Figure 4–11 The epiglottis is elevated and visualization of the vocal cords is improved by pressure on the hypoepiglottic ligament and external laryngeal manipulation. *(Courtesy of Richard M. Levitan, MD, Airway Cam Technologies Inc., Wayne, PA. Used by permission.)*

Judgment must be exercised when choosing which techniques to use. We recommend the following approach:
1. Apply cricoid pressure during RSI. Be prepared to release it during LMA placement.
2. If visualization difficulty occurs, lessen cricoid pressure.

3. If the difficulty persists, release cricoid pressure and apply the BURP or OELM maneuver in hopes of improving visualization.

Infants and Children

It is helpful to appreciate the anatomic differences between children and adults when intubating the pediatric patient (Table 4–3 and Fig. 4–12). Infants' proportionately larger heads naturally place them in the sniffing position, so a towel under the occiput is rarely necessary. The large head can even result in a posterior positioning of the larynx that prevents visualization of the vocal cords; a small towel under the child's shoulders should correct this problem. The head may also be floppy and may benefit from stabilization by an assistant. The child's increased tongue-to-oropharynx ratio and shorter neck hinder forward displacement of the tongue and, coupled with a U-shaped epiglottis, can make visualization of the glottis difficult. Consequently, direct laryngoscopy in the infant and young child is generally best performed with a straight blade:

Miller size 0 for premature infants, size 1 for normal-sized infants, and size 2 for older children. The infant's larynx lies higher and relatively more anterior. One can have an assistant lightly apply laryngeal pressure, or the clinician can use the little finger of the hand holding the laryngoscope blade for this purpose (Fig. 4–13). If no laryngeal structures are visible after laryngeal pressure, gradually withdraw the blade. Inadvertent advancement of the blade into the esophagus is a common error.

Passing the Tube. Once the vocal cords have been visualized, the final step is to pass the tube under direct vision through the vocal cords and into the trachea. Hold the tube in your right hand and introduce it from the right side of the patient's mouth. *Distraction of the cheek may greatly aid overall visualization.* Advance the tube toward the patient's larynx at an angle, not parallel with or down the slot of the laryngoscope blade. This way, the tube does not obstruct the view of the larynx until the last possible moment before the tube enters the larynx. If the patient is not chemically paralyzed,

TABLE 4–3 Comparison of the Airway in the Adult and the Child

Comparison	Child	Adult	Clinical Consequences or Adjustments for Child
Head	Proportionately larger (up to about age 10 yr)	Proportionately smaller	Child naturally in sniffing position when supine. Do not place towel under occiput; may benefit from elevation of shoulders. Large head may be "floppy," requiring assistant to hold head still during intubation.
Teeth	Easily knocked out	Stable unless decay or trauma is a factor	Teeth may be knocked out and aspirated or forced into trachea.
Tonsils or adenoids	Large and friable	Generally not a problem	Nasotracheal intubation in child may cause excessive bleeding and is not recommended. Adenoid or tonsil tissue may plug endotracheal tube or cause airway obstruction from aspiration.
Tongue	Relatively larger	Relatively smaller	Difficult to displace tongue anteriorly in child. Consider using straight blade.
Larynx	Opposite C2, C3	Opposite C4–6	More superiorly located larynx, "anterior" larynx, more difficult to visualize. Consider using straight blade.
Epiglottis	U-shaped, shorter, stiffer	Flatter, more flexible	Epiglottis more difficult to manipulate in child, may fold down and obstruct view with curved blade. Consider using straight blade.
Vocal cords	Concave upward; anterior attachment of cords lower than posterior, creating a slant	Horizontal	Concave shape does not affect intubation, but may affect ventilation. For partial airway obstruction or to break laryngospasm, consider positive-pressure ventilation with jaw-lift to open arytenoids. Anterior superior slant of the vocal cords may cause endotracheal tube to hang up on anterior commissure as it passes into larynx. Rotate tube 90° counterclockwise. Overextension of neck may cause partial airway obstruction owing to airway collapse.
Length of trachea	Relatively shorter	Relatively longer	Short trachea increases likelihood of main stem bronchus intubation. Follow formula for correct depth of placement (cm depth = 0.5 age [yr] + 12) measured from corner of mouth. Double black line on endotracheal tube should pass just beyond cords.
Airway diameter	Relatively smaller; smallest diameter is at cricoid ring	Relatively larger; smallest diameter is between vocal cords	Laryngoscope-induced trauma, edema, and foreign material will significantly alter airway diameter. Be gentle. Extremes of flexion or extension may kink airway. If trouble with bag-valve-mask ventilation, reassess degree of head flexion or extension. Cricoid pressure may cause complete airway obstruction. Endotracheal tube may pass through cords but be too large to pass through cricoid ring. If unable to pass into trachea, use next smaller tube.
Residual lung capacity	Relatively smaller	Relatively larger	Child becomes hypoxic more quickly than adult. Closely monitor O_2 saturation and avoid prolonged periods without ventilation.

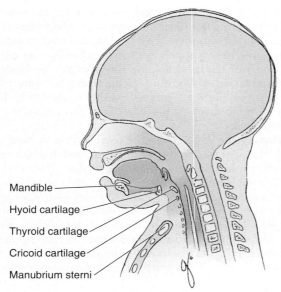

Mandible

Hyoid cartilage

Thyroid cartilage

Cricoid cartilage

Manubrium sterni

Figure 4–12 Sagittal sections of the neck of an infant shortly after birth. Note that in children, the neck is shorter and the larynx is located more cephalad. *(From Snell RS, Smith MS [eds]: Clinical Anatomy for Emergency Medicine. St Louis, Mosby–Year Book, 1993, p 16.)*

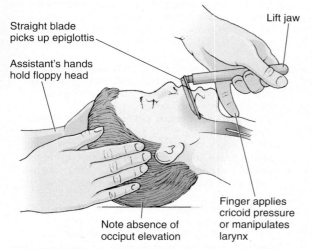

Straight blade picks up epiglottis

Lift jaw

Assistant's hands hold floppy head

Note absence of occiput elevation

Finger applies cricoid pressure or manipulates larynx

Figure 4–13 Oral intubation in a child, using a straight blade. The proportionately large, floppy head of the child may present some difficulty, and an assistant may be required to hold the child's head straight.

pass the tube during inspiration, when the vocal cords are maximally open. It enters the trachea when the cuff disappears through the vocal cords. Advance the tube 3 to 4 cm beyond this point. It is not enough to see the tube and the cords; watch the tube pass through the vocal cords to ensure tracheal placement. *Directly observing the tube pass through the cords is the "gold standard" to confirm correct placement.*

Laryngospasm. If the patient is not paralyzed, laryngospasm—the persistent contraction of the adductor muscles of the vocal cords—may prevent passage of the tube. Inadequate anesthesia is often the cause. Pretreat with topical lidocaine to decrease the likelihood of this occurring. Lidocaine, 2% or 4%, can be sprayed directly on the cords. An infrequent but

effective route for achieving tracheal anesthesia is via transtracheal puncture, injecting a bolus of 3 to 4 mL of lidocaine through the cricothyroid membrane. Laryngospasm is usually brief and often followed by a gasp. Be ready to pass the tube at this moment. Occasionally, the spasm is prolonged and needs to be broken with sustained anterior traction applied at the angles of the mandible, the jaw-lift. Do not force the tube at any time because this could cause permanent damage to the vocal cords. Consider using a smaller tube. Prolonged, intense spasm may ultimately require muscle relaxation with a paralyzing drug (see Chapter 5). The pediatric patient is far more prone to laryngospasm than an adult.[32] In a child, if vocal cord spasm prevents tube passage, a chest-thrust maneuver may momentarily open the passage and permit intubation.[33]

Positioning and Securing the Tube. Secure the ET tube in a position that minimizes both the chance of inadvertent endobronchial intubation and the risk of extubation. The tip should lie in the midtrachea with room to accommodate neck movement. Because tube movement with both neck flexion and extension averages 2 cm, the desired range of tip location is between 3 and 7 cm above the carina.[34]

The average tracheal length is between 10 and 13 cm. On a radiograph, the tip of the tube should ideally be 5 ± 2 cm above the carina when the head and neck are in a neutral position. On a portable radiograph, the adult carina overlies the fifth, sixth, or seventh thoracic vertebral body. If the carina is not visible, it can be assumed that the tip of the tube is properly positioned if it is aligned with the third or fourth thoracic vertebra. In children, the carina is more cephalad than in the adult, but it is consistently situated between T3 and T5. In children, T1 is the reference point for the tip of the ET tube.[35]

Estimate the proper depth of tube placement, before radiograph confirmation, using the following formulas, in which the *length represents the distance from the tube tip to the upper incisors in children*[36,37] *and from the upper incisors*[38] *or the corner of the mouth*[39] *in adults:*

Children: Tracheal tube depth (cm) = age (yr)/2 + 12
Adults:　　Tracheal tube depth (cm) = 21 cm (women)
　　　　　　Tracheal tube depth (cm) = 23 cm (men)

In adults, this method has been shown to be more reliable than auscultation in determining the correct depth of placement.[38] One can anticipate, however, that tall male patients will often require deeper placement, to 24 or 25 cm, and short women will often require a shallower placement of 19 or 20 cm.

Inflate the cuff to the point of minimal air leak with positive-pressure ventilation. In an emergency intubation, place 10 mL of air, and adjust inflation volume after the patient is stabilized.

After tracheal tube placement, auscultate both lungs under positive-pressure ventilation. Take care to auscultate posterolaterally because auscultation anteriorly can reveal sounds that mimic breath sounds but arise from the stomach. With the tube in position and the cuff inflated, secure the tube in place. Attach commercial ET tube holders, adhesive tape, or umbilical (nonadhesive cloth) tape securely to the tube and around the patient's head (Figs. 4–14 and 4–15). Position the tube at the corner of the mouth, where the tongue cannot expel it. This position is also more comfortable for the patient and allows for suctioning. A bite block or oral airway to prevent ET tube crimping or damage from biting is commonly incorporated into the system used to secure the tube.

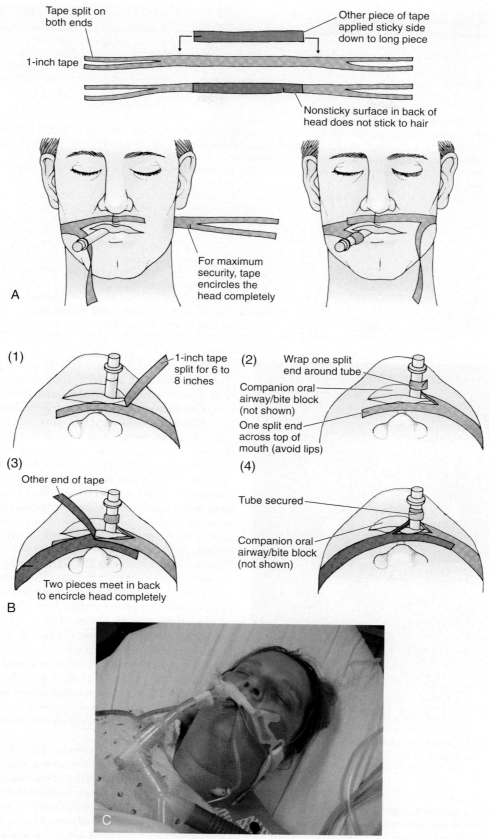

Figure 4–14 *A* and *B,* Two views of the technique for taping the tracheal tube. It is important to secure the tracheal tube properly. The method illustrated can be replaced by using a commercial holder or tracheostomy cloth tie. Avoid taping the lips. *C,* A commercial disposable tube holder is ideal and preferred to secure an ET tube without the use of messy tape.

TABLE 4–4 Assessing Proper Tube Placement

Test	Interpretation
Observe tube pass through vocal cords.	Accurate way to ensure placement; if in doubt, look again after intubation.
Auscultation of breath sounds over chest.	May be misleading, especially if only midline is examined; listen in both axillae.
Auscultation over stomach.	Gurgling indicates esophageal placement.
Condensation (fog) forms inside tube with each breath.	Quite reliable.
Observe chest rise with positive pressure and fall with release.	Generally reliable if good chest rise; may be absent in patients with small tidal volume or severe bronchospasm.
Feel air exiting from end of tube after inflation.	Reliable.
Air remains in lung after end of tube is occluded and exits when occlusion is removed.	Reliable but one may "ventilate" a closed area of esophagus.
Ask patient to speak; listen for moaning or other sounds	If tube is in proper place, no sound is possible.
Chest radiograph.	Generally reliable but can be misleading.
End-tidal CO_2 measurements.	Reliable if good persistent waveform; can be misleading with nasotracheal intubation if tip is curled supraglottically: will give positive CO_2.
Aspiration technique.	Tracheal location with patent tube if 30–40 mL of air is aspirated without resistance; probable esophageal location if unable to aspirate syringe easily or delayed bulb refill, can be misleading with nasotracheal intubation if tube curled supraglottically
Fiberoptic bronchoscope.	Reliable if tracheal rings are seen down endotracheal tube.
Lighted stylet down endotracheal tube.	Reliable if transillumination seen in low midline neck.
Ultrasound detection of tracheal tube location.	Appears reliable but not well studied.

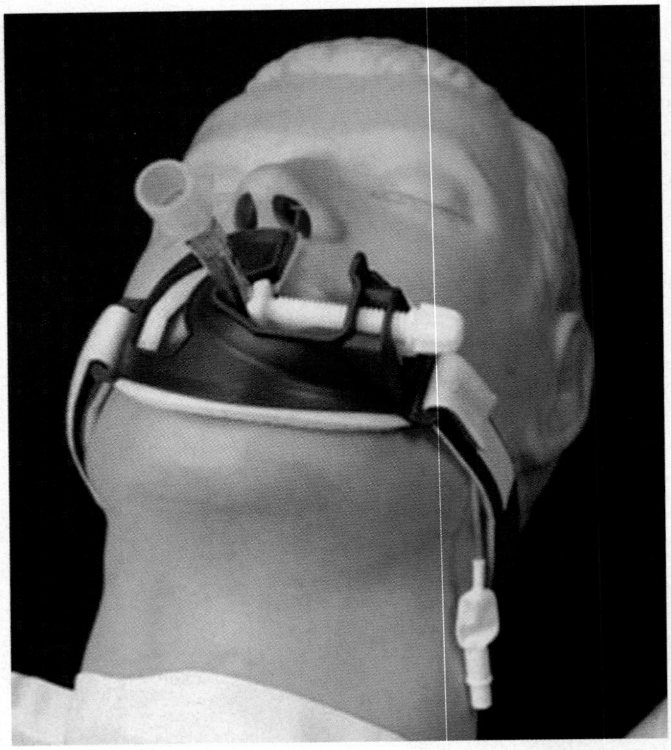

Figure 4–15 A plastic disposable ET holder firmly secures the ET tube with a small clamp. *(Courtesy of Laerdal Medical, Wappingers Falls, NY.)*

Unintentional extubation can have disastrous consequences, particularly if the patient was difficult to intubate initially. Secure the ET tube immediately after placement has been confirmed. Orotracheal intubation is associated with a higher rate of unplanned extubation than is NT intubation.[40] During transport or moving of the intubated patient, or when taking x-rays, *designate one person to tend to the ET tube to avoid accidental extubation.* Inadequate sedation is another risk factor for accidental extubation.[40] If long-acting paralytics have not been administered, consider sedation or physical restraints to prevent self-extubation in the agitated or confused patient.

Confirmation of Tracheal Tube Placement

Clinical Assessment. Confirm tracheal placement clinically *by seeing the tube pass through the vocal cords* (Table 4–4). If there is still any question, apply posterior pressure on the ET tube while the laryngoscope is still in place to expose the tube by altering the angle as it passes between the cords.[41] Absent or diminished breath sounds, *any sound or vocalization*, increased abdominal size, and gurgling sounds during ventilation are clinical signs of esophageal placement. *If the patient can moan or groan, the tube is not in the trachea!* However, esophageal placement is not always obvious. One may hear "normal" breath sounds if only the midline of the thorax is auscultated. The presence of condensation of the ET tube as a means of confirming tracheal placement may also be misleading. Blinded observers noted condensation of the ET tube during ventilation in 23 out of 27 esophageal intubations in an animal model.[42] One way to clinically assess tracheal placement after several ventilations or during spontaneous respiration is to note whether air is felt or heard to exit through the tube after cuff inflation. If the tidal volume is adequate, the exit of air should be obvious. It is important to note that when an appropriate-sized tube is placed in the trachea, the patient cannot groan, moan, or speak. Vocalization suggests esophageal placement.

Asymmetrical breath sounds indicate probable main stem bronchus intubation. Owing to the angles of takeoff of the main bronchi and the fact that the carina lies to the left of the midline in adults, right main stem intubation is most common and is indicated by decreased breath sounds on the left side. When asymmetrical sounds are heard, deflate the cuff and withdraw the tube until equal breath sounds are present. Bloch and coworkers[43] report accurate pediatric tracheal positioning if, after noting asymmetrical breath sounds, the tube is withdrawn a defined distance beyond the point at which equal breath sounds are first heard, 2 cm in children younger than 5 years and 3 cm in older children.

Esophageal Detector Device. An aspiration technique used to determine ET tube location was first described by Wee in 1988.[44] The technique takes advantage of the difference in tracheal and esophageal resistance to collapse during aspiration to locate the tip of the tracheal tube. After intubation, attach a large syringe to the end of the ET tube and withdraw the plunger of the syringe. If the tube is correctly placed in the trachea, the plunger will pull back without resistance as air is aspirated from the lungs. However, if the tracheal tube is in the esophagus, resistance is felt when the plunger is withdrawn because the pliable walls of the esophagus collapse under the negative pressure and occlude the end of the tube. Another device using the same principle as the syringe aspiration is the self-inflating bulb (e.g., Ellick device).

In the initial study conducted in the operating room, tube placement was correctly identified in 99 of 100 cases (51 esophageal, 48 tracheal).[44] The result was considered equivocal in the remaining case. That tube was removed and found to be nearly totally occluded with purulent secretions. Slight resistance was noted in 1 patient with a right main stem intubation; resistance decreased when the tube was pulled back. Before use, always check the esophageal detector device for air leaks. If any connections are loose, the leak may allow the syringe to be easily withdrawn, mimicking tracheal location of the tube.

When using the aspiration technique, apply constant, slow aspiration to avoid tube occlusion from tracheal mucosa drawn up under high negative pressure. If the tracheal tube is correctly placed, 30 to 40 mL of air can be aspirated without resistance. If air was initially aspirated and then some resistance is encountered, the tracheal tube should be pulled back between 0.5 and 1.0 cm and partially rotated. This takes the tube out of the bronchus, if it has been placed too deeply, and changes the orientation of the bevel if the tube has been temporarily occluded with tracheal mucosa. Air is easily aspirated if the tube was in the trachea, but repositioning will make no difference if the tube was in the esophagus. The syringe aspiration technique can be used before or after ventilation of the patient. Apply continuous cricoid pressure pending confirmation of proper tube placement. Inflation of the tube cuff has no effect on the reliability of the test.[45] This device is reliable, rapid, inexpensive, and easy to use.[45]

A squeeze-bulb aspirator is an alternative to the syringe technique. Attach the bulb to the ET tube and squeeze; if the tube is in the esophagus, it is accompanied by a flatus-like sound followed by absent or markedly delayed refilling. Insufflation of a tube in the trachea, however, is silent with instantaneous refill. An early study with the Ellick evacuator bulb device reported that 87% of esophageal intubations were identified.[46] A later study using a slightly different bulb device (Respironics, Murrysville, PA) found that all 45 esophageal intubations were detected.[47] The device is cheap, easy to use, and operable single-handedly in less than 5 seconds.[46] The bulb should not be used in freezing temperatures because of a loss of elasticity. Confusion may occur if the esophageal tube is tested more than once because subsequent inflations may be silent. On repeated assessments, a false-positive refilling of the bulb may occur owing to instillation of air during the first attempt. This observation has led to a recommendation that the bulb be compressed before it is attached to the ET tube. Delayed, though complete, refilling of the bulb may occur with bronchial tube placement or placement in the more pliable pediatric airway. The bulb suction modification of the aspiration technique has not been studied as thoroughly as the syringe technique.

A significant number of false positives occur with the esophageal detection devices (the tube is correctly placed in the trachea but the device suggests it is in the esophagus). These patients are almost uniformly obese. Fiberoptic evaluation found that the tracheal wall was invaginated into the ET tube owing to the negative pressure.[48] In such circumstances, if the intubation was felt to be successful, visually confirm that the ET tube went through the cords. Alternatively, if the patient has a perfusing rhythm and an expired CO_2 device is available, it should be applied. To date, there has been one reported case of unrecognized esophageal intubation undetected by the syringe aspiration technique.[49] In this case, there was marked gastric distension from forceful bag-mask ventilation.

The esophageal detection device is not reliable in confirming tracheal tube position after NT intubation because an easy aspiration of air will occur if the tube tip is located supraglottically (expired CO_2 will also be misleading). Reserve this device for tube confirmation after orotracheal intubation.

End-Tidal CO_2 Detector Devices. A high level of CO_2 in exhaled air is the physiologic basis for capnography and the principle on which end-tidal CO_2 (E_TCO_2) detectors were developed (see Chapter 2). The most commonly available devices for emergency use are colorimetric indicators, which correspond to CO_2 levels flowing through the device when placed on the tracheal tube adapter. The typical device displays opposite colors (e.g., yellow and purple) to indicate low levels of CO_2 in esophageal gas versus the high levels of CO_2 exhaled from the respiratory tree. Handheld quantitative or semiquantitative electronic CO_2 monitors are also available. It is only a matter of time, however, before all the prehospital defibrillators will have advanced monitoring capability that includes capnography.

A multicenter study of a colorimetric device demonstrated an overall sensitivity of 80% and a specificity of 96%.[50] In patients with spontaneous circulation and the tracheal tube cuff inflated, the sensitivity and specificity were 100%. The poor sensitivity (69%) seen in cardiac arrest was due to the fact that low exhaled CO_2 levels were seen in both very-low-flow states and esophageal intubation. The device must, therefore, be used with caution in the cardiac arrest victim. Levels of CO_2 returned to normal after return of spontaneous circulation. Further, colorimetric changes may be difficult to discern in reduced lighting situations, and secretions can interfere with the color change. Regardless of the monitoring device, patients in cardiac arrest should be ventilated for a minimum of six breaths before taking a reading. Otherwise, recent ingestion of carbonated beverages can result in spuriously high CO_2 levels with esophageal intubation.[51] Colorimetric changes do not rule out glottic positioning of the ET tube tip. Adequate ventilation and oxygenation may be achieved in the glottic position, but the risk remains for aspiration in the absence of a protected airway and the potential for further tube dislodgment. Glottic positioning may be difficult to detect clinically. The only signs may be persistent cuff leak or diminished chest rise with ventilation. Radiographic evidence or direct visualization confirms the diagnosis.[52]

Ultrasound Detection of Tracheal Tube Location. Some early data suggest that ultrasound may play a future role in identifying tube location after intubation. There are two reports and both are small. Nevertheless, the first study, in cadavers, had a sensitivity of 100% and a specificity of 97%.[53] The second, in the operating room, had both a sensitivity and a specificity of 100%.[54]

Comparison of Detector Devices. In the setting of spontaneous circulation, both syringe aspiration and $E_T CO_2$ detection are highly reliable means of excluding esophageal intubation. An animal study comparing these techniques with clinical assessment and measuring the speed and accuracy of tube placement determination demonstrated that both the syringe esophageal detector device and $E_T CO_2$ detection were highly accurate, approaching 100%.[55] The esophageal detector device was more rapid with determination in 13.8 seconds versus 31.5 seconds for $E_T CO_2$ detection. The detector device remained accurate when air was insufflated into the esophagus for 1 minute, simulating unrecognized esophageal placement. Clinical assessment alone yielded an alarming 30% rate of failure to identify esophageal intubation. In the setting of cardiac arrest, the aspiration method is more reliable than CO_2 detection because its accuracy is not dependent on the presence of blood flow.

An unequivocal method for determining tracheal tube location uses the fiberoptic scope. Passage of the scope through the tube with visualization of tracheal rings confirms ET placement as well as the position within the trachea. The placement of a lighted stylet down the tracheal tube and successful transtracheal illumination can also be used to determine ET placement.[56]

At present, there is no perfect device for the confirmation of ET tube placement in all situations. Be aware of the limitations of each device and ideally rely on input from multiple means of confirmation to ensure tracheal placement of the ET tube.

Complications of Intubation. Failure to achieve adequate ventilation and oxygenation is the most serious complication of tracheal intubation. The potential for hypoxia exists just before intubation as more conservative methods are attempted and then fail, during a difficult intubation when ventilation is halted for an intubation attempt, and after intubation when esophageal intubation goes undetected. Because irreversible cerebral anoxia occurs within minutes, conservative airway management maneuvers should be limited to 2 to 3 minutes; failure to achieve adequate oxygenation should lead to a quick decision to intubate.

As a guide, limit intubation attempts to the amount of time a single deep breath can be held. This is especially important in a child because the functional residual capacity of a child's lungs is less than that of an adult. Historically, the maximum recommended duration of an intubation attempt in an apneic patient has been 30 seconds, followed by a period of bag-valve-mask ventilation before intubation is attempted again. Longer intubation attempts are permissible, however, when guided by accurate data from an oxygen saturation monitor. Oxygen saturation may remain in the normal range for minutes, especially in patients who have been adequately preoxygenated. Assuming that preintubation oxygen saturations were acceptable at greater than 98%, intubation attempts should be interrupted for bag-mask ventilation if O_2 saturation drops below 92%.

Assessment of tube location is the top priority immediately after placement. The best assurance of tracheal placement is to see the tube pass through the vocal cords. Techniques to assess tube placement were discussed earlier. If esophageal intubation is discovered, *removing the tube may be followed by vomiting.* Apply cricoid pressure during tube

removal and maintain it until the intubation is successful. Keep a large-bore suction tip readily available should vomiting occur. Alternatively, leave the first tube in the esophagus to serve as temporary gastric-venting device and as a guide to intubation until tracheal intubation is achieved.

Although seldom associated with serious complications, unrecognized placement of the ET tube tip in the right main stem bronchus may cause hypoxia as well as unilateral pulmonary edema.[57] Obtain a chest radiograph soon after the intubation to confirm tube positioning. Endobronchial intubation was clinically unrecognized without a chest film in 7% of prehospital intubations in one study.[58] Persistent asymmetrical breath sounds after correct tube positioning suggests unilateral pulmonary pathology (e.g., main stem bronchus obstruction, pneumothorax, hemothorax).

Prolonged efforts to intubate can also cause cardiac decompensation. Pharyngeal stimulation can produce profound bradycardia or asystole, hence, the reason for *an assistant to follow the cardiac rhythm throughout the intubation.* Keep atropine available to reverse vagal-induced bradycardia that may occur secondary to suctioning or laryngoscopy. Prolonged pharyngeal stimulation also may result in laryngospasm, bronchospasm, and apnea.

Generally, dentures are removed for intubation, but kept in place for bag-mask verntilation. Check for loose or missing teeth before and after orotracheal intubation. Look for any avulsed teeth not found in the oral cavity on the postintubation chest film. Broken teeth are the most common complication of laryngoscopy.[59] Laceration of the mucosa of the lips, especially the lower lip, may also occur. Tracheal or bronchial injuries are rare but serious, usually occurring in infants and the elderly as a result of decreased tissue elasticity.[60]

Vomiting with aspiration of gastric contents is another serious complication that can occur during intubation. Case reports of both adult respiratory distress syndrome (ARDS) and chronic lung disease are thought to be due to the aspiration of activated charcoal.[60,61] For patients who are obtunded, at risk for seizures, or vomiting, consider tracheal intubation before the administration of activated charcoal.

There are ongoing concerns that direct laryngoscopy may cause or worsen cord injury in the patient with an unstable cervical spine injury. *The actual effects of laryngoscopy and oral intubation on worsening of extant cervical spinal cord injury are essentially theoretical, with no credible data to prove, or disprove, a true effect, or magnitude thereof.* Many anesthesiologists prefer awake fiberoptic intubation in this setting but there are no data to support one approach over another. A cadaveric study of intubation under fluoroscopy showed that direct laryngoscopy with inline immobilization, in the setting of complete C4–5 ligamentous instability, did not result in clinically significant instability.[62] The greatest degree of motion, however, occurs at the atlanto-occipital junction and decreases with each sequential interspace; studies of cervical spine instability at these higher levels have not been performed.[63] It can also be argued that cadaveric studies do not accurately depict the trauma setting, and yet this model is probably going to remain the best one available. Unless new information emerges regarding the risks of orotracheal intubation with direct laryngoscopy, *this appears to be a safe approach when performed in conjunction with in-line immobilization.*

Intubation can be complicated by a persistent air leak. This is generally caused by failure of either the cuff or the pilot balloons or by positioning the cuff balloon between the vocal cords. If the cuff balloon is leaking, replace the tracheal tube (see "Changing Tracheal Tubes," later in this chapter). If the pilot balloon is determined to be leaking, however, this can usually be remedied without changing the tube.[64] An incompetent one-way balloon valve can be fixed by placing a stopcock into the inflating valve. Reinflate the cuff and shut off the stopcock to solve the problem. If the leak involves the pilot balloon itself, or if the distal inflation tube has been inadvertently severed, cut off the defective part and slide a 20-gauge catheter into the inflation tube. Then connect the stopcock to the catheter, inflate the cuff, and close the stopcock.

Tracheal stricture used to be a significant late complication of long-term intubation with low-volume high-pressure cuffs. The standard use of high-volume low-pressure cuffs has markedly decreased the incidence of this complication.[65] Tubes with high-pressure cuffs are obsolete and should be avoided.

Conclusion

Direct laryngoscopy is the most common means of securing a definitive airway. With adequate preparation and an emphasis on preoxygenation and positioning, it is usually successful. RSI has rendered the patient much more amenable to direct laryngoscopy for emergency airway management (see Chapter 5). Once the patient is paralyzed, however, it becomes the clinician's supreme responsibility to ventilate, oxygenate, and protect the patient's airway. Mastery of direct laryngoscopy fulfills part of this obligation. Being prepared for failure and having a successful backup plan fulfills the second part. The remainder of this chapter is devoted to the adjuncts for and the alternatives to direct laryngoscopy if this approach is difficult, fails, or is otherwise not felt to be appropriate.

ADJUNCTS FOR DIRECT LARYNGOSCOPY

Tracheal Tube Introducers

If direct laryngoscopy does not bring the vocal cords fully into view, a tracheal tube introducer may be used to facilitate intubation. This adjunct is a long, thin, semirigid introducer that, with the aid of a laryngoscope, is passed through the laryngeal inlet and over which an ET tube is advanced through the cords and into the trachea. The technique, originally described over 50 years ago by MacIntosh,[66] was recommended in patients in whom visualizing the vocal cords was difficult. It has also been shown to be effective when the laryngeal inlet cannot be visualized at all.[67] It is the most common airway adjunct used in English EDs for complicated intubation.[68] Its efficacy has been demonstrated prospectively during difficult intubations in the operating room, as a pivotal component of a difficult airway algorithm in the operating room, and when compared with conventional laryngoscopy in the ED.[69-71] Despite its long history and demonstrated value, the tracheal tube introducer has seen limited use in the United States.

Equipment

A variety of tracheal tube introducers are available today (Fig. 4–16). The original adjunct was called the gum elastic bougie, or simply "the bougie," and is currently available, in reusable form, for both adults and pediatric patients (Eschmann Tracheal Tube Introducer, Portex Sims, Kent, UK). The adult size comes in two forms, a 60-cm (15-Fr) version with a short, 40° hockey-stick curve at the end and a straight one that is 70 cm. The adult version can accommodate a 5.5-mm ET tube. The pediatric version is 70 cm (10 Fr), straight, and can accommodate a 4.0-mm tube. A polyethylene introducer is also available, designed for single use, that comes only in the 60-cm version (Flextrach ETTube Guide, Greenfield Med., Austin, TX). A variation on this concept is the FROVA Introducer (Cook Critical Care, Bloomington, IN), a plastic introducer with a similar profile to the others except that it has a hollow lumen through which the patient can be ventilated when an accompanying adapter is attached.

Indications and Complications

Consider a tracheal tube introducer when a difficult airway is anticipated; it can also be helpful in all intubations in which, for whatever reason, visualization of the laryngeal inlet is limited. The trauma patient with cervical spine precautions is a typical example. The presence of blood and vomitus is rarely a significant complicating factor. Its safety record is impressive, with only two reported complications, a pharyngeal wall perforation after recent head and neck surgery[72] and atelectasis from blood clots after mild bronchial trauma,[73] despite decades of use.

Procedure and Technique

Place the patient in the sniffing position, or as the clinical circumstances dictate. Shaping the introducer may not be necessary in many cases, but with difficult laryngeal views, create a 60° bend in the distal introducer (see Fig. 4–16).[74] Ideally, tracheal tube introducer–assisted intubation is a two-person procedure (Fig. 4–17). Use the laryngoscope in the normal fashion to obtain the best possible laryngeal view. If

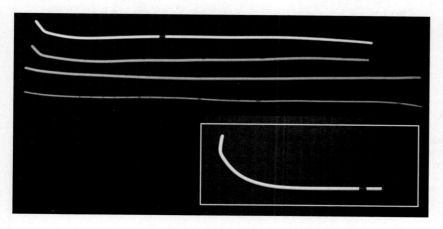

Figure 4–16 **Several types of tracheal tube introducers.** The classic introducer, the gum elastic bougie (*dark yellow*), is reusable and comes in curved- and straight-tip adult forms and a straight pediatric form. The straight bougies are 70 cm and the curved-tipped bougies are 60 cm. The blue introducer (Flextrach ETTube Guide) is polyethylene, designed for single use, and comes only in a curved-tip adult form (60 cm). The *lower right inset* demonstrates the 60° optimum curve if none of the laryngeal inlet can be seen on laryngoscopy.

the cords are in full view, proceed with the intubation using a styletted ET tube. If the view is suboptimal, ask an assistant to hand the tracheal tube introducer to you so you can place it anterior to the arytenoids and into the larynx. If only the epiglottis is visible, place the introducer, with a 60° distal bend, just under the epiglottis and direct it anteriorly. With the laryngoscope still in place and while you stabilize the introducer, ask the assistant to slide the ET tube over the introducer. Pass the tube through the larynx. Just prior to entering the larynx, rotate the tube 90° counterclockwise to avoid having the ET tube tip get caught on laryngeal structures (Fig. 4–18).[17] Withdraw the laryngoscope and confirm proper tube placement. Ask the assistant to remove the introducer.

There are a number of confirmatory findings after successful introducer placement. If any portion of the arytenoids is visible and the introducer was seen to pass anterior to them without resistance, the introducer is in the airway. Unlike

seeing an ET tube "go through the cords," when in fact the laryngeal inlet may have been momentarily obscured by the tube/balloon, the smaller-caliber introducer does not obscure the view of the glottis and thus avoids this potential pitfall. In addition to better visual confirmation, successful passage is indicated, up to 90% of the time, by feeling clicks produced by the angled tip of the introducer as it strikes against the tracheal rings.[75] An assistant will also usually feel confirmatory movement in the airway if the anterior neck is palpated. If there is still any question whether the introducer is in the airway, advance it at least 40 cm, at which point resistance should be felt as the introducer passes the carina into a main bronchus. If this is not felt, the introducer is most likely in the esophagus. Withdraw it and reattempt placement.

Several technical points should be emphasized. The first is that it is important to create a curve in the distal portion of the introducer when the laryngeal inlet is not visible. This is not uniformly appreciated even in England where the bougie is used commonly.[70] It is a mistake to think that the factory-formed curve at the tip will be sufficient to access the glottis in these situations. Although there may be some benefit to lubricating the distal aspect of the introducer, in emergency intubations, lubricating the full length of the introducer makes it slippery and hard to handle without conferring any obvious advantage. Lubricating the ET tube, conversely, remains critical for smooth passage through the vocal cords. A common error when first using the tracheal tube introducer is to remove the laryngoscope before railroading the ET tube over the introducer. This often results in difficulty placing the tube because it is displaced posteriorly by the weight of the pharyngeal soft tissue and gets hung up on the laryngeal structures. Reinsert the laryngoscope. Pull back the tube 2 cm to disengage the soft tissue. Rotate counterclockwise 90°, and then readvance. In instances in which it is difficult to get the introducer sufficiently anterior to access the laryngeal inlet, make sure that the introducer lines up with your line of vision; if the introducer enters the mouth at a significant angle above this line—most often when the clinician is too close to the patient—the introducer may be deflected posteriorly by the lip or intraoral structures without

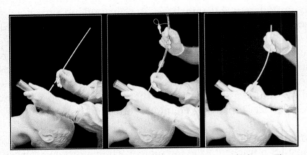

Figure 4–17 Two-person tracheal tube introducer technique. The introducer is handed to the clinician after the best glottic view has been obtained. *A,* The clinician places the introducer (the *black line,* positioned at the teeth, indicates the proper introducer depth that ensures stable positioning within the trachea while providing enough length to grasp the end of the introducer before passing the tube). *B,* An assistant passes the tracheal tube *over the introducer* as the clinician holds the introducer steady. *C,* The clinician passes the tracheal tube, with a 90° counterclockwise rotation as the tube approaches the glottis, and the assistant withdraws the introducer. (*A–C, Courtesy of Department of Emergency Medicine, Hennepin County Medical Center, Minneapolis, MN.*)

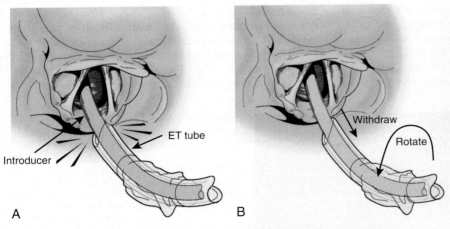
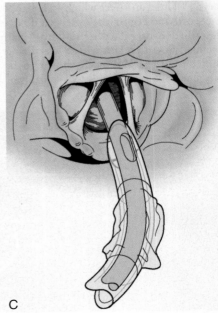

Figure 4–18 A common cause of difficulty when railroading an ET tube over a tracheal tube introducer. *A,* The ET tube tip is caught on the right arytenoid as it is being railroaded over the introducer. Corrective maneuvers: *B,* (1) The ET tube is withdrawn 2 cm to disengage the arytenoids; (2) counterclockwise rotation 90° of the ET tube to orient the bevel posteriorly. *C,* The bevel of the ET tube is facing posteriorly and allows for smooth passage through the glottis. (*A–C, Courtesy of Department of Emergency Medicine, Hennepin County Medical Center, Minneapolis, MN.*)

you being aware. This creates the impression that the introducer is "too floppy."

In the prehospital setting, where assistance might not be available, remove the laryngoscope so you can mount the ET tube onto the introducer. Once the tube is on the introducer, reinsert the laryngoscope and rotate the tube 90° counterclockwise to ensure successful passage of the tube. Mounting the tube onto the introducer and introducing them as a unit is not advised because it is often difficult to direct the introducer into the laryngeal inlet as it moves within the ET tube.

Summary

The tracheal tube introducer is a simple, inexpensive airway adjunct that is ideally suited for facilitating difficult intubation of patients in whom a portion of the laryngeal inlet can be seen. It is less effective, though still useful, in cases in which none of the inlet can be seen. Though simple in construct, there is a learning curve and attention to technical details that is important in achieving the remarkable success that can be seen with this adjunct.

LMAs in Tracheal Intubation

In the emergency setting, the LMA and the intubating laryngeal mask airway (ILMA) are excellent rescue devices for the "cannot-intubate/cannot-ventilate" situation. Both devices are valuable for rescue ventilation, but the ILMA is superior to the LMA as a conduit for intubation.[76] Thus, if there is an option between the two, the ILMA should be chosen as the rescue ventilatory device for emergency airways. The ILMA is very successful when intubating patients with known difficult airways.[77,78] In the operating room, blind intubation through the ILMA has an overall success rate of 90% and, when aided by fiberoscopy, approaches 100%.[76] It should be noted that, although it is standard practice to establish a definitive airway once ventilation and oxygenation have been achieved, both types of LMAs can be left in place in the rare instance in which intubation cannot be accomplished during the initial resuscitation.

The insertion techniques for both the LMA and the ILMA and their use as ventilatory devices have been covered in Chapter 3. This section focuses on establishing a definitive airway once these devices are in place.

Indications and Contraindications

Both the ILMA and the LMA are effective ventilatory devices in cases of difficult or impossible bag-mask ventilation. Typically, patients with a beard, severe facial injury, and morbid obesity are difficult to ventilate using a face mask. Another group of patients that can benefit from these devices are those who are difficult to intubate. In this setting, the ILMA is preferred because it is a more effective conduit for intubation. The ILMA allows blind or fiberoptic intubation with up to an 8.0-mm cuffed ET tube, whereas intubation through the classic LMA requires fiberoptic guidance and a smaller-sized ET tube.

One limitation of the ILMA is that it cannot be used in infants and small children because the smallest size, a No. 3, is not suitable for patients smaller than 30 kg. The LMA is the preferred rescue device for these patients.

LMAs are contraindicated in patients with less than 2 cm of mouth opening. They are unlikely to be successful in patients with grossly distorted supraglottic anatomy from disease processes or postradiation scarring. They are also relatively contraindicated in awake patients owing to the high risk of vomiting when gag and airway reflexes are intact.

Intubation through the ILMA

The majority of intubations through the ILMA are performed blind, using either the designated LMA ET Tube or a standard ET tube. Regardless of the tube used, it is critical that the ILMA be optimally adjusted prior to attempting blind intubation through the device.

The LMA ET Tube, also known as the LMA Fastrach, *is designed specifically for the ILMA*. There are two versions of the LMA ET Tube: a reusable and a single-use disposable. The reusable version is made of silicone and the single-use version is made of polyvinyl chloride (PVC). For purposes of blind intubation they are identical, but the cuff of the reusable LMA ET Tube is a low-volume high-pressure cuff and may not be suitable for long-term use. The cuff of the disposable version is a high-volume low-pressure cuff and is probably more suitable for long-term use. The specialized LMA ET Tubes are soft, straight, and have a midline-beveled tip. These features are designed to allow the LMA ET Tubes to emerge from the ILMA mask at an acute angle and to minimize potential injury to the vocal cords and esophagus.

Procedure and Technique

Using the LMA ET Tube. Prior to intubation through the ILMA, make sure that the patient is ventilating optimally through the device. Determine this by bagging the patient while holding the ILMA handle in the "frying-pan" position (see Chapter 3, Fig. 3–11). If there is any resistance, adjust the handle using slight rotation in the sagittal plane, until the least resistance is achieved (see step 1 of the "Chandy maneuver," Fig. 4–19A).

Prior to inserting the ET tube into the ILMA, lubricate it generously. Next, advance the tube into the ILMA airway tube with the longitudinal black line on the LMA ET Tube facing the handle of the ILMA. When the tube has advanced 15 cm, to the transverse line marked on the tube, it is an indicator that the tip is about to emerge from the ILMA mask. Just prior to advancing the tube, use the frying-pan grip and apply a slight anterior lift (not a tilt) to further align the aperture of the ILMA with the glottis (see step 2 of the "Chandy maneuver," Fig. 4–19B). Do not use a levering action. While holding the handle in this position, gently pass the tracheal tube to about 16.5 cm, or 1.5 cm beyond the transverse line. In this position, the ET tube will push the epiglottic elevating bar up and may now come in contact with the larynx or esophagus. If cricoid pressure is being applied, decrease it because it can make intubating through the ILMA more difficult. If there is no resistance, advance the tube into the trachea until the tracheal tube adapter comes in contact with the proximal end of the ILMA airway tube. Do not use force when advancing the tube.

If the ET tube does not pass into the trachea easily, withdraw the ET tube a few centimeters and readjust the ILMA position. If the tube meets resistance at about 17 cm, this may indicate a fully down-folded epiglottis or impaction of the tube tip against the anterior laryngeal wall. Rotating the tube may overcome the impaction of the tip. To correct a down-folded epiglottis, remove the ET tube and perform the "up-down maneuver," rotating the ILMA outward 5 to 6 cm without deflating the mask and then sliding it back into the hypopharynx (see Chapter 3, Fig. 3–12). If these maneu-

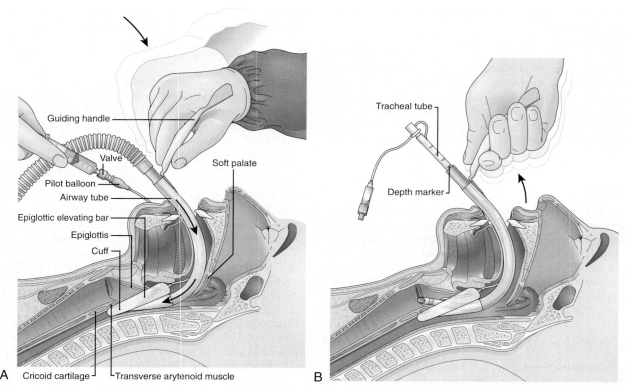

Figure 4–19 **The Chandy maneuver.** *A*, Step 1: The cuff is moved forward slightly by rotating the handle in the sagittal plane until a good seal and optimal ventilation are obtained. *B*, Step 2: Just prior to passing the tracheal tube, the handle is gently lifted anteriorly (not tilted) to better align the cuff and larynx for smooth ET tube passage.

In figure A, labels: Guiding handle, Valve, Pilot balloon, Airway tube, Epiglottic elevating bar, Epiglottis, Cuff, Soft palate, Cricoid cartilage, Transverse arytenoid muscle. In figure B, labels: Tracheal tube, Depth marker.

vers are unsuccessful, it is likely that the wrong size of ILMA is being used. Consider using a fiberoptic scope to guide intubation (also see the very detailed section, "Insertion Technique and Maneuvers Guide," on the company website: www.lmana.com).

Once the LMA ET tube has passed into the trachea, inflate the tube cuff and attempt to ventilate the patient. Check for proper tube placement using an $E_T co_2$ detector. If the tube is in the trachea, deflate the cuff of the ILMA. There is no rush to remove the ILMA; it can remain in place for an hour or longer if more pressing patient care issues need to be addressed first.

Using a Standard ET Tube. An alternative to the specialized LMA ET tube is a standard PVC ET tube. This is not recommended by the manufacturer, but it is a common practice and there are several reports in the literature supporting this practice.[79–82] The manufacturer warns that using a standard ET tube may be associated with a greater likelihood of laryngeal trauma; however, there are no reports of such trauma in the literature. In fact, the only reported death, caused by esophageal perforation during blind intubation through the ILMA, occurred with use of the designated LMA ET tube.[83] A laboratory study showed that a standard PVC ET tube exerts 7 to 10 times more pressure on distal structures than the silicone LMA ET tube.[84,85] However, the clinical relevance of this finding is unproved. Some experts suggest warming a standard PVC ET tube prior to insertion through the ILMA.[79,80,82]

Owing to the potential for injury when using a standard ET tube, use fiberoptic guidance with standard ET tubes if there is any difficulty with blind placement. If using a standard ET tube, insert the ET tube with its curvature opposite that

of the ILMA tube curvature (Fig. 4–20*B*). This allows the ET tube to exit the ILMA at a less acute angle and advance into the trachea more easily (see Fig. 4–20*C*).[82,86]

If intubation through the ILMA fails despite the recommended adjustment maneuvers and fiberoptic assistance, use a more invasive method such as a retrograde wire or a surgical airway in a controlled fashion while the patient is ventilated with the ILMA (see Fig. 4–39 for retrograde technique).[87]

Fiberoptic Intubation through the ILMA. A fiberoptic bronchoscope (FOB) can be used to verify the position of the larynx either before or during intubation. When intubating through the ILMA over an FOB, a standard ET tube is sufficient and there is no reason to use the specialized LMA ET tube. Before passing the FOB through the ILMA, advance the ET tube through the ILMA to 15 cm. At 15 cm depth, the view through the FOB should show the glottis beyond the epiglottic elevating bar. Advance the ET tube 1.5 cm before advancing the FOB. This protects the fiberoptic elements from being damaged by the epiglottic elevating bar. The view at 16.5 cm should show the vocal cords and trachea. Advance the FOB into the trachea and then railroad the ET tube over the FOB. If the vocal cords are not immediately visualized, see the LMA Fastrach Insertion Technique & Maneuvers Guide, described previously.

ILMA Removal. To remove the ILMA, deflate the cuff (Fig. 4–21*A*). Be careful not to deflate the ET tube cuff. Start by removing the ET tube adapter. Then hold the proximal end of the ET tube in place while rotating the ILMA out of the hypopharynx. As the ILMA passes over the ET tube and out of the mouth, hold the ET tube in place using the stabilizer rod provided with the ILMA (see Fig. 4–21*C*). When the ET tube pilot balloon comes in contact with the stabilizer rod,

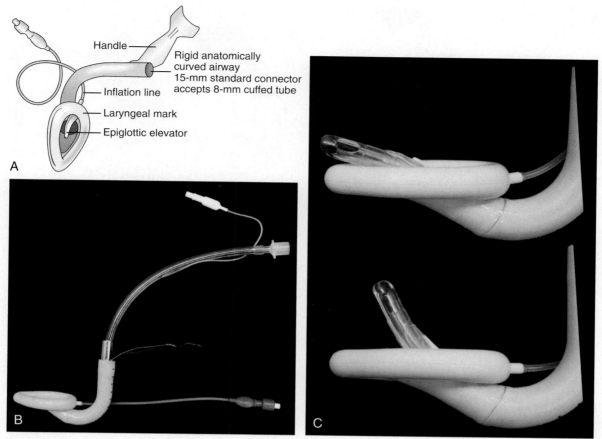

Figure 4–20 *A*, Intubating through an intubating laryngeal mask airway (ILMA) using a standard tracheal tube. *B*, The tracheal tube is inserted so the curve of the tube is opposite the curve of the ILMA. This allows the tube tip to exit the ILMA at an angle more conducive to smooth passage into the trachea. *C*, The Angle of the tracheal tube tip after normal orientation of the ET tube (*lower*) versus the correct, "reverse curve," orientation (*upper*). *(A, Courtesy of LMA North America, Inc., San Diego, CA.)*

remove the stabilizer rod to allow the pilot balloon to travel through the ILMA airway tube. Then reattach the ET adapter and resume ventilation. Adjust the ET tube depth as needed.

Intubation through the LMA. The recommended technique for tracheal intubation through the LMA employs an FOB and has a high success rate but requires a smaller ET tube and some adjustment maneuvers.[88,89] Blind intubation through a nonintubating LMA (LMA Classic or LMA Unique) has a poor success rate and is not recommended.[90–92] Using a tracheal tube introducer as a guide through the LMA is also unlikely to be successful and is not recommended.[93,94]

Fiberoptic Intubation through the LMA. Use fiberoptic guidance when intubating through an LMA (Table 4–5). After ensuring that the patient is bagging easily with the LMA, place a well-lubricated ET tube into the LMA tube and advance it about 24 cm (No. 5 LMA) so that the ET tube tip has just passed the fenestrations. Pass a lubricated FOB through the ET tube and advance it through the vocal cords. If the epiglottis is deflected downward, manipulate the tip of the FOB under the epiglottis until the vocal cords come into view. Railroad the ET tube over the FOB and into the trachea. Inflate the ET tube cuff and ventilate the patient. Check for correct ET tube placement using E_Tco_2.

Alternatively, place a hollow introducer, such as an Aintree Intubation Catheter (Cook Critical Care, Bloomington, IN; www.cookmedical.com), in conjunction with an

TABLE 4–5 Fiberoptic Bronchoscope and Endotracheal Tube Sizes (mm) for Intubation through the LMA

LMA Airway Size	LMA Classic LMA Unique	
	ET Tube (mm)	FOB (mm)
1	3.5	2.7
1½	4.0	3.0
2	4.5	3.5
2½	5.0	4.0
3	6.0 Cuffed	5.0
4	6.0 Cuffed	5.0
5	7.0 Cuffed	5.5
6	7.0 Cuffed	5.5*

*Applies to LMA Classic only, size 6 not available in LMA Unique.
ET, endotracheal; FOB, fiberoptic bronchoscope; LMA, laryngeal mask airway.
Adapted from information available on the LMA North America, Inc., website, www.lmana.com

FOB, through the LMA and into the trachea (Fig. 4–22). Remove the LMA, leaving the exchange catheter as an introducer for the ET tube, much like a conventional tracheal tube introducer.

Cricoid pressure may impede placement and intubation through the LMA.[95,96] Release cricoid pressure if necessary to accomplish these procedures.

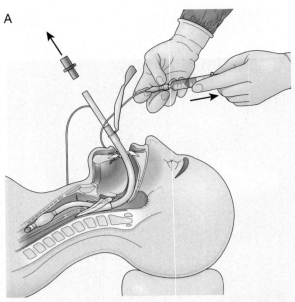

A

After achieving intubation, the intubating LMA may be left in place or removed. If left in place it should be deflated.

Removal of intubating LMA
1. Ensure patient is well oxygenated.
2. Remove TT connector.
3. Deflate mask cuff (keep TT cuff inflated).

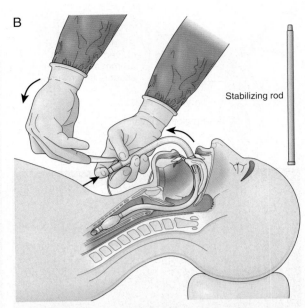

B

Stabilizing rod

Swing mask out of pharynx into oral cavity applying counter-pressure to TT with finger as shown, prior to insertion of stabilizing rod. The intubating LMA can be eased out by tapping or swinging the handle around the chin as shown. The rod can be conveniently used to measure how far the TT protrudes from the mouth before device removal to ensure it is correctly repositioned afterwards.

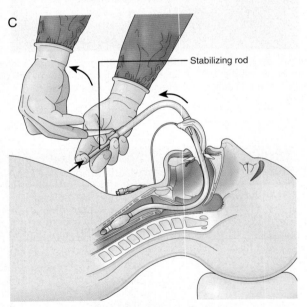

C

Stabilizing rod

Use the stabilizing rod to keep the TT in place while sliding the intubating LMA out over it until it is clear of the mouth.

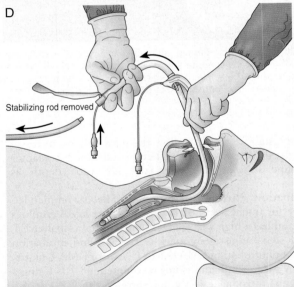

D

Stabilizing rod removed

Remove the stabilizing rod when the mask is clear of the mouth. Steady the TT to prevent accidental dislodgement.

Figure 4–21   Removal of the ILMA after successful intubation through it. *A,* The ILMA cuff is deflated and the ET tube adapter removed. *B,* The ET tube is held in place with a finger as the ILMA is rotated out of the hypopharynx. The stabilizing rod is seen on the right. *C,* Using the stabilizing rod, the ET tube is held in place as the ILMA is removed from the mouth. *D,* Remove the stabilizing rod when it comes in contact with the ET tube pilot balloon. Grasping the ET tube, complete the removal of the ILMA.

Complications when Intubating through LMAs

Although most patients can be safely intubated blindly through the ILMA, there is a small chance of injury to the larynx or esophagus, especially with multiple blind attempts. There is one case report of a death due to esophageal perforation during blind intubation through the ILMA. Consider using fiberoptic guidance if blind intubation is difficult or if the clinician is inexperienced. Intubation through a nonintubat-ing LMA is not recommended unless facilitated by an FOB.

Summary

LMAs provide an excellent means of oxygenating and ventilating when face mask ventilation is difficult or impossi-ble. In addition, the ILMA is particularly useful when manag-ing patients who are difficult to intubate with direct

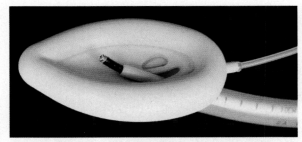

Figure 4–22 LMA as a conduit for intubation. A hollow introducer (Aintree Intubation Catheter, 60 cm) is placed though a laryngeal mask airway (LMA), and into the trachea, with the help of a fiberoptic scope. The LMA is then withdrawn, leaving the introducer in place. The tracheal tube is then railroaded over the introducer into the trachea.

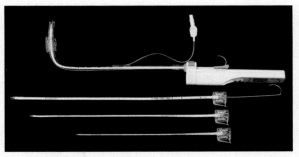

Figure 4–23 Trachlight and related stylets. The malleable stylet is bent at a 90° angle, 6.5 to 8.5 cm from the tip (marked on stylet). The smallest stylet accommodates a 2.5 internal diameter (ID) tube.

laryngoscopy. Thus, by facilitating the management of difficult/failed ventilation and difficult/failed intubation, the ILMA is an indispensable component of the difficult airway algorithm.

Esophageal-Tracheal Combitube: Replacement with an ET Tube

Combitubes placed in the esophagus generally require replacement with a tracheal tube. To do so, first deflate the proximal balloon. Ideally, empty the stomach first via a gastric tube placed through the esophageal port of the airway. Prepare suction, deflate the distal balloon, and attempt intubation. If intubation is difficult, you may need to remove the esophageal-tracheal Combitube (ETC). At this point, depending on the patient's oxygen saturation, either attempt intubation again with direct laryngoscopy or place an ILMA and ventilate the patient until definitive intubation can be performed.

Lighted Stylet Intubation

This technique uses a battery-operated lighted stylet that is placed in an ET tube and used to guide the tube into the trachea by transilluminating the soft tissues of the neck. First described in 1957 by MacIntosh and Richards,[97] it was designed for the difficult airway. It can also be useful in determining the position of the tracheal tube.[56] Early models suffered from insufficient illumination to function well in ambient light and had equipment failures that rendered them commercial failures. The Trachlight (Laerdal Medical Corp., Wappengers Falls, NY), introduced in 1995, had a brighter light source, enclosed bulb, and adjustable length and successfully addressed these problems. It is the only lighted stylet, among several available today, that has a proven track record. The Trachlight compared favorably with direct laryngoscopy in a randomized study of 950 surgical patients with a 99% overall success rate and 92% on the first attempt; reduced lighting was necessary 21% of the time.[98] In another large series, also by Hung and associates,[99] the device was 99% successful in intubating patients with difficult airways. The Trachlight is composed of a handle and a malleable optical stylet, which, in turn, is composed of an inner stiff wire stylet and an outer flexible optical element. The stylets come in adult, pediatric, and infant sizes and can accommodate down to a 2.5-mm ID tube (Fig. 4–23).

Indications and Contraindications

An excellent candidate for light-guided tracheal intubation is a patient with a difficult airway, complicated by blood and secretions, in whom direct laryngoscopy has failed. A multiple trauma patient with airway bleeding is also a good example. The patient who has been pharmacologically paralyzed and cannot be intubated with direct laryngoscopy is another example. It can also be used for routine intubations, depending on the experience and skill set of the clinician. The lighted stylet may also be helpful in successfully completing a difficult NT intubation. One advantage of this technique over NT intubation is that it can be used in an apneic patient.

Because lighted stylet intubation is a blind approach, avoid using it in patients with expanding neck masses and patients with airway compromise presumably due to a foreign body. Massive obesity is the most common cause for failure of this device because of difficulty in transilluminating the anterior neck.

Procedure and Technique

Place the patient's head and neck in the neutral or slightly extended position. If the patient is awake, spray the oropharynx and hypopharynx with lidocaine and administer sedation as indicated. Check the function of the bulb on the lighted stylet before use. Ideally, lubricate the inner wire stylet, optical stylet, and ET tube with a water-soluble agent to prepare the device for use. In practice, however, if the device is used primarily as a rescue device, it will be preassembled and only the ET tube will be lubricated. Check to make sure that the wire insert is snapped into the adjustable car on the handle, otherwise, the wire will turn freely from side to side and the tip of the tube will not be controllable as it is maneuvered within the hypopharynx.

With the Trachlight unit assembled, bend the distal tip into the shape of a hockey stick with a 90° curve beginning just proximal to the tube cuff; the obese patient with a short neck may require a bend of up to 110°. Mark the bend distance on the stylet as a 2-cm line, corresponding to 6.5 to 8.5 cm from the end of the ET tube. Use a shorter bend point in patients with short thyromental distances.[100] Stand at the patient's head. If that is not possible, then approach the patient from either side. Grasp the patient's jaw near the corner of the mouth, between the thumb, the index, and the middle fingers, and lift to elevate the tongue and epiglottis (Fig. 4–24). Turn the light on and insert the unit into the mouth in the midline, following the curve of the tongue into the oropharynx. With a rocking motion, gently advance the tip. A transilluminating glow indicates the location of the tube tip. Applying cricoid pressure may enhance the transillumina-

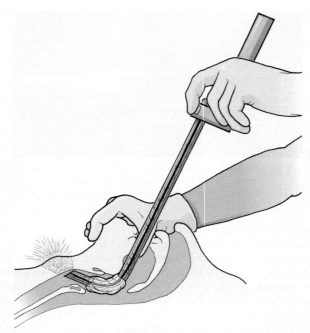

Figure 4–24 Lighted stylet intubation. Use of the Trachlight for endotracheal intubation with transillumination of the soft tissues as a guide to placement. *(Courtesy of Department of Emergency Medicine, Hennepin County Medical Center, Minneapolis, MN.)*

tion.[56] Dim the overhead lights to see the glow better in an obese patient. Positioning is optimal when a light bulb–like glow emanates from the midline just below the level of the thyroid prominence. If a more diffuse glow is seen just above this prominence, the tip may be in the vallecula. A more lateral position suggests placement in the piriform fossae. In this case, withdraw the unit 2 cm or cock it back and reposition it as indicated by the light. If you do not see a light, the tube is in the esophagus and should be pulled back. Apply external laryngeal pressure and, if necessary, extend the head slightly. In a very thin patient, it is possible to observe transillumination and still be in the esophagus. The clue is that the glow will be diffuse if the tip is in the esophagus, as opposed to the well-circumscribed glow of intralaryngeal placement. Once the tube is in the larynx, withdraw the stiff wire stylet 10 cm and advance the tube to the level of the sternal notch. Release the tube from the Trachlight, withdraw the lighted stylet, and confirm the tube's position.

Complications

Earlier reports noted complications with lighted stylets that resulted from equipment failures and lost bulbs. These technical problems have ceased since the advent of the Trachlight. No complications attributable to the Trachlight have been reported. The clear instructions to avoid using the device in patients with upper airway distortion from tumor, infection, and hematoma may be responsible for this clean record. A study of pathologic specimens showed no evidence of burn injury in the tracheal mucosa in cats intubated with the Trachlight.[101]

Summary

Lighted stylet intubation is a safe, rapid, and highly successful method that has a definite place in the management of the difficult airway. Because it is placed with the patient in a

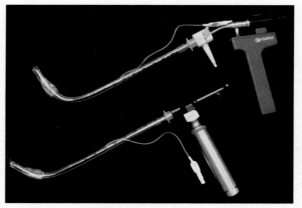

Figure 4–25 Examples of semirigid fiberoptic stylets: the Shikani *(top)* and Levitan *(bottom)*. The recommended bends when used alone *(top)* and when used with a direct laryngoscope *(bottom)* are demonstrated. The sliding adapter on the Shikani allows for various lengths of tracheal tubes.

neutral position and blood and secretions are not an impediment to success, it is especially amenable to the trauma setting. The patient who is most likely to fail lighted stylet intubation is one who is morbidly obese with a short neck. Although not overly challenging technically, practice under controlled intubating conditions is advised. Improvements in the device have made its use more practical in most settings in which emergency airway management is performed.

Semirigid Fiberoptic Stylets

A class of devices that incorporates fiberoptics into a semirigid metal or metal reinforced stylet was introduced in the late 1990s. These can be used in conjunction with direct laryngoscopy or as stand-alone intubating devices; they have been shown to require direct laryngoscopic assistance in 8% to 20% of cases and in general are more successful when used in this way.[102,103] In either case, the tip of the fiberoptic stylet, with its overlying ET tube, is passed under the epiglottis and directed through the glottis into the trachea. Visibility can be hampered by blood and secretions but less so than with flexible fiberoscopy.[104] These devices are also easier to learn how to use. The Shikani Optical Stylet and Levitan FPS Scope (Clarus Medical, Minneapolis, MN) are examples of these malleable optical stylets (Fig. 4–25). The Shikani Stylet is most often used similarly to the Trachlight, with the added feature of being able to see fiberoptically what is just beyond the tube tip. The Levitan Scope, conversely, is designed to be used with a laryngoscope, serving as a stylet for the tracheal tube while providing fiberoptic visualization if required. The Bonfils Retromolar Intubation Fiberscope (Storz Endoscopy, Culver City, CA) is rigid but otherwise structurally and functionally similar to the Shikani. The distal end of the Bonfils has a fixed curve of 40°, whereas the other scopes are malleable up to 120°. The power for the Shikani and Bonfils stylets may be supplied either by an external source or from batteries. Video cameras can be attached to the eyepiece of all of these devices but have the drawback of making them less maneuverable. The Bonfils is available with an integrated video module. The Levitan stylet is shorter than the other devices, and although conforming more to the normal length of a stylet, it currently requires that the tube be cut at 27.5 to 28 cm before mounting it on the stylet. It can accommodate down to a 5.5-mm ID tube. The Shikani stylet comes in two sizes, the adult, accommodating a 5.5-mm ID tube, and a pediatric version that goes down to a 3.5-mm ID tube. An adjustable plastic ET tube stop is located proximally on the stylet and secures the tube at the desired length as well as provides a means for directing oxygen down the tube.

The Video-Optical Intubation Stylet or VOIS (Acutonic Medical Systems AG, Baar, Switzerland) is a semirigid fiberscope that is used like a malleable stylet and attaches to the ET tube via a sliding adapter located on the more distal aspect of a 2-m length of fiberoptic cable. An external light source is required. The image is transmitted to a monitor but can also be viewed through an eyepiece. Direct laryngoscopy is used routinely with the VOIS stylet. Mannequin studies of the VOIS versus the Bullard scope and the Shikani scope versus the gum elastic boogie demonstrated greater success in Cormack and Lehane grade 3 views (see Fig. 4–4C) with the semirigid fiberoptic stylets.[105,106]

Indications and Contraindications

The semirigid fiberoptic stylets are useful when the glottis cannot be readily seen. Blood and secretions may complicate their use but less so than with flexible fiberoscopy. The Bonfils stylet, with its fixed 45° curve, is not recommended in patients with severely limited neck extension or limited mouth opening.[107]

Procedure and Technique

The semirigid fiberoptic stylet can be used with or without direct laryngoscopy. In either case, place the patient in the sniffing position. Load an ET tube onto a lightly lubricated stylet so that the ET tube extends 1 to 2 cm beyond the end of the stylet.

If the device is used alone, create an accentuated curve of between 70° and 80° at the proximal aspect of the cuff of the tube so that it can negotiate the oropharynx. Deliver high-flow oxygen down the ET tube to decrease the chance of getting blood and secretions on the optical element. Suction before intubation attempts. Grasp the mandible with the left hand and lift the jaw in order to lift the tongue and epiglottis off the posterior hypopharyngeal wall. Ask an assistant to apply a jaw-thrust or grasp the tongue with gauze and retract it anteriorly. Place the device into the mouth and, following the curve of the tongue, bring it up under the epiglottis using fiberoptic guidance. You may need to use a rocking action, similar to that used with the lighted stylet, to identify landmarks. Upon seeing the laryngeal inlet, direct the tip into the larynx. Advance the ET tube as you withdraw the stylet. If you meet resistance advancing the tube, the tip may be catching on the anterior larynx or trachea. Rotating the tube clockwise 120° at the proximal end will result in a 90° rotation at the tip and, with the bevel now anterior, allow the tube to advance without catching. It is important to remember that the direction of ET tube rotation is *clockwise* if resistance is encountered *after* going through the cords (for resistance encountered *before* the cords, which occurs with tracheal tube introducers and fiberoptic and NT intubation, rotation is *counterclockwise*).

Semirigid optical stylets can be used with direct laryngoscopy, either primarily or after encountering difficulty using the device alone. With this approach, make the angle of the distal stylet less acute, at about 35°, and introduce the device only after obtaining maximal visualization with the laryngoscope. If the epiglottis can be seen, advance the stylet tip just under it, using direct vision and being careful not to embed the ET tube tip in the supraglottic soft tissue and obscure visibility. At this point, fiberoptically guide the stylet–ET tube unit into the glottis and advance the tube off the stylet.

There have been no reported complications with semirigid fiberoptic stylets other than the failures or prolonged attempts usually related to poor visibility from blood and secretions.[102]

Summary

Semirigid fiberoptic stylets combine the features of direct and indirect laryngoscopy and provide a valuable tool when one is faced with a difficult airway. They can be used alone or in conjunction with a laryngoscope. They are considerably less expensive than rigid fiberoptic devices and easier to use than flexible scopes. To date, much of the supporting literature is case reports or relatively small series, and there are no head-to-head clinical trials with other devices. However, experience suggests that the semirigid fiberoptic stylets will play an increasing role in managing difficult intubations.

Intubation over a Flexible FOB

Flexible fiberoptic intubation is the most common technique used by anesthesiologists for known difficult airways. Physicians who perform fiberoptic intubations daily have a success rate of nearly 100% when using this technique for difficult intubations.[108] In the ED, with more difficult intubating conditions and less experienced fiberoscopists, the success rate is 50% to 90%.[109–112] The most common reason for failure of flexible fiberoptic intubation cited in the operating room is clinician inexperience.[113] In the ED, failure is most often attributed to poor visibility from blood, vomitus, and other secretions.[109–111] Mlinik and colleagues[111] found that successful ED fiberoptic intubations averaged 2 minutes whereas failures averaged 8 minutes; they recommend considering alternative approaches if intubation attempts take over 3 minutes. ED clinicians have the opportunity to develop fiberoptic laryngoscopic skills when performing diagnostic nasopharyngoscopy on ambulatory patients.

Flexible fiberoptic endoscopy is often the best method for intubating the awake patient with a known difficult airway. It can be accomplished using the nasal or oral route and is better tolerated than direct laryngoscopy. It usually provides excellent visualization of the airway and permits the evaluation of the airway before tube placement. The expense of the equipment, its fragility, and the length of time required to achieve technical proficiency are drawbacks.

FOBs are graded according to their external diameter (in millimeters). FOBs specifically designed for ET intubations are available from several companies (Pentax, Olympus, Machida, and Fujinon). A practical size for an intubating scope is about 4 mm. Although it is physically possible to pass a 4.5-mm (0.5 mm larger) tracheal tube over the scope, the fit is tight. As a rule, the tracheal tube should be about 1 mm larger than the intubating scope. The size of the working channel, the port to which suction or oxygen is applied and through which fluid or catheters may be passed, is another important dimension when evaluating FOBs. A working channel of about 2 mm is desirable to allow for adequate suction of secretions. Very thin nasolaryngoscopes, with diameters of 3.0 to 3.5 mm, have no working channel but can be used for pediatric tracheal intubation.

Indications and Contraindications

Patients with known or suspected difficult airways are good candidates for awake or semiawake fiberoptic intubation. Patients with distorted airway anatomy ranging from swelling of the mouth or tongue, upper airway abscess or infection, morbid obesity, or penetrating and blunt neck trauma are all good candidates for awake fiberoptic intubation. Patients with laryngeal tumors, especially those with a history of radiation therapy to the cervical region, may be impossible to intubate by any other nonsurgical method. The FOB can also be helpful when assessing and intubating the patient with airway obstruction from presumed foreign body aspiration. Flexible fiberoptic intubation is best used as the initial approach to tracheal intubation, but it may be used as a rescue device when other methods fail.[114] Flexible fiberoptic intubation can also be performed through an ILMA or LMA after difficult ventilation or failed intubation.

Contraindications to the nasal approach are severe midface trauma and coagulopathy. Patients likely to receive thrombolytics should also be excluded. Although there are no clear contraindications to fiberoptic orotracheal intubation, active airway bleeding and vomiting are relative contraindications because successful fiberoptic intubation is rarely achieved in these settings. If the clinician is inexperienced in fiberoptic intubation, significant hypoxia is another relative contraindication.

Procedure and Technique

Preparation of the upper airway is important for successful awake or semiawake fiberoptic intubation. Deliver local anesthetic to the upper airway by one of several methods. Nebulized lidocaine (4–6 mL of 4%) can be used to anesthetize the entire upper airway if time permits. Lidocaine (3 mL of 4%) can also be injected percutaneously through the cricothyroid membrane using a 20-gauge needle, providing anesthesia to the larynx and trachea. Some laryngeal and tracheal anesthesia can also be achieved by a transoral spray using a laryngeal tracheal anesthetic (LTA) set. Finally, lidocaine (4%) can be sprayed through the working channel of the fiberoptic scope during the procedure using the "spray as you go" technique. The maximum dose of lidocaine for airway anesthesia is 3 to 4 mg/kg (about 200 mg in an adult). Sedation for fiberoptic intubation can be accomplished with ketamine, etomidate, propofol, fentanyl, alfentenil, or midazolam (see Chapter 5). The goal of sedation is to preserve spontaneous respirations but limit patient movement and reaction to the procedure. A combination of good topical anesthesia and mild sedation allows the best chance for a successful intubation.

The optimal positioning of the neck is in extension, as opposed to the slight cervical flexion desired when using direct laryngoscopy. Extension allows for better visualization of the glottis by elevating the epiglottis off the posterior pharyngeal wall. This is especially pertinent in the comatose patient who lacks the muscle tone necessary to maintain an open airway. If problems arise with the tongue and soft tissues falling back and obscuring FOB view, apply a jaw-lift or grasp the tongue and pull it forward and away from the soft palate and posterior pharyngeal wall. This maneuver also moves the epiglottis away from the posterior pharyngeal wall, facilitating exposure of the cords. Extending the head may accomplish the same objective.

Fiberoptic intubation may be performed with the patient in the upright, semiupright, or supine positions. Stand facing the patient or at the patient's head, depending on personal preference. The upright and semiupright positions help keep pharyngeal soft tissue from obstructing the airway. Also, the upright position may be more familiar for emergency clinicians who are skilled at diagnostic nasopharyngoscopy.

The greatest impediment to successful fiberoptic intubation is the inability to visualize the larynx because blood or secretions have covered the optical element and cannot be removed. Suction actively just before FOB introduction. Once the scope is in place, suction minor secretions through the fiberoptic suction port. Significant blood and secretions, however, are best removed by high-flow oxygen through the suction port and out the tip of the scope, serving simultaneously to remove blood and secretions, defog the tip, and increase the inspired O_2 content. The setup required for oxygen insufflation should be immediately available, if not already attached to the suction port before the scope is inserted. Once the scope has entered the trachea, you may encounter difficulty advancing the ET tube. The tip of the tube most commonly catches on the right arytenoid cartilage or vocal cord. Withdraw the tube 2 cm, rotate it counterclockwise 90°, and readvance the tube to remedy the problem (see Fig. 4–18).

Nasal Approach. The nasal approach is technically easier than the oral approach because the angle of insertion allows for better visualization of the larynx with minimal manipulation of the FOB and because patient cooperation is less critical. In the unconscious patient, the tip of the scope is also less likely to impinge on the base of the tongue with a nasal approach.

First, if conditions permit, choose the most patent nostril. In the cooperative patient, determine this by simply occluding each nostril and asking the patient to identify the nostril that is easiest to breathe through. Identify the most patent nostril by direct vision or by gently inserting a gloved finger lubricated with viscous lidocaine into the nostrils. If time is not an issue, an effective method to dilate the nasal cavity and administer an anesthetic is to pass a lidocaine gel–lubricated nasopharyngeal airway (nasal trumpet) into the selected nostril. Leave this airway in place for several minutes, and introduce progressively larger trumpets.

To prepare the nose and upper airway, administer vasoconstrictors, topical anesthetics, and lubricants. Vasoconstrictors such as 0.25% or 1.0% phenylephrine drops, oxymetazoline (Afrin) spray or 4% cocaine spray limit epistaxis and ample 2% lidocaine gel in the nasal cavity help the tube negotiate the nasopharynx without complication. Hypopharyngeal anesthesia, as described previously, minimizes gagging and laryngospasm. The well-lubricated ET tube may be placed in the nostril first and the scope passed through it or the ET tube can be mounted over the scope and the scope first passed through the nostril (Fig. 4–26). The advantage of the former is that it avoids the possibility of secretions covering the scope and positions the scope near the laryngeal inlet. Disadvantages are that NT placement may cause bleeding, and in some patients, the tube may not pass easily into the nasopharynx. In some patients, the mouth is not accessible at all owing to swelling or trauma (e.g., ACE inhibitor angioedema) so the nasal route is the only option for fiberoptic intubation (Fig. 4–27A and B).

Prepare the most patent nostril and advance the ET tube until it makes the bend into the nasopharynx in the manner described under "NT Intubation." If negotiating this bend is difficult, place a well-lubricated FOB through the tube and into the oropharynx to serve as a guide for the ET tube. Once

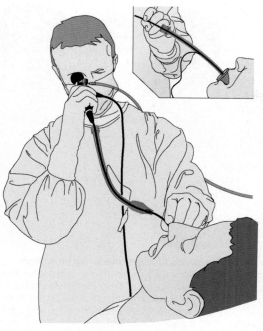

Figure 4–26   Fiberoptic intubation. The fiberoptic scope serves as a guide over which the tracheal tube is passed. *Larger image,* The nasal approach. *Inset,* Use of an oral intubating airway with the oral approach. *(Courtesy of Department of Emergency Medicine, Hennepin County Medical Center, Minneapolis, MN.)*

the tracheal tube is in the oropharynx, perform thorough oropharyngeal suctioning before introducing the scope into the ET tube. Advance the FOB toward the larynx; the epiglottis and vocal cords are seen with little or no manipulation of the tip of the FOB in 90% of patients.[91] Advance the scope and keep the cords in view by frequent minor adjustments of the scope tip.

In the comatose or obtunded patient, the tongue and other soft tissues may obscure the view of the larynx. This can be alleviated by asking an assistant to pull the tongue forward or apply a chin- or jaw-lift. Advance the scope through the larynx to the carina and pass the ET tube over the firmly held FOB into the trachea. Remember that in adults, the average distance from the naris to the epiglottis is 16 to 17 cm; if the scope has been advanced much beyond this distance and the glottis is still not seen, the scope is probably in the esophagus.[115] If the scope meets resistance at about this same level and only a pink blur is visible, the scope tip is probably in a piriform sinus; transillumination of the soft tissues may be present to confirm this as well as to indicate what corrective maneuvers are necessary.

Oral Approach. Oral fiberoptic intubation is indicated when contraindications to nasal intubation are present, the most common being severe midface trauma, or when the clinician is more comfortable with an oral approach. Skilled fiberoscopists often find the oral approach just as easy as the nasal approach. However, for the less experienced, the oral approach may be more difficult because the path of the scope is less defined by the surrounding soft tissue and the tip of the scope is more likely to impinge on the base of the tongue or vallecula. Keeping the scope in the midline and elevating the soft tissue by pulling the tongue forward or applying the jaw-

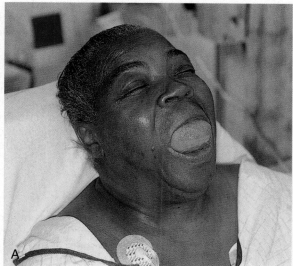

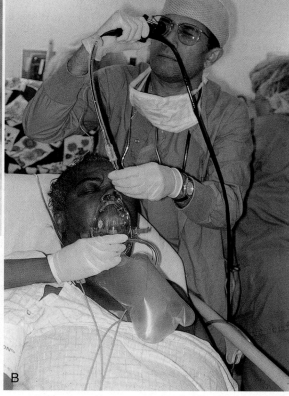

Figure 4–27   *A,* This patient with life-threatening *angiotensin-converting enzyme (ACE) inhibitor–induced angioedema* is in severe distress, and oral intubation is impossible. *B,* Fiberoptic nasotracheal (NT) intubation is a good choice, but it is very difficult, if not impossible, in a struggling patient. Ketamine anesthesia allowed for patient cooperation and supplemental oxygen.

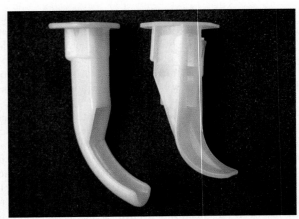

Figure 4–28 Examples of oral intubating airways. The Williams Airway Intubator (*left*) cradles the ET tube in an open, curved guide while the Ovassapian Fiberoptic Intubating Airway (*right*) positions the ET tube on the posterior surface of the intubation airway.

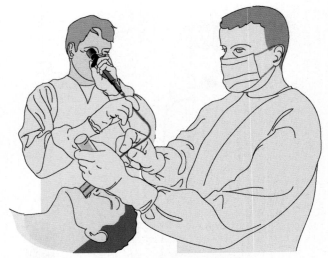

Figure 4–29 Two-person fiberoptic intubation for difficult intubation. The laryngoscopist obtains the best hypopharyngeal exposure and directs the fiberoptic tip in the direction of the glottis. The second clinician, manipulating the tip of the fiberoptic scope, directs the laryngoscopist to slowly advance the tip until it is successfully passed through the cords.

lift will minimize this difficulty. Because the oropharyngeal axis is not as well aligned with the larynx as is the nasopharyngeal axis, more scope manipulation is required when using the oral approach.

The difficulties of the oral approach can be minimized by using an oral intubating airway (Fig. 4–28). This adjunct resembles an oropharyngeal airway but is longer and has a cylindrical passage through which the FOB and tracheal tube are passed. The tip of this airway lies just cephalad to the epiglottis and ensures midline positioning and a predictable place from which to advance the scope. Make sure that the patient is either adequately anesthetized or obtunded before the oral airway is placed to minimize gagging or vomiting. Place a well-lubricated FOB, premounted with an ET tube, through the oral intubating airway and fiberoptically intubate the trachea (see Fig. 4–26, *upper right inset*). Advance the ET tube over the scope into the trachea. Occasionally. this will require the same counterclockwise maneuver as described with the nasal approach. After successful intubation, the intubating device can be left in place as a bite block or may be removed over the ET tube after removal of the tube adapter. Some oral intubating airways can be removed from the mouth without disconnecting the ET tube adapter.

An alternative approach to oral fiberoptic intubation for an anticipated difficult airway requires two clinicians. One performs direct laryngoscopy and places the tip of the fiberscope under the epiglottis and blindly advances it while the second clinician, holding the body of the scope, directs the tip fiberoptically through the cords (Fig. 4–29).

Complications

Complications of fiberoptic orotracheal intubation include hypoxia from prolonged intubation attempts, vomiting, and laryngospasm. Oxygen saturation monitoring should alert the clinician to hypoxia. Most complications seen with fiberoptically guided NT intubation are associated with passing the ET tube through the nasopharynx. Epistaxis is the most common, followed by other nasopharyngeal injuries. A rare but potentially significant complication may result if, on blind advancement of the fiberoptic scope through the ET tube, the tip of the scope exits through the Murphy eye (distal side port of the ET tube).[116] Attempts at passing the ET tube through

the larynx will fail because the tube tip, now extending off the midline, will catch on the laryngeal structures. This complication is avoided if the scope is introduced before ET tube placement.

Summary

The primary advantages of fiberoptic intubation are the ability to visualize upper airway abnormalities, to negotiate difficult airway anatomy, and to carefully perform tracheal intubation under visual guidance. Fiberoptic intubation is noninvasive and well tolerated. Its major limitation for the emergency airway is poor visibility from blood and secretions; in this setting, it is best to avoid the FOB. Procedural time can be another limitation. The FOB requires more practice than many other methods of airway management and considerable experience should be obtained before using the FOB in an airway emergency. Fiberoptic intubation is more likely to be successful if used early in the management of a difficult airway rather than as a last resort after repeated failure with direct laryngoscopy.

Rigid Fiberoptic Laryngoscopy

In the late 1980s, several rigid fiberoptic laryngoscopes were introduced that approximate the anatomy of the upper airway and provide indirect fiberoptic visualization of the laryngeal inlet. Examples include the Bullard laryngoscope (Circon Corporation, Stamford, CT), the UpsherScope (Mercury Medical, Clearwater, FL), and the WuScope (Achi Corporation, San Jose, CA). These devices offer the advantage provided by a conventional fiberoptic scope but require less training to gain proficiency in their use because alignment of the oropharyngeal and laryngeal axes is not required.[117] They are well suited for patients with potential cervical spine injury and those with limited neck mobility because no movement of the neck is necessary. Case reports also suggest their utility in patients with upper airway distortion from mass or hematoma.[107,118] These devices can also provide visual assistance with NT intubation. The Bullard and the WuScope have been shown to be superior to direct laryngoscopy when the neck must be held in neutral position.[119] The UpsherScope has been less well studied, and a problem controlling the epiglottis and difficulty inserting the tube suggests this scope may be less useful than the others.[120] The UpsherScope Ultra has been designed to address these problems. The Upsher-Scope is the simplest of these devices, and the WuScope, with three parts to assemble in addition to the fiberscope, is structurally the most complex. One potential advantage of the WuScope is that its fiberoptic element is relatively protected from blood and secretions by its tubular blade. The major difference between these devices is that the Bullard scope has a designated intubating stylet attached to the scope whereas the other devices are designed to pass the ET tube down through the blade itself. After passing the ET tube down the blade, placement into and through the larynx may be aided by using a tracheal tube introducer or a Parker Flex-It stylet (Parker Medical, Englewood, CO). The Bullard laryngoscope, the most studied of these devices, is used to represent this group.

Bullard Laryngoscope

The Bullard laryngoscope was the first anatomically shaped rigid fiberoptic laryngoscope (Fig. 4–30). In the anesthetized patient, it results in less head extension and cervical spine extension than conventional laryngoscopy.[121] It appears to be effective regardless of the patient's head and neck anatomy.[122] The addition of an intubating stylet attached along the right side of the laryngoscope has increased the ease and speed of intubation. A newer, multifunctional stylet (MFIS) has a hollow lumen that allows an introducer to be passed through it and into the laryngeal inlet and over which the tube can be advanced. Plastic tip extensions are available for the larger patient in whom the epiglottis may be difficult to elevate. The Bullard laryngoscope comes in three sizes, adult, pediatric (newborn–10 yr) and neonatal (newborn–2 yr). Its success has been demonstrated in neonates.[117]

Indications and Contraindications. The Bullard laryngoscope is indicated in patients with anticipated difficult airways who require definitive airway control. It can be used in awake or unresponsive patients.[123] Awake intubation using the Bullard laryngoscope can be performed comfortably using topical anesthesia and light intravenous sedation.[123] The Bullard scope can also be used in conjunction with NT intubation to assist in successful tube placement. Marked limitation of mouth opening is a contraindication to its use. However, because the Bullard laryngoscope follows the contour of the mouth and hypopharynx, only 2 cm of occlusal opening is necessary for the introduction of the scope and an ET tube. The laryngoscope itself requires only 6 mm of mouth opening for insertion.[124] As with all fiberoptic devices, the presence of blood, excessive secretions, or vomit is a relative contraindication owing to the propensity for obscuring the element and rendering the device useless.

Procedure and Technique. Defog the fiberoptic element prior to use, using a defogging agent or high-flow oxygen down the working port. The technique for introducing the Bullard laryngoscope blade is similar to that for direct laryngoscopy. Stand at the patient's head and open the patient's mouth while stabilizing the head. Introduce the blade into the oropharynx with the handle initially held horizontally. Rotate the handle to follow the curve of the oropharynx until it is fully vertical. Release all tension on the handle and allow to device to settle posteriorly before gently sliding it inferiorly and anteriorly to ensure that the epiglottis is lifted, although visualization of the larynx is usually possible without this maneuver. Exert only minimal force along the axis of the handle. Intubate the larynx with a styletted ET tube. With the glottis in view, advance the tube off the stylet and into the larynx. The technique is usually successful when using the Bullard intubating stylet.[122] If the multifunctional stylet is used, advance the intubation catheter into the larynx and pass the tube over it. After intubation is complete, rotate the handle forward and remove the scope. Cricoid pressure does not appear to interfere with Bullard scope success.[125]

Complications

The major difficulty in using rigid fiberoptic laryngoscopes is the inability to visualize the larynx because of blood, emesis, or secretions. Once visualized, the glottis can usually be intubated, although both accessing the inlet and passing the tube may occasionally be difficult. Another reason for failure is the inability to place the blade tip under the epiglottis,[122] although improvements in product design have minimized this difficulty. Injury due to device placement is very rare.

Summary

Rigid fiberoptic laryngoscopes are particularly useful in the management of the difficult airway resulting from limited neck movement. They may also be helpful in patients with distorted upper airway anatomy that obscure the laryngeal inlet. Each has their own minor advantages and disadvantages, but ongoing design improvements tend to mitigate these differences. When blood and excessive secretions are present, however, they suffer from the same drawback as all fiberoptic devices that have exposed optical elements at the scope tip, the frequent inability to visualize the laryngeal inlet. A possible exception is the WuScope, with its relatively protected optical element, but it has yet to be studied in this setting.

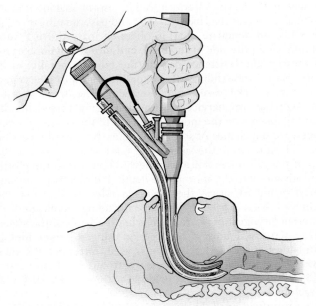

Figure 4–30 Bullard laryngoscope. An anatomically shaped laryngoscope visualizes the glottis. The tracheal tube is mounted on the attached stylet to facilitate laryngeal placement. *(Courtesy of Department of Emergency Medicine, Hennepin County Medical Center, Minneapolis, MN.)*

Video-Assisted Laryngoscopy

Video-assisted laryngoscopy transmits an image from an optical element located on the laryngoscope blade to a monitor. The optical element is often fiberoptic, although newer devices incorporate miniature video cameras on their blades. In addition to providing indirect images that may be unobtainable with direct laryngoscopy, the image is usually enhanced by magnification and a wide-angle view. Both flexible and rigid fiberoptic scopes can accept a video attachment onto the eyepiece. The primary goal of video enhancement is to improve visualization of the laryngeal inlet. When comparing laryngeal views from the video display of a Macintosh blade with that from direct laryngoscopy using the same blade, Kaplan and coworkers[126] demonstrated a 42% incidence of improvement in laryngeal view as opposed to a 3% decrease in quality. Better visualization, of course, may not translate directly into a successful intubation because a certain degree of hand-to-monitor coordination must the acquired. Another benefit of projecting the laryngeal image on a screen is that assistants who are providing external laryngeal manipulation can view the monitor and modify their maneuvers accordingly. Video-assisted laryngoscopy also has great potential as a teaching aid. The Glidescope videolaryngoscope (Verathon, Bothell, WA), first introduced in 2001, is the first of a new class of video-assisted rigid scopes that provides enhanced video views of the laryngeal inlet while being less likely to be affected by the presence of blood and secretions. It comes with a small monitor on a stand. A similar but portable model is also available. The McGrath Portable Video Laryngoscope (Aircraft Medical Ltd., Edinburgh, United Kingdom) is another device with similar characteristics but is more compact, has an adjustable blade length, and uses disposable blade covers (Fig. 4–31). It is very new and no studies have been reported on its use. The Glidescope and its use are discussed as representative of this new class of indirect video-assisted laryngoscopes.

Glidescope

The Glidescope is a video laryngoscope with a miniature camera embedded midway along the undersurface of the blade that has a 60° midblade angulation (Fig. 4–32). The blade thickness is 18 mm. The view is high resolution, wide angled, and magnified. Blood and secretions are unlikely to compromise laryngeal visualization because of the camera's orientation, its location well away from the blade tip, and its

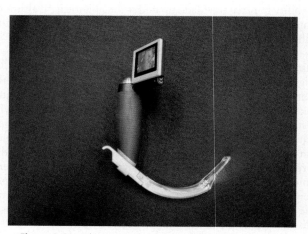

Figure 4–31 The McGrath Portable Video Laryngoscope.

antifogging technology. Visualization of the laryngeal inlet and surrounding structures is excellent. With the Glidescope, glottis visualization is usually less of a problem than placing a tube through it. Difficult laryngoscopic cases are more easily intubated with this scope than with direct laryngoscopy, but easy cases are more time consuming owing to difficulties in advancing the tube.[127] Learning to use the Glidescope is easy because the overall feel of the device is similar to that of a conventional laryngoscope. The absence of fiberoptic elements increases its durability and avoids a breakage expense often incurred with emergency flexible fiberoscopy.[111] The turnaround time for cleaning the scope with cold glutaraldehyde solution is 20 minutes.

Indications and Contraindications. The Glidescope is useful in patients in whom a difficult intubation is anticipated or in someone who cannot be intubated using direct laryngoscopy. Blood and secretions are rarely a significant problem. A contraindication is a small mouth through which the blade cannot be safely passed (opening < 2 cm). This scope is currently available only in an adult size.

Procedure and Technique. Bend a styletted tracheal tube to conform to the 60° angle of the Glidescope blade (see Fig. 4–32). Alternatively, form the tube into a J-shape and introduce it behind the tongue, bringing it anteriorly with a rolling motion, similar to the Trachlight. Grasp the Glidescope in the left hand and place it into the mouth, using the scissor technique. Under direct vision, advance it in the midline along the tongue toward the uvula. Verify its midline position on the monitor, passing the uvula as the Glidescope blade slips behind the tongue, hugging the base of the tongue. With a gentle lifting motion, place the tip of the blade in the vallecula. Elevate the epiglottis and expose the laryngeal inlet. If the inlet is not visualized well, tilt the handle back slightly to enhance exposure. Manipulate the neck externally to enhance the visualization. If more exposure is required, place the blade tip under the epiglottis and gently lift and tilt back. While attempting to optimize the laryngeal view, be careful not to place the blade too close to the laryngeal inlet because it may tip the larynx anteriorly and inferiorly, making it more difficult to access the laryngeal inlet and pass the tube through it. Once an adequate view is obtained, pass the ET tube blindly along the side of the blade and into the hypopharynx. If there is any resistance passing the tube intraorally, make sure that it is not sliding off the midline and into pharyngeal structures. Take care when advancing the tracheal tube through the oropharynx because it is being passed blindly until it appears on the monitor in front of the laryngeal inlet. Decrease the chance of soft tissue injury by carefully passing the ET tube along the side of the Glidescope.[128] When the tip of the ET tube comes into view, direct it into the glottis and advance it to the appropriate depth. If difficulty is encountered trying to access the laryngeal inlet, success may be achieved by a variety of means including application of external laryngeal pressure, increasing the bend of the stylet, using a tracheal tube introducer, or using a Parker Flex-It intubation stylet.[129] If a J-shape is used, introduce the tube from the right side of the patient and rotate it 90° and vertically into a midline position behind the tongue, similar to the Trachlight.

Complications. This is a relatively new device but injuries with its use are beginning to be reported. Fortunately, they are few and relatively minor: two cases of puncture of the right palatopharyngeal arch were reported with only one requiring surgical repair.[128]

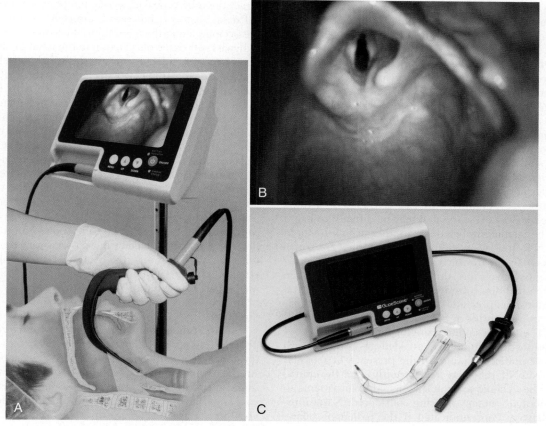

Figure 4–32 *A,* The video laryngoscope (Glide Scope/Verathon.com) provides indirect vision for intubation via a portable screen. *B,* Actual view of the vocal cords with the Glide Scope. The ET tube is guided through the cords while watching the screen. A special angulated stylet should be used. *C,* A disposable laryngoscope blade and a heated non-fogging bright light source facilitate the procedure.

Summary

Video-assisted laryngoscopy is a major advancement in the visualization of the laryngeal inlet. The Glidescope, the first device that also incorporates micro videocamera technology, is a very promising emergency airway device that provides an improved laryngeal view when compared with direct laryngoscopy while avoiding some of the problems associated with fiberoptic bronchoscopy. It has yet to be studied extensively in the setting of difficult intubation, although preliminary reports are very promising.[130] To date, the majority of intubation failures are due to inability to pass the tube through the larynx despite good or excellent glottic views.[129] Improvements in the configuration of the tracheal stylet should decrease this problem. A major conceptual difference between direct laryngoscopy and video-assisted indirect laryngoscopy is that in the former, the ET tube is guided visually through the oropharynx but may not always be seen going through the glottis. With video-assisted indirect laryngoscopy, the tube is passed blindly through the oropharynx but is normally well seen in the hypopharynx as it is advanced into the glottis. Video-assisted indirect laryngoscopy promises to be a dynamic area for advances in the management of difficult airways. Advancements need to be made in achieving tracheal intubation once the glottis is seen. Expense is a major impediment to its widespread use. Hopefully, with greater use and more competition among the manufacturers of the devices, this will become less of a factor.

NT Intubation

NT intubation was first described by Magill in the 1920s. The tube may be placed blindly or with the aid of a laryngoscope or bronchoscope. Blind NT intubation can be one of the more technically demanding airway approaches, with the outcome being heavily dependent on the skill and experience of the clinician and a certain amount of luck. The primary advantage of the blind technique is that it minimizes neck movement and does not require opening the mouth. In extenuating circumstances, it can be accomplished without an intravenous line.

General Indications and Contraindications

NT intubation is technically more difficult than oral intubation, but it has definite advantages. Blind NT intubation is possible with the patient in the sitting position, a distinct advantage when intubating a patient with congestive heart failure who cannot tolerate lying flat. In fact, patients in respiratory distress are the easiest to intubate blindly because their air hunger results in increased abduction of the vocal cords, which facilitates tube entry into the trachea.

An NT tube has advantages that extend beyond the immediate difficulties of airway control. The patient cannot bite the tube or manipulate it with the tongue. Oral injuries may be cared for without interference by the tube. An NT tube is more easily stabilized and generally easier to care for than an orotracheal tube. It is better tolerated by the patient, permitting easier movement in bed, and produces less reflex salivation than do oral tubes.

Blind Placement

Blind NT intubation is the most common form of NT intubation in the emergency setting. Danzl and Thomas[131] reported a success rate of 92% in a large series of ED patients, but success rates are highly dependent on clinician skill.

Indications and Contraindications. Patients requiring airway control who have spontaneous respirations can be considered for blind NT intubation. The typical patient is one with an anticipated difficult airway and persistently low oxygen saturation despite preoxygenation. Patients with severe chronic obstructive pulmonary disease (COPD) or asthma who have high airway pressures and may be difficult to bag if they cannot be readily intubated are another group in whom to consider NT intubation. Some other common presentations of difficult airway in which this approach can be considered are patients with a short, thick neck; the inability to open the mouth; the inability to move the neck; and oral injuries. Other conditions that preclude successful orotracheal intubation include severe arthritis or fixed deformities of the cervical spine, or ACE inhibitor–induced angioedema.

Nasal intubation should be avoided in patients with severe nasal or midface trauma. In the presence of a basilar skull fracture, an NT tube may inadvertently enter the cranial cavity.[132,133] This technique should be avoided in patients in whom thrombolytic therapy is being considered. Nasal intubation is relatively contraindicated if the patient is taking anticoagulants or has a known coagulopathy or has recently been administered thrombolytics. Apnea is the major contraindication to blind NT intubation; attempts to place the tube without respirations as a guide are futile. Blind NT intubation should be avoided in patients with expanding neck hematomas. Patient combativeness, if not controlled with sedation, is a relative contraindication. Some would argue, depending on the available alternatives, that the inability to open the mouth (such as a wired jaw) is a relative contraindication because emesis may be induced and the vomitus could not be cleared. The clinician must exercise judgment in the individual case and be prepared to use neuromuscular-blocking agents or bypass the upper airway with a surgical technique if such a complication develops.

Procedure and Technique. Place the patient in the sniffing position with the proximal neck slightly flexed and the head extended on the neck. In preparation for intubation, constrict the nasal mucosa of both nares, using either 0.25% to 1.0% phenylephrine drops, oxymetazoline (Afrin) spray, or 4% cocaine spray. Topical anesthesia of the nares, oropharynx, and hypopharynx with lidocaine spray (10%) is also indicated if time permits. If available, cocaine is ideal because it is both a vasoconstrictor and an anesthetic but caution is necessary in hypertensive patients. Choose the most patent nostril. In the cooperative patient, simply occlude each nostril and ask the patient which one is easier to breathe through. The most patent nostril can also be identified by direct vision or by gently inserting a gloved finger lubricated with viscous lidocaine into the nostrils. If time permits, a nasal airway can be passed and allowed to remain in place to physically dilate the passage. Some clinicians preemptively place this device in patients who prognosticate subsequent intubation if other interventions may fail (such as COPD exacerbations).

After preparation of the nostril, insert a well-lubricated 7.0 or 7.5 ET tube along the floor of the nasal cavity. Do not direct the tube cephalad, as one might expect from the external nasal anatomy, but rather direct it straight back toward the occiput, along the nasal floor. Twisting the tube may help to bypass soft tissue obstruction in the nasal cavity. It is sometimes recommended to orient the tube's bevel toward the septum to avoid injury to the inferior turbinate. However, such an event is rare. At 6 to 7 cm, one usually feels a "give" as the tube passes the nasal choana and negotiates the abrupt 90° curve required to enter the nasopharynx. This is the most painful and traumatic part of the procedure and must be done gently. If resistance persists despite continued gentle pressure and twisting of the tube, pass a suction catheter down the tube and into the oropharynx, which may allow successful passage of the tube over the catheter.[134] If this fails, try the other nostril. In an attempt to avoid this difficulty from the outset, use a controllable-tip tracheal tube (Endotrol, Mallinckrodt Medical Inc, St. Louis). The tube allows you to increase the flexion of the tube, facilitating passage past this tight curve. One study found that the Endotrol tube enhanced first-attempt success with blind NT intubation.[135] A study of paramedic-performed blind NT intubation reports success rates of 58% using standard ET tubes versus 72% success with directional-tip-control ET tubes.[136]

As the tube advances through the oropharynx and hypopharynx and approaches the vocal cords, breath sounds from the tube become louder and fogging of the tube may occur. At the point of maximal breath sounds, the tube is lying immediately in front of the laryngeal inlet. The tube is most easily advanced into the trachea during inspiration, when the vocal cords are maximally open. As the patient begins to breathe in, advance the tube in one smooth motion. If a gag reflex is present, the patient usually coughs and becomes stridulous during this maneuver, suggesting successful tracheal intubation. The absence of such a response should alert the clinician to probable esophageal passage. If there is a delay in advancing the tube, add oxygen to the end of the tube to increase inspired oxygen. Once the tube is in the trachea, vocalization should cease. Persistent vocalizations suggest esophageal intubation. Breath sounds coming from the tube and tube fogging are other signs of ET tube placement. Reflex swallowing during blind NT intubation may direct the tube posteriorly toward the esophagus. If this occurs, direct the conscious patient to stick out the tongue to inhibit swallowing and prevent consequent movement of the larynx. Application of laryngeal pressure may also help avoid esophageal passage.

After intubation, auscultate over both lungs while applying positive-pressure ventilation. If only one lung is being ventilated, withdraw the tube until breath sounds are heard bilaterally. The optimum distance from the external nares to the tube tip is about 28 cm in males and 26 cm in females.[137] After verification of tracheal placement, inflate the cuff and secure the tube.

Technical Difficulties

The NT tube may slide smoothly through the hypopharynx and into the trachea on the first pass. Unfortunately, this is not always the case; in an operating room series, the first attempt was successful in fewer than 50% of cases.[138] When the initial pass is unsuccessful, there are four potential locations of the tip of the tube: anterior to the epiglottis in the vallecula, on the arytenoids or vocal cords, in the piriform sinuses, or in the esophagus.

Observation and palpation of the soft tissues of the neck during attempted passage of the NT tube are helpful in finding the misplaced tube. Before reattempting placement, withdraw the tube slightly; do not remove it from the nose because this will create additional trauma to the nasal soft tissues. Keep in mind the possibility of spinal injury when considering corrective maneuvers. Any cervical maneuver that moves the neck significantly should not be used if alternatives are available. Methods for achieving success when difficulties with tube placement are encountered include the following.

Anterior to the Epiglottis. Difficulty advancing the tube beyond 15 cm or palpation of the tube tip anteriorly at the level of the hyoid bone suggests an impasse anterior to the epiglottis in the vallecula. Withdraw the tube 2 cm, decrease the degree of neck extension, and readvance the tube.

Arytenoid Cartilage and Vocal Cord. Contrary to the classic teaching,[139] studies have demonstrated a propensity for an NT tube, when placed through the right nares, to lie posteriorly and to the right as it approaches the larynx.[124,140] It is not surprising, then, that the most common obstacles to advancement of the NT tube are the right arytenoid and vocal cord. No data are available on the common obstacles encountered if the tube is placed in the left nares. If the tube appears to be hanging up on firm, cartilaginous tissue, withdraw the tube 2 cm, rotate it 90° counterclockwise, and readvance the tube. This maneuver orients the bevel of the tube posteriorly and frequently results in successful passage (Fig. 4–33). When evaluated in the ED, this maneuver was successful 73% of the time.[141] Another technique is to pass a suction catheter down the tube; it will often pass through the larynx without difficulty and the tube can then be advanced over the catheter (Fig. 4–34).[142,143]

Piriform Sinus. Bulging of the neck lateral and superior to the larynx indicates tube location in a piriform sinus. Withdraw the tube 2 cm, rotate slightly away from the bulge, and readvance. An alternate method is to tilt the patient's head toward the side of the misplacement and then reattempt the placement.[144]

Esophageal Placement. Esophageal placement is indicated by a smooth passage of the tube with the loss of breath sounds. The larynx may be seen or felt to elevate as the tube passes under it. Assisted ventilation will usually produce gurgling sounds when the epigastrium is auscultated. Withdraw the tube until breath sounds are clearly heard, reattempt passage while applying pressure to the cricoid. Increase extension of the head on the neck during placement. If attempts continue to result in esophageal misplacement, the following maneuver may result in successful tracheal intubation. From the precise point at which breath sounds are lost, withdraw the ET tube 1 cm and inflate the cuff with 15 mm of air, resulting in an elevation of the tube off the posterior pharyngeal wall and angling it toward the larynx. Advance the tube 2 cm; continued breath sounds indicate probable intralaryngeal location. At this point, deflate the cuff and advance the ET tube into the trachea (Fig. 4–35). This technique may be particularly useful in the patient with cervical spine injury because it requires no manipulation of the head or neck.[145] This maneuver, when used on the first pass in 20 patients in the operating room, was successful in 75% of cases.[138] One should bear in mind, however, that these patients were paralyzed and thus did not experience the laryngospasm that may be encountered in a breathing patient. The use of topical anesthesia is recommended. Alternatively, if a controllable-tip ET tube (Endotrol) is used, the tip can be flexed anteriorly to help avoid esophageal placement.[135] Remember that the tip is very responsive to pulling on the ring. A common mistake is to exert too much force on the ring, resulting in the tube

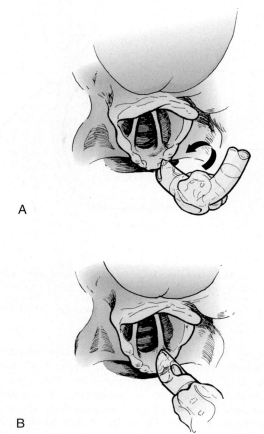

Figure 4–33 Common problem with blind tracheal tube passage through the larynx. *A,* The tip of the tube is caught on the arytenoid cartilage. *B,* Rotation of tube 90° counterclockwise orients the bevel of the tip posteriorly and allows passage into the larynx. *(A and B, Courtesy of Department of Emergency Medicine, Hennepin County Medical Center, Minneapolis, MN.)*

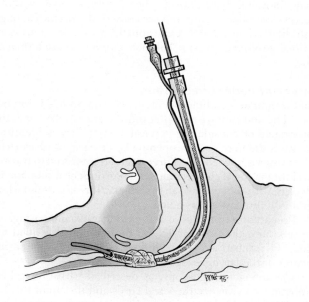

Figure 4–34 Use of suction catheter to aid in passage of nasotracheal tube caught at laryngeal inlet. The suction catheter is passed down the tracheal tube and into the trachea. The tracheal tube is then passed over the suction catheter, and the catheter is removed. *(Courtesy of Department of Emergency Medicine, Hennepin County Medical Center, Minneapolis, MN.).*

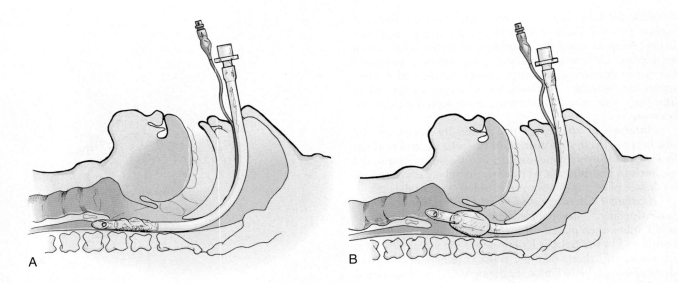

Figure 4–35 **Much skill and a lot of luck are involved with a successful blind NT intubation.** Use of tracheal tube cuff inflation may aid in nasotracheal intubation. *A*, The tracheal tube is pulled back after esophageal passage. *B*, Once breath sounds are heard, the cuff is inflated with 15 ml of air and is readvanced into the laryngeal inlet. Once seated in the inlet, the cuff is deflated and the tube is advanced into the trachea. (*A and B, Courtesy of Department of Emergency Medicine, Hennepin County Medical Center, Minneapolis, MN.*).

curling up before the larynx, and thus preventing tube advancement. There has been a case report of an Endotrol tube "kinking" at the point of sharpest curvature, causing difficulty with suctioning but no problems with ventilation.[146] Another device that allows for flexing the distal endotracheal tube is the Parker Flex-Tip stylet (Parker Medical, Englewood, CO).

Laryngospasm. Laryngospasm is a common problem that arises when NT intubation is attempted. It is usually transient. Withdraw the tube slightly and wait for the patient's first gasp to advance the tube. This is frequently successful, because the vocal cords are widely abducted during inhalation. Assess laryngeal anesthesia and, if intravenous and nebulized lidocaine have already been administered without success, consider giving transcricothyroid anesthesia (e.g., 2 mL of 4% lidocaine).[147] Occasionally, a jaw-lift is necessary to break prolonged spasm. Another option is to use a smaller tube.

Placement under Direct Vision

This technique combines elements of oral and NT intubation. The indications and precautions are similar, and the importance of considering cervical spine injury is identical. Likewise, the need for jaw opening by physical or pharmacologic means is unchanged. This method is preferred to orotracheal intubation if the presence of an orotracheal tube might interfere with the repair of an oral injury. It is also useful when blind NT intubation has failed.

Preparation of the nose and nasopharynx and passage of the tube into the oropharynx are the same as described for blind NT intubation. The technique changes with the introduction of the laryngoscope.

Use direct laryngoscopy, as described with orotracheal intubation, to visualize the vocal cords and the tip of the ET tube. With the Magill forceps in the right hand, grasp the ET tube proximal to the cuff (to avoid damage to the balloon) and direct it toward the larynx (Fig. 4–36). Ask an assistant to advance the tube gently while you direct the tip into the larynx and trachea. Cricoid pressure may facilitate the passage.

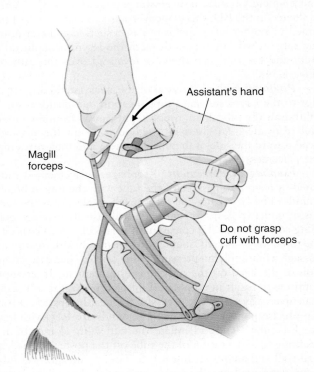

Assistant's hand

Magill forceps

Do not grasp cuff with forceps

Figure 4–36 **Nasotracheal intubation with the aid of a laryngoscope and Magill forceps.** Note that the forceps do not pull the tube—they serve to only guide the tip of the tube through the vocal cords while an assistant advances the tube. The cuff is frequently damaged if it is grasped.

Often, the larynx can be manipulated sufficiently with the laryngoscope so that the clinician can advance the tube with the right hand and guide it between the cords without using the Magill forceps. Occasionally, the natural curve of the tracheal tube guides it through the cords without any manipulation. Inflate the cuff and auscultate both lungs to ensure ventilation. When placement is satisfactory, secure the tube.

Complications

Epistaxis is the most common complication of NT intubation. However, severe epistaxis was encountered in only 5 of 300 cases reported by Danzl and Thomas.[131] Tintinalli and Claffey[148] reported severe bleeding in 1 of 71 cases and less serious bleeding in 12 others. Bleeding is usually not a problem unless it provokes vomiting or aspiration, a serious potential problem in obtunded patients with a clenched jaw or a decreased gag reflex. Other immediate complications include turbinate fracture, intracranial placement through basilar skull fracture, retropharyngeal laceration or dissection, and delayed or unsuccessful placement.[132,149,150] Complications may be minimized by selection of a smaller tube and by gentle technique.

Sinusitis in patients with NT tubes is common and can be an unrecognized cause of sepsis.[151] Rare but potentially fatal delayed complications include mediastinitis after retropharyngeal abscess[152] and massive pneumocephalus.[153]

Because most complications occur during tube advancement through the nasal passage and proximal nasopharynx, the complications of blind NT intubation and placement under direct vision are largely the same. However, retropharyngeal laceration and esophageal intubation are more of a threat in blind placement techniques because they are more likely to go unrecognized.[148] One unique problem associated with NT intubation is damage of the tube cuff with the Magill forceps.

Summary

NT intubation is being used less frequently than in the past because clinicians are increasingly comfortable using oral intubation in the patient with potential cervical spine injury. In addition, emergency clinicians frequently use paralytics to facilitate orotracheal intubation. Nevertheless, NT intubation remains an effective and potentially life-saving approach to the difficult airway and should be a dependable part of the armamentarium of all clinicians who are active in emergency airway management.

Digital Intubation

Digital intubation uses the index and middle fingers to blindly direct the ET tube into the larynx. It is particularly well adapted to the prehospital situation in which a trapped victim cannot be positioned for intubation. A prehospital series of 66 digitally intubated patients demonstrated an 89% success rate.[154]

Indications and Contraindications

Digital intubation is indicated in the deeply comatose patient whose larynx cannot be visualized and who has a contraindication to NT intubation. Advantages include speed and ease of placement, immunity to anatomic constraints and other difficulties visualizing the larynx, and little neck movement. Contraindications are primarily precautions to protect the clinician. Digital intubation should not be attempted on any patient who presents a significant risk of biting. This includes the calm and awake patient as well as the agitated patient.

Procedure and Technique

Place the patient's head and neck in the neutral position. Stand at the patient's right side, facing the patient. Introduce your left index and middle fingers into the right angle of the

patient's mouth and slide them along the surface of the tongue until the epiglottis is felt. The tip of the epiglottis should be palpated at 8 to 10 cm from the corner of the mouth in the average adult. The use of a stylet in the tube is optional; the largest reported series had good success without a stylet.[154] For the clinician with short fingers or a patient with an anterior larynx, a stylet is advantageous. If a stylet is used, place it in the tube and bend it into the form of an open J with the distal end terminating in a gentle hook. Introduce a lubricated tube from the patient's left side between the tongue and the rescuer's two fingers (Fig. 4–37). Cradle the tube between two fingers and guide the tip beneath the epiglottis. Apply gentle anterior pressure to direct the tube into the larynx. If the clinician has sufficiently long fingers, place them posterior to the arytenoids, acting as a "backstop" for the tube to both avoid esophageal passage and assist in laryngeal placement.[155] If a stylet has been used, withdraw it at this time while simultaneously advancing the tube. An alternative to using a stylet for directing the tube anteriorly is to select an ET tube with a controllable tip (Endotrol, Mallinckrodt Medical Inc., St. Louis).

A variation on the technique of digital intubation has been described for intubating a newborn.[156] In this technique, only the index finger is used to guide the tube into the larynx. Bend the end of the tube and moisten both the tube and the finger with sterile water. Use the index finger of the nondominant hand to follow the tongue posteriorly and easily palpate the epiglottis and paired arytenoids. Use the thumb of the same hand to apply cricoid pressure and steady the larynx. Hold the ET tube in the dominant hand and advance it using the nondominant index finger as a guide (Fig. 4–38). The tube snugs up (encounters subtle resistance) as it enters the trachea, and palpation of the tube through the trachea provides further confirmation of correct placement. A styletted tube, shaped

93

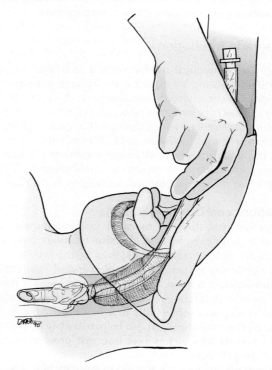

Figure 4–37 Digital intubation. The tracheal tube is cradled between the index and the middle fingers and guided into the glottic opening. (*Courtesy of Department of Emergency Medicine, Hennepin County Medical Center, Minneapolis, MN.*)

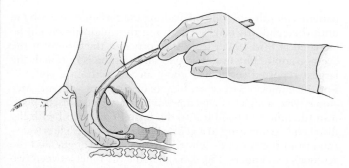

Figure 4–38 **Digital intubation in the neonate.** The tube is guided using only the index finger to palpate the epiglottis and laryngeal inlet. A stylet is optional. *(Courtesy of Department of Emergency Medicine, Hennepin County Medical Center, Minneapolis, MN.)*

in the form of a J, is usually desired until familiarity with the procedure is achieved.

Complications

The risk of esophageal intubation is always present, and being a blind procedure in deeply comatose or cardiac-arrested patients, the potential for esophageal misplacement is increased. If used in patients with a gag, induction of emesis with aspiration is a possibility. A high incidence of left main stem intubations was noted in a cadaveric study,[157] but clinical confirmation is lacking. The greatest risk seems to be to the clinician, whose fingers may be bitten.

Summary

Whereas most recent experience with digital intubation in adults has been prehospital, there is no reason why it should be confined to this setting. The majority of moribund ED patients who defy orotracheal intubation are never given a trial of digital intubation. This omission undoubtedly deprives some patients of expeditious airway management.

Retrograde Intubation

Retrograde orotracheal intubation is a technique of guided ET intubation using a wire or catheter placed percutaneously through the cricothyroid membrane or high trachea and exiting through the mouth or nose. An ET tube is then passed over this guide and advanced through the vocal cords into the trachea. Introduced by Butler and Cirillo in 1960,[158] the technique has undergone several recent modifications that have enhanced its value as a means of establishing a definitive airway when more conventional techniques have failed.

Indications and Contraindications

Retrograde intubation is indicated when definitive airway control is required and less invasive methods have failed. Indications include trismus, ankylosis of the jaw or cervical spine, upper airway masses, unstable cervical spine injuries, and maxillofacial trauma. It can be used to convert transtracheal needle ventilation (see Chapter 6) into a definitive airway. It was used successfully in a 1-month-old with developmental abnormalities.[159] It can be particularly helpful in the trauma patient with airway bleeding that prevents visualization of the glottis.[160]

Contraindications to this procedure include the availability of a less invasive means of airway control and inability to open the mouth. A relative contraindication is an apneic patient who cannot be effectively ventilated using the bag-valve mask; in this setting, it is advisable to first establish transtracheal needle ventilation (see Chapter 6) before attempting retrograde intubation or to go directly to cricothyrotomy.

Equipment

Materials include (1) local anesthetic and skin preparation materials, (2) an 18-gauge needle, (3) a 60-cm epidural catheter needle combination or an 80-cm (0.88-mm diameter) spring guidewire (J-tip preferred), (4) a hemostat, (5) long forceps (e.g., Magill) for grasping wire in pharynx, (6) an ET tube of appropriate size, (7) a syringe for tube cuff, and (8) materials for securing the tube. A prepackaged alternative is the Cook Retrograde Intubation Set (Cook Critical Care, Bloomington, IN), which also contains a sheath.

Procedure and Technique

Locate three important anatomic landmarks by palpation: the hyoid bone, thyroid cartilage, and cricoid cartilage. Prepare the skin overlying the cricothyroid membrane and anesthetize it. Next, puncture the lower half of the cricothyroid membrane with a needle directed slightly cephalad. Face the bevel also cephalad. Aspirate air to confirm needle-tip position within the lumen of the larynx. An alternative entry point is the high trachea, usually through the subcricoid space, using the same steps as described for the cricothyroid membrane.

Remove the syringe and pass the wire through the needle, advancing it until it is seen in the patient's mouth, with the help of the laryngoscope, or until it exits the nose. If the wire is found in the hypopharynx, grasp it with the Magill forceps and draw it out through the mouth. Remove the needle from the neck and secure the end of the wire at the puncture site with a hemostat. Thread the oral end of the wire in through the ET tube side port (not the end of the tube) and advance it up the tube until it can be grasped by a second hemostat. Threading the wire through the side port allows the tube tip to protrude 1 cm beyond the point at which the wire enters the larynx. Pull the wire taut and move it back and forth to ensure that no slack remains.

Advance the ET tube over the wire until resistance is met. This is the most critical point in the procedure; because this is a blind technique, it may be difficult to determine whether the tube has entered the trachea or is hung up on more proximal structures. If the ET tube has successfully passed through the vocal cords and it is being restricted by the guidewire as it traverses the anterior laryngeal wall, you should feel some caudally directed tension on the wire at its laryngeal insertion point. If this does not occur, the tip of the ET tube may be proximal to the vocal cords, either in the vallecula or the piriform sinus or abutting the narrow anterior aspect of the vocal cords. If in doubt, pull the tube back 2 cm, rotate it 90° counterclockwise, and then readvance the tube. This will usually result in successful passage through the larynx.[115] When satisfied that the tube has entered the trachea, stabilize the tube and pull out the guidewire through the mouth. Then advance the tube farther into the trachea.

The classic method of retrograde intubation, as described earlier, has undergone modifications that facilitate passage of the ET tube through the glottis. A significant advance has been the addition of a plastic sheath that is passed antegrade over the wire until it meets resistance where the wire penetrates the laryngeal mucosa (Fig. 4–39).[161] This sheath needs to be stiff enough to effectively guide an ET tube yet small

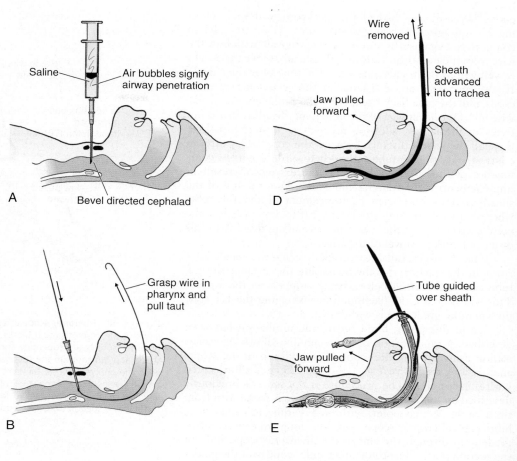

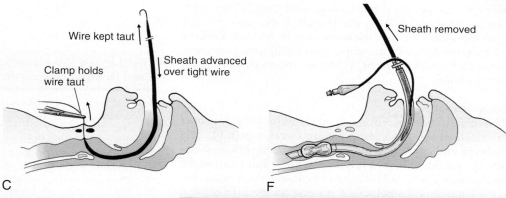

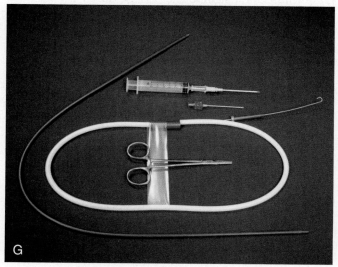

Figure 4–39 Retrograde intubation using a guidewire and antegrade sheath. *A,* Placement of a saline-filled needle through the cricothyroid membrane (*note:* the needle bevel is oriented cephalad). Aspirated bubbles of air confirm tracheal placement. *B,* Advance the J-wire directed cephalad through the translaryngeal needle. Grasp the wire in the pharynx and pull it out, long enough to advance the sheath. *C,* Grasp the wire at the neck with a clamp to keep it taut. Pass the antegrade sheath over the guidewire into trachea, *keeping both ends of the wire taut.* Note: The sheath will be stopped just below the epiglottis because the wire exits the trachea. *This is the critical portion of the procedure because only a small portion of the sheath is in the trachea. D,* Pull the jaw forward and remove the guidewire while advancing the sheath into trachea. *E,* Advance the tracheal tube over the sheath into the trachea, again with pulling the jaw forward. *F,* Removal of the sheath. *G,* A commercial retrograde intubation kit. This device has an adapter that allows ventilation throught the tube exchanger if necessary. *This kit can be used for primary intubation via laryngoscope when visualization is problematic.* The stylet is passed through the cords, ventilation is performed through the guiding stylet, then an ET tube is passed over it. (*A–F, Courtesy of Department of Emergency Medicine, Hennepin County Medical Center, Minneapolis, MN; G, courtesy of Cook Critical Care, Bloomington, IN.*)

enough to easily pass through the vocal cords without imping-ing on supraglottic or glottic structures. When the sheath comes to rest against the anterior laryngeal wall, withdraw the wire from the mouth and advance the sheath. Once the sheath is well within the trachea, pass the ET tube over the sheath. If you encounter any resistance at the arytenoids or vocal cords, pull the tube back 1 to 2 cm and rotate it counterclock-wise 90°. One advantage of the antegrade sheath is that it lies freely in the larynx, allowing for a more posterior passage through the widest distance between the cords. The wire, in contrast, pulls the ET tube anteriorly toward the narrow com-missure of the vocal cords and is more likely to result in impingement of the tube on the cords. Also, the use of the sheath permits unrestricted advancement of the ET tube, whereas a wire entering the larynx 1.0 to 1.5 cm below the vocal cords prevents the tube from advancing more than this distance before removal of the wire.

If no sheath is available, consider placing the needle infe-riorly in the trachea, thereby increasing the distance the ET tube can be advanced before being stopped by the wire.[162] This will decrease the likelihood of dislodging the ET tube tip when the guidewire is withdrawn.

Up to this point, blind retrograde intubation has been described. A modification of the technique allows for visual-ization using a fiberoptic scope.[163] In addition to the scope, an extra long guidewire (e.g., 125 cm, 0.025 cm Teflon-coated J-wire) is required. The procedure is the same as previously described up to the point at which the wire is withdrawn from the mouth. At that point, with an ET tube mounted on a lubricated fiberoptic scope, pass the long guidewire retro-gradely up through the end of the fiberoptic scope and out the suction port. Advance the fiberoptic scope over the guide-wire and through the cords, coming to rest against the ante-rior laryngeal wall (Fig. 4–40). Withdraw the wire from the suction port and advance the scope into the trachea. Slide the ET tube off the fiberoptic scope, and visualization guarantees correct ET tube placement. Withdraw the scope and auscul-tate the lungs.

Complications

The complications of retrograde intubation are largely related to cricothyroid membrane puncture (see Chapter 6). The potential for hemorrhage is minimized by taking care to punc-ture the cricothyroid membrane in its lower half to avoid the cricothyroid artery. Subcutaneous emphysema may occur, but it is of no clinical significance because no air is insufflated during this technique. A small incidence of soft tissue infec-tion is reported with translaryngeal needle procedures, but ensuring that the wire is withdrawn from the mouth rather than the neck can minimize this.

The final complication, the failure to achieve intubation, has been mitigated by the addition of the antegrade sheath over the wire.

Summary

Retrograde intubation is an underused technique for achiev-ing tracheal intubation in a patient who cannot be intubated by less aggressive means. It is more invasive than fiberoptic intubation but requires less skill. Whereas retrograde intuba-tion usually takes several minutes to complete,[155] the patient can undergo bag-mask ventilation through much of the pro-cedure. Recent modifications in the technique guarantee this method a prominent place in the management of difficult airways, particularly when active bleeding compromises the airway.

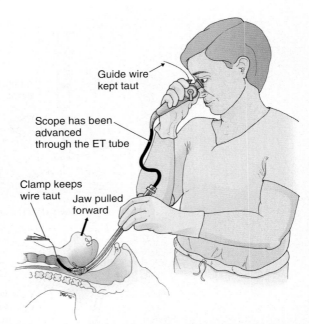

Figure 4–40 Fiberoptic scope as an aid in retrograde intubation. First, advance the scope through the ET tube. The retrograde wire (long) is placed and retrieved superiorly and threaded through the tip of the scope and out through the suction port. *A clamp and an assistant keep the proximal and distal wires taut.* The scope is then advanced until it passes through the vocal cords, stopping at the anterior laryngeal wall. The jaw is pulled forward. The wire is withdrawn through the suction port, the scope is advanced into the trachea, and the tracheal tube is advanced over the scope into the trachea. The scope is then withdrawn. *(Courtesy of Department of Emergency Medicine, Hennepin County Medical Center, Minneapolis, MN.)*

TABLE 4–6 Procedure for Changing an Orotracheal Tube Using a Salem Sump Nasogastric Tube as a Guide*

1. Cut off the proximal 6- to 8-cm flared end of an 18-Fr Salem sump nasogastric tube.
2. Test the balloon or cuff of the new tracheal tube. An 8.0-mm tracheal tube should be used. Remove the proximal adapter from the new tracheal tube.
3. Sedate the patient and restrain the hands as necessary. Preoxygenate as much as possible.
4. Lubricate the entire length of the nasogastric tube with water-soluble lubricant (K-Y, Lubrifax).
5. Advance the nasogastric tube as far as possible into the trachea through the existing tracheal tube.
6. Deflate the balloon of the existing tracheal tube and remove it. Now only the nasogastric tube remains in the trachea, to be used as a guiding stylet.
7. Thread the proximal end of the nasogastric tube through the distal end of the new tracheal tube. This is facilitated by the use of a hemostat.
8. Advance the new tracheal tube over the guide until the nasogastric tube exits through the proximal opening in the new tracheal tube.
9. Grasp the exiting nasogastric tube, have an assistant lift the patient's jaw, and advance the tracheal tube over the guide into the trachea. If resistance is encountered, rotate the tube 90° counterclockwise.
10. Remove the guide.
11. Replace the adapter on the new tracheal tube, inflate the cuff, and ventilate the patient.

*Commercial kits designed for this procedure are preferred.

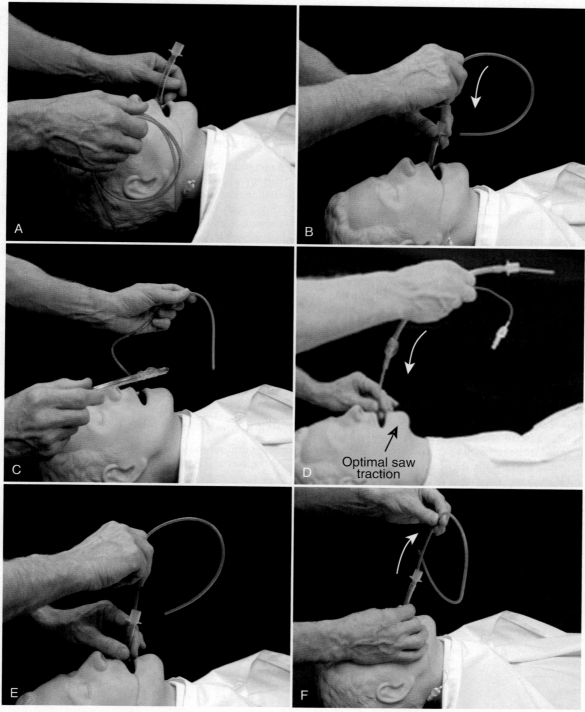

Figure 4–41 **Replacing a malfunctioning endotracheal tube.** *A,* Commercial tube exchangers are preferred though other devices are possible (see text). Shown here is an 80 cm TTX tube exchanger (Hudson Respiratory Care). Prior to tube exchange, the patient should be hyperoxygenated and sedated if necessary. *B,* The tube exchanger is passed through the defective ETT and placed deep in the airway. *C,* The defective tube is removed and the tube exchanger is left in place as a guiding stylet. *D,* The new endotracheal tube is placed over the tube exchanger and passed into the airway. A 90 degree counter-clockwise rotation of the tube and traction on the jaw will help tube passage into the laryngeal inlet; insertion of the laryngoscope may be necessary to elevate the hypopharyngeal soft tissues and facilitate tube passage. *E,* The ETT is placed to the desired depth. *F,* The tube exchanger is removed. ETT position is then confirmed.

CHANGING TRACHEAL TUBES

The tracheal tube with a leaking cuff is a vexing problem, especially if the original intubation was difficult. A method of replacing the tube without losing control of the tracheal lumen is preferred. This can be achieved by passing a guide down the defective tube, withdrawing the tube while leaving the guide in place, and introducing a new tube over the guide and into the trachea.

A number of different guides have been described (e.g., simple nasogastric tubes, 18-Fr Salem sump tubes [Table 4–6], feeding tubes), but they are poor substitutes for a designated tube exchanger such as the TTX "tracheal tube exchanger" (Hudson Respiratory Care Inc., Temecula, CA) or a similar commercially available device. The advantages of the designated tube exchanger are that, it is long enough to allow for deep placement within the airway while easily exchanging the ET tubes, it is stiff enough to prevent dislodgment when the ET tube is introduced, it is ready to use without modification, it has a printed scale to aid in determining depth of placement, and if replacement is prolonged, the patient may be oxygenated using the exchanger and wall oxygen.

Procedure and Technique

Before the procedure, sedate and restrain the patient properly. Hyperventilate the patient before placing the guide through the existing tube. Lubricate the guide and advance it into the defective tube so that it is well within the tracheal lumen (adults, 30 cm). While applying cricoid pressure (Sellick's maneuver), withdraw the defective tube over the guide, and take care not to dislodge the guide when removing the tube. Slide the replacement tube over the guide and gently advance it into the trachea (Fig. 4–41). At this juncture, it may be helpful to perform a jaw-thrust or chin-lift to facilitate passage through the pharynx. Resistance may be encountered at the laryngeal inlet or vocal cords; if this occurs, withdraw the tube 1 to 2 cm, rotate it 90° counterclockwise, and then readvance it. With the tube clearly in the trachea, remove the guide, inflate the cuff, and ventilate the patient. After correct placement has been verified, secure the new tube.

Benumof[164] described a technique in which a bronchoscope with an ET tube jacketed over the proximal end is first passed into the trachea with the defective ET tube still in place. A tube exchanger capable of jet ventilation is then passed through the defective tube. The defective tube can then be withdrawn and the new ET tube can be passed over the bronchoscope. The tube exchanger can be withdrawn once placement of the new tube is confirmed. This technique permits direct visualization of the placement of a new tube and a failsafe means to ventilate the patient should difficulties arise.

Complications are related to the time required to change the tube. A successfully performed procedure can be accomplished within 30 seconds. Laryngeal injury from forcing the guide or the tube is a possibility to consider when replacing a tube.

Conclusion

Emergency airway management in the critically ill or injured patient with acute airway compromise is one of the greatest challenges for the clinician. While the definition of a difficult airway will change as our ability to visualize the laryngeal inlet continues to improve, the challenge of the emergency airway will persist. Mastery of the basics of airway management and direct laryngoscopy, a competency in a number of guided or indirect intubation techniques, and, ultimately, the ability to perform a surgical airway, are all necessary skills before one is truly ready to assume responsibility for the emergency airway. Preparation including the mastery of technique, advance preparation of equipment, and experience in clinical decision-making are essential. Scenario visualization and advanced simulation models can provide an excellent means of practicing the difficult decision-making and technical maneuvers necessary for effective emergency airway management.

Acknowledgments

The authors would like to thank Dr. Joe Clinton for his contributions and Ben Dolan and Ed Peterson for their technical assistance with this chapter.

 REFERENCES CAN BE FOUND ON **EXPERT CONSULT**

CHAPTER 5

Pharmacologic Adjuncts to Intubation

Laura R. Hopson and Richard B. Schwartz

Endotracheal intubation in the emergency setting presents a challenge distinct from that associated with intubation of the fasted, premedicated patient in the operating room (OR). The emergency department (ED) patient is frequently uncooperative and unstable and may have medical problems that are completely unknown to the treating clinician. Within a matter of minutes, and with scant data, the clinician must assess and control the airway and diagnose and manage other life-threatening problems. Despite the clinician's familiarity with various techniques and the use of powerful medications and sedatives, *some ED patients simply cannot be readily intubated.*

In 1979, Taryle and coworkers[1] reported that complications occurred in over half of the patients intubated in a university hospital ED. They called for improved house officer training in endotracheal intubation as well as "more liberal use of the procedures and agents used in the operating room (OR), including sedatives and muscle relaxers."[1] Since this report, training programs in both critical care and emergency medicine have been greatly expanded, resulting in significant improvement in the knowledge base and expertise of clinicians providing emergent airway management.[2] Techniques and pharmacologic agents—including fiberoptic intubation, supraglottic devices, and induction and paralytic agents—that were once limited to the OR are now common in EDs. Newer pharmacologic agents allow the clinician greater ability to tailor therapy to specific clinical problems. Because of these developments, clinicians must concentrate not only on the manual skills of airway management but also on using the appropriate agents to achieve specific objectives. These objectives may include (1) immediate airway control necessitating induction of unconsciousness and muscle paralysis; (2) provision of analgesia and sedation to the awake patient; and (3) minimization of the adverse physiologic effects of intubation, including systemic and intracranial hypertension.

This chapter reviews the pharmacologic and strategic use of the drugs currently available to facilitate intubation in the ED.

RAPID-SEQUENCE INTUBATION/ INDUCTION OVERVIEW

The term *RSI* has two meanings depending upon the individual's perspective. Rapid-sequence induction (RSI) has been used by anesthesiologists to describe the sequential steps for *induction of anesthesia*, whereas in the ED, this term has been modified to rapid-sequence intubation (RSI) and is used to describe the *sequential process of intubation*. In this chapter, the abbreviation RSI shall refer to rapid-sequence *intubation*.

The steps of RSI are often described by the six "P's": preparation, preoxygenation, pretreatment and induction, paralysis, placement of the tube, and postintubation manage-

ment. This sequential technique of rapidly inducing unconsciousness (induction) combined with muscular paralysis and optimal conditions for intubation has gained broad acceptance among ED clinicians.

Preparation occurs prior to and during preoxygenation. The airway should be assessed to determine the likelihood of a difficult intubation. Simultaneously, the ED team should establish an intravenous (IV) line, place the patient on cardiac, pulse oximetry, and, when available, end tidal CO_2 monitors. They must also assemble all necessary equipment for oral intubation and desired backup methods for airway control including potential cricothyrotomy.

RSI preoxygenation is begun as soon as possible by placing the patient on 100% oxygen, for at least 2 to 3, and ideally 5, minutes. The intent is to denitrogenize the lungs and build an oxygen reserve that will last several minutes. Under optimal conditions, breathing 100% oxygen for 3 minutes has been demonstrated to *maintain acceptable oxygen saturation for up to 8 minutes in previously healthy apneic individuals.*[3] Four maximal breaths of 100% oxygen from a face mask can also maintain *acceptable saturations for 6 minutes.*[3] Comparable results may not be expected in the ED setting because of differences in the underlying health and cooperation of the patient population. Pretreatment during RSI usually occurs 2 to 3 minutes prior to the induction of unconsciousness or muscular paralysis. Although preoxygenation should be maintained for as long as practical prior to beginning intubation, the ideal situation and circumstances are not always present, and clinical judgment is the deciding factor for this portion of RSI.

Pretreatment also consists of the administration of medications to mitigate the potential untoward responses of intubation. Paralysis and induction involve the induction of an unconsciousness state with a sedative agent, followed immediately by muscle paralysis. The protocol for ED-based RSI is summarized in Table 5–1.

Endotracheal intubation and RSI have also expanded beyond the ED into the prehospital setting. Prehospital RSI protocols utilizing a sedative plus paralytic for non–cardiac arrest patients have demonstrated success rates as high as 92% to 98%.[4–7] As in the ED setting, without a full complement of medications, prehospital intubation becomes significantly more difficult, with success rates dropping to approximately 60%.[5,8] Despite these positive numbers, caution should be taken with prehospital intubation because rates of misplaced endotracheal tubes and complications by paramedics may also be much higher than previously reported.[9,10] Additionally, recent studies indicate that there may be worse outcomes for traumatic brain injury patients intubated in the prehospital setting compared with intubation in the emergency department.[10a]

PRETREATMENT AGENTS

The process of endotracheal intubation can be very painful for the patient and may induce a variety of physiologic reflexes that may have a negative impact on the patient's clinical status. Judicious use of adjunctive pharmacologic agents during RSI can potentially diminish these responses; however, the exact magnitude of their clinical effect remains undetermined and controversial.

The pressor response to stimulation of the pharynx, larynx, and trachea was first described by King and associates in 1951.[11] This reflex, mediated by the sympathetic nervous

TABLE 5–1 Rapid-Sequence Induction Protocol

1. Preoxygenate (denitrogenize) the lungs by providing 100% oxygen by mask. If ventilatory assistance is necessary, bag gently while applying cricoid pressure.
2. Assemble required equipment:
   - Bag-valve-mask connected to an oxygen delivery system.
   - Suction with Yankauer tip.
   - Endotracheal tube with intact cuff, stylette, syringe, tape.
   - Laryngoscope and blades, in working order.
   - Cricothyrotomy tray.
3. Check to be sure that a functioning, secure IV line is in place.
4. Continuously monitor the cardiac rhythm and oxygen saturation.
5. Premedicate as appropriate:
   - Fentanyl: 2–3 μg/kg given at a rate of 1–2 μg/kg/min IV for analgesia in awake patients.
   - Atropine: 0.01 mg/kg IV push for children or adolescents (minimum dose of 0.1 mg recommended).
   - Lidocaine: 1.5–2 mg/kg IV over 30–60 sec.
6. Induce anesthesia with one of the following agents administered intravenously: thiopental, methohexital, fentanyl, ketamine, etomidate, or propofol. Apply cricoid pressure.
7. Give succinylcholine 1.5 mg/kg IV push (use 2 mg/kg for infants and small children).
8. Apnea, jaw relaxation, and/or decreased resistance to bag-mask ventilations (use only when pre-RSI oxygenation cannot be optimized by spontaneous ventilation) indicate that the patient is sufficiently relaxed to proceed with intubation.
9. Perform endotracheal intubation. If unable to intubate during the first 20-sec attempt, stop and ventilate the patient with the bag-mask for 30–60 sec. Follow pulse oxymetry readings as a guide.
10. Treat bradycardia occurring during intubation with atropine 0.5 mg IV push (smaller dose for children; see item 5).
11. Once intubation is completed, inflate the cuff and confirm endotracheal tube placement by auscultating for bilateral breath sounds and checking pulse oximetry and capnography readings.
12. Release cricoid pressure and secure endotracheal tube.

RSI, rapid-sequence intubation.

system, consists of a transient increase in blood pressure and pulse rate. The stretching of the hypopharynx that occurs with laryngoscopy is the most common precipitant of the pressor response, but any manipulation of the upper airway, including nasotracheal intubation or suction, may elicit a potent response.[12–14] An increase in plasma catecholamines, including adrenaline and noradrenaline, is found in association with the pressor response.[15,16]

Considerable variation exists in the magnitude and duration of the pressor response. Studies of young healthy normotensive subjects have shown that an average increase of 20 to 25 mm Hg in mean arterial pressure occurs with laryngoscopy and intubation.[17–21] The magnitude of the response increases as the duration of the stimulus increases, reaching a peak at 45 seconds. Data from controls in several studies of patients with a broad spectrum of medical problems reveal blood pressure increases ranging from 14 to 48 mm Hg, with an average of about 30 mm Hg.[17–21] Similarly, the increase in heart rate ranges from 8 to 45 beats/min, with an average of approximately 30 beats/min. Typically, these elevations last less than 5 minutes. The magnitude of the pressor response may be increased in hypertensive patients and those with cardiovascular disease, even if the underlying hypertension is adequately controlled before intubation.

This physiologic response is probably of minimal importance in healthy patients. However, it is much more important in conditions that may deteriorate with a sudden catecholamine release, such as intracranial hemorrhage or aortic dissection. Multiple studies have evaluated interventions to pharmacologically block the pressor response, but most agents have demonstrated variable responses. *Currently, there are no proven regimens that totally abolish adverse physiologic responses to intubation, and no convincing data exist proving an ultimate or clinically consequential beneficial effect of multiple commonly used interventions.*

Lidocaine is perhaps the best known agent, but the results of these studies are inconclusive.[19,22–25] Other drugs, including thiopentone, sodium nitroprusside, labetalol, nitroglycerin, verapamil, nifedipine, clonidine, esmolol, fentanyl, sufentanil, etomidate, and magnesium have all shown variable efficacy in studies.[26–35]

Of these drugs, fentanyl and esmolol appear to be the most effective. Fentanyl effectively mitigates the hypertensive response at a dose of 200 μg.[36] Adachi and colleagues[37] found that pretreatment with 2 μg/kg of fentanyl could blunt the hemodynamic effects of tracheal tube passage, but not the hemodynamic effects of laryngoscopy. The β-adrenergic antagonist esmolol may effectively blunt the pressor response. Esmolol has a rapid onset within seconds and a very short duration of action with an elimination half-life of 9 minutes. Esmolol in doses of 1.4 to 2 mg/kg appears to be effective in blunting the pressor response.[38,39] The combination of fentanyl and esmolol also appears to act in a synergistic way to blunt the pressor response.[40]

Physical stimulation of the respiratory tract by maneuvers such as laryngoscopy, tracheal intubation, and endotracheal suctioning is commonly associated with a brief rise in intracrainal pressure (ICP). The exact mechanism responsible for this rise in ICP is unknown. One potential mechanism is the coughing and gagging that frequently follow manipulation of the upper airway and subsequent transmission of intrathoracic pressure to the cerebral circulation. An alternative explanation is that the catecholamine release that accompanies laryngoscopy causes a rise in mean arterial pressure and cerebral perfusion pressure. A small rise in ICP has also been reported after administration of succinylcholine.

Although the clinical significance of a transient rise in ICP is unknown, an intuitive concern is that it might be detrimental in patients with head trauma or already elevated ICP. A number of drugs including lidocaine, succinylcholine, and the majority of the induction agents have been studied to determine whether their use can attenuate this response.[41–47] Much of the existing clinical data are *not readily generalizable to the ED setting* because they are derived from patients in various stages of general anesthesia, often incorporating a wide variety of drug combinations and doses.

Lidocaine may be an effective agent to attenuate an ICP increase because it prevents the coughing associated with airway manipulation. It also blunts the pressor response and the resultant rise in cerebral perfusion pressure. At a dose of 1.5 mg/kg intravenously, lidocaine suppresses coughing induced by citric acid inhalation,[42] and at 2 mg/kg intravenously, it suppresses coughing associated with intubation.[43] However, studies have demonstrated conflicting results regarding lidocaine's ability to suppress the rise in ICP that follows airway manipulation.[43–46] Optimal results have been demonstrated in paralyzed patients, suggesting that paralysis alone may be the best method to suppress coughing and resultant ICP elevations during intubation.[47] Thus, the use of lidocaine to prevent coughing may have a role only when paralysis, and therefore RSI, is not an option. In the paralyzed patient, lidocaine's effectiveness is uncertain, but it may be beneficial in blunting the pressor response and, secondarily, ICP elevation. The induction of unconsciousness itself may also prevent the rise in ICP associated with intubation, so the clinical necessity for pretreatment remains unproved, although it is commonly performed. Lidocaine can also be considered as a pretreatment in the asthmatic or chronic obstructive pulmonary disease patient to prevent coughing and bronchospasm during intubation.

Succinylcholine, the most common paralytic used in RSI, has a variety of theoretical negative effects including bradycardia in children, elevated ICP, elevated intraocular pressure (IOP), elevated intragastric pressure, painful myalgias, and the potential for hyperkalemia. A number of pretreatment strategies exist to mitigate these negative effects. Prophylactic use of atropine (0.02 mg/kg) in children less than 10 years of age has been commonly accepted and is recommended by most sources; however, this practice may be called into question. Several studies indicate that *atropine may have no impact on the development of bradycardia* and that smaller doses may be as effective as the standard dose.[48,49] Challenging prior dogma, a recent review concluded that the *overall incidence of bradycardia during succinylcholine-assisted intubation is low in children (<5%), and it is not influenced by atropine.*[50] The other potential negative effects allegedly caused by succinylcholine-induced fasciculation may be limited by pretreatment with a small or "defasciculation" dose (1/10 of paralytic dose) of a nondepolarizing agent 2 to 3 minutes prior to the administration of succinylcholine. The value of using pretreatment with defasciculating doses of neuromuscular blockers (NMBs) to prevent ICP rises is also unknown.[41] This is covered in more detail under "Neuromuscular Blocking Agents," later in this chapter.

INDUCTION AGENTS

A number of diverse drugs are routinely used in the ED to induce unconsciousness prior to intubation. These include barbiturates, benzodiazepines, etomidate, ketamine, opiates, and propofol. The choice of a particular induction agent depends to a great extent on the experience and training of the clinician, the patient's clinical status, drug characteristics and institutional protocols governing use of these agents.

Considerable evidence indicates that the sedative agent selected influences the quality of intubation conditions and the rapidity of their attainment. These effects persist even when paralytic agents are utilized. Commonly used drugs and their doses are summarized in Table 5–2.

Barbiturates: Thiopental and Methohexital

The barbiturates, particularly thiopental, have been the traditional agents used for induction in the OR setting. The ultrashort-acting barbiturates thiopental and methohexital are most suited for ED RSI. However, their potential hemodynamic effects require cautious use in the ED setting. Barbiturates are central nervous system (CNS) depressants capable of producing effects ranging from mild sedation to deep coma. They do not block afferent sensory input to a significant extent and, therefore, should be used in conjunction with an analgesic agent such as fentanyl if a painful procedure is to be

TABLE 5–2 Recommended Anesthetic Doses for Rapid-Sequence Induction

Drug*	Dose
Thiopental	3–5 mg/kg IV
Methohexital	1–3 mg/kg IV
Fentanyl	5–15 µg/kg IV
Ketamine	1–2 mg/kg IV
Etomidate	0.3 mg/kg IV
Propofol	2 mg/kg IV

*Any one of these can be used before the administration of a neuromuscular blocking agent to induce anesthesia (see text).

performed. However, it is common practice to intubate patients who have received only barbiturates as the induction agent without an analgesic.

The barbiturates rapidly cross the blood-brain barrier and induce unconsciousness in less than a minute. They are rapidly redistributed and then ultimately degraded in the liver. After a single IV dose of thiopental, anesthesia lasts 5 to 10 minutes compared with 4 to 6 minutes for methohexital.[51,52] The recommended dose of thiopental is 3 to 5 mg/kg intravenously administered over 60 seconds. Methohexital is dosed at 1 to 3 mg/kg intravenously over 30 to 60 seconds.

The advantages of barbiturates as induction agents include their high potency, rapid onset, and short duration of action. They reduce cerebral metabolism and oxygen consumption and, secondarily, cerebral blood flow and ICP.[53,54] For this reason, thiopental is considered the agent of choice for anesthesia induction and maintenance of long-term anesthesia in patients with elevated ICP. Short-term use of barbiturates during RSI alone has not been clearly shown to have a protective effect on the CNS. Moreover, their use in hypovolemic patients may lead to systemic hypotension and impaired cerebral perfusion pressure that may offset any cerebral-protective characteristics.[55] Some evidence indicates that with ED RSI, thiopental may produce the best intubating conditions when used in conjunction with succinylcholine.[56]

The most significant complication of barbiturate therapy is depression of the vasomotor center and myocardial contractility, leading to significant hypotension. One study showed an average decrease in mean arterial pressures during RSI with thiopental to be 40 mm Hg.[55] This is particularly pronounced in the presence of hypovolemia or cardiovascular disease.

Barbiturates also depress the brainstem respiratory centers when given rapidly or in large doses. This effect may be accelerated by simultaneous treatment with opioids. Patients with asthma or chronic bronchitis may experience bronchospasm. Laryngospasm may occur in patients who were anesthetized lightly with barbiturates during manipulation of the upper airway. This complication usually responds to positive-pressure ventilation or neuromuscular blockade. In addition, the high pH of the barbiturate solution can cause tissue necrosis after extravascular administration and severe pain, vessel spasm, and thrombosis after intra-arterial infusion.

Etomidate

Etomidate is an ultrashort-acting nonbarbiturate hypnotic agent that has been used successfully as an anesthesia induction agent in Europe since the mid-1970s and in the United

States since 1983. A significant benefit of etomidate in the emergency setting is its lack of cardiodepressant effects.[57,58] Several case series have now demonstrated its safe and effective use in ED RSI.[59–63] Extensive experience now exists with its use for both pediatric[64] and adult patients. However, new questions are arising about long-term potential side effects.

Etomidate is a carboxylated imidazole that is both water- and lipid-soluble. The drug reaches peak brain concentrations within 1 minute of IV infusion,[65] and induces sleep within 30 seconds of administration. Its effects last less than 10 minutes after a single bolus dose.[66] Redistribution of the drug is quite rapid, which accounts for the short duration of action. Etomidate is subsequently rapidly hydrolyzed in the liver and plasma, forming an inactive metabolite excreted primarily in the urine.[65] The recommended dose is 0.3 mg/kg intravenously. There is virtually no accumulation of the drug, and anesthesia may be maintained through repeated doses.[67]

Etomidate acts on the CNS to stimulate γ-aminobutyric acid (GABA) receptors and depress the reticular activating system. It produces electroencephalographic changes similar to those produced by barbiturates as patients pass rapidly through light to deep levels of surgical anesthesia. Because etomidate has no analgesic activity,[65] it should be used in conjunction with a parenteral analgesic when painful conditions are being treated; although, as with barbiturates, it is commonly used as a sole induction agent for intubation. Etomidate decreases cerebral oxygen consumption, cerebral blood flow, and ICP, but appears to have minimal effects on cerebral perfusion pressure.[68] Most importantly in the ED setting, etomidate is characterized by hemodynamic stability without significant changes in mean arterial pressures,[58,59,62] although a slightly increased heart rate may be observed.[69] This hemodynamic stability persists even in patients with preexisting hypotension.[70]

The most common immediate side effects of etomidate are pain on injection, nausea, vomiting, and myoclonic jerks.[71] Pain on injection is reported in up to two thirds of patients. Use of a large vein, simultaneous saline infusion, and opioid premedication can reduce the discomfort in appropriate situations.[72] Myoclonic activity has been reported in about one third of cases and is believed to be caused by disinhibition of subcortical activity rather than CNS stimulation and does not represent seizure activity.[65] This sometimes dramatic effect can be avoided through use of NMBs and thus is rarely seen in the ED where paralytic agents are regularly utilized in RSI. Fleeting muscular spasms should not be misinterpreted as a seizure, and no treatment is usually necessary. If persistent, an intravenous benzodiazepine may be used.

Since the early 1980s, prolonged infusions of etomidate have been associated with suppression of adrenal function, owing to competitive enzyme inhibition during cortisol biosynthesis by the medication. When used for sedation over periods of days, the drug has been strongly linked with increased mortality in critically ill and injured patients presumably owing to insufficient cortisol production.[73,74] Increasing numbers of studies have demonstrated some degree of altered adrenal function after even a single dose of etomidate. These effects appear to persist for hours and potentially even days.[74a,74b] Studies are also raising concern about the potential consequences of these alterations. Although frank adrenal insufficiency does not appear to occur, a condition of relative adrenal insufficiency, in which there is a lack of appropriately increased cortisol production to stimulation, is linked to etomidate.[75,76] In other studies, relative adrenal insufficiency has been linked to an increased mortality rate in critically ill patients.[77,78] Although concerns have been raised regarding a causative role in this condition for etomidate and a potential for increased mortality,[79–81] to date no well-controlled studies exist to prove causality. Clearly, this is an area of ongoing research and controversy. It remains to be determined whether the benefits of predictable action and hemodynamic stability of etomidate in the critically ill patient requiring intubation in the ED are outweighed by relative adrenal insufficiency followed by potentially increased mortality. Additional areas of active investigation include the role of steroid supplementation in patients receiving etomidate. At this juncture, there is insufficient information for definitive recommendations; however, the clinician must take into account the relative advantages and disadvantages of any sedative agent prior to its use.

Ketamine

Unique among anesthetic agents and likely underused in the ED, ketamine produces a dissociative anesthesia characterized by excellent analgesia and amnesia despite the appearance of wakefulness. As a drug that is potent and relatively safe, with a rapid onset and brief duration of action, ketamine fits the profile of an agent that could be used effectively to facilitate intubation. It does, however, possess a number of pharmacologic properties that limit its use in selected circumstances.

Ketamine is a water- and lipid-soluble drug that rapidly penetrates into the CNS. Like the barbiturates, ketamine accumulates rapidly and then undergoes redistribution with subsequent degradation in the liver.[82] The recommended dose of ketamine before intubation is 1 to 2 mg/kg administered intravenously over 1 minute. Anesthesia occurs within 1 minute of completing the infusion and lasts 5 to 10 minutes. A smaller additional dose (0.5–1 mg/kg) may be given 5 minutes after the initial dose if needed to maintain anesthesia. The simultaneous administration of succinylcholine and midazolam is recommended to provide adequate muscle relaxation and to decrease the incidence of postanesthesia emergence reactions, respectively. The intramuscular dose for intubation has not been well studied, but a suggested dose is 4 mg/kg. Onset of action occurs within 2 to 3 minutes. Because of its good vascularity, the anterior thigh muscle is theoretically the preferred site for administration.

Unlike other anesthetic agents that depress the reticular activating system, ketamine acts by interrupting association pathways between the thalamocortical and the limbic systems. Characteristically, the eyes remain open, and patients exhibit spontaneous, although not purposeful, movements. Increases in blood pressure, heart rate, cardiac output, and myocardial oxygen consumption are seen, most likely mediated through the CNS. In vitro studies indicate that ketamine is a myocardial depressant, but the CNS-mediated pressor effects generally mask the direct cardiac effects,[83,84] making it potentially useful in patients with hemorrhagic shock. Respirations are initially rapid and shallow after ketamine administration, but they soon return to normal.

Other features of ketamine anesthesia include increased skeletal muscle tone, preservation of laryngeal and pharyngeal reflexes, hypersalivation, and relaxation of bronchial smooth muscle. ICP is increased, most likely as a consequence of increased cerebral blood flow,[82] thus limiting its utility in patients with intracranial pathology.

The most promising use of ketamine as an intubation adjunct has been in the setting of acute bronchospastic disease. Ketamine relaxes bronchial smooth muscle either directly, through the enhancement of sympathomimetic effects, or indirectly through the inhibition of vagal effects. Ketamine also increases bronchial secretions, which may decrease the incidence of mucous plugging commonly seen in decompensating asthmatic patients.[85] Clinical reports have demonstrated a reduction in airway resistance and an increase in pulmonary compliance that occur within minutes of ketamine administration.[86,87] *In addition, bronchospastic patients struggling to breathe and unable to tolerate oxygen masks or bronchodilators because of hypoxic encephalopathy will continue to breath deeply and rapidly under ketamine, allowing for the maximum delivery of oxygen prior to a more elective intubation* (Fig. 5–1).

The side effect that has limited the use of ketamine is its tendency to produce postanesthesia emergence reactions, a characteristic that it shares with the structurally similar drug phencyclidine (PCP). The reactions may be marked and distressing to the patient with symptoms including floating sensations, dizziness, blurred vision, out-of-body experiences, and vivid dreams or nightmares. Up to one third of patients experience such reactions. These are, however, less common in children than in adults and are rarely an issue with the doses used in the ED for intubation. Emergence reactions may be suppressed by benzodiazepines. Both diazepam and lorazepam appear to be useful in adults, but the latter is more effective, most likely owing to its enhanced amnestic effect. Midazolam, likewise, is effective in adult patients at doses of 0.07 mg/kg,[88] and may be the preferred agent because it has potent amnestic effects and a short duration of action. Studies in children fail to show a reduction in the rates of emergence reactions in pediatric patients treated with both ketamine and midazolam.[89,90]

Despite preservation of pharyngeal and laryngeal reflexes in patients sedated with ketamine, aspiration can still occur.[91,92] In addition, ketamine does not relax skeletal muscle, and production of desired intubating conditions requires the simultaneous administration of a paralytic agent, thereby removing all upper airway reflexes.

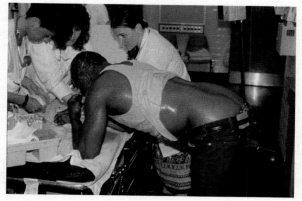

Figure 5–1 This asthmatic is diaphoretic, confused, agitated, and cannot tolerate inhaled bronchodilators. He is about to have a respiratory arrest, and cannot be preoxygenated prior to intubation. The pulse oximetry is 82–84%. Within 60 seconds following IV ketamine (100 mg) he stopped fighting but kept breathing rapidly. A nonrebreathing oxygen mask was tolerated and the oxygen saturation rose to 98%, after which he was electively intubated under controlled preoxygenated conditions. A ketamine infusion (1 mg/kg/hr) was maintained for a few hours.

Propofol

Propofol is a popular drug among anesthesiologists for OR-based induction that is ideal for ED use. Multiple reports have demonstrated the safety and efficacy of propofol for ED procedural sedation.[93–95] Although some ED clinicians now intubate using only propofol, eschewing longer-acting agents and paralysis, its role as an adjunct to intubation in the ED is undergoing evolution.

Propofol is an alkylphenol sedative-hypnotic used for induction and maintenance of general anesthesia. The drug has no analgesic activity, but it does have an amnestic effect. It produces dose-dependent depression of consciousness ranging from light sedation to coma. Propofol is a highly lipophilic, water-insoluble compound that undergoes rapid uptake by vascular tissues, including the brain, followed soon afterward by redistribution to the muscle and fat. The drug is metabolized by the liver and excreted in the urine.[96–98] After an induction dose of 2 mg/kg intravenously, unconsciousness occurs within 1 minute and lasts for 5 to 10 minutes. A smaller dose (1–1.5 mg/kg) is recommended in the elderly and when simultaneously administering other CNS depressants. Because propofol has a short duration of action and patients rapidly regain consciousness, repeat bolusing is not a practical way to maintain a desired level of sedation.[96–98] Therefore, a slow drip infusion of 3 to 5 mg/kg per hour titrated to effect is preferred.

Side effects of propofol include direct myocardial depression causing a moderate fall in blood pressure, particularly in the elderly or hypovolemic patients, and when administered simultaneously with opioids. Hypotension can be minimized with fluid loading or reversal with 5–10 mg of intravenous ephedrine. Propofol reduces cerebral blood flow and may cause mild CNS excitation activity (e.g., myoclonus, tremors, hiccups) during induction. Pain on injection occurs commonly, even when the drug is infused slowly.[96–98] Pretreating the infusing vein with 3 ml of 1% lidocaine (30 mg) injected over 30 seconds will ameliorate this pain.

Benzodiazepines (Midazolam)

The benzodiazepines are a widely used class of drugs characterized by anxiolytic, hypnotic, sedative, anticonvulsant, muscle relaxant, and amnestic effects. Several of these properties make the benzodiazepines appealing adjuvant agents for intubation, particularly when used in combination with opioids. It is important to remember that benzodiazepines do not have analgesic effects. Although they may produce excellent sedation and impair the patient's memory of an unpleasant experience, they will not prevent the pain associated with intubation.

Midazolam has, to a great extent, replaced diazepam as a preoperative sedative agent.[99,100] Midazolam is also used widely as an anesthesia induction agent, even in high-risk elderly and cardiac patients.[101–103] Compared with diazepam, the primary advantages of midazolam include a twofold increase in potency, a shorter half-life, and a lessened potential for cardiorespiratory depression. Midazolam possesses a unique imidazole ring that is stable and water-soluble in an acid medium but highly lipophilic at physiologic pH. Because it does not require suspension in propylene glycol, midazolam is not a tissue irritant. It causes minimal pain on injection, is rarely associated with phlebitis, and can be given intramuscularly when a very rapid onset of action is not required. The highly lipophilic character of the drug permits rapid accumulation in the CNS with onset of sedation in as little as 1 to 2 minutes. Rapid penetration into fatty tissue coupled with extensive binding to plasma proteins causes a prompt fall in serum levels after IV administration. This may account for the paucity of side effects outside the CNS. The half-life of elimination is 1 to 4 hours and is dependent on release of the drug from adipose tissue and protein-binding sites. The period of sedation after a single IV dose is considerably shorter. Emergence from a 0.15-mg/kg dose occurs in 15 to 20 minutes.[104]

Clinical experience using midazolam with or without fentanyl for procedural sedation is considerable and considered both safe and effective in the ED setting. The recommended dose for moderate sedation with midazolam is 0.05 to 0.1 mg/kg given in 1 mg boluses and not exceeding 2.5 mg over 2 minutes. Doses upward of 0.1 mg/kg are often needed to produce good conditions for intubation.[55,100]

Although midazolam was initially touted to be free of cardiorespiratory side effects, experience suggests that the potential adverse effects of midazolam are quite similar to those of other benzodiazepines. A small increase in heart rate is seen frequently, as is a small decrease in systolic blood pressure.[105] Changes in blood pressure may be exaggerated in the presence of hypovolemia.[106] An ED-based study reports a mean 10% decrease in systolic blood pressures and 19% of intubated patients having systolic blood pressures of less than 90 mm Hg.[107] Cardiac index and coronary artery blood flow are generally not affected. Respiratory depression may occur even at standard doses, but it most often follows rapid administration of an excessive dose. Respiratory depression is also more likely to occur in debilitated or elderly patients and in those simultaneously receiving opioids. The effects of midazolam are rapidly reversed by the administration of the benzodiazepine antagonist flumazenil. One case report has also implicated midazolam in the development of laryngospasm, which, as with respiratory depression, responded to treatment with flumazenil.[108]

Information from the National Emergency Airway Registry indicates that about 15% of patients receive midazolam as a sole induction agent during RSI. They also noted a consistent tendency to underdose the medication below the recommended 0.1 to 0.3 mg/kg level. This raises concern for patient awareness as well as for potential compromise of intubation success.[109] A study by Silivotti and Ducharme[56] of various induction agents for endotracheal intubation suggested that use of midazolam alone may be associated with suboptimal intubating conditions and increased difficulty with the performance of endotracheal intubation. In the prehospital setting, hypotension with midazolam was found to be dose related[110] and thus should be used cautiously in patients with hypovolemia or traumatic brain injury, or both. Taken as a whole, other induction agents may be preferred over midazolam alone during RSI.

Opioids (Fentanyl)

Although any of several opioids administered intravenously could be used to induce unconsciousness, fentanyl has significant advantages over other opioid agents. A synthetic opioid, it has been widely used since its introduction in 1968. Its favorable pharmacologic properties include rapid serum clearance, high potency, and minimal histamine release.[111-114] Fentanyl quickly crosses the blood-brain barrier, producing analgesia in as little as 1 to 2 minutes. Serum levels decline rapidly from peak concentrations because of extensive tissue uptake.[115,116] Unlike with morphine, the brain concentration of fentanyl falls in conjunction with the serum level. The duration of analgesic action is 30 to 40 minutes, although at high doses, a second peak of activity may be seen several hours later because of the release of the bound drug from tissue stores. Fentanyl is about 50 to 100 times as potent as morphine.[117] This unique combination of potency and short half-life permits the administration of numerous small doses that can be titrated to the desired clinical effect. Similar to other opioids, fentanyl is competitively reversed with naloxone or nalmefene.

The relative safety of fentanyl permits considerable latitude in dosing. When used as a primary anesthetic agent for major surgical procedures, doses ranging from 50 to 100 μg/kg produce minimal side effects.[118] Comparatively tiny doses produce sedation, and 3 to 5 μg/kg, given at a rate of 1 to 2 μg/kg per minute, is generally an effective analgesic dose. More rapid administration will cause greater depression of the level of consciousness. Mostert and coworkers[111] reported successful awake intubation in 99 of 103 patients who were administered an average cumulative dose of 3.7 μg/kg. Most of these patients were able to follow commands, and many recalled the events surrounding the intubation. A small percentage could not be intubated even after receiving 500 μg of fentanyl.

Larger doses, perhaps up to 25 μg/kg, may be needed to produce ideal intubating conditions, although, if given rapidly, 10 μg/kg is usually adequate. However, even this lower dose is more likely to produce unconsciousness rather than a lesser depth of sedation and it may cause a longer period of unresponsiveness than is desirable. It is preferable to use a low dose of fentanyl (2–3 μg/kg) for analgesia combined with a paralytic agent (e.g., succinylcholine) to produce adequate muscle relaxation and a sedative (e.g., midazolam) to reduce anxiety and produce amnesia for the event.

Unlike other opioids, fentanyl causes little or no histamine release, and its use is seldom associated with emesis or hypotension. It is probably the safest opioid to use in the hypovolemic patient. Fentanyl also has significantly fewer emetic effects than other opioids. Adverse effects that have been reported with fentanyl are few and primarily follow the rapid IV infusion of very large doses. Like other opioids, fentanyl may cause rigidity of the skeletal musculature, including the chest wall and diaphragm. Typically, rigidity occurs with doses in excess of 15 μg/kg, but it has also been reported with doses as low as 10 μg/kg and may also be related to too rapid administration.[111,119] The muscular rigidity may be prevented or treated with standard doses of succinylcholine or naloxone.[120] Grand mal seizures have also been reported, but are very uncommon.[121-123] Chudnofsky and associates[124] reported a complication rate of less than 1% in 841 ED patients treated with fentanyl. The most common complication was respiratory depression, and it generally occurred when fentanyl was given in combination with other CNS depressants.

NEUROMUSCULAR BLOCKING AGENTS

NMBs are used to achieve muscle relaxation for intubation. They permit complete airway control and greatly simplify visualization of the vocal cords. This is particularly important when intubation must be performed quickly under less than ideal circumstances. Sedatives may provide some muscle relaxation, but this requires that they be administered rapidly and in large doses, risking depression of the cardiovascular system. The combination of a paralytic agent and a sedative or analgesic agent is generally superior to the use of either agent alone. A 1999 report showed an 18% failure-to-intubate rate with sedative alone compared with a 0% failure rate for sedatives plus paralytics.[125] Procedural complication rates such as significant airway trauma and aspiration were also markedly higher in the group receiving sedation only.

The only absolute contraindication to the use of NMBs is the inability to manage the airway once the patient becomes apneic. Although not absolutely contraindicated, it is considered inhumane to paralyze and intubate an alert patient. A sedative or an analgesic agent should always be administered simultaneously if the patient is able to perceive pain.

NMBs are classified as either depolarizing or nondepolarizing. Depolarizing agents mimic the action of acetylcholine (ACh), producing a sustained depolarization of the neuromuscular junction during which time muscle contractions cannot occur. Nondepolarizing agents competitively block the action of ACh at the neuromuscular junction and prevent depolarization and therefore muscle contractions. NMBs in common use and their dosages and characteristics are listed in Table 5–3.

Succinylcholine

The standard depolarizing agent currently in use is succinylcholine, which was introduced in 1952. It has a chemical structure similar to that of ACh and depolarizes the postjunctional neuromuscular membrane. Administration is followed by a brief period of muscle fasciculations that corresponds to the initial membrane depolarization and muscle fiber activation. Unlike ACh, which is released in minute amounts and hydrolyzed in milliseconds, succinylcholine requires several minutes for breakdown to occur. During this time, the neuromuscular junction remains depolarized, but the muscles relax and will not contract again until the neuromuscular end plate and adjacent sarcoplasmic reticulum return to the resting state and are again depolarized. Relaxation proceeds from the small, distal, rapidly moving muscles to the proximal, slowly moving muscles. The diaphragm is one of the last muscles to relax.[126]

Succinylcholine is rapidly degraded in the serum by the enzyme pseudocholinesterase, and the duration of action of a single dose is 3 to 5 minutes. Relaxation may be maintained by repeated IV injections. Prolonged or repeated use of the drug, however, enhances its vagal stimulatory effects, which may result in bradycardia and hypotension as well as other muscarinic effects. These effects may be seen even at normal doses, particularly in children.[127] For this reason, atropine pretreatment at a dose of 0.02 mg/kg has been recommended in all small children and in adults *receiving multiple doses*, although the need and optimal dose are still in question.[48,50] Repeat dosing of succinylcholine may also produce desensitization blockade in which the neuromuscular membrane returns to the resting state and becomes resistant to further depolarization by succinylcholine.[128,129] In general, there is little need for repeated doses of succinylcholine if appropriately dosed the first time. If paralysis in excess of 3 to 5 minutes is desired, longer-acting, nondepolarizing agents such as vecuronium or pancuronium should be used.

The recommended dose of succinylcholine is 1 to 1.5 mg/kg given intravenously. Dosages at the upper end of this range may be preferred, thereby guaranteeing complete relaxation and avoiding the need for repeat dosing. Dosage calculations should also be based upon actual, as opposed to lean, body mass owing to alterations in both volume of distribution and pseudocholinesterase activity.[130] Neonates and infants require a slightly higher dose of succinylcholine (2 mg/kg intravenously) owing to their higher volume of distribution.[69,131] It is crucial that succinylcholine be administered as a rapid bolus, because slow administration may lead to incomplete relaxation. Use of a rapid 20- to 30-mL saline flush after IV administration may enhance its desired effect.

There are a number of potential adverse effects of succinylcholine use ranging from minor to life-threatening. Muscle fasciculations accompany the initial depolarization of the neuromuscular membrane. Fasciculations are most prominent in muscular patients, and emerge as deep, aching muscle pain that may last for days.[132] It is unclear whether any regimen will totally prevent succinylcholine fasciculations (seen in 73%–100% of patients) and myalgias (seen in 10%–83% of patients), and varying effects are reported with numerous interventions.[133] Interestingly, higher doses of succinylcholine may be associated with less myalgias. Traditionally, fasciculations have been prevented by preadministration of a defasciculating dose (0.01 mg/kg) of pancuronium or vecuronium, with the number needed to treat of about three patients. Interestingly, nonsteroidal anti-inflammatory drugs, magnesium, and lidocaine may also prevent these complications.[133] Fasciculations of the abdominal wall may elevate intragastric pressure and cause regurgitation of stomach contents. This is an uncommon complication that most often follows overzealous bag-mask ventilation before intubation. Distention of the stomach with air and failure to apply cricoid pressure are more likely to cause vomiting than are muscle fasciculations alone. It is also important to note that oropharyngeal manipulation of the nonparalyzed patient is far more likely to cause vomiting than are succinylcholine-induced fasciculations.

Other reported effects of muscle fasciculations include elevations of IOP and displacement of skeletal fractures or joint dislocations. The clinical significance of a transient rise in IOP in a patient with a penetrating eye injury is unknown. Paralysis will, however, prevent spontaneous motor activity such as coughing or gagging, both of which are associated with a clear risk of vitreous expulsion. The degree of elevation of IOP with administration of succinylcholine is reported to range from 3 to 8 mm Hg.[69,134–136] Blinking alone may raise IOP by 10 to 15 mm Hg, whereas more vigorous activity such as coughing, gagging, or crying may elevate the IOP by up to 70 mm Hg.[69] Although there may be theoretical advantages to using a nondepolarizing agent in patients with penetrating

TABLE 5–3 Commonly Used Neuromuscular Blocking Agents

Agent	Dose (mg/kg)	Onset (min)	Duration (min)
Succinylcholine	1.5	1	3–5
Pancuronium	0.1	2–5	40–60
Vecuronium	0.1	3	30–35
	0.25	1	60–120
Atracurium	0.5	3	25–35
Mivacurium	0.15	2–3	15–20
Rocuronium	1.0	1–1.5	30–110

eye injuries,[137] a necessary intubation using succinylcholine should never be delayed or avoided.[138]

A major consideration in the use of succinylcholine is its propensity to cause hyperkalemia. This electrolyte disturbance is believed to occur secondary to asynchronous depolarization of muscle cells and resulting cellular injury. Elevation in serum potassium occurs in normal patients after standard doses, but is typically clinically inconsequential, with increases of less than 0.5 mmol/L (mEq/L) being seen.[139] Increases in potassium are not prevented with defasciculating doses of nondepolarizing agents. Marked hyperkalemia is associated with increased extrajunctional muscle ACh receptors that develop with prolonged diseases of the neuromuscular system. Susceptibility may occur within as little as 5 to 7 days and persist indefinitely. In these cases, the hyperkalemic response may be as much as 5 mmol/L (mEq/L). These conditions include late severe burns,[140] major muscle trauma,[141] spinal cord injury, muscular dystrophy, and other upper motor neuron diseases[142,143] such as amyotrophic lateral sclerosis. These large elevations occur only in patients who have had significant tissue injury or muscle denervation for several days or weeks before the use of succinylcholine. Importantly, succinylcholine is not contraindicated in the initial management of patients with acute injuries including burns, major crush injuries, and spinal cord injuries. Succinylcholine is also not contraindicated in normokalemic patients with renal failure because the magnitude of the rise in serum potassium is the same as in patients with normally functioning kidneys.[144] A retrospective review of succinylcholine use in 38 operative cases with moderate pre-RSI hyperkalemia (5.6–7.6 mmol/L) suggests that the risk of hyperkalemia-related complications may be lower than feared.[145] In a review of over 41,000 intubations (38 patients had hyperkalemia, mean serum potassium 5.9 mmol/L), Schow and colleagues[145] concluded that it is safe to administer succinylcholine with a potassium level of 5.5 to 6.0 mEq/L. Regardless, succinylcholine is best avoided (if other equally effective pharmacologic options such as rocuronium exist) in the setting of known or suspected pre-existing hyperkalemia (e.g., renal failure patients not receiving regular dialysis or demonstrating a wide QRS complex). Concern has also been raised over the use of succinylcholine in the pediatric population owing to rare case reports of hyperkalemic cardiac arrests after administration to children with undiagnosed myopathies. Succinylcholine is currently recommended for use in pediatric patients only under emergency circumstances when the airway must be rapidly secured.[131]

Malignant hyperthermia is a rare complication with an autosomal dominant inheritance pattern that is triggered by multiple anesthetic agents including succinylcholine. Most provocative agents such as halothane are not utilized in the ED setting; therefore, it is extremely rare for the ED physician to encounter this complication. It occurs in approximately 1 in 15,000 children and 1 in 50,000 adults.[146] The clinical syndrome consists of high fever, tachypnea, tachycardia, cardiac arrhythmias, hypoxia, acidosis, myoglobinuria, and impaired coagulation. Unabated muscle contractions mediated by abnormal calcium channels are the physiologic basis for this condition.[147] Treatment includes aggressive cooling measures, volume replacement, and correction of hypoxia and acid-base and electrolyte abnormalities. Dantrolene sodium, a direct-acting skeletal muscle relaxant, is thought to be effective in reducing the muscle hypermetabolism that causes the dramatic hyperpyrexia.[148] An associated abnormal response to succinylcholine is isolated masseter spasm,[149] which can occur in isolation or portend subsequent development of malignant hyperthermia. Although rare, it has been reported in the emergency medicine literature.[150] In this condition, forcible sustained contraction of the masseter muscles occurs, preventing mouth opening and oral intubation. Management is controversial and recommendations range from bagging the patient, securing a surgical airway until the contraction abates over minutes to hours to attempting to suppress the contractions through administration of a nondepolarizing NMB.

Prolonged paralysis after administration of succinylcholine may occur in clinical conditions resulting in decreased pseudocholinesterase levels and, therefore, decreased metabolism of succinylcholine. Physiologic states in which this may occur include hepatic disease, anemia, renal failure, organophosphate poisoning, pregnancy, chronic cocaine use, advanced age, bronchogenic carcinoma, and connective tissue disorders. Patients with these conditions experience a two- to threefold increase in the duration of apnea.[151] Patients with cocaine intoxication may also experience prolonged muscle relaxation because cocaine is competitively metabolized by the cholinesterases. An inherited deficiency of pseudocholinesterase is also present in about 0.03% of the population, leading to prolonged paralysis from the administration of succinylcholine.[151]

Succinylcholine can also result in an increase in ICP; however, the magnitude and significance of the increase in ICP that occurs with succinylcholine use remains controversial.[152–156] Increases in the range of 5 to 10 mm Hg have been reported by several investigators, but other researchers have shown no increase. There is no evidence of neurologic deterioration associated with these transient elevations in ICP. Mechanisms that have been proposed to explain the elevated ICP include (1) a direct effect of fasciculations, (2) an increase in cortical electrical activity with a resultant increase in cerebral blood flow and blood volume, and (3) sympathetic postganglionic stimulation. Minton and coworkers[157] have demonstrated that pretreatment with vecuronium (0.14 mg/kg) reduces the rise in ICP after succinylcholine administration. It has been postulated that nondepolarizing blockade prevents muscle spindle firing and the increase in cortical activity that may lead to increased ICP. Pretreatment with a nondepolarizing agent may not be practical when intubation must be performed rapidly; furthermore, the dose that has been shown to be effective is itself a paralyzing dose and would obviate the need for succinylcholine. Limited studies have thus far been performed to evaluate the significance of this rise in ICP in a brain-injured human patient population. These have thus far shown no significant change in electroencephalographic activity or ICPs with succinylcholine; however, the small size of the studies limits the ability to draw conclusions about clinical outcomes.[131,158,159]

At present, questions concerning the safety of succinylcholine in the setting of acute intracranial pathology do not have clear answers. The drug has been used widely and successfully in this setting, and its continued use is supported by this experience. The very real risk of airway compromise and secondary cerebral insult due to hypoxia from delayed or failed intubation must always be weighed against the theoretical harmful effects. Succinylcholine, despite its many potential side effects, currently is the most frequently used agent for neuromuscular blockade in RSI owing to its rapid onset and offset and reliable muscle relaxation characteristics.

Nondepolarizing Agents

Nondepolarizing agents act in a competitive manner to block the effects of ACh at the neuromuscular junction. Drugs in this class include pancuronium, atracurium, vecuronium, mivacurium, and rocuronium. These drugs, particularly the intermediate-acting agents vecuronium and atracurium, have fewer side effects than succinylcholine and have the potential for reversal. They generally have longer onset and duration of action than succinylcholine, making them less attractive choices for RSI owing to the delay prior to muscle relaxation. In most instances, succinylcholine remains the agent of choice to facilitate emergency intubation, and nondepolarizing agents are indicated to maintain paralysis after intubation. However, knowledge of appropriate nondepolarizing NMBs is important for situations in which succinylcholine may be contraindicated.

Because nondepolarizing agents act competitively at the neuromuscular junction receptors, increasing the concentration of ACh may reverse their effects. Cholinesterase inhibitors such as neostigmine or edrophonium may be used, but will not be effective, until some spontaneous signs of reversal are seen. The concept of reversal is of limited clinical importance in the ED with rare exceptions, such as needing a neurologic examination on a previously paralyzed patient. When reversal is required, neostigmine 0.02 to 0.04 mg/kg is given by slow IV push. An additional dose of 0.01 to 0.02 mg/kg may be given in 5 minutes if reversal is incomplete, but the total dose should not exceed 5 mg in the adult. Atropine 0.01 mg/kg (with a minimum dose of 0.1 mg for children and a maximum dose of 1 mg for adults) should be given concurrently with neostigmine to block its systemic cholinergic effects.[160–162]

Long-acting Agents: Pancuronium

Pancuronium is an aminosteroid derivative that is primarily excreted in the urine within 1 hour of IV administration.[162] Classified as a long-acting agent, its onset and duration of action are dose-related. After a typical IV dose of 0.1 mg/kg, paralysis occurs within 2 to 5 minutes and lasts approximately 60 minutes. Paralysis may be maintained safely by repeated bolus or drip infusion. Because the effects of the drug are cumulative, repeating the original dose significantly lengthens the duration of paralysis.

Relatively few adverse effects are associated with the use of pancuronium. Many patients experience an increase in heart rate, blood pressure, and cardiac output because of the vagolytic effect of the drug. Ventricular tachycardia and severe hypertension have been reported, but are quite rare.[163,164] Pancuronium may cause histamine release that results in bronchospasm or anaphylactic reactions.[165] Prolonged paralysis may also occur, primarily in patients with myasthenia gravis or with significant impairment of renal function. One consensus panel recommends pancuronium for maintaining paralysis, except in patients with cardiac disease or hemodynamic instability, for whom they recommended vecuronium.[166]

Intermediate-acting Agents: Vecuronium, Atracurium, Mivacurium, and Rocuronium

Vecuronium and atracurium are intermediate-acting agents with an onset of action of about 3 minutes and a duration of action of 30 minutes. Mivacurium has an onset of action of 2 to 3 minutes and a duration of action of 15 to 20 minutes. Rocuronium has an onset of action within 1 to 1.5 minutes and a duration of action of 20 to 75 minutes (longer in geriatric patients). These drugs have minimal cardiovascular effects, cause little histamine release (with the exception of mivacurium),[131] and lack cumulative effects.[167]

The recommended doses of vecuronium, atracurium, mivacurium, and rocuronium are listed in Table 5–3. Use of larger doses hastens the onset of action, but greatly prolongs the period of paralysis. For example, vecuronium at a dose of 0.25 mg/kg intravenously will cause paralysis in as little as 1 minute, but the period of paralysis will last 1 to 3 hours.[168,169] Because a rapid onset of action comparable with that of succinylcholine is achieved at high doses of intermediate-acting agents, they may be used as the sole agents to facilitate intubation, particularly if a long period of paralysis is desired after intubation. However, the use of succinylcholine prior to intubation and an intermediate-acting agent at a normal dose after intubation provides rapid intubating conditions and better control over the duration of paralysis. Paralysis induced by vecuronium or atracurium may be maintained by repeat bolus or drip infusion. Unlike both pancuronium and succinylcholine, these agents have no side effects specifically related to repeated dosing in the ED. A repeated dose of 0.01 to 0.02 mg/kg of vecuronium will extend the period of paralysis 12 to 15 minutes.

Rocuronium, a structural analogue of vecuronium, is emerging as a desirable alternative agent for RSI when succinylcholine is contraindicated. At doses of 0.6 to 1.2 mg/kg, rocuronium consistently provides good to excellent intubating conditions within 1 minute of administration. The duration of action is dose-dependent, ranging from 20 to 75 minutes.[170,171] Smaller OR- and ED-based studies have demonstrated its clinical utility and safety in RSI protocols.[60,170–176] However, a 2003 Cochrane review[177] found that except when utilized in conjunction with propofol, rocuronium tended to produce inferior intubation conditions compared with utilizing succinylcholine for RSI.

AWAKE INTUBATION

An alternative to the induction of unconsciousness in patients requiring intubation is the use of local anesthetic and sedative agents in the conscious patient. The availability of relatively effective and safe induction agents such as etomidate make this a less attractive alternative than in the past, but these techniques may be desirable in specific patients such as fiberoptic intubation of the predicted difficult airway. Awake intubation offers a number of potential advantages over RSI. The natural airway is maintained along with spontaneous respiration and a degree of aspiration protection. The use of sedative agents to produce a state of mild or moderate sedation along with adequate topical anesthesia are the principal components needed for awake intubation.

Thomas[178] likened standard laryngoscopy in the awake patient to the "mouth being held open with a wrench." Awake nasotracheal intubation and fiberoptic intubation can also be an extremely unpleasant experience. The upper airway is richly innervated by sensory branches of the fifth, seventh, ninth, and tenth cranial nerves. In addition to pain fibers, there are stretch receptors that stimulate coughing and gagging reflexes with even minor airway manipulation. It is therefore essential that adequate analgesia be provided before intubation in all but the most extreme circumstances. Treatment options include topical application of anesthetic agents to the pharyngeal and tracheal mucosa and IV infusion of analgesic or sedative agents.

Local or topical anesthesia techniques may be used in patients who are awake, either in place of or as a supplement to IV analgesia or sedation. They are particularly useful as adjuncts to nasotracheal and fiberoptic intubation, but do not generally provide the degree of analgesia or relaxation desirable for traditional laryngoscopy. In addition, the time required to achieve good topical anesthesia may limit the usefulness of these techniques in emergency situations. Topical anesthesia may be achieved by direct application, by cricothyroid membrane puncture, or by inhalation of a nebulized anesthetic.

Direct Application

Achieving anesthesia of the oral and pharyngeal mucosa is a relatively simple procedure using commonly available agents such as 4% lidocaine or a combination production such as benzocaine, tetracaine, and butamben (Cetacaine). Achieving anesthesia of the hypopharynx is more difficult because optimal results require application of the anesthetic to the epiglottis and vocal cords.

This procedure begins with spraying the tongue and pharynx with a topical agent. Use of atomization devices that attach to standard syringes (e.g., Mucosal Atomization Device [MAD], Wolfe Tory Medical, Inc., Salt Lake City, UT) can provide effective drug dispersal without a forceful spray. The more forceful pressurized canister sprays commonly provoke a cough reflex. After allowing at least 2 to 3 minutes to achieve numbing of the tongue and pharynx, the epiglottis and vocal cords can be sprayed utilizing the MAD device with a malleable extension tube that allows the tip to pass around the base of the tongue to permit direct spraying of the epiglottis and vocal cords. This is generally well tolerated. An alternate method is to visualize the epiglottis and vocal cords using a laryngoscope and to directly spray with the anesthetic agent. The use of a laryngoscope to visualize the vocal cords is much more stimulating to the patient and often not well tolerated. Another alternative is percutaneous injection of an anesthetic agent into the trachea at the level of the cricothyroid membrane.[179,180]

Cricothyroid Membrane Puncture

Direct application of topical anesthesics to the subglottic region can also be achieved through cricothyroid membrane puncture. In this procedure, identify the cricothyroid membrane immediately below the thyroid cartilage. After antiseptic skin preparation, puncture the overlying tissue and membrane with a 22-gauge needle in the midline and just above the superior border of the cricoid cartilage. Take care to maintain the needle in the midline at all times to avoid injury to the recurrent laryngeal nerves. Advance the needle until air can be aspirated, indicating placement of the tip in the trachea. Inject a volume of 2 mL of 4% lidocaine rapidly. Alternatively, use 3 to 4 mL of 1% to 2% lidocaine, as used for local anesthesia, if the 4% concentration is not available. Typically, this will precipitate a cough, which distributes the anesthetic over the upper trachea, vocal cords, and epiglottis.

Nebulized Anesthesia

Nebulized anesthesia is a simple and painless technique that can be used to facilitate awake intubation when the patient's condition is stable enough to permit a several-minute delay. Deliver the anesthetic using a standard nebulizer and face mask connected to an oxygen source that delivers 4 to 8 L/min. Nebulize a volume of 4 mL of a 4% lidocaine solution over about 5 minutes. Bourke and associates[181] reported achieving consistently good topical anesthesia using this technique, although their patients were often premedicated with combinations of opioids and sedatives.

PREVENTING THE COMPLICATIONS OF INTUBATION

Numerous reports have highlighted physiologic responses to tracheal intubation and attempted to define their immediate or long-term adverse effects and to offer interventions to ameliorate potential organ injury. Whereas it is certain that intubation and adjunct medications will alter reflexes, ICP, blood pressure, and pulse rate and may induce cardiac rhythms disturbances, the *actual clinical consequences of these commonly observed changes are largely unknown*. Clinical experience suggests that most transient alterations in physiology that occur with ED intubation produce *no specific or readily documented long-term sequelae* or are often consequences that cannot be easily monitored or cannot be prevented. The prudent clinician is aware of the potential adverse effects of intubation and is cognizant of potential methods to minimize them. Most importantly, however, the careful monitoring of the postintubation milieu will guide specific interventions. Overzealous attempts to suppress those physiologic responses that normally accompany airway manipulation may be counterproductive and are to be avoided. Although it would be desirable to provide airway control under the best of circumstances and with the least amount of injury to the patient, at this juncture the ideal approach to the physiologic responses to intubation are simply unknown. Most information has been extrapolated from experimental animal models or from the anesthesia experience, but similar issues may not apply to the milieu of the ED experience. The following discussion serves as a general clinical guide to the previous considerations, but at this juncture no specific standard of care can be promulgated.

The Pressor Response

In addition to sinus tachycardia, a number of dysrhythmias have been reported after intubation. These are primarily ventricular in origin and include ectopic beats, bigeminy, and occasionally, short runs of ventricular tachycardia. Bradyarrhythmias have been reported uncommonly. Electrocardiographic changes suggestive of ischemia have been reported, particularly in patients with dramatic increases in blood pressure.[182,183] In 1977, Fox and colleagues[184] reported two patients, both of whom deteriorated after induction of anesthesia and orotracheal intubation. This report has been widely quoted as evidence that the pressor response should be prevented. However, no studies have reported comparative data and none has established a direct relationship between the response and the subsequent clinical deterioration in a large patient population. It is also unclear that attenuation of the pressor response will prevent dysrhythmias or electrocardiographic evidence of ischemia, although intuitively it is prudent to avoid sudden increases in blood pressure in unstable patients with acute cardiac or vascular disease.

Multiple studies have evaluated procedures to pharmacologically block the pressor response. Lidocaine has been the most extensively evaluated, but the results of these studies are inconclusive.[19,22–25] Although it appears that lidocaine given at 1.5 to 2 mg/kg may blunt the response, it is not clear that the reductions reported (10–15 mm Hg and 20 beats/min) are of any clinical significance. Other drugs, including thiopentone, sodium nitroprusside, labetalol, nitroglycerin, verapamil, nifedipine, clonidine, fentanyl, sufentanil, etomidate, and magnesium have shown variable responses.[26–35]

Of these drugs, fentanyl may be the most effective. It completely suppresses the pressor response at anesthetic doses of 50 µg/kg,[185,186] but considerably smaller doses may also be effective. Two studies have shown marked suppression of the response at doses of 5 to 6 µg/kg, although in both studies patients also received 5 mg/kg of thiopental.[18,20] Fentanyl has also been shown to blunt the pressor response when administered in conjunction with etomidate.[34] The 1998 SHRED (Sedatives and Hemodynamics during Rapid-Sequence Intubation in the Emergency Department) study evaluated the pressor response to RSI comparing thiopental, fentanyl, and midazolam as induction agents.[56] Midazolam, which was also associated with the poorest intubating conditions and most attempts required for intubation, showed a mean heart rate increase of 17 beats/min. Thiopental, likely due to its direct myocardial depressant and venodilatory effects, decreased mean arterial pressures by about 40 mm Hg. Fentanyl recipients maintained a relatively neutral hemodynamic profile during intubation. Use of paralytics during intubation did not appear to alter the hemodynamic response associated with each sedative agent. One study isolated the effect of laryngoscopy from the effect of tube passage into the trachea. Adachi and colleagues[37] found that pretreatment with 2 µg/kg of fentanyl could blunt the hemodynamic effects of tracheal tube passage, but not the hemodynamic effects of laryngoscopy.

It is important to note that even those studies demonstrating blunting of the pressor response failed to demonstrate that this provided any real benefit to the patients. It is likely that the pressor response is innocuous in the vast majority of patients, but it may be exaggerated and potentially harmful in the presence of preexisting hypertension and cardiovascular disease[184] or in patients with other vascular comorbidities such as esophageal varices in whom sudden changes in hemodynamics may be detrimental.[187] In addition, the pressor response may contribute to the rise in ICP that follows laryngoscopy, and therefore, it is potentially harmful in patients with intracranial pathology. Administration of lidocaine or fentanyl to blunt the pressor response is appropriate in these subsets of patients.

Intracranial Hypertension

Physical stimulation of the respiratory tract by maneuvers such as laryngoscopy, tracheal intubation, and endotracheal suctioning is commonly associated with a brief rise in ICP. The exact mechanism responsible for this rise is unknown. One potential mechanism is the coughing and gagging that frequently follow manipulation of the upper airway and

TABLE 5–4 Sample Protocol for Intubation for a Head-Injured Adult Patient*

1. Preoxygenate with 100% O_2 for 2–3 min.
2. Administer 1.5–2 mg/kg lidocaine IV.
3. Administer 0.01 mg/kg vecuronium or pancuronium (1 mg) (OPTIONAL).
4. Sedate with 3–5 µg/kg fentanyl.
5. Induce anesthesia with 0.3 mg/kg etomidate.
6. Paralyze with 1.5 mg/kg of succinylcholine.
7. Apply cricoid pressure and perform intubation.
8. Maintain postintubation analgesia and sedation.
9. Maintain paralysis if indicated (vecuronium 0.1 mg/kg).

*Benefit of this traditional protocol is unproved but can be supported if contraindications do not exist.

subsequent transmission of intrathoracic pressure to the cerebral circulation. An alternative explanation is the catecholamine release that accompanies laryngoscopy, causing a rise in mean arterial pressure and cerebral perfusion pressure. A small rise in ICP has also been reported after administration of succinylcholine. The value of using pretreatment with defasciculating doses of NMBs to prevent ICP rises is unknown.[41]

Although the exact significance of a transient rise in ICP is unknown, it is logical to assume that it may be detrimental in patients with head trauma or intracranial hypertension. A number of drugs including lidocaine, succinylcholine, and the majority of the anesthesia induction agents have been studied to determine whether their use prevents this response. Many of the existing clinical data are not particularly relevant to the ED setting because they are derived from patients in various stages of general anesthesia, often incorporating a wide variety of drug combinations and doses.

Good evidence suggests that deep general anesthesia prevents the rise in ICP associated with intubation, although depending on the drug used, anesthesia may compromise cardiovascular performance and critically reduce cerebral blood flow.[188–190] Consequently, the ideal anesthetic agents to facilitate intubation of patients with acute intracranial pathology may be those that have minimal effects on cardiovascular performance such as etomidate or fentanyl. Etomidate has been demonstrated to prevent changes in both cerebral perfusion pressure and ICP after tracheal intubation of patients with space-occupying intracranial lesions.[68]

At the present time, the clinical consequences of intubation-induced physiologic changes are not thoroughly understood, nor is the role of drugs in preventing these changes clear. Despite this lack of data, it may be intuitively reasonable to attempt to protect patients at theoretic risk. The approach outlined in Table 5–4 is recommended.

Acknowledgment

The editors and authors wish to acknowledge the contributions of Steven C. Dronen to this chapter in previous editions.

 REFERENCES CAN BE FOUND ON **EXPERT CONSULT**

CHAPTER 6

Cricothyrotomy and Transtracheal Jet Ventilation

Randy B. Hebert, Sudip Bose, and Sharon E. Mace

Few situations evoke more concern in the mind of the emergency department (ED) clinician than a patient's airway that cannot be controlled through traditional endotracheal (ET) intubation. Although the surgical airway is rarely required,[1-4] when the circumstances arise, the ED clinician may be required to perform this procedure under the most stressful and chaotic conditions that accompany an airway emergency.

Often, cricothyrotomy is a procedure of last resort. Both surgical cricothyrotomy and percutaneous transtracheal jet ventilation (TTJV) entail cricothyroid membrane puncture through the overlying skin to gain access to the airway. *These are not easy procedures, are not always successful, and can be nearly impossible in obese patients and those with other anatomic restrictions.*

Surgical cricothyrotomy refers to the technique in which the cricothyroid membrane is incised with a scalpel blade and a tracheostomy tube or modified ET tube is used to maintain the opening in the airway. *Needle* cricothyrotomy refers to the insertion of a catheter via percutaneous needle puncture of the cricothyroid membrane to allow a ventilation apparatus to be attached. As the name implies, *tracheostomy* differs from both of the other techniques in that access to the airway is gained between two of the tracheal rings inferior to the cricothyroid membrane. Other terms such as cricothyrostomy, laryngotomy, and cricothyroidotomy are sometimes used interchangeably with cricothyrotomy. Regardless of what technique is used, securing the airway is invariably the first step in any critical care algorithm.[5]

 BACKGROUND CAN BE FOUND ON EXPERT CONSULT

ANATOMY

The central structure of importance is the cricothyroid membrane, which is an elastic membrane located anteriorly and midline in the neck. The membrane is bordered superiorly by the thyroid cartilage and inferiorly by the cricoid cartilage. The lateral aspects of the cricothyroid membrane are partially covered by the cricothyroid muscles, but the central triangular portion is subcutaneous, making it an ideal location to access the airway.

Identify the cricothyroid membrane by first locating the prominent thyroid cartilage superior to it. The thyroid cartilage consists of two lateral laminae that join at an acute angle in the midline to form the laryngeal prominence, which is more pronounced in males and is commonly known as the "Adam's apple." The internal aspect of the anterior body of

the thyroid cartilage provides the attachment for the vocal ligaments. Superior to the thyroid cartilage and connecting it to the hyoid bone is the thyroid membrane, which allows for the passage of the superior laryngeal vessels and the internal branch of the superior laryngeal nerve through its laterally located foramina.

The cricoid cartilage forms the inferior border of the cricothyroid membrane and is the only completely circumferential cartilaginous structure of the larynx. It is composed of a broad posterior segment that tapers laterally to form a narrow anterior arch. The tracheal rings descend inferiorly to the cricoid cartilage.

Identify the cricothyroid membrane between the previously mentioned structures as a shallow depression measuring about 9 mm longitudinally and 30 mm transversely. If the depression is obscured by soft tissue swelling, estimate the location of the cricothyroid membrane at about 2 to 3 cm inferior to the laryngeal prominence or four fingerbreadths above the sternal notch.[14-16]

The area overlying and immediately adjacent to the cricothyroid membrane is relatively avascular and free of other significant anatomic structures. The cricothyroid arteries branch from the superior thyroid arteries and may form a small anastomotic arch traversing the superior aspect of the cricothyroid membrane. The external branch of the superior laryngeal nerve runs along the lateral aspect of the larynx and innervates the cricothyroid muscles inferior to the membrane. The isthmus of the thyroid gland most often overlies the second and third tracheal rings, although an aberrant pyramidal lobe of the gland may extend just superior to the cricothyroid membrane. The anterior attachments of the vocal cord structures are protected by the thyroid cartilage[17,18] (Fig. 6–1).

SURGICAL CRICOTHYROTOMY

Indications and Contraindications

The chief indication for surgical cricothyrotomy is the inability to secure the airway by noninvasive techniques in a patient with impending or ongoing hypoxia.[19]

Surgical cricothyrotomy, like any invasive procedure, has significant complications and should not be attempted until less invasive measures have failed. When the time and clinical situation allow, it may be appropriate to attempt to intubate multiple times or to try alternative intubation techniques. However, at some point, it becomes clear that further attempts at intubation become futile and the benefits of the surgical airway outweigh the risks the patient will incur from ongoing hypoxia.[20] In summary, when approaching a patient in respiratory distress, the clinician must have a clear algorithm in mind with a well-defined point at which attention is shifted from laryngoscopy to cricothyrotomy.

The anesthesia and emergency medicine literature are filled with attempts at identifying factors that accurately predict a difficult intubation. As the patient is being prepared for intubation, take a moment to look for external clues that intubation or bag-mask-valve ventilation may be difficult. Some clues include marked obesity, trauma, deformity of the face and neck, macroglossia, edema, or hemorrhage in and around the airway.[21-24] Table 6–1 is a list of relative indications for surgical cricothyrotomy. Use the "3-3-2 rule" to assess the adequacy of the oropharynx for intubation. If three fingers can be placed between the patient's upper and lower teeth with the mouth open, three fingers can be placed in the

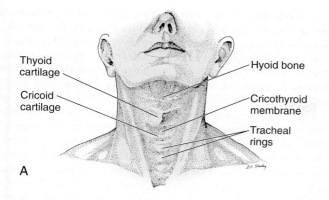

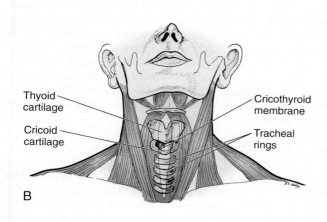

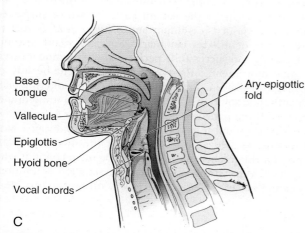

Figure 6–1 Normal adult larynx. Anatomy of the neck. *A,* Skin and superficial landmarks of the anterior neck. *B,* Muscles and cartilages of the anterior neck. *C,* Normal adult larynx. Anatomy of the neck.

TABLE 6–1 Indications for Surgical Cricothyrotomy

Failure of oral or nasal endotracheal intubation
  Massive oral, nasal, or pharyngeal hemorrhage
  Massive regurgitation or emesis
  Masseter spasm
  Clenched teeth
  Structural deformities of oropharynx (congenital or acquired)
  Stenosis of upper airway (pharynx or larynx)
  Laryngospasm
  Mass effect (cancer, tumor, polyp, web, or other mass)
Airway obstruction (partial or complete)
  Nontraumatic
    Oropharyngeal edema
    Laryngospasm
    Mass effect (cancer, tumor, polyp, web, or other mass)
  Traumatic
    Oropharyngeal edema
    Foreign body obstruction
    Laryngospasm
    Obstruction secondary to a mass effect or displacement
    Stenosis
Traumatic injuries making oral or nasal endotracheal intubation
  difficult or potentially hazardous (relative)
    Maxillofacial injuries
    Cervical spine instability
Need for prolonged intubation
Need for definitive airway during procedures on face, neck, or
  upper airway
    Laryngeal surgery
    Oral surgery
    Maxillofacial surgery
    Laser surgery
    Bronchoscopy

111

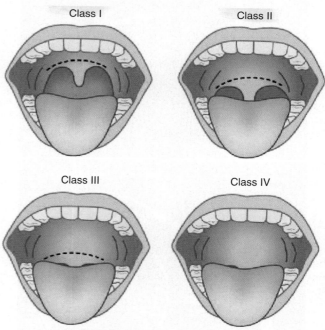

Figure 6–2 Modified Mallampati classes.

distance from the mentum to the hyoid bone, and two fingers can be placed in the space between the thyroid notch and the hyoid bone, there is sufficient space in the oropharynx to perform ET intubation.[25] Any distance shorter than that indicates a difficult intubation. Use the Mallampati score as another method to assess for a difficult intubation. It was initially developed as a preoperative examination to assess the patient's oropharynx prior to a controlled intubation in the operating room. Ask the patient to sit on the edge of the stretcher and lean slightly forward. Ask the patient to open his or her mouth as wide as possible without vocalizing. Determine the score by the degree to which the faucial pillars,

soft palate, and base of the uvula can be visualized (Fig. 6–2). Mallampati[26] concluded that the higher the score, the more difficult ET intubation would be. Unfortunately, many conditions that prohibit ET intubation also make cricothyrotomy difficult.

Given that surgical cricothyrotomy is often resorted to only after other techniques have been unsuccessful and/or the patient is not oxygenating or ventilating, most authors state that the only absolute contraindication is age. Because of the anatomic differences between children versus adults including the smaller cricothyroid membrane and the rostral funnel shaped more compliant pediatric larynx, surgical cricothyrotomy has been contraindicated in infants and young children. However, the exact age at which a surgical cricothyrotomy can be done is controversial and not well defined. Various textbooks list the lower age limit from 5 years[27] to 10 years[28] or 12 years[29] and only one of these textbooks cites any references.[30] ACLS and PALS define the infant airway as age up to 1 year, and the child airway as age 1–8 years.

Equipment

The equipment necessary to perform a traditional surgical cricothyrotomy includes a scalpel with a No. 11 blade, a Trousseau dilator, a tracheal hook, and a tracheostomy tube or modified ET tube (Fig. 6–3). Bent 18-gauge needles may substitute for tracheal hooks. In addition, the sterile tray may include a syringe and lidocaine with epinephrine for local anesthesia, sterile drapes or towels, antiseptic preparation solution, 4 × 4 sterile gauze, scissors, hemostats, and suture material.

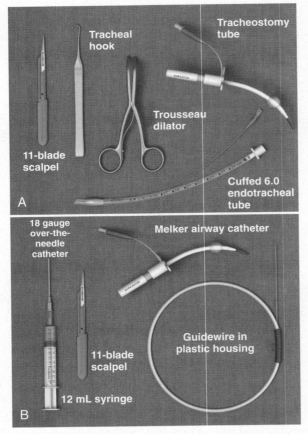

Figure 6–3 *A* and *B*, Equipment required for traditional surgical cricothyrotomy. Eighteen-gauge needles bent to 90° may be used in place of a tracheal hook. (*A and B, From Thomsen T, Setnik G [eds]: Procedures Consult—Emergency Medicine Module. Copyright 2008 Elsevier Inc. All rights reserved.*)

Given that the average adult's cricothyroid membrane is about 9 mm longitudinally and 30 mm horizontally, familiarize yourself with the dimensions of several standard tracheostomy and ET tubes in order to select the appropriate size. *Cuffed tracheostomy tubes are recommended*, and they come in various sizes. Shiley tracheostomy tubes are commonly available in most EDs. The No. 4 tube has an inner diameter of 5.0 mm and an outer diameter of 9.4 mm, and the No. 6 tube has an inner diameter of 6.4 mm and an outer diameter of 10.8 mm. Shiley tracheostomy tubes come with three parts: the cuffed outer cannula, a removable inner cannula, and a removable obturator that is solid and removed after insertion (Fig. 6–4). ET tubes are often used temporarily in place of a tracheostomy tube. ET tubes with an inner diameter of 6.0 and 8.0 mm have outer diameters of 8.2 and 10.9 mm, respectively.[31] Scalpel blades are also available in different sizes, and although a No. 11 blade is most commonly used, a No. 20 blade is recommended in some variations of the technique. Commercially available kits include the Melker Cricothyrotomy Kit for percutaneous cricothyrotomy (Melker Cricothyrotomy Kit, Cook Critical Care, Bloomington, IN) in which the Seldinger technique is used to place a cuffed or uncuffed airway catheter.

Procedure

Positioning plays a critical role in success; however, the *ideal positioning may be impossible*, based on clinical parameters. For example, hypoxic patients often cannot recline. Ketamine anesthesia does not suppress respiratory drive and may aid patient cooperation and positioning if not otherwise contraindicated. When feasible, use the supine position with the neck exposed. Unless the patient has a known or suspected cervical spine injury, it is important to *hyperextend the neck* to more readily identify the landmarks. Surgical cricothyrotomy can be safely and successfully performed with minimal cervical spine movement.[32] Preoxygenate the patient by way of bag-mask ventilation. Prepare the skin of the anterior neck with antiseptic solution and create a sterile field using drapes or towels. If the patient is awake or responding to pain, give a subcutaneous and transtracheal injection of lidocaine with epinephrine as a local anesthetic. Test the integrity of the balloon on the tracheostomy or ET tube by injecting it with 10 cc of air. Wear sterile gloves and take standard precautions by wearing a mask, goggles, and gown. All preparatory steps

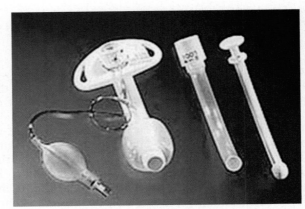

Figure 6–4 Standard Shiley tracheostomy tube with removable trocar and inner cannula.

are time permitting and depend on the urgency with which the procedure is to be performed.

Traditional Technique

Most EDs use a prepackaged kit, with or without a Seldinger apparatus. However, the "traditional" (open) cricothyrotomy technique is described here (Fig. 6–5). This technique has changed little since the original description of elective crico-

thyroidotomy by Brantigan and Grow in 1976.[12] McGill and coworkers[33] described the addition of a tracheal hook for emergency cricothyrotomy in 1982. In a follow-up report in 1989, Erlandson and associates[34] emphasized the importance of making an initial *vertical skin incision and using a relatively small (No. 4 Shiley) tracheal tube*. These modifications have generally been accepted and are commonly described as part of the traditional technique.[35]

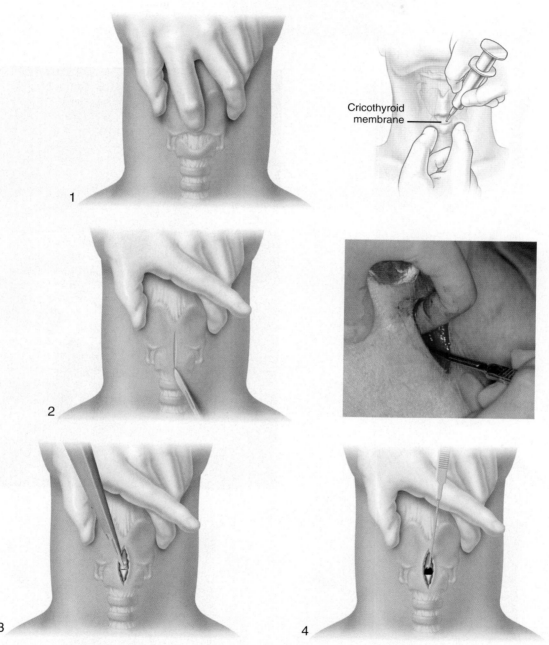

Cricothyroid membrane

Figure 6–5   Step-by-step diagram of traditional surgical cricothyrotomy. Step 1: Immobilize the larynx and palpate the cricothyroid membrane with the index finger. *Inset* to step 1: As an option to guide subsequent surgery, advance an 18-gauge needle on a syringe into the trachea, and when air is aspirated, remove the syringe and leave the needle in the trachea. Step 2: Make a *vertical* midline skin incision, 3–5 cm in length. *Inset* to step 2: Palpate the cricothyroid membrane through the skin incision to confirm anatomy. Step 3: Incise the cricothyroid membrane *horizontally*. Note that the skin incision was *vertical*. Step 4: Insert the tracheal hook and have an assistant provide upward traction. Step 5: Insert the Trousseau dilator with the blades *horizontal*, and expand the incision *vertically*. Step 6: *A,* Rotate the dilator 90° *B,* Insert the tube through the blades into the trachea. *C,* Keep the thumb on the obturator throughout the procedure. Step 7: Remove the obturator. Step 8: Replace the inner cannula and inflate the tube. *(From Custalow CB: Color Atlas of Emergency Department Procedures. Philadelphia, Elsevier Saunders, 2005.)*

Continued

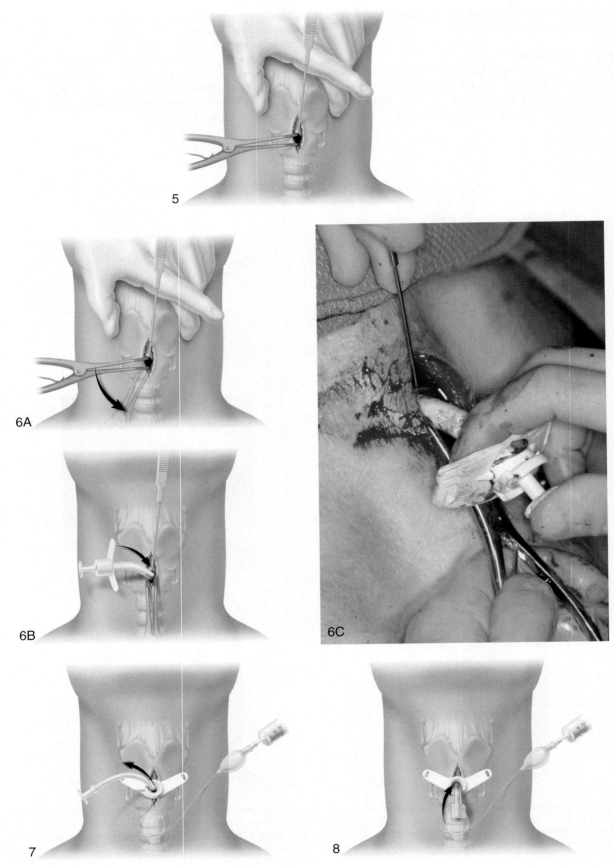

5

6A

6B

6C

7

8

Figure 6–5, cont'd

If you are right-hand dominant, stand on the patient's right side. Stabilize the larynx with the nondominant hand by grasping both sides of the lateral thyroid cartilage with the thumb and middle finger. Palpate the depression over the cricothyroid membrane with the index finger. Control the larynx throughout the procedure by stabilizing it in this manner. *At this juncture, an option is to enter the trachea through the membrane with an 18-gauge needle on a syringe (see Fig. 6–5 step 1 inset). When air is obtained, disconnect the syringe and leave the needle in place as a guide to further surgical procedures.*

Holding the scalpel with a No. 11 blade in the dominant hand, make an approximately 2- to 3-cm *vertical incision* through the skin and subcutaneous tissues (see Fig. 6–5 step 2). With the index finger of the nondominant hand, palpate the cricothyroid membrane through the incision (see Fig. 6–5 step 2 *inset*). It is important to understand that the remainder of the procedure should be performed by palpation of the anatomy, not visualization, because bleeding may obscure the field and there is no time to delay while trying to achieve hemostasis. If the cricothyroid membrane cannot be palpated, extend the initial incision superiorly and inferiorly and try to palpate again. Using the stabilizing index finger as a guide, make a *horizontal* incision of less than 1.0 cm in length through the cricothyroid membrane (see Fig. 6–5 step 3). *Note that the skin incision is vertical, but the membrane incision is horizontal.* Place the index finger into the stoma momentarily to exchange the scalpel for the tracheal hook.[36]

Using the dominant hand, place the tracheal hook into the opening in the cricothyroid membrane and grasp the inferior border of the thyroid cartilage with it. Rotate the handle cephalad and ask an assistant to provide upward traction or provide traction yourself by passing the handle of the hook to the nondominant hand (see Fig. 6–5 step 4). Use the tracheal hook to stabilize the larynx and keep it in place throughout the remainder of the procedure.

With the dominant hand, place the tips of the Trousseau dilator into the opening in the membrane with the *spreading action oriented initially in the longitudinal or vertical plane* so that the handle is facing horizontally or perpendicularly to the direction of the neck (see Fig. 6–5 step 5). It is important to note that this instrument works opposite to most ordinary instruments, such as hemostats, so that when you squeeze the handles, the blades open rather than close. This can be confusing the first time you try to use the instrument; it is worth practicing before you need it in an emergency. If this instrument is not available to you in an emergency, a Mayo scissors, a hemostat, or even the blunt end of a scalpel handle can be used to dilate the incision in the cricothyroid membrane.[37]

Dilate the incision vertically with the Trousseau dilator. There is *no need to dilate the incision horizontally* because the cricothyroid membrane is the widest (~30 mm) in this direction. Hold on to the handles of the Trousseau dilator with the nondominant hand, palm upward and *rotate the handle 90° until the handle is vertical or parallel to the neck* (see Fig. 6–5 step 6A). Perform this rotation because, if the dilator is still horizontal, the blades of the dilator prevent passage of the trachestomy tube into the trachea. Prepare the tracheostomy tube by testing the balloon, removing the inner cannula, and inserting the solid white obturator. While holding the dilator with the nondominant hand, *insert the obturator*, take the tube in the dominant hand and *insert it between the blades of the dilator* until the flanges rest against the skin of the neck (see Fig. 6–5 step 6B). Keep the thumb on the obturator throughout the procedure (see Fig. 6–5 step 6C). Carefully remove

the Trousseau dilator (see Fig. 6–5 step 7). *Insert the inner cannula* and inflate the balloon (see Fig. 6–5 step 8). Remove the tracheal hook, being especially careful not to puncture the cuff.[38,39] If a tracheostomy tube is not available, or if there is difficulty placing the tracheostomy tube into the opening in the cricothyroid membrane, try using a 6-0 cuffed ET tube cut to a shorter length. The inner–to–outer diameter ratios of tracheostomy tubes are comparable with those of ET tubes. Use of a semirigid ET tube stylet or a gum elastic bougie may facilitate the placement of an ET tube through the cricothyroid membrane into the trachea. The advantage of using the bougie is that you can get immediate confirmation that the device is inside the trachea, owing to the "washboard" vibration that the curved tip makes as it contacts the tracheal rings. The operator can modify the ET tube by cutting the distal end and replacing the adapter to the cut end (Fig. 6–6). Be careful not to cut the balloon inflation tube. If the ET tube is shortened, it is less likely to kink once it is attached to a ventilator. Advance the ET tube only about 5 cm from the tip to avoid main stem intubation. Keep in mind that standard ET tubes do not have centimeter markings at the distal end. Inserting the ET tube so that the distal cuff is about 2 cm beyond the cricothyroid membrane usually ensures proper placement.

Confirm proper placement in the same manner as with ET tube placement: end-tidal CO_2, bilateral chest movement, and breath sounds. Secure the tracheostomy tube with a circumferential tie around the neck or with sutures. Order a postprocedure portable chest x-ray.

Rapid Four-Step Technique (Brofeldt)

Brofeldt and colleagues[40] developed a rapid four-step technique (RFST) to decrease the amount of time required to establish an airway and thus reduce complications of hypoxia (Fig. 6–7). It combines aspects of traditional cricothyroidotomy and ET intubation. If you are right-hand dominant, stand at the bedside to the patient's left. Palpate the depression over the cricothyroid membrane with the nondominant hand. With the dominant hand, make a single horizontal stab incision with a No. 20 blade scalpel approximately 1.5 cm in length through the skin, the subcutaneous tissue, and the cricothyroid membrane. With the scalpel blade as a guide, pick up the cricoid cartilage with the tracheal hook and provide traction in the caudal direction to stabilize the trachea.

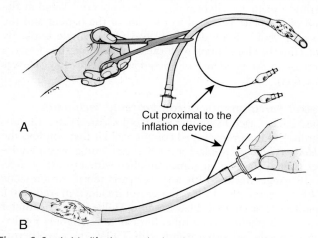

Figure 6–6 *A,* Modify the standard endotracheal tube for use in surgical cricothyrotomy. Cut the proximal ET tube end but be careful not to cut the balloon inflation apparatus. *B,* Replace the adapter on the cut end of the tube.

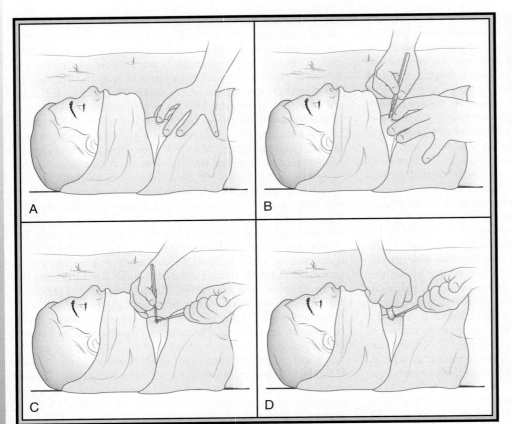

Figure 6–7 **Rapid Four-Step Technique.** *A,* Palpation. *B,* Incision. *C,* Traction. *D,* Intubation. (*A–D, Redrawn from Brofeldt BT, Panacek EA, Richards JR: An easy cricothyrotomy approach: The Rapid Four-Step Technique. Acad Emerg Med 3:1060, 1996.)*

Place a No. 4 cuffed tracheostomy tube or a 6-0 cuffed ET tube through the opening.[40] The hardest part of this modification is passing the tracheostomy tube through the smaller incision. Try advancing a gum elastic bougie (or similar introducer) into the trachea first. Then railroad the tube over the bougie with a twisting motion. The advantage of using the bougie, as noted previously, is the ease of placement and the immediate feedback (washboard feeling) of the device as it is advanced inside the trachea.

Bair and coworkers[41] modified this technique further by introducing a new device called a "Bair Claw" to replace the tracheal hook. The technique is similar to the four-step method except for advocating that the operator stand at the head of the bed instead of to the side of the patient and the use of a double-hook device instead of the single hook. By replacing the single hook with the double hook, they found a decrease in the incidence of cricoid ring fractures in cadavers (Fig. 6–8).

Melker Percutaneous Cricothyrotomy Technique

The Melker Cricothyrotomy Kit (Cook Critical Care, Bloomington, IN) is a prepackaged commercial kit that employs the *Seldinger technique* to place a tracheostomy tube over a guidewire (Fig. 6–9). The kit comes supplied with a 6-mL syringe, an 18-gauge needle with an overlying tetrafluoroethylene (TFE) catheter (the TFE catheter not included in some kits), a guidewire, a tapered dilator, and a Melker airway catheter in lieu of a tracheostomy tube. Similar to retrograde intubation or needle cricothyrotomy with TTJV, the cricothyroid membrane must be easy to identify because no initial skin incision will be made. Anatomic distortion will make locating the cricothyroid membrane with a needle more difficult.

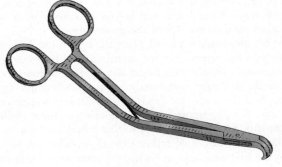

Figure 6–8 Bair Claw.

The preparation for this technique is similar to that of the other techniques. Palpate the cricothyroid membrane with the nondominant hand. With the dominant hand, attach the needle to the syringe and insert it through the cricothyroid membrane, pointing it caudally at a 45° angle relative to the skin surface. Be careful not to advance the needle too far because this may result in perforation of the posterior trachea. To help recognize when the trachea has been entered, place a small amount of saline in the syringe before the procedure. Apply gentle negative pressure while advancing the syringe. When the membrane is pierced and the trachea is entered, air will be aspirated into the syringe and bubbles will appear in the saline.

When the needle is in the trachea, pull back the syringe and needle and advance the flexible TFE catheter through the distal trachea to its hub. If the needle does not have an overlying catheter, leave the needle in place and remove the syringe. Thread the guidewire through the needle or the catheter. Once the guidewire is in place in the trachea, remove the needle or catheter. With a disposable No. 15 scalpel, make a small incision in the skin at the point at which the guidewire enters to facilitate passage of the dilator and airway catheter.

Place the gray-tipped dilator into the airway catheter and thread it over the wire as one unit. Once it is through the skin and into the trachea, advance the airway catheter to its hub

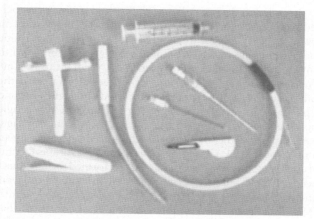

Figure 6–9 Melker Kit with Seldinger technique. *(Courtesy of Cook Critical Care, Bloomington, IN.)*

until it is flush against the neck. Remove the guidewire and dilator. Secure the kit in place with "trach tape."

Melker kits on the market differ with respect to airway catheter inner diameter and whether the airway catheter is cuffed or not. Some kits do not contain a needle with an overlying catheter[42] (Fig. 6–10).

Complications

Given that surgical cricothyrotomy is infrequently performed, under circumstances that are inherently chaotic, on a patient population who frequently has confounding medical issues and high morbidity and mortality rates, the evaluation of short- and long-term complications is difficult.[43]

Regardless of which surgical technique is used, surgical cricothyrotomies have been studied to assess what periprocedure and short-term complications occur with significant frequency. Acute complication rates have been reported between 8.7%[44] and 40%.[34] The most frequent complications are uncontrollable bleeding and misplacement of the tube.[33,45] Most bleeding is from small superficial vessels and can be controlled. Bleeding leading to significant hemorrhage can also occur as a result of the procedure. The cricoid arteries branch from the superior thyroid arteries and anastomose at the anterior superior aspect of the cricothyroid membrane. The laterally running superior thyroid arteries are more often damaged when the initial incision is broad and horizontal. To prevent hemorrhage from these vessels, make the initial incision longitudinal as in the traditional technique and maintain

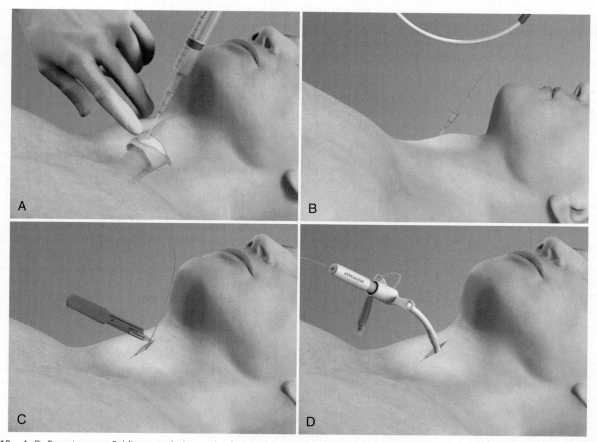

Figure 6–10 *A–D,* Percutaneous Seldinger technique cricothyrotomy using a catheter, a wire placed into the trachea, and a dilator/tube advanced over a guidewire. Make a skin incision to allow passage of the dilator. *(From Thomsen T, Setnik G [eds]: Procedures Consult—Emergency Medicine Module. Copyright 2008 Elsevier Inc. All rights reserved.)*

careful awareness of the landmarks.[46] When making the horizontal incision in the cricothyroid membrane, avoid the cricoid artery by incising the membrane at its inferior aspect. Misplacement of the tracheostomy tube or ET tube during cricothyrotomy is a concern, just as esophageal intubation is a concern with ET intubation. If the openings in the cricothyroid membrane and larynx are not carefully stabilized during the procedure, the tube may be inadvertently inserted into the subcutaneous tissue, which may be recognized by the presence of subcutaneous emphysema when attempting to ventilate the patient. It is essential to recognize this immediately to prevent the development of hypoxia. In addition, failure to detect end-tidal CO_2 and absence of breath sounds by auscultation should alert the physician to a misplaced tube. If suspected, remove the tube and reassess the airway. Misplacement of the tube during cricothyrotomy may refer to any location other than through the cricothyroid membrane, such as the larynx or trachea, but the most crucial locations are those that do not enter the airway and thus lead to hypoxia and death if unrecognized.

Many other more occult complications have been reported less frequently or have been described in case reports such as main stem bronchial intubation,[47] laryngotracheal injury,[48] tension pneumothorax,[49] and clogging of the tracheostomy tube with blood or secretions.[50] Slobodkin and associates[51] reported one case of retrograde pharyngeal intubation (Table 6–2).

Chevalier Jackson's 1921 report[11] highlighted the concern that subglottic stenosis was a major and frequent complication of cricothyrotomies. It was later refuted by Brantigan and Grow's 1976 study[13] that reported not only an overall complication rate of just 6.1% but also no occurrences of chronic subglottic stenosis as a long-term complication. Since the publication of this latter report, numerous other studies have corroborated their findings that chronic subglottic stenosis is an infrequent long-term complication of surgical cricothyrotomy.[52–56] Factors that increase the likelihood of developing subglottic stenosis include predisposing laryngotracheal pathology, prolonged time to decannulation, old age, and diabetes.[57,58]

Occurrences of long-term complications resulting in "minor airway problems" have been reported more frequently than subglottic stenosis.[59] Of these complications, subjective voice change is the most frequently reported.[60] Other reported complications include difficulty with swallowing, subjective shortness of breath, wound infection, and "noisy breathing."[61]

In order to decrease the morbidity and mortality associated with prolonged hypoxia and other factors inherent to an airway emergency, researchers have attempted to determine whether any one of the techniques is superior with regard to complication rate and time needed to secure the airway. When comparing Brofeldt and colleagues' RFST with the traditional five-step technique, Davis and colleagues[48] found an increased incidence of cricoid ring fracture when the single hook was used for cephalad traction on the cricoid cartilage, concluding that the traditional technique produced a lower complication rate. A study by Holmes and coworkers[36] comparing the same two techniques as performed by inexperienced medical students and residents on human cadavers concluded that the single-hook RFST was executed significantly faster than the traditional technique. They noted that there were more complications using the RFST but that the difference in complication rates failed to reach statistical significance. Davis and associates[62] revisited this comparison in a later study, replacing the single hook in the RFST with the double-hooked Bair Claw. The revised study showed that the airway could be secured faster using the RFST and that the complication rate was comparable, further observing that the Bair Claw did not cause any cricoid cartilage fractures.[62] Bair and colleagues' own retrospective report[63] of ED cricothyrotomy showed a lower complication rate of the RFST when compared with the traditional technique.

Similarly, consensus cannot be drawn from the literature comparing the traditional method with the percutaneous Seldinger (Melker kit) method. Some studies show no difference between time to ventilation or complication rate when the traditional technique is compared with the Seldinger technique.[64] Some studies report that the surgical method is faster than the Seldinger method,[65–68] and others conclude the opposite.[69]

Many complications of cricothyrotomy seem relatively minor compared with those caused by prolonged hypoxia. The clinician should be aware of the potential complications in order to be prepared if they do occur but not to delay performing the procedure out of fear of them. As with any invasive procedure in emergency medicine, complication rates can be reduced by maintaining a sterile field and being familiar with the techniques and anatomy.

When deciding which technique to use to perform a surgical cricothyrotomy, consider the advantages and disadvantages of each technique, the clinical scenario, equipment availability, and finally, your own comfort and familiarity with each individual technique as your guide.

Success Rates

Success rates for ED intubations are quite high (for first attempt: 90% success for all ED intubators including resi-

---

TABLE 6–2 Complications of Surgical Cricothyrotomy

Immediate or early complications
  Common
    Bleeding, hematoma
    Incorrect tube placement
    Unsuccessful tube placement
    Prolonged procedure time
    Subcutaneous emphysema
    Obstruction
  Infrequent
    Esophageal perforation
    Mediastinal perforation
    Pneumothorax, pneumomediastinum
    Vocal cord injury
    Laryngeal fracture or disruption of laryngeal cartilage
    Aspiration
Late complications
  Most common
    Obstructive problems
    Voice changes or dysphonia
    Infections
    Late bleeding
    Persistent stoma
    Subjective feeling of lump in the throat
  Infrequent complications
    Subglottic or glottic stenosis
    Tracheoesophageal fistula
    Tracheomalacia

dents, 98% success rate if an attending), with a "rescue" cricothyrotomy performed only 0.7% of the time according to the National Emergency Airway Registry.[3] For pediatric patients, the success rate for the first attempt for all ED intubators is slightly less at 85% with a rescue cricothyrotomy performed less than 1% of the time (1 of 156 patients).[70]

The success rate for cricothyrotomy similarly has been quite high (89%–100%) in most studies,[24,33,34,43,50,53,63,71] although one study found only a 62.5% success rate.[72] The incidence of failed cricothyrotomy (e.g., the tube is misplaced into pretracheal space/failed attempts) is 3.6% in the ED in one study,[63] with earlier ED studies in the 7.9% to 10% range.[33,34] In the prehospital setting, the reported cricothyrotomy failure rates are 6% to 12% for paramedics,[24,43,71] 0% for clinicians[53] and 32% to 38% for flight nurses.[63,72] One of these studies found the incidence of tube misplacement into the pretracheal space to be 3.6% in the ED versus 31.8% for the air medical transport service at the same institution.[63] In a cadaver, the first-time performance of cricothyrotomy by intensive care unit clinicians comparing a standard surgical cricothyrotomy with the Seldinger technique found successful tracheal placement in only 70% for the standard technique and 60% for the Seldinger technique.[64] In an animal model, paramedics had a 90.9% success rate using a percutaneous technique and a 100% success rate with the open surgical technique.[66]

TTJV

TTJV is a procedure in which oxygen is delivered through a catheter inserted through the cricothyroid membrane. Anatomically, the cricothyroid membrane is part of the larynx and the trachea begins at the cricoid cartilage, but the term *transtracheal jet ventilation* is generally used to refer to supplying oxygen through the cricothyroid membrane. To maintain consistency, this terminology is used in this chapter. The use of TTJV to ventilate and oxygenate a patient in a crash airway situation differs from surgical cricothyrotomy in some ways. For TTJV, the initial needle cricothyrotomy does not differ greatly from that used for the Seldinger technique variation of cricothyrotomy. *Jet ventilation* means that oxygen is administered through a small-caliber catheter, usually on the order of a 12- to 14-gauge catheter, rather than through a relatively larger-caliber tracheostomy tube. The method by which oxygen is supplied through a needle-inserted catheter has evolved over the recent years, moving from one of continuous oxygen flow, which provided adequate oxygenation but not ventilation,[73] to one of shorter bursts of oxygen flow followed by passive exhalation to resemble a more physiologic respiratory state.

Indications and Contraindications

The indications and contraindications for needle cricothyrotomy with TTJV are similar to those for surgical cricothyrotomy. Needle cricothyrotomy with TTJV can be used in place of surgical cricothyrotomy in adults in the same failed airway scenarios. Its indications include failed attempts at ET intubation with the inability to bag-mask ventilate or airway obstruction above the level of the cricothyroid membrane. Needle cricothyrotomy may be relatively indicated over surgical cricothyrotomy in adults based on the operator's experience. Much of the otolaryngology literature supports the use of TTJV as a means of nonemergent ventilation during head

and neck surgeries owing to the fact that the smaller ventilation catheter provides a relatively unobstructed field to work around.[74-76] With regard to an emergent airway situation, needle cricothyrotomy has been shown to be a successful bridge to establishing an airway via the ET route.[77] Case reports describe TTJV to be relatively indicated over the more invasive surgical cricothyrotomy when ET intubation has failed owing to copious oropharyngeal secretions. Providing temporary ventilation through the needle catheter may allow sufficient time to clear the upper airway of secretions or obstructions, giving the operator more time to establish an ET intubation.[78]

As mentioned previously, surgical cricothyrotomy is contraindicated in infants and young children. The contraindication arises from the fact that the cricothyroid membrane is too small to insert a tracheostomy tube and there is a significant risk of injury to the surrounding structures. Therefore, needle cricothyrotomy is the preferred method of securing the airway in crash airway situations in infants and young children.[79]

Absolute contraindications to needle cricothyrotomy in adults include transection of the distal trachea, because the airway would need to be established below this injury. Complete upper airway (oropharyngeal) obstruction may be considered a contraindication to needle cricothyrotomy because there is nowhere for exhaled gas to escape, thus leading to a buildup of CO_2 and increased lung volumes.[80] The operator may, therefore, elect to perform a surgical cricothyrotomy if this situation presents itself.

Equipment

The essential materials needed for TTJV include a needle with an overlying catheter, oxygen tubing, an oxygen source with a means to regulate the pressure, and a means to connect the apparatus together.

Commercial kits are available, but a standard 12- or 14-gauge angiocath attached to a 3- or 5-mL syringe normally found in the ED can be used to make the puncture through the cricothyroid membrane; then the catheter can be left in place to serve as the conduit for oxygen delivery. The larger the diameter of the catheter, the greater the oxygen flow will be, depending on the method of oxygen delivery.[81] Commercial catheters such as wire-coiled nonkinking catheters and fenestrated catheters are available as part of prearranged kits (Fig. 6–11). Larger-caliber 3.0- to 4.0-mm interior diameter percutaneous tracheal catheter devices are also available.

There are two different basic means, and thus two different armories of equipment to choose from, to deliver oxygen through the transtracheal catheter. In one method, use a standard ventilation bag to supply oxygen through the needle. This requires the constant efforts of manual bag insufflation as long as the patient is being oxygenated and ventilated this way. Attach the bag to the adapter of a 7.0-mm ET tube inserted into the back of a plungerless 3-mL syringe connected to the transtracheal catheter. Alternatively, attach the bag directly to the catheter with the adapter of a 3.5-mm pediatric ET tube.[82] An inherent problem with this setup is that the whole system is rigid. Although the transtracheal catheter itself is flexible, there is no flexibility or give from the hub of the catheter to the bag. Thus, slight movements of the bag relative to the patient may cause dislodgment of the catheter. To ameliorate this obstacle, connect standard intravenous infusion tubing directly to the transtracheal cath-

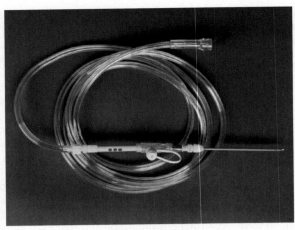

Figure 6–11 ENK oxygen flow modulator set. *(Courtesy of Cook Critical Care, Bloomington, IN.)*

eter and attach the distal cut end to a 2.5-mm ET tube attached to the bag.

In an alternative method, supply oxygen from a standard 50-psi wall source. High-pressure oxygen tubing is needed to connect the system with a manual on/off valve along with a Luer-Lok or three-way stopcock to connect the oxygen tubing to the hub of the catheter. The on/off valve can be as simple as holes placed at the end of the oxygen tubing (see Fig. 6–11) that the operator manually covers in order to control oxygen flow through the catheter and the inspiratory-to-expiratory (I/E) ratio. A pressure gauge connected to a hand-triggered jet injector may also be used to control the amount of air pressure reaching the catheter.[83] Commercial kits are available that contain prepackaged systems already assembled. Otherwise, assemble the apparatus in the ED. In an emergency situation, it is unlikely that one would be able to assemble a TTJV apparatus from individual components in a timely manner. If a prepackaged TTJV kit is not available, prepare the appropriate components from the ED ahead of time and place it with other airway supplies for easy access.

Assemble additional equipment such as antiseptic preparation solution, sterile drapes, sterile gauze, and suture material or trach tape in the kit.

Procedure

As with the surgical cricothyrotomy technique, place the patient in the supine position with the neck exposed. Prepare the skin of the anterior neck. Wear appropriate protective equipment such as sterile gloves, gown, and protective eye and face shield. Hyperextend the patient's neck unless a suspected cervical spine injury prohibits it. Infiltrate the skin with local anesthetic.

Similar to the needle insertion technique employed for guidewire-assisted surgical cricothyrotomy, locate the cricothyroid membrane with the nondominant hand by locating the thyroid cartilage and cricoid cartilage and palpating the cricothyroid membrane in the depression between these, keeping in mind that this depression will be proportionally smaller in children.

Attach a 12- to 14-gauge angiocath to a 3- or 5-mL syringe filled with 1 to 2 mL of saline or lidocaine. Once the cricothyroid membrane has been located, insert the catheter

through the overlying skin, subcutaneous tissue, and membrane directed at a 30° to 45° angle caudally. While doing so, aspirate gently with the syringe (Fig. 6–12). The cricothyroid membrane has been pierced and the airway entered when bubbles are seen in the fluid or there is an increase in the ease with which air is aspirated. Once through the membrane, hold the needle in place and advance the catheter to the hub, then remove the needle. Hold the catheter by hand until the oxygen supply is connected and appropriate placement is confirmed. Make sure that the hub of the catheter is flush against the skin to avoid air leak and then secure it with a circumferential tie around the neck. Keep one hand on the hub of the catheter until the entire procedure is completed and the airway is secured to prevent it from being dislodged.

Oxygen can be supplied to the catheter in two different ways. The choice of whether to use the ventilation bag setup or the high-flow oxygen system is determined primarily by what tidal volumes are needed to ventilate the patient. The high-flow oxygen system connects to *a wall oxygen source at full output* and provides a maximal output pressure of 50 psi. When connected through a 14-gauge catheter, a pressure of 50 psi will flow at 1600 mL/sec. Therefore, if you want to provide a tidal volume of 10 mL/kg in an 80-kg adult (800 mL/breath), you must provide 0.5 second of oxygen flow per cycle. The operator also controls the I : E ratio by letting go of the distal openings in the oxygen tubing or of the jet injector valve.[35] Commercial kits are available (Figs. 6–13 and 6–14).

With the ventilation bag, you manually inflate the lungs through the catheter. Children, especially those under 5 years old, have small total lung capacities and need smaller tidal volumes; therefore, the bag should be used instead of the jet ventilator to prevent barotrauma. Using this setup, you can control the volume of air inspired and adjust it breath-by-breath based on chest wall motion and pulse oximetry. This method is not appropriate for adults because the operator cannot both provide appropriate tidal volumes and allow enough time for exhalation[84,85] (Fig. 6–15).

Complications

As with any invasive procedures, TTJV and needle cricothyrotomy are associated with certain risks and complications. The clinician should be aware of these potential risks and balance them against the need to reverse ongoing hypoxia in a critical patient. An important and debated concern regarding TTJV is that it is regarded as only a temporizing measure, owing in part because it is labor-intensive, but more so because of its inability to provide adequate ventilation for a long period of time. It has been reported that TTJV in adults inevitably causes retention of CO_2, leading to acidemia because of poor ventilation despite adequate oxygenation. This assumption may be a remnant of earlier oxygenation techniques in which continuous low-flow "apneic oxygenation" was used without ventilation.[86] Many animal studies show that adequate ventilation, and thus normal blood pH and normal arterial CO_2 partial pressure, can be maintained with TTJV for 30 or even 60 minutes.[87-92] Factors that seem to improve ventilation are increased expiratory time[93] and high-flow oxygen source.[94] Even with regard to partial or nearly complete oropharyngeal obstruction, adequate ventilation has been achieved.[95,96] Unfortunately, none of these studies looked at ventilation for extended periods of time.

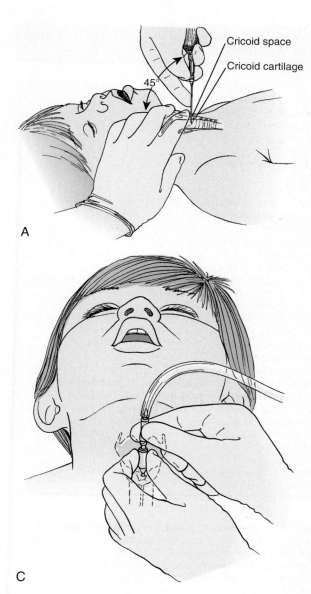

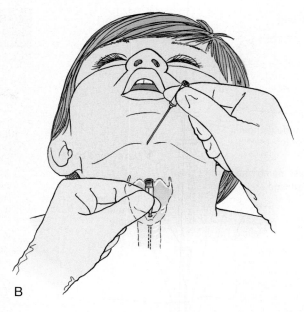

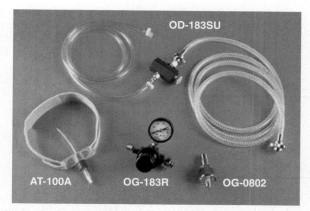

Figure 6–12 **Transtracheal jet ventilation with needle/catheter.** *A,* Puncture the cricothyroid membrane with a large needle (12–14 gauge). Aim caudally at a 45° angle. *B,* Once the airway has been entered remove the needle, leaving the catheter in the trachea. *C,* Attach a high-pressure oxygen source, such as wall oxygen, at maximal output.

Figure 6–13 Commercially available transtracheal jet ventilation (TTJV) kit (Life-Assist, Inc; Rancho Cordova, CA) with manual jet ventilator, pressure gauge, adapter, and 14-gauge angiocath with secure tie.

There have been reports of mechanical failure with the materials used for TTJV, one of which is catheter kinking.[97] A number of solutions have been proposed to prevent this from occurring. There is a commercially available wire-coiled catheter that does not kink as readily as the standard angio-cath found in the ED. One study found that if the distal 2.5 cm of the tip of the catheter is bent at 15° anteriorly and if a greater angle of insertion relative to the skin surface is used, the catheter has less of a chance of kinking while it is being advanced into the trachea.[98] It has also been proposed that a 7- or 9-French vessel dilator be used instead of an angiocath to prevent kinking.[99]

Although needle cricothyrotomy may involve less trauma to the skin surface and anterior laryngotracheal structures than surgical cricothyrotomy, the force one must apply to puncture the cricothyroid membrane is proportional to the caliber of the needle being used. Larger-bore needles carry with them a higher risk of perforating the posterior trachea.[100] Barotrauma is a significant risk associated with TTJV and occurs when there is upper airway obstruction that does not allow air to be passively exhaled. This causes an increase in

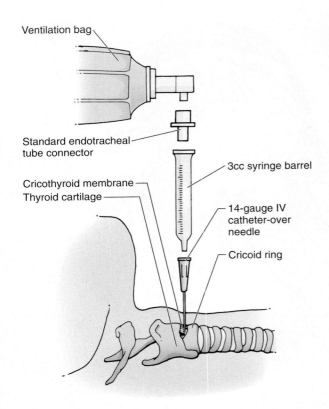

Ventilation bag

Standard endotracheal
tube connector

Cricothyroid membrane
Thyroid cartilage

3cc syringe barrel

14-gauge IV
catheter-over
needle

Cricoid ring

Figure 6–14 Homemade ventilation setup for transtracheal catheter ventilation using a ventilation bag, a standard endotracheal tube adapter, a 3-mL syringe, and a 14-gauge angiocath.

TABLE 6–3 Complications of Percutaneous Translaryngeal Jet Ventilation

Common
  Subcutaneous emphysema—most common (less occurrence if there is a "secure" fit at the skin)
  Kinking of the catheter
  Blockage or obstruction of the catheter
  Coughing (in a conscious patient)
Infrequent
  Bleeding (minor), hematoma
  Infections
  Aspiration
  Incorrect or unsuccessful catheter placement
  Prolonged procedure time
  Persistent stoma
  Subjective feeling of a "lump in the throat"
  Pneumatocele
Serious, rare complications
  Barotrauma (secondary to high airway pressures, more common with complete airway obstruction)
  Pneumothorax
  Pneumomediastinum (less occurrence if high airway pressures are avoided, and not performed with complete airway obstruction)
  Mediastinal perforation
  Esophageal perforation
  Dysphonia or voice changes (secondary to vocal cord injury, laryngeal fracture, or disruption of laryngeal cartilage)
Potential or theoretical complications (not yet commonly associated with percutaneous translaryngeal jet ventilation, although reported with tracheostomy and other airway procedures)
  Subglottic/glottic stenosis
  Tracheoesophageal fistula
  Damage to laryngotracheal mucosa (such as tracheobronchitis)
  Swallowing problems

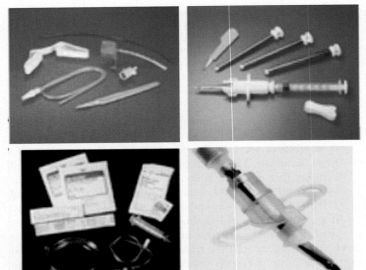

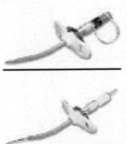

Figure 6–15 Commercially available cricothyrotomy kits. From left to right: *A*, Portex Mini-Trach II Cricothyrotomy Kit. *B*, Portex Nu-Trach Adult Cricothyrotomy Kit. *C*, Rusch, Inc. Quicktrach. *D*, Life-Assist, Inc. L/A Emergency Cricothyrotomy Kit. *E*, Ravussin. *F*, Patil Emergency Cricothyrotomy Set. *G*, Arndt Emergency Cricothyrotomy Set.

lung volumes and pressures, leading to lung injury.[101,102] Other reported complications include minor bleeding, malposition of the catheter, subcutaneous emphysema, dislodgment of the catheter, and pneumothorax.[103,104]

One would assume that a transtracheally placed catheter would not afford any airway protection against aspiration in that the diameter of the catheter is not nearly large enough to occlude the lumen of the trachea. However, a few studies have shown a decreased rate of aspiration in dog models that were ventilated with TTJV versus control animals not ventilated, suggesting some airway protection from this mode of ventilation[105,106] (Table 6–3).

Commercial hybrid kits, such as the Quicktrach, combine qualities of both cricothyrotomy and TTJV. They have the

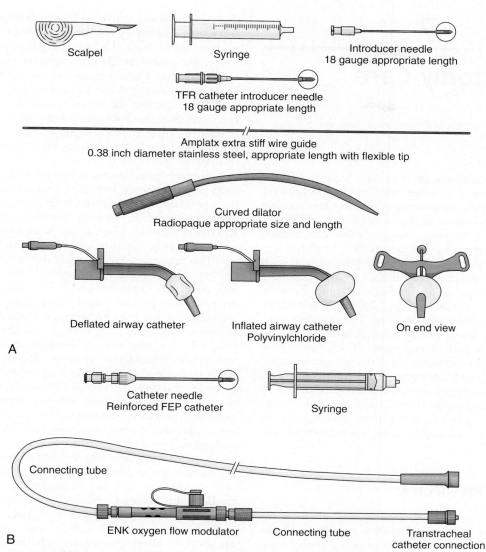

Scalpel

Syringe

Introducer needle
18 gauge appropriate length

TFR catheter introducer needle
18 gauge appropriate length

Amplatx extra stiff wire guide
0.38 inch diameter stainless steel, appropriate length with flexible tip

Curved dilator
Radiopaque appropriate size and length

Deflated airway catheter

Inflated airway catheter
Polyvinylchloride

On end view

A

Catheter needle
Reinforced FEP catheter

Syringe

Connecting tube

ENK oxygen flow modulator

Connecting tube

Transtracheal
catheter connection

B

Figure 6–16 Having a commercial kit for cricothyrotomy (Melker, Cook Critical Care) (*A*) and TTJK (ENK, Cook Critical Care) (*B*) prominently displayed in the resuscitation room or crash cart makes these techniques readily available in an emergency. (*A and B, Courtesy of Cook Critical Care, Bloomington, IN.*)

123

advantage of being relatively easy to use if the clinician is inexperienced with the technique of surgical cricothyrotomy and they may have fewer complications with regard to the actual insertion process.[107] Unfortunately, most of these transtracheal hybrid kits contain small uncuffed catheters. Studies pertaining to these hybrid kits suggest that their small caliber may prevent adequate ventilation and the lack of a cuff permits

insufflated air to escape through the oropharynx above[108] (Fig. 6-16; see also Fig. 16–15).

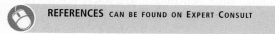

REFERENCES CAN BE FOUND ON **EXPERT CONSULT**

CHAPTER **7**

Tracheostomy Care

Kathleen A. Neacy

Advances in health care now allow patients with tracheostomies to live at home or in other relatively low technology environments including rehabilitation facilities and nursing homes. Daily medical care is delivered by a variety of caregivers, including family members, home health care nurses, patient care technicians, or lay caregivers.[1] Tracheostomy patients frequently present to the emergency department (ED) with a variety of complaints related to the care and suctioning of their tracheostomy, including displaced tube, hypoxia, respiratory distress, mucous plugs, increased secretions, bleeding, or postoperative complications. The emergency clinician's evaluation, based on the clinical scenario, should include anticipation and management of life-threatening complications as well as problems arising from routine tracheostomy care. This chapter discusses tracheostomy equipment, hygiene, suctioning, late postoperative complications, procedures, and techniques helpful in managing routine and emergent tracheostomy problems. In addition, specific pediatric tracheal suctioning techniques and considerations are reviewed.

BACKGROUND AND SURGICAL CONSIDERATIONS

Mortality associated with tracheostomy is low. Most tracheostomies are performed electively, with a postoperative complication rate of 10% to 40%.[2] The complication rate for emergent tracheotomy is severalfold higher than that reported with elective tracheostomy.[3] The elective surgical site is located between either the first and second or the second and third tracheal rings. With open tracheostomy, the anterior trachea is generally sutured to the skin until tract maturation occurs, 4 to 5 days postprocedure. Percutaneous dilational tracheostomy (PDT) eliminates the need to transport critically ill patients to the operating room. In addition, the use of blunt dissection and dilation, combined with a tightly fitting tracheostomy tube, contributes to a lower postoperative bleeding rate.[4] However, the smaller stoma created with PDT may lead to complications such as difficult replacement if it becomes dislodged in the immediate postoperative period and stomal occlusion or stenosis.

TRACHEAL ANATOMY AND PHYSIOLOGY

The lower respiratory tract begins at the vocal cords; inferior to the cords is the cricoid cartilage, encasing a 1.5- to 2-cm region known as the subglottic space. Inferior to the cricoid cartilage is the trachea. The adult trachea is approximately 10 to 12 cm in length. Forming the anterior and lateral walls of the trachea are 18 to 22 incomplete cartilaginous rings. A fibromuscular sheet completes the posterior wall, which lies anterior to the esophagus. The interior diameter of the adult trachea is approximately 12 to 25 mm; it is lined with mucosa, covered by respiratory epithelium.[5] The blood supply to the trachea comes from the branches of the inferior thyroid artery, the innominate (brachiocephalic), bronchial, and subclavian arteries. The innominate artery lies in close proximity to the tracheostomy stoma. From its origin at the aortic arch, it courses between the sternum and the anterior trachea, veering right at the sternomanubrial joint. The location of the innominate artery is important because erosion of the anterior tracheal wall can lead to a major life-threatening bleed from this artery.

The recurrent laryngeal nerve supplies innervation to most of the intrinsic laryngeal muscles and innervates the mucosa below the vocal cords. Efferent vagal fibers stimulate bronchoconstriction, mucosal secretions, and vasodilatation. Efferent sympathetic fibers of the pulmonary plexus stimulate tracheal bronchodilatation and vasoconstriction.

The upper airway, including the oropharynx and nasal passages, filters particulate matter, humidifies inspired air, and aids in the expectoration of secretions. These functions are reduced in patients with a tracheostomy.[6] Placement of a tracheostomy bypasses humidification and results in the formation of thick, dry secretions.[7] In the absence of adequate humidification, the trachea develops squamous metaplasia and chronic inflammatory changes.[8] Bronchoconstriction can result if the inspired air temperature is below the room temperature, resulting in reduced airflow. Normal mucociliary clearance is often impaired owing to increased viscosity of respiratory secretions, underlying chronic illness, and respiratory infections, particularly owing to *Mycoplasma* or viral pathogens.[9]

Tracheostomy weakens the anterior tracheal wall, allowing possible tracheal collapse. The cough mechanism, important in tracheal secretory clearance, is often blunted in tracheostomy patients.[9] Normally, the epiglottis and vocal cords close to trap air in the lungs and raise intrathoracic pressure prior to a cough. Patients with a tracheostomy tube are generally unable to generate sufficient pressure to initiate a strong cough and facilitate airway clearance.[10] Physiologic positive end-expiratory pressure (PEEP) is eliminated in patients who are unable to maintain a closed glottis.

Immune responses are often blunted in patients with tracheostomies owing to underlying illnesses, chemotherapy, or acquired immunosuppression. Pulmonary macrophage and polymorphonuclear cell functions are impaired.[9]

EVALUATION OF THE TRACHEOSTOMY PATIENT

Undertake a thorough assessment of the airway, respiratory status, and the indwelling device in all ED patients with a tracheostomy who have a respiratory complaint. Consider tube occlusion, dislodgment, or fracture. Verify snug placement of the tracheostomy tube, the presence of blood or secretions, the integrity of the skin at the tracheostomy site, and the patient's ability to speak or mentate. Perform a rapid physical examination to differentiate between tracheostomy complications and other etiologies for the basis of the patient's problem.

Obtain historical components such as the indications for tracheostomy placement, the length of time from tracheostomy to ED presentation, and previous complications. Search for other historical considerations such as planned or existing voice prosthesis surgeries, previous bleeding complications or strictures, and whether permanent tracheostomy or decannulation of the tracheostomy site is anticipated. Ask whether there have been any changes in the efficacy of home ventilator or tracheostomy care to help identify potential problems, including increased oxygen use, increased suctioning, equipment failure, or skill in out-of-hospital tube changes.

COMPLICATIONS OF TRACHEOSTOMY

The incidence of important complications after tracheostomy has been reported between 5% and 40%, with higher complication rates occurring in emergency procedures than in elective ones.[11] This section addresses only late postoperative complications because patients with immediate and early postoperative (≤4 wk postoperative) are generally hospitalized and rarely present to the ED.[12]

ED management of late postoperative tracheostomy complications requires familiarity with bleeding, obstructive, and infectious complications as well as management of tube dislodgment, equipment failure, and anatomic complications such as stenosis and tracheoesophageal (TE) fistula.

Bleeding

Bleeding complications account for 20% of ED tracheostomy presentations.[13] Minor bleeding occurs in 30% to 40% of patients, and 0.2% to 10% have massive or life-threatening bleeding complications.[5,14,15] Sources of bleeding include small superficial blood vessels at the tracheostomy site, granulation tissue, thyroid vessels, anterior jugular veins, and the bracheocephalic (innominate) artery. Bleeding from esophageal or gastric sources may present as tracheal bleeding if a TE fistula is present[5] or if the patient has aspirated blood. Erosion of a major vessel from the cuff or tip of the tube is responsible for 10% of all tracheostomy hemorrhage and for most tracheostomy-related deaths. The innominate artery is the vessel most commonly involved.[16] Thyroid artery bleeding occurs in 5% of patients during the immediate postoperative period, but rarely accounts for ED presentations.

Early bleeding, within the first 4 weeks postoperatively, is most commonly incisional. However, 85% of tracheoinnominate artery fistula bleeds are reported within the 1st postoperative month.[5] Development of a tracheoinnominate artery fistula occurs in approximately 2% of patients with tracheostomies and has a 50% to 75% mortality rate, despite identification and emergent management.[13,14] The innominate artery crosses from left to right as it moves superiorly and lies immediately anterior to the trachea at the level of the superior thoracic inlet. Risk factors for developing a tracheoinnominate artery fistula include placement of the tracheostomy stoma below the third tracheal ring, caudal migration of the tracheostomy tube from leverage on the tube, and presence of a more cephalad-coursing innominate artery, the latter occurring more commonly in thin, young patients.[13] Pressure exerted by the distal tracheostomy tube or cuff causes erosion of the anterior tracheal wall into the vessel, with subsequent bleeding. *Be alert to the possibility that brisk bleeding from the tracheostomy, hemoptysis, or a history of either complaint may signal a life-threatening bleed. Many patients experience a "sentinel" bleed hours or days before a catastrophic bleed.* Some patients report only a new cough or retrosternal pain.[16] Presume that any history or evidence of 10 mL or more of blood is arterial.

Attempt to visualize the bleeding site in stable patients. Look for a bleeding innominate artery at or below the sternal notch, in the anterior tracheal wall. If significant tracheal bleeding is present, hyperinflate the tracheal cuff in an attempt to compress the artery against the sternal wall. If this is unsuccessful, insert an endotracheal tube through the oropharynx, with the balloon positioned at the level of the upper sternum, and hyperinflate it. For continued bleeding, apply digital pressure through the tracheal stoma, compressing the anterior tracheal wall against the sternum (Fig. 7–1). Digital pressure is considered the most reliable technique to stop hemorrhage[13] and may provide control of bleeding during transport to the operating room. Emergent surgical consultation is mandatory.

Management of Minor Bleeds

Even minor bleeding from a tracheostomy site should be evaluated for a potential life-threatening event. Seemingly minor or self-limited bleeding may be a harbinger of subsequent severe hemorrhage. So-called sentinel hemorrhages, minor in nature, frequently preceed massive bleeding complications. Such potential may require an endoscopic examination for complete evaluation unless a superficial bleeding site is confirmed. Incisional bleeding or bleeding from granulation tissue is usually confined to the skin surrounding the stoma. Bloody secretions issuing from the tra-

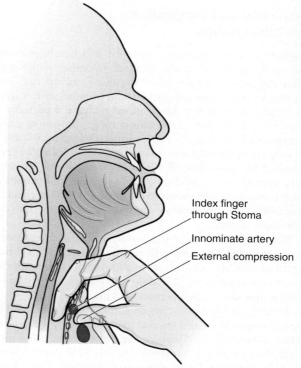

Index finger through Stoma

Innominate artery

External compression

Figure 7–1 **Control of innominate artery bleeding by digital pressure.** Be aware that minor bleeding may be a sentinel event, and a harbinger of a subsequent major hemorrhage. When major bleeding occurs and a cuffed tracheostomy tube is present, overinflation of the tube cuff may temporize (see text). When this is unsuccessful or a cuffed tube is not available, use the illustrated maneuver; digital pressure should be applied to the *anterior tracheal wall through the tracheostomy.* The index finger is placed within the trachea and then pulled against the anterior tracheal wall, allowing the airway to remain partially open. The artery is compressed between the index finger and the thumb—placed over the neck. Digital compression of the innominate artery is a temporizing procedure, until definitive (operative management) of the bleed is obtained.

cheostomy tube may represent diffuse tracheitis, rundown bleeding from the skin or thyroid, or superficial tracheal ulceration from tracheal suctioning or tracheal tube pressure. Examine the stoma site and tube gauze to help find the source and volume of blood loss. Visualize the tracheal lumen, proximal trachea, and inner stoma with a nasopharyngoscope or a small pediatric laryngoscope. It is important to differentiate superficial erosions from active bleeding. Do not disturb clots in the trachea, because this may increase the rate of hemorrhage.

Control incisional or stomal bleeding by cauterization, packing the wound with gauze, petroleum jelly,[14] or application of silver nitrate. After examination and management of minor bleeding, replace the tracheostomy tube. Following tube replacement, suction carefully to confirm resolution of superficial bleeding or to identify secondary sources of bleeding.

If stomal bleeding or intratracheal sites do not account for the bleeding, consider other sites. Place a nasogastric (NG) tube to identify gastrointestinal bleeding. Examine the nasopharynx and oropharynx for possible bleeding sources. If the patient has had radiation therapy, examine the area above the level of the tracheostomy stoma where mucosal bleeding from the therapy may be causing blood to be present in the tracheal secretions.

Obstruction and Complications from Tube Changes

Obstruction of the tracheostomy tube is a common complication; it can occur at the external opening of the tube, within the inner cannula, or at the distal end of the outer cannula. Any tracheostomy patient who presents with respiratory distress should first be assumed to have a partially or completely obstructed tracheostomy tube.[17] Improper maintenance and poor attention to routine tracheostomy care in the outpatient setting are common, and a plugged tube accounted for more than 30% of ED presentations for respiratory distress in one review.[13] Some patients and caretakers do not understand the principles of tracheostomy care and fail to routinely clean the tube or fail to understand the function of the inner cannula.

Plugging occurs most commonly with dried respiratory secretions and, less often, with blood or aspirated materials. Secretions may act as a ball valve, allowing air in but restricting outward ventilation.[5] Granuloma formation just distal to the tube may also cause obstruction.

Administer high-flow oxygen and prepare for immediate tube exchange. Manually remove obstructions at the external tracheal tube opening. Remove the inner cannula and clean off dried secretions. If no inner cannula is in place, suction the tracheostomy tube to remove obstructing plugs. Instill normal saline to loosen thick secretions with a *critical* patient, but this is no longer recommended in routine suctioning.[18,19] If evidence of obstruction persists, remove the outer tube and replace it. If the patient has persistent respiratory insufficiency despite these maneuvers, consider other etiologies for the patient's complaints.[17]

Emergency clinicians may adapt a technique described by Rumbak and coworkers[20] to evaluate a patient for obstruction, if suctioning or replacing the tube does not relieve the patient's symptoms. Prior to hospital discharge, Rumbak and cowork-

ers[20] evaluated tracheostomy patients with a trial of occluding their tracheostomy catheter with the tracheal cuff deflated. If the patient developed significant hemodynamic changes (>15% change in respiratory rate, heart rate, or blood pressure), oxygen desaturation of less than 90%, other signs of respiratory distress, or diaphoresis under observation, she or he was investigated for potentially obstructive tracheal lesions (e.g., granulation tissue, tracheal stenosis, tumor, edema). Surgical intervention or downsizing of the tracheal tube was undertaken before the patient was released. A modification of their protocol in the ED after clearing the secretions and resolution of obstructive symptoms will identify patients at risk for subsequent airway obstruction and for whom further otolaryngologic consultation is warranted.

Dislodgment

Tracheal tube displacement can occur when traction is placed on the tube, especially when it is manipulated for Ambu bag or ventilator connections. Long tracheostomy tubes can be dislodged inferiorly, causing the tip to abut the mucosal wall of the trachea or obstruct at the level of the carina. First, determine that the tube flanges rest snugly at the skin. Lateral neck x-rays may reveal that the tracheostomy tube opening abuts the anterior tracheal wall or obstructs the tracheal lumen. Gently manipulate the tube or reposition it to resolve the obstruction. Because flexion of the neck can cause downward displacement of the tube by as much as 3 to 4 cm,[14] gently extend the patient's neck to restore airflow. Secure tracheal tubes connected to respirators with tube supports or holding arms.

False Passage

Creation of a false lumen can occur during tracheal tube replacement or during repositioning of a dislodged tube. Subcutaneous air, crepitus, or distortion of the anterior neck landmarks may indicate placement of the tracheostomy tube into a soft tissue lumen anterior to the trachea. Abdominal distention after bagging may indicate tracheal tube placement through a TE fistula. Remove and replace the tracheostomy tube expeditiously if a false passage is suspected.

Equipment Failure

Cuff Problems and Tube Fracture

Fracture. Tracheostomy tubes fracture infrequently. These fractures occur most often at the juncture of the flange and the tube connection.[21] A fractured tube fragment may displace inferiorly, obstructing the tracheal lumen. To manage this problem, replace the tube if possible and consider bronchoscopy for retrieval of the tube fragment, if present.[22] Cardiac complications have been reported with aspiration of tracheostomy tubes.[22]

Tracheal Cuff Complications. Complications related to the tracheal tube cuff include cuff perforation, resulting in poor seal and increased aspiration risk; overinflation, causing pressure on or impingement of the esophageal lumen; and distention of the cuff distal to the tracheal tube, causing obstruction of the tracheal tube opening. Mucosal injury is much less common since the use of low-pressure cuffs have become standard. Pain with ventilation or swallowing, inadequate oxygenation despite correct tube placement, or presence of gastric secretions in the tracheostomy tube may indicate cuff problems. Verify appropriate inflation pressures (18–23 mm Hg) and cuff position. If the symptoms persist, replace the tube.

Infection

The long-term ventilated patient is at high risk for nosocomial pneumonia and tracheobronchitis. In general, the frequency of infection increases with the duration of mechanical ventilation, but risk is highest in the 1st week of intubation and in patients with acute illnesses. Nonventilated tracheostomy patients are at increased risk for pneumonia, tracheobronchitis, stomal infections, and soft tissue infections. Infections are common in patients with tracheostomies and account for approximately 50% of ED presentations.[13] Risk factors for systemic infection include host-defense impairment and exposure to large numbers of bacteria that bypass the upper airway defense systems. Upper respiratory secretions, in healthy patients, are colonized by normal oropharyngeal flora. In tracheostomized patients, the secretions are subject to evolution from normal flora to more virulent pathogens.[23] Most infections of the lower respiratory tract are preceded by airway colonization with enteric gram negative (EGN) bacteria. The most commonly cultured organisms from tracheostomy stomas and tubes are *Pseudomonas aeruginosa* and *Staphylococcus aureus*. Colonization rates are high in these patients, even in the absence of systemic infection. Risk factors for developing infection are numerous. The presence of the tracheostomy tube bypasses the natural protective barriers of the upper airway for filtering bacteria. Suctioning a colonized tracheostomy tube can force bacteria into the lower airways. Underlying medical conditions, impaired host-defense mechanisms, and poor nutrition all increase susceptibility to infection. Alterations in neurologic function or swallowing predispose patients to aspiration, as does maintenance of a ventilated patient in the supine position. Some degree of aspiration occurs in 65% to 85% of all patients with tracheostomies,[24] even in the presence of a cuffed tracheostomy tube. Patients undergoing chemotherapy generally have defects in neutrophil number or function. Alveolar macrophages have decreased ability to produce pro-inflammatory cytokines in response to a bacterial challenge. Impaired mononuclear cell function also contributes to the patient's decreased ability to fight bacterial infection.[23] If infection occurs, it generally involves highly resistant gram-negative or gram-positive organisms. In one study, extended postoperative prophylactic antibiotics did not decrease the rate of pulmonary infection.[25] Ventilated surgical intensive care unit patients have been reported to have a higher rate of ventilator-associated pneumonia than other intensive care unit patients[26] with *Pseudomonas* and *Staphylococcus* species being most commonly isolated in this population, with high resistance rates in these organisms. Knowledge of the patient's hospital course and previous infections can help identify and guide treatment of lower respiratory infections.

Hackeling and associates[13] reported 18 ED patients diagnosed with tracheostomy-related infections. Four had paratracheal cellulitis, and 14 were diagnosed with bronchitis, tracheitis, or pneumonia. The infectious agents cultured most frequently in tracheostomy-induced cellulitis included *S. aureus*, *Pseudomonas* species, and *Monilia*.[13] Consideration should also be given for possible *Candida albicans* in patients previously treated with one or more courses of antibiotics or underlying immunocompromised state.

Peristomal cellulitis can usually be treated with oral outpatient antibiotics. The most feared complications from cellulitis are mediastinitis, mediastinal abscess, and paratracheal abscess. Pain with breathing or swallowing or signs of systemic infection should be investigated for these complications, usually by obtaining a computed tomography (CT) scan. Deep neck infections are a risk for patients with diabetes. Huang and colleagues[27] identified different organisms and outcomes for diabetic patients with deep neck infections: *Klebsiella* pneumonia was more common in diabetic patients and *Streptococcus viridans* more common in nondiabetics.

It is essential to accurately identify infectious organisms from carefully obtained sputum samples from these patients. Obtain tracheal suctioning samples of sputum for Gram stain and culture during the patient's evaluation. Obtain blood cultures, depending on patient presentation, and institute infection control protocols. Obtain radiologic studies as indicated, including chest x-rays and CT scans for suspected soft tissue infections.

Administer systemic antibiotics in conjunction with adjuvant aerosol therapy.[28] In Hackeling and associates' review,[13] all tracheostomy patients with infections other than cellulitis were admitted for intravenous antibiotics. Depending on the patient's presentation, a cautious approach to management of infections in this population seems warranted.

Anatomic Complications and Considerations

Tracheal Stenosis and Tracheomalacia

Tracheal stenosis and tracheomalacia are late complications of tracheostomy and often present weeks to months after decannulation. Tracheal stenosis can occur at the subglottic area, stoma, or cuff.[14] Pressure on the tracheal lumen from the tracheostomy tube or cuff can cause epithelial destruction, tracheitis, ulceration, persistent inflammation, and subsequent stenosis.[14] Rigid tube systems with excessive motion and pressure points can lead to stenosis at the stoma site.[14] Cough, retained secretions, and progressive dyspnea on exertion usually herald the onset of clinically significant stenosis. Symptoms become evident when the tracheal diameter is narrowed by 50% to 75%. Stridor typically occurs when the tracheal lumen is less than 5 mm.[14]

Weakening of the tracheal cartilages from pressure necrosis may cause luminal widening and tracheomalacia. Tracheostomy tube loosening can result, as can tracheal collapse. Pediatric patients are less able to tolerate cartilaginous weakening and tracheomalacia.

Cuff overinflation and tracheal wall dilatation can be detected on chest radiography.[14] Tracheal stenosis can be accurately identified in the ED using laryngoscopy.[13] CT scans are not sensitive in detecting stenosis. Definitive diagnosis is obtained by bronchoscopy, with operative dilation of the stenosis or resection of granulomatous tissue being the most common treatment.

Relief of any associated respiratory compromise is problematic because a high-grade stenosis may make endotracheal intubation difficult or impossible. If attempts to intubate fail owing to this type of obstruction, temporizing measures can be taken while awaiting transport to the operating room. Place the patient on high-flow humidified oxygen and position the patient with the head elevated. Administer nebulized bronchodilators or racemic epinephrine if possible because this may be helpful.

TE Fistula

Early TE fistulas can occur if a puncture wound or small laceration is made in the anterior esophagus during tracheostomy surgeries. Delayed TE fistula can occur from a poorly fitting tracheostomy tube impinging on an NG tube through the common wall of the anterior esophagus. Most patients with a TE fistula present with increased secretions, pneumonia, or evidence of aspiration of gastric contents when they are on mechanical ventilation. Patients may complain of coughing after swallowing. Symptoms of a TE fistula include a persistent leak around the cuff, abdominal distention, or evidence of aspiration. The clinician may be able to auscultate breath sounds simultaneously over the lung fields and the epigastrium. Bronchoscopy or swallowing studies can aid in making the diagnosis. If a TE fistula is suspected, inflate the cuff below the level of the fistula to decrease the tracheobronchial secretions. Definitive treatment is surgical, and specialty consult is warranted.[29]

ROUTINE TRACHEOSTOMY CARE

Routine tracheostomy care is focused on maintaining a patent tube while removing respiratory secretions. Most tracheostomy tube obstructions occur from the accumulation of dried secretions at the distal tube tip or within the inner cannula. Intermittent or continuous inhalation of humidified air decreases mucus viscosity and reduces the accumulation of secretions.

The routine cleaning of the tube and inner cannula can effectively reduce accumulation of dried secretions. The inner cannula fits snugly into the tracheostomy tube and can be easily removed without disturbing tracheal tube placement. Soak it in hydrogen peroxide solution for 10 to 15 minutes and then scrub it lightly with a soft brush to remove crusted secretions.[7] Clean the tracheostomy tube flanges with dilute hydrogen peroxide if dried blood or secretions have accumulated. Thoroughly rinse all airway equipment in sterile saline before reinserting because hydrogen peroxide may cause mucosal irritation and increased tracheal secretions.[10]

Suction alone is the best way to initially remove excess secretions. Instillation of normal saline into the tracheostomy tube to loosen secretions is no longer recommended for routine suctioning. Saline and mucus are immiscible. The common practice of instilling 5 to 10 mL of sterile saline may potentially hamper oxygenation, especially during suctioning. Instilling sterile saline elicits a cough in most patients, usually preceded by forceful inspiration that may draw loose airway material and organisms into the lower respiratory tract. Dislodgment of the tube encrustations by a similar mechanism may have the same undesirable effect. For these reasons, instillation of saline for routine tracheostomy care is discouraged.[18,19,30] However, use a small amount of saline for thick secretions that do not respond to routine suctioning. The administration of supplemental oxygen can generally control any mild hypoxia associated with aspiration of the small amount of saline used to soften the thick secretions.

Enhance stomal wound care by changing the tube ties that have been contaminated with secretions, by routine cleansing of the tube flanges, and by using precut tracheostomy gauze. Loose fibers from hand-cut gauze may induce inflammatory changes at the stomal site.[10]

CHANGING A TRACHEOSTOMY TUBE

Indications

Tracheostomy tract maturation is generally completed by 5 days postoperatively. Because most tracheostomy patients who present to the ED do so beyond this timeframe,[13] routine changes of most tracheostomy tubes can be safely done in the ED. Indication for tracheostomy tube exchange include cuff rupture or leak, peritubal leak caused by tracheomalacia, complete or partial tube occlusion, or conversion to an alternate tube style (e.g., unfenestrated to fenestrated).[31] Routine cleaning of the tube also requires removal and exchange.

Few contraindications to tube exchange exist. The clinician should consider whether further tissue trauma or hemorrhage might occur as a result of the procedure[31] and anticipate possible complications, including loss of the airway, before undertaking the tube exchange. Tracheostomy tube changes should not necessarily be done on a predetermined schedule, but rather as clinical symptoms warrant.

Equipment and Setup

Tracheostomy tubes can be metal or plastic. Metal tubes are constructed of silver or stainless steel; metal tubes lack both a cuff and a 15-mm connector for attachment to a ventilator or Ambu bag. Plastic tubes are either polyvinylchloride, which softens at body temperature, or silicon, which is naturally soft and unaffected by temperature.

Tracheostomy Tube Components

Sizing. Dimensions of tracheostomy tubes are given by their internal diameter (ID), outside diameter (OD), length, and curvature. The sizes of some tubes are given by Jackson size, which refers to the length and tapering of the OD. This sizing method applies to metal tubes and most Shiley dual-cannula tracheostomy tubes. Single-cannula tracheostomy tubes are sized by the ID of the outer cannula at its smallest dimension. If an inner cannula is required for connection to a ventilator, the published ID is the ID of the inner cannula. The size of the tracheostomy tube is usually stamped on the flange of the outer cannula of the tracheostomy tube and indicates the tube's ID. In preparation for tube changes, have the tracheostomy tube in the patient's size and one or two sizes smaller available. Table 7–1 lists recommended sizes for tracheostomy tubes.

Components. Tracheostomy tubes have three standard components: the outer cannula, the obturator, and the inner cannula (Fig. 7–2). Once the tube is in place, secure the outer cannula to the patient's neck. Note that each of the two flanges of the outer cannula has a tape eyelet for tethering the tube to the patient's neck. Look for the size of the tracheostomy tube stamped on the outer cannula flange. The outer cannula is the most permanent portion of the tracheostomy tube. Leave it in place unless complications arise or a tube change is needed. The obturator is white, rounded or cone-shaped, and when inserted into the outer cannula, extends several millimeters beyond the distal port of the tube. Use the obturator to facilitate insertion of the tracheostomy tube. When it is in place, it occludes the tube lumen and no air exchange can take place. Remove the obturator once the outer

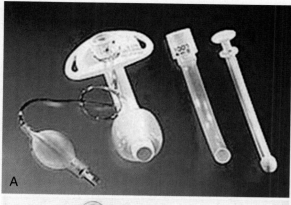

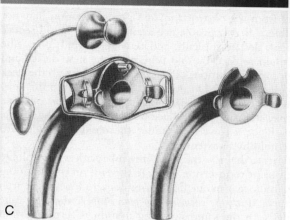

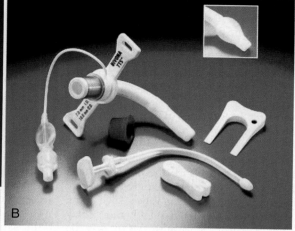

Figure 7–2 *A,* Shiley tracheostomy tube with inner cannula and obturator removed. *For normal patient use, an inner cannula should always be in place,* but some patients cannot understand this basic concept. A common cause of dyspnea is mucous plugging of the tube itself because a cannula has not been used or plugging of the smaller-diameter inner cannula, which should be removed and cleaned regularly. *B,* Bivona TTS tracheostomy tube with inner cannula in place. *Note:* The inner cannula will accept an Ambu bag when ventilation is required. If the inner cannula is not in place, the patient *cannot be bagged.* In such cases, remove and temporarily replace the tracheostomy tube with a standard endotracheal tube. *C,* A metal tube with inner cannula. The patient cannot be ventilated with positive pressure through this tube because it will not accept an Ambu bag.

129

TABLE 7–1 Tracheostomy Tube Recommended Sizes

Age	Size	Inner Diameter (mm)	Outer Diameter (mm)
Premature	00	3.1	4.5
Newborn–3 mo	0	3.4	5.0
3–10 mo	1	3.7	5.5
10–12 mo	2	4.1	6.0
13–24 mo	3	4.8	7.0
2–9 yr	4	5.0	8.5
10–11 yr	6	7.0	10.0
≥12 yr	≥6		
	8	8.5	12.0
	10	9.0	13.0

Adapted from Mullins JB, Templer JW, Kong J, et al: Airway resistance and work of breathing in tracheostomy tubes. Laryngoscope 103:1367, 1993.

cannula is seated in the tracheal lumen. Next, insert the inner cannula into the outer cannula once the obturator has been removed. Finally, using the standard 15-mm respiratory connector, attach the inner cannula to the bag-valve device or ventilator. Air exchange is accomplished through the lumen of the inner cannula. *It is imperative to note that the inner cannula contains the adapter for a standard Ambu bag. Without the inner cannula, effective ventilations cannot be maintained because a seal cannot be obtained between the Ambu bag and the outer cannula.* The inner cannula is the only portion of the tube that is routinely removed, cleaned of secretions, and replaced to provide the airway.

Tracheostomy tubes can be cuffed or uncuffed. Cuffed tracheostomy tubes are used for patients on long-term mechanical ventilation or those at risk for aspiration. In addition to preventing ventilatory volume loss during positive-pressure ventilation and reducing the risk of aspiration, inflation of the cuff prevents diversion of expired air across the vocal cords; therefore, speech is not possible with cuffed tubes. Most low-volume, high-pressure cuffs have been replaced by high-volume, low-pressure cuffs that reduce mucosal injury and the risk of tracheal erosion or stenosis,[32] although some authors advocate low-volume, low-pressure cuffs to reduce aspiration risk.[12,33] Inflate the cuff by attaching a syringe to the Luer-Lok port at the proximal end of the pilot balloon. Determine the cuff pressure by connecting the Luer-Lok port to a manometer. Recommended cuff pressures are between 20 and 25 mm Hg.[34] Assess for a leak around the cuff by auscultating over the suprasternal notch or the lateral neck.

Uncuffed tubes can be used in patients with adequate ventilatory effort who are awake and at low risk of aspiration. Depending on the size of the tracheostomy tube and how much of the tracheal diameter the tube fills, air can bypass the tracheostomy tube and be transmitted across the vocal cords. Digital occlusion of the tracheostomy, or use of specialized valves attached to the tube opening, can occlude expired air from the tracheostomy, and facilitate voice production. Certain tracheostomy tubes have single or multiple fenestrations, which allow air to be transmitted across the vocal cords. Fenestrations are generally located at the superior, posterior arch of the tracheostomy tube and are sometimes also found on the inner cannula.

Secure the tube in place by ties that tether the flange and tighten them so that one finger can be placed snugly between the tracheostomy ties and the patient's skin.

Humidifiers, Tracheal Buttons, and Endotracheal Tubes

Ventilated patients can obtain tracheal humidification from in-line humidifiers. Ambulatory patients are often fitted with a heat-moisture exchanger, which attaches to the external opening of the tracheostomy tube. These devices serve to capture the patient's own humidity on exhalation so that it can be inspired on inhalation.

Tracheal buttons are devices used during weaning to maintain stomal patency or retained permanently if decannulation is not possible. They have a hollow outer cannula and a solid inner cannula and extend from the outer skin into the tracheal lumen. Tracheal buttons can become displaced into the tracheal lumen if not correctly tethered and may become clogged with secretions.[35] Speaking valves, such as the Passy-Muir (Passy-Muir, Inc., Irvine, CA) or the Shiley Phonate (Mallinckrodt Medical, St. Louis, MO), may be present. These devices generally clip or twist on to the 15-mm coupling of the tracheostomy tube or inner cannula. Remove speaking valves before changing a tracheostomy tube.

In an emergency, if the proper-sized replacement tracheostomy tube is not available, use a standard *endotracheal* tube as a temporary replacement. Use a smaller tube than would be used for orotracheal intubation. In an adult, a 6- to 7.5-size tube may be accommodated by the stoma and trachea. Do not advance the tube more than is necessary to provide ventilation. Cautiously inflate the cuff to ensure a proper seal.

Procedure

Assemble the tracheostomy and adjunct airway supplies and equipment at the bedside before beginning the procedure. The flange on the patient's indwelling tracheostomy tube will have a size stamped on it. Prepare this size and one or two sizes smaller. Inspect the component parts prior to use. They should fit together easily, and if a cuff is present, check it for leaks. Prepare a nasopharyngoscope or red rubber catheter to facilitate tube exchange if a modified Seldinger technique is used (Fig. 7–3). Assemble additional airway equipment such as endotracheal tubes, laryngoscope, suction catheters, and oxygen at the bedside in case difficulties in tube exchange are encountered. A list of recommended equipment is outlined in Table 7–1. Use soft restraints or anxiolytic medications if needed.

Preoxygenate the patient prior to tube exchange, either by providing supplemental oxygen with a face mask applied over the tracheal stoma or by manual bagging. However, a patient who has significant tube obstruction requires immediate relief from the obstruction, and preoxygenation may not be possible.[17] If two people are available, one should secure the patient, deflate the cuff, and remove the old tube. The other should replace the old tube with the new device and assess for proper position.[36] Position the patient with the neck slightly *hyperextended*. Do not flex the neck because this may misalign the tissues and hamper attempts at tube passage. Adults may sit or lie down. Place small children in the supine position. Place a towel roll under the child's shoulders to facilitate mild hyperextension.

Lubricate the new tracheostomy tube with water-soluble lubricant prior to insertion. Deflate the cuff on the outgoing tube and remove it in one fluid movement, following the arch of the tube. *With the obturator in place*, insert the new tube smoothly, with the same sweeping motion. Use the motion of the wrist to simulate the curve of the tube as it advances (Fig. 7–4). Apply gentle pressure with an arclike motion, advancing the cannula posteriorly and downward until the flanges are flush against the neck.[36] Use a tracheal hook or a dilator to help hold the stoma open. Remove the obturator immediately and place the inner cannula inside the tube. Do

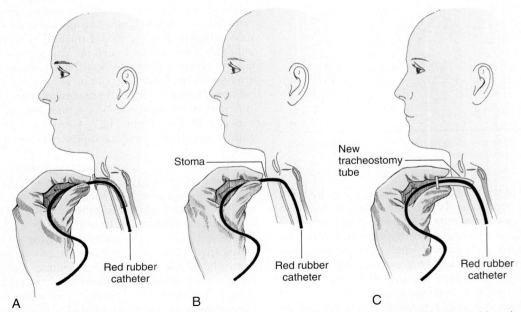

Figure 7–3   Changing a tracheostomy tube. *A*, Before the old tube is removed, a small red rubber catheter (or other guide catheter) is passed into the proximal trachea. *B*, The tracheostomy tube has been removed over the catheter, and only the catheter remains in the trachea. The catheter serves as a guide for easy and atraumatic insertion of a new tube. Note that the neck should be slightly hyperextended. *C*, A new tracheostomy tube, without the obturator, is threaded over the guide catheter; once the tube is in place, the catheter is removed. Similarly, if the tracheostomy tube has already been removed, the catheter may be passed through the stoma before a new tube is advanced. Note that an obturator or inner cannula is not used when changing a tube with this technique.

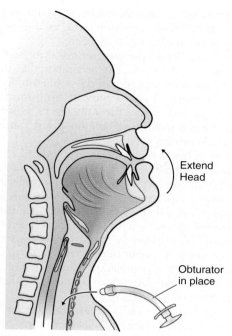

Extend
Head

Obturator
in place

Figure 7–4 The tracheostomy tube should be inserted with a gentle rocking motion of the wrist. Insertion should follow the curve of the tube, as shown. If any resistance is met during insertion, the clinician should discontinue insertion and identify the obstruction. A pediatric laryngoscope or other light source may be helpful in visualizing the tracheal lumen prior to insertion. *(Adapted from Hackeling T, Triana R, Ma O, et al: Emergency care of patients with tracheostomies: A 7-year review. Am J Emerg Med 16:681, 1998.)*

not force placement and stop the insertion if resistance is met. Creating a false passage into the soft tissue planes of the neck or posterior trachea with potentially devastating consequences is possible.

A modified Seldinger technique can also be used to replace a tube. Thread a small-diameter (≤14-Fr) red rubber catheter through the indwelling tracheostomy tube, and hold it in place while the original tube is removed.[37] Thread the new tube, without an obturator, over the catheter until it is seated in the trachea. Remove the red rubber catheter. Weinmann and Bander[31] reported a modified Seldinger technique using an airway exchange catheter that allows jet or bag ventilation into the trachea during tube exchange. This adjunct provides intratracheal oxygen delivery if hypoxemia is a threat.

If a tube is being replaced after accidental dislodgment, it may be more difficult to visualize the stoma. Insert a pediatric laryngoscope blade with a light source to assist in exploration of the wound and visualization of the airway.[13]

Following tube insertion, remove the obturator and insert the inner cannula. Note that the obturator occludes the lumen of the tube and so it should be immediately removed. Conversely, the patient can breathe normally with only the outer cannula in place. Apply tracheal tube ties with the patient's neck in slight flexion. Tighten the tethers enough so that only one finger can fit between the patient's neck and the tube tie.

Confirm correct tube placement by patient reassessment and auscultation of inspiratory and expiratory breath sounds. The clinician should be able to feel, as well as hear, breaths

coming out of the tube when it is correctly placed.[13] Visual confirmation of placement can be done by inserting a nasopharyngoscope through the tube. Visualization of the tracheal rings verifies intraluminal position.

TRACHEAL SUCTIONING

The goal of tracheal suctioning is to remove secretions or aspirated material from the upper airway in patients whose cough is impaired or in whom an artificial airway is in place. Tracheal suctioning can be performed through an orotracheal or tracheostomy tube, through a minitracheostomy in the cricothyroid membrane, or through the nasopharynx. Indications, basic procedures, and complications are similar with each technique.

Indications and Contraindications

The accumulation of secretions or aspirated material in the trachea impairs gas exchange and promotes atelectasis. Patients with obstructive pulmonary disease, bacterial infections, and pulmonary edema are prone to develop increased secretions. Patients with a decreased level of consciousness, respiratory muscle weakness, pain, or an artificial airway often have cough reflexes that are ineffective in clearing airway secretions.[38]

The primary indications for tracheal suctioning is to remove secretions in order to enhance oxygenation or to obtain samples of lower respiratory tract secretions for diagnostic tests.[17] In the ED, perform tracheal suctioning after endotracheal intubation to clear the airway of aspirated material or secretions or to enhance oxygenation in a tracheostomy patient with respiratory insufficiency.

Perform bronchopulmonary toilet when secretions are visible in the endotracheal tube or at the orifice of the tracheostomy tube. Perform tracheal suctioning when the patient has coarse rales, rhonchi, or tubular breath sounds; acute or worsening dyspnea; or arterial oxygen desaturation.[17] Suction patients when clinical symptoms warrant rather than routinely according to a predetermined schedule.[38–40]

Relative contraindications to tracheal suctioning include severe bronchospasm, which may worsen with suctioning, and persistently elevated intracranial pressure (ICP), which is exacerbated by suctioning.[39] Bronchodilators, sedatives, or paralytics may alleviate the symptoms mentioned previously. Tracheal suctioning should be undertaken with caution in patients with cardiovascular instability owing to the risk of inducing dysrhythmias. However, when oxygenation is significantly impaired, expeditious suctioning should be done using techniques that minimize these potential complications.[17]

Equipment

Suction catheters are available in different lengths, diameters, and configurations of distal ports. Choose a size whose diameter does not exceed half the ID of the tracheostomy tube. To calculate the catheter size needed, take the ID of the tracheostomy tube, divide by two, and then multiply by three to obtain the French size. For example, a size 8 tracheostomy tube would accommodate a 12-French suction catheter.[41] The OD of the catheter may be identified on the packaging as well. If the catheter is too small, it will not adequately remove secretions, and if it is too large, it will obstruct airflow around the catheter during insertion. Evacuation of airway gases by an oversized catheter may result in alveolar collapse and hypoxemia.

Catheter tips are designed to maximize removal of secretions without causing mucosal invagination and trauma. Tips may have single or multiple side ports, usually proximal to the distal tip. Coudé tips are available that allow selective suctioning of main stem bronchi. Most authors agree that mucosal injury from suctioning is related not to the tip design but to vigorous or extensive suctioning at high vacuum pressures.[10,39]

A closed-system airway encases a suction catheter in a sterile sheath attached to ventilator tubing, which allows tracheal suctioning to be performed without interrupting ventilatory support. In high-risk patients, including those requiring PEEP to maintain oxygenation, continued ventilatory support might reduce the risk of suction-induced hypoxia and dysrhythmias.[39] Closed-system catheters are reusable and are changed every 24 hours. They have not been shown to increase the risk of nosocomial pneumonia.[39]

Check suction tubing and vacuum settings before the procedure. Optimal vacuum settings should provide effective removal of secretions while minimizing mucosal trauma. Current recommendations are 60 to 80 mm Hg for infants, 80 to 120 mm Hg for children, and 120 to 150 mm Hg for adults.[39,42]

To assess suction pressures, obstruct the catheter by kinking the distal segment and simultaneously occluding the side thumb port while the catheter is attached to wall suction. Assess catheter patency by suctioning sterile saline through the catheter prior to tracheal suctioning.

Gather additional equipment helpful for nasotracheal suctioning including nasal trumpets, water-soluble lubricant, and topical anesthetic agents. Sterile sputum traps can be used if sputum samples will be sent for microbiology or cytology studies.

Procedure

Use sterile technique throughout all suctioning procedures. Inspect equipment prior to use. Unless contraindicated, elevate the head of the patient's bed to maximize diaphragmatic excursion.

Preoxygenate the patient prior to suctioning. For a non–ventilator-dependent patient, apply humidified air through a face mask placed over the tracheostomy.[7] Set the flow rate of the oxygen to 10 to 15 L/min through the face mask. For patients who are suctioned nasotracheally or through a mini-tracheostomy, place the face mask over both the nose and the mouth. Move the face mask to the mouth only for nasal insertion of the catheter. Ask the patient to take 5 to 10 deep breaths of 100% oxygen before suctioning and between aspirations.[38]

Preoxygenate ventilated patients by increasing the forced inspiratory oxygen (FI_{O_2}; to 100%), tidal volume, and respiratory rate.[10,43] Most ventilators require a 1- to 2-minute "washout" period before new FI_{O_2} levels are reached, so bag the patient just before suctioning. Deliver 4 to 10 breaths before each suctioning pass and after completing the entire procedure.

Hyperinflation and hyperventilation carry the risk of overdistention lung injury so anticipate that pneumothorax is a complication that can occur during preoxygenation.

Insert the catheter into the trachea very smoothly, without applying suction.[42] Some common terms used to describe the techniques of suctioning the trachea are

Shallow suctioning: Insert the catheter just into the hub of the tracheostomy tube to remove secretions that the patient has coughed to the opening of the tracheostomy tube.

Premeasured technique: Using a catheter with side holes close to the distal end, insert the catheter to a premeasured depth, with the most distal side holes just exiting the tip of the tracheostomy tube.

Deep suctioning: Insert the catheter deeply until resistance is met, then withdraw the catheter slightly before suction is applied. Irritation of the carina typically elicits a vigorous cough reflex, which should be allowed to subside before proceeding. Animal studies demonstrate denuded epithelium and inflammation where deep suctioning is routinely performed.[44] Consensus in the pediatric literature clearly supports using a premeasured technique to minimize mucosal trauma and granulation tissue if present,[44] and the clinician can extrapolate this to the adult population if the clinical situation supports it.

Apply suction as the catheter is withdrawn, and limit this to 10 to 15 seconds' duration. Some authors recommend intermittent application in place of continuous suctioning.[42] Gently rotate the catheter as it is withdrawn to facilitate removal of secretions. Flush the catheter with sterile saline between passes, and oxygenate the patient between suctioning attempts. Do not pass suction more than three times in succession.

Do not instill saline into the tracheal tube to elicit a cough or loosen secretions because this practice is no longer supported in the literature.[40,42] The viscosity of airway secretions does not change with saline instillation.[18] Systemic hydration and application of humidified air will decrease mucus viscosity more effectively. In addition, instillation of saline can have a detrimental effect on oxygenation, which may last up to 5 minutes postprocedure.[19] Theoretically, the cough stimulated by saline instillation may drive secretions or microorganisms into the lower airway.[18]

The recommendations presented earlier also do not address the scenario of an ED patient with a critical airway obstruction due to inspissated secretions. Of note, Hudak and coworkers[45] studied oxygen saturation and the amount of secretions suctioned, with and without saline instillation prior to suctioning. The mean weight of secretions removed increased after instillation of saline, but it was not clear whether mucus or recovered saline accounted for the increased weight. They reported no instances of oxygen desaturation as a result of saline instillation prior to suctioning. The usual instillation of 5 to 10 mL of saline is consistent with volumes infused during endotracheal drug administration, which are generally well tolerated. Nonetheless, when saline instillation is used for unusually thick secretions in a patient with respiratory symptoms, supplemental oxygen is advised.

Extract clotted blood, or other thick secretions not removed by suctioning, with a 6-French Foley catheter. Pass the catheter beyond the clotted material and inflate the catheter. Withdraw the catheter while pulling the material carefully out ahead of it.[17]

Monitor patients throughout the procedure for signs of cardiac dysrhythmias or hypoxia, and stop the procedure if either sign is evident (see "Complications of Suctioning," later). Address causes of hemodynamic instability before continuing with suctioning. However, if marked respiratory distress is presumed secondary to significant tracheal obstruction, continue with expeditious suctioning to reduce the obstruction.

Nasotracheal Suctioning Techniques

Nasotracheal suctioning has been used solely to remove secretions and avoid intubation.[46] Perform suctioning if there is audible evidence of secretions in the airway despite a patient's best cough effort. Infants with thick nasopharyngeal secretions may also benefit from nasotracheal suctioning if deep nasal suctioning does not clear the upper airway. Note that suspicion or evidence of epiglottitis or croup is an absolute contraindication to the procedure; occluded nasal passages, nasal bleeding, laryngospasm, and coagulopathy are relative contraindications.[46]

Place a nasopharyngeal airway ("trumpet") in an adult patient's nare to decrease nasal mucosal irritation and to help direct the suction catheter toward the airway. Apply topical anesthetic jelly to the nasal mucosa for patient comfort. If the patient's reflex to swallow the catheter is distressing to the patient and interfering with the procedure, ask the patient to stick his or her tongue out or manually apply traction to the tongue of a patient who is unable to voluntarily comply. Advance the catheter through the nare before attaching it to wall suction. When the catheter is properly positioned over the airway, listen for air movement from the proximal end of the catheter. Advance the catheter into the trachea until resistance is met, and then withdraw it 1 to 2 cm. Perform endotracheal suctioning as described earlier.[46] Take precautions to avoid causing mucosal injury.

Minitracheostomy Suctioning Procedures

The minitracheostomy ("minitrach") was designed to improve tracheal hygiene in patients with intact cough reflexes, normal ventilatory function, and vocalization. The minitrach serves as a small port solely for suctioning secretions. Commonly, a 4-mm indwelling, cuffless cannula is inserted through the cricothyroid membrane into the trachea. Patients who are suctioned through a minitrach are at lower risk for gagging and aspiration associated with blind endotracheal suctioning because they are able to maintain laryngeal and glottic function.[38] Because of small airway diameters, the minitrach is seldom used in children.

The technique used to suction through a minitrach is the same as that for tracheal suctioning. The smaller port size may require that smaller catheters be used. Most patients with minitrachs are decannulated before discharge from the intensive care unit and rarely present to the ED.

Complications of Suctioning

Complications that occur during or after suctioning are relatively common and can result in significant morbidity. Fortunately, most complications can be anticipated, and simple maneuvers can reduce their incidence and severity.

Hypoxemia from suctioning may be transient, but has the potential to cause increased ICP, dysrhythmias, or death. Cerebral hypoxia during suctioning may contribute to the genesis of intracerebral hemorrhage in neonates.[47] A number of factors contribute to suctioning-related hypoxia, including interruption of mechanical ventilation, aspiration of air from the respiratory tract, and suctioning-related atelectasis. Use in-line suction catheters with ventilator-dependent patients to allow continuous oxygen delivery and positive-pressure ventilation during suctioning. Size catheters appropriately (see "Procedure," earlier) to reduce the evacuation of airway gases during suctioning and to help prevent atelectasis. Limit suctioning passes to 10 to 15 seconds' duration and to only three suction passes in succession. Reoxygenate the patient between suctioning passes and after the procedure. Reduce or discontinue routine saline instillation into the trachea before suctioning.[19]

Measurements of arterial oxygen saturation may not be sufficient to assess hypoxia after suctioning. It has been shown that oxygen consumption increases during suctioning despite insignificant changes in oxygen saturation. This increase in oxygen consumption was more marked in patients who displayed a vigorous cough, agitation, or resistance to suctioning.[48]

Dysrhythmias due to suctioning may be caused by hypoxia, increased myocardial oxygen consumption, vagal stimulation, or catecholamine release. Vagal stimulation caused by suctioning or rough movement of the endotracheal tube can cause bradycardia and possible hypotension.[41] Bradycardia in the setting of hypoxia potentiates ventricular dysrhythmias, including ventricular fibrillation. Nebulized or intravenous atropine is recommended for bradycardia and can be used as pretreatment in patients at risk for bradycardia, including infants. Digoxin enhances vagal activity and may potentiate the vagal stimulation of endotracheal suctioning.[39] Sympathetic stimulation may occur as a result of hypoxia, pain, or stress of the procedure. Pain medications, anxiolytics, or preparation of the patient for the procedure may blunt the sympathetic response. Terminate suctioning immediately if any new dysrhythmia is evident.

Increased ICP during suctioning is well documented.[49–51] The theoretical risks of increased ICP include decreased cerebral perfusion pressure in patients with compromised cerebral blood flow, inducing cerebral hypoxia, worsening cerebral edema, and possibly contributing to intraventricular hemorrhage in neonates.[43,47,52] There is no common agreement on the underlying cause of increased ICP during suctioning. Mean ICP increases occur in a stepwise fashion with repeated suctioning; this effect is reversed if manual hyperventilation is extended to 60 seconds between suctioning passes.[52] Kerr and associates[43] suggested that decreases in arterial carbon dioxide pressure (Pa_{CO_2}) can minimize suctioning-induced ICP elevation and advocated increasing the rate of manual hyperventilation from 12 breaths/min to 30 breaths/min. This study demonstrated a transient decrease in Pa_{CO_2} with this rate, with a corresponding decrease in ICP during suctioning.[34] Long-term reduction in Pa_{CO_2} is not advocated. Mean arterial blood pressure also increases with suctioning, but this may be protective of cerebral oxygenation by increasing the cerebral perfusion pressure. Cerebral vasodilatation after preoxygenation has been suggested as a mechanism that maintains cerebral oxygenation, even when transient increases in ICP occur during suctioning.[43]

Vigorous coughing and increases in intrathoracic pressure are possible causes of increases in ICP. Instill lidocaine into the trachea to help suppress coughing. Pretreatment with fentanyl or thiopental has not shown a significant effect in blunting the increase in ICP during suctioning. However, intravenous lidocaine (1.5 mg/kg), intratracheal lidocaine (2 mL of 4% solution), or temporary paralysis may attenuate ICP increases in patients with severe head injury.[17] In patients

133

without evidence of increased ICP, routine pretreatment with drugs to prevent increased ICP is probably unnecessary.[17] Preoxygenation and hyperventilation are simple maneuvers that should be carried out in all patients.

Atelectasis can occur when airway gases are suctioned rapidly. To reduce this complication, choose a suction catheter that is less than half the diameter of the artificial airway and control the time and suction pressure applied during suctioning (see "Procedure," earlier). Hyperventilate after the procedure to treat suctioning-related atelectasis.[17]

Mucosal injury is a common complication of tracheal suctioning. Invagination of the mucosa into the side ports of the catheter occurs during suctioning, causing the tracheal mucosa to become denuded, edematous, and more likely to bleed. Mucosal damage also interferes with mucociliary transport. Tracheitis, indicated by blood-streaked secretions or a persistent cough, can occur as a result of frequent or improperly performed suctioning.[17] To reduce tracheitis, instill 1 mL of 1% lidocaine into the trachea.

The suctioning technique appears to be more important than the catheter-tip design in reducing mucosal injury. Suction only when clinically indicated to reduce repeated airway trauma. Limit the length of time suctioning is performed to 10 to 15 seconds and use appropriate vacuum pressures. Stop the procedure, apply positive-pressure ventilation, and use bronchodilators to help resolve this complication.[17] Sudden death has been reported during tracheal suctioning and is likely due to one or more of the complications discussed here. Make sure that cardiopulmonary resuscitation equipment and medications are available to the clinician before the procedure is initiated.[17]

Ventilating the Tracheostomy Patient

Importantly, the inner cannula serves as an adaptor to accept an Ambu bag, and positive-pressure ventilation cannot be delivered via the tracheostomy tube in the absence of the inner cannula. If such is the case, immediately remove the tracheostomy tube and replace it with a small standard endotracheal tube that will allow connection to the Ambu bag (Fig. 7–5).

TRANSESOPHAGEAL PUNCTURE FOR VOICE RESTORATION

Transesophageal puncture (TEP) has evolved into the most widely used and accepted technique for voice rehabilitation. Originally developed in the 1980s, it can be done as a primary or secondary procedure after laryngectomy or pharyngeal surgeries.

A puncture site is instrumented through the anterior esophagus and posterior tracheal wall, and the TEP prosthesis is inserted after dilation of the wound. Production of speech with TEP is similar to that of esophageal speech. The mucosa vibrate in segments of the pharyngeal esophagus resulting from airflow.

TEP Complications

Operative and immediate postoperative complications of TEP are infrequent.[53] Long-term complications include stomal stenosis, aspiration of the prosthesis, fistula leakage, TEP necrosis, and swallowing impairment. Reported infec-

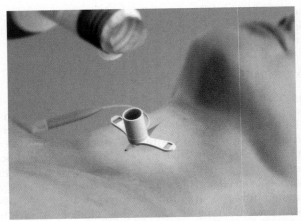

Figure 7–5 Note that the inner cannula of a tracheostomy tube will accept an Ambu bag or ventilator tube, *but if the inner cannula is missing, the patient cannot be ventilated this way.* In an emergency in which ventilation is required and the inner cannula is missing, remove the tracheostomy tube and replace it with a small standard endotracheal tube. *(From Thomsen T, Setnik G [eds.]: Procedures Consult—Emergency Medicine Module. Copyright 2008 Elsevier Inc. All rights reserved.)*

tious complications associated with TEP include deep neck abscess, aspiration pneumonia, and cervical cellulitis.[54]

Although few TEP complications are life-threatening, be aware of several considerations with this device. Thick or inspissated secretions, especially after radiation therapy, or food may accumulate above the TEP, causing airflow obstruction in the upper airway. Acute changes in voice production or decreased ability to speak warrants consideration of prosthesis dislodgment, occlusion, or erosion due to infectious etiologies, especially fungal.[55] Esophageal edema causing dysphagia and loss of TEP speech has been reported[55] and should be differentiated from other etiologies of esophageal obstruction. Ascertain the presence of TEP by history or medical records, assess airway and esophageal patency, and determine whether the patient has experienced changes or difficulties in voice production. Seek and treat for infectious complications in the ED, maintaining a high degree of suspicion for fungal etiologies. In stable patients, management of prosthesis complications can often be referred to a specialist, generally an otolaryngologist. Communication with the specialist should include consideration of prosthesis leak, dislodgment, obstruction, or infections.

TRANSTRACHEAL OXYGEN DELIVERY SYSTEMS

Low-flow oxygen administration is prescribed for patients who have adequate ventilatory function, but suffer from chronic hypoxia. Patients with chronic obstructive pulmonary disease, pulmonary fibrosis, sleep apnea,[56] lung cancer, and α_1-antitrypsin deficiency are often candidates for outpatient use of supplemental oxygen.[57,58] Traditionally, supplemental oxygen has been delivered by nasal cannula. Although technically simple, nasal cannula use has several side effects including nasal mucosa drying and epistaxis, ear discomfort, contact dermatitis from oxygen tubing,[57] and dry throat.[58] Delivery of oxygen via nasal cannula is also very inefficient because it occurs only during inspiration, and oxygen must traverse the anatomic dead space of the nares and hypopharynx.

Transtracheal oxygen catheters are small tubes that deliver oxygen directly to the lumen of the trachea for long-term home oxygen supplementation. A subcutaneous tract holds the catheter below the neck, and the catheter is inserted into the lower trachea. Low-flow oxygen (2–10 L/min) is delivered directly into the trachea through a narrow (7- to 11-Fr) catheter. Typically, an 11-cm catheter sits in the trachea with its tip 1 to 2 cm above the carina.[57] The catheter can have single or multiple distal ports for oxygen flow. The catheter is held in place by a thin band or necklace through two openings in the flange.

Transtracheal oxygen (TTO) delivery systems can be used in place of nasal cannula to enhance the efficiency of oxygenation, reduce complications, and improve patient comfort and compliance.[59]

TTO is administered through all phases of the respiratory cycle[56] and directly into the trachea, bypassing the upper airway dead spaces. For these reasons, the required oxygen flow rates are decreased, often by 50% or more.[59] Gas mixture in the distal trachea is more effective in eliminating CO_2. Clinically, these symptoms reduce the work of breathing and exertional dyspnea.[57] Physiologic benefits include reduced erythrocytosis and pulmonary vascular resistance and improved cor pulmonale, arterial oxygen tension, and exercise capacity.[60]

The surgical procedure is often done as an outpatient, under local anesthesia. Initially, a small stent is placed percutaneously into the anterior neck and replaced with a TTO catheter when the tract matures, usually in 1 to 2 weeks.[57] Dislodgment of the catheter during this time can result in tract closure within a matter of minutes. Once the transcutaneous fistula has epithelialized, the catheter may be inserted and changed safely by the patient at home. Early catheter changes may be done in the clinician's office over a guidewire if the integrity of the stoma is questionable.

Regular maintenance includes cleaning and changing the catheter. One milliliter of sterile saline is inserted into the catheter, and a cleaning rod is inserted as far as possible. The cleaning rod is inserted and removed three times to remove secretions from the catheter lumen. Catheters are changed according to manufacturer's recommendations, from twice daily to once every 2 weeks, or as needed. The stoma should be cleaned twice daily and inspected for signs of infection. All catheter maintenance procedures should be done while the patient is given supplemental oxygen by nasal cannula. Adequate humidification, cleaning, and systemic hydration reduce the incidence of mucus blockage.

Early complications (within 3 months of the procedure) occur in approximately 30% of patients[57,58] and include bleeding at the stoma, infection, pneumothorax, costochondritis,[61] ejection of the catheter from coughing,[62] and inability to replace the catheter after dislodgment. Pneumomediastinum and sudden death were reported as possible rare complications.[63] Late complications include mucus plugging, bleeding, infections, and hemoptysis[57,58,62] and occur in up to 40% of patients.[60] A mucus ball is an accumulation of inspissated mucus that adheres to the anterior and lateral surfaces of the catheter, just above the tip. Mucus balls may precipitate a cough or wheezing, but rarely result in airway obstruction.

Dyspnea or increased cough may indicate catheter obstruction by mucus or from kinking or that the catheter tip is located cephalad to the stoma. A whistling sound from the oxygen tank humidifier may indicate obstruction within the catheter or oxygen tubing. Cellulitis around the stoma, subcutaneous air, or dislodgment of the catheter should be evident on patient examination. *Candida* infections at the stoma may occur if routine broad-spectrum antibiotics are used at the stoma site and are more common in patients on systemic antibiotics or steroids or those with diabetes mellitus. Tracheal chondritis may result from bacterial infection of the cartilage. Patients with chondritis present with a deep indurated lump around the tract that may be tender but is generally not fluctuant. Treatment for chondritis includes antibiotics that cover *S. aureus* for 3 weeks.

In the ED, clean and replace the catheter if obstruction is suspected. Change the catheter by a modified Seldinger technique if the stoma tract has not healed or appears infected. Use a water-soluble lubricant for the catheter change. If changing the catheter does not relieve obstruction and the patient's airway is intact, increasing the intrathoracic pressure may help increase the force of the cough. Ask the patient to sit upright, holding a pillow to her or his abdomen, and cough forcefully after three deep inspirations. This maneuver may help mobilize secretions or small mucus plugs in the airway. Dyspnea and cough should lessen with effective removal of obstructions.

Manage bleeding complications at the catheter site with gauze packing or cauterization, if minor. If significant bleeding is identified or suspected, consult a specialist emergently and manage the airway definitively as clinically indicated. Manage skin and pulmonary infections similarly to that discussed for tracheostomy care.

TRANSTRACHEAL NEEDLE ASPIRATION

Transtracheal needle aspiration is an infrequently performed procedure used to obtain tracheal sputum samples for microbiology. It offers the advantage of providing access to lower respiratory secretions in patients for whom accurate and timely identification of infectious agents is desired. Cultures of lower respiratory tract secretions obtained by transtracheal needle aspiration are more predictive of pulmonary infection than are those obtained from expectorated washed sputum.[17] Transtracheal aspiration specimens have been shown to be useful in diagnosis of unusual pulmonary infections, including those caused by anaerobic bacteria, tuberculosis bacilii, *Aspergillus*, *Pneumocystis carinii*, and hospital-acquired and partially treated pneumonias.[17]

The primary clinical indication to perform transtracheal needle aspiration is to obtain sputum samples from patients unable to generate an adequate expectorated sample. This population may include obtunded patients or those with underlying pulmonary or neurologic illnesses that limit their ability to cough. Several contraindications to the procedure exist, including bleeding diatheses, distorted anterior landmarks, hypoxia, and the patient's inability to remain supine and cooperate with the procedure. Aspiration of sputum from patients with chronic bronchitis may yield false-positive cultures.[17]

Equipment

Commercially available intravenous catheter sets that contain an introducer needle, a J-wire guide, and tracheal catheter are available. The catheters are generally 15 to 20 cm in length and 16- to 18-gauge in diameter. An additional 10- to 50-mL syringe is needed to collect the sputum sample. Previously

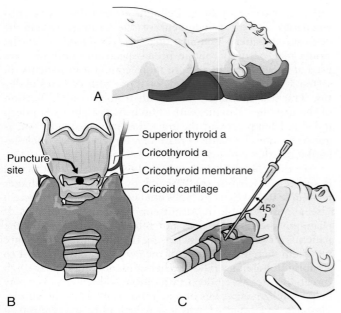

Figure 7–6 Transtracheal aspiration. *A,* Position of patient. *B,* Anatomic landmarks. *C,* Technique of puncture. The Intracath needle or J-wire introducer needle is inserted just above the cricoid cartilage through the cricothyroid membrane with its bevel up at a 45° angle to the skin. *(A–C, From Eknoyen G: Medical Procedures Manual. Chicago, Year Book Medical Publishers, 1981. Reproduced by permission.)*

discussed recommendations to limit the use of saline for sputum collection also may apply to this procedure. However, the literature does not provide data or specific recommendations regarding saline instillation for this procedure.

Procedure

The procedure is illustrated in Figure 7–6. Place the patient on a cardiac monitor and give supplemental oxygen. Cardiac resuscitation equipment should be readily available. Use sterile procedural techniques, including skin preparation and draping. Place the patient in the supine position, with a small towel or pillow between the shoulder blades, to allow full extension of the neck. Identify the cricothyroid membrane by palpation, and inject a small weal of local anesthetic subcutaneously into the skin above the membrane.

Insert the introducer needle into the trachea through the cricothyroid membrane, with the needle tip directed inferiorly. Aspirate for air through the needle to confirm intratracheal placement. Thread the guidewire through the needle, and then remove the needle. Advance the catheter over the guidewire. Attach a sterile syringe to the catheter, and aspirate sputum from the tracheal lumen with gentle suction. A small aspirate amount is suitable for analysis. After sputum has been obtained, remove the catheter, and apply direct pressure to the puncture site. Advise the patient to avoid activities that stimulate coughing for 24 hours after the procedure.[17] Antitussive medications may be helpful.

Complications

Complication rates for transtracheal needle aspiration are low and can be managed by techniques similar to those described elsewhere in this chapter. Cardiac dysrhythmias may be induced by vagal stimulation or hypoxia. Preoxygenating the patient should ameliorate hypoxia, and atropine may be required for bradydysrhythmias. Some patients develop subcutaneous emphysema, which is usually self-limiting and can be minimized by reducing the amount and force of the patient's cough. Digital pressure will control most bleeding that develops.[17]

STENTS

Tracheal stenosis is a known complication of artificial airways. Management options include surgery and placement of silicone stents in the trachea. Patients who have had successful decannulation of their tracheostomy tubes may need stents if symptomatic stenosis occurs. Indications and complications of tracheal stents are beyond the scope of this chapter, but the clinician should be aware of the possibility of these indwelling devices in patients with head and neck surgeries or previous tracheostomies.[64]

PEDIATRIC CONSIDERATIONS

Unique components of evaluation and management of pediatric patients with tracheostomies are reviewed here. Most considerations follow adult guidelines and are discussed in the appropriate sections of this chapter. A consensus article developed by the American Thoracic Society provides a comprehensive review of pediatric tracheostomy care.[44] Tracheostomy-related mortality in pediatric patients ranges from 0.5% to 3%. The main causes of death are accidental decannulation and blockage of the tracheostomy tube.[65]

Between 25% and 50% of pediatric patients with a tracheostomy will develop complications, with higher rates in patients younger than 3 years. Rates decrease with the indication for tracheostomy, with airway obstruction highest, and central nervous system disorders, respiratory distress syndrome, and congenital heart disorders less likely to have complications.[44]

Equipment

Tracheostomy tubes and catheters for suctioning, along with resuscitation medication and equipment appropriate for the pediatric population, should be available when treating pediatric tracheostomy patients.

Sizing

Pediatric tracheostomy tubes share the same components as the adult counterparts. The size of the indwelling tube is stamped on the outer cannula flange and should guide the clinician's choice of replacement tubes. Age guidelines may not be as reliable in pediatric patients because many of these patients with complex medical problems or history of prematurity may be small for their age and weight estimates by age may also be incorrect. Representative tube types and sizes are listed in Table 7–1. When the tracheostomy tube is correctly seated in the pediatric patient, it should extend at least 2 cm beyond the stoma, and no closer than 1 to 2 cm to the carina. Curvature should be such that the distal portion of the tube in situ is concentric and collinear with the trachea. Appropriate position of a replaced tube can be verified with radiographs.

Cuff

The general rule that cuffed endotracheal tubes should not be used in pediatric patients under the age of 6 does not universally apply to tracheostomy patients. Young patients who require ventilation with high pressure or who require only nocturnal ventilation or are at risk for aspiration may have cuffed tubes in place. Young infants may have a cuffed tube in place if the underlying disease (e.g., tracheal anomaly) warrants it. Replacement of these tubes should ensure that the individual's anatomic and physiologic needs are met.

Cuff pressure recommendations for pediatric patients are below 20 cm H_2O. With few exceptions, low-pressure, high-volume cuffs should be used.[44]

Humidifiers

Humidifiers are available for pediatric tracheostomy tubes; they attach to the external port. Some humidifiers have lithium-coated moisture exchangers. Systemic absorption is unlikely to cause clinical symptoms in adults but may be a consideration in pediatric patients with these devices.

Suctioning

Suctioning recommendations in pediatric patients clearly support the use of a premeasured suction catheter to reduce the rate of mucosal irritation and possible granuloma development. Exact depth of insertion in the premeasured technique helps reduce epithelial damage, if the catheter is inserted too deeply, or inadequate suctioning, if the suction catheter is not inserted deeply enough. A tracheostomy tube, the same size as the patient's, may be used to measure the depth of insertion. In children with fenestrated tracheostomy tubes, suction catheters may accidentally go through the fenestrations. If this happens repeatedly, granulation tissue may develop at the site.[44]

Complications

Granuloma formation is common in pediatric patients and most often occurs in the tracheal lumen at the superior margin of the tracheostomy or at the level of the tube tip, where mucosa can become irritated or inflamed. Definitive management of clinically significant granuloma is done by a pediatric specialist.

Pleural apices rise higher in children than in adults and may extend up into the lower neck. Intraoperative damage to the cervical pleura may result in pneumothorax or pneumomediastinum. This operative complication rarely presents in the ED, but consideration should be given to its recurrence if paratracheal tissues have been disrupted. This complication may occur from a dislodged tube that has been incorrectly placed in a false passage or if the stomal opening or tube dressings are tightly occlusive and intrathoracic pressures cause air tracking in soft tissue spaces.[65]

The most common bacterial agents that colonize pediatric tracheostomies are *P. aeruginosa* and/or *S. aureus*. Similar to adult patients, colonization does not require treatment unless signs of acute infection are present.[65] Suprastomal collapse of the anterior tracheal wall superior to the tracheostomy is very common in pediatric patients. Pressure on the tracheal rings by the tube causes inflammation, chondritis, and weakening of the cartilaginous rings. Significant collapse can hamper the patient's decannulation success. Management of massive bleeding in pediatrics patients follows recommendations given for adult patients. However, the smaller size of the tracheostomy may preclude the clinician from applying digital pressure to the bleeding site through the stoma. Conversion to a cuffed tracheostomy or endotracheal tube, with cuff inflation, may be the most expeditious temporizing measure to control arterial bleeds in these patients.

 REFERENCES CAN BE FOUND ON **EXPERT CONSULT**

CHAPTER 8

Mechanical Ventilation

Heatherlee Bailey and Lewis J. Kaplan

Initiating mechanical ventilation (MV) in the emergency department (ED) is an integral part of emergency medicine practice. However, increasing evidence holds that the manner by which human lungs are mechanically ventilated may be as deleterious as helpful.[1] The traditional view of MV as little more than a formulaic prescription that fits virtually all patients equally well should be discarded as a gross misunderstanding of pulmonary pathophysiology. Every ED clinician should embrace the firmly established paradigm of pulmonary protective ventilation and oxygenation strategies as a cornerstone of care. This chapter addresses indications for MV, new strategies for safe ventilation and oxygenation, survival advantages that accrue from such interventions, complications of positive-pressure ventilation (PPV), and advanced modes of MV. One key to providing excellent ED care is to recognize when airway control and MV are warranted.

INDICATIONS FOR MV

There are wide-ranging reasons for patients to require MV in the ED, and there are no absolute contraindications. Many time-honored indications for invasive ventilation are now identified as appropriate indications for noninvasive ventilation and are addressed later. Current indications for endotracheal intubation may be separated into several categories—emergent, urgent, delayed, and elective—based on the urgency of the airway need. *Emergent intubation* is for patients who require immediate airway protection and MV on arrival to the ED. These patients tend to be in extremis, either suffering from shock with decreased oxygen delivery ($\dot{D}o_2$) or having an absent or unprotected airway. These problems may cause hypoxemia or hypercarbia with acidosis or both. *Urgent intubation* is for patients who require assistance within the first few minutes of arrival. It is used in patients who have impending airway loss. Patients who have increased work of breathing with worsening hypoxia and rising CO_2 or those with emerging injury complexes that may compromise the airway or thoracic cage may also require urgent intubation.

Delayed intubation is for patients who are stable for the initial and secondary assessment, but then require mechanical assistance. This scenario may arise for numerous reasons including progression of the disease process despite therapy or inadequate improvement with treatment. Transport to a noncritical care area with a patient who has potential for airway loss is another reason for delayed intubation to occur.[2] More ED clinicians are facing the challenge of patients requiring delayed intubation because of increasing demands on the health care system. Patients are spending more time in the ED before admission owing to the shortage of critical care beds and appropriately trained nurses (Kaplan LJ, Medical College of Pennsylvania, Hospital Critical Care Working Group, unpublished data, 2001). This health care crisis allows the ED clinician to see these patients when they decompen-

sate due to disease progression or treatment failure (when they normally would have already been in the intensive care unit [ICU]).

Elective intubation is for patients who will require airway protection and MV to facilitate care of organ systems besides the respiratory tract. A common example is for airway control for an invasive procedure. This last category is not common in the ED. If a patient needs to leave the department for a test or for transfer to another institution and there is potential for airway compromise during the transfer/procedure, elective intubation is indicated. Emergency clinicians are acute care airway specialists and it is their responsibility to ensure patient safety.

In order to initiate and sustain appropriate MV, it is important that the ED clinician understand basic principles, standard equipment, goals, settings, and monitoring strategies for patients on MV.

BASIC PULMONARY PHYSIOLOGY

Minute Volume and Alveolar Ventilation

The volume of air that moves in and out of a patient's lungs per minute is termed the *minute volume ($\dot{V}_E$)*. $\dot{V}_E$ is the product of tidal volume ($\dot{V}_T$) and respiratory frequency or rate (f):

$$\dot{V}_E = \dot{V}_T \times f$$

$\dot{V}_T$ can be further broken down into alveolar volume ($\dot{V}_A$) and dead space volume ($\dot{V}_D$):

$$\dot{V}_T = \dot{V}_A \times \dot{V}_D$$

In healthy young persons, the anatomic dead space is accounted for by the trachea and the larger airways and is approximately 2.2 mL/kg of lean body weight. In disease states, in addition to the anatomic dead space, there is also a variable amount of "pathologic" dead space corresponding to ventilated alveoli and respiratory bronchioles that are not adequately perfused. The sum of the anatomic and pathologic dead spaces is often referred to as the *physiologic dead space*.

Alveolar minute ventilation ($\dot{V}_A$) is the product of rate times $\dot{V}_T$ minus dead space:

$$\dot{V}_A = (\dot{V}_T - \dot{V}_D) \times f$$

$\dot{V}_A$ and the rate of CO_2 production by the body ($\dot{V}_{co_2}$) determine the partial pressure of CO_2 in the alveoli ($PAco_2$), which is approximately equal to the systemic arterial CO_2 tension (Pa_{co_2}). This relationship is as follows:

$$Pa_{co_2} \approx PAco_2 = k \times (\dot{V}_{co_2} / \dot{V}_A)$$

The value of the constant (k) is 0.863 when the $PAco_2$ is measured in millimeters of mercury at 37°C saturated with water vapor. $\dot{V}_{co_2}$ is measured in milliliters per minute, and $\dot{V}_A$ is measured in liters per minute. Understanding basic pulmonary physiology is essential to understanding how to initiate MV; it ensures that the method of gas delivery meshes with the patient's underlying physiology to avoid ventilator-induced lung injury. Clinicians must also understand the basics of ventilator operation and order writing.

EQUIPMENT—STANDARD OPTIONS

Regardless of which ventilator one uses, a limited number of standard features are common to each. This discussion explores machine features and settings.

Control Mechanisms

Volume-Cycled Ventilation (VCV). With this target, the ventilator seeks to deliver a preset amount of gas. The time of gas flow is determined by the set volume ($\dot{V}_T$), flow ($\dot{Q}$), and the waveform of gas delivery (see later). When the set $\dot{V}_T$ is reached, gas flow is terminated and expiration passively begins. An advantage is that this method delivers a constant $\dot{V}_T$. Unfortunately, it does not take into account dynamic changes in lung compliance, which may alter the ability of the lung to accept delivered gas in gas-exchanging alveoli. This is the most common mode used in the United States.

Pressure-Cycled Ventilation (PCV). With this target, the ventilator alters gas flow to achieve and maintain airway pressure (P_{aw}) at a preset level for the duration of a preset inspiratory time (T_i). Gas flow is terminated when the preset change in pressure is achieved. The pressure is maintained with a variable or intermittent $\dot{Q}$ for the set T_i. Gas flow is adjusted to not exceed a set pressure limit (e.g., pressure-limited or pressure-controlled ventilation). One problem with this method is that the volume received by the patient is variable. The delivered volume is determined by the patient's lung and chest wall compliance, the airway resistance, as well as the T_i and pressure target. An advantage is that P_{aw}s are tightly managed to limit or eliminate alveolar overdistention and to reduce ventilator-induced lung injury.[3] In the setting of hypoxemia, the T_i may be increased quite precisely to increase the mean airway pressure (P_{aw}-mean) and thus oxygenation; this strategy is much more difficult, if not impossible, to manipulate using volume-cycled ventilation.

Modes

Controlled MV/Assist Control. This ventilator mode provides breaths, known as *machine breaths*, at a preset rate. If the patient tries to breathe faster than the set rate, he or she can initiate additional breaths, known as *spontaneous breaths*. In volume-cycled ventilation (VCV), the spontaneous breath receives the same $\dot{V}_T$ that is set for the machine breath, regardless of how much gas the patient wants to receive. For the patient to trigger the ventilator to initiate flow for a spontaneous breath, the P_{aw} must decrease by a preset amount below positive end-expiratory pressure (PEEP). The amount of decrease necessary to open the inflow valve is the sensitivity setting. This is typically 0.5 to 2 cm H_2O pressure. The higher the sensitivity, the greater the work of breathing required to trigger a breath.

Intermittent MV/Synchronized Intermittent MV. This ventilator mode provides breaths at a preset rate (machine breath) similar to the assist control (AC) mode. The patient can initiate an additional spontaneous breath, but receive only a spontaneous $\dot{V}_T$ that reflects the depth and time spent in inspiration. For each of these nonmandatory (i.e., spontaneous) breaths, the patient receives no support from the ventilator and has a high work of breathing. Thus, synchronized intermittent mechanical ventilation (SIMV) is typically partnered with pressure-support ventilation (PSV; see later) to aid in spontaneous breathing support and to overcome the intrinsic resistance of breathing through long tubes and the endotracheal tube with a diameter smaller than the patient's native airway. The synchronized version of intermittent mechanical ventilation (IMV) allows the ventilator to coordinate spontaneous and machine breaths to prevent it from delivering a scheduled breath on top of a spontaneous breath (excess $\dot{V}_T$ delivered) or during exhalation from a spontaneous breath (exhalation compromised by positive P_{aw}). Both conditions were a problem with the original IMV mode. This could lead to elevated P_{aw}s, alveolar overdistention, and biotrauma.[4]

Each of these modes (CMV/AC and IMV/SIMV + PSV) may be combined with either a volume target or a pressure target to achieve the desired minute ventilation (see earlier).

Continuous Positive Airway Pressure. Continuous positive airway pressure (CPAP) is another positive-pressure, spontaneously breathing mode. It is most commonly used in isolation for those with chronic obstructive pulmonary disease (COPD) or obstructive sleep apnea via a tight-fitting nasal or full face mask. In patients with an endotracheal tube (ETT) or tracheostomy tube, CPAP is typically used as a weaning mode in combination with PSV. The CPAP level when transitioning from IMV/PSV or AC mode should be the PEEP level that was being used. Reducing the CPAP below the previous PEEP may result in loss of alveolar recruitment, atelectasis, hypoxia, and an increased work of breathing.

Adjunct Ventilator Settings

Oxygen. The percentage of inspired O_2 (FI_{O_2}) is set in a range from 21% (room air; not generally indicated) to 100%. In the ED, it is common to start at 100% FI_{O_2} to ensure adequate oxygenation and titrate the FI_{O_2} down to nontoxic levels ($FI_{O_2} < 0.60$) following the oxygen saturation (SaO_2) via the pulse oximeter (SaO_2 90% $\approx$ Po_2 60 torr). In theory, placing the patient on 100% FI_{O_2} may lead to alveolar collapse due to absorption of all the O_2 in that alveolus. Recall that room air is principally N_2 mixed with O_2 and a number of inert gases. If there is only O_2 delivered to an alveolus and that O_2 is absorbed, there will be no nonabsorbed gases to keep open the alveolus. This is known as *absorption atelectasis* and leads to ventilation-perfusion ($\dot{V}/\dot{Q}$) mismatch when present. Thus, some practitioners recommend using 95% O_2 as the upper limit of FI_{O_2}.

PEEP. PEEP is the pressure in the airway at the end of exhalation. PEEP helps keep the large noncartilaginously supported airways and the smaller alveoli open to prevent collapse, atelectasis, and hypoxia at the end of expiration. The required ventilation to compensate for this triad commonly worsens lung compliance and is associated with ventilator-induced lung injury. The useful PEEP range is from 3 to 20 cm H_2O.[5] In general, most patients should be started on a PEEP of 5 cm H_2O, which is considered a physiologic level. PEEP can be increased by 3 to 5 cm H_2O every 10 to 15 minutes as needed/tolerated for patients who remain hypoxic. The initial goal is to reduce the FI_{O_2} to nontoxic levels ($FI_{O_2} < 60\%$). This goal is coming under increasing scrutiny as new information challenges the timeframe and concept of O_2-induced lung injury at FI_{O_2} levels greater than 0.6.[6]

PEEP is used to increase functional residual capacity (FRC) and move the zero pressure point of each alveolar unit more proximal in the airway so as to prevent early alveolar collapse.[7] By so doing, PEEP increases the available number of alveolar units that can participate in gas exchange. The primary effect of PEEP on gas exchange, however, is to improve oxygenation, not CO_2 removal. CO_2 clearance is rather efficient and will be well preserved in situations in which oxygenation is not. By opening one alveolar unit, the tendency of the adjacent unit is to open as well (i.e., alveolar codependency; Fig. 8–1).[8] Excessive PEEP will compromise hemodynamics. Therefore, there are two primary questions

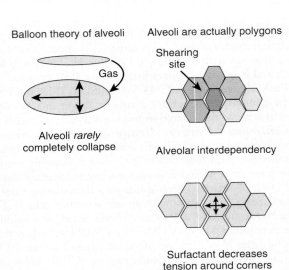

Figure 8–1 Alveolar interdependence. Note that alveoli are not round in shape; instead, they are polygons. Polygons have corners and may have two opposing surfaces that may adhere to one another via surface tension. Surfactant works to reduce this surface tension and allow alveoli to open with reduced shear stress at the junction of closed and open alveoli. Alveoli are connected via the pores of Kohn. These allow opening alveoli to pull a relatively closed alveolus open while equalizing pressure between adjacent alveoli. The central alveolus *on the right* is fairly closed in the upper diagram, but it is pulled open by its neighbors as they expand and accept gas.

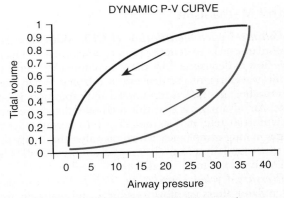

Figure 8–2 Dynamic pressure-volume (PV) loop. Note that as soon as pressure is delivered to the airway, there is an increase in measured tidal volume. The *lower arrow* denotes inspiration and the *upper arrow* indicates exhalation. This indicates that the airways are open and do not need to be forced open by increasing the pressure in the airway. If this latter case were true, then the PV loop would initially be flat along the x-axis.

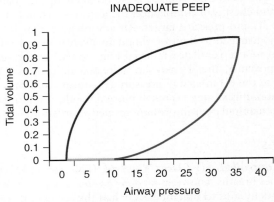

Figure 8–3 Inadequate positive end-expiratory pressure (PEEP) and the PV loop. Compare this curve with that in Figure 8–2. Note that the loop is initially flat (*lower segment*) along the x-axis. Once the airway pressure is high enough to open the alveolar units, each increase in airway pressure is matched by a corresponding increase in tidal volume.

to ask when using PEEP to augment oxygenation: What is the "optimal PEEP"? and Is the current amount of PEEP compromising the patient's hemodynamics?

There are several ways to determine the optimal PEEP. One way is to increase the PEEP until there are no longer increases in the Po_2. This method, however, may result in several untoward events. First, oxygen tension may steadily increase, but the pressure of carbon dioxide (Pco_2) may increase as well from alveolar overdistention. With overdistention, the alveolar pressure may exceed the pulmonary arteriolar pressure and actually decrease pulmonary blood flow and CO_2 clearance. Second, alveolar overdistention may increase total intrathoracic pressure and therefore diminish venous return and hence cardiac output. Third, decreased venous return may result in cerebral venous hypertension, as indicated earlier. The optimal PEEP for one organ system may be deleterious for another. For example, the optimal PEEP for ideal oxygenation may be the worst PEEP for cerebral venous drainage.

A better method of determining the optimal PEEP relies on measuring $\dot{D}o_2$ and oxygen consumption ($\dot{V}o_2$). PEEP may be increased until there is no further increase in $\dot{D}o_2$ and no increase in $\dot{V}o_2$.[9] This method does require a pulmonary artery catheter to be in place for determination of $\dot{D}o_2$ and $\dot{V}o_2$. In many institutions, the application of PEEP above 10 cm H_2O pressure in a multiply injured patient necessitates placement of a pulmonary artery catheter to make such determinations regarding oxygen extraction. An alternative is to increase PEEP until a complication of PEEP occurs (e.g., Pco_2 elevation, hypotension), and then reduce PEEP if needed (inability to tolerate hypercapnia), or expand the patient's intravascular volume to combat decreased venous return. The authors favor the placement of a pulmonary artery catheter in these situations to accurately guide therapy and know the patient's $\dot{D}o_2$ and $\dot{V}o_2$ status.

Another excellent method of determining the optimal PEEP is guided by assessing changes in plateau pressure with changes in PEEP. As PEEP is increased from a minimal level, the patient's peak airway pressure (P_{aw}-peak) as well as plateau pressure will increase by the amount of the applied PEEP. However, when the optimal PEEP for the lung units is achieved, the plateau pressure will no longer increase; in fact, as the lung is optimally recruited, the peak and plateau pressures may decrease as there is more volume of lung available to receive a set V_T. Once this level is exceeded, however, there will be further increases in plateau pressure beyond the incremental increase in PEEP as the units overdistend. Therefore, the clinician must readily identify the plateau in the plateau pressure trend. The same relationship may be displayed graphically in the dynamic pressure-volume (PV) loop (Fig. 8–2). The lower limb of the loop represents the pressure required to open the alveolar units.[10] In the absence of PEEP (or inadequate PEEP), this limb is prolonged and flattened and has an inflection point far to the right of the origin of the loop (Fig. 8–3). As PEEP is progressively increased, the inflection point travels to the left. When the optimal PEEP is achieved, there will be a rapid upstroke of the loop because the vast majority of the functional lung units are already open and ready to be ventilated (see Fig. 8–2). This strategy is known as the *open lung model* of MV.[10]

PEEP is not without untoward side effects, and increased levels of PEEP can lead to hemodynamic compromise.[11] This occurs from increased intrathoracic pressures leading to cardiac compression and collapse, principally of the right atrium. It is imperative that the patient be adequately resuscitated as volume depletion compounds this problem. Desired levels of PEEP simply may not be possible because of deleterious effects on cardiac output.

PSV. This mode augments spontaneous ventilation in the IMV/SIMV and CPAP modes. There is gas flow during inspiration for each spontaneous breath to help the patient overcome the resistance of the circuit and to achieve an acceptable $\dot{V}_T$. The range is from 0 up to 35 cm H_2O pressure; some ventilators may deliver PSV that achieves a greater range. The average starting point is 10 cm H_2O. PSV is adjusted as needed so that the spontaneous $\dot{V}_T$ approximates the set $\dot{V}_T$ for mandatory breaths. Patients placed on the combined mode of CPAP/PSV must be spontaneously breathing. PSV-based ventilation must never be combined with neuromuscular blockade agent therapy, or death from apnea, hypercarbia, and hypoxia will result. PSV is commonly used to aid in weaning from IMV-based ventilation and is frequently part of a transition strategy from IMV to CPAP.[12] In this way, PSV is used to eliminate the work of breathing improved by the ETT and the ventilator tubing. The required amount of pressure support to overcome the tube-induced resistance has been well documented (Table 8–1).[13] It is imperative not to lower the PSV during weaning below that required to overcome the resistance imposed by the diameter of the ETT or tracheostomy tube because the work of breathing may precipitously rise. Unlike AC or SIMV, PSV does not have a preset T_i. In fact, the time at which the gas flow terminates for each PSV breath is determined by an algorithm that in most older ventilators is not manipulable.

For instance, a patient breathing on CPAP/PSV on a Puritan-Bennett 7200 ventilator would have her or his maximal inspiratory flow required to achieve the set pressure-support level measured. As the patient's airways progressively fill with gas, the patient draws in gas at a slower rate, and the machine needs less of a flow rate to maintain the P_{aw}. When the machine flow rate decreases to 25% of the previously measured maximal inspiratory flow rate, all gas flow ceases. This termination occurs whether or not the patient is done inspiring. This algorithm may lead to significant patient-ventilator dysynchrony.[14] Newer ventilators, such as the Hamilton Galileo, allow user adjustment for such dyssynchrony. A common resolution using such a PSV device is either patient sedation or an increased level of pressure support so that the patient receives her or his desired amount of gas before gas flow termination.

Inspiratory-to-Expiratory Ratio. The normal inspiratory-to-expiratory (I/E) ratio in a spontaneously breathing, nonintubated patient is 1:4.[13] Intubated patients commonly achieve I/E ratios of 1:2. Shorter ratios may lead to decreased exhalation by compromising expiratory time (T_e). In its extreme form, inverse ratio ventilation (IRV), the normal pattern of breathing is reversed. A longer time is spent in inhalation to allow a longer time for oxygenation. Longer T_is allow for better matching of alveolar regional time constants.[15] The decrease in expiratory time (T_e) can lead to air trapping,

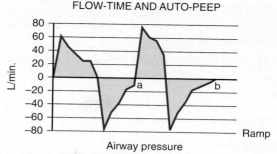

FLOW-TIME AND AUTO-PEEP

Figure 8–4 **Identifying auto-PEEP with the flow-time trace.** The x-axis is time and the y-axis is flow rate in liters per minute. Deflections above the x-axis indicate inspiration, and deflections below represent exhalation. In this example, the flow pattern is ramp (decelerating). Note that as the respiratory rate increases (decreased time for exhalation), the flow has not yet returned to baseline (a), indicating incomplete exhalation when compared to the following breath (b).

elevated P_{aw}s, and rising P_{CO_2}. These problems lead to hypercapnia, respiratory acidosis, and auto-PEEP.[15] Auto-PEEP is additional pressure that is generated within the airways from trapped gas that should have been exhaled, but for various reasons (commonly obstruction to exhalation such as COPD) was not.

Auto-PEEP can cause hemodynamic instability secondarily to decreased venous return just like high levels of PEEP.[16] Auto-PEEP may be detected in two ways: (1) evaluating the flow-time trace or (2) disconnecting the patient from the ventilator and listening for additional exhaled gas after an exhalation has already occurred.[10] The flow-time trace will demonstrate that the exhalation is not yet completed before the next breath has been initiated (Fig. 8–4). Auto-PEEP is a real potential when one initiates IRV for the management of hypoxemic respiratory failure. One can initiate IRV most easily in pressure-cycled ventilation (PCV) in which the operator sets the T_i directly. With VCV, one can achieve a similar gas delivery by adjusting the flow rate of each breath to adjust the I/E ratio; that the $\dot{Q}$ needs to be adjusted on a breath-by-breath basis makes this impractical.

Q. This is the rate of gas delivery (in liters per minute). The range of flows that can be achieved by current ventilation is from 10 to 160 L/min. Common flow settings are from 40 to 75 L/min. The higher the rate, the faster the ventilator will reach its set volume or pressure. A faster rate allows for a longer T_e, but owing to the shortened T_i, hypoxia can result. A slower rate allows for longer time in inhalation and improved oxygenation but a shortened T_e, which may lead to retained CO_2 and auto-PEEP from inadequate T_e (Fig. 8–5).

Waveforms

Square. Once the maximal inspiratory $\dot{Q}$ is achieved, the gas flow is constant until the set volume is delivered. When that point is reached, the gas flow is terminated. This waveform is best for patients with COPD and those suffering from head injury because gas delivered with this waveform allows for a longer T_e and lower P_{aw}-mean. The longer T_e is beneficial for patients with restrictive airway disease such as COPD. Spending a longer time in exhalation allows for improved venous drainage from the brain. The drawback to this waveform is an increased P_{aw}-peak, often requiring a lower $\dot{V}_T$ or $\dot{Q}$. This can lead to inadequate alveolar recruitment in patients with acute lung injury (ALI).

TABLE 8–1 Initial Ventilator Settings

Type of Ventilation	Comments
Volume-Cycled Ventilation (VCV) (Volume Set, Pressure Varies)	
Mode: SIMV	If patient is paralyzed: IMV = AC ventilation
Rate: 10–12/min	Target normal $\dot{V}_E$
$\dot{V}_T$: no acute lung injury: 10 mL/kg ventilation acute lung injury or ARDS: decrease $\dot{V}_T$: 6–7 mL/kg	Increased survivorship in ARDS with decreased $\dot{V}_T$
FI$_{O_2}$: 0.4–0.95	Titrate to Po$_2$> 60 mm Hg
PEEP: 5–20 cm H_2O pressure	Titrate to Po$_2$> 60 mm Hg and FI$_{O_2}$ $\leq$ 0.6
PSV: 10–35 cm H_2O pressure	Target $\dot{V}_T$ spont = $\dot{V}_T$ set
Waveform: decelerating ramp	Use square wave form in COPD only
P$_{aw}$-peak: <35 cm H_2O pressure	(Noted on dial on ventilator) P$_{aw}$ > 35 cm H_2O associated with lung injury
Sigh: 0–2/min	Optional—use with decreased respiratory rate to maintain alveolar recruitment
Temperature: 35°C	Not efficacious in rewarming or cooling
Q̇: start at 60 L/min (range, 45–75)	Titrate to P$_{aw}$-peak and Po$_2$
	Decrease Q̇ for hypoxemic patients
	Increase Q for patients with air hunger
Pressure-Cycled Ventilation (PCV) (Pressure set, Volume varies)	
Mode: SIMV	If patient is paralyzed: IMV = AC ventilation
Rate: 10–12/min	Decrease rate to allow longer time to exhale and to increase CO_2 clearance
PC: two thirds of prior P$_{aw}$-peak or prior plateau pressure	Titrate to P$_{aw}$-peak–$\dot{V}_T$ curve (hysteresis curve)
T$_i$: start at 2 sec and increase to increase mean P$_{aw}$ and Po$_2$	Increased T$_i$ will lead to IRV: will need heavy sedation and/or paralysis
FI$_{O_2}$: 0.4–0.95	Titrate to Po$_2$ > 60 mm Hg
PEEP: 5–20 cm H_2O pressure	Titrate to Po$_2$ > 60 mm Hg and FI$_{O_2}$ $\leq$ 0.6
PSV: 10–35 cm H_2O pressure	Target $\dot{V}_T$ spont = $\dot{V}_T$ set
Waveform: decelerating ramp	Use square wave in COPD only
Temperature: 35°C	Not efficacious in rewarming or cooling

Note:
1. Use inspiratory time-cycled PCV to precisely control I/E ratio. IRV is used to manage hypoxia but may lead to hemodynamic instability owing to decreased venous return and decreased cardiac output.
2. Best to titrate ventilator settings to the shape of the pressure-volume curve (need ventilator with a graphics package, a.k.a. "open lung model").

Special Circumstances

1. Severe acute lung injury—Consider permissive hypercapnia. If able to achieve Po$_2$ > 60 mm Hg on FI$_{O_2}$ $\leq$ 0.6, the Pco$_2$ may be allowed to be greater than 40 mm Hg if pH > 7.25. Further attempts to raise $\dot{V}_E$ to decrease Pco$_2$ may induce additional lung injury.
2. Asthma—Defect is decreased gas flow. In conventional ventilation, use higher flow rate and lower respiratory rate to allow more time for exhalation.
3. Traumatic brain injury—Do not lower Pco$_2$ < 35 mm Hg, because it may induce severe cerebral vasoconstriction and lead to cerebral ischemia. The goal is normal Pco$_2$: 35–40 mm Hg. Acceptable to hyperventilate for a patient with an acute herniation syndrome as a bridging maneuver for definitive therapy.
4. PEEP—Used to raise alveolar recruitment and increase Po$_2$ in patients with hypoxemic respiratory failure. *Caution*: Excessive PEEP can lead to hypotension from diminished venous return. Initial treatment of this hemodynamic instability is with volume replacement and lowered PEEP if possible.

AC, assist control; ARDS, acute respiratory distress syndrome; COPD, chronic olstructive pulmonary disease; FI$_{O_2}$, percent of inspired oxygen; I/E, inspiratory-to-expiratory ratio; IMV, intermittent mechanical ventilation; IRV, inverse ratio ventilation; P$_{aw}$, airway pressure; P$_{aw}$-peak, peak airway pressure; PC, pressure control (setting); Pco$_2$, pressure of carbon dioxide; PEEP, positive end-expiratory pressure (5 cm H_2O is considered physiologic); Po$_2$, pressure of oxygen; PSV, pressure-support ventilation; Q̇, flow rate; SIMV, synchronized intermittent mechanical ventilation; T$_i$, time in inspiration; $\dot{V}_E$, minute ventilation; $\dot{V}_T$, tidal volume.

Decelerating (Ramp). Once the maximal inspiratory flow is reached, the rate of gas delivery immediately begins to slow in a preprogrammed fashion. Therefore, relative to the square waveform, longer time is spent in inhalation to deliver the set $\dot{V}_T$ or achieve the target pressure, which allows for improved oxygenation. This waveform also achieves a lower P$_{aw}$-peak and a higher P$_{aw}$-mean.

Sine Wave. This is not useful in critically ill patients.

Accelerating. This is the flow pattern for neonatal gas intake and is generally not used in adult ventilation unless one must use the Siemens Servo 900 ventilator, which has only two options: square or accelerating.

Sighs. This is a large single breath or large multiple breaths, both designed to help maintain alveolar recruitment by ventilating a patient on a periodic basis at close to vital capacity. Controversy exists regarding the utility of the sigh option with regard to alveolar overdistention.[17]

Pause. Pause is a variable used on the Siemens Servo 900 ventilator to alter the I/E ratio. This is technically complex for anyone not working with ventilator setup on a daily basis.

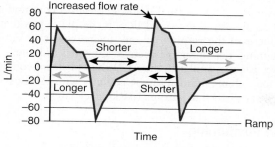

FLOW RATE: IMPACT ON T_i AND T_e

Equal V_T but different T_i and T_e

Figure 8–5 Effect of flow rate on inspiratory and expiratory times. Note that as the flow rate changes, there are corresponding alterations in the effective times for inspiration and exhalation. Deflections above the x-axis (time) indicate inspiration, and those below indicate exhalation. The delivered tidal volume for each cycle is the same, but the inspiratory and expiratory times are different.

It is much easier to directly adjust the T_i/T_e on more modern ventilators. A pause is useful to determine the plateau pressure on the Puritan Bennett 7200 or the Infrasonics Adult Star ventilator (as a point measurement). If a short pause is used to measure plateau pressure, the authors suggest no longer than 0.5 second as the pause duration; remove the pause when the measurement is completed.

NEW MODES

Airway Pressure Release Ventilation

Airway pressure release ventilation (APRV) is essentially a high level CPAP mode that is terminated for a very brief period. The CPAP level may be as high as 40 or more cm H_2O pressure. The long time during which the high-level CPAP is maintained achieves oxygenation whereas the short release period achieves CO_2 clearance (Fig. 8–6). The long time during which the high-level CPAP is present results in substantial recruitment of alveoli of markedly different regional time constants at rather low gas flow rates and lower $P_{aw}s$ (by comparison with conventional ventilation strategies). The establishment of intrinsic PEEP by the short release time enhances oxygenation. CO_2 clearance is aided by recruitment of the patient's lung at close to total lung capacity (TLC); elastic recoil creates large-volume gas flow during the release period. This is a fundamentally different mode from cyclic ventilation. This mode allows the patient to spontaneously breathe during all phases of the cycle. This mode is enabled to succeed by having a floating valve that is responsive to the patient's needs regardless of the location within the respiratory cycle. In other words, the patient is allowed to breathe in or out during the high-level CPAP phase as well as during the release phase. Accordingly, the sequence is called a *phase cycle*; there is no set inspiratory or expiratory time, and no readily identifiable respiratory rate in the traditional sense. During the high-CPAP phase, a patient may exhale 50 to 200 or more mL of gas as his or her lung volume becomes full of gas; this is not a full exhalation, and the release of excess gas should not be counted as a breath. APRV has been successfully used in neonatal, pediatric, and adult forms of respiratory failure. It is considered an alternative open lung model approach to mechanical ventilation.[18]

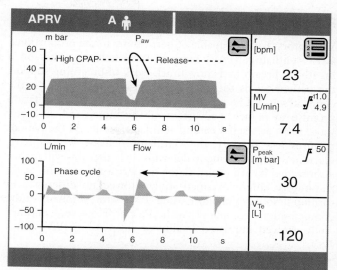

Figure 8–6 Airway pressure release ventilation (APRV)—airway pressure-time and flow-time traces. Note that the peak airway pressure (P_{aw}-high) is maintained for a long period. This phase establishes oxygenation (T_{high}). There is a short period of release when most CO_2 is cleared (T_{low}). The *bottom trace* indicates flow over time. The combined time for the T_{high} and T_{low} is known as a *phase cycle*. Note that the number of phase cycles is not the respiratory rate because patients breathe within the entirety of the T_{high}. As the release phase is initiated, the flow rate is identified as negative and is of a high rate (here ~7.5 L/min), consistent with significant alveolar recruitment. During the high continuous positive airway pressure (CPAP) phase, the patient is allowed to exhale (negative deflections on the flow-time trace). Thus, APRV is quite dissimilar from traditional cyclic ventilation. This unique mode is made possible by a floating valve system.

Given the spontaneous nature of the mode, there should be virtually no need for continuous infusions of neuromuscular blocking agents in patients placed on this mode of ventilation;[19] exceptions to this observation do occur for the management of intracranial pressure (ICP) but not for oxygenation or clearance of CO_2. This may result in a shorter length of ICU stay and a reduced incidence of prolonged neuromuscular blockade syndrome. Furthermore, because patients may be ventilated at lower $P_{aw}s$ than using cyclic ventilation, there is a reduced need for pressor support of hemodynamics to ensure $\dot{D}o_2$.[19] Moreover, there is a reduced sedative need because patients are more comfortable on this spontaneous mode than on cyclic ventilation.[19]

Hemodynamic assessment using a pulmonary artery catheter in patients on APRV has been investigated. The pulmonary artery occlusion pressure (PAOP) must be read at the middle or end of the release phase to maintain the fidelity of the reading. Reading the PAOP at any other point in the cycle will give a significantly different value by comparison with the end-expiratory reading obtained using PCV.[20] Transport of patients on APRV with a P_{aw}-high (sustained peak P_{aw}) greater than 20 cm H_2O pressure should be with the patient attached to the ventilator instead of being hand ventilated.[21] Hand ventilation is unable to match the manner of gas delivery and pressure dynamics that the patient requires. Attempts at hand ventilation, even with an appropriately set PEEP valve, are frequently complicated by unexpected hypoxemia and hemodynamic instability.

Proportional Assist Ventilation

Ventilators that are capable of performing in the proportional assist ventilation (PAV) mode will be able to assess on a breath-by-breath basis how much work of breathing support the patient needs to achieve the targets and goals that the clinician sets.[22] The unique features of this type of ventilation promise to reduce inadvertent airway injury and, in many ways, serve as a self-weaning ventilator mode. As the patient requires less support, the ventilator delivers less support. Current data are lacking to determine whether this will realize a shortened length of ventilator support for those with acute respiratory failure. A small study showed no difference in cardiopulmonary function using PAV with automatic tube compensation compared with PSV.[23] However, another study showed improved quality of sleep using PAV versus PSV.[24]

Permissive Hypercapnia

As stated, excessive P_{aw}-peak may be quite detrimental. One means of limiting P_{aw}-peak, and thereby offering protection from the trauma of ventilation, is to decrease the delivered $\dot{V}_T$ until an acceptable and less deleterious P_{aw}-peak is achieved (≤ 35 cm H_2O). However, changes in P_{aw}-peak may alter the pH-P_{CO_2} balance. If the pH is 7.25, and the patient can tolerate the elevated P_{CO_2} while still remaining well oxygenated, then the $\dot{V}_E$ is not increased. Alternatively, the f may be decreased in similar fashion, but usually not less than 8 breaths/min. This paradigm is known as *permissive hypercapnia*, and the concept represents a major departure from previously accepted tenets of MV, which mandated that MV should always achieve a normal P_{CO_2}.[25] Clearly, many patients can safely tolerate P_{CO_2} elevations that have in the past been thought to be harmful. A slower respiratory rate reduces the shear forces active across the alveolar common walls by allowing for fewer openings and closings per minute.[26] The side effect of such a rate reduction is greater time for exhalation that may lead to alveolar collapse and increased shear stress at the junction of open and closed alveoli. Nonetheless, a greater T_e helps prevent auto-PEEP, alveolar overdistention, and hemodynamic embarrassment. Likewise, a reduced $\dot{V}_T$ also helps prevent alveolar overdistention.

Although these features appear very attractive, permissive hypercapnia is not entirely benign. An elevated P_{CO_2} triggers cerebral vascular vasodilatation, which leads to increased cerebral blood flow and possible elevated ICP.[27] Increased ICP greater than 20 mm Hg can be detrimental in patients suffering from head injury or cerebral ischemia.[28] In patients with ALI complicating traumatic brain injury or stroke, such a management strategy is optimally accompanied by a measure of cerebral perfusion to evaluate for hyperemia or ICP monitoring to assess for intracranial hypertension from increased CO_2 tension.[29]

Hypercapnia also shifts the oxyhemoglobin dissociation curve to the right, leading to increased early unloading of O_2 at the tissue level. Hypercapnia also creates an acidosis that may initiate myocardial depression, dysfunction of pH-dependent enzyme kinetics, and distorted cellular metabolism.[30] Severe acidosis, pH less than 7.2, may be effectively countered by using an $NaHCO_3$ infusion. This proper intravenous infusion can be created by mixing 1 L of D_5W and 150 mEq of $NaHCO_3$, creating a sodium content similar to that of lactated Ringer's solution (130.4 mEq/L). Alternatively, if 150 mL of D_5W is removed before adding the 150 mL of $NaHCO_3$, the resultant Na^+ concentration is 150 mEq/L and approximates 0.9% normal saline solution. A common additional repair of the increased P_{CO_2} if the pH is less than 7.2 is to increase the respiratory rate to increase the $\dot{V}_E$ while maintaining the "lung protective low tidal volume." This strategy is quite similar to the ARDSNet protocol commonly used for volume ventilation of patients with ALI or acute respiratory distress syndrome (ARDS; see later).[31]

Prone Positioning

Multiple authors have proposed gravity as an effective aid in lung recruitment for those patients with severe or refractory hypoxemia.[32,33] Several studies have identified benefits in terms of increased P_{O_2} after pronation.[32,33] Prone positioning has also been shown to improve recruitment of edematous lung and reverse overinflation as compared with recruitment maneuvers, thus making aeration of the lung more homogeneous.[34] Several areas remain unresolved. It is unclear who will maximally benefit (up to one third have no benefit), how many proning cycles per day and for what duration are most beneficial, and how long to continue pronation once it has been initiated. What is clear is that chest geometry is critical in successful pronation[32] (Fig. 8–7). Patients with ovoid chests have little benefit from pronation because there are relatively equal lung volumes that exchange the superior and inferior positions when the patient is placed prone. Patients whose thoracic cage is more triangular have a greater volume of lung posteriorly (while in the supine position) that is able to

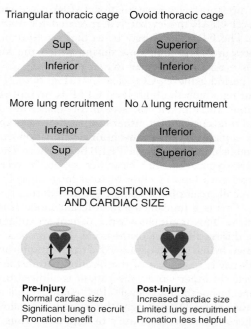

Figure 8–7 **Chest geometry and prone position.** Note that ovoid chest geometry results in equal volumes above and below the transverse axis, leading to no change in recruited lung volume with pronation. Triangular chest geometry leads to a significant increase in lung volume with prone positioning. This is by virtue of the large volume of lung that lies posterior to the transverse plane with the patient in the supine position. Increases in cardiac volume reduce the available retrocardiac lung volume and impair the effectiveness of prone positioning with regard to pulmonary recruitment.

exchange with a smaller volume of anterior lung. This patient population benefits from pronation.

Similarly, patients with small cardiac volumes benefit more than those with large volumes because there is more lung behind the heart to recruit with the pronation maneuver (see Fig. 8–7). It is quite clear that pronation is a challenging and potentially dangerous maneuver in a patient with invasive lines and an ETT in place, although no increase in unintentional extubations was noted in a study by Gattinoni and coworkers.[32] This risk of tube or catheter dislodgment or malposition is compounded by the altered hemodynamics in a patient who is not yet volume-replete, especially after trauma. A recent study of trauma and surgical ICU patients with ALI did show improvement of PaO_2/FI_{O_2} ratios, fewer ventilator days, and shorter hospital lengths of stay using a specialized bed to prone patients.[35] Given the potential for complications and the level of expertise and close monitoring required, pronation cannot be recommended as first-line therapy for hypoxemia in the ED. Instead, it is best reserved for the more controlled environment found in the ICU. Moreover, it is the author's experience that pronation use has been virtually eliminated since using APRV as the rescue mode of choice for refractory hypoxemia.

VENTILATOR ORDER GOALS

$\dot{V}_E$. $\dot{V}_E$ is the amount of gas delivered to a patient over a minute. It is calculated by multiplying the patient's respiratory rate by the tidal volume (f x $\dot{V}_T$) for patients without spontaneous breaths. It is conveniently determined by the ventilator and can be read directly for those with and without a spontaneous component to their $\dot{V}_E$. The need for $\dot{V}_E$ varies with the patient's condition, body mass, comorbidities, and acid-base status. For example, a patient who has a metabolic acidosis from diabetic ketoacidosis needs an elevated $\dot{V}_E$ to decrease Pco_2 and acutely buffer the acidosis. Thus, the emergency provider should determine what $\dot{V}_E$ range the patient will need and set the f, $\dot{V}_T$, or PCV/T_i to compensate for the increased metabolic acid load. A normal $\dot{V}_E$ is 7 to 10 L/min.

Spontaneous $\dot{V}_E$. Spontaneous $\dot{V}_E$ is the $\dot{V}_E$ derived from spontaneous breathing. During weaning, progressive increases in this parameter are expected as mandatory breaths are decreased or eliminated.

Spontaneous $\dot{V}_T$. See "Synchronized Intermittent MV" and "Pressure-Support Ventilation," earlier.

P_{aw}-peak. P_{aw}-peak is the maximum amount of reflected pressure in the patient's airway. This peak occurs during inspiration—an important concern because of the well-documented relationship of elevated P_{aw} (and volume) causing biotrauma.[4] Excessive P_{aw}-peak (>35 cm H_2O) commonly leads to alveolar overdistension and injury, causing release of inflammatory mediators and complications including pneumothoraces, pneumatoceles, pulmonary interstitial emphysema, pneumomediastinum, ALI, and ARDS. The P_{aw}-peak and alveolar overdistension are best evaluated using the PV curve, looking to abrogate any increases in P_{aw} that are not accompanied by increases in delivered volume (Fig. 8–8). Increases in P_{aw} without accompanying increases in V_T lead to a plateau of the PV curve, known as the "bird's beak" profile. This profile is a reasonable indicator of alveolar overdistension and airway injury.

Plateau Pressure. Plateau pressure is the pressure reflected from the airways once the full set volume or targeted

THE "BIRD'S BEAK" PROFILE

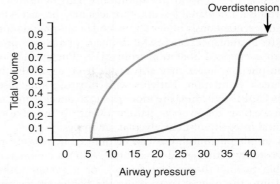

Figure 8–8 Alveolar overdistension is reflected in the increase in airway pressure without any concomitant increase in tidal volume. This PV curve pattern approximates a "bird's beak" profile.

P_{AW} AND T_i: IMPACT ON AUC

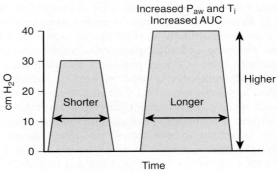

Figure 8–9 **Mean airway pressure and the pressure-time trace.** Note that the greater the maximum airway pressure and the longer the Ti, the greater the area under the curve (AUC) described by the positive-pressure (inspiratory) limb of the respiratory cycle. The increase in mean airway pressure (AUC) is the principal correlate of oxygenation in volume- or pressure-cycled ventilation.

pressure change has been achieved. It is a reflection of pulmonary compliance, airway resistance, and elastance. It is not directly manipulable, but may be affected by $\dot{V}_T$, $\dot{Q}$, PCV, T_i, and PEEP. It does provide a basis for the initiation of other modes of ventilation and is quite useful in that regard (see "Airway Pressure Release Volume," earlier).

P_{aw}-mean. The area under the pressure-over-time curve (Fig. 8–9) may be calculated and represents the P_{aw}-mean. The P_{aw}-mean correlates most closely with the achieved Po_2 in VCV or PSV modes. The longer the T_i, the greater the P_{aw}-mean. When a patient has hypoxemia and the clinician wants to change the ventilator orders, it is important to not reduce the P_{aw}-mean as a result of the change in therapy because a decreased P_{aw}-mean consistently leads to a decrease in Po_2.

COMPLICATIONS OF MV

Pneumothorax. Pneumothorax that is unassociated with trauma in a mechanically ventilated patient typically stems from alveolar overdistension (continuous or episodic), leading to alveolar rupture and escape of gas into the pleural space.[36] For patients who are on PPV, it is wise to drain the pleural space in order to prevent a simple pneumothorax from progressing to a tension pneumothorax with hemodynamic compromise. Loculated pneumothoraces may be successfully drained percutaneously under ultrasound or computed tomography (CT) guidance. Successful drainage of airspace disease leads to enchanced liberation from MV.[37] Pneumothorax or tension pneumothorax may also result from aggressive bag-valve-mask ventilation. Patients with intrinsic lung disease such as COPD or asthma are more prone to developing pneumothorax than the average patient owing to the abnormal structural integrity of their alveolar air spaces.[38]

A simple pneumothorax can be drained by surgical tube thoracostomy with a small-bore tube (24 Fr), a commercially available pneumothorax kit (Arrow), or a pigtail catheter placed into the pleural space using the Seldinger technique (see Chapter 10). Each of these catheters should be placed to a chest drainage collection unit that incorporates a water seal chamber as well as a variable suction control. Treat persistent air leaks initially with continuous suction (usually 20 cm H_2O suction) to evacuate the pleural space and promote coaptation of the visceral and parietal pleurae. Reduce suction and place the chest tube on water seal only after the resolution of the air leak. Remove the chest tube directly from water seal if there is no pneumothorax on chest film or after a test period of tube clamping and subsequent radiographic evaluation. The authors favor a 4-hour period of clamping because a recurrent pneumothorax is easier to treat by unclamping a tube than by placing a new one. Not all patients with a pneumothorax require invasive techniques to evacuate air from the pleural space. It is important to recognize that small pneumothoraces occurring in *spontaneously breathing patients* (i.e., negative-pressure ventilation) may be reevaluated in 4 to 6 hours with a repeat chest x-ray and drained only if they are expanding. This option is *not* advised for patients who are on any form of PPV because a simple pneumothorax can rapidly become a tension pneumothorax with subsequent hypotension and death. Tension pneumothoraces may be recognized by tachycardia, hypotension, elevated P_{aw}-peak (if mechanically ventilated, tachypnea if not), jugular venous distention (if not intravascularly depleted), thoracic resonance by percussion *on* the affected side, diminished or absent breath sounds *on* the affected side, and tracheal deviation *away from* the affected side. Clearly, not all signs or symptoms are present in all patients and treatment should be dictated by the patient's clinical condition.

Certain patients develop loculated pneumothoraces or fluid collections. If the collections are either single *or* immediately adjacent to one another and readily identified, they may be drained using ultrasound guidance at the bedside.[39] However, the loculations are frequently in inaccessible areas or are difficult to image with ultrasound. Therefore, CT scanning of the thorax can provide precise anatomic definition of the presence and number of loculated collections as well as a guide for the interventional radiologist. The authors have successfully used CT-guided drainage of loculated pleural collections (air and fluid) to assist weaning of head-injured patients from mechanical ventilator support.[37]

Biotrauma. *Biotrauma* refers to the self-sustaining process of lung injury from MV that follows alveolar overdistention or rupture, alveolar hypoperfusion, and repetitive shear stresses across alveolar walls. Originally, this problem was thought to be from too much pressure (barotrauma).[40] Current principles hold that elevated P_{aw}s are a straightforward reflection of excess volume delivered to a lung that cannot accept that much gas (i.e., volutrauma: excess volume is delivered).[12] When this process is active in a patient on MV, it is termed *ventilator-induced lung injury.* Lung injury is an inhomogeneous process with areas of normal lung immediately adjacent to diseased and injured segments.[41] Thus, the healthy and compliant segments with shorter regional time constants will readily accept gas, whereas their neighbors with reduced compliance and longer regional time constants will not. The end result is overdistention of the compliant segments, alveolar injury, and the liberation of inflammatory cytokines, chemokines, and activation of endothelin and arachidonic acid pathways, as well as the expression of adhesion molecules along the vascular endothelium.[4] This leads to infiltration of inflammatory cells, their destructive lysosomal enzymes, and the induction of toxic oxygen metabolites. Avoiding this inflammatory cascade is an intelligent means of protecting a patient's lungs from volume-induced lung injury. Such a notion has given rise to lung-protective ventilator strategies based on the low $\dot{V}_T$ ventilation (6–7 mL/kg body weight).[31] Several studies have reported the development of ventilator-induced lung injury in patients with normal lungs that were ventilated with larger $\dot{V}_T$s (12 ml/kg). Lung injury can develop within hours and has been linked to ventilation with large $\dot{V}_T$.[42–44] Current recommendations are for all MV to be with lower $\dot{V}_T$ than the once-standard 12 to 15 mL/kg. Patients with abnormal lungs (interstitial lung disease, lung resection, severe pneumonia, edema) and/or the presence of an ALI risk factor (sepsis, aspiration, transfusion) should be started on $\dot{V}_T$ of 6 mL/kg body weight. Those with normal lungs and no ALI risk factors should be started with $\dot{V}_T$ less than 10 mL/kg body weight.[44]

Hemodynamic Compromise. In all circumstances, the volume of venous return exactly matches the cardiac output volume. Any process that impedes venous return will decrease the available volume that establishes cardiac output. For patients on PPV, each gas delivery increases the intrathoracic pressure while exhalation decreases that pressure. Therefore, venous return principally occurs during exhalation. If the ventilator orders are constructed in such a way as to lead to increased intrathoracic pressure during exhalation, venous return will be reduced. Variables that can lead to this circumstance are increased PEEP, auto-PEEP, and IRV. Recall that venous return not only depends on a relatively negative pressure within the thoracic cavity but also relies on a sufficient amount of time for flow into the thoracic vasculature and right side of the heart. Thus, significantly high respiratory rates may compromise venous return as well. An additional untoward side effect of impaired venous return is cerebral venous hypertension from impeded venous drainage. Because there are no valves between the cerebral parenchyma and the right atrium, increased pressure on the right atrium reduces cerebral venous flow and may contribute to cerebral ischemia in patients with traumatic brain injury or stroke, especially in those with compromised systemic hemodynamics. Such patients are prone to watershed infarction; cerebral venous hypertension may increase this risk.

Ventilator-Associated Pneumonia. The association between the duration of endotracheal intubation and the promotion of pneumonia is quite clear. In fact, the likelihood of developing pneumonia is four times greater for patients in a surgical ICU than those in a medical ICU.[45] Endotracheal intubation for more than 12 hours increases the risk threefold.[45] A recent study showed that increased ED length of stay in emergently intubated blunt trauma patients was an independent risk factor for developing pneumonia. Each hour spent in the ED increased the risk of developing pneumonia by 20%.[46] Early pneumonias (<72 hr postintubation) are typically with community-acquired pathogens and may be adequately treated with American Thoracic Society (ATS) class A or B agents.[47] Late pneumonias (>72 hr) typically stem from nosocomial pathogens that may be resistant to community antibiotics.[47] Such patients need to have empirical coverage for *Pseudomonas*, methicillin-resistant *Staphylococcus aureus* (MRSA), and the other SPACE microbes (*Serratia, Pseudomonas, Acinetobacter, Citrobacter*, and Enterobactericiae). Empirical coverage for fungi is not warranted except in special circumstances (recrudescent pneumonia in a patient already on broad-spectrum antibiotics for >7 days with negative cultures; a solid organ transplant patient after implantation for >4 mo; poly-site–positive fungal cultures or fungemia). Unequivocally, clinical estimation of pneumonia is correct at best 33% of the time.[48] The most sensitive and specific test to diagnose pneumonia in a patient with a radiographic infiltrate, fever, leukocytosis, and purulent secretions is bronchoscopy and bronchoalveolar lavage (BAL) with quantitative cultures.[49] This strategy provides strong evidence of the exact pathogen(s), eliminates treating nonpathogenic microbes that are upper airway colonizers, and provides confidence in withholding antibiotic for the diagnosis of "no pneumonia," because many other diagnoses can present with a similar clinical picture (Fig. 8–10).

Nosocomial pathogens commonly have multiple resistance profiles, typically plasmid-mediated. Resistance pressure from the use of third-generation cephalosporins has led to the establishment of vancomycin-resistant enterococci (VRE) as well as extended-spectrum β-lactamase–producing (ESBL) organisms of which *Klebsiella* is the prototype.[50] Plasmid-mediated resistance to fluoroquinolones parallels the rise of ESBL-producing organisms.[51] Empirical antibiotic selection should be derived from each hospital's local antibiogram based on likely pathogens. A β-lactamase inhibitor combination paired with an aminoglycoside and vancomycin are the authors' empirical agents of choice based on their local antibiogram for ventilator-associated pneumonia. Should the reader's microbiology laboratory identify an ESBL-producing pathogen, the appropriate antibiotic class of choice is carbapenem.[52] Carbapenems consistently demonstrate excellent efficacy in eradicating ESBL-producing microbes.

ADJUNCTIVE THERAPIES

β₂-Agonists. These agents stimulate β-adrenergic receptors in bronchial smooth muscle, and induce muscle relaxation. This reduces airway resistance and improves gas flow through the conducting airways.[53] The β₂-agonists also inhibit mast cell degranulation, leading to ameliorated immune stimulation of the reactive airway. The most widely used agent in ICUs in the United States is albuterol. This agent may be administered via a side port of the ventilator circuit using a metered-dose inhaler (MDI; cost-effective). Alternatively, albuterol may be delivered by placing an in-line nebulizer device between the circuit and the ETT or on a side port on the ventilator tubing's inspiratory limb (ventilator tubing–dependent). Many patients may develop bronchoconstriction and wheezing when mechanically ventilated without a preexisting history of reactive airways disease. β₂-Agonists should be administered to patients who have poor air movement, wheezing, or both. A physiologically appropriate means of detecting and following bronchospasm is the peak-plateau gradient. A normal gradient is less than 4 cm H_2O pressure; increased values indicate increased airway resistance. The efficacy of treatment with β₂-agonists, intravenous magnesium, or diuresis may be assessed by following the changes in this gradient.

Acetylcholine Antagonists. The main utility of acetylcholine agents is to dehydrate secretions, although these agents may also block cholinergic-mediated bronchospasm. The most common agent is ipatropium bromide (Atrovent), an atropine derivative that has twice its biopotency on an equimolar basis. Ipatropium is commonly prescribed in combination with β₂-agonists every 4 to 8 hours. As with albuterol, ipatropium may be administered by MDI or nebulizer. Ipatropium is rarely used in isolation for the therapy of bronchospasm.

Mucolytics. The prototype for the mucolytic class is *N*-acetylcysteine (NAC). NAC is believed to reduce the adhesion of mucous strands to each other as well as to the luminal surface of the alveoli and larger airways. NAC may be administered by nebulizer or lavage routes but no MDI equivalent is available. NAC has the unfortunate side effect of inducing mucosal inflammation in an unpredictable fashion when used for longer than 24 hours. However, for the first 24 hours, NAC may provide significant benefit in liberating densely inspissated secretions from dependent portions of the airways.

Recruitment Maneuvers. Recruitment maneuvers are designed to apply consistent but well-regulated pressure to partly or completely closed alveoli to reintroduce gas into those segments.[54] The targeted segment(s) are those with poor compliance and long regional time constants. The area of interest is placed in a nondependent position (e.g., for left lower lobe benefit, place the left side of the patient up and the right side down), and the patient is hand ventilated using a bag-valve device attached to the ETT. An in-line pressure monitor is needed. The patient will usually require sedation to comply with the maneuver—fentanyl and midazolam are ideal. The clinician then applies pressure to the bag to achieve 35 cm H_2O pressure and holds it for 4 to 6 seconds, after which the patient is allowed to exhale. This cycle is repeated for up to 5 minutes. A second examiner listens to the area of

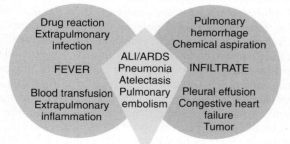

Figure 8–10 **Confounders in the diagnosis of pneumonia.** Fever, leukocytosis, radiographic infiltrate, and sputum production do not necessarily indicate the diagnosis of pneumonia. Multiple other causes should be considered as well so that one does not apply antibiotics when there is no infectious agent to address. ALI, acute lung injury; ARDS, acute respiratory distress syndrome.

FEVER PLUS INFILTRATE DOES NOT *NECESSARILY* EQUAL PNEUMONIA

Drug reaction
Extrapulmonary infection
FEVER
Blood transfusion
Extrapulmonary inflammation

ALI/ARDS
Pneumonia
Atelectasis
Pulmonary embolism

Pulmonary hemorrhage
Chemical aspiration
INFILTRATE
Pleural effusion
Congestive heart failure
Tumor

interest for an increase in breath sounds. The recruitment may be terminated when there are good breath sounds on two consecutive maneuvers. Recruitment maneuvers may be combined with chest physiotherapy for added benefit; chest physical therapy should, in general, precede the recruitment maneuver.

Bronchoscopy. See the discussion of nosocomial pneumonia under "Ventilator-Associated Pneumonia," earlier.

Bronchoscopy/BAL. With MV, the normal bacterial, viral, and secretion clearance mechanisms of the mucociliary elevator are compromised. Accordingly, excellent pulmonary toilet is required to prevent secretion impaction, atelectasis, pneumonitis, pneumonia, intrapulmonary shunt, or $\dot{V}/\dot{Q}$ mismatch. Despite seemingly adequate nursing or respiratory therapist care of a patient's airways, atelectasis, mucus plugging, and segmental or subsegmental airway obstruction and collapse may occur. Several initial maneuvers are indicated, including alveolar recruitment, chest physiotherapy, postural drainage, and aerosolized bronchodilator therapy. Frequently, these maneuvers resolve the elevated P_{aw}-peak and hypoxemia that are the markers of complications. When these initial therapies fail, a more invasive approach is warranted.

The traditional approach to clearance of inspissated secretions is therapeutic bronchoscopy. The adult flexible fiberoptic bronchoscope has an outer diameter of 3.3 mm and a working channel for suctioning of 2.5 mm. Therefore, an ETT of size 8.0 or larger is ideal because it will permit easy passage of the bronchoscope and allow for adequate MV of the patient. However, airway mucosal irritation is a powerful sympathetic stimulant. Tachycardia, systemic hypertension, and bronchospasm commonly complicate therapeutic bronchoscopy. In the setting of intracranial hypertension, the clinician must take steps to blunt any potential sympathetic stimulation. Mucosal irritation may be minimized by careful bronchoscopic technique that avoids impacting and suctioning the sidewalls. In addition, topical or systemic lidocaine will also blunt mucosal irritation. Preprocedure β-blockade with a relatively short-acting agent like esmolol will blunt the tachycardia and elevated dP/dt that accompanies heightened sympathetic tone. This will diminish any increase in cerebral blood flow that accompanies sympathetic discharge. Adjuvant therapy with narcotic analgesia, with a short-acting agent like fentanyl, will enhance sedation and ameliorate pain from mucosal injury. When these measures fail, significant sedation and cerebral protection may be achieved with cautious administration of barbiturates like sodium pentothal. Pentothal therapy may also be complicated by systemic hypotension. Alternatively, for very short procedures, etomidate is an excellent and powerful sedative that has the unique advantage of inducing diminished ICP. Thus, excellent intravenous access for fluid or inotrope administration is mandatory when using barbiturates. A postprocedure chest x-ray is indicated to assess the results of the bronchoscopy and to assess for complications such as a pneumothorax or ETT malposition.

When a specimen is obtained, examine it by Gram stain as well as culturing it for bacteria, viruses, fungi, or acid-fast bacilli when indicated. Use these results to help guide initial antibiotic therapy if the patient's clinical condition indicates infection (e.g., mucosal erythema, leukocytosis, fever, hypotension). The culture results are qualitative only and although they serve to identify which organism(s) is/are present, they do not indicate the bacterial burden. Accordingly, the utility of such results has been derided as being no more useful than an aspirate obtained by a closed-suction system. However, a closed-suction system does not allow directed suctioning of a particular side of the airway. In fact, the right side is more frequently suctioned than the left, based on the straighter geometry of the right main stem bronchus. To combat the geometry, "steerable" suction catheters are available that allow for directed lavage and suctioning. Furthermore, the suction catheter is enclosed within a sleeve that protects it from contamination during passage through the ETT and upper airways.

With both the "steerable" catheter system and therapeutic bronchoscopy, the techniques may be modified to allow for quantitative assessment of the bacterial/viral/fungal burden. The technique is called *bronchoalveolar lavage*, and relies on wedging the tip of the fluid instillation/suction catheter into a bronchopulmonary segment, instilling a known amount of fluid (usually 180 mL of normal saline in 60-mL aliquots), and recovering that fluid for analysis. An adequate recovery is greater than 50% of the instillate volume. Moreover, there are criteria for the diagnosis of infection (bacteria > 300 colony-forming units [CFU]/mL).[55] The criteria are liberalized (>500 CFU/mL) if the lavage and aspirate were performed in a larger airway such as the bronchus intermedius instead of a segmental orifice such as the superior segment of the lower lobe.

Another modality that may be useful in the diagnosis of pulmonary infection is the bronchoscopically directed "protected brush biopsy."[56] In this technique, the bronchoscope is advanced into the area of interest, and a sheathed brush is advanced through the working channel into the airway. Then the brush is extruded and worked back and forth against the airway to "biopsy" adherent microbes and airway mucosa. The brush is withdrawn into the sheath, and the entire assembly is withdrawn. The brush is then cut off and incubated in culture media. This technique has numerous advantages in that upper airway secretions may be suctioned without fear of contaminating the specimen and obtaining spurious results. By comparison, the standard BAL technique requires that the operator guide the bronchoscope into the affected region without suctioning so as to not contaminate the subsequently aspirated lavage sample. The downside to protected brush biopsy is that mucosal injury, bleeding, and pneumothorax occur more commonly than with bronchoscopically directed or steerable-catheter BAL. Regardless of the technique used, the clinician must match the sample results with the patient's clinical picture.

Gastric Content Aspiration and Pneumonia. Additional consideration is needed to avoid gastric acid blockade in patients who require prolonged intubation and MV. Gastric acid inhibition has, in some studies, been associated with a higher rate of nosocomial pneumonia than in patients who received ulcer prophylaxis with sucralfate alone.[57] It is believed that the gastric acid milieu destroys refluxed bacteria and that most nosocomial pneumonias occur because of aspiration of gastric contents. It is important to recall that aspiration may occur simply by "wicking" of gastric secretions along an indwelling nasogastric tube that stents open the upper and lower esophageal sphincters as well as by vomiting and passage of gastric contents along the sides of the cuffed ETT. Aspiration of gastric acid with intubation (the most common scenario) does not require antibiotic therapy, nor is it improved by the administration of glucocorticoids or the use of immediate bronchoscopy (unless there is large airway obstruction). The clinical syndrome of sterile gastric content aspiration is Mendelson syndrome.

Heliox Therapy. The interface of gas with airways creates a certain amount of friction. Heavier gases lead to greater amounts of friction than lighter gases. The more friction generated, the greater the work of breathing for a given gas. Severe asthma commonly entails significant work of breathing and may lead to respiratory failure from respiratory muscle fatigue. Altering the gas composition from $N_2:O_2$ to $He:O_2$ (Heliox) provides for a lighter gas that requires less work of breathing. Different percentage mixtures of $He:O_2$ are prepared and commercially available (e.g., 70% O_2 and 30% helium). Successful resolution of impending respiratory failure has been achieved using this strategy.[58] Note that this is not a commonly used therapy, but it is an important adjunct to have available when the need arises.

Negative-Pressure Ventilation. This unique mode of ventilation is best achieved using the Hayak Oscillator, a device produced in Israel. Its appearance is quite similar to a Cuirasse vest, but the driving negative-pressure source is quite different. The Hayak Oscillator features independent controls for the application of negative pressure as well as positive pressure, frequency of cycling between negative and positive pressure (inspiration and expiration), a chest physiotherapy mode for sputum expectoration (useful for those with cystic fibrosis), and a cardiopulmonary resuscitation mode. It is not widely used in the United States, but has demonstrated use in the cystic fibrosis patient population and during upper airway surgery, when an indwelling ETT would be a significant obstruction.[59]

SPECIAL TOPICS

Asthma. Fortunately, most patients with asthma are easily managed with combination therapy such as β_2-agonists, acetylcholine antagonists, and glucocorticoids. A true management challenge is the critically ill asthmatic. These patients are different from others with asthma exacerbation in that they require intubation and MV.[60] Unlike patients with many other disease states, asthmatics are not immediately improved by PPV; asthmatics often become acutely worse before any improvement from intubation and ventilation is realized. After intubation, the asthmatic's P_{aw}-peak is usually elevated. This leads to various problems including, but not limited to, early termination of a volume-cycled breath (excessive P_{aw} limiting the breath), impaired gas exchange (increased $\dot{V}_D/\dot{V}_T$), and the induction of "biotrauma" (see later). A slower respiratory rate allows for a longer time in exhalation. A prolonged T_e is essential for the patient with restrictive disease. In VCV, a lower respiratory rate with a low $\dot{V}_T$, as in the ARDSNet protocol, may be used for the management of life-threatening asthma.[31] With PCV (as discussed earlier), the set pressure may generate an inadequate $\dot{V}_T$ based on the restrictive component of the exacerbated asthma.

It is essential that bronchodilator and anti-inflammatory therapy (e.g., glucocorticoids) be pursued in conjunction with PPV for an optimal outcome.[61] A diligent search should be undertaken to discern any potential triggers (e.g., infection) that may be eliminated to hasten recovery and limit the duration of MV. Appropriate sedation is critical to ensure adequate gas exchange; it enables the patient to "synch" with the ventilator and not trigger early volume-cycled breath termination. If sedation alone is inadequate to reduce the restriction imposed by the chest wall or intra-abdominal contents, pharmacologic relaxation is then indicated (although uncommonly required). Heliox therapy has also been used with success for the failing asthmatic as a means of avoiding intubation in select patients (see "Heliox Therapy," earlier).[62] APRV has been used for severe life-threatening asthma; insufficient data are currently available to recommend this as front-line therapy. Its role may be as a salvage mode for asthmatics with refractory hypoxemia.

Ventilator-Weaning Protocols and Pathways

A well-designed weaning protocol is an invaluable aid in reducing the length of stay in the ICU. An appropriate protocol will enable the respiratory therapist and bedside nurse to initiate the weaning process each day before clinician evaluation. Computer order entry may create an ICU admission data set that automatically activates such a protocol once the entry criteria are met (i.e., the cause of respiratory failure is improving or has been eliminated, $FI_{O_2} < 0.50$, PEEP < 10 cm H_2O, and no pressors other than dopamine at < 5 $\mu g/kg$ per minute or epinephrine or norepinephrine at < 0.05 $\mu g/kg$ per minute). A ventilator pathway to chart and modify the progress of each patient through her or his MV needs is a useful tool. Such a pathway allows clinicians to regularly review a patient's progress along what would be considered a "usual course" for someone requiring MV. Deviation from this course should prompt an investigation into the cause(s). A pathway is also an excellent tool to use as a platform for quality assurance and improvement review.

Neuromuscular Blockade

Neuromuscular blocking agents are used to induce muscular paralysis for various reasons including, but not limited to, reducing P_{aw}-peaks during MV, reducing total body $\dot{V}_{O_2}$, protecting life-sustaining indwelling devices, and placing an artificial airway. Agent selection entails consideration of factors identical to those surrounding analgesic and sedative selection. Commonly used agents include pancuronium, vecuronium, and cisatracurium. All may be given by bolus or continuous infusion. Only pancuronium and vecuronium have active metabolites and reportedly result in prolonged neuromuscular blockade in some patients after cessation of drug therapy.[63] Furthermore, aminoglycosides, for instance, may potentiate the effect of neuromuscular blocking agents, thus reducing the amount of drug necessary to achieve the desired paralysis.[64] The authors prefer cisatracurium for neuromuscular blockade because it undergoes Hoffman elimination in the plasma and is therefore independent of renal or hepatic metabolism. However, the authors also rarely use neuromuscular blockade outside of the operating room except when placing an ETT.

Paralysis is commonly titrated to an effect monitored by a peripheral nerve monitor applied over the ulnar or other peripheral nerve distribution.[65] No blockade results in four twitches of the adductor pollicis muscle resulting from four supramaximal triggering stimuli; complete blockade yields no response. A common goal of blockade is use of enough agent to result in two twitches out of a "train of four." Another goal of twitch monitoring is to avoid overparalysis, to diminish the risk of prolonged neuromuscular blockade after withdrawal of the agent. If, however, zero twitches are required to achieve the goals of therapy, the monitor cannot monitor overparalysis at all. In addition, if feasible, many clinicians allow patients to emerge from paralysis once during each 24-hour period to perform a neurologic assessment and help ensure return of neuromuscular function after cessation of drug therapy. There are no data to support this practice as a preventive measure, but it seems to make intuitive sense. There is a growing trend to avoid chemical relaxation throughout the United States; chemical relaxation is rare in the European Union for patient management in the critical care arena.

The myriad potential complications of neuromuscular blockade have been described in detail in standard anesthesia texts. However, two important complications deserve mention: prolonged paralysis syndrome[63] and the polyneuropathy of critical illness.[66] The postparalysis syndrome is diffuse motor weakness associated with elevated creatine kinase levels (MM fraction) and preserved sensory nerve function on electromyography and nerve conduction velocity testing. By comparison, critical illness polyneuropathy involves both sensory and motor nerves and is less frequently associated with neuromuscular blocking agents as an etiologic cause. Critical illness polyneuropathy is believed to be principally related to the underlying disease and carries a less favorable prognosis for recovery than postparalysis syndrome. Some data implicate the aminosteroid structure of vecuronium and pancuronium in the pathogenesis of either of the complications mentioned previously by drawing a parallel between the neuromuscular blockade polyneuromyopathies discussed earlier and those identified in patients on long-term steroid regimens. However, data are currently inconclusive as to the exact etiology of the syndromes discussed earlier.

Sedation

Patients on MV commonly require some sedation, which can be provided in an intermittent bolus fashion or by continuous infusion. Clinician monitoring of the depth and adequacy of sedation is feasible in an inactive patient. When patients require sedation for agitation control, are mechanically ventilated, or are chemically relaxed, the ability of the clinician to assess the depth and adequacy of sedation is severely impaired. In addition, because the use of pharmacologic paralysis presents the external appearance of a quiet, restful patient, it is important to have some means of titrating sedation to an appropriate level. The authors favor using a modified single-lead electroencephalogram montage known as the *bispectral index* (BIS; Fig. 8–11). This device integrates a power spectrum of the coherence of electrical activity of the monitored areas of the brain and translates the information into an analog value ranging from 0 to 100.[67] Lower numbers indicate deeper levels of sedation. This device has been successfully used in the operating room to monitor and titrate the level of benzodiazepine or propofol sedation for surgical procedures.[68] Further experience is being gained in the ICU titration of therapy in pharmacologically paralyzed patients as well as monitoring serial changes after central neuraxial injury or illness that results in brain death. The authors have used BIS monitoring to decrease sedative agent usage and cost in intubated, neuromuscularly blocked and sedated patients in the critical care setting.[69] Protocol-driven sedation guidelines may decrease the duration of MV, complications, and ICU length of stay.[70]

Neonatal Ventilation

It is clear that neonatal ventilation is not simply ventilation of small adults. The vast majority of neonatal ventilation is performed as PCV, albeit with smaller volume targets than in

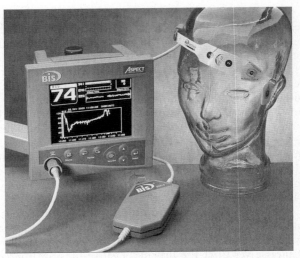

Figure 8–11 The Bispectral Index monitor (Aspect Medical, Nantucket, MA). This pole-mounted device attaches to the patient's forehead and provides a modified single-lead electroencephalogram whose power spectrum undergoes a Fourier transformation to yield a numeric representation of the level of sedation.

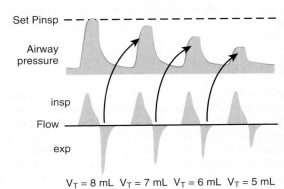

VOLUME GUARANTEE

$V_T = 8$ mL $V_T = 7$ mL $V_T = 6$ mL $V_T = 5$ mL

Figure 8–12 Volume guarantee ventilation. Note that the ventilator uses the prior breath to determine how much support is required to achieve the desired tidal volume and remain within the set pressure limit.

adults (i.e., same milliliters per kilogram of body weight but smaller changes in pressure to achieve the smaller needed volumes). Note, however, that neonatal ventilation may also be performed using VCV. Not all ventilators can deliver the small volumes required for this kind of ventilation, and special ventilators dedicated to neonatal ventilation have been developed (e.g., Babylog by Drager, Bird Ventilator). Many adult ventilators are equipped with a software package that allows the microprocessor to control pressure, flow rates, and volume in this application (e.g., Drager E4 with Neoflow, Siemens Servo 300C). Furthermore, there are hybrid modes such as pressure-support ventilation volume guarantee (PSV-VG) that combines the best of both worlds.[71] One simply sets a pressure-support limit as well as a desired volume for each breath. The ventilator then determines on a breath-by-breath basis how much pressure support is required to achieve the set target and remain within the pressure limit (Fig. 8–12). In this way, the mode is also self-weaning; as the patient's need for support decreases, the support, in fact, decreases (Fig. 8–13). Because the equipment varies at each institution,

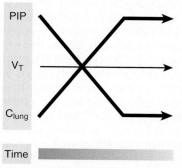

PSV + VG:
The Concept of "Autoweaning"

Figure 8–13 Pressure support volume guarantee ventilation. As the compliance of the lung (C lung) improves, the positive inspiratory pressure (PIP) decreases while maintaining a constant tidal volume ($\dot{V}_T$). When the pressure support volume is reduced to an acceptable minimum level, weaning has been achieved and the patient should be evaluated for liberation from mechanical ventilation.

clinicians are urged to familiarize themselves with the available ventilator and how to use it. Guidance from a neonatal intensivist in conjunction with a respiratory therapist is ideal.

Noninvasive Ventilation

Intubation, MV, and its sequelae may be avoided in a select group of patients suffering from acute respiratory failure by using noninvasive ventilation (NIV) techniques (see Chapter 2). It is important to recall that if the patient's physiology requires definitive airway control, NIV is not appropriate. This modality may be effectively used in patients who do not wish to be intubated (e.g., those with end-stage COPD) and in patients who need time for medical therapy to achieve its goals (e.g., those with congestive heart failure). In general, NIV is commonly used for temporary ventilatory and oxygenation support (e.g., <24 hr). Patients requiring longer acute management are optimally managed by tracheal intubation and MV.

For NIV to be used, three things must be true: the airway must be patent, the respiratory drive must be intact, and the patient must be cooperative (i.e., awake and alert). Recent studies have shown that even patients with hypercapnic encephalopathy may tolerate NIV with survival results similar to patients that were intubated and mechanically ventilated. The patients on NIV did have reduced nosocomial infections and duration of support compared with the intubated patients.[72] It is imperative that the patient understands the roles of the machine and the mask to aid with compliance and efficacy. It is essential to use the correct size mask to maintain a good seal for optimal results and to lessen the risk of injury from an inappropriately tight or ill-fitting mask. For nasal masks, there is a template to help the therapist select the most appropriate piece of equipment. The potential benefits of NIV over MV are a decrease in potential airway injury, nosocomial airway and tracheobronchial tree infection, and probably a shorter length of stay in a monitored bed or ICU.[73] Documented risks include barotrauma (volutrauma); pressure necrosis of the facial skin, subcutaneous tissue, and musculature; and gastric dilation followed by vomiting and aspiration

or hemodynamic compromise.[74] Two main types of NIV are available in the ED—CPAP and bilevel positive airway pressure (BiPAP).

CPAP

CPAP is a widely used type of noninvasive ventilatory support. This modality delivers a variable gas flow to achieve a constant P_{aw}. It is commonly used in patients with obstructive sleep apnea to prevent upper airway collapse.[75] All forms of NIV require some type of tight-fitting mask to maintain a good seal (see Fig. 3–4). The CPAP mask is a full-face mask. It must be properly fitted to the patient both for efficacy and to avoid complications (e.g., pressure necrosis). The full-face mask may be intolerable for some patients because it may induce a sense of confinement and claustrophobia. Acutely ill patients are also unable to remove the mask to eat because they are dependent on the P_{aw} for oxygenation and ventilation. For the acutely ill patient in the ED, CPAP may help reduce the work of breathing while facilitating CO_2 clearance and O_2 on-loading.

BiPAP

BiPAP is a combination of PSV and CPAP (see Chapter 3 and Fig. 3-4). The clinician can set two different pressure levels for the patient: (1) inspiratory positive airway pressure (IPAP), which is delivered during inspiration, and (2) expiratory positive airway pressure (EPAP), which is applied during exhalation. In general, IPAP exceeds EPAP. This modality is pressure limited, and flow is triggered by either the patient's inspiratory effort or a time limit between cycles.

In the patient-triggered mode, the device senses the onset of inspiration, and the preset IPAP cycle is initiated. When the patient finishes inhalation, IPAP is cycled off, and the P_{aw} is allowed to decrease to the preset EPAP level. The average starting range for IPAP is 8 to 10 cm H_2O whereas EPAP is 3 to 5 cm H_2O. Adjustments of these levels are generally made in 2–cm H_2O increments. Generally, increases or decreases in each are titrated to patient comfort (both IPAP and EPAP), SaO_2 (IPAP and EPAP), and the volume of gas that is moved (IPAP). A general approach is to increase IPAP until achieving reasonable $\dot{V}_T$ and Pco_2. If oxygenation remains inadequate, then EPAP is usually increased. Adjusting FI_{O_2} is somewhat more difficult with BiPAP than with other modes of invasive or NIV.

The BiPAP machine is connected to oxygen. It is run at the same flow rate that the patient required immediately before implementing NIV. Recall that the final FI_{O_2} is a blend of entrained room air and the bleed-in rate of O_2 from the pure 100% O_2 source (wall or tank). Each breath may therefore deliver a different final FI_{O_2}, dependent on patient comfort and the respiratory effort.

When initiating BiPAP, the initial maneuvers are similar to those for initiating CPAP. An appropriate-sized full-face mask is chosen using the guide mentioned earlier. The mask should not place direct pressure on the bridge of the nose, the lateral ala, the inferior nasal septum, or the lip. The patient can participate in his or her care by initially holding the mask in place while the therapist adjusts the settings and the patient adjusts to the sensations and pressure (airway and mask). The mask is secured in place by using adjustable Velcro straps. With the nasal mask, it is important to encourage the patient to breathe with the mouth closed; in general, nasal BiPAP is quite difficult and not recommended for the acutely ill patient. It is important to check the fit of the mask for air leaks because they diminish the efficacy of the modality in proportion to the size of the leak. It is possible to obtain near-optimal settings in about 10 minutes.

Patients undergoing NIV need close monitoring and observation.[76] Patients initiated on BiPAP therapy should not be admitted to the general medical floor; step-down–level care is a minimum whereas ICU level care is optimal. Each hospital will have admission criteria for the care of patients on NIV that is driven by both clinician and nursing protocols designed to provide safe care of patients with potentially unstable airways and respiratory dynamics. Accordingly, these patients should be initially observed on continuous SaO_2 and hemodynamic monitoring of heart rate, blood pressure, and respiratory rate. If available, continuous E_Tco_2 monitoring may be beneficial. An arterial blood gas (ABG) should be obtained after initiating BiPAP therapy to assess CO_2 clearance and pH-Pco_2 balance. Titration of O_2 flow rate may be performed using SaO_2 monitoring instead of repeat analysis of ABGs. In general, increases in IPAP will increase the V_T and lower CO_2, whereas increases in EPAP will increase FRC and increase O_2. BiPAP has been successfully used in the ED and in the postoperative ICU setting for short-term respiratory support in patients with a correctable underlying cause of their respiratory failure.[77]

Evaluation Adjuncts

The totality of the ventilator prescription interacts with the patient's pulmonary system in ways that may be assessed. The most straightforward is physical examination (see the discussion on endotracheal intubation under "Indications for MV," earlier). However, the end result of the ventilator prescription is commonly evaluated using an ABG analysis. This directly measures pH, Pco_2, and Po_2, and the remainder of the values, including base excess (deficit), are calculated from an algorithm. Additional information that is frequently available as part of the ABG analysis usually includes hemoglobin (Hgb) or hematocrit (Hct), Na^+, K^+, Ca^{2+} (ionized), glucose, and lactate.

E_Tco_2 Analysis, Capnometry, and Capnography (see also Chapter 2)

In addition, the flow pattern of exhaled gas as measured by the expired CO_2 concentration over time is evaluated by CO_2 capnometry (numeric data) or CO_2 capnography (graphic analysis).[78] Capnometry (quantitative measurement of CO_2) is a useful means of noninvasively tracking a patient's CO_2 tension. The principle behind capnometry is that the CO_2 measured at the end of a tidal exhalation (E_Tco_2) will approximate the alveolar CO_2 and thus the blood Pco_2. If the E_Tco_2 measurement and the Pa_{co_2} correlate, then changes in V_E that are designed to produce a certain Pco_2 may be followed without the need for ABG determination. In normal lungs, the E_Tco_2 is 1 to 5 mm Hg less than the Pco_2 as a consequence of heterogeneous alveolar expiratory dynamics (i.e., alveolar unit heterogeneity with regard to time constants for alveolar gas flow). E_Tco_2 measurement may be accomplished by three means: infrared spectroscopy (most common), chemical analysis (common, qualitative only), and mass spectroscopy (uncommon and expensive).

Infrared capnometry passes a narrow band of infrared light through a sample of gas and determines the CO_2 concentration by analyzing the amount of light absorbed by the CO_2. Access to exhaled gas through the ventilator circuit occurs by way of either mainstream or sidestream sampling. The mainstream sensors are directly in line with the breathing circuit and pose two hazards and one disadvantage: (1) weight and rotational torque on the ETT, (2) an increase in dead space, and (3) the need to heat the sensor to avoid condensation. Sidestream analyzers continuously obtain gas through a side port attached to the ETT and have two disadvantages: (1) the small port is easily occluded with secretions, and (2) they are slower than mainstream analyzers. Capnometry helps ensure that the ventilator is indeed connected to the patient and allows determination of dead space relative to $\dot{V}_T$ (important in patients with large anatomic dead spaces, severe lung injury, or both). However, much more information can be obtained from the graphic display of exhaled CO_2 over time (capnography).

In particular, a normal exhaled CO_2 tracing plateaus at the end of exhalation (Fig. 8–14). If there is chronic obstructive airways disease or a significant amount of air trapping from auto-PEEP, the tracing will not plateau owing to the prolonged expiratory phase required to empty the alveoli (Fig. 8–15). The presence of significant auto-PEEP may indicate increased intrathoracic pressure, impeded venous return, and thus secondary intracranial venous hypertension. Auto-PEEP may also be detected on ventilators equipped with a graphic display of flow or volume over time. However, because most ventilators in use are not so equipped, an E_Tco_2 monitor

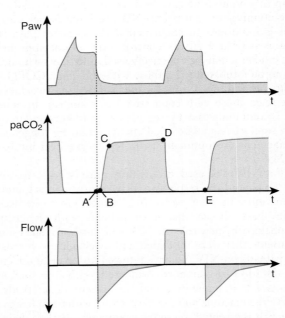

Figure 8–14 The end-tidal carbon dioxide (E_Tco_2) trace. This diagram of an E_Tco_2 capnograph represents normal exhalation flow dynamics. As exhalation progresses, the measured CO_2 rises and eventually plateaus. At the end of the plateau, immediately before the downstroke of the trace is the point at which the E_Tco_2 value is measured and reported (e.g., point D). No other values are reported on the E_Tco_2 capnometer. Thus, in the absence of the capnograph, all other information is unavailable to the clinician. Abnormalities in endotracheal tube position, blockage of the airway (complete or partial), and correct endotracheal tube placement are identifiable by evaluating the E_Tco_2 tracing. (*Reproduced with permission from Drager Medical, Hemel Hempstead, United Kingdom.*)

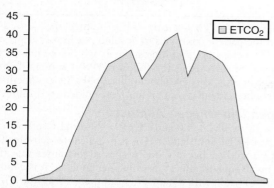

ETCO₂ AND COPD

☐ ETCO₂

Figure 8–15 The E_Tco₂ tracing in chronic obstructive pulmonary disease (COPD)—identification of auto-PEEP. In this diagram of an E_TCO₂ trace in a patient with COPD who is being ventilated at a high respiratory rate, one may detect the presence of auto-PEEP based on the abnormal expiratory flow pattern. A similar suggestion could be obtained by interrogating the flow-time trace as well.

tracing may serve as a reasonable substitute. Capnography has also been used to determine the optimal level of PEEP,[79] adequacy of cardiopulmonary resuscitation,[80] and detection of pulmonary embolus.[81] In the authors' opinions, all critically ill mechanically ventilated patients with traumatic brain injury should be attached to a capnograph/capnometer device. Infrared capnography is the current standard of care in the operating room for CO_2 detection. In the near future, estimates of metabolic rate may be available on a breath-by-breath basis using a capnometry platform.

Chemical analysis of exhaled CO_2 has been effectively used for several years to confirm endotracheal placement of artificial airways.[82] The presence of CO_2 in the exhaled gas causes a color change in the monitoring device. The device is disposable and placed between the ETT and the high-flow O_2 bag-valve unit. It does not impede ventilation. In the authors' institutions, these relatively inexpensive devices are kept in all of the airway management carts, the ICUs, and the ED and are routinely used in confirming airway placement.

Radiography. A standard portable anteroposterior chest radiograph after the initiation of MV (and ETT placement)

is the existing standard of care. It is not recommended to send a newly intubated patient requiring MV out of the ED to obtain a chest film.

RESPIRATORY THERAPY

The trained, certified respiratory therapist may be the clinician's "best friend" with regard to MV. These individuals are invaluable in helping the clinician achieve the desired goals of MV. They are generally more familiar with individual machine performance characteristics than is the typical clinician, and they are responsible for ensuring that the device is functioning properly and with appropriate alarm limits. Multiple studies have documented that respiratory therapist–driven weaning protocols achieve a more rapid liberation from MV than those driven by clinicians.[83] To achieve these results, a weaning protocol is ideally developed in a multidisciplinary fashion, activated by clinician order, and then implemented by the therapists. The clinician is again engaged when the patient either fails to progress along the pathway or has achieved extubation criteria. Only in rare circumstances is the clinician creating the settings on the ventilator—this is the purview of the respiratory therapist. If the clinician wants to manipulate the ventilator directly, advanced training and local hospital credentialing are recommended.

CONCLUSIONS

MV is a complex process that requires dedication on the part of the clinician. Usually, the least difficult aspect of initiating MV is establishing an airway. The ED clinician should recall that the early period of MV may set the tone of events related to the remainder of the patient's course on the ventilator. Optimally, the ED clinician should be familiar with the spectrum of ventilatory modes available for use in the hospital; ventilator prescriptions are not ideally managed in a "one prescription fits all" fashion. Alternatives to endotracheal intubation should be considered in select patient populations. Medical adjuncts frequently enable the clinician to manage difficult ventilation issues while optimizing pulmonary dynamics. Difficult ventilatory issues (e.g., refractory hypoxemia) may be best comanaged with a dedicated intensivist in the ED if the patient cannot be rapidly transferred to the ICU.

CASE MANAGEMENT

Placing a patient on a ventilator and managing the setup and changes in ventilation requirements are formidable tasks for any clinician. This section presents a step-by-step approach to managing two individual patients who require MV. A number of practical and logistical issues, types of ventilators, various modes of ventilation, and practical settings and subsequent changes are illustrated.

CASE 1

An 18-year-old, otherwise healthy, 60-kg female presents with an overdose of benzodiazepines. She requires intubation for airway protection and ventilatory support. There is no evidence of aspiration or an intrinsic lung problem.

VCV

Devices Reviewed
Puritan Bennet 7200, 7200a, or 7200ae or the Drager Evita 4 Pulmonary Workstation.

Target $\dot{V}_E$ 7.2 L/min
It is reasonable to assume a normal need for $\dot{V}_E$ because she has no evidence of hypoperfusion or infection, and she has not ingested any medications known to cause a metabolic acidosis that would require a higher $\dot{V}_E$ to buffer by induced hypocarbia.

Mode
Because this patient has preserved spontaneous respirations, it is reasonable to allow her to continue to do so because she is

Continued

CASE MANAGEMENT—cont'd

not presenting problems with an increased work of breathing (nonlabored respirations, no accessory muscle use, no stridor, no wheezing, and no hypoxia). This means that one must couple the SIMV mode with PSV to eliminate work of breathing increases associated with the resistance of the artificial airway. Depending on the model of 7200 ventilator, the mode settings will appear either along the bottom or at the left side (Fig. 8–16). Using the Drager E₄, the mode will appear in the lower right hand side of the touch screen (Fig. 8–17).

Rate and $\dot{V}_T$

Twelve breaths per minute and a maximum volume of 600 mL (7–10 mL/kg). These must be considered together to achieve

the desired $\dot{V}_E$. This setting will guarantee the desired $\dot{V}_E$ even if the patient continues to develop respiratory depression from the benzodiazepine ingestion. It will allow her to take additional breaths using the following PSV settings if she so desires or needs to overcome an increased CO_2 production or a metabolic acidemia from an as of yet unidentified source.

Oxygen and Oxygen Adjuncts

Start with an FI_{O_2} = 1.0 and PEEP = +5 cm H_2O pressure. As FI_{O_2} and PEEP both affect P_{O_2}, it is logical to consider their settings together. Because one wishes to guarantee that there is no hypoxemia to affect anaerobic metabolism, it is common practice to begin with a high FI_{O_2} and then reduce the FI_{O_2} to

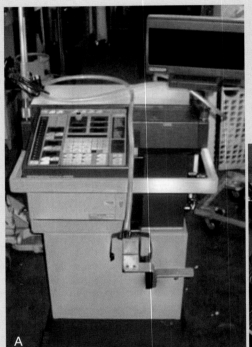

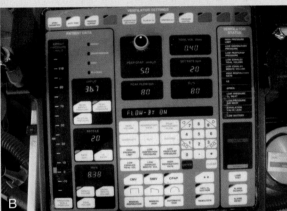

Figure 8–16 *A,* The Puritan-Bennett 7200 AE Model ventilator. The specifications of the 7200 model are shown below. This model is no longer made, but it is still one of the most commonly used ventilators in the intensive care unit. *B,* Control panel for the Puritan-Bennett 7200.

Specifications: Puritan Bennett 7200 Ventilator
Operator-selected parameters
   Tidal volume: 0.1–2.5 L
   Respiratory rate: 0.5–70 beats/min
   Maximum peak inspiratory flow: 120 L/min during mandatory breathing; 180 L/min during spontaneous breathing
Sensitivity inspiratory: 0.5–20 cm H_2O bellow PEEP
   Oxygen percentage: 21%–100%
   Plateau: 0–2 sec
   PEEP/CPAP: 0.1–2.5 L, not to exceed twice $\dot{V}_T$
   Sigh rate and frequency: 1–15 sighs/hr; 1–3 sighs/event.
Operator-selected alarm thresholds
   High airway pressure: 10–120 cm H_2O
   Low airway pressure: 3–99 cm H_2O
   PEEP/CPAP pressure: 0–45 cm H_2O
   Exhaled $\dot{V}_T$: 0–2.5 L
   Low exhaled minute volume: 0–60 L
   High respiratory rate: 0–70 beats/min
   Sigh high airway pressure: 10–120 cm H_2O, not to exceed twice high airway pressure
   Ventilatory modes: Operator selectable. Continuous mandatory ventilation (CMV); synchronous intermittent mandatory ventilation (SIMV); CPAP
   Inspiratory flow waveforms: Square, descending ramp, or sine
   Alarm control functions: Alarm silence: silences alarm for 2 min. Alarm reset: resets ventilator to prealarm state of alert.
   Parameters display: Airway pressure; exhaled volume; type of breath: assist, spontaneous, sigh, and plateau; mean airway pressure; peak airway pressure; PEEP/CPAP pressure; plateau pressure; respiratory rate; inspiratory-to-expiratory (I/E) ratio; $\dot{V}_T$; minute volume; and spontaneous minute volume.

CASE MANAGEMENT—cont'd

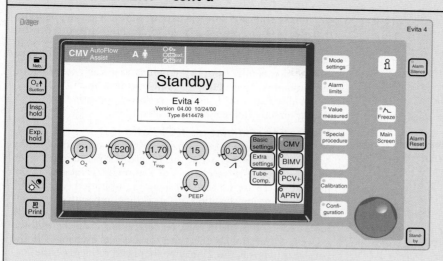

Figure 8–17   Faceplate for the Drager Evita 4 Pulmonary Workstation. Note that the liquid-crystal display (LCD) screen is colored and has controls embedded in the screen to adjust the individual mode settings. The right-hand controls on the front of the device control the kind of screen display, the silence button, and the standby button.

nontoxic levels using pulse oximetry (goal $FI_{O_2} < 0.60$). On the 7200 series, the FI_{O_2} is set using the O_2 concentration button in the central portion of the ventilator faceplate; the FI_{O_2} is directly entered using the numeric keypad followed by the "Enter" key (see Fig. 8–16). On the E_4, the FI_{O_2} is set by touching the faceplate numeric symbol for FI_{O_2} (it turns yellow), and then rotating the knob on the lower right of the ventilator faceplate to achieve the desired setting; the knob must then be pressed to signal the ventilator that you wish to accept the value (symbol reverts to green).

It is reasonable to start with a relatively low level of PEEP and evaluate the P_{O_2} that is achieved at the delivered FI_{O_2}. On the 7200, the PEEP is indicated by the "PEEP/CPAP" button (see Fig. 8–16). On the E_4, the PEEP is set directly on the faceplate using the same technique as for setting the FI_{O_2}. The evaluation of the adequacy of the set FI_{O_2} and PEEP on P_{O_2} is easily performed by assessing the Alveolar-arterial gradient (A-a gradient; normal gradient ≤50). High A-a gradients may trigger an increase in PEEP to increase FRC and P_{O_2}.

PSV

Initiate PSV at 10 cm H_2O pressure, and then titrate up or down to achieve a spontaneous breath $\dot{V}_T$ approximately equal to that of the set $\dot{V}_T$. On the 7200, the value displayed for each spontaneous breath is one breath behind what one observes in the patient. The value is displayed after depressing the $\dot{V}_T$ key in the grouping with $\dot{V}_E$ and spontaneous V_E (see Fig. 8–16); the $\dot{V}_{Tspont}$ will not display if one depresses the central keypad labeled "tidal volume," because this key gives one the set $\dot{V}_T$ and displays its figures in the liquid crystal display (LCD) bar in the middle of the faceplate (see Fig. 8–16). On the E_4, PSV is adjusted by activating the touchpad button labeled "PSV." The knob is rotated to achieve the desired setting and then depressed to accept that setting (see Fig. 8–17).

Gas Delivery Waveform

Begin with a decelerating waveform. Recall that the ramp waveform immediately begins to decrease flow after achieving the maximal inspiratory flow that one sets. This is a standard setting for the authors. The three waveforms are indicated by the three white buttons on the lower central portion of the 7200 faceplate (see Fig. 8–16); press "Enter" after selecting the waveform that is to be activated. On the E_4, the waveform may be manually selected using the setup function under "Modes," or it will be automatically selected by the E_4 using the Auto-flow feature.

Auto-flow automatically retards flow if the maximal pressure limit is achieved or increases flow if the patient desires more flow for a larger breath at that time. To manually set the waveform, Auto-flow must be disabled (not recommended).

It would not be unreasonable to start with a square waveform in this patient with normal lungs, but there is no downside to beginning with a ramp delivery pattern. The crucial information that one needs is the grouped evaluation of waveform coupled with maximal inspiratory $\dot{Q}$, and the resultant P_{aw}-peak. These data are complemented by using concomitant PV curve analysis. Because the vast majority of the 7200 ventilators are not so equipped (but instead have a separate graphic display chip and display screen), the discussion assumes that the clinician is blind to the waveforms. A later discussion under "PCV" explores the use of the PV curve and may be applied in volume ventilation as well (waveform display is standard for the E_4).

Maximal Inspiratory Flow (aka Peak Inspiratory Flow; $\dot{Q}$)

Set the initial $\dot{Q}$ at 60 L/minute. One would set a lower $\dot{Q}$ if the patient had hypoxemia ($Q = 50$ L/min) or a higher flow ($Q = 70$ L/min) if the patient had exhalation obstruction (e.g., COPD), then evaluate the resultant P_{aw}-peak. Problems generally arise if the P_{aw}-peak is too high rather than being too low. If the P_{aw}-peak is low and the patient is well oxygenated and has an acceptable CO_2 clearance for his or her current pH, then no changes are required. If the P_{aw}-peak is too high, intervention is warranted (see discussion of P_{aw}-peak). A useful paradigm is to decide if the set $\dot{V}_T$ is simply too large (base the $\dot{V}_T$ on ideal body weight, not actual or adjusted, as the lung volume is a function of the thoracic cage size and is not influenced by the addition of adipose mass). If the $\dot{V}_T$ is appropriate, reduce the flow rate by 5 L/minute and re-evaluate; repeat if necessary. If the patient is on a square waveform, change to the decelerating setting. In general, if the $\dot{Q}$ is reduced to 40 L/minute and the P_{aw}-peak remains high, then one of the following conditions are true: (1) the $\dot{V}_T$ is, in fact, too large for the available lung mass, (2) there is a tube obstruction (partial), (3) the patient has a pleural space occupying disorder (pneumo-, hemo-, hemopneumo-, or hydro-thorax), (4) the patient requires a different mode, or (5) there is a ventilator dysfunction.

Writing the Orders

The order on the chart may be best indicated as follows:

Continued

CASE MANAGEMENT—cont'd

Initiate: SIMV at 10 ventilations/min
$\dot{V}_T$ at 600 mL
FI_{O_2} at 0.95
PEEP at +5 mm Hg
PSV at +10 cm H_2O
Flow = 60 L/minute; Ramp waveform
Titrate PSV to achieve $\dot{V}_{Tspont}$ ~ 600 mL
Obtain ABG 20 minutes after initiating settings; notify clinician
with results
Obtain STAT portable chest film to verify—endotracheal tube
placement, initiation of MV; notify clinician when CXR
obtained

Pressure Controlled Ventilation

Devices Reviewed
Infrasonics Adult Star, Drager E_4 Pulmonary Workstation

Target $\dot{V}_E$
Since this is the same patient, the target remains unchanged at
7.2 L/minute. How one achieves this target is the subject of the
following discussion.

Mode
Similar to $\dot{V}_E$, the mode remains the same. On the Adult Star,
the mode is accessed in the second screen. Press the change
screen button on the lower aspect of the display console; this
will change to the second screen. Use the knob on the lower
right of the console to move from one selection to another
(selection will highlight). Then press the knob to access the
values and rotate the knob until the desired mode appears. Press
the knob again to accept. The E_4 has a mode known as PCV+.
This is already set up as an SIMV-PCV-PSV mode. The
settings are accessed under the Mode screen as in volume-
cycled ventilation discussion, and are adjusted using the touch-
rotate-press scheme reviewed earlier.

Rate
While the rate remains the same, there is no set $\dot{V}_T$. Instead,
one must set the desired pressure change above PEEP and for
the duration of that pressure change, and evaluate for the resultant tidal volume. While the goal resultant $\dot{V}_T$ may be identical
to the $\dot{V}_T$ one sets in volume ventilation, one achieves that $\dot{V}_T$
in a fashion designed to limit the P_{aw}-peak and (usually) prolong
the time spent in inspiration.

Pressure Control (PC), T_i, And $\dot{V}_T$-resultant
In this patient with normal lungs, initially set pressure control
(setting) = 20 cm H_2O pressure and T_i = 1.0 sec. The PC of 20
stems from starting with a PEEP of 5 cm H_2O pressure. Therefore, the combined P_{aw}-peak will be PC + PEEP, or 20 + 5 =
25 cm H_2O pressure. This is a safe pressure and what one might
expect as the P_{aw}-peak if the patient were on a volume-cycled
ventilation. Alternatively, one may use the upper pressure limit
of normal, 35 cm H_2O and subtract from that the amount of
initial PEEP (in this case 5 cm H_2O pressure), and then multiply the difference by 2/3. In this case the starting pressure
would be 20 cm H_2O (35 − 5 × 2/3).

For a patient who is already on MV, take the current P_{aw}-
peak, subtract the PEEP, and again multiply by 2/3. When
setting up pressure-cycled ventilation on the Adult Star, all
settings must be addressed before the mode can be activated.
Thus, one will not have a mixed group of settings at any time.
The E_4 will allow one to change screens and input settings in
a similar fashion but will not change the active ventilator settings until the operator accepts all of those mode settings.

One significant difference in pressure-cycled ventilation is
that the pressure cannot exceed 25 cm H_2O pressure (in this
example), and the amount of time in inspiration is longer than
in volume-cycled ventilation. One must then look for the tidal
volume that results from this combination. Each perturbation
in resultant $\dot{V}_T$ has multiple repair strategies in PCV.

A discussion of T_i and I/E ratio is appropriate as the T_i
setting directly influences the resultant I/E.

Inspiration: Exhalation (I/E) Ratio
A normal I/E ratio is 1:3–4 for each breath cycle in a healthy
individual. Assuming a rate of 10 breaths per minute, each
respiratory cycle is 6 seconds. For a normal I/E ratio of 1:3 at
this rate, there are 1.5 seconds spent in inspiration (T_i) and 4.5
seconds spent in exhalation (T_e). It is then imperative to evaluate the $\dot{V}_T$-resultant and $\dot{V}_E$. If these are low, the PC may be
increased. If high, the PC may be decreased. T_i may be adjusted
as well. Inspiration is the time for oxygen exchange. If the
patient is hypoxic, the T_i may be increased to increase the P_{aw}-
mean and the time spent in inspiration in an oxygen-rich environment. For patients with severe hypoxemia, such a strategy
may require inverse ratio ventilation (IRV) where the time
spent in inspiration vastly exceeds the time available for exhalation. The extreme range of pressure-controlled IRV on the vast
majority of ventilators is approximately 4:1. IRV is a distinctly
unphysiologic and uncomfortable mode on which to breathe.
Patients generally require heavy sedation and commonly in
combination with neuromuscular blockade to tolerate IRV.
The unique challenges of monitoring and achieving adequate
sedation in patients on neuromuscular blockade have been
reviewed elsewhere.[84]

Oxygen, Oxygen Adjuncts, and PSV
FI_{O_2}, PEEP, and PSV remain the same as in volume-cycled
ventilation settings.

Maximal Inspiratory Flow and Waveform
In pressure-cycled ventilation, the goal is to allow the ventilator
to adjust the flow setting in response to the patient's unique
breath-by-breath change in compliance, resistance, and elastance. Thus, setting Q at its maximal value is ideal (Start:
160 L/min; E_4: autoflow). As in volume-cycled ventilation, the
ramp waveform is ideal.

Writing the Orders
The order on the chart may be best indicated as follows:

Initiate: SIMV at 10 ventilations/min
PC at 20 cm H_2O
T_i at 1 second
FI_{O_2} at 0.95
PEEP at +5 cm H_2O
PSV at +10 cm H_2O
Flow = maximum value; Ramp waveform
Titrate PSV to achieve $\dot{V}_{Tspont}$ ~ 600 mL
Obtain ABG 20 minutes after initiating settings; notify clinician
with results
Obtain STAT portable chest film to verify endotracheal tube
placement, inititation of MV; notify clinician when chest film
obtained

Note: There is no order to notify the clinician if the $\dot{V}_T$-
resultant is less or greater than anticipated. One should be at
the bedside when ventilation is initiated and directly evaluate
to adjust the parameters. Once the appropriate settings are
achieved, then such an order is advisable as the clinician will
want to evaluate changes in the patient's dynamics.

CASE MANAGEMENT—cont'd

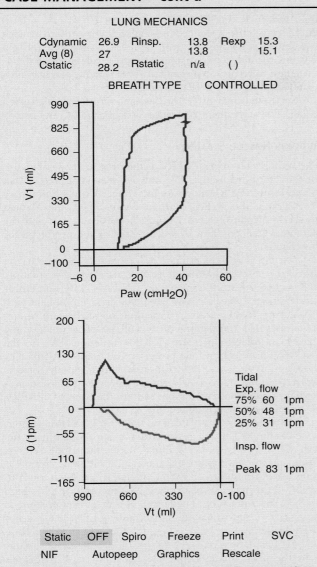

LUNG MECHANICS

Cdynamic	26.9	Rinsp.	13.8	Rexp	15.3
Avg (8)	27		13.8		15.1
Cstatic	28.2	Rstatic	n/a	( )	

BREATH TYPE   CONTROLLED

Tidal
Exp. flow
75% 60 1pm
50% 48 1pm
25% 31 1pm

Insp. flow

Peak 83 1pm

Static   OFF   Spiro   Freeze   Print   SVC

NIF   Autopeep   Graphics   Rescale

Figure 8–18   The PV curve on the Adult Star ventilator. Note that the curve is identical to the type of curve one would obtain on the E_4 with the exception of color and the ability to freeze a reference curve for comparison. Here it is accompanied by the flow-time loop as well.

Waveform Analysis (See Earlier Section on Waveforms)

It is logical to evaluate not only the achieved gas delivery volume, but how the patient's lung receives the volume. This is currently best performed by using the dynamic PV curve. Each change in ventilator prescription is best evaluated by reexamining the PV curve profile as well as the flow-time trace. On the Adult Star, the screen must be changed twice. Then rotate the knob to reach the bottom of the screen on the left. Select graphics. This will bring up the PV curve as well as the flow-time trace (Fig. 8–18). On the E_4, the graphics are accessed by selecting values measured from the righthand column of white static buttons. Then touch the field labeled loops. This will bring up the PV curve (Fig. 8–19). The green box in the upper right-hand corner of the PV-curve box will have a menu of other traces and loops—the flow-time trace is found there by selecting its label and pressing the knob.

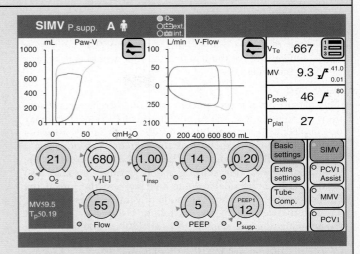

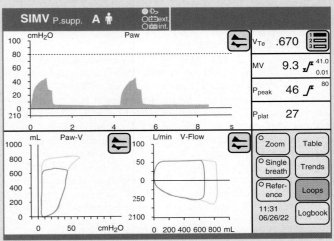

Figure 8–19   PV curve on the E_4. This display may be brought up as a solo display or integrated into other multidisplay screens, as indicated above. One accesses the menu on the lower right of the screen by activating the "values measured" button on the right of the faceplate (not the LCD screen). Then press "Loops." The device will display either a continuous set of loops or a reference and a single breath (yellow button illuminated on the appropriate green icons).

CASE 2

A 45-year-old, 70-kg male presents with high fevers, cough, and shortness of breath. The ED portable chest film demonstrates bilateral infiltrates as well as lower lobe air bronchograms. While awaiting admission to the hospital for presumed community-acquired pneumonia, the patient develops hypoxia, suffers respiratory failure, and requires urgent intubation.

Volume-Cycled Ventilation

Mode

SIMV—As before, allow the patient to breathe spontaneously when the short acting neuromuscular blockers or heavy sedative (e.g., etomidate, fentanyl, midazolam) used to facilitate intubation wears off.

Continued

CASE MANAGEMENT—cont'd

Target $\dot{V}_E$

Given the likely acidosis, this patient's $\dot{V}_E$ needs to exceed the lower limit of normal value. Thus, a target of 9.8 L/minute is a 40% increase above the baseline that one would expect for a slenderly built man.

Rate and $\dot{V}_T$

This patient has a severe pneumonia and current recomendations are to use a low $\dot{V}_T$. An initial rate of 14 is ideal and may be coupled with a normal $\dot{V}_T$ of 700 mL. It is OK to use a normal tidal volume to start as the patient does not have a history of intrinsic pulmonary disease. One must evaluate the resultant P_{aw}-peak after starting at this setting. One may also need to reduce the tidal volume and increase the rate if the P_{aw}-peak is high and no other mode of ventilation is available.

Alternatively, were one to follow Using the ARDSNet recommendations, a starting $\dot{V}_T$ of 450 to 500 mL would be ideal.[85] The required rate would be 20 breaths per minute to achieve the target $\dot{V}_E$. Recall that this strategy may not clear CO_2 as efficiently as a slower rate and a larger $\dot{V}_T$ given a larger $\dot{V}_D/\dot{V}_T$ ratio.

FI_{O_2} and O_2 Adjuncts

Begin with a high FI_{O_2} (0.95 to 1.0) to ensure adequate oxygenation. Titrate as before. Initiate PEEP at a minimum of 5 cm H_2O since one will need to maintain FRC and alveolar recruitment. Starting at a higher level may result in hemodynamic compromise in a patient who likely has intravascular volume depletion. Once the patient is volume-replete, titrate to achieve the optimal PEEP as explained earlier. It is best to start with a decelerating wave form since one may assume that the infected and collapsed segments will have much longer regional time constants than their neighboring alveolar segments. Thus, a longer T_i is ideal for alveolar recruitment. Moreover, a slow flow rate will complement the decelerating waveform and further prolong the T_i. It is reasonable to start with a $\dot{Q}$ of 50 L/minute and evaluate SaO_2 and P_{aw}-peak.

Pressure Support

Start with a higher PSV than the last patient since one may assume that the pulmonary compliance will be less than in a patient with normal lungs. Initiate PSV at 15 cm H_2O pressure and titrate as before to achieve similar V_T with the machine and spontaneous breaths.

Pressure-Cycled Ventilation

Neither the mode nor the target $\dot{V}_E$ are different. Instead of $\dot{V}_T$, one must set PC and T_i.

Rate

This is not as straightforward as in volume-cycled ventilation. A higher rate to clear CO_2 in volume-cycled ventilation will lead to reduced T_e in PCV if one is using a long T_i (see later). Thus a slower rate will allow for more time spent in recruitment, and more efficient CO_2 clearance than would be achieved with a higher rate. One must recall that the $\dot{V}_D/\dot{V}_T$ ratio also governs the efficiency of CO_2 clearance, not just the total amount of gas that is cycled in 1 minute. Thus start with a rate of 10 breaths per minute, not 14 as in volume cycled-ventilation.

PC and T_i

As described earlier, start with a PC level that is either related to the volume-cycled ventilation P_{aw}-peak or the maximal P_{aw} that one will tolerate (35 cm H_2O pressure). In this example,

use a longer T_i (start at 2.0 sec; resultant I/E at rate = 10 is I/E:1:2) given the prolonged regional time constants to manage hypoxemia, as a larger V_T will require excessive PC and lead to ventilator-induced lung injury. Progressively increase the T_i for failure to resolve hypoxemia. In this patient, one may ultimately need to employ IRV to reverse hypoxia.

Set the maximal inspiratory flow and waveform as described earlier. The subsequent evaluation is unchanged from Case 1.

Hypoxia Rescue Strategy

The authors recommend APRV as their rescue mode of choice for refractory hypoxemia. The only ventilators at present that can perform in APRV mode are the Drager Evita 4 Pulmonary Workstation, the Nellcor-Puritan Bennett 840, the Maquet (formerly Siemens) Servo i using the BiVent mode and the Hamilton Gallileo. The E_4 will be used as the prototype for this chapter.

Assume that your patient has refractory hypoxemia on either volume-cycled ventilation or pressure-cycled ventilation. The goal is to restore oxygenation in a rapid, safe, and efficacious fashion. Typically, these patients will have problems with P_{aw}s during volume-cycled ventilation, or inadequate $\dot{V}_T$ on pressure-cycled ventilation; many will be pharmacologically relaxed to tolerate pressure-cycled ventilation-IRV, or the ARDSNet protocol for lung protective ventilation. APRV represents a low-pressure, easy-to-use mode that rapidly corrects hypoxemia, and more slowly corrects hypercarbia while preserving spontaneous respiration. Indeed, the benefits of APRV are lost if the patient is chemically relaxed.[86]

Determine the P_{aw}-plateau on the prior ventilator settings as well as the PEEP. Then start APRV using a long time at the high CPAP level; APRV is found under the mode settings menu, and the settings are manipulated in the same fashion as using the other modes on the E_4 (touch, rotate knob, push to accept). If the prior P_{aw}-plateau was 28, then start with P_{aw}-high at 28 cm H_2O pressure. The length of time at that pressure is T_{high}; start at approximately 6.0 seconds (<4.5 seconds is not APRV by definition). Next, set the P_{aw}-low at 0, and the release time (T_{low}) at 0.8 seconds. Keep the FI_{O_2} at the same settings as in the prior mode. Leave the rise time at 0.20 (default setting), and activate automatic tube compensation (compensates for intrinsic tubing resistance much like PSV). These are approximate settings that need to be adjusted based on the pressure-over-time curve, the release volumes, and the patient's response.

First, recall that the time for gas flow is quite long by comparison with cyclic ventilation. Thus, release volumes may be smaller than one would desire for a V_T on conventional ventilation. Oxygenation will be enhanced despite the small volumes due to the efficiency of exchange based on exceptional alveolar recruitment. Adjusting the pressure to which the P_{aw} is allowed to drop at the end of the release phase may be done in one of two ways: setting a P_{aw}-low or adjusting the T_{low} to achieve a trace that drops to 1/3 of the amplitude of the P_{aw}-high (see Fig. 8–6). Either method is successful. If the release volumes are <5 mL/kg body weight, the authors advocate increasing the P_{aw}-high as the initial maneuver up to a maximum of 35 cm H_2O pressure. The authors have increased pressure beyond this in an awake patient who could report discomfort with no untoward consequences, but would recommend further increases in the T_{high} before exceeding 35 cm H_2O pressure.

CASE MANAGEMENT—cont'd

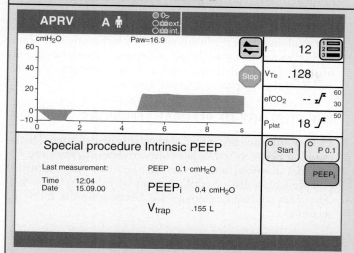

Figure 8–20   Intrinsic PEEP (PEEPi). The E$_4$ will measure the intrinsic PEEP as well as the trapped volume responsible for that PEEPi. The function is accessed by using the "special procedure" button on the right-hand side of the faceplate, activating the "start" button on the LCD screen, and then depressing the knob to initiate the procedure. In this example, the PEEPi is 0.4 cm H$_2$O pressure and represents a volume of 155 mL (0.155 L) of gas.

Next, check the intrinsic PEEP to see if the PEEPi achieved equals at least the PEEP set on the prior mode; generally, the PEEPi will be greater than the prior PEEP, mandating an evaluation of blood pressure. PEEPi is found using a special procedure button on the right of the ventilator; press start procedure to obtain the PEEPi as well as the trapped volume that has generated the intrinsic PEEP. The screen will enter freeze mode after making the measurement; remember to unfreeze it by depressing the freeze button on the right of the ventilator faceplate (Fig. 8–20).

Typically, the patient's Po$_2$ and SaO$_2$ will rise rapidly (within a few minutes of starting the mode).[19] Failure to do so has been associated with endotracheal tube malfunction, pneumothorax, and, most commonly, inadequate pulmonary blood flow associated with intravascular volume depletion or inadequate cardiac output.[19] Weaning from APRV is quite simple once the proximate cause of the hypoxemia has been corrected. The authors simply decrease the P$_{aw}$-high by 2 cm H$_2$O pressure every 2 hours until the P$_{aw}$-high = 10 cm H$_2$O pressure. If the patient is comfortable, well saturated, on minimal pressor support, and has manageable secretions coupled with an acceptable mental status, then endotracheal tube removal is appropriate.

Acknowledgment

The editors and authors wish to acknowledge the contributions of William Durston, John J. Kelly, and Barry J. Burton to this chapter in previous editions.

 REFERENCES CAN BE FOUND ON EXPERT CONSULT

CHAPTER 9

Thoracentesis

Barbara K. Blok

Thoracentesis is derived from the Greek *thorakos* (chest) and *kentesis* (to pierce). Classically, this refers to any maneuver whereby a sharp object introduces a conduit between the intrathoracic cavity and the atmosphere, allowing air or fluid to exit. Clinically, *thoracentesis* refers to the removal of fluid from the pleural space for diagnostic or therapeutic purposes. This chapter concentrates on the identification and management of fluid accumulations in the chest of patients who present to the emergency department (ED).

ANATOMY AND PHYSIOLOGY OF THE PLEURAL SPACE

During embryologic development, the lung buds grow out of a median mass of mesenchymal tissue into the future thoracic cavities. This maneuver results in the existence of two linings, the visceral pleura, which wraps the lungs, and the parietal pleura, which lines the inner surface of the thoracic cavities and meets the visceral pleura at the root of the lungs in the mediastinum. The space between the two linings is called the *pleural space*.[1]

Understanding this basic anatomy is important because it underlines the similarities and differences between the two linings, which in turn determine the physiology and pathophysiology of the pleural space. Both visceral and parietal pleurae are thin layers of connective tissue each of which is embedded with capillary beds that generate both hydrostatic and oncotic pressures. The visceral pleura is supplied by the bronchial arteries and empties into the pulmonary veins. In this system, the hydrostatic and oncotic pressures between the capillaries and the pleural space are balanced, resulting in a zero net fluid gradient across the visceral pleura in the healthy state. However, because the visceral pleura wraps the lungs, it is directly susceptible to diseases within the lung parenchyma and to fluid accumulation in the alveoli during pulmonary edema. Furthermore, because the pulmonary veins drain into the left ventricle, the presence of left ventricular failure also affects fluid flow across the visceral pleura. In contrast, the parietal pleura is supplied by the intercostal arteries and empties into the intercostal veins. Intercostal circulation reflects systemic pressure and naturally carries a higher hydrostatic pressure than the pulmonary vascular bed. As a result, a properly functioning parietal pleura generates a net gradient of about 6 cm H_2O into the pleural space. Pleural fluid generated over time is removed in bulk from the pleural space by the lymphatic system. The parietal pleura is embedded with large lymphatic stomata, which are conduits that allow fluid and particles as large as 10 μm to pass, draining the pleural space fluid in bulk through the lymphatic sinuses and into the mediastinal lymph nodes. Over the course of a day, the lymphatic system maintains a pleural space outflow of 0.1 mL/kg per hour minimum, with a 30-fold capacity of 3 mL/kg per hour.[2,3] Overall, in a healthy state, a small amount of fluid, estimated at 0.26 mL/kg of body mass, is present in the pleural space at any given time.[4]

From this design, it is clear how a variety of disease states can result in a pleural effusion simply by increasing the volume of fluid movement into the pleural space beyond the capacity of the lymphatic draining system or by decreasing the efficiency of the lymphatic draining system.

THE ETIOLOGY OF PLEURAL EFFUSIONS

Pleural effusions are either transudates or exudates. Distinguishing between transudates and exudates narrows the differential diagnosis and directs management and therapy. A comprehensive list of etiologies can be found in Table 9–1. The most common etiologies are discussed in the following sections.

 TABLE 9–1 Etiologies of Pleural Effusion
CAN BE FOUND ON EXPERT CONSULT

Transudates: Overwhelming the System

Transudates are caused by either an increase in the intravascular hydrostatic pressure or a decrease in the intravascular oncotic pressure, generating a net flow of fluid into the pleural space. These effusions are typically straw-colored and serous with very low cellular and protein content.

The most common cause of transudates is congestive heart failure (CHF). Left ventricular dysfunction leads to increased hydrostatic pressure in the pulmonary veins, resulting in an increased movement of fluid into the pleural space. When the fluid volume in the pleural space exceeds the lymphatic capacity for drainage, a pleural effusion develops. In addition, the elevated systemic hypertension associated with CHF also increases fluid flow across the parietal pleura and decreases lymphatic flow out of the thorax.[5,6] Any process that results in compromised left ventricular outflow can result in a pleural effusion including myocardial infarction, cardiomyopathy, and valvular disease.

Patients with cirrhosis are frequently hypoalbuminemic, leading to a chronic state of decreased plasma oncotic pressure. The imbalance between the hydrostatic and the oncotic forces across the pleural membrane results in an effusion.[7] In addition, experiments have shown that high volumes of ascites can stretch the diaphragm enough to allow fluid to pass through preexisting microdefects. The transdiaphragmatic communications can close spontaneously on relief of pressure and volume, although recurrent episodes usually require surgical correction and chemical pleurodesis.[8]

Exudates: Pathology of Tissues, Destroying the System

Exudates are caused by pleural inflammation, increased pleural membrane permeability, or lymphatic obstruction and therefore contain high levels of either lactate dehydrogenase (LDH), a nonspecific marker of cellular injury and inflammation, or protein.

The main mechanism of cancer-related pleural effusion is obstruction. Neoplasms can either damage functional lymph stoma in the parietal pleura or prevent outflow more distally via involvement of the mediastinal lymph nodes. Other mechanisms involving neoplasm include metastasis to the visceral pleura, increasing capillary permeability, and obstruction of the thoracic duct, creating a chylothorax.[9]

Bacterial pneumonia affects about 4 million Americans a year, 20% requiring hospitalization, and 40% of those hospitalized developing effusions.[10] A pleural effusion associated with pneumonia (bacterial or viral) or lung abscess is termed *parapneumonic effusion*.[11] In the first stage of the parapneumonic effusion, called the *exudative stage*, sterile fluid flows out from the capillaries of the visceral pleura secondary to increased permeability rendered by the surrounding inflammation or pneumonitis. When the infection and resultant inflammation continue unchecked, a simple parapneumonic effusion becomes *complicated*. This occurs initially by deposition of fibrin on the visceral and parietal pleurae resulting in loculations (the fibrinopurulent stage) and, finally, by growth of fibroblasts along the pleural surfaces forming a tough peel that encases the lung (the organizational stage).

Of the 500,000 persons who have pulmonary embolism (PE) each year, at least 30% develop a pleural effusion.[12] Therefore, when the etiology for the effusion is unclear, PE should be strongly considered. The effusion is most commonly exudative, with pulmonary ischemia and infarct leading to increased capillary permeability of the visceral pleura.[13] Occasionally, PE causes a transudative effusion by obstruction of the pulmonary vessels, leading to right-sided failure and increased hydrostatic pressures in the parietal pleura.

Traumatic Effusions: Acute and Catastrophic Destruction of the System

Esophageal rupture can result from forceful vomiting, as in the case of Boerhaave syndrome, or from instrumentation, as in the case of endoscopy, Blakemore-Sengstaken tube placement, or rigid nasogastric tube placement (Fig. 9–1A). Hemothorax can result from sharp traumatic injuries, subclavian vein or artery cannulation, PE, aortic aneurysm, and supratherapeutic levels of anticoagulant. Chylothorax develops from acute disruption of the thoracic duct, usually in the setting of trauma. These are usually large-volume effusions that accumulate over an extremely short period of time, rapidly compromising both oxygenation and circulation.

DIAGNOSIS OF PLEURAL EFFUSION

Clinical Diagnosis

The three most common symptoms related to pleural effusions are chest pain, cough, and dyspnea. The chest pain may be of several types depending on the underlying pathology. Chest pain solely from the fluid collection is often described as a "dull ache." Pleuritic chest pain is more indicative of localized irritation of the parietal pleura, which has abundant nerve fibers. Involvement of the mediastinal pleura, because of innervation of the phrenic nerve, results in chest pain with ipsilateral shoulder pain. Pain can often be referred to the abdomen via innervation of the intercostals. Cough may be due to bronchial irritation from compression of the lung parenchyma.

Because pleural effusions are a result of a large list of disease processes, the history and physical examination of the patient should involve all systems in the search for clues to the underlying disease process. The lung examination should be performed both as an evaluation of lung pathology and to determine the extent of the effusion. Large effusions can result in increased hemithorax and bulging intercostal spaces on the side of the effusion. On palpation, tactile fremitus is either reduced or completely absent over the effusion because the fluid separates the lung from the thoracic wall and absorbs the vibrations from the lung. Percussion over the effusion produces a characteristic dullness, which shifts when the patient changes position if the fluid is free flowing. In general, auscultation reveals decreased to absent breath sounds depending on the size of the effusion. Pleural rubs may be appreciated if there is pleural irritation, but are often difficult to auscultate until after fluid evacuation. Palpation, percussion, and auscultation are all useful in determining the top of the effusion. Imaging studies (plain radiographs, computed tomography [CT]) are currently used to identify and characterize pleural effusions (see Figs. 9–1 to 9–6).

Radiologic Diagnosis

Chest Radiograph

Because pleural fluid is denser than air-filled lung, a freeflowing effusion will first accumulate in the most dependent parts of the thoracic cavity, the subpulmonic space and the lateral costophrenic sulcus. Pleural effusions are usually visible on a posteroanterior chest x-ray if 200 to 250 mL of fluid is present. A lateral radiograph may define an effusion of 50 to 75 mL.

The earliest recognized sign of a pleural effusion on a chest radiograph is a *blunting of the lateral costophrenic angle*, which may be seen on either the frontal or the lateral view. With larger free-flowing effusions, the pleural fluid carries the appearance of a *meniscus*, curving downward toward the mediastinum in the frontal view and appearing "lowest" midway through the thoracic cavity on the lateral view (see Fig. 9–1B and C). The true height of the effusion corresponds to the highest portion of the meniscus. The presence of pneumothrorax or abscess may alter the meniscus appearance to more of a straight line (air-fluid level).

Occasionally, up to 1000 mL of fluid collects in the subpulmonic space and does not cause either blunting of the costophrenic angles or a meniscus appearance on the upright radiograph. This is termed *subpulmonic effusion* (see Fig. 9–1D), which should be expected if the hemidiaphragm is elevated and the dome peaks more laterally than expected on the anteroposterior radiograph. A lateral decubitus view of a patient with a questionable left pleural effusion will show free-flowing pleural fluid parallel to the x-ray table (see Fig. 9–1E).

In the diseased or scarred lung, tissue adhesions can trap pleural fluid within parietal, visceral, or interlobar surfaces. Because these adhesions anchor the fluid collection, *loculated effusions* are often described as "D-shaped" (Fig. 9–2A) and are best diagnosed with either ultrasound or CT (see later). Fluid loculated in the fissures assumes a lenticular figure (see Fig. 9–2B).

Bilateral decubitus radiographs should be obtained when a pleural effusion is seen or when a small effusion is suspected. With the side of the effusion down, a simple pleural effusion will follow gravity and layer between the floating lung and the chest wall. Unusual shapes reflect the presence of loculations, contained abscess, or masses. A lateral decubitus view

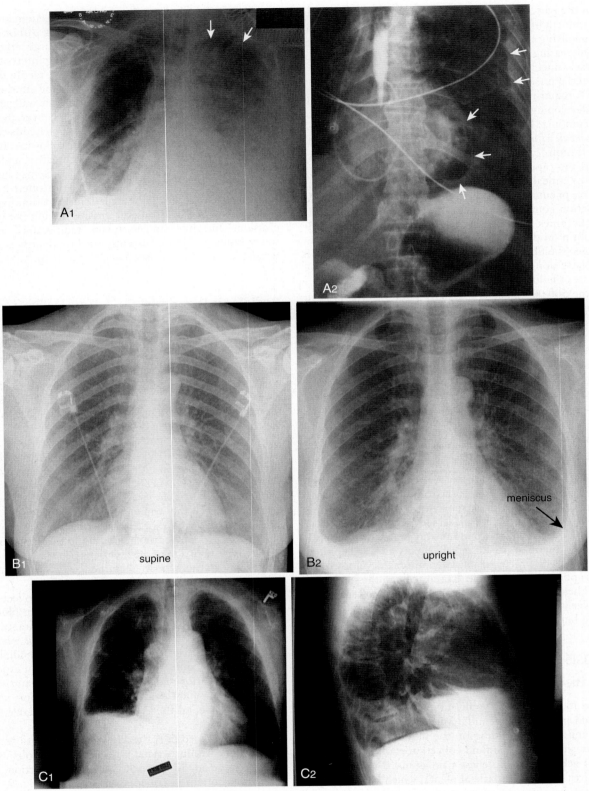

Figure 9–1 *A,* (*1*) Anteroposterior portable chest radiograph in a patient with Boerhaave syndrome and left apical pneumothorax (*arrows*). Increased density is noted over the left hemothorax as a result of a left pleural effusion. (2) Water-soluble contrast upper gastrointestinal examination shows a left pleural effusion (*closed arrows*). A retrocardiac mediastinal collection of gas and contrast medium (*open arrows*) is indicative of esophageal rupture. *B,* Bilateral pleural effusion. Supine (*1*) and upright (*2*) chest radiographs. The pleural effusion obscures the diaphragm and both costophrenic angles. It has a curvilinear upper margin concave to the lung and is higher laterally than medially. This is opposite to the findings on the supine chest radiograph in which the pleural effusion is hardly visible as a hazy opacity affecting the lower part of the thorax. Note also that the costophrenic angles *are not obscured in the supine film* and that the vascular opacities are preserved in the overlying lung. *C,* Right-sided pleural effusion. The appearance of a meniscus is best seen on the lateral radiograph. The meniscus is the highest point of the effusion for thoracentesis purposes. *D,* Right-sided subpulmonary pleural effusion. On the erect posteroanterior (*1*) and lateral (*2*) radiographs, the effusion simulates a high hemidiaphragm. Ultrasound (*3*) and computed tomography (CT) (*4*) clearly show that the effusion is located above the diaphragm. *Arrows* show the diaphragmatic area. *E,* Left lateral decubitus chest radiograph demonstrates the presence of free pleural fluid. The amount of pleural fluid can be semiquantified by measuring the distance between the two *arrows*.

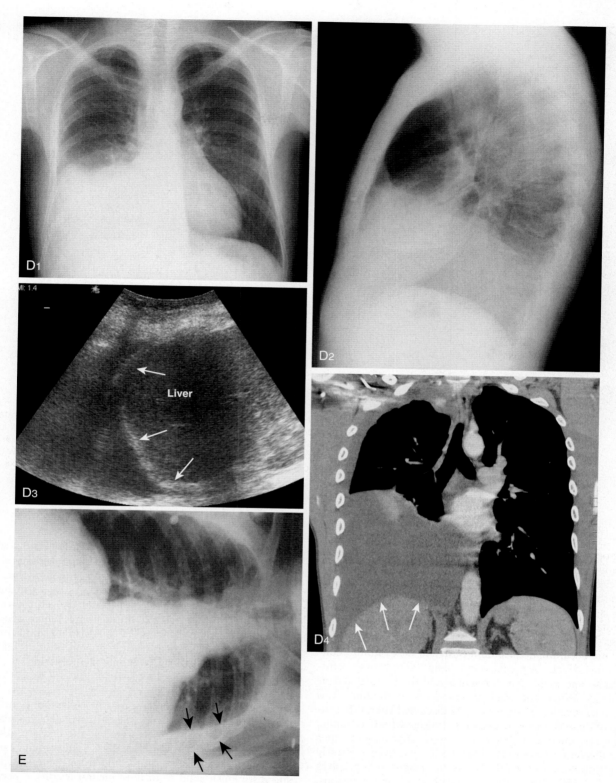

Figure 9–1, cont'd

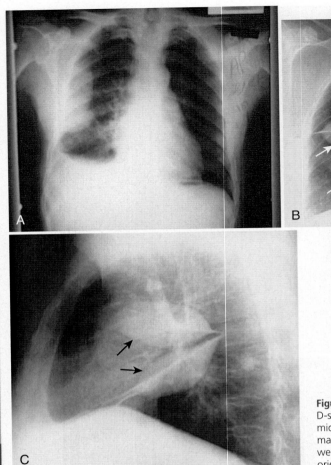

Figure 9–2 *A,* Loculated pleural effusion. This PA radiograph demonstrates the D-shaped appearance of a right-sided loculated pleural effusion (*arrows*) in the midchest. *B,* Loculated pleural effusions. Occasionally, pleural effusions (*arrows*) may become loculated in the fissures. These can be seen on the PA view (*B*) as well as on the lateral chest x-ray (*C*). These are lenticular, with a long axis oriented along either the major or the minor fissure.

on the opposite side, draws the fluid toward the mediastinum and allows visualization of the lung parenchyma to determine the presence of infiltrates or masses.

In the case of a massive pleural effusion, the entire hemithorax is opacified (see Fig. 9–3). In such films, identification of mediastinal shift is a key to identifying the underlying process. In the absence of a diseased lung or mediastinum, large fluid accumulations should push the mediastinum contralaterally. When the mediastinum is shifted toward the effusion, lungs and main stem bronchi are likely diseased and/or obstructed. When the mediastinum is fixed midline, it is likely to be invaded by tumor.[14,15] As discussed later, differentiation of these disease processes is best done with CT. Supine radiographs portray a generalized hazy appearance rather than a discrete effusion (see Fig. 9–3C), and even relatively large effusions can be subtle unless an upright radiograph is obtained. CHF often produces bilateral pleural effusions, usually first evident on the right side (see Fig. 9–4).

CT

Although thoracentesis is usually performed based on plain radiograph findings, CT is more sensitive than plain film in detecting very small amounts of effusion and can readily assess the extent, number, and location of loculated pleural effusions. Loculated lesions can appear vague on plain film. In the distinct anatomic relationships shown on cross-sectional views in CT, free-flowing pleural fluid will form a sickle shape in the most dependent regions (see Fig. 9–5), whereas loculated fluid collections will remain lenticular and relatively fixed in space. In addition, CT assesses pleural thickening, irregularities, and masses that are suggestive of malignancy and other diseases that result in exudative effusions. With intravenous contrast dye, CT differentiates lung parenchymal disease, such as lung abscess.[16] CT is also useful in the identification of mediastinal pathology and in differentiating ascites from loculated subpulmonic pleural fluid.

Ultrasound

There are definite advantages to using ultrasound for assessment of pleural effusions as well. In particular, it is easy and noninvasive and can be performed at the bedside. Although some details can be seen only with CT, ultrasound can identify fluid loculations, separate fluid from pleural thickening, and distinguish solid from fluid pleural lesions, especially in fluid collections that look solid in freeze-frame. Ultrasound can also be used to identify both pulmonic and abdominal etiologies of the pleural effusion (see Fig. 9–6).[17–19]

Magnetic Resonance Imaging

Magnetic resonance imaging (MRI) has limited use in the evaluation of pleural effusions. In extreme cases in which complex loculations hinder accurate localization of fluid collections, the multiplanar ability of MRI may provide some advantage.

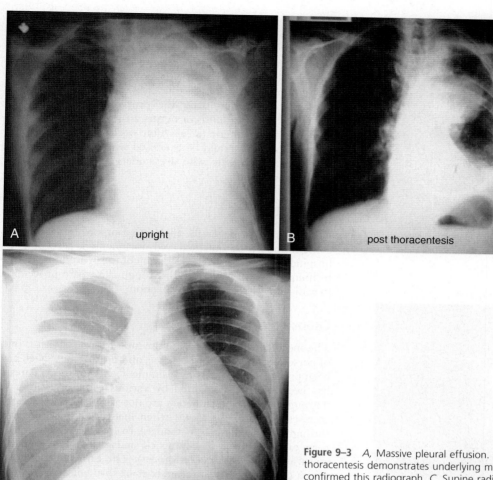

Figure 9–3 *A,* Massive pleural effusion. *B,* A repeat radiograph after thoracentesis demonstrates underlying mass. A CT scan would have prospectively confirmed this radiograph. *C,* Supine radiograph of a patient who has a large right pleural effusion. The generalized homogenous ("ground glass") increase in radiopacity of the right side of this patient is caused by posterior layering of a pleural effusion.

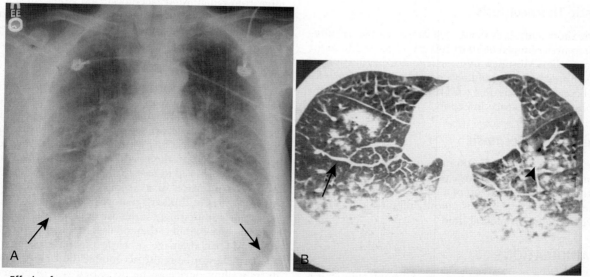

Figure 9–4 Effusion from congestive heart failure. *A,* Frontal chest radiograph in a patient with pulmonary edema shows cardiomegaly, bilateral pleural effusions (*arrows*), and central interstitial thickening, including Kerley's A lines. Note that the right effusion is slightly larger than the left effusion. *B,* High-resolution CT scan in a patient with pulmonary edema shows interstitial edema with bilateral, basilar centrilobular ground-glass opacity nodules (*arrowhead*) and smooth interlobular septal thickening (*arrow*). Bilateral pleural effusions are also present. *(A and B, Courtesy of Michael B. Gotway, MD, Department of Radiology, University of California, San Francisco.)*

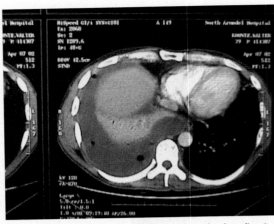

Figure 9–5 Pleural effusion. Sickle appearance of a free-flowing pleural effusion on CT scan.

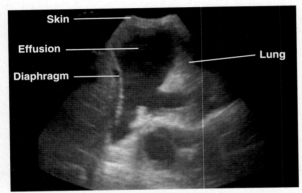

Figure 9–6 Pleural effusion. Ultrasound demonstrates the appearance of pleural fluid. *(From Thomsen T, Setnik G. [eds]: Procedures Consult—Emergency Medicine Module. Copyright 2008 Elsevier Inc. All rights reserved.)*

INDICATIONS

Diagnostic Thoracentesis

Diagnostic thoracentesis evaluates the cause of a pleural effusion and requires removal of 50 to 100 mL of pleural fluid for laboratory studies. Most new effusions require diagnostic thoracentesis. An exception would be a new pleural effusion with a clear clinical diagnosis (e.g., CHF) and no evidence for superimposed pleural space infection.

Therapeutic Thoracentesis

The usual goal of therapeutic thoracentesis is to help relieve the dyspnea associated with a large pleural effusion, but it may also aid the radiologic work-up of a patient with a large effusion. Therapeutic thoracentesis typically requires removing a much larger volume of pleural fluid.

CONTRAINDICATIONS

There are no absolute contraindications to thoracentesis. It is generally recommended that patients with severe clotting abnormalities, including a platelet count less than 50,000 or prothrombin time or partial thromboplastin time elevations of greater than twice the normal range, have platelet and/or

factor replacement prior to initiation of the procedure. Patients with mild-to-moderate abnormalities (International Normalized Ratio up to twice normal, and platelet counts of 50,000–100,000/mL^3) do not require replacement prior to the procedure.[20] All patients with coagulation abnormalities, including those with renal failure, should be watched closely for signs of bleeding after the procedure. Skin puncture through a site of cellulitis or herpes zoster should be avoided by choosing an alternate insertion site or patient position. Extreme caution should be exercised when performing thoracentesis on patients who are undergoing mechanical or manual ventilation.

PROCEDURE

Thoracentesis is generally an elective procedure. Informed consent should be obtained and documented, according to hospital policy, prior to the initiation of the procedure. Sterile technique should be followed through the entire procedure to avoid the introduction of infection.

Choosing a Technique

The specific technique and equipment for thoracentesis is one of personal choice and experience, and no specific device has been proved superior. Using a simple needle for thoracentesis has been mostly supplanted by various catheters and kits. Through-the-needle catheters are not popular because catheters can shear or break off when inadvertently withdrawn through the needle tip. A standard 16- to 18-gauge intravenous catheter, three-way stopcock, and syringe is frequently still used (Figs. 9–7 and 9–8, *inset*). The catheter technique uses a catheter that is inserted over or through a needle and subsequently left in the pleural space during fluid removal. Thoracentesis catheters are commonly marketed and sold as preassembled kits (see Fig. 9–8). Advantages of commercial thoracentesis catheters include a one-way valve that prevents air entry into the catheter during needle removal; a blunt spring-loaded safety cannula that extends beyond the sharp needle tip once the pleural space is entered, protecting the lung from puncture or laceration; and a built-in side port for fluid drainage, obviating the need for a three-way stopcock. The Safe-T-Centesis catheter drainage catheter (Fig. 9–9) is an over-the needle multiple drainage port device with a retractable intraluminal obturator designed to prevent lung injury.

Studies have attempted to determine the relative safety of the needle and catheter techniques, with varied results.[21–24] It is generally recommended that the smallest possible needle be used. With diagnostic procedures, in which only small volumes of fluid are being withdrawn, the needle technique is recommended. In therapeutic maneuvers, either technique is generally believed to be safe. The catheter technique avoids prolonged insertion of a needle in the pleural space while large volumes of fluid are removed.

Some authors suggest the use of chronic indwelling catheters (such as pigtail catheters) as a reasonable alternative for the long-term drainage of large pleural effusions. A small standard chest tube is also acceptable. One clear advantage of an indwelling device is the decreased risk of pneumothorax associated with repeated thoracentesis.[25]

For small or loculated effusions, suspicion for adhesions, the presence of relative contraindications, and in cases in which iatrogenic pneumothorax may cause significant respiratory compromise, as with severe underlying lung disease or mechanical ventilation, ultrasound guidance is recommended. Ultrasound-guided thoracentesis is associated with a significantly lower rate of complications.[22,24,26] CT-guided thoracentesis has also been used successfully for draining small pleural effusions.[27]

Patient and Equipment Preparation

The patient's identification should be confirmed and the side of the pleural effusion verified by physical examination and chest radiography. A patent intravenous line should be established prior to initiation of the procedure if indicated by the clinical scenario. A red-top tube for serum protein and LDH can be drawn at the time of intravenous line placement. For truly elective or diagnostic thoracentesis, an intravenous line is not required. Atropine should be available in the case of a vasovagal reaction during the procedure. If appropriate, oxygen saturation should be monitored by pulse oximetry and supplemental oxygen should be given as needed. A procedural time out should be taken immediately before the procedure as a final verification of the correct patient, procedure, and site. Using sterile technique, the skin is prepared with anti-

IV catheter without safety mechanism

Removable end-cap allows syringe to be attached

IV catheter with safety mechanism

Safety sheath cannot be detached; syringe cannot be attached

Figure 9–7 **Standard intravenous catheters may be used for thoracentesis (14–18 gauge).** *(From Thomsen T, Setnik G [eds]: Procedures Consult—Emergency Medicine Module. Copyright 2008 Elsevier Inc. All rights reserved.)*

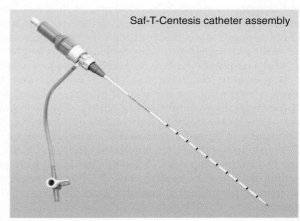

Saf-T-Centesis catheter assembly

Figure 9–9 Safe-T Centesis catheter may minimize lung injury. This comes in a kit and contains a self-sealing valve, an in-line stopcock, and a multiport pigtail catheter. *(From Thomsen T, Setnik G [eds]: Procedures Consult—Emergency Medicine Module. Copyright 2008 Elsevier Inc. All rights reserved.)*

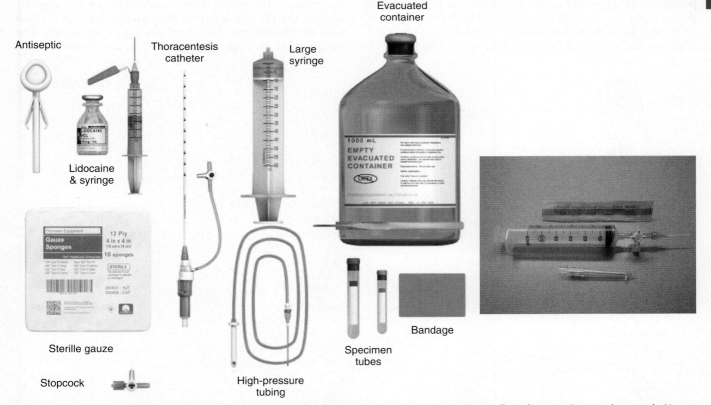

Figure 9-8 **Commercial kit for thoracentesis.** A simple set up for thoracentesis includes an over-the-needle-catheter, syringe, and stopcock. Note that the safety catheter cannot be directly attached to the syringe for aspiration, so the catheter alone is advanced slowly and a flash of fluid is sought. The catheter is then advanced over the needle, and the syringe attached to the base of the catheter. *(From Thomsen T, Setnik G [eds]: Procedures Consult—Emergency Medicine Module. Copyright 2008 Elsevier Inc. All rights reserved.)*

septic in a wide area around the thoracentesis site. Sterile towels or a sterile drape should be placed around the site.

Termination of Procedure

It is necessary to understand the end points of a procedure prior to its initiation. The most common indication for termination of thoracentesis is removal of a desired volume of fluid. For diagnostic thoracentesis, the procedure is terminated upon removal of 50 to 100 mL of fluid. For therapeutic thoracentesis, the procedure is terminated upon relief of patient dyspnea or when up to 1500 mL of fluid has been withdrawn. A maximum of 1500 mL is used to help avoid significantly negative pleural pressures, which have been associated with both symptomatic hypovolemia and the potentially fatal complication of reexpansion pulmonary edema after large-volume thoracentesis. Larger volumes may be removed if monitoring of the pleural pressures occurs, but this is not typically done in the ED setting. The procedure should also be terminated if aspiration of air occurs, indicating lung puncture or laceration, unless the needle is 20 gauge or smaller, making significant pneumothorax unlikely. Finally, a change in patient symptoms, including abdominal pain and worsening shortness of breath, should raise the suspicion for a patient complication and the procedure should be terminated.

Insertion Site and Patient Position

Figure 9–10 illustrates various patient positions for thoracentesis. Upright positioning is the desired technique for draining most pleural effusions. With this technique, the patient is positioned sitting erect on the edge of the bed with extended arms resting on a bedside table (Fig. 9–11). If the effusion is sufficiently large, the patient should be allowed to lean forward slightly while supported by the bedside table. The height of

the effusion is then located clinically by dullness to percussion and decrease in tactile fremitus. One should never rely on the chest radiograph to determine the level of effusion because the radiographic level changes with patient positioning and respiration. The thoracentesis site should be one to two intercostal spaces below the highest level of effusion in the midscapular or posterior axillary line. In all cases, the lowest level recommended is the space between the eighth and the ninth ribs, (the eighth intercostal space). Mark the designated site. If the patient is too ill to sit upright, the procedure may be performed with the patient in the lateral decubitus position with the side of the effusion down and the back at the edge of the bed. The needle insertion site in this position is the posterior axillary line. Alternatively, the patient may be positioned supine, with the head elevated as much as possible. The needle insertion site in this position is the midaxillary line. For both of these alternative positions, the fluid level must be determined clinically by dullness to percussion and a decrease in tactile fremitus and the selected site should not be lower than the eighth intercostal space.

Anesthesia and Pleural Fluid Localization

Using a 25-guage needle attached to a syringe containing 5 to 10 mL of 1% lidocaine or equivalent anesthetic, raise a skin wheal at the upper edge of the rib just below the marked intercostal space (Fig. 9–12). The upper edge of the rib is utilized to avoid accidental trauma to the neurovascular bundle, which runs at the inferior margin of each rib. With each 1 to 2 mm of needle advancement, the subcutaneous tissue and muscle are aspirated and then infiltrated with 1 to 2 mL of anesthetic. While the aspiration-infiltration process is continued, the needle is then "walked" above the superior edge of the rib and advanced through the intercostal space until the pleural space is entered (see Fig. 9–11C, inset). The needle must be held perpendicular to the chest to avoid

Figure 9–10 *A–C,* Various positionings for thoracentesis.

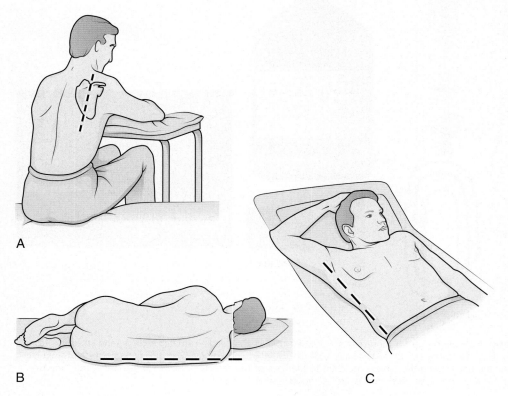

A

B

C

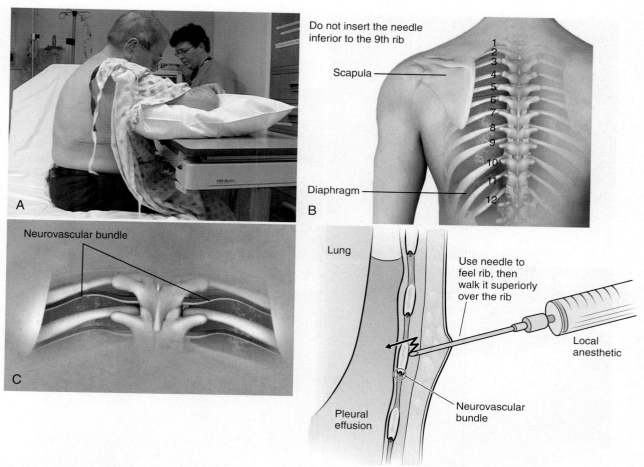

Figure 9–11 *A,* Preferred positioning for thoracentesis by the posterior approach. *B,* The inferior tip of the scapula is at the seventh rib. Do not insert the thoracentesis needle below the ninth rib. *C,* The anatomy of the neurovascular bundle mandates the needle insertion technique illustrated in the *inset. (A–C, From Thomsen T, Setnik G [eds]: Procedures Consult—Emergency Medicine Module.Copyright 2008 Elsevier Inc. All rights reserved.)*

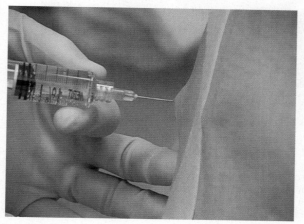

Figure 9–12 Use generous local anesthesia to anesthetize the track of the thoracentesis needle. Slowly advance the needle to touch the rib, then direct it over the rib while aspirating. With appropriate anesthesia, this procedure is minimally painful. A pop may be felt when the pleura is entered. Use this sensation to approximate the depth of the pleura when subsequently advancing the thoracentesis needle.

inadvertent trauma to the neurovascular bundle of the adjacent rib. Upon entering the pleural space, a pop may be felt and fluid should be aspirated to ensure that the pleural space has been reached. Once fluid is aspirated, *grasp the needle at the skin with the thumb and index finger and withdraw it. This allows for measurement of the proper depth of penetration needed during subsequent needle insertion.* If no fluid is encountered, this is consistent with a dry tap. A *dry tap* in the setting of a free-flowing pleural effusion indicates that either the needle is too short or the site chosen is too high or too low. A longer needle such as a spinal needle may be required for patients with significant amounts of subcutaneous tissue. If air bubbles are encountered, the lung parenchyma may have been entered and the chosen site is likely too high. If no fluid or air is encountered, the chosen site is likely too low. If a dry tap occurs during fluid localization and the patient has no new symptoms, reevaluate the patient position and fluid level, administer local anesthetic as needed, and reattempt to aspirate fluid with the needle. If the repeat attempt is unsuccessful, obtain fluid under ultrasound guidance.

Over-the-Needle-Catheter Insertion Technique

This is a preferred technique that utilizes an 8-French catheter mounted on an 18-gauge introducer needle (Fig. 9–13).

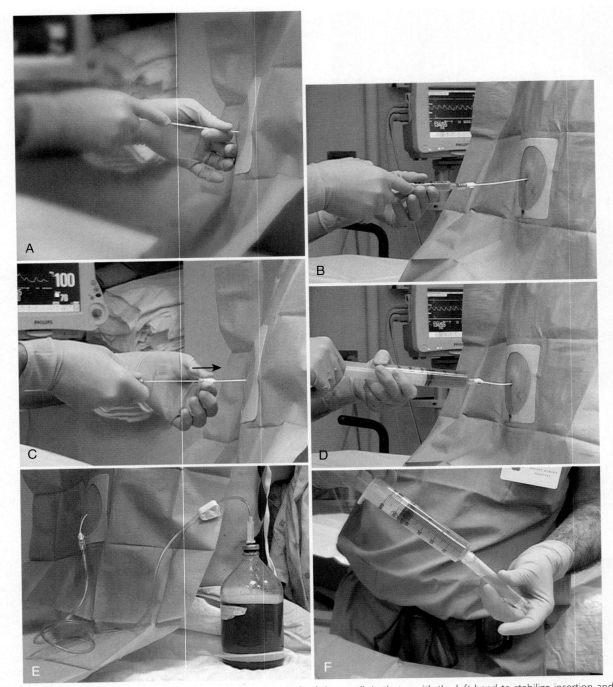

Figure 9–13 *A,* Puncture the skin with a No. 11 scalpel. Hold the shaft of the needle/catheter with the left hand to stabilize insertion and to control the advance of the device using the right hand. *B,* Attach a syringe and continue advancing and *aspirating* until the pleural space is entered. *C,* Once fluid is obtained, stop the advancement and slide the catheter over the needle into the pleural space. *D,* Confirm placement by aspirating. Attach the catheter to the vacuum drainage bottle (*E*) or use a stopcock or syringe (*F*), and place the fluid into tubes for analysis. If a stopcock is used, pay attention to avoid introducing air into the pleural space by keeping the *stop closed to the patient at all times unless draining fluid.* If cultures are taken, inoculate blood culture bottles with 10 mL of fluid *at the bedside.* To avoid errors, have an assistant transfer fluids *while the operator maintains vigilance over the procedure itself.* (*A–F, From Thomsen T, Setnik G [eds]: Procedures Consult—Emergency Medicine Module.Copyright 2008 Elsevier Inc. All rights reserved.)*

The needle-catheter unit is attached to a 10- or 20-mL syringe. A small skin pierce with a scalpel at the selected insertion site is required to ease the entry of the catheter through the skin. The depth of the pleural space as determined from the anesthetic needle is now marked by gently grasping the shaft of the needle-catheter unit with the index finder and thumb of the left hand. *This stabilizes the device and controls the*

advance. The needle-catheter unit is "walked" over the rib, through the anesthetized area into the pleural space, while constant, gentle negative pressure is applied to the syringe. As fluid is encountered, the needle-catheter unit is angled slightly caudally. The catheter is then advanced off the needle into the pleural space while holding the needle steady. The needle is withdrawn and the exposed lumen of the catheter hub is covered with a finger to prevent the entry of air. A three-way stopcock with an attached 30- to 60-mL syringe and drainage tubing is now attached to the catheter hub. Fluid is first aspirated with the syringe. The stopcock lever is then turned to prevent passage of fluid into the catheter (off to the catheter), and the fluid is expelled through the drainage tube into a sterile container or sterile vacuum bottle, where it can subsequently be transferred into appropriate specimen tubes. This process of aspirating and expelling the fluid is repeated until an adequate amount of fluid is obtained. Alternatively, fluid may be allowed to drain directly from the needle and three-way stopcock through high-pressure tubing into a vacuum bottle. The stopcock lever should be turned to prevent entry of air or fluid back into the catheter when changing bottles. If the catheter tip has multiple side ports for fluid entry, care must be taken to avoid withdrawing the catheter from chest during fluid removal, which might expose a side port and allow air entry into the pleural space. Once an indication for discontinuing the procedure has been met, the catheter is removed and the entry site is covered with a sterile bandage.

The procedure is simplified when using a commercial over-the-needle catheter. First, the self-sealing valve automatically prevents air from entering the catheter hub as the needle is removed. Second, most have a built-in stopcock, which is located either on the base of the catheter or at the end of a built-in drainage tube, obviating the need for the three-way stopcock described earlier.

TRIPLE-LUMEN CATHETER TECHNIQUE

Thoracentesis may be performed with a standard central venous triple-lumen catheter, introduced with a Seldinger technique. A stopcock is used and the procedure is the same as described previously, except that a guidewire and dilator are used, similar to the technique for venous catheterization.

PEDIATRIC PATIENTS

The indications and contraindications for performing thoracentesis are much the same in children as in adults. Positioning is also similar, but will likely require an assistant to help hold the patient and prevent patient movement. Sedation may be helpful when respiratory distress is minimal. The effusion level is again determined clinically by dullness to percussion and decrease in tactile fremitus. The needle insertion site should not be lower than the eighth intercostal space in the posterior axillary line. Any technique as described for the adult patient may be used, but the smallest possible needle or needle-catheter is recommended.

POSTPROCEDURE RADIOGRAPH

In many centers, chest radiographs are routinely obtained after thoracentesis to evaluate for procedure-related pneumothorax (Fig. 9–14). This has been shown to be unnecessary in patients who require a single needle pass, have no risk for adhesions, and have no new symptoms during or after thoracentesis.[28–30] A chest radiograph should be obtained in patients who require multiple needle passes, if air is aspirated, in those at risk for adhesions, or in those who develop any new symptoms (chest pain, dyspnea) during or after thoracentesis. In addition, it is reasonable to obtain a postprocedure radiograph

in those patients who are at risk for future decompensation from expansion of a small asymptomatic pneumothorax, including patients with severe underlying lung disease and those receiving *mechanical ventilation*.

PLEURAL FLUID ANALYSIS

Pleural fluid analysis should occur in an organized and thoughtful pattern based on clinical suspicion for a disease process. Given the impracticalities of sequential testing in the ED, some clinicians order a battery of screening tests based on the most logical etiologies. A more cost-effective approach is to collect multiple containers and have these held in the laboratory for future analysis as guided by the initial fluid evaluation and clinical suspicion.

Visual Inspection

Fluid examination in all cases begins with visual inspection. Effusions may range from clear to turbid. The presence of blood suggests trauma, malignancy, pulmonary infarct, or pneumonia.[31] White or milky fluid suggests the presence of lipids, whereas purulent, malodorous fluid indicates empyema. Pleural effusion containing food particles is highly suggestive of esophageal rupture. The odor of urine suggests urinothorax.

Distinguishing Transudate from Exudate: Light's Criteria

The next step in pleural fluid evaluation is the categorization of the fluid as exudative or transudative. The pathophysiology of each category is discussed earlier in this chapter. Table 9–1 lists the common etiologies. Light and coworkers[32] published criteria for separating transudates from exudates in 1972 based upon measurements of serum and pleural fluid protein and LDH. The value for LDH was subsequently changed to accommodate variations in assay conditions.[33] These criteria have since become known as *Light's criteria* (Table 9–2). An exception to using Light's criteria for separating transudates from exudates is in the setting of CHF treated with diuretics. Effusions in CHF are due to increased capillary hydrostatic pressure and are therefore transudates. However, it has been shown that diuretic use increases the pleural fluid protein and LDH concentrations, making the fluid appear exudative by Light's criteria.[34–36] This is hypothesized to be due to diuretic-induced shifting of fluid out of the pleural space. In the diuretic-treated CHF population with an exudate by Light's criteria, measuring the serum–to–pleural effusion albumin gradient is recommended.[34,37,38] If the serum albumin minus the pleural fluid albumin is greater than 1.2 g/dL the patient

TABLE 9–2 Transudate vs. Exudate: Light's Criteria
If at least one of the following three criteria is present, the fluid is virtually always an exudate; if none is present, the fluid is virtually always a transudate: • Pleural fluid–to–serum protein ratio > 0.5 • Pleural fluid LDH > two thirds of the upper limit of serum reference range • Pleural fluid–to–serum LDH ratio > 0.6

LDH, lactate dehydrogenase.

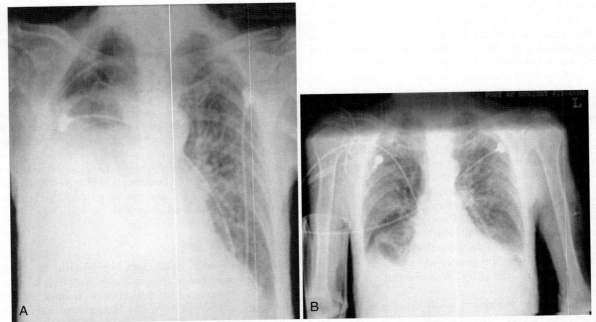

Figure 9–14 Pre- (*A*) and post-thoracentesis (*B*) chest radiographs. Postoperative films are not always routine but should be performed if air was aspirated, the patient has postprocedure chest pain or dyspnea, multiple attempts were made, or the patient is on a ventilator. (*A* and *B, From Thomsen T, Setnik G [eds]: Procedures Consult—Emergency Medicine Module.Copyright 2008 Elsevier Inc. All rights reserved.*)

likely has a transudative effusion, and no further fluid analysis is necessary.

Once a fluid is classified as transudative, it typically requires no further fluid analysis, and therapy is directed at the underlying cause of the effusion (e.g., CHF, cirrhosis).

In the presence of an undiagnosed exudative effusion, however, more extensive fluid evaluation is required.

Evaluation of Exudates

All undiagnosed exudates, at a minimum, should have pleural fluid sent for cell count with differential, glucose, and cytology[39] (Table 9–3). In regions with a high prevalence of tuberculosis (TB), adenosine deaminase (ADA) should be added to this list. Clinical suspicion for an underlying disease process should guide additional fluid evaluation.

Cell Count with Differential

In general, the presence or absence of red blood cells (RBCs) is not useful in determining the etiology of the effusion because it takes a very small amount of blood to cause a blood-tinged appearance. A grossly bloody pleural effusion or RBC count of greater than 100,000 cells/mm³ is suggestive of trauma, malignancy, pneumonia, or pulmonary infarction,[31,40] but a lack of RBCs does not exclude these diagnoses. Grossly bloody pleural fluid with a hematocrit of greater than 50% of the peripheral hematocrit often requires tube thoracostomy.

Exudates typically have a pleural fluid white blood cell (WBC) count of greater than 1000 cells/mm³, and counts may reach levels of greater than 10,000 cells/mm³, most commonly with parapneumonic effusions.[40] The differential cell count can be useful in identifying the cause of an exudative pleural effusion. A predominance of neutrophils indicates an acute process affecting the pleural surface, such as infection or pulmonary infarct. A predominance of lymphocytes is consistent with a more chronic pleural process, including malignancy, TB, PE, and viral pleuritis.[10,39] Eosinophil counts of greater than 10% often have no clear etiology, but have traditionally been associated with blood or air in the pleural space.

Culture

If infection is a concern, directly inoculate blood culture bottles *at the bedside* with 10 mL of fluid. TB cultures may be obtained from separate collection tubes.

Glucose

The concentration of glucose in exudates is extremely variable and, in general, does not correlate with any specific disease process. Routine measurement of pleural fluid glucose for exudative effusion is recommended, in that a low glucose concentration (<60 mg/dL) narrows the differential diagnosis to empyema, ruptured esophagus, complicated parapneumonic infection, malignancy, and TB.[41] Keep in mind, however, that these diagnoses are not *excluded* by a high or normal pleural fluid glucose. In addition, in exception to the just-discussed rule, patients with active rheumatoid arthritis and rheumatoid pleural effusion will commonly have an extremely low pleural fluid glucose concentration (<20–30 mg/dL).[42] Comparatively, in systemic lupus erythematosus, pleural fluid glucose levels are usually normal.[43]

Cytology

At least 50 mL of pleural fluid is typically required for cytologic evaluation. Unfortunately, the initial pleural fluid cytology is often negative in malignant pleural effusions.[40] Obtaining repeated pleural samples increases the yield of malignant cells.

TABLE 9–3 Exudates: Evaluation of the Undiagnosed Exudative Effusion

Pleural Fluid Assay	Result	Likely Diagnosis (Differential Diagnosis)
Standard Testing: Perform on All Exudative Effusions		
CBC with differential		
RBC count	Grossly bloody or >100,000 cells/mm³	Trauma, malignancy, PE, pneumonia
WBC count	>10,000 cells/mm³	Parapneumonic
Neutrophils	>50%	Acute pleural process: infection, pulmonary infarct
Lymphocytes	>50%	Chronic pleural process: malignancy, TB, PE, viral pleuritis
Eosinophils	>10%	Air or blood in pleural space
Glucose	<60 mg/dL	Ruptured esophagus, complicated parapneumonic infection, malignancy, TB, rheumatoid arthritis
Cytology	Abnormal cells	Malignancy
Selective Testing: Order if High Clinical Suspicion for Diagnosis		
ADA	>40 IU/L	TB
Gram stain and culture	Presence of organism	Pleural space infection
Amylase[57]	>100 U/L	Pancreatitis, esophageal rupture (malignancy, CABG, ruptured ectopic, TB)
Triglycerides	>110 mg/dL	Chylothorax, intrathoracic TPN infusion
Creatinine (with serum measurement)	Pleural fluid–to–serum creatinine ratio > 1	Urinothorax
Albumin (with serum measurement)	Serum–to–pleural fluid albumin gradient > 1.2 g/dL	Congestive heart failure after diuretics (exudative effusions)
Interferon γ	>140 pg/L[58]	TB (malignancy, empyema)
PCR	Presence of TB DNA sequences, TB	TB
pH	<7.2	Complicated parapneumonic effusion

CABG, coronary artery bypass graft; CBC, complete blood count; PCR, polymerase chain reaction; PE, pulmonary embolism; RBC, red blood cell; TB, tuberculosis; TPN, total parenteral nutrition; WBC, white blood cell.

Adenosine Deaminase

Pleural fluid ADA is an important screening tool in areas with a high prevalence of TB. A pleural fluid ADA above 40 U/L is highly suggestive of TB.[44–46] In the case of suspected TB, pleural fluid acid-fast bacillus staining and culture should be ordered, but these are infrequently positive.[45] Newer markers, including polymerase chain reaction and interferon γ, have been shown to be useful in the diagnosis of tuberculous pleural effusions.

Parapneumonic Effusions

Patients with suspected parapneumonic effusions warrant rapid evaluation and outcomes risk assessment based on pleural anatomy, pleural fluid bacteriology, and pleural fluid chemistry.[47] All parapneumonic effusions require at least diagnostic thoracentesis with the goal of identifying patients with complicated parapneumonic effusions. The indications for tube thoracostomy or other surgical management include large or loculated effusions, pleural thickening on CT scanning (the pleural peel), aspiration of frank pus, pleural fluid pH of less than 7.2, and positive Gram stain or culture (Table 9–4).

Pleural pH measurement gives useful information regarding pleural inflammation. Normal pleural fluid pH is approximately 7.64. Pleural fluid pH less than 7.3 indicates pleural inflammation. The differential diagnosis of pleural fluid acidosis includes not only empyema and complicated parapneumonic effusion but also malignancy, TB, esophageal rupture, and collagen vascular disease.[48] Measurement of pleural pH is essential in the evaluation of suspected parapneumonic effusions because pH is a key factor in the management algo-

rithm. The fluid must be collected anaerobically, but may be transferred from the initial 50 or 60 mL syringe into a heparinized blood gas syringe,[49] and then left at room temperature for up to 1 hour prior to laboratory analysis[50] without affecting the accuracy of the results. Because of these specifics regarding the collection and evaluation of pleural fluid pH, pleural fluid should routinely be transferred to a heparinized blood gas syringe and placed on ice while awaiting the decision for pH testing.

TABLE 9–4 Indications for Surgical Management of Parapneumonic Effusions

Effusion > 50% of hemithorax
Loculated effusion
Pleural thickening by CT
Aspiration of frank pus
Pleural fluid pH < 7.2
Positive Gram stain or culture of pleural fluid

CT, computed tomography.

COMPLICATIONS

Pneumothorax

The most frequently reported complication of thoracentesis is pneumothorax, which has a reported incidence of 4% to 19% in some studies.[23,28,51] Thoracostomy tubes were required in less than 50% of the post-thoracentesis pneumothoraces in each study. The mechanism for this complication is puncture of the lung or inadvertent air entry through the needle or catheter during the procedure. Pneumothorax should be suspected if there is aspiration of air during fluid removal or if the patient develops new symptoms during or after the procedure. Procedure-related factors appearing to contribute to pneumothorax include inexperienced operator, therapeutic taps, and use of needles larger than 20 gauge.[22,24,51,52] The risk of pneumothorax may be increased in patients with underlying chronic obstructive pulmonary disease.[53]

Cough

Cough is another frequently encountered complication. Although typically considered a minor complication resulting in only patient discomfort, it may be associated with the creation of an iatrogenic pneumothorax.[52,54] The procedure should be terminated if persistent patient coughing occurs.

Infection

As with all procedures, there is a potential risk for infection which is estimated at 2%. The risk is kept low with proper attention to patient preparation and sterile technique.

Uncommon Serious Complications

Other serious complications have been reported, but occur in less than 1% of procedures. These include hemothorax, splenic rupture, abdominal hemorrhage, unilateral pulmonary edema, air embolism, and catheter fragment left in the pleural space.[52]

Hemothorax may be suspected by a rapid accumulation or reaccumulation of pleural fluid or by a change in patient vital signs after the procedure. Hemothorax may be due to laceration of the lung or the diaphragmatic, intercostals, or internal mammary vessels. Careful attention to technique, such as *avoiding the superior portion* of the intercostal space, never puncturing medial to the midclavicular line, and not penetrating too deeply into the thorax during needle insertion, should be practiced. Hemothorax requires appropriate surgical consultation and drainage via thoracostomy tube.

Puncture of the spleen or liver through the diaphragm may result in localized organ hematoma or hemoperitoneum.[54] Clinically, this is suspected when the needle pass does not yield pleural fluid (dry tap) and is followed by a patient complaint of abdominal pain. If this diagnosis is suspected, appropriate resuscitation is the initial treatment, followed by a diagnostic imaging study, preferably CT scan. If the patient is hemodynamically unstable, bedside ultrasound and immediate surgical consultation should occur.

Through-the-needle catheters are not commonly used because the catheter may be cut or sheared off while it traverses the needle or is withdrawn.

Reexpansion pulmonary edema is a complication associated with rapid reexpansion of the lung. Symptoms include dyspnea, tachypnea, tachycardia, cough, and frothy sputum.[55] It is believed that this can be avoided by monitoring the pleural pressures carefully after 1500 mL of fluid has been withdrawn and discontinuing the procedure when the pleural pressures are greater than −20 mm Hg.[31,56] There is no proven way, however, to assure that reexpansion pulmonary edema will not occur.

 REFERENCES CAN BE FOUND ON EXPERT CONSULT

CHAPTER 10

Tube Thoracostomy

Thomas D. Kirsch

Tube thoracostomy (TT) to evacuate an abnormal accumulation of fluid or air from the pleural space is a common elective, emergent, or urgent procedure. The procedure is performed by emergency clinicians or surgeons, usually dependent on the urgency of the scenario, or local protocols. Air or fluid in the pleural space can result from a spontaneous or traumatic pneumothorax (PTX), pleural fluid accumulations from blood, malignancy, infection (empyema), or lymph (chylothorax). The first modern methods to evacuate pleural contents were developed in the 19th century, but these techniques were not widespread until 1918, when they were used to treat postinfluenza empyema. Military experience demonstrated that thoracic drainage combined with antiseptics and antibiotics reduced the mortality from thoracic trauma from 62.5% during the Civil War, to 24.6% in World War I, to 12% in World War II.[1] TT has since evolved to become a common and effective procedure.[2]

PATHOPHYSIOLOGY

The pleural space that normally separates the visceral and parietal pluerae has a thin layer of lubricating fluid separating the layers. The parietal pleura lines the interior of the chest wall. The visceral pleura covers the lungs. Under normal circumstances, a small negative pressure in the pleural space keeps the lung inflated. With inspiration, the negative intrathoracic pressure increases, leading to the expansion of the lung from an influx of air from the environment. The addition of blood, fluid, or air in the pleural space disrupts the normal pressure gradient and interferes with normal inspiratory-induced inflation, leading to the "collapse" of the lung. The degree of respiratory compromise depends on the volume of the fluid or air in the pleural space, the patient's age and baseline pulmonary status, and the integrity of the chest wall. As the amount of fluid or air increases, respiratory function worsens and produces symptoms of dyspnea with exertion and then at rest, often with pleuritic chest pain, and anxiety. Large positive-pressure accumulations associated with a tension PTX lead to severe respiratory dysfunction and cardiovascular compromise.

PNEUMOTHORAX

Because the lung remains inflated due to a negative pressure in the pleural space, a PTX results from the presence of air in the pleural space and loss of this negative pressure (Fig. 10–1). The air can enter the pleural space internally from a ruptured lung bleb, the trachea or from the outside due to a penetrating injury. A PTX often has an iatrogenic cause secondary to egress of air from puncture or rupture of the lung into the pleural space. Common causes are procedures such as subclavian venous cannulation, transthoracic biopsies, thoracentesis, positive-pressure ventilation (PPV), or cardiopulmonary resuscitation (CPR).

Spontaneous (Closed) PTX

A spontaneous PTX occurs from the rupture of a subpleural lung bleb with little or no trauma and the chest wall remains intact. Based on the presence of underlying lung disease and the approach to treatment, a spontaneous PTX can be categorized as either primary or secondary. A *primary spontaneous PTX* occurs in a patient *without* underlying lung disease. The typical patient with a spontaneous PTX is a tall, thin, 20- to 40-year-old male smoker. *Secondary spontaneous PTXs* occur in patients *with* underlying lung or pleural disease, including emphysema, chronic bronchitis, asthma, Marfan's syndrome, *Pneumocystis jiroveci* pneumonia, other pneumonias, and neoplasm. The morbidity, mortality, and long-term complications of a PTX increase for patients with underlying lung disease. Whereas a primary PTX may be selectively observed or simply aspirated, a secondary PTX often requires a more aggressive approach to management.

Common symptoms include the sudden onset of pleuritic chest pain and dyspnea with exertion or at rest. Occasionally, pain is absent and symptoms vary from mild dyspnea on excursion that the patient may ignore for days to severe dyspnea at rest. Signs and symptoms do not always correlate well with the size or cause of the lung collapse, often surprising the clinician when symptoms are investigated. Some individuals with a small spontaneous PTX may never seek medical attention, and the process will resolve spontaneously. TT is the most common treatment, but some experts recommend simple aspiration as first-line treatment for all *primary* PTXs requiring intervention.[2,3] A spontaneous PTX may rarely progress to a tension PTX. The process can be bilateral.

Traumatic Open PTX

Loss of the normal negative intrapleural pressure results in a lung collapse. An open PTX occurs when the chest wall is penetrated and the negative intrapleural pressure is lost as outside air enters the pleural space. A tension PTX may develop with even a small open chest wall defect when air enters the wound with each inspiration but is trapped during expiration by a flap that functions like a one-way valve. Each breath therefore increases the intrapleural pressure. If the diameter of the chest wound is greater than that of the trachea, then with each respiratory attempt, air moves preferentially through the chest wall opening rather than down the trachea. This is a more serious injury because, if left untreated, it can prevent any ventilation of the involved lung.

Traumatic Closed PTX

A closed PTX may also result from an injury when the chest wall is not penetrated. This usually results from a rib fracture that penetrates the lung, but can also occur when an alveolus or bleb ruptures after blunt trauma as a result of an abrupt increase in intrathoracic pressure against a closed glottis. The air leak from a closed PTX is usually self-limited, but can rarely progress to a tension PTX.

Tension PTX

A tension PTX is a life-threatening condition that requires immediate intervention. Tension PTX usually results from penetrating chest injuries. Other causes include fractures of

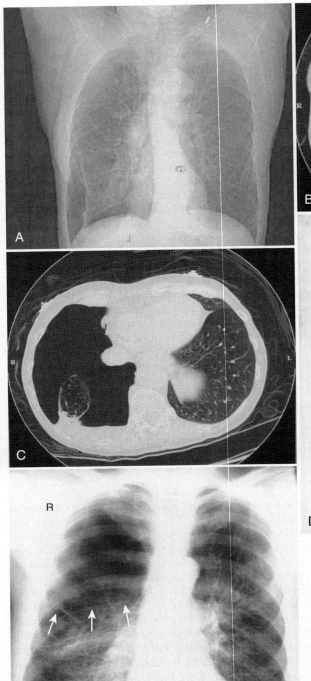

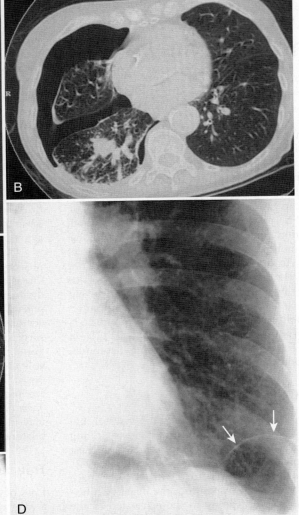

Figure 10–1 *A,* Anteroposterior chest radiograph view of a right-sided, seemingly small, simple pneumothorax (PTX). Note absence of peripheral lung markings on the right side and the distinct line indicating the edge of the collapsed lung. Although this appears to be a small PTX, it produced significant dyspnea in this patient with chronic obstructive pulmonary disease and therefore required a chest tube. *B* and *C,* Computed tomography (CT) scans show the extent of the collapse, almost 100% in some places, not appreciated on a plain x-ray. Adhesions kept part of the lung expanded. *D,* Sometimes bullae can be seen on a chest x-ray and mistaken for a PTX because their thin wall can be visualized. *E,* Larger bullae are sometimes identified only by the fact that an area on the chest x-ray does not appear to have any pulmonary vessels (*arrows*), and at the periphery, crowding of the normal lung and vessels may appear. Skin folds and the border of the scapula or external wires can also be mistaken for a PTX. A CT scan can settle these issues.

the trachea or bronchi, a ruptured esophagus, the presence of an occlusive dressing over an open PTX, and PPV. Patients *with chest or lung injuries who are undergoing PPV are at much greater risk to develop a tension PTX,* either spontaneously from lung injury due to high-pressure ventilation or when a small *PTX* is expanded by PPV. Because of this, any patient with a penetrating thoracic injury (even without immediate evidence of a hemothorax [HTX] or PTX) may be a candidate for a

"prophylactic" chest tube before mechanical ventilation. A tension PTX may develop from a simple PTX caused by CPR, but be clinically evident only after PPV has been instituted. Asthmatics or patients with emphysema may also develop a PTX, followed by tension PTX, from the high pressure required for ventilation.

A tension PTX occurs when a pulmonary or bronchial injury creates a "ball-valve" or "flap-valve" mechanism that

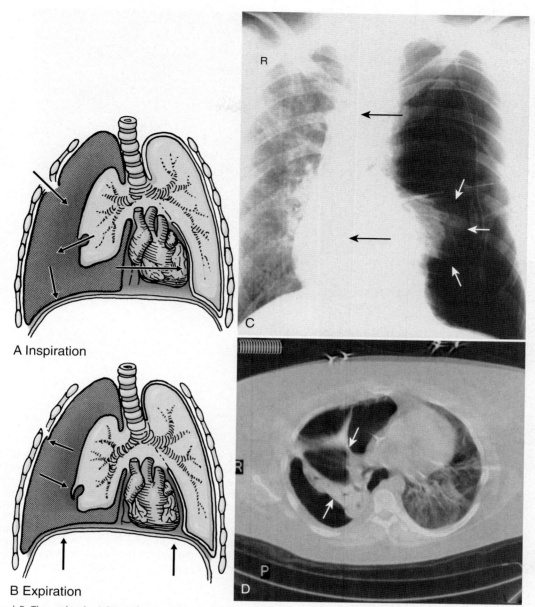

Figure 10–2 *A* and *B*, The pathophysiology of a tension PTX. During inspiration, air enters the pleural space through a one-way valve either from the outside or from the lung itself. Upon expiration, the injury/valve closes, trapping increasing amounts of air in the pleural space. Eventually, the mediastinum shifts and cardiac filling and eventually cardiac output are compromised. *C* and *D*, Tension PTX. *C*, On a posteroanterior chest x-ray, the left hemithorax is very dark or lucent because the left lung has collapsed completely (*white arrows*). The tension PTX can be identified because the mediastinal contents, including the heart, are shifted toward the right, and the left hemidiaphragm is flattened and depressed. *D*, A CT scan done on a different patient with a tension PTX shows a completely collapsed right lung (*arrows*) and shift of the mediastinal contents to the left. (*A* and *B*, From Vukich DJ, Markovchick VJ: Pulmonary and chest wall injuries. In Rosen P, Barkin RM, Braen CR, et al [eds]: Emergency Medicine: Concepts and Clinical Practice. St. Louis, Mosby-Year Book, 1988. Reproduced by permission.)

leads to the progressive accumulation of air in the pleural space. The one-way valve effect is thought to be due to the presence of a tissue flap that allows air into the pleural space but then closes with expiration and traps the air (Fig. 10–2). The increasing pressures lead to ipsilateral complete lung collapse, and if allowed to continue, impingement on the mediastinum with a shift of the heart towards the uninvolved side, restricting ventricular filling and subsequently decreasing cardiac function. This severe disruption of both respiratory and cardiac function can lead to hypotension and reduced ventilation (both hypoxia and CO_2 retention) and eventually to cardiopulmonary collapse.

Pneumomediastinum

Air in the mediastinum is termed *pneumomediastinum* (PM)[4-6] (Fig. 10–3). It is usually a benign condition that presents with nonspecific pleuritic chest or neck pain or symptoms similar to those of a pericarditis, pneumonia, pulmonary embolism, or spontaneous PTX. The most common cause is a sudden increase in intrapulmonary pressure, usually without an obvious lung alveolar rupture. Rarely, there is an associated PTX or esophageal rupture. Spontaneous PM is usually benign but Stiegmann and coworkers[4] reported a rare tension PM in which air from an alveolar rupture near the pulmonary

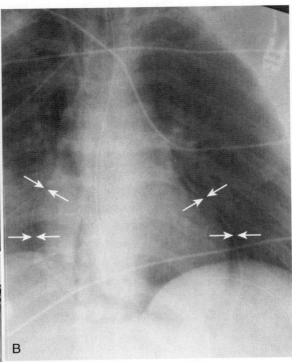

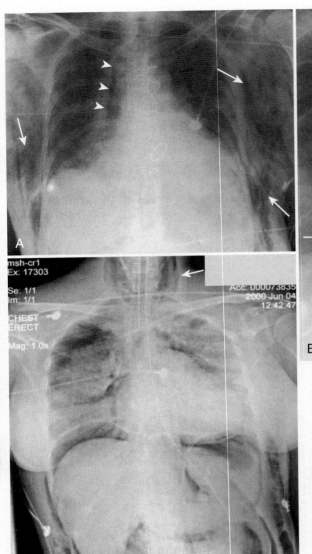

Figure 10–3 *A,* Pneumomediastinum (PM). Chest x-ray reveals extensive gas in the subcutaneous tissue (*arrows*) and outlining the mediastinal structures (*arrowheads*). *B,* Pneumopericardium. On this chest x-ray, the pericardium (*arrows*) is outlined by air between the pericardium and the heart and air in the lungs. Note that the pericardium *does not extend above the level of the pulmonary arteries*. This helps distinguish pneumopericardium from PM. *C,* Barotrauma (note air in the neck, *arrow*) as a consequence of acute respiratory distress syndrome. Note the presence of a PTX, PM, pneumopericardium, and subcutaneous air (into the neck) in this patient receiving positive-pressure ventilation (PPV). *(A–C, Courtesy of Dr. Thomas E. Stewart.)*

artery tracked to the subcutaneous mediastinal tissue where it became "trapped by scar tissue" and produced pressure on the great vessels and major airways. PM from barotrauma in a ventilated trauma patient may be very extensive and can be associated with pneumopericardium (see Fig. 10–3*C*).

The most common causes of benign spontaneous PM are inhalation drug abuse (crack cocaine or marijuana) when a Valsalva maneuver is performed to enhance drug absorption, acute asthma, blunt chest trauma, violent coughing or vomiting, or barotrauma. Often, the condition is spontaneous and no cause is found. The most common symptoms are chest pain, usually pleuritic, and neck pain, sore throat, dyspnea, or persistent cough. Vital signs, including pulse oximetry, are usually normal.

About half the time, subcutaneous emphysema, usually in the neck, can be palpated. Usually, the diagnosis is made by demonstrating air in the tissues on radiographs of the neck or chest or more readily by computed tomography (CT) scan. Lateral chest/neck radiographs are more diagnostic than anteroposterior views. This condition can be mistaken for pneumopericardium (see Fig. 10–3*B*). The classic Hamman crunch (crinkling or audible crepitance during chest ausculta-

tion) is present in only 50% to 80% of cases of PM, and is easily initially missed.

The clinical course is almost always benign, especially in young male drug inhalers, and extensive testing, hospitalization, follow-up radiographs, or antibiotics are not warranted.[5,6] A few hours of observation in the emergency department (ED) seems prudent if the symptoms are of recent onset. For the rare tension PM, decompression may be undertaken. A needle is inserted into the second or third intercostal space just lateral to the sternum and directed toward the anterior mediastinum, suggested as initial therapy in infants. Alternatively, a small incision 2 to 3 cm above the sternal notch can be made so finger dissection of the deep cervical and pretracheal fascia can be performed. A chest tube is not therapeutic.

HEMOTHORAX

A HTX is the accumulation of blood in the pleural space, caused by injuries to the heart, great vessels, or the vessels of the lungs, mediastinum, or chest wall. Bleeding from the lung parenchyma is low pressure, and is usually self-limited or ceases when a chest tube is placed. Intercostal artery, pulmonary artery, and internal mammary artery bleeding can be profuse and often requires surgical intervention.

Empyema/Effusions

An empyema is an accumulation of pus in the pleural space, usually from parapneumonic infectious effusions. Empyemas are estimated to occur in 1% to 2% of hospitalized patients with pneumonia. The remainder of empyemas result from violations of the thoracic space by surgical procedures, trauma, or esophageal perforation. *Staphylococcus aureus* is the most common isolate.

Chylothorax

Chylothorax results from an injury to the thoracic duct during central line placement, operative injury, or chest trauma. The primary thoracic duct injury is usually asymptomatic because the chyle initially collects extrapleurally and may not begin to fill the pleural cavity for 2 to 10 days. As the fluid accumulates, the patient slowly develops respiratory symptoms. The chest radiograph demonstrates a pleural effusion, and the diagnosis is made when the thoracentesis reveals a milky fluid with a high fat and lymphocyte content and 4 to 5 g/dL of protein. The definitive treatment is by either repeated thoracentesis or TT combined with parenteral alimentation until the volume of chyle decreases.

DIAGNOSIS

Symptoms

The presentation of patients with abnormal collections of fluid or air in the pleural space can range from asymptomatic to cardiopulmonary arrest. The severity of symptoms depends somewhat on the size of the PTX and especially the rapidity of accumulation, age of the patient, and the presence of an underlying lung disease. Specific symptoms range from mild dyspnea with exercise and pleuritic chest pain for small disruptions to hypotension and severe dyspnea for those with a tension PTX. A cough may also be present. Severely injured patients may be unable to relate symptoms, rendering the physical examination and chest radiograph essential to diagnose a PTX and HTX. A tension PTX must be considered in any patient with sudden respiratory or cardiac deterioration and in intubated patients who become difficult to ventilate with increased airway pressure, hypotension, or elevated central venous and pulmonary artery pressure. Conscious patients with a tension PTX will rapidly develop severe dyspnea, restlessness, agitation, and a feeling of impending doom. They are usually tachycardic and tachypnic and can quickly become hypotensive.

With a spontaneous PTX, 95% of patients complain of the sudden onset of sharp or pleuritic chest or shoulder pain, or both. Sixty percent of patients experience dyspnea, and 12% have a mild cough. Dyspnea and anxiety are more common in older patients.

The symptoms of an HTX are often similar to those of a PTX, but may be accompanied by hypotension as blood accumulation in the pleural space increases. The onset of symptoms for effusions is usually much more gradual with increasing shortness of breath and dyspnea on exertion over days to weeks, a common scenario with malignant effusions.

Physical Examination

Unstable Patients

During the initial ("ABC") phase of resuscitation, the vital signs often point to the presence of a tension PTX. This diagnosis must be considered for injured patients who are tachycardic, hypotensive, and dyspneic. Similar symptoms occur with a pulmonary embolus, pericardial tamponade, and severe pneumonia. No single examination will reliably diagnose a tension PTX, so multiple methods must be rapidly conducted. "Look, listen, and feel" is the rule. Observation of the chest wall may reveal asymmetrical chest expansion. Neck and forehead veins may be distended even if the patient is hypotensive, or the trachea may be deviated away from the side of the PTX. Auscultation may demonstrate diminished breath sounds on the injured side. In one prospective study, the sensitivity, specificity, and diagnostic accuracy of auscultation for HTX/PTX was 84%, 97%, and 89%, respectively.[7] A false-negative auscultation is more likely than a false-positive one.[7] Finally, when percussing the chest wall, there may be hyperresonance on the affected side and subcutaneous emphysema may be present. *Pulsus paradoxus* (>12 mm Hg of normal inspiratory decrease in systemic blood pressure) may be evident. For intubated patients, an early sign of tension PTX is difficulty in bagging owing to increased airway pressures.

In injured patients with apnea, hypotension, or cardiopulmonary arrest, the diagnosis and treatment of a tension PTX should be made by an immediate needle or catheter decompression thoracentesis, not by a radiograph. The diagnosis of a tension PTX is confirmed when there is a rapid improvement in the vital signs and possibly a rush of air through the needle.

Post CPR PTX. After vigorous CPR, it is not uncommon to encounter an iatrogenic PTX, from either bleb rupture from compressions, lung trauma from a broken rib, or central line placement. Rib fractures are common during CPR in patients with severe osteoporosis. A small PTX is often inconsequential, but many CPR survivors undergo PPV, and a stable PTX may be converted into a tension PTX, with cardiopulmonary deterioration. Such deterioration may be assumed to be secondary to a return of the original pathology, but a search for a treatable tension PTX must be undertaken. Subcutaneous air, decreased breath sounds, difficulty with providing ventilations, or a deviated trachea should raise suspicion for this event (Fig. 10–4).

Stable Patients

For more stable patients (and those with smaller accumulations), the physical examination is less sensitive and a chest radiograph is usually necessary for the definitive diagnosis. Physical findings may include unilaterally decreased breath sounds, tachypnea, tachycardia, decreased tactile fremitus, increased resonance with percussion, or subcutaneous emphysema, but the examination may reveal little to no abnormalities with a small PTX. A less than 20% PTX will often present with a completely normal chest examination, including equal breath sounds. Pleural fluid collections are difficult to detect by physical examination, particularly with less than 500 mL of fluid in the pleural space. Breath sounds may be decreased and percussion of the bases may be dull.

Parapneumonic empyemas often present with fever, cough, chest pain, dyspnea, and purulent sputum. The physical examination will reveal diminished breath sounds, dullness

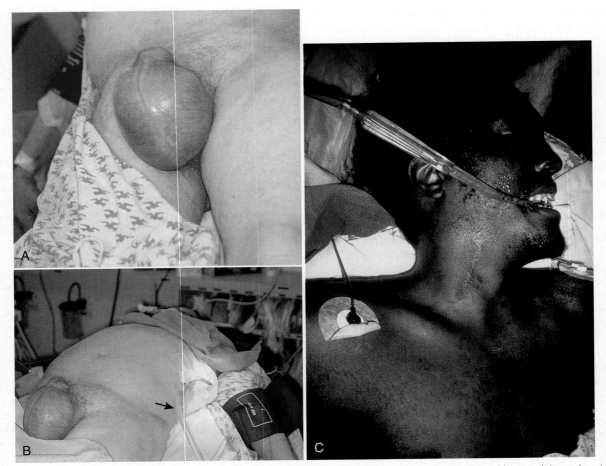

Figure 10–4 *A*, After successful cardiopulmonary resuscitation and intubation, this patient began to deteriorate, with a precipitous drop in blood pressure and a decreasing oxygen saturation. *It was believed that the cause of the initial cardiac arrest was returning.* Marked subcutaneous air was noted in the scrotum and abdominal wall, but little air was noted in the chest wall tissue. The subcutaneous air had curiously tracked via tissue planes, a distinctly unusual place for air to accumulate. *B*, A chest tube (*arrow*) quickly reversed the decompensation. *C*, This patient had a respiratory arrest from heroin injected into a neck vein (note extensive scar). After resuscitation with a bag-mask, he had a return of respiratory depression, unresponsive to naloxone, and he was very difficult to ventilate. He had a small PTX from a nick in the lung from the neck injection, and PPV turned it into a tension PTX.

to percussion, egophony, and diminished tactile fremitus on the involved side. Patients with an indwelling chest tube with an empyema will develop a fever, the pleural fluid drainage may be excessive and become purulent, and respiratory symptoms may worsen.

Radiography

Plain Radiographs
A chest radiograph is essential to diagnose a PTX in the stable patient. Unstable patients with a potential tension PTX may be diagnosed clinically or receive a portable radiograph while monitored by a clinician. The best plain radiographs for an HTX or a PTX are an *upright inspiratory* posteroanterior and lateral chest. Contrary to common belief, an *expiratory* upright posteroanterior chest radiograph is no better at detecting a PTX than the traditional upright inspiratory view. Upright is preferable to a supine chest radiograph for an HTX because even with large amounts of blood only slight *differences in the densities of the lung fields* may be found. With an upright chest radiograph 300 to 500 mL of fluid is needed to cause costophrenic angle blunting[8] (Fig. 10–5).

If there is significant clinical suspicion, then further studies are needed to rule out the presence of intrapleural fluid or air. A thoracic CT scan is the "gold standard," demonstrating many PTXs that are never visible on a plain radiograph. If this is not available, then to look for an HTX, the best additional views are bilateral decubitus chest radiographs, with the PTX expected to be seen on the side away from the table as gravity pulls down the affected lung.

On a chest radiograph, the partially collapsed lung of a PTX appears as a visceral pleural line with no pulmonary markings beyond it (see Fig. 10–1*E*). *It is easy to initially mistake large blebs for a PTX or identify the scapular border, skin folds, or indwelling lines as a PTX,* but a CT scan quickly resolves the issue. Other radiographic findings include hyperlucency of the affected HTX, a double diaphragm contour, increased visibility of the inferior cardiac border, better visualization of the pericardial fat at the cardiac apex, and possibly a depressed diaphragm. *If subcutaneous air is noted on the chest x-ray of a patient with blunt chest trauma, it can be assumed that the air came from an injured lung and that a PTX exists.*

It is difficult to accurately predict the size of a PTX on plain radiographs, and such calculations have limited clinical applicability.[9] The size is usually described as a percentage collapse, but the vagaries of the collapse can be correctly delineated only by CT. With a tension PTX, the chest radiograph reveals lung collapse with no lung markings, a depressed

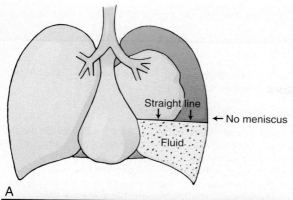

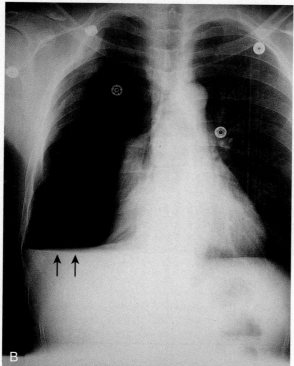

Figure 10–5 *A* and *B,* Stab wound to the chest. When accumulated fluid in the chest cavity is seen as a *straight line on an x-ray* (an air-fluid level [see *arrows*]), with no meniscus up the side, air must be present, even if a PTX cannot be seen. This poor-quality radiograph failed to show a 20% PTX found on CT, but a better plain radiograph may have also been diagnostic. If the patient is supine, these findings may not be seen.

hemidiaphragm on the affected side and a shift of the mediastinum and trachea to the opposite side. With a bilateral PTX, no mediastinal shift may be seen.

Thoracic CT Scan

CT scans of the chest are much more sensitive than plain radiographs for detecting PTXs and HTXs and more accurate to estimate the size and other characteristics of a PTX (see Fig. 10–1*A* and *C*). About 10% of trauma patients with a normal chest x-ray will demonstrate a small HTX or PTX.[10–12] The clinical significance of these small, previously undetected, occult injuries is likely not great, and it has been suggested that a small PTX seen only on CT scan may be left untreated, and simply observed, in the otherwise stable patient. Many patients with a PTX seen only on CT scan may also safely undergo PPV without the placement of a chest tube.[12]

CT scans are not routine for the diagnosis of a PTX, but are more useful for HTXs and other fluid collections. They also offer invaluable information on the etiology of such abnormalities. A CT scan may be useful when the diagnosis is unclear or when looking for small amounts of pleural fluid. CT scans are particularly useful to determine whether an empyema is loculated or draining successfully.

Ultrasound

Ultrasound has been shown to be useful in diagnosing both PTXs and HTXs. At least two ultrasonographic signs are described that are used to identify a PTX. One is the absence of the "sliding lung" sign, which is the movement of the hyperechoic line between the chest wall and the aerated lung with each respiration. The presence of the sliding lung sign effectively rules out a PTX, and its absence suggests that a PTX may be present, but confirmation with other signs is necessary. Another sign is the absence of "comet-tail artifacts," which are hyperechoic reverberation artifacts of the visceral pleural line that spread to the edge of the screen.[13]

INDICATIONS FOR TT

PTX

TT is by far the most common treatment for all types of PTXs, but controversy exists over the treatment of a small traumatic and primary spontaneous PTX. However, the American College of Chest Physicians has developed useful guidelines for the management of primary and secondary spontaneous PTXs[14] (Table 10–1).

Chest tube placement as routine initial intervention is likely not necessary in healthy patients with small primary spontaneous or isolated small traumatic PTXs in the absence of respiratory compromise, concomitant injuries, or when PPV will not be required. For a primary spontaneous PTX, a recent review concluded that there is no significant difference between simple aspiration and tube drainage with regard to immediate success rate, early failure rate, duration of hospitalization, and the 1-year success and pleurodesis.[15] Needle aspiration is associated with reduced analgesia requirements and lower pain scores compared with TT. Simple aspiration is associated with a reduction in the percentage of patients hospitalized when compared with tube drainage.

There is growing evidence that "video-assisted thoracoscopic surgery" may be the optimum treatment method for patients with an uncomplicated spontaneous PTX.[16] For patients with a simple PTX, prolonged suction is rarely required, and the tube can be simply attached to a Heimlich valve or underwater seal.[14,17] Without any intervention or continuing air leak, a small PTX will resolve over days to weeks. Supplemental oxygen will speed the reexpansion process by increasing the rate of pleural air absorption.

Most patients with a secondary spontaneous PTX have enough underlying disease to eventually require a chest tube. Patients with chronic obstructive pulmonary disease, malignancies, cystic fibrosis, and acquired immunodeficiency syndrome (AIDS)–related *Pneumocystis jiroveci* pneumonia, and tuberculosis infections are usually symptomatic enough, and have the potential for recurrence, that a TT usually cannot be avoided. Underlying infected and necrotic tissue in the AIDS patients often portends poor response to pleurodesis

TABLE 10–1 Guidelines of the American College of Chest Physicians for the Management of Primary and Secondary Spontaneous Pneumothorax

Primary Spontaneous Pneumothorax (No Underlying Lung Disease)

A clinically stable patient must have all of the following present: respiratory rate, <24 breaths/min; heart rate, >60 beats/min or <120 beats/min; normal blood pressure, room air O_2 saturation, >90%; and can speak in whole sentences between breaths.

Clinically Stable Patients with Small Pneumothoraces (<3 cm Apex-to-Cupola Distance)

Clinically stable patients with small pneumothoraces (PTXs) should be observed in the emergency department (ED) for 3–6 hr and discharged home if a repeat chest radiograph excludes progression of the PTX (good consensus). Patients should be provided with careful instructions for follow-up within 12 hr–2 days, depending on circumstances. A chest radiograph should be obtained at the follow-up appointment to document resolution of the PTX. Patients may be admitted for observation if they live distant from emergency services or follow-up care is considered unreliable (good consensus). Simple aspiration of the PTX or insertion of a chest tube is not appropriate for most patients (good consensus), unless the PTX enlarges. The presence of symptoms for longer than 24 hr does not alter the treatment recommendations.

Clinically Stable Patients with Large PTXs (≥3 cm Apex-to-Cupola Distance)

Clinically stable patients with large PTXs should undergo a procedure to reexpand the lung and should be hospitalized in most instances (very good consensus). The lung should be reexpanded by using a small-bore catheter (≤14 Fr) or placement of a 16- to 22-Fr chest tube (good consensus). Catheters or tubes may be attached either to a Heimlich valve (good consensus) or to a water-seal device (good consensus) and may be left in place until the lung expands against the chest wall and air leaks have resolved. If the lung fails to reexpand quickly, suction should be applied to a water-seal device. Alternatively, suction may be applied immediately after chest tube placement for all patients managed with a water-seal system (some consensus).

Reliable patients who are unwilling to undergo hospitalization may be discharged home from the ED with a small-bore catheter attached to a Heimlich valve if the lung has reexpanded after the removal of pleural air (good consensus). Follow-up should be arranged within 2 days. The presence of symptoms for longer than 24 hr does not alter management recommendations.

Secondary Spontaneous PTX

Clinically Stable Patients with Small PTXs

Clinically stable patients with small PTXs should be hospitalized (good consensus). Patients should not be managed in the ED with observation or simple aspiration without hospitalization (very good consensus). Hospitalized patients may be observed (good consensus) or treated with a chest tube (some consensus), depending on the extent of their symptoms and the course of their PTX. Some of the panel members argued against observation alone because of a report of deaths with this approach. Patients should not be referred for thoracoscopy without prior stabilization (very good consensus). The presence of symptoms for longer than 24 hr did not alter the panel members' recommendations.

Clinically Stable Patients with Large PTXs

Clinically stable patients with large PTXs should undergo the placement of a chest tube to reexpand the lung and should be hospitalized (very good consensus). Patients should not be referred for thoracoscopy without prior stabilization with a chest tube (very good consensus). The presence of symptoms for longer than 24 hr did not alter the panel members' recommendations.

This is meant to be a guide, and clinical judgment should always be used.
From Baumann MH, Strange C, Heffner JE, et al, and the AACP Pneumothorax Consensus Group: Management of spontaneous pneumothorax: An American College of Chest Physicians Delphi consensus statement. Chest 119:590, 2001.

and stapling, and predisposes to a persistent bronchopulmonary leak.

A catamenial PTX is a form of secondary spontaneous PTX seen in women with thoracic endometriosis, producing a lung collapse associated with menses. These may be recurrent. The issue of aspiration versus TT in these patients has not been defined. Spontaneous PTX has been described with chlomiphene citrate fertility treatment.

The underlying lung pathology of a patient with a spontaneous PTX is best initially evaluated by CT scan. Often, this is followed by diagnostic or therapeutic visual inspection of the lung and pleural space by fiberoptic thoracoscopy. Extensive evaluation is not, however, usually recommended for the first episode of a small primary PTX. When patients have recurrent spontaneous PTXs, further evaluation (CT scan, thoracoscopy) and evaluation for surgical treatment are indicated. Patients who have had one spontaneous PTX have a 30% to 50% chance of recurrence within 2 years, and after the second PTX, there is a 50% to 80% chance of a third. Surgery may be recommended for a first PTX in the following situations: life-threatening tension PTX, massive air leaks with incomplete reexpansion, an air leak persisting 4 days

after a second tube has been placed, associated HTX with complications, identifiable bullous disease, and failure of easy reexpansion in patients with cystic fibrosis.

For patients with *traumatic etiologies*, the rapidity and type of treatment depends primarily on the stability of the patient; a hypotensive patient with a tension PTX requires immediate decompression with a chest tube or needle thoracostomy, whereas a patient with normal vital signs and a small PTX may be observed. Emergent needle thoracostomy is only a temporary solution for a compromised patient owing to a PTX. Once done, a needle thoracostomy necessitates an ipsilateral TT. Other factors that modify the treatment include the patient's age, the size of the PTX, whether there are bilateral *PTXs*, and whether the current episode represents a recurrence. A chest tube is usually indicated for a PTX.

Because of the risk of a tension PTX, a chest tube should be considered for all patients with a penetrating chest injury if PPV will be used or if they will be transported a long distance for definitive care. However, CT scans of trauma victims have demonstrated that many patients with small PTXs that would have escaped detection by standard radiographs have safely undergone PPV without developing a clinically evident

TABLE 10–2 Indications for Surgery after Tube Thoracostomy Based on the Results of the Thoracostomy

Massive hemothorax, >1000–1500 mL initial drainage
Continued bleeding
>300–500 mL in 1st hr
>200 mL/hr for first 3 or more hr
Increasing size of hemothorax on chest film
Persistent hemothorax after two functioning tubes placed
Clotted hemothorax
Large air leak preventing effective ventilation
Persistent air leak after placement of second tube or inability to fully expand lung

This is meant to be a guide, and clinical judgment should always be used.

PTX. Close observation for signs of a tension PTX is necessary for patients in whom a chest tube is not placed **and** PPV is used.

HTX

TT is also used to monitor the amount and rapidity of blood output, which determines the need for additional interventions, including a thoracotomy. About three fourths of patients with a traumatic HTX can be managed by TT and volume replacement alone. The remaining patients will require immediate or delayed elective thoracotomy. The indications for surgery after an acute HTX are somewhat controversial (Table 10–2). Stable patients with a more chronic HTX (distant trauma with slow bleeding but large effusions) will usually not be approached with these surgical criteria. Early institution of blood replacement is recommended for patients with massive HTX (>2000 mL), because these are often associated with continuing hemorrhage. Autotransfusion of the shed blood is desirable if the technique is available.

Empyema

The treatment of patients with empyema depends on the severity of their infection and their underlying condition. Some patients with empyema can be treated with serial thoracenteses, but most will require continuous drainage with a TT. Thoracoscopic decortication represents definitive therapy for severe cases. Usually, a diagnostic thoracentesis is done first to assess the fluid for signs of infection. Thick pus on thoracentesis, a positive Gram stain fluid glucose less than 60 mg/dL, pH less than 7.20, or elevated lactate dehydrogenase is associated with effusions requiring chest tube drainage. Once an empyema is detected, therapy should not be delayed because the fluid can become loculated within hours. The tube is left in place until the volume of the pleural drainage becomes clear yellow and is less than 150 mL in 24 hours.

An empyema that fails to resolve on the chest radiograph within 48 hours requires chest CT scan and a careful review of antibiotic choice. Multiloculated effusions are best managed with thoracoscopic decortication.

CONTRAINDICATIONS

For unstable injured patients with a PTX or an HTX, there are no absolute contraindications to a TT. In critical patients, the placement of a chest tube is often performed empirically, because procedures to confirm the presence of, assess the extent of, or prove the absence of pathology are prohibited by logistics of the resuscitation. In the stable patient, relative contraindications include anatomic problems such as the presence of multiple pleural adhesions, emphysematous blebs, or scarring. Coagulopathic patients should be evaluated for clotting factor replacement before any invasive procedure.

TREATMENT

Treatment of a Tension PTX during a Resuscitation

Immediate decompression of the chest must be considered in all injured patients who present in extremis with unexplained hypotension, particularly those with penetrating chest injuries. The goal is to open the chest cavity quickly to allow the accumulated air to escape. This can be accomplished with a scalpel and forceps, as is done at the beginning stages of a thoracostomy, or by needle decompression (Fig. 10–6). Alternatively, a large-bore needle/angiocatheter (minimum 16 gauge) should be placed at the midclavicular second intercostal space on the side with diminished breath sounds, or both sides if unclear (Fig. 10–7). The needle should be removed, but the angiocatheter left in place to create a simple PTX.

Whether or not this is successful in improving the patient's vital signs, an open TT is then needed. If the needle decompression is not effective, an open thoracostomy can be started even without the immediate availability of a chest tube to create an exit for the air to normalize the respiratory and cardiovascular function. The technique is the same as that for a TT (see later).

Prehospital Treatment

Emergent needle decompression thoracostomy may be used in the prehospital setting or when a patient suspected of having a PTX rapidly deteriorates or presents in extremis. The needle (or catheter) may then be attached to a flutter valve (fashioned from the fingers of a surgical glove), underwater seal, or commercially available one-way (Heimlich) valve so the air can continue to escape, but blocking its influx.

A three-sided occlusive dressing is used to cover the wound of a stable patient with an open chest wound and PTX in the prehospital setting. Similar to the valve mechanisms listed previously, this dressing acts as a one-way (flap) valve but prevents the air from entering the chest cavity. In this case, the external three-sided occlusive dressings allow air to exit the pleural space while preventing air reentry through the wound. A sterile dressing, such as petrolatum-impregnated gauze that extends 6 to 8 cm beyond the wound in all directions, is used. Only three sides are taped down. Ideally, the patient is instructed to deeply inhale and then perform a Valsalva maneuver or to cough just as the dressing is placed.

ED Treatment

Equipment
Recommendations for standard instruments for a TT tray are listed in Table 10–3. The most basic needs are a scalpel, a large clamp (Kelly), and the chest tube. Because the contents of these trays vary among hospitals, emergency providers

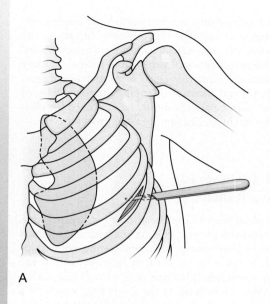

A

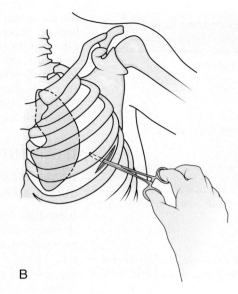

B

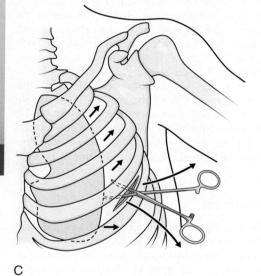

C

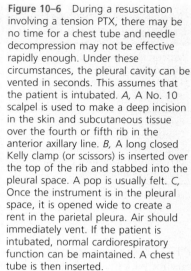

Figure 10–6 During a resuscitation involving a tension PTX, there may be no time for a chest tube and needle decompression may not be effective rapidly enough. Under these circumstances, the pleural cavity can be vented in seconds. This assumes that the patient is intubated. *A,* A No. 10 scalpel is used to make a deep incision in the skin and subcutaneous tissue over the fourth or fifth rib in the anterior axillary line. *B,* A long closed Kelly clamp (or scissors) is inserted over the top of the rib and stabbed into the pleural space. A pop is usually felt. *C,* Once the instrument is in the pleural space, it is opened wide to create a rent in the parietal pleura. Air should immediately vent. If the patient is intubated, normal cardiorespiratory function can be maintained. A chest tube is then inserted.

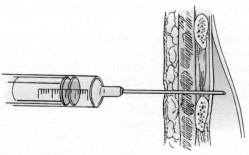

Figure 10–7 A large-bore needle/catheter combination is used to puncture the parietal pleura and establish the presence of blood or air in the pleural space. The needle can be placed anywhere in the pleural space, but traditionally, the same sites used for tube thoracostomy (TT) are used: the anterior second intercostal space in the midclavicular line or the anterior axillary line in the fourth or fifth interspace is used. The needle is placed to enter over the rib to avoid neurovascular injury. The needle is then withdrawn, leaving the catheter behind to create a simple open PTX. The procedure can be done either with or without the syringe attached to the catheter. This is only a temporary therapeutic maneuver for a tension PTX and a chest tube must also be inserted. (Redrawn from Richards V: Tube thoracostomy. J Fam Pract 6:631, 1978.)

should familiarize themselves with the trays at their facility prior to an emergency.

Chest tubes are open-ended clear plastic tubes of various diameters with a series of holes along the distal length. A radiopaque strip that is interrupted by the side ports (holes) runs along the length of the tube. This allows the provider to better visualize the tube on the postprocedure radiograph and to ensure that the side ports are within the pleural cavity. Adult tube sizes vary from 12 to 42 French, with smaller tubes used for a small PTX, and larger (a minimum of 36 Fr) for HTX and empyema. The largest possible tube should be used to drain suspected HTX. For pediatric patients, Nos. 14, 16, 20, and 24 French tubes are adequate. Before insertion, the beveled (extrathoracic) end of the tube is often cut squarely to better fit the commonly available connectors.

PROCEDURE

Before any procedure, gown, glove, mask, and goggle precautions must be used. When possible, consent should be obtained

TABLE 10–3 Recommended Equipment for Tube Thoracostomy

Procedure

Sterile drapes
10- to 20-mL syringe and assorted needles (for local anesthesia)
Local anesthetic (1%–2% lidocaine)
Antiseptic solution
No. 10 scalpel
Large clamps (Kelly)
Needle holder
Chest tubes (size appropriate)
No. 0 or 1-0 silk or similar suture
Forceps
Straight (suture) scissors
Large, curved (Mayo) scissors
Soft arm restraints

Drainage System and Tubing

Drainage apparatus with sterile water for water seal
Hard plastic serrated connectors
Sterile tubing

Dressing

Petroleum gauze or similar occlusive dressing
Gauze or similar pads
Adhesive tape—cloth-backed
Tincture of benzoin

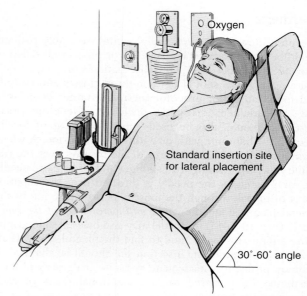

Figure 10–9 To insert a chest tube, the patient is placed semierect with the ipsilateral arm abducted as far as possible and preferably restrained. Supplemental oxygen and monitoring are recommended.

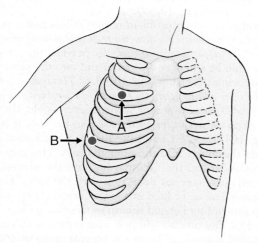

Figure 10–8 Standard sites for TT. *A,* The second intercostal space, midclavicular line is preferred for needle aspiration or catheter insertion. *B,* The fourth or fifth intercostal space, midaxillary line, lateral to the pectoralis muscle and breast tissue, is the preferred site for a chest tube, regardless of pathology. Note that placing the tube too far posteriorly will not allow the patient to lie down comfortably.

and the procedure should be conducted in the most sterile conditions that time allows.

Tube Insertion Site

The most common location for a chest tube is the mid- to anterior axillary line, usually in the fourth or fifth intercostal space (Fig. 10–8). This approach is cosmetically preferable and better tolerated than placing the tube in the anterior chest wall in the second intercostal space in the midclavicular line.

But a chest tube placed anywhere in the pleural cavity will drain blood, fluid, or air. The fifth intercostal space is approximately at the level of the nipple or the inferior scapular border in most patients, although the breast mass may lead to variance in females. The incision site should be lateral to the edge of the pectoralis major and breast tissue. To avoid penetrating the abdominal cavity, a more superior insertion site should usually be chosen because the external landmarks can be misleading. The diaphragm of a supine patient who is not taking a deep breath is much higher than suspected.

Before insertion, the tube should be held beside the chest wall with the tip of the tube at the level of the clavicle to estimate the distance the tube should be advanced from the incision site to the apex of the lung. The level of the insertion site must be sufficient to ensure that the last drainage hole on the tube will be within the pleural space. A clamp may be placed on the tube to mark the maximum length the tube is inserted to prevent the common problem of advancing the tube too far. In markedly obese patients, it is common to fail to advance the tube far enough, thereby not ensuring that the last hole is in the pleural space.

There is no evidence in adults that tube location affects the ability to drain fluid collections. As the lung expands and the pleural space becomes smaller, air and fluid that is not loculated will follow the path of least resistance and enter a functioning drainage tube, regardless of the tube's location.

Patient Preparation

Patients should be started on oxygen and placed on continuous pulse oximetry monitoring. When possible, the head of the bed should be elevated 30° to 60° (Fig. 10–9) to lower the diaphragm and decrease the risk of injury to the diaphragm, spleen, or liver. The arm on the affected side is placed over the patient's head and restrained in that position. A semierect position helps lower the diaphragm. The skin should then be cleaned with a standard surgical scrub and draped sterilely.

185

Anesthesia

The procedure can be extremely painful, so stable patients should be given parenteral analgesics or procedural sedation prior to the procedure. Unstable patients or those with severe sleep apnea should be monitored closely and considered for ketamine or propofol anesthesia rather than high-dose narcotic/benzodiazepine analgesia. Generous local anesthesia should also be used—up to 5 mg/kg of locally injected 1% lidocaine with or without epinephrine. A wheal of anesthetic is made in the area of the incision over the rib. While slowly infiltrating with a longer and larger-bore needle (19- or 21-gauge), the needle is directed over the superior aspect of the rib through the muscle, periosteum, and to the parietal pleura along the *entire anticipated track of the tube's passage* (Fig. 10–10). The needle may also be used to intermittently aspirate for air or fluid to find the pleural cavity. If air or fluid is not found, the insertion site should be changed. A common problem is inadequate systemic analgesia and local anesthesia. Be prepared to give additional doses of each throughout the procedure.

Once the tube is in place, local anesthetic may be administered through the chest tube into the pleural space to reduce the pain of the tube against the pleura. One approach for stable patients is to administer 10 mL of 0.5% bupivacaine through the chest tube while the patient is lying on the contralateral side.[18] After 5 minutes without drainage of the thorax, standard gravity or vacuum drainage is reinitiated. Parenteral analgesic agents should be used as needed to control the pain associated with the initial injury and the procedure.

Insertion

A common problem during the procedure is that the skin incision is too short to create and maintain an adequate track to insert the thoracostomy tube. The incision should be no less than 3 to 5 cm long, and there is no harm, other than slightly more scarring, in making it longer (Fig. 10–11A).

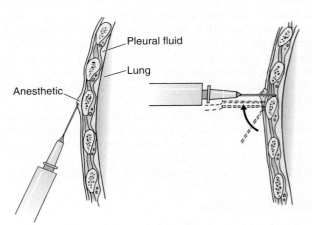

Figure 10–10 Local anesthesia is essential to reducing the pain from the insertion of a chest tube. Both the skin and the pleura should be infiltrated with a generous amount of local anesthetic. *A,* The anesthetic is first infiltrated over the rib at the site of the incision. *B,* The needle is then advanced slowly over the top of the rib while intermittently infiltrating and aspirating until the pleura is breeched and air is withdrawn. Anesthetic is then injected liberally (maximum 5 mg/kg) to cover the pleural lining. (*A and B, Redrawn from Hughes WT, Buescher ES: Pediatric Procedures, 2nd ed. Philadelphia, WB Saunders, 1980, p 234.*)

Labels in figure: Pleural fluid, Lung, Anesthetic

Traditionally, the initial skin incision is made over a rib or two lower than the intercostal space that the tube will pass through. The tube is then "tunneled" under the skin up over the next rib and then through the intercostal space. This is done to prevent air leaks, but there is no good evidence to support this. A transverse incision through the skin and the subcutaneous tissues should be made with a No. 10 blade over the rib. A large Kelly clamp is used to push and spread the deeper tissues and bluntly dissect a track over the rib. The intercostal vessels and the nerve are located on the inferior margin of each rib and must be avoided. The bluntly dissected track should pass immediately over the superior surface of the lower rib in the chosen intercostal space (see Fig. 10–11B). Firm resistance will usually be felt when the tough parietal pleura is met. At this point with the clamp closed, firm pressure must be made to penetrate the cavity. This often takes considerable force. *Penetrating the pleura is usually the most painful portion of procedure,* and extra anesthetic or analgesia may be needed at this point. To prevent penetrating too deeply, hold the clamp midshaft a few centimeters distal to the incision when resting the tip against the pleura before pushing through (see Fig. 10–11D and E). A palpable pop may be felt and a rush of air or fluid may occur when entering the pleural cavity. With only the clamp tips in the pleural cavity, the clamp is spread to make an adequate pleural entry and withdrawn (see Fig. 10–11C). *The opening in the parietal pleura should be wide enough to comfortably insert a finger and the tube; however, an extensive pleural opening should be avoided because this opening provides an egress for air. Because the pleura cannot be closed, a gapping hole predisposes to subcutaneous emphysema after the tube is secured* (Fig. 10–12).

Another common problem occurs at this point, particularly in obese patients: *the dissected track and pleural opening are lost when the clamp is withdrawn.* To prevent this, a gloved finger should be slid over the clamp and into the pleura prior to withdrawing the clamp (Fig. 10–13A). *This is done to further define the tract and to verify that the pleura has been entered and that no solid organs are present.* Whenever possible, the finger should *always be left in the pleural space* so the hole is not lost (see Fig. 10–13B and C) and the tube is passed over, under, or beside the finger into the pleural space. This step allows the clinician to feel the tube passing into the pleural cavity and avoids subcutaneous dissection with the tube. The tube can be passed alone or held in a large curved clamp, with the tube tip protruding beyond the tip of the clamp (Figs. 10–14 and 10–15). The tube should pass with little resistance; if it is hard to pass it may not be in the pleural cavity and may be passing subcutaneously (Fig. 10–16). The tube should be directed posteriorly, medially, and superiorly until the last hole of the tube is clearly intrathoracic, the marker clamp that was previously attached touches the chest wall, or resistance is felt. *Ensure that all the holes in the tube are within the pleural space.* Rotate the tube 360° to reduce the likelihood of kinking.

The tube should be attached to the previously assembled water seal or suction before the clamp is released. Asking the patient to cough and thereafter observing bubbles in the water seal chamber is a good way to check system patency.

Confirmation of Tube Placement

Multiple ways are available to confirm the location of the tube. The tube must be located in the pleural cavity such that adequate drainage can take place, without any undue bending

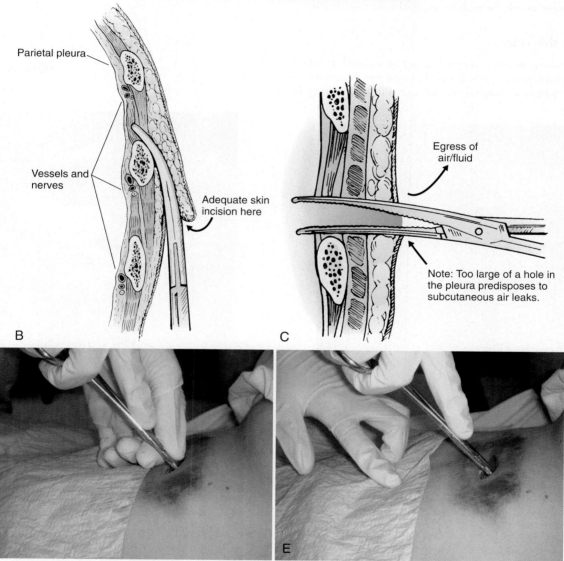

Figure 10–11 *A,* The incision should be made with a No. 10 scalpel through the skin and subcutaneous tissue over the fourth or fifth rib in the anterior axillary line. *B,* A long Kelly clamp is used to bluntly dissect over the top of the rib and then pushed into the pleural space. A "pop" is usually felt when the pleura is penetrated. *C,* Bluntly dissect to the pleural lining by pushing the closed points of the clamp forward, then spreading the tips and pulling back slightly with the points spread. Remember to dissect immediately over the rib on the superior aspect. A rush of air or fluid signifies penetration into the pleural space. Considerable force may be required when pushing through the pleura. By holding the clamp in the midsection of the curve, (*D*) the fingers will stop at the chest wall and prevent deep penetration of the tips of the clamp. To protect against inadvertent puncture of the lung when the clamp penetrates the pleural cavity, place an index finger on the distal portion of the clamp (*E*) or use the thumb and fingers of the opposite hand on the clamp to serve as a stop once the desired depth is reached. (*B, From Millikan JS, Moore EE, Steiner E: Complications of tube thoracostomy for acute trauma. Am J Surg 140:739, 1980; C, from Bricker DL: Safe, effective tube thoracostomy. ER Reports 2:49, 1981.)*

or kinking of the tube. Initially, if possible, a finger can be slid along the tube to verify that it enters the pleural cavity. Condensation on the inside of the tube and audible air movement with respirations, the free flow of blood or fluid, and the ability of the operator to rotate the tube freely after insertion are also indicators that the tube is in the pleural space. The ability to rotate the tube freely after insertion also suggests that the tube is not kinked, which can happen during tube placement. The definitive assessment of tube placement is the chest radiograph. If the tube and most proximal hole are not completely in the pleural space, the tube should be advanced *if the field has remained sterile*. If the tube is kinked or dysfunctional or the sterile field has been lost and advancement is required, a new tube should be placed in a sterile fashion through the same track. If the tube has been advanced too far, it may simply be withdrawn to the correct depth.

Securing the Tube

Once the tube position is verified, it can be secured. It is best to await radiographic confirmation before extensive efforts to secure the tube are undertaken, because adjustments may be

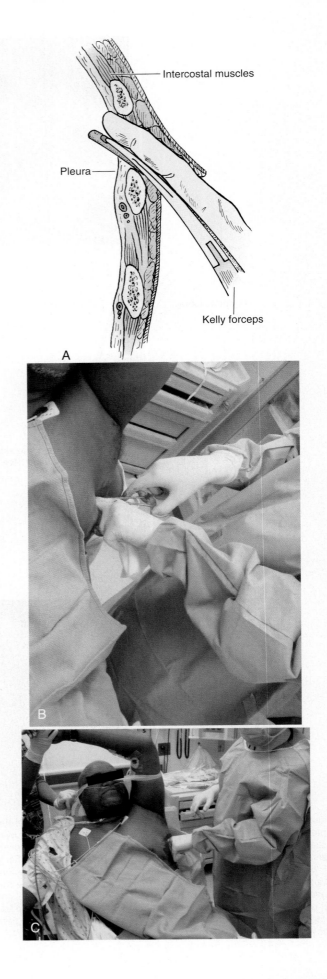

A

B

C

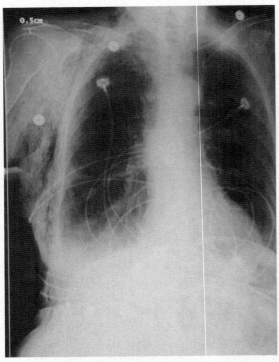

Figure 10–12 Right-sided subcutaneous emphysema after chest tube placement, *secondary to making too large a hole in the pleura, with a subsequent air leak.* It is usually benign and self-limited, but with PPV, it can be problematic. Because there is no way to close the pleura, making just the right-sized hole is the key to success.

Figure 10–13 *A and B,* After puncturing the pleural lining and spreading with the clamp, slide a gloved finger over the clamp to ensure that the pleural space has been reached and that no solid masses are present. Then, withdraw the clamp and use the finger as a guide for the chest tube to ensure entry into the pleural cavity. *C,* Once the pleural opening is found, *do not remove the finger* because the hole may be easily lost, especially in an obese patient. *(A and B, From Millikan JS, Moore EE, Steiner E: Complications of tube thoracostomy for acute trauma. Am J Surg 140:739, 1980.)*

Intercostal muscles

Pleura

Kelly forceps

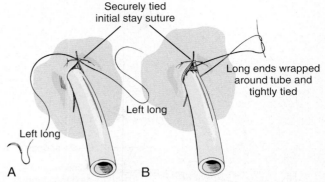

Tip of clamp grasps the chest tube

A

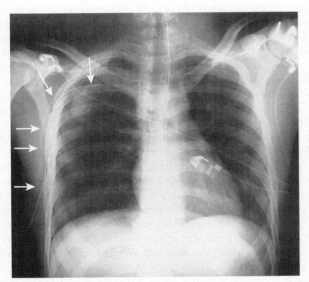

B

Figure 10–14 *A* and *B,* To reduce the risk of damage to the lung, the tube is grasped with the curved clamp, with the tube tip protruding from the jaws.

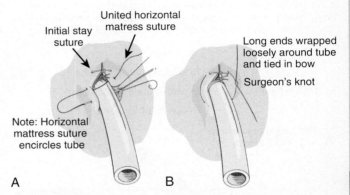

Securely tied initial stay suture

Long ends wrapped around tube and tightly tied

Left long

Left long

A   B

Figure 10–16 *A,* To secure the tube, first close the skin incision with a "stay" suture near the tube. *B,* Tie the knot securely and leave the suture ends long for wrapping around and tying the tube. Wrap the suture tightly at least twice around the tube, enough to indent the tube slightly, and tie securely.

United horizontal matress suture

Initial stay suture

Long ends wrapped loosely around tube and tied in bow

Surgeon's knot

Note: Horizontal mattress suture encircles tube

A   B

Figure 10–17 Another method to close the wound and secure the tube is with a horizontal mattress suture combined with a stay suture. *A,* A horizontal mattress suture is placed on either side (above and below) of the tube and is held only with a surgeon's knot. *B,* The loose ends are also wrapped around the tube and are tied loosely in a bow to identify the suture. This suture will be untied and used to close the skin incision after tube removal.

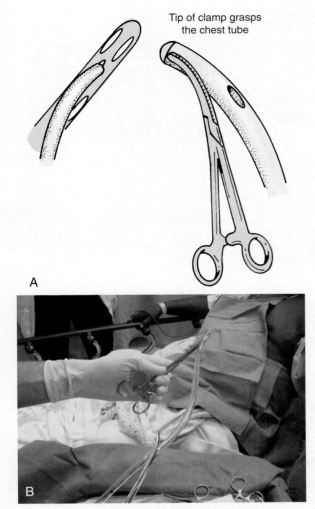

Figure 10–15 Subcutaneous placement of a chest tube (*arrows*) can occur because the tube can dissect through tissue planes with relative ease. If this tube had been directed posteriorly, the radiograph would erroneously "confirm" intrapleural placement despite the tube being subcutaneous throughout its entire course.

required. There are numerous methods to secure a tube. The usual method is to sew the tube to the skin with large 0 or 1-0 silk or nylon sutures. Nylon sutures are acceptable but must be tied tightly or they may slip on the surface of the chest tube. One common method is to use a "stay" suture in which the same suture that closes the skin incision is used to hold the tube (see Fig. 10–16). After this suture is used to close the skin incision at the site of tube insertion, the ends are left long and then wrapped tightly and repeatedly around the chest tube and tied securely. *The sutures must be tied tightly enough to indent the chest tube slightly to avoid slippage.* Longer skin incisions may require additional simple sutures to close completely.

Some clinicians use a suture technique that can both help close the skin around the tube and subsequently completely close the incision after the chest tube is removed. To do this, a *horizontal mattress suture* is placed approximately 1 cm across the incision on either side of the tube, essentially encircling it (Fig. 10–17). This is secured with a simple knot that can be easily untied so that it can be opened and retied to close the incision after the tube is removed.

After suturing the tube in place, an occlusive dressing of petrolatum-impregnated gauze should be applied where the tube enters into the skin. This may help to reduce air leaks.

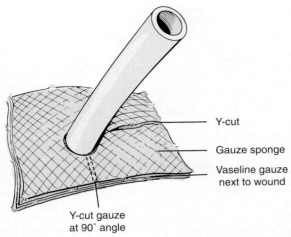

Y-cut

Gauze sponge

Vaseline gauze next to wound

Y-cut gauze at 90˚ angle

Figure 10–18 To dress the wound and reduce the risk of air leaks, an occlusive dressing should be applied. First wrap the base of the tube at the skin incision with a petroleum-impregnated dressing. A two-layer dressing of gauze sponges with a Y-shaped cut centered at the tube is shown. Place the second layer at a 90° angle to the first.

Wide tape

To skin on one side of tube

To wrap around chest tube

To skin on other side of tube

Half length of tape torn into 3 pieces

A

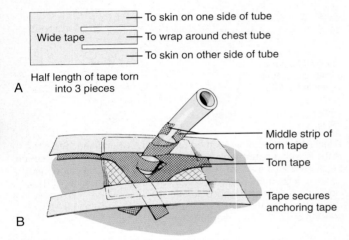

Middle strip of torn tape

Torn tape

Tape secures anchoring tape

B

Figure 10–19 One method to further secure the tube is to use wide, split cloth tape. *A,* The distal half of a 15- to 20-cm-long wide piece of tape is longitudinally split into three pieces. The two outside pieces are placed on the skin on either side of the tube, and the center strip is wrapped around the chest tube itself. *B,* This process may be repeated with a similar piece of tape placed at a 90° angle. The tape is securely anchored to the skin (benzoin is optional, but the skin must be clean and dry), and the torn tape is wrapped around the tube. Each anchoring piece is covered by another piece of tape.

The skin should then be covered with two or more gauze pads with a Y-shaped cut from the middle of one side to the center (Fig. 10–18). This dressing should be secured with wide (8- to 9-cm) cloth or elastic adhesive tape with or without benzoin.

Use approximately 10 to 12 cm of tape split into three pieces extending halfway along its length. The two outside pieces are placed on the skin on either side of the tube site, and the center section is wrapped tightly around the tube (Fig. 10–19). This is repeated with a second piece of tape placed at 180° to the first. Also securely tape the tube connections. The tube can be further secured by using tape to create a loop or stalk by wrapping it around the tube and then pressing the tape together for 1 to 2 cm before applying the tape to the chest wall (Fig. 10–20).

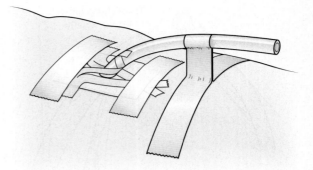

Figure 10–20 The tube can be further secured with an additional anchor system further down on the tube. Wrap a 20- to 25-cm piece of tape or elastic, adhesive dressing around the tube and seal at least 3 cm of the tape together on the side of the tube nearest the chest wall. Spread the remaining tape against the dry skin of the chest wall and secure with additional tape.

Open to atmosphere or attach to suction

Heimlich chest drain valve

To patient

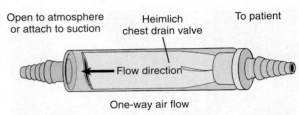

Flow direction

One-way air flow

Figure 10-21 A one-way Heimlich valve alone is often sufficient to treat a pneumothorax, but it cannot be used to treat a hemothorax.

Drainage and Suction Systems

A basic understanding of the functions of chest tube drainage systems is necessary to prevent life-threatening complications associated with their use. There are two essential components to all drainage systems: a one-way valve to allow air or fluid to drain out of the pleural space without allowing air back into the pleural space and a suction mechanism to increase the rate of drainage. The simplest drainage device is just a one-way valve without suction. This can be accomplished by either an underwater seal or with a flutter (Heimlich) valve attached to the end of the chest tube (Fig. 10–21). Normal respiration and coughing are often sufficient to create the pressure needed to remove the excess air from the pleural space, and the lung will then expand. The Heimlich valve does not require suction and has been used for outpatient therapy.

With a one-bottle underwater seal system, the intrapleural fluid or air exits under a small amount of water and collects into the single reservoir mixing with the water (Fig. 10–22*A*). The water above the tube *acts as a seal* because it is too heavy to be drawn back into the chest. It is important to remember that the intrathoracic pressure must be greater than the water pressure at the distal immersed tube to allow air or fluid to drain into the bottle. This pressure is determined by the height of the water above the exit port of the tubing. When the height is too great (the tube is too deep in the water), even coughing may not raise the intrapleural pressure sufficiently to drain the chest. To prevent inspiration from generating enough negative pressure to pull the collection bottle contents into the chest cavity, the collecting bottle must be below the patient, usually on the floor.

Suction is used initially to treat patients with a PTX or an HTX, but should be replaced by a water seal once the

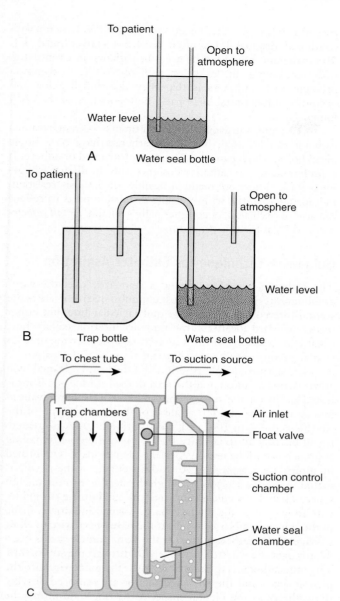

To patient

Open to atmosphere

Water level

A

Water seal bottle

To patient

Open to atmosphere

Water level

B

Trap bottle   Water seal bottle

To chest tube   To suction source

Trap chambers

Air inlet

Float valve

Suction control chamber

Water seal chamber

C

Figure 10–22 *A,* A single-bottle (water-seal) collection device. *B,* A two-bottle system. The trap reservoir proximal to the water seal keeps the accumulating drainage from affecting the water-seal pressure. *C,* This has now been replaced by a disposable system that mimics the two-bottle system (Thora Klex system, Davol, Inc.)

systems combine a two-bottle method that can be connected to suction, but with "air leak chambers" (see Fig. 10–22*C*). Bubbling in this chamber indicates the presence of an air leak, either in the drainage system itself (usually a loose tube connection) or from a large hole in the lung parenchyma. If an air leak is found, first check the system and the tube and connectors. If that does not correct the leak, check that all holes of the chest tube are within the thorax. If the air leak persists, it may be from the patient; this is usually seen only with expiration or with coughing. A continuous air leak or a leak seen during inspiration indicates a larger and possibly more significant lung injury.[19] Surgical intervention is indicated if an air leak persists for longer than 72 hours or the lung is not completely reexpanded.

When the drainage system is functioning properly, the height of the fluid level in the drainage tube fluctuates with inspiration and expiration. The absence of respiratory fluctuation or a decrease in the drainage may indicate that the system is blocked or that the lung is fully expanded. If the tube is blocked, the chest tube or collecting tubing or both can be changed, "stripped" to dislodge clots. Although replacing the tube is a complicated process, the routine use of stripping should be used sparingly because of the potentially high pressures generated. If the blockage is within the thorax, the tube can be cleared by forcing air or fluid back into the chest. The tube must be clamped distally and then compressed and stripped to force the contents proximally. *Stripping* is the opposite maneuver, in that the tube is clamped proximally and progressively compressed distally followed by a release to allow the tube to spring open. The sudden increase in negative pressure may extract clots and fluid from a more proximal location.

The drainage reservoir must remain below the level of the chest to prevent the fluid in the collection system from reentering the chest. The reservoir is usually placed on the floor or hung from the edge of the bed. Simple respirations do not generate enough negative intrathoracic pressure to pull the water in the reservoir up to the height of the chest if the reservoir is kept on the floor. The length of the tubing must be sufficient to keep the reservoir below the level of the patient, but not long enough to cause it to form dependent loops of fluid or kinks. Dependent loops collect fluid and create an additional water seal that, if large enough, requires greater intrapleural pressure to drain. If these pressures become high enough (15–25 cm H_2O), a tension PTX may result.

Occlusive clamping of chest tubes should be performed only with close monitoring because it can lead to a tension PTX in rare cases. Patients with chest tubes in place are best transported with a Heimlich valve or water seal only, not with a clamped tube. Clamping the chest tube as a trial maneuver before removal of the tube is discouraged.

Prophylactic Antibiotics

The use of prophylactic antibiotics after chest tube placement in the ED is common, but controversial, and no specific standards exist. *Multicenter trials have demonstrated no benefit.*[20,21] Routine antibiotics have no proven value in the reduction of the incidence of chest tube–associated empyema or pneumonia. If a chest tube is placed under less than ideal sterile conditions or if there is significant lung damage, prophylactic antibiotics to cover *S. aureus* may be considered, but there is a possibility of selecting out resistant organisms.

drainage and expansion are satisfactory and there are no persistent air leaks. The suction device should have high suction flow (≤20 L/min) and be able to keep the suction constant. A wall suction of 10 to 20 cm H_2O is normally used, but remember that *the amount of suction in the chest tube is dependent on the depth of water in the water seal reservoir, not on the suction from the wall valve.* When the negative pressure from the suction source exceeds the depth of the water in the chamber, air enters from the top of the third tube, causing continuous bubbling (see Fig. 10–22*B*). This prevents a further pressure increase in the chest tube. The wall suction dial can be turned down until only occasional bubbling can be detected. Vigorous bubbling does not equate with more suction.

Bottle combinations are rarely used now and many types of commercial, enclosed systems are available that essentially mimic the bottle system. Current commercial drainage

Tube Removal

Chest tubes are rarely removed by emergency clinicians. The usual indications for chest tube removal are after a chest radiograph demonstrates complete resolution of the PTX and there is no evidence of an ongoing air leak. Suction should be discontinued prior to removal, and the patient should be placed on a water seal. Clamping the tube is more controversial. Finally, most experts recommend that a repeat radiograph be completed 5 to 12 hours after suction is discontinued before pulling the tube. For empyema, the removal depends on the clinical and radiographic resolution of the infection.

To remove the chest tube, place the patient sitting upright at about 45° and remove the dressings. Prepare and drape the insertion site and follow sterile technique. If a pursestring suture was placed at the time of the insertion, only sterile scissors are needed to cut the suture. If there is no pursestring suture, suturing equipment will be needed to close the wound once the tube is removed. Additional equipment should be available to reinsert a chest tube if the lung collapses. A petrolatum- or antibiotic-impregnated gauze dressing should be prepared for covering the wound.

The pursestring suture that was previously placed should be loosened and readied for closing the wound. Then the skin loop of the suture holding the tube to the skin should be cut and removed from the skin. The tube should be clamped to prevent leakage of body fluids and then disconnected from the connecting tubing. The patient should inhale fully and perform a mild Valsalva maneuver. The tube is pulled out in one swift motion while the patient holds the breath. The pursestring suture is quickly tied and then covered with the occlusive dressing. The patient should be observed for 2 to 6 hours, with a chest radiograph obtained before discharge. Any increase in symptoms requires prompt reevaluation. After 48 hours, the dressing may be removed. Sutures may be removed in 7 to 10 days.

OTHER TECHNIQUES

Minicatheter Insertion

A less invasive alternative to traditional TT for patients with a simple PTX is treatment with a minicatheter. This technique and observation are widely used in Europe, but less so in the United States. Healthy patients with iatrogenic PTX (e.g., after central line attempts, intravenous drug injection), victims of minor nonpenetrating chest trauma, and patients with spontaneous primary PTXs are potential candidates for catheter aspiration of the PTX. Patients with underlying lung pathology, such as pneumonia, congestive heart failure, asthma, or emphysema, are generally not candidates for minicatheter use. Advantages of this technique include the ease of catheter insertion, decreased patient discomfort, less scarring, and decreased cost. The drawbacks include catheter kinking and the inability to perform video-assisted thoracoscopy through the site. After successful reexpansion of the lung, selected patients may be treated as outpatients with a Heimlich valve.

Many protocols are available for using catheter aspiration as the first step in treating simple PTXs. In general, patients with successful aspiration are observed in the ED for 4 to 6 hours after the catheter is inserted, and if a repeat radiograph shows no reaccumulation of air, the catheter is removed. After 2 more hours, another chest radiograph is obtained, and the patient is released if there is no recurrent PTX. Patients with continued residual PTX often receive a conventional TT. Minicatheters should not be used for patients on a ventilator, with continuing air leaks, or with an HTX. A common problem with catheters is that they occasionally clog and become nonfunctional in 24 to 48 hours because of the small lumen.

A 14-gauge intravenous catheter or an 8.5-French trauma catheter can be used, but these catheters have only single distal holes, which can easily become obstructed or adhere. It is preferable to use catheters designed specifically for aspirating a PTX. These are made of flexible, thrombosis-resistant, radiopaque material with multiple distal side ports to reduce the risk of occlusion. A commercially available *pigtail catheter system* is ideal for this procedure.

Guidewire Technique for Catheter Aspiration

The catheters are placed using a standard "over-the-wire" (Seldinger) technique. The most common insertion site is the second intercostal space in the midclavicular line, but either of the standard locations (the mid- to anterior axillary line, usually in the fourth or fifth intercostal space, or the midclavicular second intercostal site) can be used. The patient is placed in a semi-upright position and the skin is cleaned with an antiseptic solution and the area draped. Lidocaine is infiltrated locally for anesthesia. The guide needle is then advanced in a straight line at a 60° angle cephalad over the top of the rib (Figs. 10–23 to 10–25). Unless a straight track is created, it will be difficult to advance the floppy catheter; a tunneling approach cannot be used. When the pleural space is identified by intermittent aspiration, the advancement of the needle is halted. A guidewire is fed through the needle into the pleural space. Then the needle is removed while stabilizing the guidewire to keep it in the pleural space. A small incision is made in the skin with a No. 11 blade at the base of the wire to allow passage of the catheter through the skin. Some systems use a dilator over the wire to open the path through the soft tissues. The minicatheter is then threaded over the guidewire into the pleural space and the wire and dilator are removed, leaving the catheter in the pleural space. A twisting motion may be needed to advance the catheter through the subcutaneous tissues. The catheter should be secured to the skin with a suture and dressed. The catheter may be removed after a period of observation or the suction may be maintained for a few days. If used for a few days, the catheter will become clogged with mucus or blood, which may be cleared by injecting sterile saline through the device.

To aspirate the PTX, a three-way stopcock is attached to the catheter and the air is slowly aspirated with a 60-mL syringe until resistance is felt. Gentle wall suction can also be used, because a number of aspirations may be required until all air exits. A chest radiograph is taken to determine whether the lung is fully expanded. If residual PTX is present, further aspirations can be attempted. If air cannot be aspirated, the catheter may be kinked or blocked with soft tissue. To relieve the blockage, place the patient in the full upright position and have him or her cough or take a deep breath. Alternately, the catheter can be twisted or rotated gently.

TT IN PEDIATRIC PATIENTS

PTXs can occur in the neonatal population. They are often associated with resuscitative measures (such as mechanical

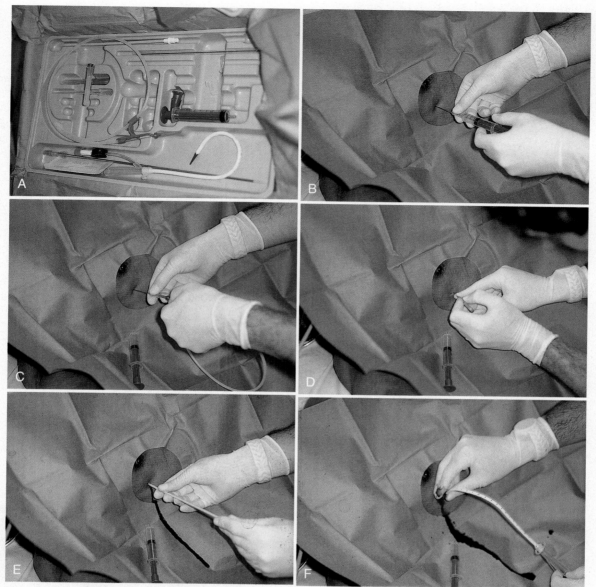

Figure 10–23 Aspiration of a pneumothorax (caused by subclavian vein catheterization) with an Arrow 14-French Percutaneous Cavity Drainage Catheterization Kit. This 23-cm pigtail multihole catheter is ideal for such purposes. Air can be aspirated from the catheter with a syringe or the catheter can be attached to suction or a Heimlich valve. This catheter is not used for patients on a ventilator, those with continuing air leaks, or those with a hemothorax. It is ideal for stable patients who have a primary PTX or a collapse that can be expected to be stable if the lung is reexpanded (such as intravenous drug use–induced, minor blunt trauma, secondary to central venous catheter insertion). *A,* Seldinger-type catheter kit demonstrates the pigtail catheter and all necessary equipment, including local anesthesia, introducing needle and syringe, scalpel, guidewire, and dilator. *B,* After generous local anesthesia, the introducing syringe is advanced in a straight line over the top of the fifth rib until air is aspirated. Unless a straight track is created, it will be difficult to advance the floppy catheter, and a tunneling approach cannot be used. *C,* The guidewire is advanced into the pleural space and the introducing needle is removed. *D,* Puncture the skin at the site of wire insertion with a scalpel. *E,* A dilator is advanced over the wire to create a track for the catheter. *F,* The pigtail catheter is advanced over the wire through the dilated tract, assuming its pigtail configuration when it is in the pleural space. A twisting motion may be needed to advance the catheter through the subcutaneous tissues. The catheter is advanced to the hilt and secured to suction. This catheter may be removed after a period of observation or the suction may be maintained for a few days. If used for a few days, the catheter will become clogged with mucus or blood, which may be cleared by injecting sterile saline through the device.

ventilation) for meconium aspiration or prematurity. For the rest of the pediatric population, trauma is the most common cause. Approximately one third of children with thoracic trauma will develop a PTX. As with adults, the physical examination of newborns and infants with PTX can be highly variable, necessitating the use of a chest radiograph for diagnosis. Ideally both anteroposterior and cross-table lateral projections are used because small PTXs may be seen only on the lateral view.

In general, TT is the treatment of choice once a symptomatic PTX is detected in infants. When signs of tension PTX are present, immediate aspiration with a plastic catheter over-the-needle device is recommended. Small PTXs (<20% of the hemithorax) in relatively asymptomatic infants (e.g., those who are without other problems and who do not require positive airway pressures) can be observed.

The technique of TT in pediatric patients is essentially the same as that for adults, but the body size and small spaces

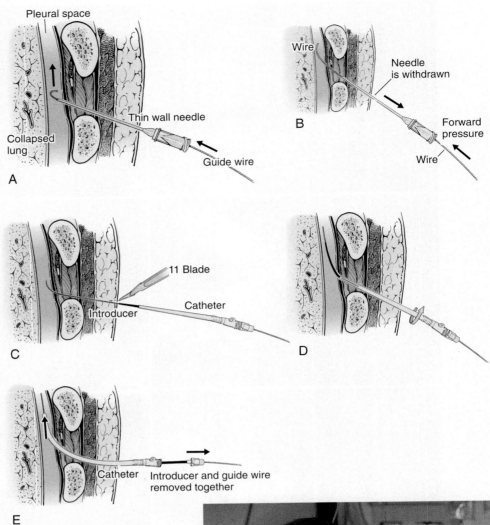

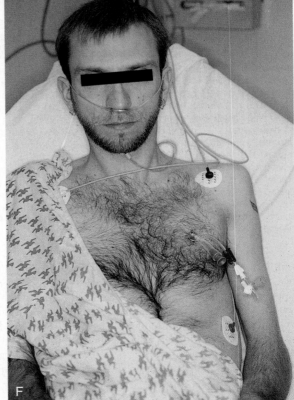

Figure 10–24 **Seldinger technique for aspiration catheter insertion.** *A*, The guidewire is passed through a needle over the rib into the pleural space. *B*, The needle is removed with the wire in the pleural space. *C* and *D*, A nick is made in the skin with a No. 11 blade, and the introducer and catheter are threaded into the pleural space. A twisting motion may be helpful. *E*, The guidewire and introducer are removed, leaving the catheter in the pleural space. *F*, This patient had a triple-lumen central line catheter to aspirate a PTX. It functioned for 2 days, then became clogged and was removed. This is not an ideal device, rather a pigtail catheter is preferred.

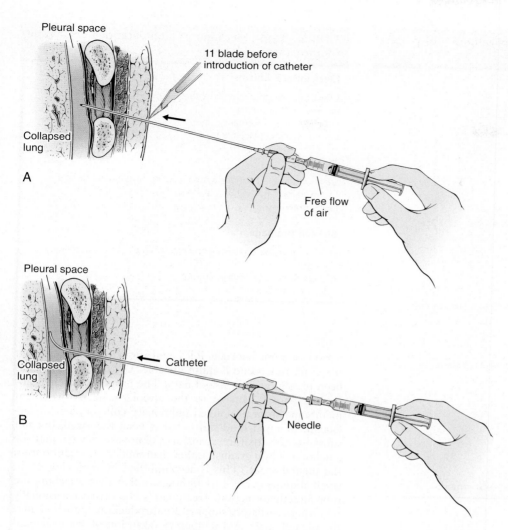

A

B

between the ribs make the procedure more difficult. The size of the tube increases with the patient's weight, starting with No. 8 to 10 Fr catheters for premature infants (Table 10–4). *Because of the risk of future breast deformities, the midclavicular approach should be avoided.* Therefore, the anterior axillary line through the fifth intercostal space should be used for newborns and infants.[22] The other important difference is that for a PTX, the tube should be directed anteriorly when inserted into the pleural space.

COMPLICATIONS

The most common complications of chest tube insertion include infection, laceration of an intercostal vessel, laceration of the lung, and intra-abdominal or solid organ placement of the chest tube (Tables 10–5 and 10–6). Subcutaneous emphysema is a common, usually benign, complication that is self-limited. This is due to making an excessively large rent in the pleura (see Fig. 10–12). Local infection at the insertion site is common and is often related to the emergent nature of the procedure. The development of palpable subcutaneous air is another complication of chest tube placement. It usually is limited to the insertion site but can become massive with PPV in a patient with continued air leak or an occluded tube.

Intercostal arteries or veins may be lacerated, but this can be minimized by using blunt dissection and carefully directing the tube just above the rib. The tube may adequately tampon-

TABLE 10–4 Approximate Pediatric Chest Tube Size by Weight	
Weight (kg)	**Chest Tube (Fr)**
<3	8–10
3–5	10–12
6–10	12–16
11–15	17–22
16–20	22–26
21–30	26–32
>30	32–40

ade such bleeding, but sometimes the incision needs to be extended to ligate the bleeding vessel. If bleeding continues, a thoracic surgeon should be consulted.

Failure of reexpansion of a PTX may be due to a mechanical air leak, but it may also indicate a bronchopleural fistula, a continued parenchymal lung leak, or a bronchial injury. A tension PTX can occur if a blockage in the drainage system at any point is associated with a continued air leak from the lung. Reinsertion or placement of a second tube may be indicated if the first tube is not functioning properly. In general, if a chest tube is not functioning properly and the patient is deteriorating, the tube should be removed and another tube inserted. Manipulating the tube by pushing it deeper into the chest cavity can lead to an increased risk of infection.

TABLE 10–5 Physical Complications of Tube Thoracostomy

Infection

Pneumonia
Empyema
Local incision infection
Osteomyelitis
Necrotizing fasciitis

Injuries—Bleeding

Local incision hematoma
Intercostal artery or vein laceration
Internal mammary artery laceration (with midclavicular line
   placement)
Pulmonary vein or artery injury
Great vessel injury

Injuries to Solid Organs or Nerves

Lung, liver, spleen, diaphragm, stomach, colon; long thoracic
   nerve, intercostal nerve

Physiologic

Allergic reactions to surgical preparation or anesthesia
Pulmonary atelectasis
Reexpansion pulmonary edema
Reexpansion hypotension

Miscellaneous

Subcutaneous or mediastinal emphysema
Persistent pneumothorax
Retained hemothorax
Recurrence of pneumothorax after chest tube removal

TABLE 10–6 Mechanical Complications of Tube Thoracostomy

Mechanical Problems

Chest tube dislodgment from chest wall
Incorrect tube position
Subcutaneous placement
Intra-abdominal placement

Air Leaks

Leaks within the drainage system (tubing or drainage device)
Last tube port not within pleural space
Leaks from skin site

Blocked Drainage

Flow of drainage contents into chest from elevation of drainage
   bottles
Kinked chest tube or drainage tubes
Clots occluding the tube

A rare complication is unilateral reexpansion pulmonary edema. The pulmonary edema ranges from mild to severe, but fatalities have been reported.[23] The condition may occur shortly after reexpansion or be delayed a number of hours. A common factor in these cases seems to be the prolonged period of time between PTX and onset of treatment, but the exact timeframe is quite variable. Usually, the PTX has been present at least 3 to 4 days. The proposed mechanisms include anoxic damage to the alveolar-capillary basement membrane from prolonged pulmonary collapse, loss of surfactant, or rapid fluid shifts. It has been theorized, but not substantiated, that reexpansion pulmonary edema may be ameliorated by a gradual, rather than sudden, evacuation from the pleural space. This is accomplished by removing air in small aliquots over 24 to 48 hours, rather than attaching the tube directly to suction. Treatment is supportive, occasionally requiring ventilatory support. Reintroduction of air back into the pleural space and temporary occlusion of the ipsilateral pulmonary artery have been other suggested, but unproven, interventions.

 REFERENCES CAN BE FOUND ON EXPERT CONSULT

CARDIAC PROCEDURES

CHAPTER **11**

Techniques for Supraventricular Tachycardias

Bohdan M. Minczak

The emergency clinician must assess patients with complaints of palpitations, heart fluttering, or rapid heart beat, often coupled with weakness, chest pain, or dizziness. The task is to determine the exact rate, rhythm, origin, and cause of the tachycardia, then "gain control" of the heart rate (HR) by directly slowing or normalizing the HR and/or treating the underlying cause. Determining the cause, origin, and rhythm of the tachycardia is often complicated by the fact that the underlying rate may be very fast (in excess of 150–300 beats/min), thus making interpretation of the electrocardiogram more difficult. Furthermore, the source(s) or pacemaker(s) producing and or facilitating the tachyarrhythmia may be in one or multiple locations: in the sinoatrial (SA) node, in one or more ectopic atrial foci, in the atrioventricular (AV) node, or in the ventricular free walls and/or septum. There may also be an abnormal conduction pathway between the atria and the ventricles. In addition, in some conditions, one or more "pacemakers" can be discharging simultaneously. To facilitate the diagnostic process, discrimination of atrial from ventricular electromechanical activity must be attempted. This chapter provides a framework to facilitate the decision making process with a focus on emergent interventions for various tachydysrhythmias.

Techniques for unmasking, identifying, and treating various forms of tachyarrhythmias are presented in Table 11–1. This chapter addresses the utility of the vagal reflex in treating and managing various pathophysiologic conditions and the use of medications and cardioversion as they apply to the treatment of various supraventricular tachycardias (SVTs). The major focus of the discussions are on the evaluation of and treatment of SVTs. A more comprehensive discussion regarding the treatment of ventricular tachycardia (VT) is provided in Chapter 12, Defibrillation and Cardioversion.

OVERVIEW/SIGNIFICANCE: ANATOMY AND PHYSIOLOGY OF SVT

Normally, the human heart beats at approximately 80 beats/min (±20 beats/min). If the HR exceeds 100 beats/min, the rate is described as a *tachycardia*. If the HR drops below 60 beats/min, it is described as a *bradycardia*. There are two general categories or types of tachycardias: supraventricular tachycardia and ventricular tachycardia. The term *supraventricular tachycardia* describes a rapid heart rhythm that has its electrochemical origin either in the atria or in the upper portions of the AV node. *Ventricular tachycardias* originate in the ventricular free walls and/or interventricular septum. VTs can quickly become unstable and require special consideration (Fig. 11–1).

SVTs can be further classified as narrow-complex (QRS duration < 0.12 sec) and wide-complex tachycardias (QRS duration > 0.12 sec). The rhythms of these dysrhythmias can be regular or irregular. Examples of narrow-complex SVTs are sinus tachycardia; atrial fibrillation (AF); atrial flutter; AV nodal re-entry; atrial tachycardia, both ectopic and re-entrant; multifocal atrial tachycardia (MAT); junctional tachycardia; and accessory pathway–mediated tachycardia. The term *wide-complex tachycardia* describes rhythms such as VT, SVT with aberrancy, or a pre-excitation tachycardia facilitated by an accessory pathway between the atria and the ventricles.

Tachycardias can be benign or can have significant physical effects on the patient. When the HR is 60 beats/min, approximately one cardiac cycle of contraction (systole) and relaxation (diastole) occurs per second. The excitation for the cardiac contraction typically originates in the SA node, the intrinsic "pacemaker" of the heart. The pacemaker impulse traverses across and depolarizes the atria causing atrial contraction or systole. Subsequently, this depolarization reaches the AV node. Upon initiating depolarization of the AV node, the conduction velocity of this depolarizing impulse transiently decreases (i.e., it undergoes "decremental conduction"), so that the ventricles can fill with blood from the antecedent atrial contraction. (*Remember*: The duration of diastole is roughly twice the duration of systole to allow for adequate ventricular filling.) *The AV node also serves as a gate/selective block to prevent an excessive number of depolarizing impulses from reaching the ventricles when the atrial rate is accelerated.*

Immediately thereafter, this depolarizing wave accelerates as it travels down the bundle of His to the Purkinje fibers, causing ventricular depolarization and contraction systole. Subsequently, the ventricles begin to relax (i.e., enter *diastole* and begin to fill with blood prior to the next depolarization).

TABLE 11–1 Diagnostic and Therapeutic Approaches to Supraventricular Tachycardias

Vagal Maneuvers

Carotid sinus massage
   Pressure on the carotid sinus
Valsalva technique
   Forced expiration of air against a closed glottis
Apneic facial exposure to cold water ("cold water diving reflex")
   Immersion of the face into cold water
Oculocardiac reflex
   The trigeminovagal reflex initiated by pressure on the eyeball

Pharmacologic Agents

Adenosine
Amiodarone
Verapamil
Diltiazem
β-Blockers including esmolol
Digoxin
Procainamide
Ibutilide

Cardioversion

Administering a synchronized shock

This describes the events of one cardiac cycle or heartbeat. The electrochemical voltage changes of these events are depicted on the electrocardiogram in the usual sequential PQRST (the P-wave indicates SA nodal depolarization, the P-R interval denotes atrial depolarization followed by AV nodal activation, and the QRS complex summarizes electrical activity during ventricular depolarization).

The discharge rate of the SA node is usually modulated by a balance of input from the sympathetic and parasympathetic nerves (i.e., the autonomic nervous system). The sympathetic input to the heart is provided via the adrenergic nerves, which innervate the atria and ventricles, and by circulating hormones such as epinephrine/norepinephrine, which are released from the adrenal gland and cause the HR to increase. The parasympathetic input to the heart is provided by the vagus nerve (cranial nerve [CN] X) fibers. These nerve fibers innervate the SA and AV nodes. Vagal output to the SA node causes slowing of the HR by decreasing the depolarization rate of the "intrinsic pacemaker" whereas vagal output to the AV node enhances nodal blockade of atrial depolarization impulses to the ventricles. Under normal physiologic circumstances, the HR is modulated to meet the metabolic needs of the body's peripheral circulation. Changes in the AV electrochemical events (i.e., rates and rhythms) are manifested as

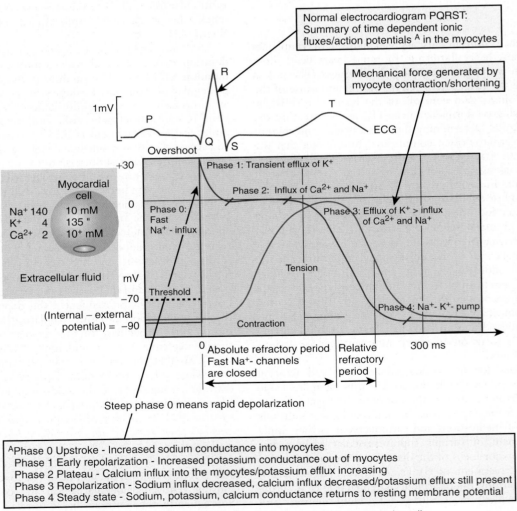

ECG AND MEMBRANE POTENTIAL OF VENTRICULAR CELLS

Figure 11–1 Electrocardiographic and membrane potential of ventricular cells.

changes in the electrocardiographic (ECG) intervals and waveforms.

As noted earlier, supraventricular tachycardic rhythms can be either sinus (i.e., originating in the SA node; sinus tachycardia) or ectopic (i.e., originating in the atrial myocytes above the ventricles). The rate of SA node discharge often varies as a result of various physiologic and pharmacologic stimuli, including fever, hypovolemia, shock, anemia, hypoxia, pain, use of cocaine, and amphetamines. These conditions often require or precipitate an increased blood flow/cardiac output (CO) to the peripheral tissues. This increase in peripheral blood flow or CO is accomplished by an increase in the HR (*Remember:* CO = HR × SV [stroke volume]). These are usually normal, benign physiologic responses to various stimuli or triggers. Direct treatment of these rhythms is usually not necessary; however, determining and treating the cause of the sinus tachycardia usually eliminates the fast HR. However, when single or multiple ectopic, spontaneously discharging foci develop in the atria or upper portions of the AV node, they can begin to "take over" or "override" the normal pacemaker activity in the heart (i.e., the SA node) and produce a rapid HR exceeding 100 beats/min. These foci may develop owing to an increased irritability/automaticity of the atrial myocytes secondary to electrolyte abnormalities, hypoxia, pharmacologic agents, or atrial stretch due to volumetric overload. If these foci are not treated/suppressed and the atrial depolarization rate proceeds to accelerate to rates greater than 150 beats/min (meaning that the heart is beating in excess of 2 beats/sec) with the impulses getting through the AV node to the ventricles, the time for diastolic filling of the ventricles will be compromised, causing a precipitous drop in SV. This will ultimately cause a drop in CO regardless of the increase in HR. Furthermore, as CO begins to drop, the mean arterial blood pressure (MABP) will drop, causing hypoperfusion of the brain and other peripheral tissues (*Remember:* MABP is the product of CO times total peripheral resistance [TPR]: MABP = CO × TRP). Treatment of this tachycardia can be achieved by pharmacologically suppressing the automaticity of the myocytes with medications (e.g., calcium channel blockers or β-blockers) and subsequently treating the underlying cause(s)—the hypoxia, electrolytes, and the like. Decreasing the hemodynamic consequences of this arrhythmia requires increasing the "blocking" of these impulses from reaching the ventricles via the AV node. This can be done by enhancing vagal input to the AV node or by pharmacologic enhancement of AV blockade. Multiple rapid depolarizations of the atria, which are conducted to the ventricles, can ultimately have a bimodal type of response; a modest increase in HR will cause an increase in CO whereas a massive increase in atrial rate with a concomitant increase in ventricular rate will cause a drop in CO. This can lead to an unstable patient with signs and symptoms such as confusion, altered mental status, or persistent chest pain. When the patient becomes unstable, immediate treatment is indicated.

In addition to areas of increased automaticity that can precipitate SVTs, a condition described as *re-entry* can also cause an SVT. Re-entry describes a condition in which a depolarization impulse is being propagated down a pathway in which some of the myocytes are still in the effective refractory period and a "unidirectional block" is present, preventing the impulse from traveling normally down this pathway. However, as the impulse travels around the area of the "unidirectional block," the tissue allows the depolarization front to travel in the opposite (antidromic) direction, back to the initial point of entry into this pathway. This allows the depolarization wavefront to restimulate the myocytes and initiate another propagated depolarization through the same tract (Fig. 11–2). If this condition is allowed to persist and these impulses stimulate the atria effectively and traverse the AV node, an SVT may develop as a result of re-entry. Suppression of this dysrhythmia can occur by terminating the conditions favoring re-entry, and the hemodynamic consequences may be attenuated by enhancing AV nodal blockade of the ventricles (e.g., through vagal stimulation, medication), thus slowing the ventricular response to this condition. Termination of the re-entry can be accomplished using either pharmacologic modification of the myocytes, rendering them refractory to depolarization impulses for a longer period of time in the stable patient, or synchronized cardioversion to uniformly depolarize the myocytes and terminate the conditions favoring the SVT.

Another situation to consider in the development and propagation of SVTs is the presence of pre-excitation or an accessory pathway between the atria and the ventricles. Arrhythmias secondary to these etiologies can be managed by the use of appropriate pharmacologic agents to either suppress the conduction through the accessory pathway or appropriately block the AV nodal transmission without enhancing conduction through the accessory pathway.

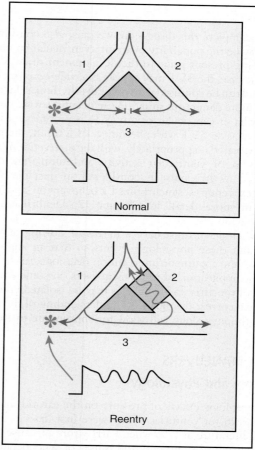

Figure 11–2 Cardiac conduction in supraventricular tachycardia (SVT). *Top,* Normal depolarization down path 1 and 2 that will "extinguish" or "cancel out" at point 3 normal depolarization/repolarization and conductance. *Bottom,* Abnormal. 1: Normal conduction; 2: delayed/slowed conduction with unidirectional block; 3: normal conduction pathway.

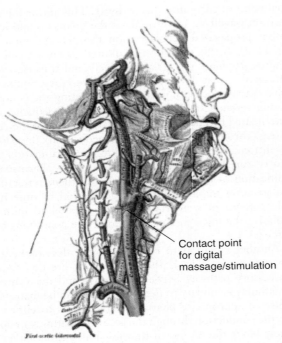

Figure 11–3 Carotid sinus.

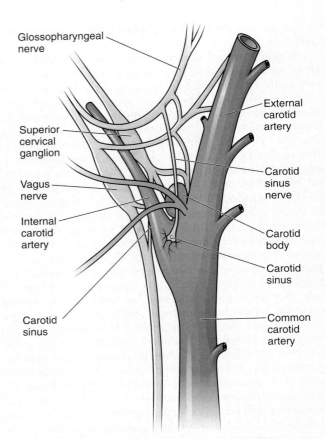

Figure 11–4 Stretch receptors of the carotid sinus.

To complete this discussion, we must also consider that there may be the possibility of an interventricular conduction delay being present prior to the development of an SVT. If this is the case, the SVT may appear as a wide-complex tachycardia and can be confused with other dysrhythmias. However, an even more dangerous situation can occur if a wide-complex tachycardia of ventricular origin (VT) is present and is misdiagnosed as an SVT with aberrancy. As a result, the patient could be treated inappropriately, with the intervention causing suppression of ventricular activity and ultimately cardiac arrest. VT with a pulse is considered an unstable rhythm that often requires synchronized cardioversion and is discussed in more detail in Chapter 12, Defibrillation and Cardioversion.

The clinician must have a means of slowing down and sorting out these physiologic events so that an appropriate diagnosis and treatment/intervention decisions can be made. With the application of vagal maneuvers, in some cases, the activity of the atria and ventricles may be isolated enough to facilitate a correct diagnosis. An understanding of the underlying pathophysiology will allow for appropriate treatment.

VAGAL MANEUVERS

Anatomy and Physiology

The physiologic effects of pressure on the carotid sinus have been known for centuries. They were first described in the medical literature in 1799 when Parry wrote a treatise entitled "An inquiry into symptoms and causes of syncope anginosa, commonly called angina pectoris."[1] He noted that pressure on the bifurcation of the carotid artery produced dizziness and slowing of the heart. The term *carotid* is derived from the Greek *karos*, meaning heavy sleep.

The bifurcation of the common carotid artery possesses an abundant supply of sensory nerve endings located within the adventitia of the vessel wall (Figs. 11–3 and 11–4). These nerves have a characteristic spiral configuration, continually intertwining along their course and eventually uniting to form the carotid sinus nerve. The afferent impulses travel from the carotid sinus via Herring's nerve or carotid sinus nerve to the glossopharyngeal nerve (CN IX) and then to the vasomotor center in the medullary area (*nucleus tractus solitarius*) of the brainstem (Fig. 11–5). The vasomotor center is composed of three distinct areas, each with a distinctive function. The vasomotor center is located bilaterally in the reticular substance of the medulla and in the lower third of the pons. The center transmits efferent impulses downward through the spinal cord and the *vagus nerve*. The efferent impulses, which originate in the medial portion of the vasomotor center, travel along the vagus nerve (CN X) to the sinus node and the AV node of the heart. The vasomotor center's medial portion lies in immediate apposition to the dorsal motor nucleus of the vagus nerve (CN X). These medial portion vasomotor center impulses decrease HRs. Efferent impulses originating in the lateral areas of the vasomotor center travel along the sympathetic chain to the heart and to the peripheral vasculature. These sympathetic impulses control either vasoconstriction or vasodilatation of the vascular system. A balance between the vasoconstriction and the vasodilatation maintains proper vasomotor tone.[2,3]

The afferent nerve endings in the carotid sinus are sensitive to MABP and to the rate of change of pressure. Research

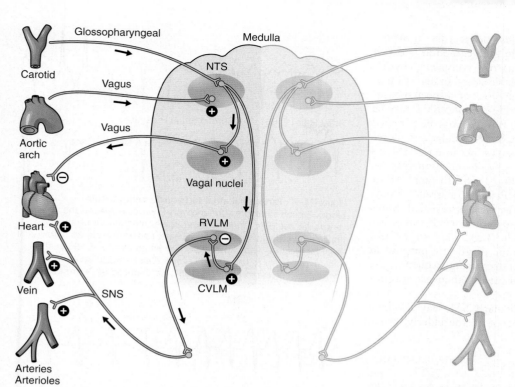

Figure 11–5 Schematic depicts the arterial baroreceptor reflex.

NTS: Nucleus of Tractus Solitarius
RVLM: Rostral Ventrolateral Medulla
CVLM: Caudal Ventrolateral Medulla
Vagal Nuclei: Dorsal motor nuclei, Nucleus Ambiguous

indicates pulsatile stimuli are more effective than sustained pressures in evoking a response. Elevated blood pressure stretches the baroreceptors, leading to increased firing of the afferent nerve endings.[2] As for low blood pressure states, the carotid sinus baroreceptors are exquisitely sensitive to low blood pressure. Hypotension causes a drop in afferent firing.[2]

The parasympathetic and the sympathetic nervous systems play independent but coordinated roles in the carotid sinus reflex. Increased firing of the carotid sinus results in reflex stimulation of vagal activity and reflex inhibition of sympathetic output. The parasympathetic effect is almost immediate; it occurs within the first second and causes a drop in HR. The sympathetic effect, which causes a drop in blood pressure through vasodilatation, becomes manifest only after several seconds.[4] The blood pressure changes may not take full effect until a minute has elapsed.[5] The changes in blood pressure and HR are independent phenomena. Epinephrine blocks the reduction in blood pressure, whereas a fall in HR is blocked by the administration of atropine.

A cerebral effect, characterized by a loss of consciousness, was once thought to be due to stimulation of the carotid sinus. However, it is seen only when sufficient pressure is exerted to occlude the more distal temporal artery pulsation and when contralateral carotid disease is present. This cerebral effect is now believed to be a result of decreased bilateral cortical perfusion.

The parasympathetic branch of the carotid sinus reflex supplies the sinus node and the AV node. The effect of the parasympathetic stimulation is to slow the HR. The SA pace-

TABLE 11–2 Potential Observations with Vagal Maneuvers in the Management of Tachydysrhythmias
1. Vagal maneuvers may slow the atrial rate in VT or complete heart block and may therefore demonstrate previously hidden P-waves or obvious (AV) dissociation.
2. Abrupt changes in the heart rate without conversion are a result of increasing AV block.
3. Gradual slowing of the ventricular rate suggests the presence of a sinus rhythm. Only rarely do vagal maneuvers decrease AV conduction in the presence of a sinus mechanism.
4. The dysrhythmias most likely to convert to sinus rhythm are PAT and paroxysmal nodal tachycardia.
5. Dysrhythmias that are associated with AV conduction defects (PAT with block, atrial flutter, and atrial fibrillation) infrequently convert to a sinus rhythm, but the ventricular rate slows. Rarely, atrial slowing will be sufficient to allow 1 : 1 AV conduction, which may actually increase the ventricular rate (Fig. 11–6).

AV, atrioventricular; PAT, paroxysmal atrial tachycardia; VT, ventricular tachycardia.

maker is more likely to be affected than the AV node, except when digitalis has been administered.[2,5,6]

Indications for Vagal Maneuvers

Vagal maneuvers are potentially useful in attempting to slow down or break an SVT. Vagal maneuvers are also indicated in settings in which slowing conduction in the SA or AV node could provide useful information (Table 11–2). These settings include patients with wide-complex tachycardia in whom carotid sinus massage (CSM) aids in the distinction between SVT and VT. CSM can elucidate narrow-complex tachycardia in which the P-waves are not visible or aid in detection of suspected rate-related bundle branch block or suspected pacemaker malfunction. After CSM, a wide-complex SVT may be converted to normal sinus rhythm, P-waves may be revealed after increased AV node inhibition, or ventricular complexes may narrow as the ventricular rate slows. Because CSM slows atrial and not ventricular activity, AV dissociation may be more easily seen, indicating VT (Fig. 11–6). In rapid AF or atrial flutter with 2 : 1 block, either P-waves or irregular ventricular activity with absent P-waves may be revealed. Sinus tachycardia may also be more apparent once P-waves are unmasked by slowing the SA node (Figs. 11–7 to 11–14). Adenosine may be used for the same diagnostic purpose in these situations as well.[7] In order of decreasing frequency, the ECG changes seen with CSM and vagal maneuvers are presented in Table 11–3.

Vagal maneuvers, and in particular CSM, may also be a useful aid to the diagnosis of syncope in the elderly. Some

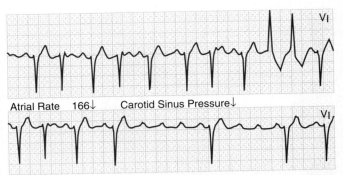

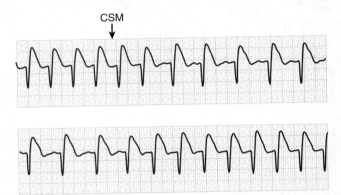

Figure 11–7 Paroxysmal atrial tachycardia with variable block. Carotid sinus pressure uncovers P-waves hidden in the ventricular complex. *Upper strip* resembles atrial flutter or atrial fibrillation with ventricular ectopic beats. *Lower strip* shows paroxysmal atrial tachycardia with variable block at an atrial rate of 166 beats/min. *(From Lown B, Levine SA: Carotid sinus—clinical value of its stimulation. Circulation 23:766, 1961. Reproduced by permission.)*

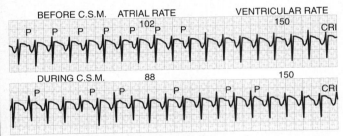

Figure 11–6 Ventricular tachycardia. Carotid sinus massage (CSM) slows atria but not ventricles, thus establishing the presence of AV dissociation, supporting the diagnosis of ventricular tachycardia. The QRS measures 0.16 sec. Note the atrial rate slowing from 102 to 88 beats/min while the ventricular rate is unaffected. *(From Lown B, Levine SA: Carotid sinus—clinical value of its stimulation. Circulation 23:766, 1961. Reproduced by permission.)*

Figure 11–8 Sinus tachycardia. The sinus P-wave is obscured within the descending limb of the T-wave. CSM transiently slows the sinus rate and exposes the P-wave. The rate then increases. The strips are continuous. *(From Silverman ME: Recognition and treatment of arrhythmias. In Schwartz GR, Safar P, Stone JH, et al [eds]: Principles and Practice of Emergency Medicine, vol 2. Philadelphia, WB Saunders, 1978. Reproduced by permission.)*

Figure 11–9 Sinus tachycardia with high-level block. *Arrows* indicate sinus P-waves. Strips IIa to IId are continuous. The basic rhythm is sinus, but marked first-degree AV block is present. High-degree (advanced) AV block associated with transient slowing of sinus rate is produced by CSS. *(From Chung EK: Electrocardiography. 2nd ed. New York, Harper & Row, 1980. Reproduced by permission.)*

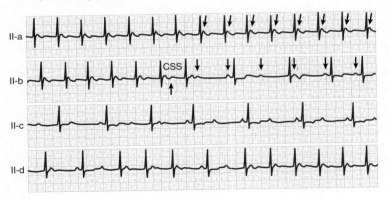

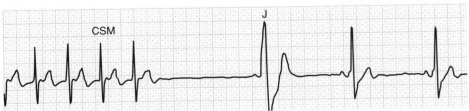

Figure 11–10 Paroxysmal atrial tachycardia. CSM abolishes the dysrhythmia and results in a period of sinus suppression with a junctional (J) escape beat. Prolonged periods of asystole may produce anxiety in the physician who is waiting for the resumption of a sinus pacemaker. *(From Silverman ME: Recognition and treatment of arrhythmias. In Schwartz GR, Safar P, Stone JH, et al [eds]: Principles and Practice of Emergency Medicine, vol 2. Philadelphia, WB Saunders, 1978. Reproduced by permission.)*

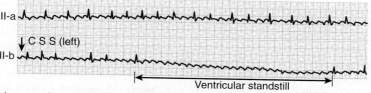

Figure 11–11   Atrial flutter. CSS *(downward arrow)* produces marked slowing of the ventricular rate in atrial flutter. Note the obvious flutter waves with an atrial rate of 300 and a long period of ventricular standstill. The strips are continuous. *(From Chung EK: Electrocardiography, 2nd ed. New York, Harper & Row, 1980. Reproduced by permission.)*

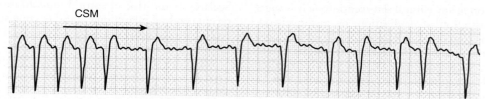

Figure 11–12   Atrial fibrillation. CSM slows the ventricular response transiently, revealing the fibrillating baseline. The ventricular rate subsequently accelerates. *(From Silverman ME: Recognition and treatment of arrhythmias. In Schwartz GR, Safar P, Stone JH, et al [eds]: Principles and Practice of Emergency Medicine, vol 2. Philadelphia, WB Saunders, 1978. Reproduced by permission.)*

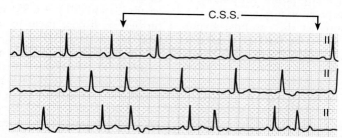

Figure 11–13   Occult premature ventricular contractions. CSM reveals ventricular extrasystoles, thereby explaining the cause of palpitation in this case. *(From Lown B, Levine SA: Carotid sinus—clinical value of its stimulation. Circulation 23:766, 1961. Reproduced by permission.)*

203

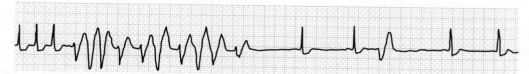

Figure 11–14 A run of ventricular tachycardia is seen immediately after a supraventricular dysrhythmia is terminated by CSM. The patient remained asymptomatic, and a normal sinus rhythm was established spontaneously within a few seconds. If asystole is prolonged, ask the patient to vigorously cough (cough CPR) or apply a precordial thump.

TABLE 11–3 Order of *Decreasing* Frequency of Electrocardiographic Changes with Vagal Maneuvers

1. Sinoatrial slowing, occurring in approximately 75% of cases and leading to sinus arrest approximately 3% of the time.
2. Atrial conduction defects, manifested by an increase in width of the P-wave on the electrocardiogram
3. Prolongation of the PR interval and higher degrees of atrioventricular block, seen in approximately 10% of cases.
4. Nodal escape rhythms.
5. Complete asystole, defined as sinus arrest without ventricular escape lasting > 3 sec, occurring in 4% of cases.
6. Premature ventricular contractions.

14% to 45% of elderly patients referred for syncope are thought to have *carotid sinus syndrome* (CSS).[6,8,9] CSS is defined as an asystolic pause greater than 3 seconds or a reduction of systolic blood pressure greater than 50 mm Hg in response to CSM. It shares many characteristics with sick sinus syndrome, suggesting that both are manifestations of the same disease. CSS causes cerebral hypoperfusion, leading to dizziness and syncope. Analysis of patients with the syndrome indicates that it results from a baroreflex-mediated bradycardia in 29% of patients, hypotension in 37%, or both in 34%.[10,11] Therefore, syncope, near-syncope, or a fall of unclear etiology in the elderly is an important indication for diagnostic CSM.[12]

Although the use of digoxin has been overshadowed by the use of other potentially less toxic agents such as calcium channel blockers and β-blockers, the clinician can still prospectively simulate the cardioinhibitory effects of digoxin on a patient by performing vagal maneuvers. This can guide use and dosage of the medication before initiating treatment/therapy with digoxin. Significant slowing or block with CSM suggests a similar sensitivity to digoxin, and a smaller loading dose should be considered.

Equipment and Setup

Prior to the initiation of any clinical intervention such as vagal maneuvers, administration of medication, or cardioversion, for SVT, if there is time, the patient should be placed on a cardiac monitor, intravenous (IV) access should be established, and a slow, keep-vein-open (KVO; 60 mL/hr saline IV) solution should be infused. The patient should also be monitored with a pulse oximeter and an indirect blood pressure monitor. Numerous antiarrhythmic medications should be readily available. A defibrillator/pacemaker should be at bedside in anticipation of a worsening dysrhythmia. The administration of oxygen is advised for the procedure, especially if conscious sedation is anticipated. The patient should be placed in the reverse Trendelenburg position if tolerated. Merely placing the patient in this position may terminate the SVT owing to increased pressure on the carotids, giving maximum carotid bulb stimulation. This position may also prevent syncope if there is a significant decrease in blood pressure or HR.

CAROTID SINUS MASSAGE

CSM is a bedside vagal maneuver technique involving digital pressure on the richly innervated carotid sinus. It takes advantage of the accessible position of this baroreceptor for diagnostic and therapeutic purposes. Its main therapeutic application is for termination of SVTs owing to paroxysmal atrial tachycardia (PAT). It also has diagnostic utility in the assessment of tachydysrhythmias and rate-related bundle branch blocks. In addition, it can provide clues to latent digoxin toxicity, as described previously, by potentiating manifestations of toxicity. It can also be used to sort out the differential diagnosis of syncope.

Returning to the use of CSM as a diagnostic technique for assessing digoxin toxicity, adverse effects/toxicity from digoxin depend more on the response of the host than on the actual digoxin level. In cases of suspected digoxin toxicity, before the level is available, or when the digoxin level is in the "normal range," CSM may be a useful diagnostic adjunct. Significant inhibition of AV node conduction associated with ventricular ectopy, especially ventricular bigeminy, should lead to the suspicion of digoxin toxicity.[1]

Other therapeutic uses of CSM have been made obsolete by current medical therapy. In 1961, Lown and Levine[1] described the dramatic effect CSM had in the 1920s on relieving acute pulmonary edema in a group of patients with hypertension and coronary artery disease. They reported: "Relief is immediate and coincides with the onset of bradycardia. In the majority, it is associated with a drop in blood pressure. The patient is promptly able to lie flat. Fear, dyspnea and chest oppression disappear." CSM also has been reported to relieve anginal pain. The technique may be useful when the diagnosis of angina is uncertain.[13] The advantage of the CSM technique

over the use of nitroglycerin is unknown. Although CSM is no longer the first approach to either pulmonary edema or angina, it remains a therapeutic or adjunct diagnostic tool in some cases or when modern pharmacologic agents are unavailable. Because adenosine may not always be readily available and cannot be used to assess the sensitivity of the carotid sinus, CSM remains a useful bedside tool.

Contraindications

CSM is *contraindicated* in the very rare patient likely to suffer neurologic or cardiovascular complications from the procedure. Patients with a carotid bruit should not have CSM because of the risk of carotid embolization or occlusion. A recent cerebral infarction is another contraindication, because even marginal reduction of cerebral blood flow may produce further infarction.

The presence of diffuse, advanced coronary atherosclerosis is associated with increased sensitivity of the carotid sinus reflex. This hypersensitivity is further augmented during an anginal attack or an acute myocardial infarction. Brown and coworkers[14] found that the degree of carotid sinus hypersensitivity was directly proportional to the severity of coronary artery disease documented by cardiac catheterization. Patients with acute myocardial ischemia or with recent myocardial infarction are already at higher risk of VT or ventricular fibrillation (VF). A CSM-induced prolonged asystole may further predispose them to these dysrhythmias. Therefore, CSM should be avoided in these patients.

Both digoxin and CSM act through a vagal mechanism to inhibit the AV node. Patients on digoxin may experience a greater inhibition of the AV node with longer AV block as a result. Patients with apparent manifestations of digoxin toxicity or known digoxin toxicity should not have CSM, because AV inhibition may be profound.[15]

Technique

This technique can be performed with or without a concomitant Valsalva maneuver. Alternatively, pressure can be applied to the abdomen by an assistant. Some clinicians prefer to place the patient supine or with the head of the bed tilted downward. The clinician should begin CSM on the patient's right carotid bulb because some investigators have found a greater cardioinhibitory effect on this side.[12,16,17] However, scientific agreement on this issue is not unanimous. Simultaneous bilateral CSM is absolutely contraindicated, because cerebral circulation may be severely compromised. Before attempting CSM, the clinician should first auscultate for carotid bruits on both sides of the neck. The presence of a bruit is a contraindication to massage.

Keeping the patient relaxed is helpful for two reasons: a tense platysma muscle makes palpation of the carotid sinus difficult, and an anxious patient will be less sensitive to CSM as a result of heightened sympathetic tone.

With the patient's head tilted backward and slightly to the opposite side, palpate the carotid artery just below the angle of the mandible at the upper level of the thyroid cartilage and anterior to the sternocleidomastoid muscle. Once the pulsation is identified, use the tips of the fingers to administer CSM for 5 seconds in a posteromedial direction, aiming toward the vertebral column. Although earlier practitioners used a longer duration of massage, a shorter period of massage minimizes the risk of complications and is adequate for diagnostic purposes in the majority of patients.[18] Pressure on the carotid sinus may be steady or undulating in intensity;

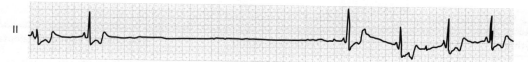

Figure 11–15 **Hyperreactive carotid sinus reflex.** Gentle pressure was applied to the carotid sinus for 3 seconds, resulting in a pause in sinus rhythm of approximately 7 seconds. This syndrome may be the cause of syncope. *(From Bigger JT Jr: Mechanisms and diagnosis of arrhythmias. In Braunwald E [ed]: Heart Disease, vol 1. Philadelphia, WB Saunders, 1980. Reproduced by permission.)*

the force, however, must not occlude the carotid artery. The temporal artery may be simultaneously palpated to ensure that the carotid remains patent throughout the procedure.

If unsuccessful, CSM may be repeated after 1 minute. If the procedure is still unsuccessful, the opposite carotid sinus may be massaged in a similar fashion. Simultaneous Valsalva maneuvers and the head-down position to enhance carotid sinus sensitivity should be done before the technique is abandoned. Importantly, *CSM should be repeated once antiarrhythmic medication has been given, and often the combination is more effective.*

Complications

Neurologic complications of CSM are rare and usually transient. In a review of neurologic complications in elderly patients undergoing this procedure, Munro and associates[19] found 7 complications from a total of 5000 massage episodes, for an incidence of 0.14%. Reported deficits included weakness in 5 cases and visual field loss in 2 others. In 1 case, the visual field loss was permanent. Patients in this study were excluded from CSM if they had a carotid bruit, recent cerebral infarction, recent myocardial infarction, or a history of VT or VF. The duration of massage was 5 seconds. Lown and Levine[1] described 1 patient with brief facial weakness during several thousand tests. Carotid emboli and hypotension have both been implicated as possible causes of the neurologic deficits. Unintentional occlusion of the carotid artery may also be responsible for some neurologic complications.

Cardiac complications include asystole, VT, or VF. A normal pause of less than 3 seconds is part of the physiologic response to CSM; a longer pause may be diagnostic of CSS. In a review of reported cases of ventricular tachydysrhythmias, five cases were described.[20] All five patients were receiving digoxin, and in several cases, VT or VF followed AV block. Digoxin is associated with more prolonged AV block resulting from CSM, perhaps leaving these patients more vulnerable.

Interpretation of Vagal Maneuvers

A pause longer than 3 seconds, or a drop in systolic blood pressure greater than 50 mm Hg in patients to whom CSM is administered while they are in a supine position, is diagnostic of CSS (Figs. 11–15 and 11–16). Patients should be supine during testing to reduce the risk of cerebral hypoperfusion.[12,21]

Although CSM is one of the better-known vagal maneuvers, a variety of other physical modalities are available to the clinician to affect a change in HR. The anticipated rhythm response to different vagal maneuvers in the setting of different underlying rhythms is shown in Table 11–4.

Valsalva Maneuver

In general, mean bradycardia changes are greatest for the Valsalva maneuver and the diving response.[2,21,22] During the

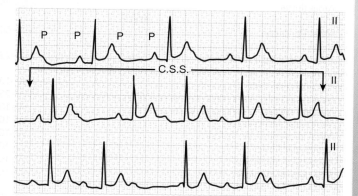

Figure 11–16 **Acceleration of ventricular rate by carotid sinus stimulation (CSS).** Continuous tracing. *Upper strip* shows 2:1 atrioventricular (AV) block: atrial rate = 102/min; ventricular rate = 51/min. The *second* and *third* strips were recorded during and after CSS, when the atrial rate was reduced to 68/min; a 1:1 response occurs. *(From Lown B, Levine SA: Carotid sinus—clinical value of its stimulation. Circulation 23:766, 1961. Reproduced by permission.)*

Valsalva maneuver (i.e., exhaling against a closed glottis or bearing down as if to defecate), intrathoracic pressures are increased, leading to increased arterial pressure, as a result of increased afterload. This increased pressure is transferred to the peripheral vascular system. Venous return to the heart is decreased, resulting in a decreased SVT. This is followed by increased venous pressure. All of these pressure changes lead to an initial increase in HR and carotid sinus pressure. As the maneuver is sustained, vagal tone is increased, leading to a compensatory decrease in SA and AV conduction. This is the expected/desired diagnostic/therapeutic response.

Contraindications

Patients must be able to cooperate with the clinician's commands. Dyspneic or tachypneic patients may not be able to hold their breath for the period of time needed to complete the maneuver.

Technique

With the patient supine; monitor in place; IV access secured; and atropine, lidocaine, and defibrillation available, have the patient take a deep breath and hold it. Instruct the patient to bear down and try to exhale without allowing the air to leave the lungs. Patient should try to hold this position for 10 to 20 seconds.[23,24] An adjunct method is to have the patient take and hold a deep breath and try to push against the clinician's hand with her or his abdomen while the clinician gently pushes on the anterior wall of the abdomen.

Apneic Facial Exposure to Cold ("Diving Response," Diving Bradycardia): Technique. This technique can be viewed as a variation on the simple Valsalva maneuver. It has been found to be useful in children who may be unable to cooperate with or be capable of performing a Valsalva maneuver. Classically, the technique consists of facial immersion,

narrow-complex tachycardias that are driven by automaticity (e.g., ectopic, multifocal, or junctional tachycardias).

Its effects on AV nodal tissue are selective in that it reduces AV conduction in tissue responsible for the tachydysrhythmia but spares normal conduction tissue.[34,38,40,41]

Indications and Contraindications. Its beneficial effects are (1) ventricular slowing of rapid AF/atrial flutter without accessory bypass conduction (2) rapid conversion of narrow-complex PSVT to sinus rhythm.[33,36,38,41,42]

Diltiazem is contraindicated in the following settings: (1) sick sinus syndrome, second-degree block, third-degree block, except in the presence of an internal pacer; (2) severe hypotension or cardiogenic shock; (3) diltiazem hypersensitivity; (4) use of IV β-blockade within a few hours of need to use diltiazem; (5) AF or atrial flutter with coexisting accessory bypass tract conduction (WPW, LGL); and (6) VT.

Dosage. An initial dose of 0.25 mg/kg can be followed by a repeat dose of 0.35 mg/kg. Maintenance infusion should be at 5 to 15 mg/hr.[15,36,38,41]

Verapamil

Verapamil is also a calcium channel blocker. This medication blocks the slow channel for calcium entry into the myocytes. Verapamil blocks not only the calcium channels in the specialized conduction tissue of the myocardium but also the contracting cells of the heart. As a result, verapamil prolongs the effective refractory period within the AV node and slows conduction.[2,40] It also has a modest effect on myocardial contractility.[2]

Indications and Contraindications. Verapamil is effective in (1) converting narrow-complex PSVT to normal sinus rhythm and (2) controlling the ventricular response in AF or atrial flutter, if the AF or atrial flutter is not complicated by the presence of an accessory bypass tract (WPW, LGL).

Verapamil should not be used in the following settings: (1) PSVT with accessory bypass tract conduction, (2) AF/atrial flutter with accessory bypass tract conduction, (3) coexistence of a sick sinus syndrome or second- or third-degree AV block unless an internal pacer is present; (4) severe left ventricular dysfunction (systolic blood pressure < 90 mm Hg), or cardiogenic shock; and (5) in patients with a known verapamil hypersensitivity.[7,33,34,38,40,41]

β-Adrenergic Blockade

β-Blockers are very useful agents for the control of ventricular response in PSVT, AF or atrial flutter, and atrial tachycardia. It is generally considered that no β-blocker offers a distinctive advantage over another because when used clinically, they all can be titrated for a desired effect on dysrhythmias, and hypertension. Examples of β blockers are atenolol, metoprolol, propranolol and esmolol. What separates the different drugs and their use is the various pharmacological characteristics which control adverse reactions, speed of onset, dosage regimes, contraindications, and drug interactions.

The electrophysiological effect of β-blockers results from the inhibition of catecholamine binding at β-receptor sites. These medications reduce the effects of circulating catecholamines and this is manifested in a decrease in HR, blood pressure, and myocardial contractility. The PR interval may be prolonged, but the QRS and the Q-T intervals are not affected. Their actions are most noted on cells that are most stimulated by adrenergic actions. Typically, these sites are the

sinus node, the Purkinje fibers, and ventricular tissue when it is stimulated by catecholamines.[2,33,34,40] These medications also have various cardioprotective effects for patients suffering from acute coronary syndromes. They exert their cardioprotective effects by decreasing myocardial workload, and hence, they decrease myocardial oxygen consumption and demand.[2] β-Blockers are useful in the treatment of narrow-complex tachycardias that originate secondary to re-entry phenomenon or an automatic focus (MAT, an ectopic pacemaker, or a junctional rhythm). These drugs can also be used to control rates in patients suffering from AF or atrial flutter, as long as ventricular function is nominal. Some representative doses of these β-blockers are (1) *atenolol* ($β_1$) 5 mg IV slowly over 5 minutes; if no effect, repeat in 10 minutes; (2) *metoprolol* ($β_1$) 5 mg IV slowly, may repeat up to 15 mg total; and (3) *propranolol* 0.1 mg/kg IV slow push divided into three equal doses at 2- to 3-minute intervals; may repeat total dose in 2 minutes. Administration rate of the drug should not exceed 1 mg/min.

In general, β-blockers should ***not*** be used in patients with a history that includes diabetes, lung diseases, bradycardias or heart blocks, use of calcium channel blockers, hypotension, or the presence of a vasospasm condition.

Propranol

Propranol is the representative drug of the β-adrenergic blockade agents. It is nonselective. It has $β_1$ and $β_2$ effects on the heart that allow for its use in controlling rapid ventricular rates. Rate slowing is caused by (1) slowing SA node impulse formation and (2) depression of myocardial contractility. The usual effects on the electrocardiogram are rate reduction and prolongation of the PR interval. The QRS and Q-T intervals are not affected. Because it is relatively nonselective (has effects on both $β_1$ and $β_2$ receptors), its contraindications are somewhat extensive.[33,40,43]

Esmolol

Esmolol is a rapid-action, short-acting $β_1$-selective (cardioselective) β-blocker. At therapeutic doses, it inhibits $β_1$-receptors located in cardiac muscle. At higher doses, the selectivity is lost and it affects $β_2$-receptors in the lung and vascular system. Esmolol is rapidly metabolized in erythrocytes and has a half-life of about 2 to 9 minutes. Its elimination half-life is approximately 9 minutes.[34,38]

Indications and Contraindications. Esmolol is indicated for the rapid conversion of SVT and the rapid control of ventricular rate in patients with non–pre-excited, AF or atrial flutter. It also has a function in rate control of noncompensated sinus tachycardia when a clinician feels the tachycardia requires slowing. It also has been proved to have a benefit as an adjunct therapy in the VT of torsades de pointes.[34,36,38,40]

Esmolol should not be used in patients with second- or third-degree heart block, or in frank heart failure. Like all β-blockers, care should be exercised when used in patients with bronchospastic disease and diabetes.

Dosage. Esmolol has a complicated dose regimen. A loading dose of 0.5 mg/kg is given over the first 1 minute. This is followed by a maintenance infusion of 50 μg/kg per minute over 4 minutes. If this is not successful, a second bolus dose of 0.5 mg/kg followed by a maintenance infusion of 100 μg/kg over 4 minutes is started. This bolus/maintenance dosing can be repeated up to a maximum infusion rate of

300 µg/kg per minute for 4 minutes.[34,38,40] Similar dosing has been recommended for children using a 100- to 200-µg/kg maintenance rate between 100-µg/kg increases in bolus doses.[34]

Procainamide

A time-honored antiarrhythmic, procainamide slows conduction and decreases automaticity and excitability of atrial, ventricular, and Purkinje tissue. It also increases refractoriness in atrial and ventricular tissue. Procainamide prolongs the Q-T interval without having much effect on Purkinje fibers or ventricular tissue.[36]

Indications and Contraindications. A long-established clinical application is in the rate management of SVT, SVT with aberrancy conduction (wide-complex SVT), AF/atrial flutter *associated with WPW conduction*, and VTs. The advantage to using procainamide is the ability to convert to the oral form when rate control is achieved.

The advanced cardiac life support (ACLS) recommended dose of procainamide is usually 20 mg/min, although in urgent situations, up to 50 mg/min can be used. Procainamide is generally used in clinical situations in which time is not a factor in patient care. Long-term management in the ED necessitates monitoring of the plasma concentrations of procainamide and the n-acetyl procainamide (NAPA) metabolite. Hypotension and conduction disturbances (torsades de pointes, heart blocks, and sinus node dysfunctions) are often signs of high plasma levels. Caution should be used in patients with histories of hypokalemia, long Q-T intervals, and torsades de pointes. Hematologic and rheumatologic disturbances are factors in long-term use. The end point of administration of the drug is when the arrhythmia is suppressed, hypotension occurs, or the Q-T duration increases by 50% of baseline or a maximum of 17 mg/kg of the drug has been administered (1.2 g in a 70-kg adult).[32]

Ibutilide

Ibutilide is a short-acting, antiarrhythmic that prolongs the refractory period of the myocardium by prolonging the duration of the cardiac action potential. This drug is useful in the management conversion of AF and atrial flutter, when the arrhythmia is present for less than 48 hours.

This medication can also be used to control HR in the face of AF or atrial flutter when calcium channel blockers and β-blockers have proved ineffective.

The dose for ibutilide is 1 mg IV over 10 minutes in a 0.1-mg/mL dilution in an adult weighing more than 60 kg. This dose can be repeated in about 10 minutes after the first dose. In patients weighing less than 60 kg, the initial dose should be 0.01 mg/kg. This drug minimally affects blood pressure and HR. However, caution should be used when using this drug in patients who have either a high potassium or a low magnesium level. The patient should be on a cardiac monitor during and after administration of the medication, Do not use this drug if the patient has a corrected Q-T interval longer than 440 msec.

Digoxin

Digoxin is a time-honored drug used for treatment of AF and atrial flutter. It is the only antidysrhythmic with inotropic characteristics. Digoxin is less useful for the emergency clinician because of its long delay of onset.

Digoxin is a cardiac glycoside found in a number of plants. Digoxin is extracted from the leaves of the *Digitalis lanata* plant. Digoxin increases intracellular Na^+ and K^+ by inhibiting Na-K-ATPase, the enzyme that regulates the quantity of Na^+ and K^+ inside the cell. An intracellular increase in Na^+ stimulates Na^+-Ca^+ exchange, leading to increased intracellular Ca^+. Digoxin effects are both direct action on cardiac muscles and indirect action on the cardiovascular system. The indirect effects are mediated by the autonomic nervous system. The results of these actions are vagomimetic effects on the SA node and the AV node.

The consequences of these actions are (1) increased force and velocity of myocardial contraction (positive inotropic effect); (2) slowing of the HR and AV nodal conduction (vagomimetic effect); and (3) decrease in symptomatic nervous system effects (neurohormonal deactivating effect).[32,33,44-47]

Indications and Contraindications. Although its use in rate control of the ventricular response in chronic AF is well established, it no longer is the mainstay of therapy for narrow-complex tachycardias. Newer agents have replaced digoxin in narrow-complex tachycardias. Its inotropic character is still widely utilized in the setting of heart failure.

Use of digoxin should be avoided in the clinical settings of sinus node disease and AV blockade. It may cause complete heart block or severe sinus bradycardia. Do not use in the presence of accessory bypass tract rhythms (WPW or LGL). It may cause a rapid ventricular response or VF. Patients with idiopathic hypertrophic subaortic stenosis, restrictive cardiomyopathy, constrictive pericarditis, or amyloid heart disease are particularly susceptible to digoxin toxicity.[48]

Dosage. The IV loading dose of 10 to 15 µg/kg, followed by individual parental dosing until the desired rate is achieved.[32–34,36,40,49–52]

SPECIAL CONSIDERATION OF ANTICOAGULATION IN AF: EVALUATION AND TREATMENT

The most common, sustained tachydysrhythmia that presents to the ED is AF. The incidence of AF in the general population is 1% to 2 %. The incidence increases with age. Approximately 1% of the population under 50 years of age have AF whereas 8.8% of the population older than 80 years have AF.[53] The connection between AF, structural heart disease, and antecedent coronary artery disease is strong. As a dysrhythmia in acute myocardial infarction, AF is relatively uncommon (11%). However, its presence is associated with a 40% mortality.[54] The long-recognized association between valvular heart disease and AF is well documented. Rheumatic valvular disease is the classic valvular disease associated with AF. However, other dysrhythmias have an association with AF: WPW, atrial tachycardia, sick sinus syndrome, and AV nodal reentrant tachycardias. Long-standing medical or cardiac conditions having strong associations with AF are hypertension, cardiac myxomas, diabetes, thyroid disease, left ventricular dysfunction, congestive heart failure, pulmonary edema, chronic obstructive pulmonary disease, and pulmonary embolism.[47,54,55]

AF was thought to be caused by abnormal pulse formation originating in the atria. In human beings, the atria as a result of disease, drug toxicity, or excessive endogenous hormones (e.g., catecholamines) trigger spontaneous automaticity of a sufficient number of atrial cells in multiple atrial sites. These firings sustain the chaotic, simultaneously firing atrial impulses that travel to the ventricles over multiple irregular routes. The transmission of these erratic low-amplitude atrial or fibrillatory f-waves through the AV node to the ventricles paints the classic ECG picture of an irregular rhythm.[54,56]

First introduced in 1959 by the Russian researchers Moe and Abildskov,[57] the hypothesis that AF was a self-sustaining rhythm, independent of multiple firing focus, was verified in 1985. At that time, an animal model was constructed showing four to six waves or "wavelets" were needed to sustain AF in a multiple circulating wave of atrial re-entry, producing the classic ECG picture. These wavelets interact to maintain the optimum atrial conditions needed to maintain sustained AF.[54]

Any adverse effects from this tachydysrhythmia are related to the disruption of the normal filling and eject components of the cardiac cycle. Classically, patients with AF present with feelings of palpitations, exertional fatigue, dyspnea on exertion, and lightheadedness. Further along in their presentation, patients respond to the fast ventricular rate and develop fluid overload, congestive failure, frank pulmonary edema, and myocardial ischemia.[54,58,59]

Treatment of symptomatic rapid AF is along three treatment fronts: (1) slowing the rapid ventricular response, (2) conversion to normal sinus rhythm, and (3) prevention of thromboembolism. This section addresses the issue of anticoagulation and prevention of thromboembolism.[38,54,59,60]

Hyperthyroidism may produce AF, occasionally in the absence of obvious signs and symptoms of thyroid storm. It is not standard to test all patients for thyroid disease before proceeding with needed or aggressive interventions, but thyroid function is a common test ordered for a complete evaluation of patients with AF. Failure to respond as expected to antiarrhythmic therapy may be a tip-off to underlying hyperthyroidism, but in subclinical cases, it would be impossible to predict this at the bedside.

CARDIOVERSION

Urgent restoration of symptomatic new-onset AF is best achieved with direct cardioversion using either the monophasic or the biphasic defibrillators. *In life-threatening or unstable presentations, patients in AF are to be immediately cardioverted because the risk of continued AF outweighs the risk of thromboembolism*[38,54,59,61] (Table 11–5). Of course, the definition of unstable/life-threatening is a clinical judgment call that must often be made with little data.

The current guidelines for treatment of symptomatic new-onset AF focus on the length of time the patient has been in AF or atrial flutter as the determining factor for the initiation of anticoagulation when confronted by the need for cardioversion to sinus rhythm. Accordingly, 48 hours or less has been determined to be the time limit that a patient with new-onset AF can be cardioverted without the need for anticoagulation. Studies have shown that staying under the 48-hour limit allows cardioversion to occur with the lowest risk for thromboembolism.[38,54,59,62] For patients who have been determined to be in AF longer than 48 hours and are not in need of urgent care need to be anticoagulated to an International Normalized Ratio (INR) of 2.0 to 3.0 for a 3-week

TABLE 11–5 Guidelines for Anticoagulation in Atrial Fibrillation

Atrial Fibrillation

I. Duration < 48 hr

Low risk for thromboembolism
Immediate electrical cardioversion if unstable
No anticoagulation necessary

II. Duration > 48 hr or Undetermined

High risk for thromboembolism
Immediate electrical cardioversion if unstable
Stable clinical situation
Warfarin: INR 2.0–3.0 for 3 wk
Cardioversion, then warfarin: INR 2.0–3.0 for 4 wk
   OR
TEE and heparinization
Left atrial appendage clot not present
Cardioversion, then continue warfarin: INR 2.0–3.0 for 4 wk
Left atrial appendage clot visualized
Continue warfarin: INR 2.0–3.0 for 4 wk, then cardioversion

INR, International Normalized Ratio; TEE, transesophageal echocardiography.
Adapted from Pelosi F, Morady F: Evaluation and management of atrial fibrillation. Med Clin North Am 85:225, 2001.

duration before cardioversion.[43] If this approach is not clinically acceptable, the patient should have a transesophageal echocardiogram (TEE) and be heparinized.

If no left atrial appendage clot is visualized on TEE, the heparinized patient should be immediately cardioverted and anticoagulated for the next 4 weeks. If a left atrial appendage clot is visualized, the patient should be anticoagulated to an INR or 2.0 to 3.0 for 3 weeks' duration and cardioverted[63-67] (see Table 11–5).

A synchronized shock (cardioversion) from a monophasic or biphasic defibrillator should be delivered with the patient sedated. Dosages for cardioverting atrial flutter are 50 to 100 J for a monophasic defibrillator; 100 to 200 J for AF. As of this writing, no specific doses are recommended for biphasic cardioversion. This topic is covered in greater detail in Chapter 12, Defibrillation and Cardioversion. Success rates with the biphasic defibrillators is reported to be approximately 94% to 95%.[68-70] An alternative treatment strategy with a reported success rate of 50% to 70% is the use of ibutilide in a bolus infusion or the use of amiodarone. Caution is recommended with the use of ibutilide in patients with prolonged Q-T intervals or severe left ventricular dysfunction. Ibutilde has a 4% risk of ventricular arrhythmia. Pretreatment of patients to be electrically cardioverted with ibutilde can increase their chances for successful conversion to nearly 100%.[32,33,40,71-74]

Amiodarone has the advantage of being effective for tachydysrhythmias when the mechanism is unclear and can be used for either wide-complex or narrow-complex tachycardias. Central venous access is advised if concentrations greater than 2 mg/mL are to be used. Amiodarone should be given as an initial bolus of 5 mg/ml over 20 to 30 minutes, followed by a maintenance infusion of 1.0 g/24 hr for a total of 48 to 72 hours.[32,34,45,49]

Other drugs with good to excellent evidence in obtaining rate control in narrow-complex AF include verapamil, diltiazem, procainamide, and β-blockers.[33,34,36,40,54]

CONCLUSIONS

The advent of β-blockers, calcium channel blockers, adenosine, amiodarone, and other effective medications to treat tachydysrhythmias—particularly the SVTs—has diminished the therapeutic use of the vagal maneuvers. However, the vagal maneuvers still remain an important diagnostic tool. These maneuvers are especially important in unmasking the underlying rhythms of narrow-complex tachydysrhythmias and in determining the presence of CSS in patients with syncope.

As for the advent of medications, which quickly and safely control the rate in tachydysrhythmias, their availability has given the emergency clinician a more varied and powerful armamentarium to be used in cardioverting these life-threatening dysrhythmias to normal sinus rhythms.

 REFERENCES CAN BE FOUND ON EXPERT CONSULT

CHAPTER 12

Defibrillation and Cardioversion

Bohdan M. Minczak

Defibrillation is an emergency procedure performed to terminate *ventricular fibrillation (VF)*. This procedure is also useful in the treatment of *pulseless ventricular tachycardia (VT)*. VF and pulseless VT are potentially lethal dysrhythmias[1-3] that require *immediate assessment and treatment*.

When VF or pulseless VT occurs, the myocytes of the ventricles become "irritable" or easily excitable. Multiple foci in the walls and septum of the heart begin to produce random, chaotic electrical discharges (Fig. 12–1). As a result, numerous cardiac cells enter into various stages of depolarization and repolarization. This activity disrupts the normal sequence of depolarization and repolarization within the myocardium. The rhythmic, sequential atrioventricular (AV) depolarization of the myocardium that originated in the sinoatrial (SA) node, the "pacemaker" of the heart, is distorted by the disorganized electrical activity from the ventricles. The surface electrocardiographic (ECG) waveforms become distorted from the normal PQRST. The electrical cardiac rhythm that is depicted on the cardiac monitor becomes a "squiggly" chaotic line (Fig. 12–2), with variable amplitude, frequency, and changing polarity. Subsequently, the mechanical activity of the ventricles becomes disorganized and the ventricles begin to contract randomly or "twitch," producing many local, disorganized weak contractions. This renders the heart incapable of ejecting blood effectively into the peripheral circulation. As a result, the victim becomes unconscious, pulseless, and apneic. This condition describes sudden cardiac arrest (SCA). Failure to treat VF/VT/SCA within the first moments after collapse renders treatment of VF/VT/SCA more difficult.[4] If defibrillation and termination of VF/VT/SCA is not accomplished within several minutes of VF/pulseless VT onset (≤4–5 min),[2] the patient is unlikely to survive neurologically intact and is very likely to suffer a fatal outcome.

SCA is a major cause of death in North America, with deaths from SCA conservatively estimated to exceed 330,000/yr.[5] SCA can strike at any time and in any place. Many of these deaths occur outside the hospital in the prehospital setting. However, a significant number of SCA events occur within the confines of the hospital; in the emergency department (ED), critical care units, non–critical care floors of the hospital, and outpatient areas. In most of these cases, VF is the underlying rhythm. Although the majority of SCA events occur in adults, SCA can also occur in the pediatric population, resulting from hypoxia, trauma, and other causes discussed later. Several rhythms are associated with SCA: pulseless VT, VF, pulseless electrical activity (PEA), and asystole. This chapter is limited to a discussion of treatment of VF and pulseless VT.

SCA/VF/VT in adults has many potential causes: SCA independent of myocardial infarction (MI), myocardial ischemia, MI, undiagnosed coronary artery disease, and electrical injuries. The use of medications such as tricyclic antidepres-

sants, digitalis, quinidine, and other proarrhythmics that cause Q-T segment prolongation and changes in the refractory period of the cardiac cycle are capable of precipitating VF. Furthermore, chest trauma, hypothermia, cardiomyopathy, profound hyperkalemia or hypokalemia, hypocalcemia, hypercalcemia, electrolyte disturbances, and various toxidromes can induce conditions favoring the development of VF. Hypoxia is another culprit that frequently precipitates VF in adults and the pediatric population. Congenital malformations of the heart and great vessels have also been associated with an increased incidence of VF in young children. Therefore, based on the multiple, potential causes of VF, the probability of a health care provider, especially a clinician charged with the care of critically ill patients, encountering SCA/VF/pulseless VT is quite high.

Prompt defibrillation is a well-documented, effective treatment for VF.[6] Defibrillation entails providing a brief "burst" of therapeutic current through the chest wall, across the myocardium, for the purpose of terminating VF. Defibrillation uniformly depolarizes a critical mass of myocardium and "stuns" the fibrillating myocardial fibers, rendering the myocytes refractory to the various chaotic stimuli. Immediately after application of the defibrillatory current, all electrical and mechanical activity is reset. As the myocytes regain their excitability, the SA node will presumptively begin to depolarize rhythmically and reinitiate pacing the heart. Subsequently, the normal, organized, sequential electrical activity of the heart resumes. Shortly thereafter, depending on the metabolic conditions of the myocardium, the mechanical pumping activity of the heart begins to return to baseline levels and circulation of blood to the vital organs slowly resumes. As a result, SCA is terminated and there is a gradual return of spontaneous circulation (ROSC).

In the last decade, much has been learned and implemented to improve survival from SCA. Defibrillators have been redesigned in order to increase the efficacy of first-shock defibrillation. New biphasic defibrillators are now touted as having a first-shock efficacy of greater than 90%.[7] Defibrillator waveforms have been modified in order to provide a configuration that defibrillates the myocardium with the least amount of energy imparted to the myocardium. This endeavor will presumptively lead to a decrease in the incidence of myocardial damage secondary to defibrillation current and decrease the incidence of nonperfusing dysrhythmias such as PEA and asystole after shock.

The characteristics of VF have been explored, yielding information regarding salient features that may serve as indicators for the timing of defibrillation. Currently available data indicate that VF has multiple phases and that defibrillation is most effective in the initial phase of VF.[8] If VF persists for several minutes, metabolic byproducts produced by VF may be building up in the myocardial tissue, rendering defibrillation more difficult. Furthermore, some of these myocardial depressants may be interfering with the contractility of the heart in the period immediately after the shock. As a result, modifications have been made in the priorities and sequence of interventions provided during the resuscitative effort of SCA/VF/pulseless VT (i.e., cardiopulmonary resuscitation [CPR] first vs. defibrillation first and immediate CPR after shock) in order to enhance the potential for successful termination of VF with subsequent increased survivability from SCA.[9]

Recent advances in electronics and computer software have further expanded the arena for defibrillation. Defibrillators manufactured today are lighter, smaller, and more portable. Integration of computer microchips and software has added sophisticated rhythm recognition to the capability of these devices. Many prehospital emergency medical services (EMS), fire departments, police departments, and even lay "first responders" who are participants in public access defibrillation (PAD) programs are providing CPR and early defibrillation to victims of SCA. As a result, the time to first shock has decreased in many venues. However, although a decrease in time to first shock has decreased and there have been many advances in technology, statistics reporting survival from SCA/pulseless VT/VF and successful defibrillation have not achieved anticipated levels.[10] A review of data from the prehospital arena has suggested that a return to the basics (e.g., good, effective CPR) may be an important therapeutic intervention that will enhance efficacy of defibrillation. This speculation occurred because it was observed that when EMS personnel responded to unwitnessed SCA calls and response times exceeded 4 to 5 minutes, victims who received several minutes (±2 min) of CPR prior to initial defibrillation demonstrated an increased rate of initial resuscitation versus those victims who were immediately defibrillated upon arrival of EMS, without prior CPR. This led to studies addressing the effect of CPR on VF.

The effects of CPR on VF have been evaluated and reported to increase the amplitude and duration of VF. In addition, performance of CPR prior to defibrillation of protracted VF (>4 min) has been suggested to increase success of VF termination by providing a nominal amount of blood flow through the coronary arteries during SCA.[11] It is currently hypothesized that this blood flow may provide substrates to the myocytes that are needed to facilitate defibrillation and

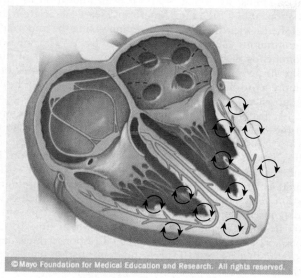

Figure 12–1 Fibrillating heart.

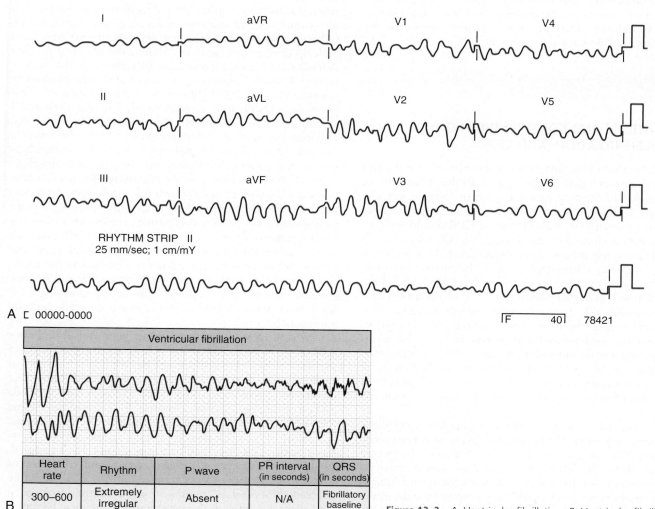

RHYTHM STRIP II
25 mm/sec; 1 cm/mV

A ⊏ 00000-0000   ⌐F   40⌐   78421

Heart rate	Rhythm	P wave	PR interval (in seconds)	QRS (in seconds)
300–600	Extremely irregular	Absent	N/A	Fibrillatory baseline

Figure 12–2 *A,* Ventricular fibrillation. *B,* Ventricular fibrillation.

that these substrates may enhance resumption of normal electromechanical activity of the ventricles after shock. In addition, byproducts of fibrillation that may be cardiac depressants may be washed away from the myocytes. As a result, defibrillation is achieved more easily. Furthermore, it has been observed that performance of CPR immediately after defibrillation facilitates the transition from SCA to ROSC by enhancing ejection of blood from the ventricle into the vasculature.

Based on these observations, the steps, sequence, and priorities of CPR have been modified to improve the efficacy of and decrease delays in providing chest compressions. Current emphasis is on increasing the number and frequency of chest compressions. This has been recommended to improve blood flow and circulation during SCA and immediately after defibrillation. Airway management and use of medications have been revised and reprioritized.

A comprehensive, in-depth review of resuscitation data has been conducted to provide an evidenced-based guide for the practice of SCA resuscitation. As a result, the American Heart Association has incorporated these new findings and released new guidelines and recommendations for resuscitation of SCA/VF/pulseless VT.[12] These new recommendations are presented later in the text. The first part of this chapter is dedicated to describing the procedure for defibrillation of VF and pulseless VT. The second part of the chapter presents current recommendations and guidelines for the treatment of VT and other supraventricular arrhythmias via cardioversion. Use of medication in the resuscitation sequences is presented where appropriate. Defibrillation and cardioversion in the pediatric population are also covered.

BACKGROUND CAN BE FOUND ON EXPERT CONSULT

214

INDICATIONS AND CONTRAINDICATIONS FOR DEFIBRILLATION (AND CPR)

As stated earlier in the text, it is well established that prompt electrical defibrillation is the most effective treatment of acute SCA/VF.[6] Starting with the onset of collapse, the survival rate for SCA/VF drops 7% to 10% for every minute of down time without defibrillation. If CPR is initiated, the survival rate declines less rapidly (i.e., 3%–4%/min of down time). If an SCA is witnessed and immediate CPR is provided, coupled with immediate defibrillation, the survival from this event has been reported to increase threefold.[22] Therefore, defibrillation is indicated whenever a patient is diagnosed with VF or pulseless VT. At times, mitigating circumstances may exist surrounding the SCA event, causing the clinician to reevaluate the sequence of interventions; however, few absolute specific contraindications to early defibrillation exist other than the presence of a pulse, absence of SCA, medical futility for the procedure, or a valid do-not-resuscitate (DNR) order. Several scenarios are provided to illustrate pertinent points.

If a patient suddenly becomes unresponsive, pulseless, and apneic (e.g., a potential victim of SCA), it is reasonable to assume that the underlying cardiac rhythm of the patient is most likely VF. Therefore, immediate action must be taken to prepare for defibrillation. A defibrillator with "quick-look" paddles or an AED should be promptly brought to the victim's side. Application of either of these devices to the

victim will provide immediate monitoring and assessment of the patient's rhythm. If there is any delay in getting a defibrillator to the victim's side, initiation of CPR is indicated. If VF or pulseless VT is diagnosed by looking at the ECG rhythm via the quick-look paddles or if the AED indicates a shockable rhythm, defibrillation must be expediently performed. Thus, witnessed SCA/VF is an indication for defibrillation and CPR. The American Heart Association has published a scientific advisory on emphasizing the importance of continuous chest compressions in SCA. The advisory recommends that bystanders who are not confident of their ability to provide conventional CPR should use hands-only (compression-only) CPR until the arrival of an AED or health care provider.[23]

If a patient is found unresponsive, pulseless, and apneic and the "down time" is unknown, it is suggested that good-quality CPR be performed while preparation is made for defibrillation. As the CPR is performed, preparation for rhythm analysis and possible defibrillation, as noted earlier, should be initiated. After performing CPR for 2 minutes, rhythm analysis should be performed. If VF or pulseless VT is diagnosed, defibrillation should be performed promptly. Data from prehospital resuscitations in which time to first shock was delayed owing to prolonged response times demonstrated that the rate of successful defibrillation increased if patients received bystander CPR prior to defibrillation.[22] A scientific evaluation of this information has proposed that CPR may enhance the defibrillation threshold by restoring substrates to the myocytes for the facilitation or resumption of normal excitation-contraction coupling. Furthermore, CPR may wash out myocardial depressants that may have built up during prolonged VF. Hence, the potential for first defibrillation shock success may increase with the performance of about 2 minutes (5 cycles of 30:2 compressions to ventilations) of CPR.[22] Therefore, administration of CPR prior to defibrillation is recommended in the prehospital setting. Data to substantiate this sequence for in-hospital resuscitation have not been presented. Thus, the issue of unknown down time, although not a definitive contraindication to immediate defibrillation, may be a factor in the clinician's decision making process regarding the resuscitation sequence. The question still remains for in-hospital resuscitation as to whether to defibrillate first or administer CPR prior to defibrillation when the down time is unknown. Other relevant questions being asked are how long the CPR should be performed prior to defibrillation and how long VF should be present before prioritizing CPR over defibrillation? Nonetheless, if the down time is unknown, initiate CPR and prepare to defibrillate as soon as possible. Consider performing CPR for a brief period before defibrillation, if deemed clinically appropriate.

Victims of SCA due to traumatic injuries usually do not survive.[24] The heart, aorta, and pulmonary arteries may have sustained injury that will prevent the resumption of normal cardiovascular function. There is a high probability that underlying hypovolemia and organ damage may preclude success of the resuscitation. However, the cause of the trauma may have been SCA with subsequent loss of consciousness. Therefore, if SCA/VF is present in the trauma patient, treatment with CPR and defibrillation should be attempted. However, if unsuccessful, then a search and treatment of the underlying cause of the trauma and the SCA should be pursued. Nonetheless, trauma is not a contraindication to defibrillation, although the resuscitative effort may be futile.

If the victim of VF/pulseless VT is a pregnant female, treatment of the mother is critical. Therefore, prompt defibrillation is indicated, using the same guidelines and sequencing as for the nonpregnant patient.[25] No harm to the fetus has been reported as a result of defibrillation. Therefore, pregnancy is not a contraindication to defibrillation.

New guidelines suggest that only one shock be administered after identification of SCA/VF.[6] After defibrillation, CPR should be resumed immediately and continued for about 2 minutes or 5 cycles, without interruptions for rhythm evaluation or pulse checks. Hence, the pulse and rhythm checks are delayed, and subsequent shocks are not recommended, but contraindicated. Administering additional shocks may indeed precipitate PEA or asystole. The administration of CPR immediately after defibrillation is indicated to enhance the mechanical function of the "stunned" heart in the immediate postdefibrillation period. This step may be modified at the discretion of the clinician in the hospital setting because of the presence of mitigating circumstances or the availability of hemodynamic monitoring devices such as Doppler devices, arterial pressure lines, or central venous pressure (CVP) monitoring.

Prior recommendations suggested delivering a "stacked" sequence of up to three shocks without interposed chest compressions if the first shock was unsuccessful in terminating VF. This was done to decrease transthoracic impedance with the monophasic damped sinusoidal (MDS) defibrillators in use (discussed later) and to deliver more current to the myocardium. However, this recommendation has been rescinded owing to lack of supporting evidence. Now with the higher first-shock efficacy (90%) in successfully terminating VF (termination of VF for 5 sec) through the use of biphasic defibrillators,[7] the recommendation to repeat a shock if the first treatment was unsuccessful is harder to justify. Furthermore, as previously mentioned, the post shock rhythms often observed after defibrillation were either asystole or PEA. These rhythms require immediate CPR as part of their treatment. Therefore, additional or multiple shocks are not recommended and are contraindicated. However, immediate CPR is recommended.

Defibrillation is also an effective treatment modality used to terminate pulseless VT. If the patient has a pulse, is stable, and has a perfusing rhythm while in VT, defibrillation is contraindicated. However, if the patient in VT becomes unstable or develops signs of poor perfusion, change in mental status, or persistent chest pain with pulmonary edema and hypotension and subsequent shock, then *synchronized cardioversion* is recommended. This procedure is addressed later. If the patient becomes unstable as a result of polymorphic VT, or becomes pulseless during the episode of VT, an *unsynchronized* shock (i.e., defibrillation) is indicated.

Patients found "down" or who have just become unresponsive can have other "rhythms present" beside VF or pulseless VT (e.g., PEA or asystole). Defibrillation is contraindicated in PEA. True asystole is NOT a shockable rhythm, and current evidence suggests that defibrillating "occult" or false asystole is not beneficial and may actually be harmful.

Patients who are found unresponsive, but who have a pulse, should obviously have their cardiac rhythm determined. However, any patient who has a pulse, fast or slow, should NOT receive defibrillation.

Some patients who succumb to SCA may have various medication-releasing patches (e.g., nitroglycerin, contraceptive hormones, antihypertensive agents, smoking-cessation adjuncts) present on their chest. Presence of these patches is NOT a contraindication to defibrillation. However, placement of the electrodes or paddles used for defibrillation should be modified to avoid contact with these items. If needed, these items should be removed prior to defibrillation to avoid current diversion from the myocardium, current arcing, sparks, and other problems.

Developments in defibrillation and computer electronics have led to the availability of implantable defibrillators (automatic implantable cardiac defibrillators [AICDs]; pacemakers) in the chest of patients who have known coronary artery disease. These patients are prone to dysrhythmias and may have episodes of VT and VF that are automatically detected and defibrillated or cardioverted. However, these devices can malfunction. If these patients present in SCA/VF, defibrillation should be performed as indicated. Presence of an AICD or pacemaker is NOT a contraindication for defibrillation. The only caveat is to avoid placement of the defibrillation paddles over the AICD or pacemaker because the current for defibrillation may be redirected away from the fibrillating myocardium and compromise termination of VF. In addition, because current from the defibrillation could enter the AICD or pacemaker, the device could be prone to future malfunction. These devices should be reevaluated after the patient has been defibrillated.

Current trends in fashion sometimes include piercing of the body in various locations. In addition, certain items of clothing and jewelry may require modification of electrode or paddle placement. The presence of metals in locations proximal to the heart or in locations on the chest should be avoided to minimize the potential for diverting the defibrillating current from the myocardium. Also, if the metal object provides a potential short circuit from the patient or leads to "ground," this object should be removed, if feasible, to avoid current diversion from the myocardium or the possibility of arcing and burns across the chest. However, the presence of these materials is NOT a contraindication to defibrillation.

In this part of the chapter on defibrillation the recommendations are intended for application to adult (>8 yr or weighing > 25 kg [55 lb]) victims of SCA/VF. If a patient is a child (e.g., 1–8 yr of age or weighing < 25 kg [55 lb]), modifications in the sequence, defibrillation energy, energy attenuation equipment, and size of defibrillation paddles must be addressed. Pediatric defibrillation details are discussed later in this chapter. If a defibrillator or AED and equipment suitable for use in children are not available, the health care provider can resort to use of a standard AED or defibrillator. Use of AEDs or defibrillation in infants less than 1 year of age is neither indicated nor contraindicated. Therefore, the age of the patient is not a contraindication, but certain modifications in the resuscitation must be considered. Pediatric defibrillation is addressed later.

As obvious from the text, defibrillation may have to be performed in various areas. Defibrillation can be an ignition source for explosion if any arcing occurs or if there are any stray or aberrant electrical discharges that occur as a result of the paddle or electrode discharge. Therefore, care should be taken to avoid defibrillation or to ensure that electrical conductivity through the patient's chest is optimal during defibrillation in an environment in which volatile explosive materials are present, such as the operating room or other areas of critical care. Some of the materials to avoid are anesthetic agents and oxygen. Therefore, a potentially explosive environment is a relative contraindication to defibrillation.[26]

When performing defibrillation, care should be taken to avoid excessive moisture on the chest or around the patient. It is unlikely that there will be any significant or dangerous current leaks from the patient onto a wet floor; however, care should be taken to avoid creating an electrical hazard. Try to ensure that the area is not wet. Thus, a wet surface is not an absolute contraindication to defibrillation. Defibrillation can be performed on ice and wet pavements.

With a high index of suspicion for the presence of VF in an unresponsive patient in early SCA, "blind" defibrillation can be life saving or it can make things worse, especially if the underlying rhythm is not determined prior to defibrillation. If the patient is indeed in VF, providing prompt early defibrillation may indeed help. If the underlying rhythm is NOT a shockable rhythm such as PEA/asystole, the resuscitation could be compromised. Shocking a patient in PEA can bring about asystole. If the patient is in asystole, things may be made worse by damaging the myocardium with electrical current, which will increase the possibility of an intraventricular conduction delay. Therefore, blind defibrillation is not recommended.[27] However, data to support or refute this are sparse.

Lastly, the defibrillation of "occult" or "false" asystole or very fine VF not detectable owing to paddle or electrode position may be considered, but is not recommended.[27] Fine VF can occasionally masquerade as ventricular standstill or asystole. This may be a function of perpendicular electrode orientation with respect to the wavefront of depolarization. When evaluating the rhythm of a patient if there is any doubt or confusion regarding the type of rhythm present, the operator should make sure that several leads are checked or that the paddles are rotated 90° from their original position to ensure that asystole is indeed present before abandoning the possibility of defibrillation. If fine VF is unmasked, provision of aggressive CPR prior to defibrillation should be considered. Also, the controls on the ECG monitor should be placed on maximal gain to ensure adequate amplification of weak signals.

DEFIBRILLATION EQUIPMENT

Preparation

Sudden cardiac death usually occurs without advanced warning and requires prompt action. To ensure an expedient response and timely intervention, it is advisable to have all of the equipment listed in Table 12–1 easily accessible, on a prearranged tray, and preferably placed on a mobile, cartlike device (Fig. 12–3) in the anticipated order of use. This equipment should always be kept in a constant state of readiness. Wherever possible, the defibrillator (Fig. 12–4), patient cables, quick-look electrode paddles (Fig. 12–5), and ECG and defibrillation electrodes and pads (Fig. 12–6) should be preconnected and labeled to facilitate application to the patient. This will provide easy access to and prompt utilization of the equipment during the resuscitation. Furthermore, members of the designated resuscitation team should check the equipment at the beginning of their clinical shifts to ensure that the equipment is fully operational and that all of the components of the cart are present and/or restocked from any prior usage. Having a list of required equipment and a log of when the cart and equipment are checked is helpful.

Intrinsic to the variability of the workplace is the potential of the health care team to encounter different types of

---

TABLE 12–1 Defibrillation Equipment

List of Materials for Defibrillation

- Defibrillator/ECG monitor
- Handheld defibrillation electrodes "quick-look" paddles
- Patient interface cables; multifunctional for ECG monitoring and defibrillation
- Electrodes and pads for ECG signal acquisition and defibrillation
- Conductive gel (*not* ultrasound gel)

Additional "Equipment" (Pertinent to VF/VT)*

ACLS Medications

- Epinephrine
- Vasopressin
- Amiodarone
- Lidocaine
- Magnesium sulfate
- Procainamide
- Atropine

Miscellaneous

- IV access equipment, central line kits, and the like

*List of suggested equipment and medications for a code cart.
ACLS, advanced cardiac life support; ECG, electrocardiographic; VF, ventricular fibrillation; VT, ventricular tachycardia.

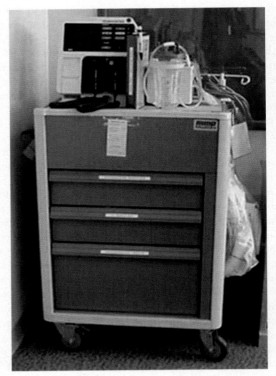

Figure 12–3 "Code cart" with defibrillation equipment.

defibrillation equipment. Input from biomedical research into the development and design of better, more effective defibrillators, capable of achieving better success with the first shock, along with competition from various manufacturers trying to increase their percentage of the health care market share by making defibrillator/monitor units more user-friendly and capable of more functions has provided a significant number of variations in defibrillator design and configuration.

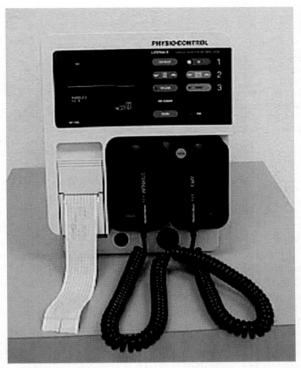

Figure 12–4 Defibrillator with paddles preconnected/paper ready.

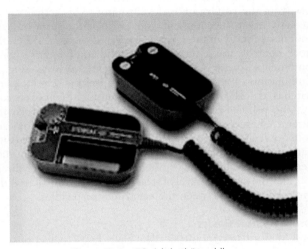

Figure 12–5 "Quick-look" paddles.

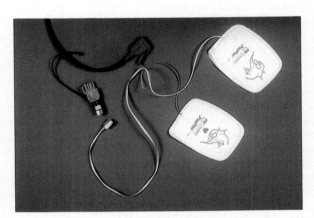

Figure 12–6 Multifunctional defibrillation pads/electrocardiographic (ECG) electrodes.

Although the basic functions and operation of all defibrillators currently in clinical use are similar, and all of these defibrillators are capable of being used for defibrillation, the layout of the controls and connections may vary significantly and cause unnecessary delays in time to first shock as the team determines how to operate the defibrillator during the resuscitation. Perceived malfunctions of equipment are often due to the operator's misuse of, or inappropriate operation of, the defibrillator controls and connections. Furthermore, differences in the type of defibrillator (e.g., waveform characteristics, discussed later) may affect the actual amount of energy delivered to the myocardium, causing unnecessary damage to the heart or causing a nonperfusing, postshock dysrhythmia if the operator is not fully aware of the equipment characteristics. Therefore, the clinician and resuscitation team or code team should become thoroughly familiar with the operation and type of equipment available in their designated patient care area. Choices and decisions made during the resuscitation may be affected by the type of equipment being used at the time. This should be done **before** the need to use the equipment suddenly arises.

Remember, the longer VF persists, the harder it is to defibrillate.

Defibrillators

Central to the procedure of defibrillation is the defibrillator. To better understand the relevance and function of the various types of defibrillators and the significance of the controls, options, and settings, a brief discussion describing the basic components of a defibrillator is provided.

Defibrillator units come in various configurations, depending on the manufacturer's design (Figs. 12–7 and 12–8; see also Fig. 12–4). Most defibrillators manufactured today are also cardiac monitors capable of displaying several ECG leads (see Figs. 12–4 and 12–7). Some units can display and provide a hard copy of a 12-lead electrocardiogram (Fig. 12–9). In addition, many defibrillator/monitors have rate alarms, computer microchips, and software to detect certain arrhythmias and the possibility of acute MI. Most defibrillator/monitors also have the capability of performing cardioversion, external pacing, pulse oximetry, telemetry, and sphygmomanometry. A comprehensive review of the various options and varieties of defibrillator monitors is beyond the scope of this chapter. Therefore, the discussion provided

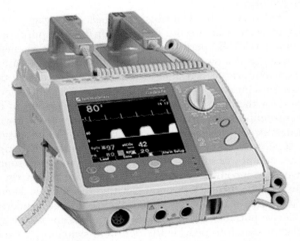

Figure 12–7 Multifunction defibrillator/monitor.

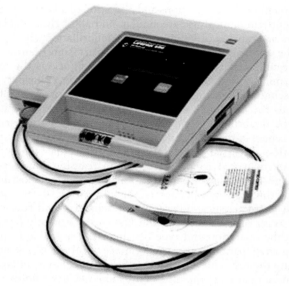

Figure 12–8 Automatic external defibrillator (AED).

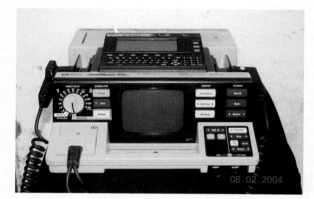

Figure 12–9 Defibrillator monitor capable of 12-lead ECG/cardioversion/pacing/limited ECG interpretation.

herein is limited to elements relevant to defibrillation and cardioversion (later in the chapter).

Basics of Defibrillator Function and Operation (Basic Controls/Switches/Components)

Defibrillation

As stated previously, defibrillation entails delivering a brief burst of current across the myocardium for the purpose of terminating VF. To perform this function, a source of energy or current and a means of producing a controlled release of this current are needed. The defibrillator is the device that serves this purpose. The defibrillator serves as the energy source for the defibrillation/cardioversion. A diagram of the patient-defibrillator circuit (Fig. 12–10) is shown to provide a visual reference regarding the components under discussion. An AC power source provides electricity to an internal transformer and power supply. The transformer and power supply convert the incoming energy to DC and store the energy in a battery. The battery holds power within the unit, even when the defibrillator is unplugged from the AC source, rendering the device portable. Some devices have a backup battery and a selector switch to provide the option of switching between alternate batteries, if the primary battery fails. When defibril-

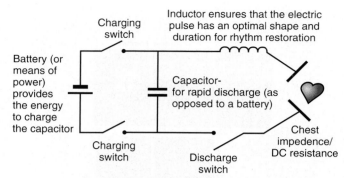

Figure 12–10 Defibrillator/patient circuit.

lation is to be performed, controls are set by the operator, which initiates a chain of events.

First, the defibrillator monitor unit must be turned on, using the appropriate selector switch or rotating dial. The electrode pads (handheld quick-look or multifunctional electrode pads) must be appropriately placed onto the chest wall of the patient, thus interfacing the patient into the defibrillator-patient circuit.

When the decision is made to defibrillate based on an assessment of the electrocardiogram, an energy level (in joules) for defibrillation is selected by the operator. This switch selects how much energy will be released during the shock. A charge switch is then activated to initiate current flow from the battery onto the capacitor. This action causes the capacitor to become charged. A capacitor stores a large amount of energy in the form of separated charges. When the shock controls are activated, electronic components and/or computer software select the appropriate pathway (e.g., a combination of resistors, inductors, capacitors, circuits, and switches) that allows release of a therapeutic amount of current into the paddles or electrodes that are interfaced with the patient. These internal controls affect the amount of energy (volts/joules/amplitude), the duration of current release (time span over which current flows through the electrodes in milliseconds), and the polarity (monophasic or biphasic) or direction that the current travels through the chest wall across the myocardium and between the electrodes or paddles.

Cardioversion Basics

Most defibrillator/monitors also have ECG detection and display devices incorporated into the device. This permits the operator to analyze the patient's rhythm and decide whether a shockable rhythm requiring intervention is present. Furthermore, the ECG device is interfaced with the defibrillator so that when shock delivery needs to be performed or synchronized at a specific time point or phase of the ECG event (e.g., during the absolute refractory period of the cardiac cycle [Fig. 12–11], discussed later), as in cardioversion, software and electronic components can be preset to discharge energy to the electrodes or paddles at the appropriate time. A selector switch designed to select the *mode* for current discharge is present on the defibrillator/monitor unit that allows the operator to either engage or disengage the ECG device from the defibrillator output circuit. This switch allows control of when the current will be delivered. Thus, when the health care provider has decided to perform defibrillation, the device is placed in the unsynchronized mode, so that the current is discharged independent of the ECG device. The current is then discharged when the operator depresses the "shock/

discharge" buttons on either the paddles or the defibrillator unit itself. If cardioversion is to be performed, the operator will select the synchronized mode or "*sync*" setting for current discharge, placing the ECG component into the discharge circuit. This will result in current being released during the

peak of the R-wave of the QRS. This synchronization is done by the defibrillator/cardioversion circuitry. This procedure is discussed in more detail in the "Cardioversion" section of the chapter.

Defibrillator Types

Defibrillators currently in use are classified by the type of shock waveforms that they produce. There are two general types of waveforms, *monophasic* and *biphasic*. These waveforms can be further classified by the rate of current drop to baseline or the actual shape/polarity of the waveform: MDS (Fig. 12–12 *left*), monophasic truncated exponential (MTE) (see Fig. 12–12 *right*), biphasic truncated exponential (BTE) (Fig. 12–13), or biphasic rectilinear (see Fig. 12–13). Several figures have been included for comparison of the waveforms (Fig. 12–14). Although no specific waveform has been proved to be superior to another regarding survival from SCA or for the return of spontaneous circulation, biphasic waveforms have been shown to be more efficient in achieving first-shock termination of VF than monophasic waveforms.[7] Of note, the amount of energy actually delivered to the myocardium by a specific waveform can differ from the actual selected

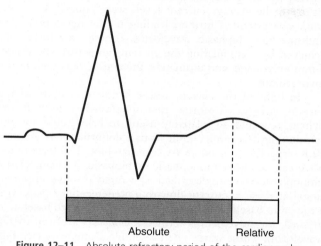

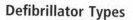

Figure 12–11 Absolute refractory period of the cardiac cycle.

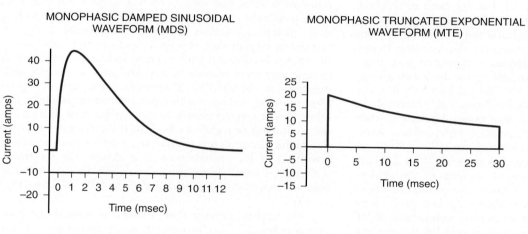

Figure 12–12 Monophasic damped sinusoidal (MDS; *left*) and monophasic truncated exponential (MTE; *right*) waveforms.

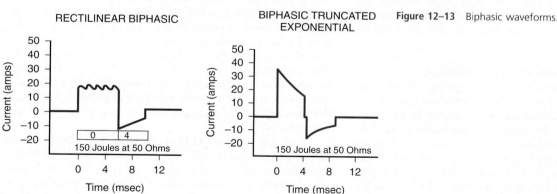

Figure 12–13 Biphasic waveforms.

Figure 12–14 Waveforms for external defibrillation.

energy level. Therefore, acquiring familiarity with the type of waveform that a particular defibrillator produces may be useful when it comes time to make the energy selection for defibrillation. A brief overview of the various waveforms is provided.

Defibrillators can also be categorized or described by their operational characteristics. Defibrillators can be described as *manual*, *semiautomated*, and *fully automatic*, based on their operational characteristics.

Biphasic Defibrillators/Energy Selection

Defibrillators manufactured today are primarily biphasic. These devices produce an output waveform that flows back and forth between the electrodes, sending the current sequentially in both directions. These devices produce either a BTE (see Fig. 12–13) waveform or a biphasic rectilinear waveform (see Fig. 12–13). A brief description of the various types of waveforms and the ascribed significance are provided for the curious reader interested in further elaboration of defibrillator wave types. These devices have been found to deliver a more successful defibrillation shock using less energy and have been found to have a better first-shock defibrillation success.[7] Although an optimal energy level for first-shock biphasic waveform defibrillation that will provide the most effective termination rate for VF has not been established, several studies have demonstrated that using relatively low energy of 200 J or less is not harmful and is as effective, if not more so, than monophasic waveform shocks using higher energy (360 J).[28] Recommendations extrapolated from these studies suggest that it is reasonable to use the lowest energy range for the termination of VF that has been shown to be effective for a given type of defibrillator. This is termed the *device-specific effective waveform dose range*. Therefore, when using a defibrillator that produces a biphasic rectilinear waveform, energy levels of 120 J are appropriate; if the defibrillator produces a BTE waveform, energy ranges of 150 to 200 J are recommended. If the operator is unaware of the device-specific effective waveform dose range, a consensus default of 200 J should be used for the initial shock. Use of the least amount of energy possible to accomplish termination of VF is currently speculated to cause less myocardial damage and precipitate fewer nonperfusing rhythms after shock delivery. These biphasic defibrillators are replacing the older monophasic defibrillators.

Monophasic Defibrillators/Energy Selection

Monophasic defibrillators were the first type introduced (generally). These devices are still available in various patient care settings, but are being phased out of production by manufacturers. Hospitals and EMS systems are replacing these defibrillators with the newer biphasic type. These defibrillators were designed to produce an MDS (see Fig. 12–12) waveform for defibrillation. When using this type of defibrillator, expert consensus suggests that an energy level of 360 J be used for the first shock.[6] These defibrillators are still capable of performing a successful defibrillation and have not been deemed inferior.

Waveforms

Until recently, modern defibrillators put out what was termed a *damped, monophasic, half-sinusoidal waveform* or a *trapezoidal truncated exponential decay* (voltage falling instantaneously) waveform, further explained later. The trapezoidal waveform

was modified to resemble a square waveform. The more square the waveform, the more effective it was for experimental defibrillation.[29] In a comparison of square waveforms and damped half-sinusoidal waveforms (voltage falling to zero gradually) for animal defibrillation, it was found that less peak current per kilogram was needed with the square waveforms, although the average current levels were equivalent.[30] This work was extended further, leading to the development of multiple new biphasic waveforms. These waveforms are achieved by manipulating the current (amperes), amplitude, duration, voltage, and ultimately, the energy delivered to the myocardium.

In light of the current research into the utility of the various energy waveforms that modern-day defibrillators deliver, it would be relatively useful to briefly describe the terminology. Current output from a defibrillator is graphed with respect to time on an x-y cartesian plot. The form of the wave can be either monophasic or biphasic. A characteristic monophasic wave is described as a rapid positive unidirectional increase in current flow to a predetermined peak with a return to baseline. If the return of the current to baseline is gradual, the waveform is termed a *damped* waveform (MDS waveform). These waves often resemble a sine wave (see Fig. 12–12). If the return of the current level to baseline is paroxysmal or sudden, the wave is an MTE waveform (see Fig. 12–12). A rapid rise in current with respect to time with a slight plateau and then a subsequent paroxysmal or sudden reversal in current flow at a predetermined time until all of the energy is delivered with a return to baseline is termed a *biphasic* waveform because of the two phases—positive and negative—in current flow. Essentially, for a biphasic waveform to occur, current travels from one pad or paddle to the other, then a reversal occurs so that current now flows from the second pad or paddle to the first. If the polarity or direction of the current flow is gradual, the wave is termed a *damped* waveform. If the current reversal is abrupt, the waveform is deemed a *truncated exponential waveform*; hence, the term *biphasic truncated exponential waveform* (BTE) (see Fig. 12–13).

The highest current flow attained is termed the *peak* energy delivered. This, however, is not synonymous with the total amount of energy delivered. Energy is delivered throughout the duration or period of the wave. The current thinking is that if there is less peak energy and a smaller amount of energy delivered to the fibrillating myocytes, there will be less damage to the heart tissue. In addition, this may decrease the perpetuation of conditions favoring VF. This suggests that these waveforms will enhance defibrillation efficacy, decrease myocardial damage, and decrease postdefibrillation arrhythmias.[31,32]

The first biphasic AED approved by the U.S. Food and Drug Administration utilized a BTE waveform.[33] Additional experiments are being done to further explore various biphasic rectilinear first-pulse waveforms. The motive behind these modifications is to find an optimal waveform that will deliver the least amount of energy to the myocardium, thus decreasing the structural damage to the myocytes[34] while achieving successful defibrillation.[24,35,36] Injury to myocardial tissue has been associated with the peak current, not the amount of energy actually delivered to the myocytes.[37] With the biphasic defibrillators, lower energy levels (150–175 J) can be used without escalating the energy up to 300 or 360 J. Experimental findings suggest that the clinical outcomes of these defibrillations are equivalent to those that used the escalating monophasic shocks.[38] However, the actual delivered energy is dependent on thoracic resistance/transthoracic impedance. Currently manufactured defibrillators are capable of determining transthoracic impedance/resistance and can actually modify the waveform and thus the amount of energy delivered across the myocardium. A more detailed discussion of transthoracic impedance is presented later in this chapter. In current clinical practice, there is little clinical difference in the effectiveness of the currently available waveforms. The trend of the future will probably be to use biphasic, impedance compensating defibrillators. Currently, monophasic defibrillators are still in use in some locations. There is no evidence to exclusively support the use of one defibrillator waveform over the other at this time.

Manual Defibrillators

Manual defibrillator/monitors are the most likely type to be found in many clinical settings. However, some of the manual defibrillators recently manufactured now have rhythm-recognition capabilities and can be configured to function as an AED with the turn of a switch or dial. This is especially helpful when there is nobody qualified present to interpret the rhythm when SCA happens in a noncritical area of the hospital. This facilitates the performance of defibrillation in various noncritical patient care areas without the presence of a clinician.

Manual defibrillators require that the operator turn on the device, select the input (e.g., the quick-look paddles or the patient ECG electrodes), place the quick-look paddles or the multifunctional ECG or defibrillation pads onto the patient's chest, and determine the type of rhythm present (e.g., VF, pulseless VT). Subsequently, the operator must select the appropriate energy level for the particular patient, based on the type of defibrillator available (monophasic or biphasic), charge the capacitor, and deliver the shock by activating the appropriate controls. If the required action is cardioversion, the operator will need to execute the steps as described previously. However, the SYNC switch needs to be activated (*MODE/SYNC*) in order to perform a *synchronized shock*. Thus, the manual defibrillator requires the setting of several controls—the input selector, the energy level, the charge button—and checking of the mode switch, followed by delivery of the shock by depressing the "Shock" controls.

Semiautomated Defibrillators

Semiautomated defibrillators or automated AEDs require that the operator turn the device on, and follow the voice and/or visual prompts provided by the device (e.g., "attach electrodes to the patient's bare chest," to "press the analyze button" on the defibrillator to initiate analysis of the rhythm, and then to either "press the shock button" or "initiate CPR" as directed by the defibrillator). Actual operation of the AED requires fewer steps and decisions by the operator. Once the AED is turned on, either the operator must place the electrodes in the appropriate position on the victim's chest and then allow the unit to analyze the underlying ECG rhythm, which was triggered by completing the patient-defibrillator circuit when the electrodes were applied to the patient's chest or the operator will be required to or prompted to depress the "*analyze*" switch. The AED will then determine whether there is a shockable rhythm present. If so the operator will be prompted to "clear" the patient for defibrillation and then she

or he will depress the shock button, delivering the defibrillatory shock to the patient. The rhythm analysis and choice of energy are done by the preprogrammed electronics intrinsic to the device. In summary, the operator need only depress the analyze switch, if specific to this type of AED, and if applicable, the operator presses the "shock" button if defibrillation is indicated (i.e., a shockable rhythm is present). Some of these devices have an optional "override" control in the module to allow a clinician or other healthcare provider to change the sequence of operation, energy levels, and so on. (These details are device-specific and can be found in the operator's manual of the particular defibrillator in use.)

Fully Automatic Defibrillators

Fully automatic defibrillators require only that the operator turn the device on and connect the electrodes to the patient. Subsequently, the defibrillator analyzes and shocks the patient, if indicated, without any further operator input, based on preprogrammed or hard-wired programs. These devices are usually provided for families of patients with known unstable cardiac arrhythmias. It is doubtful that the health care professional will encounter this type of device in a clinical or patient care setting. The only other fully automatic" defibrillators are the implantable defibrillator/pacer units or AICDs. These devices are discussed in Chapter 13 of this text.

Pads/Electrodes

The patient is placed into the defibrillation circuit or interfaced with the defibrillator/monitor via the placement of handheld paddle electrodes or self-adhesive pad electrodes onto the chest (Fig. 12–15; see also Figs. 12–5 and 12–6) and/or back (Fig. 12–16). Most, if not all, defibrillators currently have multifunctional, handheld or insulated paddles with several controls located on the handles, which can acquire the electrocardiogram and be used to deliver the defibrillation shock. The controls usually provided are for setting energy levels for the shock, a charge button for charging the capacitor remotely from the patient's side, and two "shock" buttons,

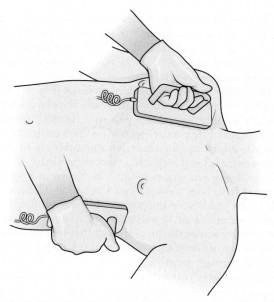

Figure 12–15 Use of quick-look paddle electrodes for rhythm (ECG) determination and defibrillation.

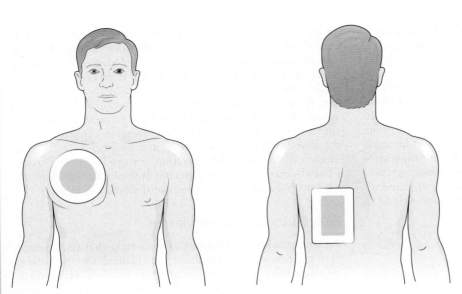

Figure 12–16 Front/back position of electrodes on patient (alternate position).

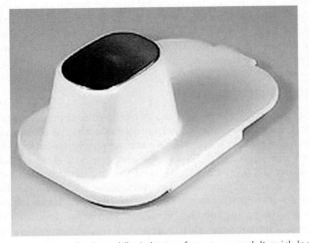

Figure 12–17 Pediatric paddles/adapters for use over adult quick-look paddles.

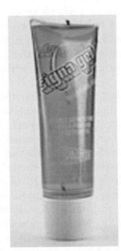

Figure 12–18 A 250-g tube of conductive gel for defibrillation.

one on each paddle, to actually deliver the shock. (*Both buttons usually have to be depressed to deliver the shock.*) (Some defibrillators also have "event-marker buttons," which allow the operator to mark an event such as administration of medication during the resuscitation.)

The paddles may have adapters on them (Fig. 12–17) for the purpose of pediatric defibrillation and the electrodes may vary in size to allow use in the pediatric patient[39] (discussed in the "Pediatric Equipment" section). When using the hand-held paddle electrodes for adult defibrillation, use of the 12-cm-diameter paddles, if available, is recommended.[40] However, pad electrodes or electrodes ranging in size from 8 to 12 cm in diameter have been shown to perform well. The goal is to use the larger paddles for the purpose of decreasing resistance or impedance at the chest wall and for providing an optimal current density across the myocardium that will be successful in terminating VF while causing minimal to no significant myocardial damage from excess current.[41] To this end, use the largest available pads or paddles that will fit on the chest wall without overlap.[41] Try to avoid using paddles that are too small in diameter, because they may cause myocardial necrosis.[42]

Conductive Materials

Use of conductive materials (Fig. 12–18) is important to lower the impedance or resistance to current flow at the electrode–chest wall interface. High impedance or resistance to current flow can compromise the amount of current actually delivered to the myocardium, leading to a failed first shock. Inappropriate use of conductive material can lead to current bridging or a short circuit and arcing of electrical current. This can cause spark production and unnecessary burns on the patient's skin. In addition, the arcing of electricity can become a possible explosion hazard, depending on the circumstances. These conductive materials need to be used when using the hand-held electrodes. There are various electrode gels on the market; these should be kept in the proximity of the defibrillator, on the prearranged cart ready to use (see Fig. 12–3) (*Do not use ultrasound gel!!*).

The mean range of impedance across the human chest wall varies from 70 to 80 ohms,[43–45] with bare skin contact yielding an impedance value of approximately 91 ± 20 ohms. With the use of saline-soaked pads, the impedance decreases to about 71 ± 11 ohms and with the conductive gel to 64 ±

15 ohms. Multiple factors affect this range of impedance (e.g., body weight, chest size, chest hair, moisture on the skin surface of the patient, paddle size [diameter], paddle contact pressure, phase of respiration, and type of conductive material used). The number of serial shocks delivered and the interval between shocks were believed to affect chest wall impedance. However, with the use of and application of biphasic defibrillation waveforms, the clinical significance of this issue has been abandoned.[46]

Self-adhesive pad electrodes now have a resistance-reducing, conductive material incorporated into the adhesive, rendering the use of a gel or other conductive material unnecessary. Firmly applying the self-adhesive electrode pads to the skin will usually be sufficient enough to minimize the impedance and allow adequate ECG acquisition and, if indicated, defibrillation.

PROCEDURE

Witnessed SCA (Fig. 12–19)

When confronted with a patient who has just become unresponsive, the emergency clinician (EC) or health care provider (HCP) should summon assistance from the ED team and follow guidelines for universal precautions. The defibrillation equipment should expediently be brought to the patient's side and preparation for immediate defibrillation should begin. *As soon as the defibrillator is available and the patient is connected to the monitor, rhythm assessment should begin.*

In the interim, as the defibrillation equipment is being turned on and the paddles or electrodes are being readied for placement on the chest, the EC/HCP should begin assessment of the patient and initiate the steps of CPR by applying the ABCs. If more than one person/HCP is present, several tasks can be performed simultaneously. The victim can be assessed by one rescuer as the equipment is readied by others and preparations are made to initiate resuscitation. If enough staff members/resuscitation team members are available, one staff member can prepare to ventilate the patient, while another positions himself or herself for possible chest compressions.

CPR

The victim's airway should be opened by using the head-tilt/chin-lift method. If cervical spine injury is suspected, the jaw-thrust maneuver should be used. Then, using the "look, listen, and feel" maneuver, the patient's airway should be evaluated by the EC/HCP. This is done by the rescuer placing her or his ear close to the victim's mouth and nose while looking down at the patient's chest to assess whether the patient is breathing. If there is no chest wall movement and no airflow is perceived to be coming through the mouth or nose, the patient is deemed to be apneic. Auscultating the patient with a stethoscope may be attempted to verify lack of air movement in the airways. If there is no evidence of breathing, ventilation must be initiated. The patient is then slowly ventilated, delivering two breaths using either a bag-valve mask (BVM) or some type of barrier device. The ventilations are interposed over 2 seconds, providing one breath/sec. The EC/HCP doing the ventilation should proceed carefully, observing for modest chest wall rise and fall, so as not to overinflate the thorax. Hyperinflation of the chest can lead to inadvertent pressurization of the esophagus, causing the lower esophageal sphincter pressures to be exceeded. This can lead to retro-grade flow of gastric contents into the esophagus, with the potential for subsequent aspiration of acid and debris into the trachea, if the airway is not adequately protected.

Next circulatory status must be determined. A quick attempt (≤10 sec) to check for a carotid pulse in the unresponsive, pulseless victim should be made. If the provider does not definitively feel a pulse, CPR should be initiated. If a pulse is absolutely present, then ventilation at 10 to 12 breaths/min or 1 breath every 5 to 6 seconds should be provided. If there is no pulse, start compressions immediately. The compression to ventilation ratio should be 30 compressions for every 2 ventilations. The rate of chest compressions should be 100 compressions/min or more. The rescuer performing the compressions should push hard and push fast. Every attempt should be made to minimize interruptions of compressions. Continue until the defibrillator is available.

Rhythm Assessment

Once the defibrillator is at the bedside, the defibrillator/monitor should be turned on and the electrodes should be placed on the patient's chest using either the quick-look paddles or the multifunctional electrode pads that can acquire ECG signals and be used concomitantly to defibrillate the patient. The handheld electrode paddles should have a conductive material such as a gel applied to the contact surface of the electrodes to decrease chest wall impedance. Care should be taken to avoid streaking the electrode gel or comparable material across the chest because this could cause electrical arcing, sparks, burns, and an electrical short circuit. This would be unfavorable for the patient and also compromise the efficacy of the defibrillation current across the myocardium, leading to an unsuccessful attempt at defibrillation. The gel is not indicated when using the multifunctional electrode pads on the chest.

The correct position for the placement of either the handheld quick-look paddle electrodes (see Fig. 12–15) or the self-adhesive pads (see Fig. 12–16) is illustrated in the depicted figures. Often, the pads are labeled with a diagram to help in placing the electrodes onto the chest wall (see Fig. 12–6). Using the patient's right side for orientation, the sternal electrode is placed just below the clavicle, just to the right of the sternum. The apical electrode is placed in the midaxillary line around the fifth or sixth intercostal space (Fig. 12–20). This approximates the lead 2 position for ECG acquisition. Once the electrodes or pads are in position, the selector dial or switch on the defibrillator monitor should be set to the appropriate position to acquire the ECG signal from the correct input source—either the handheld quick-look paddles or the multifunctional electrode pads. Errors sometimes occur when the selector switch is in the position for the patient cable and electrode pads while the operator is attempting to use the handheld paddles. (This could lead to misinterpretation of the rhythm, in which the operator perceives that the patient is in asystole, while in reality VF, pulseless VT, or some other rhythm is actually present.) (Be familiar with the operation of the switches!) In addition, the controls for gain of ECG signal should be adjusted to increase the sensitivity or gain of the ECG amplifier to ensure that fine VF is not interpreted as asystole. As the ECG rhythm appears on the monitor, a diagnosis of the type of rhythm, or lack thereof, should be made. If there is a shockable rhythm (i.e., VF or pulseless VT), defibrillation is indicated and the operator should proceed to select the appropriate energy level for the anticipated defibrillation.

223

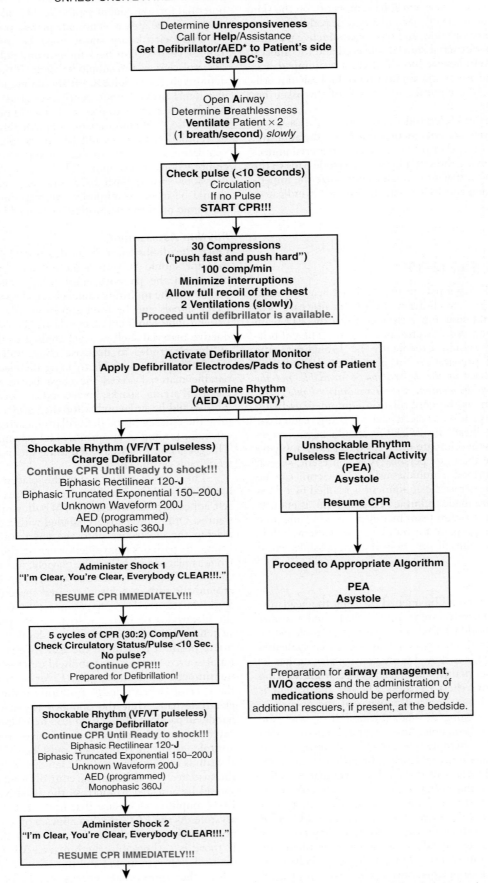

Figure 12–19 Unresponsive adult patient/witnessed sudden cardiac arrest (SCA)/ventricular fibrillation (VF)/pulseless ventricular tachycardia (VT).

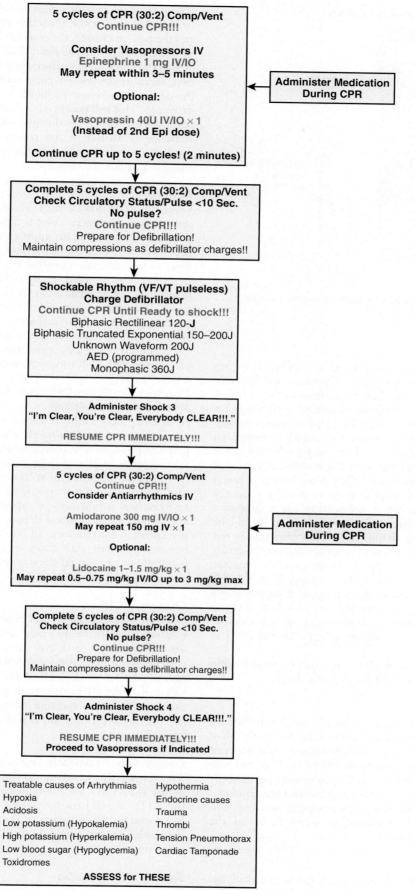

5 cycles of CPR (30:2) Comp/Vent
Continue CPR!!!

Consider Vasopressors IV
Epinephrine 1 mg IV/IO
May repeat within 3–5 minutes

Optional:

Vasopressin 40U IV/IO × 1
(Instead of 2nd Epi dose)

Continue CPR up to 5 cycles! (2 minutes)

Administer Medication During CPR

Complete 5 cycles of CPR (30:2) Comp/Vent
Check Circulatory Status/Pulse <10 Sec.
No pulse?
Continue CPR!!!
Prepare for Defibrillation!
Maintain compressions as defibrillator charges!!

Shockable Rhythm (VF/VT pulseless)
Charge Defibrillator
Continue CPR Until Ready to shock!!!
Biphasic Rectilinear 120-**J**
Biphasic Truncated Exponential 150–200J
Unknown Waveform 200J
AED (programmed)
Monophasic 360J

Administer Shock 3
"I'm Clear, You're Clear, Everybody CLEAR!!!."

RESUME CPR IMMEDIATELY!!!

5 cycles of CPR (30:2) Comp/Vent
Continue CPR!!!
Consider Antiarrhythmics IV

Amiodarone 300 mg IV/IO × 1
May repeat 150 mg IV × 1

Optional:

Lidocaine 1–1.5 mg/kg × 1
May repeat 0.5–0.75 mg/kg IV/IO up to 3 mg/kg max

Administer Medication During CPR

Complete 5 cycles of CPR (30:2) Comp/Vent
Check Circulatory Status/Pulse <10 Sec.
No pulse?
Continue CPR!!!
Prepare for Defibrillation!
Maintain compressions as defibrillator charges!!

Administer Shock 4
"I'm Clear, You're Clear, Everybody CLEAR!!!."

RESUME CPR IMMEDIATELY!!!
Proceed to Vasopressors if Indicated

Treatable causes of Arrhythmias   Hypothermia
Hypoxia   Endocrine causes
Acidosis   Trauma
Low potassium (Hypokalemia)   Thrombi
High potassium (Hyperkalemia)   Tension Pneumothorax
Low blood sugar (Hypoglycemia)   Cardiac Tamponade
Toxidromes

ASSESS for THESE

Figure 12–19, cont'd

225

DEFIBRILLATOR PAD PLACEMENT

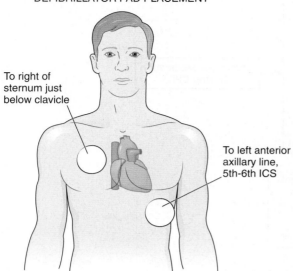

To right of sternum just below clavicle

To left anterior axillary line, 5th-6th ICS

Figure 12–20   Correct position for electrode/paddle placement.

Energy Selection

As noted previously, two major types of defibrillators are available: biphasic and monophasic. Currently, the biphasic defibrillator, which is more likely to be found in the clinical setting, produces either a biphasic rectilinear waveform or a BTE waveform (see Fig. 12–13). In addition, there are still monophasic defibrillators present that usually produce an MDS waveform (see Fig. 12–12). The energy delivered to the myocardium varies somewhat with the waveform produced by each respective defibrillator. Therefore, having a priori knowledge of the device-specific effective waveform energy range would be helpful when considering the appropriate energy level for defibrillation. This information should be posted on the respective defibrillator. However, this is not always easy to locate. Therefore, the following recommendations are made: In general, the defibrillator using the biphasic rectilinear waveform should be set to an energy level of 120 J. If a BTE defibrillator waveform is being used, energy levels of 150 to 200 J are suggested for the first shock. If the type of waveform of the biphasic defibrillator is unknown or unavailable, the consensus default energy level of 200 J is suggested.

If the defibrillator is an older monophasic model using the MDS waveform, use 360 J for the first shock.

Mode Selection

Prior to defibrillation, the operator should check to make sure that the defibrillator is set to the unsynchronized mode. Most defibrillators default into the unsynchronized mode between shocks; nonetheless, this control should be checked to make sure it is in the unsynchronized mode; otherwise, the defibrillator may not discharge when the shock buttons are depressed because it is looking for the QRS complex, which is not present in VF. This is discussed in more detail in the "Cardioversion" section later.

Defibrillate

Once the energy level has been selected and the decision has been made to defibrillate, the operator should simultaneously clear the patient for defibrillation by loudly stating "I'm clear, you're clear, everybody's clear" while the button is activated to charge the capacitor. Once the capacitor has been charged and the patient cleared, the rescuer should apply firm pressure to the defibrillation paddles (25 lb) to increase contact and deflate the lungs to the end-expiration state. This will decrease impedance at the paddle–chest wall interface. Subsequently, the defibrillation controls should be depressed and the shock delivered. This will usually be followed by a perceptible whole body muscle twitch in the patient. (If there is no obvious response or twitch of the patient, check the defibrillator controls to make sure it is in the unsynchronized mode and that the paddles are activated.)

Resume CPR

Once the shock has been delivered, the resuscitation should resume with immediate chest compressions. (These compressions should continue for approximately 5 cycles of 30 compressions to 2 ventilations or about 2 min of CPR.) This is done to facilitate the transition from SCA to ROSC after the heart has been stunned by the defibrillation and may not be functioning at optimal contractility for a few minutes after shock. If there are additional monitoring devices in place such as arterial lines or Swan catheters, this step may be modified accordingly as decided by the resuscitation team leader.

Continue CPR for approximately 2 minutes. If the rescuers become fatigued, rotate the compressor and ventilator.

Reassess the Patient/Manage Airway and Intravenous Access

After 2 minutes of CPR (5 cycles of 30:2), the patient's perfusion status or carotid pulses should be checked. If there is no palpable pulse, resume compressions immediately and prepare for delivery of a second defibrillatory shock.

As preparation for the second shock begins, the members of the resuscitation team can work on securing the airway via endotracheal intubation, laryngeal mask airway, or another appropriate device. Blood draws, and intravenous (IV) line placement, or intraosseous (IO) if applicable, should proceed, but not interfere with chest compressions. The goal is to maintain uninterrupted chest compressions and to avoid any unnecessary interruptions.

Change in CPR

Once an advanced airway has been secured, compression and ventilation cycles are no longer delivered. Now the compressor will continue to deliver compressions at a rate of 100 compressions/min *continuously*, without pausing for interposition of ventilation. The HCP/EC delivering the ventilations will provide 8 to 10 breaths/min, taking care not to overinflate the chest or to use too much force during ventilation so as not too overpressurize the airways and esophagus, potentiating reflux.

Energy Selection/Mode Selection Second Shock

The second shock energy can be the same as the one used before (i.e., 120 J for the biphasic rectilinear, 150–200 J for the BTE, or 360 J for the MDS). A higher energy level can be chosen at the discretion of the resuscitation leader. Again the mode selector should be checked to be in the unsynchronized position.

Second Defibrillation

Once the energy has been selected, the operator should charge the capacitor and CPR should be halted. The operator should clear the patient as discussed earlier and deliver the second shock.

CPR

CPR should be resumed immediately after the delivery of the second shock. This step can be modified at the discretion of the resuscitation team leader, if there is clinical evidence of ROSC or if monitoring devices are being utilized to monitor circulatory status (e.g., CVP monitor, Swan-Ganz catheter, or direct arterial line).

Unwitnessed Arrest

When the HCP/EC encounters a patient who is unresponsive and who has been down for an unknown amount of time, he or she should assess the patient, summon help, and initiate CPR immediately, if indicated. Perform CPR until the defibrillator or AED is brought to the patient's side. As preparations are being made for defibrillation, the team leader may consider performance of 5 cycles of 30:2 compressions-to-ventilations before performing defibrillation. Data from pre-hospital studies suggest that if a patient has a prolonged down time (>4–5 min), performance of CPR prior to defibrillation may facilitate first-shock defibrillation.[11] No data are currently available to support or refute this sequence in the in-hospital setting.

AED Application (see Fig. 12–19)

The presence of AEDs or semiautomated defibrillators in hospitals has increased, especially in non–critical care areas. Although AEDs are designed for lay public use, application of these devices may occur in the clinical setting. As in the algorithm, the patient must be assessed, help must be summoned, and the AED should be applied. Operation of the AED is guided by voice and visual prompts. The device must be turned on, the patient electrodes applied in the appropriate positions, the rhythm analyzed, and a shock delivered if a shockable rhythm is present. Choice of energy and rhythm determination are performed by the AED. The rescuers must integrate CPR with the shocks to enhance the potential outcome of SCA resuscitation.

Medication

Use of medication has been deemphasized, *but not abandoned*, in the current recommendations for resuscitation of SCA, VF, and pulseless VT. Therefore, if VF continues after two attempts at defibrillation with interposed CPR and there is no ROSC, CPR must be continued and the use of a vasopressor such as epinephrine (1 mg IV) or vasopressin (40 U IV) can be considered after the establishment of vascular access via IV or IO line if needed. These medications should be administered during compressions either before or after the shock, without causing *any disruption* in the continuity and speed of chest compressions.

Epinephrine (1 mg IV) can be given, CPR continued, and another shock administered, if indicated. The epinephrine (1 mg) can be repeated every 3 to 5 minutes. Another option is to give vasopressin. Vasopressin (40 U IV) can replace either the first or the second dose of epinephrine. The details of the individual drug pharmacology are given later.

If after several additional cycles of CPR, defibrillation, and administration of vasopressors, VF still persists, the use of an antiarrythmic agent such as amiodarone or lidocaine should be considered. After the first dose of amiodarone (300 mg IV/IO), a one-time subsequent dose of amiodarone (150 mg IV/IO) can be repeated or lidocaine (1–1.5 mg/kg IV/IO, first dose; followed by 0.5 to 0.75 mg/kg IV/IO) to a maximum of three doses or 3 mg/kg may be considered.

Remember that administration of IV or IO medications should be done during chest compressions, minimizing interruption of CPR. Shocks should be administered, if indicated, approximately every 2 minutes (5 cycles of CPR, 30:2 compressions-to-ventilations) after the medications have been given and circulated via chest compressions. If there is evidence of an organized rhythm on the monitor, after 2 minutes of CPR, a circulatory assessment (pulse check) should be attempted to determine whether ROSC has occurred. This step can be modified as needed by the code team leader, depending on the type of instrumentation and monitoring capabilities available during the resuscitation. Shocks should be administered as quickly as possible after compressions are held for defibrillation.

Premixing of the drugs by additional staff members, if present, may minimize interruptions in CPR. Also, flushing of the medication with 20 mL of compatible IV fluid (i.e., saline) and elevating the extremity in which the medication was pushed for 10 to 20 seconds may facilitate delivery of the medication into the circulation.

If pulseless VT or VF is associated with torsades de pointes, providers may consider administering 1 to 2 g of magnesium sulfate in 10 mL of D_5W IV or IO over 5 to 20 minutes, in a pulseless victim. If the victim has a pulse, consider administering 1 to 2 g of magnesium sulfate that has been mixed in 50 to 100 mL of D_5W as a loading dose.

Epinephrine. Epinephrine is chemically prepared and stored in aqueous solution as epinephrine hydrochloride. This medication is a catecholamine with adrenergic properties. Epinephrine stimulates both α- and β-receptors, producing what are termed *α- and β-effects.* Stimulation of the α-adrenergic receptors in the vasculature causes the vascular smooth muscle to contract (vasoconstriction). This change in vessel diameter in the coronary arteries and cerebral vasculature produces an increase in perfusion pressure in the heart and brain. Stimulation of the β-receptors in the heart ($β_1$) causes increases in heart rate and contractility, leading to an increase in myocardial workload. Furthermore, β-effects in the myocardium can lead to reduced subendocardial perfusion and ischemia. There is a dearth of evidence to support that epinephrine increases survival of SCA in humans. The use of high-dose epinephrine has showed limited results regarding early increases in ROSC and survival to hospital arrival; however, no significant changes have been manifested in survival to hospital discharge rates or to improved neurologic outcomes.

Nonetheless, epinephrine remains as a class IIb recommended drug for SCA and VF resuscitation.

Epinephrine can be given in 1 mg doses IV or IO and repeated every 3 to 5 minutes during the resuscitation of adult SCA. Higher doses may be considered when β-blocker or calcium channel blocker ingestion is an issue. If IV or IO access is unavailable, epinephrine can be given via the endotracheal tube; however, the dosage must be double the IV or IO dose.

Vasopressin. Vasopressin is a potent vasoconstrictor that causes the coronary and renal vasculature to constrict.

Because vasopressin is not an adrenergic agent, it does not have the same effect on the myocardial workload that epinephrine can have. However, scientific evaluation of this drug fails to differentiate vasopressin from epinephrine regarding clinical outcome of SCA resuscitation. There are some data to support increased survival to hospital discharge; however, the same claim cannot be made regarding improved neurologic outcomes in SCA resuscitation. However, this drug may be used once after the administration of epinephrine during the resuscitation, or it can replace the first dose of epinephrine during SCA resuscitation. The recommended dose is vasopressin 40 U IV or IO. If IV or IO access is not available, vasopressin can be administered via the endotracheal tube. However, the dose must be doubled to achieve appropriate blood levels of the drug and absorption will be obviously slower than with the IV or IO route.

Amiodarone. Amiodarone is a versatile drug that can be used to treat VF and pulseless VT resistant to defibrillation, CPR, and vasopressors. It also has usefulness in the treatment of various tachydysrhythmias, discussed later in the chapter. This medication actually blocks α- and β-adrenergic effects. In addition, amiodarone affects the kinetics of the sodium, potassium, and calcium channels. Amiodarone has been reformulated with different solvents to minimize the vasoactive or hypotensive side effects it produces. This drug has been shown to improve survival to hospital admission when compared with placebo. Data also suggest that amiodarone has a better profile for survival to hospital admission of patients in VF or unstable VT. The recommended dose of amiodarone is a 300-mg bolus IV or IO for pulseless VT and VF. A second one-time dose of 150 mg of amiodarone IV/IO may be considered if indicated.

Lidocaine. Lidocaine has been available for quite some time. It was frequently used to suppress ventricular premature beats and various arrhythmias of ventricular origin that occurred after MI. This drug affects sodium channel mechanics and suppresses ventricular irritability. Lidocaine has been used as a treatment for refractory VF in the past; however, there are no data to support its efficacy in short- or long-term outcomes. A comparison of lidocaine to amiodarone has suggested that lidocaine may cause a greater incidence of asystole after defibrillation. Furthermore, lidocaine had a lower rate of ROSC than amiodarone. In addition, amiodarone appears to have a better survival to hospital admission profile.

Nonetheless, lidocaine is an alternative antiarrhythmic that is familiar to many clinicians and has relatively few immediate side effects. It is currently considered an alternative treatment to amiodarone for refractory VF and pulseless VT. The recommended dose for lidocaine is 1 to 1.5 mg/kg IV/IO. If the first dose is unsuccessful and VF persists after defibrillation, a repeat dose of 0.5 to 0.75 mg/kg IV push may be considered at 5- to 10-minute intervals. The maximum dose should not exceed 3 mg/kg.

If IV or IO access is unavailable, lidocaine can be administered via the endotracheal tube; however, the dose must be increased by 2 to 2.5 times the IV dose.

Magnesium Sulfate. Magnesium has uses in other medical venues (e.g., obstetrics, gynecology, and possibly pulmonary medicine); however, it has been shown to be effective in the treatment of polymorphic or irregular VT (torsades de pointes) associated with a prolonged Q-T interval. This drug is not considered significantly effective in treating irregular or polymorphic VT in patients with a normal Q-T interval. If VF or pulseless VT cardiac arrest occurs in the face of torsades de pointes, 1 to 2 g of magnesium sulfate, diluted in 10 mL D_5W IV/IO can be administered. If the patient has pulses and torsades de pointes is present, consider administering 1 to 2 g of magnesium sulfate mixed with 50 to 100 ml of D_5W as a loading dose.

RECOGNITION OF VF

Characteristics of VF

ECG Characteristics (Electrocardiography and the Electromechanical Physiology)

VF is characterized on the electrocardiogram by the presence of what appears to be a chaotic, random squiggly line (see Fig. 12–2). The actual display is one of rather low-amplitude baseline undulations that are variable in both magnitude and periodicity of the waveform. Care must be taken to ensure that appropriate electrode contact with the patient is maintained and that the leads are all appropriately attached so as not to interpret VF as artifact or vice versa. Although many consider VF to represent an electrically disorganized process, electrical directionality to depolarization (i.e., wave front) can exist,[46] manifesting the characteristic VF waveform or a flat line resembling asystole, depending on monitor lead orientation. It is therefore recommended that when assessing for the presence of VF versus asystole, several ECG leads be checked, differing by 90° in orientation, and that the gain of the monitor be adjusted to the highest or most sensitive level.[47]

The resultant ECG tracing seen in VF is the resultant sum of voltage variations with respect to time from the discharge of multiple ectopic foci or induced ectopic pacemakers of the ischemic, hypoxic, electrically irritable ventricle. As the many electrical dipoles of myocyte depolarization travel through the ventricular myocardium, the randomness in the orientation of the positive leading edge of the dipoles causes the variation in the polarity of the ECG tracing. The combination of the mass of ventricular tissue undergoing VF and the sum of the dipole directions actually determines the amplitude of the undulations.

Mechanically, VF represents an uncoordinated and distinctly disorderly, ineffective contractile process. Usually the SA node depolarizes at an average rate range of 60 to 80 beats/min. Subsequently, the atria are depolarized and the electrical depolarization front traverses the AV node. The impulse is slowed through the node's, decremental conduction, to allow for adequate ventricular filling. Upon activation of the bundle of His and the Purkinje fibers, the interventricular septum and the right and left ventricular free walls contract, decreasing ventricular volume and increasing ventricular pressure so that the blood can be propelled into the elastic aorta—the stroke volume is ejected from the ventricle. The lack of an organized ventricular systole causes a compromise in cardiac stroke volume. Subsequently, cardiac output falls, resulting in lack of adequate tissue perfusion, ischemia, and hypoxemia of the target organs. If left uncorrected, VF leads to irreversible tissue damage resulting in death.

At the tissue level, VF represents a disorganization of the orderly depolarization sequence that usually occurs in the ventricles. Normally, the refractory period of depolarized muscle prevents the development of re-entrant ventricular rhythms by blocking the pathway of returning depolarization fronts. When ischemia, electrolyte disorders, cardiac drug toxicities, rapid ventricular rates, hypothermia, and certain other disorders exist, refractory periods may shorten or conduction velocities may tend to increase in certain areas of the ventricle. Wandering depolarization wave fronts can retra-

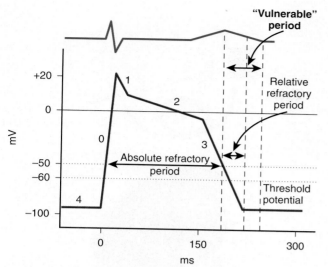

Figure 12–21 Vulnerable period of the cardiac cycle.

verse the nonrefractory areas of the ventricular myocardium, providing conditions in which a self-perpetuating ectopic focus can develop. A combination of disorders of impulse formation (automaticity) and impulse conduction (re-entry) contributes to the development of VF. The tendency for VF to occur is enhanced by, but is not entirely dependent on, premature ventricular impulses that occur during the vulnerable period of the cardiac cycle represented by early ventricular repolarization (Fig. 12–21).

Asynchronous ventricular depolarization may be confined to a small area of the ventricle if the remaining ventricle is refractory to further stimulation. Several studies have shown that a critical muscle mass is required for VF to be self-sustaining, possibly explaining why VF is so uncommon in infants undergoing resuscitation (who usually die from respiratory arrest). A large mass of muscle involved in asynchronous depolarization having a brief refractory period and a slow conduction velocity increases the tendency for the ventricles to fibrillate.

Cummins and coworkers[48,49] classified VF on the basis of average peak-to-trough wave amplitude (see Fig. 12–4). They note that the amplitude of the VF waveform is associated positively with the probability of resuming a perfusing rhythm. However, the clinical importance of coarse versus fine VF in relation to ultimate survival is unclear. Signals that have an amplitude of less than 1 mm (when the monitor is calibrated at 10 mm/mV) should be considered to indicate asystole[48,49] because countershock of such low-amplitude rhythms is only rarely associated with conversion to a perfusing rhythm.[50,51] It has been reported that as ventricular fibrillation continues in the face of ventricular ischemia or hypoxia for a time period exceeding 4 minutes, the waveform of VF changes, decreasing in amplitude and progressing to asystole.[52,53] This may be an indication that the myocytes are deteriorating and becoming unsalvageable with respect to VF unless some pharmacologic or mechanical resuscitation takes place first.[54]

A new approach to the analysis of VF is being explored. Termed *amplitude spectrum area*, this methodology may prove to have the potential of enhancing the likelihood that an electrical countershock will restore a perfusing rhythm, in a porcine model. These data, if proved useful, may allow more selective timing of shock administration and enhance the effi-

cacy of defibrillation while decreasing myocardial damage from defibrillation.[55] Human studies of out-of-hospital cardiac arrest electrocardiograms suggest that the centroid frequency and peak power frequency of the electrocardiogram depicting VF may be predictive of successful countershock.[56] However, the data to date have not led to any specific recommendations by the American Heart Association.

In summary, electrical defibrillation represents the simultaneous depolarization of sufficient ventricular tissue to render the tissue that is ahead of the VF wave fronts refractory to further electrical conduction. After generalized depolarization, the sinus node or another pacemaker region of the heart with the highest degree of automaticity can then acquire dominance of a well-ordered depolarization-repolarization sequence. Application of the defibrillation current at various time points in the cardiac cycle may affect the outcome of the countershock. A more comprehensive discussion of this topic appears in the "Cardioversion" section of this chapter.

Complications

Complications of defibrillation are soft tissue injury, myocardial injury, and cardiac dysrhythmias. Availability of multifunctional electrode pads and better applicators for electrode gels have decreased the potential for soft tissue injuries such as burns to the chest.[57] In fact, many clinicians now prefer to use the multifunctional electrode pads for ECG acquisition and for defibrillation.

Development of new, energy-efficient biphasic defibrillation waveforms, such as the BTE and the rectilinear biphasic waveform have increased first-shock success and decreased postdefibrillation dysrhythmias.[7] As a result, fewer shocks are needed to defibrillate the myocardium, and less current is applied to the myocardium, rendering less potential electrical damage to the myocytes.

Use of AEDs in PAD programs has not been reported to have produced any significant mishaps or adverse outcomes.[6]

Some older recommendations, such as the use of the precordial thump, have been retracted. This procedure has been reported to have caused asystole and/or complete heart block when applied.[58]

In addition, the use of procainamide, although not a complication, has fallen out of favor owing to long infusion times and mixed results regarding the efficacy of procainamide's effects during the acute phase of VF/pulseless VT resuscitation.[58]

PEDIATRIC DEFIBRILLATION

SCA/VF/pulseless VT is less likely to occur in children. However, 5% to 15% of pediatric and adolescent SCA events demonstrate VF in the prehospital setting. In-hospital arrests report a 20% occurrence of VF at some point during the resuscitation. Nonetheless, rapid intervention and defibrillation improve outcomes from SCA. Causes of SCA/VF/pulseless VT are more diverse.[59] Cardiac arrest usually does not occur as a result of a primary cardiac cause. Therefore, the approach to resuscitation of a pediatric patient in VF/pulseless VT may differ based on the etiology of the arrest.

VF in Children

VF is much less common in children than in adults. The etiology behind VF/SCA is most likely to be sudden infant death syndrome, respiratory compromise, sepsis, neurologic disease, and injuries.[60] Many of the injuries, such as motor vehicle crash injuries, pedestrian versus auto injuries, burns, firearm injuries, and drowning, are preventable.[61] There is an age-related pattern to the occurrence of cardiac arrest in the pediatric population: about half of the cardiac arrests that occur in children occur before the age of 1. After a child reaches 6 months of age, injuries and drowning are reported to be the major causes of death. The most common terminal rhythms reported in children under the age of 17 are PEA, bradycardia, and asystole.[62] The etiology behind these pediatric arrhythmias is most often hypoxemia, hypotension, hypoglycemia, and acidemia. In addition, focal electrical ectopy is less likely to initiate VF in the young heart. A significant myocardial mass must be unstable and fibrillating before VF becomes established. In children (from birth to 8 yr) with nontraumatic arrest, only 3% of the dysrhythmias are reported to be VF. In victims aged 8 to 30 years, the number of VF patients increases by almost sixfold (17%).[63] Several subpopulations of pediatric patients at various ages with cardiomyopathy or myocarditis or who have undergone heart surgery are at increased risk for a primary dysrhythmia.

As noted previously, the incidence of VF in cardiac arrest rhythms of pediatric patients is reported to range from 7% to 15%.[64] Others have reported that approximately 10% of reported pediatric cardiac arrest patients had VF.[65] In a retrospective out-of-hospital study of pediatric patients, VF was reported to have been found in almost 20% of the cardiac arrest victims.[64] Patients with rhythms who have been defibrillated from VF have been reported to have a higher survival to discharge rate than children who sustained asystole or PEA.[64] Therefore, there is a definite indication for early defibrillation in the pediatric population.

Procedure and Technique

The procedure for pediatric defibrillation is similar to the algorithm for adult defibrillation (see Fig. 12–19). However, a few differences must be addressed. These are discussed later.

The guidelines described later apply to children from about 1 year of age to the start of puberty. These guidelines do not apply to children younger than 1 year of age.

Pediatric SCA. When cardiac arrest occurs in a child, it is usually a terminal event of respiratory compromise or shock. The probability of SCA occurring from a primary cardiac cause is extremely low.[65] Nonetheless, it can and does occur. If prompt resuscitation occurs, the potential for a positive outcome, including preserving the patient's neurologic integrity, is quite high. To enhance the outcome of SCA resuscitation, defibrillation and CPR must be effectively integrated. The pediatric resuscitation guidelines[66] incorporated findings from a comprehensive review of the data. The revised steps for the recommended resuscitation sequence are described later.

Equipment. To perform pediatric defibrillation, a defibrillator monitor capable of energy adjustments appropriate for children is needed. If an AED is to be used, it should have an energy attenuator for adjusting the energy to the appropriate level for a child (Fig. 12–22). In addition, the quick-look electrode paddles (see Fig. 12–17) should have the appropriate adapters attached to the adult paddles to ensure appropriate contact with the chest wall without causing electrodes to

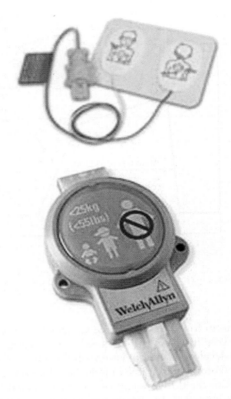

Figure 12–22 Pediatric AED energy attenuator.

overlap. If adhesive pads are used, choose the appropriate size that will not overlap. Use gels as in adults, being careful to prevent bridging across the chest wall due to streaks of conductive material that may have been carelessly applied to the chest.

Paddle/Pad Applications/Conductive Materials (The Details). To acquire the electrical rhythm and subsequently administer an effective defibrillatory shock, appropriate-sized pads and paddles must be correctly placed on the chest (see Fig. 12–19). The appropriate size and placement of the paddles or pads will ensure that the appropriate current density is delivered across the myocardium to effectively defibrillate the myocytes. Furthermore, appropriate pad or paddle size—the largest surface area possible without direct electrode-to-electrode contact—will decrease transthoracic impedance and enhance defibrillation.[67] To accomplish this, it is recommended that infant paddles be used in children weighing less than 10 kg. However, larger paddles can be used if they do not contact each other; if contact is made between the paddles, an electrical arc or short could occur.[66] In children who weigh more than 10 kg (mean age, 1 yr), it is recommended that adult pads or paddles are used (8–10 cm in diameter).[68] A conductive agent should be used to enhance skin contact and decrease transthoracic impedance. Never use dry paddles, because the resistance to current flow will be very large. However, refrain from using saline-soaked pads in children because they may cause arcing owing to the proximity of the pads on the chest. Remember that electricity will take the path of least resistance and that the current from defibrillation will travel across the chest if there is a saline bridge between the electrodes. In addition, the use of ultrasound gel and alcohol pads is discouraged because of poor electrical conductivity and potentially high impedance.[45]

The paddles or pads should be applied firmly to the chest, one to the right of the sternum, just below the clavicle (see Fig. 12–19), the other to the left of the left nipple, over the ribs (over the apex of the heart). An option when using self-adhesive pads is to place one pad just to the left of the sternum and the other over the back (see Fig. 12–16), approximating the position of the heart.[69]

Unresponsive Child. When confronted with an unresponsive child, the EC/HCP should immediately summon assistance and start the ABCs of CPR. Equipment for resuscitation should be expediently brought to the patient's side. If no help is immediately available, about 2 minutes of CPR should be done first, before leaving the patient's side. Remember, that the arrest may have been the result of respiratory compromise, and performance of CPR may ameliorate the condition.

If the victim is unresponsive to verbal and tactile stimuli, open the airway using the head-tilt/chin-lift method. If a spinal cord injury is suspected, use the jaw-thrust maneuver, without head-tilt.

Next, determine breathlessness. Look, listen, and feel for air movement from the mouth and nose while observing the victim's chest and abdomen for any signs of movement. If there is no perceivable evidence of breathing, provide two slow rescue breaths (1 breath/sec) that make the chest rise. Do not use excessive force while ventilating because this could cause regurgitation or aspiration, impede venous return to the heart, and decrease coronary blood flow as a result of increased intrathoracic pressure. After interposing the breaths, proceed to assess circulation by checking for a pulse, by either the carotid or femoral (<10 sec). If there is no palpable pulse or a very slow pulse less than 60 beats/min in very young children after 10 seconds of attempting to feel a pulse, initiate chest compressions.

Compress the lower half of the sternum, avoiding the xiphoid process. Compress the chest to approximately one third to one half the depth of the chest. The rate of compressions should be approximately 100 compressions/min. If a single rescuer is performing the compressions and ventilations, the compression-to-ventilation ratio should be 30:2. If two rescuers are available, the compression-to-ventilation ratio should be 15:2. Attempt to avoid interruptions of chest compressions.

If an adequate pulse is present, the rescuer should interpose 12 to 20 breaths/min (1 breath every 3–5 sec).

Once a defibrillator monitor or an AED is available, preparation for rhythm analysis and defibrillation, if indicated, should begin.

Rhythm Assessment. Once the defibrillator or monitor is at the patient's side, it should be turned on and the electrodes placed on the patient's chest. The positions of the electrodes on the child correspond to the positions used in the adult (see Figs. 12–15 and 12–16). If the quick-look paddles are used, carefully apply the conductive gel to the electrodes' surface. Remember that this is important to prevent arcing, burns, sparks, and other problems. If the self-adhesive multifunctional electrode pads are used, there is no need to use the conductive gel. Make sure that the input selector switch is reading from the appropriate source (i.e., paddles or pads). Adjust or increase the gain or sensitivity of the monitor so that fine VF is not missed owing to low amplitude. As the ECG rhythm appears on the monitor, the rhythm should be assessed and diagnosed. If VF or pulseless VT is present, proceed to select the appropriate energy level for the anticipated defibrillation.

Energy Selection. As mentioned earlier in the adult section of the chapter, two types of defibrillators are available: biphasic and monophasic. As of this writing, there is no specific, detailed differentiation between energy levels to be used by either type of defibrillator. However, the caveat that biphasic shocks are at least as effective as monophasic shocks and that they are less damaging to the myocardium still applies.

Based on a review of adult and pediatric animal data, when a manual defibrillator is used for the first shock attempt, an energy level of 2 joules/kg should be used, with either a biphasic or a monophasic defibrillator. If a second or subsequent defibrillation is indicated, then 4 J/kg should be used with either type.[70]

Mode Selection. Prior to defibrillation, the operator should check to make sure that the defibrillator is set to the unsynchronized mode for defibrillation. Most defibrillators default into the unsynchronized mode between shocks. Nonetheless, this control should be checked to make sure it is in the unsynchronized mode; otherwise, the defibrillator may not discharge when the shock buttons are depressed because it is looking for the QRS complex, which is not present in VF (this is discussed in more detail in the "Cardioversion" section, later).

Defibrillate. Once the energy level has been selected and the decision has been made to defibrillate, the operator should simultaneously clear the patient for defibrillation by loudly stating "I'm clear, you're clear, everybody's clear" while the button is activated to charge the capacitor. Once the capacitor has been charged and the patient cleared, the rescuer should apply firm pressure to the defibrillation paddles (25 lb) to increase contact and deflate the lungs to the end-expiration state. This will decrease impedance at the paddle–chest wall interface. Subsequently, the defibrillation controls should be depressed and the shock delivered. This will usually be followed by a perceptible whole body muscle twitch in the patient. (If there is no obvious response or twitch of the patient, check the defibrillator controls to make sure that it is in the unsynchronized mode and that the paddles are activated.)

Resume CPR. Once the shock has been delivered, the resuscitation should resume with immediate chest compressions. (These compressions should continue for approximately 5 cycles of 30 compressions to 2 ventilations or about 2 min of CPR. If two rescuers are available, use a 15:2 ratio and switch compressors when the first compressor fatigues.) This is done to facilitate the transition from SCA to ROSC after the heart has been stunned by the defibrillation and may not be functioning at optimal contractility for a few minutes after the shock. If there are additional monitoring devices in place in the hospital setting, this step may be modified accordingly as decided by the resuscitation team leader.

Continue CPR for approximately 2 minutes.

Reassess the Patient/Manage Airway/IV Access. After 2 minutes of CPR, 5 cycles of 30:2, the patient's perfusion status or carotid pulses should be checked. If there is no palpable pulse, compressions should resume immediately and preparation for delivery of a second defibrillatory shock should begin.

As preparation for the second shock begins, the members of the resuscitation team can work on securing the airway via endotracheal intubation, laryngeal mask airway, or another appropriate device. Blood draws and IV line placement, or IO if applicable, should proceed but not interfere with chest compressions. The goal is to maintain uninterrupted chest compressions and to avoid any unnecessary interruptions.

Change in CPR. Once an advanced airway has been secured, compression and ventilation cycles are no longer delivered. Now the compressor will continue to deliver compressions at a rate of 100 compressions/min *continuously*, without pausing for interposition of ventilation. The HCP/EC delivering the ventilations will provide 8 to 10 breaths/min, taking care not to overinflate the chest or use too much force during ventilation so as not too overpressurize the airways and esophagus, potentiating reflux.

Second Shock/Energy Selection/Mode. The second shock, if indicated, should occur after 2 minutes of CPR. The energy level for the second shock should be 4 J/kg. Be sure to check that the defibrillator or monitor is in the unsynchronized mode.

Immediately after the second shock, resume CPR and continue for about 2 minutes. If assessment of the rhythm and circulatory status shows continued VF/pulseless VT and no ROSC, continue CPR and consider medications such as a vasopressor (e.g., epinephrine).

Medications. If VF persists after 2 shocks, consider the use of epinephrine. The recommended dose for epinephrine is 0.01 mg/kg (1:10,000:0.1 mL/kg IV/IO). This drug can also be administered down the endotracheal tube if vascular access is unavailable at this point in the resuscitation. The endotracheal tube dose is 1:1000:0.1 mg/kg. This dosage can be repeated every 3 to 5 minutes. Medication should be given during the CPR or compression phase of the resuscitation. If another resuscitation team member is available, she or he should be designated to prepare the medication; this may decrease unnecessary interruptions in CPR compressions. After the medication has been administered and 5 cycles of CPR performed, reassess the patient. If VF is present, prepare to deliver another shock at 4 J/kg.

If VF still persists after the vasopressor is administered, an antiarrythmic should be considered. The recommended antiarrhythmics are amiodarone (5 mg/kg IV/IO) or lidocaine (1 mg/kg IV/IO). If these drugs are used, they should be flushed in with 20 mL of saline, followed by elevation of the extremity for several seconds to facilitate drug entry into the central circulation. Complete the 5 cycles of CPR and attempt to defibrillate at 4 J/kg if indicated. If no success, return to the vasopressor, epinephrine step and resume the process. At this time, the search for other causes of the VF arrest should be pursued (e.g., hypoxia, acidosis, hypovolemia, low glucose levels, hypothermia, toxins, tamponade, tension pneumothorax, thrombi, trauma).

If torsades de pointes was associated with the SCA, consider using 25 to 50 mg/kg of magnesium IV or IO up to a maximum dose of 2 g.

AEDs in Children

As mentioned previously, the incidence of VF/pulseless VT in children is low. Nonetheless, the presence of VF/pulseless VT is an indication for use of an AED or defibrillator. The age range for use of an AED or defibrillator is 1 to 8 years. No recommendations for the use of a defibrillator or AED in children under 1 year of age have been provided as of this writing.[71] A pediatric energy dose attenuator (see Fig. 12–22)

should be used to prevent delivery of too much current to the myocardium. If a pediatric dose attenuator is not immediately available, a standard defibrillator should be used at the lowest appropriate dose.

Use of the AED entails bringing the AED to the patient's side, turning the device on, following the voice or visual prompts, and connecting the electrodes to the patient. Once the patient is in the "circuit" (see Fig. 12–10), the AED will initiate the rhythm analysis automatically or the rescuer will be prompted to press a button to activate the "analyze mode" of the AED. Subsequently, the AED will diagnose the rhythm and advise a shock if indicated. The energy level and mode are all preprogrammed in the AED electronics.

Application of the AED to the aforementioned pediatric sequence is illustrated in the pediatric ALS algorithm (Fig. 12–23 and Box 12–1), which reviews clinical caveats with regard to defibrillation

CARDIOVERSION

Cardioversion is the application of DC ("shock") across the chest or directly across the ventricle to normalize the conduction pattern of a rapidly beating heart. This shock is delivered during the absolute refractory period of the ECG QRS—it is synchronized to the peak of the R-wave. *Defibrillation* refers to application of electrical energy during the nonvulnerable period to restore a fibrillating ventricle to normal sinus rhythm.

The patient with a significant tachycardia may be asymptomatic or may complain of chest pain or discomfort, lightheadedness, or shortness of breath. These symptoms are the result of altered cardiovascular physiology. Rapid cardiac rhythms allow less time for ventricular filling, resulting in reduced preload and hypotension. The reduced preload as well as the increased ventricular work caused by the rapid heart rate may also result in ventricular ischemia. Pulmonary capillary wedge pressures may also rise despite shortened filling time, owing to reduced ventricular compliance secondary to ventricular ischemia. Elevated pulmonary capillary wedge pressures can then lead to pulmonary edema.

Termination of rapid rhythms to alleviate or prevent these symptoms must occur quickly to prevent further deterioration. Persistently poor cardiac output due to rapid heart rate results in development of a lactic acidosis that further compromises cardiac function and makes cessation of the dysrhythmia even more difficult. Unchecked myocardial ischemia may lead to infarction with its attendant sequel. Drug therapy, rapid cardiac pacing, and cardioversion are the methods available to terminate tachydysrhythmias.

In many cases, DC cardioversion has specific advantages over drug therapy. The speed and simplicity of electrical cardioversion enhance its usefulness in the ED setting. Cardioversion is effective almost immediately, has few side effects, and is often more successful than drug therapy in terminating dysrhythmias. In addition, the effective dose of many antidysrhythmic medications is variable, and there is often a small margin between therapeutic and toxic dosages. Although they can often suppress an undesirable rhythm, drugs may also suppress a normal sinus mechanism or may create toxic manifestations that are more severe than the dysrhythmia being treated.

In the clinical setting of hypotension or acute cardiopulmonary collapse, cardioversion may be life saving. The key concepts in the use of this procedure include understanding

Figure 12–23 Unresponsive pediatric algorithm for pediatric VF/pulseless VT.

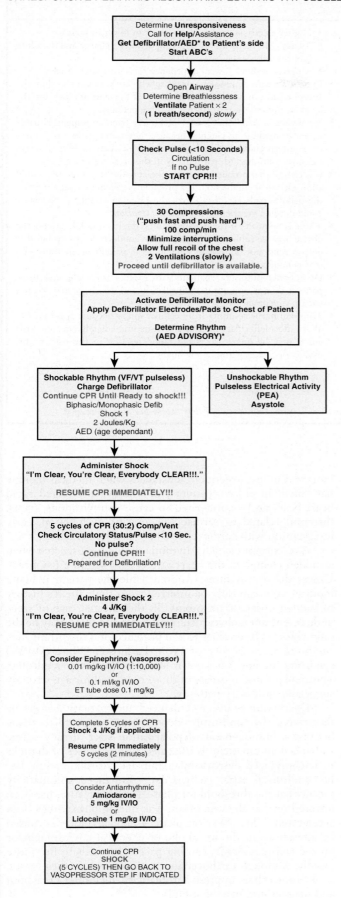

233

BOX 12-1   Caveats regarding Defibrillation

- Spontaneous defibrillation is highly unlikely and VF is lethal without prompt treatment, because the fibrillating ventricles produce no discernible cardiac output.
- Fine VF or a low-amplitude tracing may initially appear to be asystole. Asystole is not amenable to defibrillation. Therefore, a questionable rhythm should be double-checked in a second lead and the lead gain should be checked. Asystole is usually a terminal rhythm and the prognosis is grim. The prognosis is worsened, not improved, by attempts to defibrillate.
- Older defibrillators have paddles only; newer ones have either pads only or both pads and paddles. Neither has been shown to be more efficient when applied properly. Pads may be easier to apply because repeated defibrillations are easier to perform. Pads are less subject to variations, such as the pressure applied to the paddles and the required application of electrode gel or gel pads. In another respect, paddles may be safer than pads, because both paddle discharge buttons must be pressed simultaneously and the person performing the defibrillation has immediate view and control of the patient's environment.
- Be sure to have the machine in "asynchronized" or "defibrillation" mode before attempting defibrillation. The "synchronized" mode is designed to discharge after detecting an R-wave (as in the case of SVT) and, thus, cannot be used for VF.
- Maximal delivery of electrical energy is influenced by the impedance of the chest as well as by the effectiveness of the energy wave discharged. Factors affecting transthoracic impedance include:
  - Chest size. A larger chest wall absorbs more energy and thus creates more impedance.

- Higher electrical energy levels result in lower impedance.
  - A larger electrode more efficiently delivers a charge and therefore reduces impedance.
  - A previous shock lowers impedance for subsequent shocks.
- In patients with emphysema or those who are very tall and thin, the anterior pad can be placed to the right of the sternum, because the heart is often more retrosternal in these patients.
- Keep pads or paddles at least 1 inch away from an implanted pacemaker or medication patches, because these can interfere with electrical interpretation as well as discharge of current. Nitroglycerin can pose a fire hazard, particularly in the presence of oxygen.
- It is critical that no one have any contact with the patient that could allow electrical conduction. If a provider is touching a patient when the paddles/pads are discharged, the provider could be injured or could develop ventricular fibrillation. **Caution!**
- There is no need for the person holding the bag-mask to release the device because rubber and plastic do not conduct electricity, but that person must not be directly touching the patient or anything else that conducts electricity.
- Do not attempt to shock patients with asystole or PEA because these patients do not respond to defibrillation and the shock may worsen patient outcomes.[2,4]
- True skin burns resulting from cellular injury become apparent 24–48 hr after defibrillation. Skin erythema immediately after defibrillation may be due to localized blood pooling in the tissues; this usually dissipates within a few hours.

PEA, pulseless electrical activity; SVT, supraventricular tachycardia; VF, ventricular fibrillation.
From Thomsen T, Setnik G (eds): Procedures Consult—Emergency Medicine Module. Philadelphia: Saunders, 2008. Copyright 2008 Elsevier Inc. All rights reserved.

the indications for its use, the equipment involved, the importance of adequate sedation, and the concerns for health worker safety.

Background

The first successful defibrillation of the human heart was performed in 1947 by Beck and colleagues.[14] By the 1960s, electrical energy was being used to treat dysrhythmias other than VF. AC remained in vogue until 1963, when Lown and colleagues[71] advocated DC countershock as the method of choice for terminating atrial fibrillation. The use of DC significantly decreased the incidence of VF after countershock.

A brief burst of electrical current momentarily causes depolarization of the majority of cardiac cells and allows the sinus node to resume normal pacemaker function. In re-entrant dysrhythmias, such as paroxysmal supraventricular tachycardia (SVT) and VT, cardioversion restores sinus rhythm by interrupting a self-perpetuating circuit. Cardioversion is much less effective in terminating tachycardia resulting from augmented automaticity, such as digitalis-induced dysrhythmias.

Indications and Contraindications

Cardioversion is indicated whenever there is a re-entrant tachycardia causing chest pain, pulmonary edema, lightheadedness, or hypotension. This excludes those tachydysrhythmias that are known to be caused by digitalis toxicity as well as a known sinus tachycardia (i.e., known etiology). It also is

indicated in less urgent circumstances when medical therapy has failed. In elderly patients, in whom a prolonged rapid heart beat can be anticipated to cause complications, (clots, thrombi) related to cardiac ischemia or dysfunction, early intervention with cardioversion may also be beneficial.

A re-entrant tachydysrhythmia should be suspected when a sudden change in the heart rate occurs within a few beats. Unless the dysrhythmia is noted while the patient is being monitored, it can only be inferred from the patient's history of sudden onset of symptoms. In the unusual case of sinus node re-entrant tachycardia, rapid onset and offset may be the only clues.[72] Other clues to the presence of a re-entrant dysrhythmia are a history of Wolff-Parkinson-White (WPW) syndrome or another known accessory pathway syndrome. Ventricular rates in excess of those predicted for age strongly suggest an accessory pathway.

Dysrhythmias due to enhanced automaticity *will not* be terminated by uniformly depolarizing myocardial tissue because a homogeneous depolarization state already exists. Enhanced automaticity is the cause of most cases of digitalis toxicity–induced dysrhythmia, sinus tachycardia, and probably, multifocal atrial tachycardia.[73] Enhanced automaticity means that the threshold for phase 4 depolarization has been lowered or that the rate of ion leak during phase 4 has been accelerated. This effect on phase 4 depolarization is caused by alterations in the metabolic or chemical environment or on the cell membrane, causing pacemaker cells to fire more rapidly. Although cardioversion will not work in these cases, medications that suppress automaticity, including potassium and magnesium, may be useful.

TABLE 12–2 Standard Criteria to Differentiate Supraventricular Tachycardia from Ventricular Tachycardia

Rate	Too much overlap to make rate a useful criteria.
Regularity	Grossly *irregular* complexes are likely to represent one of three conductions: (1) AF with aberrancy, (2) AF with conduction through an accessory pathway, or (3) irregular form of VT. Rates > 200 beats/min with a wide-complex QRS are highly suggestive of AF with aberrancy or AF with accessory pathway conduction.
AV dissociation, fusion beats	AV dissociation during tachycardia with a wide-complex is highly suggestive of VT.
QRS axis	Preservation of normal QRS axis in a wide-complex tachycardia favors a diagnosis of SVT with aberrancy. Change in axis or extreme left or right axis deviation is often seen in VT. Abrupt change in QRS morphology is frequently seen in VT but not in SVT.
QRS duration	QRS duration > 140 msec occurs more frequently in VT than in SVT.
QRS concordance	Concordance in the precordial leads rarely is seen in SVT with aberrancy. Concordance supports a diagnosis of VT.
QRS morphology	*RBBB-shaped complex*: To distinguish RBBB aberration in SVT from VT, the presence of a triphasic pattern in V1 or a QRS pattern favors aberrancy, whereas a monophasic or biphasic QRS in V_1 or an RS or QS complex in V_6 favors VT.
	LBBB-shaped complex: SVT is suggested if the LBBB pattern has a small initial R-wave with a steeply downsloping S-wave. An initial R-wave (>30 msec) and a notched, broad (>70 msec) downslope is favorable for VT. QS complex or a QR in V_6 suggests VT.

AF, atrial fibrillation; LBBB, left bundle branch block; RBBB, right bundle branch block; SVT, supraventricualr tachycardia; VT, ventricular tachycardia.
Data from Gupta AK, Thakur RK, 2001; Yealy DM, Delbridge TR, 1998; Delbridge TR, Yealy DM, 1995.

In digoxin toxicity, cardioversion is not only ineffective; it is also associated with a higher incidence of postshock VT and VF.[74] However, for a patient with a therapeutic digoxin level, the risk of cardioversion is now thought to be no different from that of other patients.[75] Digoxin is still generally withheld for 24 hours prior to cardioversion as a precaution against inadvertently elevated levels. Pregnancy at any stage is not a contraindication to cardioversion.[76,77]

SVT with Aberrancy versus VT

Determining the rhythm is critical if the clinician is going to make the appropriate clinical or pharmacologic intervention. However, at times, SVT may manifest patterns on the electrocardiogram that look very similar to those of VT. An incorrect assessment of the electrocardiogram can prompt the clinician to implement a pharmacologic or therapeutic intervention that may result in cardiovascular collapse. Although a comprehensive discussion of SVT versus VT is beyond the scope of this chapter, some salient features to look for are presented herein to assist in the clinician's emergent decision making process.

A few caveats need to be kept in the forefront when facing the task of discriminating between SVT and VT.

First, a *wide-complex tachycardia* refers to a dysrhythmia in which the ventricles beat at more than 100 beats/min and the QRS duration is 0.12 second or more.[78–80] The originating foci for these wide-complex tachycardias can be either supraventricular or ventricular. For a supraventricular focus to produce a wide-complex tachycardia usually requires that a preexisting or new-onset intraventricular conduction block be present, resulting in increased time of depolarization. Increased heart rate or ischemia can also precipitate the appearance of a wide-complex tachycardia when it is supraventricular in origin. If the focus of the tachycardia is below the AV node, the tachycardia is considered ventricular in origin.[79] Criteria to facilitate the process of discriminating between SVT and VT were compiled by Wellens and coworkers[79] and Brugada and coworkers.[80] The Wellens cri-

TABLE 12–3 Brugada Algorithm

First reported in 1991, this algorithm was designed to aid the clinician in diagnosing lethal VT from the less urgent SVT with aberrancy conduction. Taking the standard 8- to 10-point criteria utilized by cardiology at the time, Brugada and coworkers[80] focused on four ECG criteria to aid in diagnosing VT vs. SVT with aberrancy. To differentiate VT from SVT with aberrancy, the Brugada algorithm uses the following ECG criteria. *First,* examine the ECG. Is the rhythm regular? An irregular rhythm highly suggests atrial fibrillation with aberrancy. Does the purposed dysrhythmia fit the clinical picture ascertained by the history? *Then,* ask the following questions:
1. Absence of an RS complex in all precordial chest leads?
2. RS interval (measured from the beginning of the R-wave to the deepest part of the S-wave) >100 msec in one precordial lead?
3. Atrioventricular dissociation?
4. Morphology criteria for VT present in precordial chest leads V1–2 and V6?

A single "yes" response confirms VT.
Only when none of the VT criteria is affirmed is SVT diagnosed.

ECG, electrocardiographic; SVT, supraventricular tachycardia; VT, ventricular tachycardia.
Adapted from Brugada P, Brugada J, Moht L, et al: A new approach to the differential diagnosis of a regular tachycardia with a wide QRS complex. Circulation 83:1649, 1991.

teria use several clinical data points to help determine whether the tachycardia is ventricular or supraventricular in origin.[79] The Brugada criteria extend the Wellens criteria and add a four-step decision-tree approach to the process.[80] Although the methods are not without pitfalls, a careful scrutiny of the electrocardiogram in light of the aforementioned criteria will usually lead to the appropriate diagnosis.[81]

Some of the characteristics of SVT versus VT are provided in Tables 12–2 to 12–4. Although the guidelines and criteria appear clear-cut, there are times when exceptions occur in the clinical setting.

Special Considerations: Wide-QRS-Complex Tachycardias

Wide-complex tachycardias (wide-complex SVT) are diagnostic challenges in clinical medicine. The criterion often used to define wide-complex supraventricular tachycardia (WCSVT) is a tachycardia with a QRS duration of greater than 0.12 second. It is important to differentiate the rhythm as one of the following: VT, SVT with aberrancy (left bundle branch block [LBBB] or right bundle branch block [RBBB]), or an accessory AV pathway ("pre-excitation"). The need for a proper diagnosis is obvious. Incorrect diagnosis and inappropriate treatment can be life threatening. This is especially true in misdiagnosing VT as SVT. Studies have shown that VT is often misdiagnosed, even with the ready availability of clinical and ECG criteria.[82]

Etiology

Normally, ventricular depolarization is initiated when the His bundle depolarizes both ventricles simultaneously through the bundle branches and Purkinje fibers. Normal depolarization takes place within 80 to 120 msec. Prolongation of the QRS duration happens (1) if the ventricles are activated sequentially rather than simultaneously as is the case in VT, bundle branch blocks, or accessory pathway ventricular activation (WPW, Lown-Gagong-Levine [LGL]); or (2) when His-Purkinje-myocardium conduction is slowed from ischemia, drugs, or electrolyte disturbances. Some dysrhythmias occur as a result of re-entry. There is an area of delayed conduction, due to metabolic changes in the tissue causing the depolarization front to travel at a slower speed through the myocardium. If an area proximal to the myocardium with the delayed conduction becomes reactivated, especially if there is a unidirectional block, a circular rhythm becomes established, causing the continuous firing of new ectopic focus.

Classification

Wide-complex tachycardias (QRS ≥ 0.12 sec) fall into three classifications based on mechanism: (1) VT, (2) SVT with aberrancy, and (3) pre-excited tachycardia. VT is the most common cause of wide-QRS-complex tachycardias. It is defined as three or more consecutive ventricular beats at a rate of 100 beats/min. VT is further classified as nonsustained (tachycardia lasting < 30 sec) or sustained (tachycardia that lasts > 30 sec). Sustained tachycardia usually results in hypotension or syncope and requires termination intervention.

SVT is a tachydysrthymia using the normal AV conduction system for ventricular activation. This tachycardia originates in the SA or AV node. To sustain propagation, the AV node is recruited. *Aberrancy* refers to the existence of an aberrant or nontraditional conduction mechanism resulting in a longer depolarization phase. SVTs with aberrancy by definition must result in wide-QRS-complex tachycardias. The two forms of aberrancy are fixed: a permanent bundle branch block or a functional block, which is a rate-dependent bundle branch block. The most common areas of the His-Purkinje functional block are in the left or right bundle branches. Sudden acceleration is often the initiating cause of the SVT with aberrancy. The aberrancy is maintained by a continuous, concealed, retrograde conduction pathway, which leads back into the blocked area.

For pre-excitation wide-QRS-complex tachycardias, AV conduction occurs over two circuits: (1) normal AV nodal conduction or (2) through an accessory pathway. These two pathways create the needed circuits for a re-entry circuit: the circus movement tachycardias. Aberrancy appears because of the presence of intraventricular conduction block. Pre-excited tachycardia is any tachycardia in which the ventricles are *antegradely* activated over an accessory pathway. The most common pre-excited tachycardia is atrial fibrillation with ventricular activation over an accessory pathway.

Clinical Diagnosis

The directed history on presentation may provide the most valuable clues to the diagnosis of tachydysrhythmia. The on-and-off occurrence of tachydysrhythmia in the past, the age of the patient, and the age of past occurrence all are important indicators of pre-excitation rhythms usually found in young patients. Sudden onset of tachydysrhythmia in the older coronary-prone patient or a patient with structural heart disease points more toward VTs. Symptoms associated with the tachydysrhythmia are important clues in diagnosis. The young patient often has few if any symptoms when experiencing the wide-complex or narrow-complex SVTs. The older patient may experience the entire range of cardiac symptoms. Tachydysrhythmia present for long periods often defines SVT. Patients with SVT often have recurrent tachycardias from their childhood or early adulthood. Attention must be paid to the medications the patient is using. Antiarrhythmic medications have a use-dependency property. Conduction velocity is slowed as rates increase.[83]

ECG Criteria for Differentiating VT from Wide-Complex SVT

The clinician should not attempt the differential diagnosis of wide-QRS-complex tachycardias without the use of the 12-lead electrocardiogram and extended rhythm strip. A common error is to attempt to determine the cause of a tachycardia based only on the rhythm strip. A comparison of past electrocardiograms is often helpful. Examination of the electrocardiogram should focus on the following areas: rate, regularity, AV dissociation, QRS axis, QRS duration, QRS concordance, and QRS morphology[84] (Table 12–5).

Treatment

Therapy is dictated by the specific wide-complex tachycardia and the patient's clinical presentation. The EC's initial approach must always be led, and modified if necessary, by the patient's presentation and subsequent changes. It is recommended in all cases of wide-complex tachycardias, and narrow-complex tachycardias that are producing hemodynamic instability, such that the clinician should immediately consider utilization of cardiovascular electrical cardioversion.

TABLE 12–5 Commonly Available Intravenous Medications Used for Sedation in Cardioversion

Drug	Dose	Comments
Midazolam	0.15 mg/kg	Most commonly used
		Induction occurs in about 2 min
		Small drop in blood pressure
		Flumazenil, antagonist available
Methohexital	1 mg/kg	Quicker onset than midazolam
		Shorter duration than midazolam
		Small drop in blood pressure
		Rare complication of laryngospasms
Etomidate	0.15 mg/kg	No drop in blood pressure
		Painful IV infusion
Propofol	1.5 mg/kg	Small drop in blood pressure
		Painful IV infusion
Thiopental	3 mg/kg	Painful IV infusion
Fentanyl*	1.5 µg/kg	An opiate
		Added for more sedation
		Can cause respiratory depression

*IV medications for sedation during cardioversion.

Synchronized monophasic or biphasic cardioversion is the appropriate first choice of treatment for these cases.[78]

In patients with wide-complex tachycardias who are cardiovascularly stable, the therapeutic options are more diverse. Stable, wide-complex tachycardia can always be considered VT and treated according to current VT treatment.[85] Verapamil should never be used in unknown etiology wide-complex tachycardia. A reasonable treatment protocol for stable patients may be the use of adenosine, procainamide, lidocaine, and finally, cardioversion. Amiodarone is effective for most SVTs and its use in stable unknown wide-complex SVT is both appropriate and safe.[86]

Despite the criteria listed earlier, when in doubt, the clinician should assume that the dysrhythmia is a wide-complex tachycardia and treat it as such. If it is determined not to be, the treatment should obviously be modified.

Equipment and Setup

The critical components of preparation for cardioversion are IV access, airway management equipment, drugs for sedation, and monitoring and DC delivery equipment (cardioverter).

Secure IV access is essential for delivery of sedatives, antidysrhythmics, fluids, and possibly, paralytic agents. Although many of these drugs are not used routinely, if they are needed, timing is likely to be critical. A large-bore IV catheter should be inserted and firmly taped to the patient's skin.

A significant and preventable complication of procedures involving sedation is hypoventilation leading to hypoxia. Airway management equipment includes the secure IV catheter discussed previously, working suction with a tonsil-tipped device attached, BVM apparatus, oxygen, and appropriate-sized laryngoscope and endotracheal tube. A pulse oximeter is generally recommended for patients undergoing conscious sedation. Another adjunct is continuous carbon dioxide pressure (Pco_2) monitoring. A rising Pco_2 level will be an earlier clue to hypoventilation due to sedation, because the oxygen saturation may remain normal for several minutes, especially if the patient has been preoxygenated.

Sedative medications should be ready for use in labeled syringes, with a prefilled saline syringe available for flushing the catheter. Antidysrhythmic medications for ventricular dysrhythmias (e.g., amiodarone, lidocaine) and for unexpected bradycardia (e.g., atropine) should be readily accessible.

Technique

If time permits, metabolic abnormalities such as hypokalemia and hypomagnesemia should be corrected before attempting cardioversion. At a minimum, hypoxia should be corrected with supplemental oxygen. If a patient has metabolic acidosis, compensatory hyperventilation after endotracheal intubation may be indicated prior to cardioversion. Respiratory acidosis should always be treated prior to the use of sedative drugs.

Sedation

Cardioversion may be extremely painful or terrifying, and patients must be adequately sedated prior to its use. Patients who are not adequately sedated may experience extreme anxieties and fear.[87] Several IV medications are available for sedation of patients prior to cardioversion, including etomidate (0.15 mg/kg), midazolam (0.15 mg/kg), methohexital (1 mg/kg), propofol (1.5 mg/kg), and thiopental (3 mg/kg). In addition, fentanyl (1.5 µg/kg), a synthetic opioid analgesic, is sometimes administered 3 minutes prior to induction.

Midazolam (Versed) is probably the most commonly used agent, with induction occurring about 2 minutes after a dose of about 0.15 mg/kg, or at least 5 mg for an average-sized adult. Although induction with midazolam takes slightly longer than with the other medications, it has the advantage that a commercial antagonist, flumazenil, is available for reversal if necessary. Small additional doses of fentanyl (1–1.5 µg/kg) may be added for more profound sedation. Fentanyl can cause respiratory depression, but can be reversed with naloxone. Methohexital has the advantage of quick onset and somewhat shorter duration than midazolam, but it has a rare association with laryngospasm. All the drugs except etomidate cause a small drop in blood pressure, and infusion of propofol and etomidate is painful.

In elderly patients, the pharmacodynamics and kinetics are altered by coexisting illness and polypharmacy, rather than by any intrinsic effect of old age.[88] Older patients with medical conditions such as congestive heart failure, renal failure, cancer, or malnutrition will therefore experience deeper, prolonged sedation with increased respiratory depression. Drug dose should be reduced in these patients.

Administer the anesthetic agent(s) IV over about 30 seconds and wait until the patient is unable to follow simple commands and loss of the eyelash reflex is noted. Pushing the agent too quickly may result in hypotension; pushing the agent too slowly may not allow blood levels to reach a therapeutic range, if the agent has a rapid rate of metabolism.

Cardioverter Use

Selection of synchronized or nonsynchronized mode is the next critical step. In the synchronized mode, the cardioverter searches for a large positive or negative deflection, which it interprets as the R- or S-wave. It then automatically discharges an electric current that lasts less than 4 msec, avoiding the vulnerable period during repolarization when VF can be easily induced. When the cardioverter is set to synchronize, a brief delay will occur after the buttons are pushed for discharge, as the machine searches for an R-wave. This delay may be disconcerting to the unaware operator.

If concern exists about whether the R-wave is large enough to trigger the electrical discharge, the clinician can place the lubricated paddles together and press the discharge button. Firing should occur after a brief delay. When the R- or S-wave deflection is too small to trigger firing, change the lead that the monitor is reading or move the arm leads closer to the chest.

If there is no R- or S-wave to sense, as in VF, the cardioverter will not fire. Always turn off "synchronization" if VF is noted.

Electrode Position

Electrode paddles may be positioned in two ways on the chest wall: (1) the anterolateral (or base and apex) position, with one paddle placed in the left fourth to sixth intercostal space, midaxillary line, and the other just to the right of the sternal margin in the second to third intercostal space (see Fig. 12–19), or (2) the anteroposterior position, with one paddle placed anteriorly over the sternum and the other on the back between the scapulae (see Fig. 12–16). The anterolateral position is used for emergent cardioversion, when placement of an electrode on the patient's back may not be feasible. Paddles should be pressed firmly against the skin to avoid arcing or skin burns.

Safety is a key concern in the performance of cardioversion. Any staff member acting as a ground for the electrical discharge can be seriously injured. The operator must announce "all clear" and give staff a chance to move away from the bed before discharging the paddles. Care must be taken to clean up spills of saline or water, because they may create a conductive path to a staff person at the bedside.

Energy Requirements

The amount of energy required for cardioversion varies with the type of dysrhythmia, the degree of metabolic derangement, and the configuration and thickness of the chest wall. Obese patients may require a higher energy level for cardioversion; the anteroposterior paddle position is sometimes more effective in these patients. If patients are shocked while in the expiratory phase of their respiratory cycle, energy requirements may also be lower.

VT in a hemodynamically stable patient should be treated with amiodarone 150 mg IV, and this can be repeated as needed up to a dose of 2.2 g/24 hr. If unsuccessful, cardioversion is then used. Cardioversion with 10 to 20 J is successful in converting VT in more than 80% of cases. Cardioversion will be accomplished with 50 J in 90% of cases, and conversion should be initially attempted at this energy level.[89] Cardioversion should be synchronized unless the T-wave is large and could be misread as the R-wave by the cardioverter. If the initial attempts at electrical cardioversion are unsuccessful, the energy level should be doubled, and doubled again if necessary, until a perfusing rhythm is restored. Immediately after conversion of VT, antidysrhythmic medication should be given to prevent recurrence.

Patients with pulseless VT should be initially shocked with 200 J, followed by 300 J if the first shock is not successful. Re-entrant SVTs generally respond to low energy levels. Atrial flutter, for example, usually requires less than 50 J for conversion.[17] Cardioversion of atrial flutter in the ED is indicated when the ventricular rate is not slowing in response to

pharmacologically enhanced AV node blockade or if the patient is unable to tolerate the aberrant rhythm.

The majority of patients with paroxysmal atrial tachycardia respond to adenosine. If they do not, or if urgent conversion is needed owing to a high ventricular rate, electric countershock should be administered in the synchronized mode at 50 J, and doubled if necessary.

In atrial fibrillation, the response to cardioversion is dependent on the duration of atrial fibrillation and the underlying cause. Cardioversion is successful in 90% of cases secondary to hyperthyroidism but in only 25% of cases secondary to severe mitral regurgitation.[90] However, 50% of cases revert within 6 months, especially those with long-standing atrial fibrillation.[91,92]

Most patients with atrial fibrillation do not require cardioversion in the ED unless their ventricular response is high owing to a bypass tract, as in WPW syndrome. They may also require cardioversion when sequelae of rapid ventricular contraction are present or anticipated and the ventricular rate is not responding to drug therapy aimed at slowing AV node conduction. Conversion of atrial fibrillation generally requires more energy than the re-entrant SVTs (~100 J in most cases).[93]

Complications

Complications of cardioversion may affect the patient, particularly the patient with a cardiac pacemaker, as well as health care personnel at the bedside. Patient complications are dose related and may involve the airway, heart, or chest wall, or they may be psychological.

Injuries to health care personnel with cardioversion/defibrillation include mild shock and burns. Hypoxia may result if sedation is excessive or if the airway becomes compromised. With proper preparations and precautions, airway complications can be minimized. Respirations may also be depressed by any of the anesthetic agents, and the adequacy of tidal volume must be continually assessed by either direct observation or end-tidal CO_2 monitoring. If another clinician is available, he or she should be placed in charge of monitoring the patient's airway. Routine supplemental oxygen is suggested for all patients undergoing sedation.

Chest wall burns resulting from electrical arcing are generally superficial partial-thickness burns, although deep partial-thickness burns have occurred.[94] These are preventable by adequate application of conductive gel and firm pressure on the paddles. Paddles should not be placed over medication patches or ointments, especially those containing nitroglycerin, because electrical discharge may cause ignition, resulting in chest burns.[95]

Cardiac complications after cardioversion are proportionate to the energy dose delivered. In the moderate energy levels used most commonly, the hemodynamic effects are small. At higher energy levels, however, complications include dysrhythmias, hypotension, and rarely, pulmonary edema, which may occur several hours after the countershock. A transient failure of myocardial oxygen extraction due to a direct effect on cellular mitochondria has been proposed as an explanation for some of these cardiac complications.[96]

The dysrhythmias after high-dose (~200 J) DC shocks include VT and VF, bradycardia, and AV block, in addition to transient and sustained asystole. Sustained VT or VF was reported following 7 of 99 shocks in a study of patients undergoing electrophysiologic study and requiring cardioversion for VT, VF, or atrial fibrillation.[97] These episodes occurred only in the patients with prior VT or VF. Patients with ischemia or known coronary artery disease appear to be at much higher risk for significant postshock bradycardia, with rate-support pacing required after 13 of 99 shocks in the study. Asystole requiring pacing occurred only once in 99 countershocks. Therefore, the proclivity for dysrhythmias is greater in high-dose cardioversion of an ischemic heart.

Two types of VF after cardioversion have been described. The first occurs immediately after countershock and is easily reversed by a second, nonsynchronized shock. This type of VF results from improper synchronization, with discharge of current occurring during the vulnerable period. The second variety, which is more ominous, occurs approximately 30 seconds to a few minutes after attempted cardioversion. This dysrhythmia is characteristically preceded by the development of paroxysmal atrial tachycardia with block or a junctional rhythm. In affected patients, it may be very difficult to convert the dysrhythmia to a sinus rhythm. This phenomenon occurs in patients who have been taking digitalis glycosides and is presumably a manifestation of digitalis toxicity.

In the event of VF after cardioversion, the equipment and manpower should be present for immediate defibrillation. If postcardioversion VF occurs, switch the cardioverter to "nonsynchronized" before attempting defibrillation. Electrical discharge will not occur in the "synchronized" mode, because the machine will be searching for a nonexistent R-wave.

VF is much more likely to result if depolarization occurs on the T-wave. If a patient has large T-waves in the lead selected for cardioverter sensing, the electric shock may discharge during the vulnerable period of the cardiac cycle, resulting in VF.[97] Always examine the complexes on the cardioverter monitor carefully for large T-waves and, if necessary, change the sensing lead. A randomly firing pacemaker can also be sensed by the cardioverter, resulting in countershock during the vulnerable period.[98]

Transient and intermittent ST-segment elevation has also been reported to occur (although rarely) after cardioversion, with myocardial injury or coronary vasospasm offered as possible explanations.[99]

An increase in serum enzyme levels (creatine kinase, lactate dehydrogenase, aspartate aminotransferase) may also occur after cardioversion, and the incidence has been reported to be between 10% and 70%. The enzyme rise is usually a consequence of skeletal muscle injury rather than myocardial damage. Cardioversion appears not to alter the enzyme profile of patients with MI[100]; however, some controversies exist.

Summary

In summary, cardioversion is performed on perfusing arrhythmias. The goal is not to cause VF. Therefore, during cardioversion, the shock is administered at the peak of the R-wave, during the absolute refractory period. Delivery of the shock during the relative refractory period can cause the development of a nonperfusing arrhythmia such as VF.

Cardioversion is performed to treat unstable SVT due to re-entry, unstable atrial fibrillation, and unstable atrial flutter. These arrhythmias are caused by re-entry. Delivering the shock interrupts the re-entrant focus causing these rhythms. In addition, cardioversion is recommended for the conversion or treatment of unstable monomorphic regular VT.

The recommended energy level for the treatment of atrial fibrillation is 100 to 200 J with a monophasic waveform.

If a biphasic waveform defibrillator is used, 100 to 200 J is reasonable.

As of this writing, there are no specific data to change prior energy recommendations for cardioversion. However, this may change in the near future, owing to the increasing number of biphasic defibrillators in use today.

Conversion of atrial flutter and other SVTs requires less energy. Usually, a dose of 50 to 100 J MDS is ofter sufficient. If the lower dose of 50 J is unsuccessful, increasing the dose in a stepwise fashion, using 50 to 100-J increments, is suggested.

Cardioversion may not work for multifocal atrial tachycardia or junctional tachycardias, owing to the presence of a spontaneously depolarizing automatic focus.

Treatment of VT has several variables that must be considered. The rate and morphologic characteristics must be considered. If the VT is monomorphic with a regular rate and form, but the patient is unstable, utilize 100 J with a monophasic defibrillator. If this intervention is unsuccessful, increase the energy dosage: 100 J, 200 J, 300 J, 360 J. If the patient deteriorates and becomes pulseless or synchronization is not possible, use high-energy defibrillation in the unsynchronized mode.

There are two general types of tachycardias, narrow and wide complex. Management of these tachycardias requires several steps. First, determine the patient's stability. If the patient is unstable, proceed to immediate cardioversion, with sedation if possible. If the patient is stable, obtain a 12-lead ECG reading to determine the underlying rhythm. A wide-complex tachycardia (>0.12 sec) may be VT, SVT with aberrancy, or a pre-excitation accessory pathway. Next determine whether the rhythm is regular or irregular.

Treat patients that are unstable (e.g., with hypotension, chest pain, change in mental status) with immediate cardioversion. If the patient is stable, chemical cardioversion using amiodarone 150 mg over 10 minutes may be an option. If a narrow-complex tachycardia is present and the patient is stable, attempt to determine the underlying cause (e.g., fever, dehydration, hypovolemia, shock, anemia). If possible, attempt vagal maneuvers (see Chapter 11, Techniques for Supraventricular Tachycardias) or pharmacologic cardioversion. If the patient becomes unstable, proceed to immediate cardioversion.

Use of medications can be attempted if the patient is stable and has good peripheral circulation. Medications that can be considered are amiodarone, calcium channel blockers (diltiazem, verapamil). In some cases, digitalis glycoside may be used.

Conclusions

Cardioversion is a safe and effective method of quickly terminating re-entrant tachycardia. Complications related to psychological trauma, respiratory depression, and unintentional health worker shock can be avoided with proper precautions. Adequate sedation is essential. Synchronized shock should be administered after close scrutiny of the lead used for sensing, to be sure that the R- or S-wave is significantly larger than the T-wave. Be prepared for postshock VT or VF, and if VF occurs, switch the cardioverter to "nonsynchronized" and defibrillate. Atropine and temporary pacing equipment should be available to treat postshock bradycardia, especially in patients with myocardial ischemia or MI.

239

BOX 12–2 Caveats regarding Cardioversion*

- Electrical cardioversion is much less effective in treating arrhythmias caused by increased automaticity (e.g., digitalis-induced tachycardia, catecholamine-induced arrhythmia, multifocal AT).[5]
- Patients presenting with AF or atrial flutter lasting longer than 36–48 hr are at risk for stroke from embolized thrombus originating in the left atrium. Studies have shown that patients are often unaware of the onset of AF, and thus, patients with stable AF should undergo either a 3- to 4-week course of anticoagulation treatment or TEE to rule out a clot in the left atrium before cardioversion. In the absence of contraindications, acute cardioversion of AF should be accompanied by anticoagulation therapy.
- Younger patients, patients with AF of short duration, and those with AF secondary to hyperthyroidism are more likely to convert with cardioversion. Older patients, patients with prolonged AF (>1 yr), and those with structural heart disease are less likely to convert with electrical cardioversion.[6]
- Remember, using synchronization avoids energy delivery in the early phase of repolarization when the ventricular myocardium is susceptible to VF. This is also referred to as the "R on T phenomenon."
- If there is no R-wave (e.g., in the presence of VF), the cardioverter will not discharge in synchronized mode.
- Place the paddles at least 10 cm from each other and from any internal pacemaker/defibrillator and 5 cm from the monitor electrodes. Avoid placement over a pacemaker or medicine patch because these may interfere with conduction. Nitroglycerin can pose a fire hazard if electrical arcing occurs from the paddles and so should be removed.
- Defibrillator/cardioverters default to unsynchronized mode after each electrical discharge. You must press the SYNCH button after each synchronized shock if an additional shock is indicated.

AF, atrial fibrillation; AT atrial tachycardia; TEE, transesophageal echocardiography.
From Thomsen T, Setnik G (eds): Procedures Consult—Emergency Medicine Module. Philadelphia: Saunders, 2008. Copyright 2008 Elsevier Inc. All rights reserved.

Pediatric Cardioversion

Pediatric cardioversion is similar to adult cardioversion. As previously described, the purpose of the procedure is to depolarize the myocytes completely at the most opportune time, during the peak of the R-wave, so as not to precipitate VF, and allow a slower perfusing rhythm to resume. However, the energy levels for pediatric cardioversion are different from those for the adult. In the pediatric procedure, the initial recommended energy dose is 0.5 to 1 J/kg, while the defibrillator is in the synchronized mode. If needed, a repeated cardioversion may be attempted at 2 J/kg, again while the defibrillator is in the synchronized mode! Remember to resynchronize the defibrillator after each cardioversion attempt and look for the appropriate markers on the monitor to ensure that the current is delivered at the appropriate phase of the cardiac cycle! If medication is needed, amiodarone at a dose of 5 mg/kg IV over 20 minutes or procainamide at a dose of 15 mg/kg over 60 minutes can be used. (*Do not give these drugs together!*) Box 12–2 reviews clinical caveats regarding cardioversion.

Acknowledgment

The editors and author would like to acknowledge the significant contributions to this chapter in previous editions by Steven Gazak, MD, William Burdick, MD, Jerris R. Hedges, MD, Michael Greenberg, MD, and John Krimm, DO.

 REFERENCES CAN BE FOUND ON EXPERT CONSULT

CHAPTER 13

Assessment of Implantable Devices

James A. Pfaff and Robert T. Gerhardt

Patients with implanted pacemakers or automatic implantable cardioverter-defibrillators (AICDs) are commonly seen in the emergency department (ED). Fortunately, the increased reliability of these devices has prevented a marked increase in patients presenting with true emergencies related to device malfunction, but such patients clearly have serious underlying medical problems that must be considered. Pacemaker complications are not uncommon, with rates ranging from 2.7% to 5%.[1] Many pacemakers fail within the 1st year.[2] AICD complication rates, including inadvertent shocks, occur in up to 34% of patients with the device.[3] The basic evaluation and treatment of patients with cardiac complaints who have pacemakers and AICDs are not substantially different from those of patients without the devices. However, a general knowledge of the range of problems, complications, and techniques for evaluating or inactivating pacemakers or AICDs is important for emergency clinicians. These devices are complicated so appropriate consultation, depending on the clinical situation, may be necessary.

HISTORY AND CLINICAL BACKGROUND
CAN BE FOUND ON EXPERT CONSULT

PACEMAKER CHARACTERISTICS

In essence, a pacemaker consists of an electrical pulse–generating device and a lead system that senses intrinsic cardiac signals and then delivers a pulse. The pulse generator is hermetically sealed with a lithium-based battery device weighing about 30 g with an anticipated lifetime of 7 to 12 years. A semiconductor chip serves as the device's central processing unit. The generator is connected to sensing and pacing electrodes that are placed in various locations in the heart, depending on the configuration of the pacemaker. Newer models are programmable for rate, output, sensitivity, refractory period, and modes of response,[12] and they can be reprogrammed radiotelemetrically after implantation.

Pacemakers are classified according to a standard five-letter code developed by the North American Society of Pacing and Electrophysiology/British Pacing and Electrophysiology Group (Table 13–1). Known as the NBG code, it consists of five positions or digits. The first letter designates the chamber that receives the pacing current; the second, the sensing chamber; and the third, the pacemaker's response to sensing. The fourth letter refers to the pacemaker's rate modulation and programmability, and the fifth describes the pacemaker's ability to provide an antitachycardia function. Whereas standard pacemakers generally do not have an anti-tachycardia function, AICDs do have this capability and over-drive pacing is the device's first response to tachycardia. In

normal practice, only the first three letters are used to describe the pacemaker (e.g., VVI or DDD).[13]

Pacemaker wires are embedded in plastic catheters. The terminal electrodes, which may be unipolar or bipolar, travel from the generator unit to the heart via the venous system. In a unipolar system, the lead electrode functions as the negatively charged cathode, and the pulse generator case acts as the positively charged anode, into which electrons flow to complete the circuit. The pulse generator casing must remain in contact with tissue and be uninsulated for pacing to occur. In the case of bipolar systems, both of the electrodes are located within the heart. The cathode is at the tip of the lead, and the anode is a ring electrode roughly 2 cm proximal to the tip. Bipolar leads are thicker and draw more current than unipolar leads, and are commonly preferred owing to several advantages. These include a decreased likelihood of pacer inhibition due to extraneous signals and less susceptibility to electromagnetic field interference.[14]

The typical entry point for inserting the leads is the central venous system, which is typically accessed by the subclavian or the cephalic vein. The terminal electrodes are placed either in the right ventricle or in both the right ventricle and the atrium, under fluoroscopic guidance. Proper lead placement is checked by electrocardiograms (ECGs) checking sensing and pacing thresholds.[15] The typical radiographic appearance of an implanted pacemaker is seen in Figure 13–1.

The pacemaker rate is typically programmed to pace between 60 and 80 beats/min. A significantly different rate usually indicates malfunction. When the battery is low, the rate usually begins to drop, getting slower as the battery fades. Sensing of intracardiac electrical activity is a combination of recognizing the characteristic waveforms of P-waves or QRS complexes while discriminating these from T-waves or external interfering signals, such as muscle activity or movement. The pacing electrical stimulus is a triphasic wave consisting of an intrinsic deflection, far-field potential, and an injury current, which typically delivers a current of 0.1 to 20.0 mA for 2 msec at 15 V.[16]

Pacemakers have a reed switch, which may be closed by placing a magnet over the generator externally on the chest wall; this inactivates the sensing mechanism of the pacemaker, which then reverts to an asynchronous rate termed the *magnet rate*. Essentially, *the magnet turns the demand pacemaker into a fixed-rate pacemaker*. The magnet rate is usually, but not always, the same as the programmed rate.

Several new innovations in rate regulation have been incorporated into some pacemakers. When present, the hysteresis feature causes pacing to be triggered at a rate greater than the intrinsic heart rate. When the hysteresis feature is employed in a single-chamber ventricular pacemaker, it is designed to maintain atrioventricular (AV) synchrony at rates that are lower than what would be normal for a ventricular-paced rhythm alone. To illustrate, were the hysteresis feature of the pacemaker set at 50 beats/min, an intrinsic rate under 50 beats/min would trigger ventricular pacing. Unlike a standard ventricular pacemaker, the hysteresis feature might be set to offer a ventricular pacing rate at 70 beats/min or greater once the pacer is triggered.

Rate modulation by sensor-mediated methods is an additional feature triggered and mediated by a sensed response to various physiologic stimuli. The primary application for this rate modulation feature is in the case of pacemaker patients who continue to engage in vigorous physical activity. When

TABLE 13–1 North American Society of Pacing and Electrophysiology/British Pacing and Electrophysiology Group Generic Pacemaker Code (NBG Code)

I Chamber Paced	II Chamber Sensed	III Response to Sensing	IV Rate Modulation and Programmability	V Antitachycardia Features
0—None	0—None	0—None	0—None	0—None
A—Atrium	A—Atrium	I—Inhibited	I—Inhibited	P—Antitachycardiac pacing
V—Ventricle	V—Ventricle	T—Triggered	M—Multiple	S—Shock
D—Dual	D—Dual	D—Dual	C—Communicating	D—Dual
			R—Rate modulation	

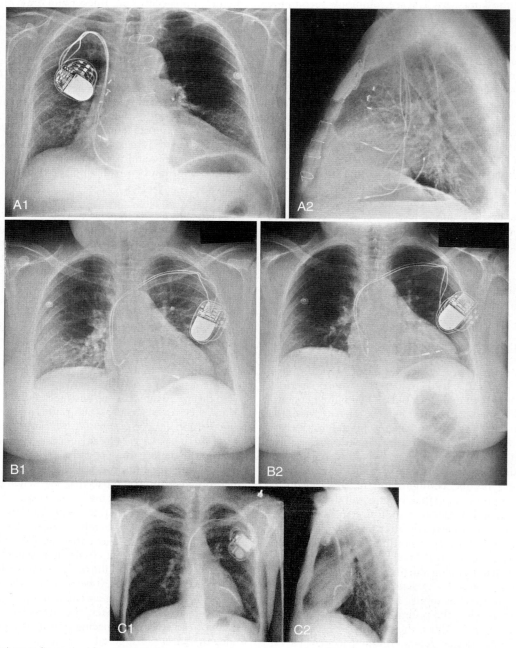

Figure 13–1 *A*, Various radiographs of an implanted pacemaker and automatic implantable cardioverter-defibrillator (AICD) show battery and lead wires. Posteroanterior (PA; *1*) and lateral (*2*) chest radiographs demonstrate a biventricular pacing system. There are three leads—the first is positioned in the right atrium, the second is in the right ventricular apex, and the third courses posteriorly in the coronary sinus and into the posterolateral cardiac vein. *B*, PA chest radiographs of a dual-chamber pacemaker. (*1*) Ventricular lead is passing through an atrial septal defect into the left ventricle. (*2*) The lead is repositioned in the right ventricular apex. *C*, A dual-chamber implantable cardioverter-defibrillator (ICD) has been implanted using active fixation leads via a transvenous approach to place the atrial lead in the systemic venous atrium and the ventricular lead across the baffle into the morphologic left ventricle.

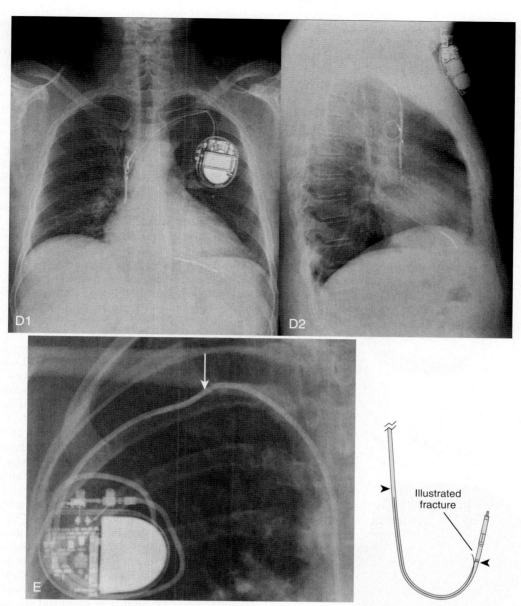

Illustrated
fracture

Figure 13–1, cont'd *D,* PA chest radiograph of a patient with a dual-chamber pacemaker (*1*). The atrial lead, originally positioned in a right atrial appendage position, is clearly no longer positioned in the right atrial appendage. Lateral view (*2*) also shows definite dislodgment of the atrial lead. *E,* Close-up view of a portion of the PA chest radiograph of a patient with a single-chamber pacemaker. The lead has fractured (a subtle finding) where it passes below the clavicle (*arrow*). The patient presented with intermittent ventricular failure to capture and intermittent failure to output on the ventricular lead. Impedance was intermittently measured at more than 9999 ohms. *Inset,* Diagram of the fracture site. *(E inset, Courtesy of Telectronics Pacing Systems, Englewood, CO.)*

present, the rate regulation feature is engaged and modulated through motion sensors installed within a pulse generator device, with a corresponding increase or decrease in pacing rate based upon the degree of motion sensed by the pacemaker device. Other physiologic sensors that may be installed as part of the pacemaker system include those designed to sense minute ventilation, Q-T interval, temperature, venous oxygen saturation, and right ventricular contractions. The latter sensors generally require that additional leads be placed.

AICD Characteristics

The basic components of an AICD include sensing electrodes, defibrillation electrodes, and a pulse generator (Fig. 13–2), which can be seen on a chest x-ray. Transvenous electrodes have obviated the prior need for surgical placement. They are inserted into the pectoralis muscle. Many transvenous systems consist of a single lead containing a distal sensing electrode and one or more defibrillation electrodes in the right atrium and ventricle.[17] Leads are inserted through the subclavian, axillary, or cephalic vein into the right ventricular apex. The left side is preferred because of a smoother venous route to the heart and a more favorable shocking vector.[18] In an effort to improve defibrillation efficiency, an additional defibrillation coil may be used.[18] Various placements of AICDs are demonstrated in Figure 13–3.

The pulse generator is a sealed titanium casing that encloses a lithium–silver–vanadium oxide battery, voltage converters and resistor, capacitors to store charges, microprocessors and integrated circuits to control the analysis of the rhythm and delivery of therapy, memory chips to store electrographic data and a telemetry module.[19] Whereas a pacemaker can draw the required voltage for its function from its component battery, the energy requirements necessary for defibrillation require a battery that is prohibitively large.[14] Subsequently, an AICD contains a capacitor that maximizes the required voltage by transferring energy from the battery prior to discharge. To achieve the required energy, AICDs use capacitors that are charged over 3 to 10 seconds by the battery and then release this energy rapidly for defibrillation.[17] The maximal output is 30 J in most units and 45 J in higher-energy units.[14] *This energy is high enough that a discharge is very obvious and often distressing to the patient.*

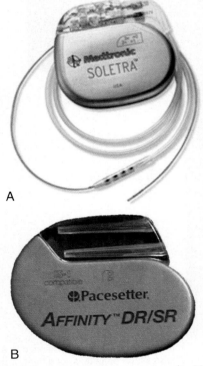

Figure 13–2 *A*, AICD. *B*, Implantable pacemaker. (*A, SOLETRA device, Courtesy of Medtronics Inc., Minneapolis, MN.*)

Most AICDs use a system in which the pulse generator is part of the shocking circuit, often described as a "can" technology, and most of them have a dual-coil lead with a proximal coil in the superior vena cava and a distal coil in the right ventricle.[20] Current flows in a three-dimensional configuration from the distal coil to both the proximal coil and the generator.[21] This dispersion of the electrical field increases the likelihood of depolarizing the entire myocardium at once, leading to successful defibrillation.[21]

AIDCs may have the same programming capabilities as pacemakers and can be single-chambered, dual-chambered or used with cardiac resynchronization therapy.[22] Single-chamber devices have only a right ventricular lead. They often have had difficulty identifying atrial arrhythmias, resulting in the *inappropriate defibrillation of atrial tachycardias.* Dual-chamber AICDs have a right atrial and a right ventricular lead and have improved ability to discriminate rhythms. In most studies, the dual devices have offered improved discrimination between ventricular and supraventricular arrythmias, decreasing inappropriate shocks due to rapid supraventricular rhythms or physiologic sinus tachycardia.[23] Approximately 50% of AICDs implanted in the United States are dual-chamber devices.[24] Cardiac resynchronization devices add an additional left ventricular lead that is placed in the coronary sinus or epicardium. In patients requiring both AICD and pacemaker functions, these devices were both placed together. The advent of technology has allowed placement of a single device that can perform both pacemaker and defibrillator functions.

AICDs use a combination of antitachycardia pacing, low-energy cardioversion, defibrillation, and bradycardic pacing in a combination also known as *tiered therapy.* They are programmed with specific algorithms that identify and treat specific rhythms. *The ventricular arrhythmias may initially be converted (or have attempts at conversion) with antitachycardic pacing as opposed to immediate defibrillation.* This *overdrive pacing* may terminate the rhythm without the need for electrical defibrillation in up to 90% of events. This is most successful for terminating monomorphic ventricular tachycardia with a rate of less than 200.[1] It is better tolerated by patients than cardioversion and reduces the risk of induced atrial fibrillation.[25] These events may be silent and not felt by the patient and only discovered by interrogating the device.

If unsuccessful, the next intervention may be low-energy cardioversion (<5 J). The device may be programmed to very

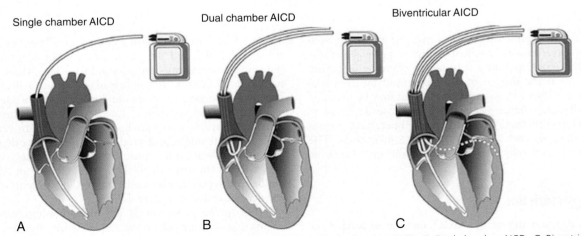

Figure 13–3 Diagrammatic demonstration of various AICD configurations. *A*, Single-chamber AICD. *B*, Dual-chamber AICD. *C*, Biventricular AICD.

low levels of electricity that, again, are better tolerated by the patient. This works best for ventricular rates greater than 150 and less than 240 beats/min.[21] This may be followed by a high-energy defibrillation. Traditionally, the energy level of the first shock is set at least 10 J above the threshold of the last defibrillation measured.[19] If the first shock fails, a backup shock may be required, but this may induce or aggravate ventricular arrhythmias (see discussion of "Pacemaker-Mediated Tachycardia," later). Unlike the proarrhythmic effects of medication, these are almost never fatal, although they may have increased morbidity.[18] Currently used biphasic waveforms have improved defibrillation thresholds.[19]

This tiered approach obviates the need for unnecessary energy requirements. The devices also have antibradycardic pacing that allows these patients to have one device instead of separate units. Additional complications associated with AICDs possessing antibradycardic pacing algorithms include a tendency toward oversensing, increased current drain, potential detection problems, and an increased incidence of hardware/software design problems.[1] At the time of insertion the amount of energy required for various AICD functioning, such as the defibrillation threshold, is determined for any given patient, and output and sensing functions can be adjusted by reprograming as needed.

INDICATIONS FOR PLACEMENT OF IMPLANTABLE PACEMAKERS AND AICDS

The most common indication for placement of a cardiac pacemaker is for the treatment of symptomatic bradyarrhythmias. Among these patients, roughly 50% of pacemakers are placed for the treatment of sinus node dysfunction (sick sinus syndrome). Other diagnoses include symptomatic sinus bradycardia, atrial fibrillation with a slow ventricular response, high-grade AV block (including Mobitz type II and third-degree AV block), the tachycardia-bradycardia syndrome, chronotropic incompetence, and selected prolonged Q-T syndromes. Although not classified as absolute indications, pacemakers are sometimes placed for the treatment of severe refractory neurocardiogenic syncope, paroxysmal atrial fibrillation, and hypertrophic or dilated cardiomyopathy. In the latter case, biventricular pacing has recently come into vogue as a viable therapeutic intervention in addition to pharmacologic management.

The 2004 American Heart Association guidelines for cardiac pacemaker implantation are summarized in Table 13–2.[26]

AICD technology is used primarily for both primary and secondary prevention in patients at risk for sudden death. Primary prevention is an attempt to avoid a potentially malignant ventricular arrhythmia in those patients identified as high risk.[27] Secondary prevention is for patients who have already had a ventricular arrhythmia and are at risk for further events. In addition, AICDs are implanted for a number of other congenital or familial cardiac conditions. Table 13–3 is a summary of class 1 indications for the placement of AICDs.[28]

PACEMAKER AND AICD RESPONSE TO MAGNET PLACEMENT

In the clinical setting, the placement of a magnet over the pulse generator of a pacemaker is a technique that might be

---

TABLE 13–2 Indications for Implantations of Cardiac Pacemakers

Absolute Indications

Symptomatic bradydysrhythmias
- Sinus nodal dysfunction
- Symptomatic sinus bradycardia
Symptomatic atrioventricular blocks
Asymptomatic Mobitz II or third-degree atrioventricular block
Atrial fibrillation with slow ventricular response
Chronotropic incompetence
Prolonged Q-T syndrome

Relative Indications

Neurocardiogenic syncope refractory to pharmacologic management
Paroxysmal atrial fibrillation
Hypertrophic cardiomyopathy
Dilated cardiomyopathy (biventricular pacing if congestive heart failure is present)

TABLE 13–3 Class One Recommendations for Automatic Implantable Cardioverter-Defibrillator Placement

Primary Prevention of SCD in Patients Who Are New York Heart Association Class II or III Who Are

1. Patients with LV dysfunction due to a prior MI who are at least 40 days post MI and have an LVEF ≤ 30%–40%.
2. Patients with nonischemic dilated cardiomyopathy who have an LVEF ≤ 30%–35%.

Secondary Prevention of SCD

1. In patients who survived VF or hemodynamically unstable VT.
2. In patients with VT with syncope who have an LVEF ≤ 40%.
3. In patients with LV dysfunction due to prior MI who present with hemodynamically unstable sustained VT to decrease mortality by reducing SCD.
4. In patients with nonischemic dilated cardiomyopathy and sustained VT.
5. In patients with hypertrophic cardiomyopathy who have sustained VT and/or VF.
6. In patients with Brugada syndrome or prolonged Q-T syndrome with previous cardiac arrest.
7. In patients with congenital heart disease with previous cardiac arrest who have had reversible causes excluded.

LV, left ventricular; LVEF, left ventricular ejection fraction; MI, myocardial infarction; SCD, sudden cardiac death; VF, ventricular fibrillation; VT, ventricular tachycardia.

---

employed either diagnostically or therapeutically by the emergency clinician. It is important to note that each pacemaker is programmed to respond in a specific fashion as determined by the manufacturer. The response to the magnet placement may vary not only by manufacturer but also by model and by the particular mode in which the pacemaker is currently operating. In most cases, manufacturers set the asynchronous baseline pacing rate in a range approximating 70 beats/min. An indicator of aging of the pacemaker, and weakening of the battery, is that this asynchronous baseline pacing rate will decrease over time as the battery approaches a point at which replacement is required.

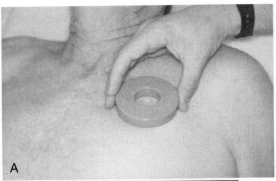

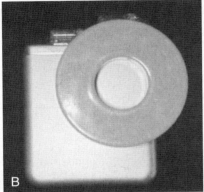

Figure 13–4 *A,* Application of a ring magnet over a pacemaker generator. *B,* Placement of a magnet on an AICD.

Keeping these provisions in mind, there are standard responses that the provider might expect to see under most circumstances. In the case of single-chamber ventricular pacemakers, the response most likely will be for asynchronous pacing (V00). In the case of dual-chamber pacemakers, the placement of a magnet usually results in dual-chamber asynchronous pacing (D00). In either case, it is important for the clinician to note that placement of a magnet over the pacemaker pulse generator *will not turn the pacemaker off.*

Placing a magnet over any of the currently available AICD models will temporarily *disable tachyarrhythmia intervention* (Fig. 13–4). An ECG before and after magnet placement should be done for comparison (Fig. 13–5). Most commercially available pacer magnets are 7 cm in size and accommodate use with most implantable devices. Each of the present models may have a slightly different response to the magnet. The magnetic field closes a reed switch in the generator circuit that will disable the recognition of tachyarrhythmia and subsequent firing of the device. There may be a variety of tones (continuous, intermittent, or silence) during activation/inactivation with the magnet, which are dependent on the manufacturer. Some devices may be programmed to not respond at all.[29] After the desired effect is obtained, the magnet should be secured to maintain inactivation.

Pacemaker and AICD patients should carry an identification card that includes information regarding manufacturer, model type, lead system, and a 24-hour emergency number to allow rapid identification of the model when it is necessary to inactivate the device. In lieu of an available device identification card, the general type, polarity, and number of ventricles involved with the implanted device may be accurately inferred by viewing an overpenetrated anteroposterior chest radiograph.

If a patient with an AICD presents with a ventricular arrhythmia, the assumption should be made that the device is inoperable and standard advanced cardiac life support (ACLS) protocols should be used to stabilize the patient.

Of further note, in some obese patients or those with heavily developed chest wall musculature, the magnetic field emitted by a single magnet device may not be strong enough to elicit the desired effect on the implanted device. As such, the clinician may find greater efficacy by employing two magnets, one on top of the other.[30]

CLINICAL EVALUATION OF PATIENTS WITH IMPLANTED PACEMAKERS AND AICDS

History

Patients generally present because their device has discharged. They will often describe a sensation of being kicked or punched in the chest, and the *sensation is not subtle.* In fact, some patients live in fear of the shock, having previously experienced it, and this is one reason for removal of the device. Ask the patient about the number of discharges and associated symptoms, including chest pain, shortness of breath, lightheadedness, palpitations, syncope, extremity edema (raising a concern for congestive heart failure or lower extremity deep vein thrombosis), or dyspnea on exertion. In addition, elicit general symptoms such as fever, chills, nausea, or vomiting, which could be indicative of infection. Inquire about medication history. Ask about the specific implanted device that they possess. Most pacemaker/AICD patients should have an identification card on their person, which will identify the manufacturer, model number, lead system, and a 24-hour emergency contact number. Sophisticated information and the prior electrical events and settings of the device can be accomplished in the ED by simply placing an external interrogating device over the unit (see Fig. 13–8).

Physical Examination

First, assess for airway patency, adequate ventilation, and cardiovascular status. The patient's mental status may also be an important clue as to the severity of his or her presentation. Perform an appropriate physical examination, emphasizing the heart and lung examination, seeking murmurs, pericardial friction rubs, and evidence of pulmonary effusion or other abnormalities. Inspect the pacemaker or AICD site for erythema or edema. Palpate the skin for evidence of obvious lead abnormalities. Examine the extremities for evidence of edema or erythema.

Radiography

The imaging modality of choice, at least initially, in a patient with implanted pacemaker or AICD complaints, is the plain chest radiograph. If the patient's stability is in question, obtain a portable anteroposterior film. In addition to the standard cardiac, pulmonary, vascular, and skeletal evaluation, this study will likely confirm the location of the pulse generator case as well as the current location of any leads. Survey the radiograph for evidence of lead fracture or displacement (see Fig. 13–1E). Compare with prior chest films. *If the patient does not have her or his device identification card in her or his immediate possession, take an overpenetrated radiograph to look for a radiopaque marker identifying the model type.*

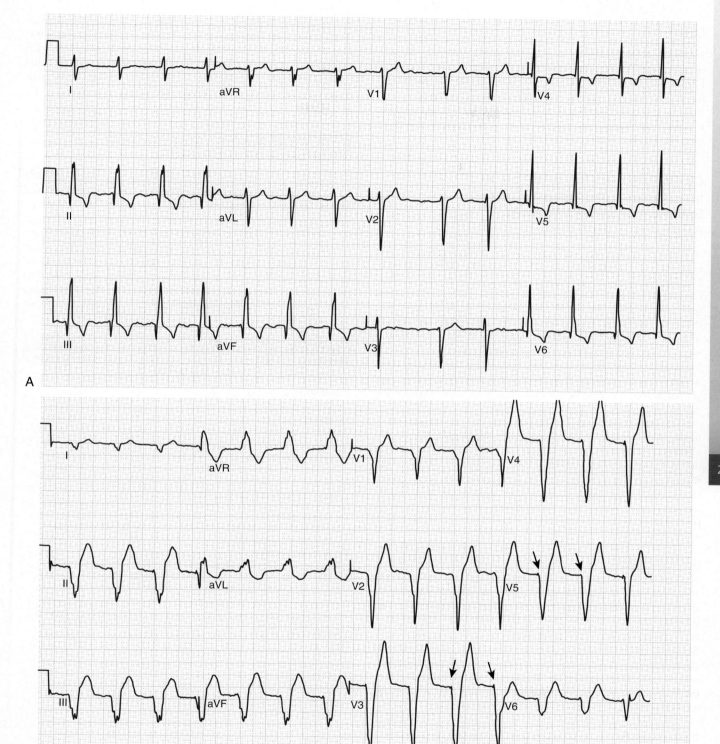

Figure 13–5 *A,* Electrocardiogram (ECG) of a patient with a nonfiring pacemaker. Intrinsic cardiac rate is 80 beats/min, and no pacemaker activity is seen. *B,* ECG of the same patient with a magnet applied over the pacemaker, producing a paced rhythm. Pacer spikes are evident (*arrows*) and the magnet rate is 85 beats/min. Note the left bundle branch bundle typical of a pacer lead in the right ventricle.

ECG

Perform an ECG seeking evidence of pacing, ectopy, and ST segment or T-wave abnormalities. A comparison ECG may be helpful. If an AICD shock has been delivered, the shock itself can cause transient electrocardiographic changes, and waiting for several minutes to repeat the ECG may identify whether the changes are a result of the discharge or due to an ongoing disease process.[31]

Cardiopulmonary Resuscitation, ACLS Interventions, and External Cardiac Defibrillation in the Implanted Pacemaker or AICD Patient

In general, ACLS interventions may be performed safely and effectively in pacemaker and AICD patients, when indicated. Cardiopulmonary resuscitation (CPR) may generally be performed in standard fashion. If an AICD is present, rescuers may notice mild electrical shocks while performing CPR; these are harmless to the rescuer. If the AICD shocks are impeding rescuer CPR performance, or if supraventricular tachycardias are noted during resuscitation, disable the AICD by applying a magnet over the corner of the device from which the leads emerge. This location is usually located easily via palpation, but may be located blindly by slowly relocating the magnet until AICD activity ceases.

External cardiac defibrillation may be performed safely in pacemaker and AICD patients with the standard expected efficacy; however, it is recommended that external paddles or defibrillator pads be placed at a location approximately 10 cm distant from the pulse generator, if possible.[32] A transcutaneous cardiac pacemaker may also be employed in a similar fashion, again with a recommendation that pacing pads be placed in anatomically appropriate locations but preferably at a distance of 10 cm from the pulse generator.

Placing the external defibrillation or transcutaneous pacemaker pads in an anteroposterior configuration is advised, because this configuration may circumvent energy shunting and shielding.[18] *Every attempt should be made to avoid application of the defibrillators directly over the device.* Use of the lowest possible energy setting for cardioversion or defibrillation is recommended. If available, biphasic cardioverter-defibrillators are further suggested.[32] In the event of successful resuscitation and return of spontaneous circulation, the pacemaker or AICD should be interrogated expeditiously by a cardiologist or electrophysiologist to ensure that no damage was sustained as a result of the resuscitation effort.

Regarding pharmacologic adjuncts, amiodarone has been reported to be more effective for treatment of potentially lethal arrhythmias in the setting of implanted device patients.[33] *Antiarrythmic medications may be required for a resistant malignant rhythm when the AICD is functioning properly, yet the arrhythmia persists* (Fig. 13–6).

Several additional considerations are unique to the setting of ACLS in the pacemaker or AICD patient. In cases of acute myocardial infarction involving areas of the myocardium in contact with the pacemaker leads, the implanted pacemaker may experience operative failure. As a result, maintain a high level of suspicion for the potential requirement of supplemental transcutaneous or transvenous cardiac pacing.

Also, in the postresuscitation setting involving the implanted pacemaker/AICD patient, it is important to main-

tain a higher index of suspicion for device lead fracture or disruption resulting from CPR. Lastly, in the postresuscitation phase, the clinician should maintain close surveillance for the development of pneumothorax, hemothorax, pericardial fusion, or other aforementioned pathophysiologic processes that could adversely affect implanted device function.

COMPLICATIONS AND MALFUNCTIONS OF IMPLANTED PACEMAKERS

Complications associated with pacemakers are listed in Table 13–4. In addition, patients with previously implanted and otherwise stable pacemakers may experience complications relating to direct or indirect trauma affecting the pulse generator or leads. Major complications of pacemaker placement or those resulting from subsequent injuries that the emergency clinician might encounter include local or systemic infections resulting from pacemaker placement, thrombophlebitis involving the transvenous route of the pacemaker leads, a venous thromboembolic event, pneumothorax or

---

TABLE 13–4 Complications of Permanent Pacemakers

Failure to Pace (No Pacemaker Activity Present)

Lead fracture
Lead disconnection
Battery depletion
Component failure
Oversensing
External interference

Failure to Sense (Constant Pacemaker Spikes despite Ongoing Intrinsic Cardiac Electrical Activity)

Lead dislodgment
Lead fracture
Fibrosis around lead tip
Battery depletion
Pacer in asynchronous mode
External interference
Low-amplitude intracardiac signal

Failure to Capture (Pacemaker Spikes but No Subsequent Cardiac Activity)

Lead dislodgment including perforation
Lead fracture
Lead disconnection
Poor lead position
Fibrosis around lead tip
Battery depletion
Metabolic abnormalities
Medications

Inappropriate Pacemaker Rate (Runaway Pacemaker)

Pacemaker re-entrant tachycardia
Resetting from external interference
Battery depletion

Other

Infections: pocket, wires
Lead displacement: cardiac perforation, tamponade, pericarditis, vascular perforation
Vascular complications: thrombosis, superior vena cava syndrome
Psychiatric: anxiety, panic attacks

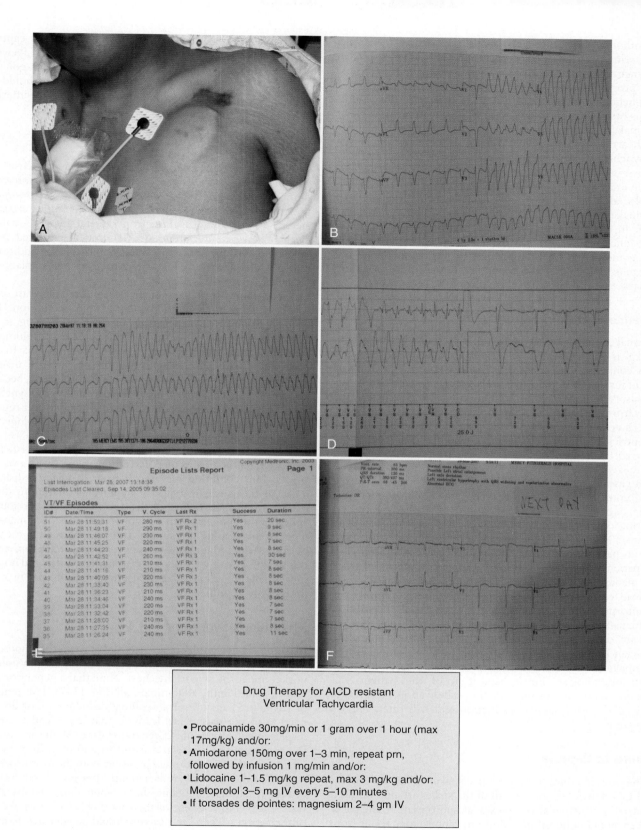

Figure 13–6 *A,* A patient with an AICD who experienced multiple discharges from an AICD due to recurrent ventricular tachycardia (VT). *B,* ECG of VT in the presence of an underlying tachycardia as the possible cause. *C,* Rhythm strip demonstrates persistent polymorphic (?torsades de pointes) VT. *D,* After attempts at overdrive pacing failed, the AICD appropriately discharges with temporary termination of VT. *E,* Interrogation of the device lists the history of over 20 episodes of recurrent VT within a few minutes. *This patient was terrified of subsequent shock because he could sense the VT and knew of the impending shock. In addition to antiarrhythmic medication, aggressive sedation is suggested to reduce catecholamine levels. F,* ECG after medical therapy with multiple medications. *Metoprolol seemed to be the deciding factor in terminating the VT in this case. G,* Current suggested medical therapy of VT in the presence of an appropriately functioning AICD.

hemothorax, pericarditis, air embolism, a localized hematoma interfering with pacemaker operation or sensing, lead dislodgment,[34] cardiac perforation, hemopericardium with possible progression to cardiac tamponade, and development of the phenomenon known as *pacemaker syndrome*. This condition is often seen in patients with single-chamber ventricular pacemakers who possess an underlying component of congestive heart failure. It is believed to be the result of the loss of AV synchrony resulting from the ventricular pacing, and may present with vertigo, syncope, hypotension, and signs specific to the exacerbation of congestive heart failure.

In addition to the complications associated with initial pacemaker placement, malfunctions of these devices may occur in the short-, intermediate-, and long-term phases of their functional life spans. Most malfunctions result from one or a combination of three primary problems: failure of the pace generator to provide output, failure to capture, or failure to sense the intrinsic cardiac rhythm.

Pacemaker Output Failure

Pacemaker generator output failure is present when no pacing "spike" is noted on the ECG despite an indication for pacing. This condition may result from battery failure, a fracture or loss of insulation in the pacer leads, oversensing of extraneous signals resulting in pacer inhibition, disconnection of the leads from the pacer generator, or in the case of dual-chamber pacer's erroneous sensing of the pacemaker's atrial signal by a ventricular sensor. The latter phenomenon is commonly referred to as *cross-talk*.[35]

Given that the reason for pacemaker implantation in most cases is for the treatment of an underlying bradycardia condition, the initial clinical management of patients with some degree of pacer output failure will usually focus on pharmacologic management aimed at restoring an acceptable intrinsic heart rate. Subsequently, a transcutaneous or transvenous pacemaker may be required to ensure stabilization of the patient. Once stabilization has been accomplished, further ED management should include a thorough secondary survey, 12-lead electrocardiographic and continuous cardiovascular monitoring, portable chest radiography to assess for condition of the pacemaker leads as well as to identify related pathology, and any other pertinent diagnostic studies. At this point, the clinician should seek to identify the type and model of the pacemaker, and should consult an available cardiologist or electrophysiologist. Final disposition of the patient will depend upon the results of the stabilization, diagnostic studies, and cardiology consultation and will often require admission.

Failure to Capture

In the case of failure to capture, pacemaker spikes are present on ECG. However, some or all of the spikes are not followed by atrial or ventricular complexes, as appropriate to the pacemaker model in question. Failure to capture may result from deterioration of lead insulation; fracture or dislodgment of the leads; electrolyte disturbances including hyperkalemia or hypocalcemia; a new condition requiring an elevated pacing threshold; acid-base disturbance; direct damage to the myocardium, which is in contact with the pacer lead's tip (such as myocardial infarction or direct trauma); or a dysfunction of the microcircuitry of the pulse generator. In addition, flecainide, a class I-C antiarrhythmic medication, has been iden-

tified as an acute cause for the rise in ventricular capture thresholds in patients with implanted pacemakers.[36] Likewise, all class-I antiarrhythmic agents (sodium channel antagonists) may affect pacer capture thresholds, and as such, should be identified as potential etiologic agents in patients suffering failure to capture.

Failure to Sense

Failure of an implanted cardiac pacemaker to sense the patient's intrinsic cardiac rhythm may be subdivided into conditions related to oversensing or undersensing. *Oversensing* is present when the pacemaker erroneously identifies extrinsic electrical signals, such as those from skeletal myopotentials or electromagnetic interference (EMI), and is inhibited from delivering inappropriate pacemaker pulse. For additional information on extrinsic EMI, refer to "EMI and Implantable Devices," later in this chapter.

The clinical management of pacemaker failure to sense will be driven largely by the patient's clinical condition. The prudent clinician will order cardiovascular monitoring, intravenous access, and a portable chest x-ray, with additional measures as dictated by the patient's presentation. In the event of symptomatic bradycardia, placement of a magnet over the pacemaker pulse generator may be indicated, because this maneuver will usually place the pacemaker in asynchronous ventricular pacing mode, restoring a stable and regular paced ventricular rhythm while a consulting cardiologist or electrophysiologist is summoned.

Undersensing is said to occur when the pacemaker fails to identify intrinsic cardiac depolarization and delivers a pacing signal. This condition may result from damage or dislodgment of the pacemaker leads, myocardial infarction, direct cardiac trauma, or failure of the pacemaker's power source, and even the application of a magnet. The initial ED management of this condition is similar to that performed in the case of oversensing. Magnet placement may also be appropriate in this setting, because it will restore a stable, regular, and normal cardiac rhythm until the pacemaker and its leads may be more thoroughly examined.

"Twiddler's Syndrome"

In some cases, implantable pacemaker patients choose to manipulate the pulse generator case within its physiologic pocket under the skin in the chest. Note that a generator may also be placed in the abdominal wall (Fig. 13–7). This practice of "twiddling" may result in coiling, dislodgment, or disconnection of the pacemaker leads. It may even lead to actual displacement of the pulse generator case. At the minimum, this may result in physical discomfort and may, in fact, precipitate cardiac arrhythmias or other complications local to the site of the pacemaker placement. After initial stabilization of the presenting complaint, these patients may require readjustment or replacement of their pacemaker devices. As part of their care, pacemaker patients should be educated to avoid manipulating their pacemakers.

Runaway Pacemaker Syndrome

This condition is seen almost exclusively in older pacemaker models, particularly as they approach the end of their battery life or when the pulse generator is damaged by radiation exposure or direct impact. The hallmark of runaway pace-

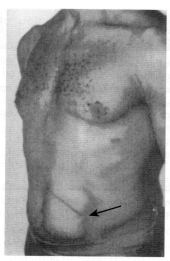

Figure 13–7 Pacemakers and AICDs may be implanted in the abdominal wall as well as the more common pectoralis muscle.

TABLE 13–5 Criteria for Electrocardiographic Diagnosis of Acute Myocardial Infarction in the Setting of Ventricular Paced Rhythm

Electrocardiographic Criterion	Sensitivity (%)	Sensitivity (%)	P
Discordant S-T segment elevation > 5 mm	53	88	.025
Concordant S-T segment elevation > 1 mm	18	94	NS
S-T segment depression > 1 mm in precordial leads V$_1$–V$_3$	2	82	NS

NS, not significant.

maker syndrome is an uncontrolled tachycardia, causing ventricular rates approaching 300 to 400 beats/min. In addition to initial attempts at stabilization, magnet placement may be attempted. However, this is often ineffective. If the patient is hemodynamically unstable in the setting of runaway pacemaker syndrome, it may be necessary to disconnect the pulse generator. To do this, identify the location of the pacer leads by physical examination or portable chest x-ray. Dissect through the skin and subcutaneous tissues, and then sever the leads with a wire cutter or similar tool.

Pacemaker-Mediated Tachycardia

In some circumstances, patients possessing implanted pacemakers or AICDs may present to the ED with symptomatic tachycardias resulting specifically as a complication of their pacemaker devices. This condition, referred to as *pacemaker-mediated tachycardia* and, alternately, as *pacemaker-induced tachycardia*, most often results from one of three clinical scenarios. In patients possessing dual-chamber pacemakers, one of the pacemaker leads may function as a pathway for either anterograde or retrograde conduction, resulting in what is referred to as an *endless loop syndrome* and thus a tachycardic arrhythmia, which may often become hemodynamically unstable. In general, patients suffering from endless loop syndrome will not have a ventricular rate greater than the maximum tracking rate of the pacemaker device. As such, this condition will rarely present with hemodynamic instability. One caveat, however, is that patients with underlying coronary artery disease who present with endless loop syndrome may experience coronary ischemia. In such a case, or in a patient who is hemodynamically unstable owing to the increased ventricular rate, application of a magnet will terminate the syndrome in most cases. Once stabilized, this condition may be prevented or at least mitigated by reprogramming the pacemaker's atrial sensor lead by an electrophysiologist.

A second presentation in patients with dual-chamber pacemakers occurs under the circumstance in which the patient experiences an intrinsic atrial tachycardia, at which point the implanted pacemaker begins to continuously discharge at its maximum preprogrammed ventricular rate. This condition may continue until the underlying atrial tachycardia is terminated by intervention.

A third instance of pacemaker-mediated tachycardia occurs in patients with AICD units possessing a backup anti-bradycardia pacing capability. It appears that in such patients, if the pacemaker feature is switched on and an ectopic ventricular stimulus is delivered after a sudden pause in the intrinsic ventricular depolarization cycle, a ventricular tachyarrhythmia may be triggered.[2,37]

Diagnosis of Acute Myocardial Infarction in the Presence of a Paced Cardiac Rhythm

Patients undergoing active ventricular pacing from an implanted pacemaker device will normally possess ECGs that resemble a left bundle branch block pattern. As a result, the electrocardiographic diagnosis of acute ischemic changes is equally challenging in both populations. Sgarbossa and coworkers[38] published a series of criteria in 1996 that offers some utility in the interpretation of ECGs in patients with active ventricular pacing, in whom acute coronary syndromes are suspected. These criteria are depicted in Table 13–5.[15]

AICD-Unique Malfunctions

Issues with sensing problems, lead migration, and battery failure are similar to pacemaker complications and most occur within 3 months after implantation.[39] A potential malfunction unique to the AICD is the inappropriate or lack of defibrillation of the device.

The AICD may not terminate ventricular arrhythmias, which may or may not be the result of device malfunction. AICD malfunction may be a result of battery depletion, component failure, undersigning, or lead malfunction. Failure-to-cardiovert/defibrillate that occurs in the setting of a functioning AICD system may be caused by inappropriate cutoff rates, failure to satisfy multiple detection criteria, completed and exhaustion of therapies, and cross-inhibition by a separate pacemaker.[18] The advent of AV, or *dual chamber AICD* devices, has improved the sensitivity of arrhythmia detection, preventing the delivery of inappropriate shocks.

Inappropriate AICD-delivered shocks occur in 20% to 25% of patients[40] and are the most common adverse events observed in AICD patients.[34] The main causes are atrial arrhythmias, sinus tachycardia, nonsustained ventricular tachycardia, lead fracture or EMI, or *electrical storm*.[40] By definition, this phenomenon occurs when three or more shocks

unchanged (Fig. 14–14).[39] Suspect LA/LL reversal when comparing two ECGs that feature changes that do not make clinical sense; if the P-QRS-T wave morphologies in lead III in the two tracings are mirror opposites, repeat the ECG with close attention to correct electrode connection.

Clues to limb electrode reversal are summarized in Table 14–3.

Precordial Electrode Misplacement and Misconnection

Unlike the limb electrodes, the precordial electrodes are more prone to misplacement, especially when variations in body habitus (e.g., obesity, breast tissue, pectus excavatum, chronic lung disease) make proper electrode placement more difficult.

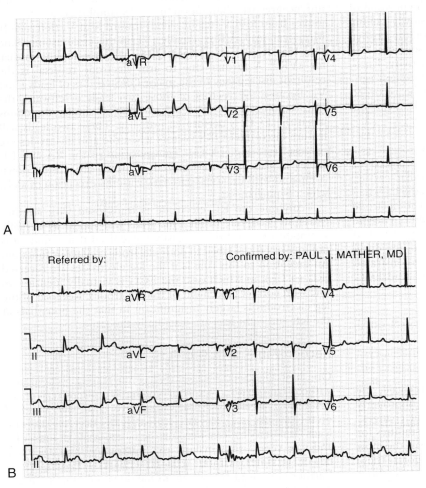

Figure 14–14 *A,* Limb lead reversal (LA ↔ LL). A patient with a history consistent with acute coronary syndrome was brought to the emergency department after this ECG was recorded in a clinic. Leads I and aVL suggest an acute high lateral infarct but, surprisingly, there are no corresponding changes in leads V5 and V6. The deep T-wave inversions in III and aVF were at first thought to be inferior ischemia or reciprocal changes (see also *B*). *B,* Correction of lead reversal (LA ↔ LL). After the leads were reconnected, this tracing reveals an acute inferior wall myocardial infarction (MI), as well as deep T-wave inversion in aVL—a harbinger of acute inferior MI. Comparing this tracing with that in *A,* note the following: lead I ↔ lead II; lead aVL ↔ aVF, and lead III is inverted. Thus, inferior changes become lateral, and lateral become inferior.

TABLE 14–3 Clues to Improper Limb Lead Connections

Reversed Leads	Old ECG Necessary for Detection?	Key Findings
LA RA	No	PQRST upside down in lead I Precordial leads normal (not dextrocardia)
LA LL	Yes	III is upside down I ↔ II; aVL ↔ aVF; aVR no change
LA RL	No	III is straight line
RA LL	No	PQRST upside down in all leads except aVL
RA RL	No	II is straight line
LL RL	Cannot detect change	Looks like normal lead placement
LA LL RA RL	No	I is straight line aVL, aVR are same polarity and amplitude *and* II is upside down III

LA, left arm; LL, left leg; RA, right arm; RL, right leg.
From Surawicz B, Knilans TK: Chou's Electrocardiography in Clinical Practice, 5th ed. Philadelphia, WB Saunders, 2001.

This may cause some variability in the amplitude and morphology of the complexes in the precordial leads. However, these changes are not usually grossly abnormal, and therefore can be difficult to detect. Variation often becomes evident when comparing the current tracing with an old ECG.[39] In such cases, it is useful to go to the bedside and examine where the electrodes were positioned relative to the recommended placement (see "Electrode Placement" earlier in this chapter). One cannot ensure, however, that the baseline ECG was done with proper electrode placement. When comparing the precordial leads on the current ECG with a baseline tracing, ST segment and T-wave changes should be viewed in the context of the relative morphologies of the associated QRS complexes. If there is a marked difference between the two tracings in the amplitude and polarity of the QRS complex in a given precordial lead, the corresponding ST-T wave changes may be due to variability in electrode placement—although cardiac ischemia cannot be completely excluded as the cause.

Misconnection of the precordial cables is usually easy to detect. The expected progression of P-, QRS, and T-wave morphologies across the precordium will be disrupted (Fig. 14–15). An abrupt change in wave morphology evolution—followed by a seeming return to normalcy in the next lead—is a good clue to precordial electrode misconnection.[39]

ARTIFACT

Electrocardiographic artifact is commonly encountered, yet not always easy to recognize. It can be attributed to either physiologic (internal) or nonphysiologic (external) sources; the former includes muscle activity, patient motion, and poor electrode contact with the skin. Tremors, hiccups, and shivering may produce frequent, narrow spikes on the tracing, simulating atrial and ventricular dysrhythmias[38,40] (Fig. 14–16). A wandering baseline featuring wide undulations, as well as other "noise" on the ECG, can often be traced to patient movement and high skin impedance, leading to inadequate electrode contact to the skin. Minimizing skin impedance and artifact may be achieved by (1) avoiding electrode placement over bony prominences, major muscles, or pulsating arteries, (2) clipping rather than shaving thick hair at electrode sites, and (3) cleaning and, most importantly, drying the skin surface before reapplying the electrode if the tracing features substantial artifact.[38,41] Nonphysiologic artifact is most often due to 60-Hz electrical interference, which is ascribable to various other sources of alternating current near the patient. This will manifest as a wide, indistinct isoelectric baseline. Other sources of nonphysiologic artifact include loose connections, broken monitor cables, and mechanical issues with the machine (e.g., broken stylus, uneven paper transport). The 60-Hz artifact due to electrical current interference can be minimized by shutting off nonessential sources of current in the vicinity as well as straightening the lead wires so that they are parallel to the patient's body in the long axis.[38,40,42]

Differentiation of artifact from true electrocardiographic abnormality is intuitively important; moreover, clinical consequences have been reported that are directly attributable to confusion of artifact with disease. Unnecessary treatment and procedures—including cardiac catheterization, electrophysio-

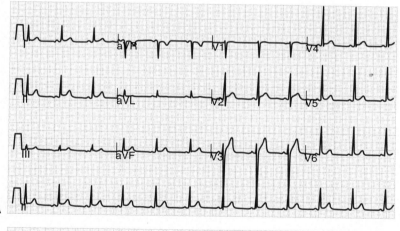

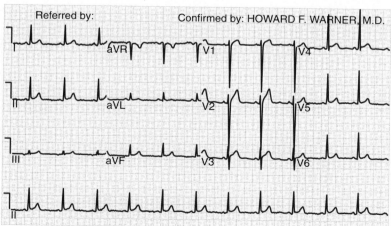

Figure 14–15 *A and B,* Precordial lead reversal (V$_2$ ↔ V$_3$). Note that the usual precordial progression of R-wave growth in leads V$_2$ and V$_3$ is disrupted in the tracing displayed in *A. B* shows a return to a normal V$_3$ transition zone.

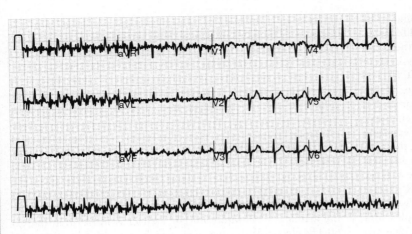

Figure 14–16 Artifact due to physiologic cause. The patient's monitor was alarming owing to a perceived heart rate of greater than 200 beats/min, and the computerized alert system called this ventricular tachycardia. The patient, who has Parkinson's disease, was without complaint. The ECG demonstrates a marked artifact, giving the appearance of atrial flutter in lead V₁.

logic testing, and even implantation of a pacemaker and an automatic defibrillator—have been reported.[43] Characteristics that may aid in differentiating artifact from dysrhythmia include absence of hemodynamic instability during the event (or even absence of any symptoms); normal QRS complexes occurring during the dysrhythmia; instability of the baseline on the tracing during and immediately after the "dysrhyth-mic" event; association with body movement; and observance of "notches" amidst the complexes of the pseudodysrhythmia which "march out" with the normal QRS complexes that precede and follow the disturbance.[44,45]

REFERENCES CAN BE FOUND ON **EXPERT CONSULT**

CHAPTER 15

Emergency Cardiac Pacing

Edward S. Bessman

The purpose of cardiac pacing is to restore or ensure effective cardiac depolarization. Emergency cardiac pacing may be instituted either prophylactically or therapeutically. Prophylactic indications include those situations in which there is high risk of atrioventricular (AV) block. Therapeutic indications include symptomatic bradyarrhythmias and overdrive pacing. Pacing for asystole has very minimal success but has been used for this condition. Several approaches to pacing exist, including transcutaneous, transvenous, transthoracic, epicardial, endocardial, and esophageal. Transcutaneous and transvenous are the two techniques most commonly used in the emergency department (ED). Because it can be instituted quickly and noninvasively, transcutaneous pacing is the technique of choice in the ED when time is of the essence. Transvenous pacing should be reserved for patients who require prolonged pacing or who have a very high (>30%) risk of heart block. Transcutaneous pacing is generally a temporizing measure that may precede transvenous cardiac pacing. Although it is not an expectation that all emergency clinicians will be adept at placing emergency cardiac pacemakers, many have mastered the techniques and are the only clinicians available to perform this life-saving procedure.

EMERGENCY TRANSVENOUS CARDIAC PACING

The transvenous method of endocardial pacing is commonly used and is both safe and effective. In skilled hands, the semifloating transvenous catheter is successfully placed under electrocardiographic (ECG) guidance in 80% of patients.[1] The technique can be performed in less than 20 minutes in 72% of patients and in less than 5 minutes in 30% of patients. However, in some instances, anatomic, logistical, and hemodynamic impediments can prohibit successful pacing by even the most skilled clinician. As with other medical procedures, it should not be performed without a thorough understanding of its indications, contraindications, and complications.[2]

However, because this is essentially a blind procedure, a certain amount of luck and chance are consequential to a successful outcome. Therefore, sometimes this procedure simply will not be successful, either because the condition is not amenable to pacing (e.g., asystole, drug overdose) or because of technical difficulties inherent with the procedure.

 BACKGROUND CAN BE FOUND ON EXPERT CONSULT

Indications

The purpose of cardiac pacing is to stimulate effective cardiac depolarization. In most cases, the specific indications for cardiac pacing are clear; however, some controversial areas remain. The decision to pace on an emergent basis requires knowledge of the presence or absence of hemodynamic compromise, the etiology of the rhythm disturbance, the status of the AV conduction system, and the type of dysrhythmia. *The clinician caring for the patient is in the best position to decide on the value, or nonvalue, of pacing, based on nuances of the clinical scenario that are not possible to unravel by any theoretical discussion.* Controversy exists throughout the literature, and this discussion *is not meant to set a standard of care for individual circumstances.*

In general, the indications can be grouped into those that cause either tachycardias or bradycardias (Table 15–3). Transcutaneous cardiac pacing (TCP) has become the mainstay of emergent cardiac pacing and is often used pending placement of the transvenous catheter or to determine whether potentially terminal bradyasystolic rhythms will respond to pacing.

Bradycardias

Sinus Node Dysfunction. Sinus node dysfunction may manifest as sinus arrest, tachybrady (sick sinus) syndrome, or sinus bradycardia. Whereas symptomatic sinus node dysfunction is a common indication for elective permanent pacing, it is seldom cause for emergency pacemaker insertion.

In acute myocardial infarction (AMI), 17% of patients will experience sinus bradycardia.[14] It occurs more frequently in inferior than in anterior infarction and has a relatively good prognosis when accompanied by a hemodynamically tolerable escape rhythm. However, sinus bradycardia is not a benign rhythm in this situation; it has a mortality rate of 2% with inferior infarction and 9% with anterior infarction.[15] Sinus node dysfunction frequently responds to medical therapy but requires prompt pacing if this fails.

Asystolic Arrest. Transvenous pacing in the asystolic or bradyasystolic patient has little value. In 1 study of 13 patients who had suffered cardiac arrest, capture of the myocardium was noted in 4 patients, but there were no survivors.[16] Transvenous pacing alone may also not be effective in postcountershock pulseless bradyarrhythmias.[17] This failure of pacing has also been demonstrated with transcutaneous pacemakers, suggesting that failure of effective pacing is primarily related to the state of the myocardial tissue.[16] Cardiac pacing may be used as a "last-ditch" effort in bradyasystolic patients but is rarely successful and is not considered standard practice. Early pacing is essential when done for this purpose if success is to be achieved[18] (see later in this section). Most importantly, given the recognition of the importance of maximizing chest compressions during cardiopulmonary resuscitation (CPR), interrupting CPR in order to institute emergency pacing is not recommended.[19]

AV Block. AV block is the classic indication for pacemaker therapy. In symptomatic patients without myocardial infarction (MI) and in the asymptomatic patient with a ventricular rate below 40, pacemaker therapy is indicated.[20]

In patients with AMI, 15% to 19% progress to heart block: approximately 8% develop first-degree block, 5% develop second-degree block, and 6% develop third-degree block.[21] First-degree block progresses to second- or third-degree block 33% of the time, and second-degree block progresses to third-degree block about one third of the time.[22]

AV block occurring during anterior infarction is believed to occur because of diffuse ischemia to the septum and infranodal conduction tissue. These patients tend to progress to high-degree block without warning, and a pacemaker is often placed prophylactically. Some patients are prophylacti-

TABLE 15–1 Four-Letter Pacemaker Code

First Letter	Second Letter	Third Letter	Fourth Letter
Chamber-Paced	**Chamber-Sensed**	**Sensing Response**	**Programmability**
A = atrium	A = atrium	T = triggered	P = simple
V = ventricle	V = ventricle	I = inhibited	M = multiprogrammable
D = dual	D = dual	D = dual (A-triggered and V-inhibited)	R = rate adaptive
O = none	O = none	O = none	C = communicating
			O = none

TABLE 15–2 History of Transvenous Pacing

Date	Investigator	Event
1700	Early investigators	First restimulation studies
1951	Callaghan & Bigelow	First transvenous approach in dogs
1952	Zoll	Transcutaneous cardiac stimulator
1958	Falkmann & Walkins	Implanted pacing wires after surgery
1959	Furman & Robinson	First transvenous pacer in humans
1964	Vogel et al	Flexible electrocardiographic catheter without fluoroscopy
1965	Kimball & Killip	First bedside transvenous pacing
1966	Goetz et al	Demand pacemaker developed
1967	Zuckerman et al	Use of demand pacemaker clinically
1969	Rosenberg et al	Semifloating pacing catheter
1973	Schnitzler et al	Balloon-tipped pacers

TABLE 15–3 Indications for Cardiac Pacing

Bradycardias

Without myocardial infarction
  Symptomatic sinus node dysfunction (sinus arrest, tachybrady [sick sinus] syndrome, sinus bradycardia)
  Second- and third-degree heart block
  Atrial fibrillation with slow ventricular response
With myocardial infarction
  Symptomatic sinus node dysfunction
  Mobitz II second- and third-degree heart block
  New left bundle branch block, right bundle branch block with left axis deviation, bifascicular block, or alternating bundle branch block
Prophylaxis: cardiac catheterization, after open heart surgery, threatened bradycardia during drug trials for tachydysrhythmias
Malfunction of implanted pacemaker

Tachycardias

Supraventricular dysrhythmias
Ventricular dysrhythmias
Prophylaxis: cardiac catheterization, after open heart surgery

cally paced on a temporary basis, even in the absence of hemodynamic compromise.

During inferior infarction, early septal ischemia is the exception and, typically, block develops sequentially from first-degree to Mobitz type I second-degree, then to third-

degree AV block. These conduction abnormalities frequently result in hemodynamically tolerable escape rhythms because of sparing of the bundle branches. The hemodynamically unstable patient who is unresponsive to medical therapy should be paced promptly. Whether and when the stable patient should be paced is unclear, but placing a transcutaneous pacer is one option that can be tried before placing a transvenous pacing catheter.

Trauma. Pacing is not a standard intervention in traumatic cardiac arrest. In selected cases, it may be considered. Several rhythm and conduction disturbances have been documented in the patient with nonpenetrating chest trauma. In these patients, traumatic injury to the specialized conduction system may predispose the patient to life-threatening dysrhythmias and blocks that can be treated by cardiac pacing.[23]

Hypovolemia and hypotension can cause ischemia of conduction tissue and cardiac dysfunction.[24] Marked bradyarrhythmias that persist even after vigorous volume replacement may rarely respond to cardiac pacing in patients with such trauma.[25]

Bundle Branch Block and Ischemia

Bundle branch block occurring in AMI is associated with a higher mortality rate and a greater incidence of third-degree heart block than uncomplicated infarction. Atkins and colleagues[26] noted that 18% of patients with MI had bundle branch block. Of these patients, complete heart block developed in 43% who had right bundle branch block (RBBB) and left axis deviation, in 17% who had left bundle branch block (LBBB), in 19% who had left anterior hemiblock, and in 6% who had no conduction block. The investigators concluded that RBBB with left axis deviation should be paced prophylactically.

A study by Hindman and associates[27] confirmed the natural history of bundle branch block during MI. In their study, the presence or absence of first-degree AV block, the type of bundle branch block, and the age of the block (new vs. old) were used to determine the relative risk of progression to type II second-degree or third-degree block (Table 15–4).

Because of the increased risk, consider pacing the following conduction blocks: *new-onset* LBBB, RBBB with left axis deviation or other bifascicular block, and alternating bundle branch block.[27] Although controversial, one author recommends prophylactic pacing for all new bundle branch blocks when MI is evident.[28]

Whether to place a transvenous pacemaker prophylactically in patients with LBBB before insertion of a flow-directed pulmonary artery catheter (PAC) remains controversial. Some researchers strongly advocate this procedure because of the

TABLE 15–4 The Influence of Different Variables on the Risk of High-Degree Atrioventricular Block in Patients with Bundle Branch Block during Myocardial Infarction

Patients	Progressing to High-Degree AVB (%)
Infarct location	
Anterior	25
Indeterminate	12
Inferior or posterior	20
PR interval	
>0.20 sec	25
≤0.20 sec	19
Type of BBB	
LBBB	13
RBBB	14
RBBB + LAFB	27
RBBB + LPFB	29
ABBB	44
Onset of BBB	
Definitely old	13
Possibly new	25
Probably new	26
Definitely new	23

ABBB, alternating bundle branch block; AVB, atrioventricular block; BBB, bundle branch block; LAFB, left anterior fascicular hemiblock; LBBB, left bundle branch block; LPFB, left posterior fascicular hemiblock; RBBB, right bundle branch block.

Reprinted by permission of the American Heart Association from Hindman MC, Wagner GS, JaRo M, et al: The clinical significance of bundle branch block complicating acute myocardial infarction. 2. Indications of temporary and permanent pacemaker insertion. Circulation 58:690, 1978.

risk of transient RBBB and life-threatening complete heart block associated with PAC placement.[29] One study notes that this risk is low in patients with prior LBBB but continues to recommend temporary catheter placement for all cases of *new* LBBB.[30] One solution to this problem is to place a transcutaneous pacemaker before catheterization as an emergency measure should heart block develop. In these cases, a temporary transvenous pacemaker can be placed in a semielective manner when needed.[31] In any event, the trend toward decreased PAC use, particularly outside of the critical care setting, makes it unlikely that this will be an issue in the ED.[32]

One final point to bear in mind regarding bradydysrythmias in the setting of AMI is that most of the investigations into the use of temporary pacing were done in the prethrombolytic era. Modern treatment of AMI is substantially different, but more recent studies, particularly of prophylactic pacing, are lacking.

Tachycardias

Hemodynamically compromising tachycardias are usually treated by medical means or electrical cardioversion. Since 1980, there has been an increasing interest in pacing therapy for symptomatic tachycardias. Supraventricular dysrhythmias, with the exception of atrial fibrillation, respond well to atrial pacing. By "overdrive" pacing the atria at rates 10 to 20 beats/min faster than the underlying rhythm, the atria become entrained, and when the rate is slowed, the rhythm frequently returns to normal sinus. A similar procedure is done for ventricular dysrhythmias.[33] Overdrive pacing is especially useful for recurrent prolonged Q-T interval arrhythmias such as

those seen with quinidine toxicity or torsades de pointes.[34] Although this is an attractive thought, there is no reported experience with these techniques in the ED. Transvenous pacing also is useful in patients with digitalis-induced dysrhythmias in whom direct current (DC) cardioversion may be dangerous or in patients in whom there is further concern about myocardial depression with drugs.[35]

Cardiac Pacing in Drug-Induced Dysrhythmias

Significant dysrhythmias can occur from excessive therapeutic medication (often in combination therapy) and from overdose of cardioactive medications. Because these drugs have direct effects on the myocardial pacemaker and conduction system cells, *cardiac pacing is usually of little therapeutic value*. Both bradycardias and tachycardias may result. Tachycardic rhythms from amphetamines, cocaine, anticholinergics, cyclic antidepressants, theophylline, and others do not benefit from cardiac pacing. Drug-induced torsades de pointes may theoretically be overdriven by pacing, but data on this technique are lacking. Any drug that affects the central nervous system (e.g., opiates, sedative-hypnotics, clonidine) may produce bradycardia. Rare causes of toxin-induced bradycardia include organophosphate poisoning, various cholinergic drugs, ciguatera poisoning, and rarely, plant toxins. Cardiac pacing is not used for bradycardias from these sources; rather, the underlying central nervous system depression is addressed.

Severe bradycardia and heart block often accompany overdose of digitalis preparations, β-adrenergic blockers, and calcium channel blockers. Although intuitively attractive, *cardiac pacing is generally not effective in serious toxin-induced bradycardias*, even though there are case reports of successes.[36-39] In β-blocker overdose, pacing may increase heart rate but rarely benefits blood pressure or cardiac output. Worsening of the blood pressure may be seen from loss of atrial contractions with ventricular pacing. Likewise, calcium channel blocker overdose and digitalis-induced bradycardia and heart block rarely benefit from cardiac pacing. Pharmacologic interventions, such as digoxin-specific Fab, glucagon, calcium, inotropic medications, and vasopressors, remain the mainstay in the treatment of drug-induced dysrhythmias. Given the lack of success of pacing, possible downsides, and the greater effectiveness of specific antidotes, it is not standard to routinely attempt transvenous cardiac pacing in the setting of drug overdose. However, as a last resort, cardiac pacing can be supported.[40]

Contraindications

The presence of a prosthetic tricuspid valve is generally considered to be an absolute contraindication to transvenous cardiac pacing.[41] Also, severe hypothermia will occasionally result in ventricular fibrillation when pacing is attempted. Because ventricular fibrillation under these conditions is difficult to convert, caution is advised when considering pacing the severely hypothermic and bradycardic patient. Rapid and careful rewarming is often recommended first, followed by pacing if the patient's condition does not improve.

Equipment

Several items are required to insert a transvenous pacemaker adequately. Like most special procedures, a prearranged tray is convenient. The usual components required to insert a transvenous cardiac pacemaker are listed in Table 15–5.

TABLE 15–5 Suggested Transvenous Cardiac Pacemaker Equipment

Pacemaker Tray*

10-mL syringe
1% lidocaine
Alcohol wipes
Povidone-iodine (Betadine)
Several gauze pads
4 sterile drapes
No. 11 scalpel blade
0.9 normal saline–2 ampules
Sterile gloves
Needle holder
Two 22-gauge needles
Scissors (suture)
Two 4-0 silk sutures on needles
Sterile basin
Introducer set (sheath, guidewire, dilator, introducer needle)

Electrical Hardware

Insulated connecting wire with alligator clamps at each end (or a male-to-male adapter)
Fresh battery and a spare
Pacing generator
Pacing catheter*
12-lead electrocardiographic machine (well grounded)

*Some or all of these components are available in prepackaged sets.

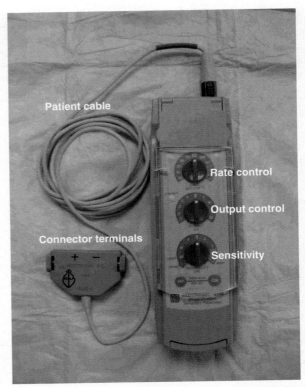

Figure 15–1 Pacemaker energy source controls and connections.

Pacing Generator

Many different pacing generators are available, but in general, they all have the same basic features. The controls frequently will have a locking feature or cover to prevent the generator from being switched off or reprogrammed inadvertently. An amperage control allows the operator to vary the amount of electrical current delivered to the myocardium, usually 0.1 to 20 mA. *Increasing* the setting *increases* the output and *improves* the likelihood of capture. The pacing control mode is determined by adjusting the gain setting for the sensing function of the generator. By increasing the sensitivity, one can convert the unit from a fixed-rate (asynchronous mode) to a demand (synchronous mode) pacemaker. The typical pacing generator has a sensitivity setting that ranges from about 0.5 to 20 mV. The voltage setting represents the minimum strength of electrical signal that the pacer is able to detect. *Decreasing* the setting *increases* the sensitivity and *improves* the likelihood of sensing myocardial depolarization. In the fixed-rate mode, the unit fires despite the underlying intrinsic rhythm; that is, the unit does not sense any intrinsic electrical activity. In the full-demand mode, however, the pacemaker senses the underlying ventricular depolarizations and the unit does not fire as long as the patient's ventricular rate is equal to or faster than the set rate of the pacing generator. A sensing indicator meter and rate control knob are also present.

Temporary pacing generators are battery operated; thus, it is always good practice to install a fresh battery whenever pacing is anticipated. An example of a pacing generator is shown in Figure 15–1.

Pacing Catheters and Electrodes

Several sizes and brands of pacing catheters are available. In general, most range from 3 to 5 French in size and are approximately 100 cm in length. Lines are marked along the catheter surface at approximately 10-cm intervals; these can be used to

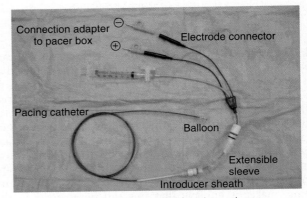

Figure 15–2 Balloon-tipped pacing catheter.

estimate catheter position during insertion. Pacing catheters differ with respect to their stiffness, electrode configurations, floating characteristics, and other qualities. For emergency pacing, the semifloating bipolar electrode catheter with a balloon tip is used most frequently (Fig. 15–2). The balloon holds approximately 1.5 mL of air, and the air injection port has a locking lever to secure balloon expansion. Before insertion, the balloon is checked for air leakage by inflating it and immersing it in sterile water. The presence of an air leak is noted by a stream of bubbles rising to the surface of the water. An inflated balloon helps the catheter "float" into the heart, even in low-flow states, but is obviously not advantageous in the cardiac arrest situation.

For all practical purposes, temporary transvenous pacing is accomplished with a bipolar pacing catheter. The terms *unipolar* and *bipolar* refer to the number of electrodes in contact with that portion of the heart that is to be stimulated.

All pacemaker systems must have both a positive (anode) and a negative (cathode) electrode; hence, *all stimulation is bipolar*. In the typical bipolar catheter used for temporary transvenous pacing, the cathode (stimulating electrode) is at the tip of the pacing catheter. The anode is located 1 to 2 cm proximal to the tip, and a balloon or an insulated wire separates the two electrodes. The distinction between the unipolar and the bipolar pacing catheter is that a bipolar catheter has both electrodes in relatively close proximity on the catheter, and both may contact the endocardium. In the bipolar catheter, the electrodes are usually stainless steel or platinum rings that encircle the pacing catheter. When properly positioned, both electrodes will be within the right ventricle so that a field of electrical excitation is set up between the electrodes. With the bipolar catheter, the cathode does not need to be in direct contact with the endocardium for pacing to occur, although it is preferable to have direct contact.

A unipolar system is also effective but is used infrequently for temporary transvenous pacing. In a unipolar system, the cathode is at the tip of the pacing catheter, and the anode is located in one of three places: (1) in the pacing generator itself, (2) more proximally on the catheter (outside the ventricle), or (3) on the patient's chest. The bipolar system may be converted to a unipolar system by simply disconnecting the positive proximal connection of the bipolar catheter from the pacing generator and running a new wire from the positive (pacing generator) terminal to the patient's chest wall. Such a conversion may be required in the unlikely event of failure of one lead of the bipolar system.

ECG Machine

An ECG machine can be used to record the heart's inherent electrical activity during pacer insertion and to aid in localization of the catheter tip without fluoroscopy. The ECG machine must be well grounded to prevent leakage of alternating current, which can cause ventricular fibrillation. Such leakage should be suspected if interference of 50 to 60 cycles/sec (Hertz) is noted on the ECG.

The ECG machine should be placed in such a manner as to allow easy visibility of the rhythm during insertion. One method is to place the machine near the level of the patient's midthorax facing the operator, on either side of the patient as logistics and operator preference allow (Fig. 15–3). Note that the operator stands at the head of the patient during internal jugular or subclavian vein passage of the catheter and at the midabdomen for femoral or brachiocephalic vein insertion. Newer patient monitors may be equipped with suitable ECG connections to allow their use in place of a stand-alone ECG machine. Because these patients will already be attached to a monitor, it may prove convenient to use the same piece of equipment to assist with pacemaker insertion.

Introducer Sheath

An introducer set or sheath is required for venous access. Some pacing catheters are prepackaged with the appropriate equipment, whereas others require a separate set. The introducer set is used to enhance passage of the pacing catheter through the skin, subcutaneous tissue, and vessel wall. The sheath must be larger than the pacing catheter in order to allow it to pass. The size of the pacing catheter refers to its outside diameter, and the size of the introducer refers to its inside diameter. Thus a 5-French pacing catheter will fit through a 5-French introducer. Introducer sheaths are available with a perforated elastic seal covering the opening

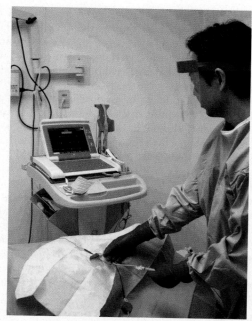

Figure 15–3 Position of an electrocardiographic (ECG) device during insertion of a pacemaker catheter through the left subclavian vein.

through which the pacing catheter is passed (pacer port). The seal allows the catheter to be manipulated while preventing blood from escaping or air from entering the vein. A side port allows the sheath to be used for central venous access. A makeshift sheath can be fashioned with an appropriate-sized intravenous (IV) catheter. For the 3-French balloon-tipped catheter, a 14-gauge, 1.5- to 2-in. IV catheter is suitable. The 4-French balloon-tipped catheter will also fit through a 14-gauge catheter or needle. However, without a seal over the hub, blood will leak from the end of the IV catheter.

Overall, the key to success with this procedure is preparation. In a typical ED, there is often a variety of vascular access kits and devices, not all of which will work well, if at all, for passing a pacing catheter. It is imperative that one examine all the components of the tray before starting the procedure and ensure that all wires, sheaths, dilators, and syringes fit as expected. Ideally, all of the equipment and accessories needed for emergency pacemaker insertion should be kept together in a designated location.

Procedure

A checklist for the preparation and initial setup of the pacing generator is shown in Box 15–1. It may be useful to have a copy of this or a similar list stored with the pacemaker to have on hand in emergent situations.

Patient Preparation

Patient instruction is an extremely important aspect of any procedure. Frequently, there is not enough time to give patients a detailed explanation or to obtain written informed consent. Nonetheless, sufficient information should be provided so that the patient feels at ease. It is always prudent to obtain and document informed consent from the patient, if possible, prior to any invasive procedure or to document that the circumstances did not allow informed consent. Patients should be assured that they will feel no discomfort after the venipuncture site has been anesthetized and that they will feel better when the catheter is in place and is functional. Continued reassurance is required during the procedure because patients are usually facing away from the operator and their faces are often covered; thus, they may be unsure of what is occurring. Sedation and analgesia should be considered when appropriate.

All operators should wear surgical masks, caps, gloves, and gowns to decrease the risk of infection before catheter placement. Patients should be prepared and draped in the usual sterile fashion. This aseptic precaution should also be explained to the patient.

Site Selection

The four venous channels that provide an easy access to the right ventricle are the brachial, subclavian, femoral, and internal jugular veins (Table 15–6). The route selected is often one of personal or institutional preference. *The right internal jugular and the left subclavian veins have the straightest anatomic pathway to the right ventricle and are generally preferred for temporary transvenous pacing.* In some centers, a particular site

---

BOX 15–1	**Checklist for Temporary Transvenous Pacing Generator***

- Insert new battery
- Turn pacemaker ON
- Set RATE (80 beats/min) OUTPUT (5 mA) and SENSITIVITY (3 mV)[†]
- Connect patient cable to pacemaker
- Open both connector terminals on patient cable
- Insert PROXIMAL (+) pin of pacing catheter into POSITIVE (+) connector terminal on patient cable
- Tighten connection firmly
- Use alligator clips to connect DISTAL (–) pin of pacing catheter to lead V_1 of ECG machine
- When catheter is in position, remove DISTAL (–) pin from V_1 and insert it into the NEGATIVE (–) connector terminal on patient cable
- Tighten connection firmly

Adjust pacemaker settings as needed to achieve proper capture and sensitivity (see text).
[†]*Guidelines only. Follow recommendations of device manufacturer if different.*
ECG, electrocardiographic.

---

is preferred for *permanent transvenous pacemaker placement,* and if possible, this site should be avoided for temporary placement.

The subclavian vein can be accessed by both an infraclavicular and a supraclavicular approach; the infraclavicular approach is most commonly reported for all temporary transvenous pacemaker insertions. This route is preferred because of its easy accessibility, close proximity to the heart, and ease in catheter maintenance and stability. The supraclavicular approach has been described in the literature for several years and has gained popularity among some clinicians.[42,43] The *left* subclavian vein is preferred because of the less acute angle traversed when compared with the right-sided approach, but either side may be used.[42,43]

The internal jugular approach may also be used. In this case, the *right* internal jugular vein is preferred because of the direct line to the superior vena cava. Problems with this approach include dislodgment of the pacemaker with movement of the head, carotid artery puncture, and thrombophlebitis.

During CPR, the use of the right internal jugular vein and the left subclavian veins for pacemaker insertion have been demonstrated to result in the highest rates of proper placement in the right ventricle.[44] The right internal jugular vein is the more direct route of the two and may be the most appropriate site.

Femoral veins, like neck veins, are compressible and easily catheterized. Problems include easy dislodgment, infection, and increased risk of thrombophlebitis.[45,46]

Brachial vein catheterization is easy to perform but results in a high incidence of infection and vessel thrombosis.[47] In addition, the catheter is easily dislodged with arm motion. This approach is seldom used in the emergency setting.

Although the left subclavian and right internal jugular veins are the preferred routes for access, in an emergency situation, the clinician should use the approach with which she or he is most experienced so as to minimize the time spent in cannulating the vein and reduce the potential for complications from the venipuncture.

Skin Preparation and Venous Access

The skin over the venipuncture site is cleaned twice with an antiseptic solution such as chlorhexidine or povidone-iodine.

TABLE 15–6 Advantages and Disadvantages of Pacemaker Placement Sites

Venous Channels	Advantages	Disadvantages
Brachial	Very safe route Vessel easily accessible, either by cutdown or percutaneous approach Compressible	Often requires cutdown Easily displaced and poor patient mobility Not reusable if cutdown technique is performed Catheter is more difficult to advance than with central or larger vessels
Subclavian	Direct access to right heart (especially via left subclavian) Rapid insertion time Good patient mobility	Pneumothorax and other intrathoracic trauma are possible Noncompressible
Femoral	Direct access to right heart Rapid insertion time Compressible	Increased incidence of thrombophlebitis Can be dislodged by leg movement and poor patient mobility Infection
Internal jugular	Direct access to right heart (especially via right internal jugular) Rapid insertion time Compressible	Possible carotid artery puncture Dislodgment with movement of the head Thrombophlebitis

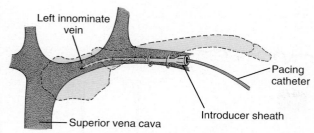

Figure 15–4 Insertion of the pacing catheter through the introducer sheath.

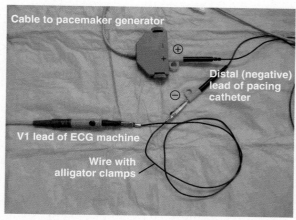

Figure 15–5 Using alligator clips to connect the pacemaker to the V_1 lead of an ECG machine.

A wide area is prepared because of the tendency for guidewires and catheters to spring from the hands of the unsuspecting operator. Similarly, wide draping is carried out in the standard manner to maintain a sterile field and to allow clear visibility of the venipuncture site.

The infraclavicular approach is used in this chapter to illustrate venous access, although the mechanics are generally the same for other vascular approaches.

Occasionally, a patient who already has a central venous line in place requires the emergent placement of a pacing catheter. An existing central venous pressure (CVP) line can be used to place the pacing catheter if the catheter lumen is large enough to accept a guidewire. The CVP line should be withdrawn 3 to 5 cm to expose an area of sterile tubing. The tubing is transected through a sterile area while being held firmly at the skin level. A guidewire can then be passed through the tubing, and the tubing can be withdrawn, leaving only the wire in the vein. The guidewire and the tubing should never be released, because embolization may result.

With the guidewire in place, a dilator and introducer sheath can then be passed together over the guidewire, as is done in the Seldinger technique. The dilator and guidewire are then removed and the pacing catheter can be passed through the introducer sheath (Fig. 15–4). One key additional step to help preserve sterility while manipulating the pacing catheter is to attach an extensible sleeve on the end of the introducer prior to inserting the pacing catheter (see Fig. 15–2). In this way, the pacing catheter can be advanced and withdrawn multiple times without fear of contamination.

Bedside ultrasound can be useful as an aid to securing central venous access and its use in the setting of emergency transvenous pacing has been reported.[48,49]

Pacemaker Placement

ECG Guidance. The patient should be connected to the limb leads of an ECG machine, and the indicator should be turned to record the chest (V) lead.

With newer ECG machines, the pacemaker may be attached to any of the V leads (usually V_1 or V_5) that are displayed during rhythm monitoring. The *distal* terminal of the pacing catheter (the cathode, or lead marked "negative", "–," or "distal") must be connected to the V lead of the ECG machine by a male-to-male connector or an insulated wire with an alligator clip on each end (Fig. 15–5). The pacing catheter is thus an exploring electrode that creates a unipolar electrode for intracardiac ECG recording. The electrocardiogram recorded from the electrode tip *localizes the position of the tip of the pacing electrode*. As the tracing on the ECG machine may be slightly delayed, advancement of the catheter after initial insertion must be carefully evaluated. If a balloon-tipped catheter is used, the balloon is inflated with air *after*

the catheter enters the superior vena cava (~10–12 cm for a subclavian or internal jugular insertion). The inflation port should be locked and the syringe left attached.

The pacing catheter should be advanced both quickly and smoothly. The V lead should be monitored, and the P-wave and QRS complex should be observed to ascertain the location of the pacing catheter tip. The use of an electrocardiogram to guide the placement of a pacing catheter is based on two concepts. First, the complex will vary in size depending on which chamber is entered. For example, when the tip of the pacing catheter is in the atrium, one will see large P-waves, often larger than the corresponding QRS complex. Second, the sum of the electrical forces will be negative if the depolarization is moving away from the catheter tip and positive if the depolarization is moving toward the catheter tip. Therefore, if the catheter tip is *above* the atrium, both the P-wave and the QRS complex will be negative (i.e., the electrical forces of a normally beating heart will be moving away from the catheter tip). As the tip progresses inferiorly in the atrium, the P-wave will become isoelectric (biphasic) and will eventually become positive as the wave of atrial depolarization advances toward the catheter tip. The electrocardiogram resembles an aVR lead initially when in the left subclavian vein (Fig. 15–6A) or midsuperior vena cava (see Fig. 15–6B). At the high right atrium, both the P-wave and the QRS complex are negative; the P-wave is larger than the QRS complex and is deeply inverted (see Fig. 15–6C and D). As the center of the atrium is approached, the P-wave becomes large and biphasic (see Fig. 15–6E). As the catheter approaches the lower atrium (see Fig. 15–6F), the P-wave becomes smaller and upright. The QRS complex is fairly normal. When striking the right atrial wall, an injury pattern with a P-Ta segment is seen (see Fig. 15–6G). As the electrode passes through the tricuspid valve, the P-wave becomes smaller and the QRS complex becomes larger (see Fig. 15–6H). Placement in the inferior vena cava may be recognized by a change in the morphology of the P-wave and a decrease in the amplitude of both the P-wave and the QRS complex (see Fig. 15–6I).

Once the pacing catheter is in the desired position, deflate the balloon by unlocking the port, observing that the syringe refills with air spontaneously, and then removing the syringe. One should avoid drawing back on the syringe because this may cause balloon rupture. If the syringe does not refill spontaneously, the operator should suspect that the balloon might be ruptured. The balloon should not be inflated and the

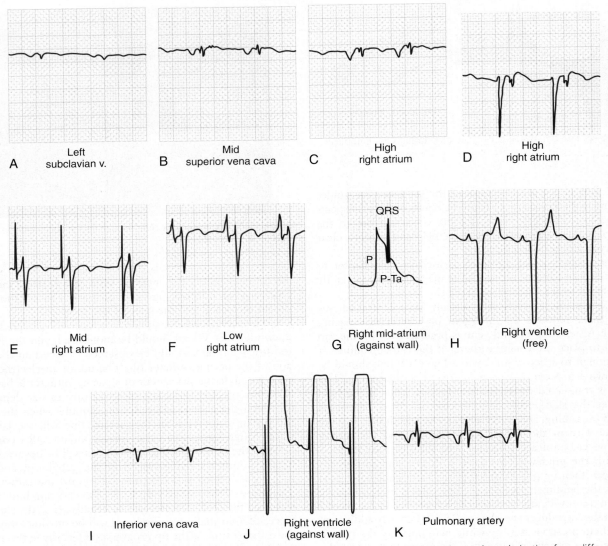

Figure 15–6 *A–K,* Intracardiac electrocardiography: Electrical signals of atrial and ventricular depolarization and repolarization from different vascular and intracardiac locations (see text). *(A–F and H–K, From Bing OH, McDowell JW, Hantman J, et al: Pacemaker placement by electrocardiographic monitoring. N Engl J Med 287:651, 1972; G, from Goldberger E: Treatment of Cardiac Emergencies, 3rd ed. St. Louis, CV Mosby, 1982, p 252.)*

pacing catheter should be withdrawn and the balloon checked for leaks. If a leak is found, a new pacing catheter should be used.

After successful passage of the catheter into the right ventricle, the tip should be advanced until contact is made with the endocardial wall. When this occurs, the QRS segment will show ST segment elevation (see Fig. 15–6*J*). Ideally, the tip of the catheter should be lodged in the trabeculae at the apex of the right ventricle; however, pacing may be successful if the catheter is in various other positions within the ventricle or outflow tract.

If the pacer enters the pulmonary artery outflow tract, the P-wave again becomes negative and the QRS amplitude diminishes (see Fig. 15–6*K*). If the catheter is in the pulmonary artery, the pacing catheter should be withdrawn into the right ventricle and readvanced. Sometimes, a clockwise or counterclockwise twist of the catheter will redirect its path in a more favorable direction. If catheter-induced ectopy develops, the catheter should be slightly withdrawn until the ectopy stops; then it should be readvanced. Occasionally, an antidys-

rhythmic drug such as lidocaine may need to be given to desensitize the myocardium. Once ventricular endocardial contact is made, the catheter is disconnected from the ECG machine and the distal lead is now connected to the negative terminal on the pacing generator. The pacing generator is then set to a rate of 80 beats/min or 10 beats/min faster than the underlying ventricular rhythm, whichever is higher. The full-demand mode is selected, with an output of about 5 mA. The pacing generator is then turned on.

The patient should be assessed for electrical and mechanical capture. Electrical capture will be manifest on the ECG monitor as a pacer spike followed by a QRS complex. If the pacer spike is seen but no QRS follows, capture is not occurring. *Mechanical capture* means that a pacer spike with its corresponding QRS triggers a myocardial contraction. This can be assessed by checking that a palpable pulse is present that is equal to the rate set on the pacemaker. If complete capture does not occur or if it is intermittent, the pacer will need to be repositioned. When proper capture occurs, the pacer should be assessed for optimal positioning. This is done by testing the thresholds for pacing and sensing and by physical examination, electrocardiography, and chest radiographs. The sequence of events is demonstrated in detail in Figure 15–7.

Catheter Placement in Low-Flow States. If the cardiac output is too low to "float" a pacing catheter or if the patient is in extremis, there may not be enough time to advance a pacing catheter using the previously described techniques. Such a situation would be asystole or complete heart block with malignant ventricular escape rhythms (although one can make a case for transcutaneous pacing in such conditions). In such emergent situations, the pacing catheter is connected to the energy source, the output is turned to the maximum amperage, and the asynchronous mode is selected. The catheter is then blindly advanced in the hope that it will enter the right ventricle and that pacing will be accomplished. The pacing catheter is rotated, advanced, withdrawn, or otherwise manipulated according to the clinical response. The right internal jugular approach is the most practical access route in this situation.

Ultrasound Guidance. As bedside ultrasound has become more widely available in the ED, new uses have been discovered. One promising technique involves using ultrasound to assist with the placement of emergency transvenous pacing catheters.[50,51] Cardiac image ultrasound may also help demonstrate whether or not mechanical capture has been achieved. The advantages of ultrasound over fluoroscopy are its safety and ready availability. Further experience will be necessary to confirm its utility.

Testing Threshold

The threshold is the minimum current necessary to obtain capture. Ideally, this is less than 1.0 mA and usually between 0.3 and 0.7 mA. If the threshold is in this ideal range, good contact with the endocardium can be presumed.

To determine the threshold, the pacing generator should be set to maximum sensitivity (full-demand mode) at 5 mA output with a rate of approximately 80 beats/min (or at least 10 beats/min greater than the patient's intrinsic rate). The current (output) should then be reduced slowly until capture is lost. This current is the threshold. This maneuver should be carried out 2 or 3 times to ensure that this value is consistent; the amperage should then be increased to 2.5 times the threshold to ensure consistency of capture (usually between 2 and 3 mA).

Testing Sensing

The sensing function should be tested in patients who have underlying rhythms. Set the rate at about 10 beats/min greater than the endogenous rhythm, place the pacemaker in asynchronous mode (*minimum* sensitivity, which is the *maximum* setting on the sensitivity voltage control), and ensure that there is complete capture. Then adjust the sensitivity control to its midposition or approximately 3 mV, and gradually decrease the rate until pacing is suppressed by the patient's intrinsic rhythm. The sensing indicator on the pacing generator should signal each time a native beat is sensed and should be in synchrony with each QRS on the ECG monitor. If the pacer fails to sense the intrinsic rhythm, increase the sensitivity (decrease the millivolts) until the pacer is suppressed. Conversely, if the sensing indicator is triggered by P- or T-waves or by artifact, decrease the sensitivity until only the QRS is sensed. Once the sensitivity threshold is determined, set the millivoltage to about half of that value.

Securing and Final Assessment

After the pacemaker's position has been tested for electrical accuracy, it must be secured in place. If a sealed introducer sheath was used, the hub should be fixed firmly to the skin with suture (e.g., 4-0 nylon or silk). A fastening suture should be sewn to the skin and the hub tied securely in place. If a plain introducer was used, it should be withdrawn to prevent leakage (Fig. 15–8) and the catheter should be sutured in place. In either case, the excess pacing catheter should be coiled and secured in a sterile manner underneath a large sterile dressing. Pacemaker function should again be assessed, and a chest film should be taken to ensure proper positioning. Ideal positioning of the pacing catheter is at the apex of the right ventricle (Fig. 15–9).

A 12-lead electrocardiogram should be obtained after transvenous pacemaker placement. If the catheter is within the right ventricle, a left bundle branch pattern with left axis deviation should be evident in paced beats (Fig. 15–10). If an RBBB pattern is noted, coronary sinus placement or left ventricular pacing due to septal penetration should be suspected.

With a properly functioning ventricular pacemaker, large cannon waves may be noted on inspection of the venous pulsations at the neck. When the pacemaker achieves ventricular capture, there may be times when the atria contract against a closed tricuspid valve resulting in a cannon wave. On auscultation of the heart, a slight murmur secondary to tricuspid insufficiency from the catheter interfering with the tricuspid valve apparatus may be evident.[52] A clicking sound heard best during expiration after each pacemaker impulse may also be noted here and is believed to represent either intercostal or diaphragmatic muscular contractions caused by the pacemaker.[53] Note that this can also be a sign of cardiac perforation.[54] On auscultation of the second heart sound, paradoxical splitting may be noted. This represents a delay in closure of the aortic valve because of delayed left ventricular depolarization.

As in any procedure, the patient should then be assessed for improvement in his or her clinical status. An evaluation of vital signs, mentation, congestive symptoms, and urinary output must be noted. In addition, complications secondary to the procedure should be sought and treated as needed.

Complications

The complications of emergency transvenous cardiac pacing are numerous[13,55] and represent a compendium of those related to central venous catheterization, those related to right-sided heart catheterization, and those unique to the pacing catheter itself (Table 15–7).

Problems Related to Central Venous Catheterization

Inadvertent arterial puncture is a well-known complication of the percutaneous approach to the venous system.[56] This problem is usually recognized quickly because of the rapid return of arterial blood. Firm compression over the puncture site will almost always result in hemostasis in 5 minutes or less.

Venous thrombosis and thrombophlebitis are also potential problems with central venous catheterization. Thrombophlebitis, which occurs early after insertion, is an uncommon complication. Thrombosis of the innominate vein is also a rare problem, with pulmonary embolism an even more

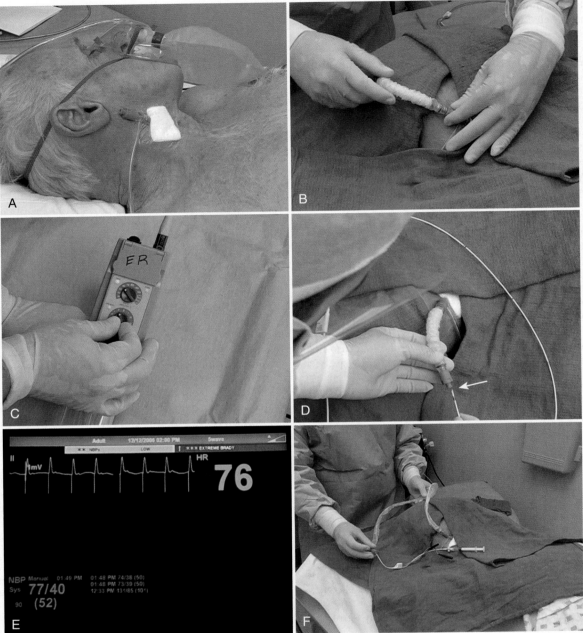

Figure 15–7 How to pass a temporary transvenous pacemaker. *Note: this is a 2-person procedure. The operator attends to pacer placement. The assistant observes the patient, the monitor, coordinates equipment, and orders appropriate drug therapy.A,* Intravenous access obtained with an introducer in *the right internal jugular vein* provides direct access to the right ventricle via the superior vena cava and right atrium. The *left subclavian vein* is the next best choice. *B,* Attach the *still-compressed* sterile sheath to the introducer hub, making sure that the connector of the sheath is firmly attached to the hub of the introducer. Open the hub of the introducer by *turning it counterclockwise to allow passage of the pacing wire.* Inflate then *deflate* the balloon on the pacing wire *before it is introduced* to test it for integrity. There is a valve that keeps the balloon inflated; it must be turned to inflate/deflate the balloon. Use 1.2–1.5 mL of air for the balloon. *C,* An assistant attaches the proximal pacing wire to the nonsterile energy source. Use the *demand mode* and turn on the pacer output to the highest level, rate about 80/min. With the balloon *deflated,* insert the pacing wire into the *still collapsed sheath* and into the hub of the introducer. *D,* Slowly advance the wire through the introducer. *Inflate* the balloon when the tip of the pacing wire is in the superior vena cava and continue to advance. Close the valve to keep the balloon inflated. *E,* Watch the electrocardiogram and look for capture, demonstrated by a wide QRS pattern after each pacer spike. The right ventricle should be encountered at 15–20 cm as noted by markings on the pacing wire. Misplacement and coiling of the wire may preclude placement into the right ventricle. If no capture is seen by 25 cm, withdraw the wire and try again—this is a blind procedure and luck plays a role. When consistent capture is seen, *deflate the balloon* and advance the wire 1–2 cm more to seat the wire in the endocardium. *F,* Tighten the valve on the sheath introducer to stop subsequent movement of the wire, and *extend the sheath its full length.* If required, suture the wire in place. Turn off the energy, then slowly turn it up to determine pacing threshold (first sign of capture). Set the output at two to three times the stimulation threshold and set the desired rate. Leave the pacer in the demand mode until stability is assured. Obtain a chest x-ray and 12-lead electrocardiogram. *(A–F, From Thomsen T, Setnik G [eds]: Procedures Consult—Emergency Medicine Module. Copyright 2008 Elsevier Inc. All rights reserved.)*

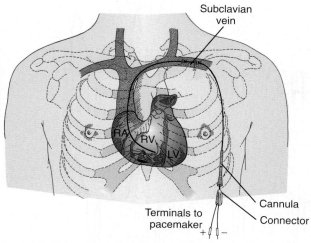

Figure 15–8 Transvenous pacer in right ventricle. LV, left ventricle; RA, right atrium; RV, right ventricle.

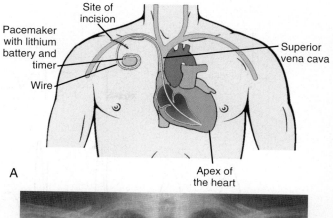

A

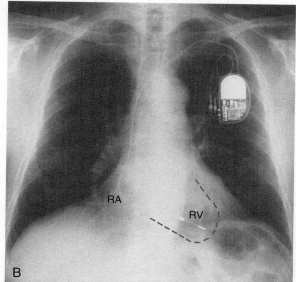

B

279

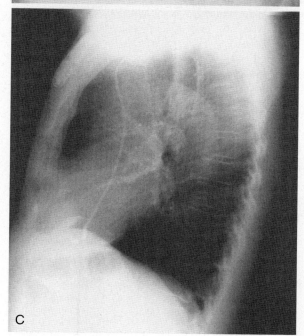

C

Figure 15–9 *A*, Schematic of proper position of pacer lead in apex of right ventricle. Normal pacemaker position in apex of right ventricle on posteroanterior (*B*) and lateral (*C*) chest films. (*A, From Chabner DA: The Language of Medicine, 6th ed. Philadelphia, Saunders, 2001.*)

uncommon event.[57] Femoral vein thrombosis, however, appears to be a much more common event associated with femoral vein catheterization.[45,58] Studies using noninvasive techniques have shown a 37% incidence of femoral vein thrombosis, with 55% of these having ventilation-perfusion scan evidence of pulmonary embolism.[58]

Pneumothorax is consistently a problem with the various approaches to the veins at the base of the neck. The decision to place a chest tube in patients with this complication depends on the extent of the air leak and the clinical status of the patient. In addition, laceration of the subclavian vein with hemothorax,[59] thoracic duct laceration with chylothorax, air embolism, wound infections, pneumomediastinum, hydromediastinum, hemomediastinum,[60] phrenic nerve injury,[61] and fracture of the guide wire with embolization[62,63] are all potential complications.[34,59]

Complications of Right-Sided Heart Catheterization

A common complication of the pacing catheter is dysrhythmia, with premature ventricular contractions being a common occurrence. One study noted a 1.5% incidence of serious dysrhythmias with a balloon-tipped catheter using ECG guidance, compared with a 32% incidence with the semirigid catheter using fluoroscopic guidance, suggesting that the balloon catheter was the preferred type of catheter.[12] Another study noted a 6% incidence of ventricular tachycardia during insertion.[45] The ischemic heart is more prone to dysrhythmias than the nonischemic heart.[64] The therapy for catheter-induced ectopy during insertion involves repositioning the catheter in the ventricle. This usually stops the ectopy; however, if after repeated attempts, it is found that the catheter cannot be passed without ectopy, myocardial suppressant therapy may be used to desensitize the myocardium.

Misplacement of the pacing catheter has been well studied. Passage of the catheter into the pulmonary artery can be diagnosed electrocardiographically by observing the return of an inverted P-wave and the decrease in the voltage of the QRS complex. Misplacement in the coronary sinus may occur and should be suspected in the patient in whom a paced RBBB pattern on the electrocardiogram is seen with right ventricular pacing (Fig. 15–11). Rarely, an RBBB pattern can be seen with a normal right ventricular position; therefore, all RBBB patterns do not represent coronary sinus pacing.[65] Further

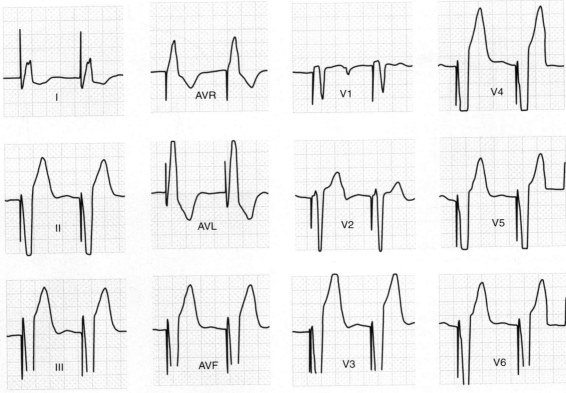

Figure 15–10 ECG pattern of right ventricular pacemaker.

TABLE 15–7 Complications of Transvenous Cardiac Pacing

Year	Reference	Patients (N)	Catheter	Route	Result
1969	Rosenberg et al[1]	111	Flexon steelwire vs. unipolar semifloating (ECG)	96 Subclavian 5 Basilic 1 External jugular	12 inconsistent pacing, 3 local infection, 2 pneumothorax, 1 subclavian artery puncture; 16% complication rate
1973	Schnitzler et al[11]	17	3-Fr bipolar semifloating balloon (ECG)	Antecubital vein	2 PVCs, stable pacing, no thrombophlebitis
1973	Weinstein et al[46]	100	6-Fr bipolar (fluoroscopy)	Femoral	2 ventricular tachycardia, 2 perforations, 2 required repositionings, 1 questionable thrombophlebitis and pulmonary embolism, 1 local infection
1973	Lumia & Rios*	142 insertions in 113 patients	Bipolar (fluoroscopy)	61 Brachial 81 Femoral	12 ventricular tachycardia and fibrillation in 9 patients, 3 perforations in 2 patients; local hematoma, abscess, and bleeding in 30%; 16.9% complication rate
1980	Pandian et al†	20	5-Fr bipolar (fluoroscopy)	Femoral	25% deep vein thrombosis
1980	Nolewajka et al[58]	29	6-Fr Cordis (fluoroscopy)	Femoral	34% venous thrombosis by venogram with 60% of these with pulmonary embolism by V̇/Q̇ scan
1981	Lang et al[12]	111	Balloon, semifloating vs. semirigid	Subclavian	Serious dysrhythmia: 1.5% balloon-tipped, 20.4% semirigid Catheter displacement: 13.6% ± 4.4 days balloon-tipped; 32% ± 1.9 days semirigid
1982	Austin et al[45]	113 insertions in 100 patients	4–7-Fr bipolar (fluoroscopy)	Brachial Femoral	Failure to sense or pace in 37%; repositioning in 37% of brachial insertions; repositioning in 9% of femoral insertions; fever, sepsis, local infection only in femoral insertions; 20% complication rate

ECG, electrocardiogram; PVC, premature ventricular contraction; V̇/Q̇, ventilation-perfusion.
*Lumia FJ, Rios JC: Temporary transvenous pacemaker therapy: An analysis of complications. Chest 64:604, 1973.
†Pandian NG, Kosowsky BD, Gurewich V: Transfemoral temporary pacing and deep venous thrombosis. Am Heart J 100:847, 1980.

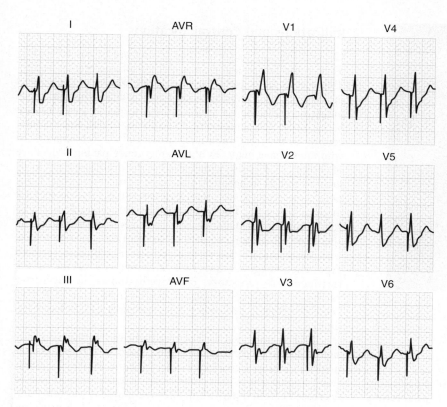

I   AVR   V1   V4

II   AVL   V2   V5

III   AVF   V3   V6

evidence for coronary sinus location can be obtained by viewing the lateral chest film. Normally, the catheter tip should point anteriorly toward the apex of the heart; however, with coronary sinus placement, the catheter tip is displaced posteriorly and several centimeters away from the sternum (Fig. 15–12). Other potential forms of misplacement include left ventricular pacing through an atrial septal defect or a ventricular septal defect, septal puncture, extraluminal insertion, and arterial insertions.[66]

Perforation of the ventricle is a well-described complication that can result in loss of capture,[67] hemopericardium, and tamponade.[68,69] Reported symptoms and signs of this problem include chest pain, pericardial friction rub, and diaphragmatic or chest wall muscular pacing.[70] At least one case of a post-pericardiotomy-like syndrome and two cases of endocardial friction rub have been reported without perforation.[71,72]

Pericardial perforation is suggested radiographically when the pacing catheter is outside or abuts the cardiac silhouette and is not in proper position within the right ventricular cavity (Fig. 15–13).[73] ECG clues include a change in the QRS and T-wave axis or a failure to properly sense. In suspected cases, a two-dimensional echocardiogram usually demonstrates the catheter's extracardiac position. Simply pulling back the catheter and repositioning it in the right ventricle can usually treat uncomplicated perforation.

During the insertion of a temporary pacing catheter when a nonfunctioning permanent catheter is in place, there is a small risk of entanglement or knotting.[74] This potential also exists with other central lines and PACs. Even without the presence of other lines, the pacing catheter can become knotted.[75] Frequently, these lines can be untangled under fluoroscopy using specialized catheters.

Local and systemic infections,[47] balloon rupture, pulmonary infarction,[76] phrenic nerve pacing,[77] and rupture of the chordae tendineae are also potential complications.[76]

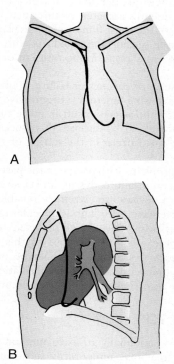

Figure 15–12 Coronary sinus position. *A*, Posteroanterior view. *B*, Lateral view. *(A and B, From Goldberger E: Treatment of Cardiac Emergencies, 3rd ed. St. Louis, CV Mosby, 1982.)*

Complications of the Pacing Electrode

The complications related to the pacing electrode can be separated into three groups: mechanical, organic, and electrical.

Mechanical failures include displacement, fracture of the catheter, and loose leads. Displacement can result in intermit-

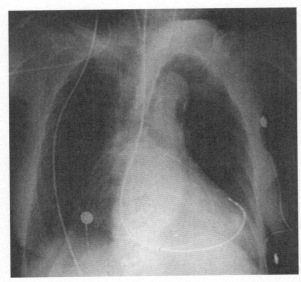

Figure 15–13 A pacing catheter that is outside or abuts the cardiac silhouette and is not properly positioned within the right ventricular cavity suggests myocardial perforation. *(From Tarver RD, Gillespie KR: The misplaced tube. Emerg Med Clin North Am 20:97, 1988.)*

tent or complete loss of capture or improper sensing, malignant dysrhythmias, diaphragmatic pacing, or perforation. Displacement should be suspected with changes in amplitude, with vector changes greater than 90°, or with a change in threshold.[78] Frequently, catheter fractures may be detected by a careful review of the chest film or may be suspected because of a change in the sensing threshold. As with displacement, catheter fractures may result in intermittent or complete loss of capture.

Organic causes of pacemaker failure result in changes in the threshold or sensing function.[79] Progressive inflammation, fibrosis, and thrombosis may result in more than a doubling of the original threshold.[80] However, this process takes several weeks and is of no concern in the setting of ED pacemaker placement.

Electrical problems with pacing in the past have included pacemaker generator failure, dysrhythmias, and outside interference. Modern devices are extremely reliable and resistant to outside interference. Although ventricular tachycardia and ventricular fibrillation have been reported to result from pacemakers, these are rare. Because of this, patients who present with such dysrhythmias should be evaluated for a nonpacemaker-induced etiology.[81] Defibrillation and cardioversion are safe in patients who have temporary pacemakers.

EMERGENCY TCP

TCP is a rapid, minimally invasive method of emergency cardiac pacing that may temporarily substitute for transvenous pacing. Electrodes are applied to the skin of the anterior and posterior chest walls, and pacing is initiated with a portable pulse generator. In an emergency setting, this pacing technique is faster and easier to initiate than transvenous pacing. Pulse generators are sufficiently portable to be used in EDs, hospital wards, intensive care units, and mobile paramedic vehicles.

BACKGROUND CAN BE FOUND ON EXPERT CONSULT

Indications and Contraindications

General indications for cardiac pacing are discussed earlier. TCP is the fastest and easiest method of emergency pacing. This technique is useful for initial stabilization of the patient in the ED who requires emergency pacing while arrangements or decisions for transvenous pacemaker insertion are being made. The equipment is readily mastered, and the procedure is fast and minimally invasive.[91,94] Refinements in equipment have made TCP the emergency pacing procedure of choice. TCP is also widely used in the prehospital environment as well as in hospital in the cardiac catheterization laboratory, operating room, intensive care units, and on general medical floors.[95–97] The technique may be preferable to transvenous pacing in patients who have received thrombolytic agents or other anticoagulants. No central venous puncture, with the attendant risk of hemorrhage, is required. Limited experience suggests that TCP also may be useful in the treatment of refractory tachydysrhythmias by overdrive pacing.[98–102] Although small pediatric electrodes for TCP have been developed, experience with pediatric TCP has been limited.[103,104]

TCP is indicated for the treatment of hemodynamically significant bradydysrhythmias that have not responded to medical therapy. *Hemodynamically significant* implies hypotension, anginal chest pain, pulmonary edema, or evidence of decreased cerebral perfusion. This technique is *temporary* and is indicated for short intervals as a bridge until transvenous pacing can be initiated or until the underlying cause of the bradydysrhythmia (e.g., hyperkalemia,[94] drug overdose[105]) can be reversed. Although generally unsuccessful, TCP may be attempted in the treatment of asystolic cardiac arrest. In this setting, the technique is efficacious only if used early after arrest onset (generally within 10 min).[106,107] TCP is not indicated for treatment of prolonged arrest victims with a final morbid rhythm of asystole.[104,108–110]

Delay from the onset of arrest to the initiation of pacing is a major problem that limits the usefulness of TCP in prehospital care. Hedges and associates[107] reported that everyday availability of pacing increased the number of patients who received pacing within 10 minutes of hemodynamic decompensation and increased long-term patient survival as well. Prehospital pacing may be most useful in the treatment of the patient with a hemodynamically significant bradycardia who has not yet progressed to cardiac arrest (e.g., heart block in the setting of AMI) or in the patient who arrests after the arrival of prehospital providers.[106,107]

In conscious patients with hemodynamically stable bradycardias, TCP may not be necessary. It is reasonable to attach electrodes to such patients and to leave the pacemaker in standby mode against the possibility of hemodynamic deterioration while further efforts at treatment of the patient's underlying disorder are being made. This approach has been used successfully in patients with new heart block in the setting of cardiac ischemia.[111] Generally, when a transvenous pacemaker becomes available, transvenous pacing is preferred because of better patient tolerance.

Equipment

Since their reintroduction, transcutaneous pacemakers have undergone rapid evolution and are now standard equipment in most EDs as well as other hospital settings and the prehospital environment. The pacemakers introduced in the early

1980s tended to be asynchronous devices with a limited selection of rate and output parameters. Units introduced more recently have demand mode pacing and more output options and are often combined with a defibrillator in a single unit. Combined defibrillator-pacers offer advantages in cost and ease and rapidity of use when compared with stand-alone devices. An example of a combined unit is shown in Figure 15–14.

All transcutaneous pacemakers have similar basic features. Most allow operation in either a fixed rate (asynchronous) or a demand mode (VVI). Most allow rate selection in a range from 30 to 200 beats/min. Current output is usually adjustable from 0 to 200 mA. If an ECG monitor is not an integral part of the unit, *an output adapter to a separate monitor is required* to "blank" the large electrical spike from the pacemaker impulse and allow interpretation of the much smaller ECG complex. Without blanking protection, the standard ECG machine is swamped by the pacemaker spike and is uninterpretable. This could be disastrous because the large pacing artifacts *can mask treatable ventricular fibrillation* (Fig. 15–15). Pulse durations on available units vary from 20 to 40 msec and are not adjustable by the operator.

Two sets of patient electrodes are usually required for operation of the device. One set of standard ECG electrodes is used for monitoring. The much larger pacing electrodes

deliver electrical impulses for pacing. Newer combined defibrillator-pacemakers can use a single set of electrodes for ECG monitoring, pacing, and defibrillation. This approach makes use of the device simpler, although the ECG waveform and analysis may be suboptimal. Provisions generally are

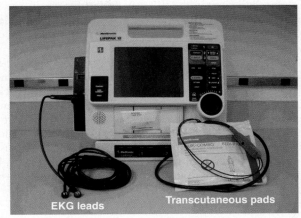

Figure 15–14 Combined pacemaker-defibrillator-ECG monitor. ECG leads are on the left. Transcutaneous pacing electrodes are connected on the right. Note that the connector for the pacing electrodes is outside of the package, allowing for rapidity and ease of use while preserving shelf life of the electrodes.

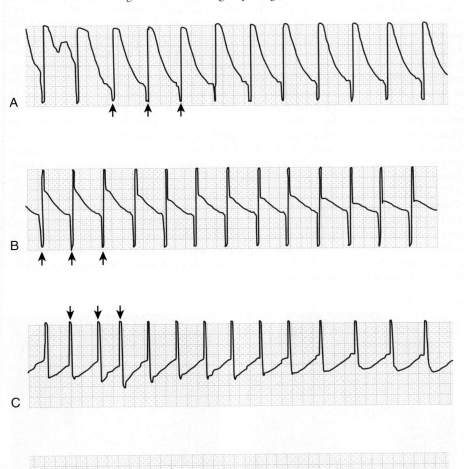

Figure 15–15 *A–C,* The top three rhythm strips are taken from a standard wall-mounted ECG monitor. They all demonstrate large pacer spikes without capture. The underlying rhythm cannot be determined and could be treatable ventricular fibrillation. *D,* The bottom rhythm strip demonstrates a tracing on the same patient with the external pacer monitor (special dampening). Note that the pacing spikes are much smaller, and it is easily seen that the underlying rhythm is asystole, without pacer capture. The presence of a T-wave after the QRS complex is a good indicator of ventricular capture.

283

made for separate ECG monitoring electrodes for use as desired by the operator.

Along with the widespread use of TCP come problems arising out of lack of equipment standardization. Pacing electrodes placed on a patient prehospital may be incompatible with the transcutaneous pacemaker used in the ED, and likewise, the equipment in the ED may differ from the in-patient units. Efforts should be made to establish a single standard for pacing electrode connectors within an institution and out to the prehospital environment if possible.

In order to facilitate setup for capture, the pacing electrodes should be connected to the pacemaker at all times. With conventional packaging, the leads are inside the packet with the pads, which means that the packet must be opened to allow connection to the pacing unit. However, exposure to the air causes the electrodes to dry out and lose their conductivity thus requiring continual replacement of the unused electrodes. Newer packaging, as shown in Figure 15–14, leaves the connectors outside of the packet, thus allowing connection to the pacemaker while preserving the shelf life of the pacing electrodes.

Technique

Pad Placement

The pacing electrodes are self-adhesive and positioned as shown in Figure 15–16. Care should be taken to avoid placing the electrodes over an implanted pacemaker or defibrillator, and any transdermal drug delivery patches should be removed if they are in the way. Excessive hair may be removed if time permits. The anterior electrode (cathode or negative electrode) is placed as close as possible to the point of maximal impulse on the left anterior chest wall, and the second electrode is placed directly posterior to the anterior electrode (see Fig. 15–16A). The posterior electrode serves as the ground. An alternative arrangement for the pacing electrodes is shown in Figure 15–16B. On females, the electrode must be placed beneath the breast. Data regarding optimum electrode placement are scarce, so selection can be made based on the clinician's preference and the patient's habitus.[112,113] Nonetheless, suboptimal capture owing to electrode placement may be rectified with a small change in electrode position. Although the polarity of the electrodes does not appear to be important for defibrillation, at least one study indicated that it might be for pacing.[114] The electrodes are labeled by the manufacturer to indicate which should be placed over the precordium; it is prudent to observe this recommendation. ECG electrodes (if used) are placed on the chest wall and/or limbs as required and connected to the instrument cable. Some clinicians prophylactically apply pacing electrodes to all critically ill patients with bradycardia to facilitate immediate TCP should decompensation occur.

There is little risk of electrical injury to health care providers during TCP. Power delivered during each impulse is less than 1/1000 of that delivered during defibrillation.[115] Chest compressions (CPR) can be administered directly over the insulated electrodes while pacing.[116] Inadvertent contact with the active pacing surface results in only a mild shock.

Pacing Bradycardic Rhythms

To initiate TCP, the pacing electrodes are applied and the device is activated. In the setting of bradyasystolic arrest, it is reasonable to turn the stimulating current to maximal output and then decrease the output as appropriate after capture is achieved. Clinicians should slowly increase the output from minimal settings until capture is achieved in patients with a hemodynamically compromising bradycardia who are not in cardiac arrest. Rate and current (output) selections are adjustable (Fig. 15–17). Generally, a heart rate of 60 to 70 beats/min will maintain an adequate blood pressure (by blood pressure cuff or arterial catheter) and cerebral perfusion.

Assessment of electrical capture can be made by monitoring the electrocardiogram on the filtered monitor of the pacing unit (Fig. 15–18). Mechanical capture is assessed by palpating the pulse as in transvenous pacing. Owing to muscular contractions triggered by the pacer, carotid pulses may be difficult to assess; palpating the femoral pulse may be easier. In addition, bedside ultrasound may prove useful in determining ventricular capture.[117,118] Ideally, pacing should be continued at an output level just above the threshold of initial electrical capture so as to minimize discomfort. One study in 16 normal male volunteers who were paced without sedation noted cardiac capture at a mean current of 54 mA (range, 42–60 mA).[119] Most subjects could tolerate pacing at their capture threshold; only 1 subject required discontinuation of pacing at 60 mA because of intolerable pain. Heller and coworkers[120] compared subjective pain perception and capture thresholds in 10 volunteers paced with five different transcutaneous pacers. Capture rates (40%–80%), thresholds (66.5–104 mA), and subjective discomfort varied from pacemaker to pacemaker.

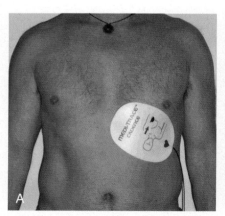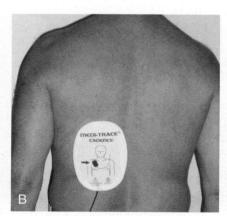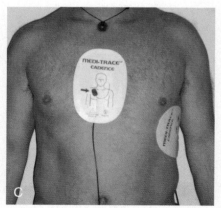

Figure 15–16   Correct placement of transcutaneous pacemaker electrodes. *A* and *B,* Anterior-posterior positions. *C,* Anterior-lateral positions (see text).

Failure to capture with TCP may be related to electrode placement or patient size. Patients with barrel-shaped chests and large amounts of intrathoracic air conduct electricity poorly and may prove refractory to capture. In one study, the scarring associated with thoracotomy was found to nearly double the pacing threshold.[121] A large pericardial effusion or tamponade also will increase the output required for capture.[122] Failure to electrically capture with a transcutaneous device in these settings is an indication to consider immediate transvenous pacer placement.

Patients who are conscious or who regain consciousness during TCP will experience discomfort because of muscle contraction.[111,119,120] Analgesia with incremental doses of an opioid agent (fentanyl seems ideal), sedation with a benzodiazepine compound, or both, will make this discomfort tolerable until transvenous pacing can be instituted.

Overdrive Pacing

Overdrive pacing[98-102] of ventricular tachycardia or paroxysmal supraventricular tachycardia is performed in patients who are stable enough to tolerate the brief delay associated with the necessary preparation for this technique. Little data exist on the efficacy or use of this procedure in the ED. The patient is sedated as explained earlier, pacing and monitoring electrode pads are placed in the standard position as detailed earlier, and brief trains (6–10 beats) of asynchronous pacing are initiated. The pacer rate must be set approximately 20 to 60 pulses/min greater than the dysrhythmia rate.[123] Generally, an impulse rate of 200 pulses/min is used for ventricular tachycardias (rate generally 150–180 beats/min), and a rate of 240 to 280 pulses/min is used for paroxysmal supraventricular tachycardias (rate commonly 200–250 beats/min).

Because rhythm acceleration is possible during overdrive pacing, it is essential that full resuscitation equipment, including a defibrillator, be available at the bedside.

Complications

The major potential complication of TCP is *failure to recognize the presence of underlying treatable ventricular fibrillation.* This complication is primarily due to the size of the pacing artifact in the ECG screen, a technical problem inherent in systems without appropriate dampening circuitry.

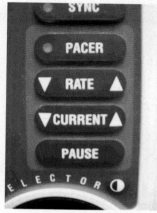

Figure 15–17 Rate and current (output) controls on a transcutaneous pacemaker.

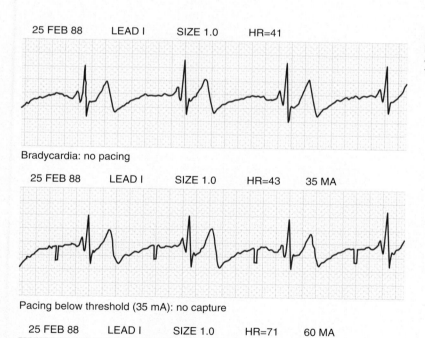

Figure 15–18 Assessing ECG capture with transcutaneous pacing. Note that the monitor has been adapted to accommodate the large pacing artifact so as not to obscure the underlying ventricular activity.

25 FEB 88   LEAD I   SIZE 1.0   HR=41

Bradycardia: no pacing

25 FEB 88   LEAD I   SIZE 1.0   HR=43   35 MA

Pacing below threshold (35 mA): no capture

25 FEB 88   LEAD I   SIZE 1.0   HR=71   60 MA

Pacing above threshold (60 mA): with capture (pacing-pulse marker⊔)

A rare complication of TCP is the induction of ventricular fibrillation. Studies of fibrillation thresholds using large precordial electrodes have shown that the longer impulse durations used in modern devices seem to decrease the chance of inducing ventricular fibrillation with TCP. Nonetheless, asynchronous TCP for tachydysrhythmias has been associated with rhythm acceleration and development of ventricular fibrillation.[101]

Studies looking at prolonged TCP in humans have not been extensive. Zoll and colleagues[87] reported 25 humans paced for up to 108 hours with impulses of 20-msec duration. Pacer-induced dysrhythmias did not occur. Leatham and colleagues[88] paced one patient for 68 hours with impulses of 20-msec duration. The patient died 2 days after pacing was discontinued. Pathologic examination revealed no evidence of pacer-induced myocardial damage. Madsen and colleagues[124] paced 10 healthy volunteers at threshold for 30 minutes and found no enzyme or echocardiographic abnormalities. TCP appears unlikely to produce cardiac injury with short-term use in the ED.

Soft tissue discomfort with the potential for injury may still occur with current transcutaneous pacemakers. Most patients are able to tolerate the discomfort, especially after sedation and analgesia. Nonetheless, prolonged use may still induce local cutaneous injury particularly in pediatric patients owing to the use of smaller electrodes.[125,126] Patients who cannot tolerate TCP or who will need long-term pacing are candidates for transvenous pacing.

 REFERENCES CAN BE FOUND ON EXPERT CONSULT

16

Pericardiocentesis

Richard J. Harper

Pericardiotomy was first performed under direct vision in 1815. Twenty-five years later, the procedure was performed blindly with a trocar on a patient with pericardial tamponade from malignancy.[1] By the end of the 19th century, the trocar-and-cannula method of pericardiocentesis was commonly used, and in 1911, the subxiphoid approach was described in writing.

Pericardiocentesis, with or without electrocardiographic (ECG) assistance, has a significant morbidity rate, reportedly 15% to 20%.[2,3] Such a procedure is, however, often required in the emergency department (ED) in life-threatening situations. The use of ultrasound to diagnose pericardial effusion and guide needle placement has become the standard for elective pericardiocentesis. It has been shown to reduce the incidence of complications (0.5%–3.7%)[4–6] and shorten the time to diagnose clinically significant effusions.[7–11] Although large pericardial effusions are a rare cause of hemodynamic instability in the ED, a lower threshold for performing bedside ultrasonography may increase the detection of effusions before they become hemodynamically significant.[8]

Even if tamponade physiology is present, ultrasound (echocardiographic) diagnosis and guidance are essential. The ECG-assisted blind pericardiocentesis technique remains an option only for truly emergent pericardiocentesis when a lengthy delay associated with obtaining and organizing ultrasound or fluoroscopic assistance could result in a poor clinical outcome, rapid deterioration, or death.

PERICARDIOCENTESIS IN PULSELESS ELECTRICAL ACTIVITY

Pulseless electrical activity (PEA) is the most common clinical scenario in which truly emergent pericardiocentesis is required. Always consider cardiac tamponade in a patient with PEA. In one series of 20 patients with PEA, 3 had tamponade requiring emergent pericardiocentesis, and another 5 had some degree of pericardial effusion.[12] Whereas blind pericardiocentesis is acceptable in PEA, ultrasonography can make the diagnosis at the bedside and increase safety by guiding the procedure.

CAUSES OF PERICARDIAL EFFUSION AND TAMPONADE

The medical literature categorizes a pericardial fluid collection as either *acute hemopericardium*, largely secondary to trauma, or *pericardial effusion* from other causes. This categorization is based on the fact that these two clinical entities differ in their time course, etiology, and treatment.

Acute Hemopericardium

The most common cause of a pericardial effusion is cardiac surgery and other cardiac procedures.[13] Although the overall incidence of this complication is low,[14,15] the frequent performance of these procedures results in a significant number of cases. The major risk factor associated with tamponade after cardiac surgery is anticoagulation. Other causes of acute hemopericardium include coagulopathies, cardiovascular catastrophes, and acute injury resulting from either blunt or penetrating trauma. All of these latter causes result in rapid accumulation of whole blood in the pericardial sac. The blood accumulates too fast for the relatively inelastic pericardial sac to stretch and accommodate the fluid. This results in cardiac tamponade from the collection of a small volume of fluid within an essentially normal pericardial size.

Penetrating Trauma

Traumatic tamponade caused by penetrating trauma may be the result of an obvious external injury such as a knife or gunshot wound, or it may be insidious, as seen with iatrogenic cardiac perforation during a cardiac or vascular procedure.

In external penetrating trauma, pericardial tamponade is most commonly the result of a stab wound.[16] Approximately 80% to 90% of stab wounds to the heart demonstrate tamponade,[16,17] compared with 20% of gunshot wounds. Stab wounds cause tamponade more often because the pericardial rent is small enough to seal and blood is trapped in the pericardial space.[16,18] Larger pericardial wounds from gunshots generally drain into the pleural space and produce a hemothorax.[19] Cardiac tamponade is often suspected with anterior chest wounds, but it is imperative to remember that any penetrating wound of the chest, back, or upper abdomen may involve the heart.

Iatrogenic causes of cardiac tamponade are relatively uncommon but well-known complications of invasive or diagnostic procedures. Pacemaker insertion (either transthoracic or transvenous) and cardiac catheterization, including valvuloplasty and angioplasty, are two of the main causes for the inadvertent penetration of cardiac chambers or coronary vessels.[20–22] Penetration of vascular structures is common during transthoracic pacemaker placement.[23] Tamponade is a complication of cardiac surgery, but it is usually anticipated. Mediastinal or pericardial drainage helps to control and prevent it.[20,24] Pericardiocentesis itself can cause tamponade by lacerating the myocardium or coronary vessels.[25,26]

Cardiac tamponade may result from perforation of the right atrium or, less commonly, of the right ventricle or superior vena cava by a central venous pressure (CVP) catheter or subclavian hemodialysis catheter.[27] The diagnosis is often delayed and, therefore, often fatal.[28] Perforation may occur during placement or, more commonly, 1 to 2 days later when the catheter erodes through tissue, particularly if a catheter made of stiff material is used or if the left internal jugular vein approach is used.[29] Tamponade from CVP line placement is seldom seen in the ED but must be considered when a patient with a CVP line suddenly decompensates. Consider tamponade when a patient deteriorates hemodynamically after an invasive diagnostic or therapeutic procedure involving the heart. To prevent this complication, be sure to place CVP catheters in the superior vena cava rather than the right atrium or ventricle.

Blunt Trauma

Blunt trauma may cause hemopericardium, often as the result of major chest injury with associated rib and sternal fractures. Cases have been reported, however, in which tamponade occurred in blunt trauma with no obvious signs of injury to the thorax.[30] Such incidents may be more common than are clinically recognized, judging by the reports of constrictive pericarditis and pericardial defects found months to years later in trauma patients who were not originally noted to have effusion. Pericardial effusion due to blunt trauma may also be a late finding, becoming symptomatic 12 to 15 days after trauma.[31]

Severe deceleration injury may cause tamponade as a result of aortic or caval injury.[32] This appears to be an uncommon development, with two case series reporting tamponade in 3.6% (1 of 28 patients) and 2.3% (1 of 43 patients) of victims of aortic injury.[33]

Theoretically, cardiopulmonary resuscitation (CPR) can cause pericardial effusion secondary to the blunt trauma of chest compressions, broken ribs, or intracardiac injections. Early studies reported pericardial effusion in 1% to 3% of CPR survivors.[34] Echocardiographic studies showed small cardiac effusions (but not tamponade) in 12% of survivors, only 4% of whom had received intracardiac injections.[35] Thus, although case reports of tamponade exist,[36,37] CPR and intracardiac drug injections are unlikely to cause significant effusion, much less tamponade.

Nontraumatic Hemopericardium

Nontraumatic but acute hemopericardium caused by a bleeding diathesis, aortic dissection, and ventricular rupture behaves much like traumatic tamponade because of its acute nature. This type of hemopericardium is less obvious in etiology than hemopericardium caused by external trauma. Tamponade from aortic dissection or ventricular rupture is usually fatal.

Bleeding diathesis may cause spontaneous bleeding into the pericardial sac. The incidence of spontaneous pericardial tamponade in anticoagulated patients has been reported to range from 2.5% to 11%.[20,38] Thrombolytic therapy has also been implicated in tamponade secondary to bleeding diathesis. In one series of 392 patients, all with large anterior myocardial infarctions, only 4 (1%) developed tamponade secondary to hemopericardium without ventricular rupture.[39]

A dissection of the ascending aorta may extend around the base of the vessel into the pericardial sac, causing rapid, and usually fatal, tamponade. This pathologic abnormality may be due to conditions such as syphilis, Marfan syndrome, or atherosclerosis. Infection may create pseudoaneurysms of the aorta, which can also present as tamponade.[40]

Ventricular rupture after myocardial infarction is a common source of acute hemopericardium. Although the prognosis is grim, survival is possible with prompt recognition and definitive treatment.[41,42]

Nonhemorrhagic Effusions

Nonhemorrhagic effusions usually accumulate slowly, allowing the pericardium to stretch and accommodate up to 2000 mL of fluid.[43] Because the effusion accumulates slowly, often over weeks to months, the circulatory system adapts, thus allowing more time for evaluation and treatment, even

in a moderately hypotensive patient.[44,45] In many cases of small nonhemorrhagic effusion, tamponade does not occur, and the effusion may resolve with treatment of the underlying disease or may be managed successfully by elective pericardiocentesis.

Many disease processes, ranging from the common to the rare (Table 16–1), can cause pericardial effusion. The cause of nonhemorrhagic tamponade may not be obvious on

TABLE 16–1 Causes of Pericardial Effusion

Neoplasm	Mesothelioma
	Lung
	Breast
	Melanoma
	Lymphoma
Pericarditis	Radiation (especially after Hodgkin's disease)
	Viral
	Bacterial
	Staphylococcus
	Pneumococcus
	Haemophilus
	Fungal
	Tuberculosis
	Amebiasis
	Toxoplasmosis
	Idiopathic
Connective tissue disease	Systemic lupus erythematosus
	Scleroderma
	Rheumatoid arthritis
	Acute rheumatic fever
Metabolic disorders	Myxedema
	Uremia
	Cholesterol pericarditis
	Bleeding diatheses
Cardiac disease	Acute myocardial infarction
	Dissecting aortic aneurysm
	Congestive heart failure
	Coronary aneurysm
Drugs	Hydralazine
	Phenytoin
	Anticoagulants
	Procainamide
	Minoxidil
Trauma	Blunt
	Major trauma
	Closed-chest cardiopulmonary resuscitation
	Penetrating
	Major penetrating trauma
	Intracardiac injections
	Transthoracic and transvenous pacing wires
	Pericardiocentesis
	Cardiac catheterization
	Central venous pressure catheter
Miscellaneous	Serum sickness
	Chylous effusion
	Löffler syndrome
	Reiter syndrome
	Behçet syndrome
	Pancreatitis
	Postpericardiotomy
	Amyloidosis
	Ascites

Data from Guberman BA, Fowler NO, Engel PJ, et al: Cardiac tamponade in medical patients. Circulation 64:633, 1981; and Pories WJ, Caudiani VA: Cardiac tamponade. Surg Clin North Am 55:573, 1975.

TABLE 16–2 Etiology of Pericardial Effusion in Two Studies*

	Krikorian & Hancock[38] (120 Patients) (%)	Guberman et al[46] (56 Patients) (%)
Neoplastic disease	—	32
Pericardial invasion	16	—
Radiation pericarditis	7.5	4
Etiology uncertain	18	—
Traumatic hemopericardium	9	—
Hemopericardium, nontraumatic	2.5	—
Rheumatic disease	12	2
Uremia/dialysis	5	9
Bacterial infection	2.5	12.5
Congestive heart failure	1.5	—
Uncertain etiology	12.5	—
Idiopathic pericarditis	13.5	14
Cardiac infarction	—	—
Iatrogenic diagnostic procedures	—	7.5
Myxedema	—	4
Aneurysm	—	4
Anticoagulation and cardiac disease	—	11
Postpericardiotomy	—	2

*Note: Various complications related to human immunodeficiency virus (HIV) infections are now probably the most common causes of large nonhemorrhagic pericardial effusions. Effusions related to bacterial, viral, and mycobacterial infections and Kaposi sarcoma and lymphoma are common.

examination in the ED, and tamponade is frequently misdiagnosed as congestive heart failure or respiratory disease. Although *neoplasm has generally been the most common underlying cause of nonhemorrhagic effusion*,[38,46] human immunodeficiency virus (HIV) has been implicated as a common etiology of large nonhemorrhagic pericardial effusion and tamponade[47,48] (Table 16–2).

HIV-related effusions have been ascribed to many opportunistic bacterial and viral infections, with mycobacterial infections being the most common.[47-49] Kaposi sarcoma and lymphoma[50,51] have caused noninfectious pericardial effusions in HIV patients. Cancer is a prominent cause of nonhemorrhagic effusions; the pericardium is involved in 20% of patients with disseminated tumors[52] and 8% of all patients with cancer.[53] There is primary pericardial involvement in 69% of acute leukemias, in 64% of malignant melanomas, and in 24% of lymphomas; however, the incidence of actual tamponade in these malignancies is not known. Of metastases to the pericardium, 35% originate in the lung, 35% in the breast, 15% in lymphomas, and less than 3% in each of the other cancers.[53] Thus, any patient who is known to have one of these malignancies should be considered at risk for tamponade. Metastasis to the heart is usually a late finding in cancer, and foci located elsewhere are usually evident.[54] Classic findings of tamponade, such as pulsus paradoxus, are frequently absent in cancer patients with tamponade, and their symptoms are usually attributed to their malignancy.[53]

Radiation pericarditis, particularly after treatment for Hodgkin's disease, is a common cause of effusion.[43] Effusion occurs in approximately 5% of those patients who receive 4000 rad to the heart.

Approximately 15% to 20% of patients on dialysis for renal failure develop pericarditis, and 35% of those with pericarditis develop tamponade.[55,56] Up to 7% of patients on chronic dialysis may have effusions, sometimes of 1 L or more.[54] Pericardial effusion in renal failure may be managed with dialysis alone in many cases.

Thirty percent of myxedema patients have pericardial effusions, but few have tamponade.[46] Most of the other etiologies listed in Table 16–1 are isolated case reports, and their exact incidences have not been determined.

Other Causes of Pericardial Tamponade

An interesting but rare cause of cardiac tamponade is pneumopericardium. Pneumopericardium is most commonly seen with pneumothorax and pneumomediastinum as a complication of respiratory therapy in infants, but it may also occur from similar barotrauma in adults.[57] Pneumopericardium also occurs spontaneously in asthma,[58] after blunt chest injury,[59,60] and even after high-speed motorcycle rides.[61] Pneumopericardium is usually benign, but tension pneumopericardium has been reported as a cause of life-threatening tamponade after blunt chest trauma.[60,62] The appearance of life-threatening pneumopericardium and tamponade has also been described immediately[63] and 6 days after penetrating chest trauma.[64]

PATHOPHYSIOLOGY OF TAMPONADE

The pericardium is a tough, leathery sac that normally contains about 25 to 35 mL of serous fluid.[65] It is not rapidly elastic, although it does demonstrate stress relaxation within minutes of increased intrapericardial pressure, providing a slight ability to accommodate sudden increases in fluid.[66] As fluid accumulates, the first 80 to 120 mL is easily accommodated without significantly affecting pericardial pressure (Fig. 16–1).[67] However, if an additional 20 to 40 mL is rapidly accumulated, the intrapericardial pressure almost doubles, thus frequently leading to sudden decompensation. With effusions that develop over weeks to months, the pericardium lengthens circumferentially to a huge size and can accommodate liters of fluid.

Pericardial compliance, which helps determine the pressure-volume response curve (Fig. 16–2),[65] varies considerably in different individuals and in various disease states. The pressure-volume relationship demonstrates hysteresis; the withdrawal of a quantity of fluid drops the pressure more than the addition of the same amount of fluid raised the pressure.

As pericardial fluid accumulates, the increased intrapericardial pressure is transmitted across the myocardial wall and causes compression of the atria, vena cava, and pulmonary veins. This reduces right ventricular filling in diastole, producing decreased stroke volume and cardiac output.[68] Pulse pressure narrows as reflex sympathetic stimulation increases. Severe tamponade is produced with intrapericardial pressures of 15 to 20 mm Hg.[69]

As stroke volume decreases, heart rate increases to maintain cardiac output. Sympathetic discharge causes both arterial and venous vasoconstriction.[69,70] Vasoconstriction increases venous pressure, which helps to restore the normal venous-atrial and atrioventricular filling gradients. These compensatory mechanisms are often effective and may permit establishment of a new homeostasis with normal cardiac output.

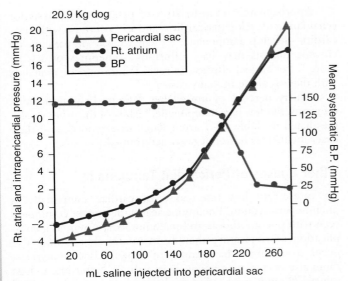

20.9 Kg dog

Figure 16–1 **Production of cardiac tamponade by injections of saline into the pericardial sac.** Although pericardial space can acutely accommodate 80 to 120 mL of fluid without a significant increase in pericardial pressure, note the steep increases in pressure and the drop in blood pressure at about 200 mL of saline. Once critical volumes are reached, very small increases cause significant hemodynamic compromise. (*From Fowler NO: Physiology of cardiac tamponade and pulsus paradoxus. II: Physiological, circulatory, and pharmacological responses in cardiac tamponade. Mod Concepts Cardiovasc Dis 47:116, 1978. Reproduced by permission of the American Heart Association, Inc.*)

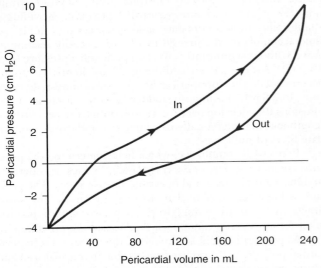

Figure 16–2 Relationship of intrapericardial pressure to volume of pericardial fluid. Note that pressure drops rapidly when a small amount of fluid is removed. (*From Pories W, Gaudiani V: Cardiac tamponade. Surg Clin North Am 55:573, 1975. Reproduced by permission.*)

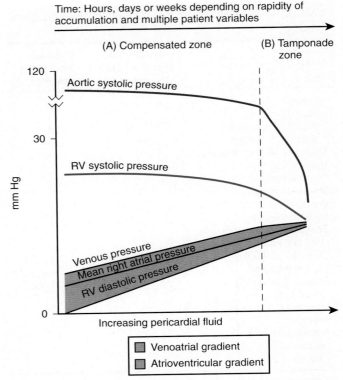

Figure 16–3 Summary of physiologic changes in tamponade. RV, right ventricle. (*From Shoemaker WC, Carey JS, Yao ST, et al: Hemodynamic monitoring for physiological evaluation, diagnosis, and therapy of acute hemopericardial tamponade from penetrating wounds. J Trauma 13:36, 1973; and Spodick D: Acute cardiac tamponade: Pathologic physiology, diagnosis, and management. Prog Cardiovasc Dis 10:65, 1967. Reproduced by permission.*)

hemorrhagic shock have five times greater coronary blood flow than animals in cardiac tamponade.[73] Severe experimental tamponade is followed by large increases in creatine kinase MB and microscopic evidence of cardiac injury resulting from ischemia.[74]

As intrapericardial pressure continues to rise, the heart's compensatory mechanisms fail. Myocardial ischemia and perhaps lactic acidosis from poor tissue perfusion may be the triggering events that disrupt the delicate equilibrium.[75] Atrial pressure rises rapidly (Fig. 16–3). The atria and pulmonary circulation, being at much lower pressure than the systemic arterial pressure, are more vulnerable to the rising intrapericardial pressure. A "pressure plateau" occurs in which right atrial pressure, right ventricular diastolic pressure, pulmonary artery diastolic pressure, and pulmonary capillary wedge pressure are virtually identical.

This equalization of pressures leads to the echocardiographic hallmark of tamponade: right ventricular collapse. At this point, hypotension is severe, bradycardia is common, and PEA may occur. Unless intrapericardial pressure is immediately decreased, pulmonary blood flow ceases and cardiac arrest follows.[75]

Total blood volume affects cardiac compensation, and it is possible to encounter a "low-pressure" cardiac tamponade.[76] The hypovolemic patient with tamponade has a decreased venous pressure, which not only decreases cardiac output but also may obscure the diagnosis because distended neck veins or an elevated CVP is not present. In a patient with a chronic pericardial effusion, the onset of hypovolemia can lower filling pressure enough to precipitate tamponade, and

With chronic effusion and in early tamponade, cardiac contractility is not affected and myocardial perfusion is normal.[68,71,72] As pressure continues to increase, coronary perfusion pressure drops; thus, in its later stages, tamponade causes myocardial ischemia. Before hypotension occurs, left ventricular blood flow has already decreased to 37%.[73] For comparable degrees of hypotension, experimental animals in conversely, providing additional volume may temporarily offset increased pericardial pressure.

Ventilation and blood CO_2 levels have significant effects on cardiac tamponade. This is of particular significance because trauma patients with tamponade may also have respiratory impairment. Pericardial pressure decreases 3 to 6 mm Hg with a hypocarbia of 24 torr and increases 2 to 4 mm Hg when the Pco_2 reaches 57 torr.[77] This degree of hypercarbia-induced pericardial pressure rise can decrease cardiac output by 25%. Similarly, fluctuations in intrapleural pressure induced by intermittent positive-pressure ventilation are transmitted to the pericardial space and can reduce cardiac output another 25%.[78] The clinical implications of these findings are that patients suspected of having tamponade should normally be allowed to breathe spontaneously under careful monitoring and should not be ventilated with positive pressure unless it is absolutely necessary, because their hemodynamic status may deteriorate precipitously.

DIAGNOSIS OF CARDIAC TAMPONADE

Patient Profile and Symptoms

Pericardial effusion is rarely diagnosed based on physical findings. In contrast, pericardial tamponade can be diagnosed based on clinical criteria, but specific clinical signs are often absent. Particularly in the setting of acute hemorrhagic tamponade, the time from the first signs of tamponade to full arrest may be brief.[79]

Classic clinical findings have been described for tamponade. However, these findings are often obvious only when the patient is unstable owing to tamponade. Ideally, tamponade is diagnosed early, when the patient suffers no more than dyspnea, weakness, or perhaps right heart failure. It is common to attribute respiratory symptoms (e.g., dyspnea on exertion) to a more common condition such as heart failure or pulmonary pathology and to overlook pericardial effusion until the classic late signs (e.g., hypotension) appear.[80]

Acute pericardial tamponade may be fatal before it is clinically recognized, and deterioration can be exceedingly rapid. Often, *therapeutic pathways must be undertaken without enough data to definitively ensure the specific diagnosis.* The condition may closely resemble tension pneumothorax, acute hemothorax, hypovolemia, pulmonary edema, aortic dissection, or pulmonary embolism. Severe right ventricular contusion can mimic the findings of tamponade.[81] The patient is often agitated or panic-stricken, confused, uncooperative, restless, cyanotic, diaphoretic, and acutely short of breath. In

the late stages, the patient is moribund. Hypotension in the presence of severe cyanosis and distended neck veins is a helpful but late finding.

Physical Signs

The classic physical findings of tamponade were first characterized by Beck in 1935.[82] He described two triads, one for acute and one for chronic compression. The chronic compression triad consists of increased CVP, ascites, and a small, quiet heart. The acute compression triad consists of increased CVP, decreased arterial pressure, and muffled heart sounds. Unfortunately, although almost 90% of patients have one or more signs,[16] only about one third demonstrate the complete triad.[75,83] The simultaneous occurrence of all three physical signs is a very late manifestation of tamponade and is usually seen most consistently shortly before cardiac arrest.

Careful hemodynamic monitoring reveals earlier changes that indicate the progression of tamponade (Table 16–3).[84] In grade I tamponade, cardiac output and arterial pressure are normal, but CVP and heart rate are increased. In grade II tamponade, blood pressure is normal or slightly decreased, and CVP and heart rate are increased. In grade III tamponade, the classic findings of Beck's acute triad occur. Although this sequence represents the natural history of acute tamponade, the time course varies. Some patients are stable at a given stage for hours; others proceed to cardiac arrest within minutes.[75,84] Unfortunately, not all patients with early tamponade respond with a predictable pattern of change in vital signs. Brown and coworkers[85] found that 6 of 18 patients with tamponade, defined through right heart catheterization, responded to tamponade with elevated systolic blood pressure. After pericardiocentesis, these patients had a marked reduction in systolic blood pressure accompanied by increased cardiac output. All of these patients had previously been hypertensive.

Pulsus Paradoxus (see also Chapter 1, Vital Signs Measurement)

Pulsus paradoxus is defined as *an exaggeration of the normal inspiratory fall in blood pressure*[70,83] (Fig. 16–4A). A paradoxical pulse (pressure) is one of the classic physical signs of tamponade, but it is not pathognomonic. It is also seen in pulmonary emphysema, asthma, labored respirations, obesity, cardiac failure, constrictive pericarditis, pulmonary embolism, and cardiogenic shock.[16,44,75] Although occasionally useful and

TABLE 16–3 Shoemaker System of Grading Cardiac Tamponade

Grade	Pericardial Volume (mL)	Cardiac Index	Stroke Index	Mean Arterial Pressure	Central Venous Pressure	Heart Rate	Beck's Triad
I	<200	Normal or ↑	Normal or ↓	Normal	↑	↑	Venous distention hypotension, muffled heart sounds usually not present
II	≥200	↓	↓	Normal or ↓	↑ (≥12 cm H_2O)	↑	May or may not be present
III	>200	↓↓	↓↓	↓↓	↑↑ (≤30–40 cm H_2O)	↓	Usually present

From Shoemaker WC, Carey SJ, Yao ST, et al: Hemodynamic monitoring for physiologic evaluation, diagnosis, and therapy of acute hemopericardial tamponade from penetrating wounds. J Trauma 13:36, 1973.

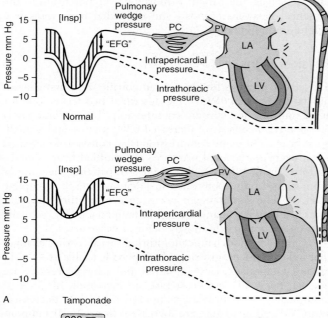

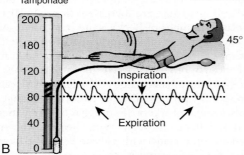

Figure 16–4 *A, top,* The normal situation in which changes in intrathoracic pressure are transmitted to both the pericardial sac and the pulmonary veins. The effective filling gradient (EFG) changes only slightly during respiration. *Bottom,* Cardiac tamponade in which changes in intrathoracic pressure are transmitted to the pulmonary veins but not to the pericardial sac. The EFG falls during inspiration. Insp, inspiration; LA, left atrium; LV, left ventricle; PC, pulmonary capillaries; PV, pulmonary veins. *B,* Normally, systolic blood pressure drops slightly during inspiration. To measure pulsus paradoxus, the patient breathes normally while lying at a 45° angle. The blood pressure cuff is inflated well above systolic pressure and slowly deflated. When the pulse is first heard only during expiration, this is the upper value. The cuff is deflated until the pulse is heard during both inspiration and expiration, and this is the lower value. The difference in the two values is the amount of pulsus paradoxus. A difference of more than 12 mm Hg is abnormal. *(A, From Bunnell IL, Holand JF, Griffith GT, Greene DG: Am J Med 25:640, 1960.)*

academically attractive, measuring the paradoxical pulse is difficult and time-consuming, and any frightened, hypotensive patient with labored breathing can demonstrate this finding (see Fig. 16–4*B*). Eschewing this test in the patient in entremis is quite acceptable.

If the difference between inspiratory and expiratory systolic blood pressures is greater than 12 mm Hg, the paradoxical pulse is abnormally high.[86] Most patients with proven tamponade will demonstrate a difference of 20 to 30 mm Hg or more during the respiratory cycle.[16,44,75] This may not be true of patients with very narrow pulse pressures (typical of grade III tamponade); they will have a "deceptively small" paradoxical pulse of 5 to 15 mm Hg. The decreased pulsus paradoxus with hypotension occurs because the paradoxical pulse is a function of actual pulse pressure, and the inspiratory

systolic pressure may be below the level at which diastolic sounds disappear.[70] For this reason, the ratio of the paradoxical pulse to the pulse pressure is a more reliable measure. A paradoxical pulse greater than 50% of the pulse pressure is abnormal.[70] Pulsus paradoxus may also be suspected from the use of pulse oximetry.[87,88] If the highest value of the upper plethysmographic peak of the pulse oximetry waveform is decreased during inspiration (ratio ≥ 1.5), pulsus paradoxus may be suspected.

Pulsus paradoxus in tamponade has been correlated with the degree of impairment of cardiac output. In atraumatic patients, a 15% pulsus paradoxus in the face of relative hypotension was found in 97% of patients with moderate or severe tamponade and only 6% of patients with absent or mild tamponade.[86] A similar study of right ventricular diastolic collapse by echocardiography found that an abnormal pulsus paradoxus had a sensitivity of 79%, a specificity of 40%, a positive predictive value of 81%, and a negative predictive value of 40%.[89]

The absence of a paradoxical pulse does not rule out tamponade. Although the mean paradoxical pulse was 49 mm Hg in one series of nonhemorrhagic tamponade,[46] 23% of the patients had a paradoxical pulse of less than 20 mm Hg, and 1 patient had no measurable paradoxical pulse. An abnormal pulsus paradoxus has been reported to be absent in tamponade when there is an atrial septal defect, aortic insufficiency, localized collections of pericardial blood, or extreme tamponade with hypotension.[76] It may also be absent when left ventricular diastolic pressure is intrinsically elevated because of poor left ventricular compliance. In traumatic tamponade, pulsus paradoxus is unreliable.[76,90–92] In one study of 197 cases of tamponade caused by trauma, only 8.6% of the diagnoses were made by finding an abnormal pulsus paradoxus.[93]

Although the absence of pulsus paradoxus rules against severe tamponade, it does not completely rule it out. Whether time is taken to determine pulsus paradoxus depends on the patient's status. If the patient is moribund or rapidly deteriorating, taking time to check this parameter is obviously poor clinical judgment.

Venous Distention

Venous distention, reflecting increased CVP, is also a late sign in cardiac tamponade (see Fig. 16–5*C*). Neck vein distention may be masked by vasoconstriction as a result of vasopressors (e.g., dopamine), intrinsic sympathetic discharge, or hypovolemia.[44,75,84,91] Neck vein distention may be obvious clinically, but the measured CVP is more reliable than the presence of venous distention. The CVP reading should take into account positive-pressure ventilation and the effects of a Valsalva maneuver. Most patients with significant tamponade will have a CVP of 12 to 14 cm H_2O or greater.[91] Hypovolemia changes the intrapericardial pressure-volume curve in tamponade and will lower the CVP reading at any given stage in the tamponade process.

Animal studies have documented that right atrial pressure can be normal in tamponade when hypovolemia is present. One case of low-pressure cardiac tamponade was reported in a patient with no jugular venous distention, no paradoxical pulse, and a right atrial pressure of 8 mm Hg.[76] Thus, although the initial CVP reading is useful and diagnostic if grossly elevated (e.g., 20–30 cm H_2O),[91,94] a series of CVP readings looking for an upward trend is the most sensitive diagnostic

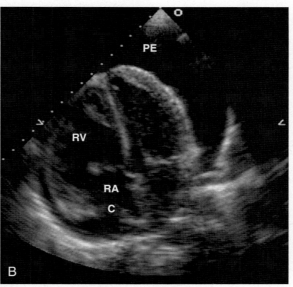

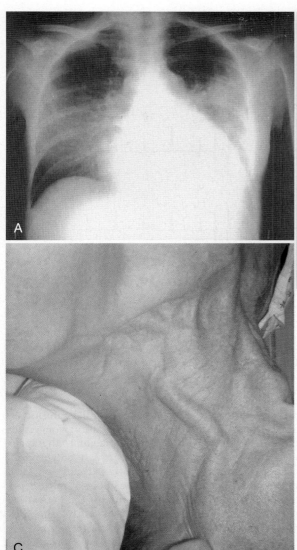

293

Figure 16–5 *A,* Chest radiograph shows an enlarged, globular cardiac silhouette ("water-bottle heart") in a patient with tamponade due to a malignant effusion. The chest x-ray has minimal value in diagnosing tamponade but is usually abnormal when significant *chronic* effusions are present. *B,* Ultrasound: Apical view of a large pericardial effusion in early ventricular diastole; marked right atrial collapse is seen. C, collapsed segment of the right atrial wall; PE, pericardial effusion; RA, right atrium; RV, right ventricle. *C,* Markedly distended neck veins may be seen with cardiac tamponade, but they are not universal, especially in hypovolemic trauma patients.

tool.[91] A rising CVP, especially when there is persistent hypotension, is extremely suggestive of tamponade in the trauma patient. In the rare case of the hypovolemic patient in whom tamponade is suspected but who demonstrates a low CVP, a fluid challenge will help clarify the situation and will also improve cardiac output, at least temporarily.[76]

Ancillary Testing

Use routine chest radiographs and electrocardiograms to increase the level of suspicion for pericardial effusion and tamponade, but make the diagnosis by noninvasive means with computed tomography (CT) or, preferably, cardiac ultrasound (Fig. 16–5*A* and *B*). If available, use bedside ultrasound because it is the fastest and most reliable for the emergency clinician to demonstrate a significant pericardial effusion, although it may not be diagnostic of tamponade.

Chest Radiographs

Chest radiographs are not useful in the diagnosis of acute traumatic tamponade because the cardiac size and shape do not change acutely. However, the radiographs may reveal other important findings such as hemothorax, bullet location, or even pneumopericardium. In the patient without trauma and with chronic effusion, a chest film often reveals an enlarged, saclike "water-bottle" cardiac shadow (see Fig. 16–5*A*). Unfortunately, it is difficult to differentiate pericardial from myocardial enlargement, and radiographs cannot be used to distinguish between simple pericardial effusion and tamponade.

Electrocardiograms

Electrocardiograms may suggest, but should not be used to diagnose, pericardial effusion or cardiac tamponade (Fig. 16–6). Most classic ECG changes, such as PR segment depression, low-voltage QRS complexes, and electrical alternans, have acceptable specificity but poor sensitivity for pericardial effusion or tamponade.[44,95,96] *Low voltage* is defined as QRS amplitude of 5 mV or less in all limb leads (or a sum of the limb lead QRS amplitude $\leq$ 30 mV), and *PR depression* is defined as depression of 1 mV or greater in at least 1 lead other than aVR. In a study correlating the electrocardiogram with echocardiographic evaluation, ECG signs had an overall sensitivity of only 1% to 17% and a specificity of 89% to

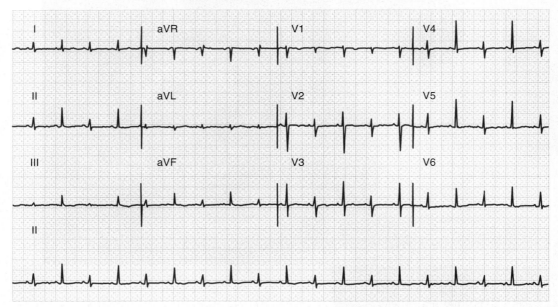

Figure 16–6 Electrical alternans may develop in patients with pericardial effusion and cardiac tamponade. Notice the beat-to-beat alternation in the P-QRS-T axis; this is caused by the periodic swinging motion of the heart in a large pericardial effusion. Relatively low QRS voltage and sinus tachycardia are also present. Overall, the electrocardiogram (ECG) has a low sensitivity for pericardial effusion or tamponade. Note that electrical alternans may be more evident in the V leads.

100% for pericardial effusion.[44] Others have demonstrated significantly higher sensitivity (i.e., in the range of 32%–68%) for voltage criteria.[97] PR segment depression is the most common ECG finding in pericardial tamponade, and low voltage is most commonly associated with a moderate to large effusion. It is important to note that none of the ECG findings differentiate tamponade from effusion.

Electrical alternans is caused by pendulum motion of the heart within the pericardial sac.[98] Alternans of the QRS complex has been seen in about 22% of medical tamponade cases[80] but in only 5% of cancer patients with tamponade.[53] Electrical alternans of both the P-wave and the QRS complex (total electrical alternans) is a rare finding, but when seen, is thought to be pathognomonic of tamponade (see Fig. 16–6).[44,99] As with electrical alternans, low voltage may be a finding associated with tamponade but not simple effusion.[100]

Echocardiography

Echocardiography is the best available tool for diagnosing pericardial effusion and has the further advantage of being noninvasive[101] (see Fig. 16–5B). Echocardiography is very sensitive in the diagnosis of pericardial effusion and tamponade.[102,103]

Patients presenting with acute and subacute cardiac tamponade usually do not display the classic triad of hypotension, neck vein distention, and muffled heart tones. Waiting for their appearance to order a confirmatory test will delay diagnosis and jeopardize the safety of the patient. Image the heart whenever a clinically significant pericardial effusion is suspected. Scenarios warranting consideration of a pericardial effusion include a patient with hypotension of unclear etiology, particularly those patients with known malignancies, recent myocardial infarction, and end-stage renal disease, as well as victims of trauma, both blunt and penetrating.[8,9,11,104,105]

Use early demonstration of a large pericardial effusion to guide further work-up, support early consultation from either cardiology or cardiothoracic surgery, and facilitate therapeutic drainage for those patients who remain hypotensive in spite of fluid resuscitation. For patients in extremis, perform pericardiocentesis immediately. Use the clinician most experienced in both sonography and aspiration of the pericardial sac to perform the procedure. For patients with large effusions who are relatively stable, management options are greater and may include a pericardial window. Consultation with either cardiology or cardiothoracic surgery is advised prior to performing aspiration on stable patients; but this is always a *clinical judgment issue best made by the clinician at the bedside*.

The disadvantages of echocardiography are that it requires ultrasound equipment and is dependent on a skilled operator who is specifically trained in echocardiography. Even when immediately available, echocardiography may take at least 5 minutes, which may be too much time for a patient who is deteriorating rapidly. If the patient is not in full arrest and ultrasound equipment is available, ultrasonography should always be used to diagnose effusion and tamponade and to guide the procedure. Pericardial fluid is relatively easy to demonstrate with bedside ultrasonography, but because many ill patients will demonstrate some pericardial fluid, bedside ultrasonography may not differentiate incidental fluid from tamponade.

Ultrasonography may also be misleading in showing loculated effusion with tamponade associated with the early period after cardiac surgery. In one series, transthoracic echocardiography failed to visualize 60% of effusions.[106] These effusions were visualized through the use of transesophageal echocardiography. It is possible to mistake an epicardial fat pad for a pericardial effusion. This may be avoided by careful attention to detail. First, the epicardial fat pad is an anterior structure. Clot in the anterior pericardial space suggests that the effusion is circumferential and, therefore, should also be seen in the dependent portion of the pericardial space. This is best demonstrated using the parasternal long-axis view. Alternatively, the probe can be aligned longitudinally so that the inferior vena cava is visualized as it enters the right atrium. The right side of the heart can be seen adjacent to the diaphragm, and blood or fluid within the pericardial sac can be readily identified as long as it is not loculated.[7] Second, the inferior vena cava should collapse when the patient sniffs; a collapse of less than 50% indicates increased intrathoracic pressure and possibly tamponade. Third, blood clotting is a dynamic process, with clots continuously forming and being broken down. If blood is present within the pericardial sac, careful examination should reveal fronds of clot waving within an anechoic (black) pericardial space. Finally, and most importantly, an anterior fat pad should not cause collapse of the right ventricular free wall. If, after careful examination, doubt still exists as to the presence of an effusion, hemodynamically stable patients should have a formal echocardiogram or CT performed.

Also, remember that fluid within the pericardial space is not always pathologic. A small (<0.5–0.9 cm) effusion may not be clinically significant, and the sonographer should exercise caution in overreading an effusion, particularly when the patient is hemodynamically stable. *The patient who is hemodynamically compromised by a pericardial effusion should have a sizable effusion with diastolic collapse of the right ventricular free wall, septal bulging, and dilatation of the hepatic veins and inferior vena cava. The heart is usually beating rapidly with hyperkinetic wall motion, and may appear to swing to and fro within the pericardial sac.* Bedside ultrasound equipment available to the emergency physician may not be technically adequate to define all of these subtle ultrasound criteria. *Pericardial fluid is the most readily seen abnormality with emergency bedside ultrasonography.*

CT

At some institutions, CT is much more readily available than echocardiography. However, it requires that the patient be transported to the site of the CT equipment and patient stability must be considered. If clinically indicated, CT is effective in defining the presence and extent of pericardial effusion in the stable patient.[107] In certain circumstances, CT can provide a more definitive diagnosis than echocardiography. In one series, eight equivocal echocardiograms were evaluated by CT.[108] Two patients thought to have pericardial effusion by ultrasonography were found by CT to have pleural effusions. Another patient with pericardial effusion by ultrasonography was found by CT to have an epicardial lipoma. CT defined three loculated pleural effusions not seen by ultrasonography. A final two patients had hemopericardium visualized by CT but not ultrasonography. In circumstances in which the patient is stable and ultrasonography produces equivocal results or is not available, CT may provide a definitive diagnosis of pericardial effusion.

INDICATIONS FOR PERICARDIOCENTESIS

There are two indications for pericardiocentesis: (1) to diagnose the cause or presence of a pericardial effusion and (2) to relieve tamponade. The former is an elective procedure and ideally should be accomplished under ultrasound guidance. The latter may be semielective and performed with ultrasound guidance or emergent and performed blindly or with ECG assistance.

Diagnostic Pericardiocentesis

The use of pericardiocentesis for diagnosis of the etiology of nonhemorrhagic effusions is widespread, although opinions of its utility vary.[43,109,110] Neoplastic cells, blood, bacteria, viruses, and chyle can be sought. Measurement of pericardial fluid pH can be helpful, because inflammatory fluid is significantly more acidotic than noninflammatory fluid.[111] When a specific etiology is suspected, additional diagnostic testing may be useful (e.g., adenosine deaminase in tuberculosis and carcinoembryonic antigen in suspected malignancy).[112]

The diagnostic accuracy of pericardiocentesis varies greatly from series to series, depending on the vigor with which a definitive etiology was sought and the prevalence of certain etiologies in the patient population under consideration. In one large series, fluid was obtained in 90% of the aspirations, but a specific etiologic diagnosis was obtained in only 24% of the fluid specimens.[38] Certain diagnoses are unlikely to be made from pericardial fluid. Pericardial fluid has been shown to give false-negative cytologic results in certain cases of lymphoma and mesothelioma.[38] In HIV patients, effusions caused by Kaposi sarcoma and cytomegalovirus have been diagnosed by pericardial biopsy after fluid studies were nondiagnostic.[113,114]

An alternative diagnostic tool is subxiphoid pericardiotomy. This technique, performed in the operating suite, obtains both fluid and a pericardial biopsy specimen. It is more likely to provide a definitive diagnosis and has been performed safely without general anesthesia.[115,116] In a prospective series of 57 patients, 36% obtained a definitive diagnosis; 40%, a probable diagnosis; 16%, a possible diagnosis; and 7% remained undiagnosed with subxiphoid pericardiotomy.[117] Although it is uncertain whether this technique is safer than ultrasound-guided pericardiocentesis, published reports show a low rate of complications in experienced hands.[117]

Regardless of technique, the need to sample small effusions or obtain pericardial tissue has been questioned. A prospective series found a diagnostic rate of 6% with pericardial fluid and 5% with pericardial tissue when a small persistent effusion was sampled for the specific purpose of diagnosis.[110] In contrast, when patients from the same population had therapeutic intervention for tamponade, the yields from fluid and tissue were 54% and 22%, respectively.[110]

The use of pericardiocentesis as a diagnostic tool in traumatic tamponade is limited. When used diagnostically to determine the presence of pericardial bleeding in trauma, the procedure has a false-negative rate of between 20% and 40%.[91,118–120] The reason for the high false-negative rate (defined as no blood aspirated) is well demonstrated by typical stab wounds of the heart.[17,121] Ninety-six percent of the patients had blood in the pericardium, but it was clotted in 41% of the patients and partially clotted in another 24%. In only 19% was the blood completely fluid and thus capable of giving a true-positive result on pericardiocentesis.

Therapeutic Pericardiocentesis

Tamponade of Uncertain Etiology

The primary reason for performing pericardiocentesis in the ED is as part of the treatment for cardiac arrest or in periar-

a continuous display during rhythm monitoring, is used. When the alligator clamp connects the base of the pericardiocentesis needle to the V lead wire, set the machine to record the V lead as the rhythm strip.

Other Equipment

The traditional needle choice is a 7.5- to 12.5-cm (3- to 5-inch), 18-gauge spinal needle with an obturator. Leave the obturator in the needle during initial passage through the skin to avoid obstruction of the needle lumen. More recently, the shorter Teflon-sheathed Intracath needle has been used. Alternatively, use a guidewire (Seldinger) technique, and insert a plastic catheter over a flexible guide or J wire. With this technique, use an 18-gauge, thin-walled needle for placement of the wire. After removal of the accompanying introducer, leave the catheter in place for prolonged drainage, if needed.[133,134]

For drainage of blood, pus, or other viscous effusions, insert a large catheter such as a No. 7- to 9-French Cordis sheath.[135] Alternatively, use the guidewire technique to insert a radiopaque, 16-gauge, flexible, fenestrated, central venous catheter, to connect to closed suction drainage and leave it in place for long periods of time.[136] Pigtail catheters with side and end holes or nephrostomy drainage catheters can also be used.[134] Maintain multilumen catheter patency by slow continuous flush with a heparinized saline solution.[134] Complete sets containing necessary equipment for placing a pigtail catheter using the guidewire technique are commercially available (see Fig. 16–9B), including sets designed for pediatric use.[137] Attach a three-way stopcock to the needle or catheter to allow removal of more than one filled syringe without moving the needle much. The continuous motion of the heart may require minor changes in needle or catheter position during the procedure. It is safer to withdraw the steel needle and put a plastic catheter in place if lengthy or repeat drainage is required.

PROCEDURE

Temporizing Measures

Consider temporizing measures while preparing for pericardiocentesis in the unstable patient or attempting to stabilize the patient while the operating suite is readied for thoracotomy or subxiphoid pericardiotomy. In the patient with suspected tamponade and without jugular venous distention, administer a fluid bolus to improve hemodynamics.[76] In the setting of nonpenetrating tamponade, a fluid challenge has been recommended.[67,138] Animal experiments have found this to be beneficial, with or without nitroprusside for afterload reduction.[139] However, a follow-up prospective evaluation in patients with tamponade found no benefit from either fluid challenge or nitroprusside; cardiac output remained unchanged at a mean of 5.1 L/min, in contrast to 9.1 L/min after pericardiocentesis.[140] In the trauma patient with penetrating cardiac injury, fluid resuscitation may produce improvement or deterioration. Animal experiments indicate that the response depends on whether fluid infusion produces recurrent bleeding from the cardiac wound.[141] Judicious volume expansion may produce temporary beneficial hemodynamic results, but this is not uniformly true.

Give vasopressors also as a temporizing measure in tamponade. Dopamine, dobutamine, norepinephrine, and isoproterenol have been evaluated. Norepinephrine produced increased cardiac output in animal models of tamponade,[142,143] but failed to increase cardiac output in patients with malignant effusion.[142] Isoproterenol increased cardiac output in animal models but detrimentally affected cardiac blood flow.[142] Both dopamine and dobutamine have produced increased cardiac output and other improvements in hemodynamics in the setting of tamponade.[31,140] Either of these agents may be helpful as a temporizing agent in tamponade, but dobutamine may be preferable on theoretical grounds because of its greater β-activity.[143]

Preparation

Check all necessary equipment and lay everything out in advance. Have full resuscitation equipment on hand, including a defibrillator. Attach the patient to a cardiac monitor and check that the intravenous line is in place and working. The nonemergent patient may require sedation, but the emergent patient is usually obtunded or unresponsive as a result of low cardiac output. Do not use sedation in these patients because of the high risk of hemodynamic or respiratory deterioration. Premedicate the patient with atropine to help prevent vasovagal reactions. When possible, determine in advance the presence of pericardial effusion and the optimal anatomic approach by echocardiography. If surgery may be needed, make sure that both operating room and surgeon are available.

If the patient's clinical condition permits, elevate the chest to a 45° angle to bring the heart closer to the anterior chest wall. If the abdomen is distended because of gastric contents or previous positive-pressure ventilation, place a nasogastric tube to decompress the stomach. Prepare the skin of the entire lower xiphoid and epigastric area with 10% povidone-iodine solution and apply sterile drapes, if time permits.

If the patient is awake, anesthetize the skin and the proposed route of the pericardial needle with 1% lidocaine. Note that the pericardium is very sensitive and should be anesthetized in patients who are awake.[133]

Blind or ECG-Guided Pericardiocentesis

Anatomic Approach

The choice of anatomic approach in the past has been governed largely by conjecture and theory, not by actual study of patients with pericardial effusion. Traditionally, the subxiphoid approach was preferred and recommended as the optimal choice (Figs. 16–10 and 16–11). However, two-dimensional echocardiography allows direct visualization in the individual patient of both the areas of maximal effusion and the location of vital structures (see Fig. 16–13). Studies of echocardiography-directed pericardiocentesis have found that the intercostal space near the heart apex is usually the best site for puncture, not the traditional subxiphoid approach.[132,135] Careful cadaver studies have corroborated this finding, demonstrating greater safety with a parasternal approach in the fifth intercostal space and showing that the greatest number of injuries (usually to the right atrium) occurred with variants of the subxiphoid approach.[23] In contrast, studies of intracardiac injection using the same routes have found an increased incidence of pneumothorax when parasternal or intracostal approaches are used (see "Complications," later in this chapter). This risk may increase with underlying lung disease. Whenever time and the patient's

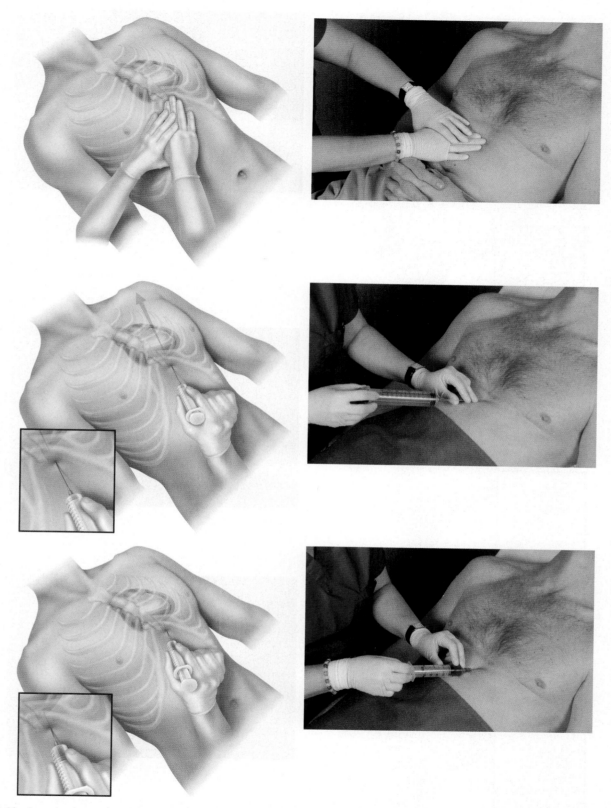

Figure 16–10 Procedural steps for pericardiocentesis (subxiphoid approach): Seldinger technique with a pigtail catheter left in the pericardial space. Local anesthesia, sedation, and analgesia are given as appropriate. *(From Custalow CB: Color Atlas of Emergency Department Procedures. Philadelphia, Elsevier Saunders, 2005, p 123.)*

Continued

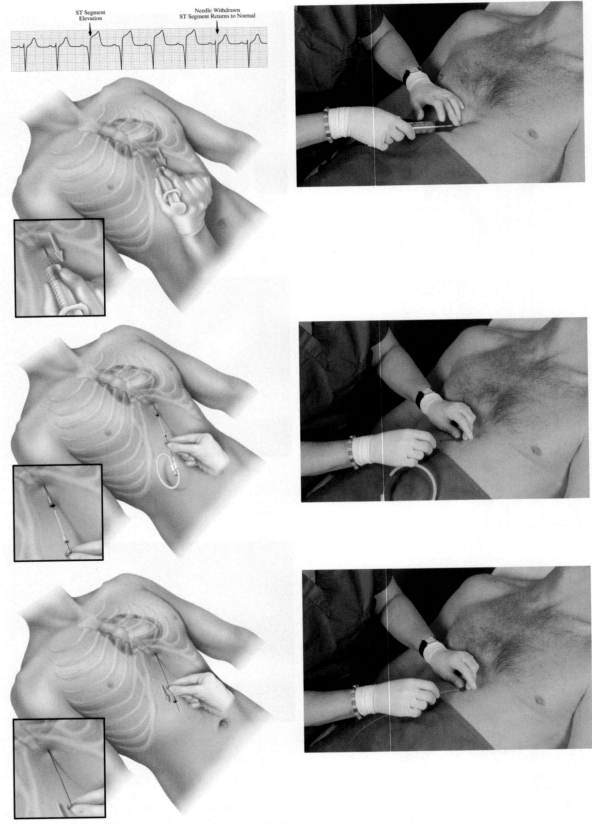

ST Segment
Elevation

Needle Withdrawn
ST Segment Returns to Normal

Figure 16–10, cont'd

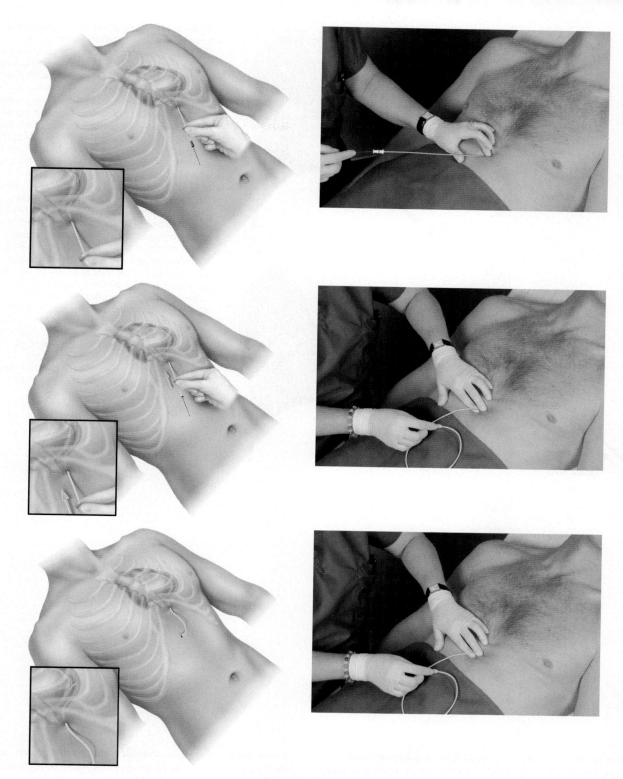

Figure 16–10, cont'd

condition permit, rely on echocardiography to define the extent of and optimal approach to pericardial effusion. When time or circumstances prevent the use of ultrasonography, the clinician should use the approach with which he or she is most familiar.

Parasternal Approach

Insert the needle perpendicular to the skin in the left fifth intercostal space medial to the border of cardiac dullness. Older texts identify the puncture site as being at least 3 to 4 cm lateral to the sternal border to avoid the internal

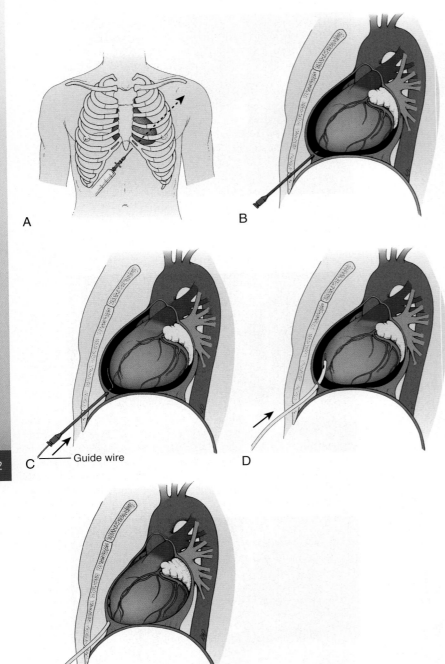

A

B

C — Guide wire

D

E

Figure 16–11 Diagram of lateral view of the technique demonstrated in Figure 16–10. Subxyphoid approach to catheter placement into the pericardial space. *A,* A short needle (16- or 18-gauge) is inserted into the left xiphocostal angle perpendicular to the skin and 3 to 4 mm below the left costal margin. After advancing the needle to the inner aspect of the rib cage, the needle's hub is depressed so that the needle points toward the patient's left shoulder. *B,* The needle is then cautiously advanced about 5 to 10 mm until fluid is reached. The fingers may sense a distinct "give" when the needle penetrates the parietal pericardium. Successful removal of fluid confirms the needle's position. *C,* The syringe is then disconnected from the needle, and the flexible tip of the guidewire is advanced into the pericardial space. The needle is withdrawn and replaced with a soft, multihole pigtail catheter (No. 6–8 Fr) using the Seldinger technique. *D,* After dilation of the needle tract, the catheter is advanced over the guidewire into the pericardial space. *E,* Once the catheter is properly positioned, aspiration of fluid should result in rapid improvement in blood pressure and cardiac output, a decrease in atrial and pericardial pressures, and a decrease in the degree of any paradoxical pulse. Electrical alternans, if present, also decreases or disappears. *(A–E, From Spodick DH: The technique of pericardiocentesis. J Crit Illn 2:91, 1987.)*

mammary artery. However, anatomic studies indicate that penetration immediately lateral to the sternum is less likely to cause this complication.[23]

Subxiphoid Approach

In the traditional subxiphoid approach, insert the needle between the xiphoid process and the left costal margin at a 30° to 45° angle to the skin (see Figs. 16–10, 16–11, and 16–13). Because the heart is an anterior structure, an angle greater than 45° may intercept the liver or stomach. In this approach, the needle enters the pericardium at the angle at which it becomes the diaphragmatic pericardium. Recommendations regarding needle aim vary widely, including among others the right shoulder, the sternal notch, and the left shoulder.[133,138] The only anatomic study conducted demonstrated that the subxiphoid approach is likely to injure the thin-walled right atrium when one aims for the right shoulder.[23] Aiming for the left shoulder directs the needle toward either the left ventricle or the anterior wall of the right ventricle.

Apical Approach

In the less commonly used apical approach, insert the needle 1 cm lateral and in the intercostal space below the apical beat, within the area of cardiac dullness. Aim toward the right shoulder.[133] If the apex cannot be palpated, insert the needle just inside the area of cardiac dullness. This area is close to the lingula and the left pleural space, and pneumothorax is more frequent; a concomitant pleural effusion may be inadvertently tapped. In theory, this technique is used because the coronary vessels are small at the apex, and if a ventricle is entered, it is the thick-walled left ventricle, which is more likely to seal off a ventricular injury. Data are insufficient to say whether these theoretical advantages are clinically important. With echocardiographic guidance, the apical approach may be more commonly used.[144]

ECG Monitoring

After the skin has been punctured but before advancing the needle, remove the obturator and attach an aspirating syringe. At this time, begin ECG monitoring. Attach a sterile electrical cord with alligator clips from the pericardial needle to any precordial lead (V lead) of the ECG machine. Record the V lead as the needle becomes an "exploring electrode." Make sure that the machine is properly tested and internally grounded. Small current leaks can induce dysrhythmias.[44] *Importantly, similar changes may be seen on the bedside ECG monitor, stressing the importance of an assistant during this procedure.* The purpose of ECG monitoring is to prevent ventricular puncture. When the needle touches the epicardium, a current-of-injury pattern, often resembling a wide-complex premature ventricular contraction (PVC) with an elevated ST segment, can be seen immediately on the electrocardiogram (Fig. 16–12). This current of injury may be local and could be missed if a lead other than a V lead is monitored or if a cardiac monitor (which has a lower frequency response than the ECG machine) is used. Usually, one notes ST segment elevation on contact with the heart or pericardium in the absence of an effusion, but a premature contraction or other ventricular dysrhythmia may also be induced by direct mechanical stimulation of the ventricular epicardium by the needle. Contact with the atrium can induce atrial dysrhythmias, marked elevation of the PR segment, or atrioventricular dissociation.[25] If there is abnormal myocardial tissue secondary to infarction, scarring, or malignant infiltration, no current of injury is generated.[26] Thus, ECG monitoring is not infallible in preventing myocardial penetration. Also, because the heart is constantly moving, it is practically impossible to merely touch the epicardium.

With continuous monitoring by electrocardiography, slowly advance the needle and syringe while gently aspirating. Although this is usually not appreciable, the needle will penetrate the pericardium at about 6 to 8 cm below the skin in adults and 5 cm or less below the skin in children.[65] The awake patient may complain of sharp chest pain as the sensitive pericardium is entered. As soon as pericardial fluid is aspirated, do not advance the needle any further. If a current of injury is seen on electrocardiography the needle is touching the epicardium and can easily lacerate myocardium or coro-

nary vessels. Withdraw the needle a few millimeters until the current of injury disappears. At this point, position the needle safely in the pericardial space, although the motion of the heart may quickly bring it back into contact with the myocardium. This is particularly a risk if the presence of a large effusion has not been demonstrated by ultrasound. If the scenario permits, use the properly placed needle to pass a wire, then catheter, into the pericardial space, rather than attempting to drain the fluid or blood with the needle alone. This is a technically difficult procedure.

Ultrasound-Guided Pericardiocentesis

Acoustic Windows

The cardiac examination is dynamic. The sonographer must identify the imaging window that provides images that best demonstrate the effusion or cardiac chamber of interest. Most frequently used are the subxiphoid and parasternal windows. It is important for the sonographer to develop expertise in using a variety of imaging windows to obtain the necessary clinical information.

Subxiphoid View

This view provides the most comprehensive information for a single view and is, therefore, the most important acoustic window for the less experienced sonographer to learn. It will readily identify a circumferential pericardial effusion and allow assessment of overall cardiac wall motion. The subxiphoid view can usually be obtained within 1 minute, and may be the only view required. To obtain the subxiphoid view, place the probe transversely at the left costal margin at the level of the xiphoid process with the beam aimed at the left shoulder (Fig. 16–13). Adjust the angle and rotation of the probe to obtain the appropriate views. The structures closest to the probe will appear at the top of the display and include the liver, diaphragm, pericardial space, and right ventricle.

Parasternal View

The next most useful view is the parasternal long-axis view. To obtain this view, place the transducer in the left parasternal area between the second and the fourth intercostal spaces. The plane of the beam should be parallel to a line drawn from the right shoulder to the left hip, with the marker pointing to the right shoulder (reverse if the image is not set for cardiac views). The parasternal view provides excellent images of the left atrium, mitral valve, left ventricle, aortic valve, and proximal ascending aorta. It is also the best view to identify small dependent collections within the pericardial sac.

Image Interpretation

The normal pericardium will appear as a single, brightly echogenic stripe adjacent to the myocardium. Fluid within the pericardial space will collect between the visceral and the

Withdraw

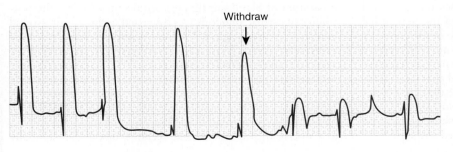

Figure 16–12 Current of injury. There is an obvious change in the ECG when the pericardiocentesis needle touches the epicardium. Following slight withdrawal (*arrow*), the ST segment elevation diminishes. This is best seen when the needle is directly attached to the ECG V lead, but may also be seen on the bedside cardiac.

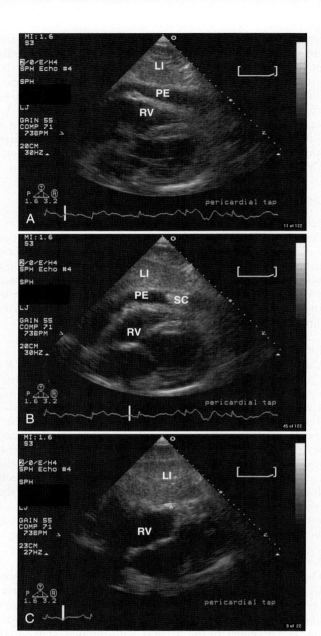

Figure 16–13   Placement of pigtail catheter in pericardial space with ultrasound assistance. Subcostal view of a small but hemodynamically significant pericardial effusion during a pericardiocentesis. *A,* The effusion. *B,* After injection of approximately 0.1 mL of agitated saline through the pericardiocentesis needle to confirm position in the pericardial space. *C,* The shaft of the pigtail catheter (*arrowhead,* two discrete parallel echogenic lines reflect the catheter walls; the echo-free area represents the catheter lumen) lying in the pericardial space after the majority of fluid has been drained. LI, liver; PE, pericardial effusion; RV, right ventricle; SC, saline contrast.

Procedure and Technique

Tsang and coworkers[145] described the technique for ultrasound-guided pericardiocentesis in 1998. The ideal site of skin puncture is where the largest area of fluid accumulation is closest to the skin surface. On ultrasound, this is demonstrated by visualizing a large anechoic area at the top of the screen (which is the body area closest to the probe) and usually corresponds to the left anterior chest wall (rather than the subcostal region). In addition to being closer to the skin surface, this approach avoids injury to the liver. Inadvertent puncture of the lung is also prevented using this approach, because air in the lung will not conduct sound waves and will prevent visualization of the heart when located immediately beneath the probe. Avoid choosing a site that might puncture either the internal mammary artery, which lies 3 to 5 cm from the parasternal border, or the neurovascular bundle located at the inferior rib border. The best site should be marked with a sterile pen.

Conform the needle trajectory and depth prior to skin puncture. Be aware that repositioning the patient will alter the position of the heart and pericardial sac within the chest and requires reassessment. Prepare the skin antiseptically and place a sterile cover over the probe. If time permits, anesthetize the selected area with 1% to 2% lidocaine, using the superior border of the adjacent rib as a landmark. Select a 16- to 18-gauge needle that is 5 to 8 cm in length. The needle should ideally have an over-the-needle sheath that allows the needle to be withdrawn after the pericardial space is entered. This helps avoid injury to the heart and other vital structures. Attach a saline-filled syringe to the needle, and gently aspirate while the needle is advanced. Keep the ultrasound probe on the chest wall immediately adjacent to the aspiration site or remove after the fluid is localized.

Once the pericardial space is entered, inject agitated saline to confirm needle placement, particularly if the pericardial fluid is grossly bloody or there is any question concerning needle position (see Fig. 16–13B). Prepare a saline echocardiographic contrast medium by using two 5-mL syringes, one with saline and the other with air, connected via a three-way stopcock to the needle catheter sheath. Rapidly inject saline between the syringes and then inject it into the sheath. Monitor the entrance of the agitated saline into the pericardial space sonographically because it appears as a brightly echogenic stream.

After confirmation of needle placement, pass a wire through the needle and a dilator (6–8 Fr Cordis) over the wire. Remove the dilator and place an introducer sheath-dilator (6–8 Fr Cordis) over the wire. Remove both the wire and the dilator and leave the introducer sheath in place. Insert the pigtail angiocatheter through the introducer sheath, and aspirate fluid to confirm placement.[145]

Fluid Aspiration and Evaluation

Aspiration of blood during pericardiocentesis raises the possibility of cardiac puncture. As discussed earlier, if ultrasound guidance is used, agitated saline "contrast" can determine ventricular versus pericardial placement. If fluoroscopy is available, inject a small amount of contrast to quickly disclose intracardiac placement. In other circumstances, the needle may need to be repositioned and the aspirate reexamined. Laboratory tests may help distinguish circulatory blood from hemorrhagic pericardial fluid. The latter should have a lower hematocrit measurement than venous blood. Substantially

parietal pericardium and will appear as a large, nonbeating, anechoic area adjacent to the ventricular myocardium. A small amount of fluid in the dependent portion of the pericardial space is normal. The sonographic appearance of the clinically significant effusion is distinct. The sonogram will reveal a hyperkinetic heart within a circumferential pericardial effusion, with diastolic collapse of the right-sided chambers. This reflects pressures within the pericardial space that are greater than the right ventricular filling pressure during diastole. The inferior vena cava will be dilated and not show respiratory variation or collapse when the patient is asked to "sniff."

different hematocrit values rule out the possibility that the needle was in a cardiac chamber. Hemorrhagic pericardial fluid usually is about 0.10 pH unit lower than simultaneously obtained arterial blood.[111] Bloody pericardial fluid may clot, particularly when bleeding is brisk, so clotting of the aspirated blood does not eliminate the possibility of a pericardial source. Nonclotting blood is indicative of defibrinated pericardial blood. Practically, however, there is rarely time for such analysis.

If an indwelling catheter is to be placed, advance a guidewire through the needle (see Fig. 16-11). Then pass a dilator over the wire to expand the needle tract. Keep the guidewire in sight and stabilized at all times. If intracardiac placement of the needle or guidewire is suspected, verify positioning by ultrasonography or fluoroscopy or by using the techniques described earlier before the needle tract is dilated. Once the tract has been dilated, place the pigtail catheter over the guidewire. If the dilator is not used, particularly with the subxiphoid approach, the pigtail catheter tip may hang in the subcutaneous tissue, making placement difficult.

After the catheter is placed, or if a decision is made to do a single aspiration, withdraw as much fluid as possible from the pericardium. The removal of even 30 to 50 mL may result in marked clinical improvement in a patient with tamponade. Place the catheter on continuous or intermittent drainage. Obtain a chest film after the procedure to rule out iatrogenic pneumothorax. Monitor the patient closely for 24 hours for signs of reaccumulating fluid or iatrogenic complications from the procedure. Repeat ultrasound examination is recommended. Diagnostic evaluation of nonhemorrhagic fluid is similar to the analysis of pleural fluid (see Chapter 9, Thoracentesis).

COMPLICATIONS

The failure of pericardiocentesis to yield fluid ("dry tap") may be considered a complication, because the procedure has failed to achieve its desired result. If a dry tap is considered a complication, it is by far the most frequent one encountered during blind pericardiocentesis. In addition, the pericardial needle can injure any organ within its reach, causing pneumothorax, myocardial or coronary vessel laceration, and hemopericardium.[124] Air embolism may be caused by air entering the heart.[146] The pericardial needle can also induce dysrhythmias from direct irritation of the epicardium or from small currents leaking from the connected ECG machine.[2]

Assessing the frequency of complications from pericardiocentesis is not straightforward. Changes in the diagnosis of effusion by ultrasonography or CT and guidance of the procedure by ultrasonography or fluoroscopy have greatly reduced the likelihood of complications.[6,144,147-149] No recent data related to complications of blind or ECG-guided emergency pericardiocentesis are available. The complication rate is expected to be quite different. For example, Wong and colleagues[3] reported that most complications occurred in patients who were found retrospectively to have no effusion. The procedure is also performed frequently in moribund patients, and distinguishing between a poor outcome resulting from a poorly performed procedure as opposed to the underlying condition can be difficult.

The use of ultrasonography will significantly minimize the risk of many of these complications, especially inadvertent puncture of the myocardium, epicardial vessels, and liver.[7,145] A summation of the results of five recent reports on echocardiographically guided pericardiocentesis[5,144,147-149] includes 564 procedures with a 98% success rate. No deaths were reported. There were 5 incidences of pneumothorax, 4 reported cardiac punctures, 1 significant dysrhythmia, 1 hemothorax, 1 pericardial-pleural shunt, and 1 instance of purulent pericarditis. Additional complications uniquely associated with ultrasonography are due to misinterpretation of the sonographic image. For example, epicardial fat pads are common in obese patients and can be misinterpreted as clot or fluid within the pericardial space.[7]

The major complications that may result from pericardiocentesis are discussed individually.

Cardiac Arrest and Death

Cardiac arrest and death is extremely rare in echocardiographically guided pericardiocentesis. In blind or ECG-guided pericardiocentesis, the patient is usually in full arrest and attribution of death to procedure or preprocedure condition is nearly impossible. For example, in one series of 52 patients, the only death occurred in a patient in cardiogenic shock who had a nonproductive pericardiocentesis and who, on postmortem examination, had severe arteriosclerotic heart disease, not tamponade.[3] An additional case of cardiac arrest (successfully resuscitated) in this series was in a patient with a nonproductive pericardiocentesis; the cause of the arrest was not discussed.[3]

In a series of 352 pericardiocenteses performed under fluoroscopic guidance, only 2 deaths resulted.[4] Ultrasonography or CT confirmation of effusion was used in all but 15 cases. The 2 deaths occurred during or after the procedure, but whether they should be attributed to the procedure is unclear. One patient with aortic rupture penetrating into the pericardial space died of cardiac arrest immediately after the puncture. The other death, in a post–myocardial infarction patient with left ventricular aneurysm, was due to ventricular fibrillation that occurred about 15 minutes after the procedure.

Cardiac Chamber, Vessel, or Lung Laceration

Cardiac chamber, vessel, or lung lacerations occur more frequently during blind or ECG-guided procedures. Nonfatal cardiac puncture, pneumothorax, suppurative pericarditis, costochondritis, and pneumoperitoneum have also been reported.[56] Most cardiac perforations occur in the right ventricle, but left ventricular[4] as well as atrial punctures have been reported.[25]

In Krikorian and Hancock's series,[38] 13 of 123 patients developed hemopericardium as a result of pericardiocentesis, 1 as a result of a lacerated coronary artery. One patient died from a punctured ventricle. Surgical control was necessary for 4 patients who developed tamponade, whereas 8 patients with hemopericardium did not develop tamponade and were managed conservatively. Several cases of induced tamponade occurred in patients with platelet counts greater than 50×10^9/L.

Guberman and colleagues[46] reported 3 right ventricular lacerations in 46 patients; 1 laceration was fatal. Wong and colleagues[3] found 5 right ventricular punctures, 4 in patients with nonproductive pericardiocentesis, but none causing any adverse sequelae. In a series of dialysis patients, 9 of 10 receiving pericardiocentesis had serious complications, including 3 deaths and 2 myocardial lacerations.[55] Duvernoy and associates[4] reported 23 penetrations (all right ventricular except 2 in which both the right and the left ventricles had been perforated), along with 4 cases of significant arterial bleeding in a series of 352 procedures.

Researchers differ in their opinions as to the adverse effects of ventricular puncture. Most ventricular punctures during the procedure occur in the lower aspect of the right ventricle. Because right ventricular pressure is lower,[65] puncture should cause less bleeding; however, the right ventricular wall is also thinner and more vulnerable to laceration. In a series of patients with ultrasound-directed pericardiocentesis, ventricular puncture still occurred in 1.5% but was without consequence owing to small needle size.[135] In another study, right ventricular laceration occurred in 1 patient despite the use of echocardiography, producing tamponade and necessitating emergency surgery.[110] Of the 23 perforations in the series by Duvernoy and associates,[4] only 3 were considered "major" complications, with 2 of the patients requiring thoracotomy.

A small number of pneumothoraces and pneumopericardia have been reported in various series but have been without clinical consequence other than drainage (Fig. 16–14). Theoretically, a tense pneumopericardium could result in tamponade. A single case of tension pneumothorax has been reported after pericardiocentesis, but a cause-and-effect relationship was unclear.[150]

Dysrhythmias

Serious dysrhythmias induced by pericardiocentesis are rare. PVCs occur commonly during the procedure and are benign in most cases. Most case series report no dysrhythmias.[3,46,56,135] Krikorian and Hancock[38] reported only 1 episode of ventricular tachycardia and several "hypotensive vasovagal reactions," which were associated with bradycardia and responded to atropine and fluid loading. Duvernoy and associates[4] reported 1 case of ventricular tachycardia and 1 case of atrial fibrillation among 352 procedures. Maggiolini and coworkers[147] reported transient third-degree heart block in a single patient.

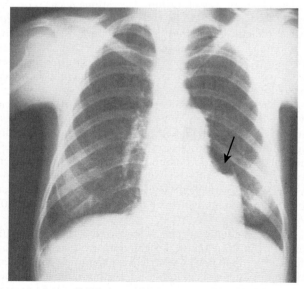

Figure 16–14 Air-fluid level (*arrow*) in the pericardial space immediately after pericardiocentesis. A minor pneumopericardium is inconsequential; a larger collection may cause tamponade.

Adverse Physiologic Consequences

There have been a few case reports of adverse consequences even when pericardiocentesis inflicts no injury. Most of these have to do with the fact that during pericardiocentesis, the stroke volume of the previously collapsed right ventricle increases 77% with the first 200 mL of fluid removed.[68] Generally, this increase in stroke volume is greater initially than that demonstrated by the left ventricle. This can have significant consequences for both right and left ventricular function. In three of six patients in whom large effusions were removed by pericardiocentesis, there was right ventricular dilatation and overload, with abnormal septal motion and either no increase in right ventricular ejection fraction or a decrease.[151] These patients returned to normal hemodynamic status slowly.

Sudden pulmonary edema also has been reported after pericardiocentesis, presumably due to a sudden increase in venous return to the left ventricle at a time when peripheral vascular resistance is still high from compensatory catecholamine secretion.[152-155] Supporting evidence for this explanation is that right ventricular stroke volume increases more after relief of tamponade than the stroke volume increase of the left ventricle.[71] Circulatory collapse with persistently low arterial blood pressure has been reported in a patient who was drained of 700 mL of clear fluid at a rate of 100 mL/min.[156] These authors suggested that ketamine anesthesia may have played a role, but the relative ischemia created by tamponade, coupled with the sudden increase in left-sided preload, created a persisting imbalance. They recommend that pericardial drainage rate not exceed 50 mL/min. Given the rare occurrence of pulmonary edema or primary cardiac compromise, it is unclear that this recommendation is justified. A case of brief profound bradycardia and rebound hypertension was reported after surgical relief of tamponade.[157] Such responses have not been noted in large series of patients receiving pericardiocentesis.

Remember that fluid within the pericardial space is not always pathologic. A small (<0.5–0.9 cm) effusion may not be clinically significant, and the sonographer should exercise caution in overreading an effusion, particularly when the patient is hemodynamically stable. The patient who is hemodynamically compromised by a pericardial effusion should have a sizable effusion (the size can vary) with diastolic collapse of the right ventricular free wall, septal bulging, and dilatation of the hepatic veins and inferior vena cava. The heart is usually beating rapidly with hyperkinetic wall motion and may appear to swing to and fro within the pericardial sac.

SUMMARY

In nontraumatic patients, tamponade should always be considered in the differential diagnosis of shock or cardiac arrest due to PEA, especially in patients who are on anticoagulants, have had recent myocardial infarction, a history of pericardial disease, malignancy, or suspected aortic dissection, or when a CVP catheter is in place. Tamponade should also be considered in the differential diagnosis when hypotension persists after closed chest CPR or attempts at cardiac pacing. Postresuscitation PEA should alert the clinician to the potential for tamponade.

In any patient with blunt or penetrating chest or upper abdominal trauma, the possibility of traumatic tamponade must also be considered. If clinical deterioration occurs in the ED pending operative care, temporizing pericardiocentesis should be considered if other therapy fails. When such a patient arrives with no obtainable blood pressure or in profound shock and unconscious, immediate thoracotomy and pericardiotomy are indicated after intubation.[123,158,159] Pericardiocentesis may cause a dangerous delay in this situation and has a low success rate.

Management of tamponade requires a sound understanding of pathophysiology, an ever-vigilant evaluation, and the knowledge of when the patient's clinical condition requires blind or ECG-guided pericardiocentesis as contrasted to the safer alternative of echocardiographically guided diagnosis and therapy.

Acknowledgment

The editors and author wish to acknowledge the contributions of Michael Callaham to this chapter in previous editions. Sarah A. Stahmer and Lisa Mackowiak Filippone developed much of the material on ultrasound in pericardiocentesis, originally contained in Chapter 67, Ultrasound-Guided Procedures.

 REFERENCES CAN BE FOUND ON EXPERT CONSULT

CHAPTER 17

Artificial Perfusion during Cardiac Arrest

Benjamin S. Abella and Lance B. Becker

Cardiopulmonary resuscitation (CPR) can be life saving when provided to a patient in cardiac arrest, particularly in conjunction with other therapies such as defibrillation or delivery of medications. In several large clinical studies, data have shown that the prompt delivery of CPR serves as an important predictor of successful outcome, increasing the chances of survival by up to twofold, whereas each minute without treatment is associated with a 10% to 15% decrease in the probability of survival.[1,2]

The quality of CPR is an important technical issue. Recent investigations have shown that CPR quality has a direct effect on patient outcome; for example, shallow chest compressions have an adverse impact on defibrillation success.[3] Owing to these and related data, emphasis has recently been placed on improving CPR quality, and such priority has been codified in consensus CPR guidelines promulgated by the American Heart Association. These guidelines are formulated through a formalized data evaluation process and updated every 5 years.[4]

Worrisome data have shown that CPR quality during actual resuscitation is endemically poor.[5,6] Specifically, chest compressions are often administered too slowly and with inadequate depth, pauses in chest compressions are too long, and hyperventilation of arrest patients is common. These deficiencies may be due to a variety of factors, including infrequent training, lack of CPR quality awareness during resuscitation, and incoherent team leadership during resuscitation efforts.[7]

CONVENTIONAL CPR

Although CPR is widely taught to health care personnel and reassessed periodically, the importance of high-quality CPR cannot be stressed enough. Quality CPR immediately before defibrillation increases the chance of successful restoration of circulation.[8] It has also been demonstrated that chest compression quality influences resuscitation drug efficacy, whereas inadequate circulation leads to minimal effects from peripherally delivered drugs.[9] Furthermore, hyperventilation is a widely prevalent problem that has been shown to dramatically compromise hemodynamics and, in animal studies, leads to reduced survival from arrest. In this section, we review the key procedural aspects of manual CPR.

Compressions

The revised 2005 resuscitation guidelines[4] emphasize the importance of chest compression quality. Focus on maintaining proper chest compression depth and rate. Compress the sternum to a depth of 1.5 to 2 inches and at a rate of 100 compressions/min (Table 17–1 provides a summary of CPR procedural recommendations). Early in resuscitation efforts, place a backboard under the victim to ensure appropriate thoracic compression. In addition, adjust the height of the bed or have the rescuer stand on top of a stepstool so that her or his entire weight above the waist can be directed on the patient's sternum. This both enhances compression depth and helps to prevent leaning on the patient's chest in between compressions, another key deficiency that has been widely observed. Extend the arms fully and place them perpendicular to the patient's chest, making sure to pull away from the chest sufficiently between compressions in order to allow for full chest recoil. Aggressively rotate rescuers (approximately every 2–3 min) to avoid deteriorating compression quality owing to exhaustion. Properly delivered compressions are highly fatiguing, and rescuer bravado often interferes with the realization of declining CPR quality over time.

Minimize pauses in chest compressions, because even short pauses can have profound effects on coronary perfusion pressure and outcomes.[10] As stated earlier, longer pauses in chest compressions before shock delivery were found to be associated with defibrillation failure.[3] Do not stop CPR for medication delivery, which can be administered simultaneously with the compressions. Keep pauses for procedures such as intubation or pulse checks to a minimum.

Ventilations

Deliver ventilations at a rate of 8 to 10 breaths/min. When using a bag-valve mask, a useful technique is to remove the rescuer's hand completely off the bag between ventilations in order to avoid unwittingly hyperventilating the patient. The team leader must be vigilant in the observation of delivered ventilations and should be ready to verbally prompt rescuers to bag at the appropriate rate.

Pulse Checks

Pulse checks tend to be performed too frequently during resuscitation efforts and to be of too long a duration. If a pulse cannot be readily felt within seconds, continue CPR immediately. There are no data suggesting that CPR is harmful to a patient with a very weak pulse, and therefore, use of Doppler ultrasound devices as pulse detectors is discouraged. If rescuers need ultrasound to find a pulse, the patient is at the very least markedly hypotensive and should probably be receiving CPR. Attempt pulse detection at the location of the carotid or femoral artery because peripheral pulse checks during profound shock or cardiac arrest states are notoriously unreliable. Often, a "pulse" can be detected during CPR itself; this phenomenon is often due to venous back-pressure during compressions and should not indicate that compressions should be stopped.

Leadership and Teamwork

Cardiac arrest resuscitations are often crowded, chaotic events filled with stress and anxiety. Establish a team protocol in these situations to maximize both calm and efficiency and ensure quality of care. Designate someone to be the leader of the resuscitation effort, and make sure all participants are clearly aware of this designation. When designated as team leader, be responsible for rhythm monitoring, giving orders for initiation and termination of chest compressions and delivery of drugs and other therapies. Situate yourself either at the head of the bed or a place where you are able to direct

TABLE 17–1 Key Procedural Elements of Manual Cardiopulmonary Resuscitation

Compressions

100 compressions/min
Depth 1.5–2 inches/compression
Release hands completely between compressions
Minimize pauses in compressions

Ventilations

8–10 ventilations/min
Avoid hyperventilation
Minimize chest compression pause for intubation

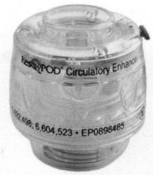

Figure 17–1 Impedance threshold device (ITD). The ITD is placed in-line between the mask or endotracheal tube and the bag-valve apparatus. This is the Res-Q-Pod, showing the flashing light indicator used to time the respiratory rate *(arrow)*. *(Courtesy of Advanced Circulatory Systems, Inc., Eden Prairie, MN.)*

the room. It is of utmost importance that, as the team leader, you do not actually deliver compressions, ventilations, or perform other specific procedures unless absolutely necessary, because you will quickly lose control of the resuscitation. Because most rescuers are unable to detect when their own compression quality is diminishing, you should observe CPR closely and order rescuer rotations throughout the duration of the arrest.[11]

New Directions: Compression-only CPR

Chest compression-only cardiopulmonary resuscitation (CC-CPR) has been shown to be possibly as effective as standard CPR in a variety of investigations among resuscitation efforts initiated by the lay public.[12,13] Compression rates of at least 100/minute are suggested. Owing to its simplicity, CC-CPR minimizes pauses in chest compressions while also maintaining proper rate and depth. It is especially useful for lay rescuers in the community who may be less experienced with standard CPR and may be uncomfortable with performance of mouth-to-mouth resuscitation. Although CC-CPR has not yet received widespread endorsement, it is likely to become a standard technique in many communities in coming years and may very well become standard for initial resuscitation in the emergency department (ED) setting as well.

ADJUNCTS TO IMPROVE CPR QUALITY

A variety of technologies have been developed to assist in the goal of improving CPR quality. Some of these tools are directly involved in improving the efficacy of chest compressions whereas others are less direct, either aiming to improve human performance or enhancing hemodynamics during chest compression delivery. This section describes some of these promising techniques.

Active Compression-Decompression CPR

Active compression-decompression cardiopulmonary resuscitation (ACD-CPR) is a variant of CPR in which the passive relaxation phase of CPR is converted into an active phase by means of a handheld suction device, improving both myocardial and cerebral circulation compared with traditional CPR.[14,15] However, not all the data surrounding these devices have been positive; there also have been studies in out-of-hospital cardiac arrest using this technique that did not find any improvements in either initial outcome or survival to

discharge, and as with many devices, there are instances when its application is impractical.[16,17]

Several different ACD-CPR devices are on the market and generally all work under similar principles (Lifestick, Montvale, NJ; LUCAS, Jolife Corp, Lund, Sweden). ACD-CPR is performed by placing the device in a midsternal position. The compression phase is similar to that of standard CPR. The decompression phase is performed to bring the chest to a fully expanded position without losing contact with it (producing ~20 lb of pressure).

Impedance Threshold Device

The impedance threshold device (ITD) is a CPR adjunct that optimizes chest compression hemodynamics via control of intrathoracic pressure. The ITD is a simple device that is placed between the endotracheal tube and the bag-valve apparatus, much like colorimetric end-tidal CO_2 detectors familiar to most ED clinicians (Fig. 17–1). The ITD contains a valve that prevents air flow through the device at less than 10 cm H_2O pressure. During resuscitation, the ITD prevents air from entering the thorax during chest wall recoil after each compression, generating a small but hemodynamically significant negative pressure within the chest. This negative pressure enhances venous return to the heart and results in an increased cardiac output with each subsequent chest compression. Studies with one model of ITD (Res-Q-Pod, Advanced Circulatory Systems, Inc., Eden Prairie, MN) have demonstrated improved hemodynamics during CPR.[18–20]

The ITD can be used during resuscitation either with mask ventilation or via an endotracheal tube and is, therefore, appropriate for both basic life support care in the field and ED resuscitation. When the device is applied, administer ventilations at a rate of 8 to 10 breaths/min as per standard resuscitation guidelines. The Res-Q-Pod ITD has a flashing light timed to prompt appropriate ventilatory rate as well. When used with a face mask, it is important to continuously maintain a tight seal between the patient's face and the mask during CPR in order to maintain ITD efficacy. This is best accomplished with a two-person ventilation technique in which one person holds the face mask and a second person squeezes the bag. If a pulse is restored, it is generally recommended to remove the ITD from the respiratory circuit at that time.

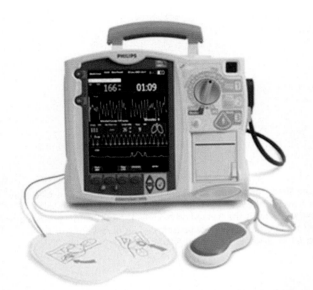

Figure 17–2 Cardiopulmonary resuscitation–sensing defibrillator. The chest compression pad with force detector and accelerometer is indicated (*arrow*). Several such devices are currently marketed; this is the MRx-QCPR. *(Courtesy of Philips Healthcare, Andover, MA.)*

Monitoring and Feedback Devices

Emphasis on CPR quality and minimizing interruptions in CPR has spurred the development of devices to monitor the quality of chest compressions and ventilations and then provide audio or visual prompts to improve performance. These devices aim to improve human delivery of CPR and, unlike ACD-CPR or the ITD, do not enhance hemodynamics or patient physiology directly.

One method of monitoring chest compressions involves applying a relatively small, external device on the patient's sternum and performing chest compressions on top of the device (Fig. 17–2). The device measures compression quality via a force detector and/or accelerometer that determines the rate and depth of chest compressions. Different versions of these CPR-quality monitoring and feedback devices are on the market. Some are incorporated into defibrillators (MRx/Q-CPR, Philips Healthcare, Andover, MA; R series with Real CPR Help, Zoll Medical Corp, Chelmsford, MA), and others are stand-alone devices applied to the chest (CPR-Ezy, Health Affairs Ltd, London, England). In recent trials, use of such a defibrillator with CPR monitoring and feedback improved CPR performance and, in one out-of-hospital trial, improved the rate of initial resuscitation.[21] Further research will be required to assess the magnitude of survival improvement these devices can offer and what training mechanisms can maximize team responses to feedback messages.

Mechanical CPR Devices

The adjuncts described previously all rely on human performance of CPR. Another general approach to improve CPR quality is to provide compressions via a mechanical device that is independent of human fatigue or performance vagaries. Such tools have been introduced in prior decades but fell out of favor owing to unwieldy design and other practical considerations. A newer generation of devices has brought the notion of mechanical CPR back to active consideration. One

such device uses a "load-distributing compression band" (Autopulse, Zoll Corp., Chelmsford, MA). The Autopulse device works via a wide band, attached to a backboard and battery-powered motor, placed across the torso. Through cycles of constriction and relaxation, the band compresses the chest in a circumferential manner at a fixed rate and "depth" consistent with resuscitation guidelines. In this fashion, pauses are also minimized by eliminating rescuer switching. Such devices have a unique role in out-of-hospital arrest, because compressions can be delivered while transporting a patient down stairs or into an ambulance. Recent studies to determine the efficacy of the Autopulse have had mixed results. Whereas initial smaller investigations looked promising, a large multicenter randomized trial was stopped early, because patients in the manual CPR arm had improved survival over those receiving care via the Autopulse.[22] A separate nonrandomized trial showed a marked improvement in survival using the device.[23] It is likely that further research will be required, and the survival benefit of such a device may very much depend on the specifics of how it is applied and used.

Another mechanical CPR device was developed in Europe (LUCAS, Jolife Corp, Lund, Sweden) and is currently being tested in clinical trials outside the United States. This device, in contrast to the band mechanism of the Autopulse, uses a piston/suction cup to compress the anterior chest, much like during manual CPR, with the suction cup providing some degree of active compression-decompression, as described earlier in this chapter.

MONITORING DURING CPR
Overview of CPR

Despite extensive research and attempts to alter the outcome of cardiac arrest, it is discouraging to realize that, at present, there are no reliable clinical criteria that clinicians can use to assess the efficacy of CPR. Although end-tidal CO_2 serves as an indicator of cardiac output produced by chest compressions and may indicate return of spontaneous circulation there is little other technology available to provide real-time feedback on the effectiveness of CPR. Pulse oximetry is not helpful during arrest. Early defibrillation has been linked to better survival rates, but no medications have been shown to improve neurologically intact survival from cardiac arrest. Despite the widespread use of epinephrine and several studies of vasopressin, no placebo-controlled study has shown that any medication or vasopressor given routinely at any stage during human cardiac arrest (pulseless VT, VF, PEA, or asystole) increases rate of survival to hospital discharge.

Arterial blood gas monitoring during cardiac arrest is not a reliable indicator of the severity of tissue hypoxemia, hypercarbia (and therefore the adequacy of ventilation during CPR), or tissue acidosis. Current evidence in patients presenting with ventricular fibrillation (VF) neither supports nor refutes the use of routine IV fluids. *There is no evidence that any antiarrhythmic drug given routinely during human cardiac arrest increases survival to hospital discharge.* There is insufficient evidence to recommend for or against the routine use of fibrinolysis for cardiac arrest.

No blood testing is considered routine nor standard during the initial stages of cardiopulmonary arrest, although early serum potassium and blood glucose monitoring are prudent if resuscitation is successful.[24]

Capnography

Whereas capnography is a common method of confirming correct endotracheal tube placement, it has also been regarded as a potential method of measuring hemodynamics and determining outcome of resuscitation efforts. Capnography measures respiratory CO_2, which is delivered to the lungs and expelled during exhalation. The highest CO_2 levels occur at the end of each exhalation, called end-tidal carbon dioxide (E_tco_2). During cardiac arrest, E_tco_2 levels fall abruptly at the onset of cardiac arrest, increase during the delivery of effective CPR, and return to physiologic levels after the return of spontaneous circulation. E_tco_2 levels correlate with cardiac output under low-flow states such as CPR.[25] Because of this relationship with cardiac output, E_tco_2 has been regarded as a likely indicator of CPR quality. During effective CPR in animal trials, E_tco_2 positively correlates with cardiac output, coronary perfusion pressure, efficacy of cardiac compression, return of spontaneous circulation, and even survival. Current research is being done to further understand the use of E_tco_2 during CPR. At the other end of the spectrum, E_tco_2 could be useful in determining when to terminate resuscitation efforts.[26]

Ultrasound Monitoring

With advances in ultrasound equipment, properly trained users can portably and accurately monitor cardiac function in real time. Preliminary studies have demonstrated that trained physicians can assess cardiac function and obtain adequate images rapidly using a subcostal approach to standard echocardiography in the cardiac arrest setting.[27] If you are adequately trained in this technology, use it during resuscitation efforts to clinically diagnose conditions such as pulseless electrical activity (PEA) and to make a global assessment of cardiac motion during CPR and pulse restoration. Use ultrasound also during arrest to rapidly diagnose and treat conditions such as cardiac tamponade. Get the ED ultrasound machine ready to use when preparing for an incoming cardiac arrest. Remember, however, that ultrasound is only a secondary diagnostic adjunct and should not interfere with the performance of high-quality CPR. Minimize interruptions to perform ultrasound and use it only during resuscitation for specific purposes (e.g., diagnosis of PEA vs. hypotensive sinus rhythm). In most cases of arrest, ultrasound is likely of little value. Finally, there is ongoing research into the use of transcranial Doppler ultrasound to determine prognosis after cardiac arrest. One preliminary study concluded that patients with severely disabling or fatal outcome could be identified within the first 24 hours using this method.[28]

CONCLUSIONS

Physicians and other health care workers have been performing CPR for over 50 years, but only since the 1990s has the full importance of CPR quality become apparent through an evidence-based approach. Chest compressions and ventilations appear deceptively easy to the newly trained, but in fact, they are highly complex skills and are difficult to perform well under stress. New technologies have been developed to assist in CPR delivery, and the use of these tools may improve the ability to save lives from cardiac arrest in the coming years.

 REFERENCES CAN BE FOUND ON EXPERT CONSULT

CHAPTER **18**

Resuscitative Thoracotomy

Michael E. Boczar and Emanuel Rivers

Trauma is the leading cause of death in people younger than 44 years old in North America.[1] Cumulative trauma mortality has a steep curve in the initial hour after injury with 50% of deaths occuring within the 1st hour.[2]

Advances in prehospital care have increased the number of patients arriving at the emergency department (ED) in various stages of shock, allowing emergency clinicians to resuscitate patients who previously would have died at the scene. Penetrating cardiac injuries are a leading cause of death in urban areas,[3] and in these patients, survival is occasionally possible if an aggressive approach using emergency department thoracotomy (EDT) is taken.

EDT is a dramatic, heroic intervention performed outside of the operating room and often in the absence of trained cardiothoracic surgeons. *It is the rare patient who survives this intervention*, but exceedingly dismal survival rates do not negate the occasional dramatic save gleaned from EDT. EDT is more common in major university centers and level I trauma centers, and there is no standard of care to support or refute that it is a procedure that must be undertaken by all emergency clinicians.

Simply stated, the performance of EDT is not a simple procedure. Merely identifying specific structures within a chest cavity filled with blood, coupled with a collapsed lung, an insured heart and major vessels, can be formidable. Finding pathology that can be reversed is even more difficult.

This chapter focuses on (1) indications and contraindications for EDT; (2) mechanism of injury; (3) prehospital/ED vital signs and outcomes that significantly influence these decisions; (4) the pathophysiology and diagnosis of disease processes that would require such an invasive procedure; and (5) the technical aspects of performing an EDT. The emergency clinician should have a systematic plan after opening the chest. In the trauma patient receiving a resuscitative thoracotomy, the clinician seeks to relieve cardiac tamponade if present; to support cardiac function (with direct cardiac compression, cross-clamping of the aorta to improve coronary perfusion, and internal defibrillation when indicated); and to control hemorrhage from the heart, pulmonary vessels, thoracic wall, and great vessels. From an organizational standpoint, each institution should have guidelines for the initiation of resuscitative thoracotomy and subsequent patient care in the ED. Ideally, an institutional plan of chest wound management after the EDT should be established with the service that will provide surgical backup when members of the surgical team cannot be on site at the time of the resuscitation. Debate regarding who should perform an EDT is not necessary. It stands to reason that whoever performs this resuscitative procedure must be credentialed for the technical and critical care aspects of patient management.

INDICATIONS AND CONTRAINDICATIONS

Chest Injuries (General)

The first successful thoracotomy was reported more than 100 years ago in a patient dying from a stab wound to the heart. Beall and coworkers[4] described using EDT ro resuscitate patients with penetrating chest injuries in 1966. The indications for EDT gradually expanded to include extrathoracic as well as blunt trauma. Survival rates vary greatly, reportedly 0% to 33%.[5] Currently, it is important to make a decision to perform EDT quickly based upon an understanding of which patients are likely to benefit from the procedure. The decision must be based on a realistic judgment that the patient has a reasonable chance of survival but cannot tolerate a delay in operative intervention.

The first decision point in determining which patients may benefit from an EDT is made in the out-of-hospital setting with the emergency medical service's (EMS) initial contact with the patient.[5] EMS providers help formulate a decision whether or not to perform an EDT, including the mechanism of injury, the site of injury, the time of injury, the time of EMS arrival, and when vital signs or cardiac electrical activity ceased. In one prehospital study of patients with penetrating chest trauma who received EDT, no patients survived to transfer out of the ED when prehospital transport times exceeded 30 minutes, whereas 63% of patients were alive in the ED when prehospital transport times were less than 30 minutes. All patients, however, subsequently died.[6]

The type of cardiac electrical activity is also helpful in determining who may benefit from EDT. Battistella and colleagues[7] reviewed 604 patients undergoing cardiopulmonary resuscitation for traumatic cardiopulmonary arrest and found that of the 204 patients in asystole, none survived. Fulton and associates[8] found that of patients in traumatic arrest, survival was improved when the patients were in ventricular fibrillation, ventricular tachycardia, or pulseless electrical activity (PEA) rather than in asystole or an idioventricular rhythm. In traumatic arrest, asystole, idioventricular rhythm, or severe bradycardia are indicative of poor outcomes or an unsalvageable patient.[1]

The mechanism of injury is of utmost importance when considering performing an EDT. Lack of an organized rhythm in an apneic, pulseless, blunt trauma victim in the field may be considered an absolute contraindication to EDT.[1] Such patients simply do not survive, regardless of the intervention. In the largest EDT series to date, Branney and coworkers[5] reviewed 868 charts of 950 consecutive patients over 23 years; no blunt trauma patient survived EDT when there were no vital signs in the field. However, 2.5% of blunt trauma patients survived EDT when vital signs were present in the field. Rhee and colleagues[9] examined 4620 cases of EDT from 24 studies over a 25-year period. The overall survival rate for blunt trauma was only 1.4%. Practice management guidelines for EDT developed by the American College of Surgeons Committee on Trauma conclude that EDT for blunt trauma patients sustaining traumatic cardiopulmonary arrest should rarely be performed.[10]

Penetrating trauma outcomes in the face of traumatic cardiopulmonary arrest are more difficult to predict. A review of 959 patients over a 26-year period of time showed that 42% (26 of 62 survivors) required prehospital cardiopulmonary resuscitation (CPR).[11] The duration of CPR ranged from 3 to 15 minutes. Twenty-two of these patients sustained penetrating trauma and 5 had asystole at the time of EDT. Patients found apneic and pulseless by EMS, but who possessed other signs of life such as pupillary response, spontaneous movement, or organized electrical activity, should be resuscitated and transported to the ED.[1]

Although survival remains the ultimate gauge of the effectiveness of EDT, it is appropriate to consider the quality of survival, specifically neurologic function. It is somewhat surprising that in general, survivors of EDT have good neurologic outcomes. Rhee and colleagues[9] reported that 280 of 303 (92.4%) patients discharged after EDT were neurologically intact. It is probably not possible to predict accurately which patients are likely to survive intact, but the Denver study[5] demonstrated that all survivors with full neurologic recovery had respiratory efforts at the scene; in 75% of these patients, respiratory efforts were still present on arrival in the ED. The presence or absence of a palpable pulse was not an absolute prognostic indicator. Sixty-six percent of long-term survivors (11 patients with penetrating trauma and 1 with blunt trauma) had no detectable pulse on arrival in the ED.[11] The first 24 hours after EDT rapidly demonstrate which patients will become long-term survivors. The San Francisco experience with 168 emergency thoracotomies for mixed trauma illustrated that most patients with fatal injuries died within 24 hours.[12] Of patients surviving the first 24 hours, 80% (33 of 41) recovered and left the hospital. Full neurologic recovery occurred for 90% of these survivors. Overall, only 2.4% (4 of 168) remained severely disabled or in a persistent vegetative state. Of these 4 patients, only 1 (0.6%) lived beyond 2 months.

Cardiac Injuries—Penetrating

Sixty to 80% of cardiac stab wounds result in pericardial effusion regardless of the presence of shock.[13] Tamponade can occur if the wound is less than 1 cm in size (depending on which chamber is involved), whereas wounds greater than 1 cm usually continue to bleed regardless of the chamber involved. Low-pressure atrial wounds usually form a thrombus before tamponade develops. The thicker-walled left ventricle may spontaneously seal stab wounds up to 1 cm in length. As little as 60 to 100 mL of blood that acutely fills the pericardium will impede diastolic filling, reduce stroke volume, reduce cardiac output, and increase catecholamine release.

The progression from compensated cardiac function to uncompensated tamponade can be sudden and profound. Although one may suspect tamponade based on well-described signs, the clinical diagnosis of pericardial tamponade in the unstable trauma patient is difficult because of the combined effect of hemorrhagic and cardiogenic shock. The classic signs of Beck's triad (distended neck veins, hypotension, and muffled heart sounds) have limited diagnostic value for acute penetrating cardiac trauma.[14] The most reliable signs of tamponade are elevated central venous pressure (CVP), hypotension, and tachycardia.

Ultrasound can identify pericardial effusion and/or tamponade. Classic ultrasound findings for tamponade include the presence of pericardial fluid with right atrial or right ventricular collapse during diastole. The focused assessment with sonography for trauma (FAST) examination is a rapid bedside screening examination to detect hemopericardium and hemoperitoneum. Rozycki and associates[15] reported a sensitivity of 100% and a specificity of 97.3% for pericardial fluid using the FAST examination (Fig. 18–1).

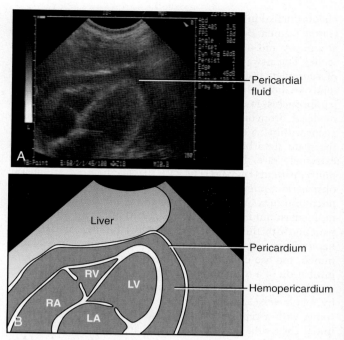

Figure 18–1 *A,* Bedside ultrasound demonstrates hemopericardium. *B,* Artist's drawing of the chambers of the heart, the pericardium and the hemopericardium as seen on the ultrasound.

Survival after EDT for penetrating cardiac wounds is also related to the mechanism of penetration. Patients with stab wounds fare better than patients with gunshot wounds. Rhee and colleagues[9] noted that 16.8% of patients with stab wounds survived to hospital discharge after EDT. Branney and coworkers[5] reported a 29% survival rate in stab wound patients with tamponade, and a 15% survival rate in those without tamponade.

Gunshot wounds, conversely, are often large injuries and unable to seal themselves; only 20% present with tamponade. Penetrating cardiac injuries from gunshot wounds are more likely to present with profound hemodynamic compromise. In addition, the increasing popularity of larger-caliber weapons has made it more difficult to resuscitate patients with gunshot wounds to the chest. Of the 112 patients with gunshot wounds to the heart in the Denver study,[5] only 2% survived neurologically intact.

Cardiac Injuries—Blunt

Blunt trauma to the heart can range from minor contusion to cardiac rupture. The most common cause of death in nonpenetrating cardiac injuries is myocardial rupture, and approximately 25% of these patients rupture the ascending aorta simultaneously.[13] Branney and coworkers[5] observed a 2% survival rate for blunt trauma patients resuscitated with EDT. Those who survived had vital signs in the field. The poor outcomes associated with this type of injury are a result of poor cardiac function caused by the myocardial contusion, even if the hemorrhage has been treated.

Pulmonary Injuries

Pulmonary injuries can be divided into three types: parenchymal, tracheobronchial, and large vessel. Parenchymal and tracheobronchial injuries rarely require EDT, being either rapidly fatal or treated initially by tube thoracostomy. Tracheobronchial injury is more common in blunt than in penetrating trauma. Bertelson and Howitz[16] reviewed 1128 patients at autopsy and only 3 had this injury, with 81% dead at the scene. The airway is usually maintained, even in the presence of a complete transection. The stiff tracheobronchial cartilage tends to hold the lumen open while the paratracheal and parabronchial fasciae preserve the relationship of the proximal to distal bronchi. Ninety percent of tracheobronchial tears occur within 2.5 cm of the carina and most commonly involve the main stem bronchi. Complete division of the trachea is extremely rare. Depending on the size and location of the injury, patients may present with massive hemoptysis, airway obstruction, pneumomediastinum, pneumothorax, or tension pneumothorax. Massive subcutaneous emphysema and pneumomediastinum are usually seen, although up to 10% of patients with this injury have no x-ray findings initially.[17] If hemorrhage is profuse, or if the site of the injury can be determined, the use of a bifid endotracheal tube or the unilateral intubation of a main stem bronchus will secure the airway.

Lacerations of the parenchyma that are not accompanied by major vessel injury generally respond to tube thoracostomy, with a reported success rate of 72% to 98%[18] If the initial chest tube drainage is more than 1500 mL,[19] or if there is persistent hypotension, immediate thoracotomy should be considered. For pulmonary injuries, survival after EDT is also related to the mechanism of injury. Branney and coworkers[5] reported 17% survival after stab wounds, 3% after gunshot wounds, and 5% after blunt trauma.

Air Embolism

Presentation

Air embolism is a complication of pulmonary parenchymal injuries and requires immediate thoracotomy if there is hemodynamic instability. The occurrence of air embolism after penetrating injuries of the lung was formerly considered a rare event.[20] The preoperative and postmortem diagnosis of air embolism is difficult, and it is likely that most air emboli are not detected. Air embolism is confirmed at thoracotomy by needle aspiration of a foamy air-blood admixture from the left or right ventricle or by visualization of air within the coronary arteries.

Air embolism may appear in either the right or the left side of the circulatory system. Involvement of the right side of the circulation is referred to as *venous* or *pulmonary* air embolism. Generally, venous air is well tolerated, but death can occur when the volume of air reaches 5 to 8 mL/kg. The rate at which air moves into the circulation and the body's position are important determinants of the volume that can be tolerated. Death usually results from obstruction of the right ventricle or the pulmonary outflow tract. Injuries of the vena cava or the right ventricle can also create portals of entry into the right circulatory system.

Air embolism involving the left side of the circulatory system is referred to as *arterial* or *systemic* air embolism. The lethal volume depends on the organs to which it is distributed. As little as 0.5 mL of air in the left anterior descending coronary artery has led to ventricular fibrillation. Two milliliters of air injected into the cerebral circulation can be fatal. The distribution of arterial air is partly a function of body position. The formation of traumatic bronchovenous fistulas creates potential entry points for air to move into the left side of the circulatory system. The only requirement is the formation of an air-blood gradient conducive to the inward movement of air. Although a lowered intravascular pressure from hemorrhage is a risk factor, the most important element in all reports of air embolism has been the use of positive-pressure ventilation.[21]

In a review of 447 cases of major thoracic trauma, Yee and coworkers[22] found adequate chart data to suggest the diagnosis of air embolism in 61 patients. About 25% of patients with air embolism have blunt trauma with associated lung injury secondary to multiple rib fractures or hilar disruption. The overall mortality is over 50%.

The diagnosis of air embolism is easily overlooked because of the similarity of the signs and symptoms to those of hypovolemic shock. Two valuable signs that were present in 36% of patients were hemoptysis and the occurrence of cardiac arrest *after intubation and ventilation*. The development of focal neurologic change, seizure, or central nervous system dysfunction in the absence of head injury is also suggestive of the diagnosis.

Management

In those at risk for air embolism, spontaneous ventilation is preferred. It is essential to rapidly control the source of the air embolism. Place the patient immediately in the Trendelenburg (head-down) position to minimize cerebral involvement and direct the air emboli to less critical organs. If the chest injury is unilateral, consider isolating the injured lung by selectively intubating the contralateral lung. If this is unsuccessful, perform a left anterolateral thoracotomy. *Flood the exposed thorax with sterile saline* and look for bloody froth created during positive-pressure ventilation in order to identify peripheral bronchovenous fistulas. Carry out a quick search for hilar injuries. If the source of the air embolism is not readily apparent, perform a contralateral thoracotomy. Once the bronchovenous communication is controlled, use a needle to aspirate residual air that commonly remains in the left ventricle and the aorta. If the patient is hypotensive, consider cross-clamping the aorta. Be aware, though, that cross-clamping the aorta before controlling bronchovenous fistulas and removing residual air may result in further dissemination of air to the heart and the brain.

Adjunctive Therapy

As mentioned, air emboli traverse capillary beds if the blood pressure is high enough. After controlling the bronchovenous fistula, produce a brief period of proximal aortic hypertension by cross-clamping the descending aorta. Maintain systemic arterial pressure with adequate fluid resuscitation. Vasopressors such as dopamine, epinephrine, or norepinephrine may be required to increase systemic pressure and facilitate the passage of air bubbles from left to right.[23]

Maintain left atrial pressure at a high level. Keep the ventilator inspiratory pressures as low as possible, and use 100% oxygen to facilitate diffusion of nitrogen from emboli. Consider high-frequency ventilation, which allows for small volumes and has been used successfully in individual patients. The most important adjunctive therapy is hyperbaric oxygen. Although it is best to begin treatment within 6 hours of traumatic insult, there are cases of success and improvement when hyperbaric oxygen has been started even 36 hours after injury.[24]

Major Vascular Injuries

Unfortunately, patients with major vessel injuries generally have a dismal prognosis and rarely survive.[10]

Blunt and Penetrating Abdominal Injury

In the setting of penetrating abdominal injury, thoracotomy with cross-clamping of the thoracic aorta has been advocated as a means to control hemorrhage from the injury, theoretically to redistribute blood flow to the brain and heart and reduce blood loss below the diaphragm. Unfortunately, aortic cross-clamping can also have detrimental effects. Kralovich and colleagues[25] studied the hemodynamic consequences of aortic occlusion in a swine model of hemorrhagic arrest. There was no difference between groups in the return of spontaneous circulation; however, the occluded aorta group experienced statistically greater impairments in left ventricular function and systemic oxygen utilization in the postresuscitation period. Branney and coworkers[5] found that 8 of 76 (10%) patients undergoing EDT for *penetrating abdominal injury* survived neurologically intact, and in general, these patients had a low survival rate. Practice management guidelines[10] suggest that EDT be performed judiciously in this group as an adjunct to definitive repair of the abdominal injury.

Open Chest Resuscitation for Nontraumatic Arrest

At present, less than 10% of CPR attempts conducted outside of hospital special care units result in survival. The first case of a human survivor of open chest CPR was reported in 1901. In 1960, Kouwenhoven published favorable survival rates using closed chest CPR in humans. After further refinement by Pearson and Redding, closed chest CPR gradually became the preferred method.

The goal of CPR is to restore coronary perfusion pressure (CPP), which is the prime determinant for return of spontaneous circulation as established in animal models. Paradis and associates[26] found that humans need a minimal CPP of 15 mm Hg to achieve a return of spontaneous circulation. Although a CPP of 15 mm Hg does not guarantee the return of spontaneous circulation, there is 100% failure of resuscitation if this CPP is not attained. Although there are a limited number of human studies on open chest CPR, the hemodynamic superiority compared to closed-chest CPR is compelling. Del Guercio and coworkers[27] measured cardiac output during both closed and open chest CPR on in-hospital cardiac arrest patients. Open chest CPR produced a mean cardiac index of 1.31 L/min per m² compared with 0.6 L/min per m² during closed chest CPR. Boczar and colleagues[28] further examined 10 patients unresponsive to closed chest CPR and measured CPP during closed-chest CPR followed by open chest CPR. The mean CPP in the closed chest group was 7.3 mm Hg versus 32.6 mm Hg in the open chest group. All patients obtained a CPP of at least 20 mm Hg at some time during their open chest CPR phase. This easily surpassed the minimal CPP required for return of spontaneous circulation.

In the setting of cardiac arrest from hypothermia, consider using open chest CPR. Cardiopulmonary or veno-veno bypass is the most rapid method of core rewarming, but is rarely immediately available. Open thoracotomy with mediastinal irrigation has been used successfully in cases of severe hypothermia with cardiac arrest. In published case reports of open chest resuscitation with direct cardiac rewarming, the patients who survived neurologically intact had 30 to 180 minutes of internal massage.[29] This provides evidence that open chest CPR can provide prolonged hemodynamic support. It should be noted that similar case reports also exist in which closed chest CPR was maintained for prolonged periods of time resulting in successful hypothermic resuscitation.[30] The rate of core rewarming can be as fast as 8°C/hr with this technique, preferentially rewarming the heart and lungs first. Heat sterile saline in a microwave oven to 40°C and then pour it slowly over the heart and into the thorax. Performing a thoracotomy for hypothermic arrest does not preclude the subsequent use of cardiac bypass.

At present, the precise indications for open chest resuscitation of nontraumatic arrest are not defined, and the procedure is not considered the standard of care. In the setting of normothermic cardiac arrest, open chest CPR may be considered. In spite of demonstrated hemodynamic superiority in both animal and human models of open chest versus closed chest CPR, outcome benefit is lacking. There are a paucity of human data evaluating the window of time during which this treatment can be effective. Consider open chest CPR in a subgroup of patients with witnessed in-hospital cardiac arrest who are without significant underlying comorbidities, who have mechanical lesions, or those for whom standard CPR may be ineffective. The prehospital cardiac arrest patient who remains without a perfusing rhythm after the initial defibrillation has a poor prognosis with conventional treatment. Whether open chest CPR has a role in the management of these patients is not established.

EQUIPMENT

Carefully select the instruments to be included in the EDT equipment tray. Including too many instruments makes the tray cumbersome and delays the procedure. Keep other nonessential instruments nearby in the resuscitation room in case they are needed for specific repair (e.g., Foley catheter tamponade of stellate cardiac wounds). The following items are essential for the thoracotomy tray:

- Scalpel with a No. 20 blade
- Mayo scissors (or long Metzenbaum scissors)
- Rib spreaders
- Gigli saw or large trauma shears
- 2 tissue forceps (10 in.)
- 2 Satinsky vascular clamps
- Large and short needle holders
- 3-0 or larger silk sutures on large-curve needle
- Teflon patches
- Suture scissors
- Aortic tamponade instrument
- Skin stapler (6-mm staples)

The following items are optional for the tray and can be supplied as needed by an assistant:

- 6 towel clips
- 4 to 6 hemostats (curved and straight)
- Metzenbaum scissors
- Right-angled clamp
- Foley catheter (20-Fr, 30-mL balloon)—sterile saline/syringe
- Chest tube (No. 30, Argyle)
- 12 lap sponges or gauze pads
- 6 towels

In addition, assemble wall suction, sterile suction tubing and tips, antiseptic solution, sterile gloves, a defibrillator with

bleeding. Then, actual reparative sutures can be accurately placed. It must be stressed that suturing the myocardium requires good technique. Excessive tension may tear the myocardium and aggravate the situation. Keys to success include using an appropriate-sized suture, getting a generous "bite" with the needle, and applying only enough tension to control the bleeding.

If exsanguinating hemorrhage is not controlled by the aforementioned methods, temporarily occlude inflow to the heart. Apply inflow occlusion intermittently for 60 to 90 seconds. During occlusion, the heart shrinks, hemorrhage is controlled, and you can place sutures in a decompressed injury. Two techniques that are useful are vascular clamping of the superior and inferior vena cava for partial inflow occlusion[40] and the Sauerbruch grip (Fig. 18–9) for occlusion of the vena cava between the ring and the middle finger of the left hand for partial inflow occlusion.[41] The Sauerbruch grip can be performed quickly with the added advantage of cradling and stabilizing the heart while you repair the wounds over either the ventricle or the left atrium. The Sauerbruch grip will interfere only with the repair of wounds involving the right atrium.

Another technique for temporarily controlling hemorrhage is to insert a Foley catheter (20 Fr with a 30-mL balloon) through a wound.[42] After inserting the catheter, inflate the balloon, clamp the catheter to prevent air embolism, and *apply gentle traction* (Fig. 18–10). Apply enough traction to slow the bleeding and provide an acceptable level to visualize and repair the wound. Excessive traction can pull the catheter out and enlarge the wound. The balloon will effectively occlude the wound internally. A pursestring suture is commonly used. When repairing the wound, be careful with the suture needle because it can easily rupture the balloon. Temporarily pushing the balloon into the ventricular lumen during needle passage is also important to prevent rupture. Use normal saline when inflating the balloon. Using air could result in air embolism if the suture needle ruptures the balloon.

Foley catheters have several advantages over other methods for controlling cardiac wounds. With the digital method, your fingertip will often slip if there is a strong heartbeat, you cannot visualize the wound during repair, and digital pressure significantly interferes with cardiac massage. Intermittent total venous inflow occlusion is an effective

method of controlling bleeding and decompressing the heart, but such control will be at the expense of a poor cardiac output. Attempt to elevate the heart for control and repair of posterior cardiac wounds often results in cardiac arrest by reduction of both venous and arterial flow. With posterior injuries, using a Foley catheter does not require continued viewing after initial placement. If bleeding can be controlled, repairs in this location should await full-volume expansion or cardiopulmonary bypass.[43] Regardless of location, the most valuable feature of the Foley catheter is that you can control hmorrhage without interfering with cardiac compression. Also, the catheter can be used for fluid infusion (see Fig. 18–10B).[44]

To initially manage wounds of the atria, use partial-occlusion clamps (Fig. 18–11). Because of the thin structure and instability of the atrial wall, you will not be able to effectively stop bleeding with digital pressure. Injuries near the caval-atrial junction are not amenable to clamping; in this location, use a Foley catheter to tamponade the wound.[42] Be careful not to obstruct atrial filling with the inflated balloon. Skin staples may also be used for closure of atrial wounds.[37]

Wounds of the septa, valves, and coronary arteries require definitive repair in the operating suite. Hemorrhage from a coronary artery can generally be controlled with digital pressure. Avoid ligation of a coronary artery whenever possible.

Control of Hemorrhagic Great Vessel Wounds

Wounds of the great vessels can be controlled with digital pressure or partial-occlusion clamps. If desired, close small aortic wounds with 3-0 silk sutures. To prevent exsanguinating hemorrhage from the left subclavian artery, try to cross-clamp the intrathoracic portion of the artery. Cross-clamping of the right subclavian artery is very difficult. For injuries of this vessel, use laparotomy pads to compress in the apex of the pleura from below and the supraclavicular fossa from above (Fig. 18–12) to prevent further bleeding as the patient is stabilized and moved to the operating suite.[36]

Aortic Cross-Clamping

For persistant hypotension (systolic blood pressure <70 mm Hg) after thoracotomy and pericardiotomy, perform temporary occlusion of the descending thoracic aorta. This maneuver can maintain myocardial and cerebral perfusion (Fig. 18–13), although Kravolich and colleagues[25] suggest that the benefit of significant improvement in CPP may be overstated. When the aorta has been injured by blunt trauma, selective clamping is necessary (Fig. 18–14). Aortic occlusion has a limited role in controlling hemorrhage below the diaphragm. When there is a tense abdomen with massive hemoperitoneum, aortic cross-clamping is clearly beneficial when applied just before laparotomy.

The aorta can be very difficult to identify in an ED, especially when collapsed from exsanguination. It lies immediately anterior to the vertebrae, actually lying on the vertebral bodies themselves. The esophagus lies anterior and slightly medial to the aorta. To expose the descending aorta, ask an assistant to retract the left lung in a superomedial direction. To achieve adequate exposure, it is sometimes necessary to divide the inferior pulmonary ligament. Identify the aorta by advancing the fingers of the left hand along the thoracic cage toward the vertebral column. Open the pleura and bluntly dissect the aorta away from the esophagus prior to clamping. To locate

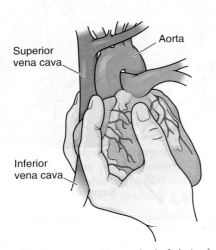

Figure 18–9 Sauerbruch maneuver. The method of choice for reducing heavy bleeding from cardiac wounds. Venous inflow occlusion is achieved by using the first and second or second and third fingers as a clamp.

In the figure labels: Superior vena cava, Aorta, Inferior vena cava

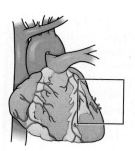

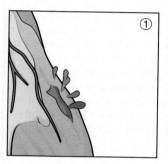 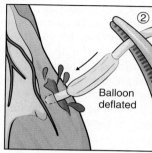 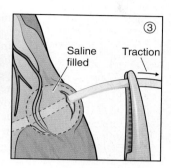

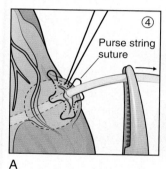 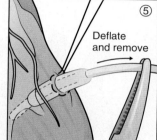 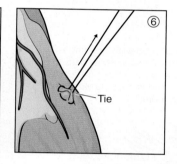

A

321

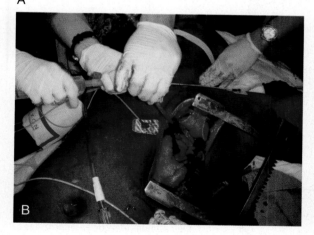

B

Figure 18–10 *A,* Serial illustration. Gentle traction on an inflated Foley catheter may control hemorrhage and allow repair. Inflate the balloon with saline, and take care not to rupture the balloon with the suture needle. This technique is particularly useful with injuries of the inferior cavoatrial junction, with posterior wounds, and during cardiac massage. Volume loading can be obtained by infusion of blood or crystalloid solutions through the lumen of the catheter. Take care to avoid an air embolus through the lumen of the catheter during placement. *B,* A Foley catheter in an atrial stab wound. Keep gentle traction on an inflated balloon and *inject saline directly into the heart via the catheter. Note how difficult it is to identify structures in the chest cavity.* The heart is collapsed and not beating, making even this organ hard to find. The aorta could not be isolated prior to stopping resuscitation efforts.

Figure 18–11 Use a partial occluding clamp in different locations for control of bleeding and subsequent repair.

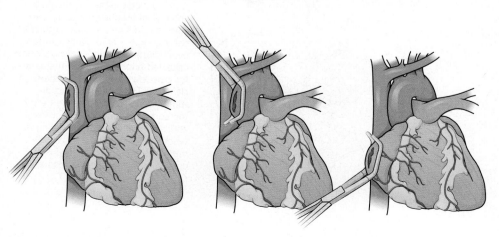

the aorta, use a DeBakey aortic clamp or a curved Kelly clamp for blunt dissection and spread open the pleura above and below the aorta (Fig. 18–15). Alternatively, if excessive hemmorhage limits direct visualization, bluntly dissect with thumb and fingertips. Separate the aorta from the esophagus, which lies medially and slightly anteriorly. It may be difficult to separate the esophagus from the aorta by feel in a hypotensive or a cardiac arrest situation. Passing a nasogastric tube from above may help to identify the esophagus. When the aorta is completely isolated, use the index finger of the left hand to flex around the vessel and apply a vascular clamp with the right hand. Check the brachial blood pressure immediately after the occlusion. If the systolic pressure is more than 120 mm Hg, slowly release the clamp and adjust it to maintain a systolic pressure of less than 120 mm Hg.[45]

Given the need for speedy intervention, the simplest and most desirable approach to aortic occlusion is to have an assistant digitally compress it or use the aortic tamponade instrument (Fig. 18–16). The aortic tamponade instrument, however, may be applied blindly to the vertebral column, permitting safe, quick, and complete aortic occlusion.[46] This technique may be most prudent when isolation of the aorta is difficult. The instrument's unique shape allows it to remain in place and to provide atraumatic occlusion with little interference in the operative field compared with digital compres-

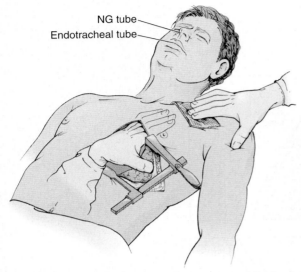

Figure 18–12 Cross-clamping for control of subclavian bleeding is difficult and time consuming. Compression with laparotomy pads in the apical pleura from below and the supraclavicular fossa from above will control hemorrhage while the patient's condition is stabilized and the patient is transported to the operating room.

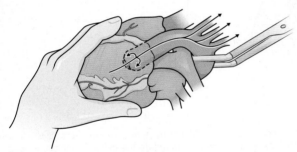

Figure 18–13 Manual cardiac massage and cross-clamping of the aorta to increase coronary and cerebral perfusion selectively.

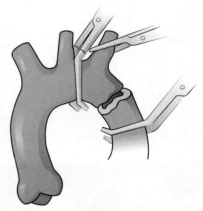

Figure 18–14 Traumatic rupture of the aorta is *usually a fatal injury*. Three clamps are required for control. Backbleeding will occur if fewer than three clamps are used.

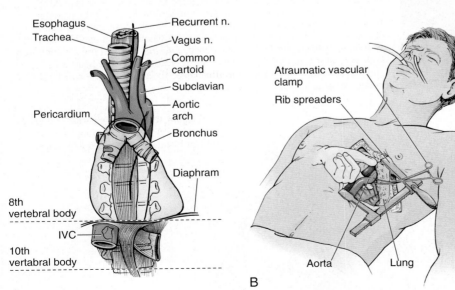

Esophagus
Trachea
Recurrent n.
Vagus n.
Common cartoid
Subclavian
Aortic arch
Pericardium
Bronchus
Diaphram
8th vertebral body
IVC
10th vertabral body

Atraumatic vascular clamp
Rib spreaders

Aorta   Lung

A   B

Figure 18–15 *A, Identification of the aorta is very difficult during emergency department thoracotomy.* If possible, first pass a nasogastric tube to help identify the esophagus. The aorta is in the posterior mediastinum, directly anterior to the vertebral bodies. The esophagus is anterior and slightly medial to the aorta. In the lower thorax, both are covered on the anterolateral surface by mediastinal pleura, which must be dissected prior to isolating the aorta for cross-clamping. *B,* Aortic cross-clamping: Using blunt dissection, spread the pleura above and below the aorta. Fully mobilize the vessel and clearly separate the esophagus before clamping. The aorta is the more posterior structure and is in contact with the vertebral bodies.

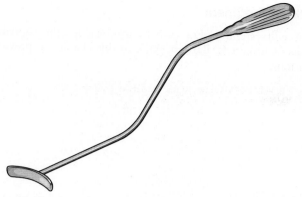

Figure 18–16 The use of a Conn aortic compressor is the method of choice for aortic occlusion because it is fast, does not interfere with the operative field, and is associated with minimal risk of injury. Alternatively, the more awkward technique of direct digital occlusion can be used. *(Courtesy of Pilling Company, Ft. Washington, PA.)*

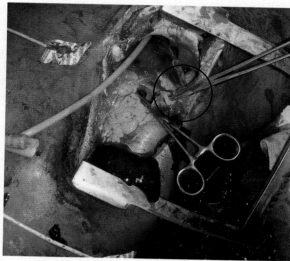

Figure 18–17 Note the sharp edges of this rib (indicated by circled clamp) fractured during an unsuccessful emergency department thoracotomy. The incidence of blood-borne diseases (e.g., human immunodeficiency virus, hepatitis) in such patients is high.

sion. The degree of occlusion can be varied by the amount of pressure exerted by the operator.

Potential complications of aortic cross-clamping include ischemia of the spinal cord, liver, bowel, and kidneys. In addition, iatrogenic injury of the aorta and the esophagus may occur. Fortunately, these complications are infrequent. The metabolic penalty of aortic cross-clamping becomes exponential when occlusion time exceeds 30 minutes.[47] Whenever possible, unclamp the aorta for 30 to 60 seconds every 10 minutes to increase distal perfusion. Perform the final release of the aorta gradually.

INTERPRETATION AND HEMODYNAMIC MONITORING

After EDT, use the systolic blood pressure after the first 30 minutes of resuscitation as a decision point for further treatment. A report of EDT for blunt and penetrating trauma demonstrates the relationship between blood pressure at 30 minutes and eventual outcome.[48] Of the 146 cases reviewed, 45 patients (31%) were transferred to the operating room after initial resuscitation and aortic cross-clamping when necessary. For those patients who survived with full neurologic recovery, the average systolic blood pressure after the first 30 minutes of resuscitation was 110 mm Hg. In those who were long-term survivors but had significant brain damage, the average systolic blood pressure was 85 mm Hg. No survivals were recorded when the mean systolic blood pressure was less than 70 mm Hg. *Transfer of these patients to the operating room for definitive repair of these mortal wounds would be futile.*

EDT IN CHILDREN

Trauma is the leading cause of death and morbidity in children over the age of 1. Just as in adults, improved transportation of injured children to the hospital has resulted in the arrival of more patients who would have been pronounced dead at the scene. Although the role of EDT has been reviewed extensively in the adult population, there is little experience and there is little data in the pediatric population. Overall survival rates in children undergoing EDT for penetrating thoracic trauma are approximately 11% to 12% and for blunt trauma 1% to 2%.[10] General consensus from the practice management guidelines for EDT use the same parameters for adults.[10]

COMPLICATIONS

A variety of significant complications occur in patients surviving EDT, but most of these are related to the primary injury rather than the thoracotomy. Techniques to avoid iatrogenic complications include noting the position of the left phrenic nerve and coronary arteries during EDT. Surprisingly, serious infection is uncommon. In a combined series of 142 EDTs, there were no reports of wound infections. It should be noted that most patients received antibiotics just before or during the procedure. As a general rule, excessive attention to antiseptic skin preparation should be avoided because it may unnecessarily delay performance of the procedure.[49] Antibiotics should be administered as soon as possible.

Another potentially serious complication of EDT is injury or disease transmission to health care workers. In an emotionally charged environment in which many clinicians are attempting to perform life-saving surgery under the harshest of conditions, it is easy to suffer a needle stick or scalpel or scissor injury. Sharp ribs can cut the clinicians quite easily (Fig. 18–17). Seroprevalence of human immunodeficiency virus (HIV) in U.S. EDs is estimated to range from 2% up to 6% to 9% in urban areas.[50] Tardiff and colleagues[50] noted an HIV-positive rate of 7.2% in their study of trauma patients presenting to their urban ED. Occupational exposure to both hepatitis B and C is of concern to health care workers, as well. Sloan and associates[51] found a 3.1% incidence of hepatitis B in trauma patients brought to their inner-city ED. Hepatitis C is now the most common viral hepatitis seen in health care workers since the advent of the hepatitis B vaccine. Approximately 2200 health care workers per year seroconvert after occupational exposure. One urban ED reported an 18% prevalence of hepatitis C in its ED patients.[52] Clearly, the risk of exposure to staff must be kept in mind, and universal precautions should be rigorously followed. Although EDT must be performed rapidly in order to be of value to the patient, excessive haste is not warranted if it threatens the health of members of the medical team.

Acknowledgment

The editors and author wish to acknowledge the contributions of Robert L. Bartlett, MD, to this chapter in previous editions.

 REFERENCES CAN BE FOUND ON EXPERT CONSULT

VASCULAR TECHNIQUES AND VOLUME SUPPORT

CHAPTER **19**

Pediatric Vascular Access and Blood Sampling Techniques

Marie M. Lozon

The tasks of sampling blood and obtaining vascular access in an infant or child can challenge and frustrate even the most skilled emergency clinician. In some instances, venous access simply cannot be obtained rapidly, making vascular access one of the most challenging clinical procedures performed during resuscitation and treatment of critically ill children. The use of invasive monitoring techniques with arterial and central venous catheters is commonplace in contemporary pediatric emergency and critical care medicine, but simple blood sampling and venous access remains a constant challenge in the emergency department (ED).

This chapter reviews the basic principles and techniques of blood sampling, as well as selection and placement of intravenous (IV) and intra-arterial catheters in infants and children, including those placed in the central circulation. The use of umbilical catheters in newborns is also reviewed. For critically ill and injured children, intraosseous (IO) access is the preferred technique if vascular access cannot be secured rapidly. IO needle placement and infusion techniques are covered in Chapter 25, Intraosseous Infusion. Although rarely required, emergency cutdown is occasionally life saving, and a section of this chapter is devoted to cutdown techniques.

PATIENT PREPARATION AND RESTRAINT

Fear and anticipation of pain associated with procedures or injections make the hospital experience traumatic for children. Before beginning any painful procedure in a child, the procedure itself and the reasons for it should be explained to the parents. In children capable of understanding, the procedure should be explained in developmentally appropriate language before starting and prior to each successive step. The use of deceptive phrases such as "This won't hurt" should be avoided. A gentle, honest explanation that the procedure will hurt a bit and saying "it is okay to cry, but not to move" will provide realistic expectations for the child and set limits as well. Depending on the situation, most parents wish to remain with their child during the procedure.[1] If they remain in the room, their role should be solely to provide comfort to the child and not to assist with any potentially painful procedure. Distracting the child with simple conversation regarding school, friends, hobbies, pets, or TV shows can also decrease the level of the child's anxiety. Despite their seeming composure, the potential for parents to faint at the sight of blood or needles should always be addressed. Parental injury under such circumstances can be a source of litigation.

The success of blood sampling or obtaining vascular access depends on proper positioning and restraint of the patient. In most cases, this requires the assistance of at least one other staff person and restraint of the extremity a joint above and below the intended insertion site. Although most of these procedures can be performed quickly, a significant amount of time may be required to perform venipuncture or vessel cannulation in neonates or young infants, during which time they can become cold from being exposed on the examination table (especially if perfusion is impaired from sepsis or hypovolemic shock). Overhead lights, warm blankets, or other warming modalities are very useful for this age group to prevent accidental hypothermia.

In recent years, products to provide topical anesthesia prior to needle sticks have become available. Parents are often aware of these products and may ask for them to be used for their children. Although theoretically attractive, such measures are often impractical in a critical situation, because these products generally require 30 to 60 minutes for adequate anesthesia. However, in the appropriate clinical setting, spending the additional time to relieve pain and anxiety is warranted. The use of lidocaine-prilocaine (also known as eutectic mixture of local anesthetics [EMLA]), L-M-X cream (ELA-Max), tetracaine base patches, and iontophoresis are reviewed in Chapter 29, Local and Topical Anesthesia.

EDs need not provide topical anesthesia/analgesia to all children requiring venipuncture or IV placement, because in skilled hands, these procedures may be done so swiftly that additional time for application of creams or iontophoresis may actually interfere with the success of the procedure and cause more distress. Each patient must be individualized and the clinician must use his or her judgment as to the best course of action. For some of the more invasive and technically difficult procedures described in this chapter, the use of procedural sedation may help reduce the trauma to the child and make the procedure easier to perform (Chapter 33, Systemic Analgesia and Sedation for Procedures). However, in critically ill or injured children, the use of sedation may not be possible.

BLOOD SAMPLING TECHNIQUES

Capillary Blood Sampling

Indications and Contraindications

Capillary blood sampling, or heel stick puncture, is a frequently used technique to obtain blood samples in young infants. In older children and adults, this technique is often used to obtain blood samples from the finger, toe, or ear lobe when repeated measurements, such as for blood glucose, are needed. Capillary blood sampling is most often indicated in a young infant when an adequate sample of blood can be obtained by the heel stick puncture technique and an alternative technique is not practical. It is also an option for obtaining "arterialized" blood for blood gas analysis when arterial access is unavailable, as in many chronically ill neonates and young infants, or when the clinician is not comfortable obtaining a percutaneous arterial blood sample.

Sampling from an area of local inflammation or hematoma should be avoided. Also, repetitive sampling from the same site may induce inflammation and subsequent scarring and hence should also be avoided. In general, heel stick sampling is not ideal for blood gas analysis (1) when the infant is hypotensive, (2) when the heel is markedly bruised, or (3) when there is evidence of peripheral vasoconstriction. It is also important to remember that capillary blood does not always produce an accurate analysis of arterial oxygen pressure (Pao_2). When the capillary oxygen pressure (Po_2) is greater than 60 mm Hg, the Pao_2 may be considerably higher, possibly putting infants receiving supplemental oxygen at risk. In this situation, the use of either transcutaneous oxygen saturation or a transcutaneous Po_2 monitor may allow adjustment of the inspired oxygen concentration until either a Pao_2 or a repeat capillary Po_2 can be obtained.[2]

Equipment and Setup

The necessary equipment for capillary blood sampling is shown in Table 19–1. A 3-mm lancet (Becton-Dickinson, Rutherford, NJ) or an automated disposable incision device (e.g., Tenderfoot, Surgicutt) should be used to perform this procedure; a scalpel blade should not be used. The use of the former devices will prevent the puncture from penetrating more than the maximum safe distance. Blood collection is performed using either heparinized capillary tubes or 1-mL Microtainer tubes with a collector attachment (Becton-

Dickinson, Rutherford, NJ). If capillary tubes are used, a clay or wax sealer will be needed to close off one end.

Technique

Although capillary blood sampling may be performed by the finger stick or heel stick methods, the latter is described. The recommended sites for heel stick puncture are the most medial and most lateral portions of the plantar surface of the heel (Fig. 19–1), but not on the curve of the heel.[3,4] This avoids penetration of the calcaneus and the risk of osteochondritis. Cautiously prewarming the foot for 5 minutes using a warm towel will produce hyperemia and will enhance blood flow. The foot is immobilized in a dependent position with one hand. After the heel is cleansed with antiseptic solution and allowed to dry, the skin is punctured with the lancet (Fig. 19–2A). Allowing the alcohol to dry will avoid falsely high glucose levels in the specimen. Although it is tempting and commonly done, *squeezing of the foot should be avoided*, because this may inhibit capillary filling and may actually decrease blood flow. Furthermore, squeezing may dilute the sample with serum or tissue fluid and make analysis less accurate. If blood does not flow freely, another puncture may be required.

The first small drop of blood is wiped away with gauze, and another drop is allowed to form. A heparinized capillary tube is placed in the drop of blood, and the proximal end of the inverted tube is allowed to fill by capillary action (see Fig. 19–2C and D). The tube (or tubes, if several tests will be needed) is sealed at one end by sticking it into clay or wax (or sealing with a specially designed cap) before the tube is sent to the laboratory (see Fig. 19–2F and G). Capillary tubes should be filled until blood reaches the demarcation line on the tube. Over- or underfilling of the tube may result in clotting or erroneous test results, or both. If 1-mL Microtainer tubes are used, the tube is held at an angle of 30° to 45° from the surface of the puncture site. The collector end is touched to the drop of blood, and blood is allowed to drain into the tube (see Fig. 19–2B). Gently tapping the tube will facilitate flow to the bottom. Once filled, the Microtainer tube is sealed using the accompanying cap (see Fig. 19–2E). After an adequate specimen is obtained, a dry dressing is applied to the puncture site.

When a heel stick is performed for arterialized blood samples, the technique used is similar to that discussed previously for routine blood sampling, with the following differences: The infant's foot must be wrapped in a warm towel for a few minutes, and the first drop of blood must be discarded while the remaining blood is allowed to flow freely into a heparinized capillary tube. The tip of the tube should be placed as near the puncture site as possible to minimize expo-

---

TABLE 19–1 Equipment for Capillary Blood Sampling

Blood collection tubes (capillary tubes or Microtainers)
Warm wet towel or diaper
Alcohol pads
Lancets or automated disposable incision devices
Clay sealer (used with capillary tubes)
Sterile bandage
Nonsterile examination gloves

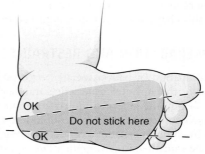

Figure 19–1 Acceptable sites for heel stick puncture (*shaded areas*).

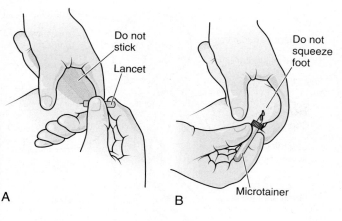

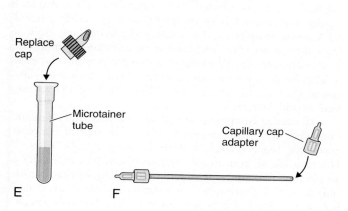

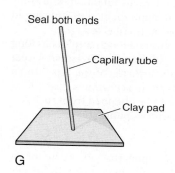

Figure 19–2 *A,* The heel stick is performed on the lateral or medial aspect of the heel. *B,* The collector end of the Microtainer is touched to the drop of blood, and blood is allowed to flow down the wall of the tube to the bottom. *C,* A heparinized capillary tube is placed in the drop of blood, and the proximal end of the inverted tube is allowed to fill by capillary action. *D,* The blood is maintained in the capillary tube using the index finger to maintain capillary tension on the end of the tube. *E,* When using a Microtainer tube, the Microtainer is capped. *F,* When using a capillary tube, the ends are capped or sealed with wax or clay. *G,* Avoid squeezing the foot, and keep the proximal end of the Microtainer below the puncture site.

sure of the blood to environmental oxygen, and the tube should be filled as completely as possible. Collection of air in the tube as well as excessive squeezing of the foot should be avoided, because this may artificially lower the Po_2. When the tube is full, the free end is occluded with the gloved finger to prevent entry of air, and both ends are plugged with clay or capped with adapters (see Fig. 19–2*D, F,* and *G*).

Complications
When properly performed, heel sticks are associated with a low incidence of complications. Lacerations should not occur when the procedure is performed with a proper incision device. Heel sticks may cause infection (local infection, bacteremia, or osteomyelitis), scarring, and calcified nodules.[5–7]

Interpretation
Studies have compared the reliability of capillary blood with that of arterial blood for determination of pH, carbon dioxide pressure (Pco_2), and Po_2.[8–11] Although the results have been variable, most investigations have documented a reasonable

correlation between arterial and capillary samples for pH and Pco_2 determinations (except when the patient is in shock or has an extremely high Pco_2). Unfortunately, the Po_2 determination has not been found to be as reliable when performed on blood obtained by capillary sampling. Most studies indicate that the capillary (heel stick) Po_2 correlates poorly with the Pao_2, especially if the Pao_2 is greater than 60 mm Hg. In nearly all situations, the capillary Po_2 is equal to or less than the Po_2, but in any individual case, one does not know how closely the capillary value approximates the arterial level. Therefore, *reliance solely on a capillary sample of blood for Po_2 measurement in an acutely sick infant is fraught with potential risks.*

Venipuncture

Indications and Contraindications
Although many laboratory tests for the small infant may be performed on blood obtained by heel sticks, larger volumes of blood may be required, making heel sticks impractical.

TABLE 19–2 Equipment for Venous Blood Sampling in Infants and Children

Tourniquet (rubber band for scalp veins and tiny infants)
A 3-, 5-, or 10-mL syringe
A 21- or 23-gauge butterfly needle
Evacuated blood tubes
Alcohol pads
Povidone-iodine swabs (if blood cultures are needed)
Sterile 2- x 2-inch or 4- x 4-inch gauze pads
Nonsterile examination gloves

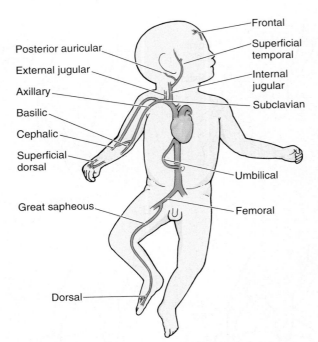

Figure 19–3 Venous access sites in the neonate and young infant. If venous access is unavailable, arterial blood may be used for most laboratory tests, including blood cultures.

Hence, venipuncture is the usual method used for obtaining larger quantities of blood from infants and children.

Venipuncture is also the recommended method to obtain blood for culture. The heel stick capillary tube procedure has been used in some centers for the procurement of blood for cultures,[12] but the technique has a significant incidence of false-positive results. In the newborn infant, blood obtained immediately after sterile insertion of an umbilical arterial or venous catheter may be used for culture; even then, some controversy exists concerning the incidence of false-positive results. If venipuncture is unsuccessful, arterial blood may also be used to obtain blood cultures. When collecting blood intended for culture, the area of venipuncture should be prepared with appropriate antiseptic solutions and allowed to dry. The blood culture collection bottle will likely state a desired volume of sample for optimal results, but 1.0 mL of blood is generally acceptable in a small infant. Iodine solutions and other detergents can irritate infant skin and should be washed off promptly after blood is collected.

Femoral venipuncture for routine blood samples has long been discouraged, especially in children younger than 1 year of age, owing to the risk of septic arthritis of the hip.[13] In an emergency setting or when few venous access sites exist, blood for laboratory analysis may have to be obtained from such less desirable venous sites or from arterial puncture.

Equipment and Setup

The equipment required for venipuncture in an infant or child is listed in Table 19–2. A small-gauge butterfly needle and syringe is usually preferred over a needle and syringe for obtaining blood in infants and young children, because it is easier to control once the vessel has been entered. Suction is also more easily controlled with the butterfly needle and syringe setup. The butterfly needle may also serve as an infusion line once adequate amounts of blood are obtained. The 23-gauge butterfly needle will generally suffice for venipuncture, regardless of age group. In older children and adolescents, a straight needle and syringe or the Vacutainer system (Becton-Dickinson, Rutherford, NJ) can be used much more easily than in infants. However, the negative pressure within the evacuated blood tube may be sufficient to collapse the punctured vein. A 3- or 5-mL syringe is less likely than a 10-mL syringe to cause vein collapse in young infants.

Technique

Like adults, the usual site for venipuncture in infants and children is the antecubital fossa. However, any reasonably accessible or easily visible peripheral vein (e.g., on the hands or feet, or scalp for very small infants) may be used (Fig. 19–3). Veins on the dorsum of the hand can be used, provid-

ing they will not be needed for IV cannulation. The external jugular and femoral veins or arterial sites are rarely needed for routine samples in the stable patient. Imaging devices (e.g., ultrasound, transillumination, or infrared devices) used to identify veins for IV catheter placement may also be used to help locate veins for venipuncture. These devices are discussed later in this chapter (see "Vascular Line Placement: Venous and Arterial").

All needed equipment should be assembled and ready for immediate use. If the situation permits, the use of a topical anesthetic (e.g., EMLA, L-M-X creams) may be offered. Drawing blood from infants and small children is usually a two-person procedure. It should be emphasized that immobilization of the extremity is mandatory and this duty should not be relegated to a family member. The butterfly needle and the syringe can be attached either before or after skin penetration. If done before, the assembly should take place out of sight of the child. To minimize the number of venipuncture attempts, the optimal site for needle insertion should be chosen after a survey of the most prominent peripheral veins. If an extremity vein is to be used, a tourniquet should be applied proximal to the selected vein; in small infants, a rubber band will serve as an adequate tourniquet, but one must be certain to remove the rubber band after venipuncture. The tourniquet should not be so tight as to impede arterial filling.

The area surrounding the chosen site of skin penetration is cleansed with antiseptic solution and allowed to dry. Slight distal traction is applied to the skin to immobilize the vein, and the needle is inserted quickly through the skin and slowly into the vein at an angle of approximately 30°, with the *bevel up* (Fig. 19–4A). Successful vessel penetration is heralded by a flashback, or flow of blood, into the butterfly tubing. *Gentle suction* is applied by slowly withdrawing the plunger of the syringe. If the required amount of blood is more than the capacity of the attached syringe, the tubing is pinched off,

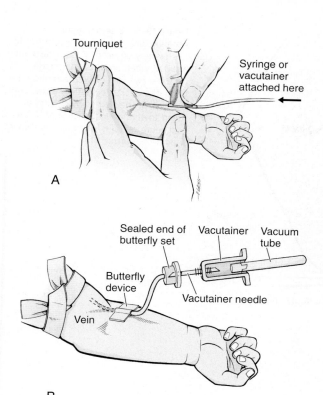

Figure 19–4 *A,* Technique for obtaining blood by antecubital venipuncture with a butterfly needle and a syringe. Once blood is obtained, the butterfly needle may serve as an infusion site. Note that this procedure often requires two persons to carry it out—one to hold the arm and insert the needle and the other to aspirate the blood. *B,* As an alternative to a syringe, a Vacutainer system may be used to apply suction. The Vacutainer needle punctures the sealed end of the butterfly set. Use of this method helps to prevent the premature clotting of blood that may occur if there is a delay in filling the collection tubes.

the filled syringe is removed, a new syringe is attached, and gentle suction is once again applied after release of the pinched tubing. After the required amount of blood is withdrawn, the needle is removed, and a sterile dressing and direct pressure are applied to the puncture site.

Suction may be applied with a Vacutainer system in which the Vacutainer needle punctures the sealed end of the butterfly device (see Fig. 19–4*B*). There are also butterfly systems available that have a second needle, occluded by a rubber shield, located at the opposite end of the butterfly tubing. Once the vein has been entered, the needle at the opposite end of the butterfly tubing is pushed through the top of a vacuum-sealed tube. In either case, if the suction is excessive, the vein will collapse and blood flow will stop.

Although peripheral sites for venous or arterial sampling are preferable, the external jugular and femoral veins may be used in infants for venipuncture during resuscitations or when peripheral sites are inadequate. The external jugular vein lies in a line from the angle of the jaw to the middle of the clavicle and is usually visible on the surface of the skin. The vein is more prominent when the infant is crying. An assistant is needed to restrain the infant in a supine position with the head and neck extended over the edge of the bed. Alternatively, a towel roll or pillow placed under the shoulders can be used. The head is turned approximately 40° to 70° from the midline (Fig. 19–5), and the skin surrounding the area to be punctured

is cleansed with alcohol or other antiseptic solution. Finger pressure just above the clavicle will help distend the jugular vein. Using a 21- to 25-gauge straight needle with a syringe or a 21- to 25-gauge butterfly needle attached to a syringe, the clinician punctures the skin and advances the needle slowly until the jugular vein is entered. The syringe is connected to the needle at all times to maintain constant negative pressure and avoid an air embolism. After the appropriate amount of blood is obtained, the needle is withdrawn and slight pressure is applied to the vessel. The infant should be placed in an upright position after the needle is removed, and slight pressure should be continued for 3 to 5 minutes. Close observation of the puncture site should follow. Use of the external jugular vein for routine venipuncture is not recommended; it should be used only when other sites prove unsuccessful or are unavailable.

The femoral vein lies medial (in most patients) to the femoral artery and inferior to the inguinal ligament (Fig. 19–6*A*). The use of femoral vessels for blood sampling is reserved for situations in which patients present in extremis and no other sampling sites are available. An assistant positions the hips in mild abduction and extension while the artery is palpated and its location identified by placing a mark on the skin just superior to the femoral triangle (see Fig. 19–6*A*). If available, ultrasound may be helpful in assessing the position of the femoral vessels. The femoral triangle is then prepared with alcohol or other antiseptic agent; a povidone-iodine or chlorhexidine scrub is also recommended when obtaining blood cultures. The technique of needle insertion is similar to that for external jugular venipuncture (see Fig. 19–5). The clinician punctures the skin and then directs the needle or catheter toward the umbilicus at a 30° to 45° angle to the skin, remaining just medial to the femoral artery pulsation (see Fig. 19–6*B*). A slight constant negative pressure is applied throughout insertion. After the needle enters the femoral vein, the desired blood samples are withdrawn, and the needle or catheter is removed (unless venous access with an IV catheter is desired). Pressure is applied to the femoral triangle for a minimum of 5 minutes, and the site is observed closely for recurrent bleeding.

Scalp veins can be very useful for venous sampling in small infants (<3 mo) when other options are not readily available.[14] The anatomic considerations and technique are discussed later (see "Peripheral Venous Catheterization: Percutaneous" and "Peripheral Venous Catheterization: Venous Cutdown"). Care should be taken with venipuncture and cannulation of scalp veins near the face, because an infiltration could have negative cosmetic consequences. Although sampling or cannulating scalp vessels may be medically necessary, parents of tiny infants are often very upset by the sight of their child's head being poked, and every effort should be made to explain the rationale for the procedure.

Complications

Complications of venipuncture include hematoma formation, local infection, injury to structures adjacent to vessels, and phlebitis. All of these complications are uncommon. Special care should be used when puncture of the external jugular vein or femoral vein is attempted. Inadvertent deep puncture in the neck can produce injury to the carotid artery, the vagus or phrenic nerves, or the apex of the lung. In the femoral triangle, injury to the femoral artery, femoral nerve, or hip capsule may occur.[13,15] However, such structures are unlikely to be injured when proper technique is used.

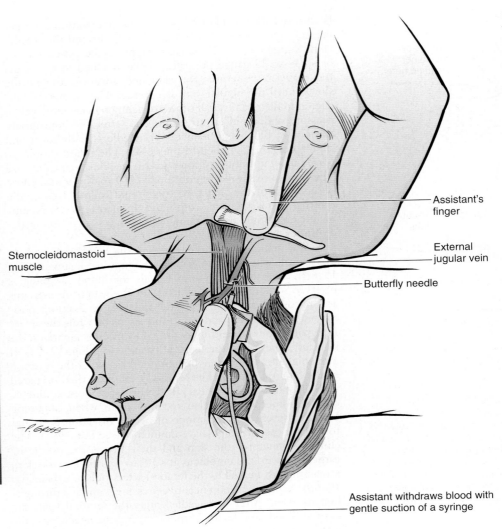

Figure 19–5 **External jugular venipuncture.** A syringe or a butterfly needle may be used. Venous distention is aided when an assistant's finger occludes the vein or when the infant cries. The neck is extended, either over the side of the bed or by placing a rolled towel under the shoulders. This procedure requires two persons. Gloves should be worn.

Assistant's finger

External jugular vein

Sternocleidomastoid muscle

Butterfly needle

Assistant withdraws blood with gentle suction of a syringe

Arterial Blood Sampling

Indications and Contraindications

Arterial blood gas evaluation provides useful information that is essentially unavailable by other means and is important for evaluation of respiratory status and acid-base equilibrium in infants or children with respiratory distress, shock, intoxication, diabetic ketoacidosis, or other metabolic derangements. Venous blood may be acceptable for tests previously performed on arterial blood, such as pH (see Chapter 20, Arterial Puncture and Cannulation). Arterial blood may also be used for routine laboratory analysis if venous blood is difficult to obtain. Possible sites for arterial blood sampling include (1) radial, brachial, temporal, dorsalis pedis, and posterior tibial arteries, (2) umbilical arteries in the newborn infant, and (3) capillaries ("arterialized").

The radial artery has several advantages that make it the most commonly used artery for blood sampling. First, its location makes it easy to palpate and puncture. The ulnar artery is more difficult to locate (and therefore puncture), making it less desirable for blood sampling. Second, no vein or nerve is immediately adjacent to the radial artery, which minimizes the risk of obtaining venous blood or damaging a nerve. This is not the case with the brachial artery, and the risk of both complications appears to be greater when this artery is used.[16] The temporal artery is also adjacent to a vein,

increasing the risk of obtaining venous blood. Another advantage of the radial artery is the presence of good collateral circulation from the ulnar artery. The brachial artery has little collateral circulation, causing many clinicians to avoid using it except in circumstances in which there are no other options.[17] Use of the ulnar artery should also be limited to preserve the collateral circulation to the hand. As a general rule, the femoral arteries should not be used for obtaining routine blood samples from the infant or child.

Transcutaneous monitoring of Po_2, Pco_2, and oxygen saturation may provide useful adjuncts to arterial sampling in many patients. Nonetheless, they do not replace intermittent arterial sampling, which remains necessary for the stabilization of infants and children and for verification of the accuracy of these noninvasive methods. Avoid puncture of an artery when infection, burn, or other damage to cutaneous defenses exists in the overlying skin. The presence of adequate collateral circulation and any potential coagulation problems should also be considered.

Equipment and Setup

The equipment required for arterial puncture in an infant or child is listed in Table 19–3. A small-gauge butterfly needle is usually preferred over a needle and syringe for arterial puncture in infants and children. As in venipuncture, a 23-gauge butterfly needle is most often used, although in new-

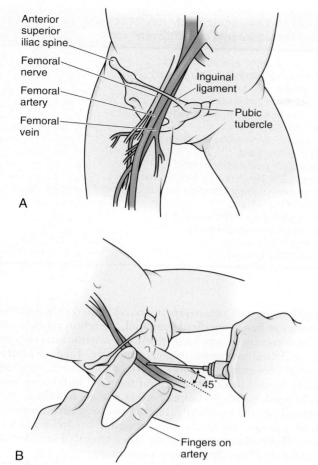

A

B

Figure 19–6 *A,* Anatomy of the femoral triangle. The vein is always medial to the artery. *B,* The needle insertion site is located one finger width below the inguinal ligament, just medial to the artery. Use the index and middle fingers to identify the course of the femoral artery. Contrary to the figure, keep both fingers proximal to the entry point of the needle to avert self-puncture. The needle is pointed medially toward the umbilicus at a 45° angle from the skin surface.

Labels in figure A: Anterior superior iliac spine; Femoral nerve; Femoral artery; Femoral vein; Inguinal ligament; Pubic tubercle

Labels in figure B: 45°; Fingers on artery

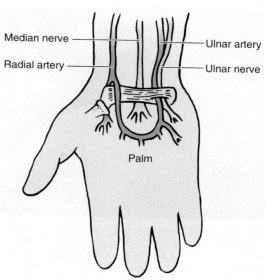

Figure 19–7 Anatomy of the volar surface of the wrist and the palm. The radial artery is preferred for sampling procedures.

Labels in figure: Median nerve; Radial artery; Ulnar artery; Ulnar nerve; Palm

---

TABLE 19–3 Equipment for Arterial Blood Sampling in Infants and Children

Heparin solution for coating syringe or prepackaged heparinized
 syringe if obtaining sample for blood gas analysis
A 1- or 3-mL syringe
A 23- or 25-gauge butterfly needle
Povidone-iodine solution
Alcohol pads
Ice-filled container (bag or cup)
Nonsterile examination gloves
Sterile 2- x 2-inch or 4- x 4-inch gauze pads

---

borns, use of a 25-gauge butterfly needle may be beneficial. Some clinicians prefer to use a 25-gauge needle connected to a syringe, but use of a butterfly allows for better control of the needle while an assistant aspirates the syringe and may also permit a larger volume of blood to be withdrawn.

Technique

Because the radial artery (Fig. 19–7) is most frequently used to obtain intermittent arterial samples from infants and chil-

dren, the technique for arterial puncture at this site will be described. (See Chapter 20, Arterial Puncture and Cannulation, for a discussion of the Allen test and the effect of heparin on blood sampling.) One should heparinize a tuberculin syringe (or use a prepackaged syringe with anticoagulant) if blood gases are being obtained. All heparin should be ejected from the syringe; a 23- or 25-gauge butterfly needle should then be attached to the syringe. The amount of heparin coating the barrel of the syringe is adequate to anticoagulate the sample; excess heparin may result in inaccurate P_{CO_2} determinations because of dilution of the blood sample.[18,19]

The clinician should hold the infant's wrist and hand in her or his nondominant hand. The child's hand is held fully supinated with the wrist slightly extended (dorsiflexed). Overextending the wrist can cause loss of arterial pulsation, which should be palpable just proximal to the transverse wrist creases. A small indentation can be made in the skin with a fingernail to mark the insertion site. The area is cleansed with antiseptic and allowed to dry. Topical anesthetic cream or an intradermal wheal of 1% lidocaine may be used if the clinical situation permits. The skin is penetrated at a 30° to 45° angle (Fig. 19–8), and while the plunger of the syringe is withdrawn, the needle is advanced slowly until the radial artery is punctured or until resistance is met (Fig. 19–9). In contrast to the procedure in adults, *it is necessary in infants to provide continuous, but gentle, suction on the plunger of the syringe* (this may require an assistant). One can be sure that the radial artery is punctured when pulsating or rapidly flowing blood appears in the hub of the needle. Some clinicians prefer to attach the syringe to the butterfly needle only after blood return is noted and suction is thereafter applied.

If resistance is met while pushing the needle deeper or no blood returns, the needle is slowly withdrawn to the point at which only the distal needle tip remains beneath the skin, and the procedure is repeated after checking the location of the pulse. Slight reorientation of the needle laterally or medially may be necessary. After the desired amount of blood is obtained, the needle is removed, and appropriate pressure is applied for 5 minutes or longer to control bleeding.

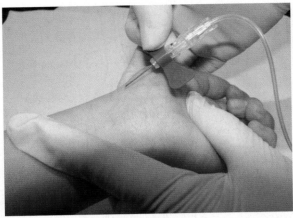

Figure 19–8 For arterial blood sampling, the needle should be inserted under the skin at a 30° to 45° angle. A butterfly needle and syringe are used if larger volumes of blood are required. The wrist is held dorsiflexed by the nondominant hand.

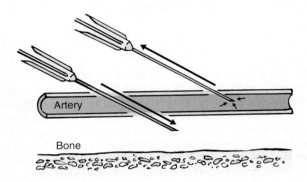

Figure 19–9 Resistance met during passage of the blood gas needle usually indicates contact with bone. The needle should be withdrawn slowly. If the needle has traversed both walls of the artery, blood will be obtained as the needle is slowly withdrawn into the arterial lumen.

Complications

The complications of radial artery puncture include infection, hematoma formation, arterial spasm, tendon injury, and nerve damage.[20,21] With the use of proper technique, however, the complication rate is extremely low. If the infant starts to cry before blood is obtained, the Po_2 and Pco_2 may not reflect the infant's true steady state. Another potential problem is the dilutional effect of heparin on the Pco_2. The heparin in the dead space of the tuberculin syringe may decrease the Pco_2 by 15% to 25% when 0.2 mL of blood is obtained and by approximately 10% with 0.4 mL of blood. This emphasizes the need for all heparin to be ejected from the dead space of the syringe *before the needle is applied*. The use of a syringe (e.g., Becton-Dickinson 1-mL U-100 insulin syringe) with minimal dead space or the use of syringes prepared with lyophilized heparin eliminates this problem (see Chapter 20, Arterial Puncture and Cannulation).[22]

VASCULAR LINE PLACEMENT: VENOUS AND ARTERIAL

Intravascular lines are indicated when access to the venous or arterial circulations is necessary. An IV line may be positioned in peripheral veins (scalp, hand, forearm, foot, ankle, axilla,

TABLE 19–4 Equipment for Peripheral Intravenous Insertion in Infants and Children

22- or 24-gauge venous catheters
Tourniquet (rubber band for infants)
IV solution and tubing
T-connector extension set
Pretorn tape ($\frac{1}{2}$-, 1-, and 2-inch)
Alcohol pads
Povidone-iodine swabs (for blood culture)
Arm or leg board
Nonsterile examination gloves
Sterile 2- x 2-inch or 4- x 4-inch gauze pads
Protective covering (container from IV catheter, T-extension set, or prefabricated cup)
IV fluid chamber with microdrip
A continuous infusion pump
Saline flush solution
3- or 5-mL syringes

thigh) or central veins (superior vena cava via the internal jugular, axillary, superficial temporal, posterior auricular, or subclavian venous approach[14,23] and the inferior vena cava via the umbilical or femoral venous approach). Likewise, intra-arterial lines may be positioned peripherally (radial, posterior tibial, dorsalis pedis, or superficial temporal arteries) or centrally (abdominal or thoracic aorta via an umbilical or a femoral artery approach). Techniques to secure access to these intravascular spaces are discussed in the following sections. Remember to consider the use of topical or intradermal anesthetics if the clinical situation warrants.

Peripheral Venous Catheterization: Percutaneous

Indications and Contraindications

In general, peripheral IV lines are indicated when the patient is unable to attain medical and nutritional goals with enteral therapy. These lines provide maintenance fluids to support adequate hydration and serve as a route for administering medications. In the acute setting, peripheral IV lines provide a route for administering resuscitative medications and fluids as well as antibiotics.

Equipment and Setup

Materials needed for placement of a peripheral IV line in an infant and child are listed in Table 19–4. The two devices most often used for peripheral IV insertion are the butterfly needle and, more commonly, a plastic over-the-needle catheter. Butterfly needles range in size from 21- to 27-gauge. Owing to their rigid nature, they tend to infiltrate very easily in the active child. As a result, butterfly needles are seldom used for infusions any longer. Rarely, they may be inserted for infusions of short duration, such as certain chemotherapeutic agents and single-dose antibiotic administration. Placement of a butterfly needle in a vein close to a flexor surface is contraindicated.

For the most part, over-the-needle catheters, such as Angiocath, Medicut, or Quikcath, are the mainstay of peripheral venous catheterization. These thin-walled, flexible catheters range in size from 14- to 24-gauge. For infants, a 22- to 24-gauge catheter will suffice in most cases. The selection of catheter size depends on the catheter's intended purpose. For example, larger-diameter catheters allow for more rapid administration of fluids in emergency situations. In general, the smallest gauge appropriate for the clinical situation should be used. The use of T-connector extension tubing connected to the catheter after insertion facilitates withdrawal of blood for specimen collection, makes flushing the catheter and maintaining patency easier (especially while taping and securing the IV line), and allows for dressing changes without disturbing the IV insertion site.[24] In recent years, traditional catheters have been replaced with similar over-the-needle catheters that have a protective cap into which the needle is retracted after cannulation to reduce needle stick injuries.

Both commercially available and homemade devices are often used to protect the IV site from a child's attempts to remove it. An arm or leg board appropriate for the size of the child should be handy to provide stabilization of the extremity after insertion. In newborns or small infants, fashioning an arm board from two tongue depressors taped together and covered with 4- x 4-in. gauze will provide the appropriate length needed. One should have primed and ready an IV fluid chamber with microdrip and a continuous infusion pump. Fluid administration in an infant must be carefully monitored. *Macrodrip tubing and liter bottles should not be used*; inadvertent infusion of large amounts of fluids in an infant may be disastrous. An infusion pump is an ideal way of limiting fluid infusion while keeping the vein open. If available, devices used to help locate veins (e.g., ultrasound, transilluminator, infrared imaging) should be on hand and ready for use.

Technique

A number of IV sites are available for placement of a peripheral IV line in the infant (see Fig. 19–3). The most common sites chosen for IV insertion in infants and children are the superficial veins of the dorsum of the hand; the antecubital fossa; the dorsum of the foot; and, in newborns and small infants, the scalp. The veins of the dorsum of the hand are the most often used. These vessels are relatively straight and lay flat on the metacarpals and therefore are stabilized easily. If the hand is chosen, one should take into consideration the age and hand preference of the patient. Veins in the antecubital fossa (cephalic and basilic veins) are easily accessible; however, their angulation across the fossa may make advancement of the catheter difficult. These veins may not be easily visible and yet may be palpable. It is recommended to select the most distal vein that is large enough to accommodate the catheter and leave the larger, more proximal veins in case (1) initial attempts are unsuccessful or (2) prolonged IV therapy may be needed and percutaneous central venous catheter placement (e.g., a peripherally inserted central catheter [PICC] line) is contemplated. Tributaries of the dorsal venous arch on the dorsum of the foot, like those on the dorsum of the hand, are relatively straight, and the extremity is easily immobilized after insertion. Because indwelling catheters in this location will prevent mobility, this site should be considered only in preambulatory patients or after attempts at other sites have been unsuccessful. The scalp veins are easy to cannulate, but their use is primarily limited to very small infants. If a peripheral vein on the hands, feet, or antecubital fossa is being used, the extremity can first be immobilized by taping it to an arm board, a padded splint, or commercially available immobilization device. The particular site is a matter of preference, and the clinician should choose the vein that appears to be the easiest to cannulate.

With few exceptions, the same techniques used for IV insertion in adults may be used in infants and children, especially in the veins of distal extremities. If a peripheral extremity is used, a tourniquet may be placed proximal to the planned site of entry. Warming the extremity is a commonly used maneuver to induce vasodilatation in the surface veins, making them easier to cannulate. Some EDs use transillumination devices commonly found in neonatal intensive care units to assist in finding veins in infants.[25,26] The Venoscope II (Venoscope LLC, Lafayatte, LA) and the Neonatal Transilluminator (Graykon Scientific, Victoria, Australia) are two such devices that work by projecting a high-intensity light into the patient's subcutaneous tissue to contrast with the surrounding tissue. The light causes the veins to contrast with the surrounding tissue, making them easier to locate.[27]

If the clinical situation allows, a topical anesthetic (e.g., EMLA or ELA-Max cream) may be applied prior to insertion. The tubing of the T-extension set should be flushed before venipuncture with a sterile IV solution, such as normal saline, to prevent air embolism. The IV catheter is directed through the skin at a 10° to 20° angle[28] and slowly advanced until blood return is noted (Fig. 19–10*A*). One then advances the catheter over the needle, into the vein. The needle is retracted or removed, depending upon the type of catheter used, and the IV line is connected to the hub of the catheter by means of a T-extension set. After 1 mL of solution is flushed through the line, the site is inspected for signs of infiltration, such as hematoma or local swelling.

The catheter is fixed to the skin with a piece of 0.5-inch tape passed over the catheter hub and fixed to the skin. A second piece of tape is placed adhesive side up and slipped under the catheter hub and crossed over the catheter hub in a V shape (see Fig. 19–10*B*). After securing the catheter with tape, some clinicians like to cover the entire area with a transparent sterile dressing such as Tegaderm (3M, St. Paul, MN) or OP Site (Smith and Nephew Medical, Massilon, OH). The tubing of the T-extension set is looped back, and a piece of tape is placed midway over the tubing and secured to skin. This ensures against accidental dislodgment if the IV tubing is suddenly pulled. The hand and forearm are securely taped to the arm board for immobilization (see Fig. 19–10*C*). A commercially available plastic dome protector, a plastic medication cup cut in half, or some other clear protective device is then taped over the catheter site (see Fig. 19–10*D*). Occasionally, the flow rate of the infusion may be positional, especially if the catheter spans a joint or the tip abuts a venous valve. Adjustment of the hand position or catheter with strategically placed sterile gauze or slight withdrawal of the catheter may be all that is required to remedy the problem.

If blood specimens are needed, one can obtain these just after IV insertion and spare the child an additional needle stick. The T-extension tubing and attached syringe should not contain any flush solution. After appropriate preparation of the insertion site and successful placement of the catheter into the vein, the T-extension tubing and syringe are connected to the hub of the catheter, and the blood is aspirated into the syringe. After the desired quantity is obtained, the syringe is removed, the T-extension tubing is connected to the IV infusion tubing, and the infusion pump is set at the desired rate. Remember to prepare the skin with povidone-iodine solution or other appropriate antiseptic if cultures are needed.

If the scalp veins are used, the area surrounding the planned site of insertion can be shaved and cleansed with an

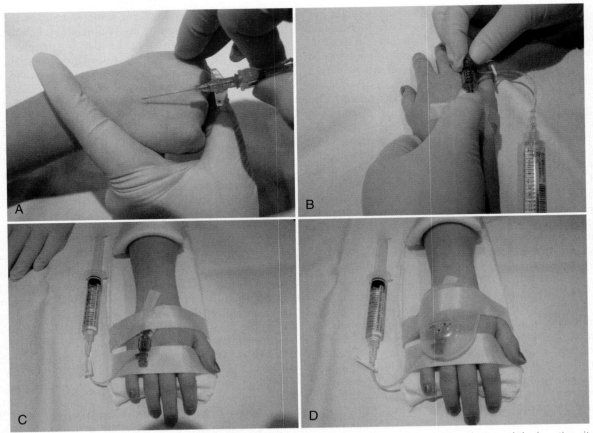

Figure 19–10 **Technique for peripheral venous catheterization.** *A,* The catheter is directed at a 10° to 20° angle toward the insertion site and advanced until blood return is seen in the catheter and hub. *B,* The stylet is removed, and the T-extension tubing is attached. Taping technique for butterfly and intravascular catheters using a crisscross pattern. *C,* The hand and forearm are secured to an arm board. *D,* Covering with the plastic wrapper from the T-extension tubing for protection.

antiseptic solution. If the child's parents become distressed at the idea of shaving their young infant's hair, trimming with small scissors so that the vessels are adequately exposed may be a reasonable compromise. Arteries and veins can usually be differentiated on the scalp because arteries are more tortuous than veins.[14] In addition, the flow of blood is away from the heart in arteries and toward the heart in veins. If an artery is entered during placement of the needle and fluid is infused, blanching will occur in the area. If this happens, the IV catheter should be removed, light pressure should be maintained for 5 minutes, and the procedure should be repeated at another site. A rubber band may be used as a tourniquet around the scalp (*never the neck*) to produce venous dilatation. One should always ensure that the rubber band is removed after venous cannulation. When removing this rubber band, it should be carefully slipped over the catheter or cut with a pair of scissors. Although cutting the rubber band with scissors is often the easiest technique, the clinician must take care to hold both cut ends to avoid having the infant "snapped" by one or both ends. Placing a piece of tape on the rubber band before placement on the scalp will facilitate lifting the rubber band away from the scalp.

If a scalp vein butterfly infusion set is used, the wings of the butterfly are grasped between the thumb and the forefinger, and the needle is introduced beneath the skin approximately 0.5 cm distal to the anticipated site of vein entrance (Fig. 19–11). The needle is advanced slowly toward the vessel until blood appears in the tubing, indicating that the vessel

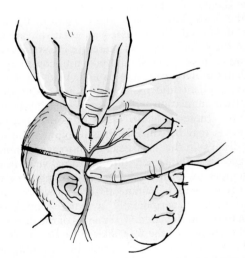

Figure 19–11 Using a rubber band as a tourniquet to distend the scalp veins, the needle is introduced approximately 0.5 cm distal to the anticipated site of the vessel puncture. Gloves should be worn.

has been entered. The tourniquet should then be removed. The needle should be flushed with 0.5 to 2 mL of IV fluid, such as normal saline, to ensure that the needle is properly in place within the vein. If infiltration occurs, as noted by a subcutaneous bump, the IV line should be removed and the process repeated at another site.

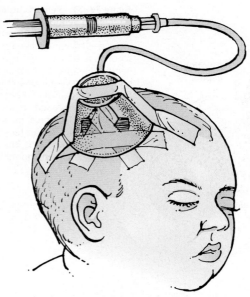

Figure 19–12 Protecting the intravenous line with a plastic medicine cup.

After the wings are secured with tape, the tubing of the butterfly set should be taped in a loop on the scalp so that it is not inadvertently pulled. A wisp of cotton may be placed under the wings of the butterfly if the infusion is positional. A small medication cup may be taped over the wings and the needle to protect the IV line (Fig. 19–12). The tubing of the butterfly set should then be connected to the tubing from the IV system. It is generally preferable to use standard over-the-needle IV catheters whenever possible, whether for extremity or scalp IV lines, because they are less likely to infiltrate and will last longer. However, a small butterfly needle that can be inserted temporarily until additional access is possible is sometimes the only option short of an IO procedure.

Vein Imaging Devices

A variety of imaging modalities, including ultrasound, transillumination, and infrared technologies, have been used to help locate peripheral veins for cannulation. In adults, there are data supporting the use of ultrasound to facilitate peripheral vein cannulation in patients with difficult access.[29,30] However, the use of ultrasound to aid in the placement of peripheral IV lines in pediatric patients is not common practice. One recently published study demonstrated that ultrasound could be used to detect peripheral veins in young children that were not "clinically apparent" (nonvisible and nonpalpable).[31] The study also found that *lack* of ultrasound visualization increased the chances of an unsuccessful placement.[31] This study suggests that ultrasound may be a useful adjunct for peripheral IV line placement in young children. However, further studies are needed to better understand its indications, applications, and limitations.

Transillumination technology uses high-intensity light near the skin to provide contrast between the subcutaneous tissues and the vessels, making them easier to see. A newer vein imaging technology, VeinViewer (Luminetx Corp., Memphis, TN) uses near-infrared technology to project an enhanced image of subcutaneous veins onto the patient's skin. The location of the venous valves and the assessment of the course of the vessel can assist the clinician in selecting the best area to be cannulated.[32] If available, these devises may help locate veins and increase the chances of successful catheter placement.

Complications

Complications of IV fluid therapy include infection;[33] injection of sclerosing agents into the subcutaneous space, with resultant necrosis and sloughing of the skin (especially in small infants);[34] air embolism;[28,35] and administration of inappropriate volumes of fluid. Because the life span of an IV needle or catheter is usually fairly short (<72 hr) in the small infant, the decision concerning elective removal and replacement of the IV system is not usually a problem. Of course, it is important to pay meticulous attention to sterility during insertion and maintenance of the IV system to decrease the risk of infection.

Peripheral Venous Catheterization: Venous Cutdown

Indications and Contraindications

With the development of small IV catheters and the rapidity and safety of IO needle placement for emergency access (see Chapter 25, Intraosseous Infusion), peripheral venous cutdowns are rarely performed in infants and children in the ED. Even in experienced hands, a saphenous vein cutdown may take more than 10 minutes and is associated with a higher rate of infection than other routes of vascular access.[36,37] Nevertheless, if peripheral venous, central venous, or IO access cannot be obtained, venous cutdowns may provide an alternative means of emergency venous access. For the purposes of illustration, the exposure and cannulation of the saphenous vein are discussed (Fig. 19–13). The same principles apply when cutdowns are performed on most peripheral veins.

Equipment and Setup

Successful venous catheterization via cutdown in infants and small children requires sterile instruments, an assistant, good lighting, and a selection of catheters. Silastic catheters, which can be obtained in 2-, 3-, and 4-French sizes (Dow Chemical Company, Midland, MI), seem to remain patent longer and can be sterilized with the instruments to make a "cutdown tray." Standard 19- to 22-gauge IV catheters (Angiocath, Deseret Medical, Inc., Sandy, UT) are also useful.

Technique

The clinician should begin with complete immobilization of the thigh, leg, ankle, and foot by taping them to a padded leg board, which in turn is attached to the table or bed where the procedure is being performed (see Fig. 19–13A). The area around the medial malleolus is prepared with antiseptic solution and draped with sterile towels. Local anesthesia should be performed (intradermal 1% lidocaine) in an area about 1 cm proximal and 1 cm anterior to the medial malleolus. No major nerves or tendons accompany the vein in this location.

A tourniquet is placed proximally on the leg and a transverse skin incision is made (usually about 2 cm in length) in the anesthetized area; a small mosquito hemostat is inserted into the wound, with the concavity of the clamp upward. The tip of the hemostat is advanced to the bone in one corner of the wound, and all tissues lying against the bone and in the subcutaneous region are "scooped up" with the hemostat (see

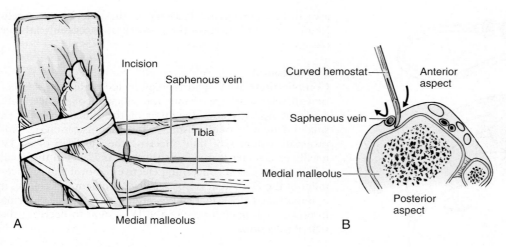

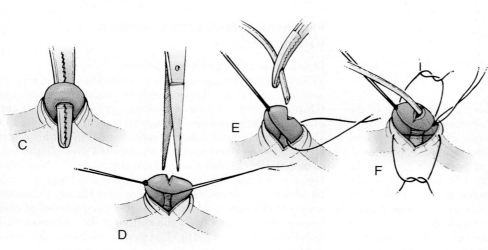

Figure 19–13 Venous cutdown (saphenous vein). *A,* Immobilization of the ankle and the site of skin incision. *B,* A curved hemostat scoops up the vein. The point of the hemostat should be kept against the bone. *C,* The vein is dissected free. *D,* With a proximal and distal tie to stabilize the vein and control bleeding, an incision is made in the upper one third of the vein. *E* and *F,* The infusion catheter is threaded into the vein lumen and advanced.

Fig. 19–13*B*). This will invariably lift the vein out of the wound along with surrounding tissues. A fine forceps or a mosquito hemostat is used to separate and remove all nonvenous structures, leaving only the saphenous vein tented over the hemostat (see Fig. 19–13*C*). To avoid injury to the vein during dissection, spread the ends of the hemostat parallel to the direction of the vein, *never* transversely.

Two 4-0 silk sutures are passed under the vein; one is pulled distally to stabilize the vein, and the other is pulled proximal to the site of venipuncture. The distal suture may be tied, but if left untied, it can still be used for stabilization of the vein. Removal of the untied distal suture after vein cannulation may allow for subsequent vein recannulation after eventual catheter removal. If the distal suture is left untied, longitudinal traction on it permits hemostasis and continued exposure of the vein above the wound. Fine scissors or a scalpel blade may be used to make an oblique or V-shaped incision (venotomy) in the anterior vein wall between the sutures (see Fig. 19–13*D*).

The Silastic catheter (prefilled with saline solution) is grasped with forceps and is advanced into the vein for a distance of 2 to 3 cm (see Fig. 19–13*E* and *F*). This is usually the most difficult and time-consuming portion of the procedure. A vein dilator or forceps may be used to hold open the venotomy incision (see Fig. 19–13*G*). Downward pull on the distal tie provides countertraction and will stabilize the vein during catheter advancement. The tourniquet is then removed, and

the proximal suture is tied around the vein with the catheter inside, taking care not to occlude the catheter by tying the suture too tight. If the distal suture was tied, the free ends of the suture can be tied around the catheter, providing additional stability. If the distal suture was not tied, it is now removed. When the distal suture is left untied, the proximal suture is still tied to secure the catheter, but the ends are left long so that the suture can be removed to allow recannulation once the infusion is removed.

Continued infusion of saline through the catheter from an attached syringe will ensure patency. The catheter is oriented into either corner of the incision, and the incision is closed with interrupted 4-0 nylon sutures. The skin suture nearest the catheter is wrapped around the catheter and tied to hold the catheter in place. Bleeding can be controlled with direct pressure. Antibiotic ointment is placed over the wound, and a sterile occlusive dressing is applied. The IV tubing is connected and taped securely to the footboard to prevent inadvertent removal of the catheter (see Fig. 19–13*H*).

Change the dressing carefully every day, using sterile technique with reapplication of antibiotic ointment. When cared for properly, catheters can remain in place for as long as 7 to 10 days. Generally, though, the catheter is replaced, using another site, after 3 to 4 days. Obviously, at the first sign of infiltration or infection, the catheter must be removed. Unfortunately, once the vein has been used for a cutdown, it is usually rendered useless for future venous cannulation.

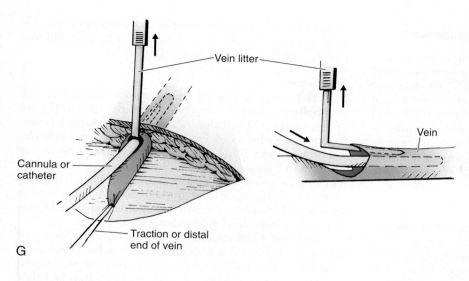

Figure 19–13, cont'd *G,* A vein lifter/dilator facilitates placement of the catheter into the vein lumen. *H,* The incision is sutured, and the catheter is secured. *(C, From Suratt PM, Gibson RS: Manual of Medical Procedures. St. Louis, CV Mosby, 1982. Reproduced by permission.)*

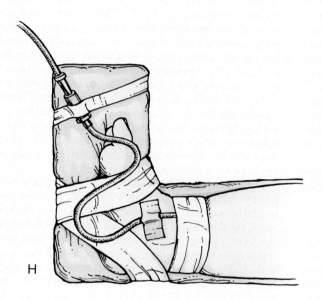

Mini-Cutdown

The cannulation of a small vein with a catheter or tube may be difficult and very time consuming if one is not experienced in the technique. As an alternative, the mini-cutdown procedure may be used. Once the vein is exposed through a skin incision and subcutaneous dissection, it is cannulated directly with a standard IV catheter (e.g., Medicut, Angiocath) rather than nicked with a scalpel (Fig. 19–14). A silk suture or hemostat may be placed under the vein to immobilize it during puncture, but with the mini-cutdown technique, the vein is not tied off after being cannulated. The catheter will not be as secure with this modification, but the technique is useful when time is critical. The vein is not destroyed with this technique. In essence, the mini-cutdown uses the percutaneous technique of cannulation, except that venipuncture is performed through a skin incision under direct visualization (see Chapter 23, Venous Cutdown).

Complications

In addition to the problems discussed with percutaneous catheter placement previously, venous cutdowns can result in wound infections and phlebitis. Adjacent structures may be

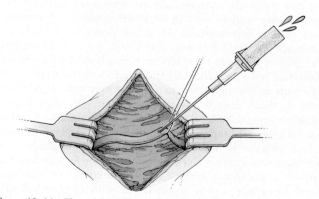

Figure 19–14 The mini-cutdown procedure using a standard intravenous catheter over-the-needle system is technically easier than the full cutdown and may be preferred in an emergency.

injured during the incision and subsequent blunt dissection. When the mini-cutdown technique without ligatures is used, extravasation of infusate may result. Light pressure on the closed wound will generally prevent continued extravasation.

Central Venous Catheterization: Percutaneous

Percutaneous placement of central venous lines has become the technique of choice of many clinicians for securing central venous access in neonates and young infants.[36] This technique has nearly supplanted the technique of cutdown for central venous catheterization, which is seldom performed in the ED any longer. Both percutaneous and venous cutdown catheterizations require central venous catheters, which can be purchased separately or within self-contained kits (e.g., Arrow International, Inc., Reading, PA; Gesco International, San Antonio, TX).

Indications and Contraindications

Percutaneous central venous cannulation is indicated to secure vascular access (1) when peripheral venous access is limited or impossible, (2) for emergency drug and fluid administration during cardiac arrest and shock, (3) when hyperalimentation and IV infusions are required for days to weeks, (4) when low-birth-weight neonates and young infants require central venous access, and (5) when precise hemodynamic monitoring is needed in a critically ill or injured child. Contraindications to percutaneous placement of central venous catheters may include an uncorrected coagulopathy; local infections or burns at insertion sites; malformations or deformations that may distort vascular anatomy; vascular insufficiency of an extremity; obstruction or compression of the access veins by tumor, abnormal vessels, hematoma, thrombus, abscess, or malformation; or absence of access veins.[15,38] Bacterial septicemia is a relative contraindication, and delaying placement of central venous access until cultures have been sterile for 48 hours has been recommended. However, this delay must be weighed against the immediate need for IV access.

Equipment and Setup

Percutaneous central venous catheterization in infants and children can be performed using any number of sterile over-the-needle catheters ranging in size from 22 to 16 gauge (the choice depends on the age of the patient) and equipment similar to that used for percutaneous peripheral venous catheterization (see Table 19–4). If insertion of a larger indwelling catheter is desired, commercially available kits are convenient because they contain most of the items needed for the procedure (Gesco International, Inc., San Antonio, TX; Arrow International, Inc., Reading, PA; Cook, Inc., Bloomington, IN). The catheters in these kits are typically made of a silicone elastomer, polyvinyl chloride, or polyethylene; some are available with an antimicrobial coating that may reduce infection rates. Catheter length is variable, and one- to three-lumen catheters are available. Rapid volume replacement, as in the case of severe dehydration or acute blood loss from trauma, is best achieved by inserting a short, large-bore catheter for the initial resuscitation and stabilization. If the patient requires hemodynamic monitoring or multiple medication infusions, the short catheter can be replaced later with a longer indwelling catheter by changing it over a wire using the Seldinger technique.

Other necessary equipment includes sterile forceps and scissors; antiseptic solution; gauze pads; sterile drapes; gowns; gloves; caps and masks; syringes (3, 5, and 10 mL); sterile transparent skin coverings (e.g., Tegaderm, 3M Company, St. Paul, MN; OP Site, Smith and Nephew Medical, Massilon, OH); Luer-Lok three-way stopcocks; 0.25 to 1.0% lidocaine; flush solution (1–2 U heparin/mL normal saline), and IV tubing with a T-connector extension. Depending on the vein to be accessed, restraint of the extremity, pelvis, or head may require a padded support, an assistant, or both.

Techniques

Percutaneous placement of central venous catheters can be accomplished using two methods that differ only in the use of a guidewire. The guidewire (Seldinger) technique is preferred when catheters are inserted into the femoral or subclavian vein. When using the basilic or cephalic vein of the forearm and antecubital space, axillary vein, or superficial temporal or posterior auricular scalp vein, many clinicians prefer to insert the catheter through an introducer needle. Details of the femoral, external and internal jugular, and subclavian and antecubital approaches follow.

Femoral Catheterization. The safety and efficacy of percutaneous femoral venous catheterization have been demonstrated.[39] Femoral venous catheterization is the central venous access route most commonly used in infants and children in emergency situations.[36] The femoral anatomy is easily learned, and the arterial pulse provides a landmark for catheter insertion. In case of inadvertent arterial puncture or venous laceration, hemostasis can be achieved by application of direct pressure. Also, femoral catheterization is less likely to interfere with emergency procedures in the region of the head, neck, and chest during medical or trauma resuscitations. Finally, the specific risks associated with subclavian and internal jugular vein catheterization (pneumothorax and carotid or subclavian artery puncture) are avoided. Risks of the procedure include thrombosis and infection; these can occur with any type of venous catheter.

Technique. The child must be adequately restrained to permit exposure of the inguinal region. In some situations, it might be necessary to sedate the child (see Chapter 33, Systemic Analgesia and Sedation for Procedures), but this should be done with caution in a child with marginal perfusion or respiratory compromise. In the last several years, experience with using real-time ultrasound to facilitate placement of central venous lines in adults has prompted a number of organizations to recommend it for widespread use.[40,41] The use of ultrasound to guide placement of central venous catheters in children has been studied, but the body of literature remains small.[42] Randomized trials comparing ultrasound-guided placement to standard "surface landmark" techniques in emergency situations have yet to be done in children. Nevertheless, the use of ultrasound to locate the femoral vasculature in children may be helpful, especially if femoral arterial pulsations are not strong, if edema makes palpation of the artery difficult, or if the artery is difficult to locate when wearing gloves. Note that during cardiopulmonary resuscitation (CPR), palpable pulsations or Doppler tones in the *femoral vein* may be detected. Hence, if the vein is not found medial to the pulsations, catheterization of the pulsating vessel during CPR may be considered as a last resort when other options for vascular access or drug delivery are unavailable. Both groins are generally prepared with antiseptic solution in the event that the initial attempt is unsuccessful.

The introducer needle supplied with the kit can be used with or without a syringe to enter the femoral vein. The femoral artery is palpated with one finger, and the needle is placed in the skin just medial to the artery. One enters the skin at a 30° to 45° angle approximately 1 cm below the inguinal ligament. The general course of the needle is in a line directed toward the umbilicus. When blood return is noted, the wire is gently passed through the needle into the proximal vein. If a syringe has been attached to the introducer needle, continuous, gentle suction is applied while the needle is inserted. When the syringe is removed to insert the wire, a sterile gloved finger is often placed over the open hub of the needle to prevent air embolus or blood loss. The wire should not meet resistance when gently introduced, and the proximal end should always be visible protruding from the hub of the needle. If there is resistance to passage of the wire, it should be removed to assess the needle's position within the vessel. If there is resistance to removal of the wire, the needle and the wire must be withdrawn together to prevent shearing off the end of the wire.[43] An alternative method that may be useful when placing the 4-French double-lumen Arrow catheter is to remove the tubing from a 21-gauge butterfly needle (Abbott Hospitals, Inc., North Chicago, IL) and use the needle to enter the vein (Fig. 19–15A). The butterfly needle is very easy to hold in a stable position and is also shorter than the needles supplied with the preassembled kits. When blood return is obtained, the wire is passed through the butterfly needle into the proximal vein.

A small incision (1–2 mm) is then made along the wire's entry point at the skin to allow passage of the vein dilator (see Fig. 19–15B) or the catheter itself. The incision is generally made with a No. 11 scalpel blade with the sharp edge of the blade pointed away from the wire. The dilator, if used, is advanced over the wire gently, then removed. The catheter, which has been flushed with saline, is advanced over the wire into the vein; and the wire is removed[44] (see Fig. 19–15C). Occasionally, it is useful to rotate and advance the dilator (or catheter) simultaneously as it enters the vein. Many times, the

dilator step is skipped in a critical situation and the catheter is placed directly after placement of the wire. Blood return is noted from the catheter ports, which are then flushed with a sterile saline solution. The catheter is subsequently secured with silk or nylon sutures (see Fig. 19–15D). A sterile transparent skin covering placed over the exit site may be used as an impermeable dressing.

This technique is useful in children as small as 1000 g. When one is placing femoral venous catheters in children smaller than 1500 g, a smaller single-lumen catheter (3 Fr or 24 gauge) should be used, because a larger catheter may occlude blood flow through the femoral vein.

External Jugular Venous Catheterization. The external jugular vein is superficial and easily visible. However, it should be used for venous access only when attempts at peripheral IV access have been unsuccessful. The external jugular vein is undesirable as a primary catheterization site during resuscitative efforts, because manipulation of the head and neck may compromise management of the airway. In addition, the success rate for central venous catheterization using the external jugular approach is lower than that with other sites owing to the acute angle of entry of the external jugular vein into the subclavian vein.[45] As a result, it is seldom if ever used to access the central circulation.

Technique. Because central venous access is not the goal of this approach, the external jugular vein is most often entered using a standard over-the-needle IV catheter. The external jugular vein lies in a line from the angle of the jaw to the middle of the clavicle and is usually visible on the surface of the skin. The vein is more prominent when the infant is crying. An assistant is needed to restrain the infant

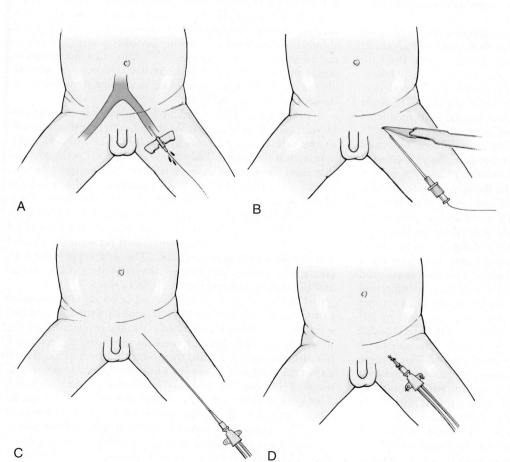

Figure 19–15 Technique for inserting a femoral venous catheter. *A,* A 21-gauge butterfly catheter is used to enter the femoral vein, and the guidewire is passed through the butterfly needle into the proximal vein. Note that the tubing has been removed from a standard butterfly set. *B,* A small incision is made alongside the wire, and the dilator is advanced over the wire and into the vein. *C,* The catheter is advanced over the wire and into the vein. *D,* The wire is removed and the catheter secured. Note that many commercial kits have a self-contained 21-gauge needle, making modification of a butterfly needle catheter unnecessary.

in a supine position with the head and neck extended over the edge of the bed. Alternatively, a towel roll or pillow placed under the shoulders can be used. The head is turned approximately 40° to 70° from the midline (see Fig. 19–5), and the skin surrounding the area to be punctured is cleansed with alcohol (or other antiseptic solution). The area may be covered with a sterile drape, and 1% lidocaine may then be infiltrated into the skin. A finger may be placed just above the clavicle to distend the jugular vein.

An 18- to 22-gauge over-the-needle catheter attached to a syringe is aligned parallel to the vein, and the skin is punctured approximately one half to two thirds of the distance from the angle of the jaw to the clavicle. The catheter is advanced slowly until the jugular vein is entered. The syringe is connected to the catheter at all times to maintain a constant negative pressure and avoid an air embolism. After the appropriate amount of blood is obtained, the catheter is advanced and secured in place and a sterile occlusive dressing is applied.

Internal Jugular Venous Catheterization.
The internal jugular veins lie within the carotid sheath containing the carotid artery and vagus nerve. The lower part of the vein lies within the triangle formed by the sternal and clavicular heads of the sternocleidomastoid muscle and becomes more lateral and anterior to the artery as it joins the subclavian vein. The right internal jugular vein is preferred over the left, because the internal jugular and innominate vein and the superior vena cava form a nearly straight line into the right atrium. This lessens the chance for pneumothorax or injury to the thoracic duct. Internal jugular vein catheterization should be performed only when central venous access is required or when attempts at peripheral venous access and external jugular access have been unsuccessful.

Technique. Three approaches (the anterior, median or central, and posterior approaches, as discussed in Chapter 22, Central Venous Catheterization and Central Venous Pressure Monitoring) to internal jugular catheterization are possible. The median or central approach is recommended in pediatric patients and is described here. The use of ultrasound to guide elective cannulation of the internal jugular vein in infants has been described, and appears to improve success rates[46,47] (see Chapter 67, Ultrasound-Guided Procedures). The child is positioned in the same fashion as that described for external jugular venous catheterization. The medial or central approach uses the apex of the angle formed by the sternal and clavicular heads of the sternocleidomastoid muscle as the puncture site. If one could imagine a line from the mastoid process to the sternal notch, the apex of the angle formed by the two muscular heads would fall approximately along the middle third of that line.[43] The skin surrounding the area to be punctured is cleansed with an antiseptic solution. The area is covered with a sterile drape, and 1% lidocaine may then be infiltrated into the skin. An 18- to 22-gauge needle attached to a syringe is introduced at the apex of the triangle at an angle of 30° downward relative to the coronal plane and directed caudad toward the ipsilateral nipple (Fig. 19–16). The needle is advanced slowly until the jugular vein is entered. The syringe is connected to the needle at all times to maintain constant negative pressure and avoid an air embolism. After blood flow is obtained, the syringe is removed, and a finger is placed over the hub of the needle. A guidewire is then inserted during a positive-pressure breath or exhalation, the needle is removed, and a catheter is introduced using the Seldinger technique. The catheter should be passed far enough to reach the supe-

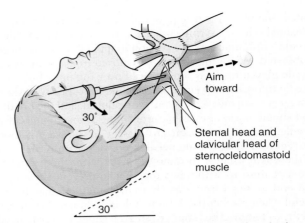

Figure 19–16 Technique for internal jugular venous catheterization (medial or central approach). The needle is inserted at the apex of the triangle formed by the sternal and clavicular heads of the sternocleidomastoid muscle. The needle is angled 30° downward relative to the coronal plane and directed toward the ipsilateral nipple. If available, ultrasound guidance is suggested.

rior vena cava/right atrium junction. The catheter is checked for blood return, the line is secured with sutures, and a sterile occlusive dressing is applied. A chest radiograph is warranted to assess the proper location of the catheter as well as to rule out pneumothorax.

Subclavian Venous Catheterization.
The subclavian vein is a popular site for central venous access in the adult patient but is used far less frequently in children. The technique is more difficult in the child because of the vessels' smaller size, as well as their more cephalad location under the clavicles. In addition, there is a high risk of pneumothorax and hemothorax, especially in younger patients and when performed during emergencies. Consequently, this approach should be considered only if other peripheral or central venous access sites are unobtainable.[36,43,48] Also, subclavian venous access may interfere with resuscitative efforts or be unavailable owing to the placement of cervical spine immobilization devices in a trauma patient.

Technique. The technique for subclavian venous catheterization differs from that for the adult in that the approach to the vein is more lateral in children. The infraclavicular approach is described. The equipment needed is the same as that used for femoral catheterization. The patient's head is turned away from the side to be punctured and a towel roll placed under the shoulders (Fig. 19–17). The right side is preferred, because the dome of the lung is more cephalad on the left side. The needle insertion site is at the distal one third of the clavicle in the depression created between the deltoid and the pectoralis major muscles. The skin is prepared with antiseptic solution, the area is covered with a sterile drape, and the skin is infiltrated with 1% lidocaine.

The finder needle is introduced bevel up and advanced slowly while negative pressure is applied with the attached syringe. The syringe and needle should be parallel to the frontal plane and directed medially and slightly cephalad, beneath the clavicle toward the posterior aspect of the sternal end of the clavicle (i.e., toward a fingertip placed in the sternal notch).[36] The needle is advanced until blood return is obtained. The syringe is then turned so that the bevel of the needle points caudad to direct the guidewire to the superior vena cava. The syringe is removed from the needle and the wire is inserted during a positive-pressure breath or natural exhalation. The needle is then removed, and the catheter is intro-

The most common sites include arm, neck, and scalp veins. The catheter is then threaded centrally. PICC lines offer several advantages over conventional peripheral IV catheters and percutaneous central venous catheters. They can remain in place for up to 3 months, sparing veins from multiple reinsertions with peripheral venous catheters; and the long-arm catheter is simpler to insert than central venous catheters and poses no risk of producing a pneumothorax or hemothorax.

Technique. The arm of the vessel to be cannulated is initially stabilized using a support board or the help of an assistant. The remainder of the procedure requires sterile technique. Povidone-iodine or other antiseptic solution is used to cleanse the skin overlying the vessel to be cannulated, and 1% lidocaine is infiltrated at the skin site to be punctured. The skin is punctured with an 18-gauge needle to ease insertion of the introducer through the skin.

The catheter to be inserted is chosen based on the size of the access vessel. Typically a 23-gauge silicone elastomer catheter with other needed accessories is used, as in a kit prepared by Gesco International, Inc. (San Antonio, TX). Advantages of this catheter include (1) a double-wing silicone adapter, which precludes the need to make homemade blunt-end adapters to fit small cannulas and simplifies the taping procedure, and (2) a breakaway introducer needle that can be peeled off the catheter, thereby precluding the need for sliding the introducer off the catheter and placing an adapter. Because the length of this catheter (33.5 cm) is longer than needed in low-birth-weight neonates and young infants, the distance from the insertion site to the superior vena cava–right atrium junction is estimated (i.e., by measuring the distance between the insertion site and the right nipple [Fig. 19–18*A*]), and the catheter is cut 1 to 3 cm longer than the estimated distance to compensate for variability between the estimated and the actual needed length of the catheter. The end of this catheter is then connected to a Luer-Lok stopcock and syringe and filled with flush solution; the catheter is then ready for use.

The 20-gauge breakaway introducer needle (Gesco International, Inc.) is also filled with flush solution and then directed slowly through the insertion site and into the access vein. When blood return occurs, the catheter is picked up approximately 1 cm from its tip and guided into the introducer needle (see Fig. 19–18*B*). The catheter is advanced in 1-cm increments until the previously estimated distance is reached (i.e., the catheter tip is at the superior vena cava–right atrium junction). The breakaway introducer needle is then withdrawn several centimeters from the insertion site before peeling the introducer off the catheter to avoid inadvertent catheter laceration. If accidental laceration occurs, blunt-end adapters should be readily available. An alternative method, the *Microintroducer technique*, introduces a guidewire through the catheter used to gain access to the vein. A small "nick" is made with a scalpel, as described previously for central venous catheters, and an introducer catheter is threaded over the wire to make a larger entry. Finally, the silicone PICC line is carefully threaded into the introducer catheter and advanced as described earlier.[53]

Immediately after catheter placement and withdrawal of the introducer needle, the clinician will be able to manipulate the position of the catheter until clotting starts to occur at the insertion site. After the sterile field is discontinued, the catheter should never be advanced. The function of the catheter is checked by withdrawing blood, by noting the presence of residual air bubbles within the catheter, or both. After the

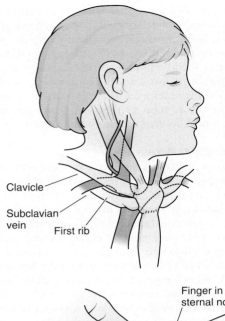

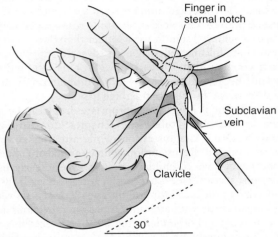

Figure 19–17 Technique for subclavian venous catheterization. The needle is inserted at the distal one third of the clavicle in the depression created between the deltoid and the pectoralis major muscles. The needle should be parallel to the frontal plane and directed medially and slightly cephalad toward a fingertip placed in the sternal notch. The patient is shown in a 30° Trendelenburg position.

Labels in figure: Clavicle; Subclavian vein; First rib; Finger in sternal notch; Subclavian vein; Clavicle; 30°

duced over the wire using the Seldinger technique as previously described for femoral catheterization. As in adults, the cardiac monitor may show a rhythm disturbance if the wire is advanced too far. Auscultation of bilateral breath sounds should be performed and a chest radiograph obtained to confirm the proper positioning of the catheter in the superior vena cava, as well as to rule out procedural complications such as pneumothorax or hemothorax. The catheter is then secured in place with sutures, and a sterile, occlusive dressing is applied.

Antecubital Access. Percutaneous insertion of central catheters by way of peripheral antecubital veins is used most frequently to obtain central venous access in patients with very small caliber vessels (e.g., low-birth-weight neonates and very young infants). These PICC lines are small Silastic catheters ranging in size from 23 to 16 gauge.[49–51] These catheters are rarely inserted as an ED procedure; more often they are placed in a stable child who will require longer-term fluid or nutritional therapy or an extended course of IV antibiotics.

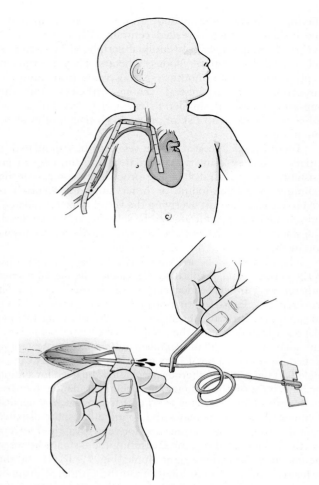

Figure 19–18 **Techniques for insertion of central catheters from peripheral veins.** *A,* A tape measure is used to determine the catheter length. *B,* Placement of the catheter through the specialized breakaway butterfly-type introducer needle.

clinician ensures that no air bubbles remain in the line, the catheter is flushed. This catheter should be "easy" to flush; if it is not, the clinician should reposition the catheter and recheck its function. If the catheter remains difficult to flush, it should be considered clotted and should be removed. Alternatively, position may be confirmed by chest radiograph and fibrinolytic therapy used, if considered appropriate.

A sterile transparent skin covering is applied, which is usually left in place until the catheter is removed. This dressing may be removed sooner, but only by clinicians who are expert in caring for these lines and only when necessary. Stabilization sutures are not routinely placed during this procedure. Occasionally, a small amount of bleeding occurs at the insertion site; this generally stops spontaneously or with gentle pressure. With the three-way stopcock in place, central venous pressure measurements and infusion of medications, IV fluids, and hyperalimentation solutions can be performed. Many clinicians at centers that frequently perform PICC insertions use sonography or fluoroscopy to increase likelihood of successful catheter placement.[52]

Complications

The incidence of complications from central venous catheterization ranges from 10% to 50%.[50,52] Infection and thrombo-

sis are the major risks associated with these catheters.[38,53] Other complications include accidental displacement, phlebitis, hemorrhage, hematoma, dysrhythmia, air embolus, vascular obstruction or perforation, right atrial perforation, and localized edema. Blood sampling from indwelling central venous lines must be performed with caution, because the risk of contamination increases each time the system is opened. Removing catheters as soon as they are no longer needed minimizes the morbidity from these complications.

Emergency Vascular Access

The first steps in managing pediatric resuscitations are to establish an adequate airway, ensure adequate ventilation, and enhance blood circulation. Maintaining or reestablishing adequate circulation often requires prompt access to the intravascular space for administration of fluids or medications, or both. However, obtaining venous access during pediatric resuscitations can challenge even the most seasoned clinician.[54,55] In a review of pediatric resuscitations by Rossetti and colleagues,[54] IV access required 10 or more minutes in 24% of the cases. The average time required for a cutdown was 24 minutes. Children who were successfully resuscitated had vascular access achieved significantly sooner than those who were not resuscitated. Emergency IV access was most prolonged in children younger than 2 years of age. This last finding is important, because the majority of cardiopulmonary arrests in children occur in this younger age group.

If no IV line is available, appropriate drugs can be given via the endotracheal tube (see Chapter 26, Alternative Methods of Drug Administration) while attempts at venous access are initiated. Resuscitation courses aimed at enhancing the emergency care of children now stress the early use of intraosseous access[36] (see Chapter 25, Intraosseous Infusion). Indeed, current dicta call for attempts at IO or central venous access concurrently with attempts at peripheral venous access when managing a child undergoing CPR or in extremis from shock. The femoral vein is usually the central vein of choice in emergencies; its consistent anatomic location and large size make it the safest and easiest central vein to catheterize. The femoral vein also can be accessed with minimal interference to resuscitative efforts.

Umbilical Vein Catheterization

Indications and Contraindications

The major indication for umbilical vein catheterization is access to the vascular system for emergency resuscitation and stabilization of the newly born. The umbilical vein may also be used for exchange transfusions and short-term central venous access in newborns. The umbilical vein may remain patent for about a week after birth (sometimes longer).[56] In the neonate who presents to the ED requiring emergency access, a peripheral vein would be preferable, but attempting to cannulate one of the umbilical vessels could be life saving. The procedure is technically easier than umbilical artery cannulation.

Equipment and Setup

The supplies and equipment for catheterization are listed in Table 19–5. The infant is placed beneath a radiant warmer (keeping the infant warm during the procedure is critical), and the extremities are restrained. Oxygen is administered as needed, and the audible beep on the cardiac monitor is turned on. The operator should wear a mask, cap, gown, and sterile

TABLE 19–5 Umbilical Vein and Artery Catheterization Equipment

Infusion solution (usually $D_{5-10}W$ with electrolytes. Some clinicians also add 1 unit heparin per milliliter of fluid to "prevent" clotting in the catheter)

Fluid chamber, IV tubing, infusion pump, filter (0.22 μm), short length of IV tubing, three-way stopcock

Umbilical artery catheter (3.5 to 5 Fr)

3-0 silk suture on a curved needle

Curved iris forceps without teeth

Small clamps, forceps, scissors, needle holder

Sterile drapes

Light source

10 mL of heparinized solution for flush (1–2 units heparin per milliliter of fluid)

Surgical cap, mask, gown, and gloves

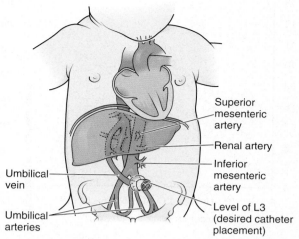

Figure 19–20 An umbilical vein catheter is directed toward the head and remains anterior until it passes through the ductus venosus into the inferior vena cava.

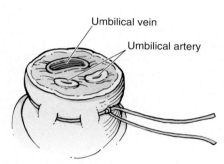

Figure 19–19 When placing an umbilical vein catheter, a pursestring suture or umbilical tape is passed around the base of the cord to provide hemostasis and to anchor the line.

gloves. Catheter length should be assessed prior to the procedure. Methods to estimate the best length for both umbilical vein and artery lines are discussed later.

Technique

Holding the umbilical stump up, the cord is scrubbed with a bactericidal solution. Pooling of liquid at the infant's side should be avoided, because this may be associated with blistering of the skin under a radiant warmer. The umbilical area is draped in a sterile fashion, with the infant's head left exposed for observation.

To provide hemostasis and to anchor the line after placement, a loop of umbilical tape or a pursestring suture is placed at the junction of the skin and the cord (Fig. 19–19). The cord is cut with a scalpel about 1 cm from the skin, and the vessels are identified. The vein is usually located at 12 o'clock and has a thin wall and large lumen. It may continue to bleed after cutting. The two arteries have thicker walls and smaller lumina, and constriction reduces bleeding after the vessels are cut. Occasionally, a persistent urachus may be mistaken for the umbilical vein, but the presence of urine should help correctly identify that structure.

The catheter (3.5 Fr [preterm infants] to 5.0 Fr [term infants]), which has been flushed with heparinized saline and attached to a three-way stopcock, is placed in the lumen of the umbilical vein and advanced gently. The catheter is advanced only 1 to 2 cm beyond the point at which good blood return is obtained. This is usually only 4 to 5 cm in a

term-sized infant. If the catheter is pushed farther than this, it may enter the *ductus venosus* and then move into the inferior vena cava, or it may enter a branch of the portal vein within the liver (evidenced by resistance at 5–10 cm).

The *inferior vena caval site* may be a desirable location in some newborn infants in whom peripheral vascular access is limited and for whom central venous access is desired for central venous pressure monitoring or infusion of medications, high concentrations of glucose (>10%), IV fluids, and hyperalimentation solutions. The catheter must be inserted approximately 10 to 12 cm in a term-sized infant to reach the inferior vena cava. Radiographs demonstrating the catheter in the liver will identify accidental entry into the portal vein. Note that an umbilical venous catheter will proceed directly cephalad (without making a downward loop) until it passes through the *ductus venosus* (Fig. 19–20).

Some practitioners use standardized graphs to estimate the length of insertion, which are based on the shoulder-to-umbilicus length (Fig. 19–21A). Such graphs are useful if stored in the drawers of the warming beds used to resuscitate newborns and small infants, along with the catheters and other equipment. Shoulder-to-umbilicus length is the perpendicular line measured from the tip of the shoulder to the horizontal level of the umbilicus. If the graph is not available, the shoulder-to-umbilicus length multiplied by 0.6 gives an approximate insertion length that will result in the tip of the catheter above the diaphragm but below the right atrium, in the inferior vena cava.[56] Formulae are also used to estimate catheter length based on birth weight,[57] but during a resuscitation, it is most prudent to gently pass the line only 4 to 5 cm in a term infant to avoid injecting hyperosmolar fluids into the portal vessels, which potentially could result in liver necrosis. Remember to account for the length of the umbilical stump in the calculation.

Air embolism may occur at the time of catheter removal if the infant generates sufficient negative intrathoracic pressure (as during crying) to cause air to be drawn into the patent umbilical vein. Therefore, caution must be used during catheter removal to ensure that the vein is promptly occluded (by tightening a pursestring suture or applying pressure on or just cephalad to the umbilicus).

343

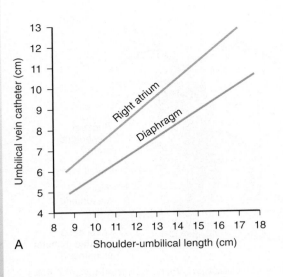

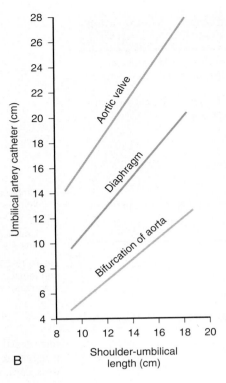

Figure 19–21 After measuring the shoulder-to-umbilicus length, a standardized graph can be used to determine the appropriate length of the umbilical venous catheter (*A*) or umbilical arterial catheter (*B*). The venous catheter should be inserted into the inferior vena cava below the level of the right atrium. The appropriate length of the arterial catheter depends on whether a "high" or "low" line is desired (see text for explanation). (*A* and B, *From The Johns Hopkins Hospital, Nechyba C, Gunn VL: The Harriet Lane Handbook: A Manual for Pediatric Home Officers, 16th ed. St. Louis, CV Mosby, 2002.*)

Complications

Complications of umbilical venous catheters include hemorrhage, infection, injection of sclerosing substances into the liver (resulting in hepatic necrosis), air embolism, catheter tip embolism, and vessel perforation.[52,58] It is most important that one follow careful technique in insertion and maintenance of catheters to minimize such complications.

Umbilical Artery Catheterization

Indications and Contraindications

Umbilical artery catheterization is a useful procedure in the care of newborn infants who require frequent monitoring of arterial blood gases and arterial blood pressure, fluid and medication administration, and exchange transfusions.[58] One of the two umbilical arteries may be cannulated for resuscitation purposes, but an umbilical vein is generally technically easier to cannulate and may be preferred in an emergency. Complications are discussed later, but one should avoid cannulating the arteries if omphalitis, peritonitis, necrotizing enterocolitis, or intestinal hypoperfusion is present.

Equipment and Setup

The equipment required for umbilical artery catheterization is identical to that used for umbilical venous catheterization (see Table 19–5). Additional equipment needed for continuous arterial pressure monitoring and infusion should be readily available. Catheter length should be estimated prior to starting the procedure. This can be done using a standard graph (see Fig. 19–21*B*) or a birth-weight regression formula.

Technique

The technique of umbilical artery catheterization is similar to that described for umbilical vein catheterization in the preceding section. After the umbilical arteries have been located,

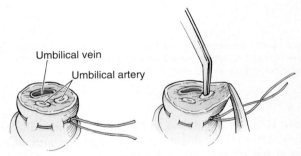

Figure 19–22 The umbilical cord is grasped with a curved hemostat near the selected artery. The umbilical artery is then dilated with a curved iris forceps.

the cord is grasped with a curved hemostat near the selected artery (Fig. 19–22). Having an assistant use two hemostats to grasp each side of the cord and slightly evert the edges can sometimes aid in exposure of the arteries. Using the curved iris forceps without teeth, one gently dilates the artery. Sometimes, repeated passes of the forceps are required because umbilical artery spasm may make the procedure difficult. A 3.5- to 5-French catheter attached to a three-way stopcock and flushed with a sterile heparinized solution may then be introduced into the dilated artery. A 3.5- to 4-French catheter is recommended for infants weighing less than 2 kg and a 5-French catheter for those weighing 2 kg or more.

When the catheter is being inserted, gentle tension should be placed on the cord in a cephalad direction, and the catheter should be advanced with slow, constant pressure toward the feet (Fig. 19–23). Resistance is occasionally felt at 1 to 2 cm and should be overcome by gentle, sustained pressure. If the catheter passes 4 to 5 cm and meets resistance, this generally indicates that a "false passage" through the vessel wall has occurred. Occasionally, one may bypass the per-

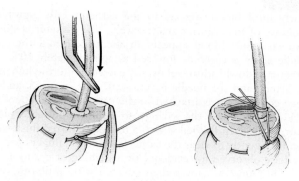

Figure 19–23 The catheter is introduced into the dilated artery and advanced toward the feet. The suture placed around the base of the cord is tied to the catheter.

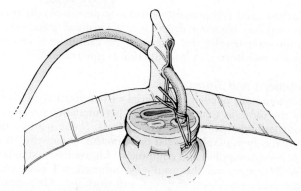

Figure 19–25 The tape is pleated above and below the catheter.

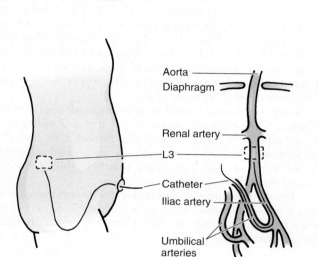

Lateral — Anterior

Figure 19–24 The umbilical artery catheter makes a loop downward before heading cephalad (schematic drawing of a radiograph interpretation).

foration by reattempting catheterization with the larger catheter.

The optimal position of the catheter tip in the descending aorta remains the subject of some debate.[59,60] If a "low line" is desired, the catheter may be advanced 7 to 8 cm in a 1-kg premature infant or 12 to 13 cm in a full-term infant. In the low position, the catheter tip should lie between L3 and L5, just above the aortic bifurcation. The renal and mesenteric vessels lie near L1, and the low position may decrease the incidence of complications owing to thrombosis in these vessels. If a "high line" is preferred, the tip of the catheter should lie above the diaphragm between T6 and T9. Graphs are available to estimate the proper catheter length for insertion of both the high and the low positions (see Fig. 19–21B). Alternatively, formulae based on birth weight may be used. These formulae may not be as accurate for babies at the extreme ends of the weight range. No unequivocal data are available to support superiority of one location over the other.

Once sterile technique is broken, the line may not be advanced. It is therefore preferable to position the catheter too high and to withdraw as necessary according to postinsertion radiographs, which will show the catheter proceeding from the umbilicus down toward the pelvis, making an acute turn into the internal iliac artery, continuing toward the head

into the bifurcation of the aorta, and then moving up the aorta slightly to the left of the vertebral column (Fig. 19–24). After it has been properly positioned, the catheter should be tied with the previously placed suture (see Fig. 19–23) and taped to the abdominal wall (Fig. 19–25).

Most unsuccessful umbilical artery catheterization attempts fail because the catheter perforates the arterial wall approximately 1 cm below the umbilical stump, where the umbilical artery begins curving toward the feet. In this instance, the catheter is advanced in the extraluminal space, and resistance is met at 4 to 6 cm.

Complications

Complications of umbilical artery catheterization include hemorrhage, infection, thromboembolic phenomena (especially to the kidneys, the gastrointestinal tract, and the lower extremities), aortic thrombosis, aortic aneurysm, vasospasm, air embolism, vessel perforation, peritoneal perforation, and hypertension.[58,61,62]

If the catheter becomes plugged or fails to function properly or if there is blanching or discoloration of the buttocks, the heels, or the toes, the catheter should be removed at once. Umbilical arteries are most easily cannulated in the first few hours of life but may provide a viable vascular route as late as 5 to 7 days of age.

Percutaneous Arterial Catheterization

Indications and Contraindications

Despite the growing use of noninvasive devices for monitoring transcutaneous oxygen and carbon dioxide, percutaneous peripheral arterial catheterization is indicated when there is a need for frequent blood gas sampling, continuous arterial blood pressure monitoring, or both. Arteries used for peripheral catheters in infants include the radial,[63] ulnar,[64] femoral,[65] temporal,[66] and posterior tibial arteries.[67]

Percutaneous radial artery catheterization has become widely accepted and has been shown to be safe in infants and children. The catheter allows for preductal blood gas determinations if placed in the right radial artery. Only the procedure for radial artery catheterization is described here, but catheterization of other vessels is similar.

Peripheral arterial catheterization is contraindicated when (1) adequate peripheral arterial samples can be obtained by percutaneous punctures, (2) circulation of the extremity to be catheterized is compromised, (3) occlusion of the vessel to be catheterized compromises extremity perfusion, (4) there is an ongoing bleeding diathesis, (5) localized infection or inflammation overlie the artery to be cannulated, and (6) intensive monitoring of line function is not available.

Equipment and Setup

The equipment needed for arterial catheterization is essentially the same as that required for percutaneous peripheral venous catheterization (see Table 19–4). Some centers use commercially available arterial line kits that come with all of the necessary supplies and equipment. Alternatively, standard 22- or 24-gauge over-the-needle IV catheters, a T-piece connector, and a three-way stopcock will work fine. One should connect the T-piece and the stopcock and then fill them with normal saline solution. An infusion pump with heparinized saline (1–5 U/mL) should be readied.[68]

Technique

The procedure should be performed with good lighting and an adequate work area, with the infant's heart and respiratory rates monitored closely. The radial artery may be palpated proximal to the transverse wrist crease on the palmar surface of the wrist, medial to the styloid process of the radius. Prior to the procedure, the artery should be compressed, and the hand and fingers are observed for color change. If blanching or cyanosis is noted (indicating poor collateral circulation), catheterization is not performed. If locating the artery by palpation is difficult, a transillumination device[69] or Doppler probe may be helpful.

The infant or child's hand and lower forearm are secured to an arm board with the wrist dorsiflexed 45° to 60° with the aid of a roll of gauze placed underneath. Care must be taken to leave the fingers exposed to assess the peripheral circulation. The radial artery is palpated at the point of maximal impulse and can be marked with a gentle indentation by one's gloved fingernail. The area over the radial artery is prepared with povidone-iodine or other antiseptic solution and washed with alcohol. Topical or local anesthetic (such as 1% lidocaine without epinephrine), or both, may be used at the planned insertion site. The catheter with needle is inserted through the skin just proximal to the transverse wrist crease at a 10° to 20° angle (Fig. 19–26). The catheter with needle is advanced

slowly until blood appears in the catheter hub, signifying puncture of the anterior arterial wall. The catheter is slowly advanced until blood appears in the needle and then the needle angle is carefully lowered to approximately 10°. The catheter is slowly advanced over the needle into the lumen of the artery, and the needle is removed. The stopcock and T-piece connector are attached to the catheter hub. The stopcock is opened to the syringe to confirm pulsatile blood return. It is then flushed with 0.5 mL heparinized flush solution very gently to clear the catheter while the fingers and the hand are observed for evidence of blanching or cyanosis.

The puncture site is then covered with antibiotic ointment, and the catheter is fixed to the skin by a thin piece of tape placed adhesive side up under the catheter hub and crossed over the catheter in a V shape. A second piece of tape is passed around and over the catheter hub and is fixed to the wrist (Fig. 19–27). A transparent sterile dressing such as Tegaderm (3M, St. Paul, MN) or OP Site (Smith and Nephew Medical, Massilon, OH) is often added for an additional layer of security and protection. A small piece of tape is used to attach the T-piece connector to the wrist area or to the splint. The fingers should be easily visible.

Only heparinized normal or half-normal saline is used for infusion. Some clinicians prefer to add 1 to 5 U of heparin/mL of infusion solution infused at a rate of 1 to 2 mL/hr. Medications, blood or blood products, amino acid solutions, IV fat solutions, and hypertonic solutions should not be infused through the catheter.

The catheter must be removed when there is evidence of blanching or cyanosis, when it is impossible to withdraw blood from the catheter, or when it becomes difficult to flush the catheter.

Complications

Complications, which have been reported with every type of arterial catheter, include hemorrhage, thrombosis, spasm, infection, scars, air embolism, retrograde blood flow, transient elevation in blood pressure with rapid (<1 sec) infusion, and nerve damage. Thrombosis or spasm may result in blanching or cyanosis of the extremity or skin.[58,70] There is potential for loss of digits, an entire extremity, or large areas of skin, as well as cerebral infarction with temporal artery catheters.[71] However, Saladino and workers[20] noted that complications from ED-placed arterial lines are uncommon and generally minor.

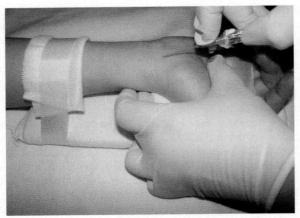

Figure 19–26 The catheter assembly is introduced into the radial artery through skin at a 10° to 20° angle. This is a smaller angle than that used for simple arterial puncture. Gloves should be worn.

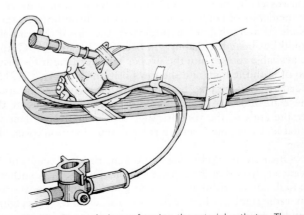

Figure 19–27 One technique of taping the arterial catheter. The arm board should be well padded and secured.

Arterial Cutdown Catheterization

Indications and Contraindications

Arterial catheterization by cutdown on the posterior tibial artery, radial artery, and temporal artery may be indicated when the need exists for frequent monitoring of arterial blood gases or blood pressure and percutaneous access is not possible.[67] Contraindications to arterial cutdowns are similar to those cited for percutaneous arterial catheterization and include (1) adequate peripheral blood gas samples can be obtained by percutaneous punctures or catheterization, (2) circulation of the extremity to be catheterized is compromised or occlusion of the vessel to be catheterized results in compromised perfusion of that extremity, (3) an ongoing bleeding diathesis, (4) localized infection or inflammation overlies the cutdown site; or (5) when intensive monitoring of line function is not available. Because of their experience with a wide variety of percutaneous vascular access techniques, emergency clinicians may find that percutaneous arterial catheterization is easier and likely to be more successful than performing an arterial cutdown.[72]

Equipment and Setup

Successful arterial cutdown catheterization in the small infant requires sterile instruments, an assistant, good lighting, and a selection of catheters. Previous clinical experience is always helpful. The equipment required for performing an arterial cutdown catheterization can be found on a cutdown tray, available in most EDs. Also needed are a 22- or 24-gauge over-the-needle catheter, T-extension connector tubing, a stopcock, a 5- or 10-mL syringe filled with flush solution (normal saline with 1–5 U heparin/mL), and silk suture ties. The operator prepares for the procedure by scrubbing and donning a mask, cap, gown, and sterile gloves.

Technique

The anatomy (Fig. 19–28) and technique for posterior tibial arterial cutdown are described in detail (Fig. 19–29). The same technique is applicable for the radial artery. The clinician stabilizes the foot in a neutral position by taping the externally rotated lower leg to a splint. The posterior tibial artery is then localized by Doppler ultrasound just posterior to the medial malleolus. The foot is prepared with a povidone-iodine or other antiseptic solution.

After subcutaneous injection of 1% lidocaine, a 5- to 7-mm transverse incision is made in the skin over the artery posterior to and at the midlevel of the medial malleolus (see Fig. 19–29A). Using blunt dissection in a vertical direction (parallel to the vessels), the tissue is separated with a small, curved forceps, and the artery is identified. The artery courses with the vein just anterior and superficial to the nerve and is usually pulsatile. Isolate the artery by sliding a small, curved forceps beneath it and gently elevating the vessel (see Fig. 19–29B). Excessive manipulation of the artery can cause spasm; if this occurs, a few drops of 1% lidocaine applied locally may result in dilation. A silk tie (without a needle) is then placed beneath the artery to stabilize it during cannulation.

At a 10° angle, a 22- or 24-gauge over-the-needle catheter is inserted bevel down into the artery over the surface of the forceps. When blood return is seen, the catheter is advanced over the stylet to its full length (Fig. 19–30). The

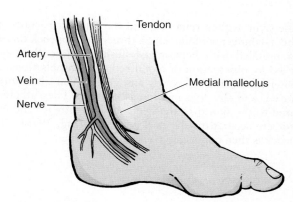

Figure 19–28 Anatomy of the posterior tibial artery and surrounding structures.

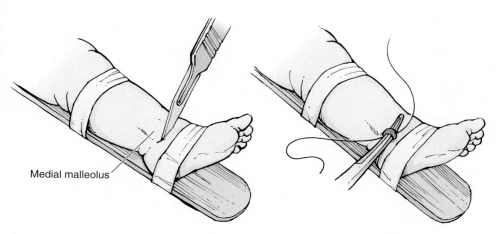

A

B

Figure 19–29 *A,* Posterior tibial artery cutdown technique. With the foot prepared and immobilized, a 5- to 7-mm incision is made in the skin posterior to and at the midline of the medial malleolus. *B,* A curved forceps and a silk suture are inserted beneath the posterior tibial artery, which courses just posterior to the medial malleolus.

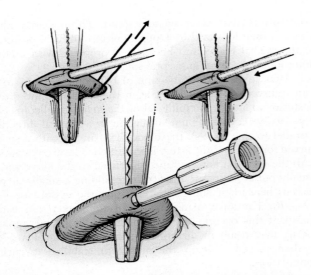

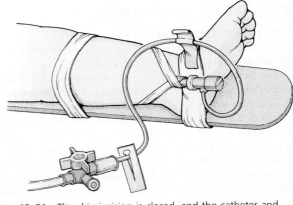

Figure 19–31 The skin incision is closed, and the catheter and connector are secured to the heel with tape.

Figure 19–30 **Technique of inserting the arterial catheter.** A silk tie is used only to stabilize the artery during cannulation. It is never tied. The catheter is inserted under direct vision without making an incision in the vessel.

needle stylet is then removed, and the catheter is connected to the T-connector tubing and a three-way stopcock that has been prefilled with heparinized flush solution. Patency is checked by observation of blood return with pulsations; the catheter is then flushed slowly and gently. The silk suture is removed, and the skin incision is sutured. The catheter is sutured to the skin over the heel, and the catheter and connector are secured to the heel with tape (Fig. 19–31). The stopcock is then connected to the infusion line.

Complications

The complications of arterial cutdown are similar to those of percutaneous arterial catheterization. They include hemorrhage, thrombosis, or spasm resulting in loss of tissue; infections; permanent scars; and nerve damage. These complications have been reported with all types of arterial cutdowns.

 REFERENCES CAN BE FOUND ON EXPERT CONSULT

CHAPTER 20

Arterial Puncture and Cannulation

Dave Milzman and Tim Janchar

Arterial puncture allows for the most accurate measure of blood sampling for true arterial blood gas (ABG) and acid-base determination. Arterial blood pressure is considered second only to heart rate as the most important vital sign. The absence of arterial blood pressure defines cardiac arrest and serves as the definitive end point of resuscitative efforts. Intra-arterial cannulation with continuous blood pressure transduction and display remains the accepted standard for comprehensive arterial pressure monitoring especially in critical patients and those on vasopressors. Intra-arterial monitoring of arterial pressure better reflects the force of systemic perfusion and is one of the most important determinants of cardiac work. Noninvasive technologies achieve near-equal performance and accuracies in most cases, but limitations need to be recognized.[1,2] Invasive modalities require expertise and sufficient support to prepare for accurate monitoring on a continual basis.

The father of Medicine, Hippocrates, was the first to suggest that the blood and arteries delivered life-giving energy to the body. Building on these ideas, the ancient Greek physician Galen first noted the existence of blood, although wrongly asserting that the heart constantly produced new blood. The idea of a pulse and pressure from circulating blood volume was not recognized until the Age of Enlightenment. The Spanish physician Severetus was among the first to accurately describe circulation in 1580 but most of his writings were destroyed when he was executed for his teachings. Soon after in 1616, William Harvey described circulation with a finite amount of blood and that the heart was the center of the circulatory system. Stephen Hales first recorded a blood pressure measurement in 1733, with a brass pipe inserted into a horse's artery and then connected to a glass conduit in which he observed blood rising and concluded that pressure was responsible. Early scientists reported utilizing surgical incision to obtain direct measurement of arterial pressure in animal models.[1,3]

J. L. M. Poiseuille first introduced the use of a mercury manometer for the measurement of blood pressure in 1828 in the severed artery of a goose. The first human measure of blood pressure was accomplished in 1847 by the kymograph developed by the German physiologist Carl Ludwig, with catheters directly inserted into the artery. Von Basch's design of the sphygmomanometer; a water-filled bag connected to a manometer, was the first to directly measure blood pressure with any accuracy. The utility of blood pressure measurement was not uniformly greeted as an innovation because older ideas on diagnoses were slow to change. Scipione Riva-Rocci did improve on the measurement by developing the prototype of the modern mercury sphygmomanometer in 1896 with an inflatable cuff placed over the upper arm to constrict the brachial artery and connected to a mercury-filled glass manometer. However, only the systolic blood pressure could be measured. The next major innovation came in 1905 when Nikolai Korotkoff described characteristic sounds heard with the stethoscope instead of palpation at certain points in cuff inflation and deflation that corresponded to systolic and diastolic blood pressure.

Advances came slowly until the space age in the 1960s introduced electrical monitoring of arterial pressure with transducers and recorders rather than mechanical devices, thus permitting mathematical waveform analysis in addition to visual analysis. More recent advances have included continuous, invasive monitoring of ABG values.[4] Such new improvements as continuous monitoring still require arterial puncture and cannulation. Currently, there are a growing number of noninvasive device and methods for accurate monitoring of arterial pressure; however, none match the proven accuracy of intra-arterial monitoring.

Arterial puncture is performed with reduced frequency mostly owing to fewer procedures and the growing acceptance of rapid venous pH in stat laboratory analysis. The traditional, macroscopic invasive approach may give way to noninvasive molecular analysis, capable of detecting changes in arterial oxygenation and perfusion before a measurable clinical presence. It is a distinct possibility that comprehensive noninvasive monitoring will be introduced and even become the standard before the next edition of this text.

INDICATIONS AND CONTRAINDICATIONS

Despite the increased use of noninvasive monitoring of respiratory functions and venous marker tests, many emergency department (ED) patients are subject to arterial puncture and some to arterial cannulation for the placement of arterial lines (Table 20–1). The use of arterial lines and continuous monitoring via the procedure is not standard in the ED, usually being performed in an intensive care setting. Nonetheless, arterial cannulation may be performed in the ED. The indications for direct arterial placement of an arterial catheter fall into three major categories[5,6]:

1. *Direct arterial blood sampling.* Catheter access removes the need for multiple arterial punctures and allows for either repeat arterial blood sampling or the placement of new sensors for continuous monitoring of blood gas and other chemistry values.
2. *Continuous real-time monitoring of blood pressure.* Patients with acute hypoperfusion and those receiving vasoactive drug infusion require the superior monitoring and moment-to-moment change detection afforded by arterial catheterization. Intraoperative and ICU care often is facilitated by arterial line placement.
3. *Failure or inability to use indirect blood pressure monitoring.* Some acutely ill patients such as those with severe burns, dialysis grafts and shunts, and morbid obesity may need ongoing perfusion monitoring that can best be accomplished by arterial catheterization.

Although acute respiratory decompensation and metabolic emergencies are the most common reasons for ABG sampling, all blood tests performed on venous blood are possible from an arterial sample. Blood cultures from an indwelling arterial line have a sensitivity and specificity equal to those of cultures obtained from a venipuncture site.[7,8] Patients with moderate respiratory decompensations may be managed without arterial puncture with continuous, noninvasive pulse oximetry, end-tidal carbon dioxide monitoring and newly

TABLE 20–1 Arterial Puncture and Cannulation

Indications	Relative Contraindications	Strict Contraindications
Blood gas sampling	Previous surgery in the area, especially cutdown	Inadequate circulation to the extremity
Continuous pressure monitoring		Raynaud's syndrome
Frequent need for blood sampling (ongoing resuscitation)	Anticoagulation, coagulopathy	Buerger disease (thromboangiitis obliterans)
Inotropic support—use of continuous infusion of vasoactive agents	Skin infection at the site, atherosclerosis	Full-thickness burns
Major surgery involving fluid shifts/blood loss and open heart procedures	Inadequate collateral flow	
Hypothermia (induced or severe exposure)	Partial-thickness burns	
Diagnostic angiography		
Therapeutic embolization		

acquired carboxyhemoglobin and methemoglobin monitoring,[9] but a role still exists for arterial blood sampling. The initial correlation between noninvasive values and acid-base status via arterial sampling is still imperative in critical illness to set a baseline or verify a trend. Metabolic and electrolyte monitoring often require additional arterial sampling, especially in patients with severe diabetic ketoacidosis who require frequent pH, electrolyte, and glucose measurements for accurate treatment.

Arterial versus Venous Analysis

Arterial sampling has been the traditional approach to evaluating acid-base abnormalities in the ill patient, especially those on a ventilator. In most ED settings, however, a *venous* pH determination may suffice for the initial or subsequent investigations of acidosis. Some still prefer to obtain an initial arterial sample, then follow the trend with venous blood analysis. Arterial versus venous blood analysis studies have demonstrated that venous blood (especially central venous blood) analyses for pH, bicarbonate, lactate, base excess, and carbon dioxide pressure (Pco_2) are within 95% limits of agreement with arterial sampling. These are relatively new data, generally extrapolated from hemodynamically stable patients, and further study may alter these initial conclusions in some subsets of patients. Arterial blood is required for an accurate oxygen pressure (Po_2) analysis.[10–12]

Arterial systolic and diastolic pressures can be continuously and accurately observed by arterial catheterization with an electromechanical pressure transducer attached to a monitor.[6] Such capabilities are routinely used in the operating room or ICU and can be useful when available in an ED for critically ill patients. Many interventions, such as the long-term use of vasoactive drugs (e.g., nitroprusside and norepinephrine), are best administered with continuous arterial pressure monitoring. The response of trauma and post–cardiac arrest patients to acute resuscitative efforts may also be more easily followed with the use of arterial catheterization.

Arterial puncture is used routinely by cardiologists and radiologists for interventional angiography. Angiography is becoming a less common indication for arterial puncture in the ED owing to advances in ultrasound, computed tomography with contrast, and rapid and routine magnetic resonance imaging with intravenous contrast. However, angiography is still considered for suspected cases of peripheral arterial trauma, suspected aortic injury, and aneurysmal or embolic disease.

Few contraindications to arterial puncture exist; none are absolute, but should always be considered on a risk-benefit evaluation. For example, post-thrombolysis, arterial cannulation should be performed only if it will provide essential data that cannot be obtained by any other method and the patient's condition requires ongoing assessments. Once a patient has received thrombolytic therapy, arterial cannulation should be avoided, but if necessary, a single arterial puncture of the readily compressible radial artery is preferred. Arterial puncture can be performed safely in patients who are anticoagulated or who have other coagulopathies, but should be undertaken with extreme caution in patients with disseminated severe coagulopathies.

There are reports of patients with complications from bleeding who require transfusion. Some patients, all of whom were anticoagulated at the time of puncture, suffered compression neuropathies secondary to hematomas as a result of arterial puncture.[13] Repeated arterial sampling in these patients should be accomplished by insertion of an indwelling cannula to minimize the number of puncture sites in the arterial wall and should be performed by only the most experienced clinicians.

The presence of severe arteriosclerosis, with or without diminution of flow, is only a relative contraindication to arterial puncture, especially when followed by cannulation. In hemodynamically precarious patients with advanced cardiovascular disease, invasive monitoring may be more valuable than most risks.[6] An alternative site should be considered if an isolated, decreased palpable pulse or bruit is felt over a selected site. Evidence of decreased or absent collateral flow in areas where flow normally exists, such as a positive Allen test (discussed later in the section on "Techniques"), should also lead one to consider an alternative site. One must avoid puncture of a specific arterial site when infection, burn, or other damage to cutaneous defenses exists in the overlying skin

EQUIPMENT: ARTERIAL PUNCTURE

Arterial Puncture with a Needle/Syringe

To obtain a single sample of arterial blood by the percutaneous method, a 3-mL syringe (preferred and most common) is attached to a needle. The needle size should vary based on puncture location and patient size and age. Most adults should have a 20-gauge, 2.5-inch needle for a femoral sample and a 1.25-inch, 22-gauge needle for a radial artery puncture. For pediatric arterial sampling, slightly shorter length needles in the range of 22 to 24 gauge should be used in the same sites as in adults.

Precoated blood gas plastic syringes (with dry lithium heparin) allow for longer shelf life and ready use and are commonly used. Such devices are designed to minimize sampling error due to heparin. If necessary, a regular syringe may be prepared with 1 or 2 mL of a heparinized saline solution (1000 IU/mL) drawn into the syringe to coat the barrel and needle. *Note that the heparin must be fully ejected through the needle immediately before puncture to minimize heparin-related errors.* Although the syringe may appear devoid of heparin, enough heparin remains in the needle and syringe to provide anticoagulation. Even dry heparin may produce ABG result abnormalities owing to a heparin-induced dilutional effect.[14] The newest blood gas and chemistry analyzers require only 0.2 mL of whole blood for accuracy, and some point-of-care devices can perform analyses on drops of blood. However, sample sizes aspirated in heparin-coated syringes with less than 1.0 mL of blood may result in heparin error to ABG values. *If 2 to 3 mL of blood are collected, heparin-related analysis problems are clinically inconsequential.* Precoated syringes require only *a minimum volume of 1 mL of blood* to prevent too large an impact of the dried heparin.

Stored heparin solution has a higher Po_2 and a lower Pco_2 than blood.[15] A dilutional effect from heparin would mean that the addition of 0.4 mL of heparin solution to a 2-mL sample of blood (dilution of 20%) will lower the Pco_2 by 16%.[14] Proper technique with dry lithium heparin–prefilled syringes, or *full ejection of excess heparin*, will prevent such problems if greater than 2 mL of blood is collected. A falsely low Pco_2 is the most clinically significant change caused by excess heparin.[14,15] *Neither Po_2 nor pH levels are significantly altered by the addition of heparin in most instances*, although a slight increase in Po_2 and a minimal decrease in pH may occur if high concentrations of heparin (25,000 IU/mL) are used.[16]

Continuous Monitoring via Arterial Catheter

The fluid-filled recording systems used with arterial cannulation have a great influence on the accuracy of pressure measurements. The frequency responses of tubing, transducers, and other components of the monitoring system influence the measurement accuracy of systolic and diastolic pressures. Failure to recognize recording system artifacts will lead to errors in pressure interpretation.[3]

Various catheter types have demonstrated similar frequency response characteristics, but some studies have found more variable effects on complication rates. There is some debate over complications due to catheter composition, such as possible increased thrombosis with Teflon catheters.[17,18] Another contributing element leading to thrombosis is catheter diameter; the incidence of thrombosis is inversely related to the ratio of vessel lumen to catheter diameter.[19,20] Thus, the risk of thrombosis decreases as the catheter diameter decreases. The incidence of thrombosis also increases with increased duration of catheter placement. The catheters coated with a combination of chlorhexidine and silver sulfadiazine have produced decreased infection rates than those of standard catheters.[21]

Puncture Site for Arterial Cannulation

There are specific recommendations relative to vessel and puncture site location. Table 20–2 lists the usual equipment for arterial cannulation, although the majority of prepackaged kits contain the most needed supplies (Fig. 20–1). Shorter catheters are ideal for peripheral artery cannulation, whereas a longer catheter using the Seldinger technique is preferable for the femoral artery

For arterial cannulation, a 16- to 18-gauge catheter should be used in adults for the femoral artery and 20 gauge in the radial artery. Small children and infants require a 22- to 24-gauge catheter, which may need to be inserted percutaneously via Seldinger or through a femoral cutdown technique. Older pediatric patients usually require 20- to 22-gauge catheters, based on the patient's size.

TABLE 20–2 Equipment for Insertion and Maintenance of an Indwelling Arterial Cannulation

Antiseptic solution
1% lidocaine (without epinephrine), usually 2–3 mL required for adequate site anesthesia, delivered by a 25- to 27-gauge needle.
10- × 10-cm dressing sponges
Arm board for brachial, radial, or ulnar cannulations
Appropriate-sized intravenous catheters
Syringes (3 cc and 5 cc for anesthesia, 5 cc for aspiration)
Pressure tubing
2 three-way stopcocks
Pressure transducer
Connecting wire
Monitor display
500- to 1000-mL bag of normal saline
Pressure blood infuser, set up with continuous flush device

Additional Equipment Required for Cutdown Insertion Technique

Scalpel blade (No. 11)
Tissue spreader, self-retaining
Two hemostats
Silk-ties 2-0, multiple
2-0 silk suture with straight needle
Needle driver with 2-0 nylon skin needle

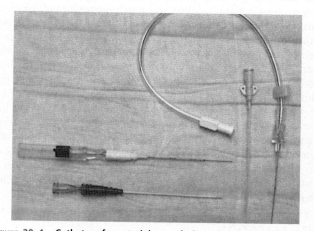

Figure 20–1 Catheters for arterial cannulation. A standard intracatheter for arterial cannulation may be used for direct vessel cannulation. Newer devices with a modified guidewire and quick-flash identifier (Arrow International, Inc., Reading, PA) or a needle with an attachable guidewire to aid cannulation are also available. *(Courtesy of J. Milzman.)*

The tubing that connects the catheter to the pressure transducer has a significant effect on monitoring system accuracy. The higher the frequency response of the entire system, the more accurate the determination of systolic and diastolic pressure; however, artifact also becomes more of a problem.[5,22] Stiff, low-capacitance plastic tubing should be used for arterial catheterization and monitoring. The electronic pressure transducer connection should be placed as close as possible to the patient and zeroed appropriately, because the frequency response of a tube is inversely related to its length.[22-24]

The pressure wave produced with each contraction is transmitted from the artery through the catheter and connecting tubing to a measuring device. The arterial fluid wave is received by an electromechanical transducer, which changes the mechanical pressure wave into an electrical signal that can be displayed on the monitor. With the use of minicomputers, various numerical values and hemodynamic parameters can be displayed or stored for future analysis. Currently, electronic transducers are most commonly used, but the technology is likely to change. The most basic system for obtaining blood pressure values uses a manometer, which has been used since antiquity as the standard reference for measuring pressure.[25] This technique may be quickly assembled if the materials are available; otherwise, except for historic purposes, the following description is superfluous for most practitioners.

A continuous method of pressure tubing flush is required to maintain the patency of the catheter lumen during intraarterial pressure monitoring. A three-way stopcock through which the tubing is intermittently flushed (a minimum of every 15–30 min) with saline is a simple, effective method. Continuous flush devices push a set amount of fluid (usually 2–3 mL/hr) through the line.[6] A typical monitoring system that includes this device is shown in Figure 20–2. The pressure transducer must be mounted at the level of the patient's heart. Current pressure monitoring setups include not only built-in stopcocks but also in-line flushing plungers to facilitate postsampling blood clearance.

Intravascular transducers were initially seen as an improvement over the external electromechanical transducer in use since the mid 1970s. The increased costs and many potential disadvantages have limited widespread use to this point. Many of the numerous brands are fragile, temperature-sensitive, of variable quality, and much more difficult to place into vessels than catheters. Anecdotal findings of fibrin deposition on these devices have been noted, but no reports have demonstrated any increased incidence of thrombus formation. The greatest advantage of these intravascular transducers is the continuous trending of arterial gas values and the elimination of potential error induced by catheters, stopcocks, and connecting tubing.[26,27] Despite obvious advantages, the use of these expensive, disposable devices has yet to penetrate many EDs. Usage of these devices is likely to happen only after the ICU and operating rooms widely adopt such devices.[4] So many transducer and monitor combinations exist that a discussion of their relative merits is beyond the scope of this chapter.

SITE SELECTION

The radial, brachial, and femoral arteries are the sites usually punctured for blood gas sampling in adults. Pediatric sites commonly used for arterial puncture include areas of the foot and the uterine artery in newborns.

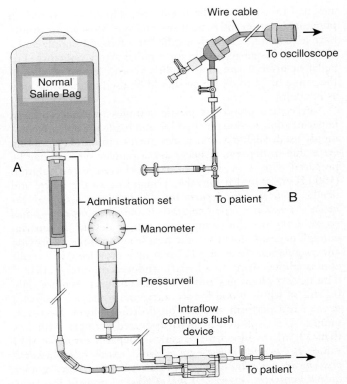

Figure 20–2 Arterial pressure monitoring systems. *A,* System for continuous flush. A 1-L bag of normal saline, pressurized to 250–300 mm Hg using a metered blood pump (not shown). The continuous flush device is set to deliver 3 mL/hr of the saline. A mechanical pressure transducer is depicted. The transducer device is a sterile, inexpensive, fully assembled monitor that can be used during patient transfer. Alternatively, the electronic transducer depicted in *B* may be used. *B,* System for manual flush. A saline flush solution can be injected manually through a syringe at the proximal or distal port. The transducer dome should be maintained at the level of the patient's heart. *(From Beal JM [ed]: Critical Care for Surgical Patients. New York, Macmillan, 1982. Reproduced by permission.)*

When an artery is cannulated for longer-term use, the potential consequence of complete blood flow loss through a vessel due to intraluminal thrombosis must be considered when choosing a site for arterial puncture. Because the most frequent complication of arterial catheterization is bleeding, the ability to control hemorrhage must also be considered. For these reasons, the radial and femoral arteries are favored owing to their good collateral blood flow and ease of compression in case of hemorrhage. Patient comfort and nursing care concerns also should be considered during site selection.

TECHNIQUES

Arterial Puncture

The arterial pulse is palpated to ascertain the location of the vessel, and the overlying skin is prepared sterilely with an antiseptic solution. The patient's skin should then be anesthetized with a wheal of local anesthetic (1% lidocaine) without epinephrine placed through a small needle (25 or 27 gauge). One study found no significant alterations in P_{CO_2} or pH from the pain or anxiety of an unanesthetized arterial puncture (Table 20–3).[28] If the patient is cooperative (with careful discussion of the procedure beforehand), in extremis,

TABLE 20–3 Parameters that Affect Interpretation of Arterial Blood Gases

Parameter	Heparin*	Air Bubble in Sample	Delayed Analysis‖
Po_2	No significant change†	Elevated	Variable¶
Pco_2	Lowered‡	No significant changes§	Elevated**
pH	Unchanged‡	No significant changes§	Lowered**

*Use only 1000 IU/mL concentration. Fill dead space of needle and syringe only and collect 3 mL of blood.
†There are reports of slight increases in Po_2 with excessive heparin.
‡The falsely lowered Pco_2 that occurs with added heparin is the most clinically significant change noted. pH may be decreased if a large volume of concentrated heparin (25,000 IU/mL) is used.
§If stored at 4°C for 20 min. Anaerobic storage at room temperature for 20 min results in no significant change.
¶Changes unpredictable at 20 min, regardless of storage method.
**Minimal changes up to 2 hr, if stored at 4°C.

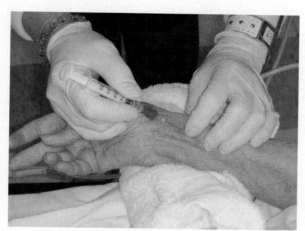

Figure 20–3 Arterial puncture. Hold the syringe like a dart, and observe for blood flow at the bottom of the syringe. The syringe-needle is held at a 30° to 45° angle and should enter with the *bevel up* and be *advanced slowly* to avoid transversing the artery. If bone is hit or no blood flows, slowly withdraw the needle and observe for blood flow. The landmark is best located by palpating the pulse using the tips of the index and middle fingers placed immediately proximal to the needle entry site and *along the course of the artery.* The needle should *not* be passed between the fingers owing to risk of operator self-injury.

or unresponsive to pain in the area to be punctured, this anesthetic infiltration may be omitted. If local anesthesia is to be performed, care must be taken to use a small amount of local anesthetic because a large wheal may obscure the pulse.

The arterial pulsation is then isolated with the index and middle fingers of the gloved, nondominant hand and the vessel course identified. The skin should be punctured through the anesthetic wheal, immediately distal to the palpated pulse under the index finger (Fig. 20–3). The older technique of placing the needle between the index and the middle finger risks self-puncture and is no longer advised. Hold the syringe like a dart, with the *bevel up*, and keep the syringe in view so blood flow can be immediately seen. The needle should be advanced slowly toward the pulsating vessel at approximately a 30° angle. A larger angle is required to puncture the deeper femoral artery. Once the needle enters the arterial lumen, the syringe plunger should be allowed to rise with the arterial pressure on its own in order to discriminate between arterial and venous sampling. As soon as blood flows, *stop needle advancement* and allow the syringe to fill. If no blood flow is

obtained, or if bone has been hit, the needle should be withdrawn slowly, because both walls of the vessel may have been punctured and the *lumen may be entered as the needle is withdrawn.* Redirection of the needle should occur only when the needle has been retracted to a location just deep to the dermis. After at least 1 to 2 mL of blood has been obtained, the needle is removed from the artery. Firm pressure is applied at the puncture site for a minimum of 3 to 5 minutes. If the patient is on anticoagulant therapy or has a coagulopathy, 10 to 15 minutes of pressure is required.

There are reports of using either a handheld Doppler or an ultrasound probe to assist in vessel location for both venous and arterial puncture and cannulation.[29] Ultrasound use is rapidly becoming standard in the clear majority of central vascular access placement procedures. The learning curve and perceived additional delay or expense may be exaggerated in some reports. Ultrasound and handheld Doppler have had increased usage owing to improved technology and decreased costs. Placement may still be attempted and accomplished with arterial palpation, but the standard is rapidly changing. The probe should be held over the artery proximal to the puncture site. An important indication of vessel identification is loss of audible pulsations with compression.

Proper handling of the sample and rapid analysis are very important. When the needle is withdrawn, it is imperative to expel any air bubbles present in the syringe to avoid false elevation of the Po_2.[30] Removal of air is neatly and easily accomplished by tapping the inverted syringe (needle pointing to the sky) to force any air to the top; then carefully and slowly depressing the syringe plunger to push out remaining air (Fig. 20–4). A gauze pad or alcohol wipe may collect any excess blood expelled with the syringe held upright and the plunger side down. The needle is removed and the syringe is capped to ensure anaerobic conditions. Air in the sample will significantly increase the Po_2 (mean increase, 11 mm Hg) after 20 minutes of storage, even if kept at 4°C. The pH and Pco_2 are not significantly altered by air bubbles if the blood is stored at 4°C for 20 minutes without significant deterioration.[16,30] If blood is stored at room temperature for longer than 20 minutes, the Pco_2 will increase and the pH will decrease, probably as a result of leukocyte metabolism. In a stored sample, the Po_2 varies to such an extent that the change is unpredictable for chemical interpretation at 30 minutes, regardless of storage method. High leukocyte or platelet counts, such as those seen in leukemic patients, may shorten acceptable storage intervals.[31,32]

In summary, ABG samples should always be kept on ice and analyzed within 15 to 20 minutes. Samples that cannot

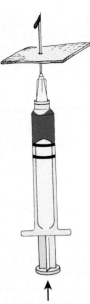

Figure 20–4 Removal of air bubbles from the syringe. Air bubbles are finger-tapped to the top of the syringe. An alcohol swab is placed over the top of the needle. The plunger is advanced to expel air while drops of blood are collected on the alcohol swab. After the bubbles are removed, the syringe is capped and sent to the laboratory.

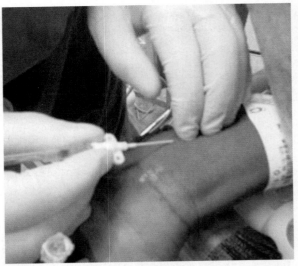

Figure 20–5 Proper technique is demonstrated by the operator for palpation of radial artery distal to the introducer needle instead of finding the pulse between two fingers. This 20-gauge 2-inch catheter over the needle wire assembly is the preferred device for rapid radial artery line cannulation. Note the small flash of blood at the hub of the catheter signaling time to advance the guidewire, once adequate flow is confirmed. *(Courtesy of M. Milzman, MD.)*

be analyzed within the timeframe should be considered faulted because they will not reflect real-time patient perfusion or oxygenation status.

PERCUTANEOUS TECHNIQUE FOR ARTERIAL CANNULATION

Direct Over-the-Needle Catheter Cannulation

Placement of an angiocatheter directly into an arterial lumen in a manner similar to placement of an intravenous catheter is the most practiced and simplest method, but it is not always successful owing to technical difficulties (Figs. 20–5 and 20–6). The only routine site for this technique is the radial artery. Although other sites, namely the femoral artery, may be attempted, use of a catheter over a guidewire using the Seldinger technique is strongly advised at most other sites (Figs. 20–7 and 20–8).

The operator should always remember to take time for proper alignment of the desired site. Delays, complications, and inability to successfully cannulate an artery often occur owing to failure to properly prepare the desired site and involved limb. An important preparatory step is to ensure that the target limb is secured flat and not rotated; any rotation could result in the desired artery being shifted from the expected anatomic position, making it more difficult to cannulate. For example, to adequately prepare the radial artery, the wrist and hand should be immobilized in mild dorsiflexion with some padding for support underneath the wrist. As usual, sterile skin preparation and local anesthetic injection using a 25-gauge or smaller needle with sufficient infiltration to ensure a painless procedure can then be performed. The subcutaneous infiltration of lidocaine or similar anesthetic may reduce vessel spasm at the time of arterial puncture.

The catheter assembly should be checked for proper movement and function. Alternatively, a 3-mL syringe with

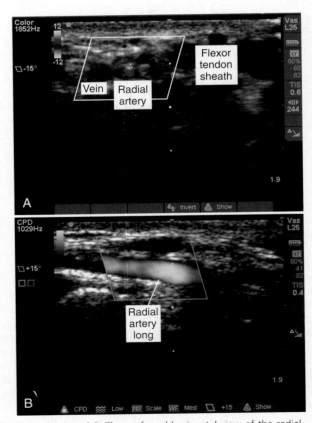

Figure 20–6 *A* and *B,* The preferred horizontal view of the radial artery for arterial line placement with color-flow Doppler. Note the flexor tendon sheath medially. Remember that the radial artery will not be compressible. *(A and B, Courtesy of Michael Antonis, MD.)*

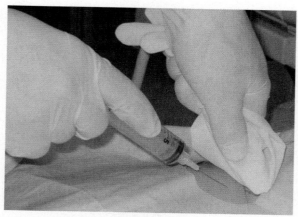

Figure 20–7 Single-person, ultrasound-guided vascular access. Usually, the operator's nondominant hand is used to hold the sterile glove–encased ultrasound probe and the syringe, which allows easy aspiration with the dominant hand. The horizontal axis is preferred for vessel identification. *(Courtesy of Michael Antonis, MD.)*

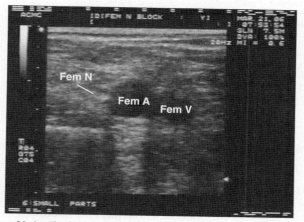

Figure 20–8 The horizontal axis view of the femoral vein, artery, and nerve from medial to lateral, respectively. *(Courtesy of Michael Antonis, MD.)*

the plunger removed could be used as a blood reservoir. The catheter is advanced toward the palpated artery at a comfortable angle for the operator, generally 30° to 45° from the skin. Making a small nick with a No. 11 scalpel or a larger-bore needle will eliminate the problem of catheter damage from kinking on the skin. The needle tip is often perceived to pierce the artery, but successful puncture is confirmed by identifying a "flash" of arterial blood flow into the needle hub and reservoir. As the needle-catheter assembly advances through the skin toward the artery, the initial flash of arterial blood is obtained by the needle alone, which protrudes beyond the catheter. For this reason, the needle-catheter should be lowered and advanced 2 mm forward to ensure that the catheter tip has cannulated the vessel, along with the needle. Confirmation of the catheter within the vessel lumen will be seen as continued arterial blood return. The catheter alone can now be advanced with care over the needle into the artery. If the catheter fails to thread, it has not properly entered the vessel lumen and should not be forced to advance without active blood return confirming placement.

When blood flow into the needle-catheter has ceased, it is likely to have pierced the backside of the artery wall. This double-puncture method is useful for cannulating small vessels, yet it is not recommended as a routine procedure to the inexperienced clinician.[5] If double puncture has occurred and blood has ceased to flow into the collection reservoir, the entire needle-catheter assembly should not be removed. Instead, simply retract the needle slightly to determine whether blood flow into the catheter can be reestablished. If blood flow occurs, gently advance the catheter. If not, the catheter should be slowly withdrawn until pulsatile blood flow reappears and then the catheter can be advanced into the artery. The important point is for the clinician to be aware whether the needle tip or the catheter is the leading edge within the vessel.[5]

Once the catheter is fully advanced into the vessel lumen, occlusive pressure is held transiently on the proximal artery to limit blood loss, and the needle is removed. A narrow-bore, low-compliance pressure tubing is then fastened to the catheter. An appropriate sterile dressing should be applied after the apparatus has been securely sutured to the wrist.

Occasionally, one will encounter difficulty advancing the catheter into the lumen. The "liquid stylet" method may aid further passage of the catheter.[33] A 10-mL syringe should be filled with about 5-mL of sterile normal saline. The syringe is then attached to the catheter hub, and 1 to 2 mL of blood should be easily aspirated to confirm intraluminal position. The fluid from the syringe is then slowly injected, and the catheter is advanced behind the fluid wave. Alternatively, a more popular method is to use a guidewire that easily passes into the vessel lumen.[34,35] This modified Seldinger technique is discussed fully in the next section.

The number of repeat attempts with additional arterial punctures increases the size of the developing hematoma and the real risk of vessel wall damage, thrombosis, and even loss of arterial flow through the vessel. Despite the added trauma, there is no reported increase in complications when both walls, rather than one, are punctured from a single cannulation attempt.[36–38]

Guidewire Techniques for Arterial Cannulation

Using a "modified" Seldinger technique can often rescue a failed over-the-needle catheter, direct cannulation attempt. If the catheter has been placed in the arterial lumen with blood return, a proper-sized guidewire may be gently passed through the catheter into the artery. The catheter should then be advanced fully into the vessel over the guidewire. The clinician is cautioned that stiffer guidewires, unlike most prepackaged ones, do not have a softer, more flexible, end tip and the vessel wall may be damaged, even perforated with excessive force. Alternatively, catheter sets are available with an attachable, catheter-contained, wire stylet that permits a modified Seldinger technique for catheter placement. The over-the-needle catheter follows the self-contained guidewire during cannulation. Numerous commercially available sets feature differing styles of guidewire and reservoir attachments to an over-the-needle catheter assembly. Most resemble the Arrow arterial catheterization system (Arrow International, Inc., Reading, PA) (Fig. 20–9). These kits are extremely practical for smaller vessels, especially radial, brachial, and axillary arteries, and have excellent success rates at first-time placement. Although some authors have suggested that guidewire-based techniques will improve arterial cannulation success rates in some patients,[35] it appears that success is more a function of operator experience and personal preference.[39]

General instructions for use of radial artery set

1. Prepare puncture site in preferred manner.
2. Peel open package and remove entire unit.
3. Remove protective shield. Trial advance and retract spring-wire guide through needle via actuating lever to ensure proper feeding. *Note:* Catheter hub wing clip can be "snapped" out of groove and removed if desired. This allows suture ring on hub to be optionally used for attachment to skin after placement.
Caution: Before insertion, actuating lever must be retracted proximally as far as possible so as not to inhibit blood flashback.
4. Puncture vessel using a continuous, controlled, slow forward motion, being careful to avoid trans-fixing both vessel walls. Blood flashback in clear hub of introducer needle indicates successful entry into vessel (A).
Caution: If both vessel walls are punctured, advancement of spring-wire guide could result in inadvertent subarterial placement.

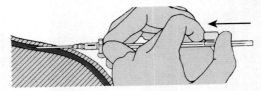

B

6. Advance the entire placement unit a maximum of 1 to 2 mm farther into the vessel.
7. Firmly hold clear introducer needle hub in position and advance catheter forward to track spring-wire guide into vessel. If difficulty is encountered during catheter advancement, a slight rotating motion of catheter hub may be helpful (C).

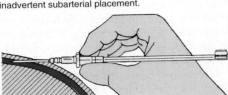

A

5. Stabilize position of introducer needle and carefully advance spring-wire guide (via actuating lever) distally as far as possible into vessel (B). Reference mark on clear feed tube indicates approximate actuating lever advancement position at which soft tip of spring-wire guide coincides with tip of needle.
Caution: If resistance is encountered while advancing spring-wire guide, *do not force feed and do not retract spring-wire guide while in vessel* (to avoid damaging wire). Withdraw entire unit and attempt new puncture.

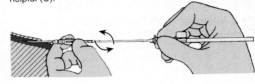

C

8. Hold catheter in place and remove introducer needle, spring-wire guide, and feed tube assembly. Free blood flow indicates successful placement in vessel.
Caution: Do not reinsert needle into catheter.
9. Attach desired stopcock, injection cap, or connecting tubing to catheter hub.
10. Secure catheter to patient in preferred manner, using wing clip or suture ring as described in step 3.
11. Cover puncture site with suitable dressing.

Figure 20–9 Step-by-step arterial cannulation, using the guidewire technique (Arrow arterial catheterization kit). *(Courtesy of Arrow International, Inc., Reading, PA.)*

Seldinger Technique

An alternative to placing an indwelling cannula is the Seldinger technique,[34] which is described in detail for venipuncture in Chapter 22, Central Venous Catheterization and Central Venous Pressure Monitoring. Overall success rates with the Seldinger, guidewire-directed technique are superior to direct arterial cannulation.[39] A few available kits are designed specifically for larger-artery cannulation, but single-lumen venous catheters with guidewires may be used if catheter size and length are appropriate for specific arteries (see the following section for guidelines). Guidewire technique should be used initially for critical patients.

A needle is percutaneously placed into the arterial lumen, as described previously. A guidewire is then placed through the needle into the vessel lumen, and the needle is removed. A catheter is then threaded over the wire, and the wire is pulled out. Although most kits have vessel dilators, especially with larger catheter sizes, caution is advised. Only the tract should be dilated, not the artery, to avoid unnecessary blood loss and excessive arterial injury.

Cutdown Technique for Arterial Cannulation

This cutdown technique is rarely practiced, but in certain circumstances, it may be used to obtain arterial access. With the increased use of ultrasound-assisted catheter placement, this technique should rarely be required. Cannulation is performed after direct visualization of the vessel. A cutdown can be performed on any artery but is most commonly reserved for distal lower limb

arteries and, rarely, the brachial. After a site has been selected, the overlying skin should be surgically prepared with an antiseptic solution. Using sterile technique, local anesthetic solution is injected subcutaneously in a horizontal line 2 to 3 cm long and perpendicular to the artery. This step may be omitted if the patient is unconscious or otherwise anesthetic at the cutdown site.

Using a scalpel with a No. 10 or 15 blade, the skin is incised along the anesthetic wheal. Underlying tissues are spread parallel to the artery with a mosquito hemostat. The pulse is palpated repeatedly throughout the procedure to ensure proper positioning. Once the surrounding soft tissue has been removed, and after exposing approximately 1 cm of the artery, it should be isolated by passing two silk sutures underneath it, using the hemostat. Strip away only enough perivascular tissue to expose the artery. Perivascular tissue will help limit bleeding at the time of catheter removal. An over-the-needle catheter device, such as that used in the percutaneous method, is then introduced through the skin just distal to the incision and advanced into the surgical site (Fig. 20–10).[33] Alternatively, a modified Seldinger guidewire setup may be used to catheterize the artery. The arterial wall is punctured with the needle tip, and the catheter is threaded into the vessel lumen. When this has been accomplished, two silk sutures, which have been used only to control the vessel, are removed, and the skin incision is closed. *The artery is not tied off as the vessel would be during a venous cutdown.* Firm pressure, as used after arterial puncture, should be applied over the cutdown site. The separation of the soft tissue during the procedure may allow considerable hemorrhage into the tissue if pressure is not applied.

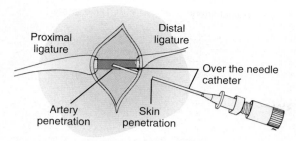

Figure 20–10 **Placement of an arterial line using the cutdown technique.** Note that the catheter enters the surgical wound percutaneously to minimize bacterial entry into the healing wound and permit better stabilization of the catheter. Catheter entry of the vessel is more parallel to the vessel than is illustrated. Ligatures are used only to *temporarily* isolate the artery and to control bleeding. *The artery should not be tied off.* The catheter is secured by suturing the hub to the skin (see Fig. 20–9).

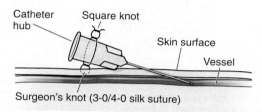

Figure 20–11 A technique for securing a vascular catheter to adjacent skin.

Local Puncture Site and Catheter Care

Once the catheter has been placed successfully, it should be advanced until the hub is in contact with the skin. The catheter is then secured by fastening it to the skin with suture material. Silk (2-0) or nylon (4-0) sutures provide the best anchoring. To accomplish this, a moderate bite of skin is taken with the needle, and a knot is tied in the suture, leaving both tails of the suture long. Take care to avoid pinching the skin too tightly. The loose ends of the suture should then be tied around the catheter at its hub. Then, after laying two ties, a second set of knots should be placed on the back portion without occluding the lumen by constriction (Fig. 20–11).

After tying the catheter in place, a drop of antibiotic ointment is applied to the puncture site,[40] and a self-adhesive dressing is applied over the area. The catheter and its connecting tubing are further secured with sterile sponges and adhesive tape. All tubing connections must be tight and secure. If the tubing becomes disconnected inadvertently, the patient may exsanguinate rapidly.

Fluid-Pressurized Systems

When successful arterial cannulation has been performed, the catheter should be attached to a pressurized fluid-filled system. A three-way stopcock is commonly interposed between the patient and the transducer for blood gas sampling and to allow flushing of the system. Flushing can be periodic or continuous at a rate of 3 to 4 mL/hr through a continuous flow device. Most institutions use normal saline in place of heparinized solution to maintain patency. There is no significant difference for patency. However, a heparinized flush solution in

pressurized arterial lines results in greater long-term accuracy of pressure monitoring, but no real difference in catheter blockage has been reported.[41]

Literature review supports the use of normal saline solution for maintaining patency of intermittent vascular catheters. In one study,[42] a change to normal saline solution as an alternative to heparinized saline solutions (2 mL 1:1000 heparin/L of saline) to maintain arterial line patency resulted in elimination of heparin-associated risks such as drug incompatibilities, thrombosis, local tissue damage, and hemorrhage. In addition, decreased potential for infections, substantial money savings, and decreased nursing time make it an attractive alternative. However, some studies found that the use of saline as a continuous flush for radial artery catheters is associated with an increased frequency of catheter occlusion and malfunctions compared with solutions containing heparin.[43,44] For short-term setups as in the ED, saline is sufficient. Later change to heparinized flush is an option depending on prevailing practice within the ICUs of the institution.

Procurement of a blood sample from the arterial catheter system is easily performed. A syringe is attached to the three-way stopcock, and blood is aspirated and discarded to clear the line. Studies examining the necessary discard volume of flush-blood solution have found considerable variation, depending on the volume of the system.[45,46] Short lengths of tubing between the catheter and the aspiration port minimize the discard volume. For a tubing length of 91 cm (36 inches), 4 to 5 mL should be aspirated[46]; for a tubing length of 213 cm (84 inches), 8 mL should be aspirated.[45] A second syringe, which has been heparinized, is then attached, and 3 mL of blood is aspirated and sent for blood gas analysis. If the blood is to be used for other tests, the second syringe does not need to be heparinized. This 4 to 8 mL of "waste" blood can be replaced intra-arterially only if institutional practice allows for this practice. Self-contained, nondetachable blood sample withdraw systems allow for less blood wasting for sampling. The stopcock and line should be flushed after sampling to avoid clotting.

SELECTION OF ARTERIES FOR CANNULATION
Radial and Ulnar

The radial artery is most frequently used for prolonged cannulation. Widespread collateral flow exists in the wrist owing to two major palmar anastomoses known as *arches* (Fig. 20–12). The superficial palmar arch lies between the aponeurosis palmaris and the tendons of the flexor digitorum sublimis. The arch is formed mainly by the terminal ulnar artery and the superficial palmar branch of the radial artery. The other major communication of these two vessels, the deep palmar arch, is formed by connections of the terminal radial artery with the deep palmar branches of the ulnar artery.[47] Some collateral flow is almost always present at the wrist, with the deep arch alone being complete in 97% of 650 hand dissections at autopsy.[48] Despite these findings, Friedman[49] noted the absence of palpable ulnar pulses in 10 of 290 (3.4%) healthy children and young adults. Interestingly, this was always a bilateral finding. Radial pulses were present in all subjects.

Before attempting radial artery cannulation, assess the adequacy of collateral flow to the hand by performing a bedside examination. This examination was originally described by E. V. Allen in 1929[50] and used to assess arterial stenosis in the hands of patients with thromboangiitis oblit-

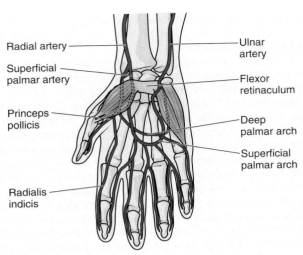

Figure 20–12 Arterial anatomy of the hand and wrist. *(From Ramanathan S, Chalon J, Turndorf H: Determining patency of palmar arches by retrograde radial pulsation. Anesthesiology 42:758, 1975. Reproduced by permission.)*

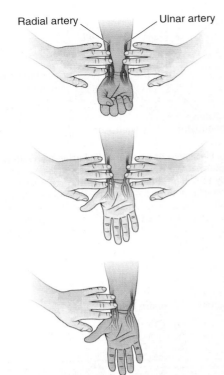

Figure 20–13 **Allen test.** Before puncturing the radial artery for cannulation, it is important to identify a competent ulnar artery should injury to the radial artery occur. This is generally not required, nor standard, for a single arterial puncture. Procedure: *(1)* The examiner compresses both arteries to occlude arterial flow, and the patient repeatedly makes a tight fist to squeeze venous blood out of the hand. Alternatively, the hand may be squeezed first, and then the arteries occluded. *(2)* The patient then extends the fingers, and the examiner observes the blanched hand. *(3)* Compression of the ulnar artery is released, and the examiner observes the hand filled with blood, signifying good flow in the radial artery. If filling does not occur within 5 to 10 seconds, radial artery puncture should not be done. If brisk filling occurs, the test is then repeated with release of the radial artery to assess radial artery patency. If both radial and ulnar arteries demonstrate patency, the wrist may be used for arterial cannulation and puncture. *(From Schwartz GR [ed]: Principles and Practice of Emergency Medicine. Philadelphia, WB Saunders, 1978, p 354. Reproduced by permission.)*

erans. The Allen test is performed to identify patients with increased risk for ischemic complications from radial artery catheterization. The procedure has seen many modifications[51,52] since originally being described in a cooperative patient. The basic Allen test is performed as follows: The examiner occludes both the radial and the ulnar arteries with digital pressure, and the patient is asked to tightly clench the fist repetitively to exsanguinate the hand. The hand is then opened, and the examiner releases the occlusion of the ulnar artery (Fig. 20–13). After 2 minutes, the test is repeated with release of the radial artery. Rubor should return rapidly to the hand with release of pressure from either vessel.

An abnormal (positive) Allen test, suggestive of inadequate collateralization, is defined as the continued presence of pallor 5 to 15 seconds after release of the artery.[19,34,52,53] If the return of color takes longer than 5 to 10 seconds, radial artery puncture should not be performed. Be careful to avoid overextension of the hand with wide separation of the digits, which may compress the palmar arches between fascial planes and give a false-positive result.[54] Time permitting, performance of some variation of the Allen test is desirable before ulnar or radial puncture for prolonged cannulation. This test is not considered mandatory or standard for one-time radial artery puncture for blood gas sampling.

The true predictive value of the Allen test is still questioned, because there are numerous reports of permanent ischemic sequelae postcannulation after a normal Allen test.[52,55,56] Notably, other studies have found no ischemic complications following radial artery catheterizations after abnormal Allen tests.[37,57] Although there are no guarantees against digital ischemia after radial artery cannulation,[58] the finding of an abnormal Allen test should result in the search for an alternative site. If available, this alternative arterial site should be used and the abnormal Allen test documented for medicolegal reasons.

Once adequate collateral flow has been ascertained, arterial puncture may be performed. At the wrist, the radial artery rests on the flexor digitorum superficialis, flexor pollicis longus, pronator quadratus and against the radius.[48] The pulsation of the artery should be isolated on the palmar surface of the wrist. The radial artery is more superficial closer to the wrist and provides a more consistent cannulation owing to fixation and less mobility. Dorsiflexing the wrist at about a 60° angle over a towel or sandbag, preferably fixing the wrist to an arm board, will also significantly help isolate the artery. This degree of preparation should be considered standard when time for setup is allowable (Fig. 20–14).[36,37]

Antegrade radial artery cannulation may be accomplished in infants and children when radial arteries are obstructed and retrograde blood flow is observed during a failed cutdown attempt at standard retrograde arterial cannulation.[59] In addition, displacement of perivascular interstitial fluid in neonates and bright light make the course of the artery visible so that under direct vision, cannulation of the artery becomes as easy as venous cannulation.[60] Doppler ultrasound use on select patients with poor peripheral pulses may facilitate percutaneous radial artery cannulations and minimize the number of punctures needed for placement.[29]

The ulnar artery is seldom used because its smaller size makes it more difficult to puncture than the radial artery. At the wrist, the ulnar artery runs along the palmar margin of the flexor carpi ulnaris in the space between it and the flexor

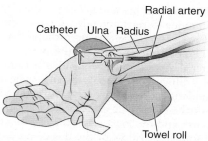

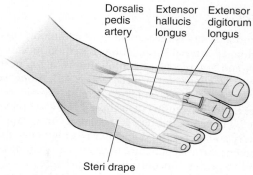

Figure 20–14 Percutaneous arterial cannulation at the wrist. The catheter unit is advanced 1 to 2 mm into the vessel lumen after blood first appears in the flash chamber. While the needle is fixed, the catheter is threaded over the needle.

Figure 20–16 A 20-gauge catheter in the dorsalis pedis artery illustrates the relationship to surrounding tendons. The catheter is secured with Steri-Drape. Splinting is not needed. *(From Johnstone RE, Greenhow DE: Catheterization of the dorsalis pedis artery. Anesthesiology 39:655, 1973. Reproduced by permission.)*

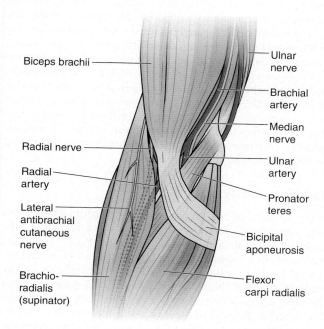

Figure 20–15 The right brachial artery and its branches. *(From Christensen JB, Telford IR [eds]: Synopsis of Gross Anatomy. New York, Harper & Row, 1972, p 304. Reproduced by permission.)*

digitorum sublimis.[48] Caution is necessary because the artery runs next to the ulnar nerve as both pass into the hand just radial to the pisiform bone. The ulnar artery can also be made more accessible with dorsiflexion of the wrist.

Brachial

The brachial artery appears safe for arterial puncture, but it does not have the anatomic benefit of the collateral circulation found in the wrist. The brachial artery begins as the continuation of the axillary artery and ends at the head of the radius, where it splits into the ulnar and the radial arteries. The preferred puncture site of the brachial artery is in or just proximal to the antecubital fossa. In this region, the artery lies on top of the brachialis muscle and enters the *fossa* underneath the bicipital aponeurosis with the median nerve occupying the medial side of the artery (Fig. 20–15). Both the radial and the axillary arteries are preferred upper extremity sites to the brachial artery. There is an increased ischemic complication risk from reduced collateral circulation as well as the necessity

of maintaining the arm in extension for puncture or prolonged cannulation. Despite all of these theoretical possibilities, the safe cannulation of the brachial artery has been demonstrated by some investigators.[61] Bazaral and coworkers[62] found only 1 minor thrombotic occurrence in more than 3000 brachial artery catheterizations over 3 years in cardiac surgery patients. A longer catheter (10 cm) is required for the brachial artery so that sufficient length is available to traverse the elbow joint.

Dorsalis Pedis

The dorsalis pedis artery continues from the anterior tibial artery and runs from approximately midway between the malleoli to the posterior end of the first metatarsal space, where it forms the dorsal metatarsal and deep plantar arteries. The lateral plantar artery, a branch of the posterior tibial, passes obliquely across the foot to the base of the fifth metatarsal. The plantar arch is completed where the lateral plantar artery joins the deep plantar artery between the first and the second metatarsals. On the dorsum of the foot, the dorsalis pedis artery lies in the subcutaneous tissue parallel to the extensor hallucis longus tendon and between it and the extensor digitorum longus (Fig. 20–16).[63]

The artery should be cannulated in the midfoot region. Although this vessel is amenable to cutdown, the vascular anatomy of the foot is quite variable. This is of no consequence if a pulse can be palpated, but Huber,[64] in his dissection of 200 feet, noted the dorsalis pedis artery was absent in 12% of patients. In 16% of patients, the dorsalis pedis artery provides the main blood supply to the toes.[65] Although the dorsal pedis and posterior tibial arteries form similar collateral foot circulation as in the hand, the nature of advancing vascular disease makes this a more difficult cannulation, with increased complication rates compared with those in the wrist. Nevertheless, this site has its major utility in pediatric monitoring cases. Attempts to predetermine collateral flow with a modified Allen test using the posterior tibial and dorsalis pedis arteries is not as easily performed in the foot as in the hand, nor are there good data to prove its validity. Monitoring problems also exist with this artery. The pressure wave obtained with an electronic transducer attached to the dorsalis pedis artery will be 5 to 20 mm Hg higher than that of the radial artery and, in addition, will be delayed by 0.1–0.2 seconds.[63]

Femoral

The femoral artery is the second most commonly used vessel for prolonged arterial cannulation. Based on its ease of cannulation and low record of complications, it has been called the vessel of choice for arterial access.[66-68] Along with the axillary artery, the femoral artery more closely resembles aortic pressure waveforms than those from any other peripheral site.[5] The femoral artery is the direct continuation of the iliac artery and enters the thigh after passing below the inguinal ligament. Arterial puncture must always occur distal to the ligament to prevent uncontrolled hemorrhage into the pelvis or peritoneum.[69] The artery may be easily palpable midway between the public symphysis and the anterior superior iliac spine. The advantage of cannulating the artery at a site just distal to the inguinal ligament is that the artery is very compressible against the fermoral head. Cannulation becomes more difficult the more distal the puncture site is from the inguinal ligament as the femoral artery splits into the superficial femoral and the deep femoral. These arteries, especially the deep femoral, can be challenging to compress if bleeding needs to be controlled. One method of locating an appropriate arterial puncture site is to place the thumb and fifth finger on the pubis symphysis and the anterior iliac spine and locate the artery underneath the middle knuckle. When puncturing this vessel, care must be taken to avoid the femoral nerve and vein, which create the lateral and medial borders, respectively (Fig. 20–17).

A longer, larger-diameter catheter is required for accurate monitoring of the femoral artery owing to the relatively greater depth at which it lies and greater vessel size. Only the Seldinger technique is recommended for this site, enabling placement of a 15- to 20-cm plastic catheter for prolonged monitoring. Use of catheter-through-the-needle or over-the-needle catheter devices should be avoided because cannulating the vessel is difficult owing to its distance beneath the skin. Leakage around the catheter can occur with catheter-through-the-needle or over-the-needle catheter devices owing to high arterial pressures and the loose fit of the cannula in the hole in the vessel wall. Regardless of the device used, the needle should enter the skin at an angle of about 45° instead of the usual 15° to 20°.

The extremely large ratio of arterial diameter to catheter diameter is thought to beneficially reduce the incidence of thrombosis, particularly total occlusion. However, occlusions have been reported with femoral cannulation for monitoring purposes.[70] A commonly postulated disadvantage of this site is the possibility of increased bacterial contamination because of its proximity to the warm, moist groin and perineum; however, no studies confirm this hypothesis.[71] The femoral area is inconvenient for any patient who is awake and mobile, or if the patient is able to sit in a chair. If the patient is that mobile, then the risk/benefit from invasive monitoring should be reconsidered. Despite theoretical difficulties, some large hospitals use femoral arterial lines almost exclusively, and the intensive care nursing staff is often more comfortable caring for these lines than those at other sites.

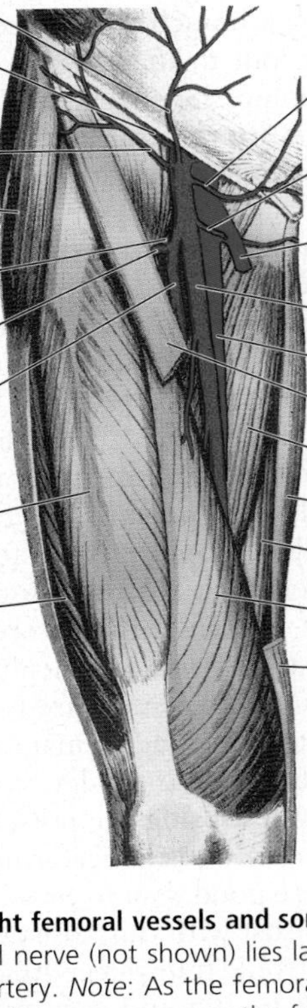

Umbilical and Temporal

In the neonate, arterial access can be accomplished for a short time through the umbilical artery. After this artery closes, the temporal artery provides a safe alternative. Prian[72] described the use of the temporal artery, noting its accessibility and the lack of clinical sequelae if it undergoes thrombosis.[72] The cutdown method should be used with a 22-gauge catheter after the artery's course has been traced with an ultrasonic flow detector. Because of the increasing accuracy of ear oximeters and the use of capillary blood gases for pH determination, prolonged arterial cannulation will become less frequent during infant care.

COMPLICATIONS OF ARTERIAL CANNULATION

Long-term arterial cannulation is safe if care is taken to avoid complications. Almost all difficulties one may encounter can be avoided or their incidence markedly decreased by adhering to a few simple principles. Reported clinical sequelae of arterial puncture and cannulation range from simple hematomas to life-threatening infections and exsanguination. Other potential complications include ischemia, arteriovenous fistula, and pseudoaneurysm formation. The incidence of complications varies with the site selection, method of cannulation, and clinician's procedural skill and experience. Early detection of complications is greatly aided by enhanced vigilance and concern of the patient's physician and nursing staff. It is difficult to compare complication rates at various sites, because most published studies have primarily used the radial artery.

No studies have compared the approach and complication rates of arterial catheters in the ED compared with the ICU or operating room uses. In a large study over 24 months, 2119 ICU patients had arterial catheters placed at admission: 52% at the radial site and 45% at the femoral site. The most

Superficial epigastric artery

Deep circumflex iliac artery

Superficial circumflex iliac artery

Tensor fasciae latae

Medial femoral circumflex artery

Lateral femoral circumflex artery

Deep femoral artery

Rectus femoris

Vastus lateralis

Superficial external pudendal artery

Deep external pudendal artery

Great saphenous vein

Femoral artery

Femoral vein

Sartorius

Adductor longus

Gracilis

Adductor magnus

Vastus medialis

Sartorius

Figure 20–17 The right femoral vessels and some of their branches. The femoral nerve (not shown) lies lateral to the artery and may be deep to the artery. *Note:* As the femoral artery becomes distal to the inguinal crease, it transverses over the femoral vein. *(From Warwick R, Williams PL [eds]: Gray's Anatomy, 35th ed. Edinburgh, Churchill Livingstone, 1973, p 676. Reproduced by permission.)*

common complication was vascular insufficiency (4%), followed by bleeding (2.1%) and infection (0.6%). No difference was reported for infection rates for femoral versus radial sites.[73] There are reports of complications from arterial puncture for procedures unrelated to long-term cannulation such as arteriography or simple arterial puncture for blood sampling as routinely performed in the ED. In a study of 2400 consecutive cardiac catheterizations over a 12-month period, complications occurred in 1.6% of patients including 17 needing vascular repair and 28 needing transfusion.[74]

A commonly encountered problem is hematoma formation at the puncture site. Zorab[75] reported this complication in 50% of catheterizations. The bruising was of minimal clinical significance in this report, but leakage can be dangerous when it occurs around the catheter or from the puncture site after the catheter is removed (Fig. 20–18). Compression neuropathy secondary to bleeding has been reported after brachial artery puncture in anticoagulated patients; in some cases, surgical decompression has been necessary.[13] The large amount of soft tissue surrounding the femoral artery makes bleeding in this area difficult to control. Large hematomas are not uncommon after femoral artery catheterization; indeed, Soderstrom and colleagues[67] reported two cases of bleeding that required transfusion after femoral puncture. More commonly, hematomas are painful, slow to resolve, and prone to infection. Multiple-site punctures and inadequate pressure applied for sufficient time account for most hematomas. Such multiple punctures should be avoided in most instances with experienced users of ultrasound-aided catheter placement. It is not acceptable for patients not in extremis to proceed with such unsuccessful invasive intervention. Furthermore, hematomas may make further procedures in the groin difficult to complete.

Thrombotic occlusion after radial arterial cannulation occurs in nearly 50% of infants and small children; however, ischemia from occlusion is rare because of collateral blood supply from the ulnar artery.[76] Insertion sites closest to the bend of the wrist increase the chances of maintaining patency. Nonpatency is four times more likely with insertion in sites 3 cm or greater above the bend in the wrist.[77] Slogoff and associates[57] described 1700 cardiovascular surgical patients who underwent radial artery cannulation without any long-term, ischemic complications, despite evidence of radial artery occlusion after decannulation in more than 25% of patients. Serious complications after radial artery cannulation are extremely rare in the absence of contributing factors such as preexisting vasospastic arterial disease, previous arterial injury, protracted shock, high-dose vasopressor administration, prolonged cannulation, or infection.[56,78]

Prevention of bleeding complications may be accomplished with frequent careful inspection of the puncture site and the use of prolonged compression after removal of the catheter or needle. Firm pressure should be maintained for 10 minutes or longer after removal of a peripheral artery catheter and longer after femoral cannulation or if the patient is anticoagulated. Five minutes of pressure is sufficient after puncture for a blood gas sample in an individual with normal coagulation. Exsanguination, a related complication, may occur if the arterial line apparatus becomes disconnected. This is more common in the obtunded or combative patient, and restraints are often required for patients with indwelling arterial cannulas. Exsanguination should not occur if tight connections are maintained throughout the system and if frequent, careful inspections of both the circuit and the patient are made.

Meticulous attention to aseptic technique is necessary during insertion and catheter maintenance to minimize the risk of catheter-related infection.[79,80] Serious infections rarely complicate arterial cannulation. Most simple interventions can reduce the risk for serious catheter-related infection. The strongest supportive evidence is from usage of full-barrier precautions during catheter insertion, specialized nursing care, and newer-generation catheters with antiseptic hubs or antimicrobial agent–impregnated catheters.[79] The incidence of catheter-related infections increases with prolonged cannulation.[71] Catheters placed with sterile technique have an extremely low rate of infection up to 96 hours. Catheters changed over a guidewire every 96 hours have an infection rate of about 10% at the radial and femoral sites.[68]

Most infections begin locally at the puncture site and remain localized, although systemic sepsis has been reported.[78] Radial and femoral sites have a similar incidence of complications, but axillary cannulations seem to have a much higher incidence of infection (although no large studies of cannulation at this site exist).[72,81] Arterial cannulas are more prone to infectious complications than other vascular catheters. Many mechanisms have been proposed for this occurrence.[80,82] The arterial pressure monitoring system usually consists of a long column of fairly stagnant fluid and is subject to frequent manipulation. Stamm and coworkers[81] found that patients were at greater risk for systemic infection if they had an arterial line and required frequent blood gas determinations than if they had the cannula alone. The sampling stopcock is a site of frequent bacterial contamination.

The risk of infection also increases as the duration of cannulation is prolonged. Older studies recommend that catheters be changed after 4 days if continued monitoring is necessary.[81,82] In addition, Makai and Hassemer[82] recommended changing the entire fluid-filled system, including transducer chamber-domes and continuous flow devices, every 48 hours. However, other risks for noninfectious concerns increase with more frequent catheter and site changes when based solely on length of catheterization of a site.

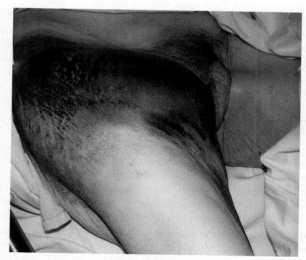

Figure 20–18 Right groin hemorrhage with resulting hematoma. The injury resulted from a failed attempt to place a right femoral artery catheter with the Seldinger technique. A large femoral hematoma is pictured here 3 days post iatrogenic injury.

Therefore, daily evaluation of the site is advised, and catheter change should not be mandatory until 7 to 8 days, if the site remains clean.

Shinozaki and colleagues[83] demonstrated a marked reduction in equipment contamination when the continuous flush device was located just distal to the transducer, as opposed to closer to the three-way stopcock used for sampling. This setup reduces the length of the static column of fluid between the sampling stopcock and the transducer. As mentioned previously, a drop of iodophor or antibiotic ointment applied to the puncture site decreases the incidence of local wound infection.[41] This technique has drawn a great deal of criticism, however. The current standard is a clean, dry dressing, not an occlusive type. An antibiotic- or silver-impregnated catheter is always recommended for long-term placements.

Thrombosis of the vessel in which the cannula is placed is another frequently encountered problem. The incidence with which this occurs varies with the method used to determine the presence of the clot. Bedford and Wollman[18] found a greater than 40% occlusion rate when radial artery catheters were left in place for longer than 20 hours. All of these occluded vessels eventually recannulized. Angiographic studies show deposition of fibrin on 100% of the catheters left in place for longer than 1 day, although clinical evidence of ischemia secondary to occlusion with thrombus present occurs in less than 1% in most studies.[84] Most reports of nonangiographic catheterizations that mention thrombosis are studies of the radial artery. Therefore, it is difficult to compare the incidence of thrombosis at other sites, although during the 176 femoral catheterizations of Soderstrom and colleagues[67] and Ersoz and associates,[85] dorsalis pedis pulses were decreased in only 2 patients, and no clinical signs of ischemia were noted. Larger catheter sizes, trauma during cannulation, and the presence of atherosclerosis have all been postulated to increase the incidence of thrombosis; however, conflicting studies abound. Downs and coworkers[20] associated tapered catheters with an increased incidence of thrombosis.

Arterial spasm after puncture (usually following multiple attempts) can predispose to thrombus formation and even lead to ischemic changes without fibrin deposition. Successful reversal of spasm after intra-arterial lidocaine, reserpine, and phentolamine has been reported, but no reliable studies of efficacy in this situation have been published.[86] Thrombosis can be minimized by decreasing the duration of catheterization, proper flushing, and using larger arteries. Surgical embolectomy or thrombectomy is rarely required because the smaller vessels that are most likely to occlude usually have good collateral circulation. A normal (negative) result on an Allen test or a similar test suggests but does not ensure adequate collateral flow.[52,58] The larger femoral artery, which has poor collateralization, rarely occludes with catheterization when used for monitoring purposes.

Another complication of thrombosis is occlusion of the catheter. Time until occlusion of radial and femoral artery catheters has been compared. Radial cannulas became occluded at an average of 3.8 days, whereas femoral cannulas occluded after 7.3 days.[68] The importance of this comparison is minimal if the clinician follows infection prophylaxis guidelines and changes arterial catheters after 4 days.

A few less common complications are easily prevented. One that occurs only with the percutaneous catheter-through-the-needle method is catheter embolization. Once the catheter has been placed through the needle, it should never be pulled back, because the end of the catheter may be sheared off by the sharp needle bevel. If this occurs, surgical removal of the catheter tip is necessary.

Skin necrosis is a complication of radial artery cannulation involving an area of the volar forearm proximal to the cannula.[87,88] Wyatt and colleagues[87] believe this is secondary to the poor blood supply of this area and stated that taking the precautionary steps described previously prevents or decreases the incidence of necrosis.

One feared complication of indwelling radial and brachial arterial catheters is the occurrence of a cerebrovascular accident secondary to embolization from flushing of the catheters.[20,89] As little as 3 to 12 mL of flush solution has shown reflux to the junction of subclavian and vertebral arteries.[67] A fatality due to air embolism from a radial artery catheter has been reported and was re-created in a primate model.[90] Although these animals are much smaller (7 kg) than an adult human, as little as 2.5 mL of air introduced at a relatively low flush rate was found to embolize in a retrograde fashion to the brain. Cerebral embolization can be prevented with the use of continuous flush systems (3 mL/hr) and by ensuring the integrity of the tubing and transducer systems to prevent air entry. In addition, small volumes (<2 mL) of intermittent flush solution should be used.

Complication rates also vary according to the method of arterial cannulation. Mortensen[91] studied the three main techniques (discussed earlier in "Techniques"), but unfortunately, most of his arterial cannulations were for angiographic purposes. The complications associated with prolonged cannulation time are therefore underrepresented. For Mortensen's series,[91] cutdown arteriotomy exhibited the lowest incidence of complications (7.7%), whereas the Seldinger technique had a complication incidence of 17.7%. Complications of percutaneous cannulation were 11.3%. Apparently, false passage of the guidewire, the catheter, or both was associated with increased intimal damage and complications. It is imperative that the wire or catheter be advanced only if no resistance is met!

In actuality, arterial puncture and cannulation are safe procedures when care is taken and basic principles are kept in mind. The operator should be skilled and should seek an atraumatic insertion. Once the monitoring system is set up, it should be manipulated as little as possible. Any handling should be performed with a flawless aseptic technique. The tubing and other fluid-filled devices should be changed every 48 hours, and catheters should be inserted into a vessel that provides a vessel-to-catheter ratio as large as possible without compromising other needs. If these principles are followed and the patient and system are carefully inspected at frequent intervals, complications of arterial puncture and cannulation can be minimized.

INTERPRETATION

An indwelling arterial catheter provides continuous blood pressure monitoring. The trend of a patient's pressure helps one assess the effect of various therapeutic interventions. The absolute systolic and diastolic pressures measured will vary at different catheter sites, with higher peak systolic pressures measured at the periphery; the pressures will also be higher when measured in the distal lower limb.[22,67] A wide variance between direct arterial pressure and pressure measured with a standard pneumatic cuff will always exist in some patients. The oscillometric blood pressure measurement can significantly underestimate arterial blood pressure. The relation between cuff size and upper arm circumference contributes substantially to the inaccuracy of this noninvasive blood pressure measurement. Such continued lack of adequate accuracy in critically ill patients underscores the need for intra-arterial catheter placement.[92]

Data averaged over a population group, however, compare fairly well.[22] For this reason, the cuff pressure and that displayed on the monitor should be compared regularly. A change in their relationship may be the first indication of difficulties with the direct measuring system. Auscultatory methods usually give a slightly lower value than direct measuring systems.

Waveform analysis may also provide an early indication of thrombosis in the arterial catheter. Many variables affect the waveform, including cardiac valvular disease, arteriosclerosis, and other peculiarities of an individual's cardiovascular system that may contribute to pulse wave reflections.[93] Waveforms may vary tremendously among patients, but after an adequate monitoring system has been established, a change in an individual's pressure wave is usually indicative of thrombosis or other malfunction in the monitoring system. A change in waveform may also indicate a change in the patient's cardiovascular status, such as a papillary muscle rupture. Once again, before making a therapeutic decision based on an electronically generated number, the patient should be rechecked with a pneumatic cuff; this device is less fallible than the electromechanical system.

Radial systolic arterial pressures poorly estimate the actual ascending aortic pressure, with more than 50% of cases reporting a difference in values of 10 to 35 mm Hg. Mean arterial pressures or even diastolic pressures were found to be highly accurate with greater than 90% of the values being within 3 mm Hg of aortic values.[94] Longer catheters have also been successfully used from radial sites to more accurately reflect central aortic pressure for cardiac surgery patients.[95]

An indwelling arterial cannula can provide valuable information about the hemodynamic status of a patient (through continuous pressure monitoring) and about the patient's respiratory and metabolic status (through intermittent sampling for blood gas analysis and other blood tests). The Pco_2 and pH of the blood can be used to define four major groups of metabolic derangement: respiratory acidosis or alkalosis and metabolic acidosis or alkalosis. Rarely will a disorder be strictly classified into one of these groups; however, a simple chart such as that shown in the Appendix helps determine the relative effects of metabolic and respiratory influence on the blood pH. (See also the discussion in the Appendix.)

A rough estimate of the contribution of respiratory factors may be made by assuming that for every 10 torr that the Pco_2 varies from 40, the pH will inversely vary 0.08 pH units from 7.4. Adequacy of blood oxygenation can be determined from the measured Po_2 of the arterial blood and from the known concentration of oxygen that the patient is inspiring. To avoid iatrogenic complications of intensive care, one must be absolutely certain that the data are from an arterial sample that has been properly analyzed before basing one's treatment decisions on the numbers obtained. Not uncommonly, one may accidentally puncture a vein when attempting to obtain an arterial blood sample. Furthermore, false readings may result if the sample is not free of air bubbles, not promptly chilled, and not analyzed within 20 to 30 minutes. Although still controversial, blood gas values that are *uncorrected* for body temperature appear more appropriate for guiding therapy in hypothermic patients.[96,97]

CONCLUSION

As intensive care knowledge and technology grow and develop, cannulation of the arterial system may decrease in frequency. Oximeters can determine the quality of blood oxygenation percutaneously and are becoming more accurate and sophisticated. Electronic sphygmomanometers are being refined for continuous indirect blood pressure monitoring. As these devices improve and noninvasive sampling methods for clinically relevant electrolytes and physiologic markers are refined, the indwelling arterial cannula may in time become considered overly invasive. The noninvasive blood pressure measurement still lacks the proven accuracy in shock states compared with invasive monitoring in all patients. In addition, in patients with obesity as well as those with vascular compromise and large burns that preclude normal cuff placement, invasive monitoring offers improved hemodynamic monitoring.

At the time of publication, the current need for frequent blood sampling for chemical and hematologic analysis remains a strong indication for its use in the most critically ill patients. Overzealous blood gas analysis may lead to iatrogenic anemia in the ICU. Multiple reports document the advantages to limiting frequent blood sampling (and its associate waste).[98-100]

Arterial puncture and cannulation are invaluable aids to the emergency and critical care clinician. Long-term catheterization is a safe procedure when the catheter is placed, maintained, and removed with care. The radial artery is the most favored location for puncture, but as more experience is gained and reported with femoral artery catheterization, the latter may become a more frequently used site. Selection of either site is associated with a low complication rate and should be determined by the skill of the clinician and the nursing team and the relative convenience and comfort of the patient. Ultrasound guidance for arterial catheter placement is rapidly becoming the standard and should be considered in every instance to reduce the need for multiple puncture attempts.

 REFERENCES CAN BE FOUND ON EXPERT CONSULT

CHAPTER 21

Peripheral Intravenous Access

Shan W. Liu and Richard Zane

Intravenous (IV) access is a mainstay of modern medicine. IV cannulation is a procedure performed by nearly all involved in the health care profession—clinicians, nurses, clinician assistants, phlebotomists, and emergency medical technicians. In the United States, more than 25 million patients have peripheral IV catheters placed per year allowing access for medication administration, fluids, and blood sampling for laboratory analysis. In small children, IV access simply may not be obtainable in a reasonable amount of time in a true emergency, but an alternate method may be attempted (cutdown, intraosseous). IV access can usually be accomplished in 2 to 5 minutes.[1–6]

INDICATIONS AND CONTRAINDICATIONS

Obtaining timely and adequate access is a major priority during a cardiac arrest and major trauma. In normal perfusion, differences in delivery times for injections centrally vs. peripherally are minimal–seconds.[7] Canine studies show that 90% of peripheral IV fluid reaches the central circulation beneath inflated pneumatic antishock garments.[8] During cardiopulmonary resuscitation (CPR), medications have been shown to reach the central circulation faster with central access than with peripheral venous access.[9] However, peripheral IV cannulation is still the *procedure of choice even during CPR because of the usual speed, ease, and safety with which it can be accomplished.*[10]

Saline locks, commonly known as heparin locks because of prior use with heparin flushes, are preferable when IV medications are needed and there are limited foreseeable fluid requirements. Saline locks cost much less than a full IV fluid and tubing assembly; approximate costs are $4.50 for saline lock, flush, needle, and angiocatheter versus $8.60 for 1 L normal saline, IV tubing, angiocatheter, and IV line kit.[10–12] Such locks are especially helpful to have when prompt vascular access may suddenly be needed. However, irrigation of the catheter requires a separate syringe and flush.[10]

In terms of contraindications to IV placement, with the risk of extravasation or suboptimal volume flow, peripheral IV lines should not be placed in extremities with massive edema, burns, sclerosis, phlebitis, or thrombosis. Furthermore, extremities on the side of radical mastectomies should also be avoided, although they can be used when an urgent condition exists and other peripheral access is not possible. Veins that drain from an area of neck trauma or an affected traumatic extremity or the side of a chest or abdominal trauma are also suboptimal because fluid or medications may not be delivered to the circulatory system. Cannulation at sites of cellulitis or extremities with shunts or fistulas should be avoided because it may cause bacteremia or thrombosis.

Blood samples for laboratory analysis are usually drawn prior to IV cannulation in order to avoid contamination with IV fluid or medication. However, studies have shown that accurate basic electrolytes and hematologic values can be drawn off peripheral IV lines when infusions are shut off at least 2 minutes, at least 5 mL of blood is wasted, and all tubes are filled to avoid inaccurate bicarbonate readings.[13–15] By adopting this technique, one can reduce the number of peripheral needle sticks, minimize trauma and sclerosis of the vein, and improve patient satisfaction.

PERIPHERAL IV CENTRAL CATHETERS

In this modern age of multiple types of IV access devices, familiarity with peripheral devices is necessary to ensure proper selection. A common option is the peripheral intravenous central catheter (PICC). It is a relatively recent addition to the IV access armamentarium and shares attributes of both central and peripheral venous access. A PICC is composed of a thin tube of biocompatible material and an attachment hub, which is inserted percutaneously into peripheral veins and advanced into a large central vein with radiographic confirmation of placement. PICCs are suitable for long-term vascular access for blood sampling and infusion of hyperosmolar solution such as total parenteral nutrition. These lines should be inserted as soon as intermediate-term access is anticipated.[16]

ULTRASOUND AND TRANSILLUMINATORS

Although more commonly used for central venous access, ultrasound machines have also been used in the placement of peripheral lines. Brannam and coworkers[17] evaluated the success rates of ultrasound-guided peripheral IV lines inserted by emergency nurses on difficult to stick patients. Of a sample of 321, the successful placement rate with the ultrasound was 87%. Keyes and colleagues[18] performed a prospective study of the success rates of peripheral cannulation with the use ultrasound by emergency clinicians. They found that of 101 enrolled patients who previously had two unsuccessful blind attempts, the rate of successful cannulation was 91%, with 73% on the first attempt. In 2% of the cases, the brachial artery was punctured. As emergency providers increase their comfort with ultrasound and as the technology becomes more affordable and available, ultrasound-guided or illumination-assisted insertion of peripheral lines will likely increase.

ANATOMY

Success of cannulation depends on familiarity with the vascular anatomy of the extremities. In the upper extremity, the veins of the hands are drained by the metacarpal and dorsal veins, which connect and form the dorsal venous arch and are excellent sites for IV therapy, comfortably accommodating 22- and 20-gauge catheters. The wrist and forearm's venous supply consists of the basilic vein, which courses along the ulna portion of the posterior forearm; it is often ignored because of its location, but can be easily accessed if the patient's forearm is flexed and the cannulator stands at the head of the patient.[19] On the radial side of the forearm, the cephalic is best known as the *intern vein*. Readily accessible, this vein can accommodate 22- to 16-gauge catheters. The median veins of the forearm course through the middle of the forearm, and accessory cephalic veins at the top radial aspect of the forearm are easily stabilized and accessible.

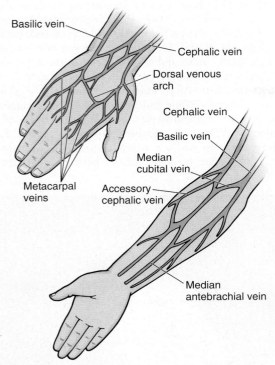

Figure 21–1 Anatomy of the veins in the hands and arms for intravenous (IV) cannulation. *(Adapted from Millam DA: How to insert an IV. Am J Nurs 79:1268, 1979.)*

The labels in the figure read: Basilic vein, Cephalic vein, Dorsal venous arch, Cephalic vein, Basilic vein, Median cubital vein, Accessory cephalic vein, Metacarpal veins, Median antebrachial vein.

The antecubital veins consist of the medial cubital, basilic, and cephalic veins and are often selected for midline catheters or blood draws. IV placement here is easy, but mobility of the arm is often subsequently restricted. The larger veins above the antecubital space, the cephalic and basilic veins, are often more difficult to see, but can be accessed if necessary without difficulty (Fig. 21–1).

The relevant lower extremity venous anatomy starts with the dorsal digital veins, which become the dorsal metatarsal veins and then form the dorsal venous arch. The arch ultimately splits into the greater saphenous vein, which travels up the medial aspect of the ankle, and the lesser saphenous vein, which courses laterally up the opposite side. These are the vascular structures most accessible for IV therapy.

The external jugular vein is formed below the ear and behind the angle of the mandible. It then passes downward and obliquely across the sternocleidomastoid and then passes under the middle of the clavicle to join the subclavian vein. It is important to note the presence of valves in the external jugular, notably about 4 cm above the clavicle, because they can significantly impede IV function.[10]

PREPARATION

Safety. In the era of human immunodeficiency virus (HIV) and hepatitis, safety of those placing IV lines cannot be overemphasized. Universal precautions must be applied to all patients, especially in emergency care settings in which the risk of blood exposure is increased and the infection status of patients is largely unknown.[20] One study showed that 11% of all hospital IV catheter injuries to health care workers occurred in the emergency department (ED).[21] Newer catheter devices have emerged to prevent inadvertent needle injuries. The

Protectiv IV Catheter safety system has a protective sleeve that encases the sharp stylet as it is retracted from the catheter. The Insyte Autoguard Shielded IV Catheter's needle is instantly encased inside a tamper-resistant safety barrel by pressing the activation button. The Saf-T-Intima IV catheter, puncture-guard winged set, Vacutainer Brand safety-lok, Shamrock safety winged needle and angel wing systems are all types of winged safety devices that have shields that advance over the needle to prevent needle exposures.[5]

Choosing Catheter Gauge. The catheter gauge will depend on the clinical scenario. The smallest gauge, shortest catheter is a 22-gauge, which is sufficient for routine maintenance fluids and routine antibiotics. A 20- or 18-gauge needle is necessary for blood product administration and a 16-gauge needle is necessary for resuscitating patients.[19]

Appropriate Site. Site selection will depend largely on the expected duration of IV therapy, the patient's activity level, the urgency of the clinical scenario, and the condition of the extremities and of the patient. When choosing a place to initiate IV therapy, the best place to start is the hand and then advance cephalad as necessary. Hand veins are appropriate for 20- to 22-gauge IV catheters. Cephalic, accessory, or basilic veins are ideal for larger-bore IV lines. Avoid veins that are not resilient and feel hard and cordlike because they are often thrombosed.[5] Deep, percutaneous antecubital venipuncture and external jugular vein cannulation are also options in the patient with difficult veins.[22]

In patients who have undergone radical mastectomy, avoid the arm on the same side as the surgery because circulation may be impaired, affecting flow and causing edema and other complications such as thrombosis.[5,19] Furthermore, whereas lower extremities veins can be useful locations for IV access and may be especially useful in the pediatric patient, they are often easily traumatized and may lead to deep vein thrombosis.[5]

Anesthesia. Prospective studies continue to demonstrate that local anesthesia, such as buffered or plain lidocaine or benzyl alcohol, significantly decrease perceived patient pain prior to IV cannulation.[23-25] Although somewhat time consuming, and sometimes as painful as cannulation itself, anesthetizing at the site of cannulation should be at least considered as part of routine IV care. Similarly, in the pediatric population, 2.5 g of EMLA (eutectic mixture of local anesthetics) can also be applied to the vein to ensure local anesthesia.[5] The main disadvantage of using EMLA is that one must wait up to an hour for anesthetic onset prior to cannulation.[26]

IV fluids and lines should be prepared as well if needed. The cap should be removed from the IV line and the tab removed from the IV bag. The IV tubing should be clamped shut and the spiked end inserted into the IV bag (Fig. 21–2). The drip chamber should be pinched and filled halfway (Fig. 21–3). The clamp should then be opened slightly to flush the IV tubing (Fig. 21–4). If saline locks are being used, the locks should similarly be flushed prior to cannulation. This can be accomplished by attaching the lock to a saline-filled syringe and flushed (Fig. 21–5).

Inspection and Positioning. After collecting supplies, and making the appropriate preparations, palpation is the next crucial step in successful cannulation. Position the patient comfortably on a flat surface. Place a 1-inch-wide tourniquet on the patient's upper arm or forearm sufficiently tight to impede venous flow but not to the extent that arterial flow is compromised. Start by placing the tourniquet under the arm

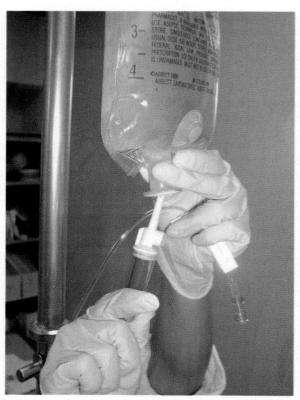

Figure 21–2 Insertion of the spiked end of the IV tubing into the IV bag.

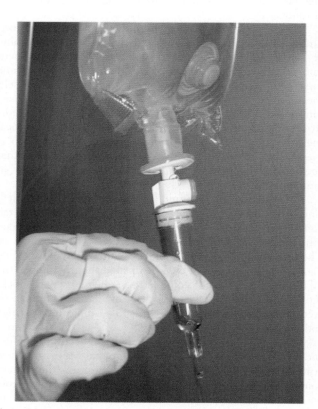

Figure 21–3 Pinching the drip chamber to fill the bulb halfway before infusing fluid.

(Fig. 21–6). Fold both ends of the tourniquet above the arm and cross the ends (Fig. 21–7). Pull the overlying end taut and tuck the middle portion below the underlying end, creating a loop (Figs. 21–8 and 21–9). After placing the tourniquet, palpate with the index and middle finger of the nondominant hand—veins are soft, elastic, resilient, and pulseless.[19]

Cannulation. After washing the hands, use gloves to clean the site with iodine and/or alcohol. Studies suggest that iodine is better as an antiseptic than alcohol in terms of fewer infections.[27] When using alcohol, allow it to dry (Fig. 21–10). Stabilize the vein without contaminating the prepared site (Fig. 21–11). Take the angiocatheter between the thumb and

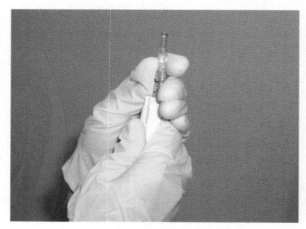

Figure 21–4 Flushing the IV tubing.

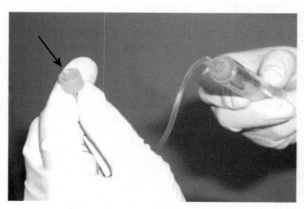

Figure 21–5 Flushing the saline lock.

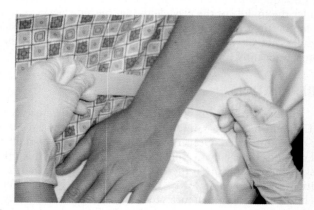

Figure 21–6 Application of the tourniquet: Place the tourniquet 3–4 cm proximal to the insertion site.

the forefinger of the dominant hand with the bevel up, angled 10° to 30° between the angiocatheter and the vein, aligned parallel to the vein. Puncture the vein (Fig. 21–12). Once a flash is seen, advance the catheter several millimeters more to ensure the catheter has entered the vein and not just the wall. Avoid advancing too far and puncturing the posterior wall; loosen the stylet and advance only the catheter (Fig. 21–13). Take the fingers anchoring the vein and occlude the vein at the tip of the catheter to prevent extravasation of blood from the angiocatheter. Remove the needle and connect the saline

lock and IV lining or syringe for phlebotomy and release the tourniquet (Figs. 21–14 and 21–15).[19]

External jugular vein cannulation deserves a special note. In the patient with otherwise little peripheral access, it should be cannulated with a simple peripheral venous catheter (16- to 20-gauge) as follows: Place patient in the Trendelenburg position to fill the external jugular. Rotate the head to the opposite side. Prepare the area as described previously, take the cannula and align it in the direction of the vein with the point aiming toward the ipsilateral shoulder. Compressing the

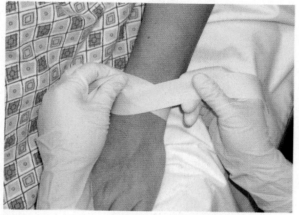

Figure 21–7 Crossing the tourniquet ends and applying tension.

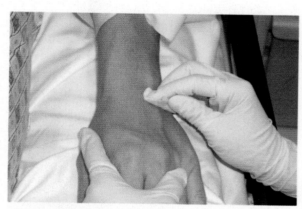

Figure 21–10 Preparing the insertion site with alcohol.

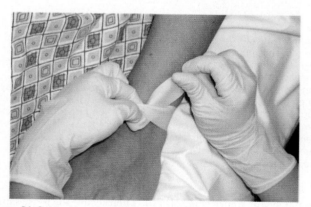

Figure 21–8 Tucking the middle portion of one end snugly under the opposite end to make a loop.

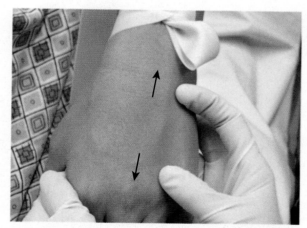

Figure 21–11 Grasping the skin and pulling it taut to apply traction.

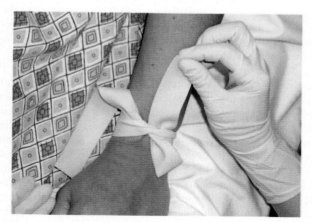

Figure 21–9 The distal portion of the tucked end is left free for one-hand release of the tourniquet.

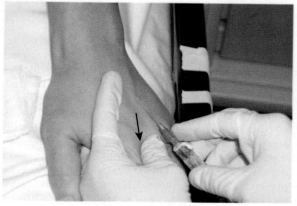

Figure 21–12 Insertion of the catheter.

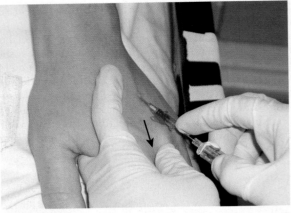

Figure 21–13 Advancing the catheter and removing the needle.

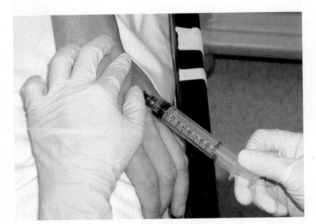

Figure 21–14 Phlebotomy.

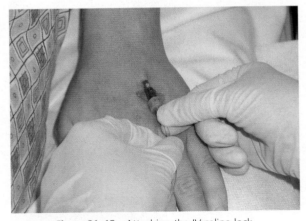

Figure 21–15 Attaching the IV saline lock.

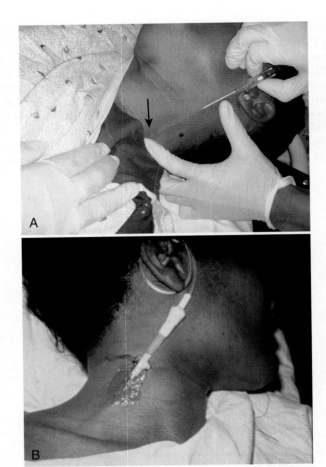

Figure 21–16 *A,* The external jugular vein may be cannulated with the same equipment, and with the same technique, as a peripheral vein. It is often used in those with no accessible peripheral veins, and is especially prominent in children. It will accept a 16- to 20-gauge angiocatheter. Flow is position-dependent and valves in the vein may be problematic and impede flow. In this case, the clinician's free hand both occludes the vein and provides skin traction for vein stabilization (*arrow*). *B,* IV catheters may be sutured in place for stability. Trendelenburg position and a Valsalva maneuver can facilitate cannulation. Air embolism is a rare potential complication with the procedure.

vein with a finger just above the clavicle may help distend the vein. Puncture midway between the angle of the jaw and the midclavicular line[10] (Fig. 21–16).

Anchoring the Device. After the IV line has been connected to the saline lock or IV tubing, anchoring the device is essential. Use a ½-inch-wide strip of tape, adhesive up, under the hub of the catheter and fold over in a bow-shaped manner (Figs. 21–17 and 21–18). This will secure the catheter and prevent lateral movement. Clear polyurethane dressings can also be used with or instead of tape (Fig. 21–19). Saline locks can be connected to needle-less hubs to prevent acci-

dental needle injury (Fig. 21–20). Then secure the loose saline lock or IV tubing with tape to prevent accidental dislodgment (Fig. 21–21). IV tubing can be similarly connected to the angiocatheter and anchored (Fig. 21–22). Commercially available securing devices can also be used. Dressings should then be signed and dated to ensure timely dressing changes.[5] Topical antibiotics or iodophor ointment should be applied to the insertion site to prevent infection.[10,28]

Maintaining Patency. An important component of IV care is maintaining patency with frequent flushing. Until recently, heparin solutions had been used to flush catheters and maintain patency but have been shown to cause problems such as hemorrhage. Studies have demonstrated that saline flushes are as effective as heparin in maintaining patency and preventing phlebitis in peripheral devices. In a meta-analysis comparing saline and heparin flushes, there was no statistical difference between the incidence of clotting and phlebitis and the duration of IV patency. With the advantage of decreased costs and avoiding complications such as bleeding or heparin-induced thrombocytopenia, heparin flushes should be replaced with saline flushes.[29–31]

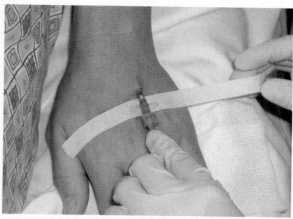

Figure 21-17 Securing the IV line down: Place the tape under the hub of the catheter, sticky side up.

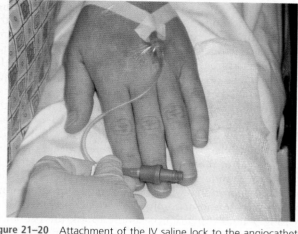

Figure 21-20 Attachment of the IV saline lock to the angiocatheter. This can be used for IV fluids or medications.

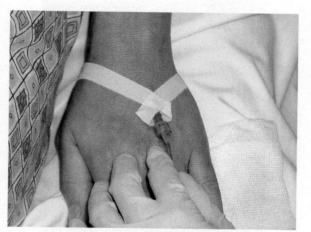

Figure 21-18 Crossing the ends of the tape over the top of the hub.

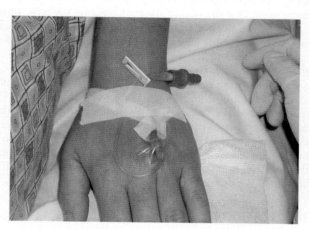

Figure 21-21 Securing the saline lock.

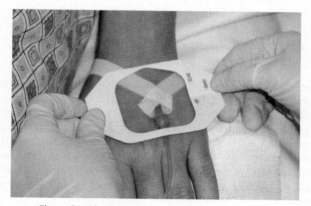

Figure 21-19 Transparent polyurethane dressing.

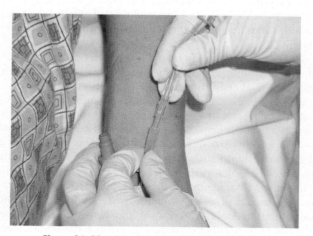

Figure 21-22 Attaching the IV tubing for infusion.

Dressing. It is not cost effective to continually redress peripheral venous catheters at periodic intervals. Sterile gauze or transparent, semipermeable, polyurethane dressings can be used and left on until removal of the catheter without increasing infection as long as the site is regularly evaluated.[32] Emerging evidence indicates that the type of securing techniques such as a device called the StatLock IV, a sterile, adhesive-backed anchor back and proprietary distal male Luer-tip

extension set, can reduce complications by decreasing mobility and the risk of dislodgment.[33]

Adjuncts. Often, patients have nonvisible and nonpalpable veins. Several older and newer adjuncts can increase the likelihood of successful cannulation.

Nitroglycerin ointment applied to the hands of patients with small-caliber veins has been shown to increase vein diameter size two to six times the original diameter and increase the rate of successful first-attempt cannulation without complications. Once the tourniquet is applied to the wrist, ¼ inch of 2% nitroglycerin is applied to a 2.5-cm-square area, left on for 2 minutes, and then rubbed off.[34] Nitroglycerin has been found to be useful and safe in the pediatric population as well.[35] Obviously, this technique should be avoided in patients with hypotension.

In the late 1980s, several small studies demonstrated the potential uses of a venous distention device—a cardboard mailing tube that was placed over the forearm with a sealed bulb at one end that would cause a vacuum within the tube. Ninety percent of the patients predetermined to be difficult to access were cannulated using this device. There were few reported complications, which were thought to be minimal such as petechiae and discomfort.[36,37] A common method of increasing venous distention is simply to ask the patient to open and close her or his fist. This causes increased blood flow into the arm or hand and distends the veins. Light tapping can also increase venous distention, although heavy tapping may cause the vein to spasm. Lowering the arm below the level of the heart can also increase venous distention. If these methods are inadequate, heat packs can be applied for 10 to 20 minutes to increase venous engorgement. This is particularly useful in the pediatric population.[5]

Percutaneous Brachial Vein Cannulation. Brachial vein cannulation is an option when attempts at peripheral IV access have failed or are contraindicated and may obviate the need for central venous access or surgical cutdown. Complications include brachial artery puncture, hematoma, and transitory paresthesias. This procedure should be performed with ultrasound guidance (Fig. 21–23) (see Chapter 67, Ultrasound-Guided Procedures).

COMPLICATIONS

Although IV placement is a common procedure, it is not without complications. Phlebitis, infiltration, infection, nerve damage, air embolism, bruising, and thrombosis are the most common complications and rarely cause significant morbidity or fatality.

Phlebitis is a common complication after IV cannulation and administration of medication, especially vancomycin, potassium, and any hyperosmolar solution or cytotoxic agents[38,39] (Fig. 21–24). IV devices facilitate infection by damaging epithelial and mucosal barriers to infection and provide microorganisms direct access to the bloodstream.[40] The most common infectious complication of peripheral IV access is a self-limited cellulitis with bacteremia, with sepsis rarely occurring. Phlebitis is described as the presence of a palpable cord accompanied by warmth, erythema, tenderness, and induration. Phlebitis will usually manifest as discomfort for the patient and necessitates removal of the catheter and its replacement on another extremity. Even with the best of care, all long-term lines eventually develop venous inflammation and, occasionally, infection at the site. Phlebitis can be reduced by minimizing trauma to the venous wall. Avoiding placement of IV lines in the lower extremities and joint sites, when possible, also decreases the incidence of IV line–related phlebitis.[5] In one study, phlebitis occurred in 15% of patients receiving IV infusions. Of these patients, 6.5% were found to have local *Staphylococcus epidermidis* colonization of the catheter.[41] Interestingly, this study also demonstrated that the increased incidence of phlebitis was not related to duration of IV placement but rather to patients with higher hemoglobin

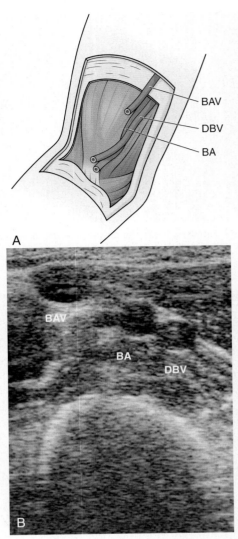

Figure 21–23 *A,* Anatomy of vessels in the anticubital fossa, noting the brachial artery (BA), basilic vein (BAV), and deep brachial vein (DBV). *B,* Corresponding ultrasound image. The vein collapses with probe pressure to distinguish it from the artery.

levels, for unclear reasons. In another study, bacteremia developed from peripherally inserted lines 0.4% of the time.[42] With such low levels of clinically significant bacteremia, some argue that routine replacement of catheters is now no longer needed.[41] The only large, prospective study investigating the incidence of phlebitis associated with peripheral IV lines required replacement of the IV lines every 72 hours.[32] Therefore, it is still standard practice to change IV lines every 72 hours.

The role of in-line filters to prevent phlebitis is controversial. It is thought that particulates from reconstituted medications, degradation products, precipitates, glass from vials, and other foreign debris all may play a part in postinfusion phlebitis. In-line filters may therefore play a role in preventing phlebitis, but given their cost, risk of clogging, and paucity of evidence supporting improved outcomes, they have not become standard of care.[43]

Usually, infiltration of a vein is a relatively minor and common complication of IV therapy. This often occurs when the catheter is dislodged from the vein during infusion.

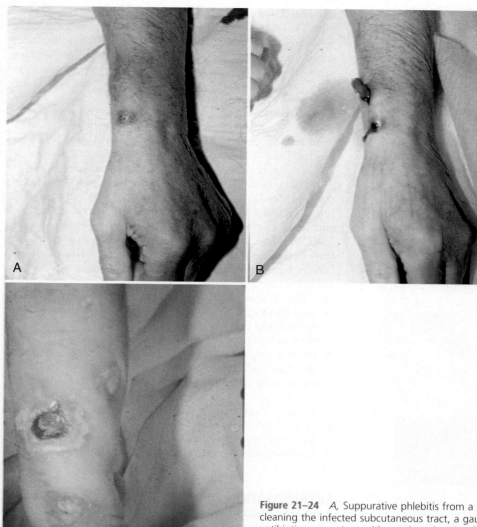

Figure 21–24 *A,* Suppurative phlebitis from a peripheral IV line. *B,* After incising and cleaning the infected subcutaneous tract, a gauze pack was placed for 24 hours, and oral antibiotics were given with good results. *C,* Infiltration of calcium chloride in an infant. Once this occurs, there is no treatment except débridement and possible skin grafting. Calcium gluconate will not cause such a reaction.

However, if the infusions are hypertonic, vasopressors, or chemotherapies, a significant risk of skin sloughing exists when infiltration and extravasation occur. In extreme cases, skin grafting may be required.[5] If dopamine extravasates, phentolamine may be used as an antidote to prevent ischemia to the local area.

Infection can be a costly and potentially devastating complication of IV therapy. Although rare with peripheral IV lines, intravascular device–related bloodstream infections are often the least recognized cause of nosocomial infection. Peripheral IV catheters are most often associated with *S. epidermidis, Staphylococcus aureus,* and *Candida* infections.[44] Infectious complications can be significantly reduced by hand-washing, wearing gloves, site preparation with iodine, and monitoring the site for signs of infection.[5]

Another rare complication of IV cannulation is nerve injury. Any peripheral nerve is potentially vulnerable to a needle-induced injury and sequelae can range from minor motor or sensory abnormality to complete paralysis. Nerve damage may come from damage from the needle, intraneural microvascular damage from hematomas, or toxic effects of the agent injected.[45] The first symptoms are often pain, numb-ness, or paresthesia. Pain may persist for years and can be debilitating. Fortunately, most simple procedures do not result in nerve injury because nerves often roll or slide away from the needle. As with all procedures, knowledge of relevant anatomy is essential. Should a patient complain of numbness or severe pain after needle puncture, injection into that site should immediately stop.[46,47]

Minor air bubbles in the line are clinically inconsequential, but a large air embolism is a significant, although exceedingly rare, complication of peripheral IV access. The symptoms are chest pain, shortness of breath, sudden vascular collapse, cyanosis, and hypotension. If air embolism is suspected, the patient must be placed in the left lateral position, ideally with Trendelenburg. Such near-fatal complications can be prevented by eliminating air from the IV tubing prior to initiating therapy and avoiding letting IV lines run dry.[5] If the air bubbles are present near the top of the IV line, tapping the tubing while holding it taut can help the trapped air escape to the top. Similarly, curling the tubing around a pen or syringe can accomplish the same goal. If the air is near the Y connector, one can use a needle and syringe to directly remove it. If all else fails and the air is between the Y connector and the patient, the tubing will likely have to be disconnected and flushed.[48]

Bruising is a common complication of IV therapy. Contrary to popular belief, flexing of the elbow after venipuncture does not prevent bruising in the antecubital site.[49] Applying direct pressure immediately after decannulation is the most useful technique to prevent bruising.

Suppurative thrombophlebitis is another extremely rare complication of peripheral IV therapy (Fig. 21–25). It most frequently occurs in patients with thermal injury, long-term cannulation with a plastic catheter, or lower extremity can-

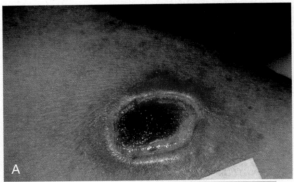
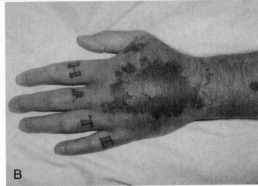
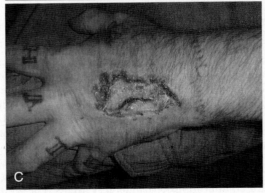

Figure 21–25 *A,* Full-thickness extravasation injury from doxorubicin extravasation, not obvious until 7–10 days after extravasation. *B,* Extravasation of phenytoin. The site 1 day after the phenytoin extravasation looks deceptively benign. A skin sough was evident in 2–3 days. Pain at the infusion site or the alarm of an infusion pump requires inspection of the IV site for extravasation when irritating solutions are infused. In this case, an unconscious patient received a concentrated phenytoin infusion for status epilepticus, but his comatose state did not allow him to complain of pain. Over a few days, a skin slough occurred, requiring many weeks to resolve. This could have been avoided with the use of a more dilute solution (i.e., no more than 2 mg/mL: phenytoin to saline solution), a central vein, or using phosphenytoin instead. *C,* Taken on follow up approximately 1 month later. *(B and C, Courtesy of Dr. Mahesh Shrestha.)*

nulation.[40] Local signs of inflammation or suppuration are often absent and can occur 2 to 10 days after catheter removal.[50] Treatment is local débridement, or in severe cases, immediate surgical excision of the entire length of the involved vein and involved tributaries. As with all the infectious complications of IV therapy, it can be prevented by meticulous aseptic cannulation technique.[51]

Thrombosis and subsequent pulmonary embolism is a rare complication of peripheral IV access and is more commonly associated with centrally placed IV catheters and central lines.[5] Although rare, thrombosis and pulmonary embolism may occur in peripheral IV lines if saline locks are not flushed or fluids are allowed to run out. Should this occur, the line should be aspirated. If there is a bloody-appearing return, discard the syringe and gently flush the saline lock and resume infusion. If there is no bloody aspirate, use 2 to 3 mL of saline to gently flush the line. If there is resistance, stop flushing immediately because there is a risk of an embolism developing. Recannulization at another site is then recommended.[52]

The Centers for Disease Control and Prevention's recommendations for IV care to prevent complications are[42]:

1. Record and date the time of the catheter insertion in an obvious location near the insertion site.
2. Do not palpate the insertion site after the skin has been cleansed with antiseptic.
3. Palpate the insertion site for tenderness daily through an intact dressing.
4. Visually inspect the site if the patient reports tenderness.
5. Wash hands before and after palpating, inserting, replacing, or dressing any intravascular access site.
6. Replace dressings when they are damp, loose, or soiled.

EXTRAVASATION OF MEDICATION AND VASOPRESSORS

Usually, infiltration of a vein is a relatively minor and common complication of IV therapy if only sterile fluid extravasates, even in large amounts. This often occurs when the catheter is dislodged from the vein during infusion. However, if the infusions are hypertonic, vasopressors, or chemotherapies, a significant risk of skin sloughing exists when infiltration and extravasation occur (Table 21–1). Pain at the infusion site or the alarm sounding on an infusion pump device requires inspection of the infusion site for extravasation. In extreme cases, skin slough with grafting may be required (see Fig. 21–2).[5] If dopamine, phenylephrine (Neo-Synephrine), or norepinephrine extravasate, phentolamine may be used as an antidote to prevent ischemia to the local area; its use is encouraged as soon as the extravasation is identified. The reversal of ischemia with phentolamine is a common technique, but its ability to totally reverse or prevent a skin slough is not gauranteed. However, if infiltration of these vasopressors occurs, the editors suggest that it be routinely used. There are no downsides to this intervention, although hypotension is a theoretical side effect because phentolamine is an α-adrenergic antagonist. To inject phentolamine, reconstitute a 5-mg vial with saline and dilute with equal parts of saline (final form: 5 mg in 2 mL). For large areas, use two vials with the contents of each vial injected 10 minutes apart, using a 25- to 27-gauge needle or a TB syringe. The entire area of skin blanching, or suspected area of extravastion, is injected with multiple small aliquots of the solution, about 0.25- to 0.5 mL each. If the IV line is still in place, inject some phentolamine through the catheter before it is removed. The procedure may be repeated in 2 to 4 hours.

Hyaluronidase is likely benign, and has been suggested in the past to ameliorate some effects of extravasation of other solutions. Although it was a common suggestion, its efficacy was not well established, and the product is not readily available. Ice or heat has varying effects to counteract any extravasation. The extravasation of IV contrast material is discussed in Chapter 36.

Extravasation of chemotherapy solutions is particularly common, and can produced full-thickness tissue slough. The patient may complain of pain and burning at the time of infusion, but skin slough may be delayed for many days. Table 21–2 lists extravasation injury from chemotherapy and some suggested treatments. Results from these interventions vary.

Injury from extravasation of phenytoin can be minimized or avoided by using dilute solutions, no more than 2 mg/mL concentration (1 g in 500 mL saline) or by using phosphenytoin instead of phenytoin. When possible, use calcium gluconate not calcium chloride in a peripheral IV line.

Bottom line: Most extravasated chemotherapy and other agents have no specific antidote or reversal agent to alter the final outcome At most extravasation sites, it may be best to avoid the empirical use of suggested treatments such as sodium bicarbonate, sodium thiosulfate, heparin, calcium gluconate, magnesium sulfate, lidocaine, cimetidine, diphenhydramine, and other chemical substances that are believed to inactivate drugs and reduce toxic effects on cells. In some experimental settings, these substances have made necrosis and ulceration worse.[53–56]

Acknowledgments

The authors wish to give special thanks to James Baab Jr. and Corey Tedrow for their assistance with photography and graphic design. Photo credits to James Baab Jr.

TABLE 21–1 Medications/Solutions That May Cause Tissue Injury When Extravasation Occurs in a Peripheral Vein*

Aminophylline	Metaraminol
Calcium chloride 10%	Mithramycin
Carmustine	Mitomycin
Chlordiazepoxide	Nafcillin
Colchicine	Neosynephrine
Crystalline amino acids 4.25%/ dextrose 10%	Nitroglycerine
	Norepinephrine
Crystalline amino acids 4.25%/ dextrose 25%	Parenteral nutrition solutions
Dactinomycin	Phenytoin†
Daunorubicin	Potassium solutions
Dextrose 10%	Propylene glycol
Dextrose 50% in water	Renografin-60
Diazepam	Sodium bicarbonate 8.4%
Dobutamine	Sodium thiopental
Dopamine	Tetracycline
Doxorubicin	Vasopressin
Epinephrine	Vinblastine
Ethyl alcohol	Vincristine
Mechlorethamine	Vindesine

*Many medications and IV solutions will cause pain and occasionally skin slough if significant amounts extravasate into soft tissues. Therefore, any complaint of pain during infusion or signs of tissue swelling should prompt an investigation for extravasation. Most extravasations have no specific therapy, so prevention is the only option. Phentolamine, injected subcutaneously to reverse vasoconstriction, is the most common technique, but its efficacy has not been well studied.

†Use a maximum concentration of 2 mg/mL of saline or phosphenytoin solution to minimize this risk.

 REFERENCES CAN BE FOUND ON EXPERT CONSULT

TABLE 21–2 Possible Antidotes for Extravasated Chemotherapeutic Agents*

Chemotherapeutic Agent	Antidote	Dose
Anthracycline	Dexrazoxane hydrochloride†	First dose, inject the equivalent of 500 mg dexrazoxane IV over 1–2 hr, second dose at 24 hr, and third dose at 48 hr.
Mechlorethamine	Sodium thiosulfate	Multiple injections in and around the area of extravasation, subcutaneous with a 25-gauge needle: 4 mL of 10% sodium thiosulfate + 6 mL water.
Vinca alkaloids (vincristine, vinblastine, and vinorelbine)	Hyaluronidase	Inject subcutaneously in and around the area of extravasation with a 25-gauge needle: 150 U (1 mL). For vinca alkaloids, apply local hot compresses.
Doxorubicin	Granulocyte macrophage colony-stimulating factor‡	Inject subcutaneously in and around the area of extravasation with a 25-gauge needle.
Doxorubicin, daunorubicin, and mitomycin	DMSO (free radical scavenger)	Apply a 50%–70% solution topically qid × 14 days. Leave uncovered.
Mitomycin	Pyridoxine‡	Inject subcutaneously in and around the area of extravasation with a 25-gauge needle.
Nonspecific	Saline	Inject subcutaneously in and around the area of extravasation with a 25-gauge needle.
Nonspecific	Corticosteroids§	Inject subcutaneously in and around the area of extravasation with a 25-gauge needle: Hydrocortisone 500 mg diluted in 500 mL saline.

*Many of these interventions are anecdotal and none are guaranteed to reverse or ameliorate tissue injury. Controversy exists surrounding the actual benefit and no randomized prospective trials have been conducted for many of the suggested regimens. Also consider elevation, surgical débridement when necessary.

†U.S. Food and Drug Administration approved for this indication.

‡Not well studied, theoretical benefit.

§Results variable, injury is not an inflammatory reaction.

CHAPTER 22

Central Venous Catheterization and Central Venous Pressure Monitoring

Bruce D. Adams, Matthew L. Lyon, and Paul T. DeFlorio

Central venous access remains a cornerstone of resuscitation and critical care in the emergency department (ED) and intensive care unit. Advanced hemodynamic monitoring, transvenous pacemakers, rapid fluid infusion, parenteral nutrition, and selected medications all require reliable central venous access. Central venous catheterization has also gained acceptance in resuscitation and treatment of the critically ill child (see Chapter 19, Pediatric Vascular Access and Blood Sampling Techniques). Fortunately the subclavian, jugular, and femoral veins have reliable relationships to easily identifiable surface landmarks and can be accessed quickly. Promising advances in technique, most notably real-time ultrasound guidance, have emerged since the early 2000s that may improve success rates and decrease complication rates.

 BACKGROUND CAN BE FOUND ON **EXPERT CONSULT**

INDICATIONS

Central venous access is indicated for several common clinical situations. If necessary, any central venous approach could be used for each one of these situations. However, experience suggests that certain approaches offer advantages over others in many clinical settings. The advantages and disadvantages of each approach are outlined in Table 22–2 and discussed in detail after the general indications.[13,14]

CVP and Oximetric Monitoring

Although somewhat supplanted by the more sophisticated flow-directed balloon-tipped pulmonary artery catheter, CVP measurement may be useful in select patients. In the specific setting of sepsis resuscitation, CVP monitoring has actually reemerged as an important component of "early goal-directed therapy."[15] Continuous or episodic measurements of the central venous oxygen O_2 saturation play a role in the aggressive treatment of septic shock.[15]

Central venous catheterization has been widely used as a vehicle for rapid volume resuscitation. It is often stated that short large-caliber peripheral catheters can be potentially as effective as central access because of the properties of Poiseuille's law (which states that the rate of flow is proportional to the radius^3 of the catheter and inversely proportional to its length). To illustrate, the gravity flow rate of saline through

a peripheral 5-cm, 14-gauge catheter is roughly twice that through a 20-cm, 16-gauge central venous catheter (CVC), with equivalent pressure heads. Consequently, the placement of large-bore peripheral catheters is generally the fastest method of volume loading. However, with the advent of thermoregulating high-volume rapid infusers, the advantages of central venous catheterization can be significant in the setting of severe hemorrhagic shock or hypothermia. Available systems can infuse blood warmed to 37°C through an 8.5-French introducer sheath 25% more rapidly than a 14-gauge peripheral intravenous (IV) line and up to 50% faster than an 18-gauge peripheral IV line.[16] The Level 1 Rapid Infuser and the Belmont FMS 2000 are examples of modern systems with infusion rates as high as 1500 mL/min.[16] Massive air embolism was a concern with early rapid infusers, but safety precautions have now been engineered to prevent this. A significant risk of these systems now is that if the catheter is misplaced, fluid or blood can be rapidly infused into the chest cavity or mediastinum with deadly consequences (Fig. 22–1).

Emergency Venous Access

The predictable anatomic locations of the subclavian and femoral veins and the speed with which they can be cannulated have prompted their use in cardiac arrest and other emergency situations. The need for a central line during cardiopulmonary resuscitation (CPR) is controversial.[17,18] When easily obtained, central venous cannulation, especially the internal jugular or subclavian route, is preferred over peripheral venous access because it provides a rapid and reliable route for the administration of drugs to the central circulation of the patient in cardiac arrest. With damage control resuscitation for thoracoabdominal trauma, the anesthesia team often requires two CVCs "one above and one below" the diaphragm.

Routine Venous Access

Patients with a history of IV drug abuse, major burns, or obesity and those requiring long-term care may have inadequate peripheral IV sites. Central venous cannulation may be indicated as a means of venous access in these patients even under nonemergent conditions.[19]

Routine Serial Blood Draws

The potential complications of CVCs do not justify their use in routine blood sampling. Lines already in place may be used for this purpose if they are properly cleared of IV fluid. A 20-cm, 16-gauge catheter contains 0.3 mL of fluid, so at least this much must be withdrawn to avoid dilution of blood samples. Furthermore, to avoid aspiration of crystalloid diluted blood from the peripheral vein, it is advised that the IV line be turned off for at least 2 to 3 minutes prior to using the catheter for a blood draw. Because of the increased risk of infectious complications, air embolus, and venous backbleeding, the IV tubing should not be repeatedly disconnected from the catheter hub. Interposition of a three-way stopcock in the IV tubing simplifies access and is an acceptable method of blood sampling in the intensive care setting, regardless of the IV site. A measurement of the oxygen level can be obtained from the SV for guidance in early goal-directed therapy of sepsis if one chooses not to place a continuous oximetric monitor.

TABLE 22–1 Central Vein Catheterization: Caveats and Helpful Hints

- Although traditional teachings recommend replacement products (such as fresh frozen plasma or platelet concentrates) before central catheterization, evidence from the literature suggests that this is not necessary. The decision to use such products should be made on a case-by-case basis.
- If there is concern about the possibility of a bleeding complication, the line should be placed in a location that allows straightforward compression (e.g., internal jugular or femoral vein). The subclavian approach should be avoided because hemorrhage in this location may require surgical intervention.
- In the case of a patient who has undergone pneumonectomy or has severe unilateral lung disease, an ipsilateral subclavian line may actually be the site of choice.
- If you are anticipating the use of a transvenous pacemaker or pulmonary artery catheter, you should use either the left subclavian vein or the right internal jugular vein. These approaches align the catheter trajectory with the superior vena cava and right atrium.
- Traditional teaching recommends that a towel be placed between the scapulae to make the scapula more prominent. However, this practice may compress the vein between the clavicle and the first rib and make catheterization difficult.[3]
- Concurrent preparation of the internal jugular insertion site during preparation for subclavian insertion allows a timely second attempt if subclavian catheterization is unsuccessful.
- If you are having trouble advancing the guidewire, withdraw it slightly, rotate it a bit, and try to readvance it.[2]
- Sometimes, resistance to insertion of the guidewire is met a third of the way in, at the junction of the subclavian and internal jugular veins. If this occurs, try increasing the degree of Trendelenburg positioning or turning the head to the ipsilateral side with the intent of compressing the internal jugular vein.
- Failure to create a large enough nick with the scalpel will result in difficult (or impossible) catheter insertion. This is especially the case with sheath introducers.
- The catheter tip should be positioned in the superior vena cava and not the right atrium. In most adults, the right atrium is 10–15 cm from the subclavian vein. Be sure that the catheter is not inserted deeper than this. Postprocedure chest radiography will assist with proper depth of placement.
- The sheath introducer is a large catheter, and a considerable amount of resistance may be encountered during advancement. A slight twisting motion at the entry site may be helpful.
- Be sure to advance the dilator and the sheath as a unit. If the sheath gets advanced ahead of the dilator, the leading edge of the sheath may kink, and proper insertion into the vessel will be impossible.
- If pneumothorax occurs and central access remains a priority, subsequent attempts should be made on the same side of the thorax as the pneumothorax to prevent the development of bilateral pneumothorax.
- Triple-lumen catheters should not be placed if rapid volume resuscitation is required. Peripheral intravenous lines with 14-gauge catheters can infuse volume twice as fast as a triple-lumen catheter can.[2] If peripheral access is not available and volume infusion is urgent, consider placing a sheath introducer.
- If the pulse cannot be palpated (e.g., cardiac arrest), divide the distance from the anterior superior iliac spine to the symphysis pubis into thirds. The artery typically lies at the junction of the medial and the middle thirds and the vein is 1 cm medial to this location.
- Excessive contralateral head rotation increases overlap of the carotid by the internal jugular and may increase the risk for arterial injury.
- Ask the patient to perform a Valsalva maneuver, or instruct an assistant to compress the patient's epigastrium to distend the IJ vein for easier identification and cannulation.
- Aggressive palpation of the carotid and femoral artery with the nondominant hand will decrease the luminal diameter of the internal jugular and femoral vein and make entry into the vessel difficult.

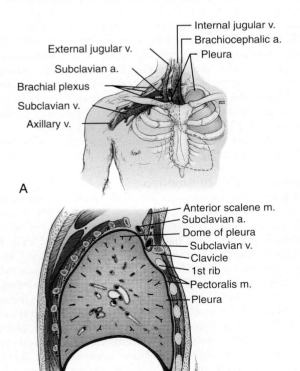

External jugular v.

Subclavian a.

Brachial plexus

Subclavian v.

Axillary v.

Internal jugular v.
Brachiocephalic a.
Pleura

A

Anterior scalene m.
Subclavian a.
Dome of pleura
Subclavian v.
Clavicle
1st rib
Pectoralis m.
Pleura

B

Figure 22–1 *A,* Anatomy of the subclavian and internal jugular veins. *B,* Sagittal section of the subclavian area. Note the position of the clavicle, subclavian vein and artery, and lung. If the needle is kept almost parallel to the clavicle, the artery and lung will not be encountered.

Infusion of Hyperalimentation and Other Concentrated Solutions

Central venous hyperalimentation is safe and reliable. Use of the subclavian infraclavicular technique frees the patient's extremities and neck; this procedure is therefore well suited to long-term applications. However, strict aseptic technique is necessary to minimize infectious complications.[20] Hyperosmolar or irritating solutions that have the potential to cause thrombophlebitis if given through small peripheral vessels are frequently infused through central veins. Examples are potassium chloride (>40 mmol/L), hyperosmolar saline, calcium chloride 10% (but not calcium gluconate, which can be safely given peripherally), 10% dextrose infusions, chemotherapeutic agents, and acidifying solutions such as ammonium chloride. Some clinicians prefer to obtain central access because of the potential harm of certain medications (e.g., phenytoin, which may result in "purple glove syndrome") and especially vasoactive substances (dopamine, norepinephrine), which may result in soft tissue necrosis should extravasation occur.

TABLE 22–2 Advantages and Disadvantages of Central Venous Access Techniques

Technique	Advantages	Disadvantages
Basilic (peripheral) puncture	Low incidence of major complications Performed under direct visualization of the vein Allows large quantities of fluid to be given rapidly	Greater incidence of minor complications of infection, phlebitis, and thrombosis Hinders free movement of arms More difficult to place catheter in correct position for CVP monitoring
IJ puncture	Good external landmarks Improved success with ultrasound Possibly less risk of pneumothorax than with subclavian puncture Bleeding can be recognized and controlled Malposition of catheter is rare Almost a straight course to the superior vena cava on the right side Carotid artery easily identified Useful alternative approach to cutdown in children younger than 2 yr	Slightly higher incidence of failures than subclavian approach More difficult and inconvenient to secure Possibly higher infectious risk than supraclavicular
Femoral puncture	Good external landmarks Useful alternative to other supradiaphragmatic approaches in patients with coagulopathies or superior vena caval trauma	Difficult to secure in ambulatory patients Generally not reliable for CVP measurement Potentially a "dirty" site Higher risk of thrombus
Infraclavicular SC approach	Good external landmarks	Unable to compress bleeding vessels "Blind" procedure Should not be attempted in children younger than 2 yr
Supraclavicular SC approach	Good external landmarks Practical method of inserting a central line in cardiorespiratory arrest	"Blind" procedure Unable to compress bleeding vessels

CVP, central venous pressure; IJ, internal jugular; SC, subclavian.

Central catheters, although safer than peripheral IV lines, are not immune to extravasation; indeed, fatal cases have been reported if the catheter becomes wedged up against the vessel wall, valves, or endocardium.[21] Strategies to avoid this complication include delivering vesicant drugs only through the distal ports or reconfirming that the proximal port is safely in the vein by aspirating blood through it.[21]

Other Indications

Other indications for central venous access include placement of a pulmonary artery catheter, transvenous pacemaker, and performance of cardiac catheterization, pulmonary angiography, and hemodialysis. The use of the pulmonary artery catheter can be valuable for determining fluid and hemodynamic status in the critically ill. It has a limited role in the ED and has drawn heavy criticism since the late 1990s and should be used only when the diagnostic benefits outweigh the potential risks.[22,23] Catheters such as the Uldall or Quinton device can be inserted within minutes, permitting emergency or short-term hemodialysis. However, these are very large and relatively stiff catheters that have been known to perforate the vena caval or atrial walls with fatal outcomes.[24,25] Extra caution should be applied in their insertion, possibly under ultrasound or fluouroscopic technique.

Relative Indications for Different Approaches

Subclavian (SV) Approaches
Subclavian venipuncture is the most frequently used means of central venous access. The infraclavicular SV approach was the first popular means of central venous access and has been widely taught during residency training for nearly half a century. It is effective, useful in many clinical situations, and relatively easy to learn. In trauma settings, it is often the best approach because a cervical collar can interfere with the IJ technique. The supraclavicular SV approach is one alternative to infraclavicular venipuncture and may be preferable during CPR because it minimizes physical interference with chest compression and airway management. The supraclavicular SV approach also avoids interference with airway management, which commonly occurs when the IJ vein is cannulated. In addition, the supraclavicular SV technique has been performed in the sitting position in patients with severe orthopnea. The left SV provides a direct route to the superior vena cava (SVC) and is the preferred site for pacemaker placement and CVP monitoring.

Internal Jugular (IJ) Approach
The IJ vein provides an excellent site for the placement of a CVC. However, there is a complication risk of 5% to 10% with serious complications occurring in about 1% of the patients.[26] Failure rates have been found to be 19.4% for landmark placed IJ catheterization when performed by a junior practitioner and from 5% to 10% by someone with extensive experience.[27] Complications of IJ vein cannulation are classified as minor or major. Major complications include laceration of neck vessels, carotid artery puncture with thromboembolism and resulting stroke, air embolism, pleural laceration with resulting pneumothorax or hemothorax, thrombosis, and infection. Minor complications include puncture of the carotid artery with hematoma formation and injury to the brachial plexus and peripheral nerves.[28] Despite these potential complications, the IJ vein is in most cases

preferred to other options for central venous access. In contrast to the SV, arterial punctures are easier to control because direct pressure can be utilized, there is a lower incidence of pneumothorax, and hematoma formation is easier to diagnose owing to the IJ vein's close proximity to the skin. In addition, the right IJ vein provides a straight anatomic path to the SVC and right atrium. This is advantageous for passage of catheters or internal pacemaker wires to the heart. Disadvantages of IJ vein cannulation over other sites include a relatively high carotid artery puncture rate and poor landmarks in obese or edematous patients.[26]

The IJ technique is useful for routine central venous access and for emergency venous access during CPR, because the site is removed from the area of chest compressions. The morbidity differences between the SV and the IJ vein approach have probably been overstated.[13,29] Catheter malposition is more frequent in the SV, but the risk of infection is probably slightly higher with IJ sites.[13,30,31] Arterial puncture is thought to be higher with IJ attempts, but the SV is not a compressible site.[13,30] Although counterintuitive, the best scientific evidence to date does not support a significant difference in the rate of pneumothorax and hemothorax.[13,30] Although there may be a slight difference in complications between the two routes, in the absence of specific contraindications, the clinician should use the technique with which he or she is most familiar. The rapid development of real-time ultrasound guidance may tip the scales toward the IJ as the preferred site.[32,33]

Femoral Approach

The cannulation of the femoral vein for central venous access has become increasingly popular, especially for venous access, infusion ports, passage of transvenous pacemakers, and pressure measurement catheters in critically ill patients.[33] The relatively simple and superficial anatomy surrounding the femoral vein affords a rapid approach to the central venous system and avoids many of the more significant complications associated with cannulation of the IJ and SV veins. These benefits are tempered somewhat by several long-term disadvantages including higher infection rates and an increased risk of venous thrombosis. Other indications for urgent femoral cannulation include emergency cardiopulmonary bypass for resuscitation purposes, charcoal hemoperfusion for severe drug overdoses, and dialysis access. The femoral area is less congested with monitoring and airway equipment than the head and neck area and the conscious patient, who is still bedridden, may turn the head and use the arms more freely without moving the central line. The femoral site is contraindicated in the ambulatory patient who requires central access.

CONTRAINDICATIONS

Contraindications to the various techniques of central venous access are shown in Table 22–3. Most listed contraindications are considered relative, and should be viewed in context with clinical conditions and available options for vascular access. Perhaps the only true absolute contraindication is insertion of catheters impregnated with antibiotic (most commonly tetracycline or rifampin) if the patient has a serious allergy to the drug.[34] Local cellulitis is a relative contraindication to any access route. Each technique is contraindicated in patients with distorted local anatomy or landmarks. Insertion of catheters through freshly burned regions, although somewhat challenging, does not have a higher incidence of infections

TABLE 22–3 Relative Contraindications to Specific Central Venous Access Routes*

General

Distorted local anatomy
Extremes of weight
Vasculitis
Prior long-term venous cannulation
Prior injection of sclerosis agents
Suspected proximal vascular injury
Previous radiation therapy
Bleeding disorders
Anticoagulation or thrombolytic therapy
Combative patients
Inexperienced, unsupervised physician

Subclavian Vein

Chest wall deformities
Pneumothorax on the contralateral side
Chronic obstructive pulmonary disease

Jugular Vein

Intravenous drug abuse via the jugular system

Femoral Vein

Need for patient mobility

*Use of this technique must be based on clinical conditions and available options for vascular access.

until approximately 3 days after the burn when bacterial colonization accelerates.[35,36] One of the more commonly encountered impediments to CVL is morbid obesity.[37] Surface landmarks are often obscured, an abdominal pannus can block the femoral access site, and deeper insertions and steeper angles are required. The IJ under ultrasound may be a safer approach under these circumstances.[37] Insertion of another catheter to the same side as a preexisting catheter risks the complication of entrapment.[38] Combativeness should be emphasized because the risk of mechanical complications greatly increases in the uncooperative victim. Sometimes, it is best to sedate and intubate critical patients before attempting central venous catheterization. Other relative contraindications include those conditions predisposing to sclerosis or thrombosis of the central veins, such as vasculitis, prior long-term cannulation, or illicit IV drug use via any of the deep venous systems.

Coagulapathy is a frequent concern surrounding CVL insertion, with the overall risk of significant hemorrhage in these patients approximating 2%. A transfusion of fresh frozen plasma is commonly used to correct existing coagulopathy. However, Segal and Dzik's review[39] concluded that if good technique is used, correction of coagulopathy is not generally required before or during the procedure. Mumtaz and coworkers[40] found that even in thrombocytopenic patients (with platelets $< 50 \times 10^9/L$), bleeding complications occurred about 3% of the time and were limited to insertion site bleeding; these were managed with additional sutures. Whereas the occasional patient may require transfusion of blood or clotting factors if a hemorrhagic complication should arise, the current literature generally has not found benefit from prophylactically correcting an abnormal International Normalized Ratio (INR) or platelet count prior to the procedure.[39–41]

SV Approach

SV access is contraindicated in patients who have undergone previous surgery or trauma involving the clavicle, the first rib, or the subclavian vessels; who have undergone previous radiation therapy to the clavicular area; with significant chest wall deformities; and with marked cachexia or obesity. However, clinicians in burn centers routinely place central catheters through burned areas. Patients with unilateral deformities not associated with pneumothorax (e.g., fractured clavicle) should be catheterized on the opposite side. Subclavian venipuncture is not contraindicated in patients who have penetrating thoracic wounds unless the injuries are known or suspected to involve the subclavian vessels or SVC. Generally, the vein on the same side of the chest wound should be cannulated to avoid the possibility of bilateral pneumothoraces. When pre-existing subclavian vessel injury is suspected, cannulation should occur on the opposite side. Formerly, subclavian venipuncture was not recommended for use in small children, but in experienced hands, it has been demonstrated to be safe.[42–44]

IJ Approach

Cervical trauma with swelling or anatomic distortion at the intended site of IJ venipuncture is the most important contraindication to the IJ approach. Neck motion is limited when the IJ line is in place, and this limitation represents a relative contraindication in conscious patients. Likewise, the presence of a cervical collar is problematic. Although bleeding disorders are relative contraindications to central venous cannulation, the IJ approach is preferred over the SV route as the IJ site is compressible. In the setting of severe bleeding diatheses, the femoral approach should be considered. Carotid artery disease (obstruction or atherosclerotic plaques) is a relative contraindication to IJ cannulation because inadvertent puncture or manipulation of the artery could dislodge a plaque. In addition, prolonged compression of the artery to control bleeding could impair cerebral circulation if collateral blood flow is compromised. If a preceding SV catheterization has been unsuccessful, the ipsilateral IJ route is generally preferred for a subsequent attempt. In this manner, bilateral iatrogenic complications can be avoided.

Femoral Vein Approach

Contraindications to femoral cannulation include known or suspected intra-abdominal hemorrhage or injury to the pelvis, groin, iliac vessels, or IVC. Palpation for the femoral pulsations in CPR is difficult and is often venous rather than arterial.[45] Ultrasound-guided catheterization under these conditions is faster, more successful, and less likely to incur inadvertent arterial puncture than the standard landmark-oriented approach.[46]

ANATOMY

SV System

The SV begins as a continuation of the axillary vein at the outer edge of the first rib (see Fig. 22–1). It joins the IJ vein to become the innominate vein 3 to 4 cm proximally. The SV has a diameter of 10 to 20 mm and is valveless. After crossing the first rib, the vein lies posterior to the medial third of the clavicle. It is only in this area that there is an intimate association between the clavicle and the SV. The costoclavicular ligament lies anterior and inferior to the SV, and the fascia contiguous to this ligament invests the vessel. Posterior to the vein, separating it from the subclavian artery, lies the anterior scalene muscle, which has a thickness of 10 to 15 mm. The phrenic nerve passes over the anterior surface of the scalene muscle and runs immediately behind the junction of the SV and the IJ vein. The thoracic duct (on the left) and the lymphatic duct (on the right) pass over the anterior scalene muscle and enter the SV near its junction with the IJ vein. Superior and posterior to the subclavian artery lies the brachial plexus. The dome of the left lung may extend above the first rib, but the right lung rarely extends this high.

Jugular System

The IJ vein begins just medial to the mastoid process at the base of the skull, running inferiorly and passing under the sternal end of the clavicle joining the SV and forming the innominate or brachiocephalic vein. The IJ vein, the internal carotid artery, and the vagus nerve course together in the carotid sheath just deep to the sternocleidomastoid muscle (SCM) at the level of the thyroid cartilage. Within the carotid sheath, the IJ vein typically occupies the anterior lateral position and the carotid artery lies medial and slightly posterior to the vein. This relationship is relatively constant, but studies have found that the carotid artery may overlap the IJ. Note that normally the IJ vein migrates medially as it nears the clavicle, where it may lie directly over the carotid artery (see Fig. 22–2B and C). Using the most common central approach (see later), the IJ tends to be more lateral than expected.[47] Furthermore, in 5.5% of those studied, the IJ vein may even be medial to the carotid artery.[48–50] The relationship between the IJ vein and the carotid artery also depends upon head position. Excessive head rotation can cause the carotid artery to rotate over the IJ vein.[28,51]

Anatomic landmarks for locating the vein include the sternal notch, the clavicle, and the SCM. The two heads of the SCM and the clavicle form a triangle that is key to understanding the underlying vascular anatomy. The IJ vein can be located at the apex of the triangle as it courses along the medial head of the SCM, occupying a position in the middle of the triangle at the level of the clavicle before it joins the SV and forms the innominate vein (Fig. 22–2). At the level of the thyroid cartilage, the IJ vein can be found just deep to the SCM.

Owing to its connection to the SV and the right atrium, the IJ vein is pulsatile. In contrast to the aorta, these pulsations are not palpable. When visualized, however, the presence of venous pulsations can give an indication of patency of the IJ vein to the right atrium. The IJ vein will also change size with respiration. Owing to the negative intrathoracic pressure at end-inspiration, blood in the IJ vein is actually drawn into the right atrium and the IJ vein's diameter shrinks. In contrast, at end-expiration, the increased intrathoracic pressure will limit blood return to the right atrium and the IJ vein's diameter will increase. Another unique characteristic of the IJ vein is its distensibility. The IJ vein will enlarge when the pressure in the vein is increased, that is, when there is obstruction of blood flow back to the right atrium as with thrombosis. This distensibility can be advantageous in the placement of central venous access. Using a head-down (Trendelenburg) position or a Valsalva maneuver will increase

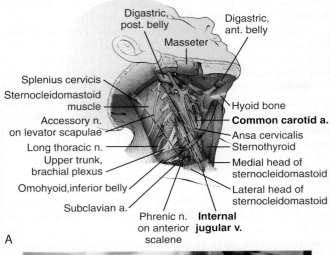

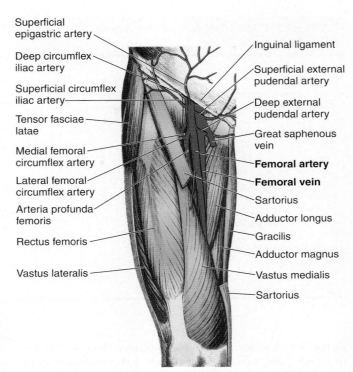

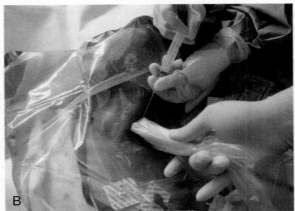

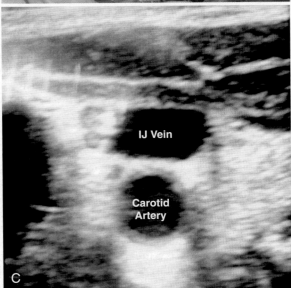

Figure 22–3 The right femoral vessels. The femoral nerve (not shown) lies lateral to the artery and may be deep to the artery. Note that distal to the inguinal ligament, the femoral artery starts to move medially and almost on top of the femoral vein. Attempts low in the groin may, without ultrasound guidance, injure the artery.

the IJ vein's diameter, increasing the likelihood of successful puncture.

Femoral System

Femoral anatomy is less complex than that of the neck and shoulder and contains fewer vital structures. The femoral vein is most easily cannulated percutaneously in patients with a palpable femoral pulse. The femoral vein is bounded cranially by the inguinal ligament, and it disappears into the large muscles of the anterior thigh as it proceeds caudally. Medially, the femoral vein abuts a robust system of lymphatics. Laterally, the vein is intimately associated with the femoral artery. The femoral nerve courses down into the leg just lateral to the femoral artery. These relationships from lateral to medial can be memorized by the pneumonic NAVEL (nerve, artery, vein, empty space, lymphatics). Note that as the femoral artery and vein course down the leg, their side-by-side relationship frequently rotates such that the femoral artery may lie on top of the vein. Therefore, to avoid arterial puncture, cannulation attempts should be kept just under the inguinal ligament (Fig. 22–3). When cannulating this vessel distally to the inguinal ligament, ultrasound guidance can be helpful to avoid arterial puncture.

TECHNIQUE AND EQUIPMENT

Preparation and organization of equipment ahead of time are imperative. Most catheters now come from the manufacturer in convenient sterile kits. We strongly recommend stocking all additional equipment such as sterile gowns, gloves, and drapes into a dedicated "central line cart" (Table 22–4). This practice has been shown to reduce the sometimes widespread

Figure 22–2 *A*, Anatomy of the internal jugular (IJ) area. Note that the vein runs nearly parallel, and lateral, to the carotid artery, but the vein is nearly over the artery at the clavicle. Ultrasound obtained during IJ catheterization (*B*) shows the IJ vein almost directly over the carotid artery above the clavicle (*C*), demonstrating the value of ultrasound-guided placement of the central venous pressure (CVP) line to avoid arterial injury.

TABLE 22–4 Materials for Central Venous Cannulation

1% lidocaine
26-gauge needle
2-mL Luer-Lok syringe (for anesthetic)
10-mL non–Luer-Lok syringe (for catheter placement)
Swabs
Preparation solution
Gloves
Drapes
Catheter device
Intravenous tubing
Intravenous solution
Needle holder
4-0 silk (or nylon) sutures
Suture scissors
Antibiotic ointment
Gauze pads
Tincture of benzoin
Cloth tape

search for supplies, improve compliance with full-barrier technique, and subsequently reduce catheter-related infections.[52,53] Maximal sterile barrier precautions with cap, face mask, sterile gowns, and gloves should be used at all times during CVC insertion.[31,54]

Some clinicians prefer to first locate the position of a central vein with a small exploratory or "finder" needle, rather than directly cannulating the vein with only the larger needle that will accommodate a guidewire or catheter. This practice is less practical for the SV approach. Although this may be desirable in some circumstances, and can minimize trauma and the complications of a larger needle, no specific standard exists. In clinical practice, this exploratory needle is seldom used in an emergency situation. The smaller introducing needles used with the Seldinger technique have largely supplanted the need for this exploratory procedure. Placing 0.5 to 1.0 ml of saline or lidocaine in the syringe before insertion allows one to expunge the small skin plug that may prevent the flash of blood signifying vessel entry. Be aware that this blood flash, when mixed with remaining clear fluid in the syringe, tends to appear brighter than usual and could be mistaken for arterial puncture.

Seldinger and Other Techniques

The most commonly used means of central venous cannulation is the Seldinger (guidewire) technique, using a thin-walled needle to introduce a guidewire into the vessel lumen. Seldinger originally described this in 1953 as a method for catheter placement in percutaneous arteriography.[50] To obtain vascular access, insert a small needle into the intended vessel. Once the introducer needle is positioned within the lumen of the vessel, thread a wire through the needle, and then remove the needle. The wire, now within the vessel, serves as a guide over which the catheter is placed. Although the Seldinger technique involves several steps, it may be performed quickly once mastered. More importantly, this technique broadens the application of central vein cannulation, permitting the insertion of standard infusion catheters, multilumen catheters, large-bore rapid infusion systems, introducer devices, and even peripheral cardiopulmonary bypass

cannulas. Given this flexibility, the use of Seldinger-type systems is advantageous, despite its greater cost.

The basic materials required for central venous cannulation are shown in Figure 22–4. The catheter may be a component in a guidewire system or of the over-the-needle variety (the other widely used method of catheter placement). To obtain central access from the basilic-cephalic system (and occasionally from the femoral vein), a through-the-needle catheter passage technique is used. This is detailed in a special section after discussion of these more common approaches.

Needle

Virtually any needle or catheter can be used to introduce a guidewire into a vessel, but there are advantages to using needles specifically designed for guidewire passage. These needles must be large enough to accommodate the desired wire, yet as small as possible to minimize bleeding complications. The needles provided with central vein catheters or introducer devices are usually thin walled, thereby maximizing lumen size relative to overall needle diameter. If a needle that is not thin walled is used, a size that is 1 gauge smaller (larger-bore) than that listed in Table 22–5 should be used. If unsure, simply test the equipment to ensure compatibility.

Standard needles may have a uniformly straight-bore lumen throughout their length. A wire passing into a straight needle may encounter an obstacle at the proximal end. The proximal end of a Seldinger needle incorporates a funnel-shaped taper that guides the wire directly into the needle (Fig. 22–5).

It is advisable to use a non–Luer-Lok or slip-tip type, because the added twisting that is required to remove a Luer-Lok syringe from the introducer needle may dislodge a tenuously placed needle. Systems now exist that permit passage of the wire without removal of the aspirating syringe by using a central tunnel in the barrel. Sometimes, the wire can become snagged at the junction of the syringe and the catheter hub. In that case, remove the syringe and insert the wire directly into the catheter hub.

Guidewire

Two basic types of guidewires are used: straight or J-shaped. The straight wires are for use in vessels with a linear configuration, whereas the J-wires are for use in tortuous vessels. Both wires have essentially the same internal design (Fig. 22–6A). The flexibility of the wire is a result of a stainless steel coil or helix that forms the bulk of the guidewire. Within the central lumen of the helix is a straight central core wire, called a mandrel, which adds rigidity to the steel coil. The mandrel is usually fixed at one end of the helix and terminates 0.5 and 3.0 cm from the other end, creating a flexible or floppy tip. Wires are also available with two flexible ends, one straight and the other J-shaped. The flexible end of the guidewire allows the wire to flex on contact with the wall of a vessel. If the contact is tangential, as in an infraclavicular approach to the SV, a straight wire is generally preferred. If the angle is more acute, as in an external jugular approach to the SV, or if the vessel is particularly tortuous or valves must be traversed, a J-shaped wire may be used. The more rounded leading edge of the J-wire provides a broader surface to manipulate within the vessel and decreases the risk of perfora-

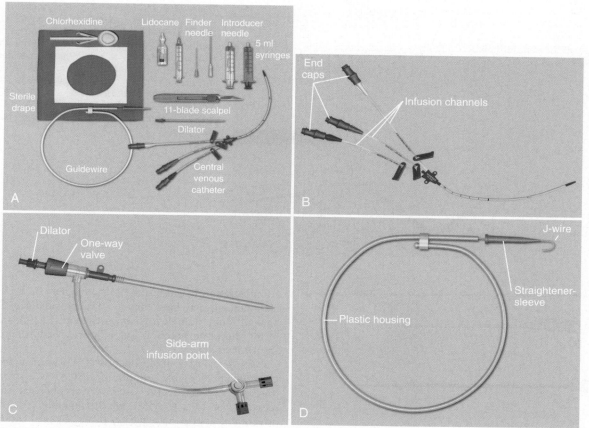

Figure 22–4   **Equipment used for central vein catheterization.** *A,* Standard commercial kit contents. *B,* Triple lumen catheter. *C,* Introducer sheath. *D,* Guidewire. *(A–D, From Thomsen T, Setnik G [eds]: Procedures Consult—Emergency Medicine Module. Copyright 2008 Elsevier Inc. All rights reserved.)*

TABLE 22–5 Needle Sizes for Venous and Arterial Catheters*	
Standard Full-Length Coil Guidewire Catheter Size (Fr)	**Needle Gauge†**
3	21
4–4.5	20
5–6.0	20–19
6–8.5	19–18

*Any size catheter from 3.0–8.5 Fr may be introduced using a 22-gauge needle if a solid wire (Cor-Flex, Cook Critical Care) is used.

†All needle gauges are for thin-walled needles only, the type supplied in central line kits.

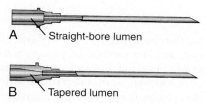

Figure 22–5   **Introducing needles.** *A,* Ordinary needle with a straight-bore lumen. *B,* Seldinger needle with a tapered lumen, allowing easy entry of the guidewire.

tion. This is especially advantageous when attempting to thread a wire through a vessel with valves. Many guidewires also contain a straight safety wire that runs parallel to the mandrel to keep the wire from kinking or shearing.

The standard size for guidewires is from 0.025 to 0.035 inch (0.064–0.089 cm) in diameter, permitting introduction through an 18-gauge thin-walled needle. A modification of this standard wire uses a bare mandrel with the flexible coil soldered to its end. This construction provides a wire with a diameter of only 0.018 inch (0.047 cm) but with the same rigidity as the larger wires. The manufacturer states that such a wire can be introduced through a 22-gauge thin-walled needle yet still guide an 8.5-French catheter (Micropuncture Introducer Sets and Trays with Cor-Flex Wire Guides, Cook Critical Care, Inc., Bloomington, IN).

It is important to emphasize that guidewires are delicate and may bend, kink, or unwind. A force of 4 to 6 pounds may cause a wire to rupture. Wires should thread easily and smoothly and never be forced. If a wire is not passing easily, withdraw the wire and the catheter as a single unit. Embolization of portions of the guidewire is possible, and sharp defects in the wire may perforate vessel walls (see Fig. 22–6*B*). However, if one encounters a good blood flash but cannot readily manipulate the wire, this may indicate that the outer wire coils may be entrapped against the proximal sharp edge of the needle bevel. The J can be straightened remotely by applying gentle force on the wire in each direction, which may allow wire retrieval.[55] Wires should be inspected for small defects such as kinks, sharp ends, or spurs before use and especially after a failed attempt.

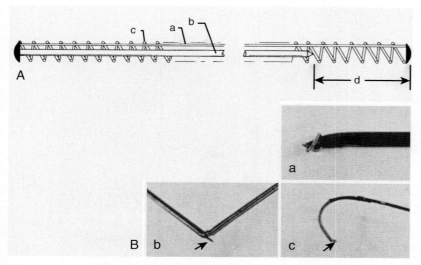

Figure 22–6 *A, Guidewire internal structure: safety wire (a), core wire (mandrel) (b), coiled wire (c), flexible tip (d). B, Flexible end of a straight-spring guidewire knotted on a vessel dilator (a), bent junction of the rigid and flexible portions of a straight-spring guidewire with protrusion of the central core (arrow) (b), partially fractured tip (arrow) of a J-spring guidewire (c). (A and B, From Schwartz AJ, Horrow JL, Jobes DR, Ellison N: Guide wires—A caution. Crit Care Med 9:348, 1981. ©1981 Williams & Wilkins, Baltimore. Reproduced by permission.)*

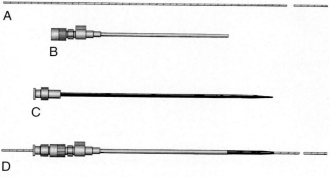

Figure 22–7 Desilets-Hoffman sheath introducer. *A, Guidewire. B, Sheath-introducer. C, Dilator. D, Assembled device.*

Catheters

A number of different catheter and introducer devices have been developed, and the method of passage into the vessel varies accordingly. The functions of catheters have become more sophisticated as well, most notably for continuous monitoring of central venous oxygen saturation and cardiac output. Generally, place single-, double-, and triple-lumen catheters by sliding the catheter directly over a guidewire into the intended vessel. Introduce larger catheters or nonlumen devices with a sheath-introducer system. Place over-the-needle catheters once intravascular placement is attained.

The Desilets-Hoffman–type sheath introducer became available in 1965 to aid in arteriography procedures that require many catheter changes. This device is commonly but incorrectly termed a "Cordis", which is actually a proprietary trade name. The sheath-introducer unit includes two parts, an inner dilator and an outer sheath (Fig. 22–7). The dilator is rigid with a narrow lumen to accommodate the guidewire. It is longer and thinner than its sheath and has a tapered end that dilates the subcutaneous tissue and the vessel defect formed by the needle. The sheath (or introducer catheter when used as a cannula for introducing Swan-Ganz catheters, transvenous pacemakers, or other devices) has a blunt end and is simply a large-diameter catheter.

Many modifications of the sheath exist, with side arms and diaphragms to aid in the placement of non-lumen devices. Care must be taken in the use of side-arm sets for rapid fluid administration because some catheters may be 8.5 French in diameter but may have only a 5-French side arm. Some sets have a "single-lumen infusion catheter" (SLIC), which performs the same function but is more easily secured to the sheath introducer.

Catheter-associated infection (CAI) is an important and generally preventable complication. CAI is associated with (but not necessarily the cause of) an increase in hospital mortality of 15% to 35%; the attributable cost of a single infection is approximately $12,000.[34,56] Special catheters have been developed to prevent bacterial contamination and line sepsis.[57,58] These catheters are impregnated with either antiseptics (silver sulfadiazine and chlorhexidine) or antibiotics (minocycline, rifampin, or cefazolin)[59-62] to reduce bacterial colonization and microbial growth. Also, heparin-coated catheters are available that prevent fibronectin binding, thereby inhibiting the formation of bacterial biofilms on the catheter's surface. These catheters can significantly decrease CAI and are cost effective when the prevalence of CAI is greater than 2%.[30] Avoid using heparin-coated catheters in patients with a history of heparin induced thrombocytopenia.[63] Minocycline- and rifampin-impregnated catheters are currently considered to be the most effective.[57] Other interventions that decrease central line infections include using full sterile barrier precautions,[31] chlorhexidine solution skin preparations,[64] and placement by experienced physicians.[31,65,66]

Guidewire Placement with the Seldinger Technique

Attach a small syringe to an introducing needle that is large enough to accommodate the guidewire (Fig. 22–8). Insert the needle and syringe together, entering the selected vessel with the needle tip. Once a free return of blood is obtained, remove the syringe, and stabilize the needle hub to prevent needle movement and displacement of the tip from the vessel. Be aware that in extremely low CVP shock states, especially with trauma, there may be no observable flash of blood. At times, detachment of the syringe from the thin-walled needle may lead to loss of the needle's intravascular position. The need to detach the syringe can be eliminated by use of the Arrow Safety Syringe. This device incorporates a hollow syringe

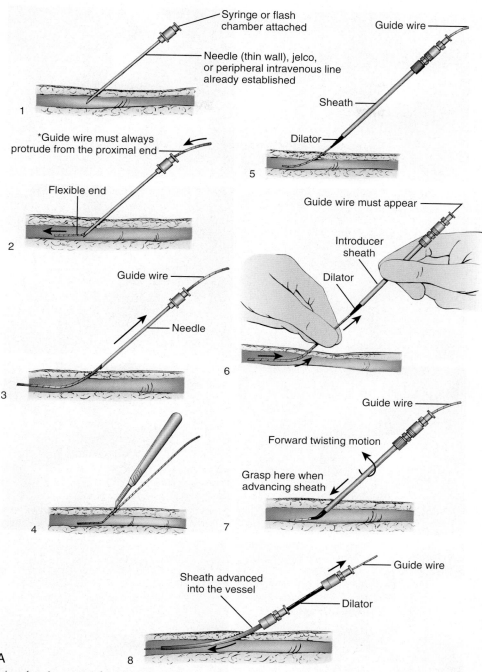

Figure 22–8 *A,* Procedure for placement of Seldinger-type guidewire catheter. *1,* Cannulate the selected vessel with a thin-walled needle, or choose an existing intravenous (IV) catheter to be changed with the wire technique. *2,* Thread the guidewire into the vessel, with the flexible end first, into the lumen of the vessel. If a J-wire is used, use the sleeve to facilitate entry into the needle (see Fig. 22–9). *3,* Remove the needle so that only the wire now exits from the vessel. *4,* Enlarge the skin entry site with a No. 11 scalpel. *5,* Thread the catheter sheath and the dilator over the wire and advance it to the skin. The wire must be visible through the back of the device. *6,* If the proximal wire is not visible, pull it from the skin through the catheter until it appears at the back of the catheter. *7,* Advance the sheath and dilator as a unit into the skin with a twisting motion. Grasp the unit at the junction of sheath and dilator to prevent bunching up of the sheath. Hold the wire (at the back of the catheter) while advancing the sheath and dilator as a unit. *8,* Once the sheath and the dilator are well within the vessel, remove the guidewire and the dilator. *B,* Placement of a central line (right subclavian vein), demonstrating the step-by-step procedure. *1,* Generous local anesthesia along the entire tract makes placement almost painless. *2,* The vein is entered (note the syringe parallel to the clavicle and the hub of the syringe flat against the chest). *3,* As soon as blood is aspirated, stop advancing the needle and stabilize the needle where it enters the skin. *4,* The most critical portion of the procedure is stabilization of the needle so it remains in the vein when the syringe is removed. Note that the hub is covered to prevent air embolism. *5,* The wire is advanced through the needle. *6,* Puncture the skin at the wire entrance to aid in advancing the catheter. *7,* Advance the vein dilator over the wire to facilitate entrance of the catheter into the vein. *Be certain the end of the wire is secured at all times (arrow).* Remove the dilator so only the wire remains. *8,* Advance the catheter over the wire (a twisting motion at the skin may help). Note that the end of the guidewire always protrudes through the distal brown port *(arrow).* *9,* Secure the catheter with staples or sutures. This catheter has the securing device integrated into the catheter; some have an optional securing guard. *10,* A catheter guard is used to maintain the catheter at a specific depth. *(B, From Thomsen T, Setnik G [eds]: Procedures Consult—Emergency Medicine Module. Copyright 2008 Elsevier Inc. All rights reserved.)*

Continued

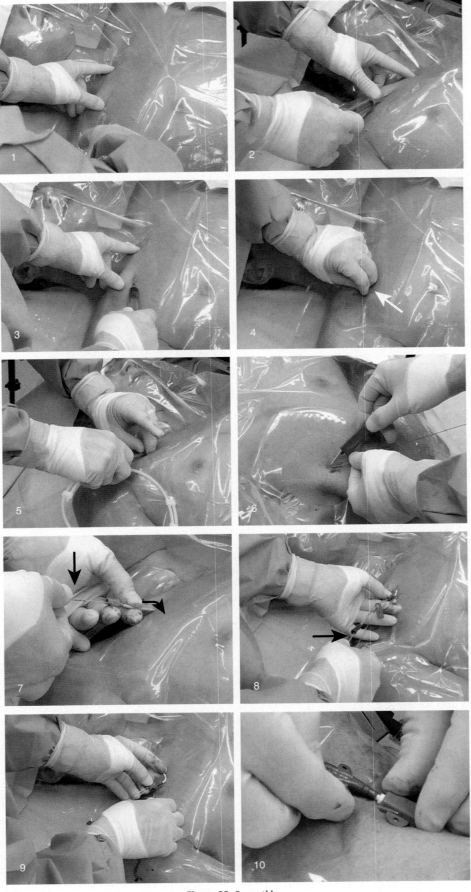

B

Figure 22–8, cont'd

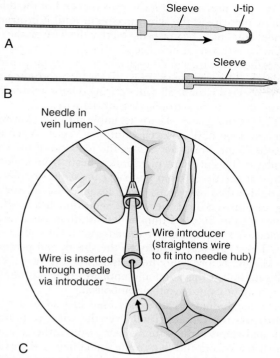

Figure 22–9 J-Wire. *A,* Plastic sleeve in the retracted position, demonstrating the J-tip. *B,* Plastic sleeve is advanced to straighten the curve to allow easy introduction into the needle hub. In an emergency, take care not to misplace or throw away the sleeve. Without it, placing the J-wire into the hub of the needle is very difficult. Some wires may have a "soft-tipped" straight end on the opposite end of the wire. These are engineered to be flexible (to avoid vessel injury) and may be used if there is difficulty passing the J end. *C,* Technique to insert J-wire into needle hub with the plastic sleeve.

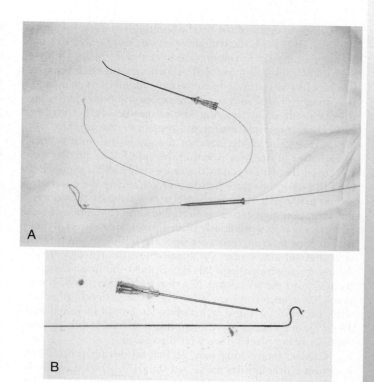

Figure 22–10 Although newer guidewires are more resistant to shearing, if a guidewire will not advance, *withdraw both the needle and the wire in one motion.* These pictures demonstrate a permanently deformed guidewire that could not be advanced. Withdrawing the wire with the indwelling introducer needle in place within a vessel may shear off a portion of the wire, resulting in systemic embolization.

385

through which the guidewire can pass directly into the thin-walled needle without detachment. This also reduces the risk of air embolism, which can occur when the needle is open to the air. It is not uncommon for the wire to get hung up at the junction of the safety syringe and the needle hub. In that case, simply remove the syringe and insert the wire directly. If the needle is removed from the syringe, cap the needle hub with your thumb before passing the guidewire to minimize the potential for air embolism.

Thread the flexible end of the guidewire through the needle. Introduce the straight wire easily by threading its flexible end into the hub of the needle. Introduce the J-wire by advancing a plastic sleeve contained in the kit to the floppy end of the wire, straightening out the J-shape. This straightened end is then introduced into the needle hub. Once the J-wire has been advanced, remove the sleeve and set it aside (Fig. 22–9). It is important not to accidentally discard this sleeve because it is difficult to insert the J-wire without it.

Thread the wire smoothly into the vein without resistance. Do not force the wire if resistance is met, but remove it from the needle and reattach the syringe and aspirate blood to confirm intravascular placement. It is important for the wire to slip easily from the needle during removal. If resistance to removal of the wire is felt, the wire and the needle should be removed as a single unit to prevent shearing of the wire and resultant wire embolism. It has been recommended by some that no wire should ever be withdrawn through the introducing needle.[54] Although there are no clinical data to support this recommendation and newer wires are stronger

and more resistant to shearing, it represents the safest course of action (Fig. 22–10). The recommendation to remove the needle and the wire as a unit is sometimes disregarded because of reluctance to abandon a potentially successful venipuncture. The clinician performing the procedure must use both caution and good judgment to determine the best course of action, but should not withdraw the guidewire against resistance. Manipulation of the wire within an introducer needle should be done only with standard coil guidewires. Solid wires (such as Cor-Flex Wire Guides from Cook Critical Care) have a small lip at the point at which the flexible coil is soldered to the wire. This lip can become caught on the edge of the needle tip, shearing off the coil portion of the wire. Solid wires must thread freely on the first attempt or the entire wire and needle assembly must be removed. Keep backup wires on hand.

Occasionally, a wire must be teased into the vessel; rotating the wire or needle often helps in difficult placements. If the wire does not thread easily, pull back slightly on the needle itself just before advancing the wire. This helps if the opening of the needle is abutting the vessel's inner wall, blocking the wire's entry, or if the vein is compressed by introduction of the needle. Changing wire tips from a straight to a J-wire or vice versa also may solve an advancement problem. If the inner lumen of a vessel is smaller than the diameter of the J, it will prevent the wire from reforming its natural shape, causing the spring in the coil to generate resistance. Any advantages of a J-wire will be negated if the wire fails to regain its intended shape. In this instance, a straight tip should be introducible without a problem. Alternatively, if the angle of entry of the needle and the vessel is more acute than was suspected, the straight wire may not be able to bend appropriately as it encounters the vessel's far wall. A J-tipped wire may be used and threaded in such a manner that the wire resumes its J-shape away from the far wall. All of these maneuvers are performed with gentle free motions of the wire within the needle. If at any time the wire cannot be advanced freely, suspect improper placement and reevaluate the attempt.

If threading easily, advance the guidewire until at least one quarter of the wire is within the vessel. The further into the vessel the wire extends, the more stable its location when the catheter is introduced. However, advancing the guidewire too far may result in ventricular ectopy secondary to endocardial irritation, myocardial puncture leading to tamponade, or entanglement in a previously placed pacemaker, internal defibrillator, or inferior vena cava filter. In both left and right IJ vein and infraclavicular SV approaches, fluoroscopic study during guidewire passage has determined the mean distance from skin to the SVC-atria junction to be 18 cm.[55] This distance has been recommended as the greatest depth of guidewire insertion for these approaches. (It should be noted that 18 cm is not necessarily the appropriate final depth for the catheter being placed—see later discussion.)

Cardiac monitoring may be helpful during central line insertions, although its use is not standard practice for most patients. Consider precautionary external pacemaker pads for patients with preexisting bundle branch blocks.[67] Any increase in premature ventricular contractions or new ventricular dysrhythmia should be interpreted as evidence that the guidewire is inserted too far, and should be remedied by withdrawing the wire until the rhythm reverts to baseline. Usually, after a moment, the procedure can be continued, with care taken not to readvance the wire. Persistent ventricular dysrhythmias require standard advanced cardiac life support (ACLS) treatment and consideration of a new vascular approach.

Occasionally, a wire threads easily past the tip of the needle and then suddenly will not advance farther. If the introducer needle demonstrated free blood return at the time of wire entry and the initial advancement of the wire met no resistance, the two options are to halt the procedure, or seek confirmation of wire position. The needle may be removed, the wire fixed in place with a sterile hemostat, and a radiograph taken to confirm the position of the wire.[56] This confirmation may be advisable if the location of a wire is suspect and the introduction of a large-sized sheath is planned. A freely advancing wire may suddenly stop once it is well within a vessel if the vessel makes an unsuspected bend or is being compressed or deviated by another structure, such as a rib or muscle. This seems especially common with the infraclavicular approach to SV and can sometimes be remedied by a more lateral approach.

Sheath Unit and Catheter Placement

Once the wire is placed into the vessel, remove the needle in preparation for passage of the catheter (see Fig. 22–8). Make a small skin incision at the site of the wire. Make the incision approximately the width of the catheter to be introduced and extend it completely through the dermis. Stabilize the guidewire at the point of the skin incision and thread the dilator/sheath assembly over the wire to a point 1 cm from the surface of the skin. Once the dilator/sheath is advanced over the wire and before it enters the skin, the wire must protrude from the proximal end of the dilator. It is very important to grasp the wire as the dilator/sheath is advanced to avoid further advancement into the circulation and potential loss of the wire. If the

wire does not protrude from the proximal end of the dilator, withdraw the wire at the skin entry point until it protrudes a sufficient amount to be grasped. Overlay the wire on the chest to allow an estimate of how deep it should go. A surprisingly long segment of wire should typically remain at proper insertion depth. The wire must always be visible protruding from the end of the dilator at all times during dilator advancement to avoid the near-catastrophic loss of the wire.

Thread the dilator/sheath assembly into the skin with a twisting motion until it is well within the vessel. When using a sheath/dilator, grasp the unit at the junction of the sheath and dilator. This prevents the thinner sheath from kinking or bending at the tip or from bunching up at the coupler end. If a rigid-walled sheath is used, advance the dilator only a few centimeters into the vessel, slide the sheath off, and advance it to its hub. If a thin-walled sheath is used, keep the introducer-sheath unit intact and advance it through the skin to the hub. This adds rigidity to the sheath and prevents it from kinking before being fully inserted in the vessel. Cover the sheath hub at this point and until attachment of the infusion tubing or cap to avoid air embolism.

If a single-lumen catheter is used instead of a sheath/dilator, pass the catheter itself over the wire to its desired depth and remove the wire. When a soft catheter is used, create a track from the skin to the vessel before the catheter can be introduced. Pass and then withdraw a separate dilator over the guidewire, after the needle is removed but before the catheter is placed. After the dilator is removed, thread the soft catheter into position over the wire. It is imperative that the guidewire protrudes from the catheter hub and that it is firmly grasped as the wire and catheter are advanced. Once the catheter is placed, gently remove the wire. Take care to maintain the desired catheter insertion length. When removing the wire from a catheter it must slip out easily. If any resistance is met, remove both the wire and the catheter as a single unit and reattempt the procedure. A common cause of a "stuck wire" is a small piece of adipose tissue wedged between the wire and the lumen of the catheter. Avoid this problem by creating a deep enough skin nick and adequate dilation of the track before inserting the catheter.

Placement of multiple-lumen catheters requires identification of the distal lumen and its corresponding hub. Find the distal lumen at the very tip of the catheter. The corresponding hub is usually labeled "distal" by the manufacturer. If there is any confusion, inject a small amount of sterile saline through each hub until it is observed exiting the distal lumen. Once the distal hub is identified, remove its cover cap to allow passage of the guidewire (remember to replace this or immediately begin infusing saline upon completion of placement). Place the catheter by threading the guidewire into the distal lumen and advancing it until it protrudes from the hub. At this point, place the device in the same manner as a single-lumen catheter. If a soft multiple-lumen device is placed, use a separate dilator to create a track over the guidewire prior to placing the catheter. An alternate method of placing multiple-lumen catheters is to thread the catheter through a standard Desilets-Hoffman sheath-introducer system. Any lumen in a multiple-lumen device that is not immediately used for an infusion must be initially flushed with saline, and with heparinized saline during longer term use.

It is important to consider the depth of catheter insertion. The SVC begins at the level of the manubriosternal junction and terminates in the right atrium, which is approximately 5 cm lower. For lines placed in the subclavian, jugular, basilic, and cephalic systems, the proper position of the catheter is in

TABLE 22–6 Formulas for Catheter Insertion Length Based on Patient Height and Approach

Site	Formula	In SVC (%)	In RA (%)
RSC	(Hgt/10) − 2 cm	96	4
LSC	(Hgt/10) + 2 cm	97	2
RIJ	Hgt/10	90	10
LIJ	(Hgt/10) + 4 cm	94	5

Hgt, patient height (in cm); LIJ, left internal jugular; LSC, left subclavian; RA, right atrium; RIJ, right internal jugular; RSC, right subclavian; SVC, superior vena cava.

From Czepizak C, O'Callaghan JM, Venus B: Evaluation of formulas for optimal positioning of central venous catheters. Chest 107:1662, 1995. Reproduced by permission.

the SVC, not the right atrium or ventricle. Therefore, thread the catheter to approximately 2 cm below the manubriosternal junction. Many commonly used catheters are long enough to reach the atrium or ventricle. For example, the standard catheters marketed for subclavian venipuncture are 20 to 30 cm long. For a subclavian catheter placed in the average adult male, 20 cm from the skin insertion site is more than sufficient to reach the SVC. Catheters 15 to 16 cm in length are recommended to avoid unintended placement to an excessive depth. Estimate the proper distance to advance the catheter by placing the catheter parallel to the chest wall before insertion. Alternatively, formulas have been developed to determine optimal insertion length based on the patient's height. One set (Table 22–6) was found to yield accurate placement in the SVC on 95% of 228 attempts.[58] Confirm proper placement by obtaining a postprocedure chest radiograph, which also rules out complications such as pneumothorax or hemothorax.

Many different catheters are currently manufactured. Although this leads to great flexibility in choice and cost, it often leads to confusion when a clinician is handed an unfamiliar catheter during an emergency. It is best to use one brand routinely and to ensure that all medical personnel are thoroughly familiar with its use.[68]

Replacement of Existing Catheters

In addition to placing new catheters, use the guidewire technique to change existing catheters. Many patients with CVCs are seriously ill and will also require subsequent pulmonary artery wedge pressure monitoring, transvenous pacemaker placement, or placement of a different catheter. The CVC that is initially inserted should have a lumen large enough to accept a guidewire and facilitate conversion to a different catheter. Use the guidewire technique to change a single-lumen CVC to a triple-lumen catheter or a sheath-introducer set. Not all commercially available CVCs will accept a guidewire.

Replacement of an existing catheter begins with selecting a guidewire longer than either of the devices to be exchanged. Use meticulous aseptic technique.[64] Insert the guidewire into the existing CVC until a few centimeters of wire are protruding from the proximal end. With one hand holding the wire securely, remove the catheter and wire as a single unit until the tip of the catheter just clears the patient's skin. Grasp the wire at the point at which it exits the skin, only then releasing the wire at the other end. Then slide the catheter off the wire, and insert the new device in the normal fashion. Exercise caution with this technique because catheter embolization can

occur, especially if a catheter is cut to allow use of a shorter guidewire for the exchange. In patients without evidence of line sepsis, exchanging the guidewire does not increase the incidence of CAIs if performed properly.[64]

Over-the-Needle Technique

An optional method for cannulation is to place an over-the-needle catheter percutaneously. Over-the-needle devices (such as the Angiocath) use a tapered plastic catheter that passes through the vessel wall into the lumen using the needle tip as a guide. There are advantages to this system. The catheter does not pass through a sharp needle, and there is less risk of shearing and resultant catheter embolization. Also, the hole made by the needle in the vessel wall is smaller than the catheter, thus producing a tighter seal. The IJ vein and SV via the supraclavicular approach are the most popular and appropriate approaches for this technique. Use these devices when rapid central venous access is required (e.g., during a cardiac arrest). The catheters are not suitable for high-volume fluid resuscitation, and they are too small for passage of a pacemaker lead. Once the clinical situation stabilizes, exchange this device for a larger central catheter via the Seldinger technique. It is convenient to keep extra wires on hand for exchanges and a 0.032-inch × 45-cm wire will fit most needs in the ED.

Prepare the skin with chlorhexidine solution. Use a longer peripheral-type catheter (such as a 16-gauge, 5¼-inch Angiocath) in an adult. Smaller-diameter devices, such as 20-gauge catheters, may be easier to pass but provide slower infusion rates. Attach the needle to a syringe, and slowly advance it into the vein with steady negative pressure applied to the syringe. This may be difficult owing to the longer length of the needle relative to the catheter. With over-the-needle catheters, the needle extends a few millimeters past the tip of the catheter. Blood return will be obtained when the tip of the needle is in the vein, whereas the catheter may actually be outside the lumen. If the needle is withdrawn before the catheter is advanced, the catheter tip will remain outside the vein. So, after the venous flash, advance the needle a few millimeters and then hold it steady while advancing the catheter into the vein. Secure the catheter and verify its placement as detailed later in this chapter.

SPECIFIC VESSEL ACCESS TECHNIQUES

If SV or IJ vein approaches are planned, prepare the skin of the area to include puncture sites for both the infraclavicular and the supraclavicular SV and IJ vein approaches. This permits the clinician to change the site after an unsuccessful attempt without repeating the preparation or having to obtain an interval chest radiograph. In this circumstance, prepare the area including the ipsilateral anterior neck, the supraclavicular fossa, and the anterior chest 3 to 5 cm past the midline and the same distance above the nipple line. Prepare for femoral access by trimming groin hairs, and then applying chlorhexidine to cover an area the breadth of, and extending 10 cm above and below, the inguinal ligament.

Each approach to central venous cannulation is described separately in the following sections. It is assumed that proper sterile procedure and any needed local anesthesia will be provided. As for any invasive task, briefly describe the procedure to awake patients, and restate each step as it is about to be performed. After the following descriptions of the common approaches to the central veins, puncture site care, placement verification, and other adjuncts to the procedure are summarized.

SV, Infraclavicular Approach

Descriptions of subclavian venipuncture often focus unduly on angles and landmarks. Indeed, the better recent studies demonstrate that some long-taught positioning maneuvers may actually hinder successful cannulation efforts.

Positioning

Place the patient supine on the stretcher with the head in a neutral position and the arm adducted at the side. Previous authors have advocated various shoulder, back, head, and arm positioning maneuvers but these take extra time and the help of an assistant and are often not helpful.[69-79]

Our consensus is that the best position for almost all infraclavicular SV attempts is the neutral shoulder position with the arm adducted.[70,72,73,79,80] Turning the head away may be helpful but is certainly not required if cervical injuries are suspected.[70,72,77] Interestingly, Jung and colleagues[81] found that at least in children, tilting the head toward the catheterization site improved catheter malposition rates. This has not been studied in adults thus far.

If unable to find the vein on several attempts, consider placing a small bump under the ipsilateral shoulder[77] or, alternately, have an assistant pull caudal traction of about 5 cm.[80] Placing the patient in a moderate Trendelenburg position (10°–20°) decreases the risk of air embolism.[72,82] The claim that this position distends the vein is somewhat controversial, but it probably does so to a small favorable degree.[70,72,74] If Trendelenburg is impractical, the SV approach is probably less affected than the IJ approach by resorting to a neutral or even an upright position.[70,72,74]

Placing a pillow under the back is commonly recommended to make the clavicle more prominent, but as the shoulder falls backward, the space between the clavicle and the first rib narrows, making the SV vein less accessible.[79] Significant compression of the subclavian vessels between these bony structures occurs as the shoulders retract, which can cause a "pinch off" of the catheter as it slides through the SV between the clavicle and the first rib.[79,83]

Venipuncture Site

The right SV is usually cannulated because of the lower pleural dome on the right and because of the need to avoid the left-sided thoracic duct. The anatomically more direct route between the left SV and the SVC is a theoretical advantage of left-sided over right-sided subclavian venipuncture. However, it has not been proved that there is a higher incidence of catheter malposition when the right infraclavicular SV approach is used. In the conscious patient, anesthetize the point of needle entry with 1% lidocaine. If possible, infiltrate the periosteum of the clavicle to make the procedure less painful. Opinions vary as to the best point of needle entry, more so than for the IJ or femoral approaches. On nonobese patients, look for the "deltopectoral triangle," which is bounded by the clavicle superiorly, the pectoralis major medially, and the deltoid muscle laterally.[75,84] The junction of the middle and medial thirds of the clavicle lies just medial to this. Further medially, the vein lies just posterior to the clavicle and above the first rib, which acts as a barrier to penetration of the pleura. This protective effect is theoretically diminished when a more lateral location is chosen. However, when approaching the vein more medially, some clinicians have difficulty puncturing the SV, dilating the tissues, and passing the J-wire. Other recommended sites of approach include lateral and inferior to the junction of the clavicle and the first rib, with the needle aiming at this junction, and entry at the site of a small tubercle in the medial aspect of the deltopectoral groove. We recommend that you puncture the skin at the lateral portion of the deltopectoral triangle and use a shallow angle of attack.[75]

Needle Orientation

Orient the bevel of the needle inferomedially in order to direct the wire toward the innominate (or brachiocephalic) vein rather than toward the opposite vessel wall or up into the IJ vein (Fig. 22–11). Align the bevel of the needle with the markings on the barrel of the syringe to permit awareness of the bevel orientation after skin puncture. You may consider making a small puncture in the skin with a No. 11 scalpel blade to avoid getting skin plugs in the needle. We suggest filling the syringe with 1 to 3 mL of 1% plain lidocaine to both anesthetize the subcutaneous tissue and flush the skin plug from the needle.

Before inserting the needle, place your left index finger in the suprasternal notch and your thumb at the costoclavicular junction (Fig. 22–12). These serve as reference points for the direction that the needle should travel. Aim the needle immediately above and posterior to the index finger. Watch for vessel entry, signaled by flashback of dark venous blood, which usually occurs at a depth of 3 to 4 cm. If the needle tip is truly intraluminal, there will be free-flowing blood. The return of pulsatile flow signifies arterial puncture. Withdraw the needle immediately. A single arterial puncture without laceration rarely causes serious harm. Using this technique eliminates the need to measure angles, to "walk" the clavicle, or to concentrate excessively on maintaining the needle parallel to the chest wall. Avoid using sweeping motions of the needle tip to prevent unseen injuries.

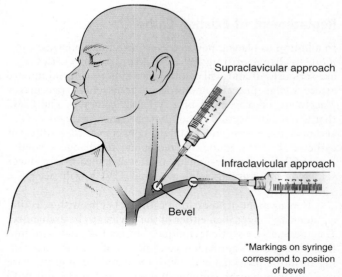

Figure 22–11 Needle bevel orientation using supraclavicular and infraclavicular venipuncture. The orientation of the needle bevel may help in positioning the catheter properly by guiding the direction of the wire during advancement. If the bevel is aligned with the markings on the syringe, the orientation of the bevel is always certain.

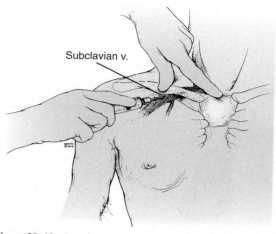

Figure 22–12 Hand position during subclavian venipuncture.

Unsuccessful Attempts

Cannulation of the SV may not succeed on the first attempt. It is reasonable to try again, but after three or four unsuccessful attempts, it is wise to move on to a different anatomic approach or allow a colleague to attempt the procedure. Use a new setup each time blood is obtained, because clots and tissue will clog the needle and mislead the clinician even if the vein has been entered successfully on subsequent attempts. If several attempts are made, inform the admitting clinician or anesthesiologist so that proper precautions are taken to identify subsequent complications. It is advisable to obtain radiographs of the chest even after unsuccessful attempts. If the initial puncture site was properly placed, use the same needle hole for subsequent attempts if possible for aesthetic reasons. If the SV route is unsuccessful on one side, attempt an IJ vein catheterization on the same side rather than an SV cannulation on the opposite side to avoid bilateral complications.

SV Approach

Positioning

The goal of the supraclavicular SV technique is to puncture the SV in its superior aspect as it joins the IJ vein. Insert the needle above and behind the clavicle, lateral to the clavicular head of the SCM. Advance it in an avascular plane, directing it away from the subclavian artery and the dome of the pleura. The right side is preferred because of the lower pleural dome, because it is the direct route to the SVC, and because the thoracic duct is on the left side. The patient's head may be turned to the opposite side to help identify the landmarks.

Needle Orientation

After the area of the supraclavicular fossa has been prepared and draped, identify a point 1 cm lateral to the clavicular head of the SCM and 1 cm posterior to the clavicle (Fig. 22–13). Alternatively, use the junction of the middle and medial thirds of the clavicle as the landmark for needle entry. This landmark had good success in a cadaveric study.[89] Anesthetize the area with 1% lidocaine. If a 3-cm-long needle is used for anesthesia, it may also be used to locate the vessel in a relatively atraumatic manner. The SV can almost always be located with this needle because of its superficial location and the absence of bony structures in the path of the needle. Advance a 14-gauge needle (or 18-gauge thin-walled needle),

following the path of the scout needle. Apply gentle negative pressure with an attached syringe.

When seeking the SV, aim the needle so as to bisect the clavicosternomastoid angle, with the tip pointing just caudal to the contralateral nipple. Orient the bevel medially to prevent the catheter from getting trapped against the inferior vessel wall. Point the tip of the needle 10° above the horizontal. Successful vessel puncture generally occurs at a depth of 2 to 3 cm.

IJ Approach

Positioning

After explaining the procedure to the patient and obtaining informed consent if applicable, position the patient. Position is critical for maximizing the success of blind (landmark technique) IJ vein cannulation. Place the patient in a supine position with the head down and turned about 15° to 30° away from the IJ vein to be cannulated. Rotate the head slightly away from the site of insertion. Rotating the head greater than 40% has been shown to increase the risk of overlapping the carotid artery over the IJ vein.[51] Occasionally, placing a rolled-up towel under the scapula helps to extend the neck and accentuate the landmarks. Stand at the head of the bed with all equipment within easy reach. This may involve moving the bed to the center of the room to allow a table or work surface to be located at the head of the bed.

Ask the patient to perform a Valsalva maneuver just prior to inserting the needle to increase the diameter of the IJ vein. If the patient is uncooperative, coordinate the insertion with respiration because the IJ vein is at its largest diameter just prior to inspiration. In the intubated patient, this relationship is reversed because mechanical ventilation increases intrathoracic pressure at end-inspiration. External abdominal compression also helps to distend the IJ vein.

Venipuncture Site

Select the venipuncture site depending on the reason for cannulation. The right IJ vein provides a more direct route to the right atrium and is advantageous when a transvenous pacer is to be placed. The left IJ vein is often more tortuous and catheters must negotiate two 90° turns at the junction of the left IJ vein with the SV and at the junction of the SV with the SVC. However, if the right IJ vein is obstructed or scarred by prior access, the left IJ vein may be accessed using the same technique. Of note, the right IJ vein has been observed to be twice the size of the left IJ vein in 34% of normal adults.[86]

Aspirate prior to injecting anesthetic so as not to inject it into the carotid artery or IJ vein. Once the infiltration is completed, use the needle to locate the IJ vein by aspirating blood into the syringe. Note the depth and angle of needle entry and use this as a mental guide to finding the IJ vein with the introducer needle. Typically, an 18-gauge 2.5-cm introducer needle attached to a syringe is used to initially puncture the IJ vein. However, this needle selection may vary depending on the central line kit used. The operator may choose from three approaches: anterior, central, and posterior.

Central Route

This approach is favored by some who believe that the incidence of cannulation of the carotid artery is decreased and the cupola of the lung avoided with this method.[86] First palpate and identify the triangle formed by the clavicle and the sternal and clavicular heads of the SCM. Use a marking pen or a local

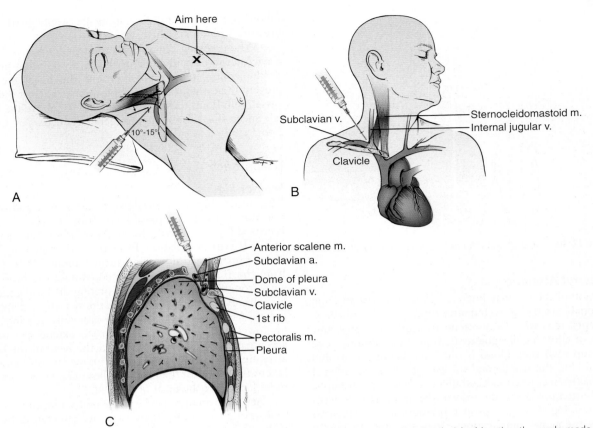

Figure 22–13 *A* and *B*, For the supraclavicular approach, the needle is inserted above and behind the clavicle, bisecting the angle made by the clavicle and the lateral border of the sternocleidomastoid muscle (clavisternomastoid angle). The point of entry is 1 cm lateral to the clavicular head of the muscle and 1 cm posterior to the clavicle. The needle traverses an avascular plane, puncturing the junction of the subclavian and IJ veins behind the sternoclavicular joint. The right side is preferred because of a direct route to the superior vena cava and the absence of the thoracic duct. The needle is directed 45° from the sagittal plane and 10°–15° upward from the horizontal plane, aiming toward the contralateral nipple. Note that the vein is just posterior to the clavicle at this juncture. *C*, Sagittal section of the supraclavicular area. As the subclavian vein passes over (and somewhat anterior to) the first rib, it is separated from the subclavian artery by the anterior scalene muscle. The dome of the pleura is posterolateral to the confluence of the great veins.

anesthetic skin wheal to mark the lateral border of the carotid pulse, and perform all subsequent needle punctures lateral to that point.

Some practitioners prefer to attempt cannulation with the catheter apparatus initially. Others use a small-gauge "locator" or scout needle to identify the vein. The smaller needle allows one to ascertain the location of the vein and helps to minimize injury to deep structures by an incorrectly placed larger needle. Using a locator needle can be time consuming in an emergency situation.

When using the scout needle technique, attach a 22-gauge, 3-cm needle to a 5- to 10-mL syringe. Insert the needle near the apex of the triangle and direct it caudally at an angle 30° to 40° to the skin. Direct the needle initially parallel and slightly lateral to the course of the carotid artery (Fig. 22–14). Estimate the course of the IJ vein by placing three fingers lightly over the course of the carotid artery as it runs parallel to the vein. The vein consistently lies just lateral to the carotid artery, albeit often minimally so. Prolonged deep palpation of the carotid artery may decrease the size of the vein, so use the three-finger technique lightly to identify the course of the artery.

Posterior and Anterior Routes

In the posterior approach, make the puncture at the posterior (lateral) edge of the SCM approximately midway between its origin at the mastoid process and its insertion at the clavicle.

The external jugular vein courses in this area and can be used as a landmark with the puncture occurring where the external jugular vein crosses the posterior-lateral border of the SCM. Be careful not to strike the external jugular vein. Advance the needle toward the suprasternal notch, just under the belly of the SCM at an angle of approximately 45° to the transverse plane. During advancement of the needle, apply pressure to the SCM in an effort to lift the body of the muscle. The vein is usually reached at a depth of 7 cm in an average-sized adult. Because the posterior approach occurs higher in the neck, there is less risk for hemothorax, pneumothorax, or carotid puncture.[87] The benefits of the posterior approach are more dramatic in obese patients, with carotid puncture occurring in 3.1% of patients versus up to 16.6% with the anterior approach.[88]

In the anterior approach, the needle puncture occurs along the anterior or medial edge of the SCM about 2 to 3 fingerbreadths above the clavicle. Insert the needle at an angle of 30° to 45° toward the ipsilateral nipple, away from the carotid pulse. If cannulation is unsuccessful, withdraw the needle to the skin and redirect it slightly toward the carotid artery.

Once the approach is chosen, slowly advance the needle toward the IJ vein. Create negative pressure with the syringe while advancing the needle. Once blood is seen, stop advancing the syringe. Evaluate the blood to determine whether it is venous or arterial. Remember that in some clinical situa-

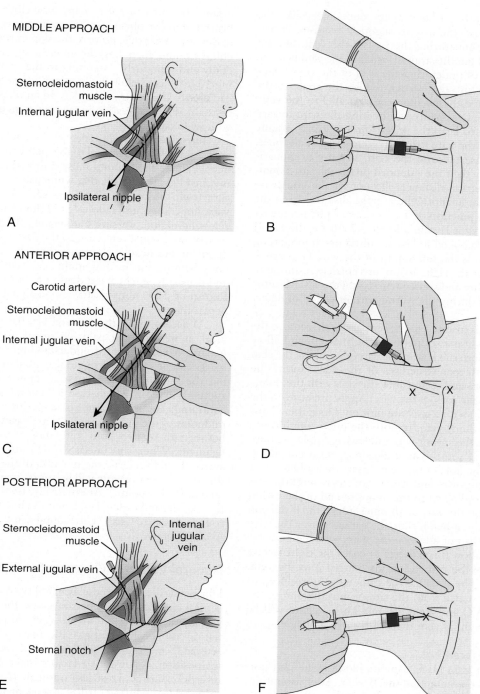

Figure 22–14   Approaches to the internal jugular vein. The patient is supine, in slight Trendelenburg position, with the neck extended over a shoulder roll and the head rotated away from the side of the approach. *A* and *B*, Middle approach. The introducer needle enters at the apex of the triangle formed by the heads of the sternocleidomastoid muscle and the clavicle and is directed toward the ipsilateral nipple at an angle of approximately 30 degrees with the skin. *C* and *D*, Anterior approach. The carotid pulse is palpated, with the course identified and marked by 2 fingers during needle placement. The artery may be slightly retracted medially. The introducer needle enters along the anterior margin of the sternocleidomastoid about halfway between the sternal notch and the mastoid process and is directed toward the ipsilateral nipple. *E* and *F*, Posterior approach. The introducer needle enters at the point where the external jugular vein crosses the posterior margin of the sternocleidomastoid and is directed under its heads toward the sternal notch.   *(From Fuhrman BP, Zimmerman JJ. Pediatric Critical Care, ed 3. St. Louis, Mosby, 2005.)*

tions, arterial blood may appear to be venous. These situations include hypoxia in which arterial blood may appear dark (like deoxygenated venous blood) or nonpulsatile (in hypotensive patients). Remove the needle from the syringe to determine whether it is pulsatile. Be careful not to allow negative intrapleural pressure to draw air into the venous system through the open needle. Because the tip of the introducer needle is beveled, lateral motions of the needle tip may cause

lacerations of the deep structures of the neck. It is therefore very important to remove the needle from the neck completely prior to any redirection of the needle.

The Seldinger technique is the preferred method of central venous catheterization. Once cannulation of the IJ vein has been confirmed, remove the syringe from the needle and place a gloved digit over the needle hub to prevent an air embolism. Insert a guidewire through the needle into the IJ vein. The guidewire has a bend at the end shaped like the letter J. This tip allows the wire to negotiate bends or curves in the vein without puncturing the wall of the vein. Do not reverse the wire and put the straight end into the vein because there is a high risk of puncturing the wall of the vein. Once the wire is inserted into the IJ vein, reduce the angle to the skin in order to make the needle nearly parallel to the vein. This allows for a higher chance of directing the wire toward the heart. Use care to keep the wire from migrating distally into the vein. Keep the wire firmly in your grasp at all times. Once the wire is inserted into the vein, advance it approximately 1 cm further than the intended dilator-sheath assembly or catheter insertion distance. Do not let the guidewire extend into the right atrium. The average distance from the insertion site to the junction of the SVC and right atrium are 16 ± 2 cm for the right IJ vein and 19 ± 2 cm for the left IJ vein. Spring-wires supplied in kits are often much longer, up to 60 cm in length. If the full length of the wire is inserted, the wire could enter the right atrium or ventricle resulting in myocardial irritability and subsequent dysrhythmias. Monitor the cardiac rhythm during the spring-wire insertion to detect cardiac irritability.

After the wire is inserted to the proper depth, remove the introducer needle. Use a scalpel to incise the skin and allow the dilator to pass into the IJ vein. Be careful to incise the skin only and not the deeper structures of the neck. Insert the dilator over the wire and feed it into the skin with the dominant hand. Follow the path of the wire. Apply pressure on the dilator near the skin with a twisting motion. Once the dilator is introduced into the IJ vein, remove the dilator but do not advance or remove the spring-wire guidewire. Apply pressure with gauze to the IJ vein because bleeding will occur owing to the dilation of the hole in the vein. Insert the catheter over the end of the spring-wire and feed it externally until the end of the wire is protruding from the opposite end of the catheter. Keep a grasp on the wire at all times. Once the distal end of the wire is firmly in hand, slide the catheter over the wire into the IJ vein. Do not advance the wire with the catheter because this may allow the catheter to enter the right atrium or ventricle. Once the catheter is introduced into the vein, remove the wire. The distance the catheter is introduced to depends on the distance from the site of introduction to the junction of the SVC and right atrium. This distance will be shorter with the right IJ vein than with the left IJ vein.

Assessing Line Placement

Once the catheter is in place, aspirate blood from each port to ensure correct placement in the IJ vein. After aspiration, flush each port with normal saline. Secure the catheter to the skin using sutures or staples, and apply a sterile dressing. After placing the IJ vein catheter, obtain a chest radiograph to rule out any complications and assess the depth the catheter has been placed. Review the chest radiograph for the presence of a pneumothorax, the direction of the catheter, the presence of a lost spring-wire, and the location of the distal end of the catheter. The optimal location of the catheter end is just proximal to the junction of the SVC and the right atrium.

Femoral Vein Approach

Positioning and Needle Orientation

Place the patient in the supine position for the femoral vein approach. This approach does not require any special positioning or tilting of the bed. Fully expose and thoroughly cleanse the area, using a soapy washcloth or surgical scrub brush to remove obvious soiling, which may be more common at this site. After this, prepare the skin of the site broadly with chlorhexidine, including the anterior superior iliac spine laterally and superiorly, extending to the midline, and continuing 10 to 15 cm below the inguinal ligament. Tape a urethral catheter to the contralateral leg. In an obese patient, have an assistant retract the abdominal pannus manually or secure it with wide tape.

Introduce the needle at a 45° angle in a cephalic direction approximately 1 cm medial to this point and toward the umbilicus. Palpate the femoral pulse 2 fingerbreadths beneath the inguinal ligament. Note that while palpating the artery, pressure from the operator's fingers can compress the adjacent vein, impeding cannulation. Avoid this anatomic distortion by releasing digital pressure but keeping the fingers on the skin to serve as a visual reference to the underlying anatomy. The depth of the needle required to reach the vein varies with body habitus, but in thin adults, the vein is quite superficial and is usually reached at a depth of approximately 2 to 3 cm. Return of dark, nonpulsatile blood signals successful venous penetration.

Whereas using the femoral arterial pulse as a guide is ideal, it may not be palpable in an obese or hypotensive patient. A more detailed understanding of the femoral landmarks can be employed to guide cannulation attempts. On all but the most grievously injured trauma patient with a disrupted pelvis (in which case a femoral approach would be contraindicated), the anterior superior iliac spine and the midpoint of the pubic symphysis are easily palpated. The line between these two bony references describes the inguinal ligament. When this line is divided into thirds, the femoral artery should underlie the junction of the medial and middle thirds. The femoral vein will lie approximately 1 fingerbreadth medial to this point.[89] Alternatively, the vascular anatomy of the region can be elucidated, and the line placed, under ultrasound guidance (see "Ultrasound-Guided Central Venous Access," later).

Femoral Catheter Placement in Cardiac Arrest

During cardiac arrest, the availability of drug delivery to the central circulation may be slower via the femoral route than via supraclavicular SV or IJ vein infusions.[90,91] Pulsations felt in the groin during CPR may be venous instead of arterial,[46] and there is a high rate of unrecognized catheter malposition.[92] These two factors make femoral central line insertion during arrest less optimal. If the pulse cannot be palpated (e.g., during cardiac arrest), divide the distance from the anterior superior iliac spine to the symphysis pubis into thirds. The artery typically lies at the junction of the medial and middle thirds and the vein 1 cm medial to this location.

Venipuncture

During needle advancement, maintain negative pressure on the syringe at all times while the needle is under the skin. Direct the needle posteriorly and advance it until the vein is entered, as identified by a flash of dark, nonpulsatile blood. If the vessel is penetrated when the syringe is not being aspirated, the blood flash may be seen only as the needle is being withdrawn. The femoral vein lies just medial to the femoral artery at the level of the inguinal ligament. It is closer to the artery than many clinicians appreciate. As the vein progresses distally in the leg, it runs closer to, and almost behind, the femoral artery (see Fig. 22–3). This anatomic fact should be considered if the cannulating needle is introduced more than a few centimeters distal to the inguinal ligament.

The basilic and cephalic venous systems are entered through the large veins in the antecubital fossa (see Fig. 22–4). Tourniquet placement aids venous distention and initial venous puncture. When veins are not visible, they may be reached with a cutdown procedure, as described in Chapter 23, Venous Cutdown. The basilic vein, located on the medial aspect of the antecubital fossa, is generally larger than the radially located cephalic vein. Furthermore, the basilic vein generally provides a more direct route for passage into the axillary vein, SV, and SVC.

CATHETER PASSAGE TECHNIQUE

Once there is a venous flashback into the syringe, detach it from the needle, and pass a catheter via the Seldinger technique or, alternatively, over or through the needle. Remove the syringe with care to avoid dislodging the needle tip from the lumen of the vein. If the syringe is tightly attached to the needle, use a hemostat to grasp and secure the needle hub during removal of the syringe. Needle tip displacement may also occur if blood specimens are drawn at this time. Hence, it is best to delay blood sampling until the catheter has been advanced. Occlude the needle hub with the thumb to avoid air embolism.

SPECIAL CONSIDERATIONS FOR THE FEMORAL AND SMALLER VESSELS
Femoral Vein Approach

Once in the femoral vein, stabilize the needle. Often, a hemostat is helpful for holding the needle during removal of the syringe. Insert a premeasured section of a 90-cm catheter using a through-the-needle system. Determine the appropriate length by holding the catheter over the patient's body and estimating the distance from the skin puncture site to the right atrium. Avoid contaminating the catheter while performing this maneuver. Once the catheter is placed, secure it with sutures and dress it in the same manner as other central lines.

In situations requiring rapid volume infusion, in the absence of intra-abdominal trauma, the femoral vein may be cannulated with a sheath introduced via the guidewire technique. The introducer will allow rapid transfusion of large volumes of blood or crystalloid solution for fluid resuscitation. The femoral vessels may also be cannulated under direct visualization using a cutdown technique (see Chapter 23, Venous Cutdown).

External Jugular Vein Approach

Central venous catheterization via the external jugular vein is time consuming and often difficult. Use of the external jugular vein for achieving central venous access requires use of a guidewire. After cannulation of the vein and intraluminal placement of the guidewire, advance the guidewire into the thorax by rotating and manipulating the tip into the central venous circulation (Fig. 22–15). Guidewire advancement is the most difficult and time-consuming portion of the procedure, and the time requirement limits the usefulness of this technique in an emergency. A small-radius J-tipped wire, a distended vessel lumen, and exaggeration of patient head-tilt, coupled with skin traction, may facilitate successful guidewire passage. Partially withdrawing the wire and twisting it 180° before readvancing the tip may also be helpful.

Basilic and Cephalic Approach

Passing a catheter into the central circulation is difficult using the basilic and cephalic routes and failure is common. The cephalic vein may terminate inches above the antecubital fossa or bifurcate before entering the axillary vein, sending a branch to the external jugular vein. The cephalic vein may also enter the axillary vein at right angles, defeating any attempt to pass the catheter centrally. Furthermore, both the basilic and the cephalic systems contain valves that may impede catheterization. Abduction of the shoulder may help to advance the catheter if resistance near the axillary vein occurs. The incidence of failure to place the catheter in the SVC ranges from a high of 40% to a low of 2%.[40,90] The greatest success rate (98%) reported was obtained with slow catheter advancement with the patient in a 45° to 90° upright position.[40] Flexible catheters were introduced into the basilic vein until the tip

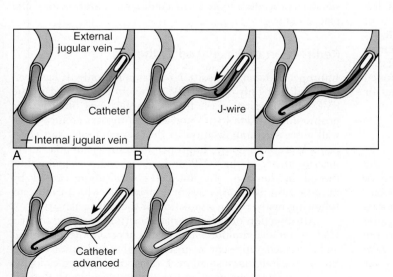

Figure 22–15 Insertion of a catheter over a wire via the external jugular vein. Successful passage may require many attempts and manipulations of the J-wire to navigate turns and valves. *(From Blitt CD, Wright WA, Petty WC: Central venous catheterization via the external jugular vein: A technique employing the J-wire. JAMA 229:817, 1974. Reproduced by permission.)*

was judged to be proximal to the junction of the cephalic and basilic veins and distal to the junction of the IJ vein with the innominate vein. The wire stylet was withdrawn 18 cm, and the catheters were advanced slowly 1 cm at a time, with 2 seconds allowed between each 1-cm insertion. The natural flexibility of the Bard catheters contributed to negotiation into the SVC when the patient was upright. This time-consuming technique is contraindicated when the patient cannot tolerate an upright position.

ASSESSING LINE PLACEMENT

Once the catheter has been passed, secure it carefully in place with one of three common techniques: suturing, staples, or an anchoring device such as the Statlock.[93,94] The Statlock may not hold well for patients with oily skin but is excellent for older patients with thin skin. Staples are somewhat faster but tend to fall out after a few days.[94] The straight suture needles found in many sets are awkward for many clinicians, so a curved needle with a driver may be helpful. Check all tubing and connections for tightness to prevent air embolism, fluid loss, or bleeding. Place a sterile dressing once secured. Because dressings are inspected and changed periodically, place a simple dressing, avoiding excessive amounts of gauze and tape. Take care to protect the skin against maceration. Transparent dressings made of polyurethane are popular and simple and yield a lower rate of catheter colonization than newer hydrocolloid dressings.[95]

Before infusing IV fluids, lower the IV fluid reservoir below the level of the patient's right atrium and check the line for backflow of blood. The free backflow of blood is suggestive, but not diagnostic, of intravascular placement. However, backflow could occur with a hematoma or a hemothorax if the catheter is free in the pleural space. A pulsatile blood column may be noted if the catheter has been inadvertently placed into an artery. Less pronounced pulsations might also occur if the catheter is advanced too far and reaches the right atrium or ventricle. Pulsations may also be noted with changes in intrathoracic pressure due to respirations, although these pulsations should be at a much slower rate than the arterial pulse. A final method of checking intravascular placement is to attach a syringe directly to the catheter hub and aspirate venous blood. It is also advisable to ensure that the catheter is easily flushed with a heparin solution, if the patient has no heparin sensitivity. This carries the additional benefit of removing air from the system. Radiographs are also always indicated to verify catheter location and assess for potential complications, except for routine femoral line placements. In an awake patient, infusing fluids via a catheter tip positioned in the IJ vein may produce an audible gurgling sound or flowing sound in the patient's ear.[93]

Radiographs

Following placement of lines involving puncture of the neck or thorax, listen to the lungs to detect any inequality of lung sounds suggestive of a pneumo- or hemothorax. Obtain a chest film as soon as possible, checking for hemothorax, pneumothorax, and the position of the catheter tip. Because small amounts of fluid or air may layer out parallel to the radiographic plate with the patient in the supine position, take the film in the upright or semi-upright position whenever possible. Proper catheter tip position is shown in Figure 22–16. Reposition misplaced catheters. In ill patients, a rotated

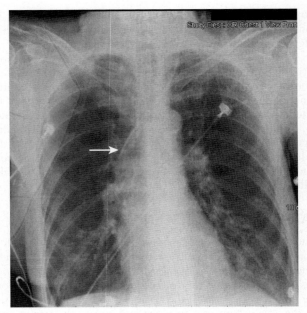

Figure 22–16 A chest film shows the proper catheter tip placement via the left IJ vein in the superior vena cava (*arrow*). The tip should not lie within the right atrium or the right ventricle.

or oblique projection on a chest radiograph may be obtained, and the clinician may be confused as to the proper position of the catheter (Fig. 22–17). In such cases, repeat the radiograph. A misplaced catheter tip is usually obvious on a properly positioned standard posteroanterior chest radiograph, but occasionally, the injection of contrast material may be required. For example, a catheter in one of the internal thoracic veins may simply appear more lateral than expected, but because of the close proximity of these veins and the SVC, malposition may not be appreciated by this subtle finding.

Postprocedure radiographs are not always warranted for routine replacement of catheters over guidewires. If such patients are stable and hemodynamically monitored, radiography may be safely deferred in the absence of apparent complications or clinical suspicion of malposition.[94] It is not standard procedure to perform a radiograph after femoral line placement.

Redirection of Misplaced Catheters

Improper catheter tip position occurs commonly. It has been reported that only 71% of SV catheters are located in the SVC on the initial chest film. Complications of improper positioning include hydrothorax, hemothorax, ascites, chest wall abscesses, embolization to the pleural space, and chest pain. More commonly, improper location yields inaccurate measurements of the CVP or is associated with poor flow caused by kinking. An unusual complication caused by improper tip position is cerebral infarction, which can occur following inadvertent cannulation of the subclavian artery.

Misdirection or inappropriate positioning of the tip of a CVC is not uncommon. These events, if promptly recognized and corrected, represent inconsequential complications. Loop formation, lodging in small neck veins, tips directed caudally, and innominate vein position are common problems. Reposition misplaced catheters as soon as logistically possible. If the

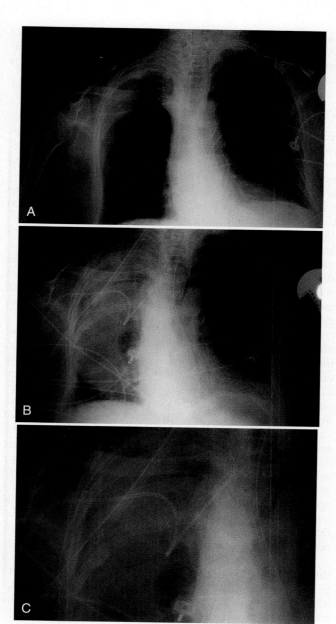

Figure 22–17 A chest radiograph should be routinely taken to assess position of a central catheter introduced via the chest or neck. *A,* In this case, a poorly positioned patient produced a rotated and oblique film, and the catheter appeared, at first glance, to be in the correct position in the right subclavian vein. The early hydrothorax was not appreciated. *B,* A repeat radiograph shows the obvious intrapleural position of the catheter, and a large hydrothorax after infusion of 2 L of saline. *C,* Close-up of the misplaced catheter.

One anecdotal strategy is to withdraw the catheter until only the distal tip remains in the cannulated vessel. This measurement is best appreciated by comparing the indwelling catheter length with another unused catheter. The clinician then simply readvances the catheter, hoping that it becomes properly positioned. Other manipulations with guidewires have been suggested, but reinsertion with another puncture is often required for the misplaced catheter to be positioned properly.

COMPLICATIONS

The medical literature is replete with reports of the complications of large vein venipuncture. Some are minor and inconsequential, such as hematoma formation, whereas others are serious and life threatening, such as hemothorax. No clinician can expect to routinely perform these procedures and be complication free. Serious complications accompany this procedure in about 15% of attempts (ranging widely from under 2% to over 25%) and the failure rate ranges up to 20%.[30] These results should not be surprising in view of the close proximity of vital structures, blind catheterization and the emergent circumstances under which the procedures are often called for. Operator skill and experience most reliably predict complication or success probability,[30] the foundations of which are an understanding of the pertinent anatomy and techniques described herein. Although we strive to limit complications, their occurrence cannot naïvely be viewed as evidence of faulty technique or substandard care. Common complications for the different approaches are summarized in Tables 22–7 and 22–8. Key injuries categorized by organ system and by approach are discussed in the sections that follow. The U.S. Food and Drug Administration has released a three-volume video entitled "CVC Complications," which was sent to all hospitals in which such catheters are placed. It is also commercially available from the Internet (at www.fda.gov).

Published rates vary widely and complication rates depend on one's definition. One 3-year retrospective review of all central catheters placed in the ED (supraclavicular SV, IJ, and femoral lines) reported a mechanical complication rate of 3.5%, or 22 of 643 lines placed.[90] Complication was defined as pneumothorax, hematoma, line misplacement, hemothorax, or any issue with the CVC (excluding infection or thrombosis) that required an inpatient consultation. In general, failure and complication rates increase as the number of percutaneous punctures increase. Malpractice claims are surprisingly uncommon accounting for less than 2% of all claims against anesthesiologists.[94] The most common liability closed claims are, in order, wire/catheter embolization, hemopneumothorax, cardiac tamponade, and carotid artery puncture.[94]

Pulmonary Complications

Pulmonary complications of subclavian and IJ venipuncture include pneumothorax, hemothorax, hydrothorax, hemomediastinum, hydromediastinum, tracheal perforation, and endotracheal cuff perforation. Pneumothorax is the most frequently reported complication, occurring in up to 6% of subclavian venipunctures.[96] Initially, the importance of this complication was minimized, but reports of fatalities caused by tension pneumothorax, bilateral pneumothorax, and combined hemopneumothorax followed.[97,98] One would expect a higher incidence of pneumothorax if the procedure were per-

catheter is being used for fluid resuscitation, the malposition may be tolerated for some time. If vasopressors or medications are infused, properly positioning the catheter tip is more critical. A number of options are available to remedy malpositioning. One strategy is to insert a 2-French Fogarty catheter through the lumen of the central line, advancing it 3 cm beyond the tip. Withdraw the entire assembly until only the Fogarty catheter is in the SV. Inject 1 cc of air into the balloon, and advance the Fogarty catheter. It is hoped that the blood flow will direct the assembly into the SVC. Deflate the balloon and advance the central line over the Fogarty catheter, which is then withdrawn.[95]

TABLE 22-7 Complications of Central Venous Access

General

Vascular

Air embolus
Adjacent artery puncture
Pericardial tamponade
Catheter embolus
Arteriovenous fistula
Mural thrombus formation
Large vein obstruction
Local hematoma

Infectious

Generalized sepsis
Local cellulitis
Osteomyelitis
Septic arthritis

Miscellaneous

Dysrhythmias
Catheter knotting
Catheter malposition

Subclavian and Internal Jugular Approaches

Pulmonary

Pneumothorax
Hemothorax
Hydrothorax
Chylothorax
Hemomediastinum
Hydromediastinum
Neck hematoma and tracheal obstruction
Tracheal perforation
Endotracheal cuff perforation

Neurologic

Phrenic nerve injury
Brachial plexus injury
Cerebral infarct

Femoral approach

Intra-abdominal

Bowel perforation
Bladder perforation
Psoas abscess

---

formed during CPR or positive-pressure ventilation. A small pneumothorax can quickly become a life-threatening tension pneumothorax under positive-pressure ventilation.

The treatment of a catheter-induced pneumothorax is controversial, but not all patients will require a formal tube thoracostomy. Some authors recommend that many stable outpatients exhibiting a pneumothorax after CVC insertion can often be successfully managed with observation alone (60% in their series) or catheter (pigtail/Heimlich valve) aspiration, reserving large tube thoracostomy for refractory cases or emergent settings.[99,100] Critically ill patients or those on mechanical ventilation will likely require invasive treatment of a catheter-induced pneumothorax.

Hemothorax may occur after SV or subclavian artery laceration, pulmonary artery puncture, or intrathoracic infu-

sion of blood. Hydrothorax occurs as a result of infusion of IV fluid into the pleural space (see Fig. 22-17). Hydromediastinum is an uncommonly reported complication that is potentially fatal.[101]

Vascular/Bleeding Complications

The most common vascular complication is inadvertent arterial puncture, which is usually easily recognized and controlled with simple compression. Rarely, an artery is lacerated to an extent that bleeding is significant and operative repair is necessary. In cardiac arrest, low-flow, or shock states, arterial puncture may not be obvious, and arterial cannulation and the intra-arterial administration of medications has occurred. When the systolic blood pressure rises, arterial pulsations become more obvious. In critically ill patients, however, this complication may escape detection for some time. The subsequent development of ischemia or thrombosis of an artery that has been cannulated or injected with detrimental medication reflects the blind nature of this procedure in an emergency.

Air embolism is a very rare, but potentially serious, complication from any central venous cannulation. Undoubtedly, minor and clinically inconsequential amounts of air enter the venous circulation during many cannulation procedures. Maintaining constant occlusion (with the operator's finger) on all needles that are located in central veins can minimize this occurrence. A 14-gauge needle can transmit 100 mL of air per second with a 5-cm H_2O pressure difference across the needle.[102] Air embolism may occur if the line is open to air during catheterization or if it subsequently becomes disconnected. The recommended treatment is to place the patient in the left lateral decubitus position to relieve air bubble occlusion of the right ventricular outflow tract.[103] If this is unsuccessful, aspiration with the catheter advanced into the right ventricle has been advocated.[104] Emergent cardiothoracic surgical consultation may also be warranted.

Catheter embolization resulting from shearing of a through-the-needle catheter by the needle tip is a serious and generally avoidable complication. Embolization can occur when the catheter is withdrawn through the needle or if the guard is not properly secured. Adverse events after embolization include arrhythmias, venous thrombosis, endocarditis, myocardial perforation, and pulmonary embolus.[54] The mortality rate in patients who did not have these catheters removed has been reported to be as high as 60%.[105] Transvenous retrieval techniques are usually attempted, followed by surgery if they are unsuccessful.[59] Entire guidewires may also embolize to the general circulation if the tip is not always secured by the operator.

Perforation or laceration of vascular structures may cause hemothorax, hemomediastinum, and volume depletion. These are rarely serious complications, but fatalities have been reported. Surgical repair is occasionally required.[60] Arteriovenous fistula formation has also been reported.[106,107]

Delayed perforation of the myocardium is a rare but generally fatal complication of central venous catheterization by any route.[108,109] The presumed mechanism is prolonged contact of the rigid catheter with the beating myocardium.[61] The catheter perforates the myocardial wall and causes tamponade either by bleeding from the involved chamber or by infusion of IV fluid into the pericardium. The right atrium is involved more commonly than the right ventricle.[82] All who insert such catheters or care for such patients should be aware

TABLE 22–8 Anatomic Structures That Can Be Injured by Central Venous Cannulation

Structure	Anatomic Relation to Vein	Error in Procedure	Injury
Subclavian Vein Cannulation			
Subclavian artery	Posterior and slightly superior, separated by scalenus anterior—10–15 mm in adults, 5–8 mm in children	Insertion too deep or lateral	Hemorrhage, hematoma, possible hemothorax
Brachial plexus	Posterior to and separated from the subclavian vein by the scalenus anterior and the subclavian artery (20 mm)	Same as with subclavian artery	Possible motor or sensory deficits of hand, arm, or shoulder
Parietal pleura	Contact with posteroinferior side of the subclavian vein, medial to the attachment of the anterior scalenus muscle to the first rib	Needle penetrates beneath or through both walls of the subclavian vein	Pneumothorax
Phrenic nerve	Same as with parietal pleura	Placement of needle above or behind the vein or by penetration of both its walls	Paralysis of the ipsilateral hemidiaphragm
Thoracic duct	Cross the scalenus anterior and enter the superior margin of the subclavian vein near the internal jugular junction	Same as with phrenic nerve	Soft tissue lymphedema or chylothorax on left
Internal Jugular Vein Cannulation			
Carotid artery	Passes with jugular vein in carotid sheath, consistently medial and deep to the vein	Insertion site too medial or needle course not directed at ipsilateral nipple	Hematoma, possible cerebral thromboembolism or airway obstruction
Phrenic nerve	Passes along anterior surface of scalenus anterior, behind the vein	Insertion too deep	Paralysis of the ipsilateral hemidiaphragm
Brachial plexus	Separated from the internal jugular by the scalenus anterior	Insertion too deep or too lateral	Possible motor or sensory deficits of hand, arm, or shoulder
Femoral Vein Cannulation			
Femoral artery	Lies lateral to the vein in the femoral triangle	Needle passed too laterally	Hematoma
Psoas muscle	Directly posterior to the artery and vein	Needle passed too deep	Hematoma, psoas abscess
Bowel	Proximal and deep to femoral vein	Needle passed too deep and above the inguinal ligament	Enterotomy, peritonitis
Synovial capsule of hip	Deep to the psoas muscle	Needle passed too deep, particularly in small children	Arthritis, septic joint

From Knopp R, Dailey RH: Central venous cannulation and pressure monitoring. JACEP 6:358, 1977.

of this deadly complication, which results in profound deterioration with hypotension, shortness of breath, and shock. Emergent echocardiography, pericardiocentesis, and operative intervention by a chest surgeon all may be required for patient salvage. This can also occur with misplacement of the CVC in the pericardiophrenic vein.[110] Fortunately, this complication is preventable by using a postinsertion chest film to confirm catheter tip position and repositioning any catheter if the tip is within the cardiac silhouette.

Catheter knotting or kinking may occur if the catheter is forced or repositioned or if an excessively long catheter is used.[62] The most common result of kinking is poor flow of IV fluids, although rare complications as severe as SVC obstruction caused by a kinked catheter have been seen.[111]

Thrombosis and thrombophlebitis occur rarely because of the large caliber and high flow rates of the vessels involved.[74] It is important to determine that the catheter tip rests in the SVC, especially during the infusion of irritating or hypertonic solutions.[111] Thrombi may also form secondary to prolonged catheter contact against the vascular endothelium. One autopsy study found a 29% incidence of mural thrombi in the innominate vein, SVC, and right ventricle of patients who had central lines in place an average of 8 days before death.[31] However, no complications were directly attributable to these small, firmly adherent thrombi.

Thoracic duct laceration is a frequently discussed complication of left-sided subclavian venipuncture; however, it is extremely uncommon, and has been reported only as a complication of IJ, not SV, cannulation.[96]

Although poorly studied, it has been promulgated that patients with a coagulopathy may experience significant bleeding from CVC placement, especially if arterial puncture/laceration has occurred. Traditionally, prophylactic blood component therapy (fresh frozen plasma, platelet infusions) has been suggested in patients with a coagulopathy prior to percutaneous placement of a CVC. Although intuitively reasonable, this concept has no support in the literature. Mumtaz and coworkers[40] challenged this concept as unproved and unnecessary, citing a 3% bleeding rate in coagulopathic patients who experienced only minor bleeding that could be controlled with digital pressure. Although central venous access may be safely performed in patients with underlying disorders of hemostasis, without correction of the coagulopathy, caution is urged. It would be prudent to target central access in patients with coagulopathies to areas amenable to arterial compression.[40]

Infectious Complications

Infectious complications include local cellulitis, thrombophlebitis, generalized septicemia, osteomyelitis, and septic arthritis.[96] The incidence of septic complications varies from 0% to 25%.[64] The frequency with which infectious complications are seen is directly related to the attention given to aseptic technique during insertion and aftercare of the catheter. For the most part, an acceptably low incidence of bacteremia using these devices has been encountered.[112] Femoral venous catheterization may be related to a greater risk of infection than subclavian catheterization. Merrer and associates[113] reported overall infectious complications from femoral versus subclavian catheters to be 19.8% and 4.5%, respectively. The most common organisms recovered from colonized femoral catheters, or involved with infectious complications from femoral catheters, were coagulase-negative staphylococci, Enterobacteriaceae, *Enterococcus* species, and *Pseudomonas aeruginosa*.[113]

Neurologic Complications

Neurologic complications are extremely rare and are presumably caused by direct trauma from the needle during venipuncture. Brachial plexus palsy and phrenic nerve injury with paralysis of the hemidiaphragm have been reported.[114,115] Infusing hypertonic medications into the internal jugular vein via a malpositioned catheter may result in a variety of neurologic complications from retrograde perfusion of intracranial vessels.[116]

SV Approaches

Although both approaches to the SV are relatively safe (Fig. 22–18), the infraclavicular SV approach is more likely to be associated with complications. In a randomized, prospective comparison of supraclavicular SV and infraclavicular SV venipuncture in 500 ED patients, complication rates were 2.0% and 5.1%, respectively.[110] The most significant complications have been pneumothorax and subclavian artery puncture; the highest incidence of pneumothorax is 2.4%.[28] Adherence to recommended techniques for supraclavicular SV subclavian venipuncture decreases the risk of these complications because the needle is directed away from the pleural dome and subclavian artery.[11] The relatively superficial location of the vein when approached from above the clavicle (1.5–3.5 cm) lessens the risk of puncture or laceration of deep structures.

Catheter tip malposition should be expected with some frequency, as high as 10% to 30% in the absence of direct imaging guidance.[117] Because of the more direct path to the SVC, the SC approach may be advantageous in this regard. For those SC series in which malposition has been reported, the overall rate is about 2% to 3%.[118,119] The highest inci-

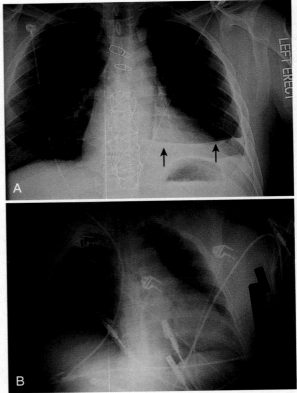

Figure 22–18 *A*, A hemopneumothorax from a left subclavian line (removed). Note the straight line of the fluid (air-fluid level) and no meniscus, indicating that a pneumothorax must be present. The edge of the partially collapsed lung can be seen, but may be difficult to appreciate. No clinician can place central venous catheters and fail to have at least some complications that are inherent to the procedure, regardless of even flawless technique. *B*, A subclavian line can easily be advanced into the internal jugular vein. Malpositioned catheters should be replaced when feasible. Infusing fluids through this line is not harmful, but if medication and vasopressors are needed, it is best to have the tip in the superior vena cava. Patients may hear a wooshing sound in the ear when fluid is infused into this catheter.

dence of malposition using the SC technique, 7%, occurred during the performance of CPR.[120]

A large case series of 178 SC attempts, often in patients with difficult anatomy, supports the high placement success (97.8%) and low significant complication rate (0.56%).[121]

IJ Approach

Many complications of IJ cannulation are similar to those of SV access. Infection, catheter malposition, thrombosis, and damage to surrounding structures are complications common to all puncture sites for central venous cannulation. The reported rates of thrombosis for IJ vein catheterizations range from 30%[122] to over 60% of patients,[123] particularly in long-term medical intensive care unit patients. Reports of significant pulmonary embolus directly attributable to an IJ catheter are very rare however.[118,123] Such wide variation in the reported incidence of complications is common, in part because of the different methods of detecting and reporting complications, variable experience with the different techniques, and the different patient populations.

The number of complications increases, especially those due to thrombosis and infection, with longer duration of catheterization and increasing severity of the patient's illness.[16]

Complications also seem to be higher with the use of the left IJ vein as opposed to the right.[49,82,83] Reported complications thought to be due at least in part to the use of the left-sided approach include mediastinal migration of the catheters and at least one instance of fatal pericardial tamponade.

One fairly common complication unique to the IJ approach is a hematoma in the neck.[124] With the IJ approach, pressure can be maintained easily on the area of swelling, and most hematomas will resolve spontaneously. If carotid arterial puncture is recognized and treated with compression, it rarely causes significant morbidity in the absence of marked athero-sclerotic disease, although arteriovenous fistulas may occur after IJ puncture.[125] Several neurologic complications unique to the IJ site of venipuncture have also been reported as a result of hematomas or direct injury. These complications include damage to the phrenic nerves, an iatrogenic Horner syndrome, trauma to the brachial plexus, and even passage of a catheter into the thecal space of the spinal canal.[116] If the carotid artery is punctured, one may again attempt IJ or SV cannulation on the same side after appropriate, prolonged (15–20 min) compression. The IJ vein valve is frequently damaged when cannulated, often resulting in its incompetence. The clinical significance of this, if any, is unknown.[126]

Arterial puncture is a contraindication to attempting the IJ route on the opposite side, because bilateral hemorrhage may occur with resultant airway compromise. The clinician should be prepared to rapidly intubate should this occur. Even in the face of a coagulopathy, however, the IJ approach has been found to be successful (up to 99.3% of cases) and safe (<1% complication rate).[127]

Femoral Approach

Some of the complications of the femoral vein approach are illustrated in Figure 22–19. Because the vital structures of the neck and chest are not at risk, complications of femoral vein cannulation are generally less severe than those of other routes to central venous access. The most common immediate complications involve bleeding from damage to either the femoral artery or the femoral vein. This can usually be managed by 10 to 15 minutes of direct pressure. Extra care should be taken in anticoagulated patients or after thrombo-lytic administration. In extreme cases in which hemostasis is not achievable through direct pressure, a vascular surgeon should be consulted.

The peritoneum can also be violated, resulting in perfo-ration of the bowel. Bowel penetration is especially likely if the patient has a femoral hernia. Injury to the bowel is usually minimal and unlikely to require specific treatment. None-theless, the potential bacterial contamination of the femoral puncture site can pose a significant problem. Aspiration of air during the placement of a femoral line necessitates removal of the catheter and reinsertion at another site. Other compli-cations include muscular abscesses, infection of the hip capsule, damage to the femoral nerve, and puncture of the bladder. The risk of these outcomes can be mitigated by strict aseptic technique, thorough assessment of landmarks, and careful control of the needle's depth. Two more complica-tions merit special mention. The first is the increased risk of catheter infection. Presumably due to anatomic association with the anogenital region, many studies have found that femoral lines become infected at significantly higher rates than IJ or supraclavicular SV lines.[113,128] Of note, some studies failed to find a statistical difference, and it is unclear how

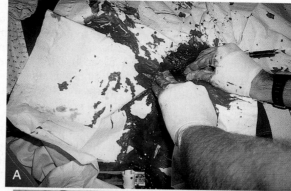

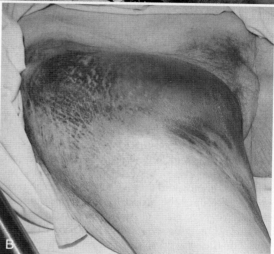

Figure 22–19 A femoral vein catheter is more prone to deep vein thrombosis and infection than a subclavian/IJ line, but it is a standard access route in the emergency department. Strict attention to sterile procedure and limiting use for a few days will negate most of the negatives of this approach. *A,* Significant hemorrhage can occur after puncture of the femoral artery, but this area is readily compressed. The femoral route may be the route of choice in the patient with a coagulopathy who requires a central line. *B,* Bleeding from catheter that was removed without adequate pressure in an anticoagulated patient.

much of the effect is due to the actual location of the line versus how it is placed and managed.

The majority of studies show that the incidence of deep vein thrombosis is also increased in lines placed via the femoral route,[113,128,129] although the clinical significance of these clots has not been definitively addressed.

Basilic-Cephalic Approaches

Cannulation of the central venous system through the arm veins also is associated with complications. Superficial infec-tions, catheter malposition and peripheral nerve injuries are somewhat common.[130,131] Cannulation of these veins requires immobilization of the entire extremity and shoulder to prevent catheter movement and kinking. Ultrasound guided tech-nique appears to improve success rates at this site.[132]

ULTRASOUND-GUIDED CENTRAL VENOUS ACCESS

Ultrasound guidance has revolutionized the cannulation of central veins. As with all anatomic structures in the human body, veins are highly variable in their location. Not surprisingly, research has demonstrated that the ability to see the internal structure's location and proximity to other structures greatly increases the safety and success rate while decreasing the time required to perform the procedure.[26,96-98] These advantages have been recognized by national organizations. In a report from the Agency for Healthcare Research and Quality, the use of ultrasound guidance was listed as one of the top 10 ways to reduce morbidity and mortality.[133] Furthermore, as this technology and technique of placement disseminates, the landmark or blind technique will become obsolete because many hospitals now require the use of ultrasound guidance for the placement of all CVCs. Currently, there is no standard mandating ultrasound-assisted cannulation of central veins, and it may not be practical in an emergency, but its use is increasing.

Ultrasound Physics

To be successful with ultrasound, the operator must have a basic understanding of the principles and physics involved in the acquisition of the image produced. Without this understanding, the operator may be confused as to the identity of certain structures, why some anatomic structures are not visible although present, and how to select the appropriate equipment for the procedure. The physics behind ultrasound can be both an enemy and an ally. Knowing these properties is the key to avoiding the pitfalls of ultrasound guidance for procedures.

Ultrasound imaging uses sound to interrogate the structures deep to the skin. Typical ultrasound machines image between 2.5 and 15 MHz. In contrast, the human hearing is in the range of 20 to 20,000 Hz. Obviously, because sound is used to make the image of the internal structures, no ionizing radiation is used. Whereas this may be obvious to the clinician, the lay person may have to be reassured that there are no known side effects or maximum dose of sound in this frequency range. For most vascular access procedures, a frequency around 10 MHz is most often used.

Sound is produced by oscillation of molecules, thereby producing a wave. As this wave propagates through material, it causes an oscillation of the molecules it is passing through. The repetitive oscillation of the molecules is called a *cycle* or a *wavelength*, that is, one full cycle results in the molecule returning to the originating place in space. *Frequency* is the measure of the amount of cycles that occur in 1 second (Fig. 22–20). Hence, the higher the frequency, the less time required between cycles. A higher frequency is equivalent to a higher energy. Hence, a 10-MHz sound wave has more energy than a 1-MHz wave.

The making of sound involves the oscillation of molecules. In the case of modern ultrasound machines, sound waves are "made" using the piezoelectric effect, or the pressure-electric effect. In this method, piezoelectric crystals are subjected to an alternating current that causes the molecules in the crystal to vibrate and produce sound waves, analogous to a speaker. The same piezoelectric crystals are also able to work in reverse, converting sound waves into an electrical current analogous to a microphone. In modern ultrasound, most images are made using a piezoelectric crystal producing sound waves then listening for the reflections of these sound waves from structures deep to the skin. This type of diagnostic ultrasound is referred to as *pulsed-echo ultrasound*. In pulsed-echo, the crystal is transmitting a minority of time. The

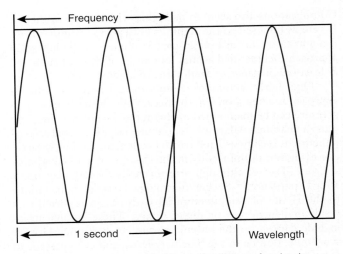

Figure 22–20 Sound is produced by the oscillation of molecules producing a wave. The repetitive oscillation of the molecules is called a *cycle* or *wavelength*, and frequency is the measure of the amount of cycles that occur in 1 sec.

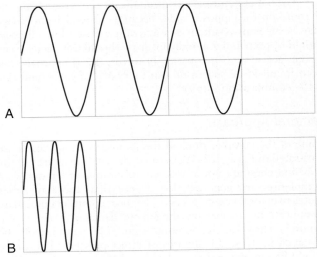

Figure 22–21 The spatial pulse length.

remaining time is spent listening for returning echoes from the transmitted sound. The length of the pulse of sound is referred to as the *spatial pulse length*, that is, wavelength times the number of cycles (Fig. 22–21). The spatial pulse length determines how close two objects can be in order to resolve (or see) a difference between them. Typically, the spatial pulse length can be changed only by changing the frequency of the probe. Therefore, as the frequency of the probe is increased, the spatial pulse length decreases, resulting in better resolution. For example, as a result of a smaller spatial pulse length, the operator may be able to detect the walls of a vessel instead of the vessel appearing as a solid line or not being seen at all. The trade-off for better resolution is that the sound waves do not penetrate the body as deeply and the deeper structures cannot be seen. Therefore, the operator must balance resolution versus depth of penetration by choosing the appropriate frequency of the probe.

As sound propagates through the body, the signal becomes weaker, which is known as *attenuation*. This loss of energy is similar to friction. When the sound strikes a surface of differing density, or impedance, some of the sound is transmitted and some of the sound wave is reflected. The reflected sound waves are what the transducer probe listens for to form an image. The amount of the wave that is reflected depends on the difference in density of the two materials at the interface between the surfaces, that is, the more dense the structure, the more sound will be reflected (Fig. 22–22). The ultrasound machine displays the reflected sound wave strength by varying the brightness on the screen. The denser the structure that reflects the sound, the greater the signal that is returned and the brighter the display on the ultrasound machine. Bone, which is very dense, appears as a bright structure, whereas blood, which is less dense, appears nearly black, having very little brightness. Owing to loss of strength as the wave propagates through the body, known as attenuation, the deeper structures reflecting sound will have less signal to reflect. Therefore, deeper structures will appear darker on the screen even if the two structures are of the same density. Most ultrasound machines allow for adjustment to correct for this property. The time gain control (TGC) allows for signals returning from deeper structures to be amplified and adjusts the brightness to account for the attenuated signal (Fig. 22–23).

Ultrasound probes vary by design, and no one transducer will fit all needs. However, for vascular access procedures, a linear probe is the best choice. In most linear probes, multiple crystals produce and receive sound. These crystals are activated one at a time in a sequential manner with the signals transmitted directly perpendicular to the face of the probe (Fig. 22–24). The typical linear probe will be around 10 MHz. This frequency balances the trade-offs between depth of penetration and good resolution. Other probes can be used for vascular access, although none provide the balanced trade-offs as effectively as a 10-MHz linear probe.

Tools and Equipment

Once an appropriate ultrasound machine and probe are selected, setting up the machine is straightforward. Specific controls and methods of adjusting the ultrasound machine will vary depending on the machine type and manufacturer. However, some basic principles will help with setup regardless of the specific machine. Specific controls are listed in Table 22–9.

Ultrasound probes are used with certain orientations by convention. Ultrasound probes usually are marked, often as a bump or a tactile protrusion on one edge of the probe (Fig. 22–25). This mark correlates to the dot or mark on the ultrasound display. Typically, the mark on the display is on the right side of the screen and the probe should be correspondingly oriented to the right side of the body or the head. Thus, ultrasound probe movements to the right correspond to movements on the screen to the right if imaging in a transverse plane. If a coronal or an axial plane is used, the probe marker points toward the head of the subject, hence the right side of the screen points toward the head. With proper orientation, probe movements will appear anatomic, that is, when objects being imaged move to the right they appear to move to the right on the ultrasound screen.

Most of the equipment and supplies for ultrasound-guided central venous access are the same supplies needed for the blind or landmark technique. Specific items needed for ultrasound guidance are sterile ultrasound gel, probe covers, and needle guides. Ultrasound gel is needed to match the impedance of the probe to the skin. Without gel, imaging is not possible. Gel must be used both under the sterile sheath

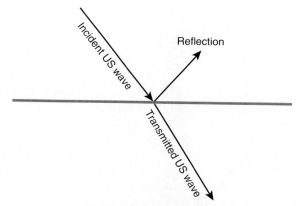

Figure 22–22 Reflection and attenuation.

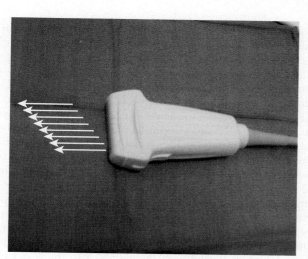

Figure 22–24 A linear probe.

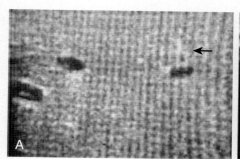
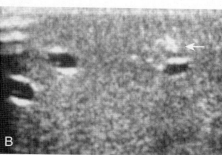
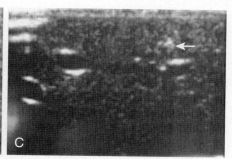

Figure 22–23 The effect of gain on an image. Arrow indicates needle tip.

TABLE 22–9 Ultrasound

Control	Function	Comment	Pitfall
Depth	Changes amount of depth displayed on screen	Adjust the depth to the minimum needed to completely visualize the structure of interest	Having too much depth displayed makes the structure of interest smaller
Gain	Adjusts the overall brightness of the image on the screen	Adjust the gain as low as possible to be able to visualize the structures of interest	As the gain is increased, contrast between different structures is lost (see Fig. 22–23)
Time gain control or near and far gain control	Adjusts the relative brightness of specific parts of the display	Adjust so that the display has similar gain and contrast from top to bottom	

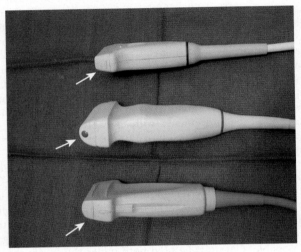

Figure 22–25 Probe indicator.

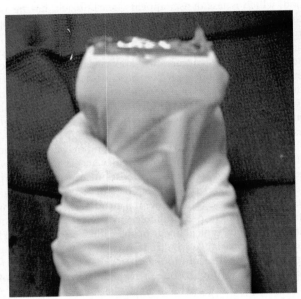

Figure 22–26 Sterile sheath or glove.

and between the sheath and the skin. Because placement of a CVC is a sterile procedure, sterile gel must be used. If sterile ultrasound gel is not available, use individually packaged lubricant. The lubricant has similar acoustic properties to ultrasound gel while being both sterile and bacteriostatic. Use sterile sheaths also because the probe itself is not sterile. If sterile sheaths are not available, use a sterile glove to cover the probe (Fig. 22–26). Needle guides may also be used to assist with ultrasound-guided vascular access (Fig. 22–27). These guides offer the advantage of providing a way of knowing the exact depth and trajectory of the needle under the ultrasound probe. However, the guide requires the use of longer needles and may prevent the cannulation of deeper veins. Further, the guides are nondisposable and are not always available. Most practitioners using ultrasound for vein cannulation prefer to use a free-hand approach. This method allows for more flexibility in the approach to the vessel and for deeper veins to be accessed. This method requires more practice, but is easy to learn.

Ultrasound Imaging

Two approaches may be used for vascular access: longitudinal and transverse. In longitudinal approach, the probe is oriented parallel to the vessel of interest and appears as a thick line. As the probe is angled side to side, sides of the vein can be visualized, aiding in the three-dimensional image of the vein and the surrounding structures. Orient the probe so that the marker is pointed toward the head or proximally. In the transverse approach, the probe is oriented perpendicular to the vein of interest. In this approach, the vein appears in its

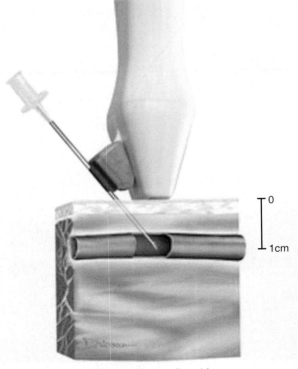

Figure 22–27 Needle guide.

short axis, that is, in a cross section or a circle. Angle the probe or move it up and down the vein in order to create a mental three-dimensional image of the vein and surrounding structures. For the transverse approach, orient the marker to the right side of the patient or object of interest.

Method of Imaging the Vessel

Regardless of which approach will be used to cannulate the vessel, begin the image acquisition with the transverse approach. Place the probe directly above the usual location of the vein. This will produce the cross-sectional view of the vein of interest. Typically, the vein, artery, and nerve will course through the tissue in a similar location. To the untrained eye, these structures may initially appear similar in appearance. Both arteries and veins will appear to be a hollow tubelike structure, if normal. Arteries typically will have a thicker wall than the vein and will appear pulsatile in most locations of the body (Fig. 22–28). Use caution when visualizing the IJ vein because this vein may also appear to pulsate. This is covered in greater detail later. Unless a thrombus is present, veins collapse when pressure is exerted by the probe. Arteries may deform but usually do not collapse unless extreme force is used (Fig. 22–29). If available, Doppler functions may be helpful in the differentiation of veins and arteries (Fig. 22–30). Color-flow Doppler displays color in relation to flow. Thus, arterial flow will appear to pulsate with color whereas a vein will appear to have no color or generally continuous color. The color displayed, red or blue, refers to direction of flow and does not identify an artery or vein. Spectral Doppler displays a visual representation of the flow within the vein or

artery. Arterial flow will be pulsatile and probably triphasic in nature. Veins will be monophasic and nonpulsatile. Nerves usually are small structures and are often not visible. However, when visualized, these structures will appear homogeneous and not appear to have a lumen, that is, they appear hollow.

Once the vein is visualized, slide the probe up and down the vein to visualize the surrounding structures and branches of the vein. Select a location in which branching of the vein will not obstruct the passage of the catheter. If a longitudinal approach will be used for the cannulation procedure, rotate the probe 90° so that the longitudinal axis is visualized. Care must be used to ensure that the vein visualized in cross section is the same vein visualized in longitudinal section. This is best accomplished by keeping the vein of interest visible on the screen as the probe is slowly rotated. If visualization of the vein is lost at any time, start again by visualizing the vein in cross section. One should not attempt to identify a vein versus an artery in longitudinal axis (Fig. 22–31).

General Technique

The technique for ultrasound-guided cannulation does not depend on the location, that is, IJ, subclavian, or femoral vein. The general technique of cannulation is discussed here and specific locations are covered later in the chapter.

The transverse approach is often felt to be easier to learn by the novice user that the longitudinal approach. However, the longitudinal approach is felt to be a safer approach and is the preferred method for ultrasound-guided cannulation.[113]

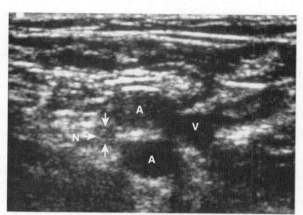

Figure 22–28 Cross-sectional view of the neurovascular bundle. A, artery; N, nerve; V, vein.

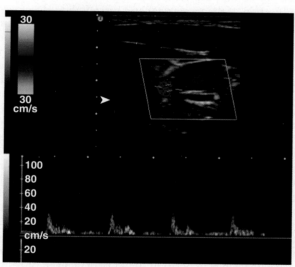

Figure 22–30 Color-flow Doppler displays color in relation to flow.

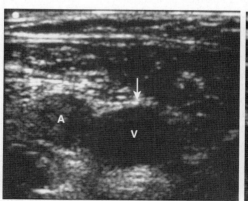
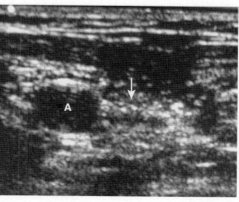

Figure 22–29 Ultrasound image of a collapsed vein due to transducer pressure.

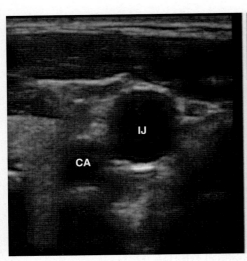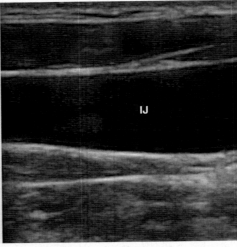

In the longitudinal approach, the entire needle is seen during the procedure. In contrast, only a cross section of the needle is seen with the transverse approach. Novice operators often mistake the cross section of the body of the needle for the tip of the needle in the transverse approach. Hence, the advantages of using ultrasound are lost because the operator does not know where the tip of the needle is located and complications may result.

Regardless of which approach is chosen for the guidance of the needle into the vein, both approaches must start with identification of the target vein and surrounding structures in short or transverse axis. In cross section, vascular structures are identified by their circular appearance with a hypoechoic, or dark, center. In contrast, nerves are smaller than the accompanying vein and artery and appear to be solid and homogeneous in appearance. Veins can be easily identified from the nearby artery by applying external pressure with the transducer. Veins collapse completely with pressure, whereas arteries may deform but usually do not collapse. Occasionally, the vein does not collapse with pressure. If this occurs, a thrombus may be present in the vein or the structure has been misidentified. If a suspected vein does not collapse with pressure, it is not an appropriate vessel for cannulation. When identifying the IJ vein, applying external pressure is not appropriate because pressure on the carotid bulb may cause bradycardia. The IJ vein may also pulsate owing to its connection to the tricuspid valve and right atria. However the IJ vein can be identified by other features. The IJ vein changes its size with change in position, Valsalva maneuver, or respiration. The IJ vein swells at the end of expiration owing to a rise in intrathoracic pressure. The carotid artery generally has a thicker wall than the IJ vein and does not change with changes in position or respiration (Fig. 22–32). If color Doppler is available, it may be used to differentiate the carotid artery from the IJ vein by the color pattern. If the identity of the vein cannot be ensured, the operator should select an alternative site, seek help from a more experienced operator, or try a different method of cannulation.

Once the vein is identified, select the cannulation approach. Using the transverse approach, keep the vein visualized in cross section for the cannulation. The probe is oriented with the right side of the probe to the right side of the vein. There is usually a marker on the probe to indicate the right side of the probe, but if there is confusion, the operator can use her or his finger to identify the right and left side of

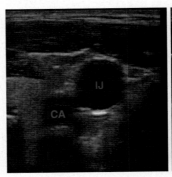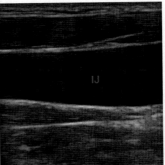

Figure 22–32 The IJ vein changes size with changes in position, Valsalva maneuver, or respiration.

the probe by seeing the motion on the ultrasound screen. Center the vein under the probe and on the ultrasound screen. Place the needle under the center of the long axis of the probe (Fig. 22–33). If the probe is centered over the vein, the needle will also be centered over the vein. Measure or estimate the depth of the vein from the screen. Also, estimate the distances to other structures such as the artery or the pleura. As the needle is advanced under the skin and probe, the needle will appear on the ultrasound screen as a bright dot and may have shadowing deep to the dot. However, with the transverse approach, the needle may be advanced without an apparent change in the needle on the screen. This is because the needle shaft is also seen in cross section. Move the probe up the vein in order to visualize the end or tip of the needle. If the tip of the needle is not visualized at all times, the needle may be passed into structures other than the vein. The key concept in using ultrasound guidance for venous access is to visualize the needle tip at all times during the cannulation. Make subtle continuous movements up and down the vein to visualize the needle tip as it approaches the vein. Guide the needle tip to the vein and visualize the puncture (Fig. 22–34).

In the longitudinal approach, after the vein has been identified, rotate the probe from the transverse position. Make this rotation carefully because the probe can easily slide off the vein and identification can be lost. If this occurs, restart in the transverse position and reidentify the vein. Errors may occur if the vein is identified in the longitudinal axis. Using transducer pressure to collapse the vein in long axis is a pitfall that may lead to misidentification of the vein. Once the vein

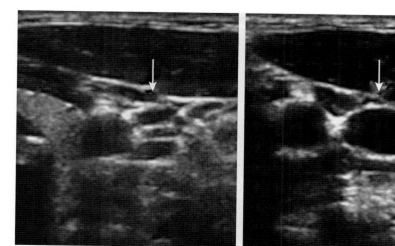

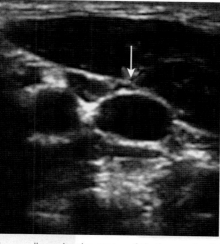

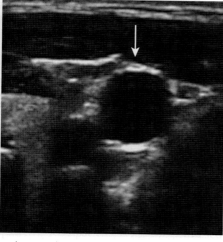

Figure 22–33 Place the needle under the center of the long axis of the ultrasound probe.

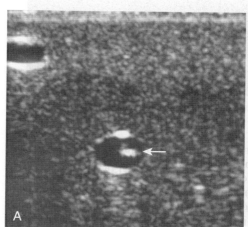

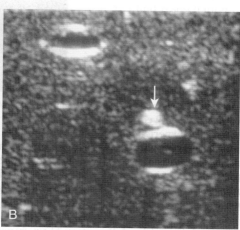

Figure 22–34 Guide the needle tip to the vein and visualize the puncture by ultrasound.

is in long axis, the vein will appear as a tube or cylinder and the needle will appear as a bright line. If the needle does not appear as a line, the probe is not exactly parallel to the needle. Insert the needle under the short face of the probe, as close to the center of the probe as possible (Fig. 22–35). After penetrating the skin, locate the needle if it is not visible on the screen. Do not advance the needle until it is located with the ultrasound and its relationship to the vein and surrounding structures is known. If the vein is visualized in its long axis and the needle is not visible, pan or tilt the probe from right to left. Once the needle is located, direct the needle back toward the vein (the same direction the probe was tilted/panned in order to visualize the vein). Once the vein and the needle are seen at the same time on the ultrasound screen, advance the needle toward the vein. If the visualization of the needle tip is lost, pan with the probe to find the tip and redirect the needle toward the vein. Visualize the needle penetrating the wall of the vein.

Many pitfalls exist when using ultrasound guidance for venous cannulation. It is very important to correctly identify the vein. This should occur only in the short or the transverse axis. Vein identity cannot be ensured from longitudinal axis without using advanced ultrasound techniques such as Doppler ultrasound. Also, visualize the needle tip throughout any advancement of the needle. This is particularly important if the transverse approach is chosen. A common mistake is to visualize the needle shaft instead of the needle tip while

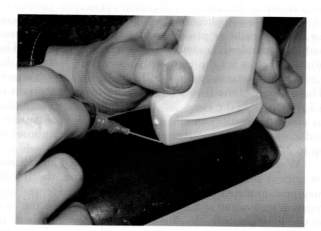

Figure 22–35 Place the needle under the center of the short axis of the ultrasound probe.

advancement is occurring. Complications such as arterial puncture or pneumothorax from pleural puncture may occur because the needle tip is not visualized and the operator has false security in the location of the needle. Also visualize the guidewire prior to dilation of the vessel (Fig. 22–36). This can be done at any point while inserting the wire to ensure that the correct vessel has been cannulated and that a posterior wall puncture has not occurred. This technique can be quite

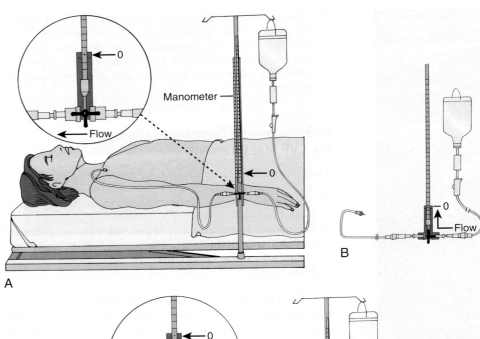

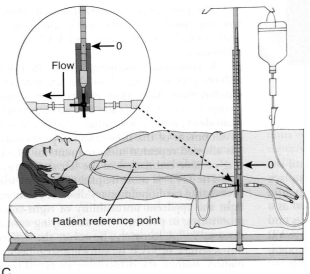

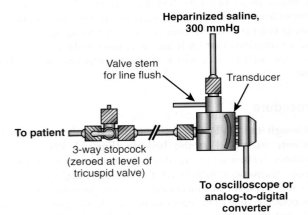

Figure 22–39 *A,* Simple manometry column used to measure CVP at the bedside. The stopcock is turned to direct the fluid flow to the patient, bypassing the manometer. This is the position that is maintained to keep the catheter patent. The tubing is always flushed before connecting it to the patient's CVP catheter. *B,* The stopcock is turned to fill the manometer to 25 cm H_2O. *C,* The stopcock is opened to the patient, and the column of water in the manometer is allowed to fall and stabilize before a reading is taken. Note that the zero mark is horizontally aligned with the tricuspid valve (midaxillary line in a supine patient).

Figure 22–40 Transducers are usually not used in the emergency department, and the stopcock/manometer is currently the CVP monitoring method of choice. For prolonged monitoring, a transducer is ideal. General configurations of an intravascular pressure transducer are shown.

the tubing will dampen the CVP wave and potentially cause underestimation of venous pressure.

After the system has been flushed, place the stopcock (with the transducer still open to air) at the level of the patient's tricuspid valve. Zero or calibrate the monitor detecting the transducer's signal. Calibrate the transducer at the level of the tricuspid valve, which can be approximated on the skin surface as a point at the midaxillary line and the fourth intercostal space.[61,110] Finally, set the stopcock so that the transducer is in continuity with the patient's venous catheter.

In spontaneously breathing patients, take readings at the end of a normal inspiration. If the patient is receiving positive-pressure ventilation, the CVP changes during the respiratory cycle are reversed, rising with inspiration and decreasing with expiration. In these patients, take readings near the end of expiration.[110] Thus, during both normal and mechanical ventilation, the lowest reading is a useful estimate of the mean CVP.

Take a reading after proper assembly of the equipment and accurate placement of the tip of the catheter have been established. To ensure optimal measurement, place the patient

TABLE 22–10 Faulty Central Venous Pressure Readings

Increased intrathoracic pressure (ventilator, straining, coughing)
Reference points in error
Malposition of catheter tip
Blocking or ball-valve obstruction of catheter
Air bubbles in circuit
Readings during wrong phase of ventilation
Readings by different observers
Vasopressors (presumed)

in the supine position. Whenever the patient is repositioned, take care to ensure that the transducer has been recalibrated to reflect the new position of the patient.

Errors in CVP Measurement

A number of extrinsic factors may alter the accuracy of the CVP reading (Table 22–10).[60,61,110] In addition to the position of the patient, these factors include changes in intrathoracic pressure, catheter tip malposition, obstruction of the catheter, and failure to calibrate or zero the line. Activities that increase intrathoracic pressure, such as coughing or straining, may cause spuriously high measurements. Make sure that the patient is relaxed at the time of the measurement and breathing normally. In mechanically ventilated patients, the CVP will be elevated to an extent directly proportional to the ventilatory pressures being delivered and inversely proportional to the mechanical compliance of the lung. Care should be exercised in interpreting filling pressures in this circumstance, because ventilator-induced elevations in CVP are not artifactual, but represent changes in the hemodynamic physiology of the patient. As in spontaneously breathing patients, CVP measurements are meaningful only in a relaxed, sedated, or paralyzed subject.

Another reason for faulty readings is malposition of the catheter tip. If the catheter tip has not passed far enough into the central venous system, peripheral venous spasm or venous valves may yield pressure readings that are inconsistent with the true CVP.

If the catheter tip has passed into the right ventricle, a falsely elevated CVP measurement is obtained. Recognition of a characteristic right ventricular pressure waveform on the patient's monitor should hopefully preclude this error. Such fluctuations may occasionally be seen in appropriately positioned CVP lines when significant tricuspid regurgitation or atrioventricular dissociation (cannon a waves) is present.[111] Inaccurate low venous pressure readings are seen when a valvelike obstruction at the catheter tip occurs either by clot formation or by contact against a vein wall. As mentioned earlier, wave damping due to air bubbles in the transducer or tubing also leads to faulty readings. Using poorly zeroed lines may result in inaccurate measurements that may be interpreted as a change in the patient's status when none has actually occurred. The transducer should be zeroed to the same level for every measurement.

Interpretation of the CVP Measurement

Because determination of the CVP can aid the clinician in assessment of the critically ill patient, it is paramount that the clinician know the normal values and the variables that may affect these values and can recognize the pathologic conditions that correlate with abnormal values. Although various ranges for normal have been reported, a summary of these values is as follows:

Low: <6 cm H_2O
Normal: 6–12 cm H_2O
High: >12 cm H_2O

In the late stages of pregnancy (30–42 wk), the CVP is physiologically elevated, and normal readings are 5 to 8 cm H_2O higher in pregnant women. A CVP reading less than 6 cm H_2O is consistent with low right atrial pressure and reflects a decrease in the return of blood volume to the right heart. This may indicate that the patient requires additional fluid or blood. A low CVP reading is also obtained when vasomotor tone is decreased, as in sepsis, spinal cord injury, or other forms of sympathetic interruption.

A CVP reading falling within a normal range is viewed in relationship to the clinical situation. A reading greater than 12 cm H_2O indicates that the heart is not effectively circulating the volume presented to it. This situation may occur in the case of either a normovolemic patient with underlying cardiac disease such as left ventricular hypertrophy (with associated poor ventricular compliance) or a patient with a normal heart who is overhydrated and overtransfused. A high CVP can also be related to variables other than pump failure, such as pericardial tamponade, restrictive pericarditis, pulmonary stenosis, and pulmonary embolus.[111]

Changes in blood volume, vessel tone, and cardiac function may occur alone or in combination with one another; therefore, it is possible to have a normal or elevated CVP in the presence of normovolemia, hypovolemia, and hypervolemia.[111] Interpret the specific CVP values with respect to the entire clinical picture. The response of the CVP to an infusion is more important than the initial reading.

Fluid Challenge

Monitoring the CVP may be helpful as a practical guide for fluid therapy.[60,61,108-110] Serial CVP measurements provide a fairly reliable indication of the capability of the right heart to accept an additional fluid load. Although the PCWP is a more sensitive index of left heart fluid needs (and in some clinical situations, PCWP measurement is essential), serial measurement of CVP can provide significant information.

A fluid challenge can help assess both volume deficits and pump failure.[109] Although a fluid challenge can be used with either PCWP monitoring or CVP monitoring, only the fluid challenge for CVP monitoring is discussed here. Slight variations in the methodology of fluid challenge are reported in the literature. Generally, administer aliquots of 50 to 200 mL of crystalloid sequentially and measure CVP levels after 10 minutes. Repeat the fluid challenge until measurements indicate that adequate volume expansion has occurred. Discontinue the fluid challenge as soon as hemodynamic signs of shock are reversed or signs of cardiac incompetence are evident.

Cardiac Tamponade

In cardiac tamponade, pericardial pressure rises to equal the right ventricular end-diastolic pressure. The pericardial pressure encountered in pericardial tamponade characteristically produces an elevated CVP.[111] The degree of CVP elevation is variable, and one must interpret measurements cautiously;

CVP readings in the range of 16 to 18 cm H_2O are typically seen in acute tamponade, but elevations of up to 30 cm H_2O may be encountered. The exact CVP reading is often lower than one might intuitively expect, and it is not uncommon to encounter tamponade with a CVP of 10 to 12 cm H_2O. A normal, or even low, CVP reading may be seen if the tamponade is associated with significant hypovolemia. An excessive rise in CVP after fluid challenge may be more important than a single reading in the diagnosis of pericardial tamponade.

Excessive straining, agitation, pneumatic antishock garment inflation, positive-pressure ventilation, or tension pneumothorax may increase intrathoracic pressure, producing a high CVP reading, and may erroneously suggest the diagnosis of pericardial tamponade. Increases in vascular tone, as seen with the use of dopamine or other vasopressors, may also elevate the CVP, mimicking tamponade and complicating volume estimation.

CONCLUSION

CVP monitoring provides useful hemodynamic monitoring information in those individuals with a relatively normal cardiopulmonary system who do not otherwise warrant PCWP monitoring.

 REFERENCES CAN BE FOUND ON EXPERT CONSULT

CHAPTER 23

Venous Cutdown

Patricia L. Lanter and Justin Williams

The venous cutdown is a time-honored, simple surgical technique that is useful in the management of seriously ill patients. It is an excellent means of venous access in children and in markedly hypovolemic patients. Complications are potentially serious but can be controlled by good surgical technique and removal of the catheter as soon as possible. Keeley[1] first described the technique in 1940, offering the procedure as an alternative to venipuncture in patients who were in shock or had small, thin veins. The increasing use of the Seldinger technique and ultrasound guidance for central venous cannulation of the internal jugular, subclavian, and femoral veins has markedly decreased the frequency of venous cutdown. Venous cutdown is no longer taught as a mandatory procedure for the Advanced Trauma and Life Support (ATLS) course, but it is optional, to be taught at the discretion of the instructor.[2] Nevertheless, the cutdown remains an excellent method of obtaining venous access in several emergent situations. Although a cutdown is mechanically simple to perform, it can only be performed rapidly and effectively with a thorough understanding of the anatomy and the procedure and its potential complications. In addition, Custalow and coworkers[3] showed that the use of animal laboratory training improved venous cutdown competency and speed.

INDICATIONS

Venous cutdown may be used as an alternative to venipuncture for critical patients in need of vascular access when less invasive options are not available. Clinical examples include small children, patients in shock, and intravenous (IV) drug abusers with sclerosed veins. In patients who are severely injured, burned, or scarred from current or previous trauma, the skin and surface anatomy may be distorted, making veins and landmarks difficult to identify. In addition, patients in asystole or pulseless electrical activity do not have palpable femoral pulses, making femoral vein catheterization difficult.

Children

Venipuncture in small children is challenging in one who is healthy and greater still in one in shock when few veins are visible. When all accessible peripheral sites, including scalp veins, have been exhausted, consider central vein catheterization, intraosseous line placement, or venous cutdown as alternative methods of venous access. The distal saphenous vein at the ankle is large enough to cannulate in most children and has a predictable anatomic location, so it may be used for venous cutdown in an emergency.[4,5]

Hypovolemic Shock

Use of the cutdown for venous access and rapid transfusion was popularized during the Vietnam War.[6] Since then, the technique has been used in certain indications for the resuscitation of patients with profound hypovolemia.[7] The flow rate for saline through a standard IV extension set cut to a length of 28 cm (12 inches) and inserted directly into the vein is 15% to 30% greater than through a 5-cm, 14-gauge catheter. The difference is greater if pressure is applied to the system. The improvement in flow rate through large-bore lines is greater for blood than for crystalloid solutions because the viscous characteristics of blood greatly impede its passage through small-bore tubing.[7] A unit of blood can be transfused in 3 minutes using IV extension tubing inserted directly into the vein. Consequently, large-bore lines placed by venous cutdown are an excellent mechanism for the treatment of severe hypovolemia.

CONTRAINDICATIONS

Venous cutdown is contraindicated when less invasive alternatives exist and when performing the procedure would cause excessive delay.[8] Although highly skilled clinicians may perform a cutdown in less than 60 seconds,[9] studies have shown that, on average, the procedure takes at least 5 to 6 minutes to complete.[10–12] The modified guidewire method described by both Shockley and Butzier[13] and Klofas[14] can decrease that time by 22%. Percutaneous insertion of large-bore catheters is the preferred method of rapid fluid infusion unless high flow rates are required or peripheral veins have collapsed. Another method of rapid fluid infusion that is technically easier and faster than cutdown is the percutaneous insertion of large-bore introducer devices into the subclavian, internal jugular, or femoral veins with or without ultrasound guidance. These devices typically use 8-French catheters with flow rates comparable with those obtained with IV tubing. For long-term venous access, the use of the subclavian and internal jugular vessels is preferable to the cutdown.

Cutdowns should be avoided when there is an infection over the site and in extremities with injuries proximal to the cutdown site. Other contraindications are relative. In the presence of coagulation disorders, impaired healing, or compromised host-defense mechanisms, the need to perform a cutdown should be weighed carefully against the potential complications.

ANATOMY

Detailed knowledge of anatomy is imperative to the success of this procedure. Veins in both the upper and the lower extremities may be used by considering accessibility and size and the clinician's experience and training. The anatomy of individual vessels and their relative merits as cutdown sites are described in the following sections.

The Greater Saphenous Vein

The greater saphenous vein is the longest vein and it runs subcutaneously throughout much of its course (Fig. 23–1). It is most easily accessible at the ankle, but may also be cannulated below the knee and below the femoral triangle. The greater saphenous vein begins at the ankle, where it is the continuation of the medial marginal vein of the foot. The vein crosses 1 cm anterior to the medial malleolus and continues up the anteromedial aspect of the leg.[15] At the level of the malleolus, the vein lies adjacent to the periosteum and is

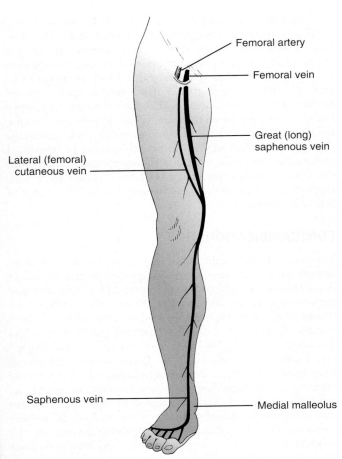

Figure 23–1   Superficial veins of the lower limb.

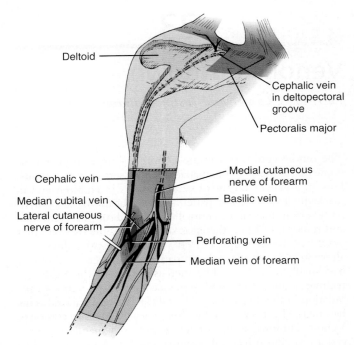

Figure 23–2   Veins of the upper limb.

accompanied by the relatively insignificant saphenous nerve, which, if transected, causes sensory loss in a small area along the medial aspect of the foot. At the ankle, the vessel can be exposed with minimal blunt dissection. The vein's superficial, predictable, and isolated location has made the distal saphenous vein the classic pediatric cutdown site.[15]

At the knee, the saphenous vein lies superficially on the medial aspect. A cutdown performed 1 to 4 cm below the knee and immediately posterior to the tibia has been described in the pediatric literature.[4] This site is distal enough to avoid interference with the performance of other resuscitative procedures, yet proximal enough to allow the passage of a long line into the central circulation.[16] However, it is seldom used for venous cutdown. Disadvantages of this site include kinking of the line as the knee is flexed and the risk of injury to the saphenous branch of the genicular artery and the saphenous nerve.[17]

In the thigh, the saphenous vein begins on the medial aspect of the knee and crosses anterolaterally as it ascends toward the femoral triangle. Proximally, it enters the fossa ovalis and joins the femoral vein. Three to 4 cm distal to the inguinal ligament, the saphenous vein is of large caliber (4–5 mm outside diameter) and is easily isolated from the surrounding fat. Also lying anteromedially in the thigh is the lateral femoral cutaneous vein, which has a smaller diameter (2–3 mm) and lies lateral to the greater saphenous vein.[18,19] The accessibility and large diameter of the greater saphenous vein in the thigh make its use an option in the treatment of profound hypovolemia.[7]

The Basilic Vein

The basilic vein is a preferred site for venous cutdown in the upper extremity. Veins of the dorsal venous network of the hand unite to form the cephalic and basilic veins, which travel along the radial and ulnar sides of the forearm, respectively (Fig. 23–2). At the level of the midforearm, the basilic vein crosses anterolaterally and is consistently found 1 to 2 cm lateral to the medial epicondyle on the anterior surface of the upper arm. The medial cubital vein crosses over from the radial side of the arm to join the basilic vein just above the medial epicondyle. The basilic vein then continues proximally, occupying a superficial position between the biceps and the pronator teres muscles. In this segment, it lies in close association with the medial cutaneous nerve, which supplies sensation to the ulnar side of the forearm. The vein penetrates the brachial fascia in the distal third of the upper arm and then occupies a deeper position.[20]

The basilic vein is generally cannulated at the antecubital fossa 2 cm above and 2 to 3 cm lateral to the medial epicondyle. It is exposed through a transverse incision on the medial aspect of the proximal antecubital fossa. The size of this vein enables it to be located easily, even in the hypotensive or hypovolemic patient; large catheters can be passed without difficulty under most circumstances. The median cubital vein is accessible through the same incision. Superficially at this level, there are no important associated structures, but the brachial artery and the median nerve are found deep to the basilic vein.

A more proximal insertion site has been recommended by Simon and colleagues[21] to avoid the network of interconnecting veins at the level of the antecubital fossa. However, in the distal third of the upper arm, there is a closer association between the basilic vein and the medial cutaneous nerve. Transection of this nerve produces sensory loss on the ulnar side of the forearm.

The Cephalic Vein

This vessel begins on the radial aspect of the wrist and crosses anteromedially, ascending toward the antecubital fossa. In the forearm, it lies in close association with the lateral cutaneous nerve, which supplies sensory innervation to the radial aspect of the forearm (see Fig. 23–2). In the antecubital fossa, it lies subcutaneously, just lateral to the midline, and then ascends in the upper arm, overlying the lateral aspect of the biceps muscle. At the shoulder, the cephalic vein lies in the delto-pectoral groove. Just below the clavicle, it passes deep to end in the axillary vein.[20]

Venous cutdown is easily performed on the cephalic vein because of its large diameter and superficial location. In the forearm, it is important to avoid the lateral cutaneous nerve. A good location is in the antecubital fossa at the distal flexor crease. Cutdown on the cephalic vein at the wrist has also been reported, but the thin skin overlying the vein at this level usually permits simple percutaneous cannulation when the vein is available for cannulation.[22] The cephalic vein may also be entered in the deltopectoral groove. The slightly deeper position and physical interference with the performance of other procedures make this approach more difficult.

The Brachial Veins

The brachial veins are small, paired vessels lying on either side of the brachial artery. In contrast to the vessels described earlier, these are not superficial and will not accommodate large cannulas. Their most superficial location is 1 to 2 cm above the antecubital fossa just medial to the biceps muscle. Palpation of the brachial pulse serves as a useful landmark. Because of its proximity, the brachial artery may be inadvertently cannulated in the pulseless patient. In addition, there is the risk of injury to the closely associated median nerve. Time-consuming blunt dissection is usually required because of the vessel's greater depth. For these reasons, brachial vein cutdown is not recommended as an emergency venous access route and should be used only in the absence of a suitable alternative.[8] This site may be acceptable when time and vessel size are not critical factors, but it is difficult to justify the deep dissection and associated risks involved.

EQUIPMENT

The materials required to perform a formal venous cutdown are shown in Figure 23–3. Perhaps the most important piece of equipment and the most difficult to find, is the vein dilator/lifter, a 90° angle plastic device used to facilitate entrance of a catheter into the cut vein. For pediatric patients, use a warming table or radiant warmer and a padded extremity board as well.

Choose a catheter based on the desired function of the venous line. When central venous pressure (CVP) monitoring is needed, choose a catheter long enough to reach the superior vena cava. The average distance from the antecubital fossa to the superior vena cava is 54 cm in the adult male. Approximate this distance by aligning the catheter over the chest with the tip at the level of the manubrial-sternal junction. Lumen size is relatively unimportant when the line is inserted for monitoring the CVP or to infuse drugs, but it is a critical factor in the treatment of hypovolemia. Short, large-bore catheters are preferred when fluid must be delivered rapidly. Silastic catheters, IV plastic tubing, or 5- or 8-French pedi-

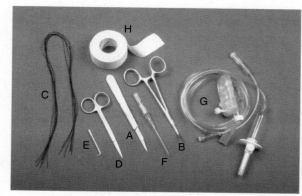

Figure 23–3 Venous cutdown tray. Note the small plastic vein dilator-lifter (E), which is especially useful in children. Equipment: A, scalpel—No. 11 blade; B, curved hemostat; C, No. 0-0 silk suture; D, iris scissors; E, plastic venous dilator; F, large-bore intravenous catheter; G, intravenous tubing, H, tape for securing catheter. *(From Custalow CB: Color Atlas of Emergency Department Procedures. Philadelphia, Elsevier Saunders, 2005, p 163.)*

 TABLE 23–1 Comparative Average Flow Rates (mL/min) for Tap Water CAN BE FOUND ON EXPERT CONSULT

 TABLE 23–2 Comparative Average Flow Rates (mL/min, 200 mm Hg Pressure) for Red Blood Cells CAN BE FOUND ON EXPERT CONSULT

 TABLE 23–3 Comparative Average Flow Rates (mL/min) CAN BE FOUND ON EXPERT CONSULT

atric feeding tubes may be used as infusion catheters in older children and adults.

Tables 23–1 through 23–3 list the flow rates of various fluids through some commonly used catheter systems. It is essential to know the relative flow rates if maximal benefit is to be obtained from the time spent performing the cutdown. Excellent flow rates can be achieved by threading IV tubing directly into the vein or by using a 5-cm, 10-gauge IV catheter. Cut sterile tubing to the appropriate length, leaving a slight bevel on the end to facilitate cannulation of the opened vein.[9,23]

TECHNIQUE

The technique of venous cutdown is essentially the same regardless of the vessel cannulated (Fig. 23–4). Prepare the skin around the incisional area with an antiseptic solution and then cover with sterile drapes. *Place a tourniquet proximal to the cutdown site* to help visualize the vein. For children, immobilize the lower leg or elbow (depending upon the cutdown site) on a padded board *before beginning the procedure* (Fig. 23–5).

In the conscious patient, give local anesthesia prior to the procedure. Make a skin incision perpendicular to the course of the vein. A longitudinal incision, although decreasing the risk of transecting neurovascular structures, may not provide sufficient exposure. Incise the skin through all of its layers until subcutaneous fat bulges through the incision. Dissect the subcutaneous tissues bluntly by spreading them gently with a curved hemostat parallel to the course of the vein and with the tips pointed downward. Bleeding is usually minimal unless

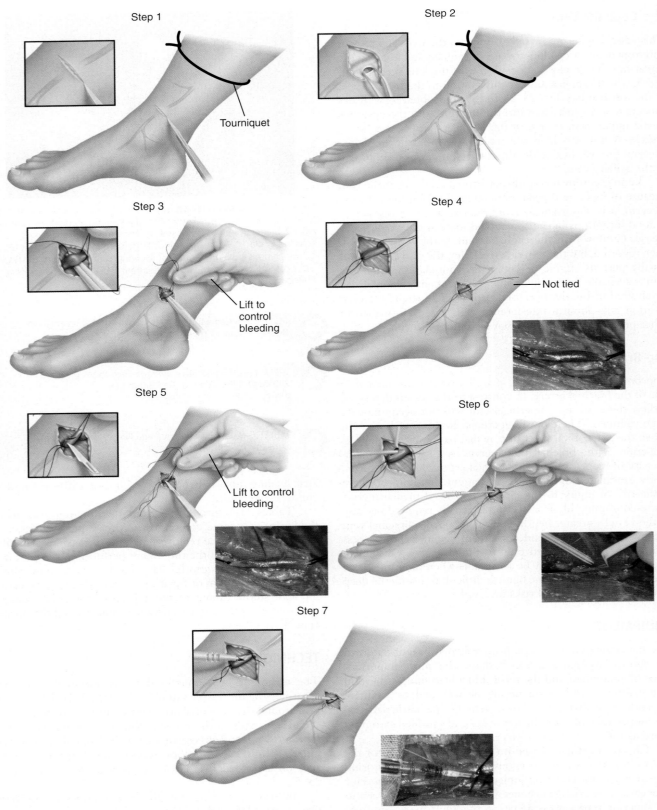

Figure 23–4 Procedural steps for venous cutdown. *Step 1*: Saphenous vein approach. The saphenous vein at the ankle can be found approximately 1 cm anterior to the medial malleolus. Place a tourniquet and use a topical antiseptic. Make a skin incision perpendicular to the course of the vein. *Step 2:* Bluntly dissect, isolate, and mobilize the vein. *Step 3*: Use a hemostat to isolate the vein and to pass the silk ties under the vein proximal and distal to the proposed cannulation site. *Step 4:* Tie the distal suture only. *Step 5:* Incise the vein while retracting the proximal ligature. Lift the proximal untied suture to control back bleeding. *Step 6:* Using the plastic venous dilator to lift the flap, advance the catheter into the vein. Attach intravenous tubing to the catheter. *Step 7:* Tie the proximal silk suture around the vein and catheter. Remove proximal suture and suture skin. *(From Custalow CB: Color Atlas of Emergency Department Procedures. Philadelphia, Elsevier Saunders, 2005, p 164.)*

the vein is nicked. Use a tissue spreader or a self-retaining retractor, if needed, to provide a wider field. Isolate the vein from the adjacent tissue and mobilize it for 1 to 3 cm.

For the standard venous cutdown technique, after mobilizing the vein, use a hemostat to pass proximal and distal silk ties under the vein for stabilization.

Tie the distal ligature after initial placement, but leave the ends long for maneuvering the vein. *Leave the proximal ligature untied to maneuver the vein to insert the catheter or tubing and to control backbleeding (by simply lifting the sutures).* Using a hemostat, elevate the vein and stretch it flat. This provides good visualization, controls the vessel, and limits bleeding when the vessel is incised. Alternatively, place gentle traction on the proximal tie to control oozing around the puncture site. Using a No. 11 blade scalpel or a pair of iris scissors, incise the vein at a 45° angle, passing through one third to one half of its diameter. If the incision is too small, the catheter may easily pass into a false channel in the adventitia. Conversely, if the incision is too large, the vein may tear completely and retract from the field.[24] If desired, make a longitudinal incision in the vein to avoid transecting the vessel, but realize that this technique makes it more difficult to identify the lumen. Be aware also that some bleeding will normally occur after the vein has merely been nicked on the surface. To perform a mini-cutdown, puncture the vein with an IV catheter and introducer needle and *do not make an incision in the vein.*

Before introducing the cannula into the vein, make a bevel in the cannula at a 45° angle. This is unnecessary if the cannula has a tapered tip. Make the bevel short, being careful not to make it sharply pointed because this may pierce the posterior wall or otherwise damage the vein. If using the rounded tip of a feeding tube, it may be more difficult to introduce, but it can be advanced less traumatically. If using an IV cannula, introduce it directly through the skin incision or through a separate stab incision.

Threading the catheter into the vein is often the most difficult and time-consuming portion of the procedure. Difficulty threading has several causes. The lumen may have been incorrectly identified, or a false passage into the adventitia may have been created. This frequently occurs and is difficult to recognize because the catheter can easily advance between layers of the vessel wall and never reach the lumen of the vein. Other causes include penetration of the posterior vessel wall, getting stuck in a venous valve, or using a catheter that is too large to cannulate the vein.

Using a plastic venous dilator can help to identify and elevate the vessel lumen, if available. Thread the small, pointed tip of the device into the vein to expose the lumen before advancing the tip of the catheter. Alternatively, bend a sterile 20-gauge needle at a 90° angle to serve as a venous dilator or elevator. A vein dilator is useful for very small veins, such as in pediatric cutdowns, but is generally unnecessary in adults. To thread large catheters in adults, grasp the proximal edge of the vessel with small forceps or a mosquito hemostat. Apply countertraction and advance the catheter. Never force a catheter that will not easily advance (Fig. 23–6).

Once the catheter is advanced into the lumen, backbleed air from the cannula and connect it to IV tubing. Tie the proximal ligature around both the vessel and the cannula. Remove the tourniquet, affix the catheter to the skin, and close the incision. Apply antibiotic ointment where the catheter passes through the skin, and dress the wound. In an emergent situation, delay skin closure, if necessary, and simply

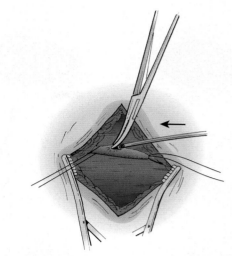

Figure 23–5 In larger veins, a mosquito hemostat can facilitate the placement of the cannula by opening the lumen and providing countertraction.

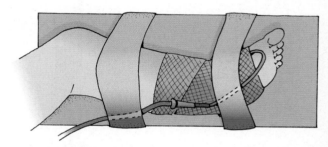

Figure 23–6 The cutdown site is securely dressed and splinted. In a child, the leg can be immobilized prior to the procedure to stabilize the site.

wrap the wound with a sterile dressing. Loop the IV tubing under the outer layers of the dressing to minimize the risk of pulling out the cannula if the external IV line is inadvertently tugged.

Mini-Cutdown

The mini-cutdown is an alternative method designed to preserve the vein and bypass the time-consuming step of placing a catheter into the vein.[25] It is preferred if time is essential. Essentially, *a deep vein is cannulized through an incision under direct vision with the same catheters used for percutaneous infusions.* Use a skin incision and blunt dissection to locate the vessel. Once identified, puncture the vein under direct vision with a standard percutaneous venous catheter. Introduce the needle through either the skin incision or a separate stab incision. If an over-the-needle device (e.g., Angiocath, Medicut) is used, withdraw the needle and discard it. With a through-the-needle device, thread the cannula into the vein, and withdraw the needle to the skin surface (Fig. 23–7). Place a guard on the needle tip, fix the catheter device to the skin, and close the incision. This method eliminates the need for tying or cutting the vein, thereby permitting repeat catheterization. Venipuncture is easier and uses the same equipment as percutaneous venous cannulation. Use the mini-cutdown in situations such as the treatment of chronically ill patients who require long-term IV therapy or in children who have a

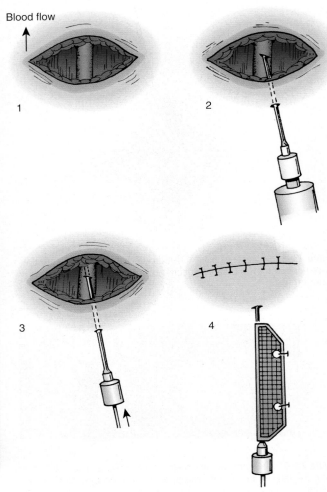

Blood flow

1

2

3

4

Figure 23–7 The mini-cutdown technique is an alternative to the venous cutdown method. The vein is cannulated under direct vision using standard percutaneous catheters. A separate entry site (shown) may be used, or the vein can be cannulated through the skin incision. Note that the vein is not tied off with this technique. A standard Angiocath IV set also may be used instead of the through-the-needle catheter shown here.

limited number of accessible veins. A simple skin incision may also permit direct visualization of veins in an obese patient and facilitate standard percutaneous venipuncture.

Hansbrough and associates[23] described a mini-cutdown procedure with a 10-gauge IV catheter (Deseret 10-gauge Angiocath). The flow rates of blood and saline with this catheter are equal to the rates obtained when IV extension tubing is placed in a vein using the more time-consuming standard venous cutdown technique. This catheter allows one to infuse a unit of whole blood in 2 to 3 minutes if high pressure and oversized IV tubing (e.g., urology irrigation tubing) are used.

MODIFIED CUTDOWN TECHNIQUE

Shockley and Butzier[13] described a further modification in which a guidewire, dilator, and sheath system is inserted after standard cutdown and venotomy. To perform this modification, set up the guidewire, dilator, and sheath system before making the skin incision. Once the vein has been incised, insert the end of the guidewire followed by the dilator

and sheath. Remove the wire and dilator, leaving the sheath. Ligatures are not usually needed with this technique. These authors found that the technique saved more than 2 minutes of time compared with the standard technique when performed by novices, and there was an increased vein salvage rate in the event of transection. Klofas[14] used a similar technique at the distal saphenous vein. He also developed a model for teaching the modified technique using wood, gauze, cast padding, and tape.

To remove catheters inserted by cutdown, cut the skin stitches holding the catheter in place and then withdraw the catheter. Control backbleeding from the proximal venous end by applying a simple pressure dressing.

COMPLICATIONS

The complications of venous cutdown include local hematoma, infection, sepsis, phlebitis, embolization, wound dehiscence, and injury to associated structures. An indirect but significant complication is deterioration of an unstable patient during a time-consuming cutdown attempt. Documentation of complications and their frequency in the literature has been sparse. Bogen[26] reported a 15% complication rate in 234 cases. Infection and phlebitis each occurred at a rate of 4%. Infectious complications may result from the introduction of pathogens during line placement, transcutaneous invasion along the course of the cannula, or deposition of blood-borne organisms on the catheter tip.[27] A clear correlation exists between the incidence of infectious complications and the length of time a catheter is left in place. Moran and coworkers[28] found that the infection rate rose from 50% to 78% when a catheter was left in place for more than 48 hours. Druskin and Siegel,[27] studying a mixed population of patients who had undergone cutdowns and others who had catheters percutaneously inserted, found that the incidence of culture-positive catheter tips rose from 0% to 52% after 48 hours.[27] In the study by Moran and coworkers,[28] *Staphylococcus albus* was the predominant organism that was isolated, but organisms more commonly thought of as pathogenic (*Staphylococcus aureus, Enterococcus spp., and Proteus spp.*) were isolated with greater frequency from cutdowns that had been in place for long periods. Rhee and colleagues[11] reported a 1.4% infection rate and 1 episode of cellulitis after 73 cutdown attempts. All catheters were removed within 24 hours.

Some evidence indicates that the rate of infectious complications decreases when a broad-spectrum topical antibiotic ointment is applied to the cutdown site. Moran and coworkers[28] found a rate of infectious complications of 18% when topical polymyxin B–neomycin-bacitracin (Neosporin) was used, compared with a 78% rate in a placebo-treated group. In this study, it was shown that topical antibiotic use resulted in only a moderate decrease (from 53% to 37%) in the incidence of phlebitis but a significant decrease (from 86% to 14%) in the incidence of phlebitis associated with positive cultures. This suggests that phlebitis is primarily a chemical or an irritative process rather than the result of infection. Whatever the cause, the incidence of phlebitis is clearly related to the duration of catheterization.[6,26,29] Early catheter removal is a key factor in the prevention of both phlebitis and the infectious complications of venous cutdown. This is especially true of lines inserted during emergency resuscitative treatment. Such lines should be removed as soon as the patient's condition stabilizes and alternative routes are in place.[7,8]

Proper attention to the details of surgical technique will limit the occurrence of minor complications, such as local hematoma, abscess, and wound dehiscence. One can avoid injury to associated structures by selecting a site in which the vein is well isolated and by specifically avoiding cutdown of the brachial vein.

FAST-FLOW FLUID WARMING SYSTEMS

The rapid infusion of crystalloid or blood products in resuscitation saves lives. Research in the early 1960s demonstrated that in patients who require large-volume blood transfusions, there were significant survival benefits when the fluids were warmed to body temperature, rather than when they were given cooled. In fact, mortality rates of patients requiring massive blood transfusion (≥3000 mL/hr) improved from 58.3% for cooled blood to 6.8% with warmed blood. Several fast fluid warming systems exist that allow infusion at rates of up to 66,000 mL/hr (Table 23–4). They serve the purpose of increasing the temperature of the administered fluid to near-physiologic temperatures, while allowing rates of fluid administration amenable to resuscitation of patients who may be losing their entire blood volume in a matter of minutes.

TABLE 23–4 Fast Flow Fluid Warming Systems CAN BE FOUND ON EXPERT CONSULT

Acknowledgment

The author and editors wish to sincerely thank Steven C. Dronen for his contributions to this chapter in prior editions.

REFERENCES CAN BE FOUND ON EXPERT CONSULT

CHAPTER 24

Indwelling Vascular Devices: Emergency Access and Management

Diann M. Krywko and Cemal B. Sozener

Indwelling vascular lines provide routes for short- and long-term infusion of antibiotics, antifungals, hyperalimentation fluids, chemotherapeutic agents, blood products, and anesthetic agents. In addition, they provide access for life-saving procedures such as hemodialysis (HD) and plasmapheresis. As of December 31, 2006, nearly 328,000 patients were receiving hemodialysis therapy[1] with three to five million central venous catheters (CVCs) being placed yearly in patients in the United States.[2] For the purpose of this chapter, all implanted devices and intermediate- to long-term catheters for vascular access are considered vascular access devices (VADs). Arteriovenous (AV) fistulas and AV grafts are included owing to their similarities to the VADs.

HISTORICAL PERSPECTIVE

A major advance, ultimately leading to the development of several types of indwelling catheters, was the introduction of Silastic (polymerized silicone rubber). This biocompatible material is an ideal substrate for intravenous (IV) catheters because it is chemically inert, antithrombogenic, rigid at room temperature, and pliable at body temperature. In 1973, Broviac and coworkers[3] used this material to develop a 90-cm x 0.22-mm indwelling right atrial (RA) catheter for total parenteral nutrition (TPN). This prototype catheter was widely used for hyperalimentation and served as a template for catheters designed for other uses. In 1979, Hickman and colleagues[4] reported experience with a 0.32-mm catheter that could be used for blood products and drug therapy for bone marrow transplant recipients. Further modification resulted in the double-lumen Hickman, a fusion of the Broviac catheter (internal diameter [ID], 1.0 mm; external diameter, 2.2 mm), and the Hickman (ID, 1.6 mm; external diameter, 3.2 mm). The increased diameter requires cannulation of a large vein, but it allows concomitant infusion of TPN through one port and IV drugs and blood products through the other. A totally implantable vascular access device (TIVAD) was first described by Fortner and Pahnke in 1972.[5] Since that time, TIVADs have become a mainstay of treatment in oncology patients. TIVADs allow less painful IV access and improve quality of life by permitting unrestricted mobility.

Temporary access for HD via an external AV shunt was pioneered by both Quinton and associates[6] and Scribner and coworkers[7] in 1960. This original shunt was composed of a loop of tubing lying on the volar forearm connecting the radial artery to a wrist vein. Although it provided effective dialysis, it was associated with a high rate of infection, thrombosis, and restriction of patient activity. Brescia and colleagues[8] then introduced the peripheral subcutaneous autogenous AV fistula in 1966. This Brescia-Cimino internal fistula used a side-to-side anastomosis (the current procedure of choice for long-term HD) connecting the radial artery to the cephalic vein in the nondominant hand. Several catheters have been developed for short-term dialysis. Erben and associates[9] described routine use of percutaneous cannulation of the subclavian vein for HD in 1969. In 1979, Uldall and coworkers[10] reported development of a single-needle, subclavian, HD catheter.

INDWELLING VADS

VADs are typically chosen based on the least invasive, smallest catheter with the lowest complication risk that will last as long as the length of therapy that is anticipated.[11] Length of therapy is often the major consideration when choosing a device. Long-term VADs consist of cuffed, tunneled RA catheters and implantable ports. Medium-term VADs include midline catheters (lasting weeks), peripherally inserted central catheter (PICC) lines (lasting months), and Silastic subclavian or jugular catheters (percutaneous multilumen catheters). Short-term devices (not reviewed in this chapter) include short peripherals, subcutaneous (butterfly), subclavian and jugular catheters, and temporary epidurals. Additional VADs include those used for dialysis as well as AV fistulas and grafts.

Cuffed, Tunneled, RA Catheters (Broviac, Hickman, Hemocath, Leonard, Raaf)

Several cuffed, tunneled, RA catheters are available, each with differences tailored to specific applications (Fig. 24–1A). The *Broviac* is an all-Silastic single-lumen catheter with a 1.0-mm ID. It is 90 cm with a thin intravascular segment (55 cm). The *Hickman*, also a Silastic catheter, has a 1.6-mm ID lumen. This allows for more frequent blood sampling without jeopardizing luminal patency.[12] Single-, double- and triple- lumen variations exist. *Hemocath/Permacath* has the largest bore of the RA catheters, 2.2 mm ID. *Quinton* Instrument Co. manufactures it for HD, plasmapheresis, long-term nutritional support, and pain control. The main advantage of the cuffed double-lumen catheter is that it can be used immediately. This has led some clinicians to consider them an alternative to AV shunts and fistulas for medium- to long-term HD.[13] However, there are several disadvantages: significant thrombosis and infection, permanent central venous stenosis or occlusion, shorter life span of 1 to 1.5 years as concluded by the Kidney Disease Outcomes Quality Initiative (K/DOQI) panel,[14] and low to inadequate flow rates. Ideally, these catheters should be used only as bridge catheters.[15]

Insertion of RA catheters is typically done in an operating or interventional radiology suite. The device is introduced via the upper anterior chest wall and tunneled subcutaneously to enter the superior vena caval system via the cephalic, subclavian, internal, or external jugular veins (Fig. 24–2A). The distal tip of the flexible catheter is advanced to the distal superior vena cava (SVC) or into the mid-RA area. The subcutaneous tunnel isolates the venous puncture site from the skin and decreases the potential for bacterial contamination. The Dacron cuffs (one near the venous entrance site and one near the skin exit site) anchor the catheter and are believed to inhibit colonization of the SVC by skin organisms.[16] However, no study has been able to support this belief. The

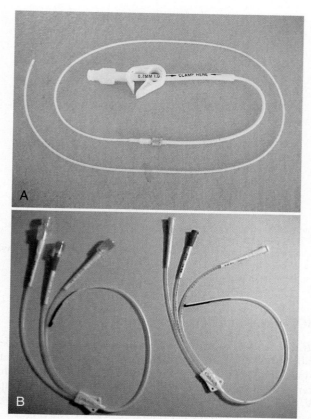

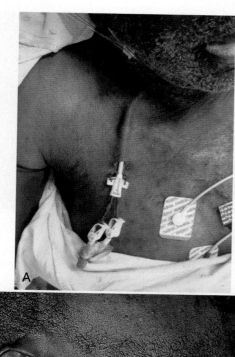

Figure 24–1 *A,* Broviac Pediatric 4.2-French Single-Lumen CV Catheter with SureCuff Tissue Ingrowth Cuff and VitaCuff Antimicrobial Cuff. *B,* The Groshong catheter has a valve to prevent backbleeding.

advantages of an RA catheter include ease of insertion and use, minimal interference with patient activity, low incidence of major complications or unintended dislodgment, ease of removal, and potential repair via a kit. Disadvantages include the need for regular maintenance and the potential for unacceptable cosmesis.

Groshong Catheters

In contrast to the Broviac and Hickmann catheters, the *Groshong* has slitlike openings just proximal to the end of the intravascular portion of the catheter (see Fig. 24–1*B*). This functions as a one-way valve to stop backbleeding and to prevent air entry and embolism from negative intrathoracic pressure. This feature obviates the need to use a heparin lock (saline may be used). In addition, external catheter clamping is not necessary. The disadvantages are high cost and requirement of pressurized infusion systems.[17]

TIVADs/Ports (Port-A-Cath, Proport, Infuse-A-Port, Mediport)

Since 1983, implanted ports have become the mainstay of treatment for long-term cancer therapy. TIVADs are tunneled RA catheters, but they differ from Broviac-Hickman catheters in that they have a subcutaneous titanium or plastic portal with a self-sealing septum (Fig. 24–3) that may be accessed by a specially designed needle (90° angled Huber needle) punctured through intact skin (Fig. 24–4). Cosmeti-

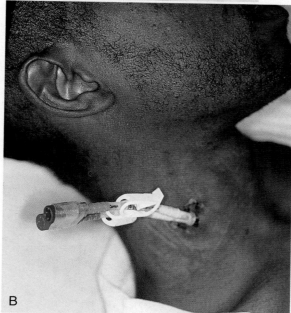

Figure 24–2 *A,* Subclavian-placed catheter with subcutaneous tunnel. *B,* Quinton dialysis catheter in the right internal jugular vein, often used until dialysis fistula is ready for use.

cally, they are superior to external tunneled catheters, require less maintenance, and afford patients greater freedom of movement and activities like swimming or bathing.

TIVADs may be inserted on an outpatient basis under local anesthesia using a subcutaneous tunnel or an open cutdown. The cutdown technique offers potential speed (mean placement time, 15 min), safety (negligible risk for pneumothorax), and low cost, with avoidance of early and late complications.[18] Placement is typically in the nondominant arm with the portal in the upper arm or chest unless there is vein occlusion or planned radiation therapy on the contralateral side.

Disadvantages of this type of device include increased cost, time-consuming insertion, the need for a specific noncoring Huber access needle, and small gauge (20–22) of the access needle, which limits fluid infusion rates and venisection.[17]

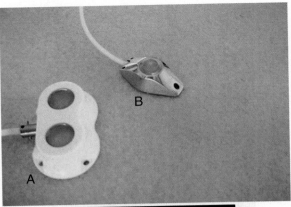

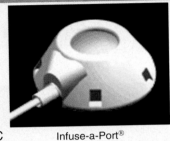

C   Infuse-a-Port®

Figure 24–3 *A,* Port-a-Cath double-lumen port (for chest placement). *B,* Port-A-Cath single-lumen port (for upper extremity placement). The Port-A-Cath system is accessed by inserting a Huber needle through the skin portal septum. *C,* Infuse-A-Port is similar to the Port-A-Cath.

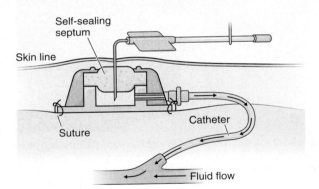

A

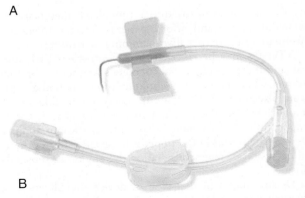

B

Figure 24–4 *A,* Porta-A-Cath system (Deltec, Inc., St. Paul, MN), This device is subcutaneous and accessed with a Huber needle introduced through the skin, into the portal septum. *B,* The Huber needle is used to access the septum, always with sterile technique.

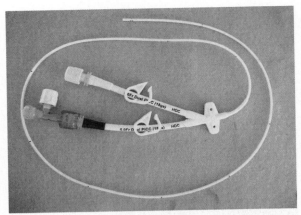

Figure 24–5 Double-lumen percutaneously inserted central catheter (PICC; 5.0-Fr, 18 gauge), is placed in the arm with the tip of the catheter in the superior vena cava. Shorter 20-cm versions (not shown) look similar, but terminate in the axillary vein, termed a midline peripheral catheter.

PICCs (Nontunneled, Noncuffed)

PICC lines are centrally placed lines that were first described in the 1970s, originally developed for the neonatal population. Subsequently, their use expanded into the adult arena and currently is used for prolonged antibiotic therapy, IV fluids, chemotherapy, TPN, and delivery of medications that are irritating to the peripheral vessels. PICCs (Fig. 24–5) are made of two substances, either polyurethane (Intracath) or silicone (Intrasil), and are radiopaque, measuring 50 to 60 cm in length with an outside diameter of 2 to 7 French. The catheter may be single- or double-lumen configuration and can be open- or close-ended or valved (e.g., Groshong). An open-ended PICC cannot prevent feedback of blood into the catheter and therefore must be flushed one or more times daily with heparinized saline. The Groshong three-way valve reduces blood backup into the catheter and therefore requires flushing as little as once a week. The most common type of PICC line in use today is the 5-French, double-lumen, closed-ended catheter.

The device selected should be based on the number of lumens necessary for therapy, recognizing that the potential for infection increases with lumen number. An access site is chosen based on many factors including the suitability of target vessels, the patient's body habitus, handedness, ability to manage self-care, comorbid conditions, the desired infusion rate, the number and compatibility of concurrent infusions, the infusate characteristics, and the estimated duration of therapy. Infusate that is hyperosmolar (TPN) or vesicant requires rapid dilution. As such, the tip must be in the SVC, where the estimated flow is 2000 mL/min. PICC lines are most frequently placed in the superficial veins proximal to the antecubital fossa (usually the basilic or the cephalic) (Fig. 24–6). However, they may also be placed by a transhepatic or translumbar approach when the SVC is thrombosed or occluded.[19]

PICC line advantages include usefulness in a wide variety of clinical situations, ease of placement, and ease of use and maintenance. They do not require surgical placement and may be placed in an outpatient setting. The PICC line is excellent vehicle for medium- to long-term IV therapy. With proper care, PICCs can remain in place for long periods, even months to years.[20]

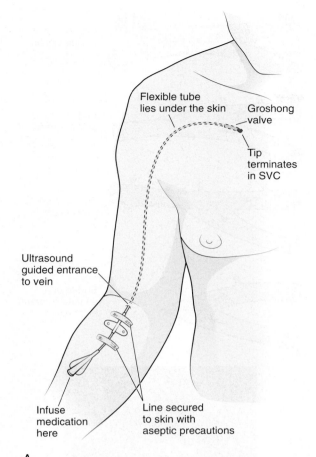

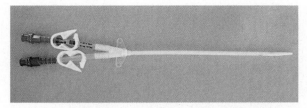

Figure 24–7 Mahurkar 11.5-Fr. × 16-cm Double-Lumen Catheter for hemodialysis, apheresis, and infusion.

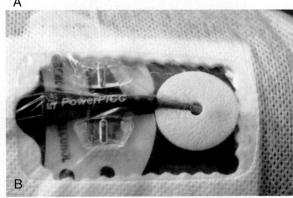

Figure 24–6 *A,* PICC line placement in the upper extremity with internal catheter tip at the superior vena cava. *B,* Most PICC lines are used for outpatient therapy, such as prolonged antibiotic therapy, so proper aseptic technique at the catheter site is essential.

Midline Peripheral Catheters

Midline catheters are often confused with PICC lines. They are also placed peripherally in the superficial veins of the antecubital fossa or upper forearm. They differ from PICCs in that these are peripheral, not central, catheters. Midlines are typically shorter (20 cm), with the tip terminating near the axillary vein. Placement above the axillary vein results in a higher risk of thrombosis and is contraindicated. They are designed for short- to medium-term use, lasting longer than a PICC. Because it does not enter the central circulation with high flow, the delivery of medication and infusion types are limited, and routine blood withdrawal is not recommended.

Differentiating between these two catheters in situ may be difficult because the outward appearance is similar. Obtaining an x-ray film for visualization of tip placement will help to determine catheter type.

HD VADs

Vascular access, which is often referred to as the Achilles heel of the renal patient, remains problematic. From the moment that the first access is created, an ongoing process is started that will end with the loss of all access possiblities if the patient survives long enough.[21] Clinical practice guidelines of the National Kidney Foundation—Disease Outcomes Quality Initiative (NKF-DOQI) recommend early AV fistula construction and avoidance of catheters for permanent or prolonged vascular access,[22] with less than 10% of permanent access in the form of catheters.[23] However, one study demonstrated that more than half of the patients began dialysis using a central catheter because a well-developed AV fistula was not available.[24] The risk of requiring three or more vascular accesses is almost double among patients who start HD using a central catheter.

Temporary Dialysis Catheters (Quinton, Mahurkar, Tessio, Vascath)

Temporary vascular access catheters (Fig. 24–7) are used for dialysis if a more permanent dialysis route (AV fistula/graft) is not available. These large-bore catheters allow for the necessary blood flow rate of 300 mL/min for dialysis. The *Quinton* catheter has two ports, one to deliver the patient's blood to the dialysis machine and another to return the blood to the patient's circulation (see Fig. 24–2B). These catheters are placed into a central vein, either internal jugular, subclavian, or femoral. The right internal jugular approach is the preferred site, even if permanent access is to be created on the right side, because it has the lowest thrombosis rate. The K/DOQI[14] recommends avoiding the subclavian vein unless no other options exist or the ipsilateral arm has no more permanent access sites. For patient comfort, a special 180° catheter can be used (Fig. 24–8). There are two avenues to place this catheter: percutaneously or surgically. Emergent percutaneous placement can be performed by the emergency clinician at the bedside. Using sterile technique and after a local anesthetic injection, place the catheter following the same procedure for placing a central line into one of the central veins.

The second technique uses a slightly larger catheter (Quinton/Hickman) and is performed in the operating room under local anesthesia with or without general sedation. This catheter is placed in much the same fashion as the tunneled

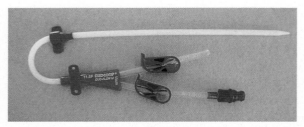

Figure 24–8 MedComp Duo-Flow Internal Jugular Vascular Catheter (11.5 Fr × 15 cm). The angle of the catheter makes it more comfortable for the patient.

RA catheters described previously. Surgically implanted catheters are preferred if more than temporary use is anticipated because they have a decreased infection risk and longer usage time.

AV Fistulas

An AV fistula is a *direct subcutaneous anastomosis of an artery and vein without prosthetic material*, and is the preferred means of vascular access for HD (Fig. 24–9). Numerous AV fistula locations are possible. However, the most recent data from the Dialysis Outcomes and Practice Patterns Study (DOPPS),[25] a prospective, observational study of HD patients across 12 countries, show a dismal prevalence rate of AV fistulas. The DOPPS study suggests that although the United States should have a fistula prevalence rate of 75%, the rate is actually 30% for native AV fistulas, 42% for grafts, and 28% catheters for dialysis patients in the United States.[15] The use of an autogenous fistula is associated with the longest period of graft patency and with relative freedom from thrombotic and infectious complications. Once a fistula matures, long-term patency is high (85% at 1 yr and 75% at 2 yr) with low infection rates compared with grafts.[26]

An autogenous AV fistula is constructed by anastomosing an artery to a vein (see Fig. 24–9), preferably a nearby one. The radial-cephalic (*Brescia-Cimino forearm*) fistula is the most frequently used (Fig. 24–10), with the brachial-cephalic and the proximal thigh being alternatives. Over time, the venous portion of the shunt is subjected to high pressure and flow becomes arterialized (hypertrophied and dilated), rendering it suitable for repeated vascular access. Full epithelialization of the shunt does not occur for 3 to 6 months.

AV Grafts

If a forearm Brescia-Cimino fistula cannot be constructed or has failed, an AV bridge graft using a donor vein or synthetic material is a well-accepted alternative. Several synthetic materials are used for grafts. Polytetrafluoroethylene (PTFE) is the most commonly used but takes 3 weeks to mature. A recently available polyurethane graft (Vectra) has the ability to be accessed within 24 hours. A standard graft is 6 to 8 mm in diameter and usually positioned in a U-shaped subcutaneous tunnel in the forearm. The graft is attached by end-to-side anastomoses to the brachial artery and antecubital vein. If no suitable antecubital vein is available, a straight bridge graft between the brachial artery and either the axillary or the basilic vein is often used. Multiple configurations are possible (Fig. 24–11). A jump graft between opposite extremities with creation of a loop across the chest or axillary artery to the iliac vein is a possibility when all other sites have been exhausted.

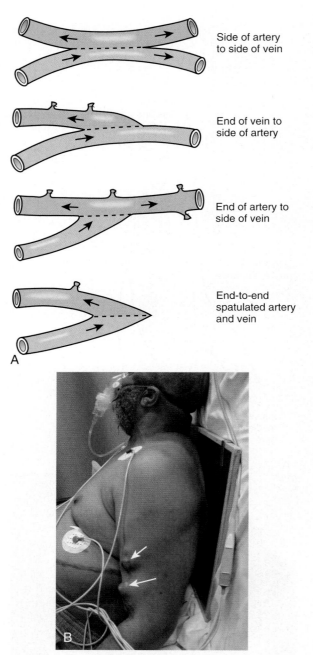

Figure 24–9 *A,* Various possible anastomotic configurations between artery and vein for autogenous fistula formation. A thrill should be palpated if this fistula is functioning. *B,* Older dialysis fistula. As demonstrated here, fistulas can develop multiple aneurysms (*arrows*) from multiple time use. Shunts made of synthetic material can develop pseudoaneurysms. *It may be difficult to distinguish a fistula from a graft by merely looking at the site.* (*A,* Adapted from Ozeran RS: *Construction and care of external arteriovenous shunts.* In Wilson SE, Owens ML [eds]: *Vascular Access Surgery.* Chicago, Year Book Medical, 1980.)

Compared with AV fistulas, AV grafts have a significantly higher incidence of thrombosis, infection, pseudoaneurysm formation, and limb loss. PTFE grafts have a low graft primary patency rate (50% at 1 yr and 25% at 2 yr).[26] However, they have a low incidence of aneurysm formation and are comparatively easy to revise. The estimated life span of a PTFE graft in clinical practice is often less than 2 years.[24]

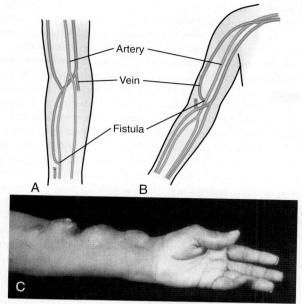

Figure 24–10 Arteriovenous fistula. *A,* Brescia-Cimino (radial-cephalic) fistula performed at the level of the wrist. *B,* Brachial-cephalic fistula performed proximal to the antecubital fossa. *C,* Multiple asymptomatic *pseudoaneurysms* resulting several years after creation of an autogenous wrist (Brescia-Cimino) arteriovenous fistula. *(B, Adapted from Rutherford RB [ed]: Vascular Surgery, 5th ed. Philadelphia, WB Saunders, 2001.)*

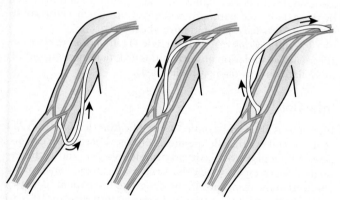

Figure 24–11 Three possible graft configurations for jump grafts in which standard sites have been used. *(Redrawn from Tilney NL, Lazarus JM [eds]: Surgical Care of the Patient with Renal Failure. Philadelphia, WB Saunders, 1982; as shown in Haisch CE: Chronic vascular and peritoneal access. In Davis JH, Sheldon GF [eds]: Clinical Surgery. St Louis, CV Mosby, 1995.)*

ACCESSING VADS IN THE EMERGENCY DEPARTMENT

When IV access is required in patients with VADs, standard methods of peripheral access should be attempted first in order to preserve the life span of the VAD and avoid complications. However, VADs, AV fistulas, and shunts may be accessed in emergency situations for phlebotomy and infusion of medications and fluids. Because of complications of infection and catheter malfunction, dislodgment and fracture, only personnel with the requisite knowledge and skill should access VADs when feasible. When VADs are accessed, antisepsis should be ensured.

The emergent need to administer parenteral medications to patients lacking other means of vascular access is the most common reason to access a VAD in the emergency department (ED). Assuming that proper access methods are used to prevent infection, the greatest risk is sludging in the catheter with resultant occlusion. *Medications should be followed by a saline flush to clear the catheter and ensure that the medication reaches the circulation.* Medications that are known to be incompatible when mixed (e.g., calcium and bicarbonate) should not be administered concurrently, even through separate ports of multilumen catheters. Blood specimens including cultures can also be obtained via VADs. Phlebotomy requires stopping infusions, appropriate catheter antisepsis, removing fluid occupying dead space in the catheter, and following the blood draw with a flush of heparinized saline.

Accessing Long-Term Venous Access Catheters[27]

The catheter (with the exception of Groshong catheters that have backflow valve protection) is first clamped to prevent air embolism. Patients usually carry their own clamps; however, a hemostat without teeth or use of sterile tape or tubing wrapped around the teeth of a hemostat will suffice in an emergency. The catheter cap is removed, and a 10-mL syringe of single-dose vial sterile water or normal saline is attached. Smaller syringes generate greater amounts of pressure for infusion, which can lead to increased intraluminal pressure and catheter rupture. Three to 5 mL of solution is injected and then withdrawn to ensure patency. More pronounced infusion might be necessary to ensure patency of Groshong catheters.

Phlebotomy is accomplished by withdrawing dead space solution, reclamping, and using a separate syringe to remove the desired amount of blood.[28] If clots are withdrawn, continue withdrawing blood until it is clot free. Bolus medications are then injected and IV solutions infused through the catheter, which is clamped whenever unattached. A 5-mL normal saline flush should be delivered between medications. On completion of either blood withdraw or medication infusion, inject 3 to 4 mL of saline to flush, then 3 to 5 mL of heparin (1000 U/mL) is injected, the line is clamped, and the cap is repositioned.[28] *Note that 1000 U/mL of heparin is used; less concentrated solutions may promote clotting.* Do not inject large amounts because it can systemically heparinize the patient. Groshong catheters need not be flushed with heparin but instead may be flushed briskly with 5 to 10 mL of saline. Multilumen central catheters have one port for each lumen and are accessed in the same manner. After antiseptic preparation is completed, access is gained by either inserting a needle or a syringe into the protective cap or removing the cap entirely. A 5-mL normal saline or sterile water flush and verification of backflow precede all subsequent procedures. Phlebotomy is performed through the proximal lumen to prevent mixture with medications being delivered through the other ports. IV infusions are delivered in similar fashion, and a normal saline flush is injected between medications. The procedure is terminated with a 3- to 5-mL heparin (1000 U/mL) flush.

Accessing TIVADS

The procedure for accessing TIVADs is unique because these devices are not external. Instead, a circular reservoir (cylinder) lies subcutaneously on the anterior chest wall. First, palpate the cylinder and then prepare the overlying skin with povidone-iodine solution. Fill a 10-mL syringe with normal saline and attach it to connecting tubing. Attach it to a 19- to 22-gauge, 90° tapered (Huber) needle. The Huber needle is a specialized needle designed for use with the TIVAD to prevent damage to the portal septum. It has a 90° bend with a slightly curved tip, opening on the side rather than on the end. Most importantly, the Huber is a noncoring needle. This avoids damage to the Silastic septum, allowing up to 2000 punctures. Do not access the TIVAD with a standard 19-gauge needle unless a code is in progress and the Huber needle is not immediately available. Apply a clamp to the connecting tubing whenever the system is open. Expel the air and insert the Huber needle through the reservoir septum. Insert the needle slowly and steadily through the diaphragm until it contacts the back of the reservoir. Be aware that although incomplete perforation of the septum will block flow, substantial pressure may also damage the back of the device and bend the needle tip. Remove the clamp slowly, and inject 5 mL of solution to ensure patency. If patency is not easily demonstrated, alteplase (recombinant tissue plasminogen activator) may be considered as a thrombolytic for catheter occlusion.[29]

Once the solution has been injected, apply gentle negative pressure to demonstrate the backflow of blood. Stabilize the Huber needle by building a 4- x 4-inch gauze pad about the needle and further reinforce it with 2.54-cm (1-inch) silk tape. First remove 8 to 9 mL of blood with a separate syringe and waste it, then perform phlebotomy through the extension tubing. If necessary, deliver IV solutions through extension tubing but realize that the rate of flow will be limited by the radius of the Huber needle. Deliver a 5-mL normal saline flush between medications. Complete the procedure with a 3- to 5-mL heparin (1000 U/mL)[28] flush and remove the Huber needle.

Accessing AV Fistulas, Shunts, and HD Catheters

AV fistulas, shunts, and Uldall and Mahurkar catheters are placed in patients who require HD and they represent the sole access for that purpose. Consequently, routine use of these sites for phlebotomy and fluid administration is strongly discouraged. In fact, *venipuncture in the same extremity as a patent AV fistula is not recommended*, except for the veins in the dorsum of the ipsilateral hand. When standard IV access cannot be obtained under emergency circumstances, however, fistulas, shunts, and catheters may all be used to administer IV solutions and medications. If possible, ascertain fistula patency by noting a bruit and palpable thrill, although these signs may not be appreciable if the patient is in extremis.

Prepare the area overlying the fistula with antiseptic solution and access the fistula with the smallest-gauge needle that is appropriate.[30] Puncture 1 to 2 cm from the anastomosis end nearest the venous side, and avoid aneurysmal sites.[30] Access AV shunts similarly by placing the smallest needle possible into the catheter, bridging arterial and venous circulations. Apply local pressure for at least 5 minutes after the procedure is completed and monitor subsequently for hemorrhage. Access Uldall and Mahurkar catheters in much the same way that multilumen central catheters are accessed. Remove or inject into the retaining cap on each arm. *Up to 5000 U of heparin is present within the two lumen*, and so it is imperative to aspirate before administering fluid or medications. After use, flush each catheter arm with 10 mL of normal saline and instill 1.5 mL of heparin solution (1000 U/mL) into each one.

COMPLICATIONS OF VADS

VADs are now sufficiently commonplace that patients with these devices will present to the ED on a regular basis. Given a complication rate of 4% to 10%,[31] it is essential that emergency clinicians are aware of these complications and their management. Fifty-two percent of reported complications are associated with health care practitioner technique; 12% are associated with device failure; 6% are related to actions taken by the patient and pathophysiologic events (such as thrombosis); and 30% have an unidentified cause.[32]

Complications of VADs include (1) infection, (2) hemorrhage and coagulation abnormalities, (3) malfunction, and (4) miscellaneous problems (Table 24–1).

Infection

Infection is the most common complication leading to VAD removal and potentially the most serious. Three main categories of infection exist: exit site, tunnel/pocket, and catheter-related bacteremia. Once the organisms spread beyond the confines of the device itself, the danger to the patient increases significantly, with an estimated case fatality rate of 10% to 20%.[24] Infectious complications include endocarditis, septic arthritis, pulmonary emboli, osteomyelitis, and spinal epidural abscess. The definitions of VAD-related infections are not uniform, making it difficult to compare results of various investigations. However, it is generally agreed that risk factors

TABLE 24–1 Complications of Indwelling Vascular Access Devices

Infection	Hemorrhage/Coagulation	Malfunction	Miscellaneous
Skin/exit site	Bleeding	Occlusion	Embolism
Reservoir/pocket	Local puncture site	Medication delivery failure	Air
Tunnel	Arterial bleeding	Precipitants	Thrombus
Catheter tip/lumen	Overheparinization	Thrombosis	Catheter fragment
Sepsis	Heparin rebound	Failure to infuse/withdraw	Arrhythmias
	Thrombosis	Pinch-off syndrome	Cutaneous Dacron cuff erosion
	Phlebitis	Steal syndrome	Catheter dislodgment
	Deep venous thrombosis	Malposition	Hyperdynamic cardiac failure
	Fibrin sheath	False aneurysms	

TABLE 24–2 Microorganisms Causing Indwelling Catheter Infection

Bacterial

Gram-Positive Cocci

Staphylococcus aureus, Staphylococcus epidermidis, Streptococcus faecalis, Streptococcus bovis, group C streptococci, and Streptococcus viridans

Gram-Negative Bacilli

Pseudomonas aeruginosa, Klebsiella spp., Acinetobacter spp., Serratia spp.

Gram-Positive Bacilli

Bacillus cereus, Bacillus laterosporus, Corynebacterium spp.

Atypical

Mycobacterium neoaurum, Mycobacterium fortuitum, Mycobacterium chelonae

Mycotic

Malassezia furfur, Malassezia pachydermatis, Aspergillus fumigatus, Aspergillus flavus, Candida albicans

---

for infection include site of insertion, hospital size, duration of catheter placement, type of catheter, and patient factors. Most studies show a lower incidence of infection for TIVADs than for external systems, presumably owing to lack of direct access of cutaneous organisms. The rates of VAD infection tend to be highest in the first 3 months after insertion, with skin flora being most common.[31,33] The rate of infection decreases significantly, reaching a plateau after 5 to 6 months.[33] The most common infecting organisms are listed in Table 24–2.

Clinical findings are unreliable in the diagnosis of infection secondary to VADs. Fever, rigors, and elevated white blood cell count may be sensitive but not specific, whereas purulent drainage at the insertion site may be specific but not sensitive. Therefore, evaluation beyond physical examination alone is essential when infection is suspected, including site purulence Gram stain, blood cultures, and catheter segment culture. In addition, transesophageal echocardiography is indicated if valvular vegetations are suspected by blood cultures that are positive for *Staphylococcus aureus*, persistent bacteremia or fungemia after catheter removal, or lack of clinical improvement.

Draw two sets of blood cultures with one set through the catheter itself and one from a peripheral site. Positive blood cultures for *S. aureus*, coagulase-negative staphylococci, or *Candida* species, in the appropriate patient setting and in the absence of another identifiable source of infection, should increase the suspicion for catheter-related bloodstream infection.[31] In most studies, blood obtained from a VAD yielding a colony count at least 5- to 10-fold greater than that for blood obtained from a peripheral site suggests a catheter-related source of infection.[34] Similarly, catheter infection should be assumed if the peripherally derived blood cultures are negative and the VAD-derived cultures are positive.[33] Not only is blood drawn from the catheter more likely to yield a positive culture, this may also occur earlier in the course of

infection. One study demonstrated that 16 of 17 patients with VAD-related infections had positive blood culture results at least 2 hours earlier from the VAD than from the peripheral blood cultures.[35]

Infusate-related bloodstream infection is uncommon and defined as the isolation of the same organism from both infusate and separate percutaneous blood cultures, with no other source of infection. When this diagnosis is suggested, cultures of the infusate should be obtained in addition to catheter and peripheral cultures.[31]

Although it had been common practice to immediately remove a VAD in the setting of acute infection, the need for removal has been called into question.[33] Remove the VAD and culture it if the patient is immunocompromised or severely ill (e.g., sepsis, shock). Remove it in a patient with sepsis and with no other source of infection. If blood cultures are positive, or if the VAD is changed over a guidewire and has significant colonization, remove and culture the catheter and place a new catheter at a new site. Without evidence of persistent bloodstream infection, or if the infecting organism is coagulase-negative *Staphylococcus* and there is no suspicion of local or metastatic complications, the VAD may be left in place.[31]

If a VAD is removed, culture it to determine the offending organism. Place the catheter in a sterile tube (red top) and send it to the laboratory for culturing. The most widely used laboratory technique for the clinical diagnosis of catheter-related infection is the semiquantitative method, in which the catheter segment is rolled across the surface of an agar plate and colony-forming units (CFUs) are counted after overnight incubation. Quantitative culture of the catheter segment requires either flushing the segment with broth or vortexing in broth, followed by serial dilutions and surface plating on blood agar. A yield of 15 CFUs or more from a catheter by semiquantitative culture, or a yield of 10^2 or more from a catheter by quantitative culture, with accompanying signs of local or systemic infection, is indicative of a catheter-related infection.[31]

HD catheters deserve special consideration. The process of HD requires several connections to the graft, thereby increasing the risk of infection. The rate of bacteremia in HD patients attributed to the graft varies from 48% to 73%. The incidence is highest when central venous dialysis catheters are used. Native AV fistulas carry the lowest risk of infection. Unfortunately, AV grafts are more commonly used in the United States.[36] As with other VAD, initiate empirical antibiotic therapy based on epidemiologic and patient factors, followed by narrowed spectrum therapy after isolation and determination of sensitivities. The most common infecting organism is *S. aureus*. There has been an association between nasal carriage of *S. aureus* in HD patients and catheter infection. Reducing carriage rates has resulted in a decreased incidence of bloodstream infections.[31]

Antimicrobial Therapy

Pending culture results, the initial choice of an antibiotic is empirical and depends on the clinical setting, site of infection, type of device, host factors (e.g., immunocompromised state), severity of illness, and whether or not the device has been removed. There are not compelling data to support either the choice of a specific empirical antibiotic or the duration of therapy for device-related infections.[31] If coagulase-negative *Staphylococcus* is the suspected organism, initiate vancomycin empirically, followed by a semisynthetic penicillin or other appropriate antibiotics as guided by sensitivity studies. When *S. aureus* is the suspected organism, give β-lactam antibiotics (e.g., penicillins, cephalosporins, carbapenems, and monobactams) for first-line therapy. In penicillin-allergic patients or those with methicillin-resistant *S. aureus* (MRSA), vancomycin is the drug of choice. In areas with significant rates of MRSA, which is becoming increasingly common, start with vancomycin followed by a semisynthetic penicillin. In the absence of significant rates of MRSA, use penicillinase-resistant penicillins, such as nafcillin or oxacillin. Provide additional coverage in immunocompromised or severely debilitated patients. Include coverage for enteric organisms as well as *Pseudomonas aeruginosa*, with a third- or fourth-generation cephalosporin (e.g., cefoperazone, ceftazidime, cefepime) or an aminoglycoside. With infections involving gram-negative bacilli, institute quinolones with or without rifampin for 14 days. If fungemia is suspected or confirmed, initiate an antifungal medication and remove the catheter. Initiate parenteral amphotericin B for patients who are hemodynamically unstable or who have received prolonged fluconazole. Initiate fluconazole when patients are hemodynamically stable, have not had recent therapy with fluconazole, or have a fluconazole-susceptible organism. Continue therapy for 14 days after the last positive blood culture and evidence of clinical improvement.[31,33,36–38]

Recommendations vary regarding exit site or tunnel or pocket infections.[31,33] Jones[33] recommended using aggressive local care in the early stages and a topical antibiotic ointment for short-term treatment. Long-term treatment should be avoided owing to the risk of *Candida* colonization.[33] Mermel and colleagues,[31] however, recommended that in patients with complicated infections, such as tunnel infection or port abscess, remove the catheter and initiate antibiotics for 7 to 10 days. Data are insufficient to make strong recommendations regarding a strict duration of antibiotic treatment; however, there are ranges of therapy that are generally agreed upon.[31,33,37] In patients who are not immunocompromised and in whom there is no evidence of complication (e.g., endocarditis, septic thrombosis/emboli, osteomyelitis), administer antibiotics for 5 to 7 days if the catheter is removed and for 10 to 14 days if the VAD is retained. After removing the catheter, treat patients with persistent bacteremia or fungemia for 4 to 6 weeks. Treat those who develop complications for 6 to 8 weeks.[31]

If the VAD is retained, consider antibiotic lock therapy (ALT). ALT is a promising area of research in VAD-related infections. Most infections in tunneled catheters originate in the hub and spread to the catheter lumen. This, combined with the deposition of fibrin, makes eradication of organisms difficult. ALT involves filling the catheter hub and lumen with a higher concentration of antibiotics and leaving them in place for extended periods of time. Studies have suggested that ALT alone may be as effective as parenteral antibiotics followed by ALT. The duration of ALT is most often 2 weeks.[31] Some recommend the use of prophylactic vancomycin lock solutions as a beneficial and cost-effective method of preventing infection in long-term tunneled and cuffed VADs.[39]

Prophylactic Measures
Antibiotic Prophylaxis during Initial Line Insertion.
Prophylaxis with vancomycin or teicoplanin during central line insertion has not consistently demonstrated reduced incidence of catheter-related bloodstream infection. Based on the limited available data, the Centers for Disease Control and Prevention (CDC) guidelines currently recommend against giving vancomycin prophylactically. This is because it is an independent risk factor for the acquisition of vancomycin-resistant enterococcus (VRE)[39] and staphylococci with reduced susceptibility to glycopeptides. Rather than using antibiotic prophylaxis, focus efforts on interventions designed to discourage the emergence of antimicrobial resistance, such as maximal barrier precautions.[40]

Impregnated Catheters.
Using antimicrobial or antiseptic-impregnated catheters or silver-impregnated collagen cuffs may be an effective intervention to reduce VAD-related bloodstream infection. Hanley and associates[41] reported beneficial results with triple-lumen catheters in an intensive care setting. These findings may be applicable to long-term tunneled or nontunneled catheters, as well as AV fistulas; but further studies are necessary. Nonetheless, the Hospital Infection Control Practices Advisory Committee of the CDC has made use of these devices a category II recommendation.[41]

Routine Line Changing.
Despite the incidence of infection and the potential complications, routine changing of VADs is not recommended. Cobb and coworkers[42] found that replacement of VADs every 3 days did not prevent infection, and in fact, doing so over a guidewire increased the risk of bloodstream infection.

Thrombus Formation

It has been estimated that from 2% to 42% of VADs are associated with deep venous thrombosis (DVT).[43] Risk factors for catheter-related DVT include the composition, diameter, and position of the VAD; elevated intraluminal pressure; turbulent blood flow; vascular calcification; endothelial injury; and increased levels of fibronectin.[43,44] Polyurethane and silicone catheters have a lower rate of VAD-related DVT than polyethylene or Teflon-coated catheters. An external diameter less than 2.8 mm has a lower incidence of DVT. Incorrect placement of the VAD in the SVC, as opposed to the junction of the SVC and the right atrium, results in a higher incidence of catheter-related DVT.[43]

DVTs may be asymptomatic and not recognized owing to the underlying condition of the patient. Luciani and colleagues[43] found that upper extremity DVT was relatively common, occurring in 11.7% of their patient population, of which the vast majority were asymptomatic (76%). They recommend routine Doppler screening for at least the first 3 months after catheter placement. Pulmonary embolism can occur with the catheter in place or days to weeks after removal.[45]

Most HD access failure (80%) is related to thrombosis, with greater than 90% of these thromboses associated with venous outflow stenosis.[15] Histologically, hyperplasia of the endothelium and fibromuscular vessel wall occurs. Over time, fibrin deposits build up on the tip of the VAD. This may continue to the point of complete occlusion, preventing infusion or aspiration from the VAD. Early detection may be enhanced by maintaining a high index of suspicion, noting prolonged bleeding after cannula withdrawal or a change in the bruit over the device, or both. Prompt consultation with a nephrologist and vascular surgeon is indicated. Systemic heparin or local thrombolytic agents, such as urokinase (both in bolus fashion and in continuous infusion), may be tried (see "Catheter Occlusion," later).

Catheter Occlusion

Catheter occlusion or low flow can be caused by improper positioning, kinking, compression of the catheter, intraluminal thrombi, extraluminal thrombi, fibrin deposits at the catheter tip, or intraluminal precipitation of infusate. *Pinch-off syndrome* occurs when the line (most often a PICC) is compressed between the clavicle and the first rib. It is manifested clinically as difficulty injecting that is posturally related.[17] Overzealous withdrawal of the syringe will collapse the catheter and cause occlusion. Chest x-ray may reveal scalloping of the catheter. Maneuvers to facilitate flow include the Valsalva maneuver, the reverse Trendelenburg position, slight tension on the catheter, placement of the catheter more laterally, IV hydration, and extension of the arms above the head.[28,46]

If these measures are unsuccessful, the occlusion may be caused by clot formation. The clinician should be familiar with local institutional recommendations for thrombolysis in the setting of recent VAD occlusion attributed to a fibrin plug. Admission and consultation are usually required. Instill 3 to 5 mL of heparin followed several minutes later by gentle aspiration; this is often successful in dislodging the clot. Atkinson and associates[47] reported good response with urokinase and follow-up tissue plasminogen activator (t-PA) when urokinase failed. For the initial treatment, instill 2 to 3 mL of urokinase (5000 U/mL) into the catheter and then aspirate 10 minutes later. If the catheter remains occluded, instill 2 mL of t-PA (1 mg/mL). Repeat the t-PA once if needed. In another protocol, instill 5000 U of urokinase and leave it to dwell for 1 hour. If unsuccessful in dislodging the clot, follow this with a 4-hour infusion with 60,000 U urokinase.

Embolization

A serious but uncommon complication of VAD use is embolization with air, catheter fragment, or thrombotic emboli.[48–50] Air emboli develop when the catheter lumen is left open to air or the catheter is fractured, perforated, or cut. The one-way valve in the Groshong catheter prevents this. Be careful to maintain a closed system by clamping the catheter appropriately to prevent air delivery into the venous circulation. Should the externalized portion of a catheter be damaged, immediately place an appropriate clamp between the damaged portion and the skin.[28] Be suspicious of air embolism if an open or damaged catheter is found in association with tachypnea and hypotension.[51] Place the patient in a left lateral decubitus and Trendelenburg position to reduce ventricular outflow obstruction by air pockets. Initiate supportive measures including high-flow oxygen.

Embolization of a catheter fragment is a potentially life-threatening complication causing acute dyspnea, palpitations, atypical chest pain, hypoxia, and atrial fibrillation. As with any embolus, sequelae include sepsis, lung abscess, dysrhythmias, vascular or cardiac perforation, and sudden death.[49] Catheter fragments may be identified radiographically or potentially by transesophageal echocardiography[52] and may be removed either surgically or using intravascular retrieval methods.

Embolization of thrombi with potential lethal sequelae may occur during routine flushing and injection of solutions through the catheter. Anderson and coworkers[53] prospectively evaluated the size and frequency of catheter thrombi in 43 patients by aspirating after a urokinase flush. Clots were noted in 40 of 43 subjects and 153 of 508 total specimens. Thrombi varied in size from small fragments to 5 cm in length. Zureikat

and colleagues[45] reported one case of pulmonary embolus associated with Broviac catheterization in a 2-month-old child.

Hemorrhagic Complications

Bleeding may be seen with any indwelling VAD or AV fistula, but is more commonly seen with nontunneled VADs or temporary dialysis catheters. It is often related to mechanical trauma, transient or preexisting thrombocytopenia, heparin rebound,[54] uremia- or drug-induced platelet dysfunction, and infection. Repeated cannulation of the fistula/graft weakens the wall of the device. Many fistulas will develop aneurysms from repeated use; synthetic grafts can develop pseudoaneurysms from frequent punctures. *Severe life-threatening hemorrhage from this high-pressure system may occur, necessitating rapid control.* The primary goal should be to control bleeding and prevent exsanguination; however, take care to minimize damage to the VAD that would prevent future use. Use full universal precautions because there is an increased risk of communicable disease (hepatitis B virus 2.4%, hepatitis C virus 7.4% in the United States) in this patient population.[55] When bleeding stops, observe the patient for 2 hours for evidence of rebleeding and to detect graft thrombosis. Treatment modalities can be divided into mechanical and correction of coagulopathy.

Mechanical

Literature addressing acute hemorrhage in the VAD patient is clearly lacking. Many of the techniques discussed are anecdotal examples used by emergency clinicians, nephrologists, and vascular surgeons informally polled at our institutions. Individual institutional guidelines, techniques, and preferences may vary; therefore, consultation with these providers is recommended when possible.

Direct Pressure. Begin management of bleeding with direct pressure. Using gloved hands, apply direct pressure with fingers and a sterile gauze bandage. For bleeding AV fistulas and shunts secondary to cannulation, apply pressure over the site of cannulation. For tunneled catheters, apply pressure over the site of vascular entry of the catheter, not the subcutaneous exit site. Note that this is not possible with subclavian VADs. Hold pressure for a minimum of 5 minutes, and then reevaluate for hemostasis. Holding direct pressure for extended periods of time or holding more diffuse pressure may cause thrombus and ultimate graft failure, which is a known and unfortunate risk. Wrapping the site with an elastic bandage for a few minutes is acceptable, but longer application in this broad manner may lead to the entire graft clotting.

Dialysis Clamps. Special self-retaining dialysis clamps may be applied over a specific bleeding site (Fig. 24–12). Be careful that the clamp does not slip off the bleeding site because the surface area of the clamp is small. Sterile gauze or *topical thrombin-impregnated gauze* is placed under the clamp. It may require 10 to 15 minutes to stop bleeding, but it is best to avoid frequent checks during the first 5 to 8 minutes to avoid disrupting hemostasis.

Suture. To adequately visualize the bleeding site (1) apply concomitant digital pressure to the proximal and distal ends of the shunt/fistula, (2) apply a pneumatic blood pressure cuff or tourniquet distal to the fistula/graft to impede the distal to proximal arterial flow, unless it is a loop graft in which case, it is applied above the device. Place a horizontal

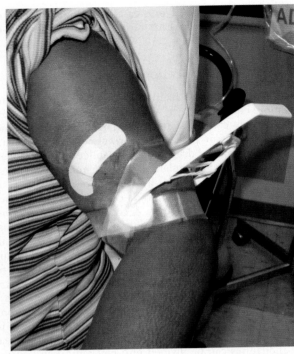

Figure 24–12 Bleeding from a dialysis graft/fistula can be massive owing to the high pressures. This dialysis graft clamp with sterile gauze (option: impregnate gauze with topical thrombin) is kept in place for about 10 minutes. Other options for a bleeding graft are discussed in the text.

mattress suture or a figure-of-eight suture using 4-0 nonabsorbable polypropylene or nylon suture at the site of bleeding. Be careful to suture as superficially as possible to prevent damage to the underlying graft or fistula. The patient may require a venogram for patency evaluation of the VAD prior to use.

Thrombogenic Agents. If major bleeding has been controlled and is minimal, oxidized cellulose hemostatic agents (Oxycell, Surgicel) may be used to achieve hemostasis. Apply these agents directly over the site of bleeding and hold them in place with gloved hands and a gauze bandage or a clamp. The disadvantage of this approach is that the agents are costly and a potential nidus for infection.

Vasoconstrictive Agents. Lidocaine (2%) with epinephrine injected subcutaneously to form a wheel using 2 to 4 mL around the site may decrease bleeding due to both vasoconstriction and local pressure. This may be used in conjunction with chemical cautery.

Chemical Cautery. Silver nitrate ($AgNO_3$), a mildly caustic and hemostatic agent, may stop residual bleeding. The agent needs to be protected from light until just before use. When ready, remove the wooden stick from the container and black plastic wrap and gently apply the gray-tipped end directly on the site. Do not apply it aggressively because this can result in dissolution or dislodgment of the formed clot.

Once bleeding is controlled, rebleeding is infrequent. It is prudent to observe the patient for 30 to 45 minutes, have her or him walk around and use the arm gently, to ensure that bleeding will not recur when discharged. If no bleeding recurs, discharge is appropriate unless other conditions preclude it.

Coagulopathy

Hemorrhage control may require treatment of an underlying coagulopathy. Perform laboratory testing to evaluate: complete blood counts (CBC), blood urea nitrogen (BUN), prothrombin time (PT), International Normalized Ratio (INR), partial thromboplastin time (PTT), and other tests depending on the patient's medical history or signs. Consult nephrology and/or vascular surgery if possible prior to reversing coagulopathy, given the potential for graft thrombosis and the need for close follow-up.

Heparin Rebound. The literature reports conflicting data regarding a bleeding phenomenon known as *heparin rebound*. It is not clear whether this occurs after a single administration of heparin or whether it requires repeated exposures such as in dialysis patients. It may account for episodes of postdialysis bleeding that are seen in the ED. This phenomenon is most likely to occur in chronic dialysis patients who are at a high risk of bleeding and therefore have heparin continuously infused into the dialyzer inlet line and protamine sulfate into the outlet line. Thus, only the blood in the extracorporeal circuit is anticoagulated. When inactive heparin-protamine complexes are metabolized during the hours after dialysis, active heparin may be released into the patient's circulation. This rebound effect may be seen up to 10 hours after dialysis.[54] It has been explained to be caused by an increase in thrombin activity after discontinuation of heparin[42,55] or as a reappearance of anticoagulant activity after adequate neutralization of heparin with protamine sulfate.[28,56-58]

Treat heparin overdose and rebound by giving protamine intravenously over 10 minutes in doses of not greater than 50 mg. One mg of protamine neutralizes 1000 U heparin. Do not administer it too rapidly, because protamine can cause hypotension. Monitor the PTT to confirm neutralization of heparin.

Uremic Platelet Dysfunction. If platelet dysfunction is suspected owing to uremia, administer desmopressin (DDAVP) or cryoprecipitate[30] to control hemorrhage. Unapproved adult dosing to control uremic bleeding is 0.3 µg/kg intravenously as a single dose or every 12 hours. Onset is 1 to 2 hours, and the duration is 6 to 8 hours after a single dose. Disadvantages include the high cost and adverse reactions including anaphylaxis, water intoxication/hyponatremia, and thrombotic events (rare).

Warfarin-Associated Coagulopathy. A medication history in addition to an elevated INR level will detect a coagulopathy associated with warfarin use. If active, serious bleeding and an elevated INR exist, consider using fresh frozen plasma as well as vitamin K (10 mg IV slow infusion).

Catheter Displacement/Migration

Catheter displacement may occur accidentally secondary to patient movement, iatrogenically, or both. Secure the catheter with sutures, sterile tape strips (with care to avoid direct contact with the catheter itself), and premanufactured devices.[20] Even with these measures, migration may still occur. In regard to TIVADs, malposition of the intravascular portion may occur with incorrect initial positioning or secondarily from forceful flushing, neck flexion, obesity, severe cough, emesis, or upper extremity movement. Malposition of the port body may occur intentionally or by unintentional manipulation of the port (Twiddler's syndrome). Obtain computed tomography of the chest to diagnose this condition. Note that surgical intervention is usually necessary.[59]

Catheter Fracture

Fracture of a VAD can occur either subcutaneously or in the externalized portion.[60] This may occur with certain physical activities such as golfing, swimming, or weightlifting, which involve repetitive and excessive motion. Subcutaneous fractures cause pain and swelling and require line removal. Fractures in the externalized portion may be repaired using commercially available kits and do not always have to be replaced.

Subclavian Steal

Vascular steal syndrome is an uncommon (1%–3% incidence) but serious complication of AV fistulas that is difficult to predict and often leads to access failure. It occurs because of a preferential flow through the low-resistance fistula at the expense of the distal circulation. The syndrome is manifested by classic arterial insufficiency symptoms with exacerbation

TABLE 24–3 Standard Intravenous Catheter Flushes*

Line	Flush Solution	Heparin Strength	Amount Per Flush	Indication
PERIPHERAL	NSS	—	1 ml saline only	• If a running IV in place—no flush necessary • If used intermittently—flush after each use
CENTRAL LINES CVP line Single lumen Double lumen Triple lumen	NSS	—	2 ml each lumen	A. If used intermittently; using a 10 ml syringe: 1. Flush with 3 ml NSS before administering any agent. 2. Flush with 5 ml NSS after medication or blood draws. 3. Each port not being used must be flushed with 3 ml NSS every 8 hr
PERIPHERAL INSERTED CENTRAL CATHETER			FOR ALL PICC'S A. Blood draw must be specifically ordered by attending physician B. Never use VACUTAINER for PICC blood draw. C. After blood is drawn or medication infused: Flush as per the below protocol	
Open ended PICCs—placed in Interventional Radiology Single lumen & Double lumen (White PICC)	NSS	NO HEPARIN When using positive pressure caps	20 ml after blood draw or TPN 5 ml routine flush every 12 hours	INTERVENTIONAL RADIOLOGY PICC's: [open ended] If used intermittently or with running IV; using 10 ml syringes: 1. Must use POSITIVE PRESSURE CAPS. 2. Flush with 20 ml NSS using (2) 10 ml syringes for each lumen 3. Pulsatile flush recommended.
Closed ended PICC with valves—Placed by IV Team—aka Groshong PICC (Blue PICC)	NSS	NO HEPARIN	20 ml after blood draw or TPN 5 ml routine flush every 12 hours	IV TEAM PICCs: No heparin needed for Groshong PICC 1. Using (2) 10 ml syringes, flush each lumen with 20 ml NSS. 2. Pulsatile flush recommended.
IMPLANTED PORT Single lumen Double lumen Chest AND arm ports	Heparin	100 units/ml 400 units Heparin per lumen	4 ml per lumen	A. If used intermittently; using 10 ml syringes: 1. Flush with 20 ml NSS after medication, TPN, or blood draw 2. Followed by 4 ml heparinized saline (100 units/ml) B. When not in use: Flush frequency = 1/mo 1. Draw-off heparin lock until blood is visualized in syringe (discard syringe) 2. Flush with 20 ml NSS 3. Flush with 4 ml heparinized saline (100 units/ml) C. Prior to deaccessing an implanted port: 1. Flush with 20 ml NSS 2. Flush with 4 ml heparinized saline (100 units/ml)
TUNNELED CATHETER (Very rarely used/seen) A. Groshong—Single lumen Double lumen B. Hickman, Broviac	NSS Heparin	— 100 units/ml 250 units Heparin per lumen	2.5 ml per lumen	A. If used intermittently; using 10 ml syringes: 1. Flush with 10 ml NSS after medication; 20 ml NSS after TPN or blood draw 2. The frequency of flushing each port is every 8 hr B. When not in use: Flush frequency = 1/wk 1. Draw-off heparin until blood is seen in syringe (discard syringe). Do this for each 2. Flush each lumen with 20 ml NSS 3. Flush each lumen with 2.5 ml heparinized saline (100 units/ml)

*If an indwelling catheter is used or manipulated in the ED, a flush solution is instilled to maintain catheter patency.
From Blackburn P, Kokotis K: BARD access systems: Vascular access device selection, insertion, and management. In Weinstein SM (ed): Plumers' Principles and Practice of Intravenous Therapy, 9th ed. Baltimore: Lippincott, 2001; Infusion Nurses Society: Infusion Therapy in Clinical Practice, 2nd ed. Philadelphia: Saunders, 2001.

during dialysis: pain, pallor, numbness, motor weakness, and diminished or absent pulses distal to the fistula.[61] This must be differentiated from the nonspecific complaints of diabetic or uremic neuropathy because it may lead to the development of irreversible neuromuscular dysfunction and tissue necrosis. The prompt recognition and correction of hand ischemia lead to increased salvage and utilization of functioning fistulas. Steal syndrome usually requires ligation or removal of the VAD with placement of a new access in the opposite extremity.

AFTERCARE INSTRUCTIONS

Before release the patient from the ED, instruct him or her regarding proper catheter care to prolong the device's lifetime[28] and to decrease morbidity and mortality. Patients may bathe and swim normally after maturation of the site; they should avoid direct pressure on the reservoir and report bruising or bleeding immediately. Long-term venous access catheters and multilumen catheters should be dressed in sterile fashion and observed daily for bleeding and signs of infection, including fever, pain, redness, swelling, and purulent drainage. VADs should be gently flushed on a routine basis.[28]

Heparin flushes are essential to prevent thrombosis (Table 24–3). Tunneled (e.g., Hickman) and nontunneled (e.g., PICC) catheters require flushing twice weekly with 5 mL of heparin (10 U/mL). TIVADs require heparin flushing every 4 weeks and after use. Generally, Groshong catheters are flushed with 5 mL of saline once weekly. Mahurkar and Uldall catheters are "flushed" during dialysis. Mahurkar catheters also are used for phoresis, in which case they are treated three times a week with normal saline and heparin, as outlined earlier. Patients should not allow phlebotomy or infusion into an extremity with a VAD or have blood pressures measured in that extremity. Signs of infection and any inability to flush an indwelling catheter should be reported immediately to a clinician.

Acknowledgment

Pino Colone, MD, coauthored this chapter in a previous edition of this text. The authors acknowledge the value of his contributions to the current chapter.

 REFERENCES CAN BE FOUND ON EXPERT CONSULT

CHAPTER **25**

Intraosseous Infusion

Kenneth Deitch

Establishing vascular access in a critically ill or injured patient can be life saving, but is often easier said than done in the emergency department (ED). Whereas this is true in both children and adults, placing an intravenous (IV) catheter in an ill or injured child can be one of the most challenging and frustrating procedures a clinician can be called upon to perform. Children have small peripheral vessels that collapse during shock, and their increased body fat makes visualization and palpation of peripheral vessels difficult. These factors often result in prolonged attempts and high failure rates.

A study of pediatric IV placement by emergency medical service (EMS) providers noted that successful placement took longer than 5 minutes in a third of the children and longer than 10 minutes in a quarter of the children.[1] In a review of vascular access success rates in pediatric cardiac arrest, the average time needed to establish percutaneous peripheral intravascular access was 7.9 ± 4.2 minutes, with only a 17% success rate.[2] In another study evaluating ED pediatric cardiac arrest, percutaneous intravascular access was successful in only 6% of patients.[3] Investigators advocate for the use of central venous lines, but these are also difficult to place in children and carry a risk of arterial injury, infection, and/or pneumothorax. Alternative routes of drug administration such as endotracheal and rectal routes, although effective in a functioning cardiovascular system, do not work as well during cardiac arrest.[4]

Peripheral IV access can also be difficult in certain adults, including those who are obese, burned, volume depleted, or in shock from any cause. This difficulty is compounded in the prehospital setting in which environmental factors and the need for rapid transport can challenge even the most skilled practitioners. In one study evaluating adult IV access in a moving ambulance, IV catheters were successfully placed in only 60% to 90% of patients and took an average of 10 to 12 minutes.[5]

Interosseous (IO) access can provide rapid, life-saving intravascular access in challenging environments and in difficult pediatric and adult patients. The American Heart Association, the American Academy of Pediatrics, and the American College of Surgeons recommend IO access in emergency situations in children when venous access is not immediately possible.[6,7] The latest edition of the Advanced Trauma Life Support Manual also notes that IO access using specially designed equipment is also possible in adult trauma patients.[6] IO access is as fast as IV access, and the success rate after failed IV attempts is high. In a retrospective study of pediatric cardiac arrest patients, time to IO access was significantly shorter than time to IV access.[8] In a similar review of intravascular access during pediatric cardiac arrest, Brunette and Fischer[2] noted that compared with central venous access and venous cutdown, IO and IV access were the fastest, but the success rate for IO access was 83% versus 17% for IV access. IO access can also be a rapid and successful technique in adults in both the hospital and the prehospital settings.[8,9] Because of

their success under difficult battlefield conditions, the military has adopted IO infusion devices for use in U.S. troops.[5]

IO access is also not always successful. In a 5-year review of prehospital IO needle placements, success rates were higher in children younger than 3 years (85%) compared with older children or adults (50%).[8] The main causes for failure were errors in landmark identification and bending of the needles. Better needle design and new devices have helped overcome problems with bone penetration (see "Equipment and Setup," later).

BACKGROUND

One of the earliest references describing the IO route was by Drinker and colleagues,[10] who in 1922 examined the circulation of the sternum and suggested it as a site for transfusion. The route was not used clinically until 1934 when Josefson,[11] a Swedish clinician, administered liver concentrate into the sternum of 12 adult patients with pernicious anemia and reported that all 12 improved. Subsequently, the technique became widespread in Scandinavian countries. In 1944, British physician Hamilton Bailey[12] described the utility of sternal IO access in blackout conditions in London during World War II.

In 1940, the technique was introduced to American clinicians by Tocantins and associates,[13,14] who described a series of animal and clinical studies that demonstrated that fluid was rapidly transported from the medullary cavity of long bones to the heart. They recommended using the manubrium in older children and adults and the upper tibia or lower femur in children age 3 or younger.[14,15] Over the next 2 decades, thousands of cases of IO infusion of blood, crystalloid substances, and drugs were reported.[16-18] The procedure was more commonly used in children because of the difficulty with other forms of IV access. Nevertheless, during the 1940s, IO infusion was also used extensively in adults, and a sternal puncture kit for bone marrow infusions was a common component of emergency medical supplies during World War II.[5,19] This resulted in over 4000 reported cases of successful IO access in wounded soldiers.[20] During this time, relatively few complications were reported, considering that the needles were often left in place for 24 to 48 hours. Heinild and coworkers in 1947[18] reviewed 982 cases of IO infusion and reported only 18 failures and 5 cases of osteomyelitis. None of the cases of osteomyelitis occurred in patients who received isotonic solutions.

With the introduction of plastic catheters and improved cannulation techniques, the need for IO infusion as an alternative route for IV access diminished, and the technique was all but abandoned. In the mid 1980s, James Orlowski brought about a renaissance in the use of IO access for pediatric resuscitation. While traveling through India during a cholera epidemic, he observed emergency health care workers using IO access to deliver fluids and medications. In 1984, he wrote an editorial, "My Kingdom for an Intravenous Line,"[21] advocating the use of IO access during pediatric resuscitation. After Orlowski's editorial, others began advocating for the use of IO access to allow rapid drug delivery during cardiopulmonary resuscitation (CPR) in children.[3,22] In 1988, IO techniques were adopted by the American Heart Association and included in the Pediatric Advance Life Support (PALS) guidelines.[7] Since then, the technique has become widespread throughout the United States and is recognized as an accepted alternative to IV access in pediatric emergencies and, increas-

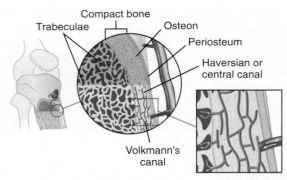

Figure 25–1 Schematic diagram illustrates the vascular anatomy of long bones with an intraosseous (IO) needle in place.

ingly, in neonatal and adult emergencies. In addition, the safety, ease, and effectiveness of the technique have led to its use for prehospital emergency care.[8,23–25]

ANATOMY AND PHYSIOLOGY

Long bones are richly vascular structures with a dynamic circulation. They are capable of accepting large volumes of fluid and rapidly transporting fluids or drugs to the central circulation. The bone, like most organs, is supplied by a major artery (nutrient artery). The artery pierces the cortex and divides into ascending and descending branches, which further subdivide into arterioles that pierce the endosteal surface of the stratum compactum to become capillaries. The capillaries drain into medullary venous sinusoids throughout the medullary space, which in turn drain into a central venous channel (Fig. 25–1). The medullary sinusoids accept fluid and drugs during IO infusion and serve as a route for transport to the central venous channel, which exits the bone as nutrient and emissary veins.[26] The medullary cavity functions as a rigid, noncollapsible vein, even in the presence of profound shock or cardiopulmonary arrest.[27] Radiographic studies have demonstrated that radiopaque dye spreads only a few centimeters in the medullary space before being transported to the venous system.[28]

Almost every drug and fluid commonly used in resuscitation has been reported in clinical and preclinical IO studies. Medications and fluids that have been administered through IO infusion are listed in Table 25–1. Crystalloid infusion studies in animals have demonstrated that infusion rates of 10 to 17 mL/min may be achieved with gravity infusion and rates as high as 42 mL/min with pressure infusions.[29–31] In a swine model of hemorrhagic shock, Neufeld and colleagues[32] found that IO delivery rates of crystalloid were similar to both peripheral and central venous administration. IO crystalloid infusions have also been shown to produce a significant increase in blood pressure in a hemorrhagic shock model in rabbits.[33] In small animals (7–8 kg), the size of the marrow cavity is the rate-limiting factor, whereas in larger animals (12–15 kg), the size of the needle determines the flow.[30] Blood under pressure can be infused approximately two thirds as fast as crystalloid fluids.[30]

Comparisons of IO and IV infusion of drugs have demonstrated that the drugs reach the central circulation by both routes in similar concentrations and at the same time (Fig. 25–2).[13,34] This holds true even during CPR, where sodium bicarbonate has been shown to provide greater buffering

TABLE 25–1 Medications and Fluids That Can Be Administered Intraosseously

Medications

Adenosine
Antibiotics
Antitoxins
Anesthetic agents
Atracurium besylate
Atropine
Calcium chloride
Calcium gluconate
Contrast media
Dexamethasone
Diazepam
Diazoxide
Digoxin
Dobutamine
Dopamine
Ephedrine
Epinephrine
Heparin
Insulin
Levarterenol
Lidocaine
Lorazepam
Mannitol
Morphine
Naloxone
Pancuronium
Phenobarbital
Phenytoin
Propranolol
Sodium bicarbonate
Succinylcholine
Thiopental
Vecuronium

Fluids

Crystalloids

Dextrose solutions
Sodium chloride solutions
Lactated Ringer's solution

Colloids

Blood and blood products
Packed red blood cells
Plasma

Data from Getschman SJ, Dietrich AM, Franklin WH, et al: Intraosseous adenosine. As effective as peripheral or central venous administration? Arch Pediatr Adolesc Med 148:616, 1994; and Sawyer RW, Bodai BI, Blaisdell FW, et al: The current status of intraosseous infusion. J Am Coll Surg 179:353, 1994.

capacity when administered by the IO route than by the peripheral IV route.[35]

Voelckel and associates[36] demonstrated that bone marrow blood flow responds to both the physiologic stress of hemorrhagic shock and vasopressors given during resuscitation after hypovolemic cardiac arrest in dogs. After successful resuscitation, bone marrow blood flow decreased after high-dose epinephrine but was maintained after high-dose vasopressin. These findings emphasize the need for pressurized IO infusion techniques during hemorrhagic shock and certain drug therapy in animal models.

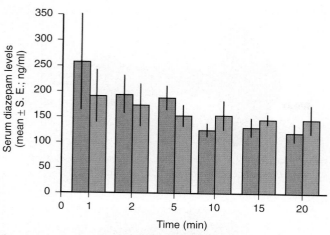

Figure 25–2 Serum diazpam levels graphed for the intraosseous (IO) (*shaded area*) and intravenous (IV) (*blackened area*) groups as a function of time when injected during normal perfusion. Initially, the IV drug level is slightly higher, but overall the difference between the two routes of administration is not significant.

INDICATIONS

When children or adults need immediate resuscitation and intravascular access cannot be quickly or reliably achieved, the IO route provides a rapid and effective means of administering drugs, fluids, and blood. Once the patient has been stabilized, percutaneous peripheral or central intravascular access may be achieved.

Because central access in adults is more readily accomplished, the primary indication for IO access is cardiac arrest in infants and young children. Unfortunately, obtaining venous access in these patients can be a difficult task even under the best circumstances. This difficulty is compounded during high-stress situations or low-flow states such as cardiac arrest. Studies have shown that IO devices provide a rapid and effective means of fluid and drug administration during pediatric CPR.[8,37] This is also true during resuscitation of critically injured infants and children, in whom IO infusion of blood, colloids, and/or crystalloids may be life saving.[6,38] IO infusion is also beneficial in the management of children with other medical conditions, including those with respiratory distress, neurologic insults, dehydration, and sepsis.[39,40]

IO access is not commonly used for premature or term infants, but it is recommended as an alternative for medication and crystalloid administration when venous access is not readily obtained.[41] IO infusion has been used with success in both premature and term infants.[42-44] In one study, 30 IO lines were placed in 20 preterm and 7 full-term neonates with a variety of illnesses (e.g., respiratory distress syndrome, perinatal asphyxia, congenital cardiac anomalies) in whom conventional venous access had failed.[44] All survived the resuscitation with no long-term effects from IO line placement. Gestational age ranged from 32 to 41 weeks and birth weight ranged from 515 to 4050 g.[44] In 1999, Abe and coworkers[45] studied the speed and ease of establishing newborn emergency vascular access using turkey bones and plastic infant legs to simulate IO access and fresh umbilical cord to simulate umbilical venous catheterization. They demonstrated that for individuals who do not frequently perform newborn resuscitation, IO placement was easier and quicker to perform than umbilical venous catheterization.

IO infusion is also indicated in adult patients in whom attempts at peripheral or central venous access has been unsuccessful. This may include adult patients with burns, trauma, shock, dehydration, or status epilepticus.[46] Multiple sites, including the illiac crest, femur, proximal and distal tibia, radius, clavicle, and calcaneus, may be used.[47-50] Of these, the tibia may be less desirable because red marrow is replaced by less vascular yellow marrow or fat by the 5th year of life. In contrast, the sternum has been advocated as the best site to establish IO access in adults because it is large and flat and can be readily located.[51] In addition, the sternum's cortical bone is thin (1–2 mm) and the marrow space relatively uniform (6–11 mm).[52]

There has also been renewed interest in IO access by the U.S. military. In addition to logistical constraints that limit the volume of isotonic crystalloid fluids available to resuscitate the injured soldier; hypotension, environmental and tactical conditions, and/or the presence of mass casualties can lead to excessive delays in obtaining vascular access.[5] The Army Institute for Research has compared several IO infusion devices including the FAST-1 Interosseous Infusion System (PYNG Medical Corporation, Richmond, British Columbia, Canada), the Bone Injection Gun (BIG; Waismed, Yokenam, Israel), the Sur-Fast Hand-Driven Threaded-Needle (Cook Critical Care, Bloomington, IL), and the Jamshidi Straight-Needle (Allegence Health Care, McGaw Park, IL).[49] Success rates for these devices were similar (94%–97%) and all were inserted in less than 2 minutes. The participants rated no one device as significantly better than the others. It was concluded that each device was easy to master and could be appropriately used during special operations when IV access could not be accomplished.[49]

In addition to serving as a route for fluid administration, the IO needle may be used for obtaining blood type, cross-match, and blood chemistry determinations from the marrow cavity. Serum electrolyte, blood urea nitrogen, creatinine, glucose, and calcium levels are very similar to those in samples obtained from an IO aspirate.[53,54] Blood gas values obtained from the IO site also are similar to those obtained from central venous sites during steady- and low-flow states in one animal model and may be an acceptable alternative to judging central acid-base status during CPR.[55] Brickman and colleagues[56] demonstrated that bone marrow aspirates obtained from an IO needle in the iliac crest could be reliably used to type and screen blood for transfusion. A complete blood cell count may not be reliable because it reflects the marrow cell count rather than the cell count in the peripheral circulation. Furthermore, the aspirated blood usually clots within seconds, even if it is placed in a tube that contains heparin.

CONTRAINDICATIONS

Relatively few contraindications to IO infusion exist. Osteoporosis and osteogenesis imperfecta are associated with a high fracture potential; therefore, unless absolutely necessary, the procedure should be avoided when these diagnoses are known. A fractured bone should be avoided because, as fluid is infused, it increases the intramedullary pressure and forces fluid to extravasate at the fracture site. This may slow the healing process, cause a nonunion of the bone, or lead to a compartment syndrome. A similar extravasation of fluid can occur through recent IO puncture sites placed in the same bone. Hence, recent prior use of the same bone for IO infusion represents a relative contraindication to IO line placement.

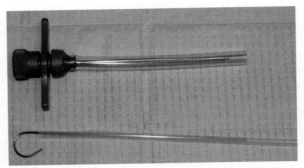

Figure 25–3 Jamshidi Bone Marrow Aspiration Needle. *(Courtesy of Cardinal Health, Dublin, OH.)*

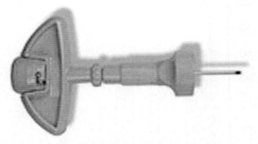

Figure 25–4 Illinois Sternal/Iliac Aspiration Needle. *(Courtesy of Monojet, Division of Sherwood Medical, St. Louis, MO.)*

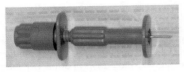

Figure 25–5 Jamshidi Disposable Sternal/Iliac Aspiration Needle. *(Courtesy of Cardinal Health, Dublin, OH.)*

Needle insertion through areas of cellulitis, infection, or burns should also be avoided.

EQUIPMENT AND SETUP

The following is a review of products currently available for IO infusion. Information regarding the use of these products is limited, and there have been few prospective studies comparing IO needles or devices in clinical practice. Until more information becomes available, practitioners are encouraged to review available products and choose those that best meet their needs.

IO Needles

Needles used for IO access range in size from 13 to 20 gauge and must be sturdy enough to penetrate bone without bending or breaking and long enough to reach the marrow cavity. Standard needles for drawing blood or administering medications are not adequate for IO infusions; generally, they are not sturdy enough to penetrate bone and do not have a stylet to prevent bone from plugging the lumen. A cadaver study of IO puncture suggests that nonstyletted needles (2.5-cm, 18-gauge phlebotomy needles and 7.6-cm, 14-gauge IV needles) enter the marrow space successfully only about half the time.[57] In the past, an 18-guage spinal needle was commonly used for children younger than 12 to 18 months. This needle, although readily available in most EDs, often bends, is too long for rapid fluid infusion, and has a greater risk of occlusion from clotted blood.[58] Very small "butterfly" needles have been used with success in preterm infants.[59]

Bone Marrow Aspiration Needle (Fig. 25–3). Bone marrow aspiration needles can be used if needles specifically designed for IO access are not available. These needles are large enough (16 gauge) to be used in older children and adults and are suitable for rapid fluid administration.

Illinois Sternal/Iliac Aspiration Needle (Monojet, Division of Sherwood Medical, St. Louis, MO) (Fig. 25–4). This needle was designed for bone marrow aspiration, but can be used for IO infusion. The needle is available in both 16- and 18-gauge sizes. It has an adjustable plastic sleeve to prevent the needle from penetrating through the opposite bony cortex. However, its long shaft and poorly designed handle make it prone to dislodgment during transport and other procedures.

Jamshidi Disposable Sternal/Iliac Aspiration Needle (Cardinal Health, Dublin, OH) (Fig. 25–5). Like the Illinois Sternal/Iliac Aspiration Needle, the Jamshidi Disposable Sternal/Iliac Aspiration Needle was designed for bone marrow

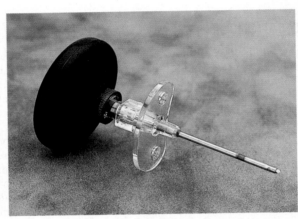

Figure 25–6 Cook IO needle. *(Courtesy of Cook Critical Care, Bloomington, IN.)*

aspiration, but it has a shorter shaft and smaller handle, which make it easier to use. It comes in either 15- or 18-gauge sizes and also features an adjustable plastic sleeve to prevent overpenetration. Once inserted, the needle protrudes approximately 2 inches from the skin, increasing the risk of accidental dislodgment. In a study using a turkey bone model, participants rated the Jamshidi needle easier to use than the Cook IO needle.[60]

Cook IO Needle (Cook Critical Care, Bloomington, IN) (Fig. 25–6). The Cook IO is specifically designed for IO insertion and infusion. It comes in a variety of sizes from 18- to 14-gauge and can be inserted to a depth of 3 to 4 cm. It has a detachable handle that reduces the risk of it being dislodged and a depth marker to help ensure proper placement.

Sur-Fast Needle (Cook Critical Care, Inc., Bloomington, IN) (Fig. 25–7). The Sur-Fast needle is also specifically designed for IO insertion and infusion. It has a threaded shaft that helps secure the needle in the bone and a detachable handle that may be reused with multiple needles. In a study by Jun and associates,[61] the Sur-Fast IO needle had a success rate similar to that of a standard bone marrow aspiration needle.

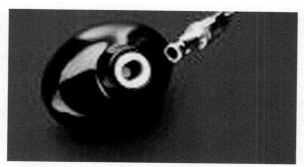

Figure 25–7 Sur-Fast needle. *(Courtesy of Cook Critical Care, Bloomington, IN.)*

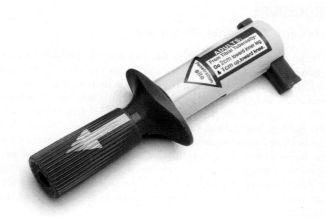

Figure 25–9 Bone Injection Gun. *(Courtesy of BIG, Waismed, Yokenam, Israel.)*

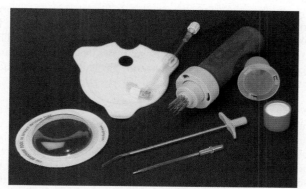

Figure 25–8 FAST-1 Intraosseous Infusion System. *(Courtesy of PYNG Medical Corporation, Richmond, British Columbia, Canada.)*

IO Devices

FAST-1 Interosseous Infusion System (PYNG Medical Corporation, Richmond, British Columbia, Canada) (Fig. 25–8). The FAST-1 Interosseous Infusion System employs an impact-driven device designed for sternal placement only. The FAST-1 has not been evaluated in the ED setting, but has been successfully used by both military and prehospital care providers.[49,62] In one prehospital care study, flow rates of 80 mL/min and 150 mL/min were obtained using gravity and a pressure bag, respectively.[63]

The device has a series of stabilizing probes that help maintain good contact with the sternum and serve as the depth control mechanism for needle insertion. These probes use the surface of the manubrium rather than the patient's skin to ensure the proper depth of insertion. Once the device is positioned against the sternum, additional pressure triggers the release of a hollow needle into the medullary space. The needle comes preconnected to IV tubing. The handle is automatically released from the stylet and infusion tubing once the needle has met its preset depth. Removal of the needle requires a threaded tool, provided with the device. The FAST-1 is larger and heavier than other IO devices, and once triggered, it cannot be reused.

BIG (Waismed, Yokenam, Israel) (Fig. 25–9). The BIG is another spring-loaded, impact-driven device that comes in both pediatric and adult sizes. Like the FAST-1 system, this device is designed for single use only. An advantage of the BIG is the ability to adjust the depth of insertion, allowing for use in different sites (e.g., tibia, humerus). However, if the device is not carefully stabilized before and during insertion, incorrect placement can easily occur. In

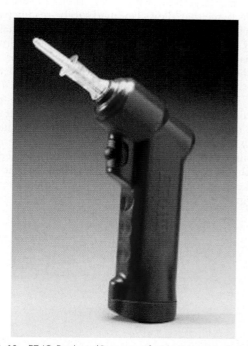

Figure 25–10 EZ-IO Device. *(Courtesy of Vida-Care, San Antonio, TX.)*

addition, there is the potential for operator and patient injury if the device is accidentally triggered or mistargeted.[62]

EZ-IO Device (Vida-Care, San Antonio, TX) (Fig. 25–10). This new handheld, battery-powered device drills an IO needle to the appropriate depth in the IO space. The EZ-IO Device allows the operator to control the pressure or force used during insertion.[64] In one study of 250 prehospital uses, successful placement was achieved in 97% of patients.[65] The authors of this study strongly recommend flushing the needle to ensure optimal flow. In another study of the EZ-IO Device, placement was successful in 118 out of 125 attempts, with an average insertion time of 4.5 seconds.[66]

TIAX Reusable IO Infusion Device (TIAX LLC, Cambridge, MA) (Fig. 25–11). TIAX has developed a compact, portable, and reusable IO infusion device for quick vascular access through the sternum of soldiers wounded in battle situations. The device is lightweight (217 g), can be operated one-handed, and has a driver/depth control system that can be used repeatedly to insert single-use IO needles. The device is currently in phase II trials.

PROCEDURE

Sites for IO Needle Placement

The patient's age and size are the two most important factors when choosing the best site for needle penetration. In infants and children younger than 6 years, the proximal tibia is the preferred site, followed by the distal tibia and distal femur. Other sites, such as the clavicle and humerus, have been used, but neither has gained popularity. In adults, the distal tibia has been the most common site for IO access. However, with the introduction of spring-loaded and drill devices, IO locations once reserved only for children are now potential sites in adults as well. In addition, the FAST-1 System makes the sternum a simple and effective location for IO access in adults.[66]

Proximal Tibia

The tibia is a large bone with a thin layer of overlying subcutaneous tissue that allows landmarks to be readily palpated, and insertion here does not interfere with airway management and CPR. On the proximal tibia, the broad, flat, anteromedial surface is used, with the tibial tuberosity serving as a landmark. The site of IO cannulation is approximately 1 to 3 cm (2 fingerwidths) below the tuberosity (Fig. 25–12A). This location is far enough from the growth plate to prevent damage but is in an area in which the bone is still soft enough to allow easy penetration of a needle. In adults, penetrating the thick bone in the proximal tibia is much more difficult and requires a 13- to 16-gauge needle. A spring-loaded device such as the BIG or a battery-powered drill such as the EZ-IO can make penetration much easier and allows the use of smaller-gauge needles.

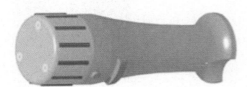

Figure 25–11 TIAX Reusable IO Infusion Device. *(Courtesy of TIAX LLC, Cambridge, MA.)*

Distal Tibia

The distal tibia, although a preferred site in adults, may be used as well in children.[58,67] The cortex of the bone and the overlying tissue are both thin. The site of needle insertion is the medial surface at the junction of the medial malleolus and the shaft of the tibia, posterior to the greater saphenous vein (see Fig. 25–12B). The needle is inserted perpendicular to the long axis of the bone or 10° to 15° cephalad to avoid the growth plate.[68]

Sternum

The sternum has several advantages over peripheral bones, including a large, relatively flat body that can be readily located by unskilled clinicians; retention of a high proportion of red marrow allowing rapid transfer of infused fluids and drugs to the central circulation; and thinner, more uniform cortical bone overlying a relatively uniform marrow space. In addition, it is less likely to be fractured in major trauma.[63] The introduction of the FAST-1 System, which allows safe and effective penetration of the sternum, has led to increased utilization and popularity of sternal IO insertion in adults.

Other Sites

The distal portion of the femur is occasionally used as an alternate site in children, but because of thick overlying muscle and soft tissue, it is more difficult to palpate bony landmarks (see Fig. 25–12C). If chosen, the needle should be inserted 2 to 3 cm above the external femoral condyles in the midline and directed cephalad at an angle of 10° to 15° from the vertical.[69] Other sites including the clavicle, humerus, and calcaneus can be used as an alternative, but these are less popular.

Site Preparation

To prepare the proximal tibia or distal femur for IO insertion, a small support such as a towel roll should be placed behind the knee. All insertion sites should be cleansed with chlorheptadine, provodone-iodine, or an alcohol-based antibacterial solution (see Fig. 25–13A). For patients with severe shock, dehydration, or cardiopulmonary arrest, local anesthesia may be considered, but is not necessary. If the patient is conscious, the skin and periosteum should be anesthetized.

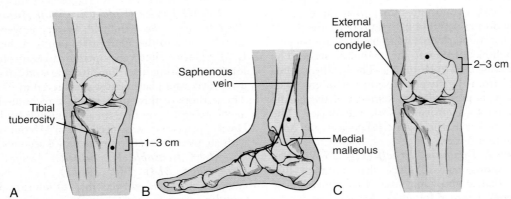

Figure 25–12 **IO insertion sites.** *A,* The proximal tibia. The IO needle is inserted 1 to 3 cm distal to the tibial tuberosity and over the medial aspect of the tibia. The bevel of the needle is directed away from the joint space. *B,* The distal tibia. The IO needle is inserted on the medial surface of the distal tibia at the junction of the medial malleolus and the shaft of the tibia, posterior to the greater saphenous vein. The needle is directed cephalad, away from the growth plate. *C,* The distal femur. The IO needle is inserted 2 to 3 cm above the external condyles in the midline and directed cephalad away from the growth plate.

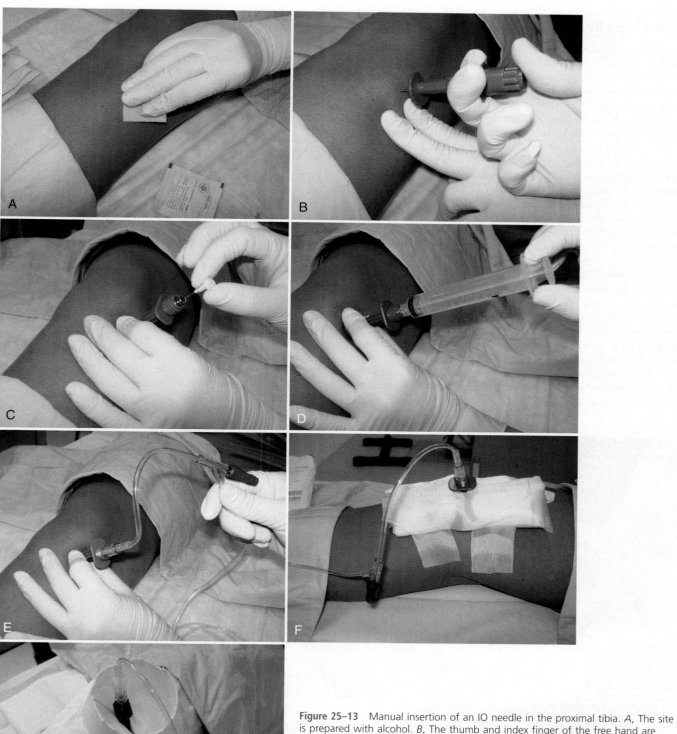
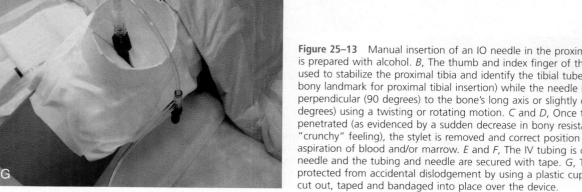

Figure 25–13 Manual insertion of an IO needle in the proximal tibia. *A*, The site is prepared with alcohol. *B*, The thumb and index finger of the free hand are used to stabilize the proximal tibia and identify the tibial tuberosity (the main bony landmark for proximal tibial insertion) while the needle is directed perpendicular (90 degrees) to the bone's long axis or slightly caudad (60–75 degrees) using a twisting or rotating motion. *C* and *D*, Once the cortex is penetrated (as evidenced by a sudden decrease in bony resistance and a "crunchy" feeling), the stylet is removed and correct position is confirmed by aspiration of blood and/or marrow. *E* and *F*, The IV tubing is connected to the needle and the tubing and needle are secured with tape. *G*, The needle can be protected from accidental dislodgement by using a plastic cup with the bottom cut out, taped and bandaged into place over the device.

Manual Needle Insertion (Fig. 25–13)

Prior to insertion, the operator's free hand (i.e., the hand not holding the IO needle) stabilizes the site and acts as a guide for identification of landmarks. For example, during proximal tibial insertion, the thumb and index finger of the free hand stabilize the proximal tibia and identify (palpate) the tibial tuberosity (the main bony landmark for proximal tibial insertion). During insertion, avoid puncturing this hand by keeping it out of the plane of insertion and clear of the puncture site. Direct the IO needle perpendicular (90°) to the bone's long axis or slightly caudad (60°–75°). Directing the needle slightly caudad will help avoid penetration of the growth plate. Advance the needle using a twisting or rotating motion, driving it into the bone and puncturing the cortex. Once the cortex is penetrated, there will be a sudden decrease in bony resistance and a "crunchy" feeling as the needle enters the marrow cavity. Penetration of the inner cortex usually occurs at approximately 1 cm. Aspiration of blood and/or marrow contents confirms correct placement. Other signs of correct placement include the needle's ability to remain upright without support and free-flowing fluid without signs of extravasation into surrounding tissue. If available, ultrasound imaging or a miniature C-arm device have also been shown to reliably confirm IO placement.[70,71]

Once proper placement is confirmed, the needle and the tubing should be secured with tape. Fastening the leg to an appropriate-sized leg board further stabilizes a lower extremity insertion site in infants and small children. The needle can be protected from accidental dislodgment by using a plastic cup with the bottom cut out, taped, and bandaged into place over the device. Commercially made shields are also available for this purpose. Remove the IO needle as soon as IV access has been secured and apply a sterile dressing over the site. Excessive bleeding can be controlled by direct pressure held over the site for 5 minutes.[72]

USE OF SPECIFIC IO DEVICES

FAST-1 (Fig. 25–14)

This device was designed specifically to penetrate the sternum and has been gaining popularity for both prehospital and military applications in which rapid, simple, and reliable IO access is required.[49,73] The FAST-1 Device is prepackaged with alcohol and iodine, and comes with a protective dressing that holds the device in place and a threaded tip remover for easy removal of the metal tip and infusion tubing.

After disinfecting the skin site on the sternum, place the target patch over the midline of the manubrium with the hole in the middle of the target approximately 1.5 cm below the sternal notch. Next, place the FAST-1 introducer in the center of the target zone. The introducer has a "bone cluster" of needles that form a circle. These needles "sense" the cortex of the sternum and help ensure the proper needle depth. Once the introducer is in position over the target zone, apply pres-

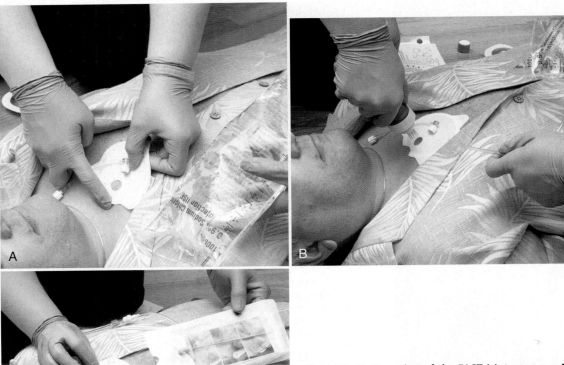

Figure 25–14 Insertion of the FAST-1 Intraosseous Device. *A,* After the overlying skin is prepared with iodine and alcohol, an adhesive target patch is placed over the midline of the manubrium with the target zone hole approximately 1.5 cm below the sternal notch. *B,* The introducer, which contains a "bone cluster" of needles, is placed in the center of the target zone. Pressure on the handle releases an inner needle upon which a plastic infusion tube with a small metal tip is loaded. The central needle advances exactly 5 mm beyond the circular cluster of needles, stopping at the cortex. The metal tip is now positioned in the cortex-medullary junction. Withdrawal of the handle leaves only the plastic infusion tube protruding from the insertion site. *C,* A plastic dome is attached via Velcro fasteners to the target patch, securing the tube in place.

sure to the handle to release an inner needle located in the center of the bone cluster. This needle has a small metal tip that is preconnected to plastic infusion tubing. After release, the central IO needle advances 5 mm beyond the circular cluster of needles, stopping at the bony cortex and positioning the metal tip at the cortex-medullary junction. At this point, withdraw the handle, leaving only the plastic infusion tube protruding from the insertion site. Marrow aspiration and rapid flow of fluid help verify position. Attach the plastic dome to the target patch via Velcro fasteners to secure the tubing in place. Removal of the infusion tube requires the use of an included threaded-tip remover. The tube can also be removed by direct pulling; however, the metal tip is sometimes left behind and must be extracted through a small incision.[49]

BIG (Fig. 25–15)

The BIG incorporates a loaded spring to facilitate penetration of the bone. To adjust the depth of insertion, remove the safety pin from one end and turn the other end clockwise or counterclockwise to reduce or increase needle depth, respectively (from the package insert). Place the BIG firmly against the skin perpendicular to the long axis of the bone (or slightly caudad) and fire the gun by applying palmar force on the back of the unit while pulling on the flanges with the middle and ring fingers. Aspiration of marrow, followed by flushing with the same syringe, and flow through the IV tubing help confirm placement. Slide the slotted safety pin into the needle to maintain stability. To remove the needle, rotate it back and forth using the small clamps provided with the unit. The site is then dressed in a manner determined by the care provider.[49]

EZ-IO Needle (Fig. 25–16)

This battery-operated "drill" can drive the IO needle through even thick bone with relative ease. The EZ-IO kit comes with the battery-operated drill and an IO needle with a stylet; the EZ-IO AD comes with a 15-gauge, 25-mm IO needle for use in patients heavier than 40 kg; the EZ-IO PD comes with a 15-gauge, 15-mm needle for use in patients lighter than 39 kg. To operate the drill, insert the needle into the driver tip and make sure it is securely seated onto the drill. Remove the safety cap from the needle and position the drill perpendicular (or slightly caudad) to the insertion site. Squeeze the trigger while applying gentle pressure to penetrate the skin. When the tip of the needle comes in contact with the bone, at least 5 mm of the IO catheter should be visible. If not, the overlying soft tissue may be too deep for the needle to enter the marrow cavity. To penetrate the bone, continue to squeeze the trigger while applying steady downward pressure until a sudden "give" or "pop" occurs, signaling entry into the medullary space. Too much pressure on the device can cause the drill to stall, preventing the needle from penetrating the cortex.

After entry into the marrow cavity, attach the EZ-connect extension set provided with the EZ-IO Kit and aspirate blood and bone marrow contents to confirm correct placement. Once catheter placement has been checked, fluids and/or medications can be infused. Attaching syringes and IV tubing directly to the IO needle can enlarge the hole in the cortex, resulting in extravasation of fluid, and should be avoided. Secure the tubing with tape and cover the area with an appropriate dressing.

COMPLICATIONS
Technical Difficulties

Technical difficulties are the most common, but these decrease as familiarity with the technique increases (Fig. 25–17). The most common mistake is to place excessive pressure on the needle during insertion and force it entirely through the bone (Fig. 25–18). Avoid this by using appropriate landmarks and keeping the needle perpendicular (or slightly caudad) to the long axis of the bone. In addition, hold the needle with the index finger approximately 1 cm from the bevel. When this finger touches the skin, the needle should be in the marrow cavity and no further pressure should be applied. Some IO needles have a mark 1 cm from the bevel (e.g., Cook IO Needle); others have a special guide or mechanism to ensure proper insertion depth of penetration (e.g., Illinois Sternal/Iliac Aspiration Needle). If available, use of these adjuncts will also help prevent overpenetration.

At times, the needle appears to be in the marrow cavity, but blood or bone marrow cannot be aspirated and fluids do not flow freely. This may occur owing to incomplete penetration of the bone or overpenetration into the opposite cortex. Incomplete penetration usually results in extravasation of fluids and can be corrected by replacing the stylet and slowly advancing the needle until successful aspiration of marrow contents and free flow of fluid occur. Penetration into the opposite cortex generally results in little or no flow. If overpenetration is suspected, pull the needle back 1 to 2 mm and check for free flow of fluids.

Fluids that initially flowed freely may stop flowing if the needle becomes clogged by clot or bone spicules. Frequently flushing the needle with 3 to 5 mL of saline will help avoid this problem. If none of these maneuvers results in free flow of fluid, the needle should be removed and reinserted in the opposite extremity (or another site) to avoid fluid extravasation through the hole left after needle removal.

Extravasation of fluid is a less common technical difficulty, but one that may be associated with a number of adverse events.[74,75] Extravasation may be caused by fluids being infused under excessive pressure and prolonged use of an IO site.[76] As noted previously, extravasation may also result from incomplete needle penetration or penetration through the opposite cortex. Even when an IO needle has been properly positioned, fluid can leak out through holes made from previous IO attempts, through an insertion site made too large from excessive "rocking" during insertion, or from an improperly secured needle that becomes loose with movement.[75,77] Interestingly, the type of needle used does not appear to influence extravasation rates.[78] Regardless of the cause, if extravasation occurs, the needle should be quickly removed and pressure should be applied to the site. Left unchecked, extravasation can lead to a number of adverse events (see "Soft Tissue and Bony Complications," later). In addition, although not directly harmful, extravasation of fluid through multiple cortical defects from previous IO attempts has been associated with lower serum levels of infused drugs.[79]

Soft Tissue and Bony Complications
Infection

A major concern for any person receiving IO infusion is infection. In the past, this concern has led clinicians to shy away from using the bone and to continue searching for other methods of vascular access. Although the potential for infection is real, its actual incidence is low. A literature review of

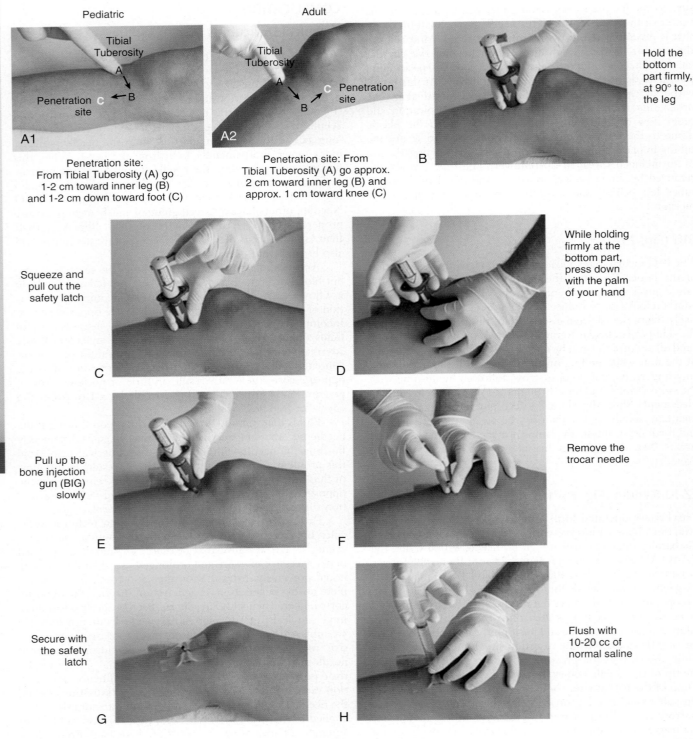

Pediatric

Tibial Tuberosity

Penetration site

A1

Penetration site:
From Tibial Tuberosity (A) go
1-2 cm toward inner leg (B)
and 1-2 cm down toward foot (C)

Adult

Tibial Tuberosity

Penetration site

A2

Penetration site: From
Tibial Tuberosity (A) go approx.
2 cm toward inner leg (B) and
approx. 1 cm toward knee (C)

B

Hold the bottom part firmly, at 90° to the leg

Squeeze and pull out the safety latch

C

While holding firmly at the bottom part, press down with the palm of your hand

D

Pull up the bone injection gun (BIG) slowly

E

Remove the trocar needle

F

Secure with the safety latch

G

Flush with 10-20 cc of normal saline

H

Use aseptic technique throughout!

Figure 25–15 Use of the bone injection gun (BIG). *A,* The site is prepared with alcohol. *B,* The thumb and index finger of the free hand are used to stabilize the proximal tibia and identify the tibial tuberosity (the main bony landmark for proximal tibial insertion) while the needle is directed perpendicular (90°) to the bone's long axis or slightly caudad (60°–75°) using a twisting or rotating motion. *C and D,* Once the cortex is penetrated (as evidenced by a sudden decrease in bony resistance and a "crunchy" feeling), the stylet is removed and the correct position is confirmed by aspiration of blood and/or marrow. *E and F,* The IV tubing is connected to the needle and the tubing and needle are secured with tape. *G and H,* The needle can be protected from accidental dislodgment by using a plastic cup with the bottom cut out and taped and bandaged into place over the device. *(A–H, Courtesy of BIG, Waismed, Yokenam, Israel.)*

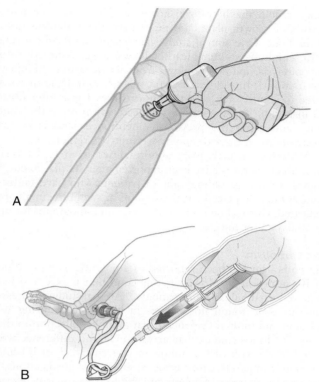

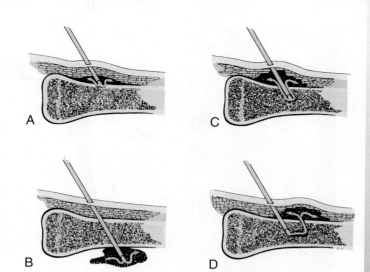

Figure 25–17 **Schematic diagram of possible problems encountered with IO infusion.** *A,* Incomplete penetration of the bony cortex. *B,* Penetration of the posterior cortex. *C,* Fluid escaping around the needle through the puncture site. *D,* Fluid leaking through a nearby previous cortical puncture site.

Figure 25–16 **Use of the EZ-IO Device.** *A,* To operate the drill, insert the needle into the driver tip and make sure it is securely seated on to drill. Remove the safety cap from the needle and position the drill perpendicular (or slightly caudad) to the insertion site. Squeeze the trigger while applying gentle pressure to penetrate the skin. When the tip of the needle comes in contact with the bone, at least 5 mm of the IO catheter should be visible. To penetrate the bone, continue to squeeze the trigger while applying steady downward pressure until a sudden "give" or "pop" occurs signaling entry into the medullary space. Too much pressure on the device can cause the drill to stall, preventing the needle from penetrating the cortex. *B,* After the needle enters the marrow cavity, attach the EZ-connect extension set provided with EZ-IO kit and aspirate blood and bone marrow contents to confirm correct placement. Attaching syringes and IV tubing directly to the IO needle can enlarge the hole in the cortex, resulting in extravasation of fluid, and should be avoided. Secure the tubing with tape and cover the area with an appropriate dressing.

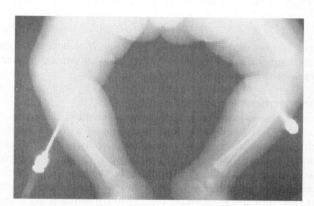

Figure 25–18 Radiograph of bilaterally misplaced IO needles with penetration through the posterior tibial cortices.

more than 4000 cases from 1942 to 1977 found a 0.6% incidence of infection.[3] Although most of the affected access sites were not placed under emergency conditions, the needles were often left in 1 to 2 days, thus increasing the likelihood of infection. A survey of more than 1000 U.S. and foreign medical schools found that the incidence of infection for IO needles placed in emergency conditions was less than 3%.[80] The most common infection is cellulitis at the puncture site, which usually responds well to antibiotics. Osteomyelitis is less common, but it also usually responds to antibiotics. Heinild and coworkers[18] reported 3 cases of osteomyelitis in 25 patients who received infusions of undiluted 50% dextrose in water ($D_{50}W$). More recently, Platt and coworkers[81] reported a case of fungal osteomyelitis and sepsis secondary to an IO infusion device.

In addition to infection, inflammatory reactions of the bone may be seen. These are most common when hypertonic or sclerosing agents are used and may produce an elevation of the periosteum with a positive bone scan (Fig. 25–19). Unlike the clinical appearance of a patient with osteomyelitis due to bacteria, a child with a sterile inflammatory reaction does not look "toxic." One hypertonic sclerosing drug that may be used during cardiac arrest is sodium bicarbonate. Heinild and coworkers[18] reported 78 cases of bicarbonate infusion with no complications. Animal studies have reported a decrease in cellularity with edema and destruction of some cells, but these changes are temporary and resolve completely in a few weeks.[82-84]

Skin Sloughing
Skin sloughing and myonecrosis have also been reported secondary to extravasation of infused fluids and medications.[85] This occurs if fluid or drugs extravasate from the puncture site into the surrounding tissues. When infusing drugs such as calcium chloride, epinephrine, and sodium bicarbonate, care should be taken to prevent dislodgment of the needle and

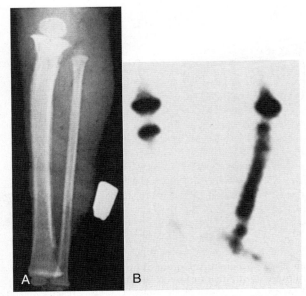

Figure 25–19 Radiograph (*A*) and bone scan (*B*) of the tibia demonstrate an inflammatory reaction 4 days after the patient received IO phenytoin and phenobarbital. The periosteum is elevated along the length of the bone, mimicking osteomyelitis on the plain film and the bone scan. A diagnosis of osteomyelitis requires either clinical evidence of infectious toxicity or positive cultures (blood or periosteal aspirate).

extravasation into the tissue. In addition, it is best to infuse such drugs only by gravity, because infusion under pressure increases the chances of extravasation.

Compartment Syndrome

Compartment syndrome may occur when fluids leak out of the bone into a closed compartment, such as the posterior compartment of the leg.[86–89] Reduce the chances of extravasation by carefully placing and securing the IO needle, limiting the number of attempts in the same bone, and removing the needle once IV access has been obtained. In addition, check the insertion site frequently, especially when fluids are being infused under pressure.

Epiphyseal Injuries

Injury of the growth plate and developmental abnormalities of the bone are ongoing concerns. These fears have not been supported in the literature, however. There have been no reports of growth plate damage or permanent abnormalities of the bone. One animal study specifically examined damage to the epiphysis; sodium bicarbonate was injected directly into the epiphysis, and no radiologic evidence of epiphyseal injury was found.[90,91] In addition, two prospective radiologic analyses failed to identify any growth abnormalities 1 year after tibial IO insertion.[92,93] By pointing the needle away from the joint space and using the previously mentioned landmarks for insertion, the danger of epiphyseal injury is remote.

Whereas growth plate abnormalities seem to be very rare, tibial fractures have been reported after IO placement.[94] Hence, follow-up radiographs of patients who have undergone IO needle placement or attempts at such placement are indicated. Cortical defects may be seen on radiographs for up to 40 days after injection.[95]

Fat Embolism

Fat embolism has been reported as a potential complication of IO insertion.[3,58] However, this condition is rare and has been reported only in adult patients.[96] Animal studies addressing this issue found no changes in blood gases during IO infusion and limited evidence of fat globule collection in the lungs.[97,98] In a swine cardiac arrest model, no difference was found in the risk of fat emboli in pigs that had an IO line inserted compared with those receiving IV medications.[99] Because the marrow in infants and children is primarily hematopoietic, this potential complication is unlikely to occur.

Pain with Infusion

Most patients undergoing IO infusion will not be in a condition to sense pain, but infusion into the bone marrow can be quite painful. Infusing 2 to 3 mL of 2% lidocaine prior to infusion has been suggested to relieve pain in the awake patient.

Acknowledgment

The author would like to sincerely thank Rachael Stanley, MD, for her contribution to this chapter in prior editions.

 REFERENCES CAN BE FOUND ON EXPERT CONSULT

CHAPTER **26**

Alternative Methods of Drug Administration

Steven J. Bauer and James H. Bryan

Endotracheal (ET) administration of select medications is a simple, rapid, and effective method of drug delivery to the central circulation. It is best reserved for situations in which a patient's condition warrants immediate pharmacologic intervention and more conventional means of drug delivery, such as by intravenous (IV) or perhaps intraosseous (IO) access, are not readily available. Such circumstances occur infrequently, and are usually in the prehospital or cardiac arrest scenario; but knowledge of the appropriate drugs and dosages that can be delivered effectively by this route may prove to be life saving.

ET drug administration dates back to 1857, when Bernard[1] demonstrated that the lung could rapidly absorb a solution of curare. In this historical experiment, he instilled the fatal solution into the upper respiratory tract of dogs by way of a tracheostomy. Over the following decades, other investigators expanded this work and demonstrated that solutions containing salicylates, atropine, potassium iodide, strychnine, and chloral hydrate were also absorbed rapidly from the lung and excreted in the urine after injection of their aqueous solutions into the tracheas of experimental animals.[2] The use of intrapulmonary medication in the treatment of lung disease gained further acceptance when studies demonstrated that the inhalation of epinephrine mist dramatically relieved the symptoms of asthma.[3]

In the late 1930s and 1940s, several important observations were made concerning ET drug therapy: (1) penicillin delivered by the ET route demonstrated a depot effect, resulting in therapeutic blood levels that lasted twice as long as those noted with intramuscular injections[4]; (2) various diluents mixed with penicillin affected both the rate and the degree of absorption from the lungs[5]; and (3) higher serum drug levels were attained with direct ET drug administration than with aerosolized administration.[5] In the 1950s, it was noted that drugs delivered endotracheally were absorbed much more rapidly than those applied to the posterior pharynx, and rapid absorption of drugs applied locally to the larynx and trachea resulted in blood levels significant enough to cause adverse anesthetic reactions.[6]

In 1967, Redding and coworkers[7] studied the use of ET administration as a route of drug delivery in a canine model of cardiopulmonary arrest. They administered epinephrine by the IV, intracardiac, and intratracheal routes, and then evaluated its effectiveness in the resuscitation of dogs that had undergone both respiratory and circulatory arrest secondary to hypoxia. Their study revealed that all three routes of drug administration were equally effective in restoring the circulation of dogs in hypoxia-induced cardiac arrest, again demonstrating that the ET route of drug delivery provides an effective window to the systemic circulation.

RECOMMENDATIONS REGARDING ET DRUG DELIVERY

In the late 1970s, Roberts and Greenberg and colleagues[8–11] revived the study of ET drug delivery with a series of laboratory experiments and clinical uses of ET epinephrine. Since that time, a number of important animal and human studies, as well as a number of case reports, have been published dealing with various aspects of ET drug administration. These investigations have addressed (1) the appropriate dose of drug to administer; (2) the effect of drug solution volume; (3) the effect of different diluent solutions; (4) the role of different ET drug delivery techniques; and (5) the effects of hypoxia, hypotension, shock, and cardiopulmonary arrest on the absorption, distribution, and efficacy of endotracheally administered drugs.

It is imperative to remember that ET drug delivery should not be the delivery method of choice. The American Heart Association (AHA) recommends that *if intravenous access is not available, then IO should be the access of choice.*[12] Although the AHA makes specific recommendations regarding the use of ET drug delivery for cardiac resuscitation (Table 26–1),[12–14] much of the literature remains controversial and is at times contradictory. It is likely, therefore, that many of these issues will continue to be the subject of future investigations.

Appropriate Dose

All investigators agree that the ET dose of a medication should be at least equal to the IV dose of the same drug given for the same indication. Most studies on the subject indicate that higher doses are needed endotracheally than intravenously. For Advanced Cardiac Life Support (ACLS) medications in adults, the AHA recommends a dose 2.0 to 2.5 times the usual IV dose.[12] This recommendation is supported by the results of a study of epinephrine administered immediately after intubation in the out-of-hospital setting[15] as well as studies of endotracheally administered lidocaine, indicating a 3-mg/kg dose was needed to obtain therapeutic serum levels.[16,17]

Studies and case reports of ET epinephrine have produced conflicting results. Some animal studies[18] and case reports[10] have shown positive effects and/or recovery from cardiovascular collapse when epinephrine was used in doses equal to recommended IV doses. In other animal[19] and human[20] studies, however, epinephrine in doses of approximately 0.02 mg/kg and 0.01 mg/kg, respectively, were shown to be unreliable in producing a physiologic response. Doses that are equivalent to IV doses may be harmful in neonates, and the current guidelines have removed the recommendation of early ET epinephrine (now Class Indeterminate) and recommend IV/IO epinephrine or a larger dose as high as 0.1 mg/kg.[14] In addition, studies using both normotensive and cardiac arrest canine models have shown that epinephrine doses of 0.01 mg/kg produce serum levels approximately one tenth that produced when the same dose is given intravenously.[9,21,22] These studies recommend increasing the ET epinephrine dose to 0.1 mg/kg and are the basis for the AHA recommendation to use a 10-fold increased dose when administering ET epinephrine to pediatric patients.[13] Some studies have shown that ET epinephrine at all doses causes a significant decrease in diastolic blood pressure immediately after instillation and that a dose of 0.3 mg/kg increased

TABLE 26–1 American Heart Association Guidelines for Tracheal Drug Administration

Guideline	Adult*	Pediatric†	Neonatal‡
Medication dose	2–2.5 times recommended IV dose	Epinephrine 0.1 mg/kg (10 times recommended IV dose) Atropine 0.03 mg/kg Lidocaine 2–3 mg/kg	Epinephrine (1 : 10,000): Consider ≤ 0.1 mg/kg (Class Indeterminate)
Total volume to instill	10 mL	5 mL	1 mL
Diluent	Normal saline or distilled water	Normal saline	Normal saline

*Adult data from American Heart Association: Guidelines 2005 for Cardiopulmonary Resuscitation and Emergency Cardiovascular Care, part 7.2: Management of cardiac arrest. Circulation 112(Suppl I):IV57, 2005.

†Pediatric data from American Heart Association: Guidelines 2005 for Cardiopulmonary Resuscitation and Emergency Cardiovascular Care, part 12: Pediatric advanced life support. Circulation 112(Suppl I):IV167, 2005.

‡Neonatal data from American Academy of Pediatrics, American Heart Association: 2005 American Heart Association Guidelines for Cardiopulmonary Resuscitation and Emergency Cardiovascular Care of Pediatric and Neonatal Patients: Neonatal resuscitation guidelines. Pediatrics 117:e1029, 2005.

diastolic blood pressure after 1 minute. This may be due to β-adrenergic blockade at lower doses.[23,24]

ET drug delivery is associated with a depot effect, with ET drugs being "stored" and released slowly over time, similar to a continuous IV drip. This presumably occurs owing to local vasoconstriction and/or lymphatic storage of the drug[8] or from pooling in the lung tissue due to poor lung perfusion.[25] With epinephrine use, the depot effect produces a potential for postresuscitative arrhythmias, hypertension, and tachycardia, with resultant increased myocardial oxygen demand. Given these conflicting data, *it seems reasonable in adults to start with a dose 2.0 to 2.5 times the usual IV dose. If this appears ineffective, higher doses may be used on subsequent administration.*

Single-Dose Volume

For ET drugs, the AHA recommends a total volume of *10 mL in adults,*[12] *5 mL in pediatric patients,*[13] and *1 mL in neonates.*[14] In studies with dogs, Mace[26] compared undiluted lidocaine to diluted lidocaine (volume, ~6.5 mL) and found significantly higher plasma lidocaine levels in the animals receiving diluted lidocaine. There were no changes in the arterial blood gas values before and after ET drug administration. In another animal study, lidocaine diluted with normal saline to volumes up to 25 mL produced no changes in arterial blood gases or clinical condition, and no change was seen in the gross anatomy or histology of the lung.[27] In contrast, a study comparing normal saline to distilled water revealed a decreased Pao$_2$ for both solutions (water producing the greatest effect), but this study used large volumes (2 mL/kg) of solution.[28]

Studies of endotracheally administered lidocaine in human subjects revealed that dilution with distilled water to a total volume of 10 mL resulted in higher plasma lidocaine levels, but also produced a decrease in arterial oxygen partial pressure (PaO$_2$) of approximately 40 mm Hg that persisted for more than 1 hour.[29] A total volume of 5 mL yielded lower plasma levels but also produced a shorter period of hypoxemia. The authors concluded that a total volume of 5 to 10 mL (in agreement with the AHA guidelines) would produce optimal results. Volume recommendations in the setting in which multiple doses of drug may be given are lacking.

It is difficult or impossible to limit the total volume of drug solution to 10 mL when using prefilled syringes. Epinephrine prefilled syringes contain 1 mg in 10 mL (1 : 10,000). Giving 2.5 times the IV/IO dose requires administration of 20 to 25 mL. It is possible to obtain epinephrine 1 : 1000 (1 mg/mL) and dilute to a total volume of 5 to 10 mL, but the higher concentration epinephrine may not be readily available during a code situation. Likewise, atropine prefilled syringes contain 1 mg in 10 mL (0.1 mg/mL). Lidocaine prefilled syringes contain 20 mg/mL (100 mg/5 mL). Again, a dose of 2 to 2.5 times the IV/IO dose could easily amount to 20 mL or more total volume in an obese patient.

Appropriate Diluent

Both normal saline and distilled water have historically been the diluents of choice for ET drug administration. The AHA ACLS Guidelines recommend either diluent, noting that "tracheal absorption is greater in lidocaine or epinephrine when the diluent is distilled water".[12] Naganobu and associates[30] reported that peak serum epinephrine levels were 13 times higher when diluted with distilled water than with normal saline. In addition, the mean arterial pressure increased significantly when diluted with distilled water but did not change significantly when diluted with normal saline. They found only minimal changes in the PaO$_2$ with either diluent and concluded that distilled water is a better diluent than normal saline. Finally, a study of ET epinephrine diluted with normal saline versus distilled water found no difference in arterial blood gases after delivery of either diluent solution.[31] In this latter canine cardiac arrest model, survival rates for ET epinephrine in either diluent were equal to the rate with IV epinephrine.

The use of saline is supported by the canine study of Greenberg and coworkers,[28] who reported that administration of normal saline via the ET route produced fewer detrimental effects on arterial blood gases than did distilled water. The safety of endotracheally administered normal saline is further supported by a study in which no changes in pulmonary status (arterial blood gas, oxygen saturation, gross anatomy, or histology) were observed in dogs given lidocaine diluted with normal saline to total volumes of between 6 and 25 mL.[27] Hence, the optimal diluent is controversial; saline may produce less pulmonary dysfunction, but distilled water appears to deliver a greater amount of drug.

Technique for ET Drug Delivery

Techniques for ET drug administration include direct instillation into the proximal end of the ET tube, administration via a catheter that extends just beyond the distal tip of the ET tube, deep endobronchial administration using a longer catheter, administration via ET tube monitoring ports, and injection through the side of the ET tube with a needle. The AHA guidelines for adults[12] recommend injecting the drug directly into the ET tube. The pediatric guidelines[13] advise against using a catheter or feeding tube, noting that these are often cumbersome and require finding the correct size to place through the ET tube. Neonatal guidelines[14] recommend either direct instillation into the proximal end of the ET tube or instillation into a 5-French feeding tube that is inserted down the ET tube. Several studies have indicated, however, that the use of a catheter or feeding tube may not be needed to enhance the drug's effectiveness. Greenberg and Spivey[32] instilled radiopaque contrast material directly into the proximal end of the ET tube and compared its distribution with that of contrast instilled via a catheter extending out the distal end of the tube. Their study revealed that both techniques were equally effective in distributing the contrast agent to the peripheral lung fields as long as instillation was followed by five rapid manual hyperventilations. Rehan and colleagues[33] demonstrated that there was no difference in the amount of drug delivered via catheter versus direct instillation in a neonatal model. Although some studies have suggested that drug absorption with direct instillation into the ET tube is inconsistent during cardiopulmonary arrest,[17,20] at least one case report has shown successful resuscitation using this method.[10] In addition, using a porcine cardiopulmonary arrest model, Jasani and colleagues[34] showed no difference in resuscitation rates or physiologic responses between epinephrine administered by direct injection into the ET tube, via a catheter extending out the distal end of the ET tube, or via a monitoring lumen built into the side wall of the ET tube. In a related study, no difference was detected in resuscitation rates or plasma epinephrine levels when epinephrine was instilled during apnea versus instillation during the ventilator inspiratory cycle.[35]

In studies in which subjects had normal perfusion, however, conflicting results have been reported. In one study using female volunteers, no difference was found in plasma lidocaine levels when the drug was administered directly into the proximal end of the ET tube versus when it was administered deeper into the trachea or lungs.[36] However, a later report by the same group[37] demonstrated significantly higher plasma lidocaine concentrations when the drug was administered directly into the proximal end of the ET tube. In direct contrast, when administered to dogs, significantly higher plasma epinephrine levels were obtained via the deep endobronchial route versus direct ET tube instillation.[38]

Given these conflicting studies, use of a catheter to enhance deep pulmonary delivery seems reasonable. However, if a catheter is not readily available, direct injection into the ET tube appears justified.

Effects of Hypoxia, Hypotension, and Cardiopulmonary Arrest

Although concern existed that medication absorption might decrease in states of hypoxia or low blood flow, studies reveal the opposite to be true. In a hemorrhagic shock model, Mace[39] demonstrated that higher plasma lidocaine levels were obtained via the ET route during shock than during nonshock states. In a lamb model, when epinephrine was administered endotracheally, higher plasma epinephrine levels were achieved during hypoxia-induced low pulmonary blood flow than during baseline, normal pulmonary blood flow.[40] Finally, higher plasma lidocaine levels were initially observed when lidocaine was administered endotracheally to dogs with hypoxemia than to dogs that were not hypoxemic.[41] However, this study did not find a difference in the pharmacokinetics of lidocaine in hypoxemic and nonhypoxemic dogs when the drug was administered via the ET route.

Despite evidence indicating that cardiopulmonary arrest does not inhibit absorption of endotracheally administered medications, other studies have indicated that ET drugs are unreliable during cardiopulmonary arrest.[17,19,20,42,43] In addition, in a neonatal ventricular fibrillation model using newborn piglets, 0.01 mg/kg ET epinephrine did not produce significant increases in serum epinephrine levels or in mean arterial pressures.[44] Whereas high-dose epinephrine has never been recommended for neonates owing to a fear of hypertension and intracranial hemorrhage, these data suggest that using the higher dosage of the recommended range (0.01–0.03 mg/kg) might be a reasonable alternative. However, the 2005 Neonatal Resuscitation Guidelines[14] discourage the routine use of ET epinephrine because 0.01 to 0.03 mg/kg appears to be ineffective. More importantly, these studies serve to emphasize that ET drug administration should not be used in lieu of attempts to obtain definitive access to the systemic circulation. ET drug administration should not be performed when more direct means of accessing the central circulation are available. The guidelines emphasize that ET administration of a higher dose of epinephrine (≤0.1 mg/kg) may be considered (Class Indeterminate), but the safety and efficacy of this practice has not been evaluated.[14]

INDICATIONS

ET drug therapy is indicated whenever there is a need for emergent pharmacologic intervention and other access, either IV or IO, is not readily available. This most frequently occurs during cardiovascular collapse. Although intuitively and experimentally attractive, randomized, controlled trials of the efficacy of ET drug therapy are lacking. Niemann and associates,[45] in a retrospective cohort study, examined the outcomes of 596 cardiac arrest patients who received IV versus ET medications. There were no survivors to hospital discharge in the 101 patients who received ET medications versus a 5% survival in patients who received IV medications. However, there were more patients who had asystole in the ET arm versus the IV arm, reflecting that these patients were already in much worse condition and survival was predictably poor.

Specific indications for the delivery of a specific drug endotracheally are the same as those for IV and IO administration. However, only a limited number of emergency drugs can be given safely and effectively by the ET route (Tables 26–2 and 26–3). Medications that have been administered endotracheally and found to be safe and effective in both experimental animal models and human studies or case reports include epinephrine,[8,10,46] atropine,[47–49] lidocaine,[36,39,41,50] and naloxone.[51,52] ET naloxone is not currently recommended in neonates.[14]

Diazepam also has been shown to be effective.[53,54] However, in one animal model, diazepam produced pneumonitis when 0.5 mg/kg was administered via the ET route.[55] Because diazepam is sparingly soluble in water, it is available

TABLE 26–2 Endotracheally Administered Drugs Shown to Be Effective Experimentally and Clinically

Atropine
Diazepam*
Epinephrine
Lidocaine
Naloxone[†]

*See text—effective, but produced pneumonitis in one animal model (Rusli et al, 1987).

[†]See text—not recommended in neonates (American Academy of Pediatrics, 2005).

TABLE 26–3 Endotracheally Administered Drugs Shown to Be Effective Experimentally but Not Proved Clinically

Flumazenil
Metaraminol
Midazolam
Propranolol
Vasopressin

only in a solution of propylene glycol, ethanol, and benzyl alcohol. It is unknown whether the reported pneumonitis was due to the direct effects of the diazepam or to that of the diluent.

In one case report, 5 mg of diazepam (i.e., ~0.1 mg/kg) was administered via a tracheostomy to an adult female, resulting in cessation of seizure activity within 2 minutes.[54] In this report, no changes in the arterial blood gas values or chest x-rays were noted over the ensuing 5 days. Additional studies are needed to resolve issues related to ET diazepam, but some authors and the AHA have removed diazepam from their list of medications that can be given safely via the ET route.[13,56,57] The rectal route may be more appropriate for this drug.

Experimental studies of vasopressin,[58,59] midazolam,[60] flumazenil,[61] propranolol,[48] and metaraminol[62] in animal models suggest that these medications also may be effective when administered endotracheally, but no clinical studies in humans have been conducted to verify these findings. Efrati and coworkers' study[59] demonstrated that ET vasopressin had greater effects on diastolic blood pressure than ET epinephrine with little effect on heart rate, but no clinical trials have evaluated its efficacy. Based on the study by Wenzel and colleagues,[58] the 2005 ACLS guidelines added vasopressin to the list of cardiac resuscitation drugs that can be administered via the ET route (in addition to lidocaine, epinephrine, atropine).[12] It is interesting to note that in the study of midazolam, no pathologic changes were seen in lung sections after midazolam administration.[60] In addition, midazolam is available commercially in aqueous solution and could, therefore, be diluted with normal saline or distilled water for ET administration. However, given that midazolam is approved for intramuscular use, it seems unlikely that ET administration would ever be necessary. Palmer and associates[61] demonstrated that therapeutic blood levels of flumazenil were obtained within a minute after ET delivery of 1 mg of drug diluted in 10 mL of saline. This is 10 times the recommended IV dose of 0.1 to 0.2 mg aliquots. The role of flumazenil by ET administration remains to be determined.

CONTRAINDICATIONS

At present, the only true contraindication to the ET delivery of an appropriate drug is the presence of another form of access to the systemic circulation through which the needed drug can be delivered rapidly and effectively, and it seems reasonable to conclude that more conventional routes of rapid and effective drug administration should be used when available. A complete list of drugs that are *contraindicated* relative to delivery by the ET method is not available. Specific emergency medications that have been shown to be ineffective or unsafe when given via the ET route include sodium bicarbonate, amiodarone, isoproterenol, and bretylium. In a study using a canine model, sodium bicarbonate was shown to inactivate lung surfactant.[63] Isoproterenol, even when given in doses 10 times the IV dose, failed to produce significant changes in arterial blood pressure or heart rate.[48] Studies of bretylium also indicate low serum levels after ET administration, even when administered at doses of 20 mg/kg.[64] Amiodarone induces pneumonitis and pulmonary fibrosis after instillation in animal studies and is, therefore, not recommended for ET administration.[65]

EQUIPMENT

For patients in need of ET drug therapy, first perform tracheal intubation. It should be noted that, in studies in which the recommended ET tube doses of medications were administered by Combitube (Kendall-Sheridan, Argyle, NY) or laryngeal mask airway (LMA; Intavent International SA, Henley-on-Thames, England), the absorption of drugs was found to be subtherapeutic.[66–68] Studies show that using epinephrine with a Combitube requires 10 times more drug than that used with an ET tube to obtain the same serum concentration and hemodynamic effects.[66] The studies of the Combitube specifically evaluated the effectiveness of the tube when it was placed in the esophagus, thus requiring medications to travel out of the side holes to reach the trachea. Presumably, a Combitube that enters the trachea directly would function equivalently to an ET tube, but no studies have been done to support this assumption.

The equipment listed here is that required to perform any of the four different techniques described. This equipment is suggested for the ideal situation and/or technique. *At no time should drug delivery be delayed while searching for the "perfect" piece of equipment.*

1. Manual bag ventilation device capable of delivering a forced inspiratory oxygen (FIO_2) of at least 50%. In circumstances in which ET drug delivery is indicated, the patient's condition almost always warrants supplemental oxygen. Although the technique may not result in any significant deterioration in respiratory function, it is still advisable to administer additional oxygen after drug delivery. Use the bag ventilation device also to deliver several rapid insufflations immediately after drug delivery to assist delivery of the drug distally, where it may be absorbed more rapidly and effectively.[32]

2. A fine-bore catheter or special ET tube to deliver the drug at or beyond the distal end of the ET tube. For adults, select a catheter that is at least 8 French in size and at least 35 cm (14 inches) in length. It should be long enough to protrude past the distal end of the ET tube. The diameter of the catheter should be large enough to allow rapid

delivery of 10 mL of solution. Several different types of tubes and catheters commonly available in the emergency department can be used for this purpose:

a. A 16-gauge central venous pressure or cutdown catheter. Most are only 30 cm in length, so shorten the proximal end of the ET tube such that the catheter can protrude past the end.

b. An 8- or 10-French polyethylene pediatric feeding tube (e.g., Argyle, St. Louis, MO). These tubes are much longer than needed so cut them to reduce dead space. Luer-Lok ends fit onto the proximal end of the tube. For neonates, use a 5-French feeding tube with a syringe and an IV adapter.

c. An 8-French (or larger) pediatric pulmonary suction catheter without the control port. Because this catheter is designed to extend past the tip of the ET tube, it is an ideal length. However, with some brands, it is difficult to attach a syringe or IV adapter lock after the suction control port is removed.

Alternatively, three ET tubes are made with built-in ports that allow instillation of drugs without removing the bag ventilation device. Unless these special tubes are used for all patients requiring intubation, the major drawback is the need to decide prior to intubation whether IV access is expected to be a problem or reintubate the patient if it is. The tubes with built-in ports are:

a. ET tubes designed for bronchoscopy (e.g., Hi-Lo Jet Tracheal Tube; Nellcor, Pleasanton, CA). These tubes have two additional ports, one used for monitoring or irrigation (opaque lumen) and one used for jet ventilation (transparent lumen). They are available in only uncuffed sizes. In a porcine cardiopulmonary arrest model, successful resuscitation using this tube was comparable with resuscitation using other forms of ET drug administration.[34] The major disadvantage to this ET tube is the need to be familiar with the specific ports prior to use. If one has never seen the tube previously, determining which port is used for irrigation could prove to be time consuming. In addition, the port requires placement of an IV adapter lock or Luer-Lok to use prefilled syringes (in which most emergency medications are now supplied).

b. ET tube with side port (ETSP; e.g., EMT Emergency Medicine Tube, Nellcor, Pleasanton, CA). This tube is designed specifically for ET drug administration but is available in cuffed sizes only. The installation lumen opens into the tube at the Murphy eye, approximately 1 cm from the end of the tube. The injection port has an IV adapter lock, which makes it amenable to use with prefilled syringes. The ETSP is not available in pediatric sizes. In addition, one study comparing the administration of lidocaine via the ETSP with administration by the proximal end of the standard ET tube, serum lidocaine measurements never reached therapeutic levels in the ETSP group, in contrast to the ET group and IV control group.[69]

c. Uncuffed tracheal tube with monitoring lumen (Nellcor, Pleasanton, CA). This tube contains a separate monitoring lumen in the wall of the tube that opens inside the distal tip. A three-way stopcock with Luer-Lok adapter provides access to the monitoring lumen. As with the other specialty tubes, the major disadvantage to this ET tube is the need to be familiar with the additional port.

3. An IV adapter lock. This can be placed as needed onto the proximal end of the irrigation lumen of the Hi-Lo Jet tracheal tube or on catheters described previously to convert them for use with prefilled syringes. This adapter is usually unnecessary if a standard syringe is used.

4. A 10- to 20-mL syringe, preferably a Luer-Lok type, large enough to deliver the desired volume of drug solution plus an additional 5 mL of air. Unfortunately (for ET drug therapy), most of the medications now prescribed for emergency situations come in prefilled syringes. This type of apparatus usually does not allow one to draw up diluent or an additional volume of air to empty the catheter of solution. In addition, depending on the manufacturer and model, some prefilled syringes have either needles or a needleless system that may require an IV adapter lock in order to utilize them for ET injection.

5. Diluent solution. As previously reviewed, deliver the drug in a final volume of 10 mL for adults, 5 mL for children, and 1 mL for neonates. Keep an adequate volume of diluent, such as normal saline or distilled water, available.

6. Medications to be instilled (see Table 26–2).

7. An 18- or 19-gauge needle to draw up the medication and to inject it. Use an 18-gauge, 8.9-cm (3.5-inch) spinal needle for direct instillation of medications into the proximal end of the ET tube.

8. Alcohol wipes for cleaning vials and injection ports.

9. Gloves, mask, and eye protection. After instillation, the solution often refluxes out of the ET tube, making blood and body fluid precautions of paramount importance.

PROCEDURE

The procedure of choice is the one that will deliver the medication to the patient in the most timely fashion. Normal saline and distilled water are both acceptable diluents in most cases.

Secure the ET tube before instilling ET medications to prevent the tube from being expelled if the patient coughs. Inflate the cuff of the tube, if present.

Direct Instillation into the ET Tube

While the patient is being ventilated, draw up the desired drug into a syringe (or use a prefilled syringe). Because no catheter is used, there is no need to draw up an additional volume of air into the syringe. Dilute the drug to a final volume of 10 mL (adults), 5 mL (children), or 1 mL (neonates) with normal saline or distilled water. Attach an 18- or 19-gauge needle. Some authors recommend using an 8.9-cm (3.5-inch) spinal needle. If using a prefilled syringe, draw up an appropriate volume of normal saline in a second syringe so that the total instillation volume (drug plus saline) equals 10 mL (adults), 5 mL (children), or 1 mL (neonates). Attach an 18- or 19-gauge needle, which will be used to flush the ET tube after drug instillation.

Interrupt the connection between the proximal end of the ET tube and the bag ventilation device. Insert the needle of the syringe into the proximal opening of the ET tube (Fig. 26–1A). Hold the proximal end of the needle with one hand to prevent loss of the needle into the tube. Discontinue cardiac compressions and inject the drug solution rapidly and forcefully. If using a prefilled syringe, flush the tube immediately with the diluent in a second syringe. If the patient makes an

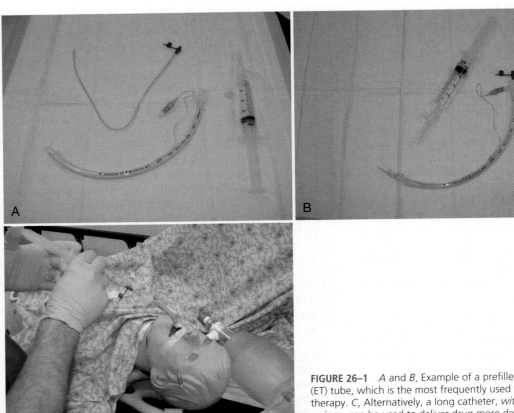

FIGURE 26–1 *A* and *B*, Example of a prefilled syringe and standard endotracheal (ET) tube, which is the most frequently used technique for drug delivery in ETI therapy. *C*, Alternatively, a long catheter, *with drug drawn into a standard syringe,* can be used to deliver drug more deeply into the lungs. Either technique is acceptable.

effort to cough, place a thumb over the opening of the ET tube to prevent expulsion of the solution. Reattach the bag ventilation device and deliver five rapid insufflations. Immediately resume chest compressions if needed.

Use of a Catheter

Using a 10 mL syringe, dilute the drug with normal saline or distilled water as needed to attain a total volume of 10 mL for adults, 5 mL for children, and 1 mL for neonates. Draw back the plunger to add 5 mL of air to the liquid in the syringe. If the drug to be delivered is in a prefilled syringe, place an IV adapter lock on the catheter if necessary to accommodate the syringe needle or needleless tip. Attach the syringe to the catheter at this time or once the catheter has been placed within the ET tube (see Fig. 26–1*B*). In addition, draw up the appropriate volume of diluent (normal saline or distilled water) plus 5 mL air into a second syringe to flush the catheter after instillation of the drug from the prefilled syringe.

Interrupt the connection between the proximal end of the ET tube and the bag ventilation device. Place the catheter within the lumen of the ET tube in such a manner that the distal end of the catheter extends approximately 1 cm beyond the distal end of the ET tube. For the catheter to reach deep enough, the proximal end of the ET tube may need to be cut to a shorter length. Hold the proximal ends of the catheter and the ET tube at all times during the procedure. If it has not already been done, attach the syringe to the catheter. If external cardiac compressions are being performed, *interrupt them during drug delivery*. Inject the drug solution rapidly and forcefully through the catheter into the trachea followed by the 5 mL of air needed to flush the catheter of any remaining

drug solution. If using a prefilled syringe, use the second syringe to flush promptly with the diluent and air. Immediately remove the syringe and catheter from the ET tube. If the patient makes an effort to cough, place a thumb over the opening of the ET tube to prevent expulsion of the solution. As soon as possible after drug delivery, reconnect the bag ventilation device with supplemental oxygen to the ET tube. Deliver five rapid ventilations to promote distal dispersion of the drug. Immediately resume chest compressions if necessary.

The air flush presumably forces out any medication adhering to the walls of the catheter's lumen. Rehan and colleagues,[33] in a neonatal model, determined that more medication was delivered with an air flush versus without an air flush when using a catheter.

Use of ET Tubes with Irrigation/ Drug Delivery Lumens

Unless these ET tubes are used for every intubation, their usefulness in emergent ET drug delivery depends on the provider's recognition prior to intubation that IV access will be problematic. If this is recognized, intubate the patient using an ET tube with monitoring/irrigation lumen (e.g., Hi-Lo Jet ET tube) or with an ETSP (e.g., EMT tracheal tube). While ventilating the patient with supplemental oxygen, draw up the required drug dose in either a 10- or a 20-mL syringe with an 18- or 19-gauge needle attached (or use a prefilled syringe). If necessary, dilute the drug with normal saline or distilled water to attain a total volume of 10 mL (adults), 5 mL (children), or 1 mL (neonates). Draw back the plunger to add

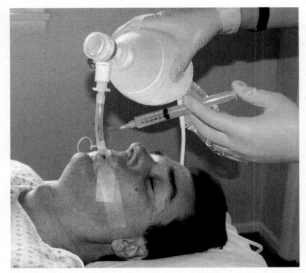

FIGURE 26–2   Method of drug injection through the ET tube wall.

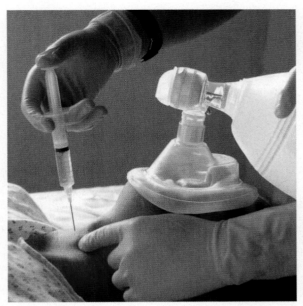

FIGURE 26–3   For endotracheal drug administration, puncture of the cricothyroid membrane may be used during bag-mask ventilation.

5 mL of air to the liquid in the barrel of the syringe. If using a prefilled syringe, draw up the appropriate volume of diluent (normal saline or distilled water) plus 5 mL air into a second syringe to flush the catheter after instillation of the drug.

Attach the syringe or insert the needle into the IV adapter lock on the ET tube monitoring/irrigation lumen (Hi-Lo Jet tube) or on the drug delivery lumen (ETSP tube). Discontinue chest compressions and rapidly and forcefully inject the drug solution during the inspiratory phase of ventilation (i.e., when the bag is squeezed). If using a prefilled syringe, use the second syringe to flush promptly with the diluent and air. Deliver five rapid hyperventilations with the bag ventilation device, and immediately resume chest compressions if necessary.

The advantage of this method of drug delivery is that it does not require interruption of the connection between the bag ventilation device and the ET tube. In addition, it offers the theoretical advantage of allowing drug delivery during the inspiratory phase of ventilation, although at least one study has shown that this is not an important factor.[35]

Injection through the ET Tube Wall

This method of drug delivery has not yet been evaluated scientifically but has been used clinically.[70,71] While the patient is being ventilated, draw up the desired drug into a syringe with an attached 18- or 19-gauge needle (or use a prefilled syringe). Dilute the drug with normal saline or distilled water to attain a total volume of 10 mL (adults), 5 mL (children), or 1 mL (neonates). No additional air needs to be added to the syringe. Insert the needle through the side of the ET tube proximally (Fig. 26–2). Discontinue chest compressions and rapidly and forcefully inject the drug solution into the ET tube during the inspiratory phase of ventilation (i.e., when the bag is squeezed). Deliver five rapid hyperventilations with the bag ventilation device, and immediately resume chest compressions if necessary. As with ET tubes with drug delivery lumens, this technique requires no interruption of the connection between the bag ventilation device and the ET tube. In addition, placing an IV adapter lock on the needle allows it to be left inserted in the ET tube for use with additional medications.[71]

Theoretically, medication can be delivered via puncture of the cricothyroid membrane while bag-valve-mask ventilations are continued. The specifics of this procedure have not been studied, but it would appear to be an option under select circumstances, based on clinical judgment (Fig. 26–3).

COMPLICATIONS

Reported complications of ET drug therapy are rare, due in part to the infrequent use of this technique. Because most patients who receive ET drug therapy are in cardiopulmonary arrest or are otherwise critically ill, it is difficult to ascertain whether an adverse outcome is the result of the therapy.

With regard to the techniques of ET drug administration, no serious complications have been reported. A theoretical complication is the loss of a needle or catheter down the ET tube, which can be prevented by specifically holding the catheter or needle while instilling the drug. Thus, the techniques of ET drug administration seem to provide a safe method of drug delivery.

After ET drug administration, well-described systemic effects of administered emergency drugs may produce adverse effects. Epinephrine administered during cardiopulmonary resuscitation has been noted in case reports to produce prolonged hypertension, tachycardia, and arrhythmias after the return of a perfusing rhythm.[10,21] It appears that these side effects are related to the depot effect, in which larger doses of drugs administered endotracheally are released slowly over time. In addition to epinephrine, atropine and lidocaine also exhibit a depot effect when administered endotracheally.[63] No serious long-term sequelae have been reported due to this effect.

A potential concern with ET drug therapy is a transient decrease in arterial oxygen content during or after drug delivery. If total volumes are maintained between 5 and 10 mL in adults, the effect on pulmonary function appears minimal. Supplemental oxygen should always be administered in an effort to improve oxygenation and offset any transient drop in arterial oxygen content that might develop.

Finally, although not technically a complication, the editor has seen a patient after cardiac arrest from a cardiac cause in which ET administered epinephrine was expelled into one eye during prehospital cardiopulmonary resuscitation, resulting in a unilaterally dilated pupil that prompted an erroneous emergency department diagnosis of brain herniation (Fig. 26–4).

 REFERENCES CAN BE FOUND ON EXPERT CONSULT

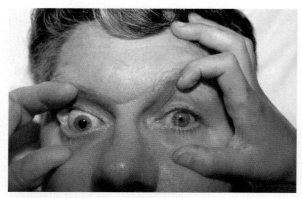

FIGURE 26–4 ET epinephrine administered during cardiac arrest can result in a unilateral fixed dilated pupil if cardiopulmonary resuscitation expels epinephrine into an eye, suggesting brain herniation. Bilateral dilated pupils from this event can erroneously prompt the diagnosis of brain death. Note the intense conjunctival vasoconstriction, secondary to epinephrine, in the affected eye compared with the unaffected eye.

CHAPTER 27

Autotransfusion

Margarita E. Pena and Charlene Babcock Irvin

Autotransfusion is defined as a "collection and reinfusion of the patient's own blood for volume replacement."[1] Autotransfusion in the emergency department (ED) is generally limited to acute hemothorax with clinically significant hypovolemia. This chapter summarizes the indications, contraindications, and complications of autotransfusion of collected pleural blood. What also follows is a detailed explanation of the available equipment and several devices that are widely used for autotransfusion.

Whereas autotransfusion is a basic technique that is theoretically possible in any ED, it is not the standard of care under all settings. Because the procedure requires familiarity with the equipment, continuing education, and quality control, it may be counterproductive to institute in a hospital that has a low trauma census or in a setting in which it will be used infrequently enough that staff education issues are problematic. Autotransfusion will be most useful in disaster and combat settings as well as in high-volume trauma centers in which the technique is used often enough to be considered routine by clinicians and ED staff.

ADVANTAGES OF AUTOTRANSFUSION

A clear benefit of autotransfusion is the immediate availability of rapidly transfused, normothermic, compatible blood that carries a decreased risk of infection from transfusion-transmissible diseases for patients who are hypovolemic from acute blood loss. There are numerous transfusion-transmissible diseases including human immunodeficiency virus (HIV), hepatitis, bacteria, parasites, and the most recently reported variant of Creutzfeldt-Jakob disease.[2,3] Although the risk for transfusion-transmissible diseases has significantly decreased in Western countries, it is still very problematic in Third World countries. Of more importance in Western countries is the immunologic transfusion reactions and post-transfusion sepsis.[4] For those patients whose religious convictions (e.g., Jehovah's Witness) prohibit transfusions with homologous blood, reinfusion of autologous blood that does not involve blood storage is an acceptable alternative.[5]

Autotransfusion provides societal benefits as well by preserving limited stores of banked blood and therefore reducing the cost of medical care.[6] Adias and coworkers[7] compared the direct costs of banked blood including donor recruitment, infectious disease testing, phlebotomy, cross-matching, administration, inventory management, and overhead expenses with the cost of autologous blood transfusion and found substantial savings per unit of autotransfusion. Furthermore, Waters[8] found that the cost per unit of cell salvaged blood decreased linearly as more units were produced. The advantages of autotransfusion are summarized in Table 27–1.

PATIENT SELECTION

Indications

In general, all victims of severe trauma, whether blunt or penetrating, should be considered potential candidates for autotransfusion. Several categories of patients for whom emergency autotransfusion is suitable have been described and are summarized in Table 27–2. Reul and colleagues[9] described the ideal candidate as a blunt or penetrating trauma victim with a hemothorax containing 1500 mL or more. Other patients who might benefit from this procedure include a hemorrhaging patient with an immediate need for transfusion but for whom insufficient homologous blood is available because of a shortage or a difficult cross-match or a patient with massive blood loss (over one whole body blood volume) for whom autotransfusion can supplement homologous replacement. O'Riordan[10] added to this list a fourth category to include those trauma patients who require blood transfusion but whose religious convictions prohibit homologous transfusion.

Contraindications

In some situations, emergency autotransfusion may pose more risk than benefit to a patient; these are summarized in Table 27–2. According to the National Blood Resource Education Program Expert Panel,[11] contraindications are limited only to active infection, gross contamination, and the possibility of malignant cells in the salvaged blood. Previous investigations have shown that even when using cell salvage systems (different from simple autotransfusion discussed here as cell salvage systems that separate and wash cells), tumor cells may be resuspended and reinfused to the patient.[12] However, more recently published work using perioperative cell salvage with cell washing suggests that the risk of dissemination of malignant disease is minimal.[13] The risk of reinfusion of tumor cells with autotransfusion as discussed here is unknown.

The matter of gross contamination from a gastrointestinal tract injury has also been disputed. An early study by Griswold and Ortner,[14] using autotransfusion without cell washing, found that despite reinfusion of massively contaminated blood, 17 of 25 patients survived without evidence of septic complications. A later study by Glover and associates[15] reported that 8 patients out of 14 survived after receiving contaminated blood. All recent work on contamination in the surgical literature used cell savers that included a cell-washing step. Several investigators believe that reinfusing limited amounts of contaminated blood from the peritoneal cavity may be done with an acceptable risk, but the current consensus is that exsanguinating hemorrhage without available homologous blood is the only acceptable indication for autotransfusion with recognized intestinal contamination.[16-18] Concurrent use of systemic antibiotics is advised.[18-20] Thus, depending on the clinical situation and the urgency for blood, it may be prudent to overrule some of these relative contraindications when there is a lack of available banked blood because the risk may outweigh the benefit.

EQUIPMENT AND MATERIALS

Issues of blood filters, vacuum suction strength, and anticoagulant addition are discussed first. Two historical techniques using standard ED materials are briefly presented for the sake of completeness. Finally, although several disposable pleural

TABLE 27–1 Advantages of Autotransfusion

Blood immediately available; no storage required.
Blood compatibility is not an issue.
Autologous blood is usually normothermic.*
No risk of transfusion transmissible disease.†
No risk of hypocalcemia or hyperkalemia.‡
Decreased risk of ARDS.§
Higher levels of 2,3-DPG compared with banked red blood cells.‖
Decreased use of banked blood.†
Decreased cost of medical care.†
May be acceptable to those religions opposed to homologous blood transfusions.¶
May be a valuable alternative to banked blood in developing countries where infected donor blood is a problem.

*Data from reference 28.
†Data from reference 6.
‡Data from references 10 and 22.
§Data from Rakower SR, Worth MH: Autotransfusion: Perspective and critical problems [editorial]. J Trauma 13:573, 1973.
‖Data from reference 52 and Schmidt H, Folsgaard S, Mortensen PE, et al: Impact of autotransfusion after coronary artery bypass grafting on oxygen transport. Acta Anaesthesiol Scand 41(8):995, 1997.
¶Data from reference 5.

TABLE 27–2 Indications and Contraindications for Autotransfusion

Indications	Contraindications (Relative)
• Hemothorax containing > 1500 mL.	• Possibility of malignant cells in the salvaged blood.
• Immediate need of transfusion and insufficient homologous blood available.	• Active infection.
• Massive blood loss.	• Gross contamination of pleural blood from gastrointestinal contents.
• Chest trauma with an urgent need for blood and the patient's religious beliefs prohibit banked blood.	• Known renal or hepatic insufficiency.

Data from references 9 and 10.

fluid collection and reinfusion devices are commercially available, two of the more common brands (Atrium and Pleur-Evac) are discussed in detail.

Atrium's website[21] includes brief educational videos that show in detail the step-by-step processes to initiate autotransfusion using their devices. They also have a 24-hour help line to assist with any questions during the setup or use of their devices (800-528-7486). Pleur-Evac has some limited information available on-line (www.teleflexmedical.com) and is available during regular business hours (919-544-8000, 8 AM–7 PM EST) to answer questions.

Blood Filters

In-line filtration is routinely used during reinfusion of blood products to reduce the danger of microembolization and resultant pulmonary insufficiency.[22–24] The relationship between the presence of microaggregates and the development of acute respiratory distress syndrome (ARDS) is controversial.[24] However, most investigators advise some form of micropore filtration. Pore size seems to be the only issue, and recommendations range from 20 to 170 μm.[25–27] The majority of investigators believe that a pore size of 40 μm minimizes the risk of microembolization without undue elevations in filtration pressures.[9,28,29] The manufacturers of the commercial devices discussed here also recommend at least a 40-μm filter size.

Vacuum Suction

Limit the level of vacuum suction in order to minimize red blood cell hemolysis.[30] The exact level at which clinically significant hemolysis occurs is uncertain, with wide variation (5–100 mm Hg) in the recommended levels.[9,25,30–33] Several commercial products recommend a starting vacuum pressure of 20 mm Hg.[21]

Anticoagulation

Blood retrieved from pleural and abdominal cavities frequently will not clot because of an absence of fibrinogen.[34] This is believed to occur because moderate rates of bleeding allow time for defibrination by contact, with serosal surfaces and by mechanical agitation from respiratory and cardiac movements. For this reason, some recommend simple reinfusion through a filter without any anticoagulant.[32,35–37] However, wounds of the great vessels may bleed at a rate that allows coagulable blood to enter the collection reservoir, clotting off the entire system.[19,32,33,38] In the ED setting in which autotransfusion is indicated owing to rapid blood loss, anticoagulation is recommended.

Although heparin anticoagulation is possible, local heparinization of the tubing and reservoir may lead to the formation of platelet microaggregates on the filter and in the line.[9,39] It also has the potential of leading to systemic heparinization that could result in further life-threatening hemorrhage in a patient who is already bleeding.[9,39,40] Therefore, the autotransfusion device manufacturers do not recommend using heparin as an anticoagulant in the trauma patient.[21]

Citrate compounds, an alternative to heparin, are frequently recommended for autotransfusion.[41] Heparin and citrate-based compounds work through different mechanisms of action. Citrates bind with the calcium ion, preventing the conversion of the protein fibrinogen into insoluble fibrin, which causes the blood to clot. Because citrate binds only with calcium, it only anticoagulates the blood it is dissolved in. Once the anticoagulated blood is infused, citrate is rapidly metabolized by the liver.

Early studies used acid citrate dextrose (ACD) as an alternative to heparin.[22] Raines and coworkers[26] found no clinical or laboratory evidence of intravascular coagulopathy after autotransfusion using ACD, even in patients who received more than 8000 mL of autologous blood. More recently, citrate phosphate dextrose (CPD) is being used because it avoids the complications of heparinization,[9] necessitates less volume as an anticoagulant, and results in less acidosis than does ACD.[9,42,43] In rare cases, excessive use of CPD can cause citrate intoxication because of chelation of calcium and subsequent cardiac dysrhythmias.[9] Use of insufficient or outdated CPD may result in clotting of collected blood.

Although anticoagulant therapy and dosage recommendations are at the discretion of the clinician, commercially available devices do offer some general guidelines. Table 27–3 lists dosage recommendations.

TABLE 27–3 ACD-A and Citrate Phosphate Dextrose Dosage Recommendations

	ACD-A Dosage Recommendations*	
Blood Volume Expected	**For 1:7, Add This Amount**	**For 1:20, Add This Amount**
Low = 140–250 mL	20–35 mL	7–12 mL
Incremental volume > 250 mL	1 mL for each 100 mL of collected blood	5 mL for each 100 mL of collected blood
Medium = 250–500 mL	40–70 mL	12.5–25 mL
High = 500–1000 mL	70–140 mL	25–50 mL

CPD Dosage Recommendations

Anticoagulant CPD solution can be added at the discretion of the clinician at a control dosage of 14 mL of CPD solution to 100 mL of collected blood (70 mL CPD/500 mL blood).

*Dosage ratios are approximate.
ACD-A, anticoagulant citrate dextrose solution A; CPD, citrate phosphate dextrose.
From A Personal Guide to Managing Chest Drainage Autotransfusion. Hudson, NH, Atrium Medical Corporation, 2004, pp 26,27; available at http://www.atriummed. com/PDF/Red%20Handbook.pdf

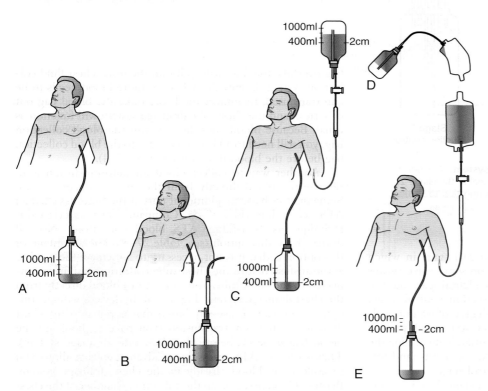

Figure 27–1 Historical technique of autotransfusion from traumatic hemothorax. *A,* Blood is collected into sterile blood collection bottle with 400 mL normal saline. *B,* After blood is collected, the chest tube is disconnected from the collection bottle. *C,* Blood is infused directly from the blood collection bottle while a new chest tube drainage bottle is connected to the chest tube. Or, *D,* blood collected from the chest tube is transferred into a sterile blood bag. *E,* Blood transferred into blood bag is infused into patient. *(A–E, From Symbas PN: Extraoperative autotransfusion from hemothorax. Surgery 84:722, 1978.)*

Historical Techniques Using Standard ED Equipment

Whereas several commercially available systems provide easy initiation of autotransfusion in the ED setting, items currently available in most EDs will also allow rapid infusion of auto-transfused blood. These systems have not been as widely tested and are not ideal compared with the commercially available systems. However, in a dire situation, such as may occur in a disaster situation or on a battlefield, it may be helpful to be aware of these less sophisticated systems.

Symbas,[44] reported on more than 400 patients autotransfused by a simplified collecting system using standard ED materials with no adverse effects attributable to this procedure (Fig. 27–1). After inserting a chest tube, establish drainage into a standard chest tube bottle containing 400 mL normal saline, maintaining suction of 12 to 16 mm Hg. Reinfuse the collected blood in the chest bottle in one of two possible ways

as shown in Figure 27–1. Consider using improvements on his historical technique, such as addition of anticoagulation and blood filters.

Schweitzer and coworkers[45] described successful autotransfusion in dogs by means of a chest tube connected to a Heimlich flutter valve (Bard-Parker, Rutherford, NJ).[46] The valve was then connected to a blood collecting bag (Fig. 27–2). Drainage was entirely by gravity without suction. This technique has never undergone any human clinical trials and, therefore, should be considered only in extremely dire circumstances.

Autotransfusion Units

All of the commercially available autotransfusion systems are based on the same three-stage system (historically called "three-bottle system") for traditional pleural fluid collection (Fig. 27–3). The first stage is for collection of pleural fluid

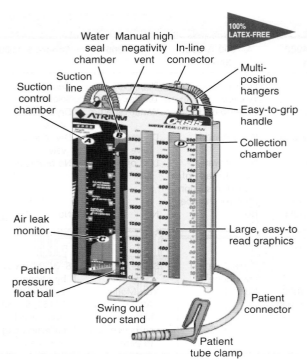

Figure 27–6 Atrium Ocean water-seal chest drain. (*Courtesy of Atrium Medical Corporation, Hudson, NH.*)

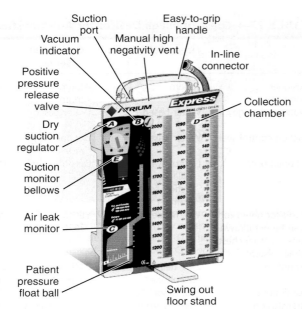

Figure 27–8 Atrium Express chest drain. (*Courtesy of Atrium Medical Corporation, Hudson, NH.*)

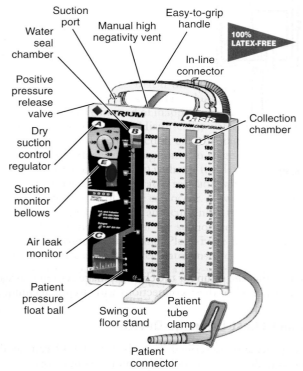

Figure 27–7 Atrium Oasis dry suction chest drain. (*Courtesy of Atrium Medical Corporation, Hudson, NH.*)

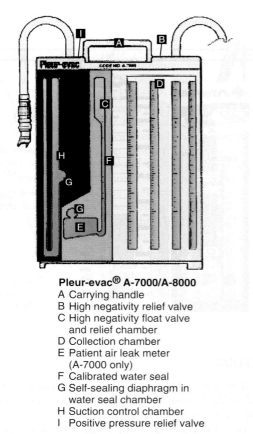

Pleur-evac® A-7000/A-8000
A Carrying handle
B High negativity relief valve
C High negativity float valve and relief chamber
D Collection chamber
E Patient air leak meter (A-7000 only)
F Calibrated water seal
G Self-sealing diaphragm in water seal chamber
H Suction control chamber
I Positive pressure relief valve

Figure 27–9 **Pleur-Evac A-7000/A-8000 chest drain.** *A*, Carrying handle. *B*, High-negativity relief valve. *C*, High-negativity float valve and relief chamber. *D*, Collection chamber. *E*, Patient air leak meter (A-7000 only). *F*, Calibrated water seal. *G*, Self-sealing diaphragm in water-seal chamber and suction control chamber. *H*, Suction control chamber. *I*, Positive-pressure relief valve. (*A–I, Courtesy of Teleflex Medical, Research Triangle Park, NC.*)

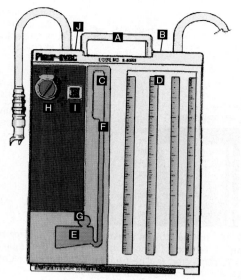

Pleur-evac® A-6000

A Carrying handle
B High negativity relief valve
C High negativity float valve and relief chamber
D Collection chamber
E Patient air leak meter
F Calibrated water seal
G Self-sealing diaphragm
H Suction control dial
I Suction control indicator window with fluorescent float
J Positive pressure relief valve

Figure 27–10   Pleur-Evac 6000 chest drain. *A*, Carrying handle. *B*, High-negativity relief valve. *C*, High-negativity float valve and relief chamber. *D*, Collection chamber. *E*, Patient air leak meter. *F*, Calibrated water seal. *G*, Self-sealing diaphragm. *H*, Suction control dial. *I*, Suction control indicator window with fluorescent float. *I*, Positive-pressure relief valve. *J*, Positive-pressure relief valve. *(Courtesy of Teleflex Medical, Research Triangle Park, NC.)*

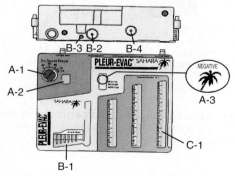

Figure 27–11   Pleur-Evac Sahara chest drain. *A-1*, Suction dial. *A-2*, Suction indicator. *A-3*, Negative-pressure indicator. *B-1*, Air leak diagnostics. *B-2*, Needleless injection site. *B-3*, Positive-pressure relief valve. *B-4*, Filtered high-negativity relief valve. *C-1*, Collection chamber. *(A–C, Courtesy of Teleflex Medical, Research Triangle Park, NC.)*

2. Close both autotransfusion blood bag clamps and remove the protective caps over the autotransfusion bag connectors.
3. Close the patient's chest tube clamp.
4. Separate the connectors between the patient's chest tube and the Ocean chest drain by depressing the connector lock.

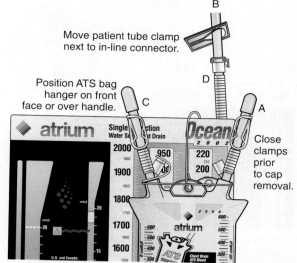

Figure 27–12   Atrium chest tube and autotransfusion system prior to connection. *A*, Female ATS connector. *B*, Patient chest tube connector. *C*, Male ATS connector. *D*, Chest tube drain connector. *(Courtesy of Atrium Medical Corporation, Hudson, NH.)*

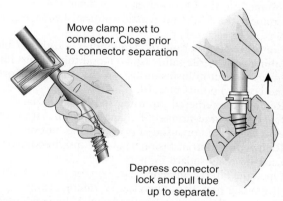

Figure 27–13   Separation of the patient chest tube and chest tube drainage system by depression of connector lock and pulling to separate. *(Courtesy of Atrium Medical Corporation, Hudson, NH.)*

5. Insert the male patient chest tube connector into the female autotransfusion bag connector.
6. Insert the male autotransfusion bag connector into the female Ocean chest drain connector.
7. Open clamps in this order (Fig. 27–14)
   a. Autotransfusion bag clamp going to Ocean chest drain.
   b. Autotransfusion bag clamp going to patient's chest tube.
   c. Patient's chest tube clamp to resume drainage. Blood will then begin to flow from the patient's chest tube into the autotransfusion blood bag.
8. When the blood bag is full (600 mL maximum), close the patient's chest tube clamp and both autotransfusion blood bag clamps.
9. Disconnect the autotransfusion blood bag connection with the Ocean chest drain connection first.
10. Disconnect the autotransfusion blood bag from the patient's chest tube connector.

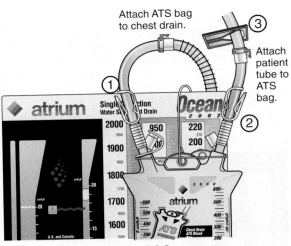

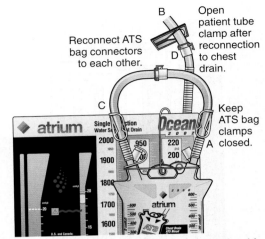

Figure 27–14 Clamp order for in-line autotransfusion. *(Courtesy of Atrium Medical Corporation, Hudson, NH.)*

Figure 27–15 In-line Atrium chest tube and ATS after blood collection. *A,* Female ATS connector. *B,* Patient chest tube connector. *C,* Male ATS connector. *D,* Chest tube drain connector. *(Courtesy of Atrium Medical Corporation, Hudson, NH.)*

11. Insert the male patient chest tube connector to the female Ocean chest drain connector.
12. Open the patient's chest tube clamp so drainage may resume into the Ocean chest drain device.
13. Connect the male and female autotransfusion bag connectors to each other.
14. Connect and preprime the blood filter and the IV blood tubing with sterile saline (spike blood tubing into filter).
15. Invert the autotransfusion bag so that the spike port (at the bottom) points upward.
16. Remove the tethered cap using sterile technique.
17. Insert the saline-primed filter spike into the autotransfusion bag spike port using a firm twisting motion.
18. Return the autotransfusion bag to an upright position and hang it on a standard IV pole.
19. Open the filtered air vent located on top of the autotransfusion bag first, then open the IV tubing clamp.
20. Evacuate all remaining air from the IV line and attach it to the patient to begin the infusion.
21. For gravity infusion, leave the air vent at the top of the autotransfusion bag open.
22. For the pressure infuser application, keep the filtered air vent closed (maximum ATS bag infuser pressure is 150 mm Hg).

Self-Filling ATS Blood Collection and Infusion Procedure

1. Identify the chest drain autotransfusion access line (at the bottom of the collection chamber of the Ocean chest drain) and close the autotransfusion access line (ATS access line) clamp (Fig. 27–15).
2. Remove the spike port cap of the ATS access line and insert the autotransfusion bag spike into the Ocean ATS access line spike port using a firm twisting motion.
3. Position the autotransfusion bag at least 2 to 4 inches below the base of the Ocean chest drain.
4. Open the clamps to the autotransfusion blood bag (on the ATS access line and on the autotransfusion blood bag).
5. Activate the autotransfusion bag spring-generated vacuum by gently bending the autotransfusion bag upward when indicated to initiate blood transfer. When activated, the self-filling autotransfusion bag will begin to fill and

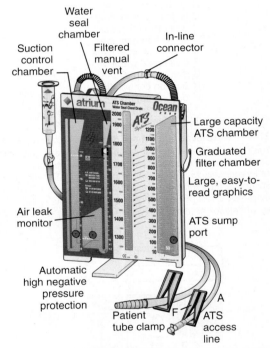

Figure 27–16 Atrium continuous autotransfusion system. *A,* ATS access line. *F,* ATS access line clamp. *(Courtesy of Atrium Medical Corporation, Hudson, NH.)*

expand as blood enters from the chest drain. Do not activate the autotransfusion bag prior to connecting it to the chest drain (Fig. 27–16).
6. Displace any air in the autotransfusion bag by gently squeezing the bag as necessary.
7. When the autotransfusion blood bag is full (700-mL-capacity bag), close the ATS access line clamp and the autotransfusion blood bag clamp.
8. Remove the autotransfusion blood bag spike from the ATS access line spike port and position the ATS access line in the holder on top of the Ocean chest drain. Keep the ATS access line clamp fully closed at all times when not in use.

9. Connect the filter to the IV blood infusion set (spike the filter with blood tubing) and preprime blood filter and IV blood tubing with sterile saline.

10. Invert the autotransfusion bag so that the spike port (at the bottom of the autotransfusion bag) points upward.

11. Remove the tethered cap using sterile technique.

12. Insert the saline primed filter spike into the autotransfusion bag spike port using a firm twisting motion.

13. Return the autotransfusion bag to an upright position and hang it on a standard IV pole.

14. Open the filtered air vent located at the top of the autotransfusion bag first, then open the IV line clamp.

15. Evacuate all remaining air from the IV line and attach it to the patient to begin the infusion.

16. For gravity infusion, leave the air vent at the top of the ATS bag open.

17. For the pressure infuser application, keep the filtered air vent closed (maximum ATS bag infuser pressure is 150 mm Hg).

Continuous Infusion

For direct reinfusion of shed autologous blood via a blood-compatible infusion pump, use a microemboli blood filter and a nonvented, blood-compatible IV administration set.

1. Spike the blood IV tubing set into the filter and prime it with sterile saline.

2. Identify the chest drain ATS access line (at the bottom of the Ocean chest drain) and close the ATS access line clamp (see Fig. 27–15).

3. Drape the ATS access line around the hanger or the patient line so that the terminal end of the ATS access line is facing the floor.

4. Remove the spike port cap on the ATS access line and insert the blood filter spike into the ATS access line.

5. Turn the filter to a spike-down position.

6. Unclamp the ATS access line and IV tubing.

7. Use a 60-mL syringe to aspirate blood through the filter and into the drip chamber of the IV tubing set.

8. When the drip chamber is one quarter full, turn the filter to the spike-up position and continue purging air from the line.

9. When purging is complete, insert the IV cassette into the pump.

10. Purge all air prior to connecting it to the patient.

11. Set pump to desired "volume to be infused" and "mL/hr."

12. Watch the infusion carefully and make sure the infusion pump is programmed to stop before all the blood in the Ocean chest drain is empty to prevent air embolism (Fig. 27–17).

Pleur-Evac Chest Drainage Devices

All Pleur-Evac models have similar designs. The method described here is for the Sahara model.

In-Line Blood Collection and Autotransfusion Procedure

1. Close the two clamps on the top of the autotransfusion bag (Fig. 27–18).

2. Attach the autotransfusion bag to the side of the chest drain device by aligning the bottom leg and the lever of the adapter with their mating receptacles on the chest drain system. Insert with a downward motion until the

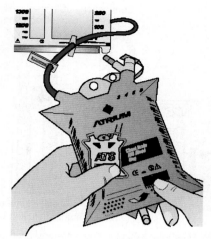

Figure 27–17 Activation of the self-filling Atrium autotransfusion bag. *(Courtesy of Atrium Medical Corporation, Hudson, NH.)*

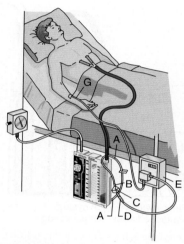

Figure 27–18 Autotransfusion connection to patient. *A,* ATS access line. *B,* End of ATS access line. *C,* Blood filter. *D,* Intravenous (IV) tubing with spike port in upward position. *E,* Blood-compatible IV infusion pump. *G,* Patient IV access. *(Courtesy of Atrium Medical Corporation, Hudson, NH.)*

lever "clicks" into position. The autotransfusion bag should be firmly attached to the chest drain device (Figs. 27–19 and 27–20).

3. Close the clamp on the patient's chest tube and disconnect the red and blue connectors separating the patient's chest tube from the chest drainage device.

4. Remove the red protective cap from the autotransfusion bag tube and connect this end to the patient's chest tube.

5. Remove the blue protective cap from the autotransfusion collection bag tube and connect this end to the chest drainage device (red connected to red and blue connected to blue).

6. Open all clamps. The autotransfusion blood bag will begin to fill.

7. To discontinue autotransfusion, first reduce excessive negative pressure using the high-negativity relief valve on the Sahara chest drain.

8. Close the clamp on the patient's chest tube, and then close both clamps on the autotransfusion bag.

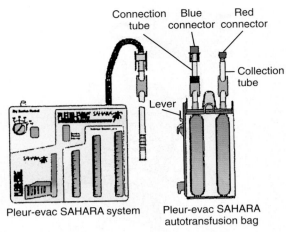

Figure 27–19 Pleur-Evac Sahara in-line autotransfusion setup. *(Courtesy of Teleflex Medical, Research Triangle Park, NC.)*

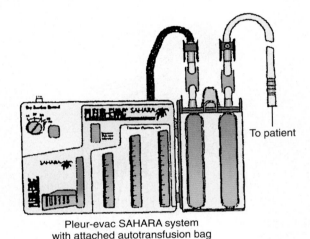

Figure 27–20 Pleur-Evac Sahara in-line autotransfusion setup with autotransfusion bag attached to the chest drain device. *(Courtesy of Teleflex Medical, Research Triangle Park, NC.)*

9. Separate the red connectors going to the patient's chest tube and the blue connectors going to the Sahara chest drain.
10. Connect the red and blue connectors on the autotransfusion bag.
11. Join the patient's chest tube red connector to the Sahara chest drain blue connector.
12. Open the clamp on the patient's chest tube so drainage from the patient to the Sahara chest drain may resume.
13. Remove the autotransfusion bag from the Sahara chest drain by depressing the lever and lifting the autotransfusion bag up.
14. Remove the adaptor bracket from the wire frame of the autotransfusion bag by twisting it slightly to disengage the bottom and then unhook the top.
15. Slide the autotransfusion bag off the wire support frame. Make sure the red and blue connectors on the top of the autotransfusion bag are secure and that the clamps on the autotransfusion bag are closed.
16. Connect the filter and IV blood tubing (spike filter with IV blood tubing spike)
17. Invert the autotransfusion bag so that the spike port points upward and remove the protective cap.

18. Insert the filter (use spike end of filter) into the spike port on the autotransfusion bag.
19. Evacuate residual air from the autotransfusion bag by opening the IV infusion set clamp, keep the autotransfusion bag inverted, and carefully squeeze all the air from the autotransfusion bag through the filter and IV line.
20. Continue to squeeze the autotransfusion bag, allowing blood to slowly prime the filter. Continue squeezing until the filter is saturated with blood and the drip chamber on the IV tubing is half full.
21. Close the IV clamp.
22. Invert the autotransfusion bag and hang it from the IV pole.
23. Open the IV infusion line clamp to carefully flush any remaining air from the blood tubing.
24. Attach the distal end of the infusion set to the patient's IV line and begin the infusion.

Continuous Infusion

1. Set up a blood-compatible IV pump.
2. Connect the filter to the IV blood tubing (spike the blood tubing into the filter), and then connect it to a bag of saline (spike the filter into the saline bag). Prime the filter and the drip chamber and the IV blood tubing with the sterile saline bag. Remove the bag of saline used to prime it.
3. Remove the blue protective cap from the autotransfusion bag and spike the autotransfusion bag with the blood filter spike.
4. Use an IV pump to prime the filter, drip chamber, and infusion line with blood.
5. If needed, depress the high-negativity relief valve on the top of the Sahara chest drain to relieve excessive negative pressure.
6. Make sure the infusion line is filled with blood and contains no air and attach it to the patient's IV catheter.
7. Make sure all the connections are secure.
8. Set the infusion rate on the IV pump.
9. Attach the Sahara drain and the autotransfusion bag to the bed rail using hangers.

Additional General Autotransfusion Information

1. Use each liner bag only once.
2. Use a new filter for each autotransfusion bag used.
3. To minimize the risk from bacterial overgrowth, do not allow collected blood to stand for prolonged periods of time before reinfusion. The American Association of Blood Banks states that there should be no more than a 6-hour shelf life between collection and reinfusion.[47] Calculate the age of the collected blood from the time of the injury. Blood reinfused after this time period is considered hazardous. Because one is performing the procedure for significant hypovolemia in the ED, the collected blood is generally transfused as soon as the collection bag is full; therefore this is usually not an issue.
4. After reinfusing a total of 3500 mL (~7 units) of autologous blood, begin giving fresh frozen plasma at a rate of 1 unit of fresh frozen plasma for every 2 units (~1000 mL) of autotransfused blood.[26]
5. If some or all of the collected blood becomes clotted in the liner bag, discard the blood.
6. To reduce the risk of an air embolism, remove all the air from the collected blood bag before hanging it for reinfusion.[48]

TABLE 27–5 Complications of Autotransfusion

Hematologic

Decreased platelet count
Decreased fibrinogen level
Increased fibrin split products
Prolonged prothrombin time
Prolonged partial thromboplastin time
Red blood cell hemolysis
Elevated plasma-free hemoglobin level
Decreased hematocrit level

Nonhematologic

Bacteremia
Sepsis
Microembolism
Air embolism
Renal insufficiency

COMPLICATIONS

In general, complications from autotransfusion are clinically insignificant if the proper technique is followed and if less than 3000 mL of blood is reinfused. Complications may be categorized as hematologic and nonhematologic (Table 27–5).

Hematologic Complications

The degree to which autotransfusion contributes to the development of a coagulopathy has still not been conclusively determined.[49] The dilemma is that severely injured trauma patients who are candidates for autotransfusion are more likely to have other independent risk factors for coagulopathy such as hypothermia and acidosis. Horst and colleagues[50] studied 154 trauma patients who received intraoperative autotransfusion and found that patients who received greater than 15 units of autologous blood and greater than 50 units of combined autologous and banked blood were found not only to have a clinically significant coagulopathy but also to be more severely injured, hypothermic, and acidotic and to have a higher mortality. This study illustrates how difficult it is to separate out the contribution of autotransfusion to coagulopathy. Finally, although coagulation test abnormalities after infusion of salvaged blood have been interpreted as evidence of disseminated intravascular coagulation, these changes likely are the result of infusion of fibrin degradation products and do not represent a consumptive coagulopathy.[51]

In general, although coagulation problems should be anticipated, they have not proved to be clinically important when volumes of autotransfused blood remain below 2000 mL in adult patients.[38] When reinfused volumes exceed 3500 mL, laboratory evidence of a dilutional coagulopathy may become evident.[26] When volumes of autotransfused blood are greater than the patient's total blood volume, animal studies suggest that there is an increased risk of a true consumptive coagulopathy.[52]

In those few patients who required a larger autotransfusion volume, a proportional decrease in platelets and fibrinogen occurred, requiring subsequent correction with fresh frozen plasma and platelets. Other investigators have confirmed these findings and have shown that elevations in pro-

thrombin and partial thromboplastin times, which were encountered routinely, were not clinically significant (usually self-corrected within 48–72 hr).[9,22,30,32] Similarly, both platelet and fibrinogen levels returned to normal by 48 to 72 hours without replacement therapy.[22,32] Because of the liver's capacity to replenish fibrinogen rapidly, the low postautotransfusion levels have not proved to be clinically significant.[9,36,38] However, some investigators believe that hepatic insufficiency is a relative contraindication to autotranfusion unless fibrinogen is supplemented.[9]

Hemolysis occurs with autotransfusion in part because of prolonged exposure of the cells to serosal linings of the traumatized body cavities.[53] Hemolysis also results from mechanical factors during collection and reinfusion such as roller pump trauma or excessive exposure to air-fluid interfaces.[9] Of note, the hematocrit falls in direct proportion to the quantity of blood transfused, averaging a decline of 10% to 20%.[9,17,44] However, nontraumatized red blood cell survival was reported to be normal in all cases studied.[26,35,45]

Recommendations regarding the volume of autologous blood that should trigger infusion of fresh frozen plasma or platelets range from ~1250 mL (25% of total blood volume in a 70-kg adult)[54] to 3500 mL.[26] Others advise reliance on laboratory tests and clinical findings rather than a volume-based protocol.[38] Prudent clinical judgment dictates application of the more liberal guidelines for replacement therapy in those patients with extensive hepatic injury, intractable shock, or ongoing losses requiring immediate surgical intervention.

Nonhematologic Complications

The theoretical risk of sepsis after the administration of potentially contaminated blood always exists within the non-sterile surrounding of the typical ED resuscitation area. Experience has shown this risk is minimal after autotranfusion from an isolated hemothorax,[22,40,55] and there is no evidence to suggest that routine prophylaxis with systemic antibiotics is beneficial in this situation. Recently, however, Dunne and associates[56] found that allogenic blood transfusion in the first 24 hours after trauma was an independent predictor of mortality (more than a fourfold increase compared with nontransfused patients) and systemic inflammatory response syndrome (two- to nearly sixfold increase).

Microemboli secondary to platelet microaggregation or fat emboli is mostly eliminated by the use of micropore filters.[9,26,30] During reinfusion of collected blood, there is usually a mild increase in screen filtration pressures indicating the formation of microemboli trapped by the filter.[30] There is no clinical evidence of pulmonary insufficiency or unexplained elevation of the alveolar-to-arterial oxygen gradient that might be attributed to the passage of microemboli beyond the micropore filter systems.[9]

As with all IV infusions, improper technique, such as applying pressure to air-containing systems, may lead to air embolism. This uncommon but often fatal complication has been associated with autotransfusion systems using automated roller pump units in which the aspirate reservoir was inadvertently allowed to run dry.[22,57–59] Air embolism with gravity or with a manually assisted technique is rare.

Infusion of large quantities of unwashed blood that contain hemolyzed red blood cells may contribute to renal failure, particularly in patients with already compromised renal function.[11] An elevated plasma-free hemoglobin is a consistent finding in patients who have received autotransfusions.[9,39,44] In the past, it was believed that elevated levels of free hemoglobin after hemolytic transfusion reactions caused renal failure by its precipitation and obstruction of renal tubules. However, more recent evidence suggests that the mechanism in this setting is independent of free hemoglobin and is instead the result of an antigen-antibody–induced intravascular coagulation that, compounded by vasoconstriction and hypotension, leads to renal ischemia.[60] Even though renal failure as a direct consequence of autotransfusion has not been reported, transient elevations in serum creatinine do occur, and in the presence of shock and systemic acidosis, acute tubular necrosis remains a potential complication.[10,56,61] Some researchers believe that renal insufficiency is only a relative contraindication to autotransfusion.[9] The clinician must judge the urgency of the need for blood and the availability of an alternate source.

CONCLUSION

Autotransfusion, a technique that is almost 200 years old, has become the subject of renewed interest in the ED setting. The previously feared hematologic, metabolic, and infectious complications have not proved to be of major clinical signifi-cance when appropriate patient selection and careful technique are followed. In addition, the use of autologous blood has several advantages over the transfusion of banked blood in the emergency patient, including immediate availability of normothermic, compatible blood; no risk of contracting a potentially life-threatening transfusion-transmissible disease; and cost effectiveness. Autotransfusion has been endorsed by the Council on Scientific Affairs of the American Medical Association.[6] Although the technique is not completely free of complications, the benefits to be gained from autotransfusing carefully selected trauma patients outweigh the relatively limited risks.

Although no generally accepted standard of care has been promulgated mandating the routine use of autotransfusion in the ED setting, many hospitals, especially trauma centers, have instituted the technique with success. Current equipment allows autotransfusion from the chest cavity to be performed relatively easily and without highly technical devices.

 REFERENCES CAN BE FOUND ON **EXPERT CONSULT**

CHAPTER **28**

Transfusion Therapy: Blood and Blood Products and Reversal of Warfarin-Induced Coagulopathy

Diane L. Gorgas

Transfusion of blood components (red cells, white cells, platelets, whole plasma, or plasma fractions) is an everyday occurrence in the practice of emergency medicine. Technical advances have made component therapy directed at specific acute and chronic pathologic conditions practical and affordable.

BACKGROUND

Red Cell Antigens and Antibodies

The first documented transfusion occurred in the early 1600s. Transfusion "medicine" had sporadic advancements for the next 3 centuries, mainly dabbling in whole blood transfusions across species. It was not until the early 1900s that Austrian Karl Landsteiner found that an individual's serum reacted with the red cells of some but not all other individuals, thereby discovering the red cell antigen-antibody system.

Red blood cell (RBC) membranes contain a series of glycoprotein moieties, or antigens, that give the cell an individual identity. Two different genetically determined antigens, type A and type B, occur on the cell surface. Any individual may have one, both, or neither of these antigens. Because the type A and type B antigens on the cell surface make the RBC susceptible to agglutination, these antigens are termed *agglutinogens*. The presence or absence of agglutinogens is the basis for the ABO blood group classification and the blood types are named accordingly as A, B, or AB. Blood type O contains neither the A nor the B agglutinogen. The relative frequencies of the different blood groups are listed in Table 28–1.

Within the 1st year of life, antibodies begin to form against the standard red cell agglutinogens not present in the individual patient. These agglutinins are γ-globulins of the immunoglobulin M (IgM) and IgG types and are probably produced by exposure to agglutinogens in food, bacteria, or exogenous substances other than blood transfusions. In the absence of type A agglutinogens (blood types B and O), anti-A antibodies, or agglutinins, spontaneously develop in the plasma. Similarly, in the absence of type B agglutinogens (blood types A and O), anti-B antibodies develop. When both A and B agglutinogens are present (blood type AB), no agglutinins are formed. Blood groups and their genotypes and constituent agglutenogens and agglutinins are shown in Table 28–2.

The reaction between red cell antigens and the corresponding agglutinins results in red cell destruction when non-compatible blood types are mixed. As many as 300 different red cell antigens have been identified, but clinically, the A and B antigens are most important, given their potential to cause transfusion reactions. With the first transfusion of ABO-incompatible blood, severe, potentially fatal agglutination can occur. The Rh system is likewise very important because there is a chance that a transfusion of Rh+ blood to an Rh− patient will result in formation of Rh antibodies. These antibodies are capable of causing severe hemolysis following a second exposure to the Rh antigen. Of the 40 antigens in the Rh system, D is the most antigenic, but others can also stimulate the production of antibodies in recipients lacking the antigen (e.g., E), thus complicating future transfusions. Other antigen systems in which antibodies could potentially cause hemolytic reactions are the Kell (K and k alleles), Duffy (Fy^a and Fy^b), Kidd (Jk^a and Jk^b), and MNS (M and N; closely linked S and s) systems. Other antigen systems are rarely of clinical importance in transfusion therapy, except in certain patient populations who may require multiple transfusions, such as sickle cell patients.

Cross-Matching

Compatibility testing, or cross-matching, involves mixing the donor's RBCs and serum with the recipient's RBCs and serum to identify the potential for a transfusion reaction. The end point of all cross-matches is the presence of RBC agglutination (either gross or microscopic) or hemolysis. Testing is performed immediately after mixing, after incubation at 37°C for varying times, and with and without an antiglobulin reagent to identify surface immunoglobulin or complement. Each unit of blood product, when properly cross-matched, can be administered with the expectation of safety.

Types of Red Cell Preparations

Whole Blood

Once commonly used to provide red cells, coagulation factors, and plasma proteins, whole blood transfusion has been replaced to a great extent by component therapy. Although intuitively an ideal transfusion agent, whole blood is seldom used except for autologous transfusions (e.g., autotransfusion) and for exchange transfusions. Whole blood is not the preferred treatment for hypovolemic shock because it can be effectively treated with crystalloids (e.g., lactated Ringer's solution), (0.9% sodium chloride), colloids (e.g., plasma protein, albumin), and packed red blood cells (PRBCs). It is not the preferred treatment for correction of thrombocytopenia, replacement of coagulation factors, or treatment of anemia.[1] The plasma of whole blood is no more effective than 5% albumin as a volume expander. In addition to providing components or fractions that are potentially unnecessary, whole blood transfusion exposes the patient to additional risk. The incidence of transfusion reactions after transfusion with whole blood is approximately 2.5 times greater than the incidence of reactions after transfusion with PRBCs.[2] In addition, whole blood contains antigenic leukocytes and serum proteins, which may produce allergic reactions (a risk of 1%). Because of the recognized advantages of component therapy, most blood banks do not stock significant quantities of whole blood. An exception to this rule may be the utility of whole blood transfusions within the field setting for military

TABLE 28–1 Frequency of Blood Groups in the General Population

Blood Groups	Frequency (%)
Type	
O	47
A	41
B	9
AB	3
Rh factor	
Rh⁻	15
Rh⁺	85

From Guyton AC (ed): Textbook of Medical Physiology, 6th ed. Philadelphia, WB Saunders, 1981.

TABLE 28–2 The Blood Groups with Their Genotypes and Constituent Agglutinogens and Agglutinins

Genotypes	Blood Groups	Agglutinogens	Agglutinins
OO	O	—	Anti-A and anti-B
OA or AA	A	A	Anti-B
OB or BB	B	B	Anti-A
AB	AB	A and B	—

From Guyton AC: Textbook of Medical Physiology, 6th ed. Philadelphia, WB Saunders, 1981.

operations in which studies have shown promising use of whole blood both for the treatment of hemorrhagic shock and for correcting trauma-induced coagulopathies.[3,4]

Group O⁻ whole blood was in the past designated the "universal donor" blood, because a recipient's naturally occurring antibodies (anti-A and anti-B) do not react with donor group O RBCs. Nonetheless, some donor serum may have a high titer of naturally occurring anti-A and anti-B antibodies capable of hemolyzing the recipient's RBCs if large quantities of blood are transfused. The significance of varying titers of anti-A and anti-B antibodies in the donor's whole blood may be essentially eliminated if packed cells are used instead of whole blood. Other RBC antigens on type O RBCs may sensitize the patient or cause antibody production, complicating future cross-matching or possibly causing future hemolytic transfusion reactions.

Approximately 25% of patients receiving a transfusion of 5 or more units of type O whole blood develop hyperbilirubinemia suggestive of a minor hemolytic reaction. Large amounts of group O whole blood may cause the patient to acquire significant amounts of anti-A and anti-B antibodies that have been passively transfused; hemolysis of RBCs may then occur when the recipient's original blood group is subsequently transfused. In a resuscitation attempt, one should continue to use group O blood if large amounts (i.e., >2 units) of whole blood have already been given.

PRBCs

PRBCs are prepared by centrifugation and removal of most of the plasma from citrate- anticoagulated whole blood. One unit of PRBCs contains the same red cell mass as 1 unit of whole blood at approximately half the volume and twice the hematocrit (70%–80%). One unit of PRBCs raises the hematocrit approximately 3% in an adult, or increases the hemoglobin level of a 70-kg individual by 1 g/dL. In children, the hematocrit rises approximately 1% for each milliliter per kilogram of packed cells. For example, if 5 mL/kg of PRBCs is transfused, the hematocrit will rise by approximately 5%. Actual changes depend on the state of hydration and the rate of bleeding. Because most of the plasma has been removed, PRBCs cause fewer transfusion and allergic reactions than whole blood.

PRBCs contain less sodium, potassium, ammonia, citrate, and antigenic protein and fewer hydrogen ions than whole blood. This may offer an advantage in patients with reduced cardiovascular, renal, or hepatic function. The rate of urticaria is still relatively high at 1% to 3% of transfusions, but the incidence of adverse reactions to packed cells is approximately one third that noted with whole blood. The benefit of increased hemoglobin must be weighed against the potential for electrolyte and acid-base imbalances after PRBC administration. Especially in cases of massive transfusion (>10 units), there is a significant risk of metabolic and respiratory acidosis and hypocalcemia, which can reach life-threatening levels. Although underlying illness or injury plays a major role in cause of death, the overall mortality of patients requiring massive PRBC transfusions is approximately 70%.[5]

Transfusion of PRBCs is indicated to provide additional oxygen-carrying capacity and expansion of volume. Packed cells are most commonly used to treat acute hemorrhage and anemia not amenable to nutritional correction. When treating acute hemorrhage, PRBCs are usually given: (1) if the hemoglobin level falls below established critical levels for that particular given patient population (see "Transfusion Thresholds," later), (2) after rapid crystalloid infusion fails to restore normal vital signs, or (3) concurrently with crystalloid infusion in the treatment of obvious life-threatening blood loss.

Washed RBCs

After centrifugation, red cells can be washed to further remove leukocytes, platelets, microaggregates, and plasma proteins. Washing reduces the titer of anti-A and anti-B antibodies, permitting safer transfusion of type O PRBCs in non-O recipients. It is specifically used to prevent allergic reactions in IgA-deficient patients.[6] Washing does not totally eliminate the risk of hepatitis. Frozen deglycerolized RBCs are also relatively free of platelets, plasma, and white blood cells, having been washed after an indefinite period of frozen storage in glycerol. Frozen and fresh RBCs function similarly; frozen RBCs provide normal levels of 2,3-diphosphoglycerate (2,3-DPG). Washed or frozen preparations should be given to patients who have had febrile (nonhemolytic) reactions to previous transfusions as a result of leukocyte antibodies or IgA sensitization. Blood bank procedures require that these be prepared to order, with routine cross-matching. Considerable delay (6 hr) may occur if the transfusion service does not have the capability to wash RBCs.

Leukocyte-Reduced RBCs

Leukocyte-reduced blood products are those that contain less than 5×10^6 leukocytes/unit, compared with standard RBC units, which contain 1 to 3×10^9 leukocytes. Reduction can be performed at the time of collection, in the transfusion laboratory, or at the bedside during transfusion. Leukocyte-reduced products are used to decrease the likelihood of febrile reactions, immunization to leukocytes, and disease transmission. They are clearly indicated for use in patients who are chronically transfused, potential transplant recipients, those who have had more than one febrile transfusion reaction in the past, and in at-risk cytomegalovirus (CMV)-seronegative patients for whom CMV-seronegative products are unavailable.[7]

Currently about 60% to 75% of the U.S. blood supply is leukoreduced.[8] Several groups advocate the use of 100% leukoreduced blood products owing to the many adverse transfusion reactions associated with leukocytes. Non-leukocyte-reduced products are virtually the exclusive method of transmission of several viruses including human T-cell lymphotropic virus (HTLV) I/II, Epstein-Barr virus (EBV), and CMV, and additionally help to reactivate and disseminate human immunodeficiency virus (HIV) and CMV. Increased rates of bacterial contamination, post-operative, and line infections have been associated with the use of non-leukoreduced products. Leukocytes lead to human leukocyte antigen (HLA) alloimmunization resulting in increased graft rejection and platelet refractoriness.[9]

Irradiated RBCs

Blood products can be irradiated to reduce the risk of graft-versus-host disease in susceptible patients. Irradiation destroys the donor lymphocytes' ability to respond to the host's foreign antigens. Irradiated products should be used for bone marrow transplant donors or recipients, directed donations from family members, HLA-matched platelets, and patients with cellular immune deficiency.[10,11] Their use is also appropriate in premature infants and in patients with leukemia or lymphoma. It is not necessary in patients undergoing chemotherapy or on steroids, or in patients with acquired immunodeficiency syndrome (AIDS) or solid tumors.

Infectious Complications of Transfusions

Although relatively uncommon, transmission of infectious diseases is the transfusion-related complication most feared by the lay public. Table 28–3 lists estimated risks of transfusion in the United States. Transmission of a wide variety of infectious diseases has been reported, but modern screening methods have sharply reduced the frequency of transmission. Viral illnesses remain the most problematic.

Between 1985 and 1999, 694 deaths associated with transfusion were reported to the U.S. Food and Drug Administration (FDA). Seventy-seven (11.1%) of these deaths were caused by bacterial contamination. However, sepsis is an uncommon occurrence because both the citrate preservative and refrigeration kill most bacteria. Concern over sepsis is responsible for the practice of completing transfusions within 4 hours and returning unused blood products to the blood bank refrigerator for future use only if they have been unrefrigerated for less than 30 minutes. Both gram-negative and gram-positive organisms are transmitted; gram-negative virulence is more commonly associated with mortality. A prospective observational study found that the rate of nosocomial infections was significantly higher in those patients receiving blood transfusion. Leukoreduction did not significantly reduce the rate of infection.[12] A multicenter study by the Centers for Disease Control and Prevention (CDC) evaluated the risks of bacterial contamination in the blood pool. Approximately 60% of the blood was examined. The results showed that the rate of bacterial sepsis is much lower than previously thought. Only 0.21 cases and 0.13 deaths per million red cell transfu-

TABLE 28–3 Estimated Risks of Transfusion per Unit in the United States

Risk	Rate
Major allergic reactions	1:100
Anaphylaxis	1:20,000–50,000
Anaphylactic shock	1:500,000
Hemolytic reaction (minor)	1:6000
Hemolytic reaction (fatal)*	1 in every 100,000 allergic reactions
Death from sepsis (RBC)†	1:5 million
Death from sepsis (platelets)†	1:500,000
Parasitic infections (Lyme, malaria, Chagas)	<1:million/data lacking
Hepatitis C‡	<1:million
Hepatitis B‡	1:140,000
Parvovirus, Creutzfeld-Jacob disease	Extremely rare/data lacking
HTLV I/II infection	1:200,000
HIV infection‡	1:2 million
West Nile virus	Extremely rare/data lacking
CMV/Epstein-Barr‡	Rare/data lacking
Acute lung injury	1:500,000
Graft-vs.-host disease	Extremely rare/data lacking
Immunosuppression	Unknown
Syphilis‡	No cases reported currently

*694 transfusion-related deaths reported to the U.S. Food and Drug Administration.
†Mandated screening for bacterial contamination.
‡All blood routinely screened.
CMV, cytomegalovirus; HIV, human immunodeficiency virus; HTLV, human T-cell lymphotropic virus; RBC, red blood cell.

sions occurred. The rate was slightly higher for platelet transfusions, with 10 cases and 2 deaths per million transfusions.[13] Mandatory screening of platelets for bacterial contaminations began in 2004 and has further reduced the rate of reported death.

Syphilis may theoretically be transmitted by transfusion, but both refrigeration and citrate markedly reduce the survival of *Treponema pallidum*. Therefore, only fresh blood or platelet transfusions are of concern for this specific infectious risk. The incubation period for syphilis transmitted by transfusion is 4 weeks to 4 months, and the initial clinical manifestation is commonly a rash. No cases of transfusion-transmitted syphilis have been recognized for many years.[14]

The risk of parasitic infection via transfusion is exceedingly low (<1:1,000,000), although prospective blood product donors who have been to an endemic region within 12 months or treated with malarial prophylaxis within 3 years are not allowed to donate blood products. Those with a history of babesiosis or Chagas disease are permanently deferred from donating. Donors with a history of Lyme disease may donate if they are symptom free and have undergone a complete treatment course.

Viruses are the organisms most likely to be transmitted by transfusion and the agents with the greatest potential to cause serious disease. Important agents include hepatitis virus, CMV, EBV, HIV, and West Nile virus (WNV).

Most blood products have the potential to transmit hepatitis. Routine testing of blood donors for hepatitis C virus (HCV) has occurred since 1991, but initial screening tests were relatively inaccurate. Since April 1999, use of the nucleic amplification technique (NAT) to detect HCV RNA has been

hemoglobin concentrations as low as 5 g/dL,[27] but that clinically almost all patients show signs of physiologic stress at hemoglobin concentrations lower than 6.[28] In addition, the optimal hematocrit with respect to oxygen-carrying capacity and viscosity in the critically ill patient is about 33%. An early influential multicenter study exploring restrictive transfusions was the Transfusion Requirements in Critical Care (TRICC) group,[29] which compared restrictive versus liberal transfusion triggers. Restrictive transfusion, as defined by Hébert and coworkers,[29] in the setting of critically ill patients, *is transfusion of RBCs if the hemoglobin drops below 7 g/dL, and maintaining hemoglobin in the 7 to 9 g/dL range.* Using restrictive transfusion triggers, numerous studies have found no increase in morbidity or mortality, with some promising results showing *lower mortality, shorter intensive care unit (ICU) length of stay, hospital length of stay, and lower ICU admission rates, particularly in the setting of trauma.*[27-30] These favorable outcome predictors were found to exist *independent of shock indices* in trauma patients such as base deficit, serum lactate level, shock index, or anemia.[30,31] Although absolute thresholds have been proposed, current practice commonly adjusts the need for transfusions based on the individual patient.[32] Particularly close attention should be paid to the understudied subset of patients undergoing or at risk for myocardial infarction or coronary ischemia, possibly applying more liberal triggers to these patients. Wu and colleagues,[33] in a U.S.-based study of Medicare patients with acute myocardial infarction, found RBC transfusions beneficial in elderly patients when hematocrit values were lower than 33%.

The disadvantage of blood administration is based on two risks in addition to its financial burden: (1) transmitted infections and (2) inflammatory response to transfusions. In general, there is concern regarding an association between transfusions and diminished organ function or death in critically ill adult patients.[34] The risk of developing systemic inflammatory response syndrome (SIRS) independently increases with the administration of more than 4 units of PRBCs.[35,36] Red cell administration can also be correlated with increased risk of development of acute respiratory distress syndrome (ARDS) and an increased mortality from ARDS.[37] The higher incidence of multiple organ failure has been correlated with blood administration as well.[38] This has been hypothesized to be linked to immunologic alterations and their effects on plasma cytokine and cytokine receptor concentrations. When these mediators were assayed in patients receiving more than 15 units of PRBCs, both levels of interleukin and soluble tumor necrosis factors were elevated.[38] It is unclear whether the use of leukocyte-reduced PRBCs can mitigate the expected inflammatory response. Post-transfusion complications did not appear to be improved with the administration of leukocyte-reduced PRBCs in a study completed by Nathens and associates,[39] but Jensen and coworkers[40] found that postoperative infection in transfused patients can be reduced by using leukocyte-depleted PRBCs. So for a number of reasons and in a number of studies, judicious and restricted administration of PRBCs for the majority of patients along with a paradigm shift to giving only the amount of red cells needed (1 unit given when only 1 unit is needed) appears to be clinically founded. By judicious employment of restrictive transfusions, the probability of a patient requiring blood can be decreased by 42% and the volume of PRBCs transfused can decrease by 0.93 unit.[41] This may be confirmed retrospectively with the knowledge that 2 total unit PRBC transfusions account for one third of all transfusions

in the setting of trauma.[42] Clinicians can expect transfusion triggers and recommendations regarding the use of leukocyte-depleted RBCs to evolve as additional studies are performed.

Another area of transfusion study focuses on the projected need for administration of PRBCs in any given patient. Knowing which patients will need blood in the first 24-hour resuscitative period based on his or her initial presentation can be helpful to allocate resources and administer blood early. Studies have correlated the base deficit with the need for transfusion, using a cut-off of −6. Those patients with a base deficit greater than −6 have a 72% chance of requiring blood, whereas those with base deficits greater than −6 have only an 18% chance of requiring PRBCs. More elaborate scales have been proposed based on easily assessable parameters. The emergency room transfusion score has evaluated a point system based on systolic blood pressure, the presence of free fluid on the FAST scan, unstable pelvic ring fracture, advanced patient age, admission from the scene, motor vehicle collision, or fall as all being predictors of future transfusion requirements.[43]

Massive Transfusions

The term *massive transfusion* is loosely defined. In the 1970s, it was considered to be the transfusion of more than 10 units of blood to an adult (equivalent to 1 volume of the patient's blood) within 24 hours. This was historically associated with dismal survival rates of less than 10%.[44] As blood banking technology and storage methods have improved, mortality associated with massive transfusions has significantly decreased. Some sources have expanded the definition of massive transfusion and are now using more than 50 units of PRBCs within the first 24 hours of resuscitation. Despite the challenges of treating the expected post-transfusion inflammatory and immunologic complications, patients requiring massive transfusions after trauma can have reasonable outcomes. Vaslef and colleagues[45] discovered that neither total blood product transfused nor the total volume of PRBC required were significant independent predictors for mortality, and in their study, 43% of patients receiving more 50 units survived the first 24 hours of resuscitation. Other institutions have reported survivability up to 65% after 48 hours of massive transfusions,[46] leading some to advocate that there is no clear threshold beyond which further administration of blood or blood products is futile.[47]

Transfusion Coagulopathy

It has been known for the past 25 years that pathologic hemostasis follows massive blood transfusions.[48-50] Coagulopathy and subsequent uncontrolled bleeding account for 40% of trauma-related deaths.[51] The exact cause of the transfusion coagulopathy is not well understood. Although such abnormalities rarely develop within the timeframe of the initial resuscitation in the emergency department (ED), an understanding of the problem leads to a more intelligent approach to transfusion practices and the anticipation of potential problems. In patients who are given a transfusion equal to 2 blood volumes, only approximately 10% of the original elements remain. The development of transfusion coagulopathy is multifactorial and largely related to tissue injury and the subsequent acidosis, the duration of shock, and hypothermia in addition to activation, consumption, and dilution of coagulation factors.[52-54] Considering the significant alteration in blood and blood products that occurs during storage, one can readily appreciate the underlying problem associated with such high-volume transfusions.

Transfusion coagulopathy is related in part to dilution of the recipient's own platelets by transfused blood, which is itself devoid of functioning platelets. Dilutional thrombocytopenia is a well-recognized complication of massive transfusion, so obtain a platelet count if more than 5 units of blood are transfused. Consider platelet therapy after the first 10 units of blood have been given, although the platelet count is the most useful parameter for estimating the need for platelet transfusions.

Disseminated intravascular coagulopathy plays a secondary role in post-transfusion bleeding. Factors V and VIII are labile in stored blood and absent in packed cells. Fibrinogen is relatively stable in stored blood but is absent in packed cells. A deficiency of most clotting factors, especially factors V and VIII and fibrinogen, occurs with massive transfusions. This deficiency probably occurs on a "washout" or dilutional basis, although the dynamics are poorly understood. Replace these factors if necessary. Specific assays for the individual factors are available, but it is more practical to measure partial thromboplastin time (PTT), prothrombin time (PT), and fibrinogen levels. Fresh frozen plasma (FFP) has been used to correct clotting factor abnormalities secondary to dilution from massive transfusions, but its effectiveness has not been firmly established. Cryoprecipitate has also been used to replace factor VIII and fibrinogen, but it is rarely required because FFP contains some fibrinogen. FFP should be infused to correct the coagulopathy as indicated by clotting studies.

Cryoprecipitate may be required if fibrinogen levels fall below 100 mg/dL and are not adequately supplemented with FFP. Although blood component therapy is best based on measured coagulopathy parameters, a general guide using 1 to 2 units of FFP for each 5 to 6 units of blood may be given empirically in the massively traumatized or bleeding patient. Clinical examination of this ratio has recently been published and found to be inadequate, in addition to the conclusion that development and severity of coagulopathy correlate with survival outcome.[55] Recently, more aggressive empirical transfusion strategies have been proposed to avoid refractory coagulopathy in trauma patients.[56] This method consists of transfusing 1 to 1.5 units of FFP for every unit of packed cells once a coagulopathy has developed, or alternatively, beginning FFP administration before plasma factor concentration drops below 50% at a FFP : RBC rate of 1 : 1.[56]

Box 28-1 is a summary of caveats regarding transfusion practices in the acutely bleeding patient

Emergency Transfusions

In an emergency or life-threatening situation, three alternatives to fully cross-matched blood exist. The preferred substitute is type-specific blood with an abbreviated cross-match. The abbreviated cross-match includes ABO and Rh compatibility. In addition, the recipient's serum is screened for unexpected antibodies, and an immediate "spin" cross-match is performed at room temperature. This abbreviated cross-match requires approximately 30 minutes. Many institutions are now using this procedure as their standard cross-match

---

BOX 28–1   Caveats Regarding Transfusion of Blood Products in the Setting of Acute Blood Loss

The total volume of blood circulating in the body is about 7% of ideal body weight in adults and 8%–9% in children. A 70-kg adult, therefore, has a total blood volume of about 5 L.

DEFINITION OF MASSIVE BLOOD LOSS
Loss of total blood volume (10 units in a 70-kg adult) in 24 hr or loss of 50% of the total blood volume over 3 hr.

GENERALIZED GUIDE TO TRANSFUSION OF RBCs*
Rarely transfuse if hemoglobin > 10 g/dL; usually transfuse if hemoglobin < 6 g/dL. In general, the aim is to keep the hemoglobin about 7–8 g/dL, hematocrit about 30%–35%, to sustain hemostasis and oxygen delivery.[†]

In critically ill patients, a restrictive transfusion policy of administering RBCs if the hemoglobin drops below 7 g/dL, and maintaining hemoglobin levels in the 7–9 g/dL range, is at least as beneficial as more liberal criteria, except, perhaps, for those patients with acute coronary ischemia.

GENERAL GUIDE TO PLATELET TRANSFUSION
Aim for platelet count ≥ 50,000/mL^3 in actively bleeding patients,[‡] but lower thresholds may be safe, especially in the absence of bleeding.

FFP
Fibrinogen levels may fall to critical level (<1 g/dL) after 150% blood volume loss; therefore, consider FFP after 1 blood volume has been

lost. Other labile clotting factors fall to 25% activity after about 200% blood loss. Transfusing 1 unit of FFP per every 5–6 units of RBCs has been traditional teaching, but decisions are best based on coagulation profiles. Preliminary evidence indicates that an FFP : RBC ratio of 1 : 1 may be more beneficial in exsanguinating hemorrhage.

CRYOPRECIPITATE§
If FFP does not raise fibrinogen levels > 1 g/dL, consider cryoprecipitate. Use in the ED is supported, but not mandated.

PROTHROMBIN COMPLEX CONCENTRATES§
Autoplex T, Proplex, and Feiba VH. All products contain factor VII but no fibrinogen. Reversal of the INR to normal is the goal. Concomitant vitamin K is used to initiate production of clotting factors that have been blocked by warfarin. Use in the ED is supported but not mandated.

RECOMBINANT FACTOR VIIA§
No strict guidelines or proven benefits exist. May consider if
1. No heparin/warfarin effect remains.
2. Surgical control of bleeding is not possible.
3. Bleeding continues despite adequate replacement of other coagulation factors (FFP, platelets, cryoprecipitate).
4. Acidosis is corrected.
   Use in the ED is supported but not mandated.

Depends on rate of blood loss and underlying medical condition. RBC transfusion likely required with 30%–40% blood volume loss.
[†]*RBCs can contribute to hemostasis by their effect on platelet margination and function.*
[‡]*This level can be anticipated by the time the patient has received 2 blood volumes of fluid or RBC transfusions, but substantial variations exist.*
§*Use in the ED is supported but not mandated, usually administered under the advice of a consultant.*
ED, emergency department; FFP, fresh frozen plasma; INR, International Normalized Ratio; RBCs, red blood cells.
Adapted from Stainsby D, MacLennan D, Thomas J, et al: Guidelines on the management of massive blood loss. Br J Haematol 135:634, 2006; and Hébert PC, Wells G, Blajchman MA, et al: A multicenter, randomized, controlled clinical trial of transfusion requirements in critical care. N Engl J Med 340:409, 1999.

for most patients. The safety and utility of the type-specific abbreviated cross-match have been demonstrated repeatedly, and transfusion reactions occur only rarely.[57]

The second preference for an alternative to fully cross-matched blood is type-specific blood that is only ABO and Rh compatible, without screen or immediate spin cross-match. The patient's ABO group and Rh factor can be determined within 2 minutes, and in an emergency, typing of the blood group and the Rh factor is all that is necessary before transfusion. Type-specific blood that is not cross-matched has been given in numerous military and civilian series without serious consequences. While the type-specific blood is being transfused, the antibody screen and the cross-match are carried out in the laboratory. The transfusion should be stopped if an incompatibility is found.

A third alternative to fully cross-matched blood is group O blood, although type-specific blood is generally preferable.[58] It is rare that a few minutes cannot safely be expended to allow the blood bank to release type-specific blood. This assumes, however, that transport of the blood specimens and other logistic issues can be resolved to make type-specific blood available within minutes. Often, this is not the case. In addition, type O blood is often stored outside of the blood bank so as to be readily available for life-threatening emergencies. Thus, despite the theoretical preference for type-specific blood in emergency situations, type O is often a reasonable and practical alternative.

One may transfuse both Rh+ and Rh− group O packed cells in patients who are in critical condition. It is a common misconception that patients who are Rh− will have an immediate transfusion reaction if given Rh+ blood. There is no particular advantage in the Rh factor determination because preformed, naturally occurring anti-Rh antibodies do not exist. Theoretically, individuals who are Rh− may become sensitized either through pregnancy or by previous transfusions, resulting in a delayed hemolytic transfusion reaction if Rh+ blood is transfused. However, this scenario is very rare and is of no great clinical significance when compared with life-threatening blood loss. Sensitization to the Rh factor is most problematic for Rh− women of reproductive age.[59] Any sensitized patient may experience a transfusion reaction if exposed again to Rh-incompatible blood. However, significant, subsequent transfusion reactions with Rh-incompatible blood in men sensitized to the Rh factor are very rare. Many advise the routine use of the more widely available O Rh+ packed cells in all patients for whom the Rh factor has not been determined, except in females of childbearing age, for whom future Rh sensitization may be an important consideration. Once resuscitated with Rh+ packed cells, patients may receive their own type without a problem. Because individuals with O Rh− blood represent only 15% of the population and the blood may be in short supply, it is reasonable to save O Rh− blood for Rh− females of childbearing potential and to use group O Rh+ packed cells routinely as the first choice for emergency transfusions. In a study of emergency blood needs, Schmidt and associates[59] reported 601 units of Rh+ type O blood transfused to 193 patients, including 8 Rh− women, before blood type was determined. No acute hemolytic reaction occurred, and no women were sensitized. A non–emergency-based study published a rate of Rh sensitization in Rh− recipients receiving Rh+ blood at about 8%, and this may be lessened if Rh immunoglobulin is given after transfusion.[60] The conclusions drawn regarding emergency administration of non–Rh-compatible blood is that Rh immune globulin prophylaxis is recommended only for Rh− women with childbearing potential receiving Rh+ blood.

If non–cross-matched blood is transfused, the laboratory should receive a plain (without a serum separator) red-top tube of venous blood from the patient as soon as possible to begin a formal cross-match procedure. Whenever possible, this should be drawn before any blood is transfused. Brickman and coworkers[61] demonstrated that bone marrow aspirates obtained by an intraosseous needle can be used for cross-matching.[61]

Rh immune prophylaxis with human immune globulins (RhoGAM) is indicated for Rh− pregnant women who may be bearing Rh+ children and may have fetomaternal transplacental hemorrhage. These events include bleeding in early pregnancy, such as spontaneous or elective abortion, ectopic pregnancy, and other potential causes of antepartum hemorrhage such as trauma. Administration of Rh immune globulin in threatened abortions is advocated by some. The product suppresses the immune response of Rh− women to Rh+ RBCs, and it is effective when given up to 72 hours after exposure to fetal erythrocytes. Dosing of Rh immune globulin is 50 µg intramuscularly (IM) for first-trimester bleeding and 300 µg IM for later bleeding.[62] In the setting of significant fetal-maternal transfusion (usually only in the third trimester), doses may be increased. In such circumstances, Rh immune globulin is prepared in the blood bank and the correct dose is suggested on an individual basis, following confirmation of Rh status, evidence of prior sensitization, and testing for fetal erythrocytes in the mother's blood by the Kleihauer-Betke assay.

Metabolic Disturbances

RBCs undergo metabolic, biochemical, and molecular changes during storage that are collectively known as the erythrocyte *storage lesion.*[63] These changes are generally subtle, but can be measured as decreased levels of 2,3-DPG, a decrease in pH, and an increase in supernatant potassium (K+) with a concurrent decrease in intracellular K+.[64] These changes may alter the performance of red cells, but have little clinical impact on patients.

Theoretically, citrate salts, which are the usual anticoagulants in donor blood, may combine with ionized calcium in the plasma, producing hypocalcemia. In clinical practice, the hemodynamic consequences of citrate-induced hypocalcemia are minimal, although the Q-T interval may be prolonged on the electrocardiogram with citrate infusion. Supplemental calcium administration is usually not necessary even during massive blood replacement as long as circulating volume is maintained, because the liver is able to remove citrate from the blood within a few minutes. Alterations in this recommendation may be necessary in the presence of severe liver disease.

Directed and Autologous Donations

The system of "directed donations," by which friends or family members may give blood to a specific individual, has been proposed to answer the concern over HIV transmission. Some believe that the blood products derived from a relative or a friend have a lower likelihood of testing positive for an HIV infection. At this time, directed donation systems are in place in some institutions, but the practice has not been widely supported. Limited studies have shown an increased association between directed donor units and infectious disease markers, malaria, and high-risk activities.[65] There is concern that directed donor products may be less safe because social pressures may limit self-deferment of high-risk donors and because clerical errors may increase owing to the increased complexity of this system. Finally, there is concern that the directed donation plan will disrupt the normal anonymous blood donor system, leaving fewer units available for other needy patients.

Although of limited clinical applicability in emergencies, autologous donations are commonplace in elective surgery. It has been suggested that up to 10% of the blood supply could be provided through this mechanism. However, current studies show that at its peak, autologous donations represented less than 2% of total blood collections and this number is declining.[66] Most appropriate applications at this time include elective cardiac, gynecologic, orthopedic, and vascular surgical cases. Benefits of this system include avoidance of exogenous blood-borne disease and sensitization. The individual can donate 1 unit of blood weekly until 3 days before surgery. Because blood can be stored up to 35 days, the donations usually begin 5 weeks before it is needed. The blood donor will require iron supplements and must maintain a hemoglobin higher than 11 g/dL.

COLLECTION AND STORAGE OF BLOOD PRODUCTS

Table 28–4 lists some characteristics of blood and its components. Whole blood is collected from donors into 500-mL plastic bags containing 63 mL of citrate phosphate dextrose (CPD) with a resultant hematocrit of 35% to 40%. Immediately after collection, sophisticated techniques permit separation of the whole blood into various components and fractions. Blood components such as FFP, PRBCs, granulocytes, and platelets are prepared from a single donor, separated, and transfused as single units. Minor blood fractions including albumin, γ-globulin, cryoprecipitate, and fibrinogen are often pooled from multiple donors. Within 24 hours, blood is essentially devoid of normally functioning platelets and some clotting factors, especially the labile factors V and VIII. Separation into individual components permits specialized storage and transfusion techniques designed to optimize the survival and availability of each component.

As is true of whole blood, PRBCs can be stored up to 21 days, although newer preservatives such as ADSOL (adenine, dextrose, saline, mannitol, and water) may allow 49-day storage. Red cell viability decreases approximately 1%/day. The storage of blood contributes to a variety of other derangements or storage lesions. Cell metabolism continues during storage, causing a mild acidosis. This acidosis is buffered effectively by the bicarbonate derived from metabolism of citrate, assuming normal hepatic function. Even in massive transfusions, acidosis is usually more the result of the disruption of normal physiologic function than the storage of blood products themselves. Levels of 2,3-DPG decrease during storage, shifting the oxygen-hemoglobin dissociation curve to the left. This shift is of small clinical significance because 2,3-DPG levels are usually normal in transfusion recipients within 24 hours of infusion. Potassium commonly leaks from red cells during storage because of a less efficient sodium-potassium adenosine triphosphatase (ATPase)–dependent pump. Most of the potassium is absorbed by the remaining blood cells, excreted by the kidney, or shifted back into the cells owing to the alkalosis produced by metabolism of the citrate in the preservative. Hyperkalemia is clinically relevant only in newborns and patients with renal impairment.

Red Cell Substitutes

Concerns over infection, the limited blood supply, the availability of blood in isolated locations, storage difficulties, and the risk of transfusion reactions have fueled interest in the development of blood substitutes that are viable in the clinical setting. This has led to a search for the ideal red cell substitute

TABLE 28–4 Characteristics of Blood and Its Components

Component	Volume	Shelf Life	Requirements for Transfusion
Whole blood	450 mL blood	21 days at 4°C	Cross-matched
ACD	63 mL anticoagulant and		
CPD	preservative		
CPD-A	35–40% hematocrit	35 days at 4°C	
	280 mL 70% hematocrit	Same as for whole blood	Cross-matched
Packed red cells concentrate washed	250 mL	1 day at 4°C	Cross-matched
	70% hematocrit		
Frozen-thawed red cells*	250 mL	? yr when frozen, 1 day after thawing	Cross-matched
	70% hematocrit		
Platelet concentrate	30 mL	5 days at 22°C	Type-specific if possible, but not essential, not cross-matched
	10^10 platelets		
Fresh frozen plasma	200–250 mL	1 year at −18°C, 24 hr after thawing[†]	ABO-compatible; random donor, not cross-matched
Cryoprecipitate	10–25 mL per bag 60–120 units of factor VIII	1 year at −18°C, 6 hr after thawing	ABO-compatible; random donor, not cross-matched
Factor IX or prothrombin concentrate	25 mL/vial	Check label	None required
Granulocyte* concentrate	400 mL	Transfuse within 24 hr at 22°C	Specific donors for each patient, cross-matched
	10^10 leukocytes		

*Special order—few hospitals have facility in house.
[†]Immediately to correct deficiency of coagulation factors.
ACD, acid citrate dextrose; CPD, citrate phosphate dextrose; CPD-A, citrate phosphate dextrose adenine.

that would fulfill these requirements. A viable blood substitute is currently not available.

Synthetic emulsions are made from fluorinated hydrocarbons, a perfluorocarbon base with particle size of 0.2 μm, thereby permitting capillary flow. These emulsions can dissolve large quantities of oxygen in a linear relation to the partial pressure of oxygen. At high inspired oxygen levels in the lungs, oxygen goes into solution and the process is reversed at the comparatively low oxygen tensions found in the tissues. The emulsions are subsequently eliminated unchanged by the lungs. A theoretical advantage of this delivery system is its ability to reach hypoxic tissue. In the setting of hypotension, capillary beds are vasoconstricted and red cells have a difficult time perfusing this tissue, even if well oxygenated. A plasma-based oxygen-carrying system may have the advantage of greater tissue penetration.[67] Research with perfluorocarbons has been directed at finding a safe short-term vehicle for oxygen delivery in the absence of available blood. It is unlikely that synthetic emulsions will be used in the long-term management of anemia or blood loss.[68] Persistent toxicity issues most likely related to complement activation problems have yet to be overcome. Modified hemoglobin solutions are biosynthetic products in which the hemoglobin molecule is altered by polymerization or encapsulation or both. This creates a product that is fully oxygen saturated at ambient forced inspiratory oxygen (FIO_2), and also mimics the sigmoidal oxygen dissociation curve. A significant advantage of modified hemoglobin solutions is the absence of antigenic characteristics of blood groups, obviating the need for compatibility testing. Currently, the developed HBOCs have an in vivo half-life of approximately 20 hours.[69] Phase II clinical trials suggest that using HBOCs attenuates the systemic inflammatory response that can be linked to multiple organ failure.[70] Phase III trials had been under way on an α-α cross-linked diasprin solution in the setting of trauma resuscitation. This trial was stopped because of increased mortality rates at both 1 week and 28 days and the multiorgan failure scores were higher in the test group than in the controls, who were resuscitated with saline only.[71] Other phase III trials on Polyheme (Northfield Laboratory, Evanston, IL) have shown promising results, even in high-volume transfusion situations with the administration of 10 to 20 units of PRBC equivalents.[72] Because hemoglobin solutions are derived from either human or bovine sources, the potential for disease transmission exists. It is possible that recombinant DNA technology will be used in the future, substantially eliminating this risk. The stability of bovine HBOCs is excellent and they can be stored at room temperature for 3 years.[73] Modified hemoglobin has been used successfully in the clinical setting, notably in cardiac and orthopedic surgery, and also in trauma resuscitation.[74]

ORDERING OF BLOOD

Ordering a type and cross-match procedure on a blood product implies that the decision has already been made to administer a transfusion. A "type and hold" or "type and screen" (no cross-match) request alerts the blood bank to the possibility that a blood product will be required for the patient so that appropriate units can be acquired and kept on hand. A type and cross-match procedure takes 45 minutes and restricts a unit of blood to a specific patient. This limits a valuable resource and should not be requested lightly. In the ED, a cross-match procedure should be considered for a

blood product only if the adult patient (1) manifests shock, (2) has symptomatic anemia (usually associated with a hemoglobin <10 g/dL) in the ED, (3) has a documented loss of 1000 mL of blood, or (4) requires a blood-losing operation immediately (e.g., thoracotomy).[75] A type and hold can safely be requested for all other situations in which a blood transfusion is considered possible during the patient's care; a desirable ratio of units cross-matched to units transfused can thus be achieved. Hooker and colleagues[76] found that the empirical trigger of prehospital hypotension (systolic blood pressure <100 mm Hg) was a useful discriminator for ordering early cross-matched blood.

The number of units requested for a cross-match procedure is determined by the size of the patient, response of the patient to the injury and subsequent emergency treatment, and presence of ongoing blood losses (e.g., arterial or massive gastrointestinal bleeding). In the majority of fatalities from massive hemorrhage, the patients die from hypovolemia rather than from lack of oxygen-carrying capacity. Table 28–5 provides specific guidelines for administering blood components.

RBC preparations for transfusion are not routinely tested for the presence of sickle hemoglobin. Donors with sickle trait are not excluded, and blood with sickle trait can be safely given to almost every patient because occlusion of blood flow caused by intravascular sickling would occur only in extreme conditions of acidity, hypoxia, or hypothermia that are unlikely to be compatible with life. Nonetheless, when transfusion is being performed in infants and patients with known sickle cell anemia, the blood bank should be alerted, and a "sickle preparation" should be requested for donor blood to avoid the infusion of sickle trait blood into such patients. In rare instances, blood from a donor with a mild variant, such as hemoglobin SC disease, has caused massive intravascular sickling and death in a hypoxic, acidotic infant.[77]

Blood Request Forms

The most important part of ordering blood components for a patient is proper identification of the patient and the intended unit of blood. Transfusion of an incorrect unit is a potentially fatal error. Most transfusion mistakes are clerical errors. Just before administering the blood, the nurse or clinician must check the identity of the numbered labels. In addition, the blood bank laboratory slip must identify the patient by name and number and contain the identification number of the unit of blood.

Usual procedures require a separate blood bank request form for each unit of RBCs or whole blood ordered. A number of units of FFP, cryoprecipitate, and platelet concentrates may be ordered on one form with proper identification (depending on individual blood bank procedures).

INTRAVENOUS ADMINISTRATION

Do not open a unit of blood unless a free-flowing intravenous (IV) access line has been established in a large-bore vein. Use a 14- to 16-gauge IV catheter if possible, both to minimize hemolysis and to ensure rapid infusion of fluid for the treatment of hypovolemia or hypotension. When a large quantity of blood must be given rapidly, administer it by means of a high-flow infusion system if possible. The purpose of a large-bore infusion line is defeated if blood is piggybacked with an

TABLE 28–5 Transfusion of Blood Products

Blood Product	Waiting Time to Receive in Emergency Department	Initial Amount to Transfuse	Expected Response in 70-kg Adult
Un–cross-matched Rh⁺ or Rh⁻ RBCs	5 min		Stabilize patient in shock
Un–cross-matched type-specific whole blood	15 min		Change in hemoglobin/hematocrit depends on hydration and rate of bleeding
Typed and screened whole blood	25 min ⎫	2–10 units, 10–20 mL/kg per hr or as needed based on clinical condition	Approximate rise of 1 g/dL hemoglobin per unit
Cross-matched whole blood	1¼ hr ⎬		Each unit raises hematocrit 2%–3%
Packed RBCs	1½ hr ⎭		In children, each mL/kg of packed cells raises hematocrit by 1%
Frozen RBCs	4–6 hr (if not prepared in house)		
Platelet concentrate†	5 min if available	1 unit/10 kg, usually 6–10 units/transfusion in an adult	Rise of 5000–10,000 platelets/mm³ per unit; 6 units usually sufficient to stop bleeding
Cryoprecipitate	20 min	1–2 bags/10 kg (7–15 bags) 10-min push, or 20–50 units/kg	Rise of 3% in factor VIII level per bag (40%–100% activity desired)
Factor IX or prothrombin concentrate	Immediately available (reconstituted powder)	10–50 units/kg	30%–100% rise in factor IX activity
FFP	40 min	1 bag/7 kg (4–10 bags for adult) 10-min push,* 3–10 mL/kg, depending on clinical condition	Correction in coagulation status; 1 unit raises all coagulation factors by 2%–3% in average-sized adult

*Administer 1 bag/4–6 units of blood transfused to replace diluted and inactivated coagulation factors. In life-threatening exsanguination, consider FFP:RBC in 1:1 replacement. Follow coagulation parameters for decision.
†Also consider thrombocytopenia as a cause of bleeding from massive transfusion.
FFP, fresh frozen plasma; RBCs, red blood cells.

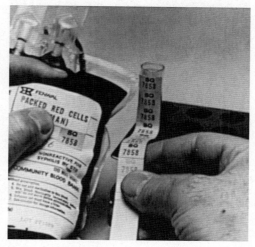

Figure 28–1 In the blood bank, cross-matched units of blood are identified with numbered labels from the patient's blood sample. *(Courtesy of Fenwal Laboratories, Deerfield, IL.)*

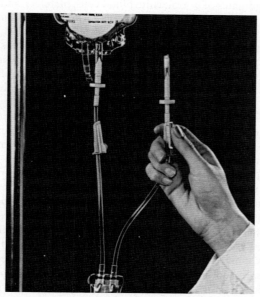

Figure 28–2 One upper adapter has been inserted into a bag containing normal (0.9%) saline. *(Courtesy of Fenwal Laboratories, Deerfield, IL.)*

18- to 20-gauge needle through a side port in the infusion tubing. For an elective transfusion, however, blood may be given through a smaller lumen. Combining hemodilution (250 mL saline to 1 unit packed RBCs) and pressurization can safely increase the flow rate through 20- and 22-gauges catheters severalfold.[78] No significant hemolysis occurs when small (21-, 23-, 25-, and 27-gauge) short needles are used for transfusion of fresh blood or packed cells in infants and children and when the maximum rate of infusion is less than 100 mL/hr.[79] For rapid infusion, however, connect the blood administration tubing directly to the infusion catheter. Monitor the infusion site for infiltration, infection, or local reactions (Figs. 28–1 to 28–4).

If the patient already has a suitable IV line in place, flush the system with a solution of normal saline before administering the blood. Do not use other IV fluids because of the risks of hemolysis or aggregation (with 5% dextrose in water)[80] or clotting (with lactated Ringer's solution).[81] Do not place any medications into the unit of blood or infusion line for the same reasons.

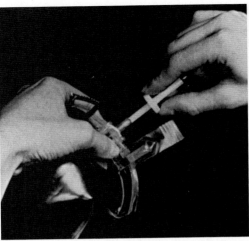

Figure 28–3   Inserting the hard plastic spike of the upper adapter. *(Courtesy of Fenwal Laboratories, Deerfield, IL.)*

Filters

Infuse all blood and blood products through an appropriate filter, such as those supplied in-line in the blood administration tubing sets. In the past, filtration was required merely to keep the IV line from becoming blocked by clots. Adverse consequences that result from infusing unfiltered blood products have since been recognized. Debris consisting of clots and aggregates of fibrin, white blood cells, platelets, and intertwined RBCs (ranging in size from 15 to 200 µm) accumulate progressively during storage of blood. The usual filter, made of a single layer of plastic with multiple 170-µm pores, traps larger particles yet allows rapid infusion of 2 to 3 units of blood before flow is obstructed. Purified components of blood plasma can be safely administered through a filter with pores as fine as 5 µm.

It has been suggested that microaggregates of debris, which could pass through a 170-µm filter, may in part contribute to the syndrome of "shock lung" seen after transfusions of many blood units in patients suffering from severe trauma and hemorrhage. Some clinicians therefore recommend using a microaggregate blood infusion filter with a mesh pore size of 40 µm when multiple units of blood are administered to a trauma victim, a patient with compromised pulmonary function, or a neonate. Microaggregate filters tend to become blocked, impeding the rate of infusion more quickly, and are not commonly required in the emergency setting. In addition, whether the infusion of microaggregates (between 40 and 170 µm in size) is in fact harmful is still an unsettled issue.[82] Replace standard filters after 2 to 3 units of blood product have been administered. Change microaggregate filters after each unit. A significant number of platelets are removed by microaggregate filters, and some advise against using these filters when platelet packs are infused. Others believe that, although platelets are removed with the microaggregate filters, the trapped platelets can be removed with saline flush without any significant loss.[83]

Rate of Infusion

One unit of whole blood can be safely administered to a hypotensive patient at a rate of 20 mL/kg per hour. In the setting of hypovolemic shock and continued hemorrhage,

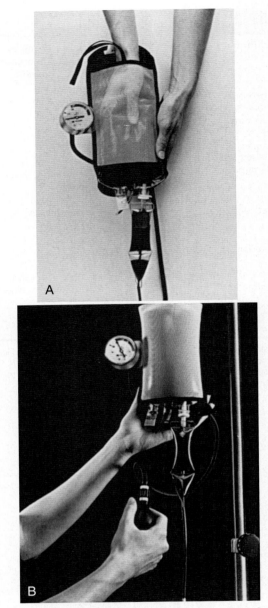

Figure 28–4   *A,* A controlled-pressure administration device for rapid infusion of blood products. *B,* A rubber bladder is pumped up, and the blood unit is squeezed uniformly against a reinforced mesh. *(A and B, Courtesy of Fenwal Laboratories, Deerfield, IL.)*

there is no limit to the transfusion rate. Multiple units may be transfused simultaneously, even under pressure. In the stable patient, administer 1 unit of whole blood (500 mL) over approximately a 2-hour period (3–4 mL/kg per hr). After this time, RBCs begin to lose metabolic activity. In addition, the unit of blood, which is an excellent culture medium, is likely to become contaminated if bacteria and fungi are allowed to grow at room temperature. Give packed cells at approximately the same rate. Give plasma products more rapidly. In a patient with a healthy cardiovascular system, administer FFP more rapidly (~15–20 min/unit) to correct coagulation deficits because the coagulant activity begins to deteriorate rapidly after 20 to 30 minutes of thawing. In patients with severe anemia and congestive heart failure, give a rapidly acting diuretic, such as furosemide (0.5 mg/kg intravenously), at the onset of transfusion to prevent circulatory overload.

If a transfusion of blood must be interrupted or delayed for any reason, return the remainder of the blood unit to the blood bank. Refrigerators in the ED or on the hospital unit should not be used to store blood products unless they are temperature controlled or continuously monitored and alarmed.

For patients in hemorrhagic shock, administer blood through two large-bore catheters at different sites if necessary. Usually, gravity provides a sufficient pressure gradient if the unit is raised above the patient to increase the rate of infusion when the clamps are wide open. Use a pressure pump (see Fig. 28–4) to make the infusion quicker.[84] Do not use a standard sphygmomanometer cuff wrapped around a unit of blood to create increased infusion pressure because the non-uniform application of pressure could burst the plastic bag containing the blood component.

If desired, dilute PRBCs with normal saline (0.9%, without dextrose) before infusion simply by opening the clamps on the upper tubes of the Y infusion set and leaving the lower (recipient end) clamps closed. Although it is generally agreed that lactated Ringer's solution should never be mixed with blood because of possible clot formation, two studies have demonstrated that a small amount of lactated Ringer's solution is compatible with blood. King and associates[85] found that 100 mL could be added to a unit of PRBCs without precipitating blood clotting, and Cull and coworkers[86] suggested that up to 150 mL of lactated Ringer's solution may be safely added as a diluent to each unit of PRBCs. Therefore, blood inadvertently mixed with a small amount of lactated Ringer's solution need not be routinely discarded. Diluting the blood, while increasing the volume, will allow for more rapid infusion by decreasing the blood viscosity, which is dependent on hematocrit. Alternatively, add approximately 200 mL of normal saline directly to the bag of PRBCs to bring the hematocrit in the blood bag to approximately 45%.

Rewarming

Blood is stored at approximately 4°C to maintain cellular integrity and to prevent the overgrowth of microorganisms. Blood products usually passively warm to 10°C by the time they are administered to the patient, unless administered under pressure. Adverse effects of hypothermia on cardiac conduction and flow rates are evident when rapid administration of a large volume of blood is performed without prewarming.

Various mechanisms have been used to warm blood to 35°C to 37°C. An ideal blood warmer should allow liberal flow rates while preventing thermal hemolysis of blood cells. Commonly used devices are bath coils that allow a plastic tube to reside in a closely regulated warm water bath and dry heat devices that allow blood to circulate through flat, thin bags sandwiched between aluminum blocks that contain electric heating elements. Both devices have relatively low flow rates and suboptimal thermal clearance.[87] Blood bag immersion in warm water baths is safe, but is considered imprecise and slow. Although much interest surrounds the use of microwave heating devices, the technique is not recommended by the Association of Blood Banks because of the risk of hemolysis. Herron and colleagues[88] advocated keeping the PRBC temperature below 50°C because they noted significant hemolysis beginning at 51°C to 53°C.

Rapid admixture warming is a promising alternative technique.[89] Mix the unit of whole blood with an equal amount of normal saline, which has been preheated to 60°C to 70°C. Once mixed, administer the product to the patient with a resultant delivery temperature of approximately 35°C. This technique combines dilution of blood product and warming into one step. Regardless of the rewarming technique used, warming refrigerated blood to body temperature decreases its viscosity two- to threefold and avoids venous spasm, thus facilitating transfusion.

Monitoring

During the first part of the transfusion of any blood product, carefully monitor the patient for evidence of a transfusion reaction. Look for signs and symptoms such as hives, chills, diarrhea, fever, pruritus, flushing, abdominal or back pain, tightness in the chest or throat, and respiratory distress. A potentially life-threatening acute hemolytic transfusion reaction in a patient who has received prior transfusions may differ clinically from a minor allergic reaction only by its effects on the patient's pulse and blood pressure. Treat an allergic reaction (hives, itching) to leukocytes or plasma proteins by administering an antihistamine (but not into the blood infusion line) and stop the transfusion.

Stop the transfusion immediately when the following signs are encountered: an increase in pulse rate, a decrease in blood pressure, respiratory symptoms, chest or abdominal discomfort, or a sensation of "impending doom." Administer normal saline to maintain blood pressure and urine output. Send samples of urine and blood to the laboratory to verify the presence of free hemoglobin. Also send the blood bank a clotted sample of blood to reassess the presence of an immune reaction. If the blood bank concludes that the reaction is a nonhemolytic allergic response, premedicate with antihistamines (diphenhydramine or hydroxyzine) and antipyretics before the next transfusion. Alternatively, use washed cells.

If a hemolytic transfusion reaction is suspected, treat the patient vigorously and promptly.[90] Most morbidity and mortality are secondary to hypotension and shock leading to cardiovascular instability, renal insufficiency, respiratory manifestations, or hemorrhagic complications of disseminated intravascular coagulation. Direct initial treatment of the hypotension by infusing 5% dextrose in saline or lactated Ringer's solution or vasopressors, if required. Determine the volume and rate of infusion by blood pressure response. Treat symptomatically with acetaminophen, a warming blanket, inhaled or subcutaneous β-agonists for bronchospasm or subglottic edema, and antihistamines.

If an acute hemolytic transfusion reaction occurs, alkalinize the urine with IV sodium bicarbonate to prevent the precipitation of free hemoglobin. Force diuresis with mannitol to maintain the urine output at 50 to 100 mL/hr. The benefit from alkalinization and diuresis in the prevention of acute renal shutdown is uncertain, although the use of these techniques is commonly advocated. After shock is controlled, assess hemostasis, respiratory function, renal function, and cardiac function to help direct later therapy of the complications; disseminated intravascular coagulation may require the administration of plasma, platelets, or fibrinogen, and acute tubular necrosis may dictate careful fluid management.

Hemolytic transfusion reactions have become unusual. They are rarely fatal and are usually attributable to an error in identification (such as can result from the treatment of two "John Doe" patients simultaneously).

Delayed, or "late," hemolytic transfusion reactions may occur days, or even weeks, after transfusion of RBCs. They are characterized by falling hemoglobin levels, jaundice, hemoglobinemia, and indirect hyperbilirubinemia.[91] This complication is usually self-limited and is not life threatening. Therapy is symptomatic, but future attempts at cross-matching for transfusions may be difficult because of the presence of RBC antibodies. Individuals so affected should wear identification tags or bracelets to alert medical personnel that prior transfusion reactions have occurred.

On completion of a transfusion, make an entry in the patient's record to indicate the type and volume of the transfusion and the presence or absence of any reaction. The progress note, the transfusion record sheet, or the transfusion laboratory slip can be used for this purpose and should be signed and dated by the clinician, in accordance with hospital policies. Discard the bag in which the blood was stored or return it to the blood bank, as individual policies dictate.

Emphasize to the patient and family how critically important any blood transfusion is to the patient's care. Suggest that the family consider arranging for replacement donations of units of blood to afford future patients the luxury of an ample, available supply of blood products.

Blood Products

Administration of Blood Components

When it has been decided that a patient needs a transfusion and the patient's condition is stable enough, ask the patient or relatives concerning any previous transfusion reactions and whether the patient abides by any religious prohibitions to transfusions. A tube of blood (~2 mL for every unit of blood product to be cross-matched) should be drawn from the patient and put into a red-topped, nonanticoagulated tube. The tube must not contain a serum separator gel. The label should be signed by the individual drawing the blood sample. This identifying signature will be used in the blood bank's cross-matching procedures.

Platelet Concentrates. Platelet concentrates are prepared by rapid centrifugation of platelet-rich plasma. Platelets are obtained by single-donor apheresis or from random donor whole blood units. HLA-matched platelets may be used when patients develop HLA antibodies from repeated random donor platelet transfusions. Platelet concentrates contain most of the platelets from 1 unit of blood in 30 to 50 mL of plasma. One unit (pack) of platelets per 7 kg of body weight will raise the platelet count by 50,000/mm³ in the absence of antibodies; therefore, 1 unit of platelet concentrate raises the platelet count by 5000 to 10,000/mm³. The usual adult dose is 6 to 10 units of platelet concentrate, depending on the clinical condition. Assuming a zero platelet level, 6 units given to a normal-sized adult should increase the platelet count to greater than 50,000 per mm³. If there is no evidence of platelet consumption, this transfusion should be adequate for 3 to 5 days. In cases of severe platelet consumption, the transfusion may be required every 6 to 24 hours. Some hospital blood banks prepare platelet concentrates regularly; in some cities, a central blood bank service, such as the American Red Cross, prepares platelet concentrates regularly and delivers units on an as-needed basis within 1 to 2 hours of the request. Platelet concentrates are viable for 5 days when kept at room temperature and gently agitated at intermittent periods or when kept in motion. They should not be refrigerated.

The issue of prophylactic platelet transfusion remains controversial. Spontaneous bleeding rarely occurs if the platelet count is greater than 10,000 to 20,000/mm³. Even in the event of surgery or trauma, excessive bleeding is uncommon in patients whose platelet count exceeds 50,000/mm³. It is generally recommended that active hemorrhage be treated with platelet transfusion if the platelet count is less than 50,000/mm³, but prophylactic transfusion may be safely withheld until the platelet count is less than 20,000/mm³ and more recent data suggest this threshold be lowered to less than 10,000/mm³.[92,93] Patients with idiopathic thrombocytopenic purpura should not receive platelets prophylactically, but they may be transfused if life-threatening bleeding occurs.

Cross-matching is unnecessary for platelet transfusion, but the donor and the recipient should be ABO- and Rh-compatible. Note that platelet concentrates contain enough RBCs to sensitize an Rh⁻ individual.

There may be a diluting effect to the platelet count that results in thrombocytopenia with massive blood transfusions. When more than 10 units of blood are transfused, the platelet count must be routinely evaluated, and platelets must be replaced accordingly. Clinically significant platelet depletion rarely occurs if less than 15 units of blood (or 1.5–2 times blood volume) have been transfused.[94]

Each 5 to 6 units of platelets contains 250 to 350 mL of plasma (~1 bag of FFP), which includes coagulation factors that may reduce the requirements of FFP. Platelets may be infused rapidly (1 unit/10 min) using specialized platelet filters.

FFP. FFP is prepared by separating plasma from the cellular components of single-donor whole blood, followed by rapid freezing and storage at 18°C or lower. Freezing preserves soluble coagulation factors of the intrinsic and extrinsic clotting systems, including the labile factors V and VIII. FFP also contains fibrinogen, although not as much as cryoprecipitate. Plasma stored for 3 months retains approximately 60% of the normal factor VIII activity and the product has a shelf life of up to 1 year. Thawed solvent-/detergent-treated plasma stored at 4°C for 6 days still contains sufficient coagulant activities of factors II, V, VII, VIII, IX, XI, and XII, fibrinogen, antithrombin, protein Cm and von Willebrand factor antigen and can be safely administered.[95] Ideally, transfused plasma should be compatible with the recipient's ABO group. Rh compatibility is not considered essential.[96] Each unit of FFP has a volume of approximately 200 to 250 mL.

Give FFP to patients with a hereditary or acquired deficiency of coagulation factors, provided that a preparation of the specific deficient factor is not available. FFP is indicated for the clotting factor deficiencies resulting from massive blood replacement. However, pathologic hemorrhage after massive transfusions is often caused by thrombocytopenia rather than by a depletion of clotting factors. More aggressive FFP replacement formulas are becoming commonplace, rather than the accepted 1 unit of FFP for every 5 to 6 units of PRBCs (see "Massive Transfusions," earlier), but plasma replacement is best dictated by evaluation of PT and PTT. Use FFP for rapid reversal of serious acute bleeding from warfarin (Coumadin) anticoagulants or for prophylaxis before surgery or an invasive procedure. Timing of the FFP administration seems to be key and this can only be facilitated by the early recognition. In a study on warfarin-related intracranial hemorrhage (ICH), each 30-minute delay in administering the first dose of FFP translated into a 20% less chance of reversing the patient's coagulopathy within the first 24 hours (a significant predictor of mortality).[97] In an emergency situation, 5 to 10 mL/kg of FFP will effect a rapid reversal of the vitamin K–dependent factors II, VII, IX, and X. As a rough guide, 1 unit of FFP increases all coagulation factor levels by 2% to 3% in the average-sized adult. In life-threatening hemorrhage from warfarin excess, factor IX concentrate (Konyne 80, Proplex, Mononine) may be used, but such therapy should not be routine because of the high incidence of hepatitis and the possibility of thrombosis with these products.[98]

FFP may be valuable in patients with other clotting abnormalities, such as a congenital deficiency of factor II, V, VII, X, XI, or XIII; von Willebrand syndrome; hemophilia A (factor VIII deficiency); hemophilia B (factor IX deficiency); or hypofibrinogenemia. However, the effectiveness is limited in severe clotting abnormalities because of the large volume that is generally required. For example, FFP may be successful in the treatment of hemarthrosis or other minor bleeding tendencies in hemophilia, but specific factor replacement is preferred. Use FFP to treat the acquired deficiency of multiple factors such as those seen in severe liver disease, disseminated intravascular coagulation, or vitamin K depletion, and for plasma exchange in thrombotic thrombocytopenic purpura or hemolytic uremic syndrome. Do not use FFP for volume expansion or to enhance wound healing.

Reactions to FFP may include fever, chills, allergic responses, HIV infection, and a risk of hepatitis similar to the risk with whole blood. Infuse FFP rapidly and give it immediately after thawing because the clotting factors are labile and rapidly loss.

Start by giving 2 bags of FFP if the PT is greater than 1.5 times normal or the activated PTT (aPTT) is greater than 1.5 times the top normal value. If the PT is less than 22 seconds or the aPTT is in the 55- to 70-second range, 1 bag of FFP may be sufficient to bring the deficit into the hemostasis range (Table 28–6). Each 5 to 6 units of platelets contain the equivalent of 1 unit of FFP, so concomitant platelet infusions may lower FFP requirements.

Cryoprecipitate. Cryoprecipitate is prepared from single-donor plasma by gradual thawing rapidly frozen plasma. This process causes precipitation of proteins rich in fibrinogen as well as factor VIII. This process yields 100 to 250 mg of fibrinogen, 80 to 100 units of factor VIII, and 50 to 60 mg of fibronectin.[6] Initially, the plasma also contains 40% to 70% of von Willebrand factor, although this degrades during storage. Cryoprecipitate is a plasma product and as such requires ABO compatibility.

Appropriate uses for cryoprecipitate include some patients with hemophilia A or von Willebrand disease, fibrinogen deficiency, congenital afibrinogenemia, dysfibrinogenemia, and factor XIII deficiency.[99,122] Cryoprecipitate is used to correct a deficiency of coagulation factor VIII (in hemophilia A and von Willebrand syndrome), factor XIII, or fibrinogen. It is of no value in the treatment of factor IX deficiency (hemophilia B). One bag of cryoprecipitate per 5 kg of body weight will raise the recipient's factor VIII level to approximately 50% of normal. The large number of units that must be given increases

TABLE 28–6 Approach to the Patient with a High INR from Warfarin Therapy

Clinical Setting	Action
INR > the therapeutic range but < 5.0; **bleeding absent**	Lower the dose or omit the next dose of warfarin. Resume therapy at a lower dose when the INR approaches therapeutic range. If the INR is only minimally above therapeutic range (≤10%), dose reduction may not be necessary.
INR 5.0–9.0; **bleeding absent***	Cease warfarin therapy; consider reasons for elevated INR and patient-specific factors. If bleeding risk is high, give vitamin K (1.0–2.5 mg orally or 0.5–1.0 mg intravenously). Measure INR within 24 hr; resume warfarin at a reduced dose once INR is in therapeutic range.
INR > 9.0; **bleeding absent†**	When there is a low risk of bleeding, cease warfarin therapy, give 2.0–2.5 mg vitamin K orally or 1 mg intravenously. Measure INR in 6–12 hr; resume warfarin therapy at a reduced dose once INR < 5.0. When there is a high risk of bleeding, cease warfarin therapy, give 1 mg vitamin K intravenously and fresh frozen plasma (150–300 mL); measure INR in 6–12 hr; resume warfarin therapy at a reduce dose once INR < 5.0.
Any clinically significant bleeding in which warfarin-induced coagulopathy is considered a contributing factor or INR > 20‡	Cease wafarin therapy, give 5–10 mg vitamin K intravenously, and fresh frozen plasma (150–300 mL); assess patient continuously until INR < 5.0 and bleeding stops. **Or** If fresh frozen plasma is unavailable, cease warfarin herapy, give 5–10 mg vitamin K intravenously, and Prothrombinex-HT (25–50 IU/kg); assess patient continuously until INR < 5.0, and bleeding stops. See text for discussion of the use of factor VIIa.

*See text for additional information on vitamin K. All references refer to vitamin K₁. High risk: elderly, history of bleeding, cancer, renal failure, anemia, hypertension, severe cardiovascular disease. Most patients can be followed as outpatients. Admit high-risk/unreliable patients.
†Admit/prolonged observation in high-risk patients/observe, repeat INR, discharge with close follow-up in very low risk patients.
‡Hospital admission.
INR, International Normalized Ratio.

the chance of exposure to blood-borne diseases—so do not use cryoprecipitate to treat HIV-negative hemophiliacs. Factor VIII concentrate is a better choice because of improved methods of viral inactivation and the availability of factor VIII prepared using recombinant DNA technology.

Mild deficiencies of factor VIII are defined as 10% to 30% of normal activity and severe deficiencies as less than 3% of normal activity. When treating bleeding, the goal depends on the site and severity of hemorrhage, but in general, aim for at least 50% of normal factor VIII activity. For life-threatening hemorrhage, aim for 100% activity. The amount of cryoprecipitate required to correct coagulation defects ranges from 10 to 20 units/kg for minor bleeding, such as hemarthrosis, to 50 units/kg for bleeding control in surgery or trauma. Guide specific replacement by laboratory assay of factor VIII activity. The half-life of factor VIII in plasma is 8 to 12 hours.

Rarely, cryoprecipitate may be required to correct significant hypofibrinogenemia (<100 mg/dL). FFP may also be used to treat mild degrees of hypofibrinogenemia.

Factor VII. Activated factor VII (rVIIa) is a recombinant DNA product that has been FDA approved to control bleeding in patients with hemophilia A or B who have inhibitors to factors VIII and IX. It works by binding to the surface of activated platelets, which then activate factor X. This then complexes with factor Va leading to thrombin burst and clot formation. Factor VII has a half-life of 2.72 hours. There is a reported thromboembolic rate of 1% to 2%.[100]

Increasingly, the product is being used in the emergency setting to control bleeding in patients who are not hemophiliacs, thus it has been dubbed the "universal hemostatic agent."[101] One multi-institutional study found that of 701 patients receiving factor VII, 92% were for off-label uses.[102] An abundance of anecdotal evidence has been reported supporting the efficacy of factor VII outside of its approved uses. In addition, several randomized, controlled trials have been performed looking at the use of rVIIa in specific settings, including ICH, gastrointestinal bleeding, and trauma. A significant consideration when contemplating the use of factor VII is cost. At an average cost per dose of $5,000 (80 μg/kg), this can be a limiting factor, especially when some studies are basing results on protocols using eight sequential doses.[103] However, when cost has been compared with adjusted quality of life with years of nontreatment, factor VII has been cost effective and sometimes cost saving.[104,105] Three general usage patterns emerging within the emergency setting are explored later.

ICH. ICH is a poor predictor of survivability and of neurologic function in a patient who has undergone an acute stroke. Risk of hemorrhage expansion within the first 24 hours is between 20% and 40% in these patients, and goal-directed therapy to minimize this risk is critical.[106] In 2005, Mayer and associates[107] published a double-blind, placebo-controlled trial that evaluated the use of rVIIa for acute ICH. They randomized 399 patients to placebo, 40 μg, 80 μg, or 160 μg/kg of rVIIa within 1 hour of a baseline computed tomography (CT) scan of the head. A repeat CT scan was performed at 24 hours. The primary outcome measured was the percentage change in volume of ICH from initial to repeat scan.

The study showed an increase in volume of the ICH of 29% in the placebo group compared with 16%, 14%, and 11% in the treatment groups, respectively. Ninety-day out-comes were also evaluated and showed a rate of death or severe disability in 69% of patients in the placebo group, and 55%, 49%, and 54% in the rVIIa groups, respectively. When looking at mortality alone, the rate was 29% in the placebo group compared with 18% in the rVIIa groups combined. In subgroup analysis, treatment was found to be more effective if given within 3 hours of symptom onset.

Other study groups have shown similar results with cessation of hematoma expansion being favorable in the factor VII treatment groups.[108] If a treatment window of 3 hours is firmly established, the impact of factor VII treatment could be felt by an estimated 15% to 20% of patients.[109,110]

Interestingly, systemic hemostasis with factor VII may not prohibit specific clot-directed therapy for stroke, as illustrated in a case report of the use of factor VII followed by successful local thrombolysis in a stroke patient.[111]

Trauma. The literature is becoming replete with submissions regarding the use of factor VII in trauma. A study by Bofford and coworkers in 2005[112] enrolled 301 ED patients presenting with major trauma who required at least 8 units of PRBCs. The treatment group received three doses of rFVIIa immediately after the 8th unit of blood had been given. Repeat doses were given at hours 1 and 3. The primary outcome measured was the total transfusion requirement, and evaluation was performed in subgroups of blunt and penetrating trauma. For blunt trauma, a small decrease was found in the transfusion requirement (7.0 units in treatment group vs. 7.5 in placebo group, $P = 0.02$), and there was a decrease in the number of patients needing massive transfusion (14% of the treatment group vs. 33% of the placebo group, $P = 0.03$). In the penetrating trauma group, the differences were not statistically significant. Other study groups have found that administration of factor VII can favorably affect the 24-hour survivability of trauma, but the patients requiring massive transfusions saw less benefit from the product.[113] The severely injured requiring massive transfusions and who develop profound coagulopathy and acidosis may not benefit at all from administration of factor VII.[114] The use of factor VII in trauma also has been tied to decreased subsequent need for other blood products, specifically PRBCs, cryoprecipitate, and platelets.[115,116]

In 2005, Raobaikady and colleagues[117] evaluated a group of 48 patients with traumatic pelvic fracture who were scheduled for large surgical repair. Patients were randomized to a dose of 90 μg/kg of rFVIIa or placebo at the time of first incision. No significant difference was found in the primary outcome measure of transfusion requirement.

Gastrointestinal Bleed. Although the data supporting the use of factor VII in gastrointestinal hemorrhage is generally more anecdotal or involving very small series of patients, early results have been favorable regarding its use. Some studies based solely on treatment of esophageal varices have been encouraging.[118] Theoretically, the cirrhotic population with bleeding esophageal varices would seem to be a tailor-made population for the use of factor VII because both coagulopathy from liver disease and bleeding are key components of the pathophysiology. A study in *Gastroenterology* in 2004[103] evaluated the use of rFVIIa in patients with cirrhosis and either melena or hematemesis. Eight doses of rFVIIa or placebo were given at timed intervals, and the rate of treatment failure was evaluated.[103] No significant differences were found in the rate of treatment failure, transfusion requirements, or mortality.

Thromboembolic Events. Of the studies just reviewed, none found a significant increase in the rate of serious adverse events, although Mayer and associates[119] did find a trend toward an increase in the rate of thromboembolic events including ischemic cardiac changes, deep venous thrombosis, and pulmonary embolism.

In summary, rFVIIa does show promise as a treatment for uncontrolled bleeding, especially in the setting of ICH. However, there is some risk of increased thromboembolism and more evidence is needed to determine the value of this treatment modality.

Factor VIII Concentrate

Human Antihemophilic Factor. Factor VIII extracted from pooled human plasma produces a concentrated stable product with a shelf life of up to 2 years. Significantly more concentrated than cryoprecipitate and available for home use, factor VIII concentrate was a major breakthrough in the treatment of hemophilia. Unfortunately, the presence of viruses in the donor pool contributed to the high prevalence of hepatitis and HIV in hemophiliacs who used earlier versions of this product. Newer products (Alphanate, Hemofil, Humate-P, Koate-DVI, Monarc-M, Monoclate-P) are produced using one or more methods to reduce viral contamination including heat treatment, pasteurization, organic solvents and detergents, gel filtration, and immunoaffinity chromatography. These methods have markedly reduced the risk of viral transmission, especially lipid-encapsulated viruses (HIV, HBV, HCV). To date, there are no reports of transmission of these viruses with the products listed earlier.

Recombinant Antihemophilic Factor. Since the gene for factor VIII production was discovered in 1984, research into recombinant genetics has aimed to provide a safer product that theoretically will be more readily available and less expensive to produce. Two recombinant DNA–derived factor VIII preparations (Recombinate, Kogenate) were approved by the FDA in 1993. More recent introductions include Bioclate, Helixate, Helixate FS, and Kogenate FS. These genetically engineered products have hemostatic activity equivalent to plasma-derived factor VIII and minimal risk of viral contamination. Because some of these products are prepared using human albumin and other animal proteins, there is potential for viral transmission. Products such as Helixate FS and Kogenate FS are prepared without human albumin, which should eliminate viral contamination. Although costlier, they are a better choice for young and newly diagnosed patients who have not already been exposed to hepatitis or HIV.[120]

Use of Factor VIII Concentrate. Administration of 1 unit of factor VIII concentrate per kilogram of body weight should increase the factor VIII activity by 2% to 2.5%. Dosage should be individualized based on the severity of bleeding, the known deficiency of factor VIII activity, and the presence of factor VIII antibodies. Factor VIII levels should be increased to 20% to 40% of normal for minor bleeds (small joint), 40% to 60% for moderate bleeds (large joint, neck, oral cavity), and 60% to 100% for life-threatening bleeds (intracranial, intra-abdominal, pharyngeal).

Antibodies develop in up to 15% of factor VIII recipients. Administration of massive doses of factor VIII has proved beneficial in overwhelming the endogenous antibody response. In addition, immunoadsorbent techniques to remove the antibody have met with some success. The general use of immunosuppressives and plasmapheresis has had limited success.

Activated prothrombin complex has been effective, but concern over the cost of preparation, the significant hepatitis risk, and the thrombogenicity associated with its use limits its application.

1-Deamino-(8-D-Arginine)-Vasopressin. A synthetic analogue of pituitary vasopressin, 1-deamino-(8-D-arginine)-vasopressin (DDAVP), has been found to stimulate the endogenous production of factor VIII in a subset of mild hemophiliacs. The exact mechanism is unknown, but treatment with 0.3 mg/kg intravenously over 15 minutes has been recommended when avoidance of the inherent risks of the factor VIII concentrate is desired.

Factor VIII Inhibitor Bypassing Activity. Factor VIII inhibitor bypassing activity (FEIBA) is a product derived from pooled human plasma containing factors II, VII, IX, and X. It promotes coagulation by bypassing the need for factors VIII and IX. FEIBA is vapor heated to achieve greater than 10 logs of reduction in all target viruses and its safety profile is favorable.[121] FEIBA is used to treat bleeding episodes in hemophilic patients with antibodies to factor VIII and is generally efficacious in this role.[122] Adverse reactions include headache, fever, chills, flushing, nausea, vomiting, and an occasional allergic reaction. The risk of thrombotic complications exists, especially in patients with liver and heart disease or those who are pregnant or breastfeeding.[122]

Factor VII in the Hemophiliac Population.

Although factor VII is being used more and more in nonhemophiliac patients, its original indication was for hemophiliacs who had developed factor VIII inhibitors and were having acute bleeding events. Study dosages for these patients were generally higher than for off-label usage (100–300 µg), but the drug was effective in controlling bleeding episodes with an acceptably low rate of thromboembolic events.[123,124]

Factor IX Concentrate.

Factor IX is prepared from pooled human plasma and is available as a lyophilized powder either as an isolated factor concentrate (Alphanine, Mononine) or as prothrombin complex concentrate, which also includes the liver-synthesized, vitamin K–dependent factors II, VII, and X (Bebulin, Konyne, Profilnine, or Proplex). Factor IX is also available using recombinant technology.

Historically, the use of factor IX concentrate has carried a very high risk of hepatitis transmission. However, improved donor screening and new methods of viral reduction have substantially reduced the risk of viral transmission. As with factor VIII concentrate, the risk of HIV and hepatitis transmission is very low using current human-derived products. Recombinant factor IX is not derived from human products and carries no risk of viral transmission.

Factor IX is indicated for the treatment of bleeding episodes in hemophilia B patients with severe deficiency of factor IX. FFP is the preferred treatment in patients with mild to moderate deficiency. Administration of 1 unit/kg body weight will increase the factor IX concentration approximately 1%. High levels of factor IX are not required to control bleeding. Levels should be increased to 15% to 25% of normal for mild to moderate bleeding and 25% to 50% of normal for more serious bleeds or before major surgery.

Hypercoagulable states have been reported after factor IX infusions, particularly with use of prothrombin complex concentrate.

Granulocyte Transfusions.

Granulocyte transfusions are indicated in severely neutropenic patients with suspected or proven bacterial infections unresponsive to appropriate treatment. They are rarely given in the emergency setting. White blood cell transfusions require prior arrangements with a large blood bank service that has the capabilities of collecting granulocytes from a suitable donor; the collection procedure takes 4 to 6 hours on a continuous-flow cell separator. Transfusions must be repeated frequently (every 12 hr) to provide a sufficient number of white blood cells to help the patient.

Blood Products for Jehovah's Witnesses. There are more than 1.5 million Jehovah's Witnesses in the United States. Based on the religious belief that the Bible prohibits blood or blood product transfusion (Acts 15:28–29), Jehovah's Witnesses do not accept transfusions of whole blood, packed cells, white blood cells, platelets, plasma, or autologous blood. Some may permit infusion of albumin, clotting factor solutions, or dextran or other plasma expanders, and intraoperative autotransfusion.[125] Although no guidelines for administration of blood products to Jehovah's Witnesses are absolute, certain recommendations can be made. Even though a transfusion may be necessary to save a patient's life and would otherwise be considered standard care, the administration of blood or blood products or both in the face of refusal after informed consent can be legally considered as battery or a violation of a patient's right to control what is done to her or his body. In the awake and otherwise competent adult, courts have ruled that clinicians cannot be held liable if they comply with a patient's directive and withhold life-saving blood administration after specific and detailed informed consent of the consequences of such an omission of treatment. The issue becomes clouded when patients are incompetent, unconscious (most Jehovah's Witnesses carry cards informing medical personnel of their religious beliefs), or minors.

In the absence of specific directives to the contrary, it is prudent to administer blood products to patients who are unconscious, judged to be incompetent adults, or minors.[126] Although case law often upholds the patient's wishes, actual damages against clinicians are difficult to document in the United States. When done under documented life-threatening circumstances, significant clinician liability would be extremely unusual. Pregnant females and significant providers for dependents have been deemed appropriate recipients of blood products against their wishes. Explicit documentation of the intent of the clinician to preserve life coupled with an accurate description of the discussion of the issue with the patient or the family and a clarification of the patient's mental capacity is mandatory. Furthermore, emergency legal assistance (e.g., court orders, appointment of a temporary guardian) should be sought immediately with rapid judicial resolution. Various clinical techniques to maximize oxygen delivery and minimize oxygen consumption should be used. Examples include limited blood draws, the use of erythropoietin and nutritional support, hypothermia, volume expansion, sedation, and oxygen.

Reversal of Warfarin-Induced Coagulopathy. Elevated International Normalized Ratios (INRs) may be encountered fortuitously or in patients with trauma or serious medical conditions. Guides to approaching and treating such patients are found in Table 28–6. In the presence of significant trauma or serious hemorrhage, any warfarin effect should be reversed. Other intervention may also be required.

To reverse warfarin, only vitamin K_1 should be used (Fig. 28–5), IV vitamin K has rarely been implicated in serious

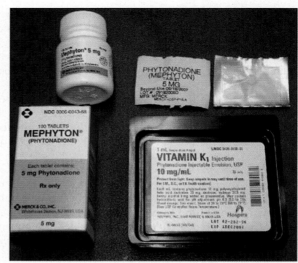

Figure 28–5 Vitamin K by the intravenous (IV) route has been implicated in serious systemic reactions and, rarely, fatalities. The oral route is universally safe and should be used when possible. If the IV route is mandated, use a dilute solution (such as 5–10 mg in 100 mL), begin with a slow rate, and be on the lookout for systemic reactions. The best remedy for a systemic reaction, likely an idiosyncratic reaction, is unknown, but general supportive measures for anaphylactoid reactions seem to work well. Vitamin K_1 can be used to reverse warfarin-induced coagulopathy, but selective use is encouraged. The IV preparation can be given orally to titrate small amounts. Tablets only are available in 5 mg strength.

anaphylactoid-like systemic reactions or, more rarely, fatalities. Oral use is universally safe, and should be used when possible. Only 5-mg tablets are available; however, the IV formulation can substitute orally for the tablets to allow for more accurate dosing. There is no strong rationale for the subcutaneous route for vitamin K. It is unclear whether any infusion protocol alleviates untoward reactions, but consider a dilute solution (e.g., 5–10 mg in 100 mL), begin with a slow rate, and monitor for systemic reactions. The best intervention for a systemic idiosyncratic reaction is unknown, but general supportive measures and protocols for anaphylaxis may be of value.

It is standard to avoid the reflex reversal of an elevated INR, especially in the absence of bleeding. Even minor bleeding can be tolerated in lieu of losing the beneficial effects of anticoagulation in select patients (e.g., those with heart valves). Use of vitamin K will render anticoagulation difficult, and it is often more prudent to simply discontinue warfarin until the INR becomes therapeutic. Usually, this takes only a few days.

Acknowledgments

The author would like to acknowledge the contributions of Jamie Treseder, MD, for her assistance and contributions in the sections on transfusion reactions, infectious complications, and factor VII therapy.

 REFERENCES CAN BE FOUND ON EXPERT CONSULT

CHAPTER **29**

Local and Topical Anesthesia

Douglas L. McGee

Local anesthetic agents are important tools used in the every-day practice of emergency medicine. This chapter describes the mechanism of action, the nuances of clinical use, and adverse reactions to anesthetics commonly used in the emergency department (ED). Detailed technical guidance for the performance of topical and infiltrative local anesthesia is provided.

BACKGROUND

The first local anesthetic was cocaine, an alkaloid in the leaves of the *Erythroxylon coca* shrub from the Andes Mountains. Early Incan society used cocaine for invasive procedures, including cranial trephination. In 1884, Koller[1] used topical cocaine in the eye and was credited with the introduction of local anesthesia into clinical practice. In the same year, Zenfel used a topical solution of alcohol and cocaine to anesthetize the eardrum, and Hall[2] introduced the drug into dentistry. In 1885, Halsted[3] demonstrated that cocaine blocked nerve transmission, laying the foundation for nerve block anesthesia. The search for alternatives to cocaine led to the synthesis of the benzoic acid ester derivatives and the amide anesthetics used today. It was not until the 1960s that a detailed understanding of the physiochemical properties, mechanism of action, pharmacokinetics, and toxicity of these agents emerged.

PHARMACOLOGY AND PHYSIOLOGY
Chemical Structure and Physiochemical Properties

Most useful local anesthetic agents share a basic chemical structure:

Aromatic segment—Intermediate
chain—Hydrophilic segment

Subtle variations of this basic structure determine each agent's main physiochemical properties: the negative log of dissociation constant (pK_a), the partition coefficient (a measurement of lipid solubility), and the degree of protein binding. Each of these properties determines the drug's potency, onset, and duration of action. Physiochemical properties are not the sole determinant of clinical activity; other factors influence the drug's effect. The intermediate chain between the aromatic and the hydrophilic segments is either an amino-ester or an amino-amide; these two chemical structures form the basis for the two main classifications of local anesthetics. Common ester-type agents include procaine, chloroprocaine, cocaine, and tetracaine. The common amide-type agents include articaine, lidocaine, mepivacaine, prilocaine, bupivacaine, and etidocaine. Different biochemical pathways metabolize each class. Esters are hydrolyzed by plasma pseudocholinesterase. Cocaine, an ester, is also partly metabolized via *N*-demethylation and nonenzymatic hydrolysis. Individuals with pseudocholinesterase deficiencies may have a greater potential for cocaine toxicity if large doses are used, although this has not been an issue when cocaine is used clinically as an anesthetic. Amides are metabolized in the liver by enzymatic degradation. Local anesthetics are poorly soluble weak bases combined with hydrogen chloride to produce the salt of a weak acid. In solution, the salt exists both as uncharged molecules (nonionized) and as positively charged cations (ionized). The nonionized form is lipid-soluble, enabling it to diffuse through tissues and across nerve membranes. The ratio of nonionized to ionized forms depends on the pH of the medium (vial solution or tissue milieu) and on the pK_a of the specific agent. The pK_a is the pH in which 50% of the solution is in the uncharged form and 50% is in the charged form. When the pH of the solution or tissue is less than the pK_a, more of the drug is ionized. When the pH increases, more of the drug is in the nonionized form. Because the nonionized form of drug can diffuse through tissues and nerves, manipulating the pH of the solution can alter a drug's diffusion properties.

Local anesthetics are available in single-dose vials or ampules and in multidose vials, with and without epinephrine. Most solutions have a pH greater than 5. Multidose vials contain methylparaben, an antibacterial preservative. Local anesthetics premixed with epinephrine also contain an anti-

TABLE 29–1 pH and Additives of Amide Local Anesthetics

Solution Content	pH (Range)	Preservative (Methylparaben)	Antioxidant
Plain, single dose	4.5–6.5	–	–
Plain, multidose	4.5–6.5	+	–
Commercial epinephrine, single dose	3.5–4.0	–	+
Commercial epinephrine, multidose	3.5–4.0	+	+
Prepared epinephrine, single dose	4.5–6.5	–	–

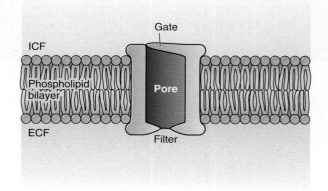

Figure 29–2 Axon membrane. *(From Wildsmith JAW: Peripheral nerve and local anesthetic drugs. Br J Anaesth 58:692, 1986. Reproduced by permission.)*

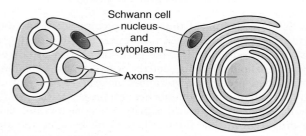

Figure 29–1 Schwann cell sheath of unmyelinated (*left*) and myelinated (*right*) nerve fibers. *(From Wildsmith JAW: Peripheral nerve and local anesthetic drugs. Br J Anaesth 58:692, 1986. Reproduced by permission.)*

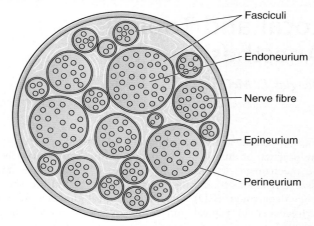

Figure 29–3 Cross-section of a peripheral nerve. *(From Wildsmith JAW: Peripheral nerve and local anesthetic drugs. Br J Anaesth 58:692, 1986. Reproduced by permission.)*

oxidant (sodium bisulfite or sodium metabisulfite) to prevent deactivation of the vasoconstrictor. These solutions must be adjusted to a more acidic pH, approximately 3.5 to 4.0, to maintain the stability of epinephrine and its antioxidant. These properties as they relate to the amide group are depicted in Table 29–1.

Nerve Structure and Impulse Transmission

Functional and Structural Components of a Peripheral Nerve

The functional nerve unit includes the nerve axon and its surrounding Schwann cell sheath. The Schwann cell (Fig. 29–1) may surround several unmyelinated axons or a single myelinated nerve fiber, forming a myelin sheath. Junctions between sheaths along the axon called *nodes of Ranvier* contain sodium channels necessary for depolarization. As myelin sheath thickness increases from autonomic to sensory to motor fibers, the nodes of Ranvier are spaced farther apart. The most important structure affecting nerve impulse transmission is the axon membrane (Fig. 29–2). The membrane is made of a double layer of phospholipids into which are embedded protein molecules that serve as channels containing pores for the movement of ions in and out of the cell. Most pores have a filter, or gate, that controls ion-specific movement and a sensor mechanism that opens or closes the gate. Bundles of nerve fibers (Fig. 29–3) are embedded in the endoneurium, which is made of collagen fibrils, and are surrounded by a cellular layer, the perineurium. The perineu-

rium functions as a diffusion barrier and maintains the composition of extracellular fluid around the nerve fibers. Surrounding the entire structure is the outer layer of a peripheral nerve, the epineurium, composed of areolar connective tissue.

The Nerve Impulse and Transmission

The inside of a nerve fiber, or axoplasm, is negative (–70 mV) at rest compared with the outside. This resting potential is the net result of the differences in ionic concentrations on each side of the axonal membrane and the forces that tend to maintain that difference. Specifically, there is a surplus of sodium extracellularly and of potassium intracellularly. The sodium channel is closed, preventing these ions from moving along their concentration gradient (out → in). Although potassium can leave the cell to follow its concentration gradient (in → out), the need to maintain electrical neutrality inside the cell prevents it from completely doing so. Potassium is in equilibrium between the concentration gradient and the electrochemical gradient, creating the negative resting potential.

The sodium channel opens when a nerve is stimulated. Sodium ions enter slowly at first until a critical threshold is reached. Sodium ions then enter the cell rapidly, along the electrochemical and concentration gradients, causing depolarization. The influx of sodium is halted when the membrane potential reaches +20 mV but potassium continues to move out of the cell, repolarizing it until the resting potential is reached. When the excitation process has been completed and the nerve cell is electrically quiet, the relative excess of sodium inside the cell and potassium outside the cell is readjusted by the adenosine triphosphate (ATP)–dependent sodium-potassium pump.

Depolarization of a portion of the nerve causes a current to flow along the adjacent nerve fiber. This current makes the membrane potential less negative and actuates the sensor to open the next sodium channel. The action potential cycle is repeated, propagating the impulse. Nerve conduction is essentially unidirectional because the sodium channel is not only closed but inactivated as well and delayed closure of specific potassium channels prevents the critical threshold from being reached in the segment just depolarized. An impulse spreads continuously down the axon in unmyelinated nerve fibers. In myelinated fibers, current flows from node to node, depolarizing intervening segments at once. This saltatory conduction causes a faster rate of impulse transmission in myelinated fibers.

Mechanism of Action

How local anesthetic agents produce nerve conduction blockade depends on the active form of the agent and specific physiologic and cellular activity.

The Active Form

Anesthetic solutions contain uncharged and charged forms. The concentration of the uncharged form increases in more alkaline milieus. Only this uncharged lipid-soluble form can cross tissue and membrane barriers. Once the uncharged drug is through a barrier, the uncharged form re-equilibrates into uncharged and charged forms in a proportion dependent on the prevailing pH. Because local anesthetics are more effective in alkaline solutions, it was originally thought that the uncharged form was responsible for conduction blockade. Alkaline solutions are currently believed to be more effective because of increased penetration through tissue barriers. The cationic charged form is responsible for the actual neuronal blockade.

The Physiologic and Cellular Basis for Neuronal Blockade

The prevention of sodium influx across the nerve membrane forms the physiologic basis for conduction blockade. Local anesthetics slow sodium influx, decreasing the rate of rise and amplitude of depolarization. If sufficient anesthetic is present and the firing threshold is not reached, the action potential is not formed. With no action potential, no impulse is transmitted and impulse conduction is blocked, resulting in local anesthesia.

How anesthetic agents prevent sodium influx is still not completely understood. It is believed that the cationic charged form blocks the action potential from inside the membrane; the agent enters the sodium channel from the axoplasmic side and binds to a receptor.[4,5] This "specific receptor" theory is well accepted and is considered the predominant mechanism in preventing sodium influx. However, this theory cannot account for the action of benzocaine and other neutral com-

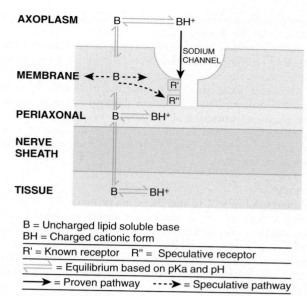

Figure 29–4 Mechanism of action of local anesthetic agents (see text for details). *(Modified from Ritchie JM: Mechanism of action of local anesthetic agents and biotoxins. Br J Anaesth 47:196, 1975. Reproduced by permission.)*

pounds or the uncharged base forms of the common local anesthetics.

In summary (Fig. 29–4), when a local anesthetic (other than benzocaine) surrounds the perineurium, it equilibrates into its uncharged and charged forms based on the tissue pH and pK$_a$. The uncharged lipid-soluble form penetrates tissue, nerve sheath, and nerve membrane to gain access to the axoplasm and re-equilibrates into both forms. The charged form enters the sodium channel and decreases sodium movement into the cell and halts nerve transmission. The uncharged base is also involved with sodium channel blockade, but the exact nature of this mechanism is unknown.

Activity Profile during Neuronal Blockade

A local anesthetic's onset, potency, and duration and its ability to produce a differential blockade in mixed nerves are a function of physiochemical properties, the physiologic environment, and to some extent, manipulation by the clinician.

Onset of Action

The pK$_a$ of an anesthetic is the primary physiochemical factor that determines onset of action. Increased tissue penetration and shortened onset of action is found in drugs with a lower pK$_a$ because more of the lipid-soluble uncharged form is present (Tables 29–2 and 29–3). Although in isolated nerve fibers onset of action directly parallels pK$_a$, other physiochemical factors influence drug activity. For example, prilocaine and lidocaine have the same pK$_a$, but lidocaine's onset is faster because of its enhanced ability to penetrate through non-nervous tissue.

The site of administration also influences the onset of action. Onset times are prolonged as the amount of interspersed tissue or the size of the nerve sheath increases because of the greater distance the agent must travel to reach its receptor. The pattern of onset for large nerves is determined by the structural arrangement of fibers. Peripheral (mantle) fibers are blocked before core fibers. Because mantle fibers innervate more proximal regions, nerve blockade proceeds in a proximal to distal progression.

Adding sodium bicarbonate to raise the anesthetic solution's pH (a technique that decreases pain on injection) yields a higher concentration of the uncharged lipid-soluble form and decreases onset time. Increasing the total dose by using a higher concentration of the same volume or a greater volume of the same concentration also shortens onset time. For most procedures performed in the ED, the onset time of most agents is short enough that manipulation to achieve shorter times is unnecessary.

Potency

The lipid solubility of an anesthetic is a primary physiochemical factor determining potency. The drug's partition coefficient, not the concentration of lipid-soluble form determined by pK_a or pH, confers its lipid solubility. Because the nerve membrane is lipid, lipophilic anesthetics pass more easily into the cell and few molecules are needed for conduction blockade (see Tables 29–2 and 29–3).

The degree of vasodilation produced by the anesthetic also affects potency because vasodilation promotes vascular absorption, reducing the amount of locally available drug. Lidocaine is more lipid-soluble than prilocaine or mepivacaine, but it produces more vasodilation. Although lidocaine is twice as potent as prilocaine or mepivacaine in vitro, it is equipotent in vivo. Although not a primary reason for its use, epinephrine, by producing vasoconstriction and making more molecules available to the nerve, increases the depth of anesthesia. Drugs more readily absorbed by fat have reduced potency. Increased concentration also increases potency.

Choosing an anesthetic for its potency is usually not necessary for any given site, because the concentration of an agent may be manipulated to make most drugs equianesthetic. For example, lidocaine, being one fourth as potent as bupivacaine, is usually used at four times the concentration (1%–2% vs. 0.25%–0.5%, respectively). For different sites and techniques, different concentrations and volumes of a given agent are needed to produce adequate blockade.

Duration

The degree of protein binding of an anesthetic primarily determines the duration of action. Agents that bind more tightly to the protein receptor remain in the sodium channel longer (see Tables 29–2 and 29–3). Like potency, the duration of action is reduced by the vasodilation produced by local anesthetics. Prilocaine, which is less protein bound than lidocaine, produces a longer duration of action because of its lesser degree of vasodilation. The duration of action also varies with the mode of administration. The duration of action is shorter when agents are applied topically.

The duration of action may be prolonged by several methods. Increasing the dose, usually by increasing the concentration, prolongs duration to limits imposed by toxic effects. Raising the pH of the anesthetic solution also has been shown to prolong duration.[6,7] The most practical way to increase duration is to use solutions that contain epinephrine.[8] Epinephrine causes vasoconstriction, decreases systemic absorption, and allows more drug to reach the nerve. The effect of epinephrine varies according to the agent. Anesthetics that intrinsically produce more vasodilation (e.g., procaine, lidocaine, mepivacaine) benefit more from epinephrine's vasoconstrictive action. The long-acting, highly lipid-soluble agents (e.g., bupivacaine, etidocaine) are less affected because they are substantially taken up by extradural fat and released slowly. In fact, lidocaine with epinephrine may be effective as long as bupivacaine without epinephrine. Generally, most ED procedures can be accomplished quickly before anesthesia wears off regardless of which drug is selected. Choose agents with a long duration of action when the procedure is lengthy or if postoperative analgesia is desired.

TOPICAL ANESTHESIA

Local anesthetic agents may be applied topically to mucous membranes, intact skin, and lacerations. There are sufficient differences among these sites to merit a separate discussion of each one. Topical anesthesia of the eye is discussed in Chapter 63, Ophthalmologic Procedures.

TABLE 29–2 Activity Profile with Primary Physiochemical Determinant

Agent	Onset: pK_a	Potency: Lipid Solubility	Duration: Protein Binding
Tetracaine	Slow	8	Long
Procaine	Slow	1	Short
Chloroprocaine	Fast	1	Short
Lidocaine	Fast	2	Moderate
Mepivacaine	Fast	2	Moderate
Prilocaine	Fast	2	Moderate
Bupivacaine	Moderate	8	Long
Etidocaine	Fast	4–6	Long

TABLE 29–3 Physiochemical Properties of Selected Local Anesthetics

Agent	Type	Site of Metabolism	pK_a	Lipid Solubility (Partition Coefficient)	Protein Binding (%)
Tetracaine	Ester	Plasma	8.5	High (4.1)	76
Procaine	Ester	Plasma	8.9	Low (0.02)	6
Chloroprocaine	Ester	Plasma	8.7	Low (0.14)	—
Lidocaine	Amide	Liver	7.9	Medium (2.9)	64
Mepivacaine	Amide	Liver	7.6	Medium (0.8)	78
Prilocaine	Amide	Liver	7.9	Medium (0.9)	55
Bupivacaine	Amide	Liver	8.1	High (27.5)	95
Etidocaine	Amide	Liver	7.7	High (141.0)	94

Note: A common way to remember the class of anesthetic (amide vs. ester): all amides have the letter "i" appearing twice in the generic name. The others are esters. Cocaine, not listed in this table, is also an ester.

Mucous Membranes

Agents and Properties

Effective anesthesia of the intact mucous membranes (not intact skin) of the nose, mouth, throat, tracheobronchial tree, esophagus, and genitourinary tract may be provided by several anesthetics (Table 29–4). Tetracaine, lidocaine, and cocaine are the most effective commonly used agents (Table 29–5). Benzocaine (14%–20%) is commonly used for intraoral or pharyngeal anesthesia. Prilocaine-phenylephrine (Prilophen) is another topical agent. The anesthesia produced is superficial and does not relieve pain that originates from submucosal structures. The onset of action may be slow, limiting the effect in urgent situations (such as passing a nasogastric tube). Agents applied topically can be systemically absorbed, and concentrated topical agents can cause toxicity.

Tetracaine solution is an effective and potent topical agent with a relatively long duration of action. It is used in concentrations from 0.25% to 1% with a recommended maximum adult dose of 50 mg. In an overdose, it has the disadvantage of severe cardiovascular toxicity without any preceding central nervous system (CNS) stimulatory phase.

Lidocaine also is an effective topical agent that is marketed in a variety of forms (solutions, jellies, and ointments) and concentrations (2%–10%). The 10% form is most effective, and minimal topical anesthesia is achieved with less potent concentrations. Lidocaine is commonly employed as the 2% viscous solution prescribed for inflamed or irritated mucous membranes of the mouth and pharynx. Patient misuse of viscous lidocaine, by repeated self-administration, can lead to serious toxicity. Topical lidocaine provides an adequate duration for most procedures, with a maximum safe dose of 250 to 300 mg.

Cocaine is an effective, but potentially toxic, topical agent applied to mucous membranes of the upper respiratory tract. Although it is an ester, hepatic metabolism occurs, as does hydrolysis by plasma pseudocholinesterase. Absorption is enhanced in the presence of inflammation. Cocaine is the only anesthetic that produces vasoconstriction at clinically useful concentrations; hence, its popularity for treating epistaxis. This major advantage is offset by its susceptibility to abuse and its toxic potential. Stimulating the CNS directly and blocking norepinephrine reuptake in the peripheral nervous system causes the toxic effects. *Cocaine should not be administered to patients who are sensitive to exogenous catecholamines or who are taking monoamine oxidase (MAO) inhibitor antidepressants.* Clinical manifestations of toxicity include CNS excitement, seizures, and hyperthermia. Central and peripheral effects of hypertension, tachycardia, and ventricular arrhythmias may be seen. Acute myocardial infarction has been reported after topical application.[9] Cocaine is commonly used as a 4% solution with a maximum safe dose of 200 mg (2–3 mg/kg). A 10% solution is available, but this concentration adds little to the topical effect while enhancing the potential for toxicity. Coronary vasoconstriction may occur with doses as low as 2 mg/kg applied to the nasal mucosa. Although the clinical effect of this is usually benign, and without electrocardiographic changes, topical cocaine should be used cautiously for patients with coronary artery disease and avoided in the elderly with known coronary disease. Should it occur, symptomatic coronary vasoconstriction can be treated with nitroglycerine (sublingual or infusion) or phentolamine (1 mg intravenously, repeated every 5 min).

Dyclonine offers advantages over other topical anesthetic agents. Dyclonine is a ketone derivative without an ester or amide linkage and may be used in patients who are allergic to the common anesthetics. Extensive experience with the topical preparation has shown it to be effective and safe.[10] Dyclonine is marketed in 0.5% and 1% solutions, with a maximum adult recommended dose of 300 mg.

Benzocaine is an ester that is marketed in its neutral form in 14% to 20% preparations (Cetacaine, Americaine, Hurricaine). Its low water-solubility prevents significant penetration of the mucous membranes, reducing systemic toxicity if applied to intact mucosa. However, it is not a potent anesthetic and has a brief duration of action. It is more allergenic

---

TABLE 29–4 Common Local and Topical Anesthetics Used in the Emergency Department

- Benzocaine spray will produce transient anesthesia of mucus membranes. Rarely, it can precipitate methemoglobinemia in standard doses. Anbesol is a popular over-the-counter benzocaine anesthetic for dental problems, such as teething.
- EMLA cream (lidocaine and prilocaine) will produce anesthesia of the intact skin but it must be in place for about 60 min to provide significant benefit. ELA-Max is another topical lidocaine preparation with a more rapid onset of action.
- "Magic mouthwash" contains equal parts of diphenhydramine elixir, Maalox, and 2% viscous lidocaine. Each 5-mL teaspoon contains < 50 mg lidocaine. It is swished, held in the mouth for 1–2 min, and expectorated.
- Viscous lidocaine (2%) may be used intraorally, but repeated use may produce systemic toxicity, especially in children. Each 5-mL teaspoon contains 100 mg of lidocaine. It should not be swallowed, but instead expectorated after holding it in the mouth for a few minutes. Viscous lidocaine is not useful for acute pharyngitis. Systemic narcotics are preferred if pain is severe.

EMLA, eutectic mixture of local anesthetics.

TABLE 29–5 Practical Agents for Emergency Department Use—Mucosal Application

Agent	Usual Concentration (%)	Maximum Dosage*		Onset (min)	Duration (min)
		Adult (mg)	Pediatric (mg/kg)		
Tetracaine	0.5	50	0.75	3–8	30–60
Lidocaine	2–10	250–300[†]	3–4[†]	2–5	15–45
Cocaine[‡]	4	200	2–3[†]	2–5	30–45

*These are conservative figures; see text for explanations.
[†]The lower dosage should be used for a maximum safe dose when feasible.
[‡]The 10% cocaine solution is best avoided because of minimal additional clinical benefit and the potential for coronary vasoconstriction in patients with coronary artery disease.

INFILTRATION ANESTHESIA

The injection of an anesthetic agent directly into tissue prior to surgical manipulation is known as *infiltration anesthesia*. Field block anesthesia is also considered a form of infiltration anesthesia, particularly because the agents, concentrations, and recommended maximum dosages are the same. A field block is created when a field of anesthesia is injected around the operative site. The injection is made proximal to or surrounding the area to be manipulated. Infiltrative anesthesia may be combined with procedural sedation (see Chapter 33, Systemic Analgesia and Sedation for Procedures) when reducing anxiety or motion is desired.

Indications and Contraindications

Infiltration anesthesia is indicated when good operative conditions can be obtained by using this technique. It may be used for the majority of minor surgical procedures such as excision of skin lesions, incision of abscesses, and suturing of wounds. Infiltration anesthesia is considered quicker and safer than nerve block and general anesthesia. Local infiltration can provide hemostasis, both by direct distention of tissue and by the concurrent use of epinephrine.

A disadvantage of local infiltration compared with nerve blocks is that a relatively large dose of drug is needed to anesthetize a relatively small area. For extensive wounds, the amount of anesthetic required may risk systemic toxicity. The maximum allowable volume can be increased by adding epinephrine, using a lower concentration of anesthetic agent, or both (Table 29–6). When large volumes are anticipated and

a nerve block is anatomically feasible, the nerve block is preferred. Infiltration is avoided for large procedures in small children and in apprehensive patients, especially those with prior adverse reactions (whether vasovagal or otherwise). Local infiltration distorts the tissues that will be incised or repaired, making it undesirable in areas requiring precise anatomic alignment (e.g., some lip repairs).

Choice of Agent

Local anesthetic agents most frequently used for infiltration are 0.5% to 1% lidocaine, 0.5 to 1% procaine, and 0.25% bupivacaine (Table 29–7). Higher concentrations are of no additional benefit. Lidocaine is most commonly used because of its excellent activity profile, low allergenicity and toxicity, user familiarity, and ready availability. Procaine is useful for patients who are allergic to amide anesthetics. Some clinicians prefer bupivacaine because of its prolonged duration. Bupivacaine may be preferred when postoperative analgesia is desired, for prolonged procedures, or even for short procedures that may be interrupted in a busy ED.

A comparison of equianesthetic doses of lidocaine and bupivacaine for infiltration anesthesia (Table 29–8) reveals the duration of action to be the major difference between the two agents. For the majority of ED procedures, it is not necessary to extend the duration of anesthesia beyond 1 hour. Plain lidocaine would seem to be a logical anesthesia choice. Patients experience a moderate amount of pain after laceration repair when the lidocaine wears off in about 1 hour.[55] Bupivacaine reduces the pain after laceration repair for at least 6 hours. This benefit of a prolonged duration of anesthesia must be weighed against the hazards of injury to an unprotected limb or the annoyance of prolonged numbness to patients who have had simple surgical procedures.

A prolonged duration of anesthesia can be achieved by adding epinephrine, sodium bicarbonate, or both to lidocaine. Epinephrine provides excellent wound hemostasis and slows systemic absorption. This latter property decreases the peak blood level, decreasing the potential for a toxic reaction, and allows a greater volume of agent to be used for extensive lacerations. The major disadvantage of epinephrine is the theoretical, but generally clinically inconsequential, damage to host defenses (Table 29–9). Bicarbonate added to the anesthetic just prior to injection decreases the pain of administration. Bupivacaine, if used with due caution, is safe and easy to use. The deciding factors are many, but some logical choices are as follows:

TABLE 29–6 Maximum Allowable Volume (Adults)

Agent	Concentration (%)	Maximum* Safe Dose (mg)	Maximum Volume (mL)
Lidocaine	0.5	300	60
	1	300	30
Bupivacaine†	0.25	175	70
Lidocaine-epinephrine	0.5	500	100
	1	500	50
Bupivacaine-epinephrine	0.25	225	90

*These are quite conservative figures for infiltration anesthesia; see text for explanation.
†Some physicians recommend 400 mg as the maximum safe dose for bupivacaine.

TABLE 29–7 Practical Agents for Emergency Department Use—Local Infiltration

Agent	Concentration (%)	Maximum Dose*†		Onset (min)	Duration‡
		Adult (mg)	Pediatric (mg/kg)		
Procaine	0.5–1.0	500§ (600)	7 (9)	2–5	15–45 min
Lidocaine	0.5–1.0	300 (500)	4.5 (7)‖	2–5	1–2 hr
Bupivacaine	0.25	175 (225)	2 (3)¶	2–5	4–8 hr

*These are quite conservative figures; see text for explanation.
†Higher maximum dose for solutions containing epinephrine appears in parentheses.
‡These values are for the agent alone; they can be extended considerably with the addition of epinephrine.
§Some authorities recommend up to 1000 mg or 14 mg/kg for procaine.
‖Some authorities recommend up to 7 mg/kg for plain lidocaine in children older than 1 yr.
¶Because of lack of clinical trial experience, drug companies do not recommend the use of bupivacaine in children younger than age 12, but bupivicaine is commonly used without problems in children.

TABLE 29–8 Comparison of 1% Lidocaine and 0.25% Bupivacaine—Infiltration Anesthesia

	Lidocaine	Bupivacaine	Advantage
Onset	2–5 min	2–5 min	Equal
Effectiveness (equianesthetic dose)	Excellent	Excellent	Equal
Duration	1–2 hr	4–6 hr	B
Infection potential	No	No	Equal
Administration pain	Less	More	L
Maximum volume*—plain lidocaine	Less	More	L
Maximum volume—epinephrine	Less	More	B
Toxic potential	Less cardiotoxic; equal CNS	More cardiotoxic; equal CNS	L

*See Table 29–6 for volume and concentration comparison.
B, bupivacaine; CNS, central nervous system; L, lidocaine.

TABLE 29–9 Epinephrine Use

Advantages	Disadvantages
1. Prolongs duration	1. Impairs host defenses—increases infection*
2. Provides hemostasis	2. Delays wound healing*
3. Slows absorption: Decreases agent's toxic potential Allows increased dose	3. Do not use for: Areas supplied by end arteries Patients "sensitive" to catecholamines
4. Increases level of blockade	4. Toxicity—catecholamine reaction†

*Based on laboratory studies and of unknown clinical importance.
†For example, in patients taking monoamine oxidase (MAO) inhibitors.

- For a wound with excessive bleeding: lidocaine with epinephrine and sodium bicarbonate.
- For an apprehensive patient: lidocaine with sodium bicarbonate.
- For anticipated prolonged postprocedure pain: bupivacaine.

Equipment

The pain of injection is reduced by use of small-gauge needles. Ideally, a 30-gauge needle is used if injection is made through the skin. If the injection is made through the cut edges of the wound, a 25- to 27-gauge needle suffices. A small-gauge needle slows the rate of injection and reduces the rate of tissue distention. A 10-mL syringe is recommended both for its ease of handling and for the relatively slow rate of injection it allows.

Technique

Once an agent has been chosen, proper administration technique minimizes pain, prevents bacterial spread, and avoids intravascular injection. Buffering, temperature manipulation, and careful infiltration reduce the pain of injection.

Buffering

Lowering the pH of an anesthetic by adding epinephrine increases pain, whereas raising the pH by adding sodium bicarbonate decreases pain dramatically. It is probable that pH is not the sole factor in producing pain, because the pain produced by various agents does not correlate strictly with the pH. Sodium bicarbonate probably works by increasing the ratio of nonionized to ionized molecules, which either renders the pain receptors less sensitive or causes a more rapid diffusion of solution into the nerve and a shorter time to anesthetic onset.

To alkalinize lidocaine, add 1 mL of sodium bicarbonate (8.4%, 1 mmol/mL) to every 10 mL of anesthetic solution. As the pH of the solution is raised, the anesthetic becomes unstable and has a decreased shelf life. It was initially recommended that buffered lidocaine be prepared just prior to use to avoid precipitation and degradation, but buffered lidocaine retains its effectiveness for 1 week and refrigeration may further increase its shelf life.[56,57] Bicarbonate may be combined with plain lidocaine for both infiltrative anesthesia[58,59] and digital nerve blocks.[60] In one volunteer study, sodium bicarbonate was effectively combined with lidocaine and epinephrine.[57]

Sodium bicarbonate can be added to bupivacaine, but the solution tends to precipitate as the pH rises. The clinical effect of this precipitation is unclear, but if it occurs, it is likely prudent to use another solution prepared with less buffer. Precipitation varies directly with the concentration of bupivacaine and the time since mixture.[61] Cheney and coworkers[62] showed that 0.05 mL of 8.4% sodium bicarbonate (measured in a tuberculin syringe) could be mixed with 10 mL of 0.5% bupivacaine without precipitation. The goal of using bupivacaine is to prolong the duration of anesthesia; this effect can also be accomplished somewhat by using buffered lidocaine (plain or with epinephrine).

Considering the amount of published literature that demonstrates that adding sodium bicarbonate to lidocaine before infiltrative anesthesia reduces the pain of injection without adverse effects, lidocaine should almost always be buffered when infiltrated in the ED.

Temperature Manipulation

Warming an anesthetic to body temperature (37°C–42°C) reduces the pain of infiltration.[63,64] Bartfield and colleagues[65] found that lidocaine warmed to 38.9°C was more painful than room temperature buffered lidocaine during intradermal injection. Brogan and associates,[66] using lidocaine warmed to 37°C, found the warmed lidocaine and room temperature buffered lidocaine to be equivalent during wound infiltration. Neither study found a synergistic effect with combined warming and buffering. Martin and coworkers[67] found warmed (37°C) lidocaine to be no less painful than buffered lidocaine. Anesthetic solutions can be warmed in a baby food warmer with thermostatic temperature control or in an IV solution warmer. Warming is not believed to adversely affect the shelf life of the local anesthetic.

Locally cooling the area to be infiltrated may provide additional pain relief. Leff and colleagues[68] demonstrated that patients receiving local infiltrative anesthesia for inguinal hernia repair had less pain when the incision area was cooled prior to infiltration. Patients were randomized to two groups that had a 1000-mL bag of saline placed over the inguinal area for 5 minutes. One group used saline bags at room temperature; the other group used saline bags cooled to 4°C. A significant decrease in pain perception was measured in the group that had the inguinal area cooled before lidocaine infiltration. Cooling of wounds in the ED prior to infiltration has not been studied.

Injection

Pain from local anesthetic injections occurs primarily from skin puncture (minimized with small-gauge needles) and during subcutaneous injection. Although patients fear the needle, there is little perceived pain merely from the needle's presence in the subcutaneous tissue. "The needle will not hurt, but the anesthetic injection will cause pain" is a correct statement. Place the injection in the *subdermal* tissues to minimize needle puncture pain and the tissue distention that occurs with *intradermal* placement. Placing the needle "up to the hub" and injecting while withdrawing along the just-created subdermal tunnel also minimizes tissue distention. After an initial injection, instead of totally withdrawing the needle from the tissue, *redirect it along another path to lessen the number of skin punctures.* Slowly injecting the smallest volume necessary reduces pain.

Because the patient barely feels a needle placed subcutaneously and skin puncture is often quite painful, *make all wound injections through the wound edge and not through the skin* (Fig. 29–6).[69] Infection spread beyond the wound margin has not been demonstrated clinically with this technique. Some clinicians may choose to inject the anesthetic through intact skin in a grossly contaminated wound. Bierman[70] described a technique of patient distraction by applying light pressure to alternate sides of the wound with one's fingers and repeated ambiguous questioning about feeling the light pressure rather than the ongoing wound injection. School-age children can be asked to count backward or say the "ABCs" to distract them during injection.

Preventing a systemic toxic reaction is best accomplished by avoiding an intravascular injection. However, for infiltration anesthesia with small-gauge needles, aspiration is usually unnecessary unless the injection is deeper than the subcutaneous area or the area to be injected contains many large vessels.

SPECIAL CONSIDERATIONS

Hematoma Block

Hematoma block has been used for many years to provide anesthesia for reduction of fractures, particularly of the distal forearm and hand. Its popularity has waned somewhat because of the fear (unproven and theoretical) of introducing infection at the fracture site and its limited efficacy. Although several studies show the hematoma block to be safe, the anesthesia it provides is not as good as that provided by the Bier block (see Chapter 32, Intravenous Regional Anesthesia). Nevertheless, there are several reasons to consider this technique.[71,72] The procedure is simple and quick to perform and does not require additional personnel. There is no need to wait for an anesthesiologist. A lower dose of anesthetic agent is required compared with that required for the Bier block (see Chapter 32,

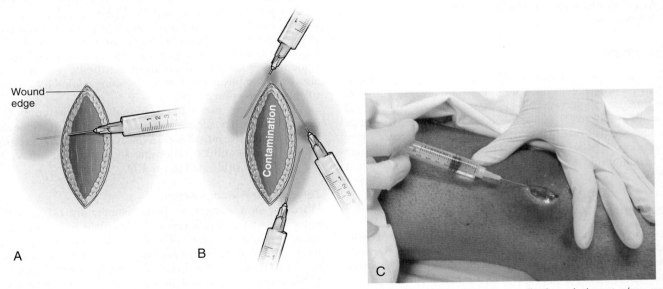

Figure 29–6 *A,* Except in the setting of gross contamination, wounds should be anesthetized by inserting the needle *through the cut edges, not through the intact skin.* Patients often will not feel a 25-gauge or smaller needle passed into the subcutaneous tissue when it is advanced slowly through the cut edge. However, pain generally occurs with tissue distention by the anesthetic, and hence, injection should be slow and deliberate. *B,* If a wound is grossly contaminated, the anesthetic may be introduced through the intact skin. The operator should limit the number of needle sticks. The needle is first introduced at a point in line with the wound and beyond the wound edge (1), and while the anesthetic is slowly injected, the needle is advanced to include one entire side of the wound (if possible) to a point well past the opposite end of the wound. The other side may be anesthetized by passing the needle through the area already infiltrated by the first injection (3), making the skin puncture painless. A 3.8-cm (1.5-inch) 27-gauge needle is a good choice. If the needle is not long enough to encompass the entire wound, the skin is painlessly punctured at a midway point that has already been anesthetized (2). *C,* Inject local anesthetic *through the subcutaneous tissue, not the intact skin.*

Intravenous Regional Anesthesia). A hematoma block is useful when the Bier block and general anesthesia are contraindicated.

Prepare the skin over the fracture site with antiseptic solution and insert the needle into the hematoma (confirmed by aspirating blood). Slowly inject from 5 to 15 mL of plain 1% lidocaine or 5 to 10 mL of plain 2% lidocaine (larger fractures require larger volumes of local anesthetic) into the fracture cavity and around the adjacent periosteum. Adequate anesthesia occurs in about 5 to 10 minutes and may last for several hours. A common error is to attempt the procedure too soon after injection. Do not perform this procedure through dirty skin or in open fractures.

Intra-articular Anesthesia

The history and physical examination of an acutely traumatized joint, such as the knee, often underestimates the severity of an injury. Instillation of 5 mL of 1% lidocaine after joint aspiration may help relieve pain and facilitate an examination, but its use is not routinely recommended.[73] Spasm and apprehension are often not relieved by local anesthesia, and the information gained usually does not influence the ED treatment plan. Intra-articular anesthesia of the knee has no effect on gait pattern or joint proprioception.[74] Postprocedure weight-bearing may be allowed without fear of producing or increasing injury if otherwise indicated. Intra-articular anesthesia may enhance elbow use after aspiration of a hemarthrosis associated with a radial head fracture.[75] The technique of administration is analogous to arthrocentesis (see Chapter 53, Arthrocentesis).

Intrapleural Anesthesia

Indications

Intrapleural anesthesia introduces local anesthetic into the pleural space (i.e., between the parietal and the visceral pleura) through an epidural catheter. The anesthetic can be introduced through a previously placed chest tube. The technique can provide relief for several conditions, primarily postthoracotomy pain; postcholecystectomy pain; and most importantly for emergency clinicians, post-traumatic chest pain (e.g., rib fractures, pneumothorax, hemothorax). This procedure not only is useful for pain relief but also facilitates turning, coughing, and deep breathing. Several studies have demonstrated improved respiratory mechanics when intrapleural anesthesia is used.[76,77] Although not unanimous, most studies show that intrapleural anesthesia is effective in providing analgesia.[78,79] Concern has been raised that intrapleural anesthesia may create a level of anesthesia below the umbilicus and make post-traumatic abdominal examinations unreliable. Until this issue is clarified, it seems prudent to rule out intra-abdominal injury before intrapleural anesthesia is used.[80]

Technique

If a chest tube is in place, it is preferable to inject anesthesia into the pleural space through the chest tube. Theoretically, the tube should be clamped for 10 to 15 minutes to allow the anesthetic to diffuse. When the tube cannot be taken off suction, or if no tube is present, the local anesthetic is injected percutaneously.[81] With the patient in the lateral position (with the affected side up), place a 16-gauge Tuohy needle 8 to 10 cm from the posterior midline in the eighth intercostal space. The needle is angled at 30° to 40° to the skin, aimed medially, bevel up, and directed just above the rib. After perforating the posterior intercostal membrane (felt as a distinct resistance), remove the stylet and attach a well-wetted, air-filled glass syringe to the Tuohy needle. Advance the needle until it enters the pleural space, denoted by the plunger being drawn down the syringe owing to the negative pressure created during inspiration. Remove the syringe and introduce an epidural catheter 5 to 6 cm into the pleural space. Remove the Tuohy needle, obtain a chest radiograph to confirm proper position, and secure the catheter.

The most commonly used anesthetic and dose is 20 mL (0.3 mL/kg) of 0.5% bupivacaine. A repeat dose every 8 hours has been shown to be safe.[82] Alternatively, 0.25% bupivicaine can be continuously infused at 0.1 to 0.2 mL/kg per hour after the bolus has been administered.[76] The solution presumably diffuses from the pleural space "back" through the parietal pleura and the intercostal muscle to reach the intercostal spaces, where it blocks the intercostal nerves. The level of anesthesia can extend from T2 to T12 and involve skin, chest, abdominal wall, and potentially the viscera if the visceral afferent fibers are blocked at the sympathetic chain in the paravertebral gutter.

Although not yet a consistently proven or a completely standardized technique, intrapleural anesthesia offers promise for patients and is a potentially valuable procedure for the emergency clinician.

COMPLICATIONS

Local Anesthetic Effect on Wounds

Wound Healing

Local anesthetics produce cytotoxic effects on cell structure and function in a dose- and time-related manner. These effects, at doses well below those used clinically, involve fibroblasts more than nervous tissue. Collagen synthesis is inhibited by lidocaine and bupivacaine.[83] Morris and Tracey[84] found that lidocaine in increasing concentrations progressively reduced the tensile strength of wounds. Epinephrine added to 1% and 2% concentrations of lidocaine further reduced tensile strength, but when epinephrine was added to distilled water or to 0.5% lidocaine, it had little effect. Several conclusions may be clinically relevant. Although it may delay anesthetic onset, lidocaine 0.5% solution, without epinephrine if possible, may be best for wound strength.

Eriksson and associates[85] found that lidocaine reduces the inflammatory response in wounds by decreasing the number of white cells and their metabolic activity. Although an inflammatory response may be beneficial in a contaminated wound, it can be detrimental in a sterile wound because of the tissue toxicity created by the release of superoxide anions, lysosomal enzymes, thromboxanes, leukotrienes, and interleukins. The clinical relevance of this is unknown. None of the concerns mentioned earlier should prohibit the use of standard anesthetics or epinephrine when their use is otherwise indicated.

Wound Infection

Although not generally appreciated, it has long been known that local anesthetics possess antimicrobial activity in vitro. Lidocaine and procaine demonstrate concentration-dependent inhibition of culture growth of most gram-negative organisms.[86–88] Gram-positive isolates are also significantly affected by lidocaine and, to a lesser extent, by procaine. Lidocaine inhibits the growth of common nosocomial pathogens including *Enterococcus faecalis*, *Escherichia coli*, *Pseudomonas aeruginosa*, and several strains of methicillin-resistant *Staphylococcus aureus* and vancomycin-resistant enterococcus.[88] Administering anesthetics before obtaining culture material, including injecting a joint prior to arthrocentesis, may give false-negative culture results and is avoided if possible. Berg and coworkers[89] demonstrated that lidocaine given prior to tissue biopsy of chronic wounds did not affect the culture results when the exposure time before culture was under 2 hours. This effect is also significant when anesthetic ointments have been applied prior to culture. EMLA cream applied before culture demonstrates powerful antimicrobial properties.[89] Furthermore, it has been shown that adding sodium bicarbonate to lidocaine greatly enhances its inhibitory effect on bacteria.[90] Although local anesthetics can interfere with culture testing, several studies show that local anesthetics, by themselves, do not appear to alter the incidence of wound infection.[91,92]

Epinephrine appears to exert a deleterious effect on host defenses, at least in animal models. Studies with infiltrated and topically applied epinephrine solutions in contaminated animal wounds show an increased potential for infection.[91,92] Epinephrine-induced vasoconstriction may contribute to tissue hypoxia, retarding the killing of *S. aureus* by leukocytes, and reducing leukocyte migration into the tissue.[93] Most clinical studies using topical anesthesia with vasoconstrictor properties (e.g., TAC mixtures) do not demonstrate significantly increased infection rates.[35,38,39,44] The concerns mentioned earlier should not prohibit the use of epinephrine for wound preparation when its use is otherwise appropriate.

Local Injuries

Injuries may result from direct application of an anesthetic agent to a nerve or from passage of a needle through soft tissue structures. Factors implicated in transient or persistent neuropathy include acidic solutions, additives, the agent itself, needle trauma, compression from hematomas, and inadvertent injection of neurolytic agents. Born[94] described a series of 49 wrist and metacarpal blocks using bupivacaine in which 8 patients developed a significant neuropathy. He postulated that damage occurred from the trapping of the drug in a confined space and recommended that whenever bupivacaine is used in this situation, it be used in low concentration and volume. Infection, hematomas, and broken needles are other local problems that can be averted by using proper technique. Erroneous needle placement also can produce complications such as pneumothorax during brachial plexus or intercostal block.

It is commonly stated that epinephrine-containing solutions injected into tissues containing end arteries can cause profound ischemia and gangrene. Given the short duration of epinephrine combined with the vasodilation that accompanies many local anesthetics (e.g., lidocaine), this cause and effect is difficult to accept and hard to substantiate. Despite admonition in most textbooks, the concept remains largely theoretical. Areas of special concern include the digits, penis, tip of the nose, or earlobe. This concern is promulgated but is certainly overrated when dilute concentrations (1:200,000) of epinephrine-containing solutions are used. Several studies have demonstrated that epinephrine-containing solutions can be safely injected into the fingers without adverse sequelae.[95,96]

A study of more that 3000 cases of elective injection of low-dose epinephrine (≤1:100,000) in the hand and fingers failed to identify a single case of digital tissue loss; phentolamine was not required to reverse vasoconstriction.[95] Because bupivacaine can be used when prolonged anesthesia is required, and because tourniquets can be used in the digits, there is little need for vasoconstrictors in the digits, although some clinicians use a dilute epinephrine solution there as well. Some authors have identified cases of digital gangrene after epinephrine injection, but other variables including hot soaks, tourniquets, and infection made it impossible to clearly link gangrene to the epinephrine alone.[97] Considering the data describing the safe use of epinephrine in fingers, perhaps the risk of tourniquets could be minimized if epinephrine was used instead.[98,99] In summary, the dogmatic admonition against the use of epinephrine-containing anesthetics in the context of ED laceration repair is not supported by scientific data. Despite a lack of evidence against its use, most clinicians tend to avoid the use of epinephrine-containing anesthetics when performing digital anesthesia. Epinephrine is best avoided in patients with peripheral vascular disease.

The use of phentolamine (Regitine), which produces postsynaptic α-adrenergic blockade, is recommended for vasoconstrictor-induced tissue ischemia. This medication is usually given by local infiltration in a dose of 0.5 to 5.0 mg diluted 1:1 with saline. If local infiltration is ineffective or limited by tension within a tissue compartment, or if the area of vasoconstriction is large, phentolamine may be given by the intra-arterial route.[100]

Systemic Toxic Reactions

Although they occur in only 0.1% to 0.4% of local anesthetic administrations, systemic toxic reactions are the most frequent serious adverse reactions encountered (Table 29–10).[101] After administration of a local anesthetic, some of the drug reaches its intended target and some is absorbed quickly into the systemic circulation. Peak blood levels are generally produced within 30 minutes. Many vagal reactions, nonspecific anxiety reactions, and sensitivity to preservatives have been attributed to "allergies" or systemic toxicity to local anesthetics. Patients may also demonstrate systemic reactions to hidden allergens that may mimic a systemic reaction, such as anaphylactic reactions to the latex in surgical gloves.

High Blood Levels
Systemic toxic reactions result from high blood levels of local anesthetic. Several factors are important in producing high blood levels, including site and mode of administration, rate, dose and concentration, addition of epinephrine, specific drug, clearance, maximum safe dosage, and inadvertent intravascular injection.

Site and Mode of Administration. Comparing the routes of administration for a given dose, the intravascular route produces the highest levels, followed by topical mucosal application, then infiltration (see Fig. 29–5). The more vascular the site, the more systemic absorption that occurs and the higher the level obtained. The following blocks are arranged in decreasing order of systemic absorption: intercostal, caudal, epidural, brachial plexus, and subcutaneous. It follows that the site of administration is an important variable in determining the safe dose of an anesthetic. For example, 400 mg of lidocaine may produce a nontoxic blood level with abdominal wall subcutaneous infiltration, but when used for

TABLE 29-10 Differentiating Systemic Adverse Reactions

Findings	Toxic Reactions	Allergy	Vasovagal	Excess Catecholamines, Anxiety[1] (Endogenous), Vasoconstrictor (Exogenous)
Relatively specific signs and symptoms	Metallic taste Tongue numbness Drowsiness Nystagmus Slurred speech Seizures* Coma Respiratory arrest*	Acute rhinitis Pruritus* Dermatitis Urticaria* Facial swelling Laryngospasm Bronchospasm*	Syncope*[2]	Headache Hypertension* Palpitations Apprehension*[3]
Overlapping signs and symptoms	Paresthesia Light-headedness Tinnitus Tremor Tachypnea Tachycardia (early) Bradycardia* Hypotension* Cardiac arrest	Light-headedness Tachycardia* Hypotension* Cardiac arrest Nausea and vomiting Dyspnea	Light-headedness Tinnitus Tachypnea Tachycardia (early) Bradycardia* Hypotension* Diaphoresis	Paresthesia* Light-headedness* Tremor Tachypnea* Tachycardia* Nausea and vomiting Dyspnea Diaphoresis

*Denotes common and significant reactions:
1. Anxiety reaction, including hyperventilation syndrome.
2. Vasovagal syncope occurs with patient upright; any loss of consciousness in the recumbent position implies a severe toxic or anaphylactic reaction.
3. Although apprehension is classically associated with anxiety and vasoconstrictor reactions, milder toxic and allergic reactions may cause patient apprehension.

an intercostal nerve block, a toxic level would likely result from this dose.

Rate. A more rapid IV injection will produce a higher blood level than a slower injection. A single topical application leads to a higher level than a dose that is fractionated over time.

Dose and Concentration. The larger the total dose, the higher the peak blood level. It is uncertain whether increasing the concentration while maintaining the total dose by decreasing the volume affects the serum level.

Addition of Epinephrine. Epinephrine produces vasoconstriction and reduces systemic absorption, thereby resulting in lower peak blood levels. Occasionally, the apprehension, tachycardia, or palpitations induced by epinephrine can be incorrectly interpreted by both clinician and patient as an "allergic" reaction.

Specific Drug. The more potent agents are more toxic on a milligram-to-milligram basis. Because anesthetics are used in equipotent doses (e.g., 1 mg bupivacaine vs. 4 mg lidocaine), they are approximately equitoxic. Blood levels achieved by a particular agent depend on the agent's absorption, distribution, and clearance from the circulation. Agents with high lipid solubility and lower protein binding (etidocaine > bupivacaine > lidocaine > mepivacaine) tend to become sequestered in tissue and have a slower absorption and lower blood levels. Agents with a greater volume of distribution or a faster clearance (etidocaine > lidocaine > mepivacaine > bupivacaine) also produce lower blood levels. Together, these effects produce margins of safety for each anesthetic, with etidocaine having the greatest safety margin, followed by bupivacaine, which is equal to or better than lidocaine.

Esters are difficult to measure in the blood because of their rapid hydrolysis by pseudocholinesterase. As a group, toxicity is inversely proportional to the rate of hydrolysis. Tetracaine is slowly hydrolyzed and is most toxic. Chloroprocaine is quickly hydrolyzed and is least toxic. Procaine falls between the two.

Clearance. The liver metabolizes amides where the clearance rate is a function of hepatic blood flow and extraction capacity of the liver. Decreased hepatic blood flow, produced by norepinephrine, propranolol, or general anesthesia, slows clearance and potentially raises drug blood levels. Decreased drug extraction, associated with congestive heart failure, cirrhosis, or hypothermia, may produce a higher blood level. Hypovolemia, which decreases hepatic flow, does not raise blood levels because it causes an offsetting decrease in absorption.

Decreased clearance of esters and an increased risk for toxicity occurs in patients with either low levels of pseudocholinesterase or an atypical form of pseudocholinesterase. Low levels occur in various disease states, including severe liver disease and renal failure, and in pregnancy. Atypical pseudocholinesterase is an inherited trait, and its presence reduces the hydrolysis rate of procaine to a greater extent than low levels do.

There are significant differences between pediatric and adult drug distribution and metabolism. Neonates exhibit both reduced levels of pseudocholinesterase and reduced hepatic metabolism, increasing the risk of toxicity. In older children, the effects of increased hepatic metabolism and a relatively larger volume of distribution increase their tolerance for higher doses.

Because lidocaine is metabolized in the liver by the cytochrome P-450 enzymes, drugs that inhibit these enzymes may slow lidocaine clearance and increase the risk of lidocaine toxicity. Although the effect of ciprofloxacin and erythromycin on infiltrated lidocaine has not been studied, these drugs decrease the metabolism of lidocaine and increase the concentration of its major metabolites when lidocaine is injected intravenously.[102–104] The clinical effect of the previously discussed phenomenon is unknown and likely of little consequence in ED wound care.

Maximum Safe Dosage. The *maximum safe dose* for a drug may be defined as the dose that produces a blood level of the drug just below the toxic level (Table 29–11). One maximum dose for an anesthetic agent appropriate for all patients and all conditions cannot be stated. A maximum safe dose cannot be based solely on the weight of a patient. In an adult, peak blood levels do not correlate well with weight, because the volume of the drug distribution is relatively constant.[105,106] As an approximation, Arthur and McNicol[107] recommended maximum dosages for children based on weight. Plain lidocaine may be used in doses of up to 4.5 mg/kg and the addition of epinephrine allows for a maximum dose of 7 mg/kg. Bupivacaine is not recommended for children younger than 12 years; although it is commonly used without adverse consequences. Furthermore, the dose should be modified according to the site and mode of administration.

Maximum safe doses as stated in package inserts should be used only as guidelines because most of them are derived from animal experiments and are based on absorption data only. Levels vary with administration site, use of a vasoconstrictor, and to some extent, the health of the patient. Levels can often be exceeded safely when the drug is accurately administered. Drugs may be toxic even within the "safe range" when inadvertently injected intravenously.

Inadvertent Intravascular Injection. Most toxic reactions are caused by inadvertent intravascular injections of anesthetics whose doses were calculated for their intended extravascular sites. For example, lidocaine 300 mg is a safe infiltrated dose that would likely cause toxicity if directly injected into the bloodstream.

Anesthetics that are injected intravascularly must pass through the lungs before they reach other organs. Lung tissue sequesters a significant amount of drug, lowering the arterial blood concentration. Anesthetics that bypass the lungs, in cases of inadvertent injection into the carotid or vertebral arteries or in patients with intracardiac right-to-left shunts, can produce CNS toxicity at low doses. Intra-arterial injections in subcutaneous end arteries about the head or neck are capable of retrograde flow into the cerebral circulation, if the injection pressure exceeds the arterial pressure. Because the blood volume in the brain is only about 30 mL at any given moment, even 1 mg of lidocaine injected into the carotid artery can theoretically produce toxic concentrations. Patients with low cardiac output or hypovolemia and preferential cerebral blood flow may suffer enhanced CNS toxicity.

Host Factors

Four factors tend to lower the body's systemic tolerance to local anesthetic agents: hypoxia, acid-base status, protein binding, and concomitant drug use.

Hypoxia. It was initially thought that local anesthetic overdose produced CNS stimulation and subsequent intracellular hypoxia, which then became the key precipitant to all toxic manifestations of the drug. It is now known that hypoxia may enhance anesthetic toxicity, but it is not the primary factor.

Acid-Base Status. Although studies of metabolic alkalosis have produced conflicting results, acidosis, particularly respiratory acidosis, can increase toxicity. The elevated CO_2 produced by respiratory acidosis crosses the blood-brain barrier, where it may act directly on the receptor and indirectly by lowering intracellular pH. The lower pH causes more drug to ionize, furthering the block in the sodium channel and increasing the potential for toxicity.

Protein Binding. Unbound drug concentration relates more closely to toxic effects than does total drug concentration (bound plus unbound) as measured in the blood. The amount of α-acid glycoprotein (AAG), the major plasma protein responsible for binding local anesthetics, is considerably decreased in neonates compared with adults. Arthur and McNicol[107] implied that low AAG levels in neonates are responsible for an increased toxic potential. Tucker and colleagues[108] list several disease states that alter AAG levels and protein binding but question whether they lead to changes in free drug concentration in vivo.

Concomitant Drugs. For years, barbiturates were used to prevent and treat local anesthesia–induced seizures. Barbiturates were found to worsen anesthetic-induced apnea and cardiovascular depression. CNS depressants are used with caution when concern exists for local anesthetic toxicity. CNS stimulants have been shown to increase anesthetic-induced excitability and are avoided. Mixtures of local anesthetics have an additive effect on toxicity. If two drugs are used at half strength, they produce the same degree of toxicity as if each were used alone at normal strength. As discussed previously, drugs that slow metabolism by inhibiting hepatic enzymes may increase the risk of toxicity.

Recognition of CNS Toxicity

The earliest manifestation of systemic toxicity is CNS stimulation resulting from blockade of inhibitory synapses. CNS

TABLE 29–11 Calculation of Anesthetic Doses

Anesthetic solutions are marketed with drug concentration expressed as percentages (e.g., bupivacaine 0.25%, lidocaine 1%). To ascertain the strength of a solution in milligrams per milliliter, consider the following:

A 1% solution is prepared by dissolving 1 g of drug in 100 mL of solution.

Therefore, 1 g/100 mL = 1000 mg/100 mL = 10 mg/mL.

To calculate the strength from the percentage quickly, simply move the decimal point one place to the right. Examples:

0.25% = 2.5 mg/mL	e.g., bupivacaine
0.5% = 5 mg/mL	e.g., tetracaine
1% = 10 mg/mL	e.g., lidocaine
2% = 20 mg/mL	e.g., viscous lidocaine
4% = 40 mg/mL	e.g., cocaine
5% = 50 mg/mL	e.g., lidocaine ointment
20% = 200 mg/mL	e.g., benzocaine

When combined in an anesthetic solution, epinephrine is usually in a 1:100,000 or a 1:200,000 dilution.

1 mL of 1:1000 epinephrine = 1 mg.

0.1 mL of 1:1000 epinephrine in 10 mL anesthetic solution = 1:100,000 dilution = 0.010 mg/mL.

0.1 mL of 1:1000 epinephrine in 20 mL anesthetic solution = 1:200,000 dilution = 0.005 mg/mL.

Some examples detailing epinephrine content:

	1:100,000	1:200,000
5 mL	0.050 mg	0.025 mg
10 mL	0.100 mg	0.050 mg
20 mL	0.200 mg	0.100 mg

Therefore, 50 mL of 1% lidocaine with epinephrine 1:200,000 contains 500 mg lidocaine and 0.25 mg epinephrine.

depression follows and is produced by direct depression of the medulla, although hypoxia may play a role. Signs and symptoms are dose-related. Potential signs and symptoms of CNS toxicity, in progressing order, are numbness of the tongue, light-headedness, tinnitus, visual disturbances, muscle twitching, convulsions, coma, and apnea. Drowsiness, commonly seen at lower doses with lidocaine, is not associated with bupivacaine or etidocaine. Tetracaine may produce apnea or cardiovascular toxicity without CNS manifestations.

Recognition of Cardiovascular Toxicity

Moderate blood concentrations of local anesthetics produce slight increases in cardiac output, heart rate, and arterial pressure because of the effects of direct peripheral vasodilation and CNS stimulation. At concentrations generally well above CNS toxicity levels, local anesthetics cause direct myocardial depression, hypotension, and bradycardia, perhaps leading to cardiovascular collapse. These agents also slow electrical conduction leading to reentry phenomenon and various supraventricular and potentially lethal ventricular dysrhythmias, especially with bupivacaine and etidocaine.

Prevention of Toxicity

Knowledge of factors contributing to toxicity guides preventive measures. Avoid esters in patients with an atypical form or a quantitative deficiency of pseudocholinesterase. Use amides with caution for patients with severe liver disease or congestive heart failure. Pay attention to maximum safe dosages, based on site, technique, epinephrine use, and patient status. Add epinephrine when possible to decrease the drug absorption rate at vascular sites. Reduce drug concentration with saline dilution to increase the volume for administration when a large area must be infiltrated. Frequently aspirate in areas of high vascularity, even though a negative aspiration may not prevent IV administration.[109] Slow infiltration is advised for safety and is also associated with less pain.

Treatment of Systemic Toxicity

Local anesthesia should not be administered without the ability to recognize and treat a toxic reaction, including having all necessary equipment and drugs readily available and being knowledgeable in their use. Despite taking all possible precautions, toxic reactions still occur, and close observation of the patient allows early detection and treatment.

Providing proper oxygenation and ventilation at the earliest sign of a reaction is the cornerstone of treatment. Encourage patients who are alert to moderately hyperventilate to lower the pressure of carbon dioxide (P_{CO_2}) and raise the seizure threshold. Intubation with high-flow oxygen and hyperventilation is performed for patients who cannot adequately ventilate. Initiate IV access and monitor vital signs and cardiac rhythm closely.

Seizures are generally self-limited but are treated if they persist or prevent adequate ventilation. Because respiratory depression secondary to toxicity may follow, low-dose lorazepam or an ultrashort-acting barbiturate (thiopental or sodium methohexital) is preferred. Intubate the patient to ensure an effective airway and prevent further lactic acidosis if seizures persist. If toxicity is caused by an ester, especially if there is an associated pseudocholinesterase problem, succinylcholine will compete with the anesthetic for the pseudocholinesterase and may increase the toxicity of both compounds.

Treat hypotension and bradycardia with fluids, leg elevation, α- and β-agonists (epinephrine, ephedrine, or dopamine), or atropine as the need dictates. Although lidocaine (with diazepam pretreatment) has been shown to be effective for bupivacaine-induced ventricular dysrhythmias, strong theoretical and experimental evidence indicates that bretylium is more effective.[110,111] However, until bretylium becomes available again, amiodarone is a reasonable alternative. High doses of atropine and epinephrine can be successful in correcting pulseless idioventricular rhythm. Cardiopulmonary resuscitation is instituted when necessary.

IV Lipid Emulsion

Recently, animal studies, case reports, and personal opinion have advocated the use of 20% lipid emulsion intravenously to resuscitate bupivacaine- and mepivacaine-related cardiac arrest, a situation that is usually fatal. Rosenblatt and associates[112] described the IV injection of 100 mL of 20% Intralipid (Baxter formulation used for hyperalimentation) followed by an infusion (0.5 ml/kg per min over 2 hr) and related this intervention to a successful resuscitation in a scenario that appeared hopeless. Picard[113] considers lipid emulsion a "crucial antidote" that should be available when local anesthetics are used for peripheral nerve blocks. It is unclear whether this intervention will prove useful for local anesthetic cardiac arrest, but initial data are encouraging.

Allergic Reactions

Allergenic Agents

True allergic reactions are rare, accounting for only 1% to 2% of all adverse reactions, but they are important to recognize because of their serious potential. Ester solutions (procaine, tetracaine), which produce the metabolite para-aminobenzoic acid (PABA), account for the great majority of these reactions. Amide solutions (lidocaine, bupivacaine) are rarely involved, and usually the preservative methylparaben (MPB), which is structurally similar to PABA, is responsible. Although pure esters and pure amides do not cross-react, amides may appear to do so if multidose vials containing MPB are used. Patients may manifest an allergic response on first contact to a local anesthetic because of previous sensitization to these agents. MPB is found in creams, ointments, and various cosmetics, and PABA is an ingredient in many sunscreen preparations. Patients who are latex-sensitive may manifest an allergic reaction incorrectly attributed to the local anesthetic.

Cell-mediated delayed reactions manifesting as dermatitis are rare; it is immediate hypersensitivity that most concerns the emergency clinician. A spectrum of signs and symptoms may occur, from rhinitis and mild urticaria to bronchospasm, upper airway edema, or anaphylactic shock. Onset may be immediate, occurring even during administration of the agent. Treat anaphylaxis in the usual manner.

The more frequent problem facing emergency clinicians is the patient who claims to have a past history of local anesthetic allergy. Most patients assume that any adverse reaction to a local anesthetic procedure is an allergy. Because allergy is rarely the cause, a careful history and a review of prior records, if available, are crucial in evaluating these patients. Procaine, trade name Novocaine, was commonly used in dentistry, and many patients who experienced many types of reactions in the dentist's office, rarely true allergy, state they are allergic to Novocaine. Procaine is no longer used in dental practice, but procaine is the local anesthetic in intramuscular penicillin preparations (procaine penicillin G).

Attempts to uncover the actual cause of the past reaction and the specific agent involved are often fruitless. Ask about the exact signs and symptoms, technique of administration, amount of drug used, and how the patient was treated. If an allergic reaction cannot be ruled out and the drug previously used is known, use an agent from the other class (whether amide or ester). Lidocaine from a dental cartridge does not contain MPB, and if this were the allergenic source, an ester agent could be used. However, if lidocaine from a multidose vial is implicated, do not use an ester because MPB may cross-react with PABA. In this case, it may be safer to use an amide without MPB or to choose an alternative (see later). In most cases, the allergen is an ester, and the patient can safely be given an amide without MPB. Single-dose ampules of 1% lidocaine without MPB, readily obtainable from a resuscitation cart, can be used for this purpose.

Uncertainty often exists regarding the specific agent involved, and the clinician must choose an alternative approach to local anesthesia. If the wounds are extensive and the risk is acceptable, procedural sedation (see Chapter 33, Systemic Analgesia and Sedation for Procedures) or general anesthesia may be used. Conversely, if minimal pain is expected and the procedure is short (e.g., one or two sutures or staples in the scalp), no anesthesia may be required. These methods may be useful, but the degree of anesthesia produced is often not sufficient. Antihistamines injected into a wound have been successfully used for many years and represent a good alternative. Local anesthetic efficacy is found in varying degrees in all antihistamines. Ketamine anesthesia may be a useful alternative in some situations and is commonly used in children.

Diphenhydramine and Benzyl Alcohol

Several studies demonstrated that 1% diphenhydramine (Benadryl) is as effective as 1% lidocaine for infiltrative anesthesia.[114–116] As long as diphenhydramine is not used at concentrations greater than 1%, potential problems of skin necrosis or significant sedation are rare. Dilute the standard 5% parenteral form to 1% concentration for subcutaneous injection (1 mL drug to 4 mL saline). The duration of action for diphenhydramine is shorter than that for lidocaine but appears to be adequate for most procedures. The injection pain of diphenhydramine exceeds that of lidocaine but can be diminished by reducing the concentration to 0.5%. At this lower concentration, the effectiveness of this agent on facial wounds is lost.[117] The addition of epinephrine to 0.5% diphenhydramine results in a more painful solution with a shorter duration of action than a standard buffered lidocaine with epinephrine solution.[118] Benzyl alcohol (0.9%) with epinephrine (1:100,000) compares favorably with diphenhydramine as an effective local anesthetic. This appears to be a useful alternative to diphenhydramine when lidocaine cannot be used but is of shorter duration than diphenhydramine.[119–121]

Skin Testing

Skin testing and progressive subcutaneous challenge doses deserve special mention because they appear to be logical and well-studied approaches. However, intradermal skin testing with local anesthetics is controversial and often of no practical benefit in the ED. False-positive results are frequently produced by local histamine release in response to needle trauma, tissue distention, or preservatives in the solution.[122] In addition, a high incidence of false-negative results can occur. It is questionable whether these low-molecular-weight drugs or their allergenic metabolites are ever capable of eliciting positive responses.[123] Other disadvantages of skin testing include its time-consuming nature and its potential hazard when even minute traces of an allergen may precipitate a serious reaction. Subcutaneous challenge testing in graduating doses has been advocated and may well eliminate many false responses, but it does not eliminate the problems of time and hazard. Swanson,[124] recognizing that allergy to pure lidocaine is extremely rare, recommended 0.1 mL as a single intradermal skin test. Although his approach eliminates the time disadvantage, the intradermal placement can still produce false responses. It would seem more reasonable to give this test dose subcutaneously while exercising due caution in the unlikely event that a patient exhibits a serious reaction.

Summary of Anesthetic "Allergy" Management

Generally speaking, the optimal approach to the patient with a presumed anesthetic allergy is to determine the specific anesthetic agent associated with a presumed allergic reaction and then use a preservative-free agent from the other class (see earlier discussion). If the agent is unknown, use an antihistamine or give 0.1 mL of preservative-free lidocaine as a subcutaneous test dose, proceeding with the full dose if no reaction occurs within 30 minutes. Given the studies mentioned earlier, the prudent choices would seem to be diphenhydramine (Benadryl) or benzyl alcohol. Epinephrine (1:100,000) can be added to both of these drugs to prolong the duration of action. Ketamine anesthesia is also an alternative.

Catecholamine Reactions

Anxiety and vasoconstrictor (epinephrine) reactions are discussed together because each produces similar manifestations caused by elevated catecholamine levels. These relatively common disorders are difficult to distinguish from each other and are generally not serious.

Excess catecholamine levels produce tachycardia, palpitations, hypertension, apprehension, tremulousness, diaphoresis, tachypnea, pallor, and on occasion, anginal chest pain. Thus, catecholamine excess may resemble the CNS stimulation phase of local anesthetic toxicity.

Catecholamine reactions are usually not caused solely by exogenous epinephrine, because if it is used in its optimal concentration (1:200,000), the maximum safe dose (0.25 mg) is rarely exceeded. However, many patients produce significant endogenous catecholamines owing to anxiety about the anesthetic approach or upcoming procedure. In this case, even the addition of small amounts of epinephrine could trigger a catecholamine reaction. Therefore, patient preparation includes proper explanation and reassurance to decrease anxiety. Exercise caution for patients who have hyperthyroidism, hypertension, or atherosclerotic cardiovascular disease, although these conditions do not contraindicate the judicious use of epinephrine-containing anesthetics. Do not give epinephrine-containing anesthetics to patients on MAO inhibitors.

Treatment of the catecholamine reaction includes stopping further drug administration; observing the patient closely; and administering α- or β-antagonists or benzodiazepine agents, if necessary, to combat severe reactions.

Vasovagal Reactions

It is not standard to monitor patients (cardiac, pulse oximetry) during routine local anesthesia procedures. Vasovagal reactions are, however, common, especially in dental procedures

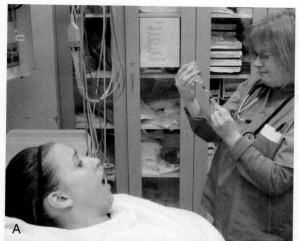

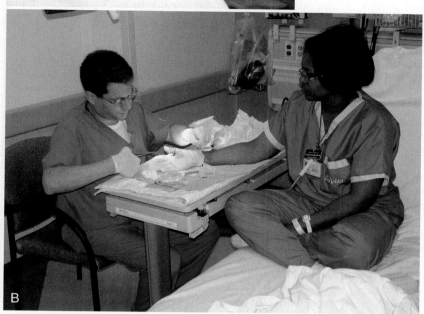

Figure 29–7 *A* and *B,* What's wrong with these pictures? *A,* Drawing up the local anesthetic with a syringe in front of the patient and (*B*) administering local anesthesia or suturing with the patient in the upright position court a vasovagal reaction. Neither is recommended.

(reported incidence, 2%–3%), during which the patient is generally in an upright position. To limit vasovagal reactions related to local anesthesia in the ED, do not draw up medication in a syringe in front of the patient, and inject only when the patient is supine (Fig. 29–7). The patient initially experiences anxiety when a triggering event, commonly the sight or sensation of needle insertion, causes a loss of sympathetic tone and an increase in vagal tone. The resultant hypotension and bradycardia may lead to syncope. Address the patient's anxiety and administer the injections with the patient recumbent as useful preventive measures. Cardiac monitoring may help identify the onset of vagally induced bradycardia when suggested by past history. Lay the patient supine and elevate the legs. Rarely, atropine is required. Should a patient lose consciousness while in a recumbent position, consider diagnoses other than vasovagal syncope, although significant bradycar-

dia, and even complete heart block, may accompany a vagal reaction in the supine patient.

SUMMARY

Emergency medicine cannot be practiced without the use of local anesthetic agents. Their effectiveness when applied topically or by infiltration makes them extremely adaptable to many clinical circumstances. A working knowledge of commonly employed agents is necessary to ensure the safe administration of these medications. Direct specific effort at maximizing the drugs' anesthetic effects while minimizing the pain of administration and risk of toxicity.

 REFERENCES CAN BE FOUND ON EXPERT CONSULT

CHAPTER **30**

Regional Anesthesia of the Head and Neck

James T. Amsterdam and Kevin P. Kilgore

Intraoral and extraoral regional anesthesia is both simple and convenient, and it lends itself for everyday use in the emergency department (ED).[1,2] Nerve blocks attain anesthesia in areas of broad distribution in the face with a minimal amount of anesthetic and resultant tissue distortion. Local anesthetic blocks are effective for closing facial lacerations, especially those of the lips, the forehead, and the midface, where the swelling caused by local infiltration may be undesirable. Local anesthetic blocks are also effective for the relief of pain, anesthesia in débridement, and diagnostic purposes.

Regional blocks are also therapeutic for both surgical procedure anesthesia and pain control for dental emergencies such as toothaches and dry sockets (see Chapter 65, Emergency Dental Procedures). Patients with dental pain who do not get relief with a regional dental block most likely do not have pain of dental origin. In cases in which the patient is thought to be seeking drugs and one wishes to avoid narcotics, a dental anesthetic block is frequently the treatment of choice.

Topical anesthetic solutions such as tetracaine-adrenaline-cocaine (TAC) solution are useful in small lacerations of the scalp and face because of the vascularity of these areas. TAC is not to be used on or near mucous membranes or the eye (see Chapter 29, Local and Topical Anesthesia). More extensive discussions of the general complications of local anesthetics and of regional anesthesia are provided in Chapters 29, Local and Topical Anesthesia, and 32, Intravenous Regional Anesthesia, respectively. Ophthalmologic anesthesia is discussed in Chapter 63, Ophthalmologic Procedures. Blocks about the ears and nasal anesthesia are discussed in Chapter 64, Otolaryngologic Procedures.

The procedures and techniques described here generally carry a low morbidity. The supraperiosteal and mental nerve infiltrations can generally be learned through reading and experimentation; more sophisticated blocks (e.g., inferior alveolar block) are best learned under the instruction of an experienced clinician, a dentist, or an oral and maxillofacial surgeon.

ANATOMY OF THE FIFTH CRANIAL (TRIGEMINAL) NERVE

The fifth cranial nerve, the trigeminal nerve, is the sensory nerve to the face (Fig. 30–1*A*) and the largest of the cranial nerves. It takes its origin from the midbrain and enlarges into the gasserian, or semilunar, ganglion. One gasserian ganglion supplies each side of the face. The gasserian ganglion is a flat, crescent-shaped structure approximately 10 mm long and 20 mm wide that divides into three branches: the ophthalmic, the maxillary, and the mandibular nerves (see Fig. 30–1*B*).

Ophthalmic Nerve

The first division, the *ophthalmic nerve* (V_1), is the smallest branch in the gasserian ganglion. It leaves the cranium through the superior orbital fissure and has five cutaneous branches. These branches are:

1. The medial and lateral branches of the supraorbital nerve, which emerge on the face through the supraorbital notch. These two sensory nerves pierce the frontalis muscle and extend to the lambdoid suture on the back of the skull.
2. The supratrochlear nerve, which is sensory to the medial aspect of the forehead just above the glabella.
3. The infratrochlear nerve.
4. The lacrimal nerve.
5. The external nasal nerve.

In addition to being sensory to the forehead, branches of the ophthalmic nerve are sensory to the cornea, the upper eyelid, structures in the orbit, and the frontal sinuses.

Maxillary Nerve

The second division, the *maxillary nerve* (V_2), is sensory to the maxilla and associated structures, such as the teeth, the periosteum and mucous membranes of the maxillary sinus and the nasal cavity, the soft and hard palate, the lower eyelids, the upper lip, and the side of the nose (see Fig. 30–1*C*). The second division exits the cranium from the foramen rotundum and ultimately enters the face through the infraorbital canal; it terminates as the infraorbital nerve. The infraorbital nerve gives sensory branches to the lower eyelids, the side of the nose, and the upper lip.

The anatomy of the maxillary nerve is rather complicated because of its numerous branches. The first branch comprises two short sphenopalatine nerves to the pterygopalatine ganglion, also called the *Meckel ganglion* or the *sphenopalatine ganglion*. The next two branches of clinical importance are the nasopalatine and the greater (anterior) palatine nerves. The nasopalatine nerve arises from the pterygopalatine ganglion, courses down along the nasal septum, and is transmitted through the anterior portion of the hard palate by way of the anterior palatine canal. This canal is located in the midline approximately 10 mm palatally to the maxillary central teeth and immediately behind the incisors. The nasopalatine nerve is sensory to the most anterior portion of the hard palate and the adjacent gum margins of the upper incisors. This nerve is rarely blocked in clinical practice, except in dental operations (Fig. 30–2).

The anterior, or great, palatine nerve arises from the pterygopalatine ganglion and passes down through the posterior palatine foramen. The posterior palatine foramen is located 10 mm palatally to the third molar and the bicuspid teeth and intermingles with the nasopalatine nerve opposite the cuspid tooth. The greater palatine nerve is sensory to most of the hard palate, as well as the palatal aspect of the gingiva. It is rarely blocked in the ED (see Fig. 30–2).

The next branch consists of the posterior superior alveolar (PSA) nerve, which courses down the posterior surface of the maxilla for approximately 20 mm, at which point it enters one or several small posterosuperior dental foramina. This nerve supplies all the roots of the third and second molar teeth and two roots of the first molar tooth. A third branch consists of the middle superior alveolar (MSA) nerve, which branches off about midway within the infraorbital canal and then courses downward in the outer wall of the maxillary sinus.

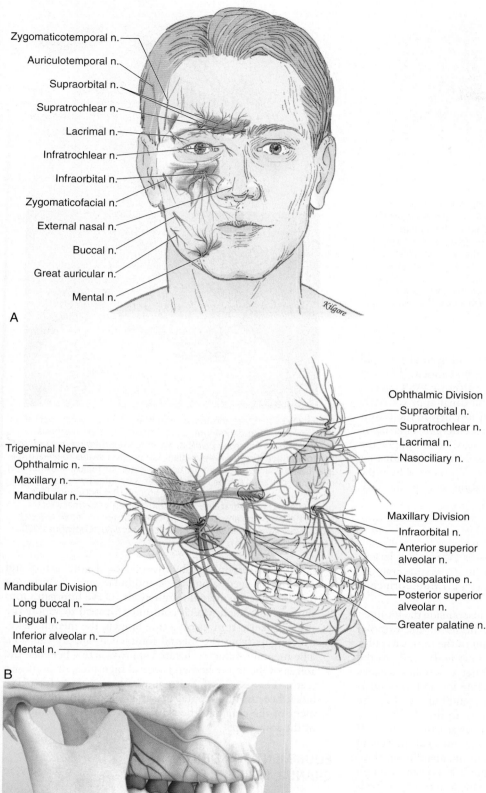

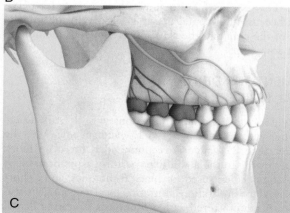

Figure 30–1 *A,* Cutaneous distribution of the trigeminal nerve (CN V). Note that the supraorbital, infraorbital, and mental foramina are all in line just medial to the pupil when the person looks straight ahead. *B,* Branches of the trigeminal nerve. *C,* Maxillary nerve branches to the upper teeth. *(A and B, Adapted from Eriksson E [ed]: Illustrated Handbook in Local Anesthesia. Philadelphia, WB Saunders, 1980; C, from Thomsen T, Setnik G [eds]: Procedures Consult— Emergency Medicine Module. Copyright 2008 Elsevier Inc. All rights reserved.)*

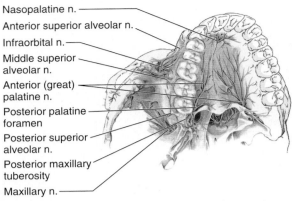

Nasopalatine n.
Anterior superior alveolar n.
Infraorbital n.
Middle superior alveolar n.
Anterior (great) palatine n.
Posterior palatine foramen
Posterior superior alveolar n.
Posterior maxillary tuberosity
Maxillary n.

Figure 30–2 The anterior one third of the palate, from canine to canine, is anesthetized by a local injection near the anterior palatine canal. There may be some overlapping branches of the anterior palatine nerve. Anesthesia of the posterior two thirds of the palate is obtained by a local injection in the area of the posterior palatine foramen. *Note:* Do not enter the foramen itself because the anesthetic may reach the middle palatine nerve and produce anesthesia of the soft palate, resulting in gagging. *(Adapted from Eriksson E [ed]: Illustrated Handbook in Local Anesthesia. Philadelphia, WB Saunders, 1980.)*

This nerve supplies the maxillary first and second bicuspid teeth and the mesiobuccal root of the first molar. The last branch consists of the anterior superior alveolar (ASA) nerve, which branches off into the infraorbital canal approximately 5 mm behind the infraorbital foramen, just before the terminal branches of the infraorbital nerve emerge. This nerve descends in the anterior wall of the maxilla to supply the maxillary central, lateral, and cuspid teeth; the labial mucous membrane; the periosteum; and the alveoli on one side of the median line. There is intercommunication among the ASA, MSA, and PSA nerves.

Mandibular Nerve

The third division, the *mandibular nerve* (V₃), is the largest branch of the trigeminal nerve. It exits from the cranium through the foramen ovale and divides into three principal branches:

1. The long buccal nerve branches off just outside the foramen ovale. It passes between the two heads of the external pterygoid muscle and crosses in front of the ramus to enter the cheek through the buccinator muscle, buccally to the maxillary third molar. The buccal nerve supplies sensory branches to the buccal mucous membrane and the mucoperiosteum over the maxillary and mandibular teeth. The cutaneous branch is the sensory nerve to the cheek.
2. The lingual nerve courses forward toward the midline. It runs downward superficially to the internal pterygoid muscle to pass lingually to the apex of the mandibular third molar. It enters the base of the tongue at this point through the floor of the mouth and supplies the anterior two thirds of the tongue, the lingual mucous membrane, and the mucoperiosteum.
3. The largest of the V₃ branches is the inferior alveolar nerve. It is sensory to all of the lower teeth, although the central and lateral incisors and the buccal aspect of the molar teeth may receive additional sensory innervation. The nerve descends, covered by the external pterygoid muscle, and passes between the ramus of the mandible and the sphenomandibular ligament to enter the mandibular

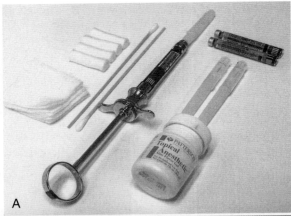

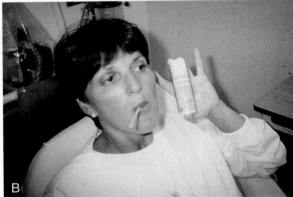

Figure 30–3 *A,* Local anesthesia—basic setup for intraoral application using an aspirating dental syringe. *B,* Topical mucosal anesthesia can *make the injection nearly painless.* Swab the *gauze-dried mucosa* with the topical agent or have the patient hold cotton swabs soaked in the agent, and wait for 1–3 min. Particularly excellent topical anesthesia of mucus membranes can be obtained after 2 minutes by applying a gel mixture of a topical anesthetics consisting of 10% lidocaine, 10% prilocaine and 4% tetracaine. (Profound, Steven's Pharmacy Costa Mesa, CA www.stevensrx.com) (*A,* From Thomsen T, Setnik G [eds]: *Procedures Consult—Emergency Medicine Module.* Copyright 2008 Elsevier Inc. All rights reserved.)

canal. It is accompanied by the inferior alveolar artery and vein and proceeds along the mandibular canal, innervating the teeth. At the mental foramen, the nerve bifurcates into an incisive branch, which continues forward to supply the anterior teeth. It gives off a side branch, the mental nerve, which exits from the mental foramen to supply the skin. The mental foramen is located approximately between the apices of the lower first and second bicuspids, or premolar teeth. This is a useful site at which to perform a nerve block because the mental nerve is sensory to the integument of the chin and the skin and the mucous membrane of the lower lip.

EQUIPMENT FOR DENTAL AND CRANIAL NERVE BLOCKS

One may easily give extraoral injections with a 3-mL Luer-Lok syringe with a 1½-inch, 25- to 27-gauge needle. A needle no smaller than 27 gauge is recommended for deep block techniques owing to the inability to perform aspiration. Generally, a long needle is used for block techniques, and a short needle is used for infiltrations. Intraoral local anesthesia is also conveniently administered with a Monoject aspirating dental syringe, which uses Carpule cartridges of anesthetic and disposable needles (Fig. 30–3A). Dental syringes are not mandatory for intraoral local anesthesia but do make the procedure simpler, particularly aspiration. Other adjuncts that are helpful in the administration of intraoral anesthesia include topical local anesthetic agents such as gels or sprays (see Fig. 30–3B).

The anesthetic agent most frequently used is 2% lidocaine with a vasoconstrictor, such as 1:100,000 or 1:50,000 epinephrine. Many other anesthetic agents, such as mepivacaine (Carbocaine) and Cetacaine (a combination of benzocaine, tetracaine, butamben, and benzalkonium), with or without vasoconstrictor agents, are also available. Bupivacaine (Marcaine) with or without epinephrine is a longer-acting anesthetic that is often ideal for the procedures performed in the ED. Bupivacaine with epinephrine is theoretically the best choice in the ED because of its longer duration of action. Because of the rich vascularity of the oral cavity, vasoconstrictors are important in sustaining the duration of anesthesia and should be used wherever possible in the absence of medical contraindications. Buffering with bicarbonate is not recommended for oral anesthesia.

GENERAL RECOMMENDATIONS

Needles no smaller than 27 gauge should be used for block techniques, because a higher-gauge needle makes aspiration difficult, possibly resulting in inadvertent intravascular injection. An intravascular injection is not problematic except that the nerve block will not be effective. Intravascular epinephrine, although used in small doses, may produce systemic symptoms (anxiety, tachycardia), but the amount of local anesthetic is inconsequential.

When an intraoral block procedure is performed, the needle should not be inserted to its full length at the hub. Should inadvertent breakage occur in such a situation, needle retrieval may be difficult. Furthermore, the direction of a needle should not be changed while the needle is deep in the tissue. One should always aspirate before injection, and inject slowly to minimize pain. A warmed anesthetic solution is also more comfortable for the patient. In addition, topical anesthetics can be placed on mucous membranes before all dental blocks to make needle puncture painless. This adjunct is greatly appreciated by the patient and suggested whenever possible (see Fig. 30–3B).

An important caveat for intraoral local anesthesia is that the injection should not be made into or through an infected area. This is especially important in inferior alveolar nerve blocks, in which tracking of an infection can be serious and difficult to treat. Trismus with inadequate oral access or direct extension of infection to parapharyngeal spaces can result. Therefore, local anesthesia should be only superficial before incision and drainage, unless a block can be performed far proximal to the site of infections.

TECHNIQUE

Topical Anesthesia

Most patients fear dental blocks greatly, and the anxiety and pain may be lessened considerably with the use of topical anesthetics applied to the mucous membranes before injection. Importantly, *the area to be injected is first thoroughly dried with gauze.* Copious saliva will wash away the anesthetic prematurely. A cotton-tipped applicator is generously coated with 20% benzocaine (Hurricane, Beutlich, Inc, Niles, IL) or 5% to 10% lidocaine, and the area of injection is painted.

The patient may hold the cotton swab in place. Anesthesia results in 2 to 3 minutes. Note that rather concentrated topical anesthetics must be used, and poor results are obtained with weaker preparations such as 2% viscous lidocaine. Cocaine (4%) is another acceptable topical anesthetic.

Supraperiosteal Infiltrations

The most common technique for intraoral local anesthesia of individual teeth is the supraperiosteal infiltration injection. This technique may supply complete relief of a toothache. The area to be anesthetized is selected and dried with gauze. A topical anesthetic, such as 20% benzocaine or 5% lidocaine ointment, is applied as described. The patient is asked to close the jaw slightly to relax the facial musculature. The mucous membrane of the area is grasped with a piece of gauze; the gauze is pulled out and downward in the maxilla and out and upward in the mandible to extend the mucosa fully and to delineate the mucobuccal fold. The mucobuccal fold is then punctured with the bevel of the needle facing the bone. The area is aspirated, and approximately 1 to 2 mL of local anesthetic is deposited at the apex (area of the root tip) of the involved tooth (Fig. 30–4). It is helpful to place a finger against the *outer* aspect of the lip overlying the injection site and apply firm and steady pressure against the lip as the local anesthetic is *slowly injected* into the supraperiosteal site.

The purpose of the injection is to deposit the anesthetic near the bone that supports the tooth. Because the anesthetic must penetrate the cortex of bone to reach the nerve of the individual tooth, the injection may fail if the solution is deposited too far from the periosteum, if the needle is passed too far above the roots of the teeth, or if the bone in the area is unusually thick or dense. If anesthesia is unsuccessful, one may also inject the palatal side. It may take 5 to 10 minutes to achieve full anesthesia with this technique, and the procedure may not be as effective for the posterior molars. Infiltration of the area around the maxillary canine and the first premolars will anesthetize the MSA and ASA nerves; lacerations of the upper lip can be treated by bilateral injection in the canine fossa areas.

Posterior or Superior Alveolar Nerve Block

Anatomy

The PSA block is used to anesthetize the maxillary molar teeth. On occasion, the maxillary first molar may not be completely anesthetized by this technique alone and may require an additional block (discussed subsequently). The landmarks for this technique are the posterior-lateral portion of the maxillary tuberosity and the second molar (see Fig. 30–5A).

Intraoral Approach

A topical anesthetic on a cotton-tipped swab is applied to gauze-dried mucosa for 60 to 90 seconds prior to introducing the needle for the nerve block.[1,3] With the patient's mouth half-open and the jaw swung toward the operator, the cheek is retracted laterally. The puncture is made in the mucosal reflection just distal to the distal buccal root of the upper second molar (Fig. 30–5). The needle is directed toward the maxillary tuberosity (i.e., upward, backward, and inward) and then along the curvature of the maxillary tuberosity to a depth of approximately 2 to 2.5 cm. On reaching this depth, the needle is aspirated and 2 to 3 mL of anesthetic solution is injected.

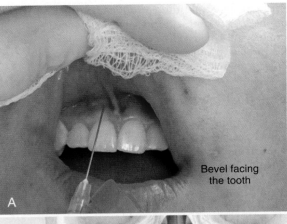

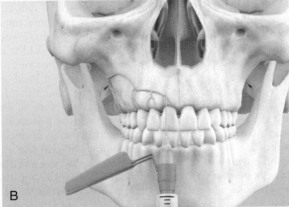

Bevel facing the tooth

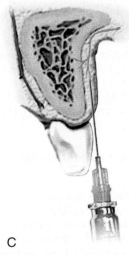

Figure 30–4 Supraperiosteal injection to numb upper individual teeth, good for an isolated toothache. Topical anesthesia is applied to the dried mucosa before injection. *A,* Supraperiosteal injection technique above the incisors for anesthesia of the upper lip or individual teeth. *B,* Diagrammatic representation of the supraperiosteal injection. *C,* The aim is to deposit the anesthetic next to the periosteum at the level of the apex (area of the root tip) of the desire tooth. The palatal side of the tooth may also be injected. *(B, From Thomsen T, Setnik G [eds] Procedures Consult—Emergency Medicine Module. Copyright 2008 Elsevier Inc. All rights reserved.)*

Complications

Complications include puncture of the pterygoid plexus and hematoma formation should the syringe not be aspirated before injection. Also, if the needle were advanced too far posteriorly, a division II block of cranial nerve V will result.

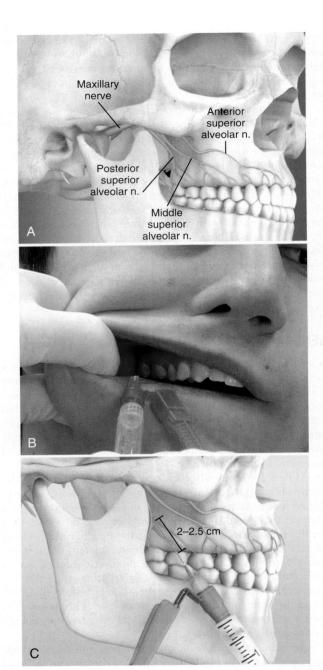

Figure 30–5 *A–C,* Posterior superior alveolar nerve block. See text for details. *(A–C, From Thomsen T, Setnik G [eds]: Procedures Consult— Emergency Medicine Module. Copyright 2008 Elsevier Inc. All rights reserved.)*

Middle Superior Alveolar Nerve Block

Anatomy

The MSA block is used to anesthetize the mesiobuccal root of the maxillary first molar in order to achieve complete anesthesia of this tooth. The landmark for this procedure is the junction between the second premolar and first molar (Fig. 30–6).

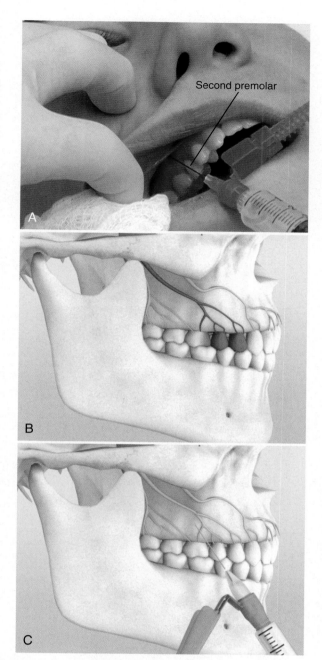

Figure 30–6 *A–C,* Middle superior alveolar nerve block. See text for details. *(A–C, From Thomsen T, Setnik G [eds]: Procedures Consult— Emergency Medicine Module. Copyright 2008 Elsevier Inc. All rights reserved.)*

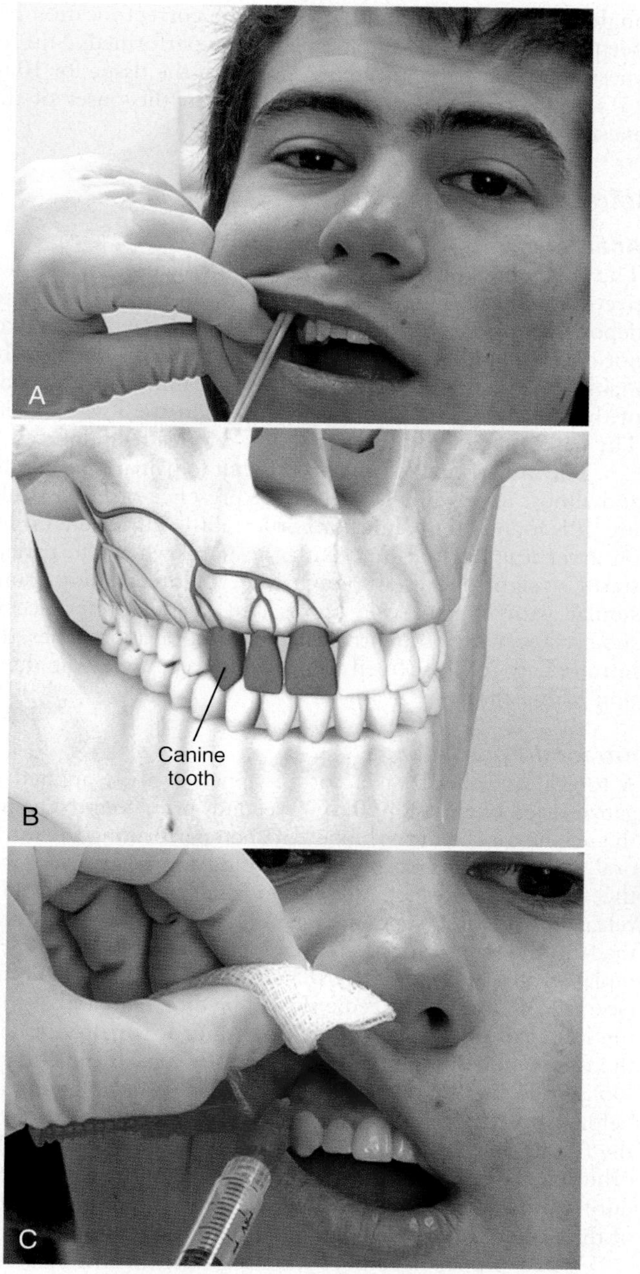

Figure 30–7 *A–C,* Anterior superior alveolar nerve block. See text for details. *(A–C, From Thomsen T, Setnik G [eds]: Procedures Consult— Emergency Medicine Module. Copyright 2008 Elsevier Inc. All rights reserved.)*

Intraoral Approach

A topical anesthetic on a cotton-tipped swab is applied to gauze-dried mucosa for 60 to 90 seconds prior to introducing the needle for the nerve block.[1,3] The cheek is retracted laterally and the puncture is made in the mucosal reflection adjacent to the mesiobuccal root area of the first molar (the space between the second premolar and the first molar) directing the needle at a 45° angle (see Fig. 30–6B). When the correct location has been determined and aspiration has been performed, 2 to 3 mL of anesthetic solution is injected. Massage of the tissue for 10 to 15 seconds after the injection will hasten the onset of the anesthesia.

Anterior Superior Alveolar Nerve Block

Anatomy
The landmark for this technique is the apex of the canine tooth (Fig. 30–7).

Intraoral Approach
A topical anesthetic on a cotton-tipped swab is applied to gauze-dried mucosa for 60 seconds prior to introducing the needle for the nerve block.[1,3] The patient is asked to close her or his jaw slightly to relax the upper lip. The lip is retracted anteriorly and the puncture is made in the mucosal reflection at the apex of the canine tooth directing the needle at a 45°

angle (see Fig. 30–7B and C). When the correct location has been determined and aspiration has been performed, 2 mL of anesthetic solution is injected. Massage of the tissue for 10 to 15 seconds after the injection will hasten the onset of the anesthesia.

Infraorbital Nerve Block

Anatomy

The infraorbital nerve block injection can be used to anesthetize the midface (Fig. 30–8A). A solution of local anesthetic deposited adjacent to the infraorbital foramen anesthetizes not only the middle and superior alveolar nerves but also the main trunk of the infraorbital nerve that innervates the skin of the upper lip, the skin of the nose, and the lower eyelid. The nasal mucosa is not anesthetized by this technique.

The infraorbital foramen is difficult to palpate extraorally and almost impossible to feel in the presence of facial swelling. It is found on the inferior border of the infraorbital ridge on a vertical (sagittal) line with the pupil when the patient stares straight ahead. Although one volunteer study found similar patient pain scale scores and overall preference in subjects receiving both intraoral and extraoral approaches, the intraoral approach seemed to provide nearly twice the duration of anesthesia.[4]

Intraoral Approach

A topical anesthetic on a cotton-tipped swab is applied to gauze-dried mucosa for 60 to 90 seconds prior to introducing the needle for the nerve block.[1,3] When performing the intraoral approach, one keeps the palpating finger in place over the inferior border on the infraorbital rim. The cheek is retracted, as in the supraperiosteal injection, and puncture is made in the mucosa opposite the upper second bicuspid (premolar tooth) approximately 0.5 cm from the buccal surface (see Fig. 30–8B). The needle should be directed parallel with the long axis of the second bicuspid until it is palpated near the foramen, a depth of approximately 2.5 cm. If the entry is too acute initially, one will encounter the malar eminence before approaching the infraorbital foramen. In addition, if the needle is extended too far posteriorly and superiorly, the orbit may be entered (see Fig. 30–8C). Therefore, the procedure should be halted if the clinician is unsure of the location of the needle or if patient cooperation is unsatisfactory.

When proper needle location has been determined and aspiration has been performed, 2 to 3 mL of solution is injected *adjacent to, but not within, the foramen*. A finger should be held firmly on the inferior orbital rim to avoid ballooning of the lower eyelid with anesthetic solution. If one is not certain of the exact location of the infraorbital foramen, one may obtain anesthesia by performing a field block. For the latter technique, 5 mL of the anesthetic solution is infiltrated in a fanlike distribution in the upper buccal fold. This technique is not as precise as a discrete nerve block but usually produces the same effect. Massage of the tissue for 10 to 15 seconds after the injection will hasten the onset of the anesthesia.

Extraoral Approach

The infraorbital foramen may also be approached from an extraoral route (Fig. 30–9A and B). The extraoral approach, of course, requires external preparation of the skin. In the extraoral approach, similar landmarks are used to locate the infraorbital foramen. The needle can be felt to pass through

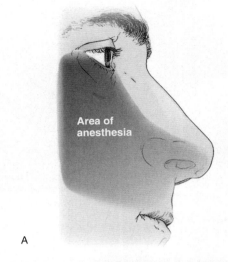

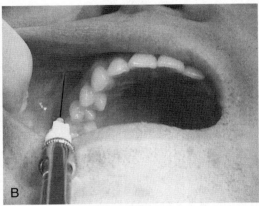

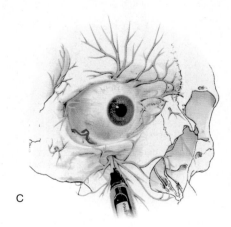

Figure 30–8 *A*, Area of anesthesia of a unilateral infraorbital nerve block. Anesthesia includes the lower eyelid and the upper lip. *B*, Intraoral approach. Lay a generous line of anesthetic in the sulcus. With the patient looking forward, this nerve is directly under the pupil. *C*, Be careful to avoid entering the orbit with this block, keep the needle tip under the orbital rim.

the skin, the subcutaneous tissue, and the quadratus labii superioris muscle. After injection, the infiltrated tissue, usually visibly swollen, should be firmly massaged for 10 to 15 seconds. Placing a finger under the eye will limit eye edema (see Fig. 30–9C).

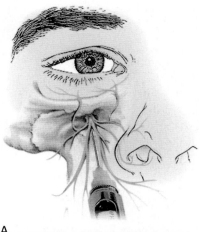

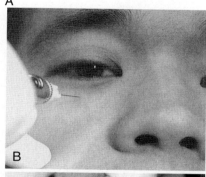

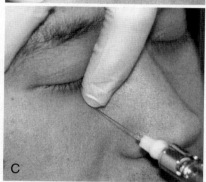

Figure 30–9 *A,* Extraoral approach for the infraorbital nerve block. This procedure is more difficult than the intraoral approach, especially when attempting to obtain anesthesia of the upper lip. *B,* Do not enter the foramen. Deposit anesthetic around the opening. *C,* While injecting, place the finger under the eyelid to minimize lid swelling. *(A–C, Adapted from Eriksson E [ed]: Illustrated Handbook in Local Anesthesia. Philadelphia, WB Saunders, 1980.)*

Care must be taken not to anesthetize the facial artery and vein, because these may lie on either side of the needle. Vasoconstrictors should be not be used with this technique to avoid vasoconstriction of the facial artery. If severe blanching of the face occurs, warm compresses should be applied to the face immediately. Local phentolamine also may be injected into the blanched area to reverse ischemia.

Inferior Alveolar Nerve Block

In the setting of extreme dental pain, the emergency clinician may find the use of the inferior alveolar nerve block and the lingual nerve block useful. This injection is somewhat more difficult than the other techniques described, and the emergency clinician is advised to view demonstrations of this pro-

cedure before attempting it. The inferior alveolar nerve block provides anesthesia to all of the teeth on that side of the mandible and desensitizes the lower lip and the chin via block of the mental nerve. This technique is primarily useful for anesthetizing patients who have sustained severe dentoalveolar trauma; those with complaints of postextraction pain, dry socket, or pulpitis (toothache); or those with periapical abscess.

Anatomy

The anatomy of the region should first be reviewed (Fig. 30–10*A*). The patient can be seated either in a dental chair or upright with the occiput firmly against the back of the stretcher, so that when the mouth is opened, the body of the mandible is parallel to the floor. Despite the use of topical anesthesia, the clinician should be ready for an unexpected quick jerk of the head when the anxious patient first feels the needle. The clinician stands on the side *opposite* the one being injected.

The technique first involves *palpation of the retromolar fossa with the index finger or thumb*. With this maneuver, the greatest depth of the anterior border of the ramus of the mandible (the coronoid notch) may be identified (see Fig. 30–10*B*). With the thumb in the mouth and the index finger placed externally behind the ramus, the tissues are retracted toward the buccal (cheek) side, and the pterygomandibular triangle is visualized (see Fig. 30–10*C*). This technique also moves the operator's finger safely away from the tip of the needle.

Approach

The gauze-dried mucosa over the area to be injected may be coated with a topical anesthetic, as described previously. When topical anesthesia has been obtained, the syringe should be held parallel to the occlusal surfaces of the teeth and angled so that the barrel of the syringe lies between the first and the second premolars on the opposite side of the mandible (see Fig. 30–11*D* and *E*). Failing to appreciate this required angle is the most common reason for failure with this nerve block. If a large-barrel syringe is used, the corner of the mouth may hamper efforts to obtain the proper angle. The angle is facilitated by carefully bending the 25-gauge needle about 30° (see Fig. 30–10*F*). Puncture is made in the triangle, at a point that is *1 cm above the occlusal surface of the molars*. If the needle enters too low (e.g., at the level of the teeth), the anesthetic will be deposited over the bony canal and prominence (lingula) that house the mandibular nerve, and not over the nerve itself.

The needle should be felt to pass through the ligaments and the muscles covering the internal surface of the mandible. One should stop when the needle has reached bone, which signifies contact with the posterior wall of the mandibular sulcus; bone *must* be felt with the needle. Failure to do so generally results from directing the needle toward the parotid gland (too far posteriorly) rather than toward the inner aspect of the mandible. This will anesthetize portions of the facial nerve. The needle should then be withdrawn slightly and aspirated, and approximately 1 to 2 mL of solution should be deposited. Three to 4 mL may be required if needle positioning is suboptimal.

In children, the angulation is not parallel to the occlusal surfaces of the teeth; instead, the barrel of the syringe must be held slightly higher, because the mandibular foramen is lower. One may anesthetize the *lingual nerve* by placing several drops of anesthetic solution while withdrawing the syringe.

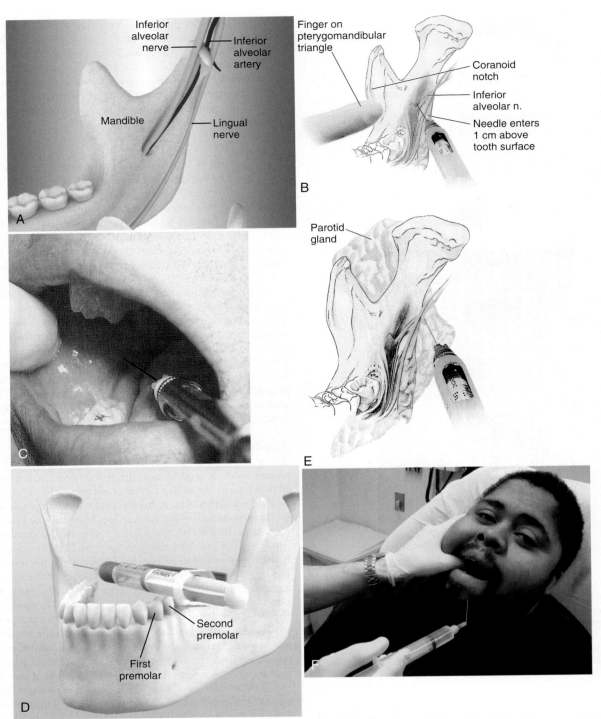

Figure 30–10 Inferior alveolar nerve block. *A,* Anatomy of the pterygomandibular triangle. *B,* The anterior border of the ramus of the mandible, the coronoid notch, is identified with the left index finger or left thumb. *C,* The ramus is grasped between an intraorally placed thumb (positioned on the coronoid notch) and an extraorally positioned index finger. The pterygomandibular triangle may then be well visualized. *D,* Note the angle of the syringe during the injection, with the barrel of the syringe overlying the first and second premolar teeth on the opposite side of the mandible. Failure to appreciate this orientation is one common cause of failure. The operator should *feel the needle contacting the bony surface of the mandible.* Also note that the injection site is 1 cm *above* the level of the occlusal plane of the molars. *E,* Directing the needle too far posteriorly during the inferior alveolar nerve block technique will result in entry into the area of the parotid gland. Anesthesia of the seventh nerve may result. This occurs because of an improper entry orientation and is corrected by following the instructions in D. *F,* To compensate for difficulty in obtaining the correct approach with a straight needle, a 25-gauge 1½-inch needle is bent 30° with the needle guard. *(A, Adapted from Eriksson E [ed]: Illustrated Handbook in Local Anesthesia. Philadelphia, WB Saunders, 1980; B–F, From Thomsen T, Setnik G [eds]: Procedures Consult—Emergency Medicine Module. Copyright 2008 Elsevier Inc. All rights reserved.)*

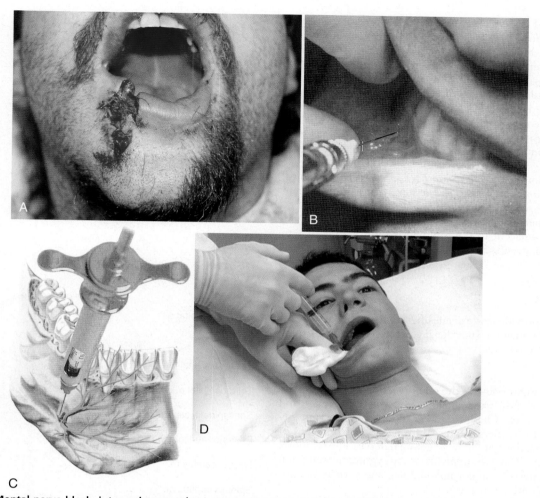

Figure 30–11 Mental nerve block, intraoral approach. *A,* A complicated lower lip laceration is an indication for this block, because it will not distort tissue. *B,* The correct supraperiosteal approach is an *infiltration* technique. *C and D,* Actual introduction of the needle into the mental foramen may produce neurovascular damage, and therefore infiltration at the foramen opening only is recommended. Use a generous amount of anesthetic and fan it out to block all branches of the nerve. *(A and D, Adapted from Eriksson E [ed]: Illustrated Handbook in Local Anesthesia. Philadelphia, WB Saunders, 1980.)*

The anterior two thirds of the tongue can thus be anesthetized. In actual practice, the lingual nerve is consistently blocked with this procedure owing to the close proximity of both nerves. One may anesthetize the *long buccal nerve* by injecting 0.2 mL of local anesthetic just distal and buccal to the last mandibular molar. Supplementing the inferior alveolar block with both the lingual and the buccal nerve blocks helps to anesthetize aberrant fibers, which may help innervate the teeth. Shortly after a successful injection, the patient will report tingling in the lower lip, however, it usually requires 3 to 5 minutes to achieve complete anesthesia.

Complications

Complications include inadvertent administration of anesthetic posteriorly in the region of the parotid gland, which will anesthetize the facial nerves. This is an annoying but relatively benign complication that will cause temporary facial paralysis (similar to a Bell's palsy) that affects the orbicularis oculi muscle and results in inability to close the eyelid. Should this occur, the eye must be protected until the local anesthetic has worn off (~2–3 hr), and the patient must be reassured. Anesthesia with bupivacaine (Marcaine) presents a more significant problem if this complication occurs, because bupivacaine anesthesia lasts from 10 to 18 hours in some patients.

Mental Nerve Block

The mental nerve is blocked by the infiltration of local anesthetic about the nerve as it exits its bony foramen. Introduction of the needle in the mental nerve foramen is to be avoided because the needle or injection of liquid into the foramen can produce neurovascular damage. Infiltration about the foramen will provide for anesthesia of the lower lip. Lacerations of the midline of the lips require administration of anesthetic about the mental nerve on each side of the face; this practice anesthetizes crossover fibers. Generally, a 1.3-cm (½-inch), 25- or 27-gauge needle on a 3-mL syringe is used.

Anatomy

The mental nerve is a continuation of the inferior alveolar nerve, which innervates the mucosa and the skin of the lower lip of the ipsilateral side of the mandible, with limited crossover of midline fibers. The nerve emerges from the mental foramen below the second premolar. Lacerations of the lower lip can be repaired with this block (Fig. 30–11*A*).

Approaches

Like the infraorbital nerve, the mental nerve may be blocked using an intraoral or an extraoral approach. Syverud and colleagues[5] found that volunteers who received intraoral topical anesthetic followed by an intraoral injection considered the technique to be less painful than the extraoral approach. Before using either approach, the mental foramen should be identified by palpation about 1 cm inferior and anterior to the second premolar. It is generally best to locate the foramen using a gloved finger placed into the labial area over the mandible. Generally, the foramen will be just medial to the pupil (while staring straight ahead) along a sagittal plane. The intraoral approach is demonstrated in Figure 30–11*B–D*.

When using the *intraoral* approach, it is best to use topical anesthesia prior to infiltration. The lower labial fold adjacent to the first or second premolar is topically anesthetized. The mental foramen is again approached at about a 45° angle, and the area adjacent to the foramen is infiltrated with 1 to 2 mL of local anesthetic and the area massaged as described previously.

Scalp Block

Scalp blocks provide surgical anesthesia for the repair of scalp lacerations, drainage of superficial scalp abscesses, and exploration of scalp wounds.

Anatomy

As shown in Figure 30–12, the scalp receives its nerve supply from branches of the trigeminal nerve (fifth cranial nerve) and the cervical plexus. The forehead is supplied by the supraorbital and supratrochlear nerves. Both nerves are branches of the ophthalmic division of the trigeminal nerve. The temporal region receives its nerve supply from the zygomaticotemporal (a V_2 branch nerve), temporomandibular, and auriculotemporal nerves (V_3 branch nerves).

The posterior aspect of the scalp is innervated by the greater auricular and the greater, lesser, and least (third) occipital nerves. The nerves that supply the posterior aspect of the scalp originate from the cervical plexus. All the nerves become superficial above a line drawn from the upper border of the external ear to the occiput and the eyebrows and converge toward the vertex of the scalp (Fig. 30–13).

Topographically, the nerves and vessels of the scalp are located in the subcutaneous tissue above the epicranial aponeurosis. From this level, they divide into small branches that extend to the deeper layers (epicranium and periosteum) (see Fig. 30–13*A*).[6]

Approaches

A scalp block can be accomplished by individually blocking each nerve that supplies the scalp, but this approach is time consuming, difficult, and cumbersome. Because the nerves on the scalp are superficially located, the scalp block can easily be performed by injecting local anesthetic agents into the subcutaneous tissue circumferentially around the area to be blocked. Injection of local anesthetic to the deeper levels is necessary only if bone is to be removed. Note that injection of local anesthetic agents only in the deeper layers without subcutaneous infiltration results in an unsuccessful block and a greater amount of bleeding during surgical intervention.[7]

In preparation for the block, a band of hair may be clipped (some clinicians prefer to shave the head, but this procedure is of unproven benefit). A band 1 cm wide and 3 cm away from the wound can be circumferentially clipped. Local anesthetics are injected in the clipped area.

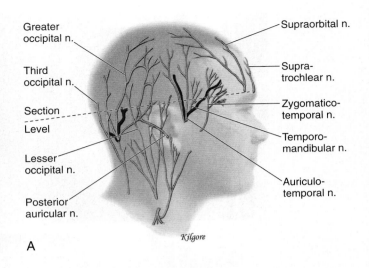

A

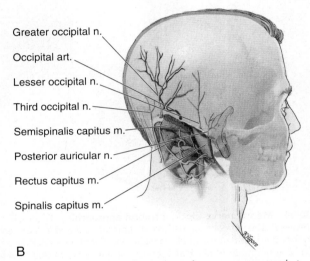

B

Figure 30–12 *A* and *B,* The sources of sensory nerve supply to the scalp.

The skin is prepared using an antiseptic solution, and a skin wheal is raised at any point along the clipped skin using a 1.3-cm (½-inch), 25-gauge needle. A 7.6-cm (3-inch), 22-gauge needle is inserted through the skin wheal into the subcutaneous tissue and advanced along the scalp circumferentially following the previously clipped area. An injection of 0.5% to 1% lidocaine or 0.125% to 0.25% bupivacaine with epinephrine (1:200,000) is used. Epinephrine should be added to the local anesthetic agent to provide vasoconstriction and to prevent excessive blood loss and local anesthetic absorption. The total dose of the local anesthetic agents should not exceed the recommended dose for the particular agent (see Chapter 29, Local and Topical Anesthesia). It may be useful to inject some local anesthetic solution into the temporalis muscle to prevent contraction of the muscle during the primary procedure.

Colley and Heavner[8] demonstrated that when bupivacaine is used, the peak plasma local anesthetic concentrations occur within 10 to 15 minutes after injection. Thus, the first 10- to 15-minute period after the injection is the most critical period for the occurrence of local anesthetic toxicity. Colley and Heavner[8] also found that despite the scalp's high vascular-

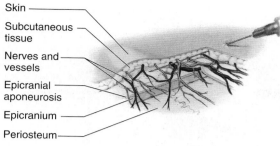

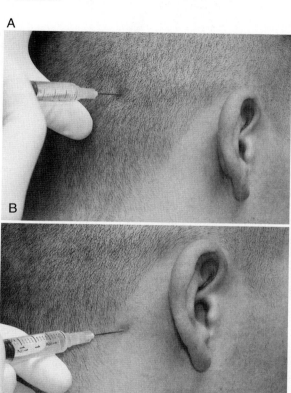

Figure 30–13 *A,* Topographic anatomy of the scalp taken above a line drawn from the upper border of the external ear to the occiput and the eyebrows. Generously infiltrating this area in a fanlike motion will block multiple sensory nerves. *B,* The greater occipital nerve is blocked on a line 3 cm lateral to the external occipital protuberance and the base of the occipital bone. *C,* The lesser occipital nerve is blocked by injection of 2–3 mL of anesthetic solution along the posterior border of the mastoid process of the temporal bone. (*A, Adapted from Eriksson E [ed]: Illustrated Handbook in Local Anesthesia. Philadelphia, WB Saunders, 1980.*)

ity, the absorption of local anesthetics from the scalp is not excessive. Considering that the toxic plasma threshold for bupivacaine is 4 µg/mL, these concentrations suggest that a scalp block using bupivacaine has a wide margin of safety, even without the use of epinephrine. When epinephrine is used with bupivacaine, its effect on absorption becomes more pronounced with concentrations of 0.125% than with those of 0.25%. This is probably because at low concentrations (0.125%), bupivacaine has a vasoconstrictor property.[9]

Greater and Lesser Occipital Nerve Block

This relatively simple block may be useful in the ED for treating occipital neuralgia and tension headaches. For occipital neuritis, a long-acting corticosteroid, such as methylprednisolone (20–40 mg) may be combined with the local anesthetic (see Chapter 52, Infection Therapy of Bursitis and Tendinitis).

Anatomy

The posterior aspect of the head is supplied by the posterior rami of the cervical nerves. Two important branches of these nerves are the greater and lesser occipital nerves. The greater occipital nerve becomes superficial on each side at the inferior border of the obliquus capitis inferior muscle and runs superiorly toward the vertex over this muscle. The nerve is located medial to the occipital artery. The lesser occipital nerve is located approximately 2.5 to 3.5 cm lateral and 1 to 2 cm caudal to the greater occipital nerve (see Fig. 30–12).[3]

Approach

It is not usually necessary to shave or clip the scalp prior to performing greater and lesser occipital nerve blocks. The greater occipital nerve can best be blocked at the nuchal line, which is in the middle of the external occipital protuberance and the mastoid process. The nuchal line is located between the insertion sites of the trapezius muscle and the semispinalis muscles. At this site, the greater occipital nerve is just medial to the occipital artery.

The occipital artery is first palpated, and a 3.8-cm, 23- to 25-gauge needle connected to a syringe that contains 5 mL of local anesthetic is inserted through the skin (see Fig. 30–13*B*). After obtaining paresthesia at the vertex, 5 mL of local anesthetic solution is injected. The lesser occipital nerve is blocked by a fanlike injection of a local anesthetic solution 2.5 to 3.5 cm lateral and 1 cm caudal to the point described for the greater occipital nerve (see Fig. 30–13*C*).[3]

This procedure is not usually associated with any complications; however, intra-arterial injections should be avoided by careful aspiration.

Ophthalmic (V₁) Nerve Block

The lateral and medial branches of the supraorbital, supratrochlear, and infratrochlear nerves may be blocked by percutaneous local injection at the point where they emerge from the superior aspect of the orbit. Anesthesia of the forehead and the scalp is achieved as far posteriorly as the lambdoid suture. Although anesthesia is easily obtained for suturing lacerations of the forehead and the scalp, the nerve block may also be used for débridement or topical treatment of burns or abrasions and for delicate lacerations of the upper eyelid. Such anesthesia is ideal for removing small pieces of glass that are embedded in the forehead from a windshield injury (Fig. 30–14).

Anatomy

The subtle supraorbital notch, which is in line with the pupil (when the patient is staring straight ahead), may be palpated along the superior orbital rim. This landmark is the site of injection for blockage of the supraorbital nerves. The supratrochlear nerve is found 0.5 to 1.0 cm medial to the notch. The infratrochlear nerve is not usually blocked but is found in the most medial aspect of the superior orbital rim. If the anesthetic is placed on the forehead proper, this block may not produce complete anesthesia of the skin of the upper eyelid if the sensory branches to the eyelid are given off before the supraorbital nerve transverses the forehead.

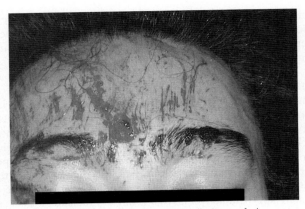

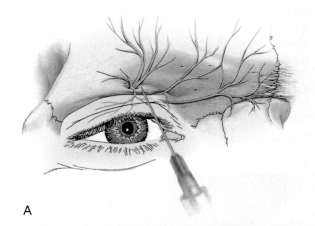

Figure 30–14 This patient had multiple small pieces of glass embedded in the forehead from a windshield injury. Removal was accomplished painlessly with bilateral supraorbital and supratrochlear nerve blocks.

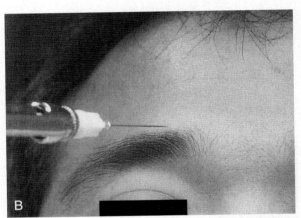

Approach

With the patient in the supine position, a skin wheal is raised. Paresthesias in the form of an electric shock sensation over the forehead are sought; these ensure a successful nerve block. One to 3 mL of anesthetic are placed in the area of the supraorbital notch. A finger or a roll of gauze should be held firmly under the orbital rim to avoid ballooning of anesthetic into the upper eyelid (Fig. 30–15*A* and *B*).

If paresthesias cannot be elicited or if the nerve block is unsuccessful, a line of anesthetic solution placed along the orbital rim from the lateral to the medial aspect will ensure block of all of the branches of the ophthalmic nerve (see Fig. 30–15*C*).

Complications

Hematoma formation or swelling of the eyelid may occur but requires only local pressure. Occasionally, ecchymosis of the periorbital region will appear the next day, and the patient should be warned of this possibility.

Although this block is infrequently used, it is easily performed and is not associated with serious side effects. Its use should be considered when anesthesia of the forehead or the anterior scalp is desired.

CONCLUSIONS

Nerve blocks about the head and neck are relatively painless when done carefully and slowly after topical mucosal anesthesia (for intraoral approaches) or local skin anesthesia (for extraoral blocks and approaches). Patients who appear anxious may benefit from sedation prior to attempting these blocks (see Chapter 33, Systemic Analgesia and Sedation for Procedures). These blocks should not be attempted in the uncooperative patient.

 REFERENCES CAN BE FOUND ON EXPERT CONSULT

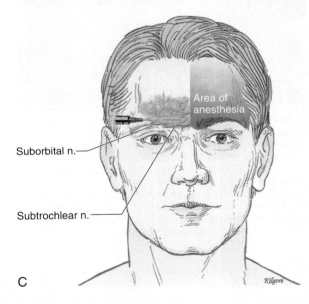

Figure 30–15 *A* and *B*, Site for local injection of the lateral and medial branches of the supraorbital nerve. It should be noted that a finger may be placed just below the margin of the superior orbital rim to avoid swelling of the eyelid. *C*, A field block of the forehead will anesthetize both the lateral and the medial branches of the supraorbital nerve as well as the supratrochlear nerves. The resultant area of anesthesia is represented by the *shaded area* of the left forehead. (*A* and *B*, *Adapted from Eriksson E [ed]: Illustrated Handbook in Local Anesthesia. Philadelphia, WB Saunders, 1980.*)

CHAPTER 31

Nerve Blocks of the Thorax and Extremities

Mark Spektor and John J. Kelly

Virtually every peripheral nerve can be blocked at some point along its course from the spine to the periphery, but digital nerve blocks of the fingers and toes are more commonly used than proximal blocks. The reasons for this are unclear but likely include a lack of experience on the part of the clinician, the time required for a block to take effect, and occasional failure to obtain adequate anesthesia. However, with proper training and experience, nerve blocks of the thorax and proximal extremities can be very useful tools for emergency clinicians. Potential applications include femoral blocks for femur fractures, ankle blocks for treatment of foot injuries and infections, intercostal blocks for rib fractures, and wrist blocks for injuries to the palm.

The preparation, technique, choice of anesthetic, precautions, and complications are similar for all nerve blocks and are described in general in the following sections. The clinician is encouraged to use the same basic techniques and precautions for all nerve blocks. Specific precautions unique to a particular nerve block are included with the description of that block. Obvious precautions, such as aspiration before injection when the needle is in close proximity to a vascular structure, are not restated in order to avoid redundancy.

GENERAL CONCEPTS

Indications

For most of the lacerations and injuries seen in the emergency department (ED), local infiltrative anesthesia is adequate and more efficient than using a nerve block (see Chapter 29, Local and Topical Anesthesia). Patients who require extensive repair and anesthesia of the entire extremity are often referred to a specialist, who may prefer to examine an unanesthetized limb. A nerve block is indicated when it will provide advantages over other techniques. Scenarios in which this requirement is met include:

- When distortion from local infiltration hampers closure (e.g., facial wounds) or may compromise blood flow (e.g., fingertip).
- When anesthesia is required over a large area and multiple injections would be painful, or the large amount of anesthetic needed for local infiltration exceeds the recommended dose.
- When a nerve block is the most efficacious form of treatment, as in an intercostal block for treating a rib fracture in a patient with chronic obstructive pulmonary disease.
- When local infiltration of the wound would be more painful than a regional nerve block, such as in the plantar surface of the foot or the palm of the hand.

- When the block is performed in order to decrease pain during finger or toe dislocation reduction.
- When extensive limb surgery or manipulation is required (e.g., extensive tendon repair) and other options are not available.

Preparation

A brief history, including drug allergies, medications, and systemic illnesses, should be taken from the patient. Specific history about allergies to local anesthetics may be prudent to elicit (see extensive discussion in Chapter 29, Local and Topical Anesthesia). Peripheral vascular, heart, and liver disease may increase the risk of severe complications. Therefore, information about the existence of these diseases should also be sought.

Instructions

The procedure—including the pain of the needle insertion, paresthesias that may be felt, and possible complications that may occur—should be explained to the patient. The possible need for additional anesthetic or alternate procedures if the initial nerve block fails should also be discussed beforehand. The patient should understand that the additional administration of anesthetic is part of the normal procedure rather than an attempt to correct an incomplete nerve block. It is not standard to obtain written informed consent for the nerve blocks performed in the ED.

Equipment

The degree of equipment preparation depends on the extent of the procedure. For a simple digital block, a 10-mL syringe, an 18-gauge needle for drawing the solution from the vial, and a 3.75-cm, 25- or 27-gauge needle for the nerve block will suffice. Note that the needle sizes given in the text are general recommendations, but for the majority of blocks, a 25-gauge needle is ideal. In addition, standard resuscitation equipment for advanced cardiac life support should be readily available any time local anesthetic agents are given.

Choice of Anesthetic

The factors influencing the choice of anesthetic agent for nerve block are similar to those for local infiltration (see Chapter 29, Local and Topical Anesthesia for extensive discussion). In general, most nerve blocks are done for the repair of painful traumatic injuries that are likely to cause pain long after the repair is complete. In such cases, anesthetics with the longest duration of action should be selected to maximize the patient's analgesia. For most of the blocks described in this chapter, 0.25% bupivacaine is suggested as the anesthetic of choice, but equal volumes of 1% lidocaine with epinephrine can be substituted. The use of epinephrine on end-organ areas is generally discouraged (e.g., toes, fingers), although the theoretical risk is largely unsubstantiated in clinical practice and recent literature.[1] Higher concentrations of lidocaine (≤2%) or bupivacaine (0.5%) are commonly used for large nerves. Ropivacaine is a relatively new amide anesthetic with a rapid onset and long duration of action (several hours). It has been reported to have fewer cardiotoxic and central nervous system effects than bupivacaine.[2,3] Care must always be taken to avoid exceeding the recommended dosages of anesthetic. Buffering the anesthetic will lessen the pain of infiltration.

Positioning of the Patient

Ideally, nerve blocks should be performed with the patient in the supine position to minimize vasovagal syncope that may occur when the patient is in an upright position. When drawing the anesthetic from the vial, do not allow the patient to see this anxiety/fear-inducing portion of the procedure.

Preparation of the Area to be Blocked

To limit the incidence of infection, the field should be prepared in an aseptic fashion before needle puncture. The antiseptic solution should be allowed to dry fully to achieve maximal antibacterial effect. Sterile drapes and gloves are not routinely required but may be considered in addition to aseptic skin preparation for the initiation of blocks that (1) are close to large joints, vessels, and nerves; (2) are located in inherently contaminated areas of the body (e.g., groin, perineum); or (3) require simultaneous palpation of the underlying structures while injecting.

Choosing the Nerves to Block

Successful anesthesia requires appropriate knowledge of anatomy. Most areas to be anesthetized have overlapping sensory innervation. Therefore, most cases require two or more nerves to be blocked. In addition, the cutaneous distribution of the various peripheral nerves differs slightly from patient to patient. A liberal margin of error should be used when determining which nerves supply the desired area of anesthesia.

Locating the Nerve

When locating a nerve to be blocked, it is best to approach it from a site with easily identifiable anatomic landmarks. The best sites are those with good structural landmarks (e.g., prominent bones or tendons) immediately next to the nerve. For example, the digital nerves are reliably found at the 2, 4, 8, and 10 o'clock positions around and just superficial to the proximal phalanx, and the median nerve lies between the palpable palmaris longus and flexor carpi radialis tendons at the proximal crease of the wrist. Nerves that course adjacent to easily palpable arteries such as in the axilla and groin are also easy to locate and are good sites for performing nerve blocks. Nerves that do not have adjacent structural or vascular landmarks are much more difficult to block.

Blocking nerves with good structural or vascular landmarks is straightforward: The landmarks are palpated, the course of the nerve in relation to those landmarks is visualized in the mind's eye, and the needle is inserted in close proximity to the nerve.

Blocking those nerves with poor landmarks, such as the radial nerve at the elbow, requires skill through practice, some degree of luck, or a nerve stimulator if such nerves are to be blocked consistently.

Nerve Stimulator

A nerve stimulator is commonly used by anesthesiologists but has never gained popularity among emergency clinicians. Its use is very acceptable but not standard.

Ultrasound

The use of ultrasound to identify injection sites for peripheral nerve blocks has been gaining popularity (see Chapter 67, Ultrasound-Guided Procedures). Ultrasonography-guided nerve blocks of the forearm nerves (median, radial, ulnar), lower extremity nerves (saphenous nerve block), and axillary plexus[4-7] have been described. Ultrasonographic guidance negates the effects of anatomic variability, provides real-time needle guidance, and allows the operator to visualize the "spread" of local anesthetic.

Paresthesia

A common technique to ensure that the needle tip is in close proximity to the nerve is to elicit a paresthesia. By touching and mechanically stimulating the nerve with movement of the needle tip, a tingling sensation or jolt known as a *paresthesia* is felt along the distribution of the nerve. In practice, the jolt of a true paresthesia is often difficult to distinguish from the "ouch" of a pain-sensitive structure. When blocking proximal nerves of the elbow or axilla, the paresthesia travels far enough away from the injection site that it can be distinguished from locally induced pain. Paresthesias at the level of the hand and wrist are much less reliably distinguished from pain. In both cases, the paresthesia is a subjective feeling that requires intelligent and cooperative patients who understand what they are expected to feel and who remain relaxed and attentive so that they are able to distinguish an "ouch" from a jolt. Before the procedure, a simple explanation of what the patient should or may feel will facilitate cooperation. Although eliciting paresthesias is generally reliable in demonstrating that the needle is close to its target, some authors feel that it may theoretically increase the rate of complications due to mechanical trauma or intraneural injection.[8-10] When a paresthesia is elicited, the needle must be withdrawn 1 to 2 mm before the anesthetic is injected. *If a paresthesia continues during the injection, stop the injection and reposition the needle.*

Injecting the Anesthetic

One strives to ensure that the anesthetic agent is not inadvertently injected into the vessels or nerve bundle. In practice, such a misplaced intravascular injection is of minimal consequence; however, small amounts of epinephrine may cause systemic symptoms, such as tachycardia or anxiety. Nerve bundle injection has the potential to cause nonspecific nerve injury. Intra-arterial injection, theoretically, is more dangerous than intravenous injection. Before injection, the syringe is aspirated to check for blood. If no blood is aspirated, the anesthetic is injected while the extremity is observed for blanching, which suggests intravascular injection. If blanching occurs, the needle should be repositioned before further injection. The onset and duration of anesthesia are greatly influenced by the proximity of the injected anesthetic to the nerve. Onset is within a few minutes if the anesthetic is in immediate proximity to the nerve. Onset takes longer or may not occur if the anesthetic must diffuse more than 2 to 3 mm, which underscores the importance of locating the nerve before injection.

More anesthetic is required if it must diffuse a large distance to the nerve. A range of suggested volumes of anesthetic is given with each nerve block description. For blocks in which a definite paresthesia is elicited or a nerve stimulator or ultrasound is used, the minimal recommended amount of anesthetic suffices. For many of the blocks of the smaller nerves, paresthesias are not easily elicited, and the anesthetic is placed in the general vicinity of the nerve. For these blocks, or when doubt exists about proximity of the needle to the nerve, larger amounts of anesthetic are recommended. This point cannot be emphasized strongly enough. *The difference between a successful and an unsuccessful block may be merely an additional 2 mL of anesthetic.* When in doubt, err on the high side of the recommended dosage. For large nerve blocks, many clinicians opt for 2% lidocaine, rather than the 1% solution that is adequate for most ED nerve blocks.

For most blocks, the onset of anesthesia occurs in 2 to 15 minutes, depending on the distance the anesthetic must diffuse to the nerve and the type of anesthetic used. One should wait 30 minutes before deciding that the block was unsuccessful.

Complications and Precautions

Complications may result from peripheral nerve blocks, but are rare in clinical practice. Most cannot be prevented by even perfect technique. General precautions include measures to minimize nerve injury, intravascular injection, and systemic toxicity. No actual statistics exist on the complication rate from nerve blocks performed by emergency clinicians. Generally, infrequently performed blocks, blocks that require high doses of anesthetic, and blocks close to major vascular structures are more likely to have complications.

Nerve Injury

Nerve injury is rare but can occur secondary to (1) chemical irritation from the anesthetic, (2) direct trauma from the needle, or (3) ischemia due to intraneural injection. Overall, the incidence of serious neuronal injury is rare, occurring in 1.9 per 10,000 blocks.[11] Given that placement of a nerve block is a blind procedure, nerve injuries do not necessarily represent an error in technique.

Neuritis, an inflammation of the nerve, is the most common nerve injury.[9,10] The patient may complain of pain and varying degrees of nerve dysfunction, including paresthesia or motor or sensory deficit. Most cases are transient and resolve completely. Supportive care and close follow-up are the mainstays of treatment. Concentrated anesthetics can produce a chemical irritation of the nerve. Emergency clinicians should not exceed recommended doses and concentrations of anesthetic (Table 31–1). In general, however, lidocaine 1% or 2% or bupivacaine 0.25% or 0.5% is safe for nerve blocks performed by the emergency clinician.

Direct nerve damage can be minimized by proper needle style, positioning, and manipulation. A short, beveled needle should be used and maneuvered so that the bevel is parallel to the longitudinal fibers. Sharp pain or paresthesia indicates that the needle is close to or in the nerve. Excessive needle movement should be avoided when the needle tip is contacting a nerve. If a 25-gauge needle is used, physical damage to a nerve should be minimal, even when directly touched by the needle tip. A 27-gauge needle is theoretically attractive, but its small size may limit aspiration testing and it may bend or break when attempting to block deep nerves.

Intraneural injection may rarely cause nerve ischemia and injury. Elicitation of a paresthesia or severe pain suggests that the needle has made contact with the nerve. *When a paresthesia is elicited, the needle must be withdrawn 1 to 2 mm before the anesthetic is injected. If the paresthesia occurs during injection, the injection is stopped and the needle must be repositioned.* Most neurons are surrounded by a strong perineural sheath through which the nutrient arteries run lengthwise. Injection directly into a nerve sheath may increase the pressure within the nerve and compress the nutrient artery. Impaired blood flow results in nerve ischemia and subsequent paralysis. Intraneural injec-

TABLE 31–1 Recommended Volumes of Anesthetic for Various Nerve Blocks

Nerve	Volume (mL)
Axillary	40–50*
Elbow	
Ulnar	5–10*
Radial	5–15*
Median	5–15*
Wrist	
Ulnar	5–15*
Radial	5–15*
Median	3–5*
Hip	
Femoral	10–30*
3-in-1	30–50*
Knee	
Tibial	5–15*
Peroneal	5–10*
Saphenous	5–10*
Ankle	
Posterior tibial	5–10*
Deep peroneal	3–5*
Saphenous, sural, and superficial peroneal	4–10*
Intercostal	5–15*
Hand	
Metacarpal and web space	2–4†
Finger	1–2†
Foot	
Metatarsal	10–15†
Web space	3–5†
Toe	2–5†

*Anesthetic: 1% lidocaine or 0.25% bupivacaine (both with epinephrine).
†Anesthetic: 1% lidocaine or 0.25% bupivacaine (both without epinephrine).
Note: For most nerve blocks performed in the emergency department, 1% lidocaine or 0.25% bupivacaine is adequate. It is also acceptable to use 2% lidocaine or 0.5% bupivacaine for larger nerves (femoral, wrist, and ankle blocks). If the stronger concentrations are used, the volume in the table should be halved.

tion is often heralded by severe pain, which worsens with further injection and may radiate along the course of innervation. The operator may notice difficulty depressing the syringe plunger. If the needle tip is in proper position, slow injection of the anesthetic should be minimally painful, and the anesthetic should go in without resistance.

Intravascular Injection

Intravascular injection may rarely result in both systemic and limb toxicity. Inadvertent intravascular injection produces high blood levels of the anesthetic. Particular care must be taken when administering large amounts of anesthetic in close proximity to large blood vessels.

Intra-arterial injection of anesthetic with epinephrine may cause peripheral vasospasm that further compromises injured tissue. Intravascular anesthetic is not toxic to the limb itself, although it may produce transient blanching of the skin by displacing blood from the vascular tree. Epinephrine, however, can cause a prolonged vasospasm and subsequent ischemia if it is injected into an artery. This is especially worrisome when anesthetizing areas with little collateral circulation, such as toes, fingers, penis, and tip of the nose. Severe epinephrine-induced tissue blanching or vasospasm may be reversed with local or intravascular injection of phentolamine (see extensive discussion in Chapter 29, Local and Topical Anesthesia).

Although vasospasm associated with epinephrine in anesthetic solutions used for nerve blocks is rare, experience in related clinical situations can help guide therapy. Roberts and Krisanda[12] used a total of 5 mg of phentolamine infused intra-arterially to reverse arm ischemia following 3 mg of epinephrine inadvertently administered into the brachial artery during cardiac resuscitation. Digital ischemia from inadvertent epinephrine autoinjection has been treated both by proximal "digital block" with 2 mg of phentolamine[13] and by local infiltration at the ischemic site with 1.5 mg of phentolamine.[14]

The route of phentolamine administration may be guided by the clinical situation. Phentolamine must reach the site of vasospasm. Arterial injection has the advantage of delivering the medication directly to the spasmed arteries. Local infiltration may be effective for ischemia of a single toe or finger. For larger areas of involvement or in instances in which local infiltration is ineffective, intra-arterial injection should be used. A dose of 1.5 to 5 mg appears to be effective in most cases,[12-14] although a total of 10 mg may be used for local infiltration. Phentolamine 5 mg can be mixed with 5 to 10 mL of either normal saline or lidocaine. The small volume of the distal pulp space may limit the infiltration dose volume to 0.5 to 1.5 mL in the fingertip. Larger volumes and dosages can be used in proximal infiltrations. For intra-arterial infusion at the radial artery in the wrist or the dorsalis pedis at the ankle, dosages of 1.5 to 5 mg of phentolamine are suitable. Slow infusion or graded dosages of 1 mg may provide enough phentolamine to reverse ischemia without excessive systemic effects such as hypotension.

Hematoma

Hematoma formation may result from arterial puncture, particularly during blocks in which a major blood vessel is being used as a landmark to locate the nerve (e.g., axillary or femoral artery). Direct pressure for 5 to 10 minutes usually controls further bleeding. Use of small-gauge needles (e.g., 25- to 27-gauge) minimizes bleeding from the punctured artery. A minor coagulopathy is not a contraindication to a nerve block.

Infection

Infection is rare and can be minimized by following aseptic technique and using the lowest possible concentration of epinephrine. Injection should be made through noninfected skin that has been antiseptically prepared. Injection through a site of infection may spread the infection to adjacent tissues, fascial planes, and joints.

Systemic Toxicity

The incidence of systemic toxicity to local anesthetics has significantly diminished in the past 30 years. Interestingly, peripheral nerve blocks have been reported to have the highest incidence of systemic toxicity.[11] Allergic reactions account for only 1% of untoward reactions[15] (see Chapter 29, Local and Topical Anesthesia, for details).

Limb Injury

Injury to the anesthetized limb can result if the patient is permitted to use the limb or is advised to use heat or cold application or to perform wound care before the anesthesia has worn off. With major nerve blocks, the patient should not be released home until sensation and function have returned.

With minor blocks, the patient may be sent home but should be properly cautioned. Care must be taken to avoid ischemia-producing compression dressings (e.g., elastic bandages), because the anesthetized area may not sense impending problems.

SPECIFIC NERVE BLOCKS

Intercostal Nerve Block

Blocking the intercostal nerves produces anesthesia over an area of their cutaneous distribution (Fig. 31–1), providing considerable pain relief for patients with rib contusion or rib fractures. Rib fractures are typically quite painful, causing the patient to splint respirations to avoid excessive movement of the injured site. The resulting hypoventilation, atelectasis, and poor expectoration may cause hypoxia or lead to pneumonia. This is particularly true in patients with preexisting pulmonary disease and minimal respiratory reserve, in whom further impairment of function may cause significant respiratory compromise.

Theoretically, anesthetizing injured ribs eases pain and facilitates deep breathing and coughing. Unfortunately, there are no controlled studies comparing intercostal blocks with oral analgesics in patients with the kinds of rib fractures that are commonly managed on an outpatient basis. However, studies do suggest that intercostal blocks may be superior to analgesics in patients who have undergone thoracotomies.[16-18] In these studies, those receiving intercostal nerve blocks had better results on pulmonary function tests, greater oxygenation, and earlier ambulation and discharge than those receiving opioid analgesics.

There are several arguments against the routine use of intercostal nerve blocks in the ED. First, rib fractures are often tolerated well in young patients, who usually require minimal oral analgesics. Second, these blocks have a relatively short duration of action. The typical duration of action of a long-acting anesthetic with epinephrine is 8 to 12 hours. However, it should be noted that patients often receive partial analgesia for up to 3 days, a period of time that cannot be

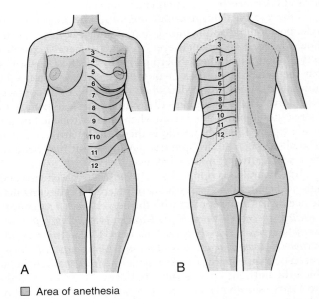

☐ Area of anethesia

Figure 31–1 Area of anesthesia and cutaneous distribution of the intercostal nerves.

attributed to the direct action of the anesthetic on the nerve. Perhaps the anesthesia reduces muscle spasm and the associated cycle of pain.

Finally, a wrongly perceived high incidence of pneumothorax and unsuccessful blocks deters many clinicians from performing intercostal nerve blocks in the ED. The true incidence of pneumothorax after intercostal nerve blocks is very low and not significant enough to prohibit the procedure. Moore[19] reported that in more than 10,000 individual rib blocks performed, the incidence of pneumothorax was less than 0.1%. However, Shanti and associates[20] reported that the incidence of pneumothorax was 1.4% for each individual intercostal nerve blocked. If more than one nerve requires blockade, the incidence of pneumothorax may be greater. The suggested approach to discussing intercostal blocks is to give patients the facts with regard to duration of analgesia and possible complications and then allow them to decide on the method for themselves. Often, they prefer oral analgesics initially but may return for further relief of pain, at which time they are more amenable to the nerve block.

Anatomy

Each thoracic nerve exits the spine through the intervertebral foramen, which lies midway between adjacent ribs. It immediately gives off the posterior cutaneous branch, which supplies the skin and muscles of the paraspinal area. The intercostal nerve then continues around the chest wall and gives off the lateral cutaneous branches at the midaxillary line (Fig. 31–2A). These branches are the sensory supply to the anterior and posterior lateral chest wall.

The intercostal nerve runs with the vein and artery in the subcostal groove (see Fig. 31–2B). The vein and artery lie *above the nerve*, and are somewhat protected by the rib during a nerve block. Posteriorly, the nerve is separated from the pleura and the lungs by the thin intercostal fascia. When blocking the nerve in the posterior aspect of the back, particular care must be taken to avoid puncture of the thin fascia and underlying lung. Fortunately, most rib fractures occur in the anterior or lateral portion of the ribs and can be blocked *in the posterior axillary line*, where the internal intercostal muscle lies between the nerve and the lung's pleura and provides a buffer for minor errors in needle placement. *Note that blocking the nerve here will anesthetize the entire course of the intercostal nerve because it is blocked before the cutaneous branches are given off.*

Technique

For adequate analgesia of most rib fractures, the lateral cutaneous branch needs to be anesthetized. Therefore, blocks are usually performed between the posterior axillary and the midaxillary line at a point proximal to the origin of this branch (see Fig. 31–2A, *arrows*). Explanation of the procedure, its benefits, and its risks, including potential pneumothorax, systemic toxicity, and ineffective block, should be done before proceeding.

A 10-mL syringe with a 3.75-cm, 25-gauge needle is used. The rib is palpated, and the area is prepared in the usual aseptic manner. The index finger of the nondominant hand is used to retract the skin at the lower edge of the rib cephalad and up over the rib (Fig. 31–3). With the syringe in the opposite hand, the skin is punctured at the tip of the finger that is retracting the skin. The syringe is held at an 80° angle with the needle pointing cephalad. The hand holding the syringe rests on the chest wall for stability. In this position, the depth of needle penetration is well controlled. The needle is slowly advanced until it comes to rest on the lower border of the rib. *The bone should be felt by the needle tip.*

At this point, the skin retraction is released. The skin returning to its natural position moves the needle shaft perpendicular to the chest wall and the needle tip to the inferior margin of the rib. The syringe is shifted from the dominant hand to the index finger and thumb of the nondominant hand. The middle finger of the same hand rests against the shaft of the needle and, by exerting gentle pressure on the shaft, walks the needle off the lower edge of the rib. Again, the palm of the hand is planted firmly on the chest wall to ensure control of the needle. With the help of the dominant hand, the needle is slowly advanced 3 mm. The needle is aspirated, and then 2 to 4 mL of anesthetic are injected while the needle is carefully moved in and out 1 mm, which ensures that the compartment containing the nerve between the internal and the external intercostal muscles is penetrated. This may also serve to minimize intravascular injections. The procedure is repeated ideally on the *two ribs above and below* to ensure that the overlapping innervation from adjacent nerves is blocked.

Although the procedure just discussed seems extensive, it takes 1 to 2 minutes to perform once the operator is familiar with the technique, and three to five intercostals can be blocked in 10 minutes total time.

Precautions

The needle must be initially placed at the lower edge of the rib. If it contacts the rib above this point, it cannot be walked off the lower edge of the rib at the proper angle. If it is inserted too low, over the intercostal space, it may be advanced too deep through the pleura and into the lung before the operator realizes the misplacement. Before inserting the needle, the depth of the bone should be estimated. If the bone is not encountered by this depth, needle position should be reevaluated. Even after the needle has been properly walked off the edge of the rib, care must be taken to avoid puncture of the pleura and lung. The depth of the intercostal groove in which the nerve runs is 0.6 cm posteriorly, diminishing to 0.4 cm anteriorly.

Because the incidence of pneumothorax is low, a chest radiograph is not routinely required after this procedure. The asymptomatic patient is observed for 15 to 30 minutes and instructed to return if problems arise. If the patient has symptoms of pneumothorax (e.g., cough, a change in the nature of the pleuritic pain, or shortness of breath), he or she should have a chest film taken before discharge.

If the clinician inadvertently causes a pneumothorax, treatment depends on the size. Many pneumothoraces from this procedure are small and require no specific intervention. Those smaller than 20% may be observed for 6 hours.[21] During this time, the patient may be administered high-concentration oxygen to help decrease the size of the pneumothorax. If the pneumothorax does not grow, the patient may be released home with arrangements for follow-up. Needle or catheter aspiration of larger pneumothoraces may be all that is needed. A chest tube is necessary if this method fails.

Nerve Blocks of the Upper Extremity

The upper extremity is supplied by the brachial plexus. Its branches—primarily the median, radial, ulnar, and musculocutaneous nerves—can be blocked at the axilla, elbow, wrist, hand, or fingers. Nerve blocks at the axilla and elbow are seldom used in the ED. Nerve blocks of the wrist are

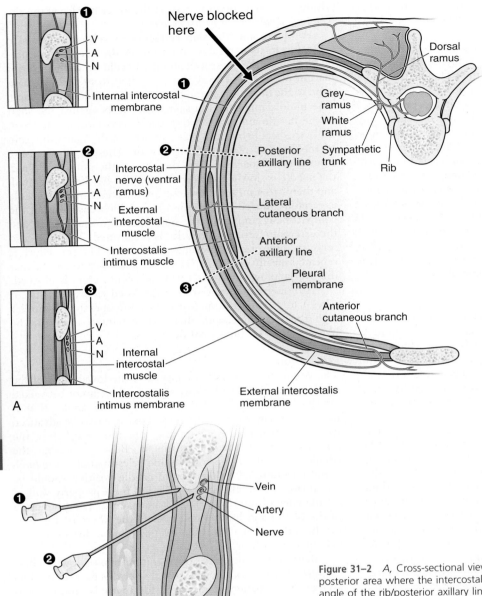

A

Nerve blocked here

- V
- A
- N

Internal intercostal membrane

Dorsal ramus

Grey ramus
White ramus
Sympathetic trunk
Rib

Posterior axillary line

Intercostal nerve (ventral ramus)

External intercostal muscle

Intercostalis intimus muscle

Lateral cutaneous branch

Anterior axillary line

Pleural membrane

Anterior cutaneous branch

Internal intercostal muscle

Intercostalis intimus membrane

External intercostalis membrane

B

Vein
Artery
Nerve

Subcostal groove

Figure 31–2 *A*, Cross-sectional view of intercostal nerve anatomy. Note the posterior area where the intercostal block is usually performed (*arrow* at the angle of the rib/posterior axillary line) so the anesthetic will also block the lateral cutaneous, lateral mammary, and anterior cutaneous branches. Note that the vein and artery lie under the inner portion of the rib, offering them protection from the anesthetizing needle. *B*, The anesthetizing needle is advanced until it touches the rib, an obvious sensation to the operator. The needle is walked down the inferior portion of the rib until it is felt to drop off the bone (see Fig. 31–3). The needle is advanced a few millimeters and a generous amount of the anesthetic is deposited (2–4 mL per rib). Too deep penetration risks pneumothorax. *(A, Adapted from Chung J: Thoracic pain. In Sinatra RS, Hord AH, Ginsberg G, Preble L [eds]: Acute Pain. St. Louis, CV Mosby, 1991.)*

performed occasionally before painful procedures or for repair of injuries to the hand. Metacarpal and digital blocks are used frequently to treat fractures, lacerations, and infections of the fingers.

Nerve Blocks at the Elbow

The median, ulnar, and radial nerves can be blocked at the elbow, providing anesthesia to the distal forearm and hand (Fig. 31–4). For most injuries extensive enough to require nerve block at the elbow, all three nerves must be blocked for successful anesthesia because of the variable and overlapping

innervation of the forearm. Furthermore, injuries to the proximal and middle forearm may require additional circumferential subcutaneous field blocks of the lateral, medial, and posterior cutaneous nerves.

Ulnar Nerve: Anatomy and Technique. The ulnar nerve can be palpated in the ulnar groove on the posteromedial aspect of the elbow between the olecranon and the medial condyle of the humerus (Fig. 31–5*A* and *B*). This nerve supplies the innervation to the small finger and ulnar half of the ring finger and the ulnar aspect of the hand (see Fig. 31–5*C*).

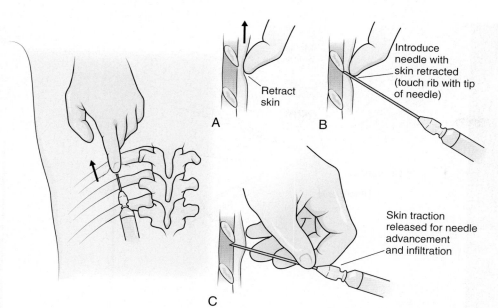

Figure 31–3 *A–C,* Method of retracting skin and the proper needle insertion site for intercostal block. See text for details.

A — Retract skin

B — Introduce needle with skin retracted (touch rib with tip of needle)

C — Skin traction released for needle advancement and infiltration

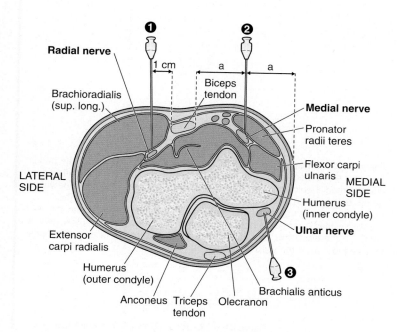

Figure 31–4 Cross-section of the elbow, looking cephalad, right arm, demonstrating (1) the median nerve, (2) the radial nerve, and (3) the ulnar nerve.

519

Radial nerve — 1 cm — Biceps tendon — a — a

Brachioradialis (sup. long.) — Medial nerve — Pronator radii teres

LATERAL SIDE — Flexor carpi ulnaris — MEDIAL SIDE — Humerus (inner condyle) — Ulnar nerve

Extensor carpi radialis — Humerus (outer condyle) — Brachialis anticus — Anconeus — Triceps tendon — Olecranon

With the elbow flexed, the nerve is palpated in the groove. A 3.75-cm, 25-gauge needle is inserted 1 to 2 cm proximal to the groove and directed toward the groove parallel to the course of the nerve. The needle tip comes to rest close to the proximal end of the groove. Care is taken to avoid blocking the nerve in the groove, where it is prone to damage. For similar reasons, a paresthesia may be elicited but is not vigorously sought. *If a paresthesia occurs during injection, slightly reposition the needle to avoid intraneural injection.* Although an elbow ulnar nerve block is common, many clinicians prefer to block the ulnar nerve at the wrist to limit the risk of injury. Once the needle tip is properly positioned, 5 to 10 mL of anesthetic is deposited. If a nerve stimulator is used, flexion of the small and ring fingers signals proximity to the nerve.

Radial Nerve: Anatomy and Technique. The radial nerve and sensory branch of the musculocutaneous nerve run together in the sulcus between the biceps and the brachioradialis muscles on the anterolateral aspect of the elbow (see Fig. 31–4). The block produces anesthesia to the lateral dorsum of the hand and the lateral aspect of the forearm (see Fig. 31–11).

The sulcus in which the nerve runs is palpated between the sharp border of the biceps muscle and the medial border of the brachioradialis muscle in the antecubital fossa just proximal to the skin crease of the elbow. Palpation is greatly facilitated by having the patient, with the elbow flexed at 90°, contract and relax these muscles isometrically so that their borders are better defined. The skin is punctured with a 3.75-cm, 25-gauge needle halfway between the muscles, or 1 cm lateral to the biceps tendon, at a point 1 cm proximal to the antecubital crease. After proper needle insertion, 5 to 15 mL of anesthetic should be injected at this depth. Because of poor landmarks and the depth of the radial nerve at the elbow, the nerve stimulator greatly facilitates the search for

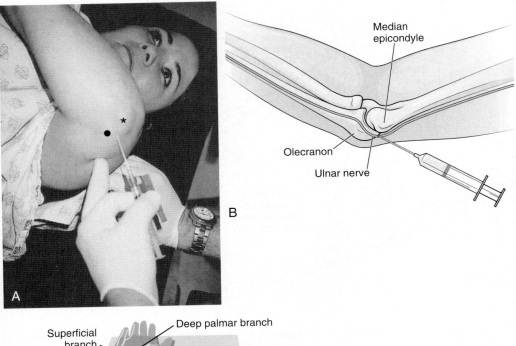

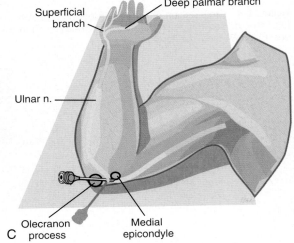

Figure 31–5 **Ulnar nerve block at the elbow.** *A,* Positioning of the patient for ulnar nerve block at the elbow. The patient is supine, the elbow flexed, and the medial epicondyle and ulnar groove are exposed. The ulnar nerve passes between the olecranon (*) and the medial epicondyle (•) of the humerus. *B,* Avoid injecting large amounts of anesthesia directly into the ulnar groove. Instead, place anesthetic proximal to the groove. *C,* The ulnar nerve's course in the distal arm, and area of anesthesia. Alternatively, the ulnar nerve may be blocked at the wrist.

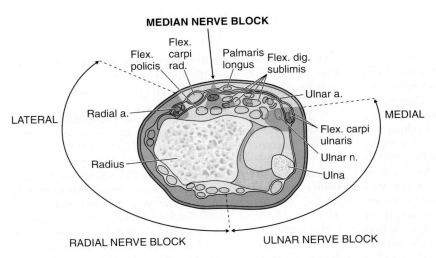

Figure 31–6 **Cross-section of the wrist looking cephalad, right wrist.** *Arrow* points to the (covered) median nerve. *Shaded triangle* depicts the area infiltrated with anesthetic. Note the relatively superficial position of the median nerve, just radial to the palmaris longus.

the nerve, which when stimulated, produces extension of the fingers and wrist.

Median Nerve: Anatomy and Technique. The median nerve runs medial to the brachial artery in the anteromedial aspect of the elbow (see Fig. 31–4). The nerve block anesthetizes the index, middle, and radial portion of the ring fingers and the palmar aspect of the thumb and lateral palm (see Fig. 31–11*C*).

The brachial artery is palpated in the flexed arm at the elbow just proximal to the antecubital crease and medial to the prominent biceps tendon. Once the anatomy is defined and marked in the flexed arm, the arm is extended to 30°. A 3.75-cm, 25-gauge needle is inserted slightly medial to the artery and perpendicular to the skin to the depth of the artery, about 2 to 3 cm, and 5 to 15 mL of anesthetic is injected. Again, the nerve stimulator facilitates the process and produces flexion of the wrist and index finger. Most commonly, median nerve blocks are performed at the wrist.

Nerve Blocks at the Wrist

The median, ulnar, and radial nerves may be blocked at the wrist, providing anesthesia to the hand. Most extensive injuries and procedures for which a wrist nerve block could be used can also be managed using local infiltration or a digital block. Compared with direct infiltration, wrist block anesthesia can have a slow and unreliable onset and can require more time to take effect if all three nerves are to be blocked. There are several circumstances, however, in which wrist nerve blocks are more advantageous than other types of blocks or anesthesia.

Diffuse lesions that can be difficult to anesthetize with local infiltration can easily be anesthetized with a wrist block. Deep abrasions with embedded debris, commonly the result of "road burn" from bike and motorcycle crashes, can be cleaned and débrided painlessly after a nerve block at the wrist. Hydrofluoric acid burns, which require treatment with numerous subcutaneous injections of calcium gluconate into the burned area, are better tolerated after a wrist nerve block. Wrist blocks are also advantageous in the severely swollen and contused hand, in which small amounts of anesthetic injected locally may increase the tissue pressure and produce further pain. Deep lacerations of the palm are very painful to anesthetize with local infiltration and will also benefit from a wrist block. In addition, burns of the hand lend themselves to nerve blocks prior to débridement.

Compared with nerves in the axilla and elbow, the nerves in the wrist are more easily located anatomically and can be blocked more reliably. All three nerves lie in the volar aspect of the wrist near easily palpated tendons. A nerve stimulator is not necessary but may be useful in locating the nerves, particularly when one is learning how to perform these blocks.

The anatomy and technique for blocking each nerve follow. Note that the median nerve lies in the midline and deep to the fascia, and the ulnar and radial nerves lie on their respective sides and have branches that wrap around dorsally. Blocking all three nerves at the wrist requires a block that when viewed end-on, roughly resembles a horseshoe straddling a horseshoe stake (Fig. 31–6).

Median Nerve: Anatomy and Technique. In the wrist, the median nerve lies just below the palmaris longus tendon or slightly radial to it between the palmaris longus and the flexor carpi radialis tendons (Fig. 31–7). Both tendons are easily palpated, but the palmaris longus may be absent in up

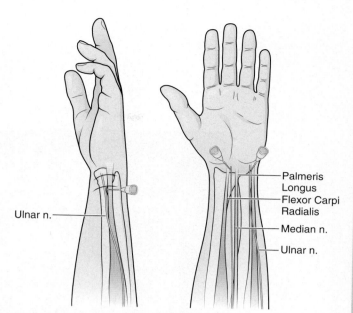

Figure 31–7 Landmarks and anatomy of the median and ulnar nerve block. The median nerve is more superficial than is often expected. It lies to the radial side of the palmaris tendon.

(Figure labels: Ulnar n.; Palmeris Longus; Flexor Carpi Radialis; Median n.; Ulnar n.)

to 20% of patients, in which case the nerve is found about 1 cm in the ulnar direction from the flexor carpi radialis tendon. The nerve lies deep to the fascia of the flexor retinaculum, but at a depth of 1 cm or less from the skin. The superficial position of the median nerve at the wrist is emphasized, because *a major cause of failure of this block is too deep instillation of the anesthetic.*

The palmaris longus tendon is located by having the patient make a fist with the wrist flexed against resistance (Fig. 31–8*A*). The site of the nerve block is selected on the radial border of the palmaris longus tendon just proximal to the proximal wrist crease. A 3.75-cm, 25-gauge needle is inserted perpendicularly and advanced slowly until a slight "pop" is felt as the needle penetrates the retinaculum and a paresthesia is produced (see Fig. 31–8*B* and *C*). If no paresthesia ensues, it may be elicited in a more ulnar direction under the palmaris longus tendon. If a paresthesia is still not elicited, 3 to 5 mL of anesthetic is deposited in the proximity of the nerve at a depth of 1 cm under the tendon. Although the nerve is surprisingly close to the skin, it is better to err slightly on the deep side of the retinaculum and continue depositing anesthetic as the needle is withdrawn, because the retinaculum is an effective barrier to a successful nerve block from a superficially injected anesthetic.

Radial Nerve: Anatomy and Technique. The radial nerve follows the radial artery into the wrist but *gives off sensory nerve branches proximal to the wrist.* These branches wrap around the wrist and fan out to supply the dorsal radial aspect of the hand

Nerve block requires an injection in close proximity to the artery and a field block that extends around the dorsal aspect of the wrist (Fig. 31–9). A 3.75-cm, 25-gauge needle is inserted immediately lateral to the palpable artery at the level of the proximal palmar crease. At the depth of the artery, 2 to 5 mL of anesthetic is injected. Another 5 to 6 mL is distributed in a subcutaneous field block from the initial point of injection to the dorsal midline. The needle must be withdrawn and repositioned to complete the block. The discomfort of numerous needle sticks is decreased if the

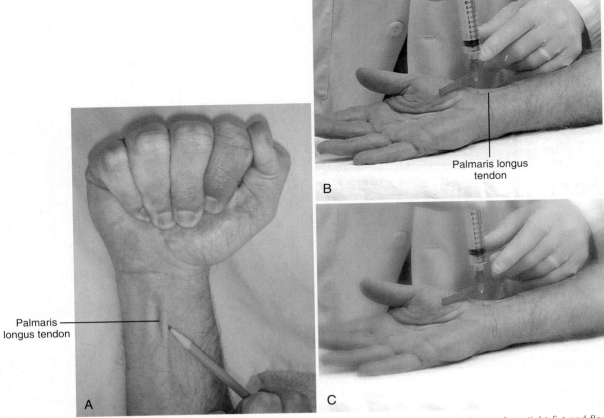

Palmaris longus tendon

Palmaris longus tendon

A

B

C

Figure 31–8 Median nerve block at the wrist. *A,* The palmaris longus tendon is found by having the patient make a tight fist and flex the wrist. This tendon may be absent in some patients. *B,* The median nerve lies slightly radial to (toward the thumb), and slightly deeper than, this tendon (see also Fig. 31–9). *C,* Use a generous amount of anesthesia, and inject with a fanlike motion to allow for some aberrations in anatomy. Note that the median nerve is not very deep, just under the retinaculum that should give a "pop" when being entered.

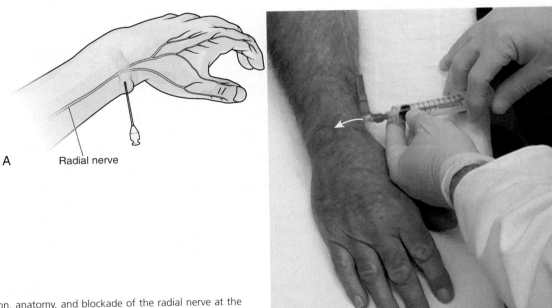

A   Radial nerve

B

Figure 31–9 *A,* Distribution, anatomy, and blockade of the radial nerve at the wrist. This nerve is only a sensory nerve at this point. *B,* A line of anesthetic is placed to encircle the radial side of the wrist. A specific nerve is not sought.

needle is repositioned to a site that has been anesthetized previously.

Ulnar Nerve: Anatomy and Technique. The ulnar nerve follows the ulnar artery into the wrist, where they both lie deep to the flexor carpi ulnaris tendon (see Figs. 31–6 and 31–10). The flexor carpi ulnaris tendon is easily palpated just proximal to the prominent pisiform bone by having the patient flex the wrist against resistance. At the level of the proximal palmar crease, the artery and the nerve lie just off the radial border of the flexor carpi ulnaris tendon; however, the nerve lies between the tendon and the artery and deep to the artery, making it difficult to approach the nerve from the volar aspect of the wrist without involving the artery.

Nerve block of the ulnar nerve can be carried out by two different approaches: lateral and volar. The lateral approach may be easier because of the reason stated previously. For the lateral approach (Fig. 31–10A), a 3.75-cm, 25-gauge needle is inserted on the ulnar aspect of the wrist at the proximal palmar crease and a wheal of anesthesia is deposited horizontally under the flexor carpi ulnaris tendon. Then the needle is directed toward the ulnar bone at a point deep to the flexor carpi ulnaris tendon, and 3 to 5 mL of anesthetic solution is injected as the needle is withdrawn.

Like the radial nerve, cutaneous nerves branch off the ulnar nerve, wrap around the wrist, and supply the dorsum of

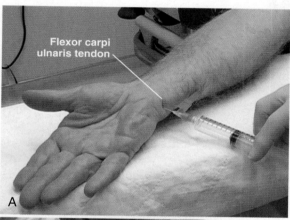

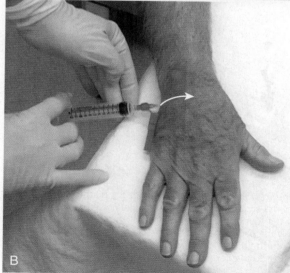

Figure 31–10 Ulnar nerve block at the wrist. This nerve can also be blocked at the elbow (see Fig. 31–5). *A,* The lateral approach (see text). *B,* Blocking the lateral cutaneous branches.

the hand. These are blocked with a 5- to 6-mL subcutaneous band of anesthetic from the lateral border of the flexor carpi ulnaris tendon to the dorsal midline (see Fig. 31–10B). Another advantage of the lateral approach is that the dorsal branches can be blocked from the same injection site.

Nerve Blocks of the Digits

The digital nerve block is one of the most useful and most used blocks in the ED. Indications for choosing it include repair of finger lacerations and amputations, reduction of fractures and dislocations, drainage of infections, removal of fingernails, and relief of pain (e.g., from a fracture or burn). The digital block is superior to local infiltration in most circumstances. Wound infiltration may be a problem in the finger that has tight skin and can accept only a limited volume of anesthetic. Administration of anesthetic into this restricted space increases the tissue pressure, impairing capillary blood flow and causing pain. Fibrous septa in the fingertip also restrict the space available for the injected substance and even limit the spread of small amounts of anesthetic.

Anatomy. Each finger is supplied by two sets of nerves. These nerves, the dorsal and palmar digital nerves, run alongside the phalanx at the 2 and 10 o'clock positions and the 4 and 8 o'clock positions, respectively (Fig. 31–11).

The principal nerves supplying the finger are the palmar digital nerves, also called the common digital nerves. These nerves originate from the deep volar branches of the ulnar and median nerves, where they branch in the wrist. The palmar digital nerves follow the artery along the volar lateral aspects of the bone, one on each side, and supply sensation to the volar skin and interphalangeal joints of all five digits. In the middle three fingers, these nerves also supply the dorsal distal aspect of the finger, including the fingertip and nailbed. Whereas many clinicians routinely block both sets of digital nerves, in the presence of normal anatomy, only the volar (palmar) branches must be blocked to obtain adequate anesthesia of the middle three fingers distal to the distal interphalangeal joint.

The dorsal digital nerves originate from the radial and ulnar nerves, which wrap around to the dorsum of the hand. They supply the nailbeds of the thumb and small finger and the dorsal aspect of all five digits up to the distal interphalangeal joints. Unlike the middle three fingers, which require blocking of only the two volar (palmar) digital nerves, all four nerves are usually blocked in the thumb and fifth finger, especially to obtain anesthesia of the fingertip and nailbed (Fig. 31–12A and B).

Technique. The digital nerves can be blocked anywhere in their course, including sites in the finger, in the web space between the fingers, and between the metacarpals in the hand. There are a variety of approaches to the nerves, including the dorsal and palmar approaches and the web space approach. Each has its merits. The technique is similar at each level.

The dorsal approach has the advantage of thinner, less pain-sensitive skin compared with volar approaches. The hand can be held firmly and flat on the table, preventing withdrawal. The disadvantage is that two injections are needed from this approach to block both volar digital nerves.

The dorsal approach can be used in the dorsum of the hand at the metacarpals, just proximal to the finger webs at the proximal end of the proximal phalanx, or distal to the web. Clinical situations may dictate which site to use; however, given equal circumstances, the preferred site is just proximal to the finger web. Here the nerve's location is more consistent

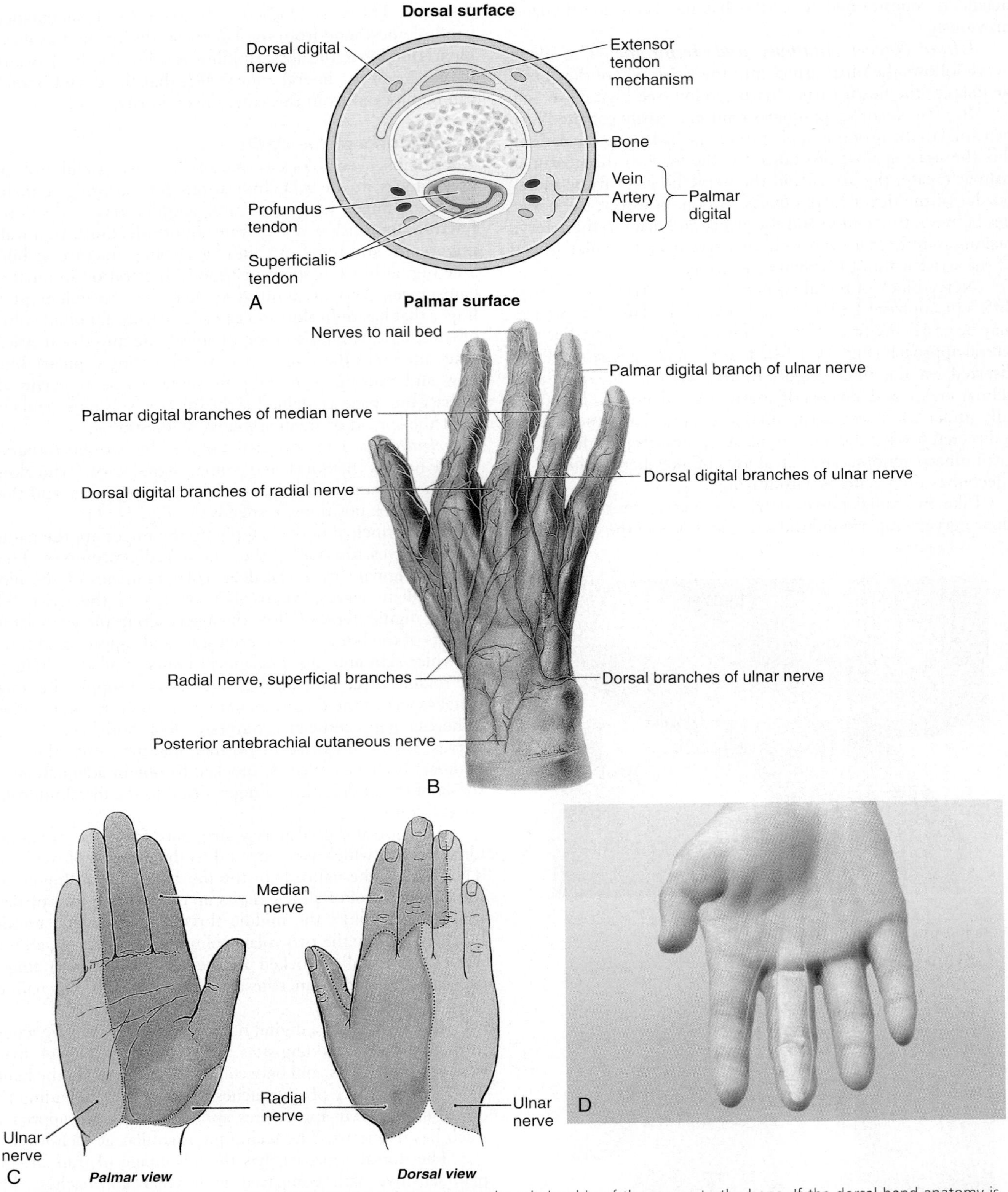

Figure 31–11 *A,* Schematic cross-section of the phalanx demonstrates the relationship of the nerves to the bone. If the dorsal hand anatomy is examined (*B* and *C*), it is obvious that in order to perform a digital block of the thumb and fifth finger, all four digital nerves (two volar, two palmar) must be blocked. *C,* Because almost the entire second, third, and most of the fourth fingers are supplied by only the palmar branch (note that each palmar nerve curves around to the dorsum from the palmar surface), only the palmar nerves must be blocked to obtain anesthesia for all but the skin of the proximal dorsal digit. The exception is the ulnar side of the fourth finger, which receives some of its distal dorsal innervation from the dorsal nerve. *D,* On the palmar aspect, the digital nerves are almost adjacent to the flexor tendon, a position that is more palmar than is usually appreciated.

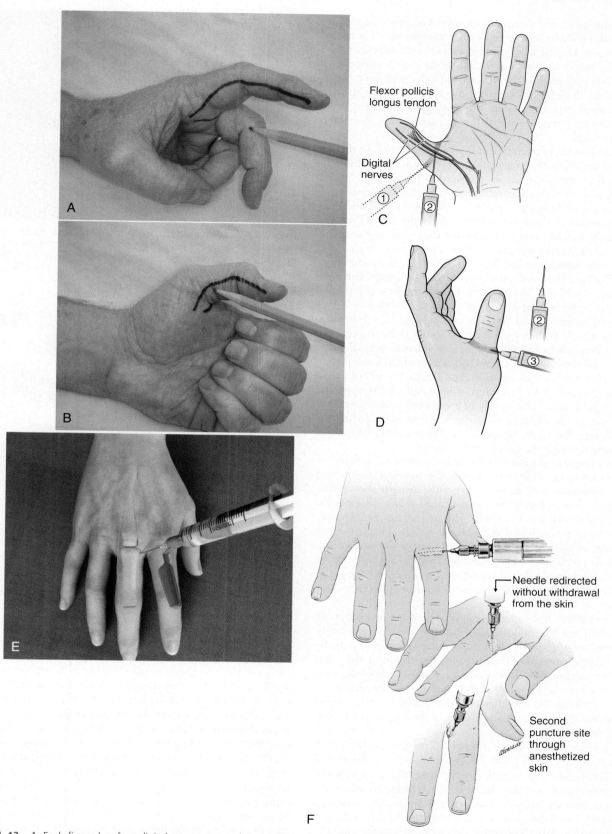

Figure 31–12 *A,* Each finger has four digital nerves: two palmar and two dorsal. The palmar nerves travel in a line connecting the top of the skin creases made by flexing the proximal interphalangeal and distal interphalangeal joints (*black line*). The nerves are more palmar than is often appreciated and are almost adjacent to the flexor tendon, so injecting the true lateral portion of the finger may miss the nerve. If the anesthesia needle is inserted at the tip of the skin creases (see probe) the nerve will be blocked. *B,* When performing a digital nerve block on the thumb, all four digital nerves must be blocked. As in the other fingers, the palmar nerve travels in a line made by connecting the top of the skin creases produced by flexing the digit (*black line*). The anesthetizing needle (see probe) must be placed almost adjacent to the flexor tendon to block the nerve. *C,* Sites of digital nerve blocks at the base of the thumb. *D,* Technique of anesthetizing the *required* second injection site to block the thumb. *E,* Block of the dorsal and volar nerve on one side of the finger using a dorsal (less sensitive) approach (see text). *F,* Another dorsal approach (see text). (*A–F, From Adriani J [ed]: Labat's Regional Anesthesia: Techniques and Clinical Applications, 3rd ed. Philadelphia, WB Saunders, 1967, p 445. Reproduced with permission.)*

than in the hand, and there is more soft tissue space to accommodate the volume of injected substance than there is in the distal finger. Digital block at the web is more efficacious in onset and requires less time to anesthesia than a metacarpal block done proximal to the metacarpophalangeal joint.[22]

Digital block requires aseptic injection technique, usually only an alcohol pad preparation is performed. Sterile gloves and drapes are not necessary, although examination gloves are recommended.

The clinician must first decide whether two or four digital nerves require blocking (see earlier discussion). Anesthesia is deposited at the positions of the appropriate digital nerves (2, 4, 8, and 10 o'clock in relationship to the bone), using a 3.75-cm, 25- or 27-gauge needle (see Fig. 31–11A). The block is performed from the dorsal surface, where the skin is thinner, easier to penetrate, and less sensitive than that of the volar surface. The needle insertion site is at the web space, just distal to the knuckle at the lateral edge of the bone (see Fig. 31–12E). Once the needle tip is subdermal, it usually contacts the bone. A wheal of 0.5 to 1 mL of anesthetic without epinephrine is injected at this level. This serves to block the dorsal digital nerve and provide anesthesia at the injection site. The needle is then passed lateral to the bone and toward the palmar surface until the palmar skin starts to tent slightly. The needle is withdrawn 1 mm and aspirated to check for an inadvertent intravenous position, and 0.5 to 1.5 mL of anesthetic is injected. This procedure is repeated on the opposite side of the finger. The result is a circumferential band of anesthesia at the base of the finger. Firm massage of the injected area for 15 to 30 seconds enhances diffusion of the anesthetic through the tissue to the nerves.

A variation of the dorsal approach is performed as follows: After injecting one side of the finger, the needle is redirected (without removing it) *across the top of the digit* to anesthetize the skin on the opposite side (see Fig. 31–12F). The needle is then withdrawn and inserted *at the site that was anesthetized*, and the block is continued as described earlier. The presumed advantage of this method is that it minimizes the pain of the second skin puncture. This procedure requires that the needle be placed across the dorsal aspect of the finger, allowing the possible disadvantage of extensor tendon puncture and trauma.

The palmar and web space approaches can be used most successfully for the middle three fingers when only a single puncture is required to block both volar nerves. This technique takes advantage of the anatomic fact that only the volar digital nerves must be blocked to obtain anesthesia of the total finger (except the proximal dorsal surface). If the thumb or fifth finger must be anesthetized, the dorsal branches must also be blocked to obtain anesthesia of the fingertip and fingernail area.

The palmar approach requires an injection in the palm, which is slightly more painful than an injection in the dorsal skin. The needle is inserted directly over the center of the metacarpal head, and anesthetic is slowly injected while the needle is advanced to the bone. At this point, the needle is withdrawn 3 to 4 mm and angled slightly to the left and right of center to block both digital nerves without withdrawing the needle (Figs. 31–13 and 31–14). To be successful, a palpable soft tissue fullness should be appreciated. The technique requires 4 to 5 mL of anesthetic.

A variation of this is particularly useful in fingertip injuries in toddlers. The finger is pinched side-to-side just distal to the proximal finger crease. This tents the skin at the finger

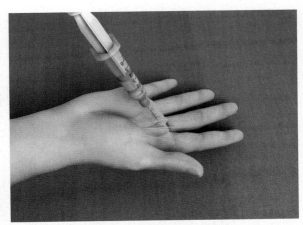

Figure 31–13   Palmar approach to the metacarpal head. After needle puncture in the midline, the needle is directed slightly to the right and left, and anesthetic is deposited along the course of both volar digital nerves. The needle is not withdrawn until both nerves are blocked. This technique blocks only the palmar nerves.

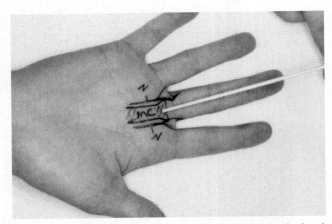

Figure 31–14   The palmar digital nerves (N) are adjacent to the head of the metacarpal (MC) in the palm. For a metacarpal head block, the anesthetizing needle punctures the palm in the middle of the MC, and anesthetic is deposited both laterally and medially, blocking both nerves with a single puncture. Injection in this area is usually more painful than injecting in the web space, but it is almost foolproof for obtaining anesthesia.

crease, which is injected subcutaneously with 0.5 to 1 mL of anesthetic. This single injection diffuses to the volar nerves and provides anesthesia to many fingertip injuries common in toddlers. With the web space approach, the patient's hand is held by the clinician in such a way that the clinician's thumb and index finger are over the dorsal and the volar metacarpal head, respectively. The clinician's third finger is used to separate the patient's fingers to expose the web space, while the fourth and fifth fingers support the finger being anesthetized (Fig. 31–15). The needle is inserted into the web space, 1 mL of anesthetic is injected, and the needle is slowly advanced until it is next to the lateral volar surface of the metacarpal head. Anesthetic is injected, and the needle is advanced slowly past the midline of the metacarpal head to the opposite digital nerve (Fig. 31–16). The operator's index finger is used to palpate a fullness as the anesthetic is injected. By redirecting the needle to the adjacent finger without withdrawing it, both fingers may be blocked with a single puncture.

Although epinephrine-containing solutions are used routinely by podiatrists in digital blocks of the toes, without

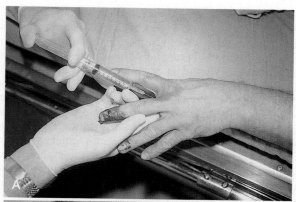

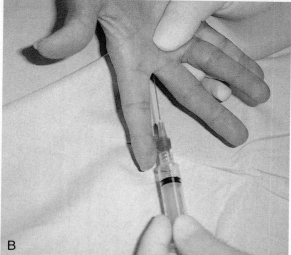

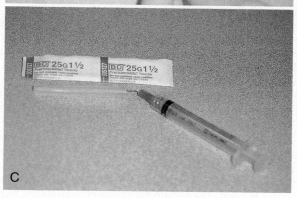

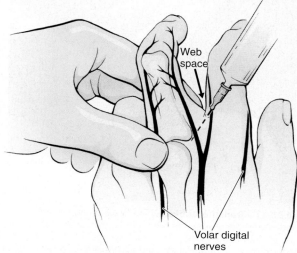

Figure 31–16 **Nerve block of the second and third digit.** After injection of anesthetic into the web space skin, the needle is advanced to the digital nerve, where it passes just lateral to the volar metacarpal head. Anesthetic is injected, and the needle is advanced to the opposite digital nerve. This procedure requires about 3–5 mL of anesthetic. If the index finger also must be blocked, the needle is redirected without withdrawal from the skin. Thus, both fingers are blocked with a single needle puncture of the less sensitive web space.

527

Figure 31–15 The web space metacarpal head block allows two of the three inner fingers to be anesthetized with a single needle puncture. *A*, Dorsal approach: The patient's second and third fingers are spread by the operator as the fingers are supported. *B*, Palmar approach: The clinician's finger palpates the patient's metacarpal head on the patient's palm while the injured finger is supported and the web space is exposed. The finger can feel the tissue distention by the anesthetic, but *care must be taken to avoid passing the needle through the skin and puncturing the operator's finger.* About 3–5 mL of anesthetic is deposited to ensure that both branches of the nerve are anesthetized. To anesthetize the adjacent finger, the needle is partly withdrawn and redirected to the other metacarpal head. *C*, Bending the needle to 30° allows easier access to the proper position without the syringe getting in the way.

morbidity, when performing a digital block, the authors advise use of anesthetics that do not contain epinephrine. The injection should go in smoothly, without resistance of the syringe plunger. Although the finger is forgiving of transient pressure from excessive anesthetic, if the injection site becomes exces-

sively tense, digital perfusion may be compromised. This concern is heightened when epinephrine-containing solutions are used. If epinephrine-containing solutions are inadvertently used for a digital block in otherwise healthy individuals without peripheral vascular disease, it is unlikely that serious ischemic injury will occur. Significant vasoconstriction generally lasts less than 60 minutes, within the time interval for which an ischemic tourniquet can safely be used in the same area.[23] However, if the entire digit remains blanched for more than 15 minutes, it is prudent to reverse the α-agonism of epinephrine with phentolamine. Using a pulse oximeter on the affected finger may help quantitate the degree of ischemia.[24] Onset of anesthesia occurs in 1 to 15 minutes and lasts for 20 minutes to 6 hours, depending on the anesthetic agent used.

Alternative Techniques

Jet Injection Technique. Jet injection for digital nerve block can be used effectively and is less painful than standard needle techniques.[25] The technique described by Ellis and Owens uses 0.15 mL of 1% lidocaine delivered by a jet injector at 2600 psi. Three injections are given to the lateral aspect of the proximal phalanx: the first, midway between the volar and the dorsal surfaces; the second, dorsal to this; the third, volar. A combined total of 0.45 mL is administered to each side of the phalanx at the 2, 3, and 4 o'clock positions and the 8, 9, and 10 o'clock positions in relationship to the bone.

The potential disadvantages of jet injection include lacerations that may occur with tangential injection. Holding the injector perpendicular to the skin avoids this problem. Thick skin associated with older age, manual labor, and male gender may require larger volumes of anesthetic.

The advantages of this technique are less pain of injection and avoidance of "needle phobia," particularly in children.

Transthecal Digital Block Technique. The transthecal block is performed by a single injection into the flexor

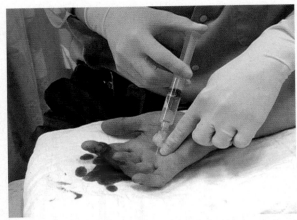

Figure 31–17 Transthecal block. The flexor tendon sheath is entered volarly just proximal to the metacarpophalangeal joint. With the use of a 25-gauge needle on a 3-mL syringe, the fluid should flow easily. Inject 2–3 mL of anesthetic and apply proximal tendon sheath pressure.

tendon sheath, which produces rapid and complete finger anesthesia. It was first described by Chiu in 1990[26] who noted rapid finger anesthesia after injection treatment of a trigger finger. Cadaver studies suggest that injected fluid diffuses out of the tendon sheath and around the phalanx and all four digital nerves.

The flexor tendon is palpated in the palm proximal to the metacarpophalangeal joint. A 25-gauge needle is attached to a 3-mL syringe and introduced at a 45° angle as it is advanced to the sheath/tendon (Fig. 31–17). Slight pressure is applied to the syringe plunger. If the sheath has been entered, the anesthetic should flow freely. If it does not, it is presumed that the tendon has been entered, and the syringe is withdrawn slowly while slight pressure is constantly applied. A total of 2 mL of anesthetic solution is injected. Smaller volumes are used in children. After the needle is removed, pressure is applied over the tendon proximally to facilitate distal spread. Average onset of anesthesia is 3 minutes.[27]

The advantage of this technique is the single injection. However, Hill and colleagues[28] found the technique to be "clinically equal" to traditional digital blocks. Other authors have stated that traditional digital block was easier to administer and produced less pain during and after injection.[29] Theoretically, the technique may increase the risk of injury to the tendon.

Complications and Precautions. The small size of the digital arteries and nerves makes intravascular or intraneural injection less likely. Inadvertent intravascular injection may cause digit ischemia from vasospasm or displacement of blood out of the capillary bed by the anesthetic. Blanching of the finger as the anesthetic is injected suggests intravascular injection. If this is observed, the injection should be discontinued. Usually the ischemia is transient and self-resolving, and serious complications are rare. Massage or topical application of nitroglycerin paste may be attempted if ischemia persists.[30] Although the incidence of vasospasm and resultant ischemia is rare and primarily occurs in patients with underlying vascular disease,[31] an anesthetic agent without epinephrine is commonly recommended. As noted earlier, if one mistakenly chooses an epinephrine-containing solution and vasospasm develops, persistent ischemia should be relieved with local infiltration of phentolamine.

Commonly, the digital nerve is lacerated or damaged by the initial injury to the finger. Careful evaluation using two-point discrimination should be performed to determine the extent of nerve injury before nerve block. Even if nerve injury is questionable, it should be documented in the chart, and the patient should be advised of the injury before the nerve block. Careful evaluation and patient education should prevent misconceptions as to the cause of the nerve injury. Although most isolated digital nerve injuries are not debilitating, they heal slowly and can be annoying to the patient. Digital nerve injury proximal to the distal interphalangeal joint may be repaired surgically. Nerve repair may be immediate when specialty consultation is available or delayed after initial simple closure.

Nerve Blocks of the Lower Extremity

Metatarsal and digital blocks in the foot are used frequently to treat ingrown toenails, fractures, and lacerations of the forefoot and toes.

Nerve Blocks of the Ankle

Nerve block of the five nerves of the ankle—the deep peroneal (anterior tibial), posterior tibial, saphenous, superficial peroneal (musculocutaneous), and sural nerves—provides anesthesia to the foot. Of all the nerve block techniques described, these are the most technically difficult and most prone to failure. Depending on the desired area of anesthesia, one or more of the five nerves are blocked. These blocks can be used in operative procedures and repair of injuries to the foot. They are particularly useful in providing anesthesia to the sole of the foot for laceration repair and foreign body removal.

A nerve block of the foot is better tolerated by the patient than local infiltration in all but the most minor procedures. The skin of the sole is thicker and more tightly bound to the underlying fascia by connective tissue septa than is skin in other parts of the body. Puncturing this skin can be difficult and is always quite painful. The fibrous septa can limit the amount and spread of anesthetic. If large amounts of anesthesia are injected, the volume of injected substance quickly exceeds the space available, possibly leading to painful distention of the tissue and circulatory compromise of the microvasculature. Local infiltrative anesthesia is adequate for treating minor injuries in which only small amounts of anesthetic are needed. For treatment of larger injuries, including incision and drainage, extensive wound care, and foreign body removal, the ankle block is better tolerated.

Anatomy. The foot is supplied by the five nerve branches of the principal nerve trunks (Fig. 31–18). Three nerves are located anteriorly and supply the dorsal aspect of the foot. Two nerves are located posteriorly and supply the volar aspect.

The anteriorly located nerves are the superficial peroneal, deep peroneal, and saphenous nerves. The superficial peroneal nerve (also called the dorsal cutaneous or musculocutaneous nerve) actually consists of multiple branches that supply a large portion of the dorsal aspect of the foot (see Fig. 31–18). These are located superficially between the lateral malleolus and the extensor hallucis longus tendon, which is easily palpated by having the patient dorsiflex the big toe. The deep peroneal nerve (also called the anterior tibial nerve) supplies the web space between the big and the second toes. In the ankle, it lies under the extensor hallucis longus tendon.

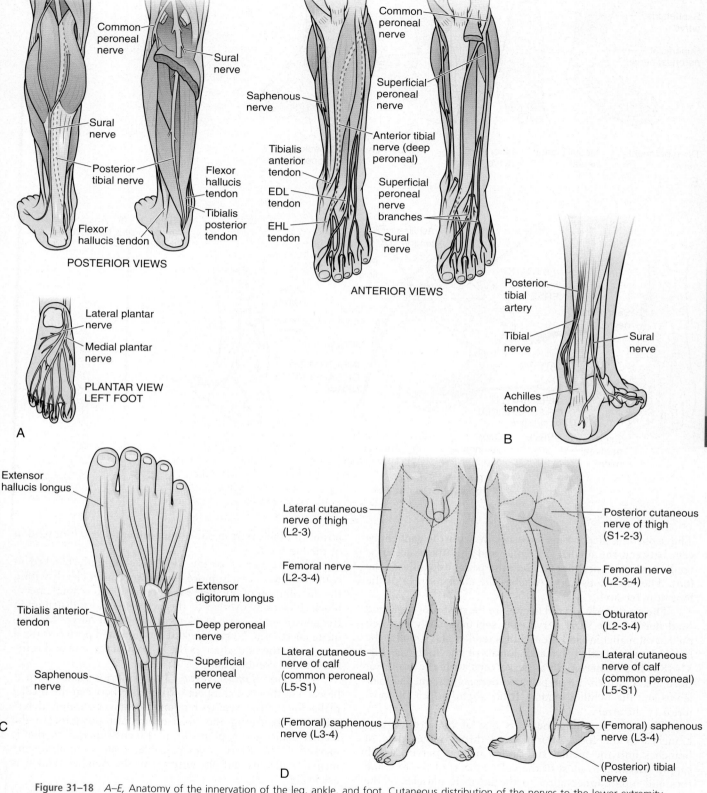

POSTERIOR VIEWS

Common peroneal nerve

Sural nerve

Sural nerve

Posterior tibial nerve

Flexor hallucis tendon

Flexor hallucis tendon

Tibialis posterior tendon

ANTERIOR VIEWS

Common peroneal nerve

Superficial peroneal nerve

Saphenous nerve

Tibialis anterior tendon

EDL tendon

EHL tendon

Anterior tibial nerve (deep peroneal)

Superficial peroneal nerve branches

Sural nerve

Lateral plantar nerve

Medial plantar nerve

PLANTAR VIEW LEFT FOOT

A

Posterior tibial artery

Tibial nerve

Sural nerve

Achilles tendon

B

529

Extensor hallucis longus

Tibialis anterior tendon

Saphenous nerve

Extensor digitorum longus

Deep peroneal nerve

Superficial peroneal nerve

C

Lateral cutaneous nerve of thigh (L2-3)

Femoral nerve (L2-3-4)

Lateral cutaneous nerve of calf (common peroneal) (L5-S1)

(Femoral) saphenous nerve (L3-4)

Posterior cutaneous nerve of thigh (S1-2-3)

Femoral nerve (L2-3-4)

Obturator (L2-3-4)

Lateral cutaneous nerve of calf (common peroneal) (L5-S1)

(Femoral) saphenous nerve (L3-4)

(Posterior) tibial nerve

D

Figure 31–18 *A–E,* Anatomy of the innervation of the leg, ankle, and foot. Cutaneous distribution of the nerves to the lower extremity.

Continued

Figure 31–18, cont'd

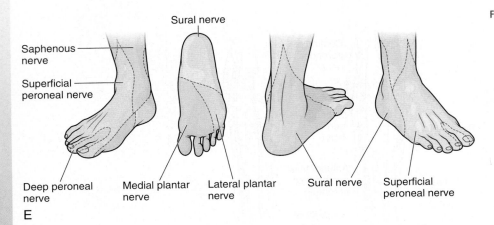

Sural nerve

Saphenous nerve

Superficial peroneal nerve

Deep peroneal nerve

Medial plantar nerve

Lateral plantar nerve

Sural nerve

Superficial peroneal nerve

E

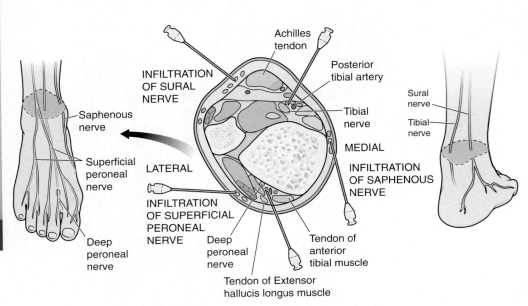

Achilles tendon

INFILTRATION OF SURAL NERVE

Posterior tibial artery

Saphenous nerve

Tibial nerve

MEDIAL

Superficial peroneal nerve

LATERAL

INFILTRATION OF SAPHENOUS NERVE

Deep peroneal nerve

INFILTRATION OF SUPERFICIAL PERONEAL NERVE

Deep peroneal nerve

Tendon of anterior tibial muscle

Tendon of Extensor hallucis longus muscle

Sural nerve

Tibial nerve

Figure 31–19 Anatomy and injection sites for nerve blocks at the ankle.

The saphenous nerve runs superficially with the saphenous vein between the medial malleolus and the tibialis anterior tendon, which is prominent when the patient dorsiflexes the foot. The saphenous nerve supplies the medial aspect of the foot near the arch.

The posteriorly located nerves are the posterior tibial and sural nerves. The sural nerve runs subcutaneously between the lateral malleolus and the Achilles tendon and supplies the lateral border, both volar and dorsal, of the foot (see Fig. 31–18). The posterior tibial nerve runs with the posterior tibial artery, which can be palpated between the medial malleolus and the Achilles tendon. It lies slightly deep and posterior to the artery.

The posterior tibial nerve is one of the major nerve branches to the foot. After passing through the ankle, it branches into the medial and lateral plantar nerves, which supply sensation to most of the volar aspects of the foot and toes and motor innervation to the intrinsic muscles of the foot.

Technique. Complete nerve block of the foot requires blocking three subcutaneous nerves and two deeper nerves (Figs. 31–19 and 31–20). Once familiar with the anatomy, the experienced clinician can anesthetize all five nerves quickly by placing subcutaneous band blocks around 75% of the ankle circumference and one deep injection next to the palpable posterior tibial artery and the other under the extensor tendon of the big toe.

The five nerves of the foot are commonly blocked in combinations of two or more. Small procedures clearly within the distribution of one nerve may require only a single nerve block. However, overlap of the nerve's sensory distribution frequently necessitates blocking a number of nerves for adequate anesthesia. Nerve block of the sural and posterior tibial nerves together anesthetizes the bottom of the foot and is the most useful combination.

Posterior Tibial Nerve. The posterior tibial nerve is blocked in the medial aspect of the ankle between the medial malleolus and the Achilles tendon. The injection site is determined by palpating the tibial artery just posterior to the medial malleolus. A point 0.5 to 1.0 cm superior to this is marked. If the artery is not palpable, a site 1 cm above the medial malleolus and just anterior to the Achilles tendon is used (Fig. 31–21).

A 3.75-cm, 25-gauge needle is directed at a 45° angle to the mediolateral plane (the needle is almost perpendicular to the skin), just posterior to the artery. At the estimated depth of the artery, approximately 0.5 to 1.0 cm deep, the needle is wiggled slightly in an effort to produce a paresthesia. If the paresthesia is elicited, 3 to 5 mL of anesthetic is injected after careful aspiration to check for inadvertent intravascular

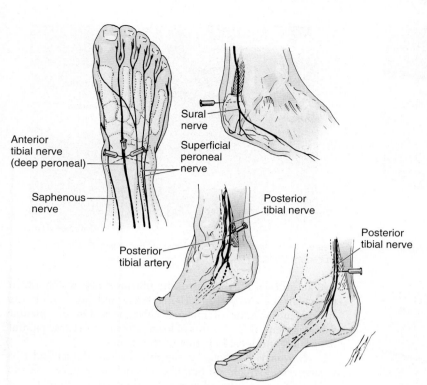

Figure 31–20 Anatomy and injection sites for nerve blocks at the ankle (lateral views). *(Adapted from Locke RK, Locke SE: Nerve blocks of the foot. JACEP 4:698, 1976.)*

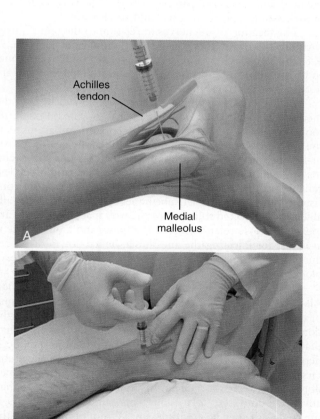

Figure 31–21 *A* and *B*, Anatomy and nerve block of the posterior tibial nerve at the ankle. *(From Thompson Procedure Consult.)*

placement of the needle tip. If no paresthesia is produced, the needle is advanced inward, again at a 45° angle, until it hits the posterior aspect of the tibia. The needle is then withdrawn slightly, about 1 mm, and 5 to 7 mL of anesthetic is injected while the needle is withdrawn another 1 cm. A rise in the temperature of the foot, due to vasodilation from loss of sympathetic tone, may herald a successful block.

Sural Nerve. The sural nerve is blocked on the lateral aspect of the ankle between the Achilles tendon and the lateral malleolus (Fig. 31–22). It lies superficially and is blocked at a level about 1 cm above the lateral malleolus. A band of anesthesia is injected subcutaneously between the Achilles tendon and the lateral malleolus using 3 to 5 mL of anesthetic.

Superficial Peroneal Nerves. The superficial peroneal nerves are blocked on the anterior aspect of the ankle between the extensor hallucis longus tendon and the lateral malleolus. They lie superficially and are blocked using 4 to 10 mL of anesthetic placed subcutaneously in a band between these landmarks (Fig. 31–23).

Deep Peroneal Nerve. The deep peroneal nerve is blocked anteriorly beneath the extensor hallucis longus tendon (see Fig. 31–23). It is blocked at a level 1 cm above the base of the medial malleolus and between the extensor hallucis longus and the anterior tibial tendons. The tendons are palpated by having the patient dorsiflex the big toe and foot, respectively. After a subcutaneous wheal is placed, the needle is directed about 30° laterally and under the extensor hallucis longus tendon until it strikes the tibia (at a depth of <1 cm). The needle is withdrawn 1 mm, and 1 mL of anesthetic is injected.

Saphenous Nerve. The saphenous nerve is blocked anteriorly between the medial malleolus and the anterior tibial tendon (Fig. 31–24). It lies superficially and is blocked with 3 to 5 mL of anesthetic injected subcutaneously between these landmarks.

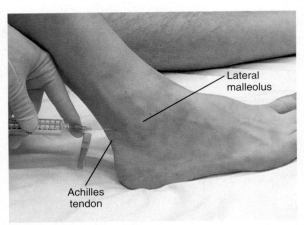

Figure 31–22 Sural nerve block at the ankle. *(From Thompson Procedure Consult.)*

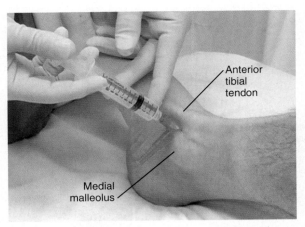

Figure 31–24 Saphenous nerve block at the ankle. *(From Thompson Procedure Consult.)*

532

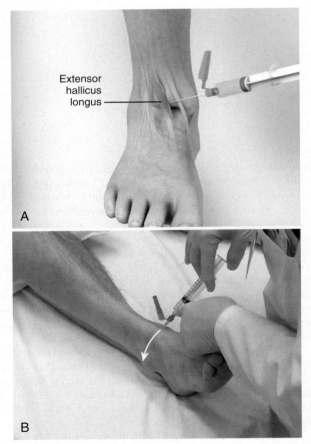

Figure 31–23 *A,* Deep and superficial peroneal nerve blocks. *B,* All nerves must be blocked to achieve anesthesia of the dorsum of the foot. *(From Thompson Procedure Consult.)*

Nerve Blocks of the Metatarsals and Toes

Like nerve blocks in the hand and fingers, nerve blocks in the foot and toes are commonly used in the ED. Indications for using these blocks include repair of lacerations, drainage of infections, removal of toenails, manipulation of fractures and dislocations, and otherwise painful procedures requiring anesthesia to the forefoot and toes.

Digital nerve blocks in the foot and toes are superior to local infiltration anesthesia in all but the most minor procedures. In the toes, the limited subcutaneous space does not accommodate enough injected material for adequate infiltra-

tive anesthesia. Furthermore, the fibrous septa, which attach the volar skin to the underlying fascia and bone, limit the spread and volume of injected substances. On the plantar surface, even small amounts of local infiltrate can cause painful distention and local ischemia of the tissues.

Anatomy. Each toe is supplied by two dorsal and two volar nerves, which are branches of the major nerves of the ankle. The dorsal digital nerves are the terminal branches of the deep and superficial peroneal nerves. The volar nerves are branches of the posterior tibial and sural nerves.

The location of the nerves in relation to the bones varies with the site of the foot. In the toes, the nerves lie at the 2, 4, 8, and 10 o'clock positions in close relationship to the bone. In the proximal foot, the nerves run with the tendons and are not in close relationship to the bones (Fig. 31–25).

Technique. The digital nerves can be blocked at the metatarsals, interdigital web spaces, or toes. The bones of the foot can be palpated easily from the dorsum and are used as the landmarks for estimating the location of the nerves. Proximally, the nerves' relationship to the bones is less consistent, making definitive needle placement and successful block less reliable. In the toes, the position of the nerves is more consistent; however, minimal subcutaneous tissue space is available for the injected solution. At the web space, the nerves are located in close relationship to the bone, and ample space is available for injecting the anesthesia; hence, for most procedures, the web space is the preferred site for the digital nerve block.

The technique for toe and metatarsal blocks is similar. All four nerves supplying each toe are usually blocked because of their sensory overlap. The blocks are performed from the dorsal surface, where the skin is thinner and less sensitive than that on the plantar aspect. A total of 5 mL of anesthetic is deposited in a fanlike pattern in the space between the metatarsal bones (see Fig. 31–25). A 1-mL skin wheal is placed dorsally between the metatarsal bones. The needle is then advanced until the volar skin tents slightly, and 2 mL is injected as the needle is withdrawn. Without removing it, the needle is redirected in a different volar direction, and the procedure is repeated. A total of 5 mL is used in each metatarsal space. Again, because of sensory overlap, two or more spaces need to be anesthetized for each toe to be blocked.

For the web space block, a site on the dorsum just proximal to the base of the toe is selected. Using a 10-mL syringe, a 3.75-cm, 27-gauge needle is inserted at the lateral edge of the bone (Fig. 31–26). A wheal is placed subcutaneously

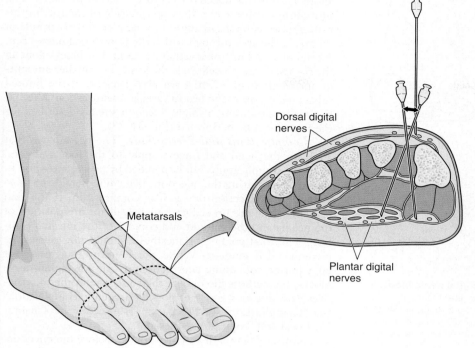

Dorsal digital
nerves

Metatarsals

Plantar digital
nerves

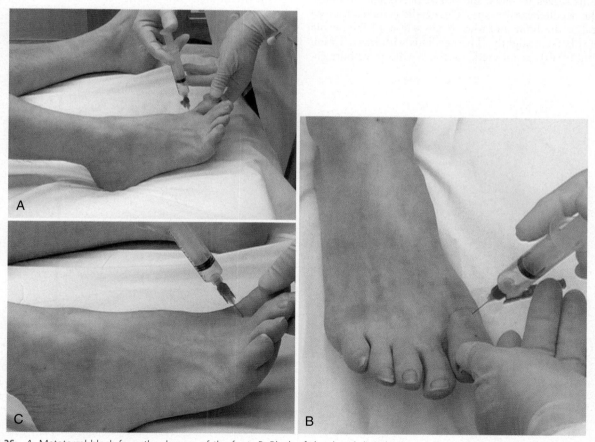

A

C

B

Figure 31–26 *A,* Metatarsal block from the dorsum of the foot. *B,* Block of the dorsal digital nerve. *C,* Penetration of the web space from the dorsum to block the plantar digital nerve (avoiding a painful injection in the bottom of the foot). *(From Thompson Procedure Consult.)*

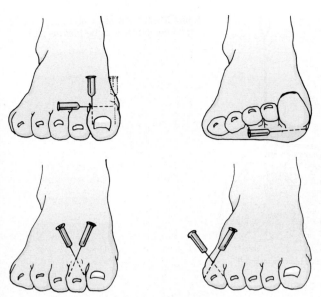

Figure 31–27. Alternative techniques of digital nerve blocks in the toes. Simply ring the base of the toe with anesthetic. After the first injection on the dorsum, the needle is going through anesthetized areas to block the rest of the toe. *(From Locke RK, Locke SE: Nerve blocks of the foot. JACEP 4:698, 1976. Reproduced with permission.)*

between the skin and the bone, using 0.5 to 1.0 mL of anesthetic. This serves to block the dorsal nerve and minimize pain at the needle insertion site. The needle is then advanced just lateral to the bone and toward the sole until the needle tents the volar skin slightly. The needle is withdrawn 1 mm, and 0.5 to 1.0 mL is injected. As the needle is withdrawn,

another 0.5 mL is injected to ensure a successful block. The procedure is repeated on the opposite side of the toe. In this manner, two columns of anesthesia are placed on each side of the toe in the area through which the four digital nerves run. A total of 2 to 4 mL of anesthetic is used. For blocks done in the toe itself, the procedure is the same, but smaller amounts of anesthetic (e.g., <2 mL) are used because of the limited subcutaneous space and fear of vascular compression. Alternative techniques using a single injection site, as described for the finger, can be performed (Fig. 31–27).

Complications and Precautions. The precautions that apply to the hand and fingers apply to the foot and toes. Ischemic complications can be avoided by paying attention to skin changes during the injection. Blanching heralds possible intravascular injection or vascular compression. If the skin blanches, halt the procedure and reevaluate the position of the needle and the amount and content of the injected solution. The total volume of anesthesia should not exceed the recommended amount. While the literature suggests that epinephrine-containing anesthetics are safe for digital nerve blocks, the authors discourage their use when other alternatives exist due to the risk of possible ischemic complications (see "Complications and Precautions" subsection and Chapter 29, Local and Topical Anesthesia).

Note any neural or vascular injuries before the injection. The close proximity of these structures to the skin and bones means that they are frequently injured. Deficits, even if questionable, should be documented in the records and brought to the attention of the patient before the nerve block.

REFERENCES CAN BE FOUND ON EXPERT CONSULT

CHAPTER **32**

Intravenous Regional Anesthesia*

James R. Roberts and Sharon K. Carney

The clinical use of intravenous regional anesthesia (IVRA) has been well established[1-3] as a safe, quick, and effective alternative to general anesthesia in selected cases requiring surgical manipulation of the upper and lower extremities. Although historically relegated to the operating room, the procedure is readily applicable to outpatient use and because of reliability, safety, and ease of use. It is now commonly used in the ED and clinic milieu. In the emergency department (ED), the technique provides quick and complete anesthesia along with muscle relaxation and a bloodless operating field. The procedure is free from the troublesome side effects associated with other regional blocks, such as the axillary block. The procedure is easily mastered and has a very low failure rate; consistently good results can be expected. It can be safely used by the operating surgeon and does not have to be administered by an anesthesiologist.[3]

The first practical use of analgesia associated with IV injection of a local anesthetic agent was described by August Gustav Bier in 1908.[4] Colbern[5] has since proposed the eponym *Bier block.* Although the procedure has been in existence for many years, the need for special equipment and a safe anesthetic agent limited its use. However, the Bier block has now gained wide acceptance as a safe and effective procedure, and several papers extol its virtues.[6-9] Although complications do exist, no reported fatalities directly attributable to the use of the Bier block *with lidocaine* have been reported. In this chapter, the techniques and complications are discussed according to their application in the ED.

INDICATIONS AND CONTRAINDICATIONS

Indications for IVRA include any procedure of the arm or leg that requires operating anesthesia, muscle relaxation, or a bloodless field, such as reduction of fractures and dislocations, repair of major lacerations, removal of foreign bodies, débridement of burns, and drainage of infection. IVRA is commonly used for extremity surgery, such as carpal tunnel surgery or tendon repair. The procedure may be carried out on any patient of any age who is able to cooperate with the clinician.

The only absolute contraindications are an allergy to the anesthetic agent and, possibly, uncontrolled hypertension. Relative contraindications include severe Raynaud's disease, Buerger's disease, or a crushed or otherwise already hypoxic extremity if further transient ischemia would be detrimental. Homozygous sickle cell disease is a theoretical contraindication, but little data exist. IVRA is best used for procedures requiring no more than 60 to 90 minutes of tourniquet time. Continuous cardiac or blood pressure monitoring are not

standard and not required unless extenuating circumstances prognosticate potential cardiovascular problems. An uncooperative patient may delay the procedure rather than contraindicate it.

EQUIPMENT

The equipment required for IVRA anesthesia consists of the following:

- 1% lidocaine (Xylocaine)*, *without epinephrine*, to be diluted to a 0.5% solution (*note*: 1 mL of 1% lidocaine = 10 mg).
- Clonidine or ketorolac if used as additives.
- Sterile saline solution as a diluent.
- 50-mL syringe/18-gauge needle.
- Pneumatic tourniquet (single or double cuff) (*note*: Do *not* use a standard blood pressure cuff) such as Zimmer A.T.S. 2000 automatic tourniquet system (Zimmer, Inc.) (Fig. 32–1).
- IV catheters (20- or 22-gauge) or a 21-gauge butterfly needle.
- Elastic bandage/Webril padding.
- 500 mL D_5W (5% dextrose in water) and IV extension tubing.

*Commercial preparations with preservatives commonly used. Lidocaine 0.5% is available.

PROCEDURE

The procedure should be explained to the patient in advance. Premedication with midazolam (Versed), diazepam (Valium), or an opioid (e.g., morphine, fentanyl) may be helpful but need not be routinely used. The only painful portions of the procedure are the establishment of the infusion catheter and the exsanguination procedure. The procedure should not be done on patients who are intoxicated or obtunded or on those with a previous reaction to a local anesthetic.

The patient need not be free of oral intake for a specific period of time before the procedure, but it is prudent to delay the procedure if the patient has just eaten a large meal. As a precaution, an option is a large-bore catheter and an IV line of D_5W in the unaffected extremity. Resuscitation equipment, including anticonvulsant drugs and oxygen, should be readily available. Cardiac and blood pressure monitoring are an option based on the clinician's assessment of the potential for cardiovascular events.

While the patient is being prepared, the lidocaine solution is readied but withheld until the injured extremity is exsanguinated and the cuff is in place and reinflated as discussed later. The standard dose of lidocaine for the arm is 3 mg/kg injected as a 0.5% solution (1% lidocaine may be mixed with equal parts of sterile saline in a 50-mL syringe). Farrell and coworkers[10] described a procedure termed the *minidose Bier block* using 1.5 mg/kg of lidocaine and reported a 95% success rate. This lower dose may decrease the incidence of central nervous system side effects and is more desirable in the ED setting. (Additional lidocaine may be infused if the initial dose is inadequate.) Lidocaine with epinephrine should *not* be used. Plain lidocaine is also available as a 0.5% solution, and as such, it can be used directly to avoid the necessity of diluting the stronger solution. Some prefer preservative-free lidocaine but most use standard lidocaine with preservatives.

*This chapter modified with permission from Roberts JR: Intravenous regional anesthesia. JACEP 6:261, 1977.

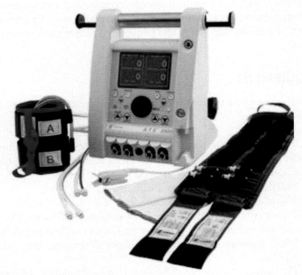

Figure 32–1 A digital-controlled double cuff system by Zimmer (A.T.S. 3000, Zimmer, Inc) allows for safe intravenous regional anesthesia (IVRA) and the ability to lessen pain from the arterial tourniquet.

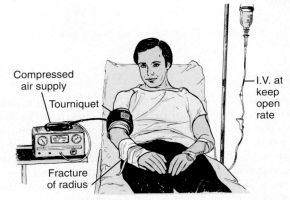

Figure 32–2 Preparation for induction of anesthesia in a patient with a fracture of the right radius. Note the precautionary intravenous (IV) line and deflated tourniquet in place. The procedure has been explained, and preoperative sedation or analgesia has been given if required. (*From Roberts JR: Intravenous regional anesthesia. JACEP 6:263, 1977.*)

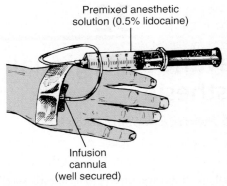

Figure 32–3 Infusion cannula securely taped in the dorsum of the hand. A butterfly needle is shown here, but a plastic catheter with the hub attached may also be used. (*From Roberts JR: Intravenous regional anesthesia. JACEP 6:263, 1977.*)

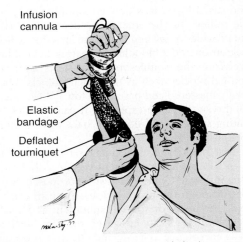

Figure 32–4 Exsanguination by elevation and elastic or esmarch bandage. The tourniquet has yet to be inflated at this point. Care must be taken not to dislodge the infusion cannula. (*From Roberts JR: Intravenous regional anesthesia. JACEP 6:263, 1977.*)

A pneumatic tourniquet with cotton padding (to prevent ecchymosis) under the cuff is applied proximal to the pathology (Fig. 32–2). *It is strongly advised that one not use a regular blood pressure cuff*, because these often leak or rupture and are not designed to withstand high pressures for any length of time. A specially designed portable double-cuff pneumatic system, such as that marketed by Zimmer Corporation, is ideal.

The anesthetic is premixed in the syringe. The tourniquet is inflated, and a plastic catheter or a metal butterfly needle is placed in the superficial vein, as close to the pathologic site as possible, and securely taped in place (Fig. 32–3). It is usually desirable to use a vein on the dorsum of the hand, but importantly, the injection site should be at least 10 cm distal to the tourniquet to avoid injection of anesthetic proximal to the tourniquet. The hub remains on the catheter to avoid backbleeding or the syringe is attached to the butterfly tubing. This catheter will be the route of injection of the anesthetic agent.

The tourniquet is deflated, and the extremity is exsanguinated so that when the anesthetic agent is injected, it will fill

the vascular system. Exsanguination may be accomplished by either of two methods. Simple elevation of the extremity for a few minutes may be adequate, but wrapping the extremity in a distal-to-proximal direction with an elastic bandage or Esmarch bandage, being careful not to dislodge the infusion needle, significantly enhances the exsanguination (Fig. 32–4). Wrapping may be painful; this step can be eliminated if it causes too much anxiety to the patient. If the wrapping procedure is not done, the extremity should be elevated for at least 3 minutes. During the wrapping procedure, care must be taken not to dislodge or infiltrate the infusion catheter.

With the extremity still elevated, the tourniquet is inflated to 250 mm Hg (or 100 mm Hg above systolic pressure), the arm is placed by the patient's side, and the elastic exsanguination bandage is removed. In a child, the tourniquet is inflated to 50 mm Hg above systolic pressure. In elderly obese patients with calcified peripheral vessels, arterial occlusion may not be achieved safely.[11] In the leg, cuff pressures of 300 mm Hg are suggested, or approximately twice the systolic pressure measured in the arms.

The 0.5% lidocaine solution is then slowly injected into the infusion catheter at the calculated dose. Note that the solution is placed in the arm in which circulation is blocked, *not* in the precautionary keep-open IV line on the unaffected side. At this point, blotchy areas of erythema may appear on the skin. This is not an adverse reaction to the anesthetic agent, but merely the result of residual blood being displaced from the vascular compartment, and it heralds success of the procedure.

In 3 to 5 minutes, the patient will experience paresthesia or warmth, beginning in the fingertips and traveling proximally, with final anesthesia occurring at the elbow. Complete anesthesia ensues in 10 to 20 minutes, followed by muscle relaxation. Note that adequate analgesia may exist even though the patient can still sense touch and position and has some motor function. If the "minidose" technique (1.5 mg/kg of lidocaine) does not provide adequate anesthesia, an additional 0.5 to 1 mg/kg may be infused at this time. Additional lidocaine was required in 7% of cases in one series using the minidose regimen.[10] The clinician should be patient, however, and wait a full 15 minutes before infusing additional lidocaine. Alternatively, if analgesia is slow or inadequate, an extra 10 to 20 mL of *saline* solution may be injected to supplement the total volume of solution to enhance the effect. *Do not exceed a 3-mg/kg total dose of lidocaine.* For obese patients, a maximum of 300 mg of lidocaine is suggested for the arm, and no more than 400 mg for the leg. Data for very obese patients do not exist. The infusing needle is then withdrawn, and the puncture site is tightly taped to prevent extravasation of the anesthetic agent. The surgical procedure or manipulation is performed, including postreduction x-ray films and casting or bandaging (Fig. 32–5).

Anesthesia from a fingertip-to-elbow direction seems to occur irrespective of the site of anesthetic infusion, but selecting an injection site near the site of pathology may provide more rapid anesthesia at a lower dosage.

On completion of the procedure, deflation of the tourniquet may be *cycled* to prevent a bolus effect of any lidocaine that may remain in the intravascular compartment. The cuff is deflated for 5 seconds and reinflated for 1 to 2 minutes. *This action is repeated two or three times.* This is likely only required if the cuff has been inflated for less than 30 minutes. A single deflation is often performed if the cuff has been inflated for more than this time period.

If the tourniquet has been in place for less than 30 minutes, an increase in transient lidocaine-related side effects may be seen if the cycled deflation has not been used because adequate tissue fixation of the lidocaine probably has not occurred. This may result in a higher peak plasma lidocaine level, with increased side effects. If the surgical procedure is completed rapidly and the 3-mg/kg limit of lidocaine has been infused, the tourniquet should remain inflated until 20 to 30 minutes has elapsed, and only then should it be deflated using the cycling technique. It is reasonable to use a 20-minute cutoff if the minidose technique is used or a total of 200 mg of lidocaine or less has been used because this dose is equal to a commonly administered antiarrhythmic IV bolus.

Sensation returns quickly when the tourniquet is removed, and in 5 to 10 minutes, the extremity returns to its preanesthetic level of sensation and function. Many patients describe a transient intense tingling sensation after cuff deflation. After 30 minutes of observation, the patient may be discharged (Table 32–1). If the procedure takes longer than 20 or 30 minutes, many patients complain of pain from the tourniquet, because the tourniquet is not inflated over an anesthetized area. The use of a double-cuff tourniquet may alleviate the problem of pain under the cuff. A wide tourniquet cuff (14 cm) is less painful than a narrow tourniquet (7 cm) when the cuff is inflated 10 mm Hg above the loss of arterial pulse.[12] The reason for pain under the tourniquet is unknown, but this can be a limiting parameter because most patients begin to feel significant discomfort after 30 minutes if only a single cuff is used. Tourniquet pain can be significantly reduced, and tourniquet time extended, by adding ketorolac to the lidocaine anesthetic (see below).

In the double-cuff system, two separate tourniquets are placed side by side on the extremity. One is termed the *proximal cuff*, and the other is called the *distal cuff*. The proximal cuff is inflated at the beginning of the procedure, and anesthesia is obtained under the deflated distal cuff. When the patient begins to feel pain under the proximal cuff, the distal cuff is first inflated over an already anesthetized area, and the pain-producing proximal cuff is then deflated. One must be certain to inflate the distal cuff before the proximal cuff is

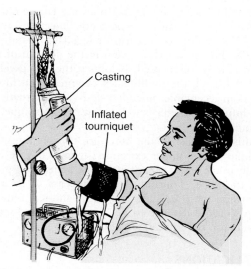

Figure 32–5 A cast is applied under anesthesia. Because the tourniquet is portable, postreduction radiographs may be obtained without losing anesthesia. *(From Roberts JR: Intravenous regional anesthesia. JACEP 6:263, 1977.)*

Labels on figure: Casting; Inflated tourniquet

TABLE 32–1 Intravenous Regional Anesthesia: Step-by-Step Procedure

Begin intravenous (IV) line in uninvolved extremity.

Draw up 0.5% lidocaine (1.5–3 mg/kg).*

Place padded tourniquet, and inflate upper cuff.

Insert small plastic IV cannula near pathologic lesion and secure.

Deflate tourniquet.

Elevate and exsanguinate extremity.

Inflate tourniquet (250 mm Hg), and remove exsanguination device. Inflate the proximal cuff only, if a double-cuff system is used.

Infuse anesthetic solution.

Remove infusion needle, and tape site.

Perform procedure.

If pain is produced by the application of the tourniquet, first inflate the distal cuff, then deflate the proximal cuff.

After the procedure has been carried out, deflate the cuff for a few seconds, then reinflate it for 1 min. Repeat three times. Do not deflate the cuff if total tourniquet time is less than 20 to 30 min.

Observe for possible reactions.

*Commercial preparations with or without preservatives are acceptable.
From Roberts JR: Intravenous regional anesthesia. JACEP 6:263, 1977.
Reproduced with permission.

released; otherwise, the anesthetic will rapidly diffuse into the general circulation.

There are no specific post procedure cautions but it is suggested that driving be prohibited for 6 to 8 hours and the patient leave with a responsible adult.

MECHANISM OF ACTION

Some of the anesthesia is undoubtedly related to the ischemia produced by the tourniquet, but most of the anesthesia is secondary to the anesthetic agent itself. Although the exact mechanism by which anesthesia is produced is unknown, the site of action of the anesthetic may be at sensory nerve endings, neuromuscular junctions, or major nerve trunks.[13] Contrast studies have demonstrated that the anesthetic agent does not diffuse throughout the entire arm, yet anesthesia of the entire limb is obtained. For example, when the anesthetic agent is injected into the elbow and kept in that region with both distal and proximal tourniquets, anesthesia of the entire arm develops.[14] Evidence indicates that the local anesthetic does not simply diffuse from the venous system into the tissue but travels via vascular channels directly inside the nerve. Regardless of where the anesthetic is infused, the fingertips are the first area to experience anesthesia, suggesting that the core of the nerve is in contact with the anesthetic agent initially. After release of the tourniquet, a considerable amount of the drug still remains in the injected limb for at least 1 hour.[15] This would suggest that at least a portion of the anesthetic leaves the vascular compartment and becomes tissue fixed.

PROCEDURAL POINTS

Anesthetic Agent

Using 0.5% plain lidocaine at a dose of 1.5 to 3 mg/kg is preferred for the upper extremity. For procedures in the leg, 150 ml of 0.25% lidocaine (375 mg) has been used with a thigh cuff. The greater volume can augment drug distribution in the larger lower extremity. Other agents have been used without demonstrable advantage and are not recommended.[16] Bupivacaine (Marcaine, Sensorcaine) is *contraindicated* because of the potential for serious cardiovascular and neurologic complications.[17,18]

Some authors have suggested the use of ketorolac (60 mg) or clonidine (0.15 mg if the IV preparation is available) in addition to the lidocaine.[19,20] These additives are mixed with the lidocaine and injected into the operative arm. Both have been shown to be safe, and they decrease the need for postoperative analgesics and antiemetics. Tourniquet time is prolonged with these agents, as pain under the tourniquet is the main reason for discontinuing the procedure. Opiates have not been found helpful when added to the lidocaine.

Dunbar and Mazze[8] showed that patients with IVRA actually had significantly lower plasma lidocaine concentrations than patients with axillary block or lumbar epidural anesthesia for similar procedures. Peak plasma concentrations are reached 2 to 3 minutes after deflation of the tourniquet, and side effects are minimal if the deflation is cycled after the surgical procedure. The plasma half-life of lidocaine is approximately 60 seconds (see the excellent detailed discussion of pharmacokinetics by Covino[21]), but the drug demonstrates a theoretical three-compartment model similar to a direct IV infusion once the tourniquet is released.[22] Peak blood levels are related to the duration of vascular occlusion and to the concentration of the anesthetic.[21,22]

Postrelease peak plasma lidocaine levels decrease as the time of vascular occlusion (tourniquet time) increases. If the tourniquet is inflated for at least 30 minutes and the deflation-reinflation technique is used when the procedure is finished, plasma concentration of lidocaine should be approximately 2 to 4 µg/mL, below the 5- to 10-µg/mL level at which serious reactions occur.[8] Tucker and Boas[22] demonstrated a peak plasma lidocaine level of 10.3 µg/mL after a 10-minute period of vascular occlusion, compared with 2.3 µg/mL if the tourniquet was inflated for 45 minutes.

More dilute solutions of lidocaine are associated with lower peak lidocaine levels. When equal doses of lidocaine are used, the peak arterial plasma levels are 40% lower when the 0.5% solution is used than when the 1% solution is used.[22] For example, after 10 minutes of vascular occlusion, the peak plasma concentration of lidocaine has been demonstrated to reach 10.3 µg/mL with the 1% solution, compared with only 5.6 µg/mL when the drug was given under similar circumstances as a 0.5% concentration.[22]

Exsanguination

Many clinicians consider exsanguination of the extremity before injection of the anesthetic agent essential for success. Others do not believe that it is a critical factor. Exsanguination by simple elevation of the extremity should be done in all cases, but in certain cases, one should consider avoiding the painful wrapping of the extremity with an elastic or Esmarch bandage. (Note that applying an Esmarch wrap over a fracture site is usually quite painful.) A pneumatic splint, such as the type used for prehospital immobilization, is also a reasonable alternative to painful wrapping. The process of exsanguination is believed to allow for better vascular diffusion of the anesthetic.

Site of Injection

Anesthesia is usually obtained no matter where the local anesthetic is injected, but some evidence indicates that the procedure is more successful when the anesthetic is injected distally. Sorbie and Chacho[23] noted the following failure rates associated with specific sites of anesthetic injection: antecubital fossa, 23%; middle of forearm or leg, 18%; hand, wrist, or foot, 4%. For most cases, a vein in the dorsum of the hand or foot is most often used. If local pathology precludes the use of the hand, the midforearm or antecubital fossa of the elbow is an acceptable, albeit less desirable, alternative as long as the infusion catheter is well below the tourniquet to avoid systemic injection.

Although most of the literature stresses the use of this technique on the upper extremity, it may also be used successfully in the leg. It cannot, however, be used for procedures above the knee. Tourniquet pain appears to be a limiting factor when the procedure is used on the leg. One must be certain to avoid damage to the peroneal nerve by using the tourniquet in the midcalf area only.

COMPLICATIONS

Although IVRA is both safe and simple, one should not be lulled into complacency, because complications do occur and are usually related to equipment failure or mistakes in the technique.

Anesthetic Agent

Serious complications seldom occur if proper attention is paid to technique. True lidocaine allergy is very rare. Other reactions to lidocaine are rare and are usually systemic reactions from high blood levels.[8,18,24] High levels may result from miscalculation of dosages, from too-rapid release of the tourniquet before the anesthetic has become tissue fixed ("bolus effect"), or rarely, from advancement of the infusion catheter proximal to the tourniquet, resulting in direct IV infusion.[25] To emphasize the safety of this procedure, it should be noted that the dose of lidocaine used in the minidose technique is similar to an IV bolus routinely given to patients with significant cardiovascular disease in the presence of ventricular dysrhythmias.

Generally, the central nervous system effects of lidocaine are minor, resulting in mild reactions such as dizziness, tinnitus, lethargy, headache, or blurred vision. This should not occur in more than 2% to 3% of patients and requires no treatment.[8] Transient hypotension and bradycardia may occur and are usually self-limited. Convulsions may occur but are extremely rare.

The most common complication relating to the anesthetic agent is rapid systemic vascular infusion, which occurs when a blood pressure cuff explodes or slowly leaks, resulting in both loss of anesthesia and high blood levels.[26] Similar complications may occur if the cuff is deflated before 20 to 30 minutes after the induction of anesthesia. Both complications are the result of a bolus effect of the anesthetic, resembling an IV injection.

Van Neikerk and Tonkin[24] reported 3 seizures in a series of 1400 patients. Auroy and colleagues[27] reported 23 seizures in 11,229 cases, with no cardiac arrest or fatalities, deeming IVRA safer than general anesthesia or peripheral nerve blocks. Seizures are generally not recurrent and are treated with oxygen and anticonvulsant drugs. Transient cardiovascular reactions, such as bradycardia and hypotension, are possible with large doses of lidocaine. Vasovagal reactions do occur. If resuscitation equipment is available and a precautionary IV line is started in the opposite arm, there should not be any serious sequelae.

One case of cardiac arrest for 15 seconds after the use of 200 mg of lidocaine has been reported, but the actual clinical scenario may have been a vasovagal reaction rather than a true cardiac arrest.[28]

Additional Complications

Thrombophlebitis can occur following IV administration of anesthetics, and the formation of insignificant amounts of methemoglobin with the use of prilocaine hydrochloride (Citanest) has been reported.[29] Methemoglobinemia also can theoretically occur with lidocaine but has not been reported. Bupivacaine offers no benefit over lidocaine, has been associated with deaths, and should be avoided.[30]

A particularly bothersome problem has been the infiltration of the infusion catheter during exsanguination, resulting in tissue extravasation of the anesthetic agent. Also, some leakage of anesthetic has occurred after the infusion needle has been removed. Both problems may result in poor anesthesia but may be minimized if a small, well-secured plastic infusion needle is used instead of a metal scalp vein ("butterfly") needle and if the puncture site is tightly taped after withdrawal of the catheter.

This procedure cannot be used in manipulations or operations in which the pulse must be monitored as a guide to reduction (e.g., supracondylar fractures of the humerus), because the tourniquet occludes arterial flow. The use of the Bier block in patients with sickle cell disease is not well documented. It should be used with caution until the ischemic effect of the tourniquet on the red blood cells of such patients has been clarified. In all patients, the tourniquet time should not exceed 90 minutes. Ischemia for less than that amount of time is not associated with serious sequelae.

An excellent summary of very favorable experience with IVRA of both the arm and leg in 1900 outpatients is available in the Brown reference.[31]

 REFERENCES CAN BE FOUND ON **EXPERT CONSULT**

Systemic Analgesia and Sedation for Procedures

Steven M. Green and Baruch Krauss

Procedural sedation and analgesia (PSA) is the use of analgesic, dissociative, and sedative agents to relieve the pain and anxiety associated with diagnostic and therapeutic procedures performed in various settings. PSA is an integral element of emergency medicine residency and pediatric emergency medicine fellowship curricula, and graduates of these programs are skilled in the practice of PSA. Emergency clinicians are skilled in resuscitation, vascular access, and advanced airway management, permitting them to effectively recognize and manage the potential complications associated with PSA.

The most common clinical errors associated with PSA in a recent study of all practitioners were *delayed recognition of respiratory depression and respiratory arrest, inadequate monitoring, and inadequate resuscitation*[1,2]—mistakes that are unlikely for emergency clinicians. The safety of PSA techniques by emergency clinicians has been well documented in numerous series in both children[3-6] and adults.[3,7] Successful and safe application of PSA requires careful patient selection, customization of therapy to the specific needs of the patient, and careful patient monitoring for adverse events. Emergency clinicians must ensure that all patients receive pain relief and sedation commensurate with their individual needs during any procedure.

TERMINOLOGY

The progression from minimal sedation to general anesthesia represents a nonlinear continuum that does not lend itself to division into arbitrary stages. Low doses of opioids or benzodiazepines induce mild analgesia or sedation, respectively, with little danger of adverse events. If, however, clinicians continue administering additional medication beyond this initial level, progressively altered consciousness ensues with a proportionately increased risk of respiratory and airway complications. If further medications are administered, the patient will advance along this continuum until protective airway reflexes are lost and general anesthesia is ultimately reached. This sedation continuum is not drug-specific, in that varying states from mild sedation to general anesthesia can be achieved with virtually all nondissociative PSA agents (e.g., opioids, benzodiazepines, barbiturates, etomidate, propofol).

In 1985, the American Academy of Pediatrics (AAP)[8] and National Institutes of Health (NIH)[9] issued guidelines for the management and monitoring of children receiving sedation for diagnostic and therapeutic procedures in response to the growing use of opioids and sedative-hypnotic agents in the outpatient setting and a number of sedation-related deaths. In these documents, three levels of sedation were defined (conscious sedation, deep sedation, general anesthesia) to create a common language for describing drug-induced alterations in consciousness (Table 33–1). A key development in the field of PSA has been the revision of the original terminology and the adoption of clearer descriptions of varying types and degrees of sedation (see Table 33–1). Although historically popular, the widely misinterpreted and misused term "conscious sedation" has fallen into disfavor,[10] labeled as "confusing,"[11] "imprecise,"[12] and an "oxymoron,"[10,11] and has been replaced with the term *moderate sedation*.[13]

Despite improvements in PSA terminology, the system is imperfect and there is still no objective way to assess sedation depth. Levels of responsiveness remain at best crude surrogate markers of respiratory drive and retention of protective airway reflexes. This is especially true for all levels of sedation in young children (infants and toddlers) who do not understand or are unreliable in following verbal commands. Although respiratory depression and respiratory arrest can be quickly detected using standard interactive and mechanical monitoring, there is no safe and practical way to assess the status of protective airway reflexes. There are currently insufficient data to determine whether deep sedation is associated with impairment of protective reflexes, or whether such danger is encountered only when "pushing" deep sedation to a point at which it approaches or reaches general anesthesia.

PSA GUIDELINES

Prior to the promulgation of PSA guidelines by specialty societies and governmental agencies, clinicians simply administered sedatives in varied clinical settings and applied individual judgment as to the need for specific monitoring devices and supporting personnel. Since 1985, at least 27 sets of PSA guidelines have been published,[14] each crafted for the unique and differing settings in which PSA is practiced. Naturally, not all are in agreement.[5] The intent of each of these guidelines is to better standardize the manner in which PSA is performed in order to enhance patient safety. Those most pertinent to emergency clinicians are from the American College of Emergency Physicians,[3] the AAP,[15] and the American Society of Anesthesiologists (ASA).[12,16]

In the early 1990s, the Joint Commission on Accreditation of Healthcare Organizations (JCAHO), an independent, not-for-profit organization that evaluates and accredits hospitals in the United States, took a special interest in PSA, with the central theme that the standard of sedation care provided should be comparable throughout a given hospital. Thus, patients sedated in the emergency department (ED) should not receive a significantly different level of attention or monitoring than those sedated for a similar-level procedure in the operating room or in the endoscopy suite. To ensure this, the JCAHO requires specific PSA protocols that apply consistently throughout each institution. These hospital-wide sedation policies will vary from site to site based upon the specific needs and expertise available within each institution. In 2001, the JCAHO released new standards for pain management, sedation, and anesthesia care.[13]

At each hospital accreditation survey, the JCAHO will see whether practitioners practice PSA consistently with their hospital-wide sedation policy, and whether they provide sufficient documentation of such compliance. Clinicians must be familiar with their hospital's sedation policies and should work with their medical staff to ensure that such policies are suitably detailed, but yet reasonable and realistic. Unduly restrictive policies do a disservice to patients by discouraging appropriate use of analgesia and anxiolysis. Most hospitals pattern their sedation policies after the JCAHO standards and

TABLE 33–1 Procedural Sedation and Analgesia Terminology and Definitions

General

- **Analgesia***: Relief of pain without intentional production of an altered mental state such as sedation. An altered mental state may be a secondary effect of medications administered for this purpose.
- **Anxiolysis***: A state of decreased apprehension concerning a particular situation in which there is no change in a patient's level of awareness.
- **Procedural sedation and analgesia (PSA)**[3]: A technique of administering sedatives, analgesics, and/or dissociative agents to induce a state that allows the patient to tolerate unpleasant procedures while maintaining cardiorespiratory function. PSA is intended to result in a depressed level of consciousness but one that allows the patient to maintain airway control independently and continuously. Specifically, the drugs, doses, and techniques used are not likely to produce a loss of protective airway reflexes.

Current Sedation State Terminology

- **Minimal sedation (anxiolysis)**[13]: A drug-induced state during which patients respond normally to verbal commands. Although cognitive function and coordination may be impaired, ventilatory and cardiovascular functions are unaffected.
- **Moderate sedation (formerly conscious sedation)**[13]: A drug-induced depression of consciousness during which patients respond purposefully to verbal commands, either alone or accompanied by light tactile stimulation. Reflex withdrawal from a painful stimulus is not considered a purposeful response. No interventions are required to maintain a patent airway, and spontaneous ventilation is adequate. Cardiovascular function is usually maintained.
- **Dissociative sedation**[17]: A trancelike cataleptic state induced by the dissociative agent ketamine characterized by profound analgesia and amnesia, with retention of protective airway reflexes, spontaneous respirations, and cardiopulmonary stability.

- **Deep sedation**[13]: A drug-induced depression of consciousness during which patients cannot be easily aroused but respond purposefully after repeated or painful stimulation. The ability to independently maintain ventilatory function may be impaired. Patients may require assistance in maintaining a patent airway and spontaneous ventilation may be inadequate. Cardiovascular function is usually maintained.
- **General anesthesia**[13]: A drug-induced loss of consciousness during which patients are not arousable, even by painful stimulation. The ability to independently maintain ventilatory function is often impaired. Patients often require assistance in maintaining a patent airway, and positive-pressure ventilation may be required because of depressed spontaneous ventilation or drug-induced depression of neuromuscular function. Cardiovascular function may be impaired.

Original AAP/NIH Terminology[8,9]

- **Conscious sedation:** A medically controlled state of depressed consciousness that (1) allows protective reflexes to be maintained; (2) retains the patient's ability to maintain a patent airway independently and continuously; and (3) permits appropriate response by the patient to physical stimulation or verbal command (e.g., "open your eyes").
- **Deep sedation:** A medically controlled state of depressed consciousness or unconsciousness from which the patient is not easily aroused. It may be accompanied by a partial or complete loss of protective reflexes, and includes the inability to maintain a patent airway independently and respond purposefully to physical stimulation or verbal command.
- **General anesthesia:** A medically controlled state of unconsciousness accompanied by a loss of protective reflexes, including the inability to maintain a patent airway independently and respond purposefully to physical stimulation or verbal command.

AAP, American Academy of Pediatrics; NIH, National Institutes of Health.
*From Sacchetti A, Schafermeyer R, Gerardi M, et al: Pediatric analgesia and sedation. Ann Emerg Med 23:237, 1994.

definitions. It is important to note that the unique ketamine dissociative state does not fit into the existing JCAHO definitions of sedation and anesthesia.[17] A ready solution is assigning a distinct definition for "dissociative sedation" (see Table 33–1).

The JCAHO[13] requires that PSA practitioners who are permitted to administer deep sedation must be qualified to rescue patients from general anesthesia. Emergency clinicians will typically perform all levels of sedation except general anesthesia. Moderate sedation suffices for the majority of procedures in adults and cooperative children, although it will not be adequate for extremely painful procedures (e.g., hip reduction, cardioversion). Deep sedation can facilitate these, but at greater risk of cardiorespiratory depression than moderate sedation. Moderate sedation is frequently insufficient for effective anxiolysis and immobilization in younger, frightened children, with deep or dissociative sedation typically appropriate alternatives.

EVALUATION PRIOR TO PSA

The practice of PSA has three essential components performed in sequence: the initial presedation evaluation, sedation during the procedure, and postprocedure recovery and patient discharge from the ED. In all but the most emergent situations, a directed history and physical examination should precede PSA. If this evaluation suggests additional risk, the advisability of sedation should be reconsidered. High-risk cases may be better managed in the more controlled environment of an operating room.

Presedation assessments are a JCAHO requirement, and most hospitals have developed specific forms to facilitate consistent documentation of the involved items. Except in emergency situations, the risks, benefits, and limitations of any PSA should be discussed with the patient (or their parent or guardian) in advance and verbal agreement obtained. Formal written informed consent is not required as a standard of care (unless a local institutional requirement), although documentation, as discussed earlier, is essential.

General. Clinicians should assess the type and severity of any underlying medical problems. This is usually best documented by the standard ED medical record, history and physical examination, and nursing notes. Another tool used for this purpose is the ASA's physical status classification that is used for preoperative risk stratification (Table 33–2). Current medications and allergies should be verified. It is advisable to inquire regarding prior adverse experiences with PSA or anesthesia.

TABLE 33–2 American Society of Anesthesiologists' (ASA) Physical Status Classification

ASA Class	Description	Examples	Suitability for Sedation
1	A normal healthy patient	Unremarkable past medical history	Excellent
2	A patient with mild systemic disease—no functional limitation	Mild asthma, controlled seizure disorder, anemia, controlled diabetes mellitus	Generally good
3	A patient with severe systemic disease—definite functional limitation	Moderate to severe asthma, poorly controlled seizure disorder, pneumonia, poorly controlled diabetes mellitus, moderate obesity	Intermediate to poor; consider benefits relative to risks
4	A patient with severe systemic disease that is a constant threat to life	Severe bronchopulmonary dysplasia, sepsis, advanced degrees of pulmonary, cardiac, hepatic, renal, or endocrine insufficiency	Poor, benefits rarely outweigh risks
5	A moribund patient who is not expected to survive without the operation	Septic shock, severe trauma	Extremely poor

From Krauss B, Green SM: Sedation and analgesia for procedures in children. N Engl J Med 342:938, 2000.

Airway. The airway should be inspected to determine whether there are abnormalities (e.g., severe obesity, short neck, small mandible, large tongue, trismus) that might impair airway management. Previously described assessments such as Mallampati scoring or the distance between the chin and the hyoid bone can be considered.

Cardiovascular. Cardiac auscultation should be performed to assess for rhythm disturbance or other abnormality. In patients with known cardiovascular disease, their degree of reserve should be evaluated, because most PSA agents can cause vasodilatation and hypotension.

Respiratory. Lung auscultation should be performed to assess for active pulmonary disease, especially obstructive lung disease and active upper respiratory infections that may predispose the patient to airway reactivity.

Gastrointestinal. Because pulmonary aspiration of gastric contents is a dreaded complication of vomiting when protective airway reflexes are impaired, clinicians should assess the time and nature of the last oral intake. A four-step assessment tool to stratify presedation aspiration risk and identify prudent limits of targeted sedation is shown in Figure 33–1,[18] although it has not yet been validated.

More conservative guidelines from ASA for elective surgery or procedures in healthy patients specify an age-stratified fasting requirement of 2 to 3 hours for clear liquids and 4 to 8 hours for solids and nonclear liquids.[19] Despite this, they acknowledge that *"the literature provides insufficient data to test the hypothesis that preprocedure fasting results in a decreased incidence of adverse outcomes"* in PSA.[12,16] The concept of preprocedure fasting is logistically difficult or impossible for emergency clinicians, who have no control over patients' oral intake prior to ED presentation. In actual practice, emergency clinicians routinely perform safe PSA on patients noncompliant with the ASA elective procedure fasting guidelines.[18–20] Procedures can sometimes be delayed for a number of hours; however, this must be balanced with prolongation of pain and anxiety for the patient, inconvenience for the patient and family, and expenditure of room space and other finite ED resources. In addition, many ED procedures require urgent if not immediate attention (e.g., débridement and repair of animal bite wounds, acute burn management, arthrocentesis for suspected septic arthritis, reductions of joint dislocations, lumbar puncture in the uncooperative septic patient, hernia reduction, eye irrigation for ocular trauma or chemical burns,

cardioversion in the hemodynamically unstable patient). Although uncommon, there may be occasions in which nonfasting patients requiring urgent procedures with a substantial depth of sedation may be more safely managed in the operating room with endotracheal intubation to protect the airway.

Selecting agents less likely to produce vomiting, such as opting for fentanyl over morphine/meperidine, may decrease the aspiration potential. Concomitant antiemetic administration is an unproven adjunct, but a common consideration. In summary, *common sense should apply and clinical judgment should prevail, but it is standard for PSA to be performed in the ED on patients in the nonfasting state.*

Hepatic/Renal. The implications of delayed metabolism or excretion of PSA agents in infants younger than 6 months of age, in the elderly, and in the presence of hepatic or renal abnormality should be carefully evaluated.

PERSONNEL AND INTERACTIVE MONITORING

The most important element of PSA monitoring is close and continuous patient observation by an individual capable of recognizing sedation complications. This person must be able to continuously observe the patient's face, mouth, and chest wall motion, and equipment or sterile drapes must not interfere with such visualization. This careful observation will allow prompt detection of adverse events such as respiratory depression, apnea, partial airway obstruction, emesis, and hypersalivation.

PSA personnel should understand the pharmacology of analgesic and sedative agents and their respective reversal agents and be proficient at maintaining airway patency and assisting ventilation if needed. PSA requires a minimum of two experienced individuals, most frequently one clinician and one nurse or respiratory therapist. The clinician typically oversees drug administration and performs the procedure, while the nurse or respiratory therapist continuously monitors the patient for potential complications and documents medications administered, response to sedation, and periodic vital signs. The nurse or respiratory therapist may assist with minor, interruptible tasks; however, their ability to remain focused on the patient's cardiopulmonary status must not be impaired. An individual with advanced life support skills should be immediately available, a requisite easy to fulfill in the ED setting.

Standard-risk patient[a]

Oral intake in the prior 3 hours	Procedural urgency[b]			
	Emergent procedure	*Urgent procedure*	*Semi-urgent*	*Nonurgent*
Nothing	All levels of sedation	All levels of sedation	All levels of sedation	All levels of sedation
Clear liquids only	All levels of sedation	All levels of sedation	Up to and including brief deep sedation	Up to and including extended moderate sedation
Light snack	All levels of sedation	Up to and including brief deep sedation	Up to and including dissociative sedation: nonextended moderate sedation	Minimal sedation only
Heavier snack or meal	All levels of sedation	Up to and including extended moderate sedation	Minimal sedation only	Minimal sedation only

Higher-risk patient[a]

Oral intake in the prior 3 hours	Procedural urgency[b]			
	Emergent procedure	*Urgent procedure*	*Semi-urgent*	*Nonurgent*
Nothing	All levels of sedation	All levels of sedation	All levels of sedation	All levels of sedation
Clear liquids only	All levels of sedation	Up to and including brief deep sedation	Up to and including extended moderate sedation	Minimal sedation only
Light snack	All levels of sedation	Up to and including dissociative sedation: nonextended moderate sedation	Minimal sedation only	Minimal sedation only
Heavier snack or meal	All levels of sedation	Up to and including dissociative sedation: nonextended moderate sedation	Minimal sedation only	Minimal sedation only

Procedural sedation and analgesia targeted depth and duration

Increasing potential aspiration risk ↓

- Minimal sedation only
- Dissociative sedation; brief or intermediate-length moderate sedation
- Extended moderate sedation
- Brief deep sedation
- Intermediate or extended-length deep sedation

Brief: <10 minutes
Intermediate: 10–20 minutes
Extended >20 minutes

543

Figure 33–1 Prudent limits of targeted depth and length of emergency department (ED) procedural sedation and analgesia (PSA) based on presedation assessment of aspiration risk.

a. Higher-risk patients are those with one or more of the following present to a degree individually or cumulatively judged clinically important by the treating clinician:

- Potential for difficult or prolonged assisted ventilation should an airway complication occur (e.g., short neck, small mandible/micrognathia, large tongue, tracheomalacia, laryngomalacia, history of difficult intubation, congential anomalies of the airway and neck, sleep apnea).
- Conditions predisposing to esophageal reflux (e.g., elevated intracranial pressure, esophageal disease, hiatal hernia, peptic ulcer disease, gastritis, bowel obstruction, ileus, tracheoesophageal fistula).
- Extremes of age (e.g., >70 yr or <6 mo).
- Severe systemic disease with definite functional limitation (i.e., American Society of Anesthesiologists [ASA] physical status ≥ 3).
- Other clinical findings leading the emergency physician [EP] to judge the patient to be at higher than standard risk (e.g., altered level of consciousness, frail appearance).

b. Procedural urgency:

- Emergent (e.g., cardioversion for life-threatening dysrhythmia, reduction of markedly angulated fracture or dislocation with soft tissue or vascular compromise, intractable pain or suffering).
- Urgent (e.g., care of dirty wounds and lacerations, animal and human bites, abscess incision and drainage, fracture reduction, hip reduction, lumbar puncture for suspected meningitis, arthrocentesis, neuroimaging for trauma).
- Semi-urgent (e.g., care of clean wounds and lacerations, shoulder reduction, neuroimaging for new-onset seizure, foreign body removal, sexual assault examination).
- Nonurgent or elective (e.g., nonvegetable foreign body in external auditory canal, chronic embedded soft tissue foreign body, ingrown toenail). (From Green SM, Roback MG, Miner JR, et al: Fasting and emergency department procedural sedation and analgesia: A consensus-based clinical practice advisory. Ann Emerg Med 49:454, 2007.)

During deep sedation, the individual dedicated to patient monitoring should be experienced with this depth of sedation and have no other responsibilities that would interfere with the advanced level of monitoring and documentation appropriate for this sedation level.[15] Individual hospital-wide sedation policies may have additional requirements for how and when deep sedation is administered, based on their specific needs and available expertise.

For situations in which sedation is initiated by the intramuscular, oral, nasal, inhalational, or rectal routes, it is not mandatory to have intravenous (IV) access, although this may be preferred based upon anticipated depth of sedation or comorbidity or for the convenience of additional drug titration. When sedation is performed without IV access, an individual skilled in initiating such access should be immediately available—again, a requisite easy to fulfill in the ED setting.

EQUIPMENT AND MECHANICAL MONITORING

The routine use of mechanical monitoring has greatly enhanced the safety of PSA. With current technology, oxygenation (via pulse oximetry), ventilation (via capnography), and hemodynamics (via blood pressure and electrocardiogram [ECG]) can all be monitored noninvasively in nonintubated, spontaneously breathing patients.

Pulse Oximetry

PSA mechanical monitoring should include continuous pulse oximetry with an audible signal. Pulse oximetry measures the percentage of hemoglobin that is bound to oxygen and is not a substitute for monitoring ventilation, because there is a variable lag time between the onset of hypoventilation or apnea and a change in oxygen saturation of hemoglobin molecules.

Capnography

Capnography is not currently a requirement or standard for all PSA in the ED, but it is a very useful technique that provides a continuous, breath-by-breath measure of respiratory rate and CO_2 exchange. Importantly, capnography can detect the common adverse airway and respiratory events associated with PSA.[21-33] Capnography is the earliest indicator of airway or respiratory compromise and will manifest an abnormally high or low end-tidal carbon dioxide (E_Tco_2) well before pulse oximetry detects a falling oxyhemoglobin saturation, especially in patients receiving supplemental oxygen. Early detection of respiratory compromise is especially important in infants and toddlers who have smaller functional residual capacity and greater oxygen consumption relative to older children and adults.[34,35] Capnography provides a nonimpedance respiratory rate directly from the airway (via oral-nasal cannula). This is more accurate than impedance-based respiratory monitoring, especially in patients with obstructive apnea or laryngospasm, in whom impedance-based monitoring will interpret chest wall movement without ventilation as a valid breath.

Both central and obstructive apnea can be almost instantaneously detected by capnography. Loss of the capnogram, in conjunction with no chest wall movement and no breath sounds on auscultation, confirms the diagnosis of central apnea. Obstructive apnea is characterized by loss of the capnogram, chest wall movement, and absent breath sounds. The absence of the capnogram in association with the presence or absence of chest wall movement distinguishes apnea from upper airway obstruction and laryngospasm. Response to airway alignment maneuvers can further distinguish upper airway obstruction from laryngospasm.

Capnography appears more sensitive than clinical assessment of ventilation in detection of apnea. In a recent study, 10 of 39 patients (26%) experienced 20-second periods of apnea during procedural sedation and analgesia. All 10 episodes of apnea were detected by capnography but not by the anesthesia providers.[36]

As the amplitude of the capnogram is determined by E_Tco_2 and the width is determined by the expiratory time, changes in these parameters affect capnogram shape. Hyperventilation (increased respiratory rate, decreased E_Tco_2) results in a low-amplitude and narrow capnogram, whereas classical hypoventilation (decreased respiratory rate, increased E_Tco_2) results in a high-amplitude and wide capnogram. Acute bronchospasm results in a capnogram with a curved ascending phase and upsloping alveolar plateau. An E_Tco_2 greater than 70 mm Hg, in patients without chronic hypoventilation, indicates respiratory failure.

Two types of drug-induced hypoventilation occur during PSA.[24] Bradypneic hypoventilation (type 1), commonly seen with opioids, is characterized by an increased E_Tco_2 and an increased arterial carbon dioxide pressure ($Paco_2$). Respiratory rate is depressed proportionally greater than tidal volume resulting in bradypnea, an increase in expiratory time, and a rise in E_Tco_2, graphically represented by a high-amplitude and wide capnogram.

Bradypneic hypoventilation follows a predictable course with E_Tco_2 increasing progressively until respiratory failure and apnea occur. Although there is no absolute threshold at which apnea occurs, patients without chronic hypoventilation with E_Tco_2 greater than 70 mm Hg are at significant risk.

Hypopneic hypoventilation (type 2), commonly seen with sedative-hypnotic drugs, is characterized by a normal or decreased E_Tco_2 and an increased $Paco_2$ as airway dead space remains constant (e.g., 150 mL in the normal adult lung) and tidal volume is decreasing. Tidal volume is depressed proportionally greater than respiratory rate, resulting in low tidal volume breathing that leads to an increase in airway dead space fraction (dead space volume/tidal volume). As tidal volume decreases, airway dead space fraction increases, which in turn results in an increase in the $Paco_2 - E_Tco_2$ gradient. Even though $Paco_2$ is increasing, E_Tco_2 may remain normal or be decreasing, graphically represented by a low-amplitude capnogram.

Hypopneic hypoventilation follows a variable course. It may resolve over time as sedatives redistribute from the central nervous system to the periphery, it may progress to periodic breathing with intermittent apneic pauses (which may resolve spontaneously or progress to central apnea) or directly to central apnea.

The low tidal volume breathing that characterizes hypopneic hypoventilation increases dead space ventilation when normal compensatory mechanisms are inhibited by drug effects. Minute ventilation, which normally increases to compensate for an increase in dead space, does not change or may decrease. As minute ventilation decreases, arterial oxygenation decreases. If minute ventilation decreases further, oxygenation is further impaired. However, E_Tco_2 may initially be high (bradypneic hypoventilation) or low (hypopneic hypoventilation) without significant changes in oxygenation, particularly if supplemental oxygen is given. Therefore, a drug-induced increase or decrease in E_Tco_2 does not necessarily lead to oxygen desaturation and may not require intervention.

ECG Monitoring

Although continuous ECG monitoring cannot be considered mandatory nor standard of care in the absence of cardiovascular disease, such monitoring is simple, inexpensive, and readily available.

Bispectral Index Monitoring

The bispectral index (BIS) is a monitoring modality that uses a processed electroencephalogram signal to quantify anesthetic or sedation depth. A BIS value of 100 (unitless scale) is considered complete alertness, 0 is no cortical activity at all, and the range of 40 to 60 is believed to be consistent with general anesthesia. Although this technology has been widely used to monitor depth of sedation in the operating room, the ASA has judged that its clinical applicability for this purpose "has not been established."[37] Whereas PSA research has demonstrated statistical associations between BIS and standard sedation scores, these studies have also noted unacceptably wide ranges of BIS values at various depths of sedation.[21,36–42] Thus, whereas BIS is correlated with sedation depth in aggregate groups, it lacks sufficient capacity to reliably gauge such depth in individual patients and, therefore, cannot currently be recommended for ED PSA.

Resuscitation Equipment and Supplies

The sedation area should include all necessary age-appropriate equipment for airway management and resuscitation, including oxygen, a bag-valve mask, suction, and drug reversal agents. A defibrillator should be available for subjects with significant cardiovascular disease.

Vital Signs

Vital signs should be periodically measured at individualized intervals, in most cases including measurements at baseline, after drug administration, on completion of the procedure, during early recovery, and at completion of recovery. During deep sedation, it is advisable to assess vital signs every 5 minutes. Patients are at highest risk of complications 5 to 10 minutes after IV medications and during the immediate postprocedure period when external stimuli are discontinued.

SUPPLEMENTAL OXYGEN

Currently, substantial practice variation exists with regard to the use of supplemental oxygen during PSA. Its premise is a logical one—increasing systemic oxygen reserves should naturally delay or perhaps avert hypoxemia should an airway or respiratory adverse event occur. However, the price paid for this well-intentioned safeguard is the loss of pulse oximetry as an early warning device.[12,15,21] Hyperoxygenated patients will desaturate only after apnea is prolonged—indeed, the time required for preoxygenated apneic adults and adolescents to desaturate to 90% averages more than 6 minutes.[43,44]

In the current PSA literature, there is only a single controlled trial of supplemental oxygen, and this study found no differences in the rates of hypoxia and respiratory depression with this intervention.[23] Larger studies are needed, including those in deeply sedated patients[21]; however, in the interim, supplemental oxygen cannot be considered mandatory and remains an option best left to clinician preference. If oxygen is administered, and capnography is not available, continual visual inspection of chest wall motion and air movement is especially important.

DISCHARGE CRITERIA

All patients receiving PSA should be monitored until they are no longer at risk for cardiorespiratory depression (Table 33–3). To be discharged, they should be alert and oriented (or returned to age-appropriate baseline) and vital signs should be stable. Many hospitals have chosen to use standardized recovery scoring systems similar to those used in their surgical postanesthesia recovery areas (Table 33–4). Although no generally accepted minimum durations for safe discharge have been established, one large ED study[45] found that in children with uneventful sedations, no serious adverse effects occurred more than 25 minutes after final medication administration. This suggests that in most cases, prolonged observation beyond ½ hour is unlikely to be necessary.

All patients should leave the hospital with a reliable adult who will observe them after discharge for postprocedural complications. It is desirable to document the name of the individual on the hospital record. Written instructions should be given regarding appropriate diet, medications, and level of activity (Tables 33–5 and 33–6). Even though patients may appear awake and able to comprehend instructions, they may not remember details once they leave the ED.

To be eligible for safe discharge, children are not required to demonstrate that they can tolerate an oral challenge (most PSA agents are emetogenic and forcing fluids postsedation can lead to emesis before and/or after discharge), nor are they required to walk unaided. The AAP guidelines require only that "the patient can talk (if age-appropriate)" and "the patient can sit up unaided (if age-appropriate)."[15] When infants and young children are discharged after their evening bedtime, it is particularly important to caution parents to position the

TABLE 33–3 Postsedation Complications

Complication	Etiology
Delayed awakening	Prolonged drug action
	Hypoxemia, hypercarbia, hypovolemia
Agitation	Pain, hypoxemia, hypercarbia, full bladder
	Paradoxical reactions
	Emergence reactions
Nausea and vomiting	Sedative agents
	Premature oral fluids
Cardiorespiratory events	
Tachycardia	Pain, hypovolemia, impaired ventilation
Bradycardia	Vagal stimulation, opioids, hypoxia
Hypoxia	Laryngospasm, airway obstruction, oversedation

From Krauss B, Brustowicz R (eds): Pediatric Procedural Sedation and Analgesia. Philadelphia, Lippincott Williams & Wilkins, 1999, p. 145.

TABLE 33–4 Sample Recovery Scoring Systems

Steward Recovery Score

Consciousness

Awake	2
Responding to stimuli	1
Not responding	0

Airway

Coughing on command or crying	2
Maintaining good airway	1
Airway requires maintenance	0

Movement

Moving limbs purposefully	2
Nonpurposeful movements	1
Not moving	0

Modified Aldrete Score

Vital Signs

Stable	1
Unstable	0

Respirations

Normal	2
Shallow respirations/tachypnea	1
Apnea	0

Level of Consciousness

Alert, oriented/returned to preprocedural level	2
Arousable, giddy, agitated	1
Unresponsive	0

Oxygen Saturation

95%–100% or preprocedural level	2
90%–94%	1
<90%	0

Color

Pink/preprocedural color	2
Pale/dusky	1
Cyanotic	0

Activity

Moves on command/preprocedural level	2
Moves extremities/uncoordinated walking	1
No spontaneous movement	0

Sedation Score	Action
>8	Consider discharge if no score = 0
7–8	Vital signs q20min
4–6	Vital signs q10min
0–3	Vital signs q5min—consider further evaluation if prolonged

From Krauss B, Brustowicz R (eds): Pediatric Procedural Sedation and Analgesia. Philadelphia, Lippincott Williams & Wilkins, 1999, p. 157.

TABLE 33–5 Sample Adult Disposition Instructions after PSA

1. Do not drive or operate heavy machinery for 12 hr.
2. Eat a light diet for the next 12 hr.
3. Take only your prescribed medications as needed, including any pain medication you were discharged with. Avoid alcohol.
4. Do not make any important decisions or sign important documents for 12 hr. You may be forgetful owing to medications that were administered.
5. If you experience any difficulty breathing or persistent nausea and vomiting, return to the emergency department.
6. You should have a responsible person with you for the rest of the day and during the night.

TABLE 33–6 Sample Pediatric Disposition Instructions after PSA

Your child has been given medicine for sedation and/or pain control. These medicines may cause your child to be sleepy and less aware of his or her surroundings, making it easier for accidents to happen while walking or crawling. Because of these side effects, your child should be watched closely for the next few hours. We suggest the following:

1. No eating or drinking for the next 2 hr. Infants may resume half normal feedings when they are hungry.
2. No playing for 12 hr that requires normal coordination, such as bike riding or jungle gym activities.
3. No playing without an adult to watch and supervise for the next 12 hr.
4. No baths, showers, cooking, or use of potentially dangerous electrical appliances unless supervised by an adult for the next 12 hr.

If you notice anything unusual about your child, call us for advice or return to the emergency department for reevaluation.

child's head in the car seat carefully. Significant forward flexion might cause airway obstruction if the child falls asleep on the way home.

GENERAL PRINCIPLES

Therapeutic mistakes resulting in inadequate analgesia and sedation include using the wrong agent, the wrong dose, the wrong route and frequency of administration, and poor use of adjunctive agents. With proper training and technique, adequate PSA can be provided under almost any circumstance. Understanding titration principles is critical to providing safe and effective PSA. Clinicians must have a thorough knowledge of the pharmacokinetics, dosing, administration, and potential complications of the PSA agents they use. Onset time from injection to initial observed effect must be appreciated, especially when using drugs in combination, to avoid stacking of drug doses resulting in oversedation.

The correct agent (or combination of agents) and the route and timing of administration depend on the following factors: How long will the procedure last? Will it be seconds (e.g., simple relocation of a dislocated joint, incision and drainage of a small abscess, cardioversion), minutes (e.g., complex fracture manipulation for reduction, breaking up loculations in a large abscess and then packing it), or prolonged (e.g., complex facial laceration repair)? How likely is it that the procedure will need to be repeated (e.g., fracture reduction)? Can topical, local, or regional anesthesia be used as an adjunct? Does the patient require sedation only for a noninvasive diagnostic imaging study?

Prior to drug administration, every effort should be made to minimize a patient's anxiety and distress, particularly in children. The emotional state of a patient on induction strongly correlates with the degree of distress on emergence and in the immediate days after the procedure.[46-49] Emergency clinicians must avoid being pressured by consultants to cut corners or rush PSA. Incorporating into the presedation preparation a discussion with the consultant about the sedation plan and the length of time required to safely prepare and sedate the patient can avoid the risks associated with a hurried sedation.

For pediatric PSA, clinicians should appreciate the adult doses of the sedation agents they are administering as the maximum thresholds. Understanding that the initial dose of midazolam for PSA in a 100-kg patient on a milligram-per-kilogram basis is far less than the 0.1 mg/kg used in a child is essential to avoid unexpected mishaps in drug dosing.

ROUTES OF ADMINISTRATION

For nondissociative agents, IV titration to patient response is the best method of obtaining rapid and safe analgesia and/or sedation. It is important to wait the appropriate time for the medications to produce the intended effect before adding more doses. When using opioids, doses administered in 2- to 3-minute increments—observing for side effects such as miosis, somnolence, decreased responsiveness to verbal stimuli, minimally impaired speech, and diminished pain on questioning—are appropriate initial end points. For sedative-hypnotics, similar incremental dosing and end points such as ptosis (rather than miosis), somnolence, slurred speech, and gaze alteration should be sought. Repeated doses may be given in a titrated fashion based on the patient's response during the procedure.

Oral, transmucosal (i.e., nasal, rectal), and intramuscular (IM) routes are more convenient means of administration because IV access is not necessary. However, they are much less reliable for timely dose titration to a desired response. New drug delivery systems are expanding the effectiveness and ease of use of these routes of administration. The refinement of intranasal drug delivery has significantly increased the efficacy of this route of administration.[50,51] Prior to the development of metered-dose atomizers, the degree of absorption and effectiveness of intranasal drug administration were operator dependent. Further, new drug formulations with concentrations appropriate for intranasal administration are becoming available for study.[52,53]

The main advantage of these other routes is for pediatric patients in whom IV access may be problematic or for procedures that may require only minimal sedation in conjunction with the use of local anesthetics. These routes are also advantageous for simple sedation for diagnostic imaging.

With the exception of ketamine, agents administered intramuscularly have erratic absorption and a variable onset of action. As such, prolonged preprocedural and postprocedural observation may be necessary. When required, the IM route offers little advantage over oral or transmucosal administration.

Another PSA route is via inhalation using nitrous oxide. This gas can be either delivered by a demand-flow system using a handheld mask or delivered to young children by a continuous-flow system under close clinician supervision using a nose mask.

Because individual needs may vary widely, application of arbitrary ceiling doses of analgesic and sedative regimens is unwarranted. The true ceiling dose of an agent is that which provides adequate pain relief or sedation without major cardiopulmonary side effects such as respiratory depression, apnea, bradycardia, hypotension, or allergic reactions.

There are two absolute PSA contraindications: severe clinical instability requiring immediate attention and refusal by a competent patient. Relative contraindications include hemodynamic or respiratory compromise, altered sensorium, or inability to monitor side effects (e.g., magnetic resonance imaging without remote monitoring). However, even in many of these circumstances, appropriate agents can be given to provide analgesia and sedation while minimizing the chances for further deterioration. Although safely sedating patients at the extremes of age is challenging and requires additional care as well as reductions in drug dosing owing to decreased drug metabolism and excretion, age is not a contraindication to PSA.

DRUG SELECTION STRATEGIES

The majority of nonpainful or minimally painful ED procedures in older children and adults can be performed without systemic sedation and analgesia. Skilled practitioners can frequently combine a calm, reassuring bedside manner with distraction techniques, careful local or regional anesthesia, or both.[54-56] Many procedures, however, cannot be technically or humanely performed without PSA. These situations can be divided into three categories.

Insufficient Analgesia. Despite a cooperative patient, for some procedures, it is impossible to achieve effective pain control with local or regional anesthesia. Examples of procedures requiring systemic PSA include fracture reductions, dislocation reductions, large loculated abscess incision and drainage, wounds that require scrubbing such as "road rash," cardioversion, bone marrow aspiration/biopsy, and extensive burn débridement.

Insufficient Anxiolysis. Despite effective local or regional anesthesia, some patients will be so frightened that procedures cannot be technically or humanely performed without PSA. Young children requiring laceration repair are frequently terrified, and older children and adults may be highly anxious in anticipation of laceration repairs in sensitive and/or personal regions (e.g., face, genitalia, perineum).

Insufficient Immobilization. Despite effective local or regional anesthesia and anxiolysis, PSA may be indicated to prevent excessive motion during procedures that require substantial immobilization (e.g., repair of complex facial lacerations, diagnostic imaging studies). Immobilization is most commonly an issue with young children and the mentally challenged.

General Considerations. Clinicians must therefore customize their drug selection (e.g., anxiolysis, sedation, analgesia, immobilization) based upon the unique needs of the patient and their individual level of experience with specific agents (Table 33–7). A risk-benefit analysis should be performed before every sedation (Table 33–8). The benefits of reducing anxiety and controlling pain should be carefully weighed against the risks of respiratory depression and airway compromise. Factors influencing the extent of pharmacologic management are listed in Table 33–9. Some general

TABLE 33–7 Procedural Sedation and Analgesia Indications and Sedation Strategies*

Clinical Situation	Indication	Procedural Requirements	Suggested Sedation Strategies
Noninvasive procedures	CT Echocardiography Electroencephalography MRI Ultrasonography	Motion control Anxiolysis	Comforting alone Chloral hydrate PO (in patients < 3 yr of age) Methohexital PR Pentobarbital PO, IM, or IV Midazolam IV Propofol or etomidate IV
Procedure associated with low pain and high anxiety	Dental procedures Flexible fiberoptic laryngoscopy Foreign body removal, simple IV cannulation Laceration repair, simple Lumbar puncture Ocular irrigation Phlebotomy Slit-lamp examination	Sedation Anxiolysis Motion control	Comforting and topical/local anesthesia Midazolam PO/IN/PR/IV Nitrous oxide
Procedures associated with high level of pain, high anxiety, or both	Abscess incision and drainage Arthrocentesis Bone marrow aspiration/biopsy Burn débridement Cardiac catheterization Cardioversion Central line placement Endoscopy Foreign body removal, complicated Fracture/dislocation reduction Hernia reduction Interventional radiology procedures Laceration repair, complex Paracentesis Paraphimosis reduction Sexual assault examination Thoracentesis Thoracostomy tube placement	Sedation Anxiolysis Analgesia Amnesia Motion control	Propofol or etomidate IV ± fentanyl Ketamine IM/IV Midazolam and fentanyl IV

*There is no universally accepted or clinically correct dose, medication, or combination. Many regimens are acceptable. This table is intended as a general overview. Sedation strategies should be individualized. Although the pharmacopoeia is large, clinicians should familiarize themselves with a few agents that are flexible enough to be used for the majority of procedures. In all cases, it is assumed that practitioners are fully trained in the technique, appropriate personnel and monitoring are used as detailed in this chapter, and specific drug contraindications are absent.

CT, computed tomography; MRI, magnetic resonance imaging.
Modified from Krauss B, Green SM: Sedation and analgesia for procedures in children. N Engl J Med 342:938, 2000.

TABLE 33–8 Risk-Benefit Analysis for Procedural Sedation and Analgesia

- Why is PSA needed in the first place? Is the procedure very painful, frightening, or requiring extreme cooperation?
- Are the risks of PSA appropriate for the procedure involved?
- If a child, do the parents or guardian consent to the use of PSA?
- How long will the procedure take? If it is a short procedure, is it worth the added risk and expense to the patient? If it is a longer procedure, is there an appropriate agent that can be titrated to allow adequate PSA throughout the entire length of the procedure?
- Are there significant side effects that limit a particular drug's usefulness?
- Are there enough nurses and support personnel present to safely allow the use of PSA?
- What is the recovery period for a given agent? Are there enough treatment areas and staff in the ED to allow adequate observation during recovery?
- When did the patient last eat? Is a delay in waiting for a sufficient fasting time worth the time lost in performing the procedure?

ED, emergency department; PSA, procedural sedation and analgesia.
From Krauss B, Brustowicz R (eds): Pediatric Procedural Sedation and Analgesia. Philadelphia, Lippincott Williams & Wilkins, 1999, p. 294.

drug selection strategies are discussed later and shown in Table 33–7.

Minor Procedures in Cooperative Adults and Older Children. These procedures can usually be managed with topical, local, or regional anesthesia. Systemic PSA is typically unnecessary, although mild anxiolysis (e.g., nitrous oxide, oral midazolam) can make these patients more comfortable.

More Complex Procedures of Longer Duration in Cooperative Adults and Older Children. Supplementation of topical, local, or regional anesthesia with either nitrous oxide or IV midazolam and fentanyl permits customization of sedation depth and pain relief to the specific needs of each patient.

Procedures in Uncooperative Adults or the Mentally Challenged. Essentially all procedures in uncooperative adult-sized patients are difficult without systemic PSA. Depending upon operator experience, IV midazolam/fentanyl, IV propofol/fentanyl, IV etomidate/fentanyl, or IM/IV ketamine/midazolam may be used in these situations. Midazolam and fentanyl can be titrated intravenously to a relatively deep level of sedation, although, as discussed previously, the risk of adverse effects increases with sedation depth.

TABLE 33–9 Factors Influencing the Extent of Pediatric Pharmacologic Management

Age

Selected drugs and routes of administration have age limitations and are not recommended above or below a certain age (e.g., demand flow nitrous oxide in children < 5 yr old, nasal and rectal routes of administration in children > 6 yr old).

Time of Day

A toddler presenting at naptime or at 9 PM who is tired and sleepy will usually require a smaller dosing and possibly a lower level of procedural sedation and analgesia (PSA) than required at 9 AM. Young children presenting with facial lacerations at night, after their normal bedtime, may only require topical anesthesia and a quiet room for 20–30 min to achieve a painless laceration repair while the child sleeps.

Fasting Status

Young children can be extremely difficult and uncooperative when hungry and/or tired. In anticipation of PSA many children are kept NPO from the time they are triaged in the ED. This can further increase hunger and irritability, especially if the child waits 1–2 hr to be seen by a clinician.

Staffing and Equipment Availability

Staffing availability can affect the use and timing of sedation and is especially important in busy EDs with multiple sedations occurring concurrently and in smaller units that are set up for only one sedation at a time.

Location of the Injury

Injuries located in areas of cosmetic concern (especially on the face) or near sensory organs (e.g., ears, eyes, mouth, nose) will often require a high degree of agitation control and a concomitant level of PSA.

Previous Medications

An accurate history of prior medication administration is important in situations in which a child is referred from another facility, because this can affect the type and timing of PSA agents that can be given. In particular, a child may have received opioids or sedative/hypnotics prior to transfer and may still be sedated on arrival, necessitating an adjustment in the PSA regimen.

Level of Anxiety

The level of anxiety of both the child and the accompanying adult(s) must be accurately assessed. Children manifest anxiety in many different ways, and emergency clinicians must be facile at recognizing the varying expressions of anxiety, especially in young children. A child with a facial laceration quietly sitting on the stretcher during the initial examination will not necessarily be a calm and cooperative patient during laceration repair (infants and toddlers). The nursing assessment at triage of the state of the child and accompanying adult(s) can be very helpful in some cases in determining the need of PSA. The child who was frightened and uncooperative in triage may be calm and compliant during a procedure. Unfortunately, the reverse is also true. When confronted by an extremely anxious child, ED personnel should ascertain what the parents have told the child about the upcoming procedure. Many parents, in the hope of lessening their child's anxiety, will tell the child that she or he will get a "shot" or a "needle" and that the procedure will "only hurt for a minute." This type of parental preparation, especially in young children who do not have the cognitive abilities to mediate their anxiety, often results in a significant increase in the child's anxiety and a decrease in their ability to cooperate, especially if the child has had a previous negative experience with a procedure in the ED. It is also important to assess the parent's level of anxiety, because this will determine the degree to which they can assist during the procedure. An extremely anxious parent or a parent who must take care of other siblings during the procedure will find it difficult to assist in distracting the child or otherwise helping her or him to cope with the procedure.

Previous Experience

Childrens' previous experience in hospitals can greatly affect their response to the current situation. Direct experience is not the only way to create anxious, frightened, and uncooperative patients, though. Images from television, stories from peers, or prior witness of a sibling being forcibly restrained for a laceration repair can leave a powerful and lasting impression. This type of influence should be especially suspect in children whose anxiety seems out-of-proportion in the present situation. Eliciting from the parents a history of a previous difficult experience in the ED can be a decisive factor in determining the degree of sedation required. Children who have had a recent unpleasant laceration repair, and who now present with a new laceration, may well require PSA as opposed to simple anxiolysis (either pharmacologic or nonpharmacologic) had there been no previous trauma.

Child's Behavior at Routine Primary Care Visits

Inquiring into how a child behaves during routine primary care visits can yield important information on how the child reacts to stressful situations, how cooperative he or she will be with the anticipated procedure, and whether pharmacologic management is needed. Children who cry but hold still when vaccinated may be more compliant than children who are described by their parents as being "afraid of doctors" or "wild" during visits to the primary care physician.

ED, emergency department; PSA, procedural sedation and analgesia.

Ketamine (typically with coadministered midazolam when used in adults) can also provide the profound analgesia and immobilization necessary to perform painful procedures. However, in adults, there is a risk of unpleasant hallucinatory recovery reactions. Ketamine should be used with extreme caution in older adults, because its sympathomimetic properties may aggravate underlying coronary artery disease or hypertension. Occasionally, procedures in extremely uncooperative adults or the mentally challenged are best managed in the operating room with general anesthesia.

Minor Procedures in Uncooperative Older Children and in Young Children. Minor procedures (e.g., small lacerations, IV cannulation, venipuncture, superficial foreign body removal) in uncooperative children can frequently be managed by skilled practitioners using a combination of nonpharmacologic techniques (e.g., distraction, guided imagery, hypnosis, comforting, breathing techniques) in conjunction with topical anesthesia, careful local anesthesia, and when necessary, brief forcible immobilization (by personnel or a restraining device). In other cases, supplementing nonpharmacologic techniques with topical or local anesthesia and anxiolysis with oral midazolam may be sufficient to permit successful wound repair. Although oral administration is most popular and least invasive, the nasal or rectal routes can also be used depending upon operator experience and preference.

Major Procedures in Uncooperative Children. Major painful procedures (e.g., fracture reduction, large loculated abscess incision and drainage, arthrocentesis of a major joint) require systemic PSA. Options include IM/IV ketamine, IV propofol/fentanyl, IV etomidate/fentanyl, or IV fentanyl/midazolam. Ketamine may be the best option in such children, because dissociative sedation can consistently provide the immobilization and analgesia while maintaining protective airway reflexes and upper airway muscular tone.

PHARMACOPEIA

There is no universally correct or preferred medication or drug regimen. Many options are acceptable and successful. The best choice is an agent whose pharmacologic properties are familiar to the operator, is used frequently by the operator, is easily titrable, and has a short duration of action or is readily reversible. All drugs should be given in adequate doses, because underdosing opioids or sedatives provides no useful purpose. Dosing recommendations for PSA drugs are shown in Table 33–10, with specialized protocols for midazolam/fentanyl, propofol, and ketamine shown in Tables 33–11, 33–12, and 33–13, respectively. Individual agents are discussed in the following section.

Sedative-Hypnotic Agents

Chloral Hydrate

Pharmacology. Chloral hydrate is a pure sedative-hypnotic agent without analgesic properties. When administered orally, the average time to peak sedation is approximately 30 minutes, with a recovery time of an additional 1 to 2 hours.[57,58] Residual motor imbalance and agitation may persist for several hours beyond this.[59] Rectal administration is erratically absorbed and therefore not recommended.

Adult Use. The use of chloral hydrate is limited to diagnostic imaging studies in children. It has no current uses in adults.

Pediatric Use. Chloral hydrate is widely used as a sedative to facilitate nonpainful outpatient diagnostic procedures such as electroencephalograms[58] and computed tomography (CT) or magnetic resonance imaging (MRI) scanning.[60-64] IV Pentobarbital appears to be more effective for the latter indication than chloral hydrate,[65] although many centers prefer chloral hydrate in younger children (e.g., <18 mo) simply to avoid the need for IV access.[61,62,65]

Adverse Effects. Despite a wide margin of safety, chloral hydrate can cause airway obstruction and respiratory depression, especially at higher doses (75–100 mg/kg).[1,58,61,63,64] The incidence was 0.6% in one large series.[58] There is no known dosage threshold of chloral hydrate below which this potential complication can be consistently avoided,[1,63] and accordingly, standard interactive and mechanical monitoring precautions apply to chloral hydrate as they do to other PSA agents.

Because it is a halogenated hydrocarbon, overdoses of chloral hydrate can be arrhythmogenic, producing ventricular dysrhythmias. *β-Blockers may be most effective in terminating ventricular arrhythmias.* Despite reports of potential carcinogenicity, the AAP has judged that the evidence is currently insufficient to avoid single doses of chloral hydrate for this reason alone.[66]

Midazolam

Pharmacology. Benzodiazepines are a group of highly lipophilic agents that possess anxiolytic, amnestic, sedative, hypnotic, muscle relaxant, and anticonvulsant properties. They lack direct analgesic properties and, thus, are commonly coadministered with opioids. Caution must be exercised when using benzodiazepines and opioids together, because the risks of hypoxia and apnea are significantly greater than when either is used alone.[67]

Midazolam is by far the most common benzodiazepine used for PSA, and is preferred over the longer-acting lorazepam and diazepam. The time to peak effect for midazolam is approximately 2 to 3 minutes when given intravenously. Unlike diazepam, midazolam and lorazepam are water-soluble, making parenteral administration less painful and mucosal absorption faster. *Midazolam is readily reversed with flumazenil*, and individuals undergoing PSA with midazolam are good candidates for this antidote should reversal be required.

Adult Use. Midazolam can be effectively used for moderate and deep sedation through careful IV titration to effect, typically together with fentanyl (see Table 33–11).

Pediatric Use. The advantage of midazolam over other benzodiazepines for pediatric PSA is its short duration of action, reversibility, and availability in multiple routes of administration. Midazolam may be used for the same indications and manner as in adults. Some children require larger doses than would be typical for adults on a milligram-per-kilogram basis,[68] and paradoxical responses (e.g., hyperexcitability) are not uncommon.[59,69,70] Midazolam does not reliably render a child motionless, and thus methohexital or pentobarbital is generally preferred for neuroimaging.[65,71,72]

To avoid the need for IV access in frightened children, midazolam has been alternatively administered via the IM,[73] oral,[69,74-78] intranasal,[74,79-82] and rectal[83,84] routes. However, the inability to effectively titrate using these routes dictates that a reliable depth of sedation cannot be predictably or regularly achieved. Thus, these non-IV routes are primarily reserved for pure anxiolysis and/or mild sedation for minimally painful procedures. Respiratory depression can also occur via these routes.[78]

TABLE 33–10 Procedural Sedation and Analgesia Drug Dosing Recommendations*

Drug	Clinical Effects	Indications	Adult Dose†	Pediatric Dose	Onset (min)	Duration (min)	Comments
Sedative-Hypnotics							
Choral Hydrate (Noctec)	Sedation, motion control, anxiolysis. No analgesia. Not reversible.	Diagnostic imaging (age < 3 yr).	Not recommended.	PO: 25–100 mg/kg, after 30 min may repeat 25–50 mg/kg. Maximum total dose: 2 g or 100 mg/kg (whichever is less). Single use only in neonates.	PO: 15–30	PO: 60–120	Effects unreliable if age >3 yr. Avoid in patients with significant cardiac, hepatic, or renal disease. Rectal absorption is erratic. May produce paradoxical excitement. Because drugs cannot be titrated with the oral route, monitor closely for oversedation.
Etomidate (Amidate)	Sedation, motion control, anxiolysis. No analgesia. Not reversible.	Procedures requiring sedation and/or anxiolysis.	Sedation: 0.1 mg/kg IV; repeat if inadequate response.	Not FDA approved in children.	IV: <1	IV: 5–15	Adverse effects include respiratory depression, myoclonus, nausea, and vomiting. Adrenocortical suppression occurs, but is rarely of clinical significance.
Midazolam‡ (Versed)	Sedation, motion control, anxiolysis. No analgesia. Reversible with flumazenil.	Procedures requiring sedation and/or anxiolysis.	IV: Initial 1 mg, then titrated to max 5 mg. IM: 5 mg or 0.07 mg/kg IM.	IV (0.5–5 yr): Initial 0.05–0.1 mg/kg, then titrated to max 0.6 mg/kg. IV (6–12 yr): Initial 0.025–0.05 mg/kg, then titrated to max 0.4 mg/kg. IM: 0.1–0.15 mg/kg. PO: 0.5–0.75. mg/kg IN: 0.2–0.5 mg/kg. PR: 0.25–0.5 mg/kg.	IV: 2–3. IM: 10–20. PO: 15–30. IN: 10–15. PR: 10–30.	IV: 45–60. IM: 60–120. PO: 60–90. IN: 60. PR: 60–90.	Reduce dose when used in combination with opioids. May produce paradoxical excitement. Because drugs cannot be titrated with the PO/PR/IN routes, monitor closely for oversedation.
Methohexital (Brevital)	Sedation, motion control, anxiolysis. No analgesia. Not reversible.	Diagnostic imaging.	Anesthesia induction IV: 1 mg/kg (less for sedation, **caution, limited research**).	PR: 25 mg/kg. IV (**caution, limited research**): 0.5–1 mg/kg.	PR: 10–15.	PR: 60.	Avoid in patients with temporal lobe epilepsy or porphyria. Because drugs cannot be titrated with the PR route, monitor closely for oversedation.

Continued

TABLE 33–10 Procedural Sedation and Analgesia Drug Dosing Recommendations—cont'd

Drug	Clinical Effects	Indications	Adult Dose[†]	Pediatric Dose	Onset (min)	Duration (min)	Comments
Pentobarbital (Nembutal)	Sedation, motion control, anxiolysis. No analgesia. Not reversible.	Diagnostic imaging.	Not recommended.	IV: 1–6 mg/kg, titrated in increments of 1–2 mg/kg to desired effect. IM: 2–6 mg/kg, maximum 100 mg. PO/PR (<4 yr): 3–6 mg/kg, maximum 100 mg. PO/PR (>4 yr): 1.5–3 mg/kg, maximum 100 mg.	IV: 3–5. IM: 10–15. PO/PR: 15–60.	IV: 15–45. IM: 60–120. PO/PR: 60–240.	May produce paradoxical excitement. Avoid in patients with porphyria. Because drugs cannot be titrated with the PO/PR routes, monitor closely for oversedation.
Propofol (Diprivan)	Sedation, motion control, anxiolysis. Not reversible.	Procedures requiring sedation and/or anxiolysis.	Load 1 mg/kg IV; may administer additional 0.5 mg/kg doses as needed to enhance or prolong sedation.	Load 1 mg/kg IV; may administer additional 0.5 mg/kg doses as needed to enhance or prolong sedation.	IV: <1	IV: 5–15	Frequent hypotension and respiratory depression. Avoid with egg or soy allergies.
Thiopental (Pentothal)	Sedation, motion control, anxiolysis. No analgesia. Not reversible.	Diagnostic imaging.	Not recommended.	PR: 25 mg/kg.	PR: 10–15.	PR: 60–120.	Avoid in patients with porphyria. Because drugs cannot be titrated with the PR route, monitor closely for oversedation.
Analgesic[§]							
Fentanyl (Sublimaze)	Analgesia. Reversible with naloxone	Procedures of moderate to severe pain.	IV: 50 µg, may repeat q3min, titrate to effect.	IV: 1 µg/kg/dose, may repeat q3min, titrate to effect.	IV: 3–5.	IV: 30–60.	Reduce dosing when combined with midazolam.
Dissociative Agent							
Ketamine (Ketalar)	Analgesia, dissociation, amnesia, motion control. Not reversible.	Procedures of moderate to severe pain or requiring immobilization.	Limited experience in ED setting. IV: 1–1.5 mg/kg slowly over 1–2 min, may repeat 1/2 dose q10min prn.	IV: 1.5 mg/kg slowly over 1–2 min, may repeat 1/2 dose q10min prn. IM: 4–5 mg/kg, may repeat after 10 min (full or 1/2 dose without additional atropine).	IV: 1. IM: 3–5.	IV: dissociation 15; recovery 60. IM: dissociation 15–30; recovery 90–150.	Multiple contraindications.‖ Risk of unpleasant hallucinations/dreams if age > 15 yr (rare if younger), which may be blunted with midazolam. Hypersalivation can be minimized with concurrent atropine 0.01 mg/kg IM/IV (minimum 0.1 mg, maximum 0.5 mg).

Inhalational Agent

Nitrous oxide (Nitronox)	Anxiolysis, analgesia, sedation, amnesia (all mild).	Procedures requiring mild analgesia or sedation (age > 4 yr).	Preset mixture with minimum 40% O_2 self-administered by demand valve mask (requires cooperative patient).	Preset mixture for cooperative child; continuous-flow nasal mask in uncooperative child with close monitoring.	<5.	<5 following discontinuation.	Requires specialized apparatus and gas scavenger capability. Several contraindications.¶ Synergistic effect with recent opioids or sedative-hypnotics—use with caution in this setting.

Reversal Agents (Antagonists)

Naloxone (Narcan)	Opioid reversal.	Opioid toxicity.	IV/IM: 0.4–2 mg.	IV/IM: 0.1 mg/kg/dose up to maximum of 2 mg/dose, may repeat q2min prn.	IV: 2.	IV: 20–40. IM: 60–90.	If shorter acting than the reversed drug, serial doses may be required.
Flumazenil (Romazicon)	Benzodiazepine reversal.	Benzodiazepine toxicity.	IV: 0.2 mg, may repeat q1min up to 1 mg.	IV: 0.02 mg/kg/dose, may repeat q1min up to 1 mg.	IV: 1–2.	IV: 30–60.	If shorter acting than the reversed drug, serial doses may be required. Do not use in patients receiving chronic benzodiazepines, cyclosporine, isoniazid, lithium, propoxyphene, theophylline, tricyclic antidepressants.

*Alterations in dosing may be indicated based upon the clinical situation and the practitioner's experience with these agents. Individual dosages may vary when used in combination with other agents, especially when benzodiazepines are combined with opioids.

†Use lower doses in geriatric patients and those with significant cardiopulmonary disease.

‡Midazolam is preferred to other benzodiazepines (e.g., diazepam, lorazepam) for PSA due to its shorter duration of action and multiple routes of administration.

§Fentanyl is preferred to other opioids (e.g., morphine, meperidine) for PSA due to its faster onset, shorter recovery, and lack of histamine release.

‖Generally accepted contraindications to ketamine: Age <3 months; history of airway instability, tracheal surgery, or tracheal stenosis; procedures involving stimulation of the posterior pharynx; active pulmonary infection or disease (including active upper respiratory infection); cardiovascular disease including angina, heart failure, or hypertension; significant head injury; CNS masses, hydrocephalus; glaucoma or acute globe injury; psychosis; porphyria; thyroid disorder or thyroid medication.

¶Generally accepted contraindications to nitrous oxide: Pregnancy (patient or personnel); preexisting nausea/vomiting; trapped gas pockets (e.g., middle ear infection, pneumothorax, bowel obstruction).

ED, emergency department; FDA, U.S. Food and Drug Administration; IV, intravenous; IM, intramuscular; IN, intranasal; PO, oral; PR, rectal.

Adapted from Krauss B, Green SM: Sedation and analgesia for procedures in children. N Engl J Med 342:938, 2000.

TABLE 33–11 Procedure for Moderate to Deep Sedation with Intravenous Midazolam and Fentanyl

Caveats

- Do not consider this procedure if you lack experience with the drugs or do not have the time to perform procedural sedation and analgesia (PSA) properly. Do not attempt this procedure if the pulse oximeter, suction, oxygen, or bag-mask are not working, the IV is not secured, or the room is too small or not set up for PSA.
- This is a two-person procedure, one to monitor the patient and one to perform the procedure.
- Individual response to the drugs is variable and dependent upon the patient's underlying physiologic state and the presence of concomitant drugs/medication.
- Maximum drug effect occurs 2–3 min after administration. Proceed slowly and patiently, allowing the medication to take full effect before giving the next dose.
- Have naloxone and flumazenil immediately available for oversedation and/or respiratory depression.
- If the patient seems overly sedated, begin the procedure. The pain of the procedure often stimulates respiration and lessens sedation.

Contraindications—Absolute (Risks Essentially Always Outweigh Benefits)

- Active hemodynamic instability.
- Active respiratory distress or hypoxemia.

Contraindications—Relative (Risks May Outweigh Benefits)

- Respiratory depression or altered level of consciousness.
- Anticipated difficulty if ventilatory assistance should become necessary (e.g., facial deformity or trauma, small mandible, large tongue, trismus).

Protocol

- Establish IV access.
- Connect appropriate monitoring equipment to the patient. Routine supplemented oxygen is commonly used but not always mandated.
- Pulse, respiratory rate, blood pressure, and level of consciousness should all be recorded initially, and periodically throughout the procedure depending on the depth of sedation.
- Suction equipment, oxygen, a bag-valve-mask, and reversal agents should be immediately available. An age-appropriate resuscitation cart with oral and nasal airways, endotracheal tubes, and a functioning laryngoscope must be nearby.
- The order of the drugs is one of personal preference. The ratio of analgesia to sedation is determined by the nature of the procedure. Some procedures require primary analgesia and secondary anxiolysis/sedation (e.g., abscess incision and drainage, bone marrow aspiration, arthrocentesis, burn débridement, central catheter placement). In this case, administer fentanyl first. Others require primary anxiolysis/sedation with secondary analgesia (e.g., lumbar puncture, simple foreign body removal); administer midazolam first.
- Administer local anesthesia if indicated after PSA initiated (this often serves to help gauge effectiveness of systemic analgesia).
- Perform the procedure. Additional doses of fentanyl or midazolam may be required if further pain or anxiety are noted based on the response and length of the procedure.
- If hypoxemia, oversedation, or slowed respirations are seen during or after the procedure, the patient should be first stimulated while oxygen is applied and the airway repositioned. If the patient's response is insufficient, assist ventilations with a bag-valve-mask. Reversal agents should be considered if there is not a prompt response to assisted ventilation.
- Continue close observation until the patient is awake and alert, and release the patient with a friend, parent, or relative only after a sufficient discharge score has been attained.

Adverse Effects. When administered by skilled practitioners using standard precautions (see Table 33–11), the safety profile for midazolam is excellent.[5,6,84] However, when administering benzodiazepines, one must maintain continuous vigilance for respiratory depression.[1,59,67,84,85] Such respiratory depression is dose-dependent and greatly enhanced in the presence of ethanol or other depressive drugs, especially opioids. These effects are exaggerated in the elderly. Deaths from undetected apnea have occurred,[67] underscoring the critical role for continuous interactive and mechanical monitoring.

Benzodiazepines induce minimal cardiovascular depression. Although hypotension can occur, it is rare when the agents are carefully titrated. One reason midazolam is ideal for painful procedures is its significant amnesic effect. Even though patients appear to feel pain during the procedure, it is often not remembered.

Pentobarbital

Pharmacology. Pentobarbital is a barbiturate capable of profound sedation, hypnosis, amnesia, and anticonvulsant activity in a dose-dependent fashion. It has no inherent analgesic properties. When carefully titrated intravenously, sedation is evident within 5 minutes with a duration of approximately 30 to 40 minutes.[71]

Adult Use. Pentobarbital has no advantage over midazolam for adult PSA and is rarely used for this purpose.

Pediatric Use. Pentobarbital is the IV sedative of choice in many centers for diagnostic imaging in children.[62,65,71,86,87] It is regarded as superior to midazolam[65,71,72] or chloral hydrate[65] for this indication. Pentobarbital, like midazolam, is available in multiple routes of administration.

Adverse Effects. Like other barbiturates, pentobarbital can lead to respiratory depression and hypotension, because it is a negative inotrope.[62,65,71,72]

Ultrashort-Acting Sedative-Hypnotic Agents

Ultrashort-acting sedatives (i.e., propofol, etomidate, thiopental, methohexital) can rapidly produce potent sedation when administered intravenously, and all exhibit rapid awakening (<5 min) after drug discontinuation. ED use of these agents—propofol in particular—for a variety of common short, painful procedures has expanded dramatically in recent years, because their brief yet profound obtundation creates superlative conditions.

Substantial controversy surrounded the early administration of these agents for ED PSA.[88] Proponents have cited their extremely rapid onset and recovery as enormous advantages over other sedatives. Critics have cited the level of continuous vigilance required to achieve a desired effect while simultaneously avoiding significant cardiopulmonary depression, because these agents can exhibit rapid swings in levels of consciousness. Research including thousands of ED patients for propofol and hundreds for etomidate has subsequently

TABLE 33–12 Procedure for Deep Sedation with Propofol

Indications

- Brief, painful procedures for which deep sedation is indicated, including fracture and dislocation reductions, incision and drainage of abscesses, cardioversion, tube thoracostomy, and central line placement.

Contraindications

Absolute (Risks Essentially Outweigh Benefits)

- Known or suspected allergy to soy or eggs.

Higher Relative Risk Patients:

- Patients > 55 yr of age, debilitated, or with significant underlying illness (i.e., ASA physical status score 3 or 4) are at an increased risk of propofol-induced hypotension and other complications. When the benefits of using propofol outweigh the risks, administer lower doses more slowly. Patients should ideally have their volume status optimized before receiving propofol.
- Because there is no clear consensus on optimal fasting time prior to sedation, decision making should balance the relatively low probability of aspiration with the patient's underlying risk factors, the timing and nature of recent oral intake, the urgency of the procedure, and the depth and length of required sedation.

Personnel

- The minimum personnel present during deep sedation should be an emergency clinician and an ED nurse. Most institutions also use a separate emergency clinician who is solely dedicated to drug administration and patient monitoring.

Presedation

- Physicians should perform a standard presedation assessment, with special attention on the potential for airway management during deep sedation.
- Suction, airway, and resuscitation equipment should be immediately available.
- Unless precluded by the urgency of the procedure, IV analgesia is recommended in addition to propofol for painful procedures.

Propofol Administration: General

- Propofol induces sedation approximately 30 sec after bolus injection, with typical resolution of clinical effects within 6 min.
- The most common ED dosing is with an initial bolus dose of 1 mg/kg followed by 0.5 mg/kg every 2–3 min as needed to achieve or maintain the desired level of sedation. This dosing applies to both adults and children.
- Propofol is typically titrated to slurring of speech and/or lid ptosis depending on the depth of sedation and degree of relaxation needed for the procedure.

Interactive And Mechanical Monitoring

- Patients should have their airway patency, oxygen saturation, electrocardiographic tracing, and level of consciousness continuously monitored.
- The optional addition of end-tidal carbon dioxide monitoring (capnography) can provide warning of impending airway and respiratory complications before clinical examination or pulse oximetry.
- Although proof of its benefit is thus far lacking, the administration of supplemental oxygen throughout propofol sedation may decrease the need for or duration of assisted ventilation should respiratory depression or apnea occur. Such oxygen administration will also delay the detection of airway or respiratory adverse events by pulse oximetry.

Potential Adverse Effects

- Respiratory depression or apnea leading to assisted ventilation (0%–3.9%).
- Transient hypotension (2.2%–6.5%).
- Emesis (0%–0.5%).
- Pain with injection (2%–20%).

Recovery And Discharge

- Patients receiving propofol should be monitored until they have returned to their baseline mental status.
- Qualified personnel should accompany patients who require transport prior to recovery.

ASA, American Society of Anesthesiologists; ED, emergency department.
From Miner JR, Burton JH: Clinical practice advisory: Emergency department procedural sedation with propofol. Ann Emerg Med 32:249, 2007. Epub 2007;February 5.

demonstrated that the safety profiles of these agents are the same or better than other agents in the PSA pharmacopoeia.[21] An additional dedicated clinician (separate from the individual performing the procedure) is generally considered advisable to oversee medication administration.[89]

Propofol

Pharmacology. Propofol is becoming an agent of choice for PSA in the ED because of its efficacy and safety profile (Fig. 33–2). When administered by IV bolus, the onset of action is typically within 30 seconds. The half-life for blood-brain equilibration is approximately 1 to 3 minutes, and clinical effects typically resolve within 5 to 7 minutes. Longer procedures can be facilitated by repeat dosing. Patients are typically awake and alert within 15 minutes after discontinuation. Propofol exhibits inherent antiemetic and perhaps euphoric properties, and patient satisfaction is typically high. Propofol should be avoided in patients with known or suspected allergy to eggs or soy products.[22,89–95]

Adult and Pediatric Use. Deep sedation can be reliably achieved in both adults and children using a single loading dose of propofol intravenously. Repeat bolus dosing is pre-

ferred, but an IV drip can be administered as needed to enhance or prolong sedation.[22,89–95]

Adverse Effects. Transient apnea and respiratory depression can occur with propofol but typically resolve spontaneously before intervention is necessary. Reported rates of assisted ventilation range from 0% to 4.6%.[89] Similarly, transient hypotension (by direct negative inotropy as well as arterial and venodilatation) is common but typically resolves spontaneously without treatment. Injection site pain is noted less frequently in the ED setting than in the operating room, where higher doses are typically administered.[22,89–95] Administering 2 to 3 ml of 2% lidocaine slowly into the vein prior to propofol infusion will lessen injection pain.

Propofol has been reported to cause an antimuscarinic or an atropine-like syndrome (agitation, tachycardia, confusion, hallucinations) that can be reversed with physostigmine. This syndrome may accentuated by the concomitant use of anticholinergic agents, such as meperidine and promethazine.[96] Transient movement disorders (dystonia, masseter spasm, seizure-like movements) have rarely been reported with propofol.[97]

TABLE 33–13 Procedure for Dissociative Sedation with Ketamine

Caveats

- Do not consider if you are not experienced with ketamine or if you do not have time to perform such sedation properly. Do not attempt the procedure if the pulse oximeter, suction, oxygen, or bag-mask are not working, or the room is too small or not set up for PSA.
- This is a two-person procedure, one to monitor the patient and one to perform the procedure. Both must be knowledgeable regarding the unique characteristics of ketamine.
- Ketamine is best suited for (1) short, painful procedures, especially those requiring immobilization (e.g., complex facial laceration, burn débridement, fracture reduction, abscess incision and drainage, central line placement, colonoscopy, tube thoracostomy) or (2) examinations judged likely to produce excessive emotional disturbance (e.g., pediatric sexual assault examination).

Contraindications—Absolute (Risks Essentially Always Outweigh Benefits)

- Age < 3 mo (suggestive evidence of higher risk of airway complications).
- History of airway instability, tracheal surgery, or tracheal stenosis (presumed but insufficient evidence of higher risk of airway complications).
- Known or suspected psychosis, even if currently stable or controlled with medications (supportive evidence of exacerbation potential).

Contraindications—Relative (Risks May Outweigh Benefits)

- Age 3–12 mo (higher risk of airway complications).
- Procedures involving stimulation of the posterior pharynx (moderately higher risk of laryngospasm).
- Active pulmonary infection or disease, including upper respiratory infection or asthma (moderately higher risk of laryngospasm).
- Known or suspected cardiovascular disease including angina, heart failure, or hypertension (exacerbation due to sympathomimetic properties of ketamine). Avoid ketamine in patients with ED blood pressures ≥ 140/90 mm Hg. Avoid ketamine in older adults with risk factors for coronary artery disease.
- Head injury associated with loss of consciousness, altered mental status, or emesis (elevated intracranial pressure with ketamine).
- Central nervous system masses, abnormalities, or hydrocephalus (elevated intracranial pressure with ketamine).
- Glaucoma or acute globe injury (elevated intraocular pressure with ketamine).
- Porphyria, thyroid disorder, or thyroid medication (enhanced sympathomimetic effect).

Protocol

- IV access is unnecessary in children receiving IM ketamine. IV access is desirable in adults to permit prompt treatment of unpleasant recovery reactions should they occur.
- Connect appropriate monitoring equipment to the patient.
- Pulse, respiratory rate, blood pressure, and level of consciousness should all be recorded initially, and periodically throughout the procedure depending on the depth of sedation.

- Suction equipment, oxygen, a bag-valve-mask, and reversal agents should be immediately available. An age-appropriate resuscitation cart with oral and nasal airways, endotracheal tubes, and a functioning laryngoscope must be nearby.
- Educate accompanying family regarding the unique characteristics of the dissociative state, especially if they will be present during the procedure and/or recovery.
- Adults and children of verbal age should be encouraged to "plan" specific, pleasant dream topics in advance of sedation (believed to decrease unpleasant recovery reactions).
- Option: May coadminister atropine 0.01 mg/kg (minimum, 0.1 mg; maximum, 0.5 mg) either IV just prior to ketamine, or draw up and have atropine by the bedside. For IM injection, mix with ketamine in the same syringe (hypersalivation suppression). Glycopyrrolate is an acceptable alternative at equipotent doses.
- Option: Ondansetron (0.15 mg/kg to a maximum dose of 4 mg) at the time of ketamine administration may reduce vomiting.
- Benzodiazepine coadministration is unnecessary in children to blunt emergence reactions; however, such drugs should be readily available to treat rare unpleasant recovery reactions should they occur. Midazolam may also be used to attain preprocedural anxiolysis prior to ketamine administration, especially in frightened toddlers and early-school-age children. Benzodiazepine prophylaxis should be considered in adults owing to their higher baseline risk of unpleasant reactions and to enhance cardiovascular stability. Midazolam 0.05–0.1 mg/kg (2–4 mg) slowly IV is an example of such pretreatment.
- Ketamine is not administered until the clinician is ready to begin the procedure, because onset of dissociation typically occurs within 5 min.
- Ketamine is administered as a single IM injection or IV loading dose, and there is no benefit from routine attempts to titrate to effect.
- When administered IM, give 4–5 mg/kg with atropine mixed in the same syringe. Repeat ketamine dose (full or half dose IM without additional atropine) if sedation is inadequate after 5–10 min (unusual) or if additional doses are later required.
- When administered IV, give a loading dose of 1.5 mg/kg IV over 1–2 min. 100 mg is a typical adult dose. IV administration more rapidly than over 1–2 min produces high central nervous system levels and has been associated with respiratory depression. Additional incremental doses of ketamine may be given (0.5 mg/kg) if initial sedation is inadequate, or if repeated doses are necessary to accomplish a longer procedure. Repeat doses of atropine are generally unnecessary.
- Adjunctive physical immobilization may be occasionally needed to control random motion.
- Adjunctive local anesthetic may be needed for incomplete analgesia, although this is unusual.

Route of Administration	IM	IV
Advantages	No IV access necessary Slightly faster recovery	Ease of repeat dosing
Peak concentrations and clinical onset	5 min	1 min
Typical duration of effective dissociation	15–30 min	10–15 min
Typical time from dose to discharge	60–140 min	50–110 min

Whenever possible, minimize lighting, noise, and physical contact during recovery until wakefulness is well established. Advise family to not stimulate the patient prematurely.

ED, emergency department; PSA, procedural sedation and analgesia.

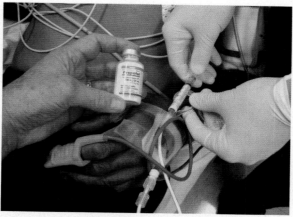

Figure 33–2 Propofol is emerging as an agent of choice for painful ED procedures. It is safe, effective, and very short acting. It can be cautiously combined with the short-acting narcotic fentanyl. All the safety caveats for PSA apply.

Etomidate

Pharmacology. When administered by IV bolus, the onset of action is typically within 30 seconds, and patients are typically awake and alert within 30 minutes after discontinuation.

Adult Use. Deep sedation can be reliably achieved using single loading doses.[98-101] Repeat dosing can be administered as needed to enhance or prolong sedation. Etomidate may be somewhat less effective overall than propofol and, given its additional adverse effect of myoclonus, appears a less desirable choice than propofol for deep sedation.[21,38]

Pediatric Use. There is significantly less published experience with etomidate in children for ED PSA; however, the safety and efficacy profiles appear similar to those in adults.[102,103]

Adverse Effects. The primary adverse effects of etomidate are respiratory depression, myoclonus, nausea, and vomiting.[97,103,104] Respiratory depression has been reported to be less with propofol PSA than with methohexital, fentanyl/midazolam, or etomidate.[105] Myoclonus is generally benign but can be disconcerting and can interfere with the procedure. It consists of transient jerking or twitching movements that can be mistaken for seizure activity. Transient adrenal suppression occurs with etomidate in septic patients but appears to lack clinical significance for single doses when used for ED PSA.[21,89,106]

Thiopental and Methohexital

Pharmacology. Because of their lipid solubility, barbiturates are rapidly absorbed rectally. When given intravenously, both thiopental and methohexital produce sedation within 1 minute. Clinical recovery is rapid (~15 min), reflecting the rapid redistribution from the central nervous system to the periphery.

Adult Use. There is limited published experience using these IV barbiturates for ED PSA,[107] and propofol or etomidate would appear a better choice.

Pediatric Use. Rectal thiopental and methohexital can reliably produce sedation suitable for CT or MRI scanning.[108-113] Respiratory depression is unusual when using typical doses (see Table 33–10) but can occur.[108,109,111-113] There is limited published experience using these IV barbiturates for ED PSA,[107] and propofol would appear a better choice.

Adverse Effects. Barbiturates cause potent respiratory depression; in one ED report, apnea occurred in 10% of the patients.[114] Barbiturates can frequently cause hypotension at typical IV doses, so their use should be avoided whenever possible in patients with volume depletion or cardiovascular compromise.

Analgesic Agents

Fentanyl

Fentanyl is the most common opioid used for PSA owing to its rapid onset, brief duration, rapid reversibility by naloxone, and lack of histamine release.[7] It is often combined with other agents, such as propofol, etomidate, and midazolam, to provide additionl effect and pain relief. Fentanyl is immediately reversed with naloxone should excessive sedation or respiratory depression occur. The longer-duration opioids, morphine and meperidine, are preferred for nonprocedural or preprocedural pain control and are frequently given initially for acute analgesia followed by fentanyl to facilitate the needed procedure. Although longer-acting opioids can be readily used for analgesia during PSA, they will be associated with longer recovery times and a higher incidence of histamine-related effects (e.g., nausea/vomiting, hypotension, pruritus). Fentanyl lacks these effects and therefore is preferred.

Pharmacology. Fentanyl is 75 to 125 times more potent than morphine and has no intrinsic anxiolytic or amnestic properties. A single dose given intravenously has rapid onset (<30 sec), with a peak at 2 to 3 minutes and brief clinical duration (20–40 min). This increase in potency and onset of action is in part related to its greater lipid solubility, which facilitates its passage across the blood-brain barrier. The effects of fentanyl can be rapidly and completely reversed with opioid antagonists (e.g., naloxone, nalmefene).

Adult Use. Because of its pharmacokinetics, IV fentanyl is an ideal agent when analgesia is required for painful procedures; it can be easily and rapidly titrated.[7] As anxiolysis and sedation do not occur at low doses (1–2 μg/kg), the concurrent administration of a pure sedative, most commonly midazolam, is advisable, especially in children (see Table 33–11).

Pediatric Use. The combination of fentanyl and midazolam remains a popular PSA sedation regimen in children, with a strong safety and efficacy profile when both drugs are carefully titrated to effect.[6,84,115,116] Any necessary level of mild to deep sedation can be achieved using these agents.

Fentanyl is also available in an oral transmucosal preparation. Although this novel and noninvasive delivery route obviates the need for IV access, titration is difficult and efficacy is variable.[117] Furthermore, the incidence of emesis is high (31%–45%),[117,118] and consequently, this formulation has never become popular for PSA.

Adverse Effects. Like all opioids, fentanyl can cause respiratory depression.[6,7,84,115,116] When used for PSA, standard interactive and mechanical monitoring is required. Because the opioid effect is most pronounced on the central nervous system respiratory centers, apnea precedes loss of consciousness. If apnea should occur, verbal or tactile stimulation should be attempted prior to administration of opioid antagonists. As discussed earlier, *caution must be exercised when using benzodiazepines and other PSA agents and opioids together, because the risks of hypoxia and apnea are significantly greater than when either is used alone.*[5,67]

In the absence of significant ethanol intoxication, hypovolemia, or concomitant drug ingestion, hypotension is rare, even with very large doses of fentanyl (doses of 50 µg/kg are common in adult and pediatric cardiac surgery). Because of its safe hemodynamic profile, fentanyl is an ideal analgesic agent for use in critically ill or injured patients. In addition, nausea and vomiting are rare compared with analgesia with morphine or meperidine. A commonly observed reaction to fentanyl is nasal pruritus, and patients frequently attempt to scratch their noses during the procedure.[7]

A rare side effect of fentanyl with potential for respiratory compromise is chest wall rigidity. This complication has not been problematic in the ED and is related to higher doses (>5 µg/kg as a bolus dose) than those used for PSA and has not been reported in any ED series.[6,7,115,116] If it should occur, chest wall rigidity usually can be reversed with opioid antagonists and/or positive-pressure ventilation. Equipment for urgent pharmacologic paralysis should be available if reversal and positive-pressure ventilation are unsuccessful.

Diamorphine

Diamorphine is a nasal opioid that is currently available in the United Kingdom, Australia, New Zealand, and Canada but not the United States.[50,51,119] Diamorphine has an onset and duration of action similar to that of morphine; however, its higher water solubility permits potent doses to be delivered in the small (0.1 mL) volumes necessary for comfortable intranasal administration. In two studies of children and teenagers with fractures, intranasal diamorphine 0.1 mg/kg provided a similar level of analgesia with faster onset than IM morphine 0.2 mg/kg. Intranasal spray administration was better tolerated than the injection, and there were no adverse events.[50,51,119] Diamorphine may prove to be a useful initial analgesic for children and teenagers with acute pain, although, practically, an IV line would most likely be established to permit titration to full pain relief and PSA for any needed procedures (e.g., fracture reduction). The role for diamorphine in adults remains to be determined.

Other Short-Acting Opioids

Sufentanil, alfentanil, and remifentanil are other short-acting opioids that have a potential role in PSA. Currently, however, there is insufficient published experience to warrant their routine use. Although intranasal sufentanil 0.75 µg/kg appeared promising in one small pediatric trial,[120] in another, doses of 1.5 µg/kg resulted in oxygen desaturation in 8 of 10 children studied.[80] This low toxic-therapeutic ratio and inability to titrate would appear to limit the utility of intranasal sufentanil. In the one published report of IV remifentanil with midazolam for PSA, there was an unacceptably high incidence of hypoxemia.[121] Currently, there does not appear to be a clinically important advantage to these drugs compared with fentanyl.

Ketamine

Pharmacology. Ketamine produces a unique state of cortical dissociation that permits painful procedures to be performed more consistently and effectively than with other PSA agents. This state of "dissociative sedation" is characterized by profound analgesia, sedation, amnesia, and immobilization (Fig. 33–3) and can be rapidly and reliably produced

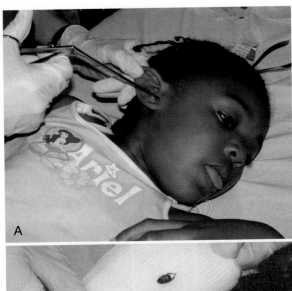
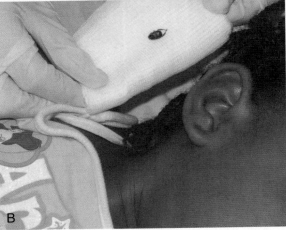

Figure 33–3 *A*, A child undergoing insect removal from the ear under ketamine. No child, or adult, can cooperate for this painful procedure, and general anesthesia is often the other option to ketamine. The blank stare is common. *B*, Insect successfully, and atraumatically, removed.

with IV or IM administration.[17] Ketamine has been widely used worldwide since its introduction in 1970 and has demonstrated a remarkable safety profile in a variety of settings.[4,6,122–124] In 1999, the JCAHO confirmed that ED ketamine administration is fully compliant with its standards when administered according to protocol.[125] Clinicians administering ketamine must be especially knowledgeable about the unique actions of this drug and the numerous contraindications to its use (see Table 33–10).

Ketamine differs from other PSA agents in several important ways. First, it uniquely preserves cardiopulmonary stability. Upper airway muscular tone and protective airway reflexes are maintained. Spontaneous respiration is preserved, although when administered intravenously, ketamine must be given slowly (over 1–2 min) to prevent respiratory depression. Second, it differs from other agents in that it lacks the characteristic dose-response continuum to progressive titration. At doses below a certain threshold, ketamine produces analgesia and sedation. However, once a critical dosage threshold (~1–1.5 mg/kg intravenously or 3–4 mg/kg intramuscularly) is achieved, the characteristic dissociative state abruptly appears. This dissociation has no observable levels of depth, and thus, the only value of ketamine "titration" is to maintain the presence of the state over time. Finally, the dissociative state is not consistent with formal definitions of moderate sedation, deep sedation, or general anesthesia (see Table 33–1) and, therefore, must be considered from a different perspective than agents that exhibit the classical sedation continuum.[14,17]

Ketamine is most effective and reliable when given intravenously or intramuscularly. Ketamine has a one arm-brain circulation time when given intravenously, with onset of dissociation noted within 1 minute and effective procedural conditions lasting for about 10 to 15 minutes. When given intramuscularly, the same effect is achieved within 5 minutes, with effective procedural conditions for about 15 to 30 minutes. The typical duration from dosing until dischargeable recovery is 50 to 110 minutes when given intravenously, and 60 to 140 minutes when given intramuscularly.[122,126]

Like the benzodiazepines, ketamine undergoes substantial first-pass hepatic metabolism. As a result, oral and rectal administration results in less predictable effectiveness and requires substantially higher doses. Clinical onset and recovery are substantially longer than when given parenterally, and thus, these routes are rarely used in the ED.[83,127]

Ketamine can induce salivation and to combat this, some have coadministered an anticholinergic. Atropine is most commonly chosen in emergency medicine owing to its ready familiarity to clinicians and nurses, although glycopyrrolate is an equally acceptable but not superior alternative (see Table 33–13). The clinical effects of salivation are usually inconsequential, and many clinicians forgo the routine coadministration of atropine or glycopyrrolate.

Adult Use. Ketamine is widely and successfully used in adults throughout the developing world for both minor and major surgery, particularly in areas lacking resources for inhalational anesthesia.[122,123,128,129] Hallucinatory so-called emergence reactions have been reported in up to 30% of adults receiving ketamine (although rare in children) and can be fascinating and pleasurable or, alternatively, unpleasant and nightmarish.[122] Concurrent benzodiazepines are believed to blunt but not entirely eliminate such reactions in adults,[122,123,128,129] and apprehension regarding such unpleasant recoveries has limited the popularity of ketamine administration in the developed world for adults.

One study reported success administering dissociative doses (2 mg/kg intravenously) of ketamine with concurrent midazolam (0.07 mg/kg intravenously) to 77 ED adults to facilitate painful procedures (e.g., abscess incision and drainage, fracture reduction). There were no moderate or severe emergence reactions, and only 5 patients experienced mild reactions.[130] Furthermore, there appears to be no reason to avoid standard dissociative doses when ketamine is administered to adults. In a 1996 study using subdissociative doses (0.2 mg/kg intravenously) for the goal of bronchodilation in the treatment of acute asthma, three of six adults suffered dysphoric reactions.[131]

Ketamine presents potential risks to patients with coronary artery disease, because it is sympathomimetic and produces mild to moderate increases in blood pressure, heart rate, and myocardial oxygen consumption. The actual risk remains unclear owing to limited experience in adults with known coronary artery disease.[128]

Given the available data, it would appear appropriate for emergency clinicians to carefully transpose their experience with ketamine into selected adult situations. Careful patient selection can help minimize potential adverse events (see Table 33–13).[128,130]

Pediatric Use. Ketamine is an ideal agent to facilitate short, painful procedures in children. The safety and efficacy of ketamine for this indication have been widely documented.[4,6,122,126] The IM route is simple and effective. Venous access is unnecessary, and atropine can be concurrently administered in the same syringe.[4] IV administration is attractive because a lower cumulative dose can be used and recovery is faster than with the IM route. The primary caution is that with this route, ketamine must be administered slowly (each dose over 1–2 min) or respiratory depression and transient apnea can occur.[126]

Unpleasant recovery reactions are uncommon in children and teenagers and are typically mild when they do occur.[132,133] There is no evidence of any benefit from the prophylactic administration of concurrent benzodiazepines in children,[132,133] and their role should be confined to treating preprocedural anxiety or unpleasant reactions if they should occur.

Adverse Effects. In the largest published ED series (1022 patients), the following adverse airway events were noted: airway malalignment (0.7%), transient laryngospasm (0.4%), and transient apnea or respiratory depression (0.3%). All were quickly identified and treated, and there were no sequelae.[4]

Vomiting was noted in 6.7% from the same series, and in most cases, it occurred well into recovery.[4] The incidence was age-related, occurring in 12.1% of children aged 5 years or older, and 3.5% in those younger than 5 years.[124] There was no evidence of aspiration[4]; indeed, in 30 years of regular use, there have been no documented reports of clinically significant ketamine-associated aspiration in patients without established contraindications. Delayed vomiting may occur after discharge, and patients should be advised of this possibility. Because of its unique preservation of protective airway reflexes, ketamine may be preferred over other agents for urgent or emergent procedures when fasting is not ensured.[4,5,122] Vomiting may be associated with higher doses (a cumulative dose of ketamine over 7 mg/kg), and may be reduced by concomitant benzodiazepine administration. Ondansetron prophylaxis (0.15 mg/kg up to a maximum of 4 mg IV) at the time of ketamine administration has been demonstrated to significantly reduce vomiting in children undergoing procedural sedation with ketamine in the ED.[134]

Mild agitation (whimpering or crying) during recovery was noted in 17.6% of children from the same series, with more pronounced agitation in 1.6%. The incidence was age-related, with agitation occurring in 12.1% of children aged 5 or older, and 22.5% in those younger than 5.[124] Only 2 of 1022 children had reactions that treating clinicians judged severe enough to require treatment, and both children responded promptly to small doses of midazolam.[4] Another study quantified the degree of recovery agitation using a 0- to 100-mm visual analog scale; the median rating of recovery agitation was a 5, likely below the threshold of clinical importance.[132]

The prophylactic use of benzodiazepine to lessen this reaction is often suggested, but the actual benefit is uncertain and individual practice varies. Severe emergence reactions are rare and may be ameliorated by keeping the patient in a quiet and undisturbed environment during recovery.

Ketamine-Propofol Combination (Ketofol) for PSA in the ED

The combination of ketamine and propofol ("Ketofol") for PSA, especially in children, has recently been studied, with promising results.[135] This combination has been used in anesthesiology for some time, but only recently has been studied in the ED. The drugs are combined for synergic effect, and to reduce any potential adverse effects of either drug used alone. The actual benefit and safety of this combination in the ED is still undergoing clarification at the time of this publication, but it appears safe and effective in initial reports. Careful observation for respiratory depression is required, and the precautions listed for both agents should be stringently observed.

The ketamine/propofol combination is touted to produce less total sedation, faster recovery, and fewer side effects than either medication used alone. When used in combination for procedural sedation, the initial IV doses of ketamine and propofol are approximately half of the doses of the drugs used individually. As a general conservative guideline, the initial suggested regimen is combining 0.5 mg/kg of ketamine and 0.5 mg/kg of propofol, with an additional 0.25–0.5 mg/kg of propofol, titrated every 2–3 minutes for effect. Some also use additional ketamine (0.25–0.5 mg/kg) with the subsequent propofol dose.

The regimen by Sharieff et al[136] consists of IV ketamine (0.5 mg/kg) followed by IV propofol (1 mg/kg) one minute later as the initial infusion. A second dose of ketamine (0.25 mg/kg) and/or propofol (0.5 mg/kg) can be used for supplementation of PSA if required.

The regimen by Willman et al[137] consists of a 1:1 mixture of propofol (10 mg/ml) and ketamine (10 mg/ml: *note concentration*) given IV in 1 to 3 ml aliquots at the discretion of the clinician. This protocol required a mean dose of 0.75 mg/kg of both ketamine and propofol.

Nitrous Oxide

Pharmacology. Inhaled nitrous oxide provides anxiolysis and mild analgesia. It is commonly dispensed at concentrations between 30% and 50%, with oxygen composing the remainder of the mixture. Nitrous oxide quickly diffuses across biologic membranes and accordingly has a rapid onset of action (30–60 sec). Maximum effect occurs after about 5 minutes, and the clinical effect wears off quickly upon discontinuation. At typical PSA concentrations, there is preservation of hemodynamic status, spontaneous respirations, and protective airway reflexes.[138-141] Nitrous oxide is widely used in dentistry at higher concentrations.[142]

Nitrous oxide has an excellent safety profile; however, as a sole agent, it cannot reliably produce adequate procedural conditions.[138-141] Given its relatively weak analgesic properties, in many cases, nitrous oxide needs to be supplemented with an IV opioid and/or local or regional anesthesia.

Adult and Cooperative Child Use. The safest method of nitrous oxide administration is via a self-administered demand-valve mask (Fig. 33–4).[139-141] Patients must generate a negative pressure of 3 to 5 cm H_2O within the handheld mask or mouthpiece to activate the flow of gas. They can thus self-titrate themselves by inhaling at will through the mask. Naturally, this will be effective only when the patient is cooperative. This technique provides a built-in fail-safe in that if

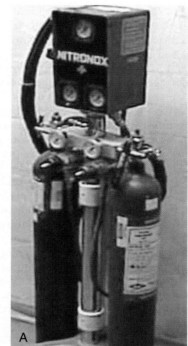

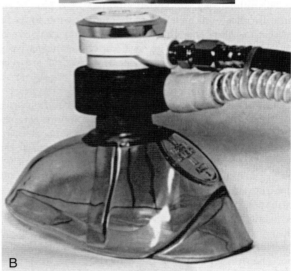

Figure 33–4 *A,* A demand-flow nitrous oxide/oxygen system. *B,* Example of a free mask for a nitrous oxide system. The patient must hold the mask in contact with the face. (*A, Courtesy of Nitronox delivery system by Matrx Medical, division of Henry Schein. matrx2@aol.com*)

patients become somnolent, the masks will fall from their faces and gas delivery will cease.

Nitrous oxide can be used as an adjunctive anxiolytic during mildly painful procedures or during local or regional anesthesia administration for other procedures. It may also be administered during difficult or high-anxiety procedures such as pelvic examinations or during attempts at difficult IV access.

A double-tank system is commonly used to deliver the nitrous oxide and oxygen mixture. The system relies on a mixing valve preset to deliver a fixed ratio and will deliver gas only when oxygen is flowing. The double-tank system contains a fail-safe device that automatically stops the flow of nitrous oxide when the oxygen supply is depleted.

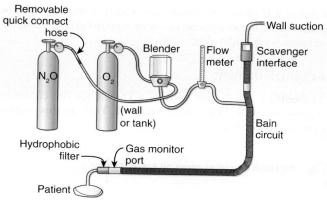

Figure 33–5 Nitrous oxide/oxygen continuous-flow system.

Uncooperative Child Use. The primary limitation of self-administration is that it is ineffective in uncooperative patients, including most frightened young children. Continuous-flow nitrous oxide has been used in this population via a mask strapped over the nose or over the nose and mouth (Fig. 33–5).[143–146] Nitrous oxide can effectively produce moderate or deep sedation when administered in this manner; however, this technique necessitates an additional clinician dedicated to continuous gas titration to avoid oversedation. In addition, it appears that the continuous-flow technique is associated with a higher rate of emesis (10%)[143–146] than self-administration (0%–4%),[138–141] which may be a potential hazard if a mask is strapped tightly over the child's mouth.[144]

Adverse Effects and Precautions. A number of generally minor adverse effects may be seen, including nausea, dizziness, voice change, euphoria, and laughter.[138–141] Nitrous oxide should be avoided in closed-space disease such as bowel obstruction, middle ear disease, pneumothorax, or pneumocephaly. Because of its property of high diffusibility, it has potential to increase the size of the closed space. This should be unlikely for short-term use in typical PSA concentrations.

A scavenging system must be in place to collect exhaled nitrous oxide, and care must be taken to ensure compliance with occupational safety regulations. Care should also be taken to avoid nitrous oxide exposure in pregnant ED staff members because nitrous oxide is a known teratogen and mutagen.

Although the potential for abuse by ED staff exists, such abuse should be rare if simple steps are taken. As with other agents, a strict protocol of accountability should be in place. A simple locking device can be added to the cylinders of gas. In addition, the delivery valve or mouthpiece may be locked in the same location as controlled substances.

Other PSA Agents

Historically, a popular PSA cocktail was the IM combination meperidine, promethazine, and chlorpromazine (DPT, Dem compound). However, this regimen cannot be titrated, is frequently ineffective, and is associated with prolonged recovery times.[147,148] Its use can no longer be recommended.

Antagonists

Reversal agents should not be routinely administered after administration of opioids or benzodiazepines for PSA, but rather should be reserved for rare situations of oversedation or significant respiratory depression. The downside of reversal agents is that one must wait for the antagonist to dissipate before one can analyze residual PSA agent effect, with the caveat that long-acting PSA agents may last longer than the administered antagonist. Serious resedation after antagonism is usually not an issue with fentanyl or midazolam, but caution is advised, especially when large doses of PSA agents, and large doses of antagonists, have been used. Obviously, the length of observation varies with the dose of antagonist that has been administered.

Naloxone

Naloxone is an antagonist that competitively displaces opioids from opiate receptors. It rapidly reverses the analgesic and respiratory depressant effects of opioids. It may be administered intravenously, intramuscularly, subcutaneously, or even sublingually if needed,[149] and dosing has been standardized for infants and children.[150] Naloxone will not induce systemic opioid withdrawal symptoms in a patient without preexisting physiologic dependence. However, some patients will experience nausea with opioid reversal, and those patients with persistent pain after their procedure will be quite uncomfortable. Rapid reversal also may lead to return of anxiety and sympathetic stimulation. If the situation permits, careful titration of small amounts of naloxone (0.1 mg aliquots intravenously) may permit partial rather than complete reversal. The only absolute contraindication to the use of naloxone is administration to a neonate born to an opioid-dependent mother owing to the risk of precipitating life-threatening opioid withdrawal. Length of observation is dose-related, but usually no more than 60 to 90 minutes postreversal will be sufficient if no more than 1 mg IV naloxone has been administered.

Nalmefene

Nalmefene is a long-acting opioid antagonist with a duration of action significantly longer than naloxone.[151] Nalmefene may be given intravenously, intramuscularly, or subcutaneously, although IV is the preferred route.[151,152] Intravenously, it can be titrated in incremental doses of 0.25 µg/kg every 2 to 5 minutes until the desired effect is attained. Although either naloxone or nalmefene will reverse analgesia due to opioids, naloxone is the preferred agent. For ED PSA, short-acting opioids such as fentanyl are commonly used and administration of a reversal agent with a duration of action as prolonged as that of nalmefene does not confer any additional benefit. Furthermore, nalmefene would interfere with postprocedure opioid pain control.

Flumazenil

Flumazenil is a benzodiazepine antagonist that can promptly reverse benzodiazepine-induced sedation and respiratory depression.[1,14,153,154] In the setting of PSA, flumazenil is a safe and effective method of reversing oversedation caused by benzodiazepines. It is not routinely used to reverse PSA because of the potential for resedation, and many clinicians prefer to allow patients to recover on their own. Flumazenil has not been shown to substantially decrease the time of observation in the ED required of a patient undergoing PSA. Flumazenil lowers the seizure threshold and may rarely lead to life-threatening seizures. It should be avoided in settings of known benzodiazepine dependence, seizure disorder, cyclic antidepressant overdose, and elevated intracranial pressure.[151]

HEALING BY FIRST INTENTION

HEALING BY SECOND INTENTION

FIGURE 34–1 Steps in wound healing by first intention (*left*) and second intention (*right*). Note large amounts of granulation tissue and wound contraction in healing by second intention.

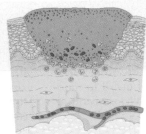
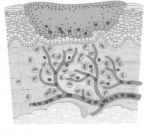

— Scab

24 hours

— Neutrophils
— Clot

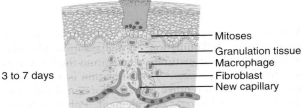
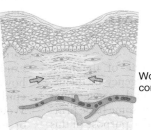

3 to 7 days

— Mitoses
— Granulation tissue
— Macrophage
— Fibroblast
— New capillary

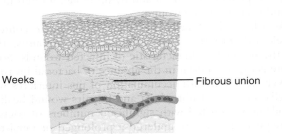

Weeks

— Fibrous union

Wound contraction

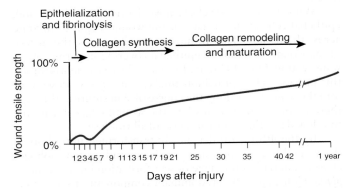

FIGURE 34–2 Graphic representation of the various phases of wound healing. Note that the tensile strength of scar tissue never reaches that of unwounded skin. Displayed values of tensile strength are approximate and demonstrate the general concept of wound healing.

Decisions regarding the optimal time for suture removal and the need for continued support of the wound with tape are influenced by (1) wound tensile strength, (2) the period of scar widening, and (3) the cosmetically unacceptable effect of epithelialization along suture tracks. Scars are quite red and noticeable at 3 to 8 weeks after closure. However, the appearance of a scar should not be judged before the scar is well into its remodeling phase. The cosmetic appearance of wounds 6 to 9 months after injury cannot be predicted at the time of suture removal.[8] Therefore, any scar revision should be postponed until 6 to 12 months after injury.

One of the most important factors in predicting the cosmetic result of a wound is its location.[9] In general, wounds on concave surfaces heal with better cosmetic results than wounds on convex surfaces. Other factors that affect cosmesis include wound size, wound depth, and skin color.[10] Small, superficial wounds in lax, light-colored skin, especially in areas in which the skin is thin, result in less noticeable scars. Wounds on convex surfaces look better after primary closure than after secondary healing. Static and dynamic forces, and the propensity toward keloid formation, may influence the long-term cosmetic appearance of wounds more than the surgical skills of the clinician who repaired the wound.[8] Repigmentation occurs over 3 to 5 years, even in large wounds that heal by secondary intention.[10]

INITIAL EVALUATION

The approach to the management of a particular wound, and the decision to close a wound immediately or after a period of observation, is based primarily on factors that affect the risk of infection. History and physical examination should be directed toward identifying those factors. Some wounds may appear benign but conceal extensive and devastating underlying tissue damage. The discovery that an extremity wound was produced by a roller or wringer device, a high-pressure injection gun, high-voltage electricity, heavy and prolonged compressive forces, or the bite of a human or a potentially rabid animal radically alters the overall management of the affected patient. The American College of Emergency Physicians' "Clinical Policy for the Initial Approach to Patients

Presenting with Penetrating Extremity Trauma" provides a useful approach to the evaluation of all wounds.[11]

History

In the initial evaluation of a wound, the clinician should identify all the extrinsic and intrinsic factors that jeopardize healing and promote infection. These include the mechanism of injury, the time of injury, the environment in which the wound occurred, and the patient's immune status.

Wound Age

In general, the likelihood of wound infection increases with time to definitive wound care.[12] A delay in wound cleaning is the most important factor and may allow bacteria contaminating the wound to proliferate. A delay of only a few hours in treatment of a heavily contaminated wound can result in infection. In contrast, some evidence suggests that wounds in highly vascular regions such as the face and scalp can be closed without increased risk as long as 24 hours after injury.[13] Contrary to popular belief, the "golden period"—the maximum time after injury that a wound may be safely closed without significant risk of infection—is not a fixed number of hours.[14]

Many factors affect infection risk, and closure decisions should not be based solely on temporal considerations. All data accumulated in the initial evaluation, both historical and physical, must be considered when making the decision to close a wound in a particular patient.[12] In addition, the techniques of wound care in and of themselves may extend the golden period; with skillful cleaning and débridement, a clinician can sometimes convert a contaminated wound into a clean wound that can be safely closed.[5]

Other Historical Factors

Other factors that affect wound healing or the risk of infection include the patient's age and state of health. Patient age appears to be an important factor in host resistance to infection; those individuals at the extremes of age—young children and the elderly—are at greatest risk.[12,15] Infection rates are reported to be higher in patients with medical illnesses (e.g., diabetes mellitus, immunologic deficiencies, malnutrition, anemia, uremia, congestive heart failure, cirrhosis, malignancy, alcoholism, arteriosclerosis, arteritis, collagen vascular disease, chronic granulomatous disease, smoking or chronic hypoxia, renal and liver failure), in obese patients, and in those taking steroids or immunosuppressive drugs or receiving radiation therapy. Shock, remote trauma, distant infection, bacteremia, retained foreign bodies, denervation, and peripheral vascular disease also increase wound infection rates and slow the healing process.[6,12,15–17]

In most instances, the clinician cannot totally negate infection risks, but can favorably affect the rate and extent of infection with adequate wound care. Unfortunately, simply prescribing antibiotics in the hope that infection will somehow be averted is an unrealistic expectation.

Additional information pertinent to decision making in wound management includes:

- *Current medications* (specifically, anticoagulants and immunosuppressive drugs).
- *Allergies* (especially to local anesthetics, antiseptics, analgesics, antibiotics, and tape).
- *Tetanus immunization status.*

- *Potential exposure to rabies* (in bite wounds and mucosal exposures).
- *Potential for foreign bodies* embedded in the wound, especially when the mechanism of injury is unknown or was associated with breaking glass or vegetative matter.[18]
- *Previous injuries and deformities* (especially in extremity and facial injuries).
- *Associated injuries* (underlying fracture, joint penetration).
- *Other factors* (availability for follow-up, patient understanding of wound care or compliance).

Physical Examination

All wounds should be examined for amount of tissue destruction, degree of contamination, and damage to underlying structures. The examiner should wear clean or sterile gloves and avoid droplet contamination from the mouth. Wounds should be examined under good lighting and after bleeding is controlled. It may be necessary to create a bloodless field with the use of tourniquets. Distal perfusion and motor and sensory function should be assessed and documented during the evaluation of extremity wounds and before the use of anesthetics.

Mechanism of Injury and Classification of Wounds

The magnitude and direction of the injuring force and the volume of tissue on which the force is dissipated determine the type of wound sustained. Three types of mechanical forces—shear, tension, and compression—produce soft tissue injury. The resulting disruption or loss of tissue determines the configuration of the wound. Wounds may be classified into six categories:

1. *Abrasions.* Wounds caused by forces applied in opposite directions, resulting in the loss of epidermis and possibly dermis (e.g., skin grinding against road surface).
2. *Lacerations.* Wounds caused by shear forces that produce a tear in tissues. Little energy is required to produce a wound by shear forces (e.g., a knife cut). Consequently, little tissue damage occurs at the wound edge, the margins are sharp, and the wound appears "tidy." Tensile and compressive forces also cause separation of tissue. The energy required to disrupt tissue by tensile or compressive forces (e.g., forehead hitting a dashboard) is considerably greater than that required for tissue disruption by shear forces, because the energy is distributed over a larger volume. These lacerations have jagged, contused, "untidy" edges; consequently, they have a higher risk of infection.[15]
3. *Crush wounds.* Wounds caused by the impact of an object against tissue, particularly over a bony surface, which compresses the tissue. These wounds may contain contused or partially devitalized tissue.
4. *Puncture wounds.* Wounds with a small opening and whose depth cannot be entirely visualized. Puncture wounds are caused by a combination of forces.
5. *Avulsions.* Wounds in which a portion of tissue is completely separated from its base and is either lost or left with a narrow base of attachment (a flap). Shear and tensile forces cause avulsions.[19]
6. *Combination wounds.* Wounds with a combination of configurations. For example, stellate lacerations caused by compression of soft tissue against underlying bone create wounds with elements of crush and tissue separation; missile wounds involve a combination of shear, tensile, and

compressive forces that puncture, crush, and sometimes   débridement of compound fractures, neurorrhaphy, vascular

TABLE 34–1 Summary of Agents Used for Wound Care

Agent	Biologic Activity	Tissue Toxicity*	Systemic Toxicity*	Potential Uses	Comments
Povidone-iodine surgical scrub (Betadine 7.5%)	Virucidal; strongly bactericidal against gram-positive and gram-negative organisms	Detergent can be toxic to wound tissues	Painful to open wounds; other reactions extremely rare	Hand cleanser	Iodine allergy possible; systemic absorption of iodine from burns, open wounds; not routinely used in open wounds
Povidone-iodine solution (Betadine 10%)	Same as povidone-iodine scrub; virucidal, bactericidal	Minimally toxic to wound tissues at full strength; 1% solution has no significant tissue toxicity	Extremely rare	Wound periphery cleanser; diluted to 1% for wound irrigation	Probably the safest and most effective product currently available; iodine is the active agent, povidone is the carrier molecule; iodine allergy possible; systemic absorption of iodine from burns, open wounds; dilute 10:1 (saline:Betadine) if used to irrigate wounds
Chlorhexidine gluconate (Hibiclens)	Strongly bactericidal against gram-positive organisms, less strong against gram-negative bacteria	Ionic detergent can be toxic to tissue/cellular components; eye and inner ear toxicity	Extremely rare	Hand cleanser	Generally avoid use in open wounds; not for use in eye/ear
Polaxamer 188 (Shur-Clens; Pluronic F–68)	No antibacterial or antiviral activity	None known; does not inhibit wound healing	None known	Wound cleanser (particularly useful on face)	Nonionic detergent used for its cleansing properties; nontoxic even with intravenous use; will not damage eye/cornea; lack of antibacterial properties limits use
Hexachlorophene (pHisoHex)	Bacteriostatic against gram-positive bacteria, poor activity against gram-negative bacteria	Detergent can be toxic to wound tissues	Possibly teratogenic with repeated use	Alternative hand cleanser; not used on open wounds	Systemic absorption causes neurotoxicity
Hydrogen peroxide	Very weak antibacterial agent	Toxic to tissue/red cells	Extremely rare	Wound cleanser adjunct; very weak antiseptic properties	Breaks down to water and oxygen; foaming activity useful to remove debris/coagulated blood

*Based largely on in vitro studies/animal data. The true harm (or benefit) of these products for routine ED use is theoretical and likely of minimal clinical consequence for most wounds.

tion; there is no standard volume per length of wound. Irrigation should continue until all visible, loose particulate matter has been removed. A potential complication of wound irrigation is that infectious material can be splashed into the face of the clinician, even when the tip of the irrigation device is held below the wound surface. A plastic cup device that fits on the end of a syringe (ZeroWet Splashield, Zerowet, Inc., Palos Verdes Peninsula, CA) can be used to contain the splatter (Fig. 34–4). The wound should be positioned to allow continuous drainage of fluid during irrigation by any method. Warmed irrigant solutions are comfortable for patients, even after the wound is anesthetized.[43]

In the event that a commercially prepared device is unavailable, a simple method to reduce splatter is to pierce the base of a small medicine cup with a large-bore needle. The cup can be placed upside down to cover the area to be irrigated and the syringe with the 19-gauge needle can be inserted through the base (Fig. 34–5).

Antibiotic Solutions for Irrigation
A variety of antibiotic solutions have been instilled directly into wounds or used as irrigation solutions, including ampicillin, a neomycin-bacitracin-polymyxin combination; tetracycline; penicillin; kanamycin; and cephalothin. Although there

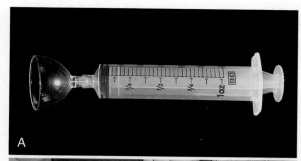

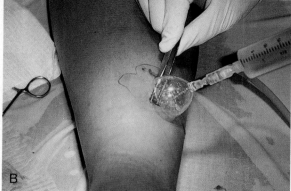

FIGURE 34–4 *A,* ZeroWet Splashield attached to end of a syringe. This irrigating device shield is held near or against the skin, and the tip of the syringe directs the irrigating solution via a high-pressure laminar flow nozzle. No needle is required. *B,* This protective shield allows forceful irrigation without splatter of infectious fluids. Note that the clinician is *holding the laceration open with forceps to allow irrigation of the deep structures.* The margins of this small puncture-like laceration were extended to allow for better irrigation (see also Fig. 34–25*C*).

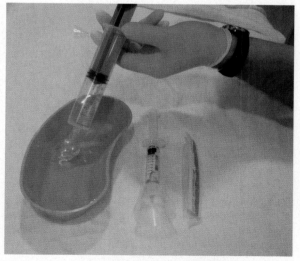

FIGURE 34–5 Fill the irrigating syringe by drawing irrigating fluid through the splash protector. Also, a makeshift splash protector is a syringe passed through a hole in a medicine cup. A plastic intravenous catheter may be attached to the irrigating syringe.

have been no reports of topical sensitization or toxic tissue levels of the antibiotic, studies have found inconsistent effectiveness in reducing infection rates.[44–47] The indications for antibiotic solutions in cleaning wounds have not been defined, and this practice is not considered standard.

Recommendations for Cleaning the Wound

The prerequisites of any wound cleaning technique are a calm or sedated patient, satisfactory anesthesia, and a thorough cleaning of the skin surface adjacent to the wound. The primary goal of wound cleaning is to rid the wound of major contaminants and infective doses of bacteria. Two strategies are recommended. The contaminated or "dirty" wound can be irrigated, or both scrubbed and irrigated, with a 1% povidone-iodine solution (Betadine preparation, not Betadine scrub). This should be followed by flushing with a 0.9% saline solution. As an alternative, the wound can be scrubbed with pluronic polyols and irrigated with a normal saline solution. Only pluronic polyols or saline should be used near the eyes. Scrubbing should be performed with a soft, fine-pore sponge, and high-pressure techniques should be used for all irrigation. The use of hydrogen peroxide on open wounds is discouraged. Either gentle scrubbing with poloxamer and normal saline high-pressure irrigation or irrigation alone appears to be a satisfactory method for cleaning minimally contaminated wounds.

A sterile bottle of saline solution is often used to irrigate the wounds of multiple patients until the bottle is empty. However, once the bottle is opened, bacterial contamination occurs quite rapidly.[48] Only solutions in bottles opened within the past 24 hours should be used to irrigate wounds.[48,49] Patients frequently irrigate their wounds with tap water before presentation. Many clinicians routinely irrigate wounds, especially extremity wounds, with tap water instead of sterile saline, with infection rates that are comparable with that of saline irrigation[50–53] (Fig. 34–6). The advantage of using tap water is that large volumes of irrigant can be quickly applied to an open wound. The disadvantages of this technique are that irrigation pressures are difficult to control, and the patient may faint if allowed to stand at a sink. If tap water is used to irrigate nonextremity wounds, it can also be delivered through a syringe at the bedside.

Preparation for Wound Closure

Before débridement or wound closure, the wound must be prepared and draped. Body hair should generally be left intact, because preoperative wounds that were shaved demonstrated higher infection rates.[16,54–56] For wounds in hair-bearing areas, hair can be removed by clipping if it interferes with the procedure.[55] Stubborn hairs that repeatedly invade the wound during suturing can be coated with petrolatum jelly or water-soluble ointments to keep them out of the field. Eyebrows should not be shaved, because critical landmarks needed for exact approximation would be lost. Although shaved eyebrows will grow back eventually, shaving produces an undesirable cosmetic effect.

The skin surface adjacent to the wound (not the wound itself) can be disinfected with a standard 10% povidone-iodine or chlorhexidine gluconate (Hibiclens) solution. The solution is painted widely on the skin surrounding the wound but should not seep into the interior of the wound itself.

After hand washing, the clinician and any assistants involved in the procedure must wear sterile or clean gloves.[57] *Sterile gloves are not required, and their use does not decrease infection rates.* Face masks are recommended, especially for any clinician with a bacterial upper respiratory infection. Because droplets of saliva may leak even from around the edges of a face mask, talking in proximity to the wound should be

569

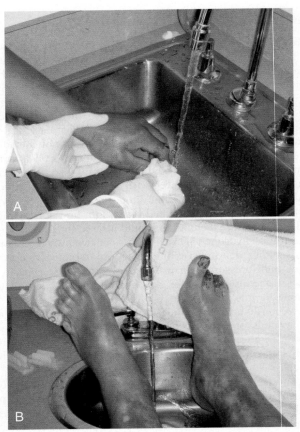

FIGURE 34–6 *A,* Tap water and nonsterile gloves are commonly used to copiously irrigate wounds of the extremities, taking advantage of volume and force parameters from the faucet. The laceration has been anesthetized before cleaning. Be mindful of the potential for the patient to faint. *B,* For foot wounds, the patient is placed on a stretcher and wheeled to the sink.

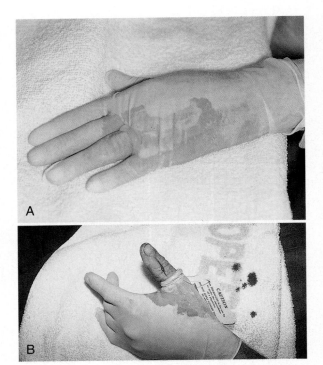

FIGURE 34–7 *A* and *B,* A nonsterile clean glove on the hand with the finger cut out, instead of an annoying drape, and a finger tourniquet to provide a bloodless field make examination and suturing of a wound easier. Prior to suturing the hand is placed on a clean towel.

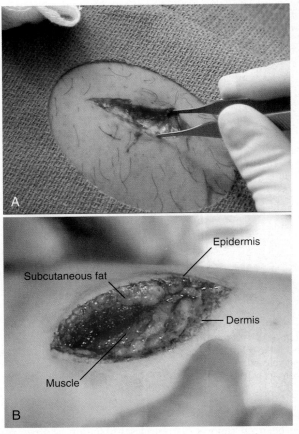

FIGURE 34–8 *A,* The depths of the wound are examined for injured structures, foreign bodies, and extent of injury. *B,* Anatomy of a deep laceration. *(A and B, From Thomsen T, Setnik G [eds]: Procedures Consult—Emergency Medicine Module. Copyright 2008 Elsevier Inc. All rights reserved.)*

avoided.[58] A single fenestrated drape or multiple folded drapes are placed over the wound site. A sterile glove may be used to provide a sterile field for a hand wound in lieu of a fenestrated drape (Fig. 34–7). The area to be sutured can be exposed by cutting the glove, and the extremity can be placed on a sterile towel. This technique provides a clean field without the need to continually adjust the drape or to operate through a small opening.

The entire depth and the full extent of every wound should be explored in an attempt to locate hidden foreign bodies, particulate matter, bone fragments, and any injuries to underlying structures that may require repair (Fig. 34–8). The clinician should avoid the temptation to initially explore wounds with a finger in search of a foreign body or to assess wound characteristics (Fig. 34–9). Embedded glass, metal fragments, or sharp pieces of bone may cut the clinician and cause a significant exposure to blood-borne infections. Direct visualization with good lighting in a bloodless field, exploration with a metal probe, and the use of radiographs are much safer approaches to wound exploration. Despite these measures, lacerations through thick subcutaneous adipose tissue are treacherous, because large amounts of particulate matter can be totally obscured in deeper folds of tissue. Unless a careful search is undertaken, these contaminants may be left in the depths of a sutured wound, and infection usually follows. Some clinicians are reluctant to extend lacerations to properly clean or explore them; however, opening the wound to permit

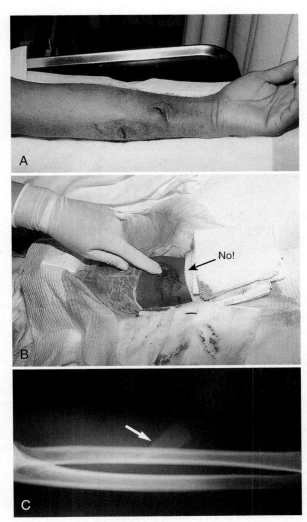

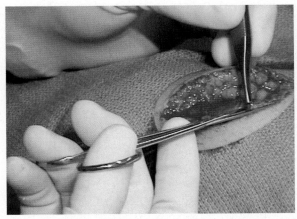

FIGURE 34–10 Sharp débridement (here with scissors, but a scalpel is also used) is the best way to remove devitalized tissue and create a more cosmetic result . Alternatively, the skin is first sharply incised with a scalpel for a clean edge, and then the rest of the subcutaneous tissue is removed with scissors. *(From Thomsen T, Setnik G [eds]: Procedures Consult—Emergency Medicine Module. Copyright 2008 Elsevier Inc. All rights reserved.)*

FIGURE 34–9 *A,* This patient punched out a window, a setup for retained glass. *B, Do not explore this laceration with a finger. C,* Instead, use radiographs and instruments to search for foreign bodies (*arrow* defines a large piece of glass that could cut the examining finger). Many patients are unaware of the presence of surprising large FBs in a deep wound, although they should be questioned about the possibility or sensation of retained material.

adequate visualization may be needed for successful wound exploration.

Débridement

Débridement of foreign material and devitalized tissue is of undisputed importance in the management of the contaminated wound. With this technique, the clinician can remove tissue embedded with foreign matter, bacteria, and devitalized tissue that otherwise impairs the ability of the wound to resist infection and prolongs the period of inflammation. Débridement also creates a tidy, sharp wound edge that is easier to repair and results in a more cosmetically acceptable scar.

If the wound already is clean and the edges are viable, sharp débridement may not improve the outcome. Irregular wounds have greater surface areas than do linear lacerations. Because skin tension is distributed over a greater length, the scar width is usually less in jagged wounds than if the wound is converted to an elliptical defect with tidy edges. If the edges are devitalized or contaminated, the wound edges must be débrided (Fig. 34–10). To avoid a wide scar in this situation, the wound can be undermined.

Excision. Excision is the most effective type of débridement, because it converts the contaminated traumatic wound into a clean wound. If significant contamination occurs in areas in which there is a laxity of tissues, and if no important structures, such as tendons or nerves, lie within the wound, the entire wound may be excised[5] (Fig. 34–11). Complete excision of grossly contaminated wounds such as animal bites allows primary closure of such wounds with no greater risk of infection than in relatively uncontaminated lacerations.[31]

When a puncture wound is excised, the axis of the excision should be made parallel to a wrinkle, a skin line, or a line of dependency or facial expression. The long axis of this lenticular-shaped excision should be three to four times as great as the short axis (Fig. 34–12). The clinician may plan this type of excision by premarking the skin with a surgical marking pen or by making a superficial "scoring" mark (cutting only down to the epidermis) around the wound with the blade of a No. 15 scalpel. Tension should be placed on the surrounding skin with a finger or a skin hook. With the clinician's hand steadied on the table or on the patient, the No. 15 blade is used to cut through the skin at right angles, or at slightly oblique angles, to the skin surface. If complete excision of the entire depth of the wound is not necessary, the tissue scissors may be used to cut the edge of the wound, following the path premarked in the epidermis by the scalpel blade. If a complete excision is desired, the incision on each wound edge should be carried past the deepest part of the wound. The wedge of excised tissue should be removed carefully, without contaminating the fresh wound surface.

Excision should be planned carefully; excessive removal of tissue can create a defect that is too large to close. Wounds of the trunk, the gluteal region, or the thigh are amenable to excision. In contrast, simple excision of a wound of the palm or the dorsum of the nose will make approximation of the resulting surgical wound edges difficult. In hair-bearing areas of the face, particularly through the eyebrows, the incision should be angled parallel to the angle of hair follicles to avoid linear alopecia (Fig. 34–13).

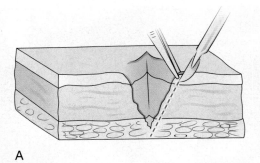

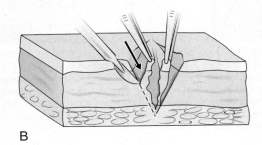

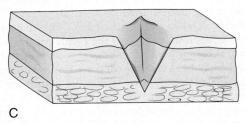

FIGURE 34–11 *A–C,* Complete excision of a wound. Grossly contaminated wounds may be excised and sutured primarily.

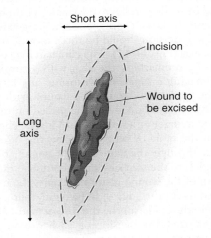

FIGURE 34–12 The long axis of an excision around a wound should be three to four times as great as the short axis.

Selective Débridement. Complete excision is impossible for most wounds because of insufficient skin elasticity, and selective débridement must be used.[5,21] Stellate wounds and wounds with an irregular, meandering course have greater surface areas and less skin tension per unit length than do linear lacerations. In some cases, excision of an entire wound would result in the loss of too much tissue (i.e., produce a gaping defect and excessive tension on the wound edges

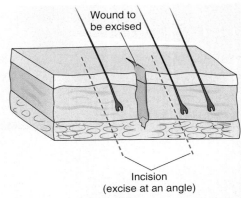

FIGURE 34–13 Excision through an eyebrow. Use an angled incision to remove tissue in the eyebrow, thus avoiding further injury of hair follicles.

when closed). This problem can be avoided with selective débridement and approximation of the irregular wound edges. This technique involves sharp débridement of devitalized or heavily contaminated tissue in the wound piece by piece and eventual matching of one edge of the wound with the other. Selective débridement is time consuming but preserves more surrounding tissue.

Identifying devitalized tissue in a wound remains a challenging problem. Tissue with a narrow pedicle or base, especially distally based, narrow flaps on extremities, is unlikely to survive and should be excised. Sometimes, a sharp line of demarcation distinguishes devitalized skin and viable skin, but in most wounds, usually only a subtle bluish discoloration is present. A clinician can predict tissue viability by comparing capillary refill of injured tissue with that of adjacent skin. If circulation is adequate, viable tissue also becomes hyperemic after the release of a proximal tourniquet.

In heavily contaminated wounds, especially those with abundant adipose tissue, all exposed fat and all fat impregnated with particulate matter should be removed. The subcutaneous adipose tissue attached to large flaps or to avulsed viable skin should be débrided before reapproximation of the wound; removal of this fatty layer allows better perfusion of the flap or the graft. Contaminated bone fragments, nerves, and tendons are almost never removed. Every effort should be made to clean these structures and return them to their place of origin, because they may be functional later.[59] Fascia and tendons perform important functions despite potential loss of viability. If they can be cleaned adequately, these tissues should not be débrided. They may be left in wounds as free grafts and covered by viable flaps of tissue.[60]

Instruments usually required for débridement include two fine single- or double-pronged skin hooks, a scalpel with a No. 15 blade, tissue scissors, hemostats, and a small tissue forceps. The jagged wound edges are stabilized with skin hooks or forceps, and the scalpel or scissors are used to cut away devitalized tissue from one end of the wound to the other. After débridement or excision, the wound should be irrigated again to remove any remaining tissue debris.

Control of Hemorrhage

Hemostasis is essential at any stage of wound care. Persistent bleeding obscures the wound and hampers wound exploration and closure. If bleeding is not a problem before wound débridement, it may becomes a complication during cleaning or after the wound edges are excised. Hematoma formation in a sutured wound separates wound edges, impairs healing, and risks dehiscence or infection.

Several practical methods of achieving hemostasis are available. Sustained direct pressure with gloved fingers, gauze sponges, or packing material, combined with elevation, is usually effective in immediately controlling a single bleeding site or a small number of sites until cut ends of vessels constrict and coagulation occurs. In a patient with multiple injuries and several urgent problems, hemorrhage can be controlled temporarily with a compression dressing. Several absorptive sponges are applied directly over the bleeding site, and these are secured in place with an elastic bandage (e.g., Ace wrap) or elastic adhesive tape (Elastoplast). Pressure is provided by the elasticity of the bandage. The bleeding part should be elevated. Wound care can then be deferred while the clinician attends to more pressing matters.

Although simply crushing and twisting the end of a small vessel with a hemostat avoids the introduction of suture material into the wound, this method provides unreliable hemostasis. Ligation of the vessel with fine absorbable suture material is preferred. Bleeding ends of vessels are clamped with fine-point hemostats, providing immediate hemostasis. Because nerves often course with these vessels, all clamping should be done under direct visualization. The tip of the hemostat should project beyond the vessel to hold a loop of a ligature in place (Fig. 34–14). While an assistant lifts the handle of the hemostat, a synthetic absorbable 5-0 or 6-0 *absorbable* suture is passed around the hemostat from one hand to the other. The first knot is tied beyond the tip of the hemostat. Once the suture is securely anchored on the vessel, the hemostat is released.[61,62] Three knots are sufficient to hold the ligature in place. The ends of the suture should be cut close to the knot to minimize the amount of suture material left in the wound.

Vessels with diameters greater than 2 mm should be ligated. Those smaller than 2 mm that bleed despite direct pressure can be controlled by pinpoint, bipolar electrocautery. A dry field is required for an effective electrical current to pass through the tissues; if sponging does not dry the field, a suction-tipped catheter should be used. Trauma is minimized by using fine-tipped electrodes to touch the vessel or by touching the active electrode of the electrocautery unit to a small hemostat or fine-tipped forceps gripping the vessel.[3] The power of the unit should be kept to the minimum level required for vessel thrombosis. Self-contained, sterilizable, battery-powered coagulation units are alternatives to electrocautery. These devices cauterize vessels by the direct application of a heated wire filament. Although these units may damage more surrounding tissue than electrocautery units, they are compact, simple, and well suited for use in the ED (Fig. 34–15).

A cut vessel that retracts into the wall of the wound may frustrate attempts at clamping, ligation, or cauterization. Bleeding should be controlled first by downward compression on the tissue. A suture is passed through the tissue twice, using a figure-of-eight or horizontal mattress stitch, and then tied. This stitch will constrict the tissue containing the cut vessel (Fig. 34–16).

Large superficial varicosities may spontaneously bleed or bleed from minor trauma. Such varicosities may bleed profusely, especially when the patient stands up and increases venous pressure. A simple figure-of-eight suture will halt bleeding (Fig. 34–17).

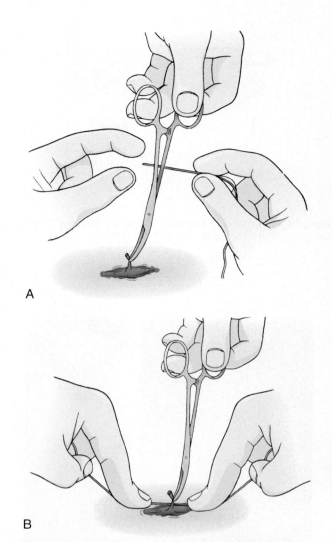

A

B

FIGURE 34–14 *A*, When one attempts to tie off a bleeding vessel, the tip of the hemostat should project beyond the clamped vessel. The handles of the hemostat are raised by an assistant as a ligature is passed under them. *B*, The ligature thread stretched between the index fingertips is carried under the projecting tips of the hemostat.

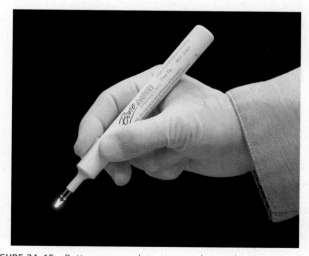

FIGURE 34–15 Battery-powered cautery can be used to coagulate minor subcutaneous bleeders.

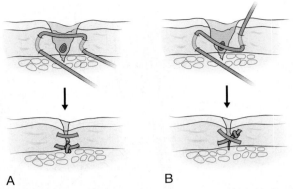

FIGURE 34–16 Ligation of a retracted, bleeding vessel. *A,* Horizontal mattress technique. *B,* Figure-of-eight technique.

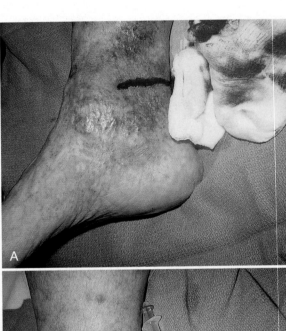

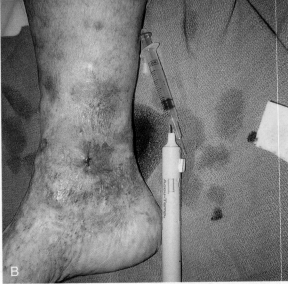

FIGURE 34–17 *A,* This elderly patient experienced massive spontaneous bleeding from a ruptured varicose vein. Blood loss was substantial, and recurrent when she walked. *B,* After cautery, a figure-of-eight suture was placed and bleeding stopped. Simple cautery *without suturing* is not always effective. A pressure dressing is applied after hemostasis is verified by walking.

Epinephrine is an excellent vasoconstrictor. Topical epinephrine (1:100,000) on a moistened sponge can be applied to a wound to reduce the bleeding from small vessels. Combined with local anesthetics, concentrations of 1:100,000 and 1:200,000 prolong the effect of the anesthetic and provide some hemostasis in highly vascular areas. Vasoconstrictors should be used only in situations in which widespread small vessel and capillary hemorrhage in a wound is not controlled by direct pressure or cauterization. Hemostasis of a specific vessel may be obtained by directly injecting the soft tissues around the base of the bleeder with a small amount of lidocaine/epinephrine solution, even though the wound has been previously anesthetized. The combination of pressure and vasoconstriction may halt bleeding long enough for the vessel to be ligated or cauterized or allow the wound to be closed and a compression dressing applied.

Fibrin foam, gelatin foam, and microcrystalline collagen may be used as hemostatic agents. Their utility is limited in that vigorous bleeding will wash the agent away from the bleeding site. Their greatest value may be in packing small cavities from which there is a constant oozing of blood.[61]

Clinicians should not spend excessive time attempting to tie off several small bleeding vessels while the patient slowly exsanguinates. In highly vascular areas, such as the scalp, it is sometimes best to suture the laceration after wound exploration and irrigation, despite active bleeding; the pressure exerted by the closure will usually stop the bleeding (Fig. 34–18). If bleeding is too brisk to permit adequate wound evaluation and irrigation, hemorrhage can often be controlled by clamping and everting the galea or dermis of each wound edge using hemostats. Raney clamps, or a large hemostat, are an excellent way to stop scalp bleeding, and they are used during neurosurgery procedures. The edge of the entire scalp is compressed and all bleeding from the edges will stop (Fig. 34–19). In the majority of simple wounds with persistent but minor capillary bleeding, apposition of the wound edges with sutures, followed by a compression dressing, provides adequate hemostasis.

Tourniquets

If bleeding from an extremity wound is refractory to direct pressure, electrocauterization, or ligation, or if the patient presents with exsanguinating hemorrhage from the wound, a tourniquet placed proximal to the wound can be used to control the bleeding temporarily. Tourniquets also are helpful in examining extremity lacerations by providing a bloodless field. However, they can cause injury in three ways:

1. They can produce ischemia in an extremity.
2. They can compress and damage underlying blood vessels and nerves.
3. They can jeopardize the survival of marginally viable tissue.

Although problems rarely develop from tourniquets used in routine wound care, potential problems can be minimized if (1) a limit is placed on the total amount of time that a tourniquet is applied and (2) excessive tourniquet pressures are avoided. It is also imperative that all tourniquets be removed before releasing the patient; a small tourniquet may be overlooked if it is covered by a bulky dressing.

A single-cuff tourniquet (sphygmomanometer cuff) placed around an arm or a leg effectively stops distal venous or arterial bleeding without crushing underlying structures. The length of time that a tourniquet may remain in place is limited by the development of pain underneath and distal to

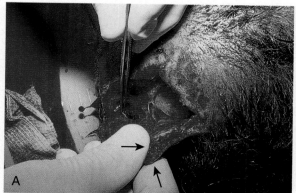

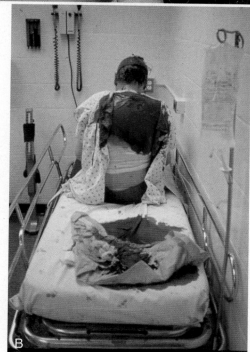

FIGURE 34–18 *A,* Scalp lacerations may bleed profusely, and arterial vessels may not retract if they are in tough fibrous tissue. This clamp was applied to crush a small pumping artery. Placing large (3-0 nylon) sutures, *incorporating all scalp layers,* defined as all tissues between the thumb and index finger (*arrows*), is preferred to attempting to cauterize or ligate small bleeders. *B,* This patient's pressure dressing fell off while in a back hall stretcher, and he experienced significant blood loss from a large scalp laceration. His intoxication prevented him from supplying his hemophilia history.

the tourniquet. This occurs within 30 to 45 minutes in a conscious patient, well within the limits of safety.[15]

Before application of the tourniquet, the injured extremity should be elevated and then manually exsanguinated to prevent persistent venous oozing. An elastic bandage (e.g., Ace wrap or Esmarch) may be wrapped circumferentially around the extremity, starting distally and moving in a proximal direction. A cuff 20% wider than the diameter of the limb is placed around the arm proximal to the wound and inflated to 250 to 300 mm Hg, or 70 mm Hg higher than the patient's systolic blood pressure, and the tubing is clamped. The bandage is then removed, and the extremity is lowered. Because tourniquets impair circulation and may produce neurapraxia, their use in the ED should be limited to a maximum of 1 hour.

Tourniquets on digits have a greater potential for complications. The maximum tourniquet time that is safe for a finger may easily be exceeded. Also, finger tourniquets can exert excessive pressures over a small surface area at the base of the finger and injure digital nerves or cause pressure necrosis of digital vessels. For this reason, simple rubber bands should not be used as tourniquets. A 0.5-inch Penrose drain placed around the base of a finger and stretched to no more than two thirds of its circumference provides safe and effective hemostasis. Pressure under a Penrose drain ranges between 100 and 650 mm Hg, but it can be easily controlled.[63] A few millimeters of difference in total stretch makes a large difference in the pressure applied by this type of tourniquet.[64] Tourniquet pressures of only 150 mm Hg are needed for hemostasis in digits (Fig. 34–20).

A latex rubber surgical glove placed over a patient's cleaned hand also can serve as a finger tourniquet. The tip of the glove covering the injured digit is removed, and the latex rubber is then rolled proximally along the patient's finger to form a constricting band at the base. Another advantage of this technique is that contamination of the wound during closure is less likely. Rolled surgical gloves produce pressures ranging from 113 to 363 mm Hg, depending on the thickness, the amount of glove finger removed, the number of rolls, and the size of the glove in relation to the size of the patient's hand.[64] Commercial ring-shaped exsanguinating digit tourniquets are available (Tourni-cot [Mar-Med Company]) (Fig. 34–21). There is a danger of forgetting to remove such a small tourniquet and of accidentally incorporating it in the dressing.

These techniques provide bloodless fields in which to examine, clean, and close extremity wounds. The maximum tourniquet time on a finger should not exceed 30 to 45 minutes.[63,64] Débridement of questionably devitalized tissue in a wound is best accomplished without a tourniquet or pharmacologic vasoconstriction, because bleeding from tissues is often an indication of their viability.[59]

CLOSURE

The various techniques of wound closure are presented in Chapter 35, Methods of Wound Closure. The remainder of this chapter addresses issues related to wound management (e.g., secondary closure, wound dressings, antibiotic use, aftercare instructions, and suture removal).

Open versus Closed Wound Management

Wounds that heal spontaneously (i.e., by secondary intention) undergo much more inflammation, fibroplasia, and contraction than those whose edges are reapproximated by wound closure techniques.[7,65] During wound healing, contraction covers the defect, but it may result in deformity (contracture) or loss of function. Left to itself, the healing process may be unable to close a defect completely in areas in which surrounding skin is immobile, such as on the scalp or in the pretibial area[7] (Fig. 34–22). Exposed tendons, bone, nerves, or vessels may desicate in an open wound. If the patient is careless with an otherwise adequate dressing that covers an open wound, the wound may be further contaminated.[66] Surgical closure of wounds minimizes inflammation, fibroplasia, contracture, scar width, and contamination.

However, surgical closure of wounds can cause complications. Closure of contaminated wounds increases the probability of wound infection, with impaired healing, dehiscence,

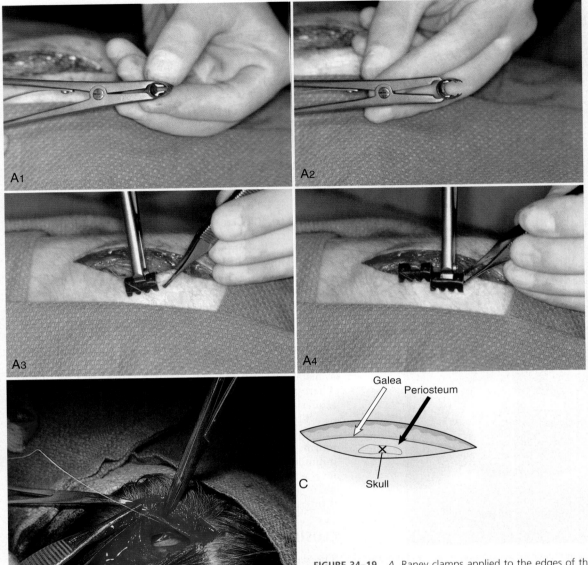

Galea
Periosteum

C

Skull

FIGURE 34–19 *A,* Raney clamps applied to the edges of the scalp will stop bleeding. 1. Load the clip onto the applicator 2. Lock the handles of the applicator to open the clip. 3. Slide the clip onto the wound edge 4. Release the clip by unlocking the applicator. *B,* A hemostat placed on the scalp edge can be similarly used on a single bleeder. *C,* Note that the suture will incorporate *all layers of the scalp.* Both the galea (↔) and the periosteum are identified (➡), with exposed skull (x). The periosteum is not sutured (also see Fig. 35–58). *(A, From Custalow CB. Color Atlas of Emergency Department Procedures. Philadelphia: Elsevier Saunders, 2005; p. 136–137.)*

and sepsis as possible complications. For instance, raised pretibial flap lacerations in elderly patients often necrose when sutured but survive and heal well by secondary intention if taped back into position.

Sutures in themselves are potentially detrimental to healing and can increase the risk of infection.[67] Each suture inflicts a small intradermal incision, damaging surface epithelium, dermis, subcutaneous fat, blood vessels, small nerves, lymphatics, and epithelial appendages such as hair follicles, sweat glands, and ducts. Once divided and separated by a stitch, these appendages usually undergo inflammation and resorption.[68] Each suture is another piece of foreign material that provokes inflammation.[7] When a suture is removed, bacteria that have settled on the exposed portion of the suture are pulled into the suture track and deposited there.[68]

The clinician must estimate the risk of infection. If the wound is judged to be clean or is rendered clean by scrubbing, irrigation, and débridement, it may be closed. If the wound remains contaminated despite the best of efforts, it must be left open to heal by secondary intention. If the status of the wound is uncertain, delayed primary closure is another available option.

Delayed Primary or Secondary Closure

There is a common misconception that all wounds must be either sutured within a few hours or left open and relegated to slow healing and an unsightly scar. If there is a substantial risk that closure of a particular wound might result in infection, the decision to close or to leave the wound open can be

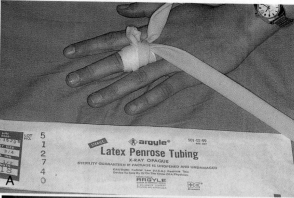

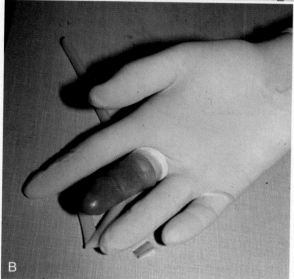

FIGURE 34–20 *A,* Use of a Penrose drain for a finger tourniquet, placed over padding. *B,* Use of a sterile glove to provide a clean field and serve as a finger tourniquet. The distal end of the glove is clipped, and the glove finger is rolled proximally over the digit. A Penrose drain is also incorporated into this tourniquet.

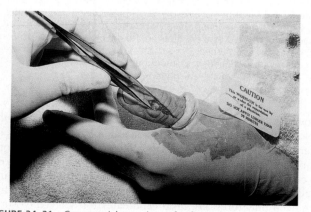

FIGURE 34–21 Commercial tourniquet for finger lacerations (Tourni-cot Mar Med Company). Various sizes are available. The accompanying warning tag has been left exposed to remind the operator of the tourniquet device. Note how the tendon injury can be seen once a bloodless field is obtained.

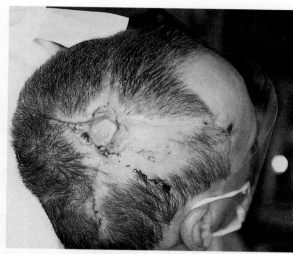

FIGURE 34–22 In areas in which the skin is immobile, as in the scalp, wounds left open may not heal.

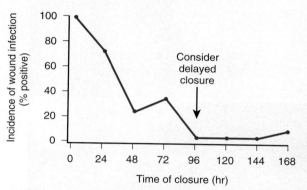

FIGURE 34–23 Incidence of wound infection over time when delayed closure is performed. Delayed closure is best accomplished on the fourth or fifth day to minimize the risk of infection. *(From Edlich RF, Thacker JG, Rodeheaver GT, et al: A Manual for Wound Closure. St. Paul, MN, 3M Medical Surgical Products, 1979. Reproduced by permission. © 1979 by Minnesota Mining and Manufacturing Company.)*

postponed. After cleaning, wounds left unsutured appear to have a higher resistance to infection than do closed wounds. The condition of the wound after 3 to 5 days will then determine the best strategy (Fig. 34–23).

Although cleaning and débridement should be accomplished as rapidly as possible, there is no urgency in closing a wound. Edlich and associates[20] point out that "the fundamental basis for delayed primary closure is that the healing open wound gradually gains sufficient resistance to infection to permit an uncomplicated closure." Despite its effectiveness, delayed primary closure is a technique that remains largely unappreciated and likely underused by many clinicians (Fig. 34–24).

Open wound management is usually an outpatient procedure. The technique consists of the usual careful cleaning and débridement, followed by packing of the wound with sterile, saline-moistened, fine-mesh gauze. The packed wound is covered by a thick, absorbent, sterile dressing. Depending on the specifics of the wound and the ability of the patient to perform his or her own wound care, the packing may be changed daily at home or in the ED or the wound may be left undisturbed for several days. Sterile saline-soaked packing is

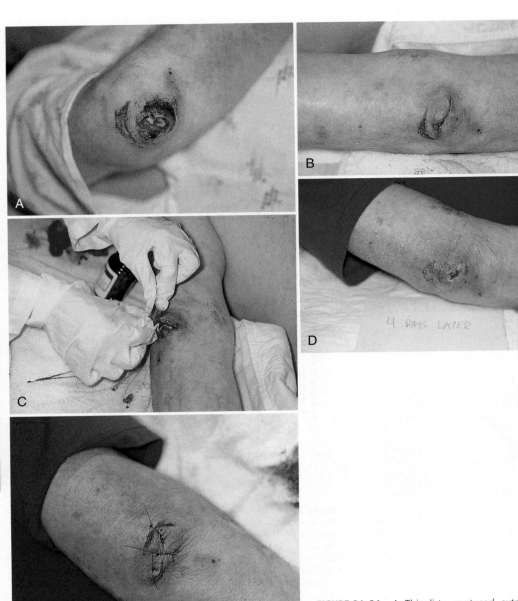

FIGURE 34–24 *A,* This dirty, contused, extremity wound, now 18 hr old, is an ideal candidate for a delayed primary closure. *B,* At presentation, the wound is anesthetized, scrubbed, irrigated, and sharply débrided. *C,* The wound is packed with sterile gauze and covered by a dry dressing. No antibiotics were prescribed and the wound was left undisturbed. *D,* Four days later, the packing is removed, and the wound is minimally débrided. *E,* Interrupted sutures are placed as though this is a fresh, clean wound. At suture removal 10 days later, only a linear scar was evident.

standard, and there is no need to impregnate wounds with antiseptics. Prophylactic antibiotics are occasionally prescribed, but their use is neither mandatory nor of proven benefit. On the 4th or 5th postoperative day, the wound is reevaluated for closure. If no evidence of infection is present, the wound margins can be approximated (delayed primary closure), or the wound can be excised and then sutured (secondary closure) with minimal risk of infection. Because the wound is closed before the proliferative phase of healing, there is no delay in final healing, and the results are indistinguishable from those of primary healing.

Certain wounds should almost always be managed open or by delayed closure (Fig. 34–25). These include wounds that are already infected and those heavily contaminated by soil, organic matter, or feces. Also included in this category are wounds associated with extensive tissue damage (e.g., high-velocity missile injuries, explosion injuries of the hand, or complex crush injuries) and most bite wounds. Deep or contaminated lacerations to the bottom of the feet, such as those occurring when the patient steps on an unknown object while wading in a stream or running through a field, or wounds that are deep punctures, are ideal candidates for delayed closure. Some are never sutured but left open for primary healing. Human bite wounds (extending past the dermis) should probably never be closed and are *often opened or extended further for cleaning.* Clinicians disagree as to which animal bite wounds may be closed initially. Most would suture cosmetically deforming injuries, including facial bites, and bite wounds that can be completely excised.[69] Others would suture nonextremity dog bites.[70] In severe soft tissue injuries, delayed

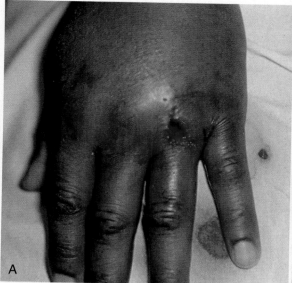

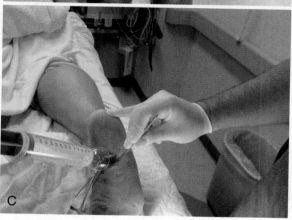

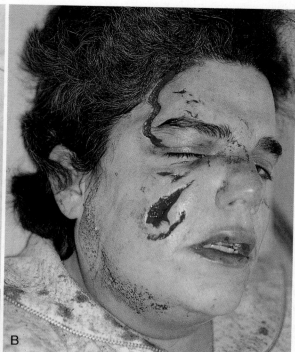

FIGURE 34–25 *A,* Human bites are never closed primarily and are often opened and extended to facilitate cleaning and a search for other injuries, such as fragments of teeth. *B,* Dog bites in a cosmetic area may be closed primarily. This is best closed in the operating room by a surgeon with a lot of time to correctly prepare the wound. *C,* This wound on the bottom of the foot, sustained by stepping on an unknown object, while running in a stream, should not be closed but should be left open to heal primarily. Note that an assistant holds the wound open and pressure irrigation is applied. This was initially a much smaller puncture wound that was extended for cleaning, and initially packed open.

579

closure allows time for nonviable tissue to demarcate from uninjured tissue. Débridement can then be accomplished with maximal preservation of tissue.[66]

PROTECTION

Dressings

At the conclusion of wound repair, dried blood on the skin surface should be wiped away gently with moistened gauze to minimize subsequent itching, and the wound should be covered with a nonadherent dressing. Depending on the specifics of the wound and the type of repair, a dressing can consist of a simple dry gauze pad or a complex multilayer dressing. Some wounds, such as sutured scalp lacerations, do not routinely require any dressing. Various specialized (and expensive) synthetic dressings are available, including vapor-permeable adhesive films, hydrogels, hydrocolloids, alginates, synthetic foam dressings, silicone meshes, tissue adhesives, barrier films, and collagen-containing dressings. However, little data exist to support their use over readily available, properly applied gauze dressings on acute, traumatic wounds managed in the ED.

Function of Dressings

Dressings serve various functions. They protect the wound from contamination and trauma, absorb excess exudate from the wound, immobilize the wound and the surrounding area, exert downward pressure on the wound, and improve the patient's comfort.[14,71,72] Occlusive dressings on burns or abrasions maintain a moist environment and prevent painful exposure of the wound to the air and dehydration of the wound surface.[73] Sutured wounds are particularly susceptible to infection from surface contamination during the first 2 days after wound repair. Dressings protect the wound from contamination during this vulnerable period.

One of the primary functions of a gauze dressing is to *absorb the serosanguineous drainage that exudes from all wounds.* Absorbent dressings also reduce the development of stitch abscesses to some extent. Surface sutures produce small indentations at their points of entrance; tiny blood clots and debris overlie these indentations, allowing bacterial growth at the site. Small "stitch abscesses" can develop; these are initially undetectable but are nevertheless destructive to epithelium. Stitch abscesses rarely infect the entire wound but can slightly increase the width of the scar and produce noticeable, punctate suture marks.[14]

The most common type of dressing is constructed in three layers: a nonadherent contact layer, an absorbent layer, and an outer wrap (Fig. 34–26).[74] Ideally, this dressing provides nonadherence without maceration. The optimal appearance of an abrasion or an open wound under a dressing is a moist red surface with capillary and epithelial growth.

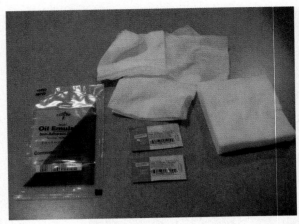

FIGURE 34–26 A common three-layer dressing, consisting of antibiotic ointment, Adaptic, and gauze.

Contact Layer: Dry, Semiocclusive, and Occlusive Dressings

Wounds covered with permeable dressings such as plain gauze tend to dry out. Whereas this is acceptable for dressing sutured wounds, drying of the wound surface damages a shallow layer of exposed dermis, which impedes epidermal resurfacing of abrasions, burns, and incisions.[72] Wound desiccation results in further epidermal necrosis, crust formation, and increased inflammation.[75,76] Coarse weaves of gauze, usually available in the form of multilayered pads, absorb blood and exudate, but the dressing will adhere if the interstices of the fabric are relatively large. Capillaries, fibrin, and granulation tissue will penetrate and become enmeshed in the material. If the proteinaceous exudate from the wound dries by evaporation, the scab usually clings to the dressing.[74,75] Some clinicians use this effect to "débride" the wound when the gauze is removed. However, it may also destroy healing tissue, particularly the new epithelium. Although débridement of the wound with wet-to-dry dressings is quick, careful débridement with surgical instruments is more controlled and less traumatic.

Adherence to the wound can be prevented if the dressing is nonabsorbent, occlusive, or finely woven. If the wound is kept moist by covering it with an occlusive film or nonadherent covering soon after wound management, and if the film is left in place for at least 48 hours, the epidermis will migrate over the surface of the dermis faster than when a dry scab is allowed to form.[77–79] Protection of wounds that are healing by secondary intention with occlusive or semiocclusive dressings has several advantages,[10] including more rapid healing, less pain from air exposure, better cosmetic result, few dressing changes, and protection from bacteria.

Petrolatum gauze (e.g., Adaptic, Xeroform, Betadine, Aquaflo) is commonly applied next to the wound surface to prevent the wound from sticking to the dry gauze in the absorbent layer and to protect the regenerating epithelium (Table 34–2). (Nonadherent material should always be used to cover skin grafts.) Some clinicians use fine-mesh gauze (41–47 warp threads/inch^2) rather than petrolatum gauze on abrasions, especially on those wounds that are heavily contaminated, because removal of this type of dressing débrides only the small tufts of granulation tissue that become fixed in the mesh pores, leaving a clean, even surface. Once a healthy, granulating surface is present and reepithelialization is pro-

ceeding, nonporous dressings can be used.[75] Fine-mesh gauze also is used next to exposed tissue in wounds being considered for delayed primary closure; a protective and absorptive bulky dressing is placed on top of the wound.

Various polyurethane-derived membranes—such as Epilock (Derma-Lock Medical Corporation), Op-Site (Smith and Nephew, Ltd.), Tegaderm (3M), Bioclusive (Johnson & Johnson), and Primaderm (ACCO, Inc.); those with soluble collagen or gelatin backing, such as DuoDerm (Convatec) and Biobrane (Woodroof Laboratories); products with hydrogels, such as Vigilon[75]; and other occlusive dressings, such as Dermicel (Johnson & Johnson), and Telfa (Kendall)—provide an occlusive effect. One fear of using occlusive dressings is that microorganisms will proliferate in the moist environment beneath the occlusive film and increase wound infection rates.[72,80] However, occlusive dressings such as DuoDerm actually serve more as a barrier to external pathogenic bacteria.[81] Although skin bacteria under occlusive dressings can multiply,[82] even chronic wounds contaminated with large numbers of bacteria are routinely treated with occlusive dressings successfully.[83]

Adhesive-backed dressings (e.g., DuoDerm and Op-Site) may adhere to an open wound and remove new epidermis, macerate skin, or produce a thick eschar. The wound then must epithelialize underneath the eschar.[84] These dressings do not allow exudate to drain out the edges of the dressing. Between dressing changes, the wound should be coated with petrolatum or an antibiotic ointment before these products are applied.[10] Epilock has the advantage of thermally insulating the wound by virtue of its thickness, but unlike Tegaderm and Op-Site, it is opaque and does not allow inspection of the underlying wound surface.[85] Because Epilock allows drainage of exudate, it is better tolerated by patients if the overlying gauze bandage is changed daily. Wounds covered with certain occlusive dressings or with silver sulfadiazine (Silvadene [Marion Laboratories]) applications appear to be blanketed with pus; this exudate actually represents the beneficial proliferation of macrophages and polymorphonuclear leukocytes.[79,85]

Absorbent Layer

When dressing wounds with considerable drainage, sufficient gauze should be used to cover the wound and to absorb all of the drainage. Any dressing should be changed whenever it becomes soiled, wet, or saturated with drainage. Once a dressing becomes moist, pathogens can pass through it to the underlying wound.[72] Consequently, a dressing that is used to absorb exudate or débride the wound must be changed more frequently than one designed solely to occlude. Absorbent dressings on draining wounds can be changed daily to avoid bacterial overgrowth beneath the dressing.[7,75] Fluid accumulating under an occlusive dressing should be aspirated or the dressing changed every 1 to 2 days during the 1st week or until the exudate no longer accumulates.[86]

Outer Layer

Bleeding may persist despite attempts to provide good hemostasis. Compressive dressings may be helpful in preventing hematoma formation and eliminating dead space within a wound. They are particularly useful in wounds that have been undermined extensively and in facial wounds, in which subcutaneous capillary bleeding and swelling can exert tension on fine skin sutures and jeopardize skin closure. Pressure dressings should be used to immobilize skin grafts. Surgical tape can serve as a pressure dressing in areas such as fingertips on which bandages cannot be easily applied.

Pressure dressings should be applied to all ear lacerations to prevent hematoma formation and subsequent deformation and destruction of cartilage. The ear should be enveloped in the dressing so that pressure from the outer bandage is distributed evenly across the irregular surface of the pinna. Moistened cotton is packed into the concavities of the pinna until the cotton is level with the most lateral aspect of the helical rim. Square pieces of gauze cut to fit the curvature of the ear are placed behind (medial to) the pinna. Several more gauze squares are placed on the lateral surface of the ear; the packing is then secured in place with a circumferential head bandage. The bandage must not encompass the opposite ear because it would just as easily cause pressure necrosis of that ear if left unprotected

Traumatic wounds are bandaged to compress or immobilize the wound or to secure and protect the underlying dressing. Most bandaging is performed on extremities, on which dressings are difficult to secure with tape alone. Rolls of cotton (Kerlix; Kling stretch gauze) are well suited for this purpose. The bandage is wound around the extremity, advancing proximally with circular, overlapping turns. Care should be taken to avoid allowing wrinkles in the bandage, which will later create pressure points, or making loose turns that shorten the effective life of the dressing. When joint surfaces are crossed, the cotton is anchored distally with several turns, unrolled obliquely across the joint several times in a figure-of-eight pattern, and anchored proximally by two complete turns. This process is repeated until the bandage is securely in place. The ends of the bandage are fastened to the skin by strips of adhesive tape.

Bandages over the forearm and the lower extremities are particularly prone to slippage because of the constant motion of these parts and because of the marked changes in extremity diameter over a short distance. The roll of bandage can be rotated 180° after each circular turn, producing a reverse spiral and reducing the bandage's mobility (Fig. 34–27). The dressing of a single digit can be covered with a finger cut from a glove (Fig. 34–28).

Certain chemically treated wide-mesh weaves have the properties of cling and stretch, holding snugly in place but expanding if edema develops.[74] An elastic cotton roll (Kerlix) allows the bandage to conform to body contours, provides some mobility to bandaged joints, and permits the wound to swell without the circumferential bandage constricting the extremity. The inelastic Kling bandage better immobilizes the part. Rigid immobilization with plaster splints or braces is needed to protect wounds in mobile areas, such as around large joints.

Most scalp wounds do well when left uncovered. Daily showering is encouraged for sutured scalp lacerations to

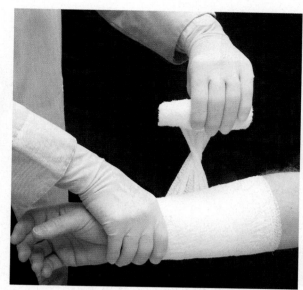

FIGURE 34–27 Snugness of the bandage is increased by 180° rotation of the bandage roll after each circular turn to create a reverse spiral.

remove debris. If a dressing is necessary, it must be held in place by a bandage. The outer layer of dressings should be changed when it becomes externally contaminated or saturated with exudate or when inspection and wound cleaning are required.

Dressings vary in their absorbency, adhesiveness, occlusiveness, opacity, and insulating properties. Further research may identify types of dressings best suited for different phases of the healing wound. Currently, a two- or three-layer dressing is used for most traumatic wounds; the choice of material for the contact layer is determined by the characteristics of the individual wound.[87]

Splinting and Elevation

Immobilization of wounds and sutured lacerations may be used to enhance healing and to provide patient comfort (Fig. 34–29). *Immobilization of an injured extremity promotes healing* by protecting the closure and by limiting the spread of contamination and infection along lymphatic channels. Wounds overlying joints are subjected to repeated stretching and movement, which delays healing, widens the scar, and could possibly disrupt the sutures.[20] Short-term splints are almost always beneficial for lacerations that overlie joints and are frequently necessary for protection of wounds involving fingers, hands, wrists, the volar aspects of forearms, the extensor surfaces of elbows, the posterior aspects of legs, the plantar surfaces of feet, and the extremities when skin grafts have been applied. A plaster or aluminum splint may be incorporated into a bandage to reduce the mobility of the part.

Elevation of injured extremities is important in all but trivial injuries. Elevation limits edema formation and allows more rapid healing.[20] Elevation also reduces throbbing pain. Patients given this information are often more motivated to elevate the extremity as instructed. Slings can be used to elevate wounds involving the forearm or the hand. A pillow may be wrapped around an injured hand to promote elevation at home (see Fig. 34–29A). With severe injuries, elevation begins in the ED (see Fig. 34–29B).

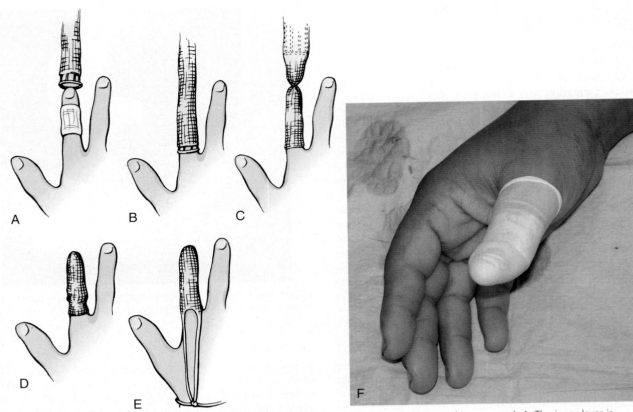

582

FIGURE 34–28 Tube gauze finger dressing, applied loosely. *Throbbing pain under this dressing mandates removal. A*, The inner layer is nonadherent gauze or whatever is required for soft tissue care. The middle layer is 2- x 2-inch gauze sponges wrapped circumferentially and held in place with a small strip of tape. *B*, Begin No. 2 tube gauze at the base of the finger. It is useful to hold this end with one finger while the tube gauze applicator is pulled toward the fingertip. A twisting motion firms the wrap about the digit; generally about 90° is necessary. Excessive stretch or twisting can compromise circulation. *C*, When the fingertip is reached, make a 360° twist, but avoid placing a constricting twist around the finger itself. *D*, Pass the applicator toward the finger base with an additional 90° twist. Repeat once more; thus, three layers are in place. *E*, Cut enough gauze to reach the base of the finger, and tape it there. As an alternative, pull the final layer beyond the tip, leaving it long enough to reach to and around the wrist (about three times the finger length). Split this gauze into two strands; bring them dorsally to the wrist, knot, and loosely wrap around the wrist. *F*, For a distal finger dressing, covering the gauze with a finger cut from a clean glove provides protection from dirt and wetness.

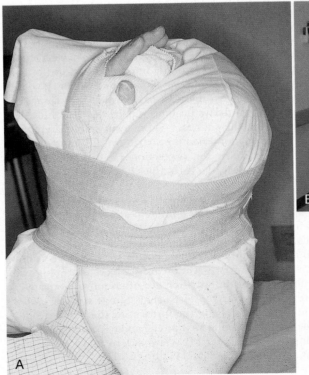

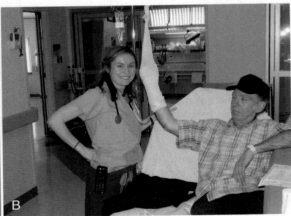

FIGURE 34–29 *A*, A pillow wrapped around a bandaged hand promotes elevation at home. Note that this sutured hand laceration also has a plaster splint for comfort. In general, immobilization promotes healing. *B*, Elevation of a severe hand injury in the ED while awaiting the surgeon.

Ointments

The safety and efficacy of topical antibiotic preparations used on wound surfaces are unproved, and no universal standard exists. Many clinicians routinely suggest the use of antibiotic ointments over sutured wounds, whereas others opt for a simple dry dressing. Use of a triple-antibiotic preparation containing neomycin, bacitracin, and polymyxin provides a broad spectrum of protection against infection in abrasions without systemic absorption and toxicity or the emergence of resistant strains of bacteria. There is some evidence that Neosporin ointment, Silvadene cream, and Mupirocin (Bactroban, GlaxoSmithKline, London) (as well as their inert bases and vehicles) either improve wound healing or slightly reduce infection rates.[88] Although there is a risk of allergic sensitization or contact dermatitis by preparations containing neomycin, it is uncommon unless the ointment is used repeatedly (Fig. 34–30).

One obvious benefit from the use of topical antibiotics is that ointments prevent adherence of the wound surface to the dressing. Ointments can also be used to reduce the formation of a crust that covers and separates the edges of the wound. Lacerations surrounded by abraded skin are especially predisposed to coagulum formation. In such cases, the patient can be instructed to cleanse the wound frequently and to follow the cleansing with an application of ointment during the first few days.[20]

Stronger topical corticosteroids have detrimental effects on healing. Application of 0.1% triamcinolone acetonide in an ointment retards healing in wounds by as much as 60%, whereas hydrocortisone probably does not interfere with epithelialization.[89] Some clinicians believe that single and low doses of oral corticosteroids probably have no effect on wound healing but that repeated, large doses of steroids (≥40 mg of prednisone per day) inhibit healing, particularly if used before the injury or during the first 3 days of the healing phase.[90] There is some evidence that topical vitamin A may reverse some of the anti-inflammatory and immunosuppressive effects of corticosteroids.[91]

The exact value of ointments in the treatment of lacerations has yet to be determined. However, their routine use after wound cleaning does encourage patient inspection of the wound. Ointments should not be used on wounds closed with tissue adhesive because the ointment will dissolve the adhesive.

Wound Cultures

Cultures taken at the time of wound preparation and closure in the ED serve no useful purpose and are not recommended. Results of such cultures cannot logically guide future antibiotic selection. It is not necessary to routinely culture all infected wounds presenting after closure, unless the patient is immunocompromised or methicillin-resistant *Staphylococcus aureus* is suspected.

Systemic Antibiotics

Most traumatic soft tissue injuries sustain a low level of bacterial contamination[66]; thus, uncomplicated wound infection rates in ED patients range from 2% to 5%, *regardless of clinician intervention*. In a number of clinical studies of relatively uncontaminated and uncomplicated traumatic wounds (which represent the majority of wounds managed in the ED), prophylactic antibiotics administered in various routes and regimens did not reduce the incidence of infection.[92–98] Studies of antibiotic prophylaxis for animal bite wounds have produced variable results, and no large study providing stratification of the many prognostic factors has been done.[99]

Even after multiple studies on the use of prophylactic antibiotics for ED wounds, there is no clear practice standard.[100] Because no benefit has been established through multiple attempts with numerous antibiotic regimens, one would intuit that they have no benefit. In most soft tissue wounds in which the level of bacterial contamination after cleaning and débridement is low, antibiotics are not recommended. Heavily contaminated wounds (such as wounds in contact with pus or feces), infection often develops despite antibiotic treatment. Nevertheless, antibiotics may have marginal benefit when the level of contamination is overwhelming or if the amount of questionably viable tissue left in the wound is considerable (e.g., with crush wounds). Antibiotics may be considered for extremity bite wounds, puncture-type bite wounds in any location, intraoral lacerations that are sutured, orocutaneous lip wounds, wounds that cannot be cleaned or débrided satisfactorily, and highly contaminated wounds (e.g., those contaminated with soil, organic matter, purulence, feces, saliva, or vaginal secretions). They may also be considered for wounds involving tendons, bones, or joints; for wounds requiring extensive débridement in the operating room; for wounds in lymphedematous tissue; for distal extremity wounds when treatment is delayed for 12 to 24 hours; for patients with orthopedic prostheses; and for patients at risk of developing infective endocarditis.[20]

Whereas some consider prescribing prophylactic antibiotics in immunocompromised patients (diabetics and others), a true benefit has not been consistently demonstrated in any subset. The downside is the selecting out of resistant organisms, and many resistant strains now encountered in clinical practice (patients and in the community) have been linked to the excessive use of needless antibiotics. It seems most prudent to eschew routine antibiotic prophylaxis and opt for meticulous wound care, close follow-up, and the selective use of antibiotics in proven infection. Other disadvantages of routine antibiotic use include needless expense and potential side effects (e.g., rash, anaphylaxis, diarrhea, vomiting). If antibiotics are considered useful in a specific case, they should be

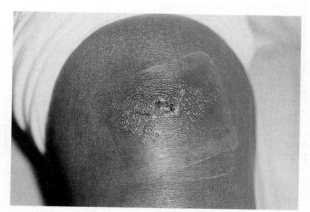

FIGURE 34–30 This patient used a neomycin-containing ointment on a minor wound and developed redness, swelling, pruritus, and skin changes. The patient thought it was an infection, but it was a contact dermatitis from the neomycin. Plain bacitracin ointment will not cause this relatively common reaction. Bacitracin or silvadene are alternative topicals, but any preparation is likely of minimal value.

given as soon as possible after wounding and continued for only 2 to 3 days in the absence of a developing infection. If the infection risk is high enough to warrant antibiotics, delayed primary closure may also be considered.

Many patients have difficulty in determing infection in their wounds and mistake the normal healing process for infection; therefore, in high-risk patients (a clinical judgment), mandatory follow-up would appear to be the best tactic.[101]

The choice of antibiotic, particularly for bite wound prophylaxis, is as controversial as the indications for usage.[102] Many species of bacteria cause animal bite wound infections, making complete coverage impossible.[103] Antibiotic regimens vary with the species of the biter and with evolving bacterial resistance. The duration of antibiotic prophylaxis also is in question. It is common practice to provide antibiotics for 72 hours. (See additional comments on animal bites at the end of this chapter.)

Immunoprophylaxis

Although tetanus is rare, it still occurs in the United States and is a preventable disease. Therefore, any wound should be assessed for its potential to cause tetanus, and prophylaxis should be considered in the ED. About 70% of Americans older than 6 years have protective levels of tetanus antibodies.[104] Levels declined as age increased, and elderly women had the lowest levels of protection. Hispanics (and likely other immigrants) were most likely to have inadequate immunity. Hence, efforts at preventing tetanus should be especially addressed in immigrants and the elderly. The Centers for Disease Control and Prevention's recommendations for tetanus prophylaxis are listed in Figure 34–31.[105]

When patients are questioned about their tetanus immunization status, they should be asked whether they completed the primary immunization series, and if not, how many doses have been given. Patients who have not completed a full primary series of injections may require both tetanus toxoid

and passive immunization with tetanus immune globulin. Tetanus immune globulin will decrease, but not totally eliminate, the subsequent development of clinical tetanus. Tetanus and diphtheria immunizations are often given together. The preferred preparation for active tetanus immunization in patients 7 years of age and older is 0.5 mL of tetanus toxoid (plus the lower, adult dose of diphtheria toxoid); the dose of tetanus immune globulin is 250 to 500 units given intramuscularly.[104]

Mild local reactions consisting of erythema and induration are common (~20%) after tetanus toxoid injections; occasionally, they are accompanied by a fever and mild systemic symptoms. Reactions are about twice as common if diphtheria immunization is coupled with tetanus immunization. This is a hypersensitivity reaction, not an infection, and does not represent an absolute contraindication to further immunizations. A minor febrile illness, such as an upper respiratory infection, is not a reason to delay immunization. Although serious reactions are rare, some patients with high antibody levels develop a hypersensitivity reaction of tenderness, erythema, and swelling, or serum sickness. Generalized urticarial reactions and peripheral neuropathy have also been reported.[106] The only absolute contraindication to tetanus toxoid is a history of anaphylaxis or a neurologic event. In such cases, tetanus immune globulin can be given safely. Pregnancy is not a contraindication to either toxoid or immune globulin, although some suggest that the toxoid be used with caution during the first trimester. Given the excellent amnestic response to the toxoid, it is likely that the primary immunization series, coupled with intermittent boosters, conveys immunity for most of one's life. However, a significant percentage of elderly patients fail to develop protective antitoxin antibody titers after 14 days when given tetanus toxoid boosters.

Treatment decisions are based on the differentiation between clean and contaminated wounds. Whereas any break in the skin can harbor *Clostridium tetanii*, traditional definitions of tetanus-prone wounds include injuries more than 6

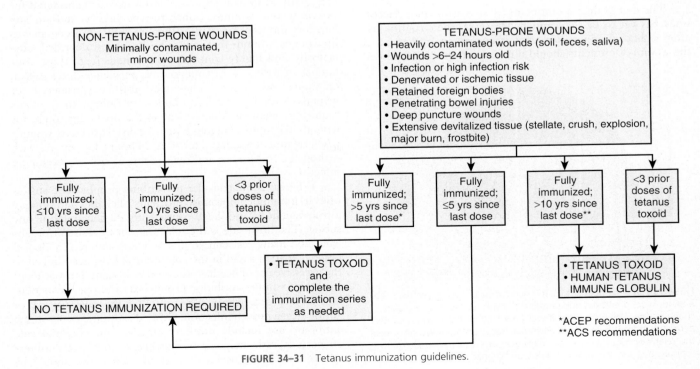

FIGURE 34–31 Tetanus immunization guidelines.

hours old; wounds contaminated by feces, saliva, purulent exudate, or soil; wounds with retained foreign bodies or containing devitalized or avascular tissue; established wound infections; penetrating abdominal wounds involving bowel; deep puncture wounds; and wounds caused by crush, burns, or frostbite.

Tetanus can develop despite prior immunization, and it can result from chronic skin lesions and apparently minor or clean wounds.[107] In 10% to 20% of cases, no prior wound can be identified. Patients' recall of past immunizations is imperfect, and immunity may be, on rare occasions, inadequate after a complete series of tetanus toxoid.[108] Tetanus boosters given more frequently than advised increase the incidence of adverse reactions to subsequent injections. However, the benefits of overtreatment seem to outweigh the risks.

PATIENT INSTRUCTIONS

Successful wound healing is partly dependent on the care given to the wound once the patient leaves the ED. Patient satisfaction depends not only on the cosmetic result but also on the expectation of that result.[10] Both are reasons why the patient should receive thorough and clear instructions.

The patient should be informed that no matter how skillful the repair, any wound of significance produces a scar. Most scars deepen in color and become more prominent before they mature and fade. The final appearance of the scar cannot be judged before 6 to 12 months after the repair.[8] Some wounds heal with wide, unattractive scars despite ideal management and closure. Wounds more likely to have significant scars are those that cross perpendicular to joints, wrinkle lines, or lines of minimum tension (Kraissel lines); that retract more than 5 mm; and that are over convexities or in certain anatomic locations (e.g., anterior upper chest, back, shoulders) where hypertrophic scars are common. A wound crossing a concave surface may result in a bowstring deformity; one crossing a convexity may leave a scar depression. To avoid these complications, a Z-plasty procedure can be done at the time of initial wound management, or the scar can be revised later. The patient should be told to expect suboptimal outcomes in these situations.[24]

Patients may experience dysesthesias in or around a scar, particularly about the midface. Gentle rubbing or pressing on the skin may relieve the symptoms. If wounds extending to subcutaneous levels lacerate cutaneous nerves, patients may be bothered by hypoesthesia distal to the wound. Dysesthesia and anesthesia usually resolve in 6 months to 1 year.[10]

After 48 hours, the patient may remove the dressing in uncomplicated wounds and check for evidence of infection: redness, warmth, increasing pain, swelling, purulent drainage, or the "red streaks" of lymphangitis. Not all patients are able to identify these signs, often overlooking an early infection or overcalling infection in the presence of normal healing. Patients with complicated or infection-prone wounds should be examined in 2 to 3 days by a clinician or nurse.[109] Patients should be informed that sutures themselves do not cause pain. A painful wound is often a sign of infection or suture reaction, and pain should prompt a wound check. If there is no sign of infection after 48 to 72 hours, the patient can care for the wound until it is time for removal of the sutures.

Because the wound edges are rapidly sealed by coagulum and bridged by epithelial cells within 48 hours, the wound is essentially impermeable to bacteria after 2 days.[14,110] The patient should be instructed to protect the wound by keeping the dressing clean and dry for 24 to 48 hours. In this initial period, the dressing should be changed only if it becomes externally soiled or soaked by exudate from the wound. If possible, the injured part should be kept elevated.

A daily gentle washing with mild soap and water to remove dried blood and exudate is probably beneficial, especially on areas such as the face or the scalp,[109,111] but vigorous scrubbing of wounds should be discouraged. Patients may bathe with sutures in place, but not immerse the wound for a prolonged time. Although diluted hydrogen peroxide can be used to remove blood from the skin surface, it should not be repeatedly used as a cleaning agent on the healing wound itself.[35] Generally, a wound should be protected with a dressing during the 1st week, and the dressing should be changed daily. If the wound is unlikely to be contaminated or traumatized, it may be left uncovered. Sutured scalp lacerations are usually left open, and showering is encouraged.

If an injured extremity or finger is protected by a splint, it should be left undisturbed until the sutures are removed. Patients with intraoral lacerations can be instructed to use warm salt water mouth rinses at least three times a day.

Swimming is often prohibited while sutures are in place. There are no data supporting this admonition. In general, showering and bathing are quite acceptable in the presence of sutured wounds. Common sense should prevail in making such decisions.

Patients may ask about the efficacy of various creams and lotions (e.g., vitamin E, aloe vera, cocoa butter) in limiting scar formation. At this time, there are no data to evaluate the use of these substances. Their use is acceptable and may prompt some patients to participate in wound inspection and cleaning more regularly.

SECONDARY WOUND CARE

Reexamination

Patients with simple sutured wounds may be released with appropriate instructions for home care and told to return for suture removal at an appropriate time. High-risk wounds such as bite wounds and other infection-prone wounds should be examined in 2 to 3 days for signs of infection. All wounds should be inspected if the patient experiences increasing discomfort or develops a fever or believes that the wound is infected.[71] Wounds being considered for delayed primary closure are evaluated in 4 to 5 days.[112]

Wounds in which extensive dissection of subcutaneous tissue has been performed may develop an intense inflammation similar in appearance to a low-grade, localized cellulitis. It is rarely necessary to open these wounds. The removal of one or two stitches may relieve some of the tension caused by mild swelling. With daily cleansing using water and a mild soap and with application of warm compresses, this type of wound reaction should subside within 24 to 48 hours.[71]

A wound that has become infected should be evaluated for the presence of a retained foreign body. Also, in most sutured wounds that become infected, the sutures must be removed to allow drainage. If a wound exhibits a minor infection, a few sutures, or all of them, may be removed, but grossly infected wounds should be packed open to allow for further drainage. Infection around a suture can lead to the formation of a stitch mark.[113] Infected wounds should be treated with daily cleansing, warm compresses, and antibiotics. Wounds that have been opened should be left to heal by

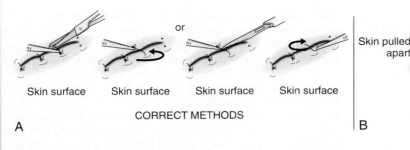

CORRECT METHODS

Skin surface   Skin surface   Skin surface   Skin surface

A

Skin pulled apart

Skin surface

INCORRECT METHOD

B

FIGURE 34–32 Technique for suture removal. Pull should be toward the wound line (*A*) rather than away from it (*B*), which causes the wound to tear apart. After suture removal, support of the wound with surgical tape (Steri-Strips) may be advisable if tension or minor dehiscence is present.

secondary intention, which involves wound contraction, granulation tissue formation, and epithelialization.

Most wound infections can be treated in the outpatient setting with oral antibiotics and follow-up, but each case is individualized. Lymphangitis does not mandate intravenous antibiotics or hospitalization.

Suture Removal

The optimal time for suture removal varies with the location of the wound, the rate of wound healing, and the amount of tension on the wound. Certain areas of the body such as the back of the hand heal slowly, whereas facial or scalp wounds heal rapidly. Speed of wound healing is affected by systemic factors such as malnutrition, neoplasia, or immunosuppression. Therefore, only general guidelines can be given for the timing of suture removal. At the time that suture removal is being considered, one or two sutures may be cut to determine whether the skin edges are sufficiently adherent to allow removal of all the sutures.[5] Removing sutures too early invites wound dehiscence and widening of the scar, whereas leaving sutures in longer than necessary may result in epithelial tracts, infection, and unsightly scarring.[114]

Percutaneous sutures stimulate an inflammatory reaction along the suture track. Factors that determine the severity of stitch marks include the length of time skin stitches are left in place, skin tension, the relationship of the suture to the wound edge, the region of the body, infection, and tendency for keloid formation.[113,115] The skin of the eyelids, palms, and soles and the mucous membranes seldom show stitch marks. In contrast, oily skin and the skin of the back, the sternal area, the upper arms, the lower extremities, the dorsum of the nose, and the forehead are likely to develop the permanent imprints of suture material on the skin surface.[113]

If sutures are removed within 7 days, generally no discernible needle puncture or stitch mark will persist.[115] However, at 6 days, the wound is held together by a small amount of fibrin and cells and has minimal strength.[68] The tensile strength of most wounds at this time is adequate to hold the wound edges together, but only if there are no appreciable dynamic or static skin forces pulling the wound apart.[5] Minimal trauma to an unsupported wound at this point could cause dehiscence. The clinician should decide on the proper time of suture removal after weighing these various factors. If early suture removal is necessary (such as on the face), wound repair can be maintained with strips of surgical skin tape. The key to wound tensile strength after suture removal is an adequate deep tissue layer closure.

Some general guidelines exist for suture removal. Sutures on the face should be removed on the 5th day after the injury or alternate sutures should be removed on the 3rd day and the remainder on the 5th day. On the extremities and the anterior aspect of the trunk, sutures should be left in place for approximately 7 days to prevent wound disruption. Sutures

on the scalp, back, feet, and hands and over the joints must remain in place for 10 to 14 days, even though permanent stitch marks may result.[113] Some clinicians recommend the removal of sutures in eyelid lacerations as early as 72 hours to avoid epithelialization along the suture tract, with subsequent cyst formation.[116]

Removing sutures is usually relatively simple. The wound should be cleansed, and any remaining crust overlying the wound surface or surrounding the sutures should be removed. The skin is wiped with an alcohol swab. Each stitch is cut with a scissors or the tip of a No. 11 scalpel blade at a point close to the skin surface on one side. The suture is grasped on the opposite side with forceps and is pulled across the wound (Fig. 34–32). The amount of exposed suture dragged through the suture tract is thereby minimized. It is difficult to remove sutures with very short ends. At the time of suture placement, the length of the suture ends should generally equal the distance between sutures to permit easy grasping of the suture during subsequent removal while avoiding entanglement during the knotting of adjacent sutures.

Once the skin sutures are removed, the width of the scar increases gradually over the next 3 to 5 weeks unless it is supported. Support is provided by previously placed subcutaneous stitches that brought the skin edges into apposition or by the application of skin tape. A nonabsorbable subcuticular suture can be left in place for 2 to 3 weeks to provide continued support for the wound. Although complications such as closed epithelial sinuses, cysts, or internal tracts can occur from prolonged use of this stitch, they are unusual and can be avoided by the placement of a buried subcuticular stitch using an absorbable suture.[14]

Small stitch abscesses may occur in wounds in which sutures remain more than 7 to 10 days. Localized stitch abscesses generally resolve after removal of the sutures and application of warm compresses and without antibiotics.

If time and effort have been invested in a cosmetic closure of the face, the repair should be protected with skin tape after the skin sutures have been removed. Wound contraction and scar widening continue for 42 days after the injury.[68] Because the desired result is a scar of minimal width, the tape can be used as long as 5 weeks after suture removal. With exposure to sunlight, scars in their first 4 months redden to a greater extent than surrounding skin. In exposed cosmetic areas and when prolonged exposure to the sun is anticipated, appropriate sun protection strategies should be used (hat) or consideration of the use of a sunscreen containing para-aminobenzoic acid (PABA).

COMPLICATIONS

There are several reasons why wounds fail to heal; some are related to decisions made at the time of wound closure, and others are consequences of later events. Some of the impediments to healing include ischemia or necrosis of tissue, hematoma formation, prolonged inflammation caused by foreign material, excessive tension on skin edges, and immunocompromising systemic factors. A primary cause of delayed healing is wound infection. Wound cleaning and débridement, atraumatic and aseptic handling of tissues, and the use of protective dressings minimize this complication. Inversion of the edges of a wound during closure produces a more noticeable scar, whereas skillful technique can convert a jagged, contaminated wound into a fine, inapparent scar. The patient's actions also affect wound healing. Delay in seeking treatment for an injury may significantly affect the ultimate outcome of the wound. Furthermore, in the first few days after an injury, the patient must take responsibility for protecting the wound from contamination, further trauma, and swelling.

Infection is probably the most common cause of dehiscence. If the patient is careless or unlucky, reinjury can reopen a wound despite the protection of a thick dressing. If the suture size is too small, the stitch may break. A stitch that is too fine or tied too tightly may cut through friable tissue and pull out. Knots that have not been tied carefully may unravel. The suture material may be extruded or absorbed too rapidly. Finally, if a stitch is removed too early (i.e., before tissues regain adequate tensile strength), the wound loses needed support and falls open. If the wound edges show signs of separating at the time of suture removal, alternate stitches can be left in place and the entire length of the wound supported by strips of adhesive tape.

The final appearance of a scar is determined by several factors. Infection, tissue necrosis, and keloid formation widen a scar. Wounds located in sebaceous skin or oriented 90° to dynamic or static skin tension lines result in wide scars.

Miscellaneous Aspects of Wound Care

Traumatic wounds are created by a wide variety of mechanisms, and clinicians must sometimes adjust wound management techniques to match special circumstances.

Puncture Wounds

The approach to specific puncture wounds is discussed in other sections, but a few caveats are repeated here. By definition, the entire depth of a puncture wound cannot be entirely visualized. As a consequence of its narrow configuration, it is usually impossible to completely clean a puncture wound. In fact, it may be counterproductive to attempt to do so in some areas of the body. Attempting to irrigate the track of a puncture wound by inserting a needle into the depths of the wound and forcibly injecting irrigating solution has the potential to disseminate contamination and increase soft tissue swelling. Unfortunately, if gross contamination remains in a puncture wound, it is unlikely that antibiotics will prevent or totally treat an infection. This leaves the clinician with the reality that many puncture wounds usually do quite well with minimal intervention, whereas others do quite poorly because of their inaccessibility to wound cleaning techniques. "Coring out" a puncture wound with a conical excision is an option if gross contamination or infection is present. A more effective method of exposing the length of the puncture wound (and concealed foreign bodies) is to incise the skin and cutaneous tissue over the tract, *converting a puncture into a linear laceration.* The success of this method depends on the depth of the puncture wound, the thickness of adipose tissue, and the presence of underlying structures.

It may be impossible to predict the outcome of most puncture wounds on the first encounter. These limitations, and the importance of reevaluation of the wound in 2 to 3 days, should be discussed with the patient.

Gunshot Wounds

A subset of gunshot wounds may be definitively handled in the ED, with outpatient follow-up. Studies by Ordog and colleagues[117,118] documented a very low infection rate in gunshot wounds treated with standard wound care on an outpatient basis, even when the missile was left in place and minor fractures were present. Because most gunshot wounds are puncture wounds, minimal deep wound cleaning is possible. Superficial soft tissue wounds with entrance and exit wounds in proximity may be débrided by passage of a sterile gauze back and forth through the wound track (Fig. 34–33).

Animal Bites

Many aspects of the treatment of animal bites are controversial and no universal standards exist. Most bites are caused by dogs or cats that are family pets. Numerous organisms can be cultured from the infected bite wound caused by a dog or cat, and cultures may guide antibiotic therapy.[103] Wound cultures taken at the time of an animal bite are worthless. The gram-negative rod *Pasteurella multocida*, as well as *S. aureus* and *Streptococcus viridans*, are common culprits in bite wound infections. Cat bites, which are usually puncture wounds that cannot be completely cleaned, frequently become infected with *Pasteurella*. The incidence of infection after thoroughly cleaned dog bite lacerations may not be significantly greater than lacerations in general. Consequently, some clinicians have advocated the primary closure of large dog bite lacerations that are centrally located on the body; however, markedly contused lacerations are good candidates for delayed primary closure (see Fig. 34–25B).

The use of prophylactic antibiotics for animal bites is controversial (see earlier discussion). The best way to approach bite wounds is simply to adhere to the basic principles of wound care. No specific intervention has been demonstrated to be superior for the preparation of bite wounds. Care should be taken to search for underlying fractures or tooth fragments in deep animal bites. When a wound results from the bite or scratch of either a wild or a domestic animal, prophylaxis against rabies also must be considered (Tables 34–3 and 34–4).

Serious Wound Infections

Most wound infections are easily recognized and can be treated in the outpatient setting with oral antibiotics, suture removal, a consideration for a retained foreign body, and a common sense follow-up schedule. Systemic complaints (fever, malaise, nausea), worsening infection in follow-up, an unreliable patient, or an immunocompromised patient may prompt impatient treatment. Some infections, such as a subgaleal infection in a scalp laceration, can be quite serious and require prompt aggressive therapy (Fig. 34–34).

Digital Nerves. Numbness in the area of digital innervation, concomitant injury to a digital artery (flash/pulsating bleeding), or an electric shock sensation when exploring a laceration should alert the clinician to a possible digital nerve injury. If there is uncertainty about nerve injury, the diagnosis can be established at the time of a follow-up visit. However,

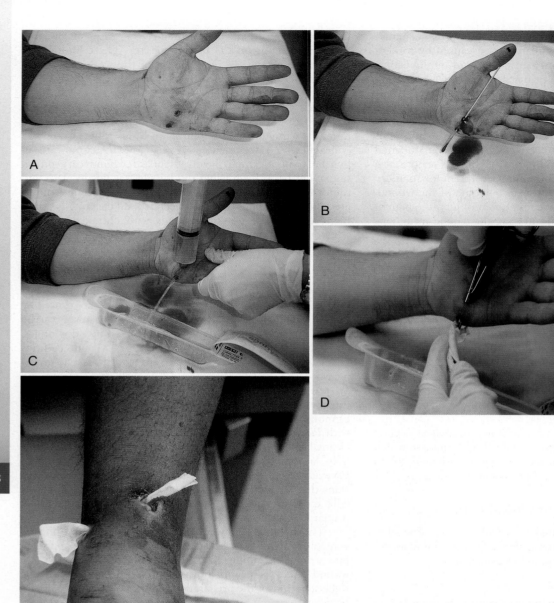

FIGURE 34–33 Patients with minor gunshot wounds may be treated as outpatients, even when bullet fragments remain and there are minor fractures. *A* and *B,* This through-and-through injury traversed the hypothenar eminence. No bullet remained and no bones were involved. *C,* Usually, it is impossible to irrigate a puncture wound, but in this case, note the saline at the exit site. *D,* After the entrance wound is débrided of the powder burn, an instrument is passed through the wound. The instrument grasps gauze packing and pulls it into the wound. The gauze was pulled *back and forth to débride the wound tract*. Clean packing is then similarly placed. *E,* For a similarly cleaned gunshot wound of the leg, the gauze pack is left in the track for 48 hr. No antibiotics were given, the pack was removed at wound check in 48 hr, and the patient did well.

lacerations of digital arteries that impair distal circulation must be identified early during the initial evaluation.

Débridement of hand and finger lacerations should be minimal, and wound preparation should be gentle yet thorough. Digital nerves that are transected distal to the metacarpophalangeal joint may be candidates for surgical repair. It is unclear at which point along the course of a digital nerve a transection can be repaired successfully, so proper referral to a hand specialist is essential. Often, injuries proximal to the distal interphalangeal joint are not repaired, but many other factors will influence operative decisions. Repair of a digital

nerve will frequently result in return of good sensory function (but it takes months), and repair can prevent painful neuromas from developing. Most hand surgeons will not repair digital nerves at the time of initial presentation. Instead, they advise wound cleaning, skin closure, splinting, and outpatient follow-up in 24 to 36 hours, followed by delayed nerve repair.

Accidental Soft Tissue Injection with an EpiPen

An EpiPen provides self-injected subcutaneous epinephrine (0.3 or 0.15 mg) for emergency treatment of anaphylaxis.

TABLE 34–3 Rabies Postexposure Prophylaxis Guide—July 1999

The following recommendations are only a guide. In applying them, take into account the animal species involved, the circumstances of the bite or other exposure, the vaccination status of the animal, and the presence of rabies in the region. Local or state public health officials should be consulted if questions arise about the need for rabies prophylaxis.

Animal Species	Condition of Animal at Time of Attack	Treatment of Exposed Person*
Domestic		
Dog and cat	Healthy and available for 10 days of observation.	None, unless animal develops rabies.† Local wound healing should be included under the treatment of exposed person for each category.
	Rabid or suspected rabid.	RIG‡ and HDCV.
	Unknown (escaped).	Consult public health officials. If treatment is indicated, give RIG‡ and HDCV.
Wild		
Skunk, bat, fox, coyote, raccoon, bobcat, and other carnivores	Regard as rabid unless proved negative by laboratory tests.§	RIG‡ and HDCV.
Other		
Livestock, rodents, and lagomorphs (rabbits and hares)	Consider individually. Local and state public health officials should be consulted on questions about the need for rabies prophylaxis. Bites of squirrels, hamsters, guinea pigs, gerbils, chipmunks, rats, mice, other rodents, rabbits, and hares almost never call for antirabies prophylaxis.	

*All bites and wounds should immediately be thoroughly cleansed with soap and water. If antirabies treatment is indicated, both rabies immune globulin (RIG) and human diploid cell rabies vaccine (HDCV) should be given as soon as possible, regardless of the interval from exposure. Local reactions to vaccines are common and do not contraindicate continuing treatment. Discontinue vaccine if fluorescent antibody tests of the animal are negative.

†During the usual holding period of 10 days, begin treatment with RIG and HDCV at first sign of rabies in a dog or cat that has bitten someone. The symptomatic animal should be killed immediately and tested.

‡If RIG is not available, use antirabies serum, equine (ARS). Do not use more than the recommended dosage.

§The animal should be killed and tested as soon as possible. Holding for observation is not recommended. Vaccination may be discontinued if immunofluorescence tests of the animal are negative.

From Leads from Centers for Disease Control and Prevention: Human rabies prevention—United States, 1999: Recommendations of the Advisory Committee on Immunization Practices (ACIP). MMWR Morb Mortal Wkly Rep 48(RR-1), 1999. Available at http://www.cdc.gov/mmwr/preview/mmwrhtml/00056176.htm

TABLE 34–4 Rabies Postexposure Prophylaxis Schedule, United States

Vaccination Status	Treatment	Regimen*
Not previously vaccinated	Local wound cleansing	All postexposure treatment should begin with immediate thorough cleansing of all wounds with soap and water.
	RIG	20 IU/kg of body weight; if anatomically feasible, up to half the dose should be infiltrated around wounds and the rest administered IM in gluteal area; Note: RIG should not be administered in the same syringe or into the same anatomic site as vaccine, because RIG may partially suppress active production of antibody. No more than the recommended dose should be given
	Vaccine	HDCV or RVA, 1 mL, IM (**deltoid area**†), one each on days 0, 3, 7, 14, and 28.
Previously vaccinated‡	Local wound cleansing	All postexposure treatment should begin with immediate thorough cleansing of all wounds with soap and water.
	RIG	RIG should not be administered.
	Vaccine	HDCV or RVA, 1 mL, IM (deltoid area†), one each on days 0 and 3.

*These regimens are applicable for all age groups, including children.

†The deltoid area is the only acceptable site of vaccination for adults and older childen. For younger children, the outer aspect of the thigh may be used. Vaccine should never be administered in the gluteal area.

‡Any person with a history of preexposure vaccination with HDCV or RVA, prior postexposure prophylaxis with HDCV or RVA, or previous vaccination with any other type of rabies vaccine and a documented history of antibody response to the prior vaccination.

HDCV, human diploid cell rabies vaccine; IM, intramuscularly; RIG, rabies immune globulin; RVA, rabies vaccine, adsorbed. Four formulations of three inactivated rabies vaccines are currently licensed for preexposure and postexposure prophylaxis in the United States.

From the Recommendations of the Immunization Practices Advisory Committee. MMWR Morb Mortal Wkly Rep 40(RR-3):1, 1991.

Occasionally, the device is inadvertently discharged, usually into a finger, and intense distal vasospasm is produced (Fig. 34–35). The patient presents with a blanched finger and minor sensory disturbances. The natural history of untreated vasospasm is unknown, and although ischemia may last for an hour or two, likely it is self-limited given the pharmacology of epinephrine. Digit amputation from this event has not been reported. Nonetheless, clinicians may be faced with an obviously ischemic finger, and intervention is considered. Local heat and nitroglycerine ointment have been tried, but are of no proven benefit. Placing a pulse oximeter on the finger tip can indicate the degree of resultant hypoxia, an indirect

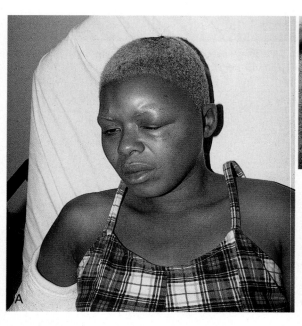

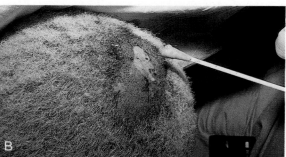

FIGURE 34–34 Scalp lacerations rarely become infected because of the excellent blood supply to the area. *A,* This patient presented with a painful swollen area under a sutured scalp laceration and impressive forehead and facial swelling from a laceration on top of the head. It was originally thought to be a hematoma. *B,* Removal of sutures revealed frank pus and an extensive subgaleal abscess, requiring drainage and intrvenous antibiotics. This infection can drain into the brain, face, neck, or mediastinum.

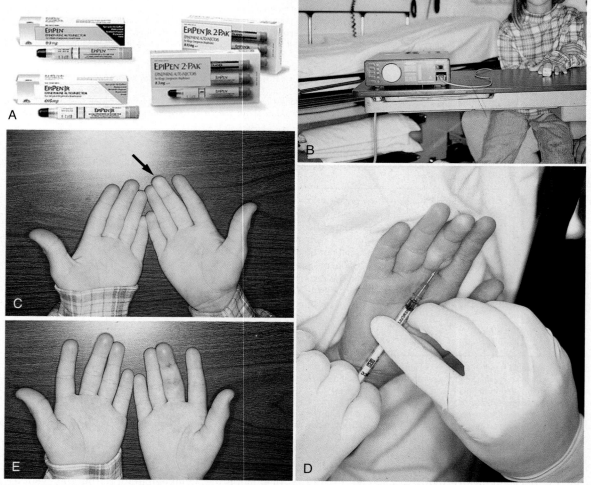

FIGURE 34–35 *A,* The EpiPen and EpiPen, Jr. Each injector issues only one dose of epinephrine, each one delivers a total volume of 0.3 mL. The adult version injects 0.3 mg of epinephrine (it contains epinephrine in a 1 : 1000 concentration so there is 1 mg of epinephrine in 1 mL of volume). The EpiPen, Jr., injects a similar 0.3-mL volume but uses a 1 : 2000 dilution of epinephrine, so only 0.15 mg of epinephrine is delivered with the injection. Accidental discharge of an EpiPen into a finger will usually cause intense distal vasoconstriction. *B,* A pulse oximitry probe on the affected digit assesses circulation and response to treatment. *C,* A blanched finger from an EpiPen injection on the volar surface of the third finger (*arrow*). *D,* Infiltration of phentolamine: lidocaine at the site of epinephrine injection. *E,* A hyperemic finger results in 5–10 min. No further injections should be required.

quantification of ischemia, and can likewise be used to assess reversal therapy.

Injecting the digit with the α-adrenergic antagonist phentolamine (Regitine) will immediately and permanently reverse the ischemia and can be safely initiated in the ED. A 5-mg vial of phentolamine is reconstituted and diluted 1:1 with lidocaine 1% plain or saline:phentolamine. Inject a small aliquot of the mixture with a 25- to 27-gauge needle. Either a digital block or directly injecting the reversal agent into the site of epinephrine injection has been described. Injecting the actual site of penetration is intuitively the best option, but no studies have been performed. Within 5 to 10 minutes, the ischemia is reversed, and no further action is required.[119,120]

 REFERENCES CAN BE FOUND ON EXPERT CONSULT

CHAPTER **35**

Methods of Wound Closure

Richard L. Lammers

Once the decision to close a wound has been made, the clinician must select the closure technique best suited for the location and configuration of the wound. The most commonly used techniques include use of tape, tissue adhesive, metal staples, and sutures. All traumatic wounds should be cleaned, and wounds containing devitalized tissue should be débrided before closure (see Chapter 34, Principles of Wound Management).

Self-inflicted wounds can present to the emergency department (ED) with a vague or inaccurate history. Characteristic self-mutilation patterns are depicted in Figure 35–1. No specific treatment is required other than recognizing these patterns of injury

WOUND TAPE

Surgical tape strips are now routinely used to close simple wounds. Tape strips can be applied by health care personnel in many settings, including EDs, operating rooms, clinics, and first aid stations. Advantages include ease of application, reduced need for local anesthesia, more evenly distributed wound tension, no residual suture marks, minimal skin reaction, no need for suture removal, superiority for some grafts and flaps, and suitability for use under plaster casts. One main advantage of wound tapes is their greater resistance to wound infection compared with standard sutures and wound staples.[1-4]

Background and Tape Comparisons

Currently, there are several brands of tapes with differing porosity, flexibility, strength, and configuration. Steri-Strips (3M Corporation, St. Paul, MN) are microporous tapes with ribbed backing. They are porous to air and water, and the ribbed backing provides extra strength. Cover-Strips (Beiersdorf, South Norwalk, CT) are woven in texture and have a high degree of porosity. They allow not only air and water but also wound exudates to pass through the tape. Shur-Strip (Deknatel, Inc, Floral Park, NY) is a nonwoven microporous tape. Clearon (Ethicon, Inc, Somerville, NJ) is a synthetic plastic tape whose backing contains longitudinal parallel serrations to permit gas and fluid permeability. An iodoform-impregnated Steri-Strip (3M Corporation) is intended to further retard infection without sensitization to iodine.[3] Other tape products include Curi-Strip (Kendall, Boston), Nichi-Strip (Nichiban Co., Ltd, Tokyo), Cicagraf (Smith & Nephew, London), and Suture Strip (Genetic Laboratories, St. Paul, MN).

Scientific studies of wound closure tapes provide some comparisons of products. Koehn[5] showed that the Steri-Strip tapes maintained adhesiveness about 50% longer than Clearon tape. Rodeheaver and coworkers[6] compared Shur-Strip, Steri-Strip, and Clearon tape in terms of breaking strength, elongation, shear adhesion, and air porosity. The tapes were tested in both dry and wet conditions. The Steri-Strip tape was found to have about twice the breaking strength of the other two tapes in both dry and wet conditions; there was minimal loss of strength in all tapes when wetted. The Shur-Strip tapes showed approximately two to three times the elongation of the other tapes at the breaking point, whether dry or wet. Shear adhesion (amount of force required to dislodge the tape when a load is applied in the place of contact) was slightly better for the Shur-Strip tape than for the Steri-Strip tape and approximately 50% better than for the Clearon tape. Of these three wound tapes, the investigators considered Shur-Strips to be superior for wound closure.

One comprehensive study of wound tapes compared Curi-Strip, Steri-Strip, Nichi-Strip, Cicagraf, Suture Strip, and Suture Strip Plus.[7] All tapes were 12 mm wide except for Nichi-Strip, which was 15 mm. Each tape was compared for breaking strength, elongation under stress, air porosity, and adhesiveness. Curi-Strip, Cicagraf, and Steri-Strip exhibited equivalent dry breaking strengths. However, when wet (a condition that can occur in the clinical setting), Cicagraf outperformed all tapes. All of the tested tapes had similar elongation-under-stress profiles with the exception of Suture Strip Plus. This tape did not resist elongation under low or high forces. Excessive elongation may allow wound dehiscence. Nichi-Strip was the most porous to air, and Cicagraf was almost vapor-impermeable. Nichi-Strip and Curi-Strip had the best adherence to untreated skin. When the skin was treated with tincture of benzoin, however, Steri-Strip dramatically outperformed all other products. When all study parameters were considered, Nichi-Strip, Curi-Strip, and Steri-Strip achieved the highest overall performance rankings.

Indications

The primary indication for tape closure is a superficial straight laceration under little tension. If necessary, tension can be reduced by placing deep closures. Areas particularly suited for tape closure are the forehead, chin, malar eminence, thorax, and nonjoint areas of the extremities. Tape also may be preferred for wounds in anxious children when suture placement is not essential. In young children who are likely to remove tapes, tape closures must be protected with an overlying gauze bandage.

In experimental wounds inoculated with *Staphylococcus aureus*, tape-closed wounds resisted infection better than wounds closed with nylon sutures.[2] Tape closures work well under plaster casts when superficial suture removal would be delayed. Tape closures effectively hold flaps and grafts in place, particularly over fingers, the flat areas of the extremities, and the trunk (Fig. 35–2).[3,4] Wounds on the pretibial area are difficult to close, especially in the elderly because of tissue atrophy. Wound tapes provide an alternative to suture closure in this situation. Tape closures can be applied to wounds after early suture removal, particularly on the face, to maintain wound edge approximation while reducing the chance of permanent suture mark scarring. Finally, because of the minimal skin tension created by tapes, they can be used on skin that has been compromised by vascular insufficiency or altered by prolonged use of steroids.

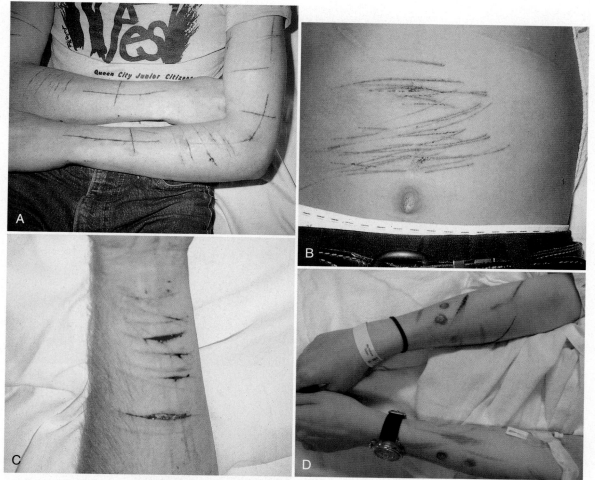

Figure 35–1 *A–C,* These patients had minor lacerations and were brought to the emergency department (ED) simply for tetanus prophylaxis or for other vague or unrelated reasons. Obviously, these are classic self-inflicted wounds, representative of serious underlying psychiatric issues, requiring further evaluation. *D,* These cigarette burns are also self-inflicted, but the patient initially stated that she burned them on grease while cooking.

Contraindications

Tape closures have disadvantages. Tape does not work well on wounds under significant tension or on wounds that are irregular, on concave surfaces, or in areas of marked tissue laxity. In many cases, tape does not provide satisfactory wound edge apposition without concurrent underlying deep closures. Tape does not stick well to naturally moist areas, such as in the axilla, the palms of the hands, the soles of the feet, and the perineum. Tape also has difficulty adhering to wounds that will have secretions, copious exudates, or persistent bleeding. They are of little value on lax and intertriginous skin, in the scalp, and in other areas with high concentration of hair follicles. Tape strips are also at risk for premature removal by young children.

Tapes should not be tightly placed circumferentially around digits because they have insufficient ability to stretch or lengthen. If placed circumferentially, the natural wound edema of an injured digit can make the tape act like a constricting band, which can lead to ischemia and possible necrosis of the digit. Semicircular or spiral placement techniques should be used if digits are to be taped.

Equipment

For a simple tape closure, the required equipment includes forceps and tape of the proper size. Most taping can be done in the ED with ¼-x 3-inch strips. In wounds larger than 4 cm, however, ½-inch-wide strips provide greater strength. Most companies manufacture strips up to 1 inch wide and up to 4 inches long.

Procedure

Proper wound preparation, irrigation, débridement, and hemostasis must precede tape closures. Fine hair may be cut short or shaved, and the area of the tape application is thoroughly dried to ensure proper adhesion. Attempting to apply tapes to a wet area or over a wound that is slowly oozing blood will usually result in failure of the tapes to stick to the skin. On fingers, tapes can be applied to a wound that is kept dry by a tourniquet temporarily placed at the base of the finger (see Fig. 35–2G).

The technique of applying tapes is shown in Figure 35–3. After the wound has been dried, a liquid adhesive such as

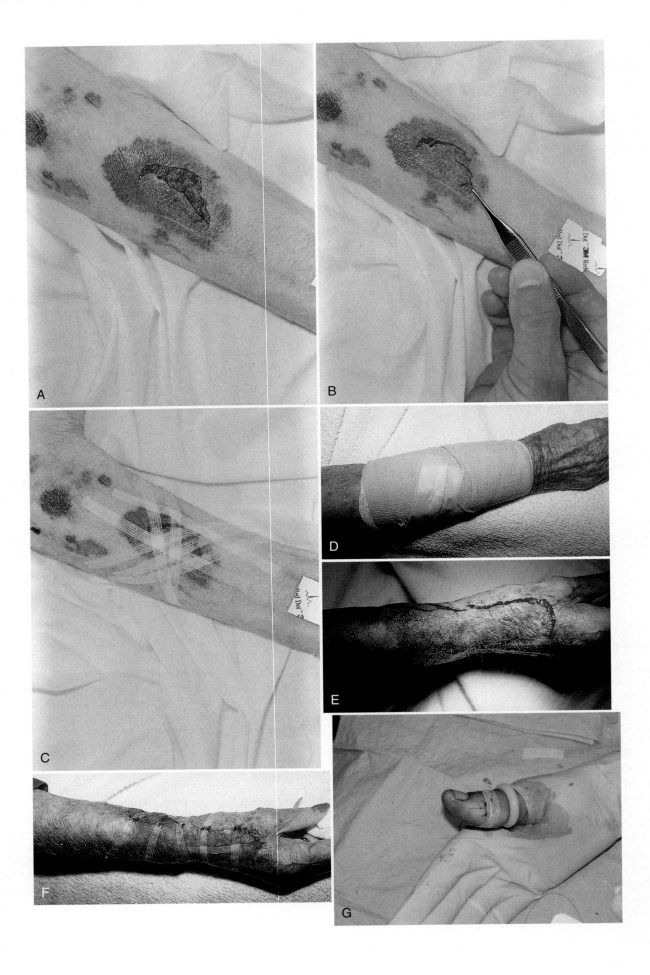

Figure 35–2   *A,* A skin avulsion in the elderly following minor trauma is an ideal wound to close with closure tapes, as such injuries cannot be closed with sutures. The goal is to provide approximation of the avulsed skin and apply pressure to avoid skin flap movement or fluid accumulation under the avulsion. Tissue glue can augment this procedure. An elderly woman who was on steroids had extremely thin skin and suffered a skin avulsion that could not be replaced with sutures. *B,* The skin edges are uncurled, stretched, and anatomically replaced. *C,* The wound should heal when closure tapes keep the skin in place. Tissue glue (Dermabond®) was also dabbed on various parts of the edges, allowing for fluid egress. *D,* A compression dressing, such as an elastic bandage or a Dome paste (Unna) boot dressing, can be applied to minimize flap movement and decrease fluid buildup under the flap. *E* and *F,* Large avulsion replaced with Steri-Strips and tissue glue. Tape should be placed in a semicircular or spiral pattern on digits to avoid constriction. *G,* After suturing this proximal-based flap, Steri-Strips are applied under a tourniquet, compressing the flap to arrest flap motion and lessen fluid buildup.

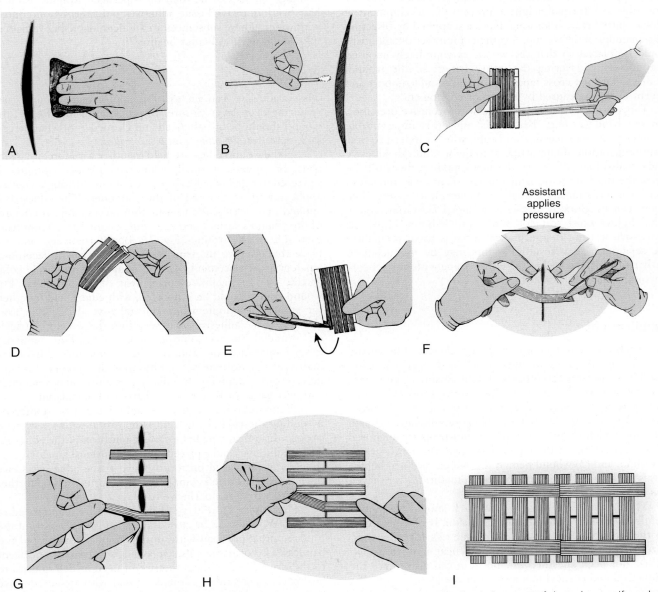

Figure 35–3   Proper technique for application of tapes for skin closure. *A,* After wound preparation (and placement of deep closures, if needed), dry the skin thoroughly at least 2 inches around the wound. Failure to dry the skin and failure to obtain perfect hemostasis are common causes of failure of tapes to stick to the skin. *B,* If desired, apply a thin coating of tincture of benzoin around the wound to enhance tape adhesiveness. Benzoin should not enter the eye, as it causes pain if it seeps into an open wound. *C,* Cut the tapes to the desired length before removing the backing. *D,* The tapes are attached to a card with perforated tabs on both ends. Gently peel the end tab from the tapes. *E,* Use forceps to peel the tape off the card backing. Pull directly backward, not to the side. *F,* Place half of the first tape at the midportion of the wound; secure firmly in place. *G,* Gently but firmly appose the opposite side of the wound, using the free hand or forceps. If an assistant is not available, the operator can approximate the wound edges. The tape should be applied by bisecting the wound until the wound is closed satisfactorily. *H,* Wound margins are completely apposed without totally occluding the wound. *I,* Additional supporting tapes are placed approximately 2.5 cm from the wound and parallel to the wound direction. Taping in this manner prevents the skin blistering that may occur at tape ends.

tincture of benzoin or Mastisol can be applied to the skin adjacent to the wound to increase tape adhesion.[2] All tapes come in presterilized packages and can be opened directly onto the operating field. Tapes should be handled with gloved hands. With backing still attached, tapes are cut to the desired length or long enough to allow for approximately 2 to 3 cm of overlap on each side of the wound. After the end tab is removed, the tape is gently removed from its backing with forceps by pulling straight back. Do not pull to the side, because the tape will curl and will be difficult to apply to the wound. One half of the tape is securely placed at the midportion of the wound. The opposite wound edge is gently but firmly apposed to its counterpart. The second half of the tape is then applied. The wound edges should be as close together as possible and at equal height to prevent the development of a linear, pitted scar. Additional tapes are applied by bisecting the remainder of the wound. A sufficient number of tape strips should be placed so that the wound is completely apposed without totally covering the entire length of the wound. Finally, additional cross tapes are placed to add support and prevent blistering caused by unsupported tape ends.[1]

Taped wounds are not covered with occlusive dressings. Adhesive bandages (e.g., Band-Aids) and other impermeable dressings promote excessive moisture, which can lead to premature separation of tape strips from the wound. An adhesive bandage also may adhere to the tapes, pulling them off the skin at the time of the dressing change. Tapes may remain in place for approximately 2 weeks or longer, if necessary. The patient can be allowed to clean the taped laceration gently with a slightly moist, soft cloth after 24 to 48 hours. However, if excessive wetting or mechanical force is used, premature tape separation may result. Patients may be instructed to gently trim curled edges of the closure tape with fine scissors to avoid premature loss of the tape.

Complications

Complications are uncommon with tape closure. The wound infection rate in clean wounds closed with tape compares favorably with rates for other standard closures.[1] However, some investigators believe that tape closure leads to inferior cosmetic results.[8] Premature tape separation occurs in approximately 3% of cases.[6] Other complications include (1) skin blistering, which occurs if the tape is not properly anchored with the cross strip or the tape is stretched too tightly across the wound, and (2) wound hematoma, which results if hemostasis is inadequate. Tape may loosen prematurely over shaved areas as hair grows back.

When tincture of benzoin is used, it should be applied carefully to the surrounding, uninjured skin. If spillage occurs into the wound, the wound is at higher risk for infection.[9] Benzoin vapors cause pain when applied near an open wound that has not been anesthetized. Benzoin can also injure the conjunctival and corneal membranes of the eye.

Summary

Modern tape products and techniques serve a valuable role in minor wound management of ED patients. Tape closure in selected wounds is as successful as suture closure.[1,10] Closure tapes should be considered for superficial wounds in cosmetically unimportant areas and for wounds on relatively flat surfaces that are too wide for simple dressings but do not require sutures.

TISSUE ADHESIVE (TISSUE GLUE)

Tissue adhesive (also called tissue "glue") provides a simple, rapid method of wound closure. Tissue adhesive has been approved for use in the United States since 1998. Two types of tissue adhesives are available: N-2-octylcyanoacrylate (Dermabond, Ethicon, Inc) and N-butyl-2-cyanoacrylate (Indermil, Tyco Healthcare Group LP). Dermabond and Indermil are packaged in sterile, single-use ampules. These bonding agents can be used on superficial wounds, even in hair-bearing areas. Tissue adhesives polymerizes on contact with water. These substances are biodegradable but remain in the wound until well after healing.[11]

Procedure

Tissue adhesive can be used to approximate wounds not requiring deep-layer closure. In preparation for closure, the wound should be anesthetized and cleaned and, when necessary, débrided. *Bleeding must be controlled.*

As the wound edges are held together with forceps, gauze pads, or fingers, a small, cylindrical plastic container is squeezed to expel droplets of tissue adhesive through a cotton applicator tip at the end of the container. The adhesive is applied in at least three to four thin layers along the length of the wound's surface and extending about 5 to 10 mm from each side of the wound (Fig. 35–4). Alternatively, one can place the adhesive in strips perpendicular to the laceration (analogous to placement of closure tapes). The purple color of the solution facilitates placement of the droplets. The wound edges should be supported, with edges held together, for at least 1 minute while the adhesive dries. The low-viscosity tissue adhesives may seep into the wound or trickle off rounded surfaces during application. This tendency toward migration or "runoff" can be minimized by using high-viscosity adhesives,[12] positioning the wound horizontally, or slowly applying the adhesive. Runoff can be contained with wet gauze or by creating a barrier of petrolatum.

Wound closures with tissue adhesive can be reinforced by pulling the wound edges into apposition with a few strips of porous surgical tape before the application of the adhesive. Tissue adhesive can be placed on top of surgical tape, but tape should not be placed on top of dried tissue adhesive. Once the adhesive has dried completely, the closure can be further protected with a nonocclusive bandage.

The primary advantage of tissue adhesive is the speed of closure. Wounds can be closed in as little as one sixth of the time required for repair with sutures. Application is rapid and painless. Use of tissue adhesive avoids suture marks adjacent to the wound and reduces the risk of needle stick injuries to health care personnel. Wounds closed with tissue adhesive have less tensile strength than sutured wounds in the first 4 days,[13,14] but 1 week after closure, the tensile strength and overall degree of inflammation in wounds closed with tissue adhesive were equivalent to those closed with sutures.[11,15] Cosmetic results are similar to those obtained with suture repair.[14,16–22] Tissue adhesive serves as its own wound dressing and has an antimicrobial effect against gram-positive organisms.[23,24] The material sloughs off in 5 to 10 days, thereby

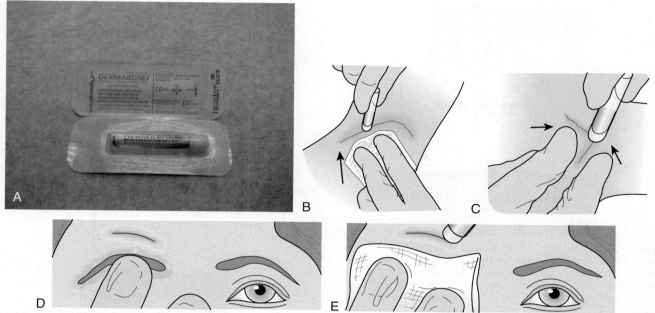

Figure 35–4 *A,* Tissue adhesive, 2-octylcyanoacrylate, comes in a variety of commercially available dispensers. *B,* To apply tissue adhesive (glue), the laceration must be dry. High-viscosity glue limits runoff. *C,* Bring the edges together, using a gauze pad or fingers, and apply glue in a few layers, with drying between applications. Do not get the glue in the eyes. *D,* Near the eye, keep the patient supine and *tilt the head* to avoid eye contamination and apply a layer of petroleum jelly as a barrier to the glue entering the eye. Do not apply the jelly to the area where the tissue adhesive must adhere. *E,* Alternatively, use a gauze barrier. If the adhesive enters the eye or lids, wipe it off with the gauze and flush with saline. Lids glued shut may be loosened with antibiotic ointment/petroleum jelly. If unsuccessful, tell the patient to shower normally and the eye will open in a few days as the glue sloughs off the lid. Note: *Glue that touches a latex glove, gauze, or plastic instrument (but not vinyl gloves or metal instruments) will glue them to the patient.*

597

saving the patient from a clinician visit. Ointments or occlusive bandages should not be placed on wounds closed with tissue adhesive.

Complications

Percutaneous sutures provide a more secure immediate closure than tissue adhesive.[11] Although tissue adhesive is classified as nontoxic and does not cause a significant foreign body reaction, it should not be placed within the wound cavity.[14,15] If hemostasis is inadequate or an excessive amount of adhesive is applied too quickly, the patient can experience a burning sensation or sustain a local burn from the heat of polymerization. After polymerizing, tissue adhesive can fracture with excessive or repetitive movement. Although gentle rinsing is permitted, if the adhesive is washed or soaked, it will peel off in a few days, before the wound is healed.[14]

If the clinician's gloved fingers, gauze, or plastic instruments contact the tissue adhesive during application, the glove may adhere to the patient's skin. Tissue adhesive can be removed with antibiotic ointment, petrolatum jelly, or more rapidly with acetone.[22] Indermil must be stored under refrigeration.

One risk involving the use of tissue adhesive is its ease of use—clinicians may fail to adequately clean wounds before closure with tissue adhesive.[25] Tissue adhesive should not be used to close infected wounds. If the wound edges cannot be held together without considerable tension, tissue adhesive should not be used.[22] Tissue adhesive should not be used near the eyes, over or near joints, on moist or mucosal surfaces, or on wounds under significant static or dynamic skin tension.

See Figure 35–4 for information on managing eyelids that are accidentally glued shut.

WOUND STAPLES

Background

Automatic stapling devices have become commonplace for closure of surgical incisions and traumatic wounds. Clinical studies of patients with stapled surgical incisions have found no significant differences between stapling and suturing when infection rates, healing outcome, and patient acceptance are compared.[26–31] Wound stapling and nylon suture closure of skin compared favorably in wound tensile strength, complication rates, patient tolerance, efficiency of closure, scar width, color, general appearance, suture or staple marks, infection rates, and cost. In animal models, staples cause less wound inflammation and offer more resistance to infection in contaminated wounds.[32–35]

The most significant advantage of wound stapling over suturing is speed of closure. On average, stapling is three to four times faster than suturing traumatic wounds.[36–38] When clinician time and cost of instruments are considered, the cost difference between stapling and suturing is minimal[37] or favors stapling.[36,39]

Indications and Contraindications

The indications for stapling are limited to relatively linear lacerations with straight, sharp edges located on an extremity, the trunk, or the scalp. Staples may be especially useful for

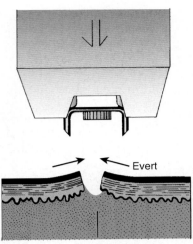

Figure 35–5 The skin edges must be approximated and everted by hand or with forceps before they are secured with staples. Failure to evert the wound edges is a common error that may cause an unacceptable result. *(Adapted with permission from Edlich RF: A Manual for Wound Closure. St. Paul, MN, 3M Medical-Surgical Products, 1979. Reproduced by permission.)*

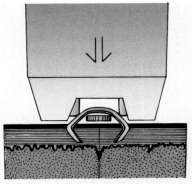

Figure 35–6 When the stapler handle is squeezed, a plunger advances one staple into the wound margins. *(From Edlich RF: A Manual for Wound Closure. St. Paul, MN, 3M Medical-Surgical Products, 1979. Reproduced by permission.)*

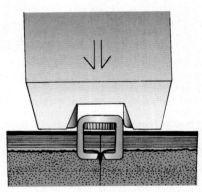

Figure 35–7 An anvil automatically bends the staple to the proper configuration. *(From Edlich RF: A Manual for Wound Closure. St. Paul, MN, 3M Medical-Surgical Products, 1979. Reproduced by permission.)*

superficial scalp lacerations in the agitated or intoxicated patient. Because of their superficial placement in the adult scalp (usually above the galea), staples are not recommended for deep scalp lacerations. Staples may not provide the same hemostasis that is possible with deep sutures. They should not be placed in scalp wounds if computed tomography head scans are to be performed because staples produce scan artifacts. Similarly, staples should not be used if the patient is expected to undergo magnetic resonance imaging, because the powerful magnetic fields may avulse the staples from the skin surface. As they are currently configured and manufactured, staples should not be used on the face, neck, hands, or feet.

Equipment

Standard wound care should precede wound closure. In many cases, when débridement and dermal (deep) closures are unnecessary, only tissue forceps are needed to assist in everting wounds.

Many stapling devices are commercially available. The most versatile and least expensive stapler is the Precise (3M Corporation). Different units that hold between 5 and 25 staples can be purchased. The 10-staple unit will suffice for most lacerations. Other devices include the Proximate 11 (Ethicon, Inc), Cricket (US Surgical, Irvine, CA), and Appose (Davis & Geck, Columbus, OH).

Procedure

Whenever necessary, deep, absorbable sutures are used to close deep fascia and to reduce tension in the superficial fascia and dermal layers. Before stapling, the wound edges should be everted, preferably by a second operator. The assistant precedes the operator along the wound and *everts the wound edges with forceps or pinches the skin with the thumb and forefinger.* Stapling flattened wound edges may precisely place the staple but results in wound inversion. Once the edges are held in eversion, the staple points are gently placed across the wound (Fig. 35–5). When the stapler handle or trigger is squeezed, the staple is advanced automatically into the wound and bent

to the proper configuration (Figs. 35–6 and 35–7). The operator should not press too hard on the skin surface in order to prevent placing the staple too deeply and causing ischemia within the staple loop. When properly placed, the crossbar of the staple is elevated a few millimeters above the skin surface (Fig. 35–8). A sufficient number of staples should be placed to provide proper apposition of the edges of the wound along its entire length. After the wound is stapled, an antibiotic ointment may be applied to minimize dressing adherence, and a sterile dressing is applied. If necessary, the patient can remove the dressing and gently clean the wound in 24 to 48 hours. *Scalp lacerations can be cleansed by showering within a few hours.*

Removal of staples requires a special instrument made available by each manufacturer of stapling devices. The lower jaw of the staple remover is placed under the crossbar (Fig. 35–9), and the handle is squeezed (Fig. 35–10). This action compresses the crossbar and bends the staple outward, thereby releasing the staple points from the skin. Many primary care physicians do not routinely stock the instrument. If the patient is referred for office removal of staples, the patient can be given a disposable staple removal device. Motivated patients can remove their own staples if given the removal device. The interval between staple application and removal is the same as that for standard suture placement and removal. Staples can cause significant scarring if left in place for too long (Fig. 35–11).

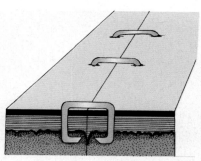

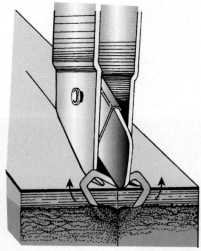

Figure 35–8 Allow a small space to remain between the skin and the crossbar of the staple. Excessive pressure created by placing the staple too deep causes wound edge ischemia as well as pain on removal. Note that the staple bar is 2 to 3 mm above the skin line. *(From Edlich RF: A Manual for Wound Closure. St. Paul, MN, 3M Medical-Surgical Products, 1979. Reproduced by permission.)*

Figure 35–10 When the handle is squeezed gently, the upper jaw compresses the staple and allows it to exit the skin. *(Adapted from Edlich RF: A Manual for Wound Closure. St. Paul, MN, 3M Medical-Surgical Products, 1979. Reproduced by permission.)*

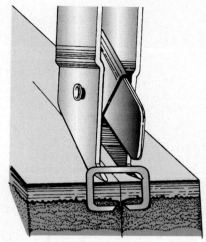

Figure 35–9 Patients should be supplied with a staple remover when being referred to an office for removal or for self-removal. The lower jaw of the staple remover is placed under the crossbar of the staple. *(From Edlich RF: A Manual for Wound Closure. St. Paul, MN, 3M Medical-Surgical Products, 1979. Reproduced by permission.)*

Complications

Patient acceptance and comfort and wound infection and dehiscence with staple-closed wounds are equal to those of sutured wounds. However, removal of staples can be somewhat more uncomfortable than removal of sutures.

A common error during staple insertion is failure to evert the skin edges before stapling (see Fig. 35–11). Eversion avoids the natural tendency of the device to invert the closure. Eversion may be accomplished with forceps or by pinching the skin with the thumb and index finger, a procedure that requires some practice. Staples do cause marks in the skin similar to sutures. In patients who tend to scar more easily, the resulting scar from the staples may be more pronounced than that produced by sutures, especially if the staples are left in place for prolonged periods.

Wound stapling achieves results that are generally comparable with those of sutures for the closure of traumatic, linear lacerations in noncosmetic areas, such as the scalp, trunk, and extremities. Stapling is much faster than suturing. Wound stapling does not differ significantly from suturing in terms of cost, infection rates, wound healing, and patient acceptance. Cosmesis does, however, suffer, especially if the staples are left in too long (see Fig. 35–11*D* and *E*).

SUTURES

In the United States, most traumatic wounds are closed by suturing.

Equipment

Instruments

In addition to the instruments used for débridement, a needle holder and suture scissors are required for suturing. The mechanical performance of disposable needle holders distributed by different surgical instrument companies varies considerably.[40] The size of the needle holder should match the size of the needle selected for suturing—that is, the needle holder should be large enough to hold the needle securely as it is passed through tissue, yet not so large that the needle is crushed or bent by the instrument.

Instruments used to débride a grossly contaminated wound should be discarded and replaced by fresh instruments for the closure. Instruments covered with coagulated blood can be cleansed with hydrogen peroxide, rinsed with sterile saline or water, and then used for suturing.

Suture Materials

A wide variety of suture materials are available. For most wounds that require closure of more than one layer of tissue, the clinician must choose sutures from two general categories: an absorbable suture for deeper, subcutaneous (SQ) layer and a nonabsorbable suture for surface (percutaneous) closure.

Sutures can be described in terms of four characteristics:
1. Composition (i.e., chemical and physical properties).
2. Handling characteristics and mechanical performance.
3. Absorption and reactivity.
4. Size and retention of tensile strength.

Composition. Sutures are made from natural fibers (cotton, silk), from sheep submucosa or beef serosa (plain gut, chromic gut), or from synthetic materials such as nylon (Dermalon, Ethilon, Nurulon, Surgilon), Dacron (Ethiflex, Mersilene), polyester (Ti-Cron), polyethylene (Ethibond),

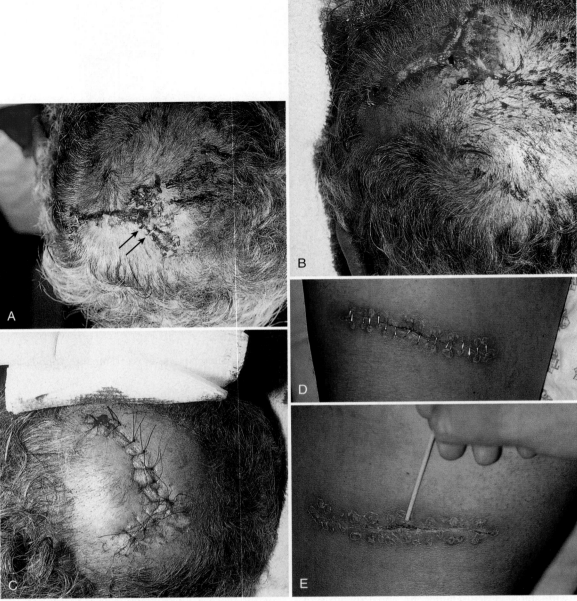

Figure 35–11 *A,* A very poor result occurred when staples (some marked with *arrows*) were used to close this deep scalp laceration. The wound edges were not everted, sections of the skin overlapped significantly, poor hemostasis was obtained, and the galea could not be closed by the superficial staples. The patient did not wash the hair as instructed. Three days later during a wound check, the staples were removed (*B*), and the laceration was closed with 3-0 interrupted nylon sutures (*C*). The clinician should attempt to obtain a cosmetic closure on all scalp lacerations, because as patients lose their hair, a previously hidden, unsightly scar emerges. In general, staples should not be used to close full-thickness scalp lacerations, especially wounds that are actively bleeding. *D,* A sloppy stapling on an extremity with *wound edge inversion* rather than *eversion*. *E,* The staples were kept in too long, giving a poor cosmetic result.

polypropylene (Prolene, Surgilene), polyglycolic acid (Dexon), and polyglactin (Vicryl, coated Vicryl). Stainless steel sutures are rarely, if ever, useful in wound closure in the ED setting because of handling difficulty and fragmentation. Some sutures are made of a single filament (monofilament); others consist of multiple fibers braided together (Table 35–1).[41]

Handling and Performance. Desirable handling characteristics in a suture include smooth passage through tissues, ease in knot tying, and stability of the knot once tied (Table 35–2). Smooth sutures pull through tissues easily, but knots slip more readily. Conversely, sutures with a high coefficient of friction have better knot-holding capacity but are difficult

to slide through tissues. Smooth sutures will loosen after the first throw of a knot is made, and a second throw is needed to secure the first in place. However, the clinician may want to tighten a knot further after the first throw is made. This is difficult with rougher types of sutures.

Multifilament sutures have the best handling characteristics of all sutures, whereas steel sutures have the worst. In terms of performance and handling, significant improvements have been made in the newer absorbable sutures. Gut sutures have many shortcomings, including relatively low and variable strength, a tendency to fray when handled, and stiffness despite being packaged in a softening fluid.[42,43] Multifilament synthetic absorbable sutures are soft and easy to tie and have few problems with knot slippage. Polyglactin 910 (coated Vicryl) sutures have an absorbable lubricant coating. The "frictional drag" of these coated sutures as they are pulled through tissues is less than that of uncoated multifilament materials, and the resetting of knots after the initial throw is much easier. This characteristic allows retightening of a ligature without knotting or breakage and with smooth, even adjustment of suture line tension in running subcuticular stitches.[44] Synthetic monofilament sutures have the troublesome property of "memory"—a tendency of the filament to spring back to its original shape, which causes the knot to slip and unravel. Some nonabsorbable monofilament sutures are coated with polytetrafluorethylene (Teflon) or silicone to reduce their friction. This coating improves the handling characteristics of these monofilaments but results in poorer knot security.[43]

Three square knots will secure a stitch made with silk or other braided, nonabsorbable materials, and four knots are sufficient for synthetic, absorbable, and nonabsorbable monofilament sutures.[45] Five knots are needed for the Teflon-coated synthetic Tevdek.[46] With the use of coated synthetic suture materials, attention to basic principles of knot tying is even more important. An excessive number of throws in a knot weakens the suture at the knot. If the clinician uses square knots (or a surgeon's knot on the initial throw, followed by square knots) that lie down flat and are tied securely, knots will rarely unravel.[47]

Absorption and Reactivity. Sutures that are rapidly degraded in tissues are termed *absorbable*; those that maintain their tensile strength for longer than 60 days are considered *nonabsorbable* (see Table 35–1). Plain gut may be digested by white blood cell lysozymes in 10 to 40 days; chromic gut will last 15 to 60 days. Remnants of both types of sutures, however, have been seen in wounds more than 2 years after their placement.[42,45,48] The Ethicon catgut is rapidly absorbed within 10 to 14 days but with less inflammation than that caused by chromic catgut.[49] Vicryl is absorbed from the wound site within 60 to 90 days[42,45] and Dexon, within 120 to 210 days.[50,51] When placed in the oral cavity, plain gut disappears after 3 to 5 days, chromic gut after 7 to 10 days, and polyglycolic acid after 16 to 20 days.[52] In contrast, SQ silk may not be completely absorbed for as long as 2 years.[45] The rate of absorption of synthetic absorbable sutures is independent of suture size.[50]

Sutures may lose strength and function before they are completely absorbed in tissues. Braided synthetic absorbable sutures lose nearly all of their strength after about 21 days. In contrast, monofilament absorbable sutures (modified polyglycolic acid [Maxon, Davis & Geck] and polydioxanone [PDS, Ethicon]) retain 60% of their strength after 28 days.[53,54] Gut sutures treated with chromium salts (chromic gut) have a prolonged tensile strength; however, all gut sutures retain tensile strength erratically.[42,45] Of the absorbable types of sutures, a wet and knotted polyglycolic acid suture is stronger than a plain or chromic gut suture subjected to the same conditions.[43,55]

Polypropylene remains unchanged in tissue for longer than 2 years after implantation.[56] In comparison testing, sutures made of natural fibers such as silk, cotton, and gut are the weakest; sutures made of Dacron, nylon, polyethylene, and polypropylene are intermediate in tensile strength; and metallic sutures are the strongest.[43] The comparison of suture strength versus wound strength is a measure of the usefulness of a suture. Catgut is stronger than the soft tissue of a wound

601

TABLE 35–1 Examples of Suture Materials

Absorbable Sutures	Nonabsorbable Sutures
Monofilament	
Plain gut	Dermalon (nylon)
Chromic gut	Ethilon (nylon)
PDS (polydioxanone)	Prolene (polypropylene)
Maxon (polyglyconate)	Silk
	Steel
	Surgilene (polypropylene)
	Tevdek (Teflon-coated)
Multifilament	
Dexon (polyglycolic acid)	Ethibond (polyethylene)
Coated Vicryl (polyglactin)	Mersilene (braided polyester)
	Nurulon (nylon)
	Surgilon (nylon)
	TiCron (polyester)

TABLE 35–2 Characteristics of Suture Materials

Suture Material	Knot Security	Tensile Strength	Tissue Reactivity	Duration of Suture Integrity (days)	Tie Ability (Handling)
Absorbable					
Surgical gut	Poor	Fair	Greatest	5–7	Poor
Chromic gut	Fair	Fair	Greatest	10–14	Poor
Coated Vicryl	Good	Good	Minimal	30	Best
Dexon	Best	Good	Minimal	30	Best
PDS	Fair	Best	Least	45–60	Good
Maxon	Fair	Best	Least	45–60	Good
Nonabsorbable					
Ethilon	Good	Good	Minimal		Good
Prolene	Least	Best	Least		Fair
Silk	Best	Least	Greatest		Best

Modified with permission from Hollander J, Singer A: Laceration management. Ann Emerg Med 34:351, 1999.

for no more than 7 days; chromic catgut, Dexon, and Vicryl are stronger for 10 to 21 days; and nylon, wire, and silk are stronger for 20 to 30 days.[57]

All sutures placed within tissue will damage host defenses and provoke inflammation. Even the least reactive suture impairs the ability of the wound to resist infection.[56] The magnitude of the reaction provoked by a suture is related to the quantity of suture material (diameter x total length) placed in the tissue and to the chemical composition of the suture. Among absorbable sutures, polyglycolic acid and polyglactin sutures are least reactive, followed by chromic gut. Nonabsorbable polypropylene is less reactive than nylon or Dacron.[43,58,59] Significant tissue reaction is associated with catgut, silk, and cotton sutures. Absorbable polyglycolic acid sutures are less reactive than those of nonabsorbable silk.[60] Highly reactive materials should be avoided in contaminated wounds.

The chemical composition of sutures is a factor in early infection. The infection rate in experimentally contaminated wounds closed with polyglycolic acid sutures is less than the rate when gut sutures are used.[56] However, other authors have compared plain gut and nonabsorbable nylon sutures for skin closures in children and found comparable cosmetic results and infection rates.[61] Lubricant coatings on sutures do not alter suture reactivity, absorption characteristics, breaking strength, or the risk of infection.[44,56] Multifilament sutures provoke more inflammation and are more likely to produce infection than monofilament sutures if left in place for prolonged periods.[62,63] Monofilament sutures elicit less tissue reaction than do multifilament sutures, and multifilament materials tend to wick up fluid by capillary action. Bacteria that adhere to and colonize sutures can envelop themselves in a glycocalix that protects them from host defenses,[64] or they can "hide" in the interstices of a multifilament suture and, as a result, be inaccessible to leukocytes.[62] PDS provides the advantages of a monofilament suture in an absorbable form, making it a good choice as a subcuticular stitch. Polypropylene sutures have a low coefficient of friction, and subcuticular stitches with this material are easy to pull out.[65]

Size and Strength. Size of suture material (thread diameter) is related to the tensile strength of the suture; threads of greater diameter are stronger. The strength of the suture is proportional to the square of the diameter of the thread. Therefore, a 4-0 suture of any type is larger and stronger than a 6-0 suture. The correct suture size for approximation of a layer of tissue depends on the tensile strength of that tissue. The tensile strength of the suture material should be only slightly greater than that of the tissue, because the magnitude of damage to local tissue defenses is proportional to the amount of suture material placed in the wound.[45,66]

Synthetic absorbable sutures have made the older, natural suture materials unnecessary for most wound closures. Polyglycolic acid (Dexon) and polyglactin 910 (coated Vicryl) have improved handling characteristics, knot security, and tensile strength. Their absorption rates are predictable, and tissue reactivity is minimal.[67,68] The distinct advantages of synthetic nonabsorbable sutures over silk sutures are their greater tensile strength, low coefficient of friction, and minimal tissue reactivity.[56,67] They are extensible, elongating without breaking as the edges of the wound swell in the early postoperative period.[66,67] In contrast with silk sutures, synthetics can be easily and painlessly removed once the wound has healed. The monofilament synthetic suture Novofil has elasticity that allows a stitch to enlarge with wound edema and to return to

its original length once the edema subsides. Stiffer materials lacerate the encircled tissue as the wound swells.[69]

The suture materials most useful to emergency clinicians for wound closure are Dexon or coated Vicryl for SQ layers and synthetic nonabsorbable sutures (e.g., nylon or polypropylene) for skin closure. Fascia can be sutured with either absorbable or nonabsorbable materials. In most situations, 3-0 or 4-0 sutures are used in the repair of fascia, 4-0 or 5-0 absorbable sutures in SQ closure, and 4-0 or 5-0 nonabsorbable sutures in skin closure. Lips, eyelids, and the skin layer of facial wounds are repaired with 6-0 sutures, whereas 3-0 or 4-0 sutures are used when the skin edges are subjected to considerable dynamic stresses (e.g., wounds overlying joint surfaces) or static stresses (e.g., scalp).

Needles

The eyeless, or "swaged," needle is used for wound closure in most emergency centers (Fig. 35–12). Selection of the appropriate needle size and curvature is based on the dimensions of the wound and the characteristics of the tissues to be sutured. The needle should be large enough to pass through tissue to the desired depth and then to exit the tissue or the skin surface far enough that the needle holder can be repositioned on the distal end of the needle at a safe distance from the needle point (Fig. 35–13). Although it is tempting to use the fingers to grasp the needle tip to pull the needle through the skin, this practice risks a needle stick. The clinician should either reposition the needle holder or use forceps to disengage the needle from the laceration.

In wound repair, needles must penetrate tough, fibrous tissues—skin, SQ tissue, and fascia—yet should slice through these tissues with minimal resistance or trauma and without

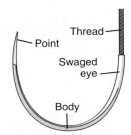

Figure 35–12 The eyeless, or "swaged," needle. *(From Suture Use Manual: Use and Handling of Sutures and Needles. Somerville, NJ, Ethicon, Inc, 1977, p 29. Reproduced by permission.)*

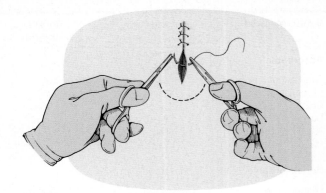

Figure 35–13 The needle should be large enough to pass through tissue and should exit far enough to enable the needle holder to be repositioned on the end of the needle at a safe distance from the point.

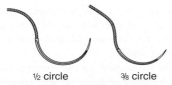

½ circle   ⅜ circle

Figure 35–14 One half and three eighths circle needles, used for most traumatic wound closures.

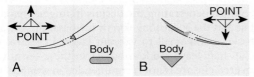

Figure 35–15 Types of needles. *A,* The conventional cutting needle has two opposing cutting edges, with a third edge on the inside curvature of the needle. The conventional cutting needle changes in cross-section from a triangular cutting tip to a flattened body. *B,* The reverse cutting needle is used to cut through tough, difficult-to-penetrate tissues such as fascia and skin. It has two opposing cutting edges, with the third cutting edge on the outer curvature of the needle. The reverse cutting needle is made with the triangular shape extending from the point to the swage area, with only the edges near the tip being sharpened. *(From Suture Use Manual: Use and Handling of Sutures and Needles. Somerville, NJ, Ethicon, Inc, 1977, p 31. Reproduced by permission.)*

bending. The type of needle best suited for closure of SQ tissue is a conventional cutting needle in a three eighths or one half circle (Fig. 35–14). Double-curvature needles (coated Vicryl with PS-4-C cutting needles, Ethicon) may be easier to maneuver in narrow, deep wounds. For surface closure, a conventional cutting-edge needle permits more precise needle placement and requires less penetration force (Fig. 35–15).[70,71]

Suturing Techniques

Skin Preparation
Before suturing, the clinician should ensure adequate exposure and illumination of the wound, with the patient placed at an appropriate height. The clinician should assume a comfortable standing or sitting position at one end of the long axis of the wound.

The skin surrounding it is prepared with a povidone-iodine solution and covered with sterile drapes. Some surgeons do not drape the face but prefer to leave facial structures and landmarks adjacent to the wound uncovered and within view. A clear plastic drape (Steri-Drape, 3M Corporation) can be used to provide a sterile field and a limited view of the area surrounding the wound. If no drapes are used on the face, the skin surrounding the wound should be widely cleansed and prepared. Wrapping the hair in a sheet or placing the patient's hair in an oversized scrub hat prevents stray hair from falling into the operating field

Closure Principles
There is a tendency to overuse sutures for minor lacerations that will heal nicely with no intervention. Therefore, before suturing, one must assess the need for the procedure (Fig. 35–16).

Three principles apply to the suturing of lacerations in any location: (1) minimize trauma to tissues, (2) relieve tension

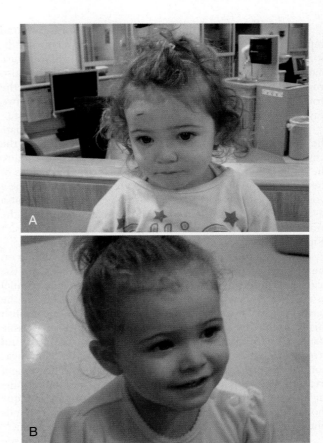

603

Figure 35–16 There is a tendency to overuse sutures. *A,* This child sustained a superficial forehead laceration just through the epidermis. The swelling accentuated the defect. Treatment was simply keeping the laceration clean. *B,* Four months after the injury, an excellent result was obtained. As the laceration was healing, it became red and more noticeable, *as do all scars,* but eventually faded.

exerted on the wound edges by undermining and layered wound closure, and (3) accurately realign landmarks and skin edges by layered closure and precise suture placement.

Minimizing Tissue Trauma. The importance of careful handling of tissue has been emphasized since the early days of surgery. Skin and SQ tissue that has been stretched, twisted, or crushed by an instrument or strangled by a suture that is tied too tightly may undergo necrosis, and increased scarring and infection may result. When the edges of a wound must be manipulated, the SQ tissues should be lifted gently with a toothed forceps or skin hook, avoiding the skin surface.

When choosing suture sizes, the clinician should select the smallest size that will hold the tissues in place. Skin stitches should incorporate no more tissue than is needed to coapt the wound edges with little or no tension. Knots should be tied securely enough to approximate the wound edges but without blanching or indenting the skin surface.[72]

Relieving Tension. Many forces can produce tension on the suture line of a reapproximated wound. Static skin forces that stretch the skin over bones cause the edges of a new wound to gape, and they also continuously pull on the edges of the wound once it has been closed. Traumatic loss of tissue or wide excision of a wound may have the same effect. The best cosmetic result occurs when the long axis of a wound happens to be parallel to the direction of maximal skin tension; this alignment brings the edges of the wound together.[69]

Muscles pulling at right angles to the axis of the wound impose dynamic stresses. Swelling after an injury creates additional tension within the circle of each suture.[72] Skin suture marks result not only from tying sutures too tightly but also from failing to eliminate underlying forces distorting the wound. Tension can be reduced during wound closure in two ways: undermining of the wound edges and layered closure.

Undermining. The force required to reapproximate the wound edges correlates with the subsequent width of the scar.[73] Wounds subject to significant static tension require the undermining of at least one tissue plane on both sides of the wound to achieve a tension-free closure. To undermine a wound, the clinician frees a flap of tissue from its base at a distance from the wound edge approximately equal to the width of the gap that the laceration presents at its widest point (Fig. 35–17).

The depth of the incision can be modified, depending on the orientation of the laceration to skin tension lines and the laxity of skin in the area. A No. 15 scalpel blade held parallel to the skin surface is used to incise the adipose layer or the dermal layer of the wound. The clinician also can accomplish this technique by spreading scissors in the appropriate tissue plane. Undermining allows the skin edges to be lifted and brought together with gentle traction.[74] Potential complications of this procedure include injury to cutaneous nerves and creation of a hematoma under the flap.[57] Because undermining may harm the underlying blood supply, this technique should be reserved for relatively uncontaminated wounds when no other methods adequately relieve wound tension.[70]

Layered Closure. The structure of skin and soft tissue varies with the location on the body (Fig. 35–18). Most wounds handled in an ED require approximation of no more than three layers: fascia (and associated muscle), SQ tissue, and skin surface (papillary layer of dermis and epidermis).[75] The presence of "dead space" (or unapposed edges) within a wound may fill with blood or exudate and enhance the development of infection. Closure of individual layers obliterates this dead space.

Separate approximation of muscle and SQ layers hastens the healing and return of function to the muscle. However, the fascia, not muscle, should be sutured. Muscle tissue itself is too friable to hold a suture. Layered closure is particularly important in the management of facial wounds; this technique prevents scarring of muscle to the SQ tissue and consequent deformation of the surface of the wound with contraction of the muscle. If a deep, gaping wound is closed without approxi-

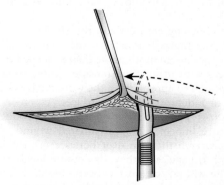

Figure 35–17 The technique of undermining is underused and can markedly improve cosmetic results by relieving wound tension. The scalpel is used to find an appropriate site; a natural plane often exists at the epidermis-dermis junction.

mation of underlying SQ tissue, a disfiguring depression may develop at the site of the wound. Finally, layered closure provides support to the wound and considerably reduces tension at the skin surface.

Several exceptions exist to the general rule of multilayered closure. The adipose layer of soft tissue should not be closed separately. A "fat stitch" is not necessary, because little support is provided by closure of the adipose layer, and additional suture material may increase the possibility of infection.[2,76] Scalp wounds are generally closed in a single layer. For lacerations penetrating the dermis in fingers, hands, toes, and feet and in the sebaceous skin of the nasal tip, the amount of SQ tissue is too small to warrant layered closure; in fact, SQ stitches may leave tender nodules in these sensitive locations. Layered closure is not recommended in wounds without tension, those with poor vascularity, and those with a moderate or high risk for infection. With single-layer closure, the surface stitch should be placed more deeply.[57]

Suture Placement

SQ Layer Closure. Once fascial structures have been reapproximated, the SQ layer is sutured. Although histologically the fatty and fibrous SQ tissue (hypodermis) is an extension of (and is continuous with) the reticular layer of the dermis,[77] suturing of these layers is traditionally referred to as a *SQ closure*. One approach is to close the length of this layer in segments, placing the first stitch in the middle of the wound and bisecting each subsequent segment until the closure of the layer has been completed.[41] This technique is useful in the closure of wounds that are long or sinuous, and it is particularly effective in wounds with one elliptical and one linear side. The needle is grasped by the needle holder close to the suture end. The clinician can suture more rapidly if the fingers are placed on the midshaft of the needle holder rather than in the rings of the instrument (Fig. 35–19).

The suture enters the SQ layer at the bottom of the wound (Fig. 35–20*A*) or, if the wound has been undermined, at the base of the flap (see Fig. 35–20*B*), and exits in the dermis. Once the suture has been placed on one side of the wound, it can be pulled across the wound to the opposite side (or the wound edges pushed together) to determine the matching point on the opposite side. The needle is then advanced into this point. The needle should enter the dermis at the same depth as it exited from the opposite side, pass through the tissue, and exit at the bottom of the wound (or the base of the flap). The edges of the wound can be closely apposed by pulling the two tails of the suture in the same direction along the axis of the wound (Fig. 35–21). Some clinicians place their SQ suture obliquely rather than vertically to facilitate knot tying. When the knot in this SQ stitch is tied, it will remain inverted, or "buried," at the bottom of the wound. Burying the knot of the SQ stitch avoids a painful, palpable nodule beneath the epidermis and keeps the bulk of this foreign material away from the skin surface. Most emergency clinicians construct knots using the instrument tie technique. Hand and instrument knot-tying techniques are described and illustrated in wound care texts.[78,79]

Once the knot has been secured, the tails of the suture should be pulled taut for cutting. The scissors are held with the index finger on the junction of the two blades. The blade of the scissors is slid down the tail of the suture until the knot is reached. With the cutting edge of the blade tilted away from the knot, the tails are cut. This technique prevents the scissors from cutting the knot itself and leaves a tail of 3 mm, which protects the knot from unraveling.[80] The entire SQ layer is sutured in this manner.

After the SQ layer has been closed, the distance between the skin edges determines the approximate width of the scar in its final form. If this width is acceptable, surface sutures can be inserted.[81] Despite undermining and placement of a sufficient number of SQ sutures, on occasion a large gap between the wound edges may persist. In such cases, a horizontal dermal stitch may be used to bridge this gap (see Fig. 35–40).

Surface Closure. The epidermis and the superficial layer of dermis are sutured in a single layer with nonabsorbable synthetic sutures. The choice of suture size, the number of sutures used, and the depth of suture placement depend on the amount of skin tension remaining after SQ closure.

If the edges of the wound are apposed after closure of deeper layers, small 5-0 or 6-0 sutures can be used simply to match the epithelium of each side. Wounds with greater tension and separation should have skin stitches placed closer

to each other and closer to the wound edge; layered closure is important in such wounds. If the wound edges remain retracted or if SQ stitches were not used, a larger-size suture placed deeply may be required.

The number of sutures used in closing any wound will vary with the wound location, the amount of tension on the wound, and with the degree of accuracy required by the clinician and patient. For example, sutures on the face would probably be placed between 1 and 3 mm apart.[62] Unless the wound edges are uneven, sutures should be placed in a mirror-image fashion such that the depth and width are the same on both sides of the wound.[45] In general, the distance between each suture should be approximately equal to the distance from the exit of the stitch to the wound edge.[41,78]

Skin closure may be accomplished with sutures placed in segments (Fig. 35–22) using the appropriate number of sutures (Fig. 35–23). When suturing the skin, right-handed operators should pass the needle from the right side of the wound to the left. The needle should be driven through tissue by flexing

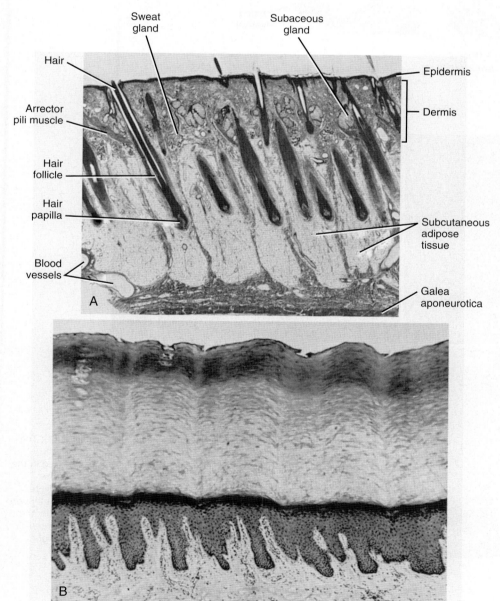

Figure 35–18 Variation in the structure of skin. *A,* Section of the skin of the scalp, x15. *B,* Skin of the human fingertip, illustrating a very thick stratum corneum. Hematoxylin and eosin, x65. *C,* Section of human sole perpendicular to the free surface, x100. *D,* Section through human thigh perpendicular to the surface of the skin. Blood vessels are injected and appear black. Low magnification. *(A, Courtesy of H Mizoguchi; C and D, after AA Maximow. From Bloom W, Fawcett DW: A Textbook of Histology, 10th ed. Philadelphia, WB Saunders, 1975. Reproduced by permission.)*

Continued

Labels in figure A: Sweat gland, Subaceous gland, Hair, Epidermis, Arrector pili muscle, Dermis, Hair follicle, Hair papilla, Subcutaneous adipose tissue, Blood vessels, Galea aponeurotica

Figure 35–18, cont'd

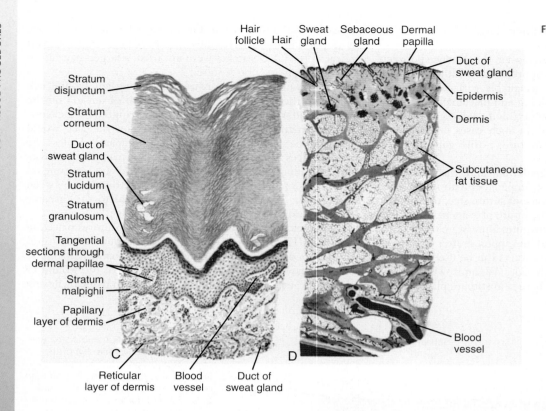

Stratum disjunctum

Stratum corneum

Duct of sweat gland

Stratum lucidum

Stratum granulosum

Tangential sections through dermal papillae

Stratum malpighii

Papillary layer of dermis

Reticular layer of dermis

Blood vessel

Duct of sweat gland

Hair follicle   Hair   Sweat gland   Sebaceous gland   Dermal papilla

Duct of sweat gland

Epidermis

Dermis

Subcutaneous fat tissue

Blood vessel

C   D

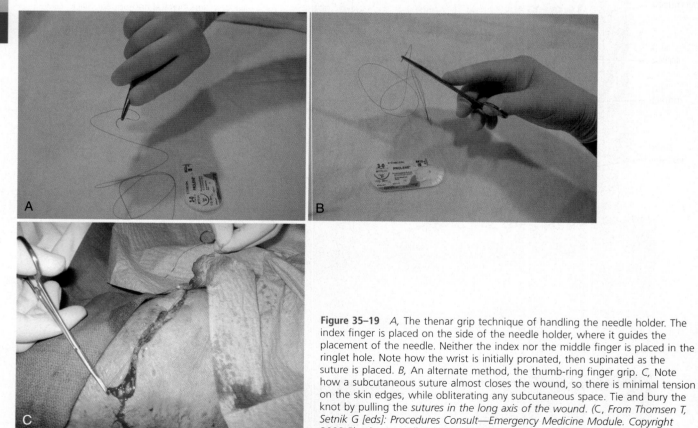

A   B

C

Figure 35–19 *A,* The thenar grip technique of handling the needle holder. The index finger is placed on the side of the needle holder, where it guides the placement of the needle. Neither the index nor the middle finger is placed in the ringlet hole. Note how the wrist is initially pronated, then supinated as the suture is placed. *B,* An alternate method, the thumb-ring finger grip. *C,* Note how a subcutaneous suture almost closes the wound, so there is minimal tension on the skin edges, while obliterating any subcutaneous space. Tie and bury the knot by pulling the *sutures in the long axis of the wound. (C, From Thomsen T, Setnik G [eds]: Procedures Consult—Emergency Medicine Module. Copyright 2008 Elsevier, Inc. All rights reserved.)*

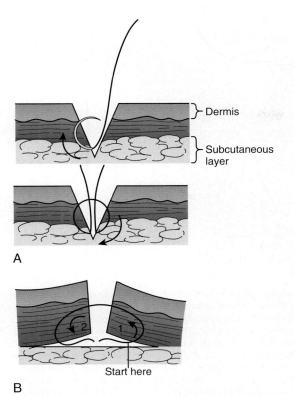

Figure 35–20 *A and B,* Inverted subcutaneous stitches.

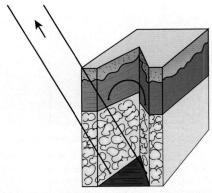

Figure 35–21 The two tails of the subcutaneous suture are pulled in the same direction, tightly apposing the edges of the wound.

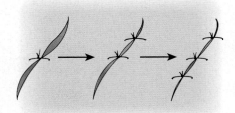

Figure 35–22 Closure of the surface of the wound in segments rather than from one end. Place the first suture in the center of the wound for a straight suture line.

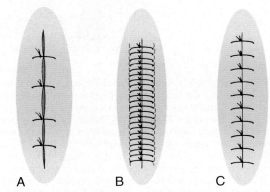

Figure 35–23 *A,* Too few stitches used. Note gaping between sutures. *B,* Too many stitches used. *C,* Correct number of stitches used for a wound under an average amount of tension.

607

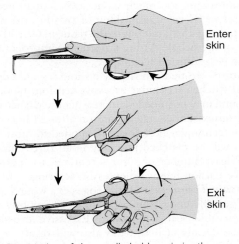

Figure 35–24 Motion of the needle holder mimics the curve of the needle. Rotate the wrist (pronate) so the needle enters the skin perpendicularly, not at an angle, as the wrist supinates. This helps evert the wound edge. *(From Anderson CB: Basic surgical techniques. In Klippel AP, Anderson CB [eds]: Manual of Outpatient and Emergency Surgical Techniques. Boston, Little, Brown, 1979. Reproduced by permission.)*

the wrist and supinating the forearm; *the course taken by the needle should result in a curve identical to the curvature of the needle itself* (Fig. 35–24). *The angle of exit for the needle should be the same as its angle of entrance so that an identical volume of tissue is contained within the stitch on each side of the wound* (Fig. 35–25).

Once the needle exits the skin on the opposite side of the wound, it is regrasped by the needle holder and advanced through the tissue; care should be taken to avoid crushing the point of the needle with the instrument. Forceps are designed for handling tissue and thus should not be used to grasp the needle. The forceps can stabilize the needle by holding the needle within the tissue through which the needle has just passed. An assistant can keep excess thread clear of the area being sutured or the excess can be looped around the clinician's fingers. If the point of the needle becomes dulled before

all of the attached thread has been used, the suture should be discarded.

Complications. Sutures act as foreign bodies in a wound, and any stitch may damage a blood vessel or strangulate tissue. Therefore, the clinician should use the smallest size and the least number of sutures that will adequately close the wound.[56] However, if spaced too widely, surface stitches will leave a "crosshatch" pattern of marks.

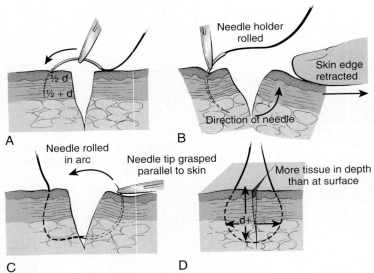

Figure 35–25 The simple suture. *A,* Hold the needle pointing down by excessively pronating the wrist so that the needle tip initially moves farther from the laceration as the needle penetrates deeper into the skin. (See also Fig. 35–19.) Drive the needle tip downward and away from the cut edge, into the subcutaneous layer. *B,* Advance the needle into the laceration. The needle tip is directed toward the opposite side at the same level by rolling the needle holder. The arc of the needle pathway is controlled by retracting the skin edge. This method incorporates more tissue within the stitch in the deeper layers of the wound than at the surface. As an alternative, if a small needle is used in thick skin or the distance across the wound is great, the needle can be removed from the first side, remounted on the needle holder, and advanced to the opposite side. *C,* Advance the needle upward toward the surface so that it exits at the same distance from the wound edge as on the contralateral side of the wound. Grasp the needle behind the tip and roll it out in the arc of the needle. *D,* The final position, with more tissue in the depth than in the surface. The distance from each suture exit to the laceration is half the depth of the dermis. (*A–D, Redrawn from Kaplan EN, Hentz VR: Emergency Management of Skin and Soft Tissue Wounds: An Illustrated Guide. Boston, Little, Brown, 1984, p 86. Reproduced by permission.*)

Encompassing too much tissue with a small needle is a common error. Forcefully pushing or twisting the needle in an effort to bring the point out of the tissue may bend or break the body of the needle. Using a needle of improper size will defeat the best suturing technique.

If sutures are tied too tightly around wound edges or if individual stitches are under excessive tension, blood supply to the wound may be impeded, increasing the chance of infection, and suture marks may form even after 24 hours.[45,82]

If the techniques described are applied to most wounds, the edges will be matched precisely in all three dimensions, using the least number of sutures required to appose edges and relieve tension but avoid excessive scarring.

Eversion Techniques. If the edges of a wound invert, or if one edge rolls under the opposite side, a poorly formed, deep, noticeable scar will result. Excessive eversion that exposes the dermis of both sides also will result in a larger scar than if the skin edges are perfectly apposed, but inversion produces a more visible scar than does eversion. Because most scars undergo some flattening with contraction, optimal results are achieved when the epidermis is slightly everted without excessive suture tension (Fig. 35–26). Wounds over mobile surfaces, such as the extensor surfaces of joints, should be everted. In time, the scar will be flattened by the dynamic forces acting in the area.

Numerous techniques can be used to avoid inversion of the edges of the wound. If the clinician angles the needle obliquely away from the laceration, a surface stitch can be placed so that it is *deeper than it is* wide[74] and the stitch encircles more tissue in the SQ layer than at the surface. If this "bottle-shaped stitch" is intended to produce some eversion of the wound edges, the stitch must include a sufficient amount of SQ tissue (see Fig. 35–25D).

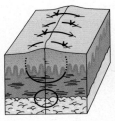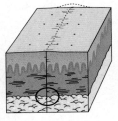

Sutures placed   Sutures removed

Figure 35–26 Skin edges that are slightly *everted* will gradually flatten to produce a level wound surface when the sutures are removed. An inverted wound catches the light in a shadow and is more visible. In addition, eversion allows subcutaneous tissue to heal. (*From Grabb WC: Basic technique of plastic surgery. In Grabb WC, Smith JW [eds]: Plastic Surgery: A Concise Guide to Clinical Practice. Boston, Little, Brown, 1979. Reproduced by permission.*)

Eversion can be accomplished by lifting and turning the edge of the wound outward with a skin hook or fine-tooth forceps before insertion of the needle on each side (Fig. 35–27). Eversion can also be obtained simply by pressing on the skin adjacent to the wound with a closed forceps (or thumb and a finger as long as a needle stick is avoided) (Fig. 35–28).

Vertical mattress sutures are particularly effective in everting the wound edges, and they can be used exclusively or alternated with simple interrupted sutures (Fig. 35–29).[83] In wounds that have been undermined, an SQ stitch placed at the base of the flap on each side can in itself evert the wound (Fig. 35–30).

Interrupted Stitch. The simple interrupted stitch is the most frequently used technique in the closure of skin. It consists of separate loops of suture individually tied. Although the

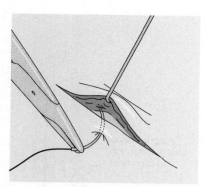

Figure 35–27 The use of a forceps or skin hook to evert the wound edge. This technique allows the operator to see the needle path, ensuring that the proper depth has been reached, and promotes eversion of the skin edges.

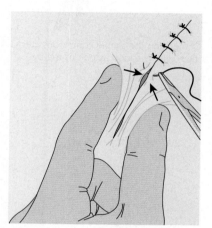

Figure 35–28 Eversion of the wound edge by thumb and finger pressure *kept away from the needle to avoid a needle stick. (From Converse JM: Introduction to plastic surgery. In Converse JM [ed]: Reconstructive Plastic Surgery: Principles and Procedures in Correction, Reconstruction, and Transplantation, vol 1, 2nd ed. Philadelphia, WB Saunders, 1977. Reproduced by permission.)*

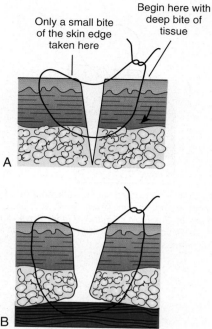

Figure 35–29 The vertical mattress suture is the *best technique for producing skin edge eversion. A,* The usual type of mattress suture for approximating and everting wound edges. *B,* "Tacking" type of vertical mattress suture, extending into deep fascia to obliterate dead space under wound. Note that only a small bite of skin is included on the inner suture. *(Modified from Converse JM: Introduction to plastic surgery. In Converse JM [ed]: Reconstructive Plastic Surgery: Principles and Procedures in Correction, Reconstruction, and Transplantation, vol 1, 2nd ed. Philadelphia, WB Saunders, 1977. Reproduced by permission.)*

609

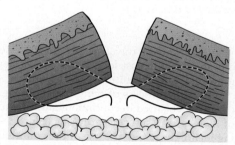

Figure 35–30 Deep dermis suturing technique. The suture enters the base of the flap, is brought up into the dermis, and exits just proximal to the wound edge along the base of the flap to be tied and cut. *(From Stuzin J, Engrav LH, Buehler PK: Emergency treatment of facial lacerations. Postgrad Med 71:81, 1982. Reproduced by permission.)*

tying and cutting of each stitch are time-consuming, the advantage of this method is that if one stitch in the closure fails, the remaining stitches continue to hold the wound together (Fig. 35–31).

Continuous Stitch. A continuous stitch is an effective method for closing relatively clean, low-risk wounds that are under little or no tension and are on flat, immobile skin surfaces. In a continuous, or "running," stitch, the loops are the exposed portions of a helical coil tied at each end of the wound. A continuous suture line can be placed more rapidly than a series of interrupted stitches. The continuous stitch has the additional advantages of strength (with tension being evenly distributed along its entire length), fewer knots (which are the weak points of stitches), and more effective hemostasis. This stitch will accommodate mild wound swelling. The continuous technique is useful as an epithelial or "surface" stitch in cosmetic closures; however, if the underlying SQ layer is not stabilized in a separate closure, the continuous surface stitch tends to invert the wound edges.

The continuous suture technique has some disadvantages. This technique cannot be used to close wounds overlying joints. If a loop breaks at one point, the entire stitch may unravel. Likewise, if infection develops and the incision must

be opened at one point, cutting a single loop may allow the entire wound to fall open. The simple continuous stitch has a tendency to produce suture marks if used in large wound closures and if left in place for more than 5 days.[72] However, if all tension on the wound can be removed by SQ sutures, stitch marks are seldom a problem.

Among the variations of the continuous technique, the simple continuous stitch is the most useful to emergency clinicians (Fig. 35–32). An interrupted stitch is placed at one end of the wound, and only the free tail of the suture is cut. As suturing proceeds, the stitch encircles tissue in a spiral pattern. After each passage of the needle, the loop is tightened slightly, and the thread is held taut in the clinician's nondominant

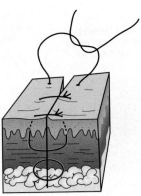

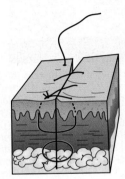

Figure 35–31 Simple interrupted stitch. Additional throws in a partially tied knot are not shown. *(From Grabb WC: Basic techniques of plastic surgery. In Grabb WC, Smith JW [eds]: Plastic Surgery: A Concise Guide to Clinical Practice. Boston, Little, Brown, 1979. Reproduced by permission.)*

Figure 35–32 Simple continuous stitch. *(From Grabb WC: Basic techniques of plastic surgery. In Grabb WC, Smith JW [eds]: Plastic Surgery: A Concise Guide to Clinical Practice. Boston, Little, Brown, 1979. Reproduced by permission.)*

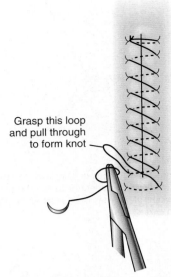

Grasp this loop and pull through to form knot

Figure 35–33 Completing the simple continuous stitch. A series of square knots is tied, with the loop as one of the ties.

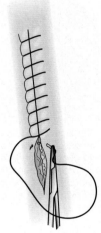

Figure 35–34 Continuous interlocking stitch. *(Modified from Suture Use Manual: Use and Handling of Sutures and Needles. Somerville, NJ, Ethicon, Inc, 1977. Reproduced by permission.)*

hand. The needle should travel perpendicularly across the wound on each pass. The last loop is placed just beyond the end of the wound, and the suture is tied, with the last loop used as a "tail" in the process of tying the knot (Fig. 35–33). A locking loop may be used in continuous suturing to prevent slippage of loops as the suturing proceeds (Fig. 35–34). The interlocking technique allows the use of the continuous stitch along an irregular laceration.[74]

Continuous Subcuticular Stitch. Nonabsorbable sutures used in surface closure outlast their usefulness and must be removed. On occasion, wounds require an extended period of support, longer than that provided by surface stitches. Some patients with wounds that require skin closure are unlikely or unwilling to return for suture removal. Some sutured wounds are covered by plaster casts. On occasion, the patient (child or adult) is likely to be as frightened and uncooperative for suture removal as for suture placement. Surface sutures are more likely to produce stitch marks in children because the wounds are under greater tension than those in adults. The continuous subcuticular (or "dermal") suture technique is ideal for these situations; the wound can be closed with an absorbable subcuticular stitch, obviating the need for later suture removal. In patients prone to keloid formation, the subcuticular technique can be used in lieu of surface stitches, which avoids disfiguring stitch marks. Buried, absorbable subcuticular stitches do not appear to provoke more inflammation than percutaneous running stitches with mono-

filament nylon.[71] Because stitch marks are not a problem, a nonabsorbable subcuticular suture can be left in place for a longer period than a surface suture.[83]

Although this technique is commonly used in cosmetic closures, closure of the subcuticular layer alone may not alter the scar width.[84] This technique does not allow for perfect approximation of the vertical heights of the two edges of a wound,[85] and in cosmetic closures, it is often followed by a surface stitch. The subcuticular stitch requires a 4-0 or 5-0 suture made of either absorbable material or nonabsorbable synthetic monofilament. An absorbable suture can be "buried" within the wound, whereas a nonabsorbable suture is used for a "pull-out" stitch. The absorbable synthetic monofilament suture PDS (Ethicon) is designed for subcuticular closure. It passes through tissues as easily as nonabsorbable monofilament sutures and is absorbed if left in the wound.

Before the subcuticular stitch is begun, the SQ layer should be approximated with interrupted sutures to minimize

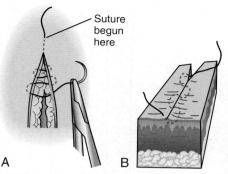

Figure 35–35 Pull-out subcuticular stitch. For deep wounds, first place interrupted sutures to relieve tension on skin edge. The suture is introduced into the skin in line with the incision, approximately 1–2 cm away. *(From Grimes DW, Garner RW: "Reliefs" in intracuticular sutures. Surg Rounds 1:46, 1978. Reproduced by permission and from Grabb WC: Basic techniques of plastic surgery. In Grabb WC, Smith JW [eds]: Plastic Surgery: A Concise Guide to Clinical Practice. Boston, Little, Brown, 1979. Reproduced by permission.)*

tension on the wound. The pull-out subcuticular stitch is started at the skin surface approximately 1 to 2 cm away from one end of the wound. The needle enters and exits the dermis at the apices of the wound (Fig. 35–35). Bites through tissue are taken in a horizontal direction, with the needle penetrating the dermis 1 to 2 mm from the skin surface. These intradermal bites should be small, of equal size, and at the same level on each side of the wound.[68,83] Each successive bite should be placed 1 to 2 mm behind the exit point on the opposite side of the wound so that when the wound is closed, the entrance and exit points on either side are not directly apposed (Fig. 35–36). Small bites should be taken to avoid puckering of the skin surface, and the stitch should not be accidentally interlocked. Some clinicians prefer to place a fine (6-0) running skin suture on the surface, in addition to the subcuticular suture, for meticulous skin approximation. The skin suture is removed in 3 to 4 days to avoid suture marks.

If the subcuticular stitch is used on lengthy lacerations, it is difficult to remove the suture. The placement of "reliefs," consisting of periodic loops through the skin every 4 to 5 cm along the length of the stitch, facilitates later removal (see Fig. 35–36). The suture is crossed to the opposite side, and the needle is passed from SQ tissue to the skin surface. The suture is carried over the surface for approximately 2 cm before reentering the skin and SQ tissue. The subcuticular stitch is then continued at approximately the point at which the next bite would have been placed had the relief not been used.

At the completion of the stitch, the needle is placed through the apex to exit the skin 1 to 2 cm away from the end of the wound. The stitch should be tightened by pulling each end taut. If reliefs have been used, pulling on the reliefs will take up any slack in the stitch. The clinician can secure the two ends of the stitch by taping them to the skin surface with wound closure tape, by placing a cluster of knots on each tail close to the skin surface, or by tying the two ends of the suture to each other over a dressing. Laxity of the subcuticular stitch will occur as tissue swelling subsides 48 hours after wound closure. The stitch can be tightened at this time.

Subcuticular closure can be accomplished by using absorbable sutures that do not penetrate the skin. The closure is begun with a dermal or SQ suture placed at one end of the wound and secured with a knot. After placement of the continuous subcuticular stitch from apex to apex, the suture is

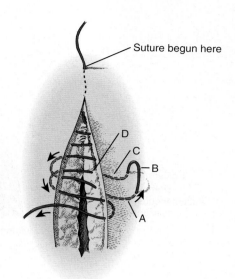

Figure 35–36 In constructing the relief to facilitate suture removal, the suture is crossed to the opposite side, going into the subcuticular area beneath the skin for approximately 2 cm before exiting (*A*). The suture is then carried over the epidermis for approximately 2 cm (*B*) and then back under the dermis again (*C*). Reentry is made into the wound area (*D*) at approximately the same location where the next "bite" would have been placed had the relief not been used. *(From Grimes DW, Garner RW: "Reliefs" in intracuticular sutures. Surg Rounds 1:47, 1978. Reproduced by permission.)*

pulled taut, and a knot is tied using a tail and a loop of suture (Fig. 35–37). The final knot can be buried by inserting the needle into deeper tissue; the needle exits several millimeters from the wound edge. By pulling on the needle end, the knot disappears into the wound.[67] The advantage of this technique is that there are no suture marks in the skin.

Nonabsorbable subcuticular sutures can be left in place for 2 to 3 weeks, thus providing a longer period of support than surface sutures, without the problem of stitch marks.[72] If skin sutures are used in conjunction with the subcuticular stitch, they are removed in 3 to 4 days. A subcuticular closure in itself is stronger than a tape closure. If the subcuticular technique is used exclusively to approximate the skin surface, skin tape can be applied to correct surface unevenness and to provide a more accurate apposition of the epidermis.

The primary disadvantage of the subcuticular stitch is that it is time-consuming, especially when supporting surface stitches are used. Another, faster method that avoids penetrating the skin is the interrupted subcuticular stitch (Fig. 35–38).[83] Wounds with strong static skin tension may benefit from a few interrupted dermal stitches placed horizontally to the skin surface instead of a continuous subcuticular stitch.

Mattress Stitch. The various types of mattress stitches are all interrupted stitches. The *vertical mattress stitch* is an effective method of everting skin edges (Fig. 35–39; see also Fig. 35–29). The vertical mattress stitch may be used to take a deep bite of skin, eliminating the need for a layered closure in areas where excessive tension does not result. If the superficial loop is placed first, the tails can be pulled upward while the deep loop is placed, ensuring wound eversion in less time than with the traditional technique.[86]

The *horizontal mattress stitch* is an SQ stitch that is oriented 90° to the interrupted SQ stitch described previously. The horizontal mattress stitch apposes skin edges closely

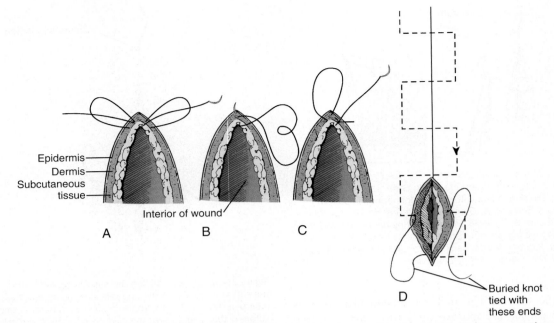

Epidermis
Dermis
Subcutaneous
tissue

Interior of wound

A   B   C

D   Buried knot
tied with
these ends

Figure 35–37 Subcuticular closure without epidermal penetration. *A,* The initial knot is secured in the dermal or subcutaneous tissue. *B,* The short strand is cut, and the needle is inserted into the dermis at the apex of the wound. *C,* The needle in the dermis, close to the corner of the wound and exiting the wound at the same horizontal level. *D,* After the subcuticular stitch has been completed, a knot is tied with the tail and the loop of the suture. (A–D, *Modified from Stillman RM: Wound closure: Choosing optimal materials and methods. ER Rep 2:43, 1981.*)

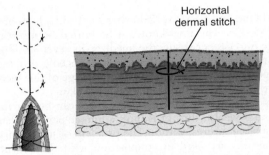

Horizontal
dermal stitch

Figure 35–38 Interrupted subcuticular stitch (also called a horizontal dermal stitch). Absorbable sutures are used. (A vertical suture also closes the deep tissue.)

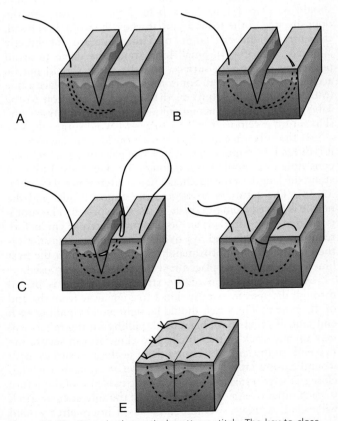

A   B

C   D

E

Figure 35–39 Steps in the vertical mattress stitch. The key to close apposition and exact alignment of edges is to place the inner sutures very close to the suture line (wound edge).

while providing some degree of eversion (Fig. 35–40).[72] The horizontal mattress suture may be ideal for areas where eversion is desirable but there is little SQ tissue.

The *half-buried horizontal mattress stitch* is particularly useful in suturing the easily damaged apex of a V-shaped flap (Fig. 35–41). In the execution of the "corner stitch," the suture needle penetrates the skin at a point beyond the apex of the wound and exits through the dermis. The corner of the flap is elevated, and the suture is passed through the dermis of the flap. The needle is then placed in the dermis of the base of the wound and returned to the surface of the skin. All dermal bites should be placed at the same level. The suture is tied with sufficient tension to pull the flap snugly into the corner without blanching the flap.[72,87] If the tip of a large flap with questionable viability may be further jeopardized by postoperative swelling, a cotton stent can be placed underneath the knot of the corner stitch. The cotton absorbs the tension produced by swelling.

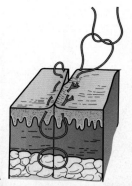

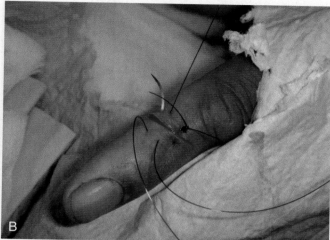

The only disadvantage of the horizontal and vertical mattress stitches is that they cause more ischemia and necrosis inside their loops than either simple or continuous stitches.[88]

Figure-of-Eight Stitch. The figure-of-eight stitch is useful in wounds with friable tissue, on the eyelids where the skin is too thin for buried sutures, or in areas in which buried sutures are undesirable (Fig. 35–42).[89] This stitch reduces the amount of tension placed on the tissue by the suture, allowing the stitch to hold in place when a simple stitch would tear through the tissue. The disadvantage of this technique is that more suture material is left in the wound. A vertical variation of the figure-of-eight stitch is sometimes used to approximate close, parallel lacerations (Figs. 35–43 and 35–44).[90] Another technique involves a vertical mattress stitch.

Correction of Dog-Ears. When wound edges are not precisely aligned horizontally, there will be excess tissue on one or both ends. This small flap of excess skin that bunches up at the end of a sutured wound is commonly called a *dog-ear*. This effect also occurs when one side of the wound is more elliptical than the opposite side, or when an excision of a wound is not sufficiently elliptical because it is either too straight or too nearly circular.[41,83]

If a dog-ear is present, it can be eliminated on one side of the wound in the following manner: The flap of excess skin is elevated with a forceps or skin hook, and an incision is carried at an oblique angle from the apex of the wound toward

613

Figure 35–40 *A,* Horizontal mattress stitch. *B,* The dorsum of the hand, foot, or finger is an ideal place for a horizontal mattress suture to evert the wound edges. The relatively thin skin in these areas precludes the use of vertical mattress sutures. (A, *From Grabb WC: Basic techniques of plastic surgery. In WC, Smith JW [eds]: Plastic Surgery: A Concise Guide to Clinical Practice. Boston, Little, Brown, 1979. Reproduced by permission.*)

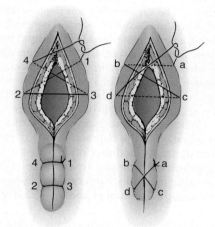

Figure 35–42 Figure-of-eight stitch, two methods. *(Modified from Dushoff IM: About face. Emerg Med 6:11:1974. Reproduced by permission.)*

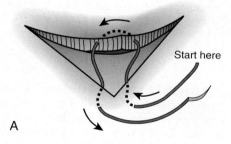

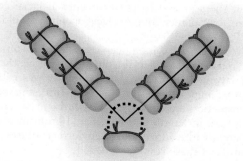

Figure 35–41 *A* and *B,* Corner stitch: Approximation of a flap with a half-buried horizontal mattress stitch, followed by interrupted sutures for the rest of the wound.

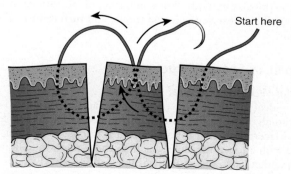

Figure 35–43 Vertical figure-of-eight suture technique. This can be used to close parallel lacerations. *(From Mitchell GC: Repair of parallel lacerations [letter]. Ann Emerg Med 16:924, 1987.)*

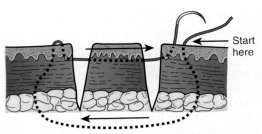

Figure 35–44 Technique for closure of parallel lacerations in which the central tissue island has an intact base. *(Redrawn from Samo DG: A technique for parallel lacerations. Ann Emerg Med 17:297, 1988.)*

the side with the excess skin. The flap is then undermined and laid flat. The resulting triangle of skin is trimmed, and the closure is completed (Fig. 35–45A).[81,87] An alternative method consists of carrying the incision directly from the apex, in line with the wound. The flap of excess tissue is pulled over the incision while skin hooks are used to retract the extended apex of the wound. Excess tissue is excised, and the remainder of the wound is sutured.[83] If dog-ears are present on both sides of one end of the wound, the bulge of excess tissue can be excised in an elliptical fashion, and the wound can be closed (see Fig. 35–45B).[87]

Stellate Lacerations. The repair of a stellate laceration is a challenging problem. Usually a result of compression and shear forces, these injuries contain large amounts of partially devitalized tissue. The surrounding soft tissue is often swollen and contused. Much of this contused tissue cannot be débrided without creating a large tissue defect. Sometimes tissue is lost, yet the amount is not apparent until key sutures are placed. In repairing what often resembles a jigsaw puzzle, the clinician can remove small flaps of necrotic tissue with an iris scissors; large, viable flaps can be repositioned in their beds and carefully secured with half-buried mattress stitches. If interrupted stitches are used to approximate a thin flap, small bites should be taken in the flap and larger, deeper bites in the base of the wound. A modification of the corner stitch can be used to approximate multiple flaps to a base (Fig. 35–46). Thin flaps of tissue in a stellate laceration with beveled edges may be more easily repositioned and stabilized with a firm dressing.[72]

Closure of stellate lacerations cannot always be accomplished immediately, especially if there is considerable soft tissue swelling. It may be best in some instances to consider delayed closure or revision of the scar at a later date. In complicated lacerations, inexact tissue approximation may be all that is possible initially. For small stellate lacerations, it may be possible to excise the lesion totally and turn it into a linear repair.

Repair of Special Structures

Facial Wounds (General Features)

The ideal result in the repair of a facial laceration is an extremely narrow, flat, and inapparent scar. Facial and forehead lacerations that follow natural skin creases or lines will heal with a less noticeable scar than those that are oblique or perpendicular to the natural wrinkles of the skin (Fig. 35–47). In addition to basic wound management, a few additional techniques can be used to achieve satisfactory cosmetic results.

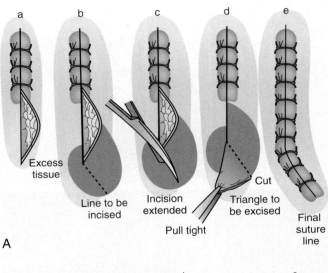

A

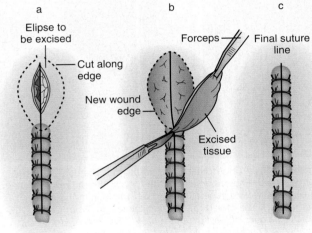

B

Figure 35–45 *A,* Correction of a dog-ear. *B,* Excision of bilateral dog-ears. *(A, From Dushoff IM: A stitch in time. Emerg Med 5:1, 1973. Reproduced by permission.)*

Although necrosis of partially devitalized wound edges contributes to wide scars, facial skin with apparently marginal circulation may survive because of excellent vascularity. SQ fat, which in other locations may be débrided thoroughly, *should be preserved if possible in facial wounds* to prevent eventual sinking of the scar and to preserve normal facial contours. Therefore, débridement of most facial wounds should be conservative[75] (Fig. 35–48).

A *layered closure* has long been considered essential in the cosmetic repair of many facial wounds. However, the importance of layered closures in facial wounds was called into question by Singer and associates.[91] These investigators found similar cosmetic outcomes and scar widths in facial wounds less than 3 cm in length and less than 10 mm in width that were repaired with and without deep dermal sutures. Further confirmation of these results is needed.

If a layered closure is undertaken, approximation of the dermis with a SQ stitch, or with a combination of SQ and subcuticular stitches, should bring the wound edges together or within 1 to 2 mm of apposition—close enough that the use of additional sutures seems almost unnecessary.[81] If an SQ

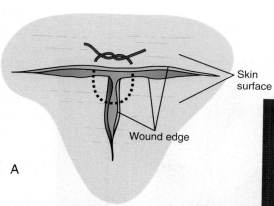

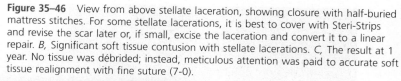

Figure 35–46 View from above stellate laceration, showing closure with half-buried mattress stitches. For some stellate lacerations, it is best to cover with Steri-Strips and revise the scar later or, if small, excise the laceration and convert it to a linear repair. *B*, Significant soft tissue contusion with stellate lacerations. *C*, The result at 1 year. No tissue was débrided; instead, meticulous attention was paid to accurate soft tissue realignment with fine suture (7-0).

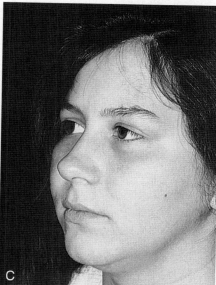

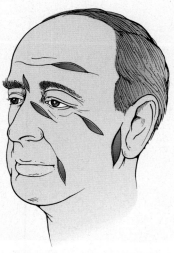

Figure 35–47 Lacerations following natural skin lines (shown here) heal with a less noticeable scar than those that are oblique or perpendicular to natural lines (or wrinkles).

stitch is the only stitch used to close the deeper layers, it should pass through the dermal-epidermal junction, or within 1 to 2 mm of the skin surface, without causing a dimpling effect. The stitch should be tied snugly by pulling the two ends of the suture in the same direction (see Fig. 35–19).

In cosmetic areas, the surface stitch should not be used to relieve a wound of significant tension. The surface stitch on the face is most appropriately used to match the epidermal surfaces precisely along the length of the wound. If the wound edges are separated more than about 2 to 4 mm after closure of the SQ layer, a 5-0 or 6-0 subcuticular suture can be used to eliminate the tension produced by this separation and to provide prolonged stability. An alternative approach is the use

of a few *guide stitches* to hold sections of the wound together before definitive closure with surface stitches. Guide stitches allow the surface sutures to be placed with little tension on each individual stitch, they match irregular edges, and they protect the SQ stitches from disruption. The first guide stitch is placed at the midpoint of the wound, and subsequent guide stitches bisect the intervening spaces. Once the definitive surface stitches have been placed, the guide stitches, if slack, can be removed. Because a needle damages tissue with each passage through the skin, guide stitches should be used only when necessary.

In a straight laceration, better apposition during surface closure is achieved if the wound is stretched lengthwise by finger traction or with skin hooks. When the needle is placed on one side of the wound, if that side is higher than the opposite side, a shallow bite is taken. The needle is used to depress the wound edge to the proper height, after which the needle "follows through" to the other side, pinning the two sides together. If the first side entered is lower, the needle is elevated when entering the second side to match the epithelial edges.

If the skin edges are apposed closely by the SQ stitch or a subcuticular stitch, a small, shallow *"epithelial" stitch* can be used in lieu of the standard, deeper, surface stitch to correct discrepancies in vertical alignment.[74] Precise alignment of wound edges is achieved by inserting the needle as close to the edge as possible without tearing through the tissue. A 6-0 synthetic nonabsorbable suture is an excellent material for this stitch. A continuous stitch is preferable because it can be placed quickly, but interrupted stitches are acceptable. Epithelial stitches should be spaced no more than 2 to 3 mm apart and should encompass no more than 2 to 4 mm of tissue.[74] Once skin closure is complete, final adjustments in the tension on a continuous suture line are made before the end of the stitch is tied. If any level discrepancies persist, interrupted

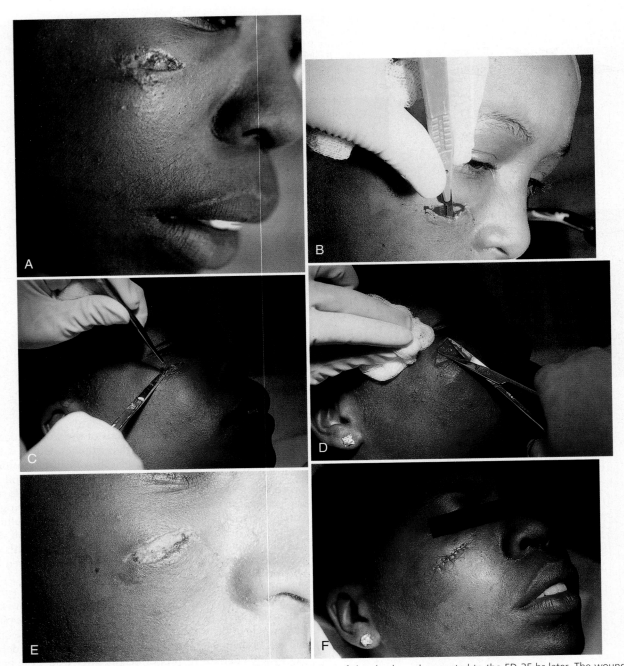

Figure 35–48 *A,* This woman was punched in the face, suffered a laceration of the cheek, and presented to the ED 35 hr later. The wound was not infected, but it had contracted and was beginning to heal by granulation. Under local anesthesia, the wound was opened, irrigated, minimally débrided, and the skin edges were trimmed. *B,* Using a No. 15 blade, a 1-mm-deep incision was made in the skin along the edges of the wound border. *C,* The incised edges were then cut away using tissue scissors. *D,* The wound was undermined to relieve tension on the skin. *E,* The wound is clean, undermined, and ready to close *F,* The wound was closed with 6-0 interrupted sutures that were removed in 5 days. No antibiotics were used, and only a small linear scar resulted.

sutures or tape can be used to flatten these few irregularities. The disadvantages of epithelial stitches are that they are time-consuming and add more suture material to the wound. Level discrepancies can often be corrected with surgical tape.

Surgical tape is useful as a secondary support, protecting the surface stitch from stresses produced by normal skin movements (Fig. 35–49). Facial wounds have a tendency to swell and place excessive stretch on a surface stitch. This can be minimized by applying a pressure dressing and cold compresses to the wound after closure. Surgical tape can serve to a limited extent as a small pressure dressing. In simple, low-

tension facial wounds, wound closure with surgical tape provides results that are equivalent to closure with tissue adhesive.[92]

Forehead

Although the forehead is actually a part of the scalp, lacerations in this region are treated as facial wounds. Vertical lacerations across the forehead are oriented 90° to skin tension lines, and the resulting scars are more noticeable than those from horizontal lacerations. Midline vertical forehead lacerations may result in cosmetically acceptable scars with standard closure techniques; uncentered lacerations may benefit from S-plasty or Z-plasty techniques during the initial repair or during later revision of the scar.

Superficial lacerations may be closed with skin stitches alone, but deep forehead lacerations must be closed in layers. Significant periosteal defects should be approximated before the closure of more superficial layers. If skin is directly exposed to bone, adhesions might develop that in time may limit the movement of skin during facial expressions. The frontalis muscle fascia and adjacent fibrous tissue should be closed as a distinct layer; if left unsutured, the retracted ends of this muscle will bulge beneath the skin. If the gap in a muscle belly is later filled with scar tissue, movement of the muscle pulls on the entire scar and makes it more apparent.[75]

A U-shaped flap laceration with a superiorly oriented base poses a difficult problem. Immediate vascular congestion and later scar contraction within the flap produce the "trap-door" effect, with the flap becoming prominently elevated (Fig. 35–50). This effect can be minimized by approximation of the bulk of SQ tissue of the flap to a deeper level on the base side of the wound; the skin surfaces of the two sides are apposed at the same level (Fig. 35–51). A firm compression dressing helps eliminate dead space and hematoma formation within the wound. Despite these efforts, secondary revision is sometimes necessary.[72] Often, swelling of the flap resolves

over a 6- to 12-month period. Because flap elevation can be quite disconcerting, the clinician should forewarn the patient and family about a possible trap-door effect.

When a forehead laceration borders the scalp and the thick scalp tissue must be sutured to thinner forehead skin, a horizontal or vertical mattress stitch with an intradermal component can be used (see Fig. 35–51B).[83]

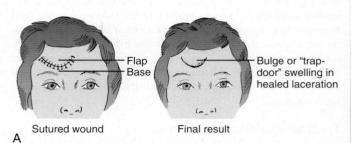

A

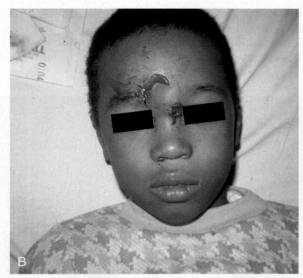

Figure 35–50 *A*, Elevation of a forehead flap. The "trap-door effect" is a natural healing process of elliptical or round lacerations. Patients should be advised of this phenomenon. *B*, This flap-type laceration of the forehead will heal with a puffed-up center (trap door), even under the best of circumstances. (*A, From Grabb WC, Kleinert HE: Technics in Surgery: Facial and Hand Injuries. Somerville, NJ, Ethicon, Inc, 1980. Reproduced by permission.*)

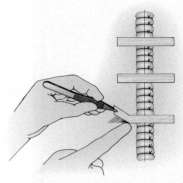

Figure 35–49 Wound closure tape can be used to provide additional support while sutures are in place and after they are removed. This may be especially useful in cosmetic areas, such as the face.

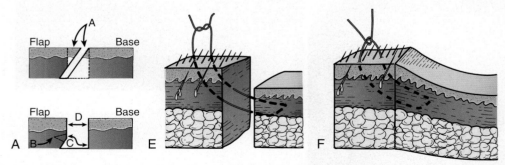

Figure 35–51 Repair of a U-shaped flap laceration with a superiorly oriented base to minimize the trap door effect. *A*, Excision of edges. *B*, Undermining. *C*, Approximation of subcutaneous tissue on the flap to subcutaneous tissue at a deeper level on the base. *B* and *C*, When a laceration in the thin skin of the forehead borders the thicker skin of the scalp, a horizontal mattress suture with an intradermal component can enhance healing by bringing tissues to the same plane. These figures show eversion of thinner skin to obtain adequate approximation with thicker scalp tissue. *D–F*, Skin closure. (*E and F, From Converse JM: Introduction to plastic surgery. In Converse JM [ed]: Reconstructive Plastic Surgery: Principles and Procedures in Correction, Reconstruction, and Transplantation, vol 1, 2nd ed. Philadelphia, WB Saunders, 1977. Reproduced by permission.*)

Note that even a minor forehead contusion or laceration may bleed subcutaneously and, in a few days, *produce blackness around the eyes* (Fig. 35–52). Patients should be forewarned about this. So-called raccoon eyes were once thought to represent a fracture, and although associated with fractures, this is usually a common benign finding, albeit occasionally a striking one.

Windshield injuries to the forehead can be problematic (see Fig. 35–52C) to the extent that multiple superficial cuts harbor small glass particles and the injuries do readily not lend themselves to suture closure. Supraorbital blocks can be used to anesthetize the forehead while the clinician meticulously looks for glass in each skin defect, often feeling pieces only with forceps or a small hemostat. Some pieces of glass are best felt, others are appreciated as shining objects under a good light source.

Eyebrow and Eyelid Lacerations

Jagged lacerations through eyebrows should be managed with little, if any, débridement of untidy but viable edges. The hair shafts of the eyebrow grow at an oblique angle, and vertical excision may produce a linear alopecia in the eyebrow, whereas with simple closure, the scar remains hidden within the hair.

If partial excision is unavoidable, the scalpel blade should be angled in a direction parallel to the axis of the hair shaft to minimize damage to hair follicles.

Points on each side of the lacerated eyebrow should be aligned precisely; a single percutaneous stitch on each margin of the eyebrow should precede SQ closure. The edges of the eyebrow serve as landmarks for reapproximation; therefore, the eyebrow must not be shaved, because these landmarks will be lost. Shaved eyebrows grow back slowly and sometimes incompletely, and shaving them often results in more deformity than the injury itself. Care must be taken not to invert hair-bearing skin into the wound.[85]

The thin, flexible skin of the upper eyelid is relatively easy to suture. A soft 6-0 suture (or smaller) is recommended for closure of simple lacerations. Traumatized eyelids are susceptible to massive swelling; compression dressings and cool compresses can be used to minimize this problem.

The emergency clinician must recognize complicated eyelid lacerations that require the expertise of an ophthalmologist. Lacerations that traverse the lid margin require exact realignment to avoid entropion or ectropion. Injuries penetrating the tarsal plate frequently cause damage to the globe (Fig. 35–53A). A deep horizontal laceration through the

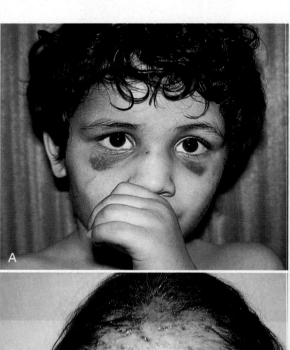
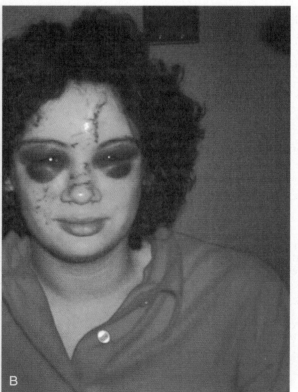
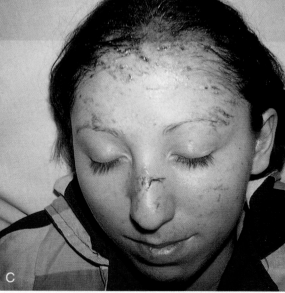

Figure 35–52 Raccoon eyes. *A,* Patients should be informed that minor forehead or nasal bridge trauma can produce benign blackness around the eyes in a few days. *B,* Most often benign, this phenomenon can be impressive. *C,* Under bilateral supraorbital nerve blocks, multiple small lacerations from this windshield injury are explored with a metal instrument and good lighting to remove tiny pieces of glass. Most superficial cuts can be left alone, others sutured with 6-0 nylon sutures (a clinical call as to which require closure).

DIRECT CLOSURE OF A MARGINAL EYELID LACERATION

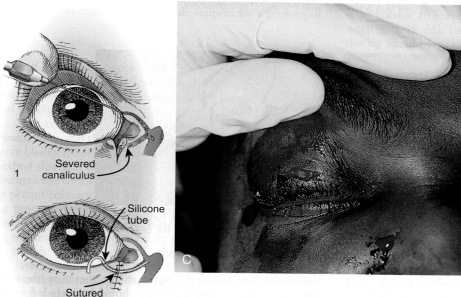

Placement of intial margin suture	Partial-thickness lamellar sutures in the tarsus	Margin sutures tied through skin sutures

Orbicularis muscle — Tarsus — Skin

Eyelid retractors — Tarsus sutures

Skin sutures

A

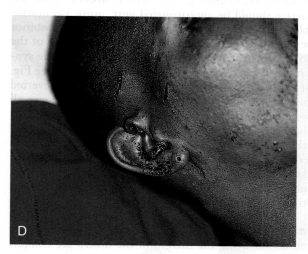

Severed canaliculus

Silicone tube

Sutured canaliculus

1

2

B

C

D

Figure 35–53 *A,* A laceration of the eyelid margin is a complicated repair usually done by an ophthalmologist or plastic surgeon. The principles of repair are demonstrated here: *1,* The suture is placed precisely in the plane of the meibomian glands at the eyelid margin, approximately 2 mm from the wound edges and 2 mm deep. This placement should provide adequate margin eversion. *2,* Partial-thickness lamellar sutures are placed across the tarsus and tied anteriorly. *3,* The anterior skin and muscle lamella are closed with fine sutures, and these are tied over the long marginal sutures to prevent corneal touch. *B,* A method of identifying and repairing the canaliculus. This repair is best left to the ophthalmologist, but the emergency clinician must recognize the potential for a canaliculus injury. *C,* Deep laceration of the left upper lid with herniation of orbital fat. For fat to prolapse, the orbital septum (and potentially the globe itself) must have been perforated. This is a wound requiring operating room exploration and repair. *D,* Lacerations of the ear require a special repair aimed at covering cartilage and preventing hematoma formation. With this through-and-through laceration of the margin of the pinna, the cartilage is trimmed just enough to allow the skin to be approximated to cover all exposed cartilage. Sutures are not used in the cartilage itself for this laceration, but the edges are approximated by skin sutures incorporating the perichondrium. The repair is easiest if the *posterior* pinna is sutured first. An ear compression dressing should be used to prevent hematoma (see Chapter 64 for discussion of anesthesia and dressing for this injury).

Continued

CHAPTER **36**

Foreign Body Removal

Daniel B. Stone and Matthew R. Levine

FOREIGN BODY REACTIONS

Many soft tissue foreign bodies (FBs) must be removed because of either infection or FB reaction. Some FBs produce an inflammatory reaction or infection a few days after introduction into the body; other objects may not cause problems for weeks, months, or even years, often flaring up for no apparent reason. The primary factors in the extent of tissue reactions are contamination and whether the material is inert versus reactive with human tissue. Reactive FBs, such as wood, will always produce inflammation eventually, whereas inert FBs, such as bullets, rarely do. Some inert FBs may carry dirt particles, pieces of clothing, or other sources of bacterial contamination. Expeditious removal may be necessary, even if the FB itself is relatively small and unlikely to cause a reaction.

A purulent bacterial infection may develop in the presence of any FB, but not in all cases. Karpman and coworkers[1] found a 15% infection rate (*Staphylococcus aureus* and Enterobacteriaceae) in a series of 25 patients treated for cactus thorn injuries of the extremities. Certain thorns (black thorns, rose thorns), redwood and Northwest cedar splinters, toothpicks, hair, and stingray or sea urchin spines are noted for their ability to initiate chronic FB reactions. Sea urchin spines and other marine FBs are covered with slime, calcareous material, and other debris that commonly initiate an FB granuloma. The inflammatory reaction seen with cactus thorns may be an allergic reaction to fungus found on the cactus plant.

Many FB reactions are thought to result from an inflammatory response to organic material or they may represent infection from bacteria introduced at wounding. Clinically evident reactions may be delayed for weeks or even years after injury (Fig. 36–1). The chronic infection or inflammatory reaction may not be accompanied by the production of pus, but it may be quite painful or result in loss of function. FBs may also be associated with the formation of a chronic pseudotumor, development of a sinus tract, or evidence of osteomyelitis-like lesions of bone and soft tissue.[2] Organic material has also been noted to induce chronic tenosynovitis, chronic monarticular synovitis, and chronic bursitis.

Rapidly traveling projectiles with considerable inherent heat (e.g., bullets) are less likely to cause infection but are more apt to cause other difficulties. Damage to surrounding areas can occur during passage through tissue. Rarely do retained lead FBs, such as bullets or shotgun pellets, leach out lead into the general circulation and produce systemic lead poisoning (Fig. 36–2). If this process occurs, it may take years to develop and can cause vague or nondescript symptoms (e.g., fatigue, arthralgia, headache, or abdominal pain) many years after the initial injury. Elevated blood lead levels are more likely to occur if bodily fluids such as joint, pleural, peritoneal, or cerebrospinal fluids bathe the lead. Bullets retained in muscle or other soft tissues are not likely to produce any sequelae related to their lead content. However,

Farrell and colleagues[3] reported unsuspected elevated lead levels in patients with retained lead fragments who presented to the emergency department (ED) with a variety of complaints. Lead levels of up to 50 µg/dL were reported. Levels greater than 45 µg/dL are generally considered an indication for chelation therapy. The relation between the retained lead and the presenting symptoms was unclear, but this report verifies the observations of others that retained lead FBs in selected areas can significantly elevate blood lead levels and may produce symptomatic plumbism.

DIAGNOSIS

Bedside Evaluation

A history and physical examination appropriate for the clinical scenario should initially be performed. It is important to determine the exact mechanism of injury and whether the specific characteristics of the foreign material are known. Some scenarios may be particularly suspicious for a retained FB, such as stepping on broken glass. Occasionally, an FB initially was removed before ED arrival. A patient who experiences a sharp, sudden pain in the foot while walking barefoot across a carpet may have a sewing needle or toothpick embedded, rather than a "sprained foot" (Fig. 36–3). An abscess or cellulitis that recurs or wounds that do not heal as expected should always be investigated for retained FBs.[2,4] Certain mechanisms of injury, such as punching or kicking out a window or stepping on an unknown object while walking in a field or stream, are highly suggestive of a retained FB. Most lacerations from metal objects do not contain foreign material, but if the patient states that considerable force was applied during injury and the instrument is not available for inspection, radiographic imaging may be warranted. Occasionally, as a knife encounters the bone, the tip of the knife's blade may break off.

In old injuries, a thorough history of the type of foreign material and method of introduction is warranted. However, a hasty or extensive exploration for the foreign material that may or may not still exist is not recommended. The initial history should also include any unusual medical problems that would preclude use of adequate local anesthesia, such as allergy to local anesthetics, bleeding diathesis, and medical problems (including diabetes mellitus, vascular disease, uremia, or a compromised immune status) that might lead to unusual or more difficult wound management. Finally, *enough time, a proper space and equipment, and especially a cooperative and willing patient are essential for success.* Attempting to remove an FB in an intoxicated, drugged, mentally retarded, or overtly uncooperative patient is obviously self-defeating. Few FBs cannot wait for a repeat examination when the patient is able to be properly examined, often on a follow-up visit a few days later.

Because the patient's perception of an FB sometimes correlates with the presence of an FB, it is suggested that the clinician ask the patient if he or she thinks a wound may harbor foreign material. Steele and associates,[5] however, found that the positive predictive value of patient perception was only 31%, with a negative predictive value of 89%.

Many, but not all, retained FBs will produce pain when the patient moves the injured area or when the wound edges are palpated or depressed. It is prudent to carefully palpate the periphery of all wounds to elicit such tenderness. Superficial FBs may be palpated through the skin, but surprisingly

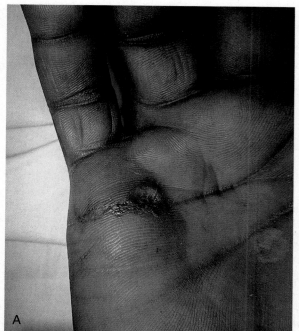

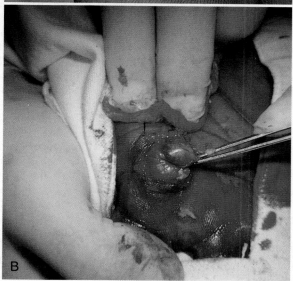

Figure 36–1 This foreign body (FB) granuloma developed after the FB was stable for 6 mo. There was no gross infection and the mass was dissected en mass.

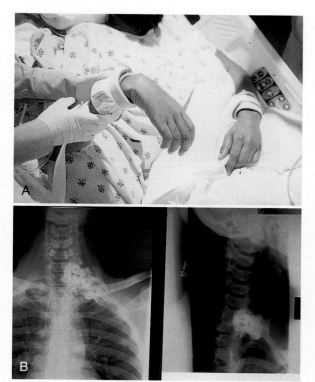

Figure 36–2 Most lead FBs are well tolerated, but if a bullet is bathed in synovial, pleural, peritoneal, or cerebrospinal fluid, the lead may leach out over time and produce a significant elevation in blood lead levels. Symptoms are often vague, and the relation between the retained lead and the patient's clinical scenario may be difficult to sort out. *A,* This patient had chronic neurologic findings, including wrist drop, and was wheelchair bound. *B,* The symptoms were due to chronic lead poisoning from a 20-year-old retained bullet.

635

large FBs may be found in seemingly minor wounds without much external evidence. Whereas puncture wounds are more likely than wide, gaping lacerations to contain an FB, the external characteristics of the wound do not yield firm evidence as to the presence or absence of an FB.

Superficial FBs, such as splinters, bullets, or embedded glass, may be palpated if they are near the skin surface. Deeper FBs must be localized by other techniques. A metal probe may identify the FB by feel or sound. Because glass is difficult to identify by sight in soft tissue, touching it with metal causes a characteristic grating sound. Because of the increasing incidence of human immunodeficiency virus (HIV), probing a wound with a gloved finger to locate or identify an FB is strongly discouraged (Fig. 36–4) because sharp objects can easily penetrate a gloved finger, exposing the clinician to blood-borne diseases such as HIV and hepatitis.

Exploration is an important part of the bedside evaluation, whether done initially or after further imaging studies (Figs. 36–5 to 36–7). This requires adequate pain control, good lighting, proper equipment, a bloodless field, and a cooperative patient to visualize as much of the wound as possible. Some authors have suggested injecting the entrance wound with methylene blue to outline the track of the FB.[6] The blue line of injected dye is followed into the deeper tissues. This technique is of limited value, because the track of the FB often closes tightly and does not allow passage of the methylene blue.

It is not uncommon to serendipitously encounter soft tissue FBs, even though their presence was not suggested by history. Anderson and coworkers[7] reported that clinicians who initially treated a series of hand injuries did not suspect FBs in 75 of 200 consecutive cases.

Imaging Techniques

A variety of imaging techniques may detect and localize FBs. Whenever there is an index of suspicion for a retained FB as a result of the history, mechanism of injury, patient complaint, or examination, attempts should be made to visualize the FB. Modalities available include plain radiographs, ultrasound (US), computed tomography (CT), magnetic resonance imaging (MRI), and fluoroscopy (Fig. 36–8).

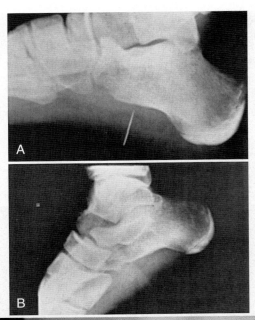

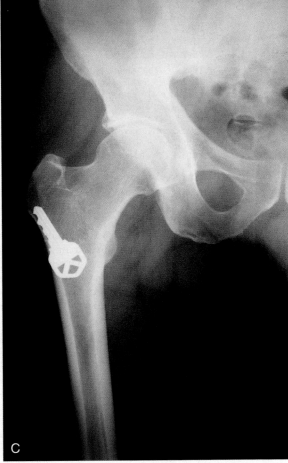

Figure 36–3 *A,* A common FB of the foot is a splinter, toothpick, pin, or needle that is impaled while walking barefoot on a carpet. This sewing needle was obvious, but some FBs may be mistaken for a simple puncture wound, heel spur, contusion, or tendinitis. *B,* Postoperative radiographs demonstrate complete removal. *C,* This patient fell, landed on a metal pipe, and suffered a deep laceration to the thigh. A radiograph was taken to rule out a fracture, and the key was seen but thought to be an artifact (i.e., an item left on the backboard). During the examination, the key was found embedded in the wound. It had been in the patient's pants pocket and was forced into the wound by the pipe during the injury.

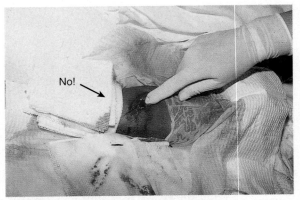

Figure 36–4 What's wrong with this picture? Although historically suggested as a useful technique to find FBs, probing the depths of a wound with a gloved finger may result in a puncture wound in the operator. The practice is strongly discouraged because of the prevalence of hepatitis and human immunodeficiency virus infections.

Plain Radiography

Many emergency clinicians mistakenly believe that in the absence of adipose tissue, if the base of the wound can be clearly visualized and explored, an FB can always be ruled out. Although this is commonly true, Avner and Baker[8] detected glass by routine radiographs in 11 of 160 wounds (6.9%) that were inspected and believed by the clinician to be free of glass. Orlinsky and Bright[9] found the reliability of exploration to be related to wound depth. Only 2 out of 133 superficial wounds that were deemed adequately explored had an FB on plain films, but 10 out of 130 wounds beyond the subcutaneous fat had FBs despite negative explorations. Clinicians evaluating for FBs should keep low thresholds for ordering plain films, unless they feel certain after thorough exploration of the superficial wounds that no FB is present.

Plain radiographs are readily available, are easily interpreted, and cost significantly less than CT, US, or MRI.[10] The ability of plain films to detect FBs in soft tissues depends on the object's composition (relative density), configuration, size, and orientation. Multiple projections may be required. Metallic objects, such as pins, bullets, and BBs, are readily visualized. It is a common misconception that glass must contain lead to be visualized on a plain radiograph. *Almost all glass objects in soft tissue (bottles, windshield glass, light bulbs, microscope cover slips, laboratory capillary tubes) are at least somewhat radiopaque and can be detected by plain radiographs, unless they are obscured by bone (see Fig. 36–5).*[10,11] Very small glass fragments (<1 mm) may be more difficult to detect by this technique, but plain films have been demonstrated to be highly sensitive for detecting glass greater than 1 mm in size.[12] The absence of a glass FB on multiple projections is strong, although not absolute, evidence that glass is not contained in a wound. Other nonmetallic objects readily visualized include teeth, bone, pencil graphite, asphalt, and gravel.[10,13] Aluminum, which has traditionally been deemed radiolucent, can occasionally be visualized on plain films if the object is projected away from underlying bone. Ellis[14] demonstrated that pure aluminum fragments as small as 0.5 × 0.5 × 1 mm could be identified in a chicken wing model simulating a human hand or foot. Ellis[14] cautioned that other aluminum FBs, such as pull tabs from cans, may not be visualized in other parts of the body such as the esophagus or stomach.

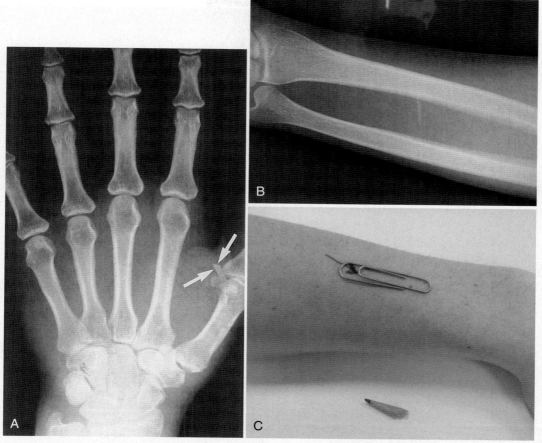

Figure 36–5 *A, Almost all glass is visible on plain radiograph, regardless of lead content.* If glass is superimposed on bone it may be missed, so multiple projections are viewed. Plain film radiography shows sharp corners characteristic of glass. Proximity of the FB to the bone may be deceiving. *B,* This pencil point broke off in the forearm. Graphite, but not wood, is radio-opaque. *C,* Place an arrow and paperclip over the puncture site and take an x-ray (multiple views are essential) to confirm the orientation of the FB. Remove the paperclip and use the arrow to guide the surgical exploration based on radiographic findings.

637

Certain FBs are radiolucent and will not usually be visualized by plain film radiography. Vegetative materials, such as thorns, wood, splinters, and cactus spines, are radiolucent and not readily visualized by plain radiographs. These materials absorb body fluids as they sit in situ and become isodense with the surrounding tissues. Because of their varying chemical composition and density, plastics may or may not be visible on plain films.[15]

Detection of FBs on plain films can be enhanced by requesting that the technician use an underpenetrated soft tissue technique.[16] *Multiple views should always be obtained when attempting to visualize an FB because many clearly radiopaque objects are obscured by superimposed bone on one view but are quite obvious when viewed from another angle.* Digitized radiographs may be manipulated to enhance identification of a suspected FB. Plain films may provide indirect evidence of the presence of an FB if one sees trapped or surrounding air, a radiolucent filling defect, or secondary bony changes such as periosteal elevation, osteolytic or osteoblastic changes, or pseudotumors of bone.[16]

Besides simply diagnosing FBs, radiographs can also be used to estimate the general location, depth, and structure of radiopaque FBs. If one strategically attaches a marker (needle or paper clip) to the skin surface at the wound entrance before taking a radiograph, the FB will be seen in relation to the entrance wound. This also helps to identify the path that leads to the FB and the relative distance from the surface to the FB.[17] Needles at two angles may also be used to aid localization (Fig. 36–9).

The liberal use of plain film radiography makes sound medicolegal practice. A review of 54 wound FB claims against 32 physicians from 22 institutions found glass, a radiopaque material, to be the most common material. However, only 35% of the cases involving glass had plain films. Cases with a glass FB without an x-ray ordered were associated with unsuccessful defense (60%) and higher indemnity payments.[18]

US

Most soft tissue FBs are hyperechoic on US. For this reason, US has become the modality of choice for imaging radiolucent FBs such as wood and thorns. If in place for more than 24 hours, most FBs will be surrounded by a hypoechoic area corresponding to granulation tissue, edema, or hemorrhage (see Fig. 36–8). This area may aid in making the diagnosis.[19] Metal will leave a linear trail of echoes deep to the FB, referred to as the "comet-tail artifact." A wooden object leaves an acoustic shadow without artifact.[20,21] The technique requires a high-frequency transducer (at least 7.5 MHz, such as an endovaginal probe) because most FBs are small and superficial. A spacer may be needed to adjust the "focal zone"—where

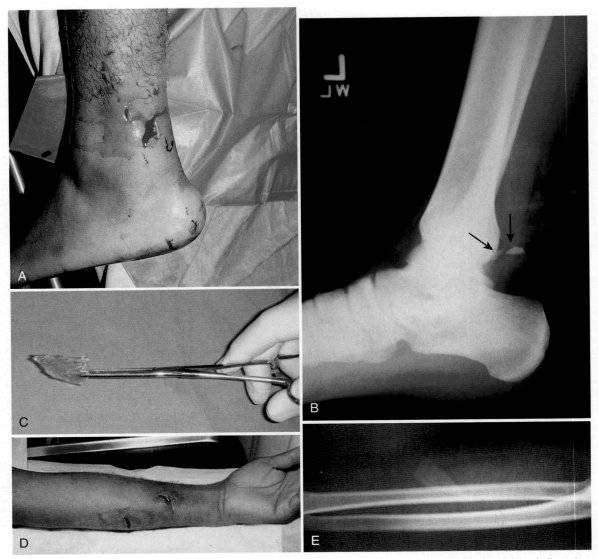

Figure 36–6 *A*, This intoxicated patient kicked out a window and sustained seemingly minor puncture wounds. He did not believe that glass was in the wound, there was little pain, and no FB could be palpated externally. A radiograph (*B*) revealed a large shard of glass (*arrows*) deeply embedded in the wound (*C*). A large shard of glass was removed, but only after 20 min of exploration. *D*, Another classic scenario for a retained glass FB is putting the arm through a window. A FB was not suspected or sensed by the patient or clinician. *E*, When a radiograph was taken a large shard of glass is readily detected. Despite its size, removal was difficult and time consuming.

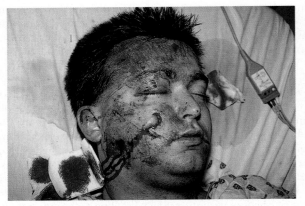

Figure 36–7 A windshield forehead injury usually harbors multiple retained pieces of glass that are difficult to find. Probing with a needle or forceps to feel or hear contact with the fragments may help find them. A supraorbital nerve block is ideal to facilitate probing.

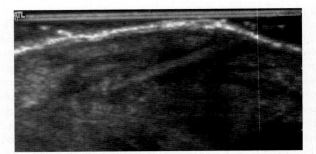

Figure 36–8 Ultrasound shows a wood FB with characteristic acoustic shadowing deep to the FB. *Wood FBs may become less echogenic over time.*

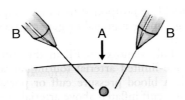

Figure 36–9 When a small entrance wound (A) is noted but the FB is not seen, noninvasive localization is preferable to blind probing. Metal markers taped to the skin or needles inserted close to the FB under local anesthesia (B) and radiographed at different angles provide a guide to FB localization and extraction. (*Reproduced from Hospital Medicine, © January 1981, with permission of Cahner's Publishing Co.*)

the beam is the narrowest and the signal intensity is the highest. If the FB is deep, a lower frequency transducer may be needed to penetrate deeper, but may miss small FBs.[22]

Advantages of US include low cost, no ionizing radiation, the ability to define the object in three dimensions, and real-time bedside imaging that may be used during removal.[16] Many studies report that US is highly sensitive for FB detection in adequately trained personnel, either radiologists, technicians, or emergency physicians.[9] It is difficult to cite a precise sensitivity or specificity owing to the wide variation in these studies with regard to FB size, material, location, operator experience, and model used in these studies.[23–25] US may be particularly difficult in the hand or foot, where there are many echogenic structures and webspaces.[26] As with all US studies, accuracy is operator-dependent. The presence of air in surrounding tissue may result in false-positive results.[26] False-positives may also occur in the presence of scars, calcification, sutures, and sesamoid bones.[23] Imaging may also be limited when the FB is adjacent to bone.[19,21]

CT

Because CT depends on x-ray absorption, it generally visualizes the same materials detected on plain films.[13] CT, compared with US, however, is more costly and exposes the patient to ionizing radiation. CT, however, can detect subtle differences in soft tissue densities and may detect FBs not readily visible on plain films.[10] Wood is unlikely to be visible initially on CT. By 1 week, the wood absorbs surrounding blood products and may become higher in attenuation than muscle and fat. It may then appear on CT as a linear area of increased attenuation. It is best seen on a wide window setting, such as a bone window.[27] Because it produces a better three-dimensional image of tissue than plain films, CT can visualize objects embedded in or behind bone.

MRI

Although MRI is expensive and not as readily available to emergency clinicians as plain films and CT, it may be superior to CT in detecting small, nonmetallic, radiolucent FBs, such as plastic, particularly in the orbit.[28] MRI may not visualize wood. Wood appears as a linear signal with associated inflammation and looks hypointense compared with muscle on T_1- and T_2-weighted sequences, appearing as a signal void.[27] Plastic is more easily visualized with MRI than with CT. MRI cannot be used for metallic objects and gravel, which contain various ferrometallic particles that produce signal artifacts on MRI.[10] Metallic objects, in addition to producing a high degree of artifact on MRI, have a theoretical risk of shifting

within the magnetic field and causing structural damage to adjacent structures. This is of little importance in superficial extremity wounds, but it is particularly important when evaluating FBs in the eye, brain, or deep structures of the neck, face, or extremities. FBs may be difficult to differentiate from other low-signal structures, such as tendon, scar tissue, and calcium, on MRI.[29]

Fluoroscopy

More recently, portable, low-power, C-arm fluoroscopy has become available in some EDs, particularly for orthopaedic reductions. Its use has also been reported for removal of BB pellets, metal, glass, and coins from patients.[30] Like radiography, fluoroscopy can visualize objects that are radiopaque but not radiolucent like wood and plastic[30,31] By using correct technique and shielding, radiation scatter to imaging personnel is minute, less than 0.0001 roentgen/hr.[32] Fluoroscopy also offers the advantage of real-time bedside imaging.[30,32] Fluoroscopic image-intensifying equipment may be used to follow a wound's entrance, localize the material, grasp the FB, and remove it without making a larger incision. Ariyan[33] described a technique in which two needles are placed in the soft tissue from opposite directions, pointing toward the FB. The extremity is rotated while the clinician watches the image under the image intensifier to obtain a three-dimensional effect. An incision is placed perpendicular to the plane of the needles, and the object is removed. Although the technique to use fluoroscopy is relatively easy to learn, the lack of instruction and availability are the major limitations to its use in the ED.[32–34]

General Imaging Approach

A reasonable initial approach for localizing nonvisualized FBs in the ED is to obtain multiple-projection plain radiographs with a soft tissue technique. This technique will visualize the majority of FBs, especially metal and glass. US should be considered for objects known to be radiolucent, such as wood or thorns. The role of CT and MRI for FB evaluation in the ED is limited, but they are the definitive tests in confusing cases. For suspected intraorbital or intracranial FB, CT is recommended. CT or MRI is also warranted *when a previously negatively explored wound exhibits recurrent infection, poor healing, or persistent pain*. CT or MRI may be the appropriate initial test for patients with nonspecific swelling to define FBs and alternative possible diagnoses such as abscesses, masses, or other inflammatory processes.[27] Bedside US and fluoroscopy (for radiopaque FBs) may be used to guide difficult FB extractions if initial removal attempts are unsuccessful, if the proper equipment and experienced personnel are available.

FB REMOVAL

Removal Decisions

One should judiciously evaluate and manage each FB scenario individually. The composition and location of an FB, as well as the patient's medical status and vocational/avocational activities, greatly affect decision making related to FB removal. The history, physical examination, and localization techniques available will determine the best time and place for FB removal. Reactive material, such as wood, should be removed immediately when accessible because retained wood will invariably lead to inflammation and infection. Other inert materials, such as glass or plastic, may often be removed on

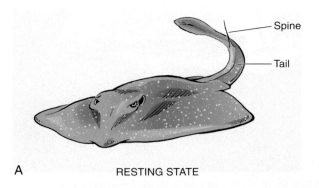

A   RESTING STATE

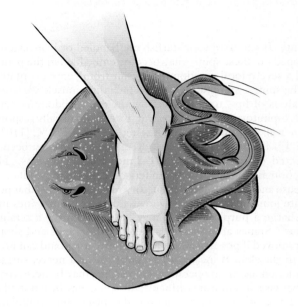

B   STINGRAY ATTACK

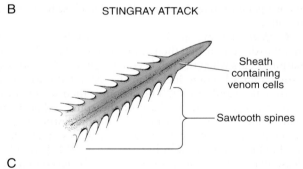

C

Figure 36–21 *A,* Stingray resting on the bottom of the ocean, usually covered by a layer of sand. *B,* An unsuspecting victim steps on the stingray, and the whiplike tail impales the foot (even through a heavy boot) with one or more spines. The spine has backward-facing barbs covered by a sheath with venom-containing cells (*C*), causing a toxic envenomation and the potential for multiple FBs.

serrated spines. Portions of the spine may become buried in the victim's skin. Each spine is covered with a sheath containing venom glands, and in addition to immediate toxin-induced pain, pieces of the spine or sheath may remain embedded in the wound. These fragments, although often difficult to locate, do not dissolve and must be removed. Persistent pain and inflammation, even weeks to months after the attack, mandate consideration of a retained FB, but a *persistent and difficult-to-treat irritative process can occur in the absence of a*

retained spine or sheath. Immediate local and systemic reactions occur as a result of injection of a complex toxin. Systemic reactions may be severe and can include muscle cramps, vomiting, seizures, hypotension, arrhythmias, and (rarely) death.[58]

Treatment consists of irrigation with saline followed by hot water immersion at 43.3°C to 46.1°C (110°F–115°F) for 30 minutes to 1 hour in order to inactivate the heat-labile toxin. Local digital blocks without vasoconstrictors provide effective analgesia for hand wounds. All wounds should be explored and débrided, and all remnants of the spine and integumentary sheath removed.[52] Wounds should heal by secondary intention. The venom can cause significant local tissue necrosis, and surgical débridement may be required.

Antibiotic Therapy. Prophylactic antibiotic therapy for marine injuries is common, although there are no convincing data to support or refute the practice. Unlike other soft tissue infections, marine injuries become infected with unusual gram-negative organisms, particularly *Vibrio* species. Although there are few studies evaluating the effects of specific antibiotics, it is recommended that quinolones, trimethoprim-sulfamethoxazole, tetracyclines, third-generation cephalosporins, or aminoglycosides be used in lieu of penicillin, ampicillin, erythromycin, or first-generation cephalosporins.[53] It is always difficult to differentiate chronic inflammation caused by toxins and foreign material from true infection, and often surgical exploration is required in persistent cases. Tetanus prophylaxis should be administered as per routine recommendations.

Cactus Spines

The sizes of cactus spines fluctuate considerably. The difficulty of removal is generally inversely proportional to the FB size.[59] Larger embedded cactus spines are managed like wood splinters and sea urchin spine FBs. More advanced imaging techniques (US, CT, or MRI) may be required for localization of deeply embedded spines.

Deeply embedded cactus spines generally produce granulomatous reactions, and infections are rare.[1] Dermatitis from embedded cactus spines is a well-described phenomenon. Hence, efforts to remove deeply embedded spines should be made after carefully weighing the benefit and potential harm related to a deep exploration, especially in a sensitive location.[59] Using forceps, superficially embedded, medium- to large-sized cactus spines are best removed by direct axial traction of each spine. Smaller spines (glochids) may be difficult and tedious to remove individually. Adherent facial mask gel application and removal of spines en masse with the mask are recommended (Fig. 36–22). Depilatory wax melted in a microwave oven and applied warm, commercial facial gels, and household glue (Elmer's Glue-All [Borden, Inc., Columbus, OH]) have all been recommended for this purpose.[59–62] Over-the-counter "home use" facial mask gels are not adherent enough to be effective without multiple (eight or more) applications.

Ring Removal

Frequently, a ring must be removed to prevent laceration of tissue or vascular compromise. The use of thorough lubrication (a water-soluble lubricant [e.g., K-Y jelly]) and a circular motion with traction on the ring are usually sufficient. However, the string-wrap method or physically cutting off the ring may be necessary. Preferably, all rings should be removed before edema is extensive enough to cause pain or vascular compromise.

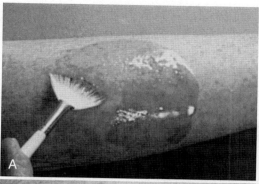

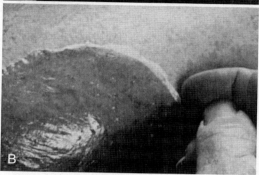

Figure 36–22 *A,* A thousand or more glochids affixed to the skin by contact with a single pad of polka dot cactus. *B,* To remove them, professional facial gel is spread with a fan brush, spread thin at the edges. *C,* The gel rollup is started by picking at the edge with the fingernails. When the gel is peeled off, all of the very small spines come with it. (*A–C, From Lindsey D, Lindsey WE: Cactus spine injuries. Am J Emerg Med 6:362, 1988. Reproduced by permission.*)

String-Wrap Method. An occasional patient can remain calm during this procedure, but if swelling is significant or the digit has been traumatized, anesthesia is necessary (Fig. 36–23). A proximal digital or metacarpal block provides sufficient anesthesia and helps to minimize tissue distention at the ring site. Before ring removal, a wide Penrose drain is wrapped circumferentially in a distal-to-proximal direction to reduce soft tissue swelling, and the wrap should remain in place for a few minutes to reach the maximum effect. Some nonanesthetized patients panic during the procedure because of increasing pain due to compression and unwinding.[63]

A 20- to 25-inch piece of string, umbilical tape, or thick silk suture is first passed between the ring and the finger. Shorter lengths are discouraged, because one may need to repeat the wrapping procedure midway. If there is marked soft tissue swelling, the tip of a hemostat may be passed under the ring to grasp the string and pull it through. The distal string is wrapped clockwise around the swollen finger (proximal to distal) to include the proximal interphalangeal (PIP) joint and the entire swollen finger. The wrapping starts next to the ring. The wrap should be snug enough to compress the swollen tissue. Successive loops of wrap are placed next to each other to keep any swollen tissue from bulging between the strands. When the wrapping is complete, the proximal end of the string is carefully unwound in the same clockwise direction, forcing the ring over that portion of the finger that has been compressed by the wrap. The PIP joint is the area that is most difficult to maneuver and causes the most pain to the patient.

Occasionally, the finger must be rewrapped if it was not carefully done initially. It is not uncommon to produce abra-sions or other trauma to the skin during this procedure. If the finger with the ring is lacerated or there are underlying fractures, it is prudent to cut off the ring instead of attempting this technique.

Certain rings are made of extremely hard materials such as tungsten carbide or ceramic. In these cases, cracking the material with standard vice-grip pliers can break the ring. Place the pliers on the ring and adjust the jaws to fit tightly, then remove and readjust, increasing the tension with each subsequent adjustment. Continue until the material cracks and falls apart. Some rings may be lined with a metal band. A standard ring cutter can then be used to remove the band.

Ring Cutter. A ring cutter should be used when there is excessive swelling or other methods fail (Fig. 36–24). Power devices are available. The ring cutter has a small hook that fits under the ring and serves as a guide for a saw-toothed wheel that cuts the metal. The cut ends of the ring are spread using large hemostats (e.g., Kelly clamps), and the ring is removed. If the tension is too great to spread the ring, another cut 180° apart from the original ring cut can be performed. This will allow the ring to fall off in two pieces. A jeweler can subsequently repair cut rings.

Body Piercing and Removal

The art of body piercing predates most history books. Over the last decade, an enormous increase in the practice of body piercing has occurred. With these piercings have come the complications associated with the practice.[64] For centuries, the ears were the most common place. Today, the lips, tongue, eyebrow, nose, navel, nipples, and genital areas have become sites of body piercing. To date, there are a limited number of studies on postpiercing infections in areas other than the ears. Three major types of jewelry are used: (1) barbell studs, which are straight bars with a ball threaded onto both ends; (2) labret studs, which are straight bars with a ball threaded on one end and a disk permanently fixed on the other end (more commonly used on the lips); and (3) a captive bead ring, which consists of a bead with small dimples on opposite sides, held "captive" by tension from both sides of an incompetent ring. The bead ring is a variation of this: One bead is permanently fixed to one end, and an opening is made by removing the free end of the ring.[65]

The most common reason for removal is infection. Other symptoms such as bleeding, edema, allergic reaction, and keloid formation may prompt removal. Occasionally, tongue piercings must be removed to permit intubation. In order to remove the barbell- and labret-type studs, hold the bar with forceps and unscrew the bead on the other end. To remove the captive bead ring, hold the ring on both sides of the captive bead to release the tension on the bead. This will dislodge the bead from the ring, which is holding it in place. If the jewelry is near the mouth or nose, care must be taken to prevent aspiration of the bead. The microbiology of infections related to body piercing has not yet been determined. However, organisms such as *Staphylococcus epidermidis* and *S. aureus*, along with *Pseudomonas aeruginosa*, have been commonly implicated pathogens. Other infectious complications from body piercing such as septic arthritis, endocarditis, hepatitis B and C, and HIV have been reported.[66,67]

Most commonly, however, local wound infections predominate and can be managed with warm compresses, antibacterial soap, and topical antibacterial ointment once the FB is removed. The possibility of leaving the piecing in place while treating the infection has yet to be studied.

649

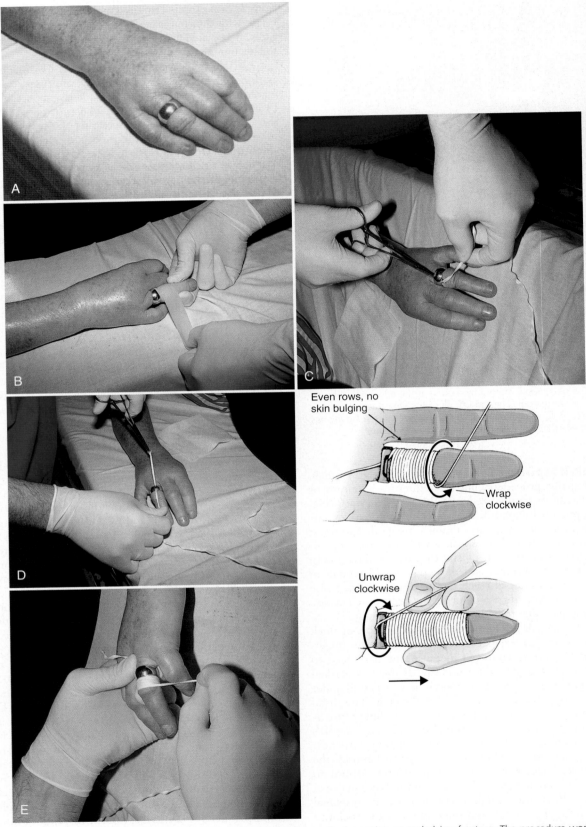

Even rows, no
skin bulging

Wrap
clockwise

Unwrap
clockwise

Figure 36–23 String removal technique for a tight ring. *A,* Note the absence of a laceration or underlying fracture. The procedure works best with a smooth ring. A digital or metacarpal block is suggested. *B,* Edema is lessened by compression of the finger with a Penrose drain left tightly wrapped for 3–5 minutes. *C,* Slide a small hemostat under the ring, grab a long piece of umbilical tape, and pull a short portion under the ring. *D,* The long distal section is the *winding* or *compressing* portion, the short proximal portion is the *unwinding or removal* section. *E,* Begin winding the distal piece either clockwise (*inset*) or counterclockwise (*photograph*) to compress the skin distal to the ring (see details in inset).

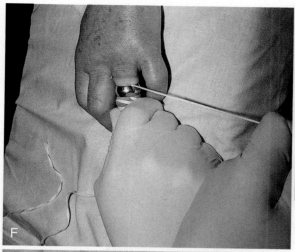

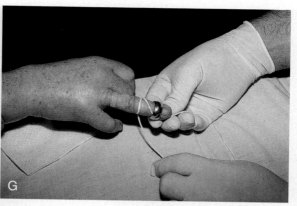

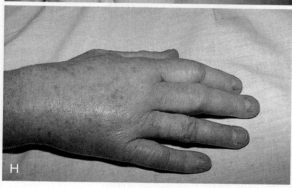

Figure 36–23, cont'd *F* and *G*, The ring is removed by unwrapping the proximal tape *in the same direction it was wrapped*. The most difficult area to negotiate is the proximal interphalangeal joint. You may have to repeat the wrapping procedure to totally remove the ring. *H*, Ring removed with only minor skin abrasions.

Postoperative Suture Removal

FBs in the form of nonabsorbed suture material are frequently encountered in the postoperative period. Drainage, localized pain, tenderness, and inflammatory reaction along the suture line are characteristic of a retained FB (suture abscess). In this instance, probing the wound with a sterilized needle bent in the shape of a crochet hook is frequently successful. Hooking the suture material through the sinus tract and removing it allows the wound to heal over the tract.

Tick Removal

The early removal of ticks is recommended, because the hard tick of the Ixodid family is likely to transmit disease. Rocky Mountain spotted fever, Lyme disease, tularemia, and ascending paralysis are among the many infections identified as tick-borne diseases. It is important to note that the rate of disease transmission before 48 hours of attachment is exceedingly small.[68] Tick removal of Ixodid ticks is difficult because the mouth parts become cemented within 5 to 30 minutes of contact with the host's skin (Fig. 36–25). Removal will become more difficult the longer the tick is attached. Inadequate or partial removal of the tick may cause infection or chronic granuloma infection. Traditional and folk methods of forcing the tick to disengage (e.g., the use of petroleum jelly, fingernail polish, a hot match, or alcohol) are not advised. Removal by mechanical means is recommended.[69] Nonmechanical means of tick removal can cause the tick to regurgitate, increasing the possibility of infectious transmission.

Straight or curved forceps or tweezers is the recommended method of removal. If these instruments are not available, a gloved hand will suffice. Grasp the tick as close to the patient's skin surface as possible and gently apply steady axial traction (see Fig. 36–25B). Take care not to squeeze or

crush the tick body because this may expel infective agents. Do not twist or jerk the tick in order to prevent the mouth parts from breaking off during extraction. If mouth parts are left behind after removal of the body, they may be removed with tweezers. If one is still unable to remove the mouth parts, excision under local anesthesia will be needed to prevent local infection.

Many patients have great anxiety over subsequent tick-borne diseases after tick removal. Some studies have demonstrated that single-dose doxycycline (200 mg) may prevent the development of Lyme disease.[68] However, prophylactic antibiotic treatment of all tick bites is not recommended. When patients are in areas where the incidence of Lyme disease is high or when a partially engorged deer tick in the nymphal stage is discovered on their body, they are more likely to benefit from prophylaxis. Regardless of whether prophylaxis is given, patients should be instructed on the symptoms and signs of Lyme disease and encouraged to return or seek medical evaluation.

Zipper Entrapment

The skin of the penis may become painfully entangled in a zipper mechanism. Unzipping the zipper frequently lacerates the skin and increases the amount of tissue caught in the mechanism. Although the clinician may anesthetize the skin and excise the entrapped tissue, a less invasive method may be useful.

Cutting the median bar between the faceplates of the zipper mechanism remains the most common method. The interlocking teeth of the zipper then fall apart when the median bar (diamond or bridge) of the zipper is cut in half (Fig. 36–26) and the skin is subsequently freed. A bone cutter or wire clippers and a moderate amount of force may be

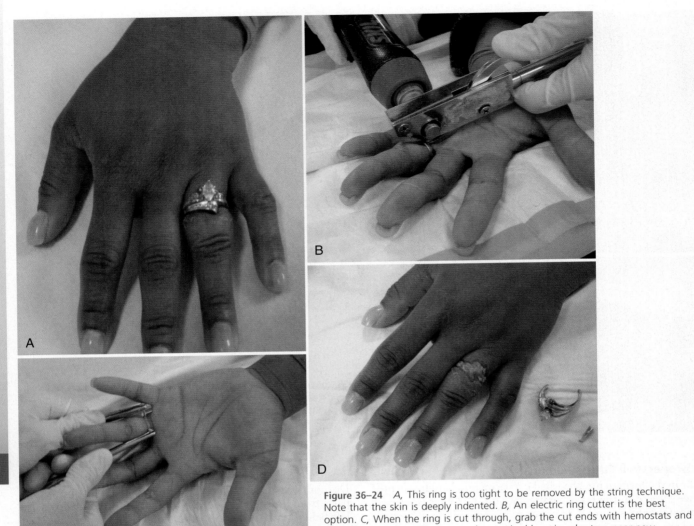

Figure 36–24 *A,* This ring is too tight to be removed by the string technique. Note that the skin is deeply indented. *B,* An electric ring cutter is the best option. *C,* When the ring is cut through, grab the cut ends with hemostats and separate the sides. This ring can be repaired by a jeweler to a near-new condition. *D,* Note the macerated tissue under the ring.

Grasp the head, not the body

Figure 36–25 Ticks should be removed as soon as possible to minimize the transmission of tick-borne pathogens and to limit their fixation to the skin by a secreted cement compound. *A,* This engorged tick has been attached for about a day and has burrowed under the skin. Most home remedies are worthless. *B,* A recommended approach is to grasp the tick with forceps near its head where it enters the skin (avoid the soft body) and gently pull it out. Some advise twisting the head counterclockwise, but this has not objectively been found to be more effective. If pieces of the tick remain, they should be dug out.

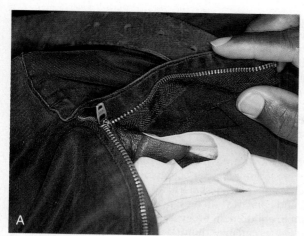

Figure 36-26 *A*, When loose skin is caught in the teeth of a zipper (*B*), one can release it quickly and without risk to the patient by cutting the diamond that holds the slider together with a bone cutter or a pair of wire clippers. *C* and *D*, Alternatively, the zipper teeth can be separated by cutting the cloth between the teeth, either above or below the zipper head. The head is then moved forward or backward. Local anesthesia may be injected in to the incarcerated skin if this procedure is painful. (*A–C*, From *Emergency Medicine, October 15, 1982, p. 215. Used by permission.*)

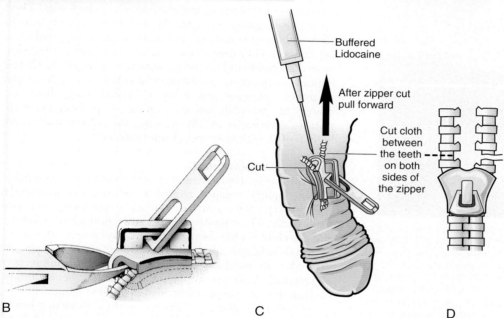

Buffered
Lidocaine

After zipper cut
pull forward

Cut cloth
between
the teeth
on both
sides of
the zipper

Cut

B

C

D

required to break the bar. The addition of mineral oil followed by traction has been demonstrated with some success. Patients with penile lacerations warrant urologic follow-up to assess for urethral injury.

Infiltration of Radiographic Contrast Material

The infiltration of high-osmolality intravenous contrast material has the potential to cause skin necrosis, but the use of low-osmolality dye has essentially eliminated this problem (Fig. 36–27). The use of high-pressure dye injectors, with the technologist out of the room, calls for a careful inspection of the intravenous site prior to injection. Once contrast material has infiltrated, no intervention has been demonstrated to ameliorate local reactions, which are usually mild. It is best to resist the temptation to use excessive heat or cold, and injection of steroids or other agents have no known benefit. Low-osmolality dye usually is totally resorbed in a few days, with no serious consequences. The progress of the dye's egress may be followed with radiographs.

Taser Darts

The Thomas A. Swift Electric Rifle, or "Taser," is a conducted electrical weapon used in many areas by police to

subdue violent patients (see Chapter 71, Physical and Chemical Restraint). The Taser fires two barbed electrodes on long copper wires (Fig. 36–28*A*). The barbs attach to skin or clothing and create an arc that delivers an electrical jolt that causes overwhelming pain and involuntary muscle contraction that incapacitates the subject. The electricity is such high frequency that it is believed to stay near the surface and not penetrate to internal organs. The barbs are designed not to penetrate deeper than 4 mm, and police are taught to remove them by stretching surrounding skin and tugging sharply (see Fig. 36–28*B*). If this fails, cutting down on the dart after local anesthesia should facilitate removal.[70,71] Patients may need medical evaluation after ED removal of the darts for the underlying state of agitation that required Taser usage, electrical injury complications, injury from the fall after incapacitation, and injury from the barb, especially if struck in mouth, eye, neck, or groin. Most patients do well with minimal intervention and proper wound management, if the patient is not unduly agitated and the Taser did not involve the critical areas of the body just mentioned.

Human/Animal Bite FBs

The most common FB in a human bite is a piece of tooth. These FBs can be difficult to find and may not be appreciated

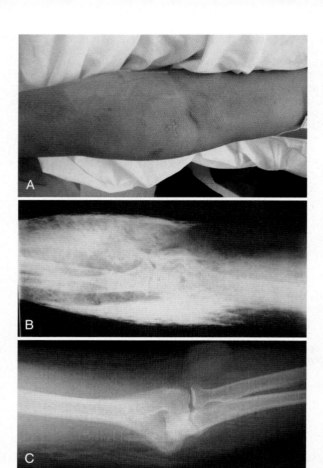

Figure 36–27 The entire volume (100 ml) of nonionic low-osmolality contrast material (Isovue) for a computed tomography (CT) scan was pressure-injected into the antecubital soft tissue when the intravenous line infiltrated. High-volume injections are automatically controlled and the technician is not in the room to stop it. *A,* There was only mild pain, but considerable soft tissue swelling, and most of the redness and the blistering occurred when the technician taped an unprotected ice pack directly to the skin, causing near frostbite. *B,* X-ray evidence of the infiltration. *C,* Within 36 hr, the dye was absorbed, without further treatment. No skin necrosis occurred as has been seen when older ionic high-osmolality agents infiltrate. There is no known proven way to ameliorate potential soft tissue injury.

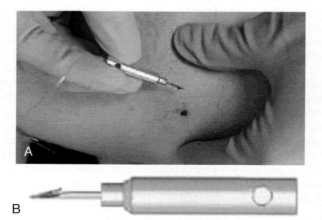

Figure 36–28 *A* and *B,* Barbed Taser darts can be removed by a quick pull or through a small incision made over the barb.

if the patient lies about the injury, denying a bite wound. Usually, the bite puncture is small and not easily cleaned or visualized. The puncture can be widened by a formal incision to aid in cleaning and for an evaluation of the tendon integrity, joint capsule, fracture, or FB (Fig. 36–29*A*). Occasionally, small pieces of teeth can become embedded in a wound, such as with dog, cat, or snake bites (see Fig. 36–29*B*). Radiographic detection is variable, and often exploration is the only alternative.

Pyogenic Granuloma (Lobar Capillary Hemangioma)

A pyogenic granuloma is a benign acquired polypoid, friable vascular lesion of the skin (hand, neck, foot, fingers, and trunk) and mucous membranes (Fig. 36–30). They are common in children; in pregnancy, the lesion is termed *Epulis gravidarum* (pregnancy tumor). The cause is unknown; they are not due to infection, and they are not granulomas. They grow rather rapidly over a few weeks, occasionally are associated with minor trauma, and have a glistening dark red appearance. They may bleed. There is some association with topical retinoids and the protease inhibitor indinavir. Histologically, a pyogenic granuloma is a hemangioma. A variety of topical therapies (silver nitrate, cryotherapy), laser, or cautery are available, but removal by sharp dissection with primary suturing is usually curative. Recurrence may be as high as 40% with nonsurgical intervention.[72]

Hair-Thread Tourniquet

Hair or thread fibers adherent to infant clothing occasionally become tightly wrapped around a child's digits or genitals (Fig. 36–31).[73] If these are left in place, amputation may eventually occur. The offending fibers may be difficult to visualize, and the child is often brought for evaluation only after signs of distal ischemia appear. Occasionally, the fiber can be grasped with toothless forceps or a small hemostat and unwrapped. More commonly, fibers cannot be identified because they are deeply embedded in swollen tissue.

A No. 11 blade can be used to cut the constricting bands under a regional nerve block.[74] It may be difficult to identify individual hairs that are deeply embedded in a swollen digit and even more difficult to assess the success of the intervention. Often, multiple hairs are involved. Because the bands may be quite deep, the incision should avoid known neurovascular tracts. Barton and coworkers[73] recommend a dorsal, rather than lateral, incision on the digits. If the soft tissue of the distal digit has been rotated after a circumferential dermal laceration from the tourniquet, the distal tissue can be realigned with the proximal tissue and two dorsolateral sutures placed or tissue adhesive glue applied to maintain the digit in alignment.

Generally, conservative wound care is sufficient once the band has been removed. Application of an antibiotic ointment may enhance healing and allow easier removal of serous drainage from the circumferential laceration. Clinical reassessment in 24 hours will indicate whether any constricting bands remain.

DISPOSITION MANAGEMENT

Tetanus

Wounds with FBs should be considered contaminated wounds, and tetanus status should be updated according to recommendations for patients with contaminated wounds.

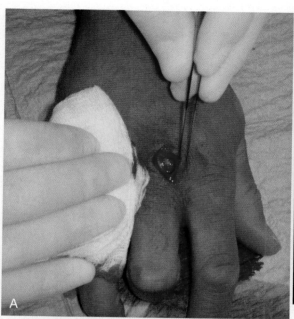

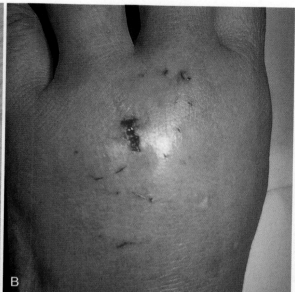

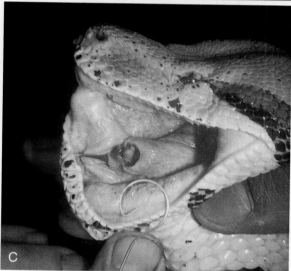

Figure 36–29 *A,* This human bite puncture wound was enlarged with an incision to aid in cleaning and a search for an FB, usually a piece of tooth. *B,* The bite of a boa constrictor, although not poisonous, may contain small tooth fragments (*C*). As with cat and dog bites, radiographic evaluation is variable and exploration may be required.

Antibiotics

There is no consensus or standard for antibiotic use after wound FB removal. Antibiotics may be indicated for immunocompromised patients, but there are no data to support the routine use of antibiotics in any subset of patients for wounds that have been thoroughly cleaned and from which all foreign material has been removed. Prophylaxis may be considered if there was excessive time between injury and removal, obvious contamination, or when the ability to adequately clean a wound is suspect. However, under these circumstances, it is more prudent to opt for an open wound and a delayed closure.

If prophylactic antibiotics are prescribed, traditionally a first-generation cephalosporin or a penicillinase-resistant penicillin have been first-line choices. For patients with contraindications to penicillins and cephalosporins, and with the increasing incidence of community-acquired methicillin-resistant *S. aureus* in many areas, clindamycin, trimethoprim/sulfamethoxazole, or tetracycline may provide appropriate coverage.[75] However, infections associated with FBs are not likely to be from methicillin-resistant *S. aureus*. Under certain circumstances, alternative antibiotics may be indicated. For infected plantar punctures through the shoe, a fluoroquinolone to cover *P. aeruginosa* would be appropriate coverage, although most such infections are complex or involve extensive débridement and intravenous antibiotics. Saltwater marine FBs may be contaminated with *Vibrio* species, usually sensitive to tetracyclines, aminoglycosides, or third-generation cephalosporins, whereas freshwater FBs are more likely to harbor *Aeromonas hydrophila*, which can be covered with tetracyclines.

Discharge Instructions

The patient should be informed that despite every effort, there can be no absolute guarantee that all foreign material has been identified or extracted, regardless of whether some or any FB was removed during initial exploration. The prudent clinician should always suggest close follow-up and should

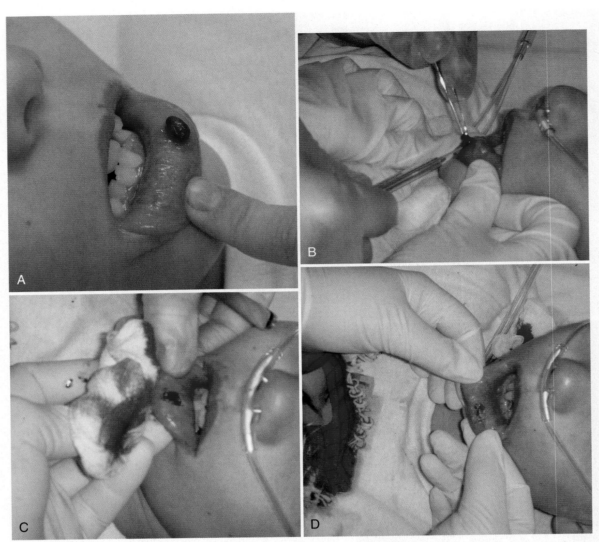

Figure 36–30 *A–D,* Pyogenic granulomas removed by sharp dissection under ketamine anesthesia and primary suturing.

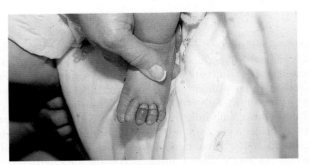

Figure 36–31 This child has multiple hairs compromising the circulation to two toes. The hairs are deeply embedded in the skin creases and cannot be visualized. The only way to ensure removal of the constriction is to cut the depth of the folds with a scalpel blade (using a dorsal incision to avoid the neurovascular bundle) and attempt to extricate individual fibers. Return of circulation should be obvious by temperature and color change in the affected digit(s), before it is assumed that all of the fibers have been cut.

leave open the option that an occult FB may still remain in any wound. Discharge instructions should also include signs and symptoms of problems related to the possibility of any retained material. Some centers routinely add this caveat on all discharge instructions for patients treated for lacerations or soft tissue defects. Patients should be assured that additional steps may be undertaken should the presence of foreign material be subsequently suspected.

Acknowledgment

The authors and editors wish to thank Ted Koutouzis for contributions to this chapter in previous editions

REFERENCES CAN BE FOUND ON **EXPERT CONSULT**

CHAPTER 37

Incision and Drainage

Kenneth H. Butler

Incision and drainage in the emergency department (ED) is most commonly done for soft tissue abscesses. Similar techniques are used for foreign body excision (see Chapter 36, Foreign Body Removal) and drainage of hematomas and seromas (discussed at the end of this chapter). Much of this chapter deals with cutaneous abscesses, which account for 1.8% of ED visits.[1] In contrast to most bacterial diseases, which are usually described in terms of their etiologic agent, cutaneous abscesses are best described in terms of their location.

The emergence and predominance of methicillin-resistant *Staphylococcus aureus* (MRSA) as the cause of cutaneous abscess during the past several decades necessitated major revisions in long-standing guidelines for antibiotic administration. In light of this significant etiologic change, MRSA should be considered as a cause in most skin abscesses, and aggressive cellulitis, until proven otherwise.

ABSCESS ETIOLOGY AND PATHOGENESIS

Localized pyogenic infections may develop in any region of the body. They usually are initiated by a breakdown in the normal epidermal defense mechanisms, with subsequent tissue invasion by normal resident flora. Thus, an abscess is likely to be caused by the flora indigenous to that area. An exception is direct inoculation of extraneous organisms, as occurs during a mammalian bite.[2]

Staphylococcal strains, which are normally found on the skin, produce rapid necrosis, early suppuration, and localized infections with large amounts of creamy yellow pus—the typical presentation of an abscess. Group A β-hemolytic streptococcal infections, conversely, tend to spread through tissues, causing a more generalized infection characterized by erythema and edema, a serous exudate, and little or no necrosis—the typical presentation of cellulitis. Anaerobic bacteria, which proliferate in the oral and perineal regions, produce necrosis with profuse brownish, foul-smelling pus[3] and may cause both abscesses and cellulitis.

Normal skin is extremely resistant to bacterial invasion, and few organisms are capable of penetrating intact epidermis. In the normal host with intact skin, the topical application of even very high concentrations of pathogenic bacteria does not result in infection. The requirements for infection include a high concentration of pathogenic organisms, such as occurs in the hair follicles and their adnexa; occlusion, which prevents desquamation and normal drainage, creating a moist environment; adequate nutrients; and trauma to the corneal layer, which allows organisms to penetrate.[4] Trauma may be the result of abrasions, hematoma, injection of chemical irritants, incision, or occlusive dressings that macerate the skin. The presence of a foreign body can potentiate skin infections, enabling a lower number of bacteria to establish an infection. For example, abscesses occasionally develop at suture sites in otherwise clean wounds. In addition, abscesses

can develop at any site used for body piercing. "High" ear piercings (through the cartilage of the pinna) seem to be at particular risk of infection because of the avascularity of the auricular cartilage.[5]

When favorable factors are present, the normal flora of cutaneous areas can colonize and infect the skin. In persons performing manual labor, the arms and the hands are infected most frequently. In women, the axilla and submammary regions are frequently infected because of minor trauma from shaving and contact with garments and because of the abundance of bacteria in these areas. Intravenous (IV) drug users may develop infections anywhere on the body, although the upper extremities are most commonly affected.[6,7] Deep soft tissue abscesses can be caused by addicts' attempts to access deep venous structures when peripheral venous access sites are exhausted.[8] In addition, areas with compromised blood supply are more prone to infection because normal host cell-mediated immunity is not as available.[4]

Infections in the soft tissue often begin as cellulitis. Some organisms cause necrosis, liquefaction, and accumulation of leukocytes and debris, followed by loculation and walling off of pus, all of which result in the formation of one or more abscesses. The lymph tissues may be involved, producing lymphangitis and subsequent bacteremia. As the process progresses, the area of liquefaction increases until it "points" and eventually ruptures into the area of least resistance. This may be toward the skin or the mucous membrane, into surrounding tissue, or into a body cavity. If the abscess is particularly deep seated, spontaneous drainage may occur, with persistence of a fistulous tract and the formation of a chronic draining sinus. This development, or the recurrence of an abscess previously drained, should suggest the possibility of osteomyelitis, a retained foreign body, or the presence of unusual or drug-resistant organisms.

Bacteriology of Cutaneous Abscesses

The microbiology of skin and soft tissue abscesses is related to their location. *Staphylococcus pyogenes* and *S. aureus* colonize the skin all over the body and thus can be isolated from any spot. Various organisms can contribute to an infection, and the offending species is determined by location on the body.

In 2002, Brook[9] compiled the findings of more than 15 bacteriologic studies of 676 polymicrobial abscesses. *S. aureus* and group A β-hemolytic streptococci were the most prevalent aerobes in skin and soft tissue abscesses and were isolated in specimens from all body sites. Gastrointestinal and cervical flora (enteric gram-negative bacilli and *Bacteroides fragilis*) were found most often in intra-abdominal, buttock, and leg lesions. Group A β-hemolytic streptococci, pigmented *Prevotella*, *Porphyromonas* species, and *Fusobacterium* species—all normal residents of the oral cavity—were most commonly found in lesions of the mouth, head, neck, and fingers.

In a study of the bacteriology of cutaneous abscesses in children, Brook and Finegold[10] found aerobes (staphylococci and group A β-hemolytic streptococci) to be the most common isolates from abscesses of the head, neck, extremities, and trunk, with anaerobes predominating in abscesses of the buttocks and perirectal sites. Mixed aerobic and anaerobic flora were found in the perirectal area, head, fingers, and nailbed. This study found an unexpectedly high incidence of anaerobes in nonperineal abscesses. Anaerobes were found primarily in areas adjacent to mucosal membranes (e.g., the mouth), where these organisms tend to thrive, and in areas that are easily contaminated (e.g., by sucking fingers, which causes nailbed and finger infections or bite injuries).

Parenteral drug users develop somewhat atypical abscesses. The injection of a cocaine/heroin mixture ("speed-ball") may predispose users to abscesses by inducing soft tissue ischemia.[11] Bergstein and coworkers[7] found anaerobes in 143 of 243 isolates from 57 drug-abusing patients. Abscesses at the site of injection tend to contain predominantly staphylococcal and streptococcal species. However, some drug users lick their needles prior to injection for "lubrication," which might account for the presence of unusual oral pathogens as *Eikenella corrodens* in injection-site abscesses.

If an unexpected or atypical organism is found in an abscess culture, the clinician should consider an underlying process not readily apparent from the history or physical examination. A typical finding is tuberculosis or fungal isolates in immunocompromised patients (e.g., those with diabetes or acquired immunodeficiency syndrome [AIDS]). Finding *Escherichia coli* suggests an enteric fistula or even self-inoculation of feces in some patients with a psychiatric illness such as Munchausen syndrome. Recurrent abscesses without an obvious underlying cause could indicate clandestine drug use. What appears to be a typical recurrent abscess may be a manifestation of an underlying septic joint or, rarely, metastatic or primary cancer (Fig. 37–1).

Special Considerations

Parenteral drug users, insulin-dependent diabetics, hemodialysis patients, cancer patients, transplant recipients, and individuals with acute leukemias have an increased frequency of abscess formation compared with the general population. At presentation, the patient might emphasize an exacerbation of the underlying disease process or an unexplained fever, leaving symptoms of an abscess as a secondary complaint. In this situation, the abscesses tend to have exotic or uncommon bacteriologic or fungal causes and typically respond poorly to therapy.[12-15] The patient with diabetes-induced ketoacidosis should be evaluated extensively for an infectious process; a rectal examination should be included with the physical examination to rule out a perirectal abscess. This also holds true for patients with abnormal cell-mediated immunity. The increased frequency of abscess formation among diabetic patients and parenteral drug users has several causes: intrinsic immune deficiencies, an increased incidence of *Staphylococcus* carriage, and frequent needle puncture, which allows access by pathogenic bacteria.[16]

Abscesses in parenteral drug users yield no bacterial growth if they are the result of the injection of necrotizing chemical irritants. Drug users frequently use veins of the neck and the femoral areas, producing abscesses and other infectious complications at these sites.[17] Any abscess near a vein of the antecubital fossa or dorsum of the hand should alert the clinician to possible IV drug use; however, substance users may also inject directly into the skin ("skin popping"), causing cutaneous abscesses distant from veins (Fig. 37–2).

A foreign body may serve as a nidus for abscess formation. Because IV drug users frequently break needles off in skin toughened by multiple injections, the clinician should maintain a high index of suspicion for retained needle fragments. If an abscess is recurrent or if the patient is a known or suspected IV drug user, radiographs or other techniques should be considered to search for foreign bodies, an underlying septic joint, or osteomyelitis.[18]

Community-Acquired Methicillin-Resistant *Staphylococcus aureus*

First acknowledged in the 1960s as a cause of infection in patients in health care settings, MRSA has now become the most common identifiable cause of *community-acquired* skin and soft tissue infections in many metropolitan areas in the United States. The spread of this category of organism is considered an epidemic, and it is a very virulent and aggressive organism.[19,20]

Virulent CA MRSA causes rapid and destructive soft tissue infection due to the presence of two bacterial toxins elaborated by the omnipresent VSA-300 and VSA-400 strains. The Panton-Valentine leukociden (PVL) enhances tissue necrosis, and phenol soluble modulin (PSM) is toxic to neutrophils. A small pustule can become a large abscess in 24 to 48 hours (Fig. 37–3). Such lesions are often mistaken for a spider bite or drug use because of their rapid progression and seemingly spontaneous onset in otherwise healthy persons.

In 1980, the spread of MRSA from hospitals into communities became evident, primarily among individuals with known risk factors (Table 37–1). More recently, community-acquired infections have occurred more frequently, even in people without known risk factors. Community-acquired strains of methicillin-resistent *S. aureus* (CA-MRSA) may be more virulent than hospital-acquired MRSA, but they tend to be susceptible to a broader array of antibiotics.[21]

In an assessment of the prevalence of MRSA across the United States, Moran and colleagues[22] compiled data from adults who sought treatment for acute skin and soft tissue infections in EDs in 11 American cities in August 2004. *S. aureus* was isolated from three fourths of the 422 patients who met study criteria. Seventy-eight percent of the *S. aureus* isolates were resistant to methicillin. MRSA was isolated from 59% of the patients in the study. The prevalence of MRSA ranged from 15% to 74% among the participating EDs (Table 37–2). MRSA was the most common identifiable cause of skin and soft tissue infections in all but 1 of the EDs.

Frazee and associates,[21] reporting from an ED in northern California, found that half of the 137 patients in their study were either infected with or colonized by MRSA. Three fourths of all *S. aureus* isolates were MRSA. In addition, 76% of cases met a strict clinical definition of CA-MRSA.

Based on a review spanning 15 years (1990–2004), Crum and coworkers[23] documented the emergence of distinct community-acquired strains of MRSA genetically unrelated to nosocomial isolates from the same community (military medical facilities in San Diego). This observation suggests that the community-based strains did not emerge from nosocomial strains. In this study, the incidence of CA-MRSA increased steadily from 1990 to 2001 and then dramatically in 2002 and each year thereafter.

MRSA has also emerged as a sexually transmitted disease. Roberts and colleagues[20] described their treatment of two patients who came to their urban ED with abscesses likely transmitted by heterosexual oral-genital contact. Both tested positive for MRSA. In a retrospective chart review, Roberts and colleagues[20] found that 18% of the 524 subcutaneous abscesses treated in their urban ED in 2006 were confined to the genital area. Almost three fourths of the 272 outpatient wound cultures performed on that year's patient population were positive for MRSA.

This trend of increasing prevalence of MRSA holds true across the country and throughout the world.

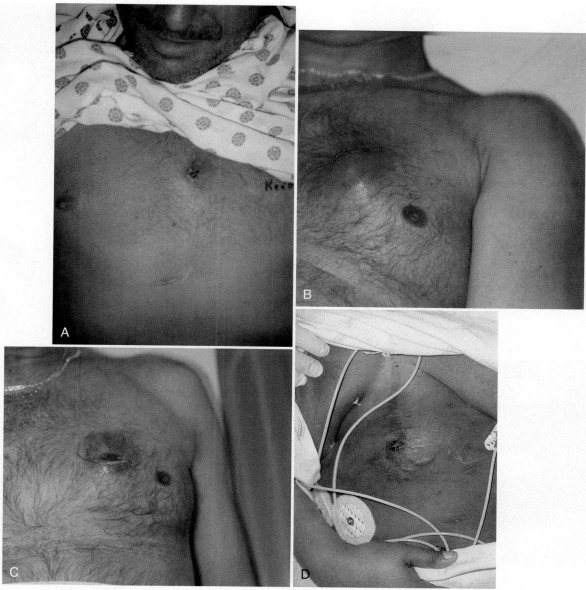

Figure 37–1 An abscess that appears in an atypical place or recurs after initial treatment is successful should raise the possibility of rare or underlying conditions. *A,* This intravenous (IV) drug user had an "abscess" of the chest wall drained in various emergency departments (EDs) several times over a 2-month period, and it seemed to initially respond to drainage and antibiotics. He still manifested an area of cellulitis, minor fluctuance, and continued drainage near the center of the chest. This is an atypical place for a simple cutaneous abscess. Magnetic resonance imaging demonstrated osteomyelitis and an abscess of the sternoclavicular joint that was draining to the skin, simulating a recurrent cutaneous abscess. He required extensive surgical débridement and prolonged antibiotics. The etiologic organism was never ascertained, but pseudomonas is often present. *B,* This patient has a large "abscess" of the lateral chest wall that initially drained unusual gelatinous material, not frank pus. *C,* At follow-up 3 days later, the abscess was much improved. The contents of the abscess had been sent for pathologic analysis because it had an unusual consistency and it demonstrated a highly undifferentiated soft tissue malignancy. The fluid was sterile. Normally, analyzing or culturing the contents of an abscess will not yield helpful information, but in this case, the unusual consistency of the collection prompted further analysis. *D,* This patient had a sternotomy for bypass surgery a few months ago. She had been sporadically treated for a minor wound infection but then presented with a draining fluctuant mass at the inferior border of the sternum. This is the external manifestation of extensive sternal osteomyelitis.

MANIFESTATIONS OF CUTANEOUS ABSCESSES

The diagnosis of cutaneous abscess formation is usually straightforward. The presence of a fluctuant mass in an area of induration, erythema, and tenderness is clinical evidence that an abscess exists. An abscess may appear initially as a definite tender soft tissue mass, but in some cases, a distinct abscess may not be readily evident. If the abscess is quite deep, as is true of many perirectal, pilonidal, and breast abscesses, the clinician may be misled by the presence of a firm, tender, indurated area without a definite mass. To confirm the diagnosis of early abscess via the presence of pus, needle aspiration can be performed.[24] This approach also may identify a mycotic aneurysm or an inflamed lymph node simulating an abscess. A specific entity commonly mistaken for a discrete abscess is the sublingual cellulitis of Ludwig angina (see Chapter 65, Emergency Dental Procedures).

Parenteral injection of illicit drugs can produce simple cutaneous abscesses that unpredictably advance to extensive necrotizing soft tissue infections. The emergency clinician

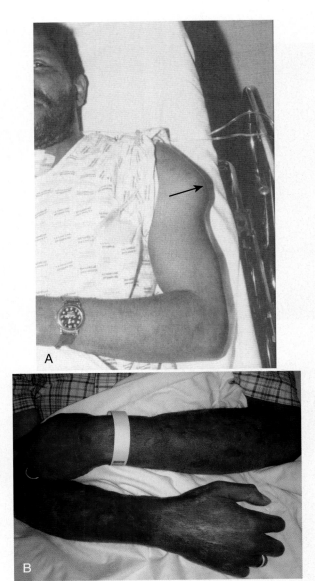

Figure 37–2 *A,* This patient presented with a large abscess of the deltoid area (*arrow*) and could offer no explanation for it. This is a typical scenario for a drug user who injects directly into the skin. *B,* The characteristic circular skin lesion from "skin popping" found on the arms confirmed the clinical suspicion. Even though a drug screen was positive for opioids, the patient denied drug use and attributed the leg lesions to frequent trauma on the job.

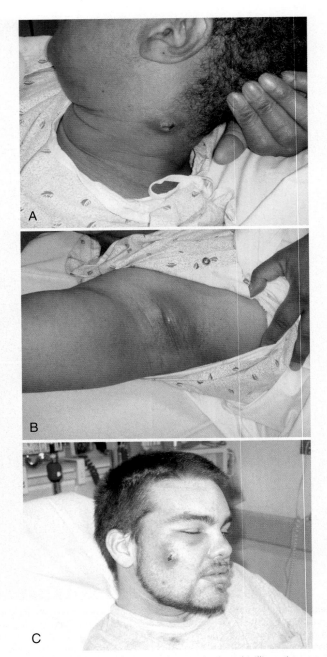

Figure 37–3 Examples of community-acquired methicillin-resistant *Staphylococcus aureus* (CA-MRSA) infections. These are aggressive infections that can spread rapidly. The patient often describes a small pustule that becomes an abscess in 24–48 hr. Patients often believe this is a spider bite because of its rapid onset in an otherwise healthy person with no other reason for the lesion.

must maintain a high index of suspicion to avoid missing this potentially life-threatening condition.[6] Cellulitis and abscess formation may lead to bacteremia and sepsis, especially in the immunocompromised patient.

The pain of an abscess often brings the patient to the hospital before spontaneous rupture. However, the patient can present with a draining abscess that appears to have undergone spontaneous rupture and is manifesting a self-cure. The patient may have punctured the abscess in an attempt to drain it. In most cases, a formal incision, drainage, and packing procedure will be helpful in eliminating the process, even though copious drainage will not be encountered. Although no formal drainage may be required after the spontaneous rupture of a simple cutaneous abscess, conditions such as a perirectal abscess, Bartholin gland abscess, and breast abscess are usually best managed with further drainage and packing.

IMAGING
Diagnostic Bedside Sonography

Abscesses often begin as cellulitis; therefore, the two conditions may coexist, leading to missed diagnoses and unnecessary invasive procedures.[25] In more than half of patients considered unlikely to have an abscess based on clinical examination, fluid can be detected on ultrasound examination.[26]

Imaging studies are usually not done for soft tissue infections unless an underlying foreign body is suspected. The soft tissue ultrasound examination is technically uncomplicated and can be performed in less than a minute. By definition, subcutaneous abscesses are located superficially and are therefore amenable to interrogation using the highest-frequency setting on the linear probe. This yields high-resolution images unaffected by body habitus, and detection of these superficial infections is less dependent on operator ability than is ultrasound assessment of deeper structures.

The technique of soft tissue ultrasound is straightforward.[25] The transducer is placed on the skin at the region of erythema or swelling (Fig. 37–4). The gray scale appearance of the abscess is a heterogenic, anechoic, or hypoechoic mass containing a variable amount of internal echoes. Abscesses tend to be spherical with poorly defined borders (Fig. 37–5). Compression of the abscess with the transducer may demonstrate movement or swirling of pus. Fragile structures such as arteries, veins, and nerves may also be visualized. In comparison, cellulitis appears on ultrasound as thickening and diffuse hyperechogenicity of the subcutaneous fat, with obliteration of the interface between echogenic fat and dermis ("cobblestoning") (Fig. 37–6).

Ultrasound-Guided Needle Aspiration

Radiologists have performed needle aspiration of abscesses for some time, and now emergency clinicians are becoming more comfortable with the procedure. High-resolution ultrasound technology is being used to facilitate various "blind" procedures done in the ED (e.g., joint aspiration and central line placement).

For ultrasound-guided drainage of a cutaneous abscess, a high-resolution probe (5 or 7.5 MHz) is suggested. Maintain sterility throughout the procedure. Place the sterile transducer over the main body of the abscess, and insert the needle through the skin adjacent to the transducer. Adjust their relative relationships depending on the depth and location of the abscess cavity. Guide the needle—seen as a bright artifact—directly into the abscess. Watch the abscess cavity collapse as pus is drained out. Scan the entire area of suspected abscess to capture unexpected extensions. Be sure to drain all pockets.

LABORATORY FINDINGS

A complete blood count (CBC), blood cultures, Gram stain, and culture are not standard of care for the treatment of straightforward cutaneous abscess in the ED. Theoretically, a culture will identify an unusual or a resistant organism should incision and drainage not be curative; therefore, some clinicians will opt for cultures to address that subsequent possibility.

The majority of patients with an uncomplicated cutaneous abscess will have a normal CBC count and will not experience fever, chills, or malaise. Therefore, in the absence of extenuating circumstances, it is not standard to analyze blood cultures from patients with typical cutaneous abscesses because laboratory test results do not lead to a specific therapeutic path. Perhaps an exception is a blood or urine glucose determination to assess diabetes in patients with relevant clinical scenarios. An abscess may produce leukocytosis, depending

---

TABLE 37–1 Risk Factors for Methicillin-Resistant _Staphylococcus aureus_

Contact sports
Previous antibiotic use
Day care attendance
Health care worker
Diabetes mellitus
Hospitalization
Invasive indwelling devices
Mechanical ventilation
Endotracheal tube
Intravenous drug abuse
Hemodialysis
Immunosuppression
Chronic illness
Previous isolation of MRSA
Sexual contact

MRSA, methicillin-resistant _Staphylococcus aureus_.
Based on Cohen PR, Grossman ME: Management of cutaneous lesions associated with an emergency epidemic: Community-acquired methicillin-resistant _Staphylococcus aureus_ skin infections. J Am Acad Dermatol 51:132, 2004.

TABLE 37–2 Bacterial Isolates from Purulent Skin and Soft Tissue Infections in U.S. Emergency Departments*

Site	Patients (_N_)	MRSA[†]	MSSA	Other Bacteria[‡]	No Bacterial Growth
Albuquerque	42	25 (60)	10 (24)	3 (7)	4 (10)
Atlanta	32	23 (72)	4 (12)	3 (9)	2 (6)
Charlotte	25	17 (68)	0	4 (16)	4 (16)
Kansas City, MO	58	43 (74)	6 (10)	4 (7)	5 (9)
Los Angeles	47	24 (51)	6 (13)	8 (17)	9 (19)
Minneapolis	28	11 (39)	4 (14)	9 (32)	4 (14)
New Orleans	69	46 (67)	11 (16)	9 (13)	3 (4)
New York	20	3 (15)	8 (40)	5 (25)	4 (20)
Philadelphia	58	32 (55)	12 (21)	12 (21)	2 (3)
Phoenix	30	18 (60)	8 (27)	4 (13)	0
Portland, OR	13	7 (54)	2 (15)	3 (23)	1 (8)

*Thirty-one cultures, including 10 cultures from which MRSA was isolated, were polymicrobial. Because of rounding, percentages may not total 100.
[†]$P < .001$ for the test for homogeneity of MRSA prevalence across sites.
[‡]Other bacterial isolates were as follows: MSSA (17%), _Streptococcus_ species (7%), coagulase-negative staphylococci (3%), and _Proteus mirabilis_ (1%).
MRSA, methicillin-resistant _Staphylococcus aureus_; MSSA, methicillin-susceptible _Staphylococcus aureus_.
From Moran GJ, Krishnadasan A, Gorwitz RJ, et al, for the EMERGEncy ID Net Study Group. Methicillin-resistant _S. aureus_ infections among patients in the emergency department. N Engl J Med 355:666, 2006.

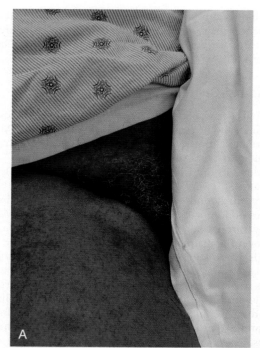

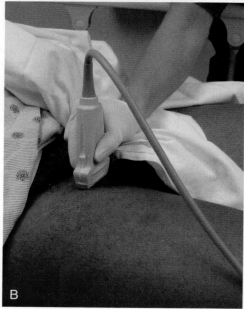

Figure 37–4 An ultrasound probe may differentiate abscess from cellulitis and guide drainage procedures.

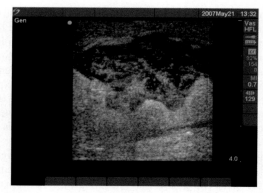

Figure 37–5 Subcutaneous abscesses can be identified by their mixed echogenic appearance. *(Image courtesy of Brian D. Euerle, MD, Department of Emergency Medicine, University of Maryland School of Medicine, Baltimore, MD.)*

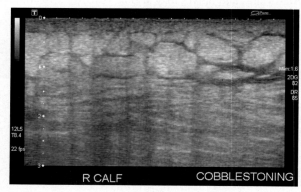

Figure 37–6 Ultrasound image (8.0-MHz linear probe) of cellulitis shows "cobblestoning." *(Courtesy of John Christian Fox, MD, RDMS, Department of Emergency Medicine, University of California, Irvine.)*

on the severity and duration of the purulent process; however, the presence or absence of leukocytosis has virtually no diagnostic or therapeutic implications. Bacteremia may occasionally manifest as a peripheral abscess resulting from septic emboli, usually producing clinical characteristics dissimilar to those associated with cutaneous abscesses. The cutaneous abscess itself rarely produces the bacteremia.

Gram stain is not indicated in the care of uncomplicated simple abscesses. However, patients who appear "toxic" or immunocompromised and those who require prophylactic antibiotics (see "Prophylactic Antibiotics," later in this chapter) may benefit from Gram stain and cultures. Gram stain results have been shown to correlate well with subsequent culture results, so in compromised hosts, the test can

be used to direct antibiotic choice.[27,28] Anaerobic infections should be suspected when multiple organisms are noted on Gram stain, when a foul odor is associated with the pus, when free air is noted on radiographs of the soft tissue, and when no growth is reported on cultures.[12]

In uncomplicated abscesses, routine culture of pus is unnecessary because of the expected prompt response to surgical therapy and the polymicrobial nature of abscess formation. However, culturing the abscess contents might provide useful information when MRSA is suspected; when managing complicated cases; for recurrent, unusual, or atypical abscesses; and in immunosuppressed patients. This information could be useful if the patient responds poorly to initial surgical drainage, if secondary spread of the infection occurs, or if bacteremia develops.[29] When obtaining a specimen for culture, it is best to aspirate the pus with a needle and syringe before incision and drainage. The material should be cultured for aerobic and anaerobic bacteria. A "sterile" culture from a specimen collected with a standard cotton swab after incision is frequently the result of improper anaerobic culture technique. There is a general misconception that foul-smelling pus is a result of *E. coli*. This foul odor is actually caused by the presence of anaerobes; the pus of *E. coli* is odorless.

The discovery of solid or suspicious material in an abscess should prompt laboratory investigation (i.e., histology). Malignancy may mimic cutaneous abscess (see Fig. 37–1*B* and *C*).

INDICATIONS AND CONTRAINDICATIONS

Surgical incision and drainage is the definitive treatment of a soft tissue abscess;[25] antibiotics alone are ineffective. The drainage of a suppurative focus results in a marked resolution of symptoms in most uncomplicated cases. In the initial stages, only induration and inflammation may be found in an area destined to produce an abscess. Premature incision, before localization of pus, will not be curative and theoretically may be deleterious, because extension of the infectious process and, rarely, bacteremia from manipulation can result. In some cases, the application of heat to an area of inflammation may ease pain, speed resolution of the cellulitis, and facilitate the localization and accumulation of pus. Nonsurgical methods are not a substitute for surgical drainage and should not be continued for more than 24 to 36 hours before the patient is reevaluated.

ANCILLARY ANTIBIOTIC THERAPY

The usefulness of administration of antibiotics remains unproved for prophylaxis against and treatment of uncomplicated, and adequately drained cutaneous abscesses; routine antibiotics are not standard of care. *No data definitively demonstrate the need for antibiotic therapy in conjunction with incision and drainage of uncomplicated cutaneous abscesses in healthy, immunocompetent patients without valvular heart disease.* The practice of prescribing antibiotics if there is "significant surrounding cellulitis" is a vague concept and is not supported by prospective data and "significant" is difficult to quantify. *The specific value of concomitant antibiotics in the immunocompromised patient, although intuitively attractive and commonly practiced, is also unproved.* If antibiotics are prescribed, they should be given for 2 to 3 days only, and their continuation should be reassessed at the first follow-up visit. Because the bacteriology of abscesses is complicated and multifactorial, no single specific antibiotic can be generically recommended. Most clinicians use antibiotics considered effective for "soft tissue infections," but this concept is vague and ultimately clinically useless.

Conflicting results have been reported from the few investigations into a relationship between incision and drainage of cutaneous abscesses and bacteremia. For example, in 1985, Fine and associates[30] concluded that incision and drainage of cutaneous abscesses is *often* accompanied by transient bacteremia. They compared blood culture results from specimens obtained before and at 1 minute, 5 minutes, and 20 minutes after incision and drainage procedures in 10 patients with soft tissue infections. None of the blood cultures obtained before incision and drainage was positive; however, 6 patients had at least one positive culture after the procedure. Eleven of the 30 postprocedure cultures yielded growth. In contrast, in 1997, Bobrow and coworkers[31] concluded that incision and drainage of a localized cutaneous abscess is *unlikely* to result in transient bacteremia in afebrile adults. Their study involved 50 patients with localized cutaneous abscesses. Blood samples were collected before and at 2 and 10 minutes after incision and drainage. In addition, specimens from the wound were collected after drainage. None of the blood cultures was positive, even though 64% of the wound cultures were positive, primarily for *S. aureus.* Bobrow and coworkers[31] noted that prophylactic antibiotics should be given to patients at high risk for bacterial endocarditis. In a discussion of the differences between these findings and those reported by Fine and associates,[30] Bobrow and coworkers noted that Fine and associates' cultures were obtained from indwelling, heparinized IV catheters, a practice that allows ample opportunity for contamination. Further, half of the patients in Fine's group had perirectal abscesses, and if those abscesses involved mucosal surfaces, the risk of bacteremia could have been increased.

Prophylactic Antibiotics

Prophylaxis for Endocarditis

The precise risk for endocarditis after incision and drainage of cutaneous abscess remains unknown, and it is impossible to predict which patients will develop this infection and which particular procedure will be responsible. However, because bacteremia clearly occurs with manipulation of infected tissue, it is generally agreed that patients at risk for cardiac complications related to transient bacteremia should be treated with appropriate antibiotics within the hour preceding the procedure.

Guidelines issued by the American Heart Association in 2007 recommend antibiotic prophylaxis for procedures on the respiratory tract or involving infection skin, skin structures, or musculoskeletal tissue only in patients with cardiac conditions that carry the highest risk of adverse outcome from infective endocarditis.[32] Those conditions are listed in Table 37-3. Most skin infections are polymicrobial, but only staphylococci and β-hemolytic streptococci are likely to cause infective endocarditis. Therefore, the therapeutic regimen should include an agent active against those organisms, such as an antistaphylococcal penicillin or a cephalosporin. For patients who cannot tolerate a β-lactam or who have, or may have, an MRSA infection, vancomycin or clindamycin can be substituted.

Two clinical situations deserve special mention. First, because of the frequent incidence of valvular damage among IV drug users, prophylactic antibiotics may be indicated before the incision and drainage of abscesses in these patients; however, no standard of care exists. It is prudent to inquire about prior endocarditis or ascultate for a heart murmur if IV drug abuse is known, and administer antibiotics under these circumstances. Second, any patient with a documented history of endocarditis must receive prophylactic antibiotics before the incision and drainage procedure.

TABLE 37-3 Cardiac Conditions with the Highest Risk of Adverse Outcome from Endocarditis

Prosthetic cardiac valve
Previous infective endocarditis
Congenital heart disease (CHD)*
    Unrepaired cyanotic CHD, including palliative shunts and conduits
    Completely repaired congenital heart defect with prosthetic material or device, whether placed by surgery or by catheter interventions, during the first 6 mo after the procedure†
    Repaired CHD with residual defects at the site of or adjacent to the site of a prosthetic patch or prosthetic device (which inhibits endothelialization)
Cardiac transplantation, with development of cardiac valvulopathy

*Except for the conditions listed previously, antibiotic prophylaxis is no longer recommended for any other form of CHD.
†Prophylaxis is recommended because endothelialization of prosthetic material occurs within 6 mo after the procedure.
From Wilson W, Taubert KA, Gewitz M, et al: Prevention of infective endocarditis. Circulation 116:1736, 2007.

Because cutaneous abscesses may result from active endocarditis and prophylactic antibiotics may obscure subsequent attempts to identify the causative organism, two or three blood cultures (aerobic and anaerobic) should be obtained from those at risk for endocarditis before antibiotic therapy. Patients with the diagnosis of mitral valve prolapse have traditionally been included for treatment with prophylactic antibiotics. The indication for this is unclear. The risk of an allergic reaction may outweigh the benefits of treatment in this group,[33] and clinical judgment is required. Kaye[34] suggested prophylaxis only for patients who have a holosystolic murmur secondary to mitral valve prolapse.

Prophylaxis for Bacteremia in Other Conditions

Immunocompromised patients may benefit from the prophylactic administration of antibiotics in preparation for incision and drainage of cutaneous lesions. In contrast to patients with endocarditis risks, immunocompromised patients are at risk for septicemia secondary to brief bacteremia. IV drug users have a high incidence of diseases associated with human immunodeficiency virus (HIV),[35-37] and the treating clinician must anticipate various degrees of immunodeficiency among them. Because no specific standard of care is agreed upon, clinical judgment must guide the use of antibiotics in these situations.

No specific guidelines have been offered for the antibiotic regimen to be used before incision and drainage of infected cutaneous tissue in patients at risk for conditions other than endocarditis. Choice of antibiotics is based on the organism anticipated to cause the bacteremia. Although the location of the abscess will give some clue to the organism involved, most abscesses contain multiple strains of bacteria. Not all bacteria are potent pathogens, so their mere presence does not predict their role in subsequent morbidity. Because *Staphylococcus* continues to be the most common cause of abscess, a broad-spectrum antistaphylococcal drug is indicated.[38] Prophylaxis should consist of a single IV dose given half an hour prior to incision and drainage. A first-generation cephalosporin or penicillinase-resistant penicillin is a good initial choice. Vancomycin may also be considered. Others may prefer cefazolin (Ancef, Kefzol), 1 g intravenously, for adults. This regimen covers staphylococcal and streptococcal species, many gram-negative organisms, and many anaerobes.

Management of Cutaneous CA-MRSA Infections

At the current time, standards of care for CA-MRSA infections treated in the ED are evolving and subject to controversy owing to lack of data. Simple cellulitis is usually not CA-MRSA related, but necrotizing fasciitis may be caused by this organism. When cutaneous CA-MRSA infection presents as an *abscess*, incision and drainage remain the mainstay of therapy. CA-MRSA skin and soft tissue infections have occasionally been observed to persist, worsen, or recur despite incision and drainage, especially when additional systemic antimicrobial therapy is withheld or concurrent treatment is initiated with an antibiotic to which the bacterium is not susceptible. CA-MRSA is somewhat contagious and can be associated with infection appearing within other family members and close contacts. Antibiotic therapy, in addition to appropriate surgical intervention, may be helpful to limit the spread of infection. As of this writing, however, the Center for Disease Control and the Infectious Disease Society of America recommend incision and drainage alone, *without antibiotics*, for

most patients with a simple cutaneous abscess, and use of an antibiotic effective against MRSA *only if the abscess is persistent or recurrent*.[38a] However, as guided by clinical judgment, after incision and drainage of suspected or confirmed CA-MRSA skin abscesses, initiation of empirical or culture-guided therapy with a systemic antimicrobial agent is an acceptable alternative conservative therapeutic approach.[39]

Bacterial culture may be performed at the initial visit, especially if widespread surgical intervention, such as inpatient incision and drainage, or poor response to initial therapy can be intuitively anticipated. The choice of empirical antibiotic therapy should be guided by tolerability, ease of administration, cost, and efficacy. The duration of oral antibiotics therapy depends on the severity of the infection, the therapeutic response, and the host factors, although a minimum of 10 to 14 days of therapy is usually necessary. Treatment for 2 or 3 weeks may be needed in severe cases, in patients who are slow to respond, and in vulnerable hosts.[39]

In geographic areas with high rates of outpatient MRSA infections, orally administered non–β-lactam antibiotics to which most strains of MRSA are susceptible (e.g., trimethoprim-sulfamethoxazol, clindamycin, or tetracycline) should be used initially for empirical treatment of uncomplicated skin and soft tissue infections.[39]

In most areas, clindamycin, cephalosporins or fluoroquinolones are acceptable first line empiric choices for cellulitis.[39a] For presumed or confirmed cutaneous CA-MRSA infection, trimethoprim-sulfamethoxazole (one or two double-strength tablet [160 mg/800 mg] every 12 hr in adults, with dose adjusted for patients with renal insufficiency) has been recommended as either monotherapy or in combination with rifampin (600 mg daily in adults). Some have recommended higher doses of trimethoprim-sulfamethoxazole, such as 2 DS tablets given every 12 hours, until response can be evaluated. When the rate of inducible clindamycin resistance is high in the community, trimethoprim-sulfmethoxazole may be the preferred empirical treatment for CA-MRSA.[39,40]

Clindamycin (300–450 mg q 6 hr in adults), as either monotherapy or in combination with rifampin (600 mg daily in adults), is also useful to treat presumed or confirmed cutaneous CA-MRSA infection. Rifampin alone is not used. In contrast to trimethoprim-sulfamethoxazole, clindamycin is usually active against β-hemolytic streptococci. Clindamycin has been associated with the adverse effect of pseudomembraneous colitis.[39]

CA-MRSA isolates may also be susceptible to tetracycline. Minocycline (100 mg q 12 hr in adults) and doxycycline (100 mg q 12 hr in adults) are inexpensive, well-tolerated, long-acting tetracyclines that have excellent oral bioavailablity and possess greater antistaphylococcal properties than tetracycline.[39,41,42]

A relatively unstudied, but a common and currently accepted strategy for patients with soft tissue infections (especially CA-MRSA infections) that are borderline, by clinical judgment, for hospital admission and therapeutic intravenous antibiotics, is to administer a single dose of an intravenous antibiotic in the ED, followed by oral antibiotics and close outpatient follow-up. When a CA-MRSA infection is likely, IV vancomycin, or linezolid are reasonable options. Oral linezolid may be as effective as the IV form. Newer antibiotics aimed at CA-MRSA infection are currently in development. For non-CA-MRSA soft tissue infection (such as cellulitis), using a cephalosporin or fluoroquinolone for this strategy is reasonable. Whether or not this strategy is superior to

TABLE 37–4 Strategies to Eradicate CA-MRSA Carrier States in Patients with Recurrent CA-MRSA Soft Tissue Infections

Recurrent CA-MRSA soft tissue infections have been linked to a carrier state in the affected individual, with the nose and skin as areas that the bacteria colonize. It may be difficult to totally or permanently eradicate colonization, and *there are no proven methods to accomplish this.* The following strategies have been used in an attempt to eradicate the carrier state in individuals with recurrent CA-MRSA soft tissue infections. The appropriate time to implement these procedures is not known, but it would be reasonable to institute first line techniques if more than 2–3 episodes of proven CA-MRSA infection are documented.

First Line

Apply 1 cm of mupirocin (Bactroban) ointment (an intranasal form is available) to the anterior nares 3 times a day for 7 days. (1) plus
Daily total body wash with (4%) chlorhexidine (Hibiclens) for 5–7 days. (2)

Second Line

Obtain a culture to ascertain sensitivities to various antibiotics
Repeat mupirocin and chlorhexidine as above
Rifampin 300 mg twice a day, PLUS, if sensitivities dictate, trimethoprim/sulfamethoxazole DS or doxycycline (100 mg) twice a day for 1 to 2 weeks. (3)

Note: For multiple recurrent infections consider infectious disease expert consultation.
(1) May cause burning, pruritis, dry membranes, erythema. Avoid long term use. *Do not substitute bacitracin.*
(2) May cause skin and eye irritation. Apply for 5 minutes, rinse thoroughly.
(3) Do not use rifampin alone since resistance may develop. Can cause orange color to urine/tears, and stain contact lenses. Adjust dose for renal impairment. Do not use in hepatic impairment.

simply beginning appropriate well absorbed oral antibiotics is unknown.

An approach to *recurrent* CA-MRSA soft tissue infections is outlined in Table 37–4.

Therapeutic Antibiotics

In contrast to prophylaxis before surgery, the routine use of therapeutic oral antibiotics after incision and drainage of simple cutaneous abscesses in otherwise healthy patients with no immunocompromise *appears to have no value, and their empirical use cannot be scientifically supported.* Llera and Levy[43] performed a randomized, double-blind study to compare outcomes of patients treated with a first-generation cephalosporin after drainage of cutaneous abscesses in the ED with those who received a placebo. They found no significant difference in clinical outcome between the two groups and concluded that antibiotics are unnecessary in individuals with normal host defenses. This confirmed previous less well controlled studies.[44-46] It should be noted that high-risk patients were often excluded from these studies. The immunocompromised patient has not been adequately studied in this situation and is therefore often given antibiotics empirically, but this practice, although common, has not been supported by rigorous prospective studies.

Patients with cutaneous abscesses often have concomitant disease processes that may warrant the consideration of par-

enteral or oral antibiotics. Most abscesses have a defined surrounding area of erythema and induration, but this may not necessarily qualify as "significant surrounding cellulitis." Whereas cellulitis or lymphangitis often accompanies abscesses, and therapeutic antibiotics may have theoretical value under these circumstances, this concept is difficult to quantify and not well addressed nor supported in the literature. Cellulitis and lymphangitis usually subside after the draining of the abscess itself. Meislin[47] noted that pathogen identification in cases of cellulitis without abscess can be difficult, and empirical antibiotics may be helpful. IV drug users who present with an abscess and fever require parenteral antibiotic therapy after blood cultures have been drawn until bacterial endocarditis can be ruled out.[48] Obviously, patients who are clinically septic require immediate IV antibiotics as well as aggressive surgical drainage of pus. By administering IV ampicillin/sulbactam (2 g/1 g) every 6 hours, Talan and colleagues[49] achieved 100% eradication of pathogens from major abscesses in hospitalized IV drug users and non–drug users.

As a general guideline, therapeutic antibiotics may be considered following abscess drainage for immunocompromised patients (e.g., patients with AIDS or diabetes, patients receiving chemotherapy or steroids, transplant recipients, and alcoholic patients) and for the immunocompetent patient with "significant" cellulitis, lymphangitis, or systemic symptoms, such as chills or fever. Although it has not been studied, it is reasonable to also give antibiotics prophylactically, before surgery, to all patients who will obviously be given therapeutic antibiotics. As with prophylactic antibiotics, a first-generation cephalosporin or semisynthetic penicillin is a reasonable therapeutic choice unless the specific abscess site dictates alternative therapy. The ideal duration of therapeutic antibiotics is unknown. As a general guideline, immunocompromised patients should receive antibiotics for 5 to 7 days and immunocompetent patients for 3 to 5 days after the procedure, depending on the severity of the condition and clinical response at follow-up.

Facial abscesses should be handled carefully and checked frequently. Any abscess above the upper lip and below the brow may drain into the cavernous sinus, and thus manipulation may predispose to septic thrombophlebitis of this system. Treatment with antistaphylococcal antibiotics and warm soaks after incision and drainage has been recommended pending resolution of the process. Areas not in this zone of the face can be treated in a manner similar to that used for other cutaneous abscesses.

INCISION AND DRAINAGE PROCEDURE

Procedure Setting

Definitive incision and drainage of soft tissue abscesses is performed in either the ED or the operating room (OR). When abscesses are drained in the ED, some centers prefer to use a special area to avoid contamination of general treatment rooms.

The choice of the locale for the procedure depends on a number of important factors. The location of the abscess may dictate management in the OR. Large abscesses or abscesses located deep in the soft tissues require a procedure involving a great degree of patient cooperation, which might be achieved only under general or regional anesthesia. Proximity to major neurovascular structures, such as in the axillae or antecubital fossa, may necessitate specific management. Infections of the hand (with the exception of distal finger infections) have traditionally been managed in the OR because of the many important structures involved and the propensity for limb-threatening complications.

Lack of adequate anesthesia is the most common limiting factor in ED incision and drainage. The current increased use of ED procedural sedation (see Chapter 33) has changed prior OR cases to ones that can be well managed in the ED. If the clinician believes the abscess cannot be fully incised and drained because of inadequate anesthesia, the patient should be taken to the OR for management under general anesthesia. In addition to limiting proper drainage, it is inhumane and unethical to subject a patient to extreme pain when alternatives are available.

Equipment and Anesthesia

A standard suture tray provides adequate instruments if a scalpel and packing material are added. Although sterility is impossible during the procedure, one should avoid contamination of surrounding tissue. Some clinicians prefer to use an obligatory skin scrub with an antiseptic solution, but the value of this step is dubious.

It is often quite difficult to obtain local anesthesia by direct infiltration because of the poor function of local anesthetic agents in the low pH of infected tissue. Furthermore, the distention of sensitive structures by a local injection is quite painful and, hence, poorly tolerated by most patients. Skin anesthesia is usually possible, but total anesthesia of the abscess cavity itself generally cannot be achieved. If a regional block can be performed (see Chapters 30, Regional Anesthesia of the Head and Neck, 31, Nerve Blocks of the Thorax and Extremities, and 32, Intravenous Regional Anesthesia), this type of anesthesia is preferred. Alternatively, a field block may be used. It should be noted that infected tissue is very vascular, and local anesthetics are quickly absorbed. Strict adherence to maximum safe doses of local anesthetics is required.

The skin over the dome of an abscess is often quite thin, making skin anesthesia difficult. If a 25-gauge needle is carefully used, one can often inject the dome of the abscess subcutaneously. The anesthetic solution spreads over the dome through the subcutaneous layers into the surrounding skin and provides excellent skin anesthesia. If the needle is in the proper plane (best accomplished by holding the syringe parallel, rather than perpendicular, to the skin), the surrounding skin blanches symmetrically during infiltration without having to reposition the needle (Fig. 37–8). In the extremely anxious or uncomfortable patient, the judicious use of preoperative sedation (see Chapter 33, Systemic Analgesia and Sedation for Procedures) with IV opioids and sedatives or nitrous oxide makes the procedure easier for both patient and clinician. If adequate anesthesia cannot be obtained and pain limits the procedure, the patient should be treated under general anesthesia. Ketamine may be an option in the ED setting.

Some clinicians recommend the use of topical ethyl chloride or Fluori-Methane spray for the initial skin incision, but although this is an attractive concept to patients, the pain relief offered by these agents is variable and fleeting. Ethyl chloride is also highly flammable. These vapocoolant sprays may be useful to provide momentary anesthesia for local anesthetic injection or for the initial skin incision if the injection or incision is made immediately after blanching of the skin. In general, however, these agents are of minimal benefit for a stand-alone anesthetic agent for all but the smallest of superficial abscesses (e.g., purulent folliculitis).

Incision

One should make all incisions conform with skin creases or natural folds to minimize visible scar formation (Fig. 37–9). Extreme care should be taken in such areas as the groin, the posterior knee, the antecubital fossa, and the neck, so that vascular and neural structures are not damaged.

A No. 11 or 15 scalpel blade, held perpendicular to the skin (see Fig. 37–7), is used to nick the skin over the fluctuant area, and then a simple linear incision is carried the total length of the abscess cavity (see Fig. 37–8). This will afford more complete drainage and facilitate subsequent breakup of loculations. *Attempting to drain an abscess with an inadequate incision is counterproductive and makes packing changes more difficult.* A cruciate or X incision and an elliptical skin excision are to be avoided in the routine treatment of cutaneous abscess. The tips of the flaps of a cruciate incision may necrose, resulting in an unsightly scar (Fig. 37–10). A timid "stab" incision may produce pus but is generally not adequate for proper drainage. The scalpel is used only to make the skin incision and is not used deep in the abscess cavity.

Exceptions to this rule regarding aggressive incision are abscesses in cosmetic areas, in areas under significant skin tension (e.g., extensor surfaces), and in areas with extensive scar tissue (e.g., sites of multiple prior drainage procedures). In these special circumstances, a stab incision or simple aspiration alone may be attempted initially, with the goal of limiting tissue injury and resultant scar formation. Use of this less aggressive approach requires that the patient be counseled that multiple decompressions (e.g., via needle aspiration) or delayed aggressive incision and drainage may be required. The abscess will need to be reassessed in 24 to 48 hours to determine whether additional intervention is needed.

Wound Dissection

Following a standard incision, the operator should probe the depth of an abscess to assess the extent of the abscess and ensure proper drainage by breaking open loculations (see Fig. 37–8D). An ideal instrument for this procedure is a hemostat wrapped in gauze (or a cotton swab for small abscesses), which is placed into the abscess and swirled around to all sides of the cavity (see Fig. 37–8E). Traditionally, the operator's gloved finger has been suggested as an ideal way to assess the depth of the abscess cavity and to break up loculations, but this is a potentially dangerous practice that should be avoided unless it is certain that the abscess contains no sharp foreign body. Of particular concern is the abscess caused by skin-popping of IV drugs. These abscess occasionally harbor broken needle fragments (Fig. 37–11). In addition, patients who engage in this practice have a high incidence of hepatitis and HIV infection. Clinicians are often surprised at the depth or extent of abscesses discovered during probing. Sharp curettage of the abscess cavity is usually not required and may produce bacteremia.[44] Although tissue probing is usually the most painful aspect of the technique and total local anesthesia is difficult to attain, this portion of the procedure should not be abbreviated. If pain persists, additional local anesthetic can be *administered through the cut skin edges*, and into deeper

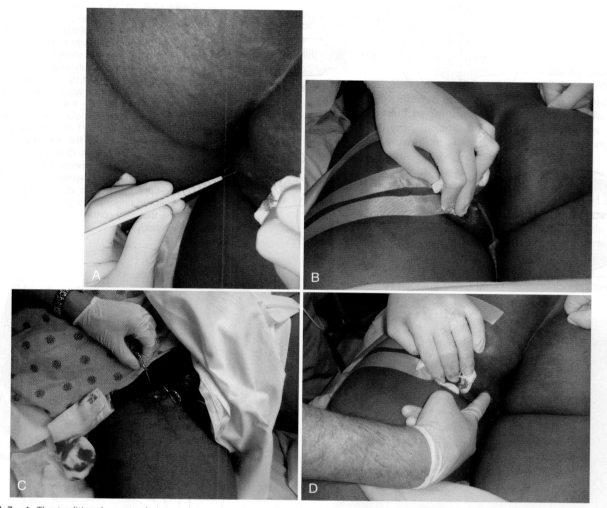

Figure 37–7 *A,* The traditional way to drain an abscess is to incise the skin with the scalpel held perpendicular to the skin. *B,* The egress of pus signifies that the cavity has been entered and the scalpel is no longer used. The skin incision is large enough to allow ready drainage. A puncture incision is not adequate. *C,* The subcutaneous tissue is probed with a hemostat that is opened in the base of the abscess. *D,* If no sharp foreign body is possible, a finger may be used to identify and open the cavity and aid in drainage.

tissues, to provide additional anesthesia (Fig. 37–12). If the procedure is limited because of pain, the use of appropriate analgesia/anesthesia is mandated. Failure to adequately pack the abscess on the first visit makes follow-up packing changes more problematic.

A blunt-end suction device can be used to extract copious pus from large or deep abscesses, while also assisting in loculation breakup (Fig. 37–13).

Wound Irrigation

Following the breaking up of loculations, some clinicians advocate copious irrigation of the abscess cavity with normal saline to ensure adequate removal of debris from the wound cavity. Although it may seem intuitively to be a helpful step, irrigation of the abscess cavity has not been experimentally demonstrated to significantly augment healing or affect outcome. Hyperemic tissue may bleed profusely, but bleeding usually stops in a few minutes if packing is used. Abscesses of the extremities can be drained with the use of a tourniquet to provide a bloodless field.

Packing and Dressing

After irrigation, a loose packing of gauze or other material is traditionally placed gently into the abscess cavity to prevent the wound margins from closing and to afford continued drainage of any exudative material that may otherwise be trapped. Although the specifics of packing have not been well studied, and some advocate nonpacking of abscesses, routine packing is usually performed. The packing material should make contact with the cavity wall so that, upon removal, gentle débridement of necrotic tissue will occur spontaneously. A common error is to attempt to pack an abscess too tightly with excessive packing material. In essence, the pack merely keeps the incision open, and its main purpose is not to absorb all drainage—a dressing accomplishes this goal. Care must be exercised to ensure that the packing does not exert significant pressure against the exposed tissue and lead to further tissue necrosis. Some prefer to use plain gauze, some use gauze soaked in saline or povidone-iodine, and some use gauze impregnated with iodine (iodoform). For large abscess cavities, gauze pads (without cotton backing) are ideal

ated 48 hours after the procedure, with the first packing change occurring at this time. Some wounds warrant closer monitoring. Diabetic patients or other patients with impaired healing capacity, mental impairment, or physical disabilities may require a home care nurse or admission for more frequent wound care/packing changes. Wounds that are at high risk for complications, such as those about the face or hands or those with significant cellulitis, require close follow-up, ideally by the same examiner. The patient should be encouraged to play an active role in wound care. During the first follow-up visit, the compliant and able patient should be taught to change the packing and dressing. If this is anatomically impossible, a friend or family member can be instructed in the technique. If long-term packing or complicated wound care is required, referral to wound care centers, rather than multiple repeat ED visits, may be more practical.

The technique of packing change is usually one of personal preference (Fig. 37–15). It should be emphasized that patients often fear a repeat visit and expect significant pain with subsequent wound care, especially if the initial incision

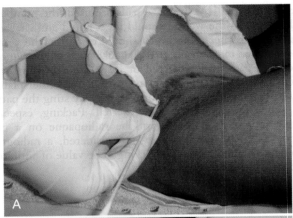
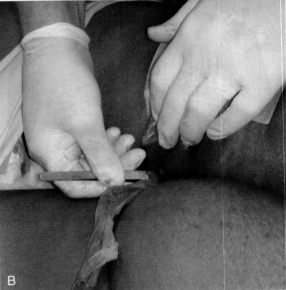

Figure 37–14 *A,* The traditional packing material is ¼- to ½-inch gauze. *B,* A 4- × 4-cm gauze pad, soaked in povidone-iodine (Betadine), can be used to pack a large abscess, but be careful to avoid losing or forgetting about packing material in the base of a large abscess.

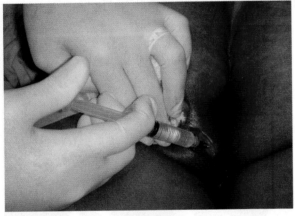

Figure 37–12 If pain persists while an abscess is being drained, the clinician pulls open the skin and injects additional anesthetic into subcutaneous tissue under direct vision.

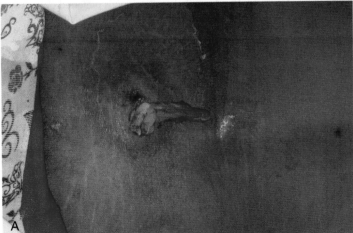
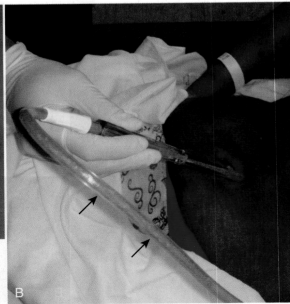

Figure 37–13 *A,* This large abscess is draining copious pus. *B,* A tonsil suction device is used to both break up loculations and extract pus. Note copious pus in tubing (*arrows*).

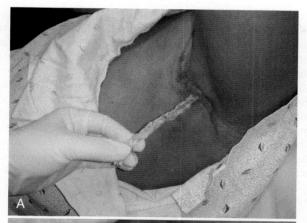

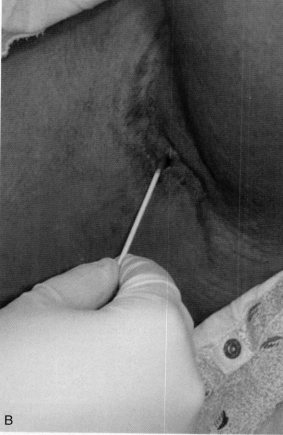

Figure 37–15 *A,* Packing gauze is removed from the abscess on the first wound check. If drainage is present, the abscess is repacked. *B,* Small abscesses can be cleaned with a cotton swab swirled in the cavity that is left open. This care can be continued at home.

the packing is removed, the wound is inspected for residual necrotic tissue. The cavity may be irrigated with saline before replacing the pack if there is significant exudate, but this is often not required because the packing absorbs most debris.

The frequency of packing or dressing changes is also clinically guided. Some wounds require multiple packing changes, and other wounds require only the initial packing. In all facial abscesses, the packing should be removed after only 24 hours, at which time warm soaks should be started. Wounds large enough to require packing should be repacked at least every 48 hours (occasionally daily for the first few visits) until healing continues in a deep-to-superficial direction. Large wounds that are allowed to close superficially will create an unsterile dead space that will potentiate the formation of recurrent abscesses. After the first few days (and in the motivated and compliant individual), an alternative to packing is to have the patient clean the base of the abscess three times a day with cotton swabs soaked in peroxide. This promotes drainage, produces gentle débridement, and keeps the incision open. After cleaning, the abscess can be irrigated with tap water and a dry dressing applied.

In general, once healthy granulation tissue has developed throughout the wound and a well-established drainage tract is present, the packing may be discontinued. The patient should then be instructed to begin warm soaks of the wound.[50] Gentle hydrostatic débridement may be performed by the patient in the shower at home: the patient holds the skin incision open and directs the shower or faucet spray into the abscess cavity. Wet-to-dry normal saline dressing changes should then follow until healing is completed. When all signs of infection (e.g., erythema, drainage, pain, and induration) have resolved and healthy granulation tissue is present, the patient may be discharged from medical care.

Complicated wounds that require prolonged care are best followed by a single clinician and should not be routinely referred back to the ED for prolonged wound care. Large perirectal or pilonidal abscesses are some conditions meeting that definition. These patients should receive early referral to their primary care clinician or specialist. Wound care centers or physical therapy departments are ideal outpatient follow-up mechanisms. Wounds in cosmetically important areas may require revision once healing is complete. Patients should be informed of this possibility early on in their care.

In select cases in which extensive or prolonged drainage occurs or if the patient is unable to return for proper follow-up care, a catheter system of drainage may be preferred.[51,52] After incision, a balloon-tipped or flared-tip catheter is placed into the abscess cavity, and pus is allowed to drain continuously through the catheter lumen. This technique has been most successful in pilonidal and Bartholin gland abscesses, but the technique is applicable to any abscess not on the face.

SPECIFIC ABSCESS THERAPY
Staphylococcal Diseases

The *Staphylococcus* bacterium is a ubiquitous pathogen that frequently colonizes the nose, skin, perineum, and gut. The umbilicus of neonates is also commonly colonized. Staphylococci grow on the skin and thrive particularly well in hair follicles, causing boils (furuncles), wound infections, and occasionally, carbuncles. The pathogenesis of staphylococcal disease is a complex host-bacteria interaction. *S. aureus* invades the skin by way of the hair follicles or an open wound and

drainage was difficult. Therefore, the specifics of packing change should be addressed before release home after the initial drainage procedure. Ideally, the initial procedure was accomplished without undue pain to allay subsequent fears. Some clinicians suggest that an oral opioid be taken 30 to 40 minutes before the next visit or the use of local anesthesia or parenteral analgesia if significant pain is anticipated. Removal of packing material is often painful, but if the packing is moistened with saline before removal, it may be less traumatic. If the original incision was of the proper length, loculations were adequately removed, and packing was adequate, subsequent packing changes will be considerably easier. Once produces local tissue destruction followed by hyperemia of vessels. Subsequently, an exudative reaction occurs, during which polymorphonuclear cells invade. The process then extends along the path of least resistance. The abscess may "point" or form sinus tracts. The process can disseminate by invasion of vessels and thus can infect other organs. Most cases of staphylococcal osteomyelitis, meningitis, and endocarditis occur by this mechanism.[53,54]

Folliculitis represents a small abscess occurring at the root of a hair. Local measures, including warm compresses and antibacterial soaps and ointments, are the usual treatment. Systemic antibiotics may be required if multiple sites are involved or the patient is a chronic staphylococcal carrier.

Furuncles, or boils, are acute circumscribed abscesses of the skin and subcutaneous tissue that most commonly occur on the face, neck, buttocks, thigh, perineum, and breast and in the axilla. Carbuncles are aggregates of interconnected furuncles that frequently occur on the back of the neck (Fig. 37–16). In this area, the skin is thick, so extension occurs laterally rather than toward the skin surface. Carbuncles may become large and can cause systemic symptoms and complications. They are found in increased frequency among diabetics; all patients with a carbuncle should be evaluated for this underlying disease. Treatment should consist of surgical drainage and administration of systemic antibiotics. Large carbuncles may be impossible to drain adequately in the ED. Carbuncles usually consist of many loculated pockets of pus, so simple incision and drainage is often not curative. Occasionally, wide excision and skin grafting are required.

Most recurrent staphylococcal skin infections are caused by autoinfection from skin lesions or nasal reservoirs. Prevention is directed at eliminating the organism. This is accomplished by application of bacitracin to the nares and by good hygiene, including frequent cleansing with antibacterial soap. If these measures are unsuccessful, systemic oral antistaphylococcal treatment is instituted for 2 to 3 weeks. Detection and treatment of infection in family members may be necessary.[53,54]

S. aureus produces suture abscesses. A suture abscess is often misdiagnosed as a wound infection, but in fact, it is a local nidus of inflammation or infection, or both, caused and potentiated by suture material. Such an abscess usually appears after sutures have been in place for 3 to 5 days, with single or multiple discrete areas of redness and tenderness noted at the site of suture penetration of the skin. Simply removing the suture (a drop of pus may be expressed) and providing warm compresses and topical antibiotic ointment is usually all that is required. Wide opening of the wound and systemic antibiotics are seldom required. When the suture is buried, a small incision should be followed by probing of the wound with a small hook or bent needle (see Chapter 35, Methods of Wound Closure) to snare the suture for its removal.

Hidradenitis Suppurativa

Hidradenitis suppurativa (Greek; *hidros*, sweat; *aden*, gland) is a chronic, relapsing, inflammatory disease process affecting the apocrine glands in the axilla, the inguinal region,[55] and the perineum (Fig. 37–17). Its prevalence is 0.3% to 4% in industrialized countries; most affected individuals are young women.[56] The condition results from occlusion of the apocrine ducts by keratinous debris, which leads to ductal dilatation, inflammation, and rupture into the subcutaneous area. Secondary bacterial infection ensues, leading to abscess formation and scarring. This chronic recurring process leads to draining fistulous tracts, which involve large areas and are not amenable to simple incision and drainage procedures (Fig. 37–18).[57]

Genetic factors may play some role in hidradenitis suppurativa.[58] Fitzsimmons[59] proposed a single dominant gene transmission. Individuals of African descent appear to have an increased incidence compared with Caucasians. Because apocrine glands become active during puberty, it is rare to find hidradenitis suppurativa in the pediatric population.[55] Onset after menopause is rare. B-Mode ultrasound images reveal larger hair follicles in affected individuals than in controls.[60]

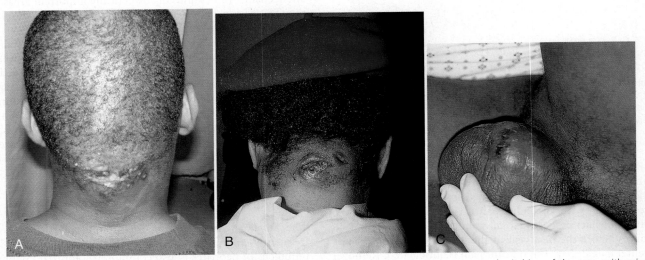

Figure 37–16 *A* and *B*, A carbuncle is a complicated abscess on the nape of the neck. The first symptom may be itching of the area, with minor skin changes mistaken for a nondescript rash. It is very common in diabetics. Carbuncles are usually caused by *Staphylococcus aureus*, including CA-MRSA. Because of its many crypts and loculations, and intercommunicating small abscesses, simple incision and drainage are often not readily curative. When fluctuance is appreciated, incision is indicated. One should avoid multiple small incisions because tissue circulation may be compromised. Antibiotics may augment healing of this abscess, but wide surgical excision may be required. *C*, A scrotal abscess from CA-MRSA in a diabetic patient.

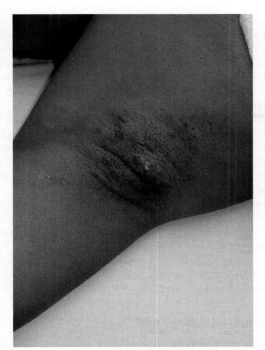

Figure 37–17 Axillary abscesses are common and recurrent. CA-MRSA is an increasing cause.

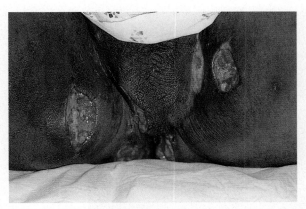

Figure 37–18 Hidradenitis suppurativa of the groin or axilla is a complicated series of abscesses that may not be amenable to simple incision and drainage. In this patient, with involvement of the groin, extensive surgery was required to excise recurrent infection.

Women are affected more frequently than men. Shaving and depilation have frequently been suggested as causes of this discrepancy; however, this theory was not supported in a study that compared the frequency of these behaviors in patients with hidradenitis suppurativa and a group of controls.[61] Obesity is associated with a higher incidence of the disease.[62] Excessive dermal folds provide dark, wet, and warm areas that are ideal for the proliferation of bacteria. Antiperspirants and deodorants may decrease wetness and bacterial overgrowth, but they can produce inflammatory responses that exacerbate the disease process.

The bacteriology of acute abscess formation in hidradenitis suppurativa reflects organisms seen in other soft tissue abscesses. *Staphylococcus* is the most commonly isolated organism,[63] with *E. coli* and β-hemolytic *Streptococcus* being other important pathogens. In the perineal region, enteric flora are often found. Many of these abscesses have multiple isolates, and anaerobic bacteria are frequently found. CA-MRSA is an increasing cause of such abscesses.

Hidradenitis suppurativa begins as a single inflammatory event involving an apocrine gland, which progresses to frank suppuration and, at this stage, is no different from a simple furuncle. The clinical entity is distinguishable only in its chronic scarring phase. By then, the lesion exhibits multiple foci coupled with areas of induration and inflammation that are in various stages of healing. Progression of the process reveals coalesced areas of firm, raised violaceous dermis. The lesion is usually markedly tender.

Initial outpatient management of an acute suppurative lesion usually involves intervention. Any fluctuant area requires drainage as described in the section titled "Incision and Drainage Procedure." In cases of extensive cellulitis, a broad-spectrum, antistaphylococcal antibiotic should be used. Unfortunately, hidradenitis suppurativa cannot be cured with localized incision and drainage. If incision and drainage is required for relief of a secondary abscess, it should be made clear to the patient that this procedure does not cure the underlying disease.[64] The chronic nature of the disease produces multiple areas of inflammation and subcutaneous fistulous tracts that induce routine recurrences. The patient must be informed of this unfavorable prognosis and should be referred to a dermatologist or surgeon for long-term care.

Milder forms of the disease are initially treated with conservative measures. Many different approaches have been tried, with only limited degrees of success. Few controlled studies of treatment strategies have been performed. Patients are often counseled to lose weight, refrain from shaving, stop using deodorants, and improve personal hygiene. The benefits of these efforts are unknown. Oral antistaphylococcal antibiotics are most commonly used, with varying results.[65] There have been reports of success with topical clindamycin[66,67] and laser therapy,[68] but these treatments have not been studied in a controlled setting and require further investigation. Dermal infection results from breakdown of the normal host-defense mechanism, which occurs with irritation, traumatic injury, or inflammation, coupled with the availability of concentrated opportunistic bacteria. Therefore, the clinician must institute therapies that will decrease bacterial availability without causing further injury to the affected dermis.

Advanced stages of the disease are managed with wide or local excision and primary or delayed closure (see Fig. 37–18).[69,70] Skin grafting may be warranted.[71] Combination therapy (clindamycin/rifampicin[72]) and the administration of tumor necrosis factor–α inhibitors (infliximab, adalimumab[73,74]) have been successful in treating a few intractable cases. Despite such radical approaches, many patients experience recurrences of this challenging and distressing disease.

Breast Abscess

Most breast abscesses occur in women who are not in the puerperium.[75,76] Breast infections are caused by normal skin bacteria, which enter through a break or crack in the skin, usually the nipple. The infection becomes established in the parenchymal tissue, causing pain and swelling.

A breast abscess in its early stages, when cellulitis predominates, can be difficult to diagnose. In equivocal cases, antibiotics may be curative. Cellulitis may progress to frank abscess formation. Women with this condition may be quite ill and appear toxic.

The estimated incidence of inflammatory processes of the breast (mastitis) among lactating women ranges from 2% to 33%.[77] The infection is usually precipitated by milk stasis after weaning or missed feedings. The cause is usually bacterial invasion through a cracked or abraded nipple by *S. aureus* or streptococci originating from the nursing child. Manifestations are redness, heat, pain, fever, and chills. Treatment consists of antistaphylococcal antibiotics, continued breast emptying with a breast pump, and application of heat. It is important to encourage continued breast emptying to promote drainage. Nursing can be continued with the noninfected breast.[78]

Ultrasound-guided needle aspiration is becoming the standard of care for most breast abscesses. Compared with incision and drainage, aspiration causes less scarring, does not interfere with breast feeding, and does not require general anesthesia.[79] Christensen and associates[80] recommend that ultrasound-guided drainage should replace surgery as first-line treatment for uncomplicated puerperal and nonpuerperal breast abscesses. The emerging treatment parameters are these: ultrasound-guided needle aspiration for abscesses less than 3 cm in diameter and ultrasound-guided catheter drainage for abscesses 3 cm in diameter or larger.[78,81] As seen on ultrasound images, breast abscesses are inhomogeneous, hyperechoic masses (Fig. 37–19).

Recurrent abscesses are a common, troublesome complication after traditional treatment with incision, drainage, and antibiotics.[82,83] Fortunately, the reported recurrence rates associated with ultrasound-guided aspiration/drainage procedures is quite low.[80,81] Patients with persistent recurrences need to be managed by a surgeon for total excision of the involved area.

Although breast abscess is rarely a harbinger of malignancy, it could be the initial presentation of a metastatic process.[84-86] After needle aspiration or catheter drainage, the aspirate should be sent for culture and cytology, and a postdrainage mammogram and ultrasound scan should be done to eliminate concerns over missing a malignancy.[87]

Breast abscesses may be a complication of breast implants inserted under appropriate medical care[88] as well as via illicit cosmetic procedures.[89] The infection has also been associated with nipple piercing.[90]

A breast abscess in a man is an unusual occurrence. Malignancy and underlying bone or joint infection should be considered (see Fig. 37–1).

Bartholin Gland Abscess

The Bartholin glands (the greater vestibular glands) are located at the 4 and 8 o'clock positions on each side of the

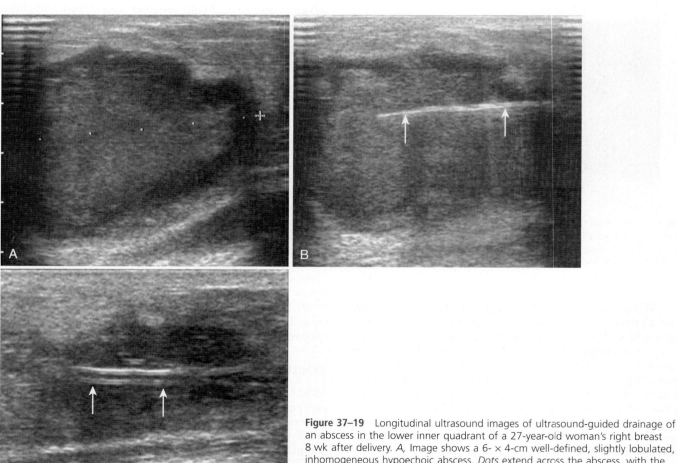

Figure 37–19 Longitudinal ultrasound images of ultrasound-guided drainage of an abscess in the lower inner quadrant of a 27-year-old woman's right breast 8 wk after delivery. *A*, Image shows a 6- × 4-cm well-defined, slightly lobulated, inhomogeneous hypoechoic abscess. *Dots* extend across the abscess, with the *cursor* at one margin of the abscess. *B*, Image shows a 7-Fr pigtail catheter containing trocar (*arrows*) in the abscess cavity. *C*, Image obtained after trocar removal and aspiration of 70 mL of pus. *Parallel lines* represent catheter walls (*arrows*). (A–C, From Ulitzsch D, Nyman MKG, Carlson RA: *Breast abscess in lactating women: US-guided treatment. Radiology 232:904, 2004.*)

vestibule of the vagina. These mucous-secreting glands maintain the moisture of the vaginal mucosa. When the ostium becomes blocked by inflammation or trauma, fluid cannot drain, leading to the formation of a cyst. If the cyst becomes infected, a painful abscess may develop.

Asymptomatic cysts (no pain, no discharge) frequently occur from duct blockage and retention of secretions. Symptomatic cysts (vulvar pain, dysparenuria, and discomfort while walking or sitting) can be managed with warm sitz baths and compresses. Cysts cause swollen and tender labia and a fluctuant, grape-sized mass that can be palpated between the thumb and the index finger. The more typical ED presentation is a painful, sometimes debilitating, abscess requiring surgical intervention.

The most common procedure for treating a Bartholin abscess is insertion of a drainage catheter, as described by Word in 1968.[91] This single-barreled, sealed-stopper, balloon-tipped catheter serves as initial and long-term therapy (Fig. 37–20). In his original description, Word reported only 2 recurrences in 72 lesions, both of which were treated successfully with a second catheter. No patient required marsupialization. The procedure involves fistulization of the duct cavity by a 1-inch catheter with an inflatable balloon tip.[92] Although not a traditional incision and drainage procedure, the technique permits continued drainage of the gland.

In preparation for insertion of the catheter, place the patient in standard dorsal lithotomy position and drape the perineum. Cleanse the area with povidone-iodine solution. If an anesthetic is deemed necessary for patient comfort and cooperation, lidocaine can be infiltrated just external to the hymen ring, where the distal duct opening should be located (at the 5 or 7 o'clock position).[93] Make a small incision into the mucosa. Use the scalpel or a hemostat to puncture the

abscess cavity (Fig. 37–21). (It can be difficult to enter this deep abscess cavity.) Failure to obtain frank pus or to appreciate the "pop" of entering the abscess usually prognosticates failure of the procedure. Stabilize the abscess with the thumb and forefinger, hold the hemostat in place, and skewer the abscess onto the hemostat. Pushing the hemostat into the immobilized abscess is technically more difficult (see Fig. 37–21E). Make a stab incision large enough to accommodate the catheter but small enough to prohibit the inflated balloon from being extruded. Once the abscess has been entered (signaled by a palpable pop or the free flow of pus), place the deflated balloon in the abscess cavity. Using a 25-gauge needle to minimize the hole in the stopper, fill the balloon with 2 to 4 mL of water (not air). Persistent pain indicates that too much fluid has been used. Most abscesses drain for a few days, and the Word catheter often falls out within a week. Ideally, the device is left in place for 2 to 4 weeks to allow fistula formation, so follow-up is required. If the catheter falls out prematurely, it should be replaced quickly to fulfill the time needed for fistulization. Some clinicians do not reinsert the catheter if healing has progressed significantly after the first drainage procedure.

Standard incision and drainage can give the patient immediate relief, but this procedure is not recommended because the abscess recurrence rate is so high.[94] But if a Word catheter is not available, incision and drainage can be performed, with the caveat that the clincian and the patient must appreciate the likelihood of unfavorable long-term outcome. The incision is made over the medial surface of the introitus (on the mucosa, not on the skin) on a line parallel to the posterior margin of the hymenal ring. The abscess cavity is slightly deeper than most cutaneous abscesses, so the clinician must be certain to enter the actual abscess cavity to achieve

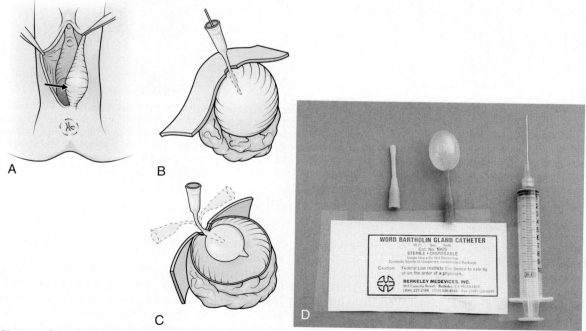

Figure 37–20 Use of the Word catheter for outpatient drainage of a Bartholin gland abscess. This is a fistulization procedure rather than a standard incision and drainage. *A,* A stab incision is made on the mucosal surface. A catheter is inserted into the cyst cavity (*B*) and filled with 3–4 mL of water (*C*). *D,* Inflatable bulb-tipped catheter. *Left,* Uninflated. *Right,* Inflated with 4 mL water. (*A–C, From Word B: Office treatment of cyst and abscess of Bartholin gland. JAMA 190:777, 1964; D, from Word B: Office treatment of cyst and abscess of Bartholin gland duct. South Med J 61:514, 1968. Reproduced with permission.*)

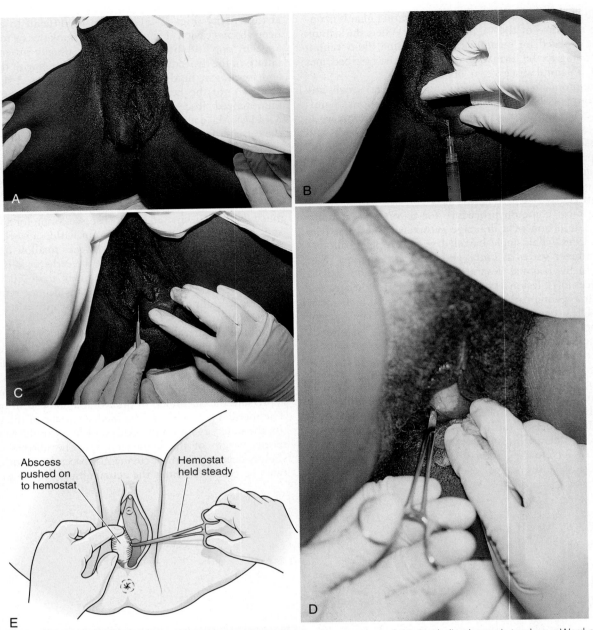

Figure 37–21 *A,* An alternative to formal incision, drainage, and packing for the treatment of this Bartholin abscess is to place a Word catheter. *B,* The abscess is stabilized with the thumb and index finger, and a local anesthetic is injected into the mucosal (not skin) surface. *C,* A stab incision is made with a scalpel. Copious pus drainage signals entrance into the abscess cavity. *D,* The abscess is punctured with a hemostat. Deep abscesses may be difficult to puncture. *E,* It is technically easier to enter the Bartholin gland abscess cavity if the hemostat is held steady and the abscess, held with the thumb and index finger, is skewered onto the hemostat. Attempting to puncture the deep immobilized abscess by stabbing with the hemostat may be more difficult. A palpable pop when entering the abscess or drainage of frank pus is expected, and confirm the diagnosis and proper technique.

complete drainage. This is most easily accomplished by inserting a hemostat through the mucosal incision and spreading the tips of the instrument in the deeper soft tissue.

After the contents have drained, the abscess is packed for 24 to 48 hours, and sitz baths are started thereafter. Broad-spectrum antibiotics are not required after routine incision and drainage, but they can be prescribed for patients with significant cellulitis and for those in whom an actual abscess has not yet formed. If the abscess recurs, more definitive therapy in the form of marsupialization or complete excision of the gland may be required; however, these procedures are

not performed initially and, when chosen, should be done in an OR.

Alternative treatment strategies have been explored. Gennis and coworkers[95] designed a rubber ring catheter (the Jacobi ring) from an 8-French T-tube threaded with 2-0 silk suture material. The catheter enters and exits the abscess through separate incisions, forming a closed ring when the suture ends are tied. The device was tested in a randomized study involving 38 women, 25 of whom received a ring catheter and 13 of whom receive a Word catheter. The catheters were rated similarly in terms of successful placement, abscess

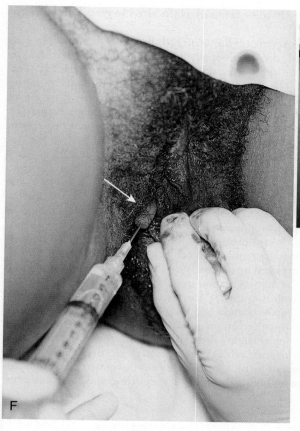

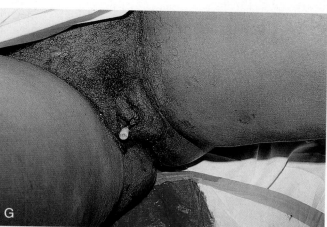

Figure 37–21, cont'd *F,* The catheter (*arrow*) is placed to its hilt into the abscess cavity, and the balloon is filled with 3–4 ml saline. Use a 25-gauge needle to fill the balloon. *G,* The catheter is left in place for 2–4 wk to form a fistula. Antibiotics are of no proven value once drainage is performed, but practice varies.

resolution (all resolved within 3 wk), and recurrence rates (no recurrences at 6 mo and 2 [1 in each treatment group] at 1 yr). However, the ring catheter outperformed with Word catheter in patient satisfaction.

Empirical antibiotics are indicated only for patients with frank abscess and local cellulitis. No growth is obtained on more than 80% of cultures from Bartholin cysts and a third of cultures from abscesses.[96] Cultures that are positive typically show polymicrobial growth, usually anaerobes, especially *Bacteroides* species and other colonic bacteria. Much less often, *Neisseria gonorrhoeae* is cultured from the abscess cavity. Chronic low-grade inflammation from gonococcal infections has been implicated as a causative factor in cyst formation and occasionally in the development of an abscess; therefore, the antibiotic chosen should provide coverage for *N. gonorrhoeae.* It is reasonable to take cervical and anal cultures for gonorrhea from women with Bartholin gland abscesses because of the association of these infections with sexually transmitted disease,[97] but one need not routinely treat patients for gonorrhea unless the clinician suspects that it is present. At the current time, CA-MRSA infections of the Bartholin glands are uncommon.

Particular care must be taken when treating pregnant women with Bartholin gland abscess, because they are at high risk for complications. The development of sepsis in a pregnant woman after marsupialization of an abscess has been reported.[98] Postmenopausal women presenting with what appears to be a Bartholin gland abscess should be referred to a gynecologist to rule out malignancy. A vulvar abscess in an HIV-positive woman should raise suspicion for Kaposi sarcoma.[99]

Pilonidal Abscess

Pilonidal sinuses are common malformations that occur in the sacrococcygeal area. The cause of the sinus formation is unclear; the malformation may occur during embryogenesis. Pilonidal cyst formation is thought to be secondary to blockage of a pilonidal sinus. The result of this obstruction is repeated soft tissue infection, followed by drainage and partial resolution, with eventual reaccumulation. The blockage is most commonly the result of hairs in the region, and the lesion may in part be a foreign body (hair) granuloma. Although pilonidal sinuses are present from birth, they usually do not manifest clinically until adolescence or the early adult years. Pilonidal abscess formation most commonly affects young (often white) adults. The sinuses and cysts are lined with stratified squamous epithelium and, after excision, may be found to contain wads of hair and debris. When cultured, pilonidal abscesses generally yield mixed fecal flora with a preponderance of anaerobes.[100] Poor hygiene and repeated trauma (called "Jeep bottom" in World War II) may precipitate acute infection. At the current time, CA-MRSA infections are not common.

The patient with a pilonidal abscess will seek care for back pain and local tenderness. On physical examination, the area is found to be indurated. Frank abscess formation may not be appreciated in this deep abscess. One will usually see barely perceptible dimples or tiny openings at the rostral end of the gluteal crease (Fig. 37–22). A hair or slight discharge may be noticed at the opening. One may find a more caudal cyst or abscess, possibly with a palpable sinus tract connecting the two. The sinus and cyst may be draining chronically, or

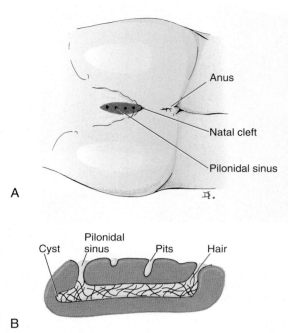

Figure 37–22   Pilonidal sinus. *A,* Sinuses occur in the midline some 5 cm above the anus in the natal cleft. *B,* Longitudinal section shows sinuses and pits. *(A and B, From Hill GJ II [ed]: Outpatient Surgery, 3rd ed. Philadelphia, WB Saunders, 1988. Reproduced with permission.)*

they may become infected as the size increases and blockage occurs.[101]

Treatment of the acutely infected cyst is the same as previously discussed for any fluctuant abscess: All hair and pus should be removed, and the lesion should be packed (Fig. 37–23). The abscess cavity may be quite large, necessitating a lengthy incision to ensure complete drainage. It may take many weeks for the initial incision to heal. The area may be repacked at 2- to 4-day intervals as an outpatient procedure, although some prefer to discontinue packing after the 1st week. Antibiotic therapy is not usually required.

Simple incision and drainage is usually not curative; therefore, the patient should be referred to a surgeon for removal of the cyst and sinus after the inflammatory process has resolved. Small abscesses may be incised and drained as an outpatient procedure performed under local anesthesia, but the disease process is often extensive, and general anesthesia may be required to achieve complete drainage. One is often surprised by the extent of the cyst cavity and the volume of pus encountered upon initial incision.

Closure strategies for these potentially large wounds vary. Gencosmanoglu and Inceoglu[102] concluded that a modified lay-open technique is superior to excision with primary closure for chronic pilonidal sinuses in regard to morbidity and recurrence rates. When primary closure is chosen, the administration of a broad-spectrum regimen of antibiotics (e.g., preoperative infusion of cefuoxime and metronidazole

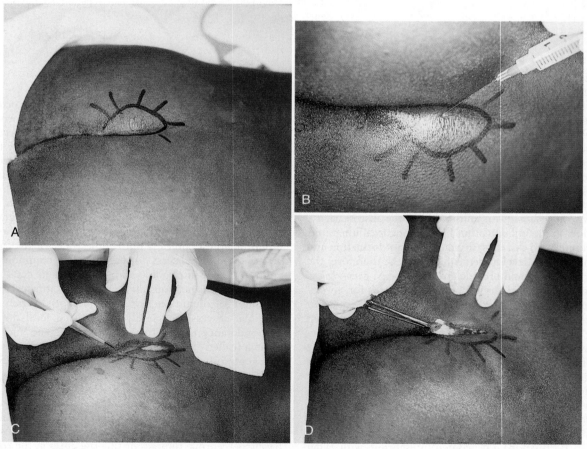

Figure 37–23   *A,* A pilonidal abscess can be quite extensive (induration *outlined by marker*), but it may be difficult to feel fluctuance because of the depth of the infection. *B,* Local anesthesia and conscious sedation make the initial ED incision and drainage successful. *C,* A deep incision yields copious pus and occasionally other debris such as hair. *D,* The abscess cavity is packed open. When infection and inflammation have subsided, definitive treatment may include wide excision of the sinus and its lateral tracks. Antibiotics are of no proven value following adequate surgical drainage, but practice varies.

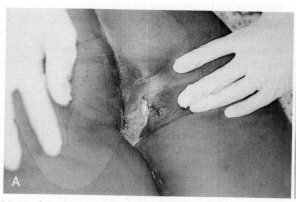
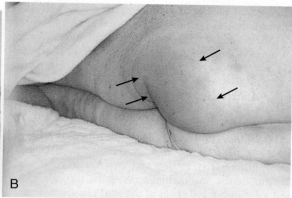

Figure 37–24 *A,* If a perirectal abscess spontaneously ruptures and drains, a formal incision, drainage, and packing should still be performed. *B,* A deep, poorly localized perirectal abscess of this size simply cannot be adequately drained in the ED. *Arrows* outline the area of induration. This patient requires extensive drainage under general anesthesia. A computed tomography scan may further evaluate the location of the abscess. Broad spectrum intravenous antibiotics may be started in the ED prior to definitive surgical intervention.

followed by 5 days of oral co-amoxiclav[103]) offers protection against wound infections.

Perirectal Abscesses

Most anorectal infections originate in the cryptoglandular area located in the anal canal at the level of the dentate line. Abscesses within these glands can penetrate the surrounding sphincter and track in a variety of directions, leading to larger abscesses within the perianal, intersphincteric, ischiorectal, and supralevator spaces. A small number of anorectal abscesses have a noncryptoglandular etiology such as Crohn's disease, atypical infection (e.g., tuberculosis, lymphogranuloma venereum), malignancy, or trauma.[104]

Perirectal infections can range from minor irritations to fatal illnesses. Surprisingly clandestine infections often occur in diabetics. Successful management depends on early recognition of the disease process and adequate surgical therapy. Small abscesses can be initially managed on an outpatient basis with simple incision and drainage, described previously. Because of the morbidity and mortality associated with inadequate treatment of these conditions, patients with large and deep abscesses should be promptly admitted to the hospital for evaluation and treatment under general or spinal anesthesia (Fig. 37–24).

It is important to understand the anatomy of the anal canal and the rectum in order to appreciate the pathophysiology of these abscesses and their treatment (Fig. 37–25). The mucosa of the anal canal is loosely attached to the muscle wall. At the dentate line, where columnar epithelium gives way to squamous epithelium, there are vertical folds of tissue, called the *rectal columns of Morgagni,* which are connected at their lower ends by small semilunar folds called *anal valves.* Under these valves are invaginations termed *anal crypts.* Within these crypts are collections of ducts from anal glands. These glands are believed to be responsible for the genesis of most, if not all, perirectal abscesses. These glands often pass through the internal sphincter but do not penetrate the external sphincter.

The muscular anatomy divides the perirectal area into compartments that may house an abscess, depending on the direction of spread of the foci of the infection (Fig. 37–26).[101,105]

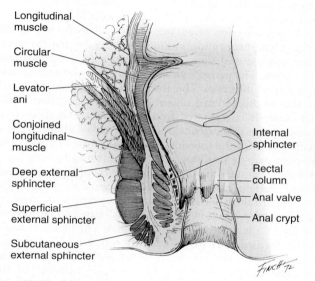

Figure 37–25 Schematic coronal section of the anal canal and the rectum. *(From Schwartz SI, Lillehei RC [eds]: Principles of Surgery, 2nd ed. New York, McGraw-Hill, 1974. Reproduced with permission.)*

Longitudinal muscle
Circular muscle
Levator ani
Conjoined longitudinal muscle
Deep external sphincter
Superficial external sphincter
Subcutaneous external sphincter
Internal sphincter
Rectal column
Anal valve
Anal crypt

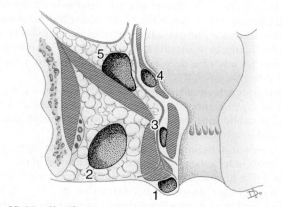

Figure 37–26 Classification of perirectal abscesses. *1,* Perianal. *2,* Ischiorectal. *3,* Intersphincteric. *4,* High intramuscular. *5,* Pelvirectal. *(From Hill GJ II [ed]. Outpatient Surgery, 3rd ed. Philadelphia, WB Saunders, 1988. Reproduced by permission.)*

The circular fibers of the intestinal coat thicken at the rectum–anus junction to become the internal anal sphincter. The muscle fibers of the levator ani fuse with those of the outer longitudinal fibers of the intestinal coat as it passes through the pelvic floor. These conjoined fibers are connected by fibrous tissue to the external sphincter system, which consists of three circular muscle groups.

Pathophysiology

As described previously, the anal glands are mucus-secreting structures that terminate in the area between the internal and the external sphincters. It is believed that most perirectal infections begin in the intersphincteric space secondary to blockage and subsequent infection of the anal glands. Normal host-defense mechanisms then break down, followed by invasion and overgrowth by bowel flora.[106]

If the infection spreads across the external sphincter laterally, an ischiorectal abscess is formed. If the infection dissects rostrally, it may continue between the internal and the external sphincters, causing a high intramuscular abscess. The infection may also dissect through the external sphincter over the levator ani to form a pelvirectal abscess.[105]

When infection of an anal crypt extends by way of the perianal lymphatics and continues between the mucous membrane and the anal muscles, a perianal abscess forms at the anal orifice. The perianal abscess is the most common variety of perirectal infection. The abscess lies immediately beneath the skin in the perianal region at the lowermost part of the anal canal. It is separated from the ischiorectal space by a fascial septum that extends from the external sphincter and is continuous with the subcutaneous tissue of the buttocks. The infection may be small and localized or it may be very large, with a wall of necrotic tissue and a surrounding zone of cellulitis.[53] Perianal abscesses may be associated with a fistula in ano. The fistula in ano is an inflammatory tract with an external opening in the skin of the perianal area and an internal opening in the mucosa of the anal canal. The fistula in ano is usually formed after partial resolution of a perianal abscess, and its presence is suggested by recurrence of these abscesses with intermittent drainage. The external opening of the fissure is usually a red elevated piece of granulation tissue that may have purulent or serosanguineous drainage on compression. In many cases, the tract can be palpated as a cord. Patients with anal fistulas should be referred for definitive surgical excision.[105]

Ischiorectal abscesses are fairly common. They are bounded superiorly by the levator ani, inferiorly by the fascia over the perianal space, medially by the anal sphincter muscles, and laterally by the obturator internus muscle. These abscesses may commonly be bilateral, and if so, the two cavities communicate by way of a deep postanal space to form a "horseshoe" abscess.[53]

Intersphincteric abscesses are less common. They are bounded by the internal and external sphincters and may extend rostrally into the rectum, thereby separating the circular and longitudinal muscle layers.

Causes of perirectal abscesses other than the cryptoglandular process have been documented but are fairly rare. It is believed that hemorrhoids, anorectal surgery, episiotomies, or local trauma may cause abscess formation by altering local anatomy and thus destroying natural tissue barriers to infections.[106–108] Perirectal abscesses may serve as a portal of entry for organisms responsible for necrotic soft tissue infections such as Fournier's gangrene.[109]

Physical and Laboratory Findings

A perianal abscess is generally not difficult to diagnose. The throbbing pain in the perianal region is acute and is aggravated by sitting, coughing, sneezing, and straining. There is swelling, induration, and tenderness, and a small area of cellulitis is present in proximity to the anus. Rectal examination of the patient with a perianal abscess reveals that most of the tenderness and induration is below the level of the anal ring. Deeper abscesses may be difficult to localize. A computed tomography scan may be obtained to provide definitive diagnosis and to further evaluate complicated cases.

Patients with ischiorectal abscesses present with fever, chills, and malaise, but at first, there is less pain than with the perianal abscess. Initially on physical examination, one will see an asymmetry of the perianal tissue; later, erythema and induration become apparent. Digital examination reveals a large, tense, tender swelling along the anal canal that extends above the anorectal ring. If both ischiorectal spaces are involved, the findings are bilateral.

Patients with intersphincteric abscesses usually present with dull, aching pain in the rectum rather than in the perianal region. No external aberrations of the perianal tissues are noted, but tenderness may be present. On digital examination, one frequently palpates a soft, tender, sausage-shaped mass above the anorectal ring; if the mass has already ruptured, the patient may give a history of passage of purulent material during defecation.[106,107]

Diagnosis of pelvirectal abscesses may be very difficult. Usually, fever, chills, and malaise are present, but because the abscess is so deep-seated, few or no signs or symptoms are present in the perianal region. Rectal or vaginal examination may reveal a tender swelling that is adherent to the rectal mucosa above the anorectal ring.

Laboratory findings usually do not aid in the diagnosis. Kovalcik and colleagues[106] found that less than 50% of their patients had a white blood cell count greater than $10.0 \times 10^9/$ L. Cultures of perirectal abscesses usually show mixed infections involving anaerobic bacteria, most commonly *B. fragilis* and gram-negative enteric bacilli. Currently, CA-MRSA infections are not common.

Treatment

Successful management of perirectal abscesses depends on adequate surgical drainage. Complications from these infections may necessitate multiple surgical procedures, prolong hospital stay, and result in sepsis and death. Bevans and associates[108] retrospectively studied the charts of 184 patients who were surgically treated over a 10-year period. These patients were evaluated primarily to identify the factors that contributed to morbidity and mortality. Initial drainage was performed under local anesthesia in 38% of the patients and under spinal or general anesthesia in 62%. The authors identified three key factors in excessive morbidity and mortality: (1) a delay in diagnosis and treatment, (2) inadequate initial examination or treatment, and (3) associated systemic disease. They believed that the only way to effectively examine and adequately drain all but superficial well-localized perirectal abscesses was under spinal or general anesthesia. This assessment was supported by evidence of an increased incidence of recurrence and of sepsis and death in patients treated with local anesthesia. Drainage of deep abscesses under local anesthesia generally does not allow drainage of all hidden loculations. In addition, local anesthesia is not adequate for treatment of associated pathologic conditions.

Small, well-defined perianal abscesses are the only perirectal infections that lend themselves to outpatient therapy. All other perirectal abscesses require hospitalization for definitive therapy. The result of incision and drainage is almost immediate relief of pain and rapid resolution of infection. Indications for inpatient drainage are failure to obtain adequate anesthesia, systemic toxicity, extension of the abscess beyond a localized area, or recurrence of a perianal abscess. Recurrence may be caused by the presence of a fistula in ano.

A perianal abscess is drained through a single linear incision over the most fluctuant portion of the abscess in a manner previously described for other cutaneous abscesses. It is extremely painful to probe a perianal abscess and to break up loculations, so liberal analgesia is advised. The patient may begin sitz baths at home 24 hours after surgery. Packing is replaced at 48-hour intervals until the infection has cleared and granulation tissue has appeared. This usually occurs within 4 to 6 days. Antibiotics are generally not required.

Use of de Pezzer catheters in anorectal abscesses has been described as an alternative to traditional incision and packing. In a series of 91 patients treated in this manner, Kyle and Isbister[110] found equivalent rates of subsequent fistula surgery, less need for general anesthesia, and a shorter postoperative hospital stay compared with patients treated with traditional incision and packing. Beck and coworkers[111] reported successful use of catheter drainage in 55 patients with ischiorectal abscess. Owing to the complexity of ischiorectal abscesses, this technique is probably best left to the surgeon providing ongoing care.

Perirectal abscesses are currently recognized as a fairly common cause of fever in the granulocytopenic patient. These abscesses have a different bacteriologic profile: *Pseudomonas aeruginosa* organisms are isolated most frequently. These patients present later because pain develops later in the course, and fever may be the first manifestation. Therefore, any patients who are granulocytopenic with vague anorectal complaints, especially those with fever, should be examined carefully for perirectal abscesses. Any abscess that is found should be drained immediately under appropriate anesthesia, and extensive IV antibiotic coverage should be initiated.

Patients who present with a spontaneously ruptured perirectal abscess may appear to have experienced a self-cure, but under most circumstances, they should undergo formal incision, drainage, and packing. Treatment should be individualized.

Infected Sebaceous Cyst

A common entity that appears as a cutaneous abscess is the infected sebaceous cyst. Such infections are increasingly caused by CA-MRSA. Sebaceous cysts, caused by obstruction of sebaceous gland ducts, may occur anywhere on the body. The cyst becomes filled with a thick, cheesy, sebaceous material, and the contents frequently become infected. Sebaceous cysts can be quite large and may persist for many years before they become infected. When infected, they clinically appear as tender, fluctuant subcutaneous masses, often with overlying erythema.

The initial treatment of an infected sebaceous cyst is simple incision and drainage. The thick sebaceous material must be expressed, because it is too thick to drain spontaneously (Fig. 37–27A). An important difference exists between infected sebaceous cysts and other abscesses. A sebaceous cyst has a definite pearly white capsule that must be excised to prevent recurrence (see Fig. 37–27B and C). Traditionally, in the presence of significant inflammation, it is preferable to drain the infection initially and remove the shiny capsule on the first follow-up visit or a later visit, when it may be more easily identified. Alternatively, the entire cyst can be removed at the time of initial incision. At the time of capsule removal, the edges are grasped with clamps or hemostats, and the entire capsule is removed by sharp dissection with a scalpel or scissors. After excision of the capsule, the area is treated in the same manner as a healing abscess cavity. Simple drainage without excision of the capsule often leads to recurrence.

Kitamura and colleagues[112] reported a randomized study of 71 patients treated with either traditional incision and drainage or primary resection of the cyst, followed by irrigation and wound closure. In this study, the patients treated with primary resection had faster healing, fewer days of pain, and less scarring.

Paronychia

A paronychia is an infection localized to the area around the nail root (Fig. 37–28). Paronychias are common infections probably caused by frequent trauma to the delicate skin around the fingernail and the cuticle. These infections have also been linked to "insults" induced by nail cosmetics (mechanical trauma, irritant reactions, and allergic reactions)[113] and to a number of occupations (e.g., hair cutting and meat handling).[114] When a minor infection begins, the nail itself may act like a foreign body. Usually, the infectious process is limited to the area above the nail base and underneath the eponychium (cuticle), but occasionally, it may spread to include tissue under the nail as well, forming a subungual abscess. Lymphadenitis and lymphadenopathy are usually not seen. Generally, a paronychia is a mixed bacterial infection. *Staphylococcus* is commonly cultured from these lesions; however, anaerobes and numerous gram-negative organisms may be isolated.[115] Paronychias in children are often caused by anaerobes, and it is believed that this is the result of finger sucking and nail biting. Occasionally, a group A β-hemolytic infection will develop in a paronychia in a child with a streptococcal pharyngitis who engages in thumb sucking.[116,117]

A paronychia appears as a swelling and tenderness of the soft tissue along the base or the side of a fingernail (Fig. 37–29). Pain, often around a hangnail, usually prompts a visit to the ED. The infection begins as a cellulitis and may form a frank abscess. If the nailbed is mobile, the infectious process has extended under the nail, and a more extensive drainage procedure should be performed. Although no comparative trials of surgical management versus oral antibiotics have been performed,[118] some general guidelines for management of paronychia have become established in clinical practice. If soft tissue swelling is present without fluctuance, remission may be obtained from frequent hot soaks (six to eight times a day) and a short course of oral antibiotics (3–4 days).[115] Incision will be of no value at this early cellulitic phase. Antibiotic treatment for localized infection is summarized in Table 37–5. If significant cellulitis is present, a broad-spectrum antistaphylococcal antibiotic (cephalosporin or semisynthetic penicillin) may be tried. The digit should be splinted and elevated.[117–119] One should never rely solely on antibiotic therapy once frank pus has formed.

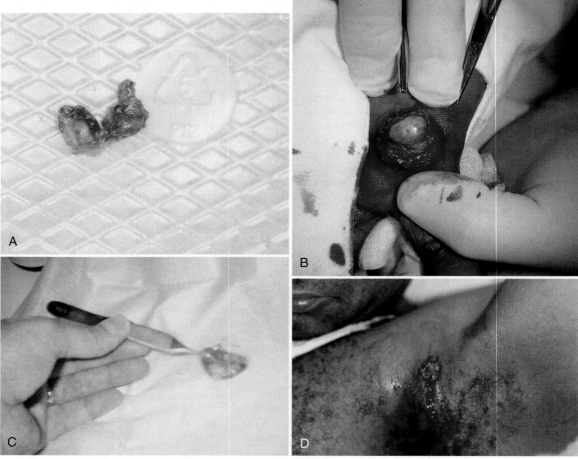

Figure 37–27 *A,* The thick, cheesy sebaceous material of a sebaceous cyst must be expressed after incision. The shiny capsule of this infected sebaceous cyst is unpunctured and easily visible (*B*) and was removed in its entirety on the initial visit (*C*). Capsule removal may be easier on a follow-up visit when inflammation has subsided. *D,* Capsule spontaneously expelled during first packing change.

TABLE 37–5 Common Hand Infections, Usual Offending Organisms, and Appropriate Therapeutic Regimens

Condition	Most Common Offending Organisms	Recommended Antimicrobial Agents	Comments
Paronychia	Usually *Staphylococcus aureus* or streptococci; *Pseudomonas,* gram-negative bacilli, and anaerobes may be present, especially in patients with exposure to oral flora.	First-generation cephalosporin or antistaphylococcal penicillin; if anaerobes or *Escherichia coli* is suspected, oral clindamycin (Cleocin) or a β-lactamase inhibitor such as amoxicillin-clavulanate potassium (Augmentin).	Incision and drainage should be performed if infection is well established. If infection is chronic, suspect *Candida albicans.* Early infections without cellulitis may respond to conservative therapy.
Felon	*S. aureus,* streptococci	First-generation cephalosporin or antistaphylococcal penicillin.	Incision and drainage should be performed if infection is well established. Oral antibiotic therapy usually is adequate.
Herpetic whitlow	Herpes simplex virus.	Supportive therapy.	Antivirals may be prescribed if infection has been present for <48 hr. For recurrent herpetic whitlow, suppressive therapy with an antiviral agent may be helpful. Consider antibiotics if secondarily infected. Incision and drainage are contraindicated.

Adapted from Clark DC: Common acute hand infections. Am Fam Physician 68:167, 2003.

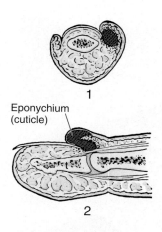

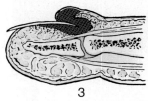

Eponychium
(cuticle)

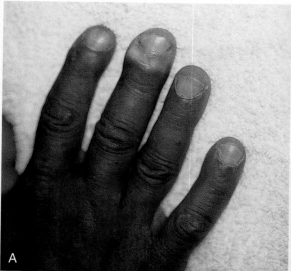

Figure 37–28 Paronychia. *1,* The site of the abscess at the side of the nail. *2,* The infection has extended around the base of the nail. It has raised the eponychium but has not penetrated under the nail. *3,* End stage of paronychia, with a subeponychial and subungual abscess. *(From Wolcott MW [ed]. Ferguson's Surgery of the Ambulatory Patient, 5th ed. Philadelphia, JB Lippincott, 1974. Reproduced with permission.)*

When a definite abscess has formed, drainage is usually quickly curative. A number of invasive operative approaches have been suggested. Actual skin incision or removal of the nail is rarely required, and neither procedure should be the initial form of treatment. One can invariably obtain adequate drainage by simply lifting the skin edge off the nail to allow the pus to drain. This is usually curative because a paronychia is not a cutaneous abscess per se, but rather a collection of pus in the potential space between the cuticle and the proximal fingernail. Drainage may be accomplished without anesthesia in select patients[120] but frequently requires a digital nerve block. After softening the eponychium by soaking, advance a No. 11 blade, scissors, or a 21- to 23-gauge needle parallel to the nail and under the eponychium at the site of maximal swelling (Fig. 37–30).[118,119,121] Pus rapidly escapes, with immediate relief of pain. A tourniquet placed at the base of the finger may limit bleeding and aid the clinician in determining the exact extent of the infection during the drainage procedure.

If more than a tiny pocket of pus is present, fan the knife tip or needle or spread the scissors under the eponychium, keeping the instrument parallel to the plane of the fingernail. When a large amount of pus is drained, a small piece of packing gauze is slipped under the eponychium for 24 hours to provide continual drainage. Cultures are generally not indicated. Antibiotics are frequently prescribed, although they are not essential if drainage is complete or if the surrounding area of cellulitis is minimal. An alternative to systemic antibiotics is to keep the operative site bathed in antibiotic ointment.

683

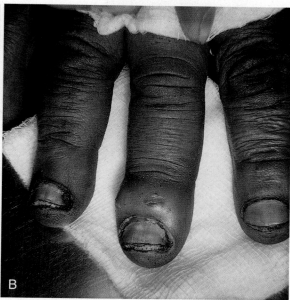

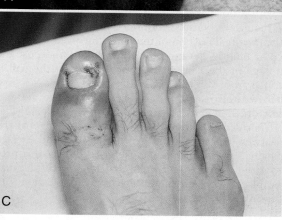

Figure 37–29 A paronychia may occur with obvious pus localization between the eponychium (cuticle) and the nail. Actual pus may be seen under the skin (*A*) or the area is swollen and tender (*B*). A paronychia can also occur in the toe (*C*). This is not a true cutaneous abscess but rather a collection of pus in a potential space. Actual skin incision is not required if eponychial elevation results in adequate drainage.

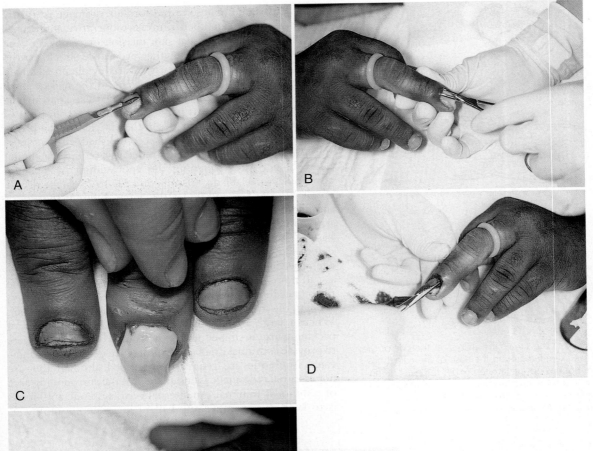

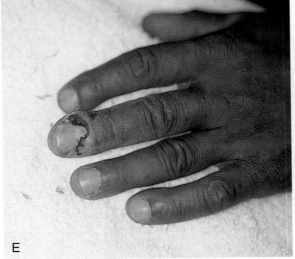

Figure 37–30 An initial treatment method for a well-localized paronychia. After a digital nerve block, the eponychium (cuticle) is elevated at the area of greatest fluctuance, and no actual skin incision is made. A tourniquet can be used to limit bleeding and facilitate drainage. *A,* A sharp instrument (an 18-gauge needle, scissors or a No. 11 blade) is held parallel to the nail and advanced until pus is drained. *B,* A hemostat or scissors is placed into the base and all margins of the pus collection and spread in a fanlike fashion to open the abscess. *C* and *D,* The entire pocket is opened to break up loculations and create a cavity. *E,* A small packing is placed for 2 days. At recheck, a new pack may be placed or the cavity left open to heal. Note that some skin may slough. Actual incision of tissue or removal of the nail is reserved for complicated or resistant infections and is not first-line therapy. Post drainage antibiotics are of no proven value, but practice varies.

After anesthesia has worn off, the patient may be started on frequent soaks in warm tap water at home. In most cases, the patient may easily remove the packing. At 24 to 36 hours, the finger is soaked in hot water and the gauze pulled out; a repeat visit to a clinician is not required if healing is progressing. Once the packing is removed, the area is covered with a dry, absorbent dressing. An antibiotic ointment may be applied to the site for a few days. The benefit of antibiotic ointments in reducing infection is unproved, but instructing the patient concerning the detailed use of the ointment may prompt soaking. In addition, the ointment helps keep the bandage from sticking.

If the infection has produced purulence beneath the nail (subungual abscess), a portion of the nail must be removed or the nail trephined to ensure complete drainage. As an alternative to nail removal, a hole may be placed in the proximal nail with a hot paper clip. A large opening or multiple holes are required to ensure continued drainage. Most commonly, the proximal portion of the nail is involved. This may be treated by bluntly elevating the eponychium to expose the proximal edge of the nail. The proximal third of the nail is then elevated from the nailbed and resected with a scissors. The distal two thirds of the nail is left in place to act as a physiologic dressing and to decrease postoperative pain (Fig. 37–31). If purulence is found below the lateral edge of the nail, the affected part may be gently elevated and excised longitudinally.[120,122] Care must be exercised during this procedure to avoid damage to the nail matrix. A wick of gauze should be placed beneath the eponychium for 48 hours to ensure continued drainage.

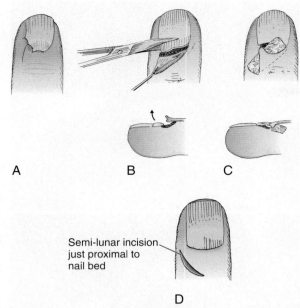

Semi-lunar incision just proximal to nail bed

Figure 37–31 *A–C,* Aggressive treatment of recurrent paronychia or subungual abscess includes removal of a portion of the proximal nail and incision of the eponychium. *D,* Some physicians prefer to use a semilunar incision proximal to the eponychium rather than directly incising and potentially injuring the cuticle permanently. These aggressive therapies are seldom required and are not first line interventions.

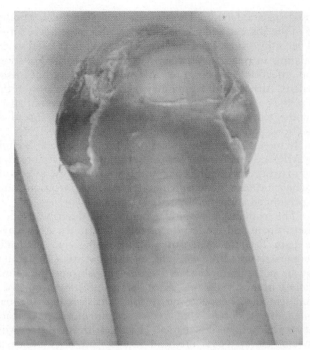

Figure 37–32 A well-developed felon. In this advanced case, the patient had little pain at the time of presentation. The distal phalanx was almost completely resorbed, owing to pressure and inflammation and chronic osteomylitis. This infection is extensive and warrants consultation with a hand specialist.

Most paronychia resolve in a few days, and one to two postoperative visits should be scheduled to evaluate healing and reinforce home care. For compliant patients with a small paronychia, home care alone may suffice after the initial drainage. Clinical infection lasting longer than a few weeks should prompt evaluation for osteomyelitis of the distal phalanx, a well-known but rare complication of even a properly drained paronychia.

Patients occasionally present to the ED complaining of a chronic, indolent paronychial infection. These seldom respond to ED intervention. Frank purulence is seldom present, and conservative treatments are often unsatisfactory. Many causes of this frustrating condition have been described, including fungal, bacterial, viral, and psoriatic conditions. Patients with chronic paronychia unresponsive to therapy should be screened for malignancy.[123] Treatment modalities are varied, and controlled studies evaluating the various techniques are lacking. Meticulous hand care, oral and topical antimicrobial medications, and occasionally aggressive surgical intervention have been suggested.[119,124] These patients should be referred to a dermatologist or hand surgeon because of the prolonged treatment required.

Herpetic Whitlow

Herpetic whitlow is an extremely contagious infection of the distal phalanx caused by the herpes simplex virus (type 1 or 2). Inoculation occurs through a discontinuity in the skin.[122] Health care providers exposed to oral secretions (e.g., dental hygienists and respiratory therapists) and patients with other herpes infections are most commonly infected.[124–129] After a 2-day to 2-week incubation period, the infected individual may experience prodromal signs and symptoms such as fever, malaise, lymphadenitis, and axillary lymphadenopathy. In the affected finger, the infection is characterized by tenderness

followed by throbbing pain (out of proportion to physical findings), edema, and erythema. Vesicles containing clear, bloody, or cloudy fluid then form, marking the most infectious stage of the process. These lesions are typically quite painful but are self-limited and resolve in 2 to 3 weeks. Incision and drainage of a herpetic whitlow is contraindicated because it may induce a secondary bacterial infection and delay healing.[130–133] Treatment is symptomatic, consisting of splinting, elevation, and analgesia as needed. Antiviral agents effective against herpes infections (acyclovir, famciclovir, or valacyclovir) can shorten the course of the disease if given early (see Table 37–4). After accidental needle stick in health care workers, oral famciclovir may be used as a preventative.[134] Infection recurs in 30% to 50% of cases, but the initial infection is usually the most severe.

Consideration must be given to preventing spread of the infection. An occlusive dressing decreases the chance of viral transmission, but health care providers with herpetic whitlow should limit, and perhaps even refrain from, patient contact, especially until all lesions have crusted over and viral shedding has stopped.[126–128] Compliance with universal precautions will decrease the likelihood of patient-to-provider transmission.

Felon

A felon is an infection of the pulp of the distal finger (Fig. 37–32). The usual cause is trauma with secondary invasion by bacteria. A felon may develop in the presence of a foreign body, such as a thorn or a splinter, but often a precipitating trauma cannot be identified. An important anatomic characteristic of this area is that many fibrous septa extend from the volar skin of the fat pad to the periosteum of the phalanx; these subdivide and compartmentalize the pulp area. When an infection occurs in the pulp, these structures make it a closed-space infection. The septa limit swelling, delay pointing of the abscess, and inhibit drainage after incomplete surgical decompression. Pressure may increase in the closed space, initiating an ischemic process that compounds the infection. The infection can progress to osteomyelitis of the distal phalanx. Although the septa may facilitate an infection in the pulp, they also provide a barrier that protects the joint space and the tendon sheath by limiting the proximal spread of infection.

In most cases, the offending organism is *S. aureus*, including MRSA;[135] mixed infections and gram-negative infection also may occur. A felon is one of the few soft tissue infections in which a culture may be helpful, because the infection could be prolonged and osteomyelitis is a concern.

The patient developing a felon will describe gradual onset of pain and tenderness of the fingertip. In a few days, the pain becomes constant and throbbing and gradually becomes severe. In the initial stages, physical examination may be quite unimpressive, because the fibrous septa limit swelling in the closed pulp space. As the infection progresses, swelling and redness become obvious. Occasionally, one may elicit point tenderness, but frequently, the entire pulp space is extremely tender. The patient characteristically arrives with the hand elevated over the head because pain is so intense in the dependent position. Cessation of pain indicates necrosis and nerve degeneration.

During the early stages of cellulitis, a felon may be controlled by treatment consisting of elevation, oral antibiotics (see Table 37–4), and warm water or saline soaks. For more developed felons, proper treatment consists of early and complete incision and drainage.[122] Antibiotics alone are not curative once suppuration has occurred. Delaying surgery may result in permanent disability and deformity. Most surgeons routinely administer broad-spectrum antibiotics to patients for 5 to 7 days after surgical incision. MRSA infections can be treated with vanocmycin, 1 g twice a day, or linezolid, and may require weeks until resolution.[135] Oral linezolid may allow outpatient treatment.

A minor felon usually can be drained on an outpatient basis using a digital nerve block (Fig. 37–33). A long-acting anesthetic (bupivacaine) will prolong anesthesia. A tourniquet (1.25 cm Penrose drain) should be used to allow incision into a bloodless field.

Surgical drainage must be performed carefully to avoid injury to nerves, vessels, and flexor tendons. Most felons can be managed with a limited procedure, but many surgical options have been advocated, none of which has been proven superior for all circumstances.[122] Traditional incisions ("hockey stick" or "fish mouth") have a propensity for complications such as sloughing of tissue and postoperative fat pad anesthesia or instability and are rarely used. The preferred initial treatment is a simple longitudinal incision over the area of greatest fluctuance,[136,137] which may occur laterally or along the volar surface (Fig. 37–34). Frank pus may be encountered during incision, but usually only a few drops are expressed. One more often drains a combination of necrotic tissue and interstitial fluid. A foreign body should be sought even if the history is not known. A potential drawback to an incision in the middle of the fat pad is the production of a scar in a very sensitive and commonly traumatized area. The incision must not extend to the distal interphalangeal crease because of the danger of injuring the flexor tendon. The subcutaneous tissue is bluntly dissected using a hemostat to provide adequate drainage. A gauze pack may be placed in the wound for 24 to

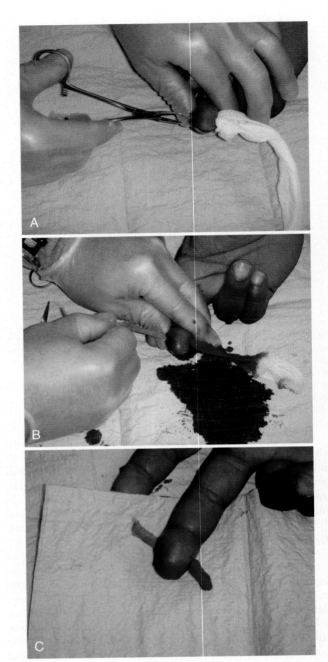

Figure 37–33 Drainage of a felon. Gauze is grasped by the hemostat (*A*) and pulled through the incision (*B*). *C*, The edges are trimmed. Repeat packing usually requires a digital block anesthesia. Post drainage antibiotics are usually given.

48 hours to ensure continued drainage. Recurrent or more severe infections may require a more aggressive approach by a hand specialist.

No matter which incision is made, it must not be carried proximal to the closed pulp space because of the danger of entrance into the tendon sheath or the joint capsule. The patient should be rechecked in 2 to 3 days. A snug dressing, splinting and elevation, and adequate opioid analgesics are prerequisites for a successful outcome.

On the first postoperative visit, a digital block may again be induced and any packing removed. The incision is irrigated copiously with saline, and any additional necrotic tissue is removed. At this time, the drain may be replaced for 24 to 48 hours if there is continued drainage, but usually it can be

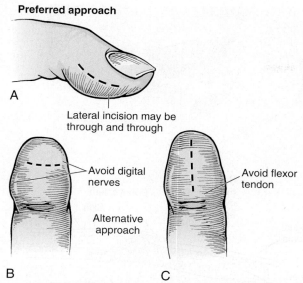

Preferred approach

A

Lateral incision may be through and through

Avoid digital nerves

Alternative approach

B

Avoid flexor tendon

C

Figure 37–34 The preferred initial incision for draining a felon is made directly into the area of most fluctuance. More aggressive incisions should be reserved for complicated cases, because they have a greater morbidity and require more complicated wound care. *A*, The unilateral longitudinal approach is a good first choice. Some prefer a similarly located through and through incision (see Fig. 37–33). Fat pad incisions are acceptable but may be associated with a painful scar in an area that is often traumatized. The transverse fat pad incision should not injure digital nerves (*B*), and the longitudinal fat pad incision should avoid the flexor tendon (*C*).

removed and a dressing reapplied. Soaking may be advised. At the first revisit, the sensitivities of the bacterial cultures are checked, and a decision to continue or change antibiotics is made. Most felons are treated empirically with antibiotics for at least 5 days. A broad-spectrum cephalosporin is a reasonable choice, pending cultures (if done). Antibiotics against MRSA should also be considered.

Some clinicians advocate radiographic evaluation for retained foreign bodies at the initial visit as well as a baseline evaluation of the bone for subsequent evaluation of osteomyelitis. Other clinicians reserve radiographs for wounds not showing significant improvement in 5 to 7 days. Evidence of osteomyelitis, however, may not be found radiographically for several weeks after the appearance of the lesion. Persistent infections require more radical incision and drainage and may require IV antibiotics. After adequate drainage, osteomyelitis may respond surprisingly well to outpatient antibiotic therapy, achieving almost complete regeneration of bone if incision and drainage have been adequate.

Fingertip infections can be stubborn. Difficult or persistent cases require evaluation and care by a hand surgeon. In these cases, early consultation is advisable to avert catastrophic complications such as loss of function or amputation.

SEROMA AND HEMATOMA DRAINAGE

Although most incision and drainage procedures are performed for decompression of purulent collections, drainage of sterile hematomas or seromas may be required in the ED. In general, the same principles used for formal drainage of pus in the soft tissues apply to drainage of a sterile fluid collection, and hence, one can directly apply the principles of this chapter to the drainage of sterile fluids. In addition, when

a sterile fluid collection is drained, the operator has the option of primarily closing the incision site after wound irrigation (see Chapters 34, Principles of Wound Management, and 35, Methods of Wound Closure, for wound management techniques). Drainage of a soft tissue hematoma is generally best postponed several days after an initial injury to permit hemostasis and to minimize the risk of hematoma reaccumulation after drainage. The procedure is generally reserved for those soft tissue hematomas that are large and painful (secondary to tissue distention) and are expected to either resolve slowly or result in soft tissue deformity if not drained. Seromas and hematomas rarely become infected if the overlying skin remains intact. It is best to avoid needle aspiration because this procedure rarely drains the collection completely, and it has the potential to introduce infection into a good culture medium in a closed space. If a hematoma becomes infected, it should be treated as a cutaneous abscess.

Although it is tempting to drain a small seemingly fluctuant noninfected hematoma that has persisted for many days, a conservative nonoperative approach is usually best. A persistent mass after trauma usually causes concern in patients, so a thorough explanation should be provided. Most hematomas will resolve, albeit slowly (weeks), and incision often is disappointing in its yield (unless the hematoma is large and superficial) and leaves a scar. Drainage of a subungual hematoma represents a special case of hematoma drainage.

Subungual Hematoma

Subungual hematomas are typically caused by hitting a fingertip with a hammer, slamming a finger in a door (Fig. 37–35), or dropping a weight on a foot. The patient's main concern is getting relief from the terrible throbbing pain that increases with the pressure under the nail.

When describing the injury, the clinician should estimate the percentage of nailbed covered by the hematoma and discuss associated trauma to the nail margins or surrounding tissue. The examination should include tests of the extensor and flexor tendons, of circulation by capillary refill, and of the sensitivity of the area.[138]

If fracture of the distal phalanx is suspected (if the fingertip is unstable or the mechanism of injury suggests fracture), anteroposterior and lateral x-ray films should be obtained. Radiographs differentiate tendinous from bony mallet-type injuries. Crush injuries are associated with three types of distal phalanx fractures: longitudinal, transverse, and comminuted. If the fracture is angulated or displaced, unstable or intra-articular, or involves a third or more of the articular surface, the patient should be referred to a hand surgeon.[138] Because trephination in patients with a distal phalanx fracture converts a closed fracture into an open one, there is concern about infectious and cosmetic complications. In the two studies that examined this possible association,[139,140] with fracture subsets totaling 26, no infections occurred. *The presence of an underlying fracture does not contraindicate nail trephination for fear of changing a closed fracture into an open one.*

Nail removal is unnecessary as long as the nail margins and nail are intact.[140] If the nailbed is significantly lacerated or the edges of the nail are unstable, the nail should be removed and the nailbed repaired (see further discussion in Chapter 35, Methods of Wound Closure). *Simple trephination of an uncomplicated subungal hematoma, even if it involves the entire subungal area, gives a good result, functionally and cosmetically.*[141] Trephination should be considered if the hematoma

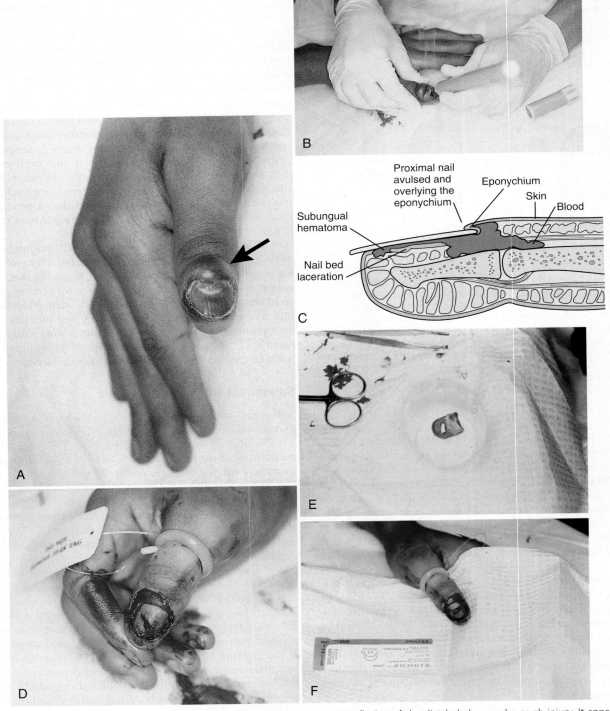

Figure 37–35 *A,* This patient slammed his finger in a car door, sustaining an acute flexion of the distal phalynx and a crush injury. It appears to be a simple subungual hematoma, but note the blood in the paronychial space (*arrow*). There is a communication between the nailbed laceration and the eponychium. *B,* All of the blood did not drain when the nail was trephinated. *C,* Blood accumulated in this area because the base of the fingernail has been avulsed from its origin and now lies between the eponychium (cuticle) and the skin. This is appreciated when the skin is débrided. Note the white avulsed base of the fingernail just under the skin. The closed nature of the injury causes the confusion. With the nail removed, the nail bed laceration can be seen and repaired. *D,* The old trephined nail can now be replaced in its original position to keep the eponychial space open, or that space can be packed with gauze for a few weeks to discourage scar formation and subsequent nail deformity. To keep open the eponychial space and protect the nail bed, the original avulsed nail (*E*) is placed under the cuticle and (*F*) sutured in place for 2 weeks. A new nail will push out the old one in 2 to 3 weeks and the old nail is discarded. Note drainage hole in original nail.

covers more than half the intact nail, or if smaller and painful.

Prophylactic antibiotics are not necessary for patients with uncomplicated subungual hematoma that have been trephinated. For more serious injuries, a slight risk of infection exists, but in most cases, rigorous wound cleaning and careful soft tissue repair constitute adequate treatment.[142,143]

Methods of Trephination

All methods of trephination require aseptic technique. The nail should be cleaned thoroughly and the digit placed in a sterile field. Universal precautions should be followed because the fluid under the nail is under pressure and can spurt.[138] The practitioner must ensure that adequate analgesia has been administered; anesthesia is not always required but a digital block can be used to calm an anxious patient and is commonly performed.

Hot cautery is the most common form of trephination, usually done with a paper clip that has been straightened and heated in a flame. The hot end is placed on the nail above the center of the hematoma and gentle pressure is applied until the nail is breached and the hematoma expressed. A "give" is felt as the instrument passes through the nail. The pressure should be stopped at this point to avoid damage to the nail bed. Blood rapidly exits, and the blackened nail regains its normal color (Fig. 37–36). The blood usually remains fluid for 24 to 36 hours and is easily expressed with slight pressure. Multiple holes may be needed for continued drainage. Hot

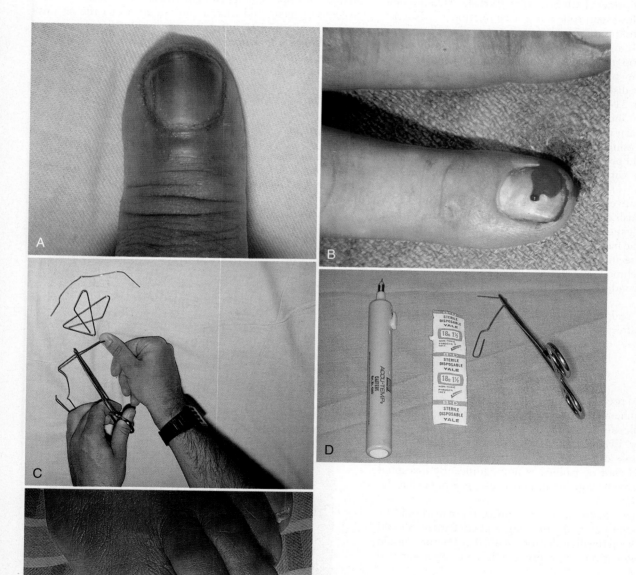

Figure 37–36 *A,* Subungual hematoma with a totally blackened nailbed. Do not remove this intact nail even though the nail bed is lacerated or there is a total hematoma and underlying minor tuft fracture. In this example, the blood accumulated only under the nail, not in any paronychial areas. *B,* After trephination, blood flows freely from the puncture site and the blackness totally disappears. *C* and *D,* An adequately sized drainage hole may be placed in the nail with a heated paper clip or 18-gauge needle. The hole should be large enough to allow continued drainage of blood. A small piece of the nail can be removed by cautery. Small holes tend to clog and inhibit drainage. *E,* Inadequate drainage of a subungual hematoma with a hole that is too small.

cautery trephination should not be used on artificial nails because they are flammable.[144]

Hot cautery with a paper clip is easy to perform, but hematomas treated in this way tend to reform. A cold lancet has the benefits of reducing pain immediately as well as reducing the likelihood of infection.[145]

A portable hot-wire electrocautery unit can be used, but it is difficult to obtain an adequate drainage hole without adapting the instrument. It can be modified to burn a larger hole by "fattening" the end of the wire loop and rotating the device slowly as the nail is penetrated or by removing a small rectangle of nail. In addition to being convenient, the cautery device is desirable because the wire stays hotter longer, enhancing nail penetration.

The PathFormer (Path Scientific, Carlisle, MA) is a new device that allows controlled nail trephination ("mesoscission") and therefore minimizes patient discomfort during the procedure.[146] It uses electrical resistance in the nailbed as feedback to stop and retract the drill when it penetrates the nail plate. The nailbed, with its blood supply and nerve endings, is not disturbed.

An 18- or 21-gauge needle can be rotated between the thumb and the index finger while gentle pressure is applied so that the sharp end of the needle corkscrews through the nail.[147] When using a needle, the give is harder to feel, so the clinician should proceed slowly until blood is drawn. Because the hole made with a needle is small, a second hole may be required.

An alternative needle-based approach is being used by a group of Turkish dermatologists. Kaya and associates[148] used extra-fine, 29-gauge insulin syringes for evacuation of hematomas. After the nail is trimmed, the needle is inserted parallel to the nail plate and advanced to the distal edge of the hematoma. This technique is especially effective for small hematomas of the second, third, and fourth toenails, which are hard to trephine.

A No. 11 scalpel blade can be used to score and then cut through the affected nail. This approach is painful for the patient because the hole is usually larger than what is required.

Outcome

It is difficult to predict the fate of the fingernail after drainage of a subungual hematoma. Obviously, there must be a nail bed laceration if bleeding occurs, but with a stable nail bed, repair is unnecessary. Even if there is a small tuft fracture, most do well with simple drainage. Some patients will lose the nail, but if the nail root or nailbed is not significantly disrupted and the nail remains implanted, a normal-appearing nail is the usual final result.

After a hematoma has been drained, the nail should be cleaned thoroughly and a dry dressing applied. Patients should be advised to keep the digit dry for 2 days. Any fracture should be splinted and given appropriate follow-up at a surgical clinic.

Conditions with Similar Appearance

One condition that may be mistaken for a simple subungual hematoma is the closed avulsion of the base of the fingernail that occurs in conjunction with a subungual hematoma from a nailbed laceration. A common mechanism is slamming a finger in a car door, with sudden flexion of the distal phalynx in conjunction with a crush injury of the nailbed. The nail itself is usually stable, so generally no repair of the nailbed

appears to be required. However, if the subungual hematoma extends past the confines of the nailbed, such as in the paronychial space (under the skin of the cuticle), there must be a communication between the nailbed and this space. This produces a paronychial hematoma, in which blood occupies the space where pus would be in an infectious paronychia (see Fig. 37–35). When this condition is present, the avulsed proximal portion of the fingernail overlies the nail fold of the cuticle, but is appreciated only after the overlying skin is opened. An open reduction (replacement) of the nail must be performed. The replaced nail often grows normally, but a lost or deformed nail is possible. Repair of the nailbed laceration is optional at this juncture but may not be required if the nail is stable. Once the injury is anatomically aligned, splinting and soaking follow that for a simple subungual hematoma. These injuries rarely become infected, and there is no evidence that the prophylactic use of antibiotics is necessary.

Subungual hematomas can be manifestations of diseases such as Kaposi sarcoma and melanoma. These conditions should be considered when no trauma has occurred and when physical examination findings are not consistent with a simple subungual hematoma.

MUCOCOEL

Sometimes mistaken for infection, a mucocoel of the mucous membranes of the mouth is a nontender pearl-colored small lump that is felt by the patient's tongue. It is a plugged saliva

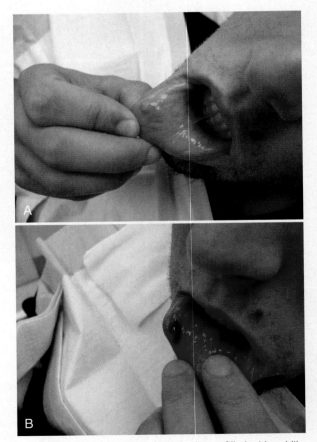

Figure 37–37 A mucocoel is a nontender lump, filled with gel-like substance, that often appears on the mucosa of the lip. Lidocaine with epinephrine is injected locally. *A,* The entire structure is excised. *B,* The operative site is left open and heals rapidly. Simple aspiration of the mucocoel usually is not curative.

gland, and it becomes evident when it fills up with gel-like substance. Occasionally, the patient will squeeze it to express the gel, but it may return unless excised. Under local anesthesia, the entire mass is removed by sharp dissection with a scalpel. The ulcer is left open and will heal quickly (Fig. 37–37).

Acknowledgments

The author acknowledges the significant contributions of Todd M. Warden, Mark W. Fourre, and Howard Blumstein to this chapter in previous editions. He thanks Linda J. Kesselring, MS, ELS, technical editor/writer in the Department of Emergency Medicine at the University of Maryland School of Medicine, for copyediting the manuscript.

 REFERENCES CAN BE FOUND ON EXPERT CONSULT

CHAPTER **38**

Burn Care Procedures

Courtney A. Bethel and Anthony S. Mazzeo

Each year in the United States, some 2 million people suffer a burn-related injury. Typical victims are children younger than 5 years of age or young adults who are exposed to fire or hot or corrosive substances.[1] Fortunately, 95% of these burns are classified as minor and are amenable to outpatient management, with most patients completing their treatment course within 2 weeks.

The classification of burns is based on three criteria:[2] depth of skin injury, percentage of body surface area involved, and source of injury (thermal, chemical, electrical, or radiation). The seriousness of a burn injury is determined by the characteristics and temperature of the burning agent, the duration of exposure, the location of injury, the presence of associated injuries, and the age and general health of the victim (Table 38–1).

The American Burn Association defines minor burns as uncomplicated partial-thickness burns of less than 5% of the total body surface area (TBSA) in children (<10 yr old) or the elderly (>50 yr old) or less than 10% TBSA in adults, or full-thickness burns less than 2% TBSA.[3] Moderate or major burns include injuries that involve a greater TBSA, as well as burns to areas of specialized function, such as the face, hands, feet, or perineum. More serious burns also include those due to a high-voltage electrical injury or those with associated inhalation injuries or other major trauma.

The TBSA burned may be estimated in a number of ways. It is more common to overestimate the size of a burn than to underestimate it. In adults, the "rule of nines" is a useful rule of thumb, but the formula is only a guide and must be modified for children who have proportionately larger heads and smaller legs (Fig. 38–1). The Lund and Browder charts are another (more precise) guide to estimating the percentage of TBSA burned (Fig. 38–2). For smaller or multiple burns, one can rapidly estimate the TBSA burned by using the area of the patient's palm as approximately 1.25% TBSA.

Throughout the course of history, clinicians have experimented with burn therapies to relieve pain and promote healing. Many treatment regimens and useless home remedies have been successful, largely owing to the fact that minor burns generally do well with a modicum of intervention and common sense wound care. Although little has changed in the care of minor ambulatory burns over the past 20 years, the treatment of major burns, the development of sophisticated burn centers, increased knowledge of burn wound physiology, and the prevention of infection have significantly altered the care of seriously burned patients.

WOUND EVALUATION

Emergency clinicians should be aware that the depth of a burn wound cannot always be determined accurately on clinical grounds alone at the time of presentation and that burn injury is a dynamic process that may change over time, particularly during the 24 to 48 hours after the burning process has been arrested. It is common, for example, for a seemingly minor or superficial burn to appear deeper on the second or third return visit (Fig. 38–3). This phenomenon is not a continuation of the burning process but is considered to be a pathophysiologic event related to tissue edema, dermal ischemia, or desiccation.[4]

First-degree burns involve the epidermis only. The skin is reddened but is intact and not blistered. This injury ranges from mildly irritating or even pruritic to exquisitely painful. Minor edema may be noted. Causes include ultraviolet light (as in sunburn) and brief thermal "flash" burns. First-degree burns frequently blister within 24 to 36 hours, so the patient should be instructed appropriately. Often, the skin begins to flake or peel within 5 to 10 days, but healing eventually occurs with no scarring.

Second-degree burns involve the entire epidermis and extend into the dermis to include sweat glands and hair follicles. *Superficial partial-thickness burns* involve only the papillary dermis. These burns are pink, moist, and extremely painful. Blisters may be present or the skin may slough. The burn blanches with pressure, and mild to moderate edema is common. Hair follicles are often noted to be intact. This is the most common depth of minor burn seen in the emergency department (ED). The usual causes are scalds, contact with hot objects, or exposure to chemicals. Barring infection or repeated trauma, these burns heal completely without scarring in about 2 weeks. Areas of first- and second-degree burns may be sensitive to subsequent sunburn, windburn, and skin irritation for months after the original injury appears healed.

Deep partial-thickness burns extend into the reticular dermis and appear as mottled white or pink. There is obvious edema and sloughing of the skin, and any blisters are usually ruptured. Blanching is absent. These burns are generally not painful initially, but pressure can be perceived. Within a few days, however, these burns can become exquisitely painful. This type of burn can easily be converted to a full-thickness injury by further trauma or infection. Partial-thickness burns heal by reepithelialization from dermal appendages, including hair follicles, sebaceous glands, and sweat glands.

In *full-thickness burns*, coagulation necrosis extends into the subcutaneous (SQ) tissues. These burns may appear in a variety of colors but are usually dry, pearly white, or charred. They are initially painless, with a leathery texture. Marked edema and decreased elasticity may necessitate escharotomy when circulation is compromised. Exposure of the skin to temperatures in excess of 77°C for more than 3 to 4 seconds generally causes a full-thickness injury. Although initially painless, in a few days these deep burns can become painful. Chemical burns often produce full-thickness injuries affecting a small or scattered surface area. Flame burns produce full-thickness injuries in less than 2 seconds if the temperature of the flame exceeds 500°C. Generally, any burn wound that is not reepithelialized or does not possess dense epidermal budding by 14 days after the burn should be considered a full-thickness injury.[4]

Fourth-degree burns extend deeply into SQ tissue, muscle, fascia, or bone. These burns are characteristically caused by contact with molten metal, flame, or high-voltage electricity.

TABLE 38–1 Characteristics of Burns, by Depth

Classification of Burn	Etiology	Appearance	Sensation	Time to Complete Healing	Scarring
First Degree					
• Superficial epidermal layers	• Sunburn, other UV exposure • Short flash flame burns	• Dry, red • Blanches with pressure	• Present • May be quite painful	• 3–7 days	• No
Second Degree					
• Varying depth, blisters, or bullae formation • Dermal appendages spared (e.g., sweat glands, hair follicles) • Includes entire epidermis and some portion of the dermis					
Superficial partial thickness	• Water scald • Longer flash burn	• Blisters, peeling skin • Blanches with pressure • Skin red/moist under blisters	• Painful • Exposure to air and temperature is painful	• 7–21 days	• Unusual if no infection and proper follow-up • Pigment change may be seen • Burned area may be sensitive to frostbite, windburn, sunburn for many months • Itching may be problematic for weeks after healing
Deep partial thickness	• Flame • Water immersion • Oil, grease, hot foods (e.g., soup)	• Variable color • Wet or waxy dry, does not blanch • Blisters easily removed, skin peeling off	• Pressure only	• >21 days	• Severe; risk of contracture
Third Degree					
• Loss of all skin elements; thrombosis and coagulation of vessels	• Flame, steam, oil grease • Immersion, scald • Caustic chemical, high voltage	• Leathery appearance, white or charred dry, inelastic; blanching with pressure • May be present under blisters	• Deep pressure only	• Never heals • Requires grafting	• Very severe, high risk of contracture

UV, ultraviolet.
Modified after Clayton and Solem, Postgrad Med 97:151, 1995; and Morgan et al, Am Fam Physician 62:2015, 2000.

HISTOPATHOLOGY OF BURNS

One thermal wound theory describes three zones of injury in burns:[5]
1. Zone of coagulation: dead, avascular tissue that must be débrided.
2. Zone of stasis: injured tissue in which blood flow is impaired. Desiccation, infection, or mechanical trauma may lead to cell death.
3. Zone of hyperemia: minimally injured, inflamed tissue that forms the border of the wound. The hyperemia usually resolves within 7 to 10 days but may be mistaken for cellulitis.

Histologically, full-thickness burns are characterized by confluent vascular thrombosis involving arterioles, venules, and capillaries. Edema due to loss of microvascular integrity results not only from the effects of direct thermal injury but also from the release of vasoactive mediators. The increase in vascular permeability is linked to complement activation and histamine release. Histamine increases the catalytic activity of the enzyme xanthine oxidase, with resultant production of hydrogen peroxide and hydroxyl radicals. These by-products increase the damage to dermal vascular endothelial cells and result in progressive vascular permeability.[6]

TABLE 38–2 American Burn Association's Grading System for Burn Severity and Disposition of Patients*

	Type of Burn		
	Minor	**Moderate**	**Major**
Criteria	<10% TBSA burn in adult <5% TBSA burn in young or old <2% full-thickness burn	10%–20% TBSA burn in adult 5%–10% TBSA burn in young or old 2%–5% full-thickness burn High-voltage injury Suspected inhalation injury Circumferential burn Concomitant medical problem predisposing patient to infection (e.g., diabetes, sickle cell disease)	>20% TBSA burn in adult >10% TBSA burn in young or old >5% full-thickness burn High-voltage burn Known inhalation injury Any significant burn to face, eyes, ears, hands, feet, genitalia, or joints Significant associated injuries (e.g., fracture, other major trauma)
Disposition	Outpatient management	Hospital admission	Referral to burn center

*Burn, partial-thickness or full-thickness burn, unless specified; young, patient < 10 yr of age; adult, patient 10–50 yr of age; old, patient > 50 yr of age.
TBSA, total body surface area (percentage) affected by the injury.
Adapted with permission from Hospital and prehospital resources for optimal care of patients with burn injury: Guidelines for development and operation of burn centers. American Burn Association. J Burn Care Rehabil 11:98, 1990; with additional information from Hartford CE: Care of outpatient burns. In Herndon DN (ed): Total Burn Care. Philadelphia, WB Saunders, 1996, p 71.

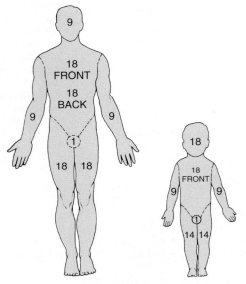

Figure 38–1 The "rule of nines" for estimating percentage of area burned. (As a rough guide, the area covered by the individual's palm is approximately 1.25% the total body surface area [TBSA].) The rule of nines is a rough estimate of the TBSA burned. Note that adults and children are different. This formula frequently overestimates the extent of a burn in clinical practice. See Fig. 38–2 for a more accurate method of determining the TBSA burned for children.

The cellular debris and denatured proteins of the eschar provide a substrate for the proliferation of microorganisms. The devitalized tissue (eschar) sloughs spontaneously, usually as a result of the proteolytic effect of bacterial enzymes. The greater the degree of wound bacteriostasis, the greater the delay in sloughing.

Partial-thickness burns result in incomplete vascular thrombosis, usually limited to the upper dermis. The dermal circulation is gradually restored, usually over several days, resulting in a significant interval of relative ischemia. The eschar in deep partial-thickness burns is thinner than in a full-thickness burn and sloughs as a result of reepithelialization rather than bacterial proteolysis.

OUTPATIENT VERSUS INPATIENT CARE

One of the first steps in minor burn care is to select patients for whom outpatient care is appropriate (Table 38–2). Generally, there are no "unnecessary" initial admissions for patients with burn injuries. Candidates for outpatient treatment are generally adults and children who meet the minor burn criteria detailed earlier. *Clinical judgment is always the most reasonable way to decide on where the burn patient would be best cared for, and there is considerable latitude in this decision.* Persons who have deep burns of the hands, face, feet, neck, or perineum; burns resulting from abuse or attempted suicide; burns involving other significant trauma or inhalation injuries; or electrical burns should generally be managed as inpatients.

Poor candidates for outpatient care of even minor burns include those who have concomitant medical problems such as diabetes mellitus, peripheral vascular disease, congestive heart failure, and end-stage renal disease; patients who are using steroids or other immunosuppressive agents; patients who are very young or very old; those who are mentally retarded; alcoholics; the homeless; those who are malnourished; and any individual with a suspect or unacceptable home support system. Inpatient treatment should be considered under these circumstances even though the burn might be considered "minor" by TBSA formulas. Pain control, the ability to obtain follow-up, the capacity to understand home care, and the overall social situation must influence the final decision.[7]

PROCEDURE

Initial Care of Major Burns

The care of major burns is not within the scope of this chapter. Such patients should be cared for in a formal burn unit. The initial resuscitation of a burn victim follows standard practices, with attention to airway, breathing, and cardiovascular support; and attention to carbon monoxide and cyanide poisoning, associated trauma, and fluid resuscirtation. Fluid resuscitation formulas are included for completeness (Box 38–1).

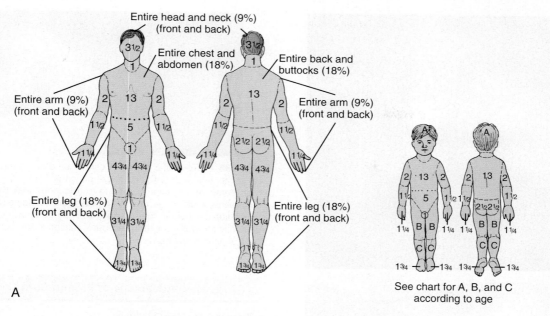

AGE	Birth–1 yr	1–4 yr	5–9 yr	10–14 yr	15 yr	Adult
Head	19	17	13	11	9	7
Neck	2					
Ant trunk	13					
Post trunk	13					
R buttock	2½					
L buttock	2½					
Genitalia	1					
R U arm	4					
L U arm	4					
R L arm	3					
L L arm	3					
R hand	2½	6½	8	8½	9	9½
L hand	2½	6½	8	8½	9	9½
R thigh	5½	5	5½	6	6½	7
L thigh	5½	5	5½	6	6½	7
R leg	5					
L leg	5					
R foot	3½					
L foot	3½					

B   BODY AREA

Figure 38–2 *A,* The Lund and Browder charts are somewhat more accurate than the rule of nines in estimating the TBSA burned. *B,* The proportion of TBSA of individual areas, according to age. Compared with adults, children have larger heads and smaller legs. Other areas are relatively equivalent throughout life. The rule of nines is not accurate in determining the percentage of TBSA burned in children.

BOX 38–1	**Emergency Department Burn Fluid Resuscitation**

FIRST 24 HOURS
Fluid of choice: lactated Ringer's

Adults
2 to 4 ml/kg/% BSA burned (excluding first-degree burns)
One half of fluid to be infused in the first 8 hours after the injury
One half of fluid to be infused over the next 16 hours

Pediatrics
4 ml/kg/% BSA burned (excluding first-degree burns)
One half of fluid to be infused in the first 8 hours after the injury
One-half of fluid to be infused over the next 16 hours
Add normal maintenance fluids to burn resuscitation fluid

The above calculations are only a guide. Adjust fluids to maintain urine output of 0.5 ml/kg/hr in adults and 1 ml/kg/hr in children.

Initial Care of the Minor Burn Victim

Prompt cooling of the burned part is an almost instinctive response and is one of the oldest recorded burn treatments, having been recommended by Galen (AD 129–199) and Rhazes (AD 852–923).[4] Room-temperature tap water irrigation, immersion, or compresses (20°C–25°C) are optimal in obtaining pain relief and providing some measure of protection for burned tissues without the problems of hypothermia that iced solutions can cause.[8,9] First aid telephone advice from the emergency clinician includes immediately immersing the wound in room-temperature or slighly cooled tap water. Whereas immediate cold water immersion may limit the extent of a burn if performed immediately and provide significant pain relief, packing the wound in ice must be avoided.

All involved clothing and jewelry (such as rings), along with any gross debris, should be removed from the burned area. Chemical burns to the skin or eyes require prolonged

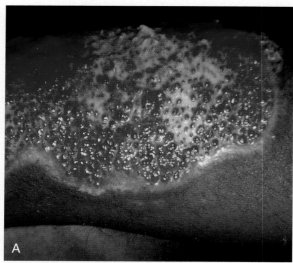

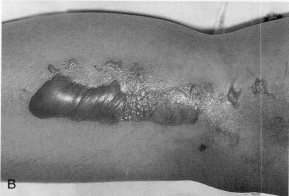

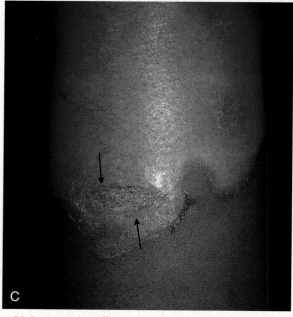

Figure 38–3 It may be difficult to accurately assess the depth or severity of a burn on the first visit. *A,* This is a full-thickness burn that will not heal without a skin graft. *B,* This blistered hot water burn is likely second degree, but full-thickness burns can develop under blisters. *C,* At 2 wk, a second-degree burn and small area of third-degree burn (*arrows*).

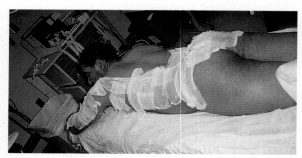

Figure 38–4 To cool a burn that cannot be easily immersed in water, cover the area with unfolded gauze pads that have been soaked in room-temperature saline. Continue to frequently soak the gauze with cool saline or tap water drawn up in a syringe. Adding a few ice chips to the liquid is helpful, but do not cover the burn with ice. Towels are generally too bulky for this procedure. Narcotics are the best way to control pain in any burn.

TABLE 38–3 Advantage of Prompt Burn Cooling

Reduction or cessation of pain
Elimination of local hyperthermia
Inhibition of postburn tissue destruction
Decreased edema
Reduced metabolism and toxin production

---

tap water irrigation. The burn should otherwise be covered with a moist, sterile dressing—nonmentholated shaving cream makes an excellent temporary covering for out-of-hospital use if a dressing is not available.[10] Common home remedies such as butter, grease, or petrolatum usually do not adversely influence subsequent care, but they are best avoided.[11]

In the ED and prehospital phase, appropriate analgesics, usually narcotics, are the best way to control pain and should not be forgotten in the initial phase of burn care. The burned area may be immediately immersed in room-temperature water or covered with gauze pads soaked in room-temperature water or saline (Fig. 38–4). The gauze may be kept cool and moist to provide continued pain relief; the patient will quickly let the clinician know when additional cooling is required. Many clinicians use sterile saline for cooling, but it has no proven benefit over tap water, even when the skin is broken. It is acceptable to add ice chips to water or saline to lower the temperature. However, immersion of burned tissue in ice or ice water should be avoided because ice immersion increases pain and risks frostbite injury or systemic hypothermia.

The potential benefits of burn cooling are listed in Table 38–3. It is unlikely that the clinician can favorably affect the burned tissue with any intervention in the ED, and many patients seek medical advice after initial cooling may have been helpful. With the exception of pain relief and removal of debris, the benefits of burn cooling are experienced only if the burn is cooled promptly, within the first 3 minutes after injury, making home care important.[12,13]

Minor burns are considered tetanus-prone, and tetanus toxoid should be administered if the patient is unsure of tetanus immunization status or when it has been more than 10 years since the last immunization. Nonimmunized patients should receive human tetanus immune globulin, 250 units intramuscularly, along with tetanus toxoid, and a booster injection of toxoid in about 3 weeks.

Definitive Care of the Minor Burn

Few areas in medicine are fraught with as much mysticism, personal bias, and unscientific dogma as the care of the minor burn wound. Many clinicians are rigidly committed to a specific ritual or approach merely because "it is the way it's done" in a specific institution or because the clinician has had success with a particular therapy in the past. In reality, the plethora of successful regimens attests to the fact that almost any non-injurious approach results in a favorable outcome. Many misconceptions probably arise because the issues associated with major thermal injury are often erroneously extrapolated to the minor burn wound. Most minor outpatient burns do very well, regardless of therapy, and it is difficult to do anything wrong if common sense is evoked.

Minor burns are not associated with immunosuppression, hypermetabolism, or increased susceptibility to infection.[14] Many complications seen in minor burn care result from overtreatment of the injury rather than undertreatment. Examples include too-vigorous dressing changes that may peel off newly formed skin and secondary infections or pseu-domembrane formation that results from topical or systemic antibiotic use.

Burn Dressings

Open Burn Care. Burns are cared for using two general methods: open or closed. In the open method, a burn wound dressing is not used. The area is left open to the air and is washed two or three times per day, followed by application of a topical agent. This is the preferred method for managing burns of the face and neck and is an excellent way to manage minor hand burns, because it allows continuous inspection and range of motion exercises. The open method is impractical in young active persons, in children, or in other individuals in whom wound contamination is likely. Although many burns may be treated with this method, many patients prefer a dressing over a wound for cosmetic reasons.

Simple Closed Dressing. The closed burn treatment method involves a dressing, of which there are various types. This is the method of choice for managing most minor burns treated in the ED. Wound preparation and basic bandaging should include the following steps (Fig. 38–5):

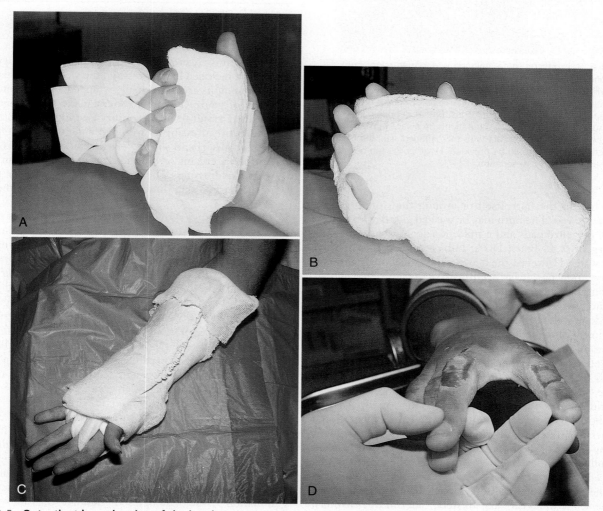

Figure 38–5 Outpatient burn dressing of the hand. Patients with serious hand burns should be admitted to the hospital, but minor burns can be treated in the outpatient setting. After application of an antibiotic ointment or a dry, nonadherent dressing, *the fingers are separated* with fluffs in the web spaces (*A*), and the entire hand is enclosed in a position of function (*B*) (here with the help of a roll of Kerlix). *C,* If the wrist is involved, a removable plaster splint may be applied over the dressing. *D,* The result of a minor burn to the hand when the fingers were not wrapped individually. Initially, there were only a few blisters, but this patient now has second-degree skin loss due to an improper burn dressing that caused maceration of normal skin between the fingers. Not only were the fingers incorrectly wrapped together in one gauze wrap, but the first wound check was incorrectly scheduled in 6 days, too long for the first wound check in a hand burn.

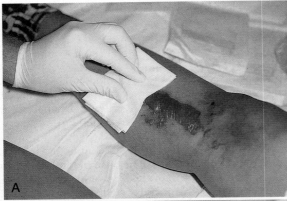
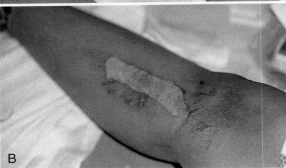

Figure 38–6 It is difficult to do anything wrong with minor burn blisters, and many regimens are acceptable. Eventually, however, blisters will have to be débrided. An expeditious and relatively painless way to débride a burn is to use a dry gauze pad to grasp the dead skin (A) and peel it off (B). Meticulous instrument débridement is often time-consuming and stressful to the patient. Be aware that pain occurs when air comes in contact with the débrided skin and prophylactic analgesia should be provided. Large burns can be débrided under procedural sedation.

TABLE 38–4 General Approach to Blisters in Minor Burns*

If Treated < 48 Hr after the Burn

1. Leave all intact blisters alone.
2. If blisters have ruptured, treat them as dead skin and débride them completely.
3. Needle aspiration is generally not advised but may be used to decompress large burn blisters that appear ready to burst.

On Follow-up, or > 48–72 Hr after the Burn

1. Débride large (>5 cm in diameter) intact blisters and all blisters that have ruptured. Large, firm blisters of the palms and soles may be left intact longer. Do not aspirate blisters.
2. Do not débride small or spotty blisters until they break, or until 5–7 days after the burn.

Five to 7 Days after the Burn

1. Débride all blisters completely.
Note: Intact blisters provide significant pain relief. Be prepared for an exacerbation of pain immediately after débridement. Prophylactic analgesia is recommended.

*All blisters and burned skin are débrided in the presence of infection.
Note: Multiple approaches to blisters are acceptable, and practice varies considerably.

1. The hair in the burn itself or around the wound should not be shaved. The burn may be washed gently with a clean cloth or gauze pads and a mild nonalcohol-based soap or detergent (e.g., Ivory, Dove, Hibiclens) and then flushed with water. However, the benefit of this seemingly rational intervention has never been proved, and this step should be minimal. There is no need to vigorously wash a minor wound with strong antiseptic preparations (such as povidone-iodine [Betadine] and others).[15]
2. Obviously sloughed skin should be débrided. This may be accomplished with scissors and forceps, but an expeditious and effective (and often painless) method is to use a dry 10- x 10-cm gauze pad (Fig. 38–6) to quickly débride loose skin. Meticulous and time-consuming instrument débridement is often quite stressful to the patient. Analgesia should be provided for any painful débridement. Some clinicians prefer to débride a wound on a subsequent follow-up visit when the wound has matured and reached its full extent, thereby hoping to subject the patient to this procedure only once.
3. In the absence of infection, intact blisters are often left alone at the first visit (see "Blisters," later in this chapter). Ruptured blisters are usually débrided as soon as they are recognized (Table 38–4). All sloughed skin and blisters are débrided if infection is present.
4. A fine-mesh gauze or a commercial nonadherent gauze such as Adaptic or Aquaphor is applied to the dry burn wound.
5. The burn is covered with loose gauze fluffs. If fingers and toes are included in the dressing, the web spaces are padded and the digits are individually wrapped and separated with strips of gauze. Failure to individually wrap fingers and toes may result in further injury (see Fig. 38–5D).
6. The entire dressing is wrapped snugly (but not tightly) with an absorbent, slightly elastic material such as Kerlix.
7. Antibiotic creams or ointments may be used as an option with this dressing. The topical antibiotic may be applied to the burned skin directly or impregnated into the gauze after step 3.

Burn dressings should enhance healing. Much is made of specific dressings and dressing materials, but no single approach has proven superior efficacy. The most important characteristic of a dressing is that it is capable of controlling fluid balance. To accelerate healing, a burn dressing should be designed to keep the wound surface moist but avoid pooling of fluids.[16] The best material for this purpose is a generous amount of simple dry gauze applied over a nonadherent dressing or topical preparation. The outer dressing layer should be porous to permit the evaporation of water from the absorbent dressing material. Some clinicians prefer to eschew a nonadherent portion of the dressing so that subsequent dressing removal aids in minor débridement.

Biologic Dressings. Biologic dressings are natural tissues, including skin, that consist of collagen sheets containing elastin and lipid. They are not routinely used in emergency care of minor wounds. Benefits of biologic dressings include a reduction in surface bacterial colonization, diminished fluid and heat loss, prevention of further wound contamination, and prevention of damage to newly developed granulation tissue. Examples of biologic dressings include cadaveric human skin and commercially available porcine xenograft or collagen sheets.

Synthetic Dressings. Synthetic dressings are manufactured in various forms. Film-type dressings have a homogeneous structure and are usually polymers. Because these dressings are nonpermeable, problems with retention of wound exudates have occurred. Some second-generation dressings have been developed to address these problems. These products include Tegaderm, Vigilon, DuoDerm, Biobrane, Op-Site Omniderm, Sildimac.[17] These preparations have theoretical benefits under certain circumstances, but none has proven superior performance over simple gauze dressings for minor outpatient burns. These products are most often used by burn centers and have little applicability for minor burns discharged from the ED. For patients admitted or transferred to a burn center, simple gauze dressings are appropriate. Some burn centers prefer that topical agents not be applied before transfer so the full extent of the burn can be immediately assessed.

Specific Clinical Issues in Minor Burn Care

Analgesia. Pain is a much-feared feature of any burn injury. *Pain relief by the appropriate and judicious use of narcotic analgesics is of paramount importance in the initial care of all burn patients.* Prehospital narcotics are very appropriate when standard contraindications do not exist. Analgesia should be provided before extensive examination or débridement is performed. Inadequate analgesia is probably the most common ED error in the treatment of burn injuries. This error is most common in children. Parenteral narcotic analgesics have been erroneously relegated to pain control in only major burns, but it is suggested that narcotics be generously administered in the initial treatment of even minor painful burns.

Parenteral opioids (fentanyl, 1–2 μg/kg, or morphine, 0.1–0.2 mg/kg) are usually required, especially if painful procedures such as débridement and dressing changes are planned. We prefer to use intravenous (IV) opioids (occasionally supplemented with a short-acting benzodiazepine such as midazolam) for all painful procedures. For complicated débridement or dressing changes, adequate analgesia and sedation (see Chapter 33, Systemic Analgesia and Sedation for Procedures) is strongly advocated.

Regional or nerve block anesthesia is an excellent alternative when practical, and when feasible, nitrous oxide analgesia may be used. Ketamine may also be a reasonable alternative. Oral opioids may be inappropriate for initial treatment of significant pain but can be used for continued outpatient analgesia. Local anesthetics may be injected in small quantities when appropriate, such as for the débridement of a deep ulcer or other small burn. Topical analgesics have no role in burn care. A properly designed dressing will do much toward preventing further discomfort after release home; however, home burn care and dressing changes may be quite painful. For this reason, an adequate supply of an oral opioid analgesic should be provided, and responsibility should be encouraged in analgesic use.

Edema. Minor burns lead to immediate inflammation mediated by the release of histamine and bradykinins, causing localized derangements in vascular permeability, with resultant burn wound edema. This edema is harmful in several ways. First, the increase in interstitial fluid increases the diffusion distance of oxygen from the capillaries to the cells, increasing hypoxia in an already ischemic wound. Second, the edema may produce untoward hemodynamic effects by a purely mechanical mechanism: compression of vessels in muscular compartments. Third, edema has been associated with the inactivation of streptococcicidal skin fatty acids, thus predisposing the patient to burn cellulites.[18]

The successful management of burn edema hinges on immobilization and elevation. Most patients are unfamiliar

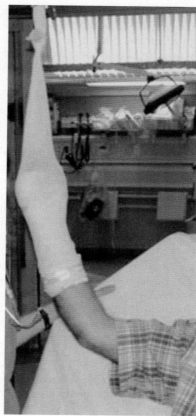

Figure 38–7 Elevation of a burned hand should begin in the emergency department (ED). After a properly applied hand dressing is applied, the arm is suspended from an intravenous (IV) pole with stockinette. A plaster/fiberglass splint may also be incorporated into the dressing.

with the medical definition of elevation and are not aware or convinced of its value. Patient education in this regard is critical; however, certain burns (e.g., burns in dependent body areas) are prone to edema, despite everyone's best intentions. It is for this reason that lower extremity burns in general, and foot burns in particular, are prone to problems. Major burns of the hand should be elevated while the patient is still in the ED. This is most readily accomplished by hanging the injured hand from an IV pole, with stockinette used to support the bandaged hand (Fig. 38–7).

Use of Topical Preparations/Antimicrobials. Minor burns result in insignificant impairment of normal host immunologic defenses, and burn wound infection is usually not a significant problem. Topical antimicrobials are often used; however, some believe these agents may actually impair wound healing.[19] Although the procedure is of unproven value, many clinicians routinely use antibiotic creams or ointments on even the most minor burns. Most patients expect some type of topical concoction, so a discussion of their use, or nonuse, is prudent.

Topical antimicrobials were designed for the prevention and care of burn wound sepsis or wound infection, primarily in hospitalized patients with major burns, and there is no convincing evidence that their use alters the course of first-degree burns and superficial partial-thickness injuries. As noted, the burn dressing is the key factor in minimizing complications in all burns. Nonetheless, topical antimicrobials are often soothing to minor burns, and their daily use prompts the patient to look at the wound, assess healing, perform prescribed dressing changes, or otherwise become personally involved in her or his care. Keep in mind that if a topical antimicrobial is used, its effectiveness is decreased in the presence of proteinaceous exudate, necessitating regular dressing changes if the antimicrobial benefit of topical therapy is to be realized. In reality, once-daily dressing changes are most practical and are commonly prescribed, and there are no data to indicate that this regimen is inferior to more frequent dressing changes.

All full-thickness burns should receive topical antimicrobial therapy because the eschar and burn exudate are potentially good bacterial culture media, and deep escharotic or subescharotic infections may not be easily detected until further damage is done. All deep partial-thickness injuries likewise benefit from the application of a topical antimicrobial. As stated, this intervention can await definitive therapy in a burn unit.

Criteria for choosing a specific topical agent include in vitro and clinical efficacy, toxicity (absorption), superinfection rate, ease and flexibility of use, cost, patient acceptance, and side effects. Note that there are no firm scientific data that convincingly support the use of any specific topical antimicrobial in minor outpatient burns.

Specific Topical Agents

Silver Sulfadiazine (Silvadene). This poorly soluble compound is synthesized by reacting silver nitrate with sodium sulfadiazine. It is the most commonly used topical agent for outpatients, and it is well tolerated by most patients. It has virtually no systemic effects and moderate eschar penetration, and it is painless on application. Although silver sulfadiazine is commonly used, many burn specialists prefer plain bacitracin ointment as the topical of choice because of its cost, equal efficacy, and good patient acceptance.

Silver sulfadiazine is available as a "micronized" mixture with a water-soluble white cream base in a 1% concentration that provides 30 mEq/L of elemental silver. It does not stain clothes, is nonirritating to mucous membranes, and washes off easily with water. It may be used on the face, but such use may be cosmetically undesirable for open treatment. Its broad gram-positive and gram-negative antimicrobial spectrum includes β-hemolytic streptococci, *Staphylococcus aureus* and *Staphylococcus epidermidis*, *Pseudomonas* spp., *Proteus* spp., *Klebsiella* spp., Enterobacteriaceae spp., *Escherichia coli*, *Candida albicans*, and possibly Herpesvirus hominis.

Silver sulfadiazine often interacts with wound exudate to form a pseudomembrane over partial-thickness injuries. The pseudomembrane is often difficult and painful to remove. Except for term pregnancy and in newborns (i.e., owing to possible induction of kernicterus), there are no absolute contraindications to the use of silver sulfadiazine. Allergy and irritation are unusual, although there is a potential cross-sensitivity between silver sulfadiazine and other sulfonamides.

Other Topical Preparations. Mafenide acetate (Sulfamylon), gentamicin, chlorhexidine, povidone-iodine, and silver nitrate are products that have been replaced with newer topicals, but they are mentioned for historical interest. These products are not used in modern burn therapy, although they are generally acceptable alternatives.

BROAD-SPECTRUM ANTIBIOTIC OINTMENTS. Many nonprescription topical antimicrobials are used for minor burn therapy despite data attesting to specific benefits. Included are bacitracin zinc ointment, polymyxin B–bacitracin (Polyspo-

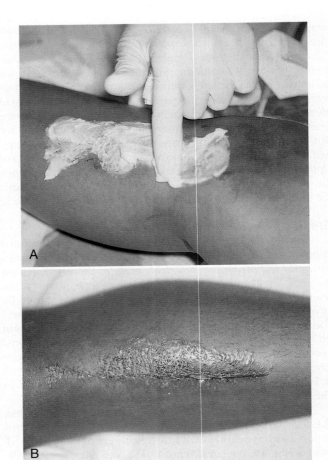

Figure 38–8 *A*, The most popular topical burn preparation is Silvadene cream. Although commonly used on minor burns, it likely has little beneficial effect on healing, and minor burns rarely become infected. Nonetheless, Silvadene is a standard intervention that at least causes the patient to look at the burn and become involved in dressing changes. *B*, Some clinicians suggest inexpensive topical antibiotic ointments (such as bacitracin and polymyxin B sulfate, neomycin sulfate [Neosporin]) for all outpatient burns. They are commonly used on face and neck burns. *Bacitracin is preferred* because a *contact dermatitis*, such as is noted in this abrasion, can occur from the neomycin portion of some topicals.

rin), and nitrofurazone (Furacin). These are all soothing, cosmetically acceptable for open treatment (such as on the face), and effective antiseptics under burn dressings. Some researchers caution against agents containing neomycin because of a potential for sensitization (Fig. 38–8). Although commonly applied by patients without adverse effects, we advise against the use of topicals that contain neomycin (Neosporin) because of the potential for contact dermatitis. The editors suggest plain bacitracin ointment as the routine topical agent, although Silvadene is a very acceptable, albeit expensive, alternative.

ALOE VERA CREAM. Aloe vera cream is commercially available in a 50% or higher concentration with a preservative. It exhibits antibacterial activity against at least four common burn wound pathogens: *Pseudomonas aeruginosa*, *Enterobacter aerogenes*, *S. aureus*, and *Klebsiella pneumoniae*. Heck and coworkers[20] compared a commercial aloe vera cream with silver sulfadiazine in 18 patients with minor burns. Healing times were found to be similar, and there was no increase in wound colonization in the aloe vera group as compared with the patients treated with silver sulfadiazine. Other authors have promulgated the use of aloe gel preparations for minor burns.[21] Aloe vera cream is an acceptable, inexpensive option for open or dressed outpatient care of minor burns.

HONEY. Honey has long been advocated as an inexpensive and effective topical for minor outpatient burns. The physicochemical properties of honey (osmotic effect, pH) give this product antibacterial and anti-inflammatory properties that support its use. It may be superior to silver sulfadiazine with regard to minor burn wound healing. Honey is not widely used, but it has been promulgated as a safe, effective, and inexpensive dressing for the management of outpatient burn wounds.[22-24]

CORTICOSTEROIDS. High-potency topical steroid preparations have no beneficial effects on the rate of healing, or limitation of scarring, of thermal burns. Although likely not harmful, their use is not supported.[25]

FOLLOW-UP CARE OF MINOR BURNS

The specifics of outpatient follow-up of minor burns are controversial and often based on clinician preference and personal bias rather than on firm scientific data. Follow-up should be individualized for each patient and should be based on the reliability of the patient, the extent of the injury, the frequency and complexity of the dressing changes, and the amount of discomfort anticipated during a dressing change. Often, fast-track sections of the ED are used for burn checks that require only a few visits. Physical therapy departments or wound care centers have excellent facilities to follow outpatient burns with periodic clinician oversight.

If a topical antibiotic agent is used, the dressing should be changed daily with removal and reapplication of the topical preparation. The wound should be rechecked by a clinician after 2 to 3 days and periodically thereafter, depending on compliance, healing, and other social issues. If a dry dressing is opted for, follow-up every 3 to 5 days is usually adequate. The purpose of any burn dressing changes or home care regimen is defeated if the patient cannot afford the material or is not instructed in the specifics of burn care. Many EDs supply burn dressing material on patient release. (A complete pack includes antibiotic ointment/cream, gauze pads [fluffs], an absorbent gauze roll, a sterile tongue blade to apply cream, and tape.) Providing limited supplies of the items necessary for dressing changes may enhance compliance to follow-up if the patient has to return for additional supplies. Writing a prescription and merely stating that the dressing should be changed daily is often futile.

Daily home care can be performed by the patient with help from a family member or visiting nurse (Table 38–5). The dressing may be removed each day and gently washed with a clean cloth or a gauze pad, tap water, and a bland soap. Sterile saline and expensive prescription soaps are not required. A tub or shower is an ideal place to gently wash off burn cream. The affected area may be put through a gentle range of motion during dressing changes. After the burn is cleaned, the patient inspects it, with the hope that complications can be recognized and prompt further follow-up. After complete removal of the old cream, a new layer is applied with a sterile tongue blade and covered with absorbent gauze.

If the undermost fine-mesh gauze of a dry dressing is dry and the coagulum is sealed to the gauze, the patient should simply reapply the overlying gauze dressing. If the wound is macerated, the fine-mesh gauze should be removed and the wound cleaned and redressed. The patient is instructed not to remove a dry adherent fine-mesh gauze from the underlying crust. When epithelialization is complete, the crust will separate, and the gauze can be removed at that time. Dryness in healing skin may be treated with mild emollients such as Nivea (Beiersdorf, Inc., Norwalk, CT) or Vaseline Intensive Care lotion (Chesebrough Ponds, Inc., Greenwich, CT). Natural skin lubrication mechanisms usually return by 6 to 8 weeks.[14] Excessive sun exposure should be avoided during wound maturation because this may lead to hyperpigmentation. When the patient is outdoors, a commercially available sun block should be used. Exposure of the recently healed burned area to an otherwise minor trauma (chemicals, heat, sun) may result in an exaggerated skin response. Pruritus is common and may be treated with oral antihistamines or a topical moisturizing cream.

Outpatient Physical Therapy for Burn Care

When the hospital's outpatient physical therapy department or wound care center is equipped to treat minor burns, it is prudent to consider this option if more than a few ED/fast-track follow-up visits are expected. Many centers make available daily or periodic burn treatment, consisting of dressing changes, whirlpool débridement, and range of motion exercises. An additional advantage is that medically trained personnel evaluate the burn daily, thereby decreasing clinician visits and enabling identification of problems before serious complications develop. Generally, all that is required from the clinician is to write a prescription for "burn care and dressing changes" and set up the appointment.

Burn Healing

Follow-up care will in part be guided by expectations of burn healing and observed healing. The following discussion is intended to serve as a general guide. However, burn healing is different from that of other wounds.[2] The timing is often variable, but it is proportional to burn depth. The inflammatory phase lasts 3 to 7 days (at times longer) and, if the burn is severe enough, is accompanied by the release of histamine and bradykinins, along with complement degradation. This degradation of complement may lead to immunologic, coagulation, and metabolic aberrations.

Within 1 to 3 weeks, neovascularization of the burn occurs, accompanied by fibroblast migration. Macrophages

---

TABLE 38–5 How to Change a Burn Dressing at Home: Patient Instructions

1. Take pain medicine ½ hr before dressing change if you find dressing changes to be painful.
2. If the burn is on the hand, foot, or other area that is difficult to reach, have someone help you.
3. Have all materials available. Gloves may be worn.
4. Remove the dressing and rinse off all burn cream or ointment with tap water, under a shower, or in the bathtub. The area can be gently washed with mild soap and a clean cloth or gauze pads.
5. Look at the burn and assess the healing, blistering, and amount of swelling. Note any signs of infection.
6. Gently exercise the area through range of motion.
7. Apply the burn ointment with a sterile tongue blade.
8. Cover the cream with fluffed-up gauze.
9. Wrap the area in bulky gauze.
10. Repeat this dressing change daily.

begin to replace the tissue neutrophils. Collagen production begins, but the molecules are often laid down in random fashion, leading to a scar. Reepithelialization follows, but the presence of necrotic tissue and eschar impedes all aspects of wound healing. The amount of scar tissue produced is directly related to healing time. Burns requiring fewer than 16 days to heal generally do not scar excessively.[2]

Healing in superficial partial-thickness burns occurs within 10 to 14 days. After healing, the new epithelial layer tends to dry easily and crack. Using bland, lanolin-containing creams for 4 to 8 weeks after healing alleviates this problem. Deep partial-thickness burns heal by reepithelialization from the wound edge and from residual dermal elements. Healing is slow and often unsatisfactory, frequently taking longer than 3 weeks, producing an unstable epithelium that is prone to hypertrophic scarring and contractures. This is a particular problem in burns that extend across joints. Burns that take longer than 2 to 3 weeks to heal are prone to infection; hence, topical antimicrobials should be used. Because these burns often heal in complicated fashion, they should be considered for referral to expedite early excision, grafting, and physical therapy.

SPECIAL MINOR BURN CARE CIRCUMSTANCES

Blisters

The management of blisters in minor burns is controversial. In reality, there is little one can do wrong when it comes to a clinical approach to blisters in minor burns. Management arguments are generally theoretical or emotional or based on local tradition; the ultimate outcome of a minor burn is rarely determined by how one deals with blisters. Intact blisters do offer a physiologic dressing that rarely becomes infected; however, most large blisters spontaneously rupture after 3 to 5 days and eventually require débridement. When the integrity of the blister is breached, the fluid becomes a potential culture medium. Clinical choices include débridement, aspiration, or simply leaving the blister intact.

Some studies suggest that intact burn blisters may allow for reversal of capillary stasis and less tissue necrosis.[2] Madden and colleagues[26] showed that burn exudate (as contained within intact blisters) is beneficial for the stimulation of epidermal cell proliferation.

Swain and associates[27] demonstrated that the density of wound colonization with microorganisms was much lower in minor burns with blisters left intact. They also found that 37% of patients with aspirated blisters experienced a reduction in pain versus none of those whose blisters were unroofed. Other investigators believe that undressed wounds with débrided blisters have additional necrosis secondary to desiccation, which can convert a partial-thickness burn to a full-thickness injury.[3] Finally, intact blisters clearly provide some pain relief, as evidenced by a sudden increase in pain immediately after débridement. Increased pain should be anticipated and analgesia offered as appropriate when débridement is necessary. We suggest the guidelines in Table 38–4 as a general approach to burn blisters.

Minor Burn Infections

Prophylactic systemic antibiotics are not warranted in the routine treatment of outpatient burns. It may be difficult to separate the erythema of the injury or healing process from cellulitis, but minor burns rarely become infected, with infection rates well under 5%.[28] There are bacteria on the skin at all times—normal skin usually harbors nonvirulent pathogens such as S. epidermidis and diphtheroids. Therefore, all burns are contaminated but not necessarily infected. Thermal trauma results in a coagulative necrosis. Therefore, burn wounds contain a variable amount of necrotic tissue, which if infected, acts much as an undrained abscess, preventing access of antibiotics and host-defense factors.

The microbial flora of outpatient burns varies with time after the burn. Shortly after injury, the burn becomes colonized with gram-positive bacteria such as S. aureus and S. epidermidis. After this period of time, there is a gradual shift toward inclusion of gram-negative organisms, 80% of which originate from the patient's own gastrointestinal tract.[4] Common organisms seen on days 1 to 3 include S. epidermidis, β-hemolytic streptococci, Bacillus subtilis, S. aureus, enterococci, Mima polymorpha, Enterobacter spp., Acinetobacter spp., and C. albicans. One week after the burn, these organisms may be seen along with E. coli, P. aeruginosa, Serratia marcescens, K. pneumoniae, and Proteus vulgaris.

Anaerobic colonization of burn wounds is rare unless there is excessive devitalized tissue, as occurs in a high-voltage electrical injury.[29] For this reason, routine anaerobic cultures are generally unnecessary in an assessment of infective organisms that produce minor infections.

A healing burn may produce a leukocytosis and a mild fever in the absence of infection, especially in children. Early (days 1–5) burn infections are generally caused by gram-positive cocci, especially β-hemolytic streptococci. Streptococcal cellulitis is characterized by marked, spreading erythema extending outward from the wound margins. Despite the plethora of organisms and the presence of some gram-negative pathogens noted in superficial burn cultures, first-line treatment in the normal host is oral penicillin, 1 to 2 g/day. Alternatives include erythromycin, cephalosporins, and dicloxacillin.

Effective topical treatment at the time of initial burn care and subsequent dressing changes is meant to delay bacterial colonization, maintain the wound bacterial density at low levels, and produce a less diverse wound flora. Because outpatient management of burns should be attempted only when the risk of infection is minimal, the use of systemic antibiotics is unnecessary for minor burns, even in the setting of delayed treatment, diabetes, and steroid use.[30] Unnecessary antibiotic use may select out resistant organisms. Antibiotics in the management of minor burns have been recommended for patients undergoing an autograft procedure.[31] There are no data on the use of antibiotics as prophylaxis for patients with burns in the setting of valvular heart disease.

In minor burn care, wound cultures are not required or recommended. It is useless, for example, to culture blister fluid in the patient who presents for emergency care immediately after a thermal injury. Cultures are necessary only when overt infection develops, especially when this occurs while a topical or systemic antibiotic is being used. Cultures may also be of benefit when the infected wound is old, when hygiene is poor, or when there are old abrasions nearby.[32] Swab surface cultures are generally eschewed. Although they may adequately reflect wound flora, falsely sterile cultures are relatively frequent. These cultures do not reflect deep burn flora and give no quantitative information.

Sterile wound biopsy for culture is most satisfactory for the assessment of intraescharotic, subescharotic, or invasive infections and allows for quantification of bacterial flora.

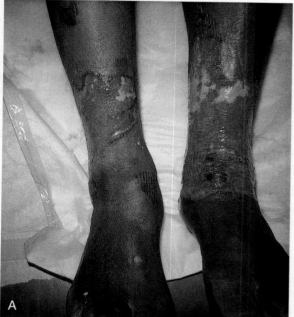

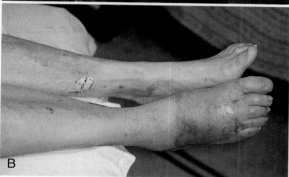

Figure 38–9 Burns of the feet are specialized burns that require a careful evaluation and an individualized treatment plan, even if the burn surface area is relatively small. It is difficult for most patients to provide ideal burn care at home when the feet are involved. *A,* It is tempting to initially treat this seemingly minor superficial second-degree foot burn in an outpatient setting, but the patient's compliance and social situation must be ideal for a successful outcome. Hospitalization until home health care can be established is prudent. *B,* An example of a foot burn that is a potential disaster, in this case due to a late presentation in a diabetic.

Foot Burns

Despite their relatively small surface area, foot burns tend to heal poorly, usually owing to excessive edema; therefore, they are formally categorized as major burns. Foot burns are the most common burn category to fail outpatient therapy and subsequently require admission and inpatient care (Fig. 38–9). Zachary and coworkers[33] reported on a series of 104 patients with foot burns. No patient admitted on the day of injury developed burn cellulitis; in contrast, 27% of delayed-admission patients had cellulitis. Their study also noted a higher incidence of hypertrophic scarring and need for skin grafting in the delayed-admission group. Overall, fewer days of hospitalization were required for the initially admitted group.

Specific problems in the care of foot burns include pain, wound drainage, difficulty in changing dressings without help, inability of even motivated patients to comply with requirements for elevation, and prolonged convalescence. Hospital admission allows for splinting, intensive local burn care, physical therapy, and bedrest with elevation, which minimizes edema. For these reasons, initial admission is advised for all but the most minor of foot burns.

Hand Burns

Because of their functional importance, hand burns can be a devastating injury, despite involvement of a relatively small TBSA. Hand function is critical, regardless of whether the patient is dealing with loss of use during healing, later limitation by scar contractures, a long-term appearance change, or loss due to amputation.[34]

As with other burns, the depth and extent of the burn determine the severity of the injury. The entire surface of one hand represents only 2.5% TBSA, yet even small burns can cause a disproportionate functional loss. Deep partial- or full-thickness hand burns, even if quite small, often warrant referral for early excision and grafting in order to limit scarring and maintain function. The skin on the dorsum of the hand is thinner than that on the palm and is more susceptible to burn injury but must remain flexible to allow for finger motion. Any exposed tendon or bone, such as may be seen with an electrical burn, constitutes a true fourth-degree injury, which requires either flap closure or amputation in order to heal the wound.

Many of the issues complicating outpatient management of foot burns are relevant to the care of hand burns. After initial burn cooling, the wound should be gently cleansed with mild soap. Any loose skin or ruptured blisters should be gently débrided, rinsed, patted dry, and covered with a topical antimicrobial agent and a nonadherent, bulky gauze dressing. The fingers should be carefully separated and bandaged individually. Small, intact blisters that do not interfere with hand function should be left intact to serve as a biologic dressing. Elevation of the hand is very important in the first few days after a burn injury in order to minimize edema. Deep partial- or full-thickness burns to the dorsum of the hand should be splinted after bandaging to avoid the development of contractures or a boutonnière deformity.

Hospital admission should be considered for significant hand burns, particularly full-thickness injuries and circumferential burns involving the digits (Fig. 38–10). If outpatient treatment is attempted, the patient must be given comprehensive instructions and should have the resources available to perform daily dressing changes and range of motion exercises of the fingers and wrist during these dressing changes. An initial follow-up visit should be arranged in 48 to 72 hours, but the patient should be encouraged to return if there is development of a burn cellulitis, worsening pain, fever, or lymphangitis. Ideally, the patient should be seen twice in the 1st week after injury and once a week after that until the burn is healed.

Facial Burns

Facial burns commonly result from unexpected ignition flash burns (e.g., from a stove, oven, or charcoal grill) or from car radiator accidents (Fig. 38–11).[35,36] Facial burns from these sources usually do well, but often result in singeing of facial hair, significant edema, and pain. However, facial burns from these etiologies may rarely produce airway problems and require skin grafting. Concurrent globe or corneal injury is quite rare owing to protective blinking reflexes. If the eye is burned, it is usually in the setting of a life-threatening concomitant burn injury.[37] Burns to the eyelids can cause

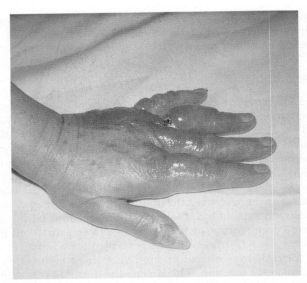

Figure 38–10 This badly burned hand requires referral to a surgeon or burn center and should not definitively be handled in the ED. Note the very tight ring.

significant scarring. Fluorescein staining and slit-lamp examination may be used to confirm the diagnosis of suspected corneal injury. The treatment of a corneal injury involves irrigation, topical ophthalmic antibiotic ointment, and consideration of eyepatching versus protective soft contact lens (see Chapter 63, Ophthalmologic Procedures). Referral to an ophthalmologist is usually prudent. Facial burns are otherwise treated in the usual fashion and with an open (no dressing) technique. Patients are instructed to wash the face two or three times a day with a mild soap and then apply a thin layer of antibiotic ointment, such as bacitracin zinc. There are no compelling reasons to avoid silver sulfadiazine on the face, but by tradition, bacitracin ointment has become the preferred topical agent. Car radiator burns result from the combination of a hot liquid and steam burn. Antifreeze does not produce a caustic injury, nor is it systemically absorbed. Neck burns are treated similarly.

All patients presenting with head or neck burns should be carefully evaluated for a concomitant inhalation injury. Such patients may present with direct evidence of injury, such as oral burns, blisters, soot, or hyperemia, a history of being in an enclosed space, or with indirect evidence, such as dyspnea, wheezing, arterial hypoxemia, or an elevated carboxyhemoglobin level. The definitive diagnostic test for inhalation injury is fiberoptic bronchoscopy.[38] Flash ignition burns to the face do not pose a problem with carbon monoxide poisoning, and inhalation injuries are generally not a consid-

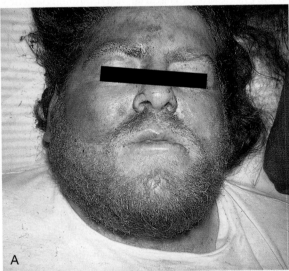

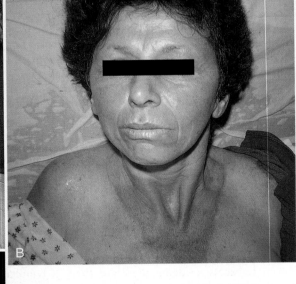

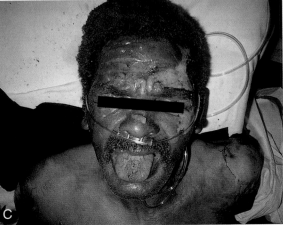

Figure 38–11 *A,* Flash burns to the face from lighting a gas stove. These burns are painful and may cause edema, but usually they do well. Note the singed facial hair. The eyes are usually protected by rapid reflex blinking, and carbon monoxide poisoning and pulmonary burns are not an issue. Most can be handled in the outpatient setting with bacitracin ointment and no dressing. Pain control may be problematic unless opioids are prescribed. *B,* Facial and neck burns when a radiator cap was removed and the victim was sprayed with steam and hot antifreeze. *C,* This patient has a severe facial burn with smoke inhalation, evidenced by the soot in the pharynx and singed nasal hairs. Tracheal intubation is in the near future for this patient.

eration. Inpatient care should be considered for all patients with significant facial burns. Outpatient pain control may be difficult in facial burns, the degree of edema may be difficult to predict, and home care can be problematic. There are no universally agreed-upon standards for admission versus outpatient treatment of facial burns.

Corneal contact burns, as from accidental contact with a curling iron, often present rather dramatically, with opacified, "heaped-up" corneal epithelium. Despite their appearance, the end result is usually excellent. Treatment is the same as for a corneal abrasion.[39]

Abuse of Children and Elderly Individuals

Recognition of the possibility of deliberate abuse by burning in the pediatric and geriatric populations is essential. In addition, children younger than 2 years old have a thinner dermis and a less well-developed immune system than do adults. Elderly patients (>65 yr) likewise tolerate burns poorly. These two populations are the most prone to abuse, often by family members (Fig. 38–12). For these reasons, both groups of patients often require inpatient care.[9]

The majority of abused children are 18 to 36 months old, and for unknown reasons, the majority are male.[19] Immersion burns are a common type of abuse. These are characterized by circumferential, sharply demarcated burns of the hands, feet, buttocks, and perineum. Cigarette burns and burns from hot objects such as irons should be obvious. Contact burns on "nonexploring" parts of the child also warrant suspicion. A delay in seeking treatment may be a tip-off that a burn resulted from abuse. Self-inflicted burns are characteristic, especially cigarette burns, of psychiatric disease (see Fig. 38–12E).

Burns in Pregnancy

There is little information in the literature concerning the special problems of the pregnant burn victim. Ying-bei and Ying-jie[40] reported on 24 pregnant burn patients representing a wide range of burn severity. Complications of the burn injuries included abortion and premature labor, although all patients in this series with burns covering less than 20% TBSA did well and delivered living full-term babies.

As the resistance of pregnant women to infection is lower than that of nonpregnant women, control of burn wound infection is paramount. Gestational age appears to have no direct bearing on prognosis. Silver sulfadiazine cream should be avoided near term because of the potential for kernicterus.

SPECIFIC BURNING AGENTS

Hot Tar Burns

Asphalts are products of the residues of coal tar commonly used in roofing and road repair. These products are kept heated to approximately 450°F. When spilled onto the skin, the tar cools rapidly, but the retained heat is sufficient to produce a partial-thickness burn. Fortunately, full-thickness burns are unusual. Cooled tar is nonirritating and does not promote infection. When cooled tar is physically removed, the adherent skin is usually avulsed (Fig. 38–13). Careless removal of the tar may inflict further damage on burned tissues. Agents such as alcohol, acetone, kerosene, or gasoline have been used to remove the tar, but these are flammable

and may cause additional skin damage or toxic response secondary to absorption.

There is no great need to meticulously remove all tar at the first visit. Obviously devitalized skin can be débrided, but adherent tar should be emulsified or dissolved rather than manually removed (Fig. 38–14). Polyoxyethylene sorbitan (Tween 80 or polysorbate 80) is the water-soluble, nontoxic, emulsifying agent found in Neosporin and several other topical antibiotic creams. Note that the cream formulations, not the ointments, contain the most useful tar dissolvers. The creams contain a complex mixture of ethers, esters, and sorbitol anhydrides that possess excellent hydrophilic and lyophilic characteristics when used as nonionic, surface-active emulsifying agents. With persistence, most tar may be removed (emulsified) on the initial visit.

Another household product (De-Solv-It multi-use solvent) also appears logical for topical ED use.[41] The De-Solv-It product has a surface-active moiety that wets the chemical's surface and emulsifies tar and asphalt. Because the latter product is itself a petroleum-based solvent, it should be applied only briefly, and the operator should wear gloves and protective eyewear during application. It should be used only for external exposure to tar or asphalt.

Many clinicians prefer instead to emulsify the majority of tar on an outpatient basis. A generous layer of polysorbate-based ointment can be applied under a bulky absorbent gauze dressing. The patient is then released home, and the residual tar is easily washed off after 24 to 36 hours (Fig. 38–15). A number of dressing changes may be required. Once the residual tar is removed, the wound is treated like any other burn.

Shur-Clens, a nontoxic, nonionic detergent, also works well for tar burn wound cleansing, as do mineral oil; petrolatum; and Medisol (Orange-Sol, Inc, Chandler, AZ), a petroleum-citrus product. Butter-soaked gauze has been suggested as an emulsifier of tar.

Chemical Burns

Chemical burns usually occur in the workplace, and the offending substance is usually well known. More than 25,000 chemicals currently in use are capable of burning the skin or mucous membranes. Commonly used chemical agents capable of producing skin burns are shown in Table 38–6.

Injury is caused by a chemical reaction rather than a thermal burn.[42] Reactions are classified as oxidizing, reducing, corrosive, desiccant, or vesicant or as protoplasmic poisoning. The injury to skin continues until the chemical agent is physically removed or exhausts its inherent destructive capacity. The degree of injury is based on chemical strength, concentration, and quantity; duration of contact; location of contact; extent of tissue penetration; and mechanism of action.

Immediate flushing with water is recommended for all chemical burns, with the exception of those caused by alkali metals. Flushing serves to cleanse the wound of unreacted surface chemical, dilute the chemical already in contact with tissue, and restore lost tissue water. Leonard and colleagues[43] clearly demonstrated that patients receiving immediate copious water irrigation for chemical burns showed less full-thickness burn injury and a 50% or greater reduction in time of hospital stay.

Acid and Alkali Burns

Alkalis cause saponification and liquefactive necrosis of body fats. Alkaline burns are penetrating and cause much tissue

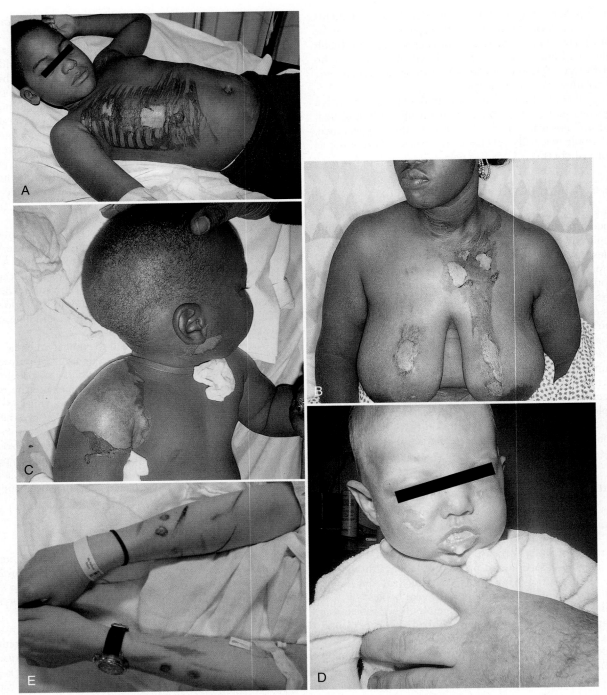

Figure 38–12   Burns can be a manifestation of child abuse, spouse abuse, or abuse of the elderly. *A,* Abuse burns from contact with a hot metal grate, from a child allegedly falling. *B,* This burn was the result of spouse abuse, caused by throwing hot soup during an argument. Domestic abuse is often initially denied but the delayed presentation to the hospital was a clue. *C,* Burns of the face and neck are common when a toddler pulls hot liquid from a stove. This case was never proved to be child abuse, but burns in young children often are due to abuse, especially if they are in atypical places. Although the body surface area of this burn is relatively small, the patient's age and the burn's location, coupled with the possibility of child abuse, require that this child be hospitalized. *D,* This infant received a severe blistering sunburn at the beach despite being in the shade most of the day. Reflections of sunlight from the sand and water can injure the delicate skin of an infant, who should have sunscreen applied. *E,* Self-inflicted cigarette burns in a psychiatric patient.

destruction. With acid burns, tissue coagulation produces a thick eschar that limits the penetration of the agent. Desiccant acids, such as sulfuric acid, create an exothermic reaction with tissue water and can cause both chemical and thermal injury. With extensive immersion injuries, acids may be systemically absorbed, leading to systemic acidosis and coagulation abnormalities.

Chemical burns may be excruciatingly painful for long periods of time. Discomfort can be out of proportion to what one might expect from the depth or extent of the burn.

The emergency care team should remove all potentially contaminated clothing. Any dry (anhydrous) chemical should be brushed off the patient's skin. The involved skin should be irrigated with large amounts of water under low pressure. Any

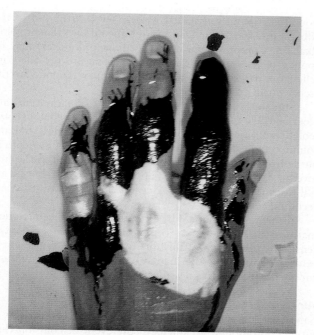

Figure 38–13 There is no compelling reason to remove all tar on the first visit. Physical removal of cooled tar usually results in avulsion of the underlying skin. Skin that is obviously loose should be débrided, but adherent tar is best liquefied with an emulsifying agent. Neomycin cream, not ointment, is a suggested emulsifier, but others are acceptable (see text). Final removal may be delayed for several days to permit loosening of the tar. Frequent dressing changes using an emulsifying agent can be performed by the patient, removing the tar over a few days.

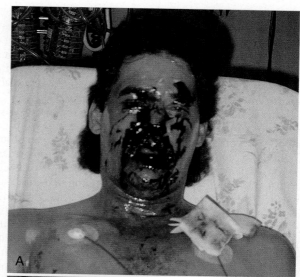

TABLE 38–6 Commonly Used Acids and Alkalis	
Acids	**Alkalis**
Picric	Sodium hydroxide
Tungstic	Ammonium hydroxide
Sulfosalicylic	Lithium hydroxide
Tannic	Barium hydroxide
Trichloroacetic	Calcium hydroxide
Cresylic	Sodium hypochlorite
Acetic	
Formic	
Sulfuric	
Hydrochloric	
Hydrofluoric	
Chromic	

Figure 38–14 Tar stuck to the face (*A*) can be emulsified with various agents and a lot of patience and persistence (*B*). Fortunately, tar burns are usually not full-thickness burns.

remaining particulate matter should be carefully débrided during irrigation.

Strong alkali burns may require irrigation for 1 to 2 hours before the tissue pH returns to normal. Some recommend that after extensive irrigation, if the burn continues to feel "slippery" or tissue pH has not returned to normal, chemical neutralization may be helpful.[44,45] Given that any heat of neutralization will be carried away with the irrigation solution,[46] prompt irrigation with a dilute acid (e.g., vinegar; 2% acetic acid) may hasten neutralization and patient comfort.

Wet Cement Burns

The major constituent of Portland cement, an alkaline substance, is calcium oxide (64%), combined with oxides of silicon, aluminum, magnesium, sulfur, iron, and potassium.

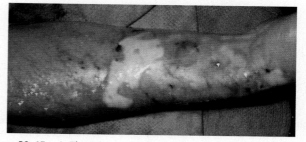

Figure 38–15 *A,* There is no need to remove all the tar on the first visit. *B,* This extremity was covered with an emulsifying agent and with gauze, and the residual tar was washed off easily 36 hr later.

There is considerable variability in the calcium oxide content of different grades of cement, with concrete having less and fine-textured masonry cement having more.[43] The addition of water exothermically converts the calcium oxide to calcium hydroxide ($Ca(OH)_2$), a strongly corrosive alkali with a pH of 11 to 13. As the cement hardens, the calcium hydroxide reacts with ambient carbon dioxide and becomes inactive.

Both the heat and the $Ca(OH)_2$ produced in this exothermic reaction can result in significant burns. Because of its low solubility and consequent low ionic strength, a long exposure to $Ca(OH)_2$ is required to produce injury. This usually occurs when a worker spills concrete into his or her boots or kneels in it for a prolonged period. The burn wound and the resultant protein denaturation of tissues produce a thick, tenacious, ulcerated eschar. Concrete burns are insidious and progressive. What may appear initially as a patchy, superficial burn may in several days become a full-thickness injury requiring excision and skin grafting.[47] The pain of these burns is often severe and more intense than the appearance of the wound might suggest (Fig. 38–16). Interestingly, many workers are not warned of the dangers of prolonged contact with cement, and because initial contact with cement is usually painless, exposure may not be realized until the damage is done.

Treatment is as follows: Any loose particulate cement or lime is brushed off, contaminated clothing is removed, the wound is copiously irrigated with tap water (the pH of the effluent is tested and irrigation continued if the effluent is still alkaline). Compresses of dilute acetic acid (vinegar) may be applied to neutralize the remaining alkali and provide pain relief after irrigation, and antibiotic ointment is applied to the eschar during the early postburn period.

Sutilains ointment (Travase, Flint Pharmaceuticals, Deerfield, IL) is often recommended because it contains proteolytic enzymes and helps speed eschar separation, but any common topical burn preparation is acceptable. The depth of burns from wet cement can be difficult to assess in the first several days. If it becomes apparent that the burns are full-thickness burns, early excision and skin grafting are recommended.

Cement burns should be differentiated from cement dermatitis, which is far more common. The latter is a contact sensitivity reaction, probably due to the chromates present in cement. The contact dermatitis can initially be treated as a superficial partial-thickness burn.

Air Bag Keratitis/Thermal Burns

Safety legislation has mandated increased use of air bags to protect automobile occupants in the event of collision (Fig. 38–17). Burns from air bags can be thermal, friction, or chemical. The automobile air bag is a rubberized nylon bag that inflates on spark ignition of sodium azide, yielding nitrogen gas, ash, and a small amount of sodium hydroxide. Within seconds, the superheated air is vented, and this can produce a thermal burn if it contacts an extremity, face, or upper torso.[48,49] If the air bag ruptures, the alkaline contents of the bag are dispersed as a fine, black powder that usually causes no problems unless the eyes are exposed. Patients present with clinical evidence of a chemical keratoconjunctivitis, including photophobia, tearing, redness, and decreased visual acuity. The tear pH is usually elevated, and there may be a small amount of particulate material in the fornices.[50]

The severity of an ocular alkaline burn is related to the duration of exposure and the concentration and pH of the chemical. For this reason, prompt, copious irrigation of the eyes with frequent assessment of tear pH is essential to prevent or minimize the injury (see Chapter 63, Ophthalmologic Procedures). A rising pH suggests that trapped particulate matter is releasing additional chemical. Corneal edema and conjunctival blanching are signs of serious injury and necessitate immediate ophthalmologic consultation.

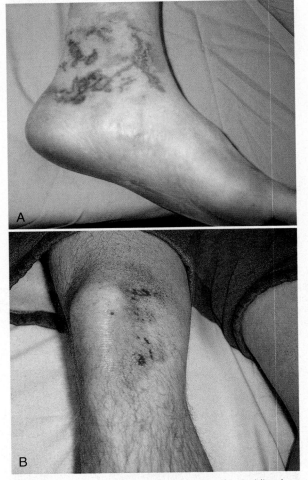

Figure 38–16 Alkali burns from wet cement develop insidiously, are extremely painful, and are frequently full-thickness injuries. They are most common on the feet when cement leaks over the top of the boots (*A*) or from kneeling in wet cement while working (*B*). The alkali can penetrate clothing.

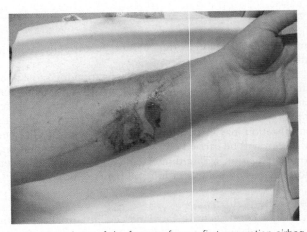

Figure 38–17 A burn of the forearm from a first generation airbag can be a combination of friction and chemical. They are usually minor.

Hydrocarbon Burns

Hydrocarbons are capable of causing severe contact injuries by virtue of their irritant, fat-dissolving, and dehydrating properties. Cutaneous absorption may cause even more dangerous systemic effects. Gasoline, the usual agent involved, is a complex mixture of C_4 to C_{11} alkane hydrocarbons and benzene; the hydrocarbons appear to be the major toxic agent. Lead poisoning caused by either absorption through intact skin or burns from leaded gasoline exposure have been previously reported but are currently quite rare because unleaded gasoline has virtually replaced the leaded version for most purposes.[51]

Depth of injury is related to the duration of exposure and concentration of the chemical agent. Gasoline immersion injuries resemble scald burns and are usually partial thickness.[52] Occasionally, gasoline-injured skin exhibits a pinkish-brown discoloration, possibly related to dye additives. A common source of exposure is a comatose patient from a motor vehicle crash who had been lying in a pool of gasoline.

The lungs are the usual site of systemic absorption and are often the only major route of excretion. The resultant high pulmonary concentrations may lead to pulmonary hemorrhages, atelectasis, and adult respiratory distress syndrome. Treatment of hydrocarbon burns includes removal of contaminated clothing, prolonged irrigation or soaking of the contaminated skin, early débridement in significant burns caused by lead-containing gasolines (to reduce systemic lead absorption), and use of topical antibiotic ointments.

Phenol Injury

Phenol is a highly reactive aromatic acid alcohol that acts as a corrosive. Carbolic acid, an earlier term for phenol, was noted to have antiseptic properties and was used as such by Joseph Lister in performing the first antiseptic surgery. Hexylresorcinol, a phenol derivative, is in current use as a bactericidal agent. Phenols, in strong concentrations, cause considerable eschar formation, but skin absorption also occurs and can cause systemic effects such as central nervous system depression, hypotension, hemolysis, pulmonary edema, and death. Interestingly, phenol acts differently from other acids in that it penetrates deeper when in a dilute solution than when in a more concentrated form.[42] Therefore, irrigation with water is suboptimal for phenol burns, but because water commonly is readily available, it is frequently used for irrigation.

Full-strength polyethylene glycol (PG 300 or 400) is more effective than water alone in removing phenolic compounds and should be obtained and used after water irrigation has begun. Polyethylene glycol is nontoxic and nonirritating and may be used anywhere on the body. When immediately available, polyethylene glycol can be used to remove the surface chemical before water irrigation (and chemical dilution) is begun.

Hydrofluoric Acid Injury

Hydrofluoric acid (HFA) is one of the strongest inorganic acids known; it has been widely used since its ability to dissolve silica was discovered in the late 17th century.[53] Currently, HFA is used in masonry restoration, glass etching, and semiconductor manufacturing; for control of fermentation in breweries; and in the production of plastics and fluorocarbons. It is also used as a catalyst in petroleum alkylating units. It is available in industry as a liquid in varying concentrations up to 70%. It is also readily sold in home improvement and hardware stores. Significant concentrations of HFA are present in many home rust-removal products, aluminum brighteners, automobile wheel cleaners, and heavy-duty cleaners in concentrations of less than 10%. Despite its ability to cause serious burns, unregulated and poorly labeled HFA products are recklessly used on a regular basis in the home and in small businesses. The public and many clinicians are generally unaware of the potential problems with this acid (Fig. 38–18).

Although HFA is quite corrosive, the hydrogen ion plays a relatively insignificant role in the pathophysiology of the burn injury. The accompanying fluoride ion is a protoplasmic poison that causes liquefaction necrosis and is notorious for its ability to penetrate tissues and cause delayed pain and deep tissue injury. This acid can penetrate through fingernails and cause nailbed injury. With home products, the unwary user does not realize that the substance is caustic until the skin (usually the hands and fingers) is exposed for a few minutes to hours, at which time the burning begins and becomes

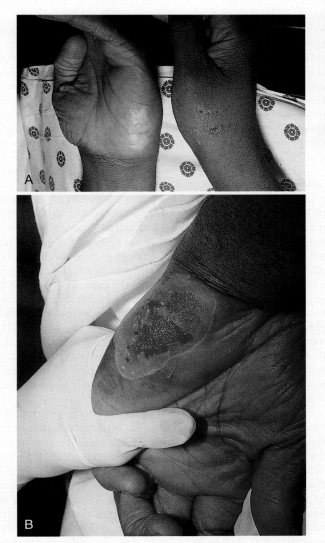

Figure 38–18 *A,* Initially, this very painful hydrofluoric acid (HFA) burn of the thenar and hypothenar eminence appeared minimal. *B,* Despite infiltration with calcium gluconate, a deep burn developed 3 days later.

progressively worse. At this point, the damage is done and the absorbed HFA cannot be washed off. With higher-strength industrial products, symptoms are almost immediate.

The initial corrosive burn is due to free hydrogen ions; secondary chemical burning is due to the tissue penetration of fluoride ions. Fluoride is capable of binding cellular calcium, resulting in cell death and liquefaction necrosis. The ionic shifts that result, particularly shifts of potassium, are believed to be responsible for the severe pain associated with HFA burns.

In high concentrations, the fluoride ions may penetrate to the bone and produce demineralization. Skin exposure to concentrated HFA involving as little as 2.5% TBSA can lead to systemic hypocalcemia and death from intractable cardiac arrhythmias; it has been calculated that exposure to 7 mL of anhydrous HFA (HFA gas) is capable of binding all of the free calcium in a 70-kg adult.[54,55] If the hands are exposed, the acid characteristically penetrates the fingernails and injures the nailbed and cuticle area. As with most caustics, the pain is generally out of proportion to the evident external physical injury. HFA burns produce variable areas of blanching and erythema, but rarely are blisters or skin sloughing seen initially. Skin necrosis and cutaneous hemorrhage may be noted in a few days.

Immediate treatment should begin with copious irrigation with water. Another approach is to wash the area with a solution of iced magnesium sulfate (Epsom salts) or a 1 : 500 solution of a quaternary ammonium compound such as benzalkonium chloride (Zephiran) or benzethonium chloride (Hyamine 1622). Magnesium and calcium salts form an insoluble complex with fluoride ions, preventing further tissue diffusion. Although frequently recommended, topical preparations are often ineffective in limiting injury or controlling pain.

If there is no or only minimal visible evidence of skin injury and minimal pain, the burn may be dressed with topical calcium gluconate paste. This is not commercially available in the United States but is easily compounded in the pharmacy by mixing 3.5 to 7 g of pulverized calcium gluconate with 5 oz of a water-soluble lubricant such as K-Y Jelly. This will form a thick paste with a calcium gluconate concentration of 2.5% to 5.0%. Some have suggested dimethyl sulfoxide as a vehicle to aid in skin penetration of the calcium. Plastic wrap (e.g., Saran Wrap) is used over a standard dry burn dressing to cover the calcium paste on the limbs; a vinyl or rubber glove is used over the paste when used on the hands. The wound should be completely redressed and the paste reapplied every 6 hours for the first 24 hours. As with most topical treatments of HFA burns, calcium gluconate is only minimally effective in relieving pain, and its value is likely overestimated in the literature.

A digital or regional nerve block with long-acting bupivacaine is an excellent way to provide prolonged pain relief if the hands are involved, but this does nothing to ameliorate the injury. In most cases, oral opioids are required. If bullae or vesicles have formed, these should be débrided to decrease the amount of fluoride present, and the wound should then be treated as any partial-thickness burn. Burns with HFA of less than 10% strength will heal spontaneously, usually without significant tissue loss, but pain and sensitivity of the fingertips may persist for 7 to 10 days. In addition, the fingernails may become loose.

The presence of significant skin injury or intense pain implies penetration of the skin by fluoride ions. This scenario is particularly common with exposure to HFA solutions in concentrations of 20% or greater, but tissue injury can occur with prolonged exposure to less concentrated products.

Initial treatment of a more concentrated exposure begins as described earlier and includes immediate débridement of necrotic tissue to remove as much fluoride ion as possible. After this, a 10% solution of calcium gluconate (note: avoid calcium chloride for tissue injections) is injected intradermally and subcuticularly with a 30-gauge needle about the exposed area, using about 0.5 mL per square centimeter of burn. Pain relief should be almost immediate if this therapy is adequate. Because the degree of pain is a measure of the effectiveness of treatment, the use of anesthetics, especially by local infiltration, may be deleted if the burn is on the arm or leg. HFA can penetrate fingernails without damaging them. Soft tissue can be injected without prior anesthesia, but if the fingertips or nailbeds are involved, they may be injected after a digital nerve block has been performed (Fig. 38–19). Before anesthesia and prior to injecting calcium, the patient can outline the affected areas with a pen to ensure accurate injection of the antidote (see Fig. 38–19B). Although some investigators recommend that the fingernails be removed routinely, we strongly advise against this unless the nails are very loose or there is obvious necrosis of the nailbed. Fingers are best injected with a 25- or 27-gauge needle (a tuberculin syringe works well).[56] Nails frequently become loose in a few days, but often, they return to normal and do not require removal, particularly when lower-concentration nonindustrial products are involved.

Although calcium gluconate infiltration is somewhat effective, the technique has certain limitations. Injections are painful, and the calcium gluconate solution itself causes a burning sensation. Because of the volume restrictions, not enough calcium may be delivered to bind all the free fluoride ions present. For example, 0.5 mL of 10% calcium gluconate contains 4.2 mg (0.235 mEq) of elemental calcium, which will neutralize only 0.025 mL of 20% HFA.

Several authorities have advocated intra-arterial calcium infusions in the treatment of serious HFA burns of the extremities.[54,57] Although very effective, this technique is not recommended for burns secondary to dilute HFA (i.e., concentrations < 10%), because morbidity is usually quite mild. When using this technique, 10 mL of 10% calcium gluconate is diluted in 50 mL of a 5% dextrose and water solution. The dilute solution is given by a slow infusion into an arterial catheter. It is unclear which artery best delivers the calcium to injured tissues. If only the radial three digits are involved, probably only the radial artery need be cannulated. Otherwise, a percutaneous catheter is inserted into the brachial artery. However, some investigators have advocated the use of the radial artery in all cases, and because the arterial supply of the hand is interconnected, this may be a reasonable recommendation.[58] The radial artery is usually more easily cannulated than is the brachial artery. When the arterial access has been accomplished, the solution is slowly infused over 4 hours. At this point, the catheter is left in place, and the patient is observed. If pain returns at any time over the next 4 hours, the infusion is repeated. If the patient is pain-free over the 4-hour observation period, the burn is dressed, and the patient is released home. This technique may be initiated in the ED, but many clinicians are reluctant to cannulate an artery and infuse calcium in the ED. Such patients require hospitalization, or a burn center referral, for further evaluation and observation.

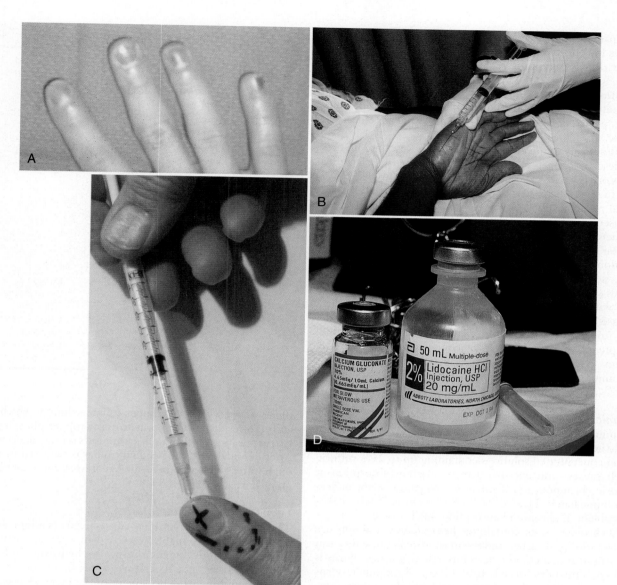

Figure 38–19 HFA burns to the fingertips are extremely painful, despite minimal clinical findings, initially manifesting only hyperemia and minor ecchymosis. HFL can penetrate the intact fingernail, producing a significant injury to the nailbed. *A,* The area of burn can be injected with calcium gluconate minimally diluted with plain lidocaine. *B,* Using a small-gauge needle, generously infiltrate the entire area of the burn, *C,* Before performing digital block anesthesia in order to painlessly infiltrate the fingertips with calcium gluconate, the patient outlines the painful areas with a felt-tip marker to ensure accurate placement of the antidote. In the treatment of HFA burns, topical therapy is often ineffective. Calcium gluconate may be injected subcutaneously with a 25- to 27-gauge needle *into the nailbed via the fat pad under a digital nerve block*. Fingernails should not be removed routinely if burns are mild, such as those seen with household products containing less than 10% concentration of the acid. Intra-arterial calcium infusions are often quite successful in relieving pain and limiting necrosis. *D,* Calcium gluconate is combined with a small amount of lidocaine for injection.

Advantages of the intra-arterial method are elimination of the need for painful SQ injections and avoidance of the volume limitations of the SQ route while providing substantially more calcium to neutralize the fluoride. Disadvantages of intra-arterial calcium therapy include the possibility of local arterial spasm (which can be treated with vasodilators such as phentolamine or removal of the catheter), local arterial injury or thrombus, and the long duration of treatment required.

Infusing calcium into the general venous circulation is of no benefit for HFA burns. Some authors have advocated the use of regional IV calcium gluconate, similar to the method used with the Bier block for regional anesthesia.[59] Case reports have noted variable success, but this technique has neither been well studied nor rigorously compared with other options. This method would be useful only for upper extremity burns. To perform regional calcium therapy, an IV catheter is placed in the dorsum of the hand on the involved extremity. The arm is partially exsanguinated by elevation or wrapping with an elastic bandage, or both. A Bier block tourniquet, or a heavy-duty blood pressure cuff, is applied proximal to the burn and inflated to 20 to 30 mm Hg above systolic pressure to stop blood flow to and from the arm. Slow deflation of a regular blood pressure cuff may thwart success of the procedure, and the use of a specialized tourniquet is recommended. Then, 10 mL of 10% calcium gluconate, diluted with 30 to 40 mL of saline, is infused into the venous catheter, and the solution is kept in the arm by the tourniquet for 20 to 30 minutes.

Some patients cannot tolerate arm ischemia for this period, limiting the effectiveness of this procedure. Theoretically, the calcium diffuses out of the venous system and into the injured tissues. After 20 to 30 minutes, the cuff is deflated and normal circulation to the extremity is achieved. It may require 10 to 20 minutes after tourniquet deflation before the patient experiences pain relief. This procedure is safe, but its efficacy is variable.

HFA burns to the eye are potentially devastating injuries that deserve special mention. Ophthalmologist referral is mandatory. Ocular exposure to liquid or gaseous HFA will result in severe pain, tearing, conjunctival inflammation, and corneal opacification or erosion. Complications include decreased visual acuity, globe perforation, uveitis, glaucoma, conjunctival scarring, lid deformities, and keratitis sicca. Optimal therapy for ocular HFA burns, other than initial irrigation, is unknown. Irrigation may be performed with water, isotonic saline, or magnesium chloride.[60] We advise copious saline irrigation. Topical antibiotics and cycloplegics, along with light pressure patching, are also recommended. The use of topical steroids has been advocated by some in order to lessen corneal fibroblast formation, but other attempted therapies such as subconjunctival injections of calcium gluconate and ocular irrigation with quaternary ammonium compounds have been associated with additional injury.[61]

Chromic Acid Injury

Chromium compounds are used extensively in industry, mainly in metallic electroplating. Chromic acid is commonly used in concentrated solutions containing up to 25% sulfuric acid. It causes sufficient skin damage to allow absorption of the toxic chromium ion if intensive irrigation is not undertaken immediately. Heated (60°C–80°C) chromic acid makes the problem of chromium absorption much worse.

Dichromate salts containing hexavalent chromium are the most readily absorbed and the most toxic because they can cross cell membranes. The mortality rate from these burns is very high if the burn exceeds 10% TBSA. Chromium absorption leads to diarrhea, gastrointestinal bleeding, hemolysis, hepatic and renal damage, coma, encephalopathy, seizures, and disseminated intravascular coagulation.

Treatment includes immediate excision of the burned tissues to lessen the total body dichromate burden. Wounds should be washed with a 1% sodium phosphate or sulfate solution and dressed with bandages soaked in 5% sodium thiosulfate solution. These actions reduce the hexavalent chromium ion to the less well absorbed trivalent form.[62]

Chelation therapy with ethylenediaminetetraacetic acid should be instituted, and IV sodium thiosulfate and ascorbic acid given. Hemodialysis, peritoneal dialysis, or exchange transfusion may be indicated.

Phosphorus Burns

White phosphorus is a translucent, waxy substance that ignites spontaneously on contact with air. For this reason, it is usually stored under water. It is used primarily in fireworks, insecticides and rodenticides, and military weapons.

Phosphorus causes both thermal burns from the flaming pieces and acid burns, which result from the oxidation of phosphorus to phosphoric acid. The burns classically emit a white vapor with a characteristic garlic odor.[63]

These burns are treated first with immersion in water, followed by débridement of any gross debris. The wound is then washed with a 1% copper sulfate solution, which reacts with the residual phosphorus to form copper phosphate; the latter appears as black granules and allows for easy débridement. After débridement, the residual copper is removed by a thorough water rinse, and the wound is dressed and treated as any other burn.

Elemental Alkali Metal Burns

The commonly encountered alkali metals (sodium, lithium, and potassium) are highly reactive with water and with water vapor in air, producing their respective hydroxide with liberation of hydrogen gas. Therefore, water should never be used for extinguishing or débridement of the metal. A class D fire extinguisher or plain sand may be used for smothering the fire, followed by application of mineral oil or cooking oil to isolate the metal from water and allow safe débridement. The burn is then treated as an alkali burn.

Magnesium burns in a less intense fashion but otherwise acts as do other alkali metals. These burns may be particularly injurious, however, because if all of the metallic debris is not removed, the small ulcers that form will slowly enlarge until they become quite extensive.

The initial topical treatment for unusual chemical burns is outlined in Table 38–7.

EMERGENCY ESCHAROTOMY

Full-thickness burns result in an eschar that is inelastic and may become restrictive. During fluid resuscitation and as a direct result of transcapillary extravasation of fluid from thermal injury, intracellular and interstitial edema progresses. As the soft tissues become edematous and pressure rises under the unyielding eschar, first venous and then lymphatic, capillary, and ultimately arterial flow to the underlying and distal unburned tissue may be compromised. Full-thickness and extensive partial-thickness circumferential extremity burns are most likely to impede peripheral blood flow. Circumfer-

TABLE 38–7 Chemical Burn Treatment

Water lavage	Chromic acid	Tannic acid
	Potassium permanganate	Tannic acid
	Cantharides	Sulfosalicylic acid
	Lyes (hydroxide salts)	Trichloracetic acid
	Chlorox	Cresylic acid
	Dichromate salts	Acetic acid
	Pieric acid	Formic acid
Calcium salt infection	Oxalic acid	
	Hydrofluoric acid	
Oil immersion	Sodium metal	
	White phosphorus	
	Mustard gas	
Avoid water lavage	Sodium metal	
	Potassium metal	
	Lithium metal	
Specific approaches	Sodium metal	Excision
	Lyes (hydroxide salts)	Weak acid lavage (vinegar)
	Hydrofluoric acid	Calcium gluconate injection
	White phosphorus	Copper sulfate solution

entential chest burns may restrict chest wall movement, impairing ventilation, and circumferential neck burns may result in tracheal obstruction. In such cases, immediate escharotomy may be indicated.

On occasion, because of high-volume fluid resuscitation, noncircumferential and deep partial-thickness burns require surgical decompression to prevent complications of nerve or muscle damage. Once signs and symptoms of vascular impairment are present, the clinician must act quickly to prevent tissue hypoxia and cellular death. This pathophysiology may manifest itself within a timeframe that mandates that the emergency clinician must intervene. Frequent reassessment of capillary refill, Doppler signals, pulsoximetry, and compartment pressure measurments may detect developing ischemia. Escarotomy is rarely required in the ED, especially when resuscitative measures are being perfomred. The reluctance of non–burn specialists to perform an adequate escharotomy is illustrated by the report of Brown and associates,[64] who found that 44% of pediatric burn cases were inadequately decompressed before arrival at a referral burn unit.

It is not standard of care that emergency clinicians be skilled in emergency escarotomy, nor can it be expected that this procedure will be done in the ED. The technique is described here for those circumstances when escarotomy is considered by the non–burn specialist.

Indications

The indications for escharotomy are based on clinical examination, compartment pressure, or both. A high index of suspicion and a low threshold for intervention are essential for a successful outcome. Skin temperature and palpation of pulses are unreliable and imprecise indicators of adequacy of circulation because of peripheral vasoconstriction and local edema. The patient with circulatory embarrassment significant enough to warrant escharotomy may complain of deep aching pain, progressive loss of sensation, or paresthesias, but these parameters are difficult to quantitate in the severely burned, sedated, or mechanically ventilated patient. However, motor activity and peripheral pulses may remain intact despite severe underlying muscle ischemia. In the series by Brown and associates,[64] peripheral pulses were present in 74% of the limbs that required decompression. Muscle compartments with pressures in excess of 30 mm Hg should be decompressed. Measurements should be taken before and after escharotomy to ensure adequate decompression.

In the patient with absent distal arterial flow (as determined by Doppler ultrasonic flowmeter) but an otherwise adequate blood pressure, immediate escharotomy is indicated. Bardakjian and coworkers[65] suggested that an oxygen saturation below 95% in the distal extremity as demonstrated by pulse oximetry (in the absence of systemic hypoxia) also is a reliable indicator of the need for emergency escharotomy.

Technique of Escharotomy

Because full-thickness burns are insensible to pain and involve coagulation of superficial vessels, no anesthesia is needed. Deep partial-thickness burns may still possess pain sensation, and escharotomy may be performed with local anesthesia or systemic analgesia. A properly executed escharotomy releases the eschar to the depth of the SQ fat only. This results in minimal bleeding, which can be controlled by local pressure or electrocautery. These incisions, although limb- or life-

saving, are potential sources of infection for the burn patient and should be treated as part of the burn wound. The wounds should be loosely packed with sterile gauze impregnated with an appropriate topical antimicrobial such as silver sulfadiazine cream. Fasciotomy, which involves a deeper incision, may be needed for thermal or electrical burns.

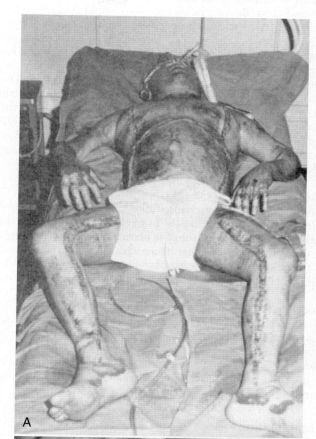
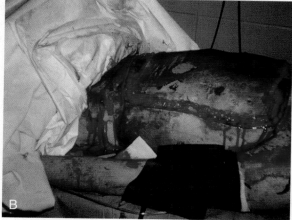

Figure 38–20 *A,* The circulatory embarrassment caused by edema beneath the encircling full-thickness burns of the legs of this patient was relieved by escharotomy incisions placed in the midmedial line of each limb. The restriction of the ventilatory excursion of the chest wall caused by the encircling full-thickness truncal burns was relieved by escharotomies placed in both anterior axillary lines and by a costal margin escharotomy. *B,* Compression of the abdominal contents and restriction of diaphragmatic excursion by the constricting deep abdominal wall burns were relieved by placement of escharotomy incisions in the lateral abdominal wall bilaterally. *(From Davis JH, Drucker WR, Foster RS, et al: Clinical Surgery. St. Louis, CV Mosby, 1987.)*

Limbs

Under sterile conditions, the lateral and medial aspects of the involved extremity are incised with a scalpel or electrocautery 1 cm proximal to the burned area, extending to 1 cm distal to the involved area of constricting burn (Fig. 38–20). The incision is carried through the full thickness of skin only and results in immediate separation of the constricting eschar to expose SQ fat. Because joints are areas of tight skin adherence and potential vascular impingement, incisions should cross these structures (Fig. 38–21). Care must be taken to avoid vital structures, such as the ulnar nerve at the elbow, the radial nerve at the wrist, the superficial peroneal nerve near the fibular head, and the posterior tibial artery at the ankle. The incision should extend to the great toe medially and the little toe laterally in circumferential burns of the feet and to the thenar and hypothenar aspects of the hands (see Figs. 38–20 and 38–21). Improvements in color, sensation, Doppler flow signal strength, and oximetry values indicate adequate release.

Chest

Full-thickness circumferential chest or upper abdominal burns may impair respiration. For release of this eschar, the incision should extend from the clavicle to the costal margin in the anterior axillary line bilaterally, avoiding breast tissue in females, and may be joined by transverse incisions, resulting in a chevron-shaped escharotomy.

Neck

Neck escharotomy should be performed laterally and posteriorly to avoid the carotid and jugular vessels.

Penis

Penile escharotomy is performed midlaterally to avoid the dorsal vein.

Complications

Complications of escharotomy include bleeding, infection, and damage to underlying structures. Complications of inadequate decompression include muscle necrosis, nerve injury (such as foot drop), and even amputation of the limb. Systemic

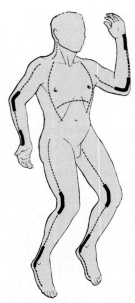

Figure 38–21 Preferred sites for escharotomy incisions. *Dotted lines* indicate the escharotomy sites. *Bold lines* indicate areas where caution is required because vascular structures and nerves may be damaged by escharotomy incisions. *(From Davis JH, Drucker WR, Foster RS, et al: Clinical Surgery. St. Louis, CV Mosby, 1987.)*

complications of inadequate decompression include myoglobinuria and renal failure, hyperkalemia, and metabolic acidosis.

CONCLUSION

Patients with circumferential or nearly circumferential burns should be evaluated for deep tissue ischemia. Emergency clinicians should not hesitate to perform an escharotomy before transfer of the patient to the burn center if there is evidence of reduced perfusion.

 REFERENCES CAN BE FOUND ON **EXPERT CONSULT**

GASTROINTESTINAL PROCEDURES

CHAPTER 39

Esophageal Foreign Bodies

David W. Munter

Patients with foreign bodies (FBs) lodged in the esophagus commonly present to the emergency department (ED) for evaluation and treatment. Objects may be accidentally or purposefully swallowed. Patients may present with a sensation of a recently passed FB, minor irritation, life-threatening airway obstruction, or other significant complications. Because of the anatomic and physiologic features of the esophagus, FBs in this area of the gastrointestinal tract present unique clinical issues to the clinician.

GENERAL FEATURES

Anatomy

The esophagus is a muscular tube, from 20 to 25 cm in length. There are three anatomic areas of narrowing in which FBs are most commonly entrapped (Fig. 39–1): the upper esophageal sphincter, which consists of the cricopharyngeus muscle; the crossover of the aortic arch in the midesophagus; and the lower esophageal sphincter (LES). *The LES is the narrowest point of the esophagus and of the entire gastrointestinal (GI) tract.*

Epidemiology

Patients with retained esophageal FBs generally fall into one of these categories: pediatric patients, psychiatric patients, prisoners, and adults who either are edentulous or have underlying esophageal pathology.

Children account for 75% to 85% of esophageal FBs seen in the ED, with the peak incidence at ages 18 to 48 months.[1–9] The incidence is equal in boys and girls. Inquisitive children frequently place objects in their mouths, and unintentional swallowing is common. As a result, children most commonly ingest coins, buttons, marbles, beads, screws, or pins.[1,2,4,9–13] Unlike adults, children who have entrapped FBs do not normally have underlying esophageal disorders.[14]

Patients with an anatomic abnormality of the esophagus or a motor disturbance are more prone to entrapment of FBs.[12,15,16] Anatomic abnormalities include strictures, webs, rings, diverticuli, and malignancies. Motor disturbances include achalasia, scleroderma, and esophageal spasm. Adults who have dentures or underlying esophageal anatomic or motor abnormalities may accidentally ingest food boluses, chicken or fish bones, glass, toothpicks, fruit pits, or pills while in the act of eating.[13]

Prisoners and psychiatric patients ingest a wide variety of objects, some of which may be quite unusual: spoons, razor blades, pins, nails, or practically any other object.[12,15]

Complications

Impacted FBs of the esophagus must be removed or dislodged. The timeframe under which this mandate must be carried out varies widely and depends on many circumstances. In general, however, the esophagus does not tolerate FBs well, or for prolonged periods of time, being prone to pressure, edema, necrosis, infection, and eventually perforation. FBs can transit the esophagus in a matter of seconds or minutes or may adhere to the mucosa. Retained objects may become less symptomatic after time, and the clinician must resist the urge to allow esophageal FBs to "pass by themselves" or "dissolve." Once FBs become stuck in the mucosa, *they may become less symptomatic but they rarely pass on their own.* The one exception may be in children with coins, especially those lodged at the LES. Approximately one third of these coins may pass spontaneously within 24 hours, and some authors have advocated an observation approach, although this is more poorly accepted by parents.[17–20]

A wide array of complications can arise from retained esophageal FBs (Table 39–1). These include benign mucosal abrasions, lacerations, esophageal stricture,[21] and necrosis from corrosive agents such as button batteries. Esophageal perforation[22–27] can lead to life-threatening conditions such as retropharyngeal abscess,[28] mediastinitis, pericarditis, pericardial tamponade,[29] pneumothorax, pneumomediastinum, tracheoesophageal fistula, and vascular injuries including to the subclavian vein and the aorta.[20,30,31] Complications are more common when FBs are entrapped for longer than 24 hours[2,32] and when they are sharp.[33] An estimated 1500 deaths occur annually from esophageal FBs, primarily from complications of esophageal perforation.[9]

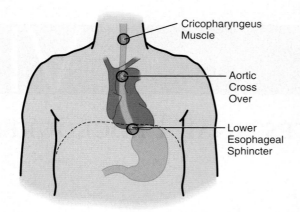

Figure 39–1 Blunt esophageal foreign bodies (FBs) are most commonly lodged at one of three anatomic areas of narrowing: the cricopharyngeus muscle, the level of the aortic crossover, and the lower esophageal sphincter (LES).

TABLE 39–1 Complications of Esophageal Foreign Bodies

Airway compromise due to tracheal compression
Aspiration pneumonia
Esophageal necrosis
Esophageal perforation
Esophageal stricture
Failure to thrive
Mediastinitis
Mucosal abrasion
Paraesophageal abscess
Pericarditis/pericardial tamponade
Pneumothorax
Pneumomediastinum
Retropharyngeal abscess
Tracheoesophageal fistula
Vascular injury including aortic perforation
Vocal cord paralysis

Clinical Presentation

An esophageal FB impaction usually presents acutely, particularly in adults who have a clear history of ingestion. Children also commonly remember an ingestion, but some will have a vague presentation or history. As many as one third of children with proven esophageal FBs are asymptomatic on presentation[20,34–36]; therefore, a high index of suspicion is indicated, especially in a child who was seen with an object in his or her mouth that disappeared. This is especially true if there was transient coughing or gagging, even though the actual ingestion was not witnessed. Poor feeding, irritability, fever, stridor, cough, wheezing, and aspiration can all be caused by an underlying esophageal FB in a child, especially young infants.[15,37–39]

Dysphagia is a common presenting complaint in esophageal FBs. Drooling is suggestive of a high-grade obstruction, and the complete inability to handle oral secretions is a sign of complete obstruction. Infants with a clandestine esophageal FB can present with wheezing, or chronic cough. They may appear to have bronchospasm and may be treated for asthma. Stridor from an FB can mimic epiglottitis.

TABLE 39–2 Level of Entrapment of Esophageal Foreign Bodies

Level	Pediatric (%)	Adult (%)
Cricopharyngeus muscle	74	24
Aortic crossover	14	8
Lower esophageal sphincter	12	68

The esophagus is well innervated proximally, and patients typically can accurately localize FBs in the oropharynx or upper third of the esophagus. However, scratches or abrasions of the esophagus can create a persistent FB sensation. Upper esophageal FBs often cause gagging or vomiting. In rare cases, an upper esophageal FB can impinge upon the trachea, especially in children, mimicking infection by creating wheezing, stridor, or frank respiratory distress. The lower two thirds of the esophagus is not as well innervated, and FBs in this location typically cause vague symptoms of discomfort, fullness, or nonlocalizing pain. Swallowed coins that lodge in the lower esophagus of children may cause no overt symptoms until feeding is attempted.

The location of retained esophageal FBs is age related (Table 39–2). Children more typically have entrapped objects in the upper esophagus at the level of the cricopharyngeus muscle, whereas adults more commonly have entrapments at the LES.[18,38,40–42]

Evaluation

The most useful aspect of the evaluation is the history. The time of the ingestion, size and shape of the ingested object, and any current symptoms should be ascertained. The physical examination is frequently normal in patients with esophageal FBs, unless they present with complete obstruction. In this case, they will be drooling, spitting, and unable to handle oral secretions. Even though a patient may be asymptomatic on presentation, transient coughing or gagging should raise the index of suspicion for an esophageal FB. An examination of the oropharynx, neck, respiratory system, cardiac system, and abdomen is essential in the evaluation of potential complications.

After attending to life-threatening conditions such as airway compromise, the goal of the ED evaluation is to localize the FB to determine what, if any, interventions need to be undertaken to remove it or assist its transit into the stomach. Once an FB passes into the stomach, it has a greater than 90% likelihood of passing through the entire GI tract without any further problems.[33] Even large, irregular, and seemingly dangerous FBs will often transit the entire GI tract with relative ease.

RADIOLOGY OF ESOPHAGEAL FOREIGN BODIES
Background

Radiographic imaging of a patient with a suspected esophageal FB is a common practice and is particularly useful for the detection of radiopaque FBs. Traditionally, the inability to quickly identify the object by physical examination encouraged the use of plain radiography in attempts to verify and localize the retained FB. Plain radiography limitations require that other diagnostic approaches be considered as well.

Indications

Interactive, verbal patients can provide valuable information about the ingested culprit and can typically localize the retained body with reliable accuracy.[43] In these cases, the diagnostic work-up should be tailored to the localization of symptoms and the ingested material. However, nonverbal patients including preschool children and those who are senile or debilitated warrant a low threshold for screening radiography in cases with a suspicious history. Examples include a child seen with an object in the mouth that "disappeared" or a patient with symptomatology suggestive of an esophageal FB such as drooling, gagging, or unexplained respiratory symptoms.

Plain Radiographs

Plain radiographs reliably verify and localize radiopaque FBs such as glass and metal of sufficient size and are indicated as the main method of radiologic evaluation for these objects.

Unfortunately, many ingested FBs are nonopaque including non bony foods, plastic, wood, and aluminum. Some pull tabs from beer cans may be seen if oriented in the coronal plane. A magnetic metal detector has been reported to help localize radiolucent aluminum pull tabs.[44,45] Calcification of fish and chicken bones is often incomplete, and cooking alters bone structure, making them radiolucent on plain films. The degree of bony calcification varies with fish species and between different samples of the same species, thus preventing useful guidelines.[46–49] For these reasons, *plain films provide little substantive evidence in the majority of cases of fish or chicken bone dysphagia.* They detect only 25% to 55% of endoscopically proven bones and carry a high rate of false-negative and false-positive interpretations.[43,48–53] Because of the lack of diagnostic value for detecting bones, *many clinicians do not routinely order plain radiographs, opting initially for computed tomography (CT) scan in those cases for which radiographic evaluation is required.*[54]

When used, a complete oropharyngeal radiograph series includes the nasopharynx to the lower cervical vertebra in both lateral and anteroposterior views. Optimum quality radiographs are mandatory. Patients should be positioned upright with the neck extended and the shoulders held low. Soft tissue technique enhances the discrimination of weak radiopaque FBs. Phonation of "eeeee" during radiography prevents motion artifact from swallowing, distends the hypopharynx, and enhances soft tissue landmarks. As previously mentioned, FBs are most frequently entrapped at one of three locations in the esophagus: the cricopharyngeus muscle (Fig. 39–2), the aortic crossover (Fig. 39–3), and the LES (Fig. 39–4).

Plain radiography of the neck is limited by the radiographic properties of ingested materials and the complicated anatomy of the upper aerodigestive tract. The tongue base, palatine and lingual tonsils, vallecula, and pyriform recesses are common regions of entrapment for small, sharp objects and deserve careful interpretive attention (Fig. 39–5). Superimposition of the mandible contributes to suboptimal resolution of this region on lateral neck films.[55] Calcified airway cartilages often masquerade as FBs and contribute to false-positive rates as high as 25%.[43,48,50,52,56–58] Normal ossification of airway cartilages begins in the 3rd decade and progresses with age.[59] The typical curvilinear contour and well-defined margins of bony FB fragments may help distinguish them

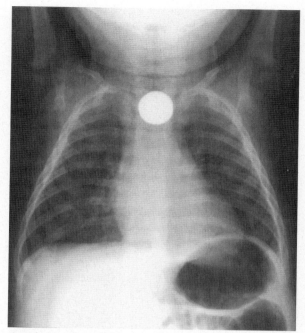

Figure 39–2 Posteroanterior (PA) radiograph of an esophageal FB (coin) lodged at the level of the cricopharyngeus muscle. This is the most common area of the esophagus to harbor a coin in children. Coins remaining in the upper tract are usually removed unless there is steady progression with observation. This coin would likely be symptomatic in an infant, causing respiratory distress, drooling, wheezing, and perhaps stridor. *Note:* Chance of spontaneous passage, about 20%–25%.

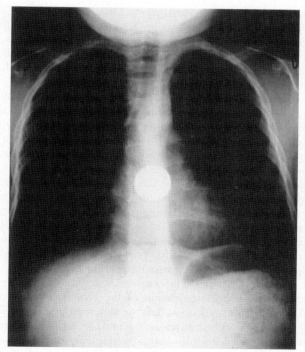

Figure 39–3 PA radiograph of an esophageal FB (coin) lodged at the level of the aortic crossover. *Note:* Chance of spontaneous passage, about 20%–25%.

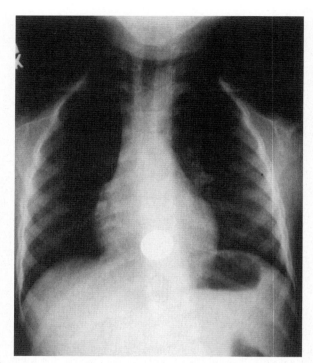

Figure 39–4 PA radiograph of an esophageal FB (coin) lodged at the level of the LES. Coins in this area are most likely to pass and be favorably manipulated by medication (see Table 39–3). *Note:* Chance of spontaneous passage, about 25%–60%; chances increase with prolonged observation. *(From Waltzman ML, Baskin M, Wypij D, et al: A randomized clinical trial of the management of esophageal coins in children. Pediatrics 116:614, 2005; and Soprano JV, Fleisher GR, Mandl KD: The spontaneous passage of esophageal coins in children. Arch Pediatr Adolesc Med 153:1073, 1999.)*

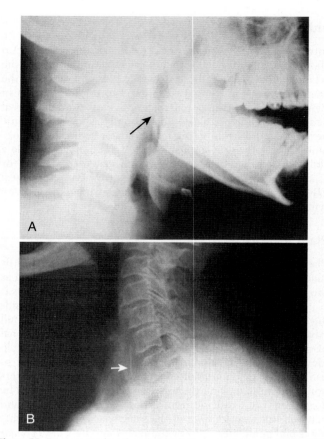

Figure 39–5 *A,* Lateral neck radiograph shows a chicken bone (*arrow*) lodged in the pharynx with associated soft tissue swelling. Plain radiographs have poor diagnostic accuracy for detecting bones in the esophagus, and they are often eschewed in favor of a computed tomography (CT) scan if radiographic evaluation is deemed necessary. *B,* Chicken bone in the lower esophagus where it is more readily seen on radiograph.

from normal laryngeal calcifications. Orientation of bony FBs is variable. The C6 vertebra approximates the level of the cricopharyngeus, a common site of FB impaction. Increased prevertebral soft tissue width, air within the cervical esophagus, and soft tissue emphysema are rare indirect findings that may help identify radiolucent objects.[49,60]

Posteroanterior (PA) and lateral views of the chest evaluate the remainder of the esophagus. Both projections are indicated to identify multiple objects and those FBs visible in only one plane. Esophageal FBs typically lie in the vertical plane and are differentiated from airway bodies or calcifications by their location posterior to the tracheal air column on lateral radiographs. As a rule, flat objects such as coins perch in the coronal plane in the esophagus and in the sagittal orientation in the trachea. Intraesophageal air and air-fluid levels represent indirect evidence of esophageal obstruction and may aid in verification of radiopaque FBs. Soft tissue swelling, extraluminal air, and aspiration pnuemonitis can occasionally help identify complicated impactions radiographically.

In children, a nasopharynx-to-anus film is frequently obtained, allowing visualization of the entire nasopharynx, throat, and esophagus, as well as the abdomen in case the FB has passed into the stomach or beyond. Radiation exposure can be minimized if adult-sized radiograph cassettes are used. Swallowed coins or other FBs may become lodged in the nasopharynx, usually after gagging or vomiting, and could be missed if this area is not included on the radiograph. In adults, if neck or chest films are negative, abdominal films are sometimes obtained for reassurance of the presence of the FB in the stomach.

Contrast Esophagograms

Background

The contrast esophagogram is a test with limited utility in the ED as a routine intervention to evaluate for an esophageal FB. It may be considered when plain radiographs are negative, but the esophagogram has largely been replaced by CT and endoscopy for FB evaluation. This technique uses swallowed contrast to help identify the presence and location of an impacted radiolucent FB, the degree of obstruction, underlying anatomic abnormalities, and the presence of perforation. A variation of this technique is to have the patient swallow contrast-soaked cotton pledgets. This technique uses smaller contrast loads and may identify impacted FBs by impeding progression of the cotton or by tagging sharp irregular objects with radiopaque cotton threads as the bolus passes. Theoretically, this variation might interfere less with follow-up endoscopy owing to attenuated contrast loads. Unfortunately, liquid contrast ingestion yields overall results no better than those of plain film radiography. More importantly, contrast may interfere with the detection and extraction of FBs at endoscopy (barium) and may increase the risk of aspiration pneumonitis (diatrizoate meglumine and diatrizoate sodium [Gastrografin]).[49,61,62] Therefore, routine, serial contrast esophagograms after negative plain radiography for patients with known or suspected FBs are unnecessary for diagnostic purposes in most cases. Selective use is reasonable, but CT or endoscopy is the intervention with the best, and most cost-effective, yield.[63]

Procedure

Esophagograms couple voluntary ingestion of enteric contrast (Gastrografin or barium) and plain radiography. Immediately after ingestion, erect and horizontal radiographs are performed at right-angle projections (PA and lateral or right and left anterior oblique). In addition to anatomic abnormalities, radiolucent FBs may be identified by contrast delineation or filling defects within the contrast column (Fig. 39–6).

The initial choice of contrast agent is debated and should be individualized depending on the threat of aspiration and perforation. Other logistical concerns, listed later, have relegated this test to minimal use in the ED. Water-soluble Gastrografin is indicated first in most cases of suspected perforation because it causes less mediastinal inflammation when extravasated; however, it can cause a severe chemical pneumonitis if aspirated and is relatively contraindicated in patients with a complete esophageal obstruction.[12] Patients without evidence

of complete esophageal obstruction are instructed to swallow progressively larger aliquots of contrast agent up to approximately 50 mL. If these films are normal, the procedure is repeated with half-strength and then full-strength barium to delineate small esophageal injuries. Note that water-soluble contrast (Gastrografin) causes more pulmonary reaction than barium when inadvertently aspirated and should be used in small aliquots if aspiration or complete esophageal obstruction is a concern. Contrast esophagograms coupled with fluoroscopy are seldom used in acute esophageal FB impactions, although slowed progression or abnormal peristalsis may suggest a retained FB or an anatomic abnormality. Barium interferes with endoscopy and should not be used when endoscopy is anticipated.

CT

Noncontrast CT of the neck and mediastinum is an easy, rapid, cost-effective, and noninvasive means of detecting or ruling out upper GI FBs (Fig. 39–7)[48,49,51,54] and has garnered support in the clinical setting of suspected FB entrapment.[64-66] CT further excels at localization and characterization of the

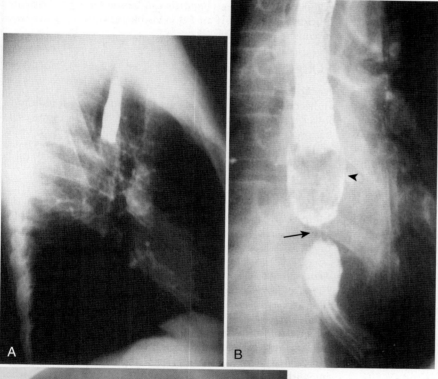

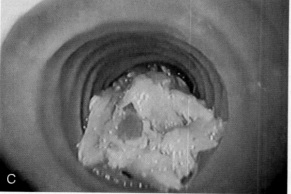

Figure 39–6 *A,* Barium swallow demonstrates a complete esophageal obstruction in the proximal to midesophagus. *B,* Barium esophagogram demonstrates a large piece of meat lodged above an esophageal stricture (peptic). Many patients with lodged meat have underlying esophageal pathology. *C,* Bolus of meat seen in the distal esophagus with endoscope. The scope provides removal and esophageal evaluation simultaneously. This young person had a ringed esophagus as his pathology.

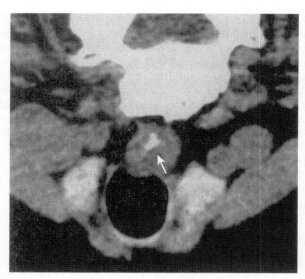

Figure 39–7 CT demonstrates an esophageal FB.

impacted FB and identification of associated complications such as perforation.[49,64,67–69]

CT clearly provides improved diagnostic utility for fish bone FB over that of plain radiography with or without barium.[48,49,51,54] Using CT in cases with high clinical suspicion of a retained FB has the potential to reduce the number of unnecessary endoscopies.[51]

Conclusions

Diagnostic radiography for esophageal FB requires case individualization. Plain radiographs clearly assist the clinician in two situations: (1) screening of children, senile adults, and nonverbal patients with a history or symptoms suspicious for purposeful or inadvertent FB ingestion that *can be assumed to be radiopaque*, and (2) localization of known radiopaque ingestants to clarify the necessity and means of FB extraction. Conversely, attempts to verify radiolucent bodies, including bones, by plain radiographs are often misleading. Contrast esophagograms may be used in special situations but have largely been replaced by CT and direct endoscopy. The utility of CT to exclude fish bones and other FBs is effective when initial routine plain films are avoided.[63]

VISUALIZATION OF ESOPHAGEAL/ PHARYNGEAL FOREIGN BODIES

Direct Pharyngoscopy

Background

Direct visualization of the oropharynx is simply a physical examination using a light source and aided by a tongue blade. This examination is limited to visualizing only the upper oropharynx, tonsils, tonsillar pillars, and in some cases, the tip of the epiglottis. In many cases, an FB such as a fish bone can be visualized and then removed with forceps.

Indications

Direct visualization is indicated in most patients who have an FB sensation in the oropharynx or upper neck. The only contraindication is a patient with potential airway obstruction.

Procedure

The supplies needed for a direct visualization are a light source and a tongue depressor. Although penlights are traditionally used for this purpose, a fiberoptic headlight or a head mirror reflecting a bright light source is superior for a thorough examination. When using a headlamp, position the lamp on the examiner's forehead between the eyes, and focus the beam at a distance of approximately 2 ft. Test the position by focusing the beam on the examiner's thumbs held together at a comfortable working distance. When using a head mirror, position it with the central hole over the examiner's dominant eye. Position the light source behind one shoulder of the patient, where it will be reflected by the head mirror into the oropharynx.

For the best direct visualization, place the patient in a sitting position, with the examiner standing. Examine the entire visible oropharynx using a tongue depressor to carefully depress the base of the tongue and provide better visualization of the pharyngeal wall, tonsils, and tonsillar pillars. Having the patient apply gentle but firm traction to her or his own tongue can also aid exposure. Ask the patient to assume a "sniffing" position with the neck slightly flexed and the head extended. Use a topical anesthetic on the pharyngeal mucosa to minimize discomfort and gagging when using the tongue blade. The tip of the epiglottis can be seen in some patients, especially children. If an FB is visible, grasp the object with forceps to remove it.

Indirect Laryngoscopy

Background

Indirect laryngoscopy is an examination of the middle and lower oropharynx using a mirror. This technique allows evaluation of the epiglottis, vallecula, arytenoids, arytenoid folds, and vocal cords. Indirect visualization requires experience with the procedure and a cooperative patient. This technique has been largely replaced by endoscopy.

Indications

Indirect visualization can be used in patients who have an FB sensation in the oropharynx or upper neck, with the exception of those with airway compromise.

Procedure

Prepare for the procedure by assembling a light source (headlight or head mirror), a laryngeal mirror, a topical anesthetic agent, and a gauze pad to hold the patient's tongue (see Chapter 64, Otolaryngologic Procedures). Place the patient in a sitting position leaning slightly forward, as described for direct pharyngoscopy. Anesthetize the oropharynx by spraying with topical anesthetic. Warm the laryngeal mirror either in warm water or a mirror warmer (to prevent fogging) and check the temperature on the back of your hand. Stand in front of the patient and grasp the tongue with the gauze pad. Pull lightly on the tongue while having the patient open his or her mouth widely. Insert the mirror without touching the tongue. Elevate the uvula and soft palate slightly with the mirror if necessary, but avoid the pharyngeal wall. If the patient cannot tolerate this maneuver without gagging, instill more topical anesthetic and reattempt. Evaluate the base of the tongue, epiglottis, vallecula, arytenoids, arytenoid folds, and vocal cords. Use forceps to remove a visible FB. If unable to extract a visible FB, obtain otorhinolaryngology or gastroenterology consultation for endoscopy and removal.

Nasopharyngoscopy

Background

Careful visualization of the oropharynx and hypopharynx is vital in the evaluation of patients presenting with complaints of FB sensation. Although a significant proportion of complete evaluations will not discover any abnormalities, the combination of direct, indirect, and flexible endoscopic nasopharyngoscopy is simple, fast, and curative in those with an identifiable FB,[43,55,70] thereby reducing the need for rigid esophagoscopy and general anesthesia in these patients.

Indications and Contraindications

Indications for this procedure span the scope of clinical situations necessitating thorough visual examination of the pharynx and proximal esophagus, including patients with FB sensation and acute pill and postprandial food dysphagia.

Croup is quoted as the sole absolute contraindication to flexible nasopharyngoscopy.[71] The risk-to-benefit ratio of endoscopy should be considered in patients with coagulopathy or severe bleeding diathesis, although the risk of initiating significant hemorrhage is low. Medication allergy precludes the use of some topical agents.

Equipment

Nasopharyngoscopy is best accomplished via a 3- to 6-mm external diameter flexible fiberoptic nasopharyngoscope (see Chapter 64, Otolaryngologic Procedures). Scope side ports enable suction, anesthetic injection, and FB extraction via forceps, but are not mandatory. Traditional scopes require an external light source whereas some newer-generation fiberoptic scopes include battery-powered, self-contained light sources. Inexpensive adapters enable a laryngoscope handle to double as an endoscopy light source. The endoscope eyepiece should be adjusted to accommodate the operator's visual acuity. Yankauer suction and angled McGill forceps or a Kelly clamp should be available to retrieve identified FBs orally. Topical cocaine, phenylephrine (Neo-Synephrine), oxymetazoline (Afrin), and liquid or viscous lidocaine may be used for anesthesia and vasoconstriction, but are not necessities.

Procedure

Nasopharyngoscopy is generally well tolerated, but patients should have a clear understanding of the examination procedure before initiation. Discuss the procedure with the patient and include potential complications and alternatives.

Topical anesthesia is recommended for patient comfort but is not mandatory.[43,55] Examine the nares and choose the one with the least anatomic resistance for endoscopy. Cotton balls or pledgets soaked with 10% cocaine or a combination of 0.05% oxymetazoline (Afrin) and 2% lidocaine (Xylocaine) provide nasal mucosal anesthesia and vasoconstriction within minutes. Viscous 2% to 4% lidocaine applied by a cotton-tipped applicator is an alternative anesthetic. Atomized 2% lidocaine (Xylocaine) or topical benzocaine spray (20% Hurricane spray, Cetacaine) can be used to further anesthetize the hypopharynx. Patients may complain of discomfort or globus sensation after anesthesia and may require explanation and reassurance. Patients only rarely need an antisialogogue, such as glycopyrrolate. Others may need mild sedation with a short-acting benzodiazepine.

Ask the patient to sit upright in a chair with posterior headrest support to prevent movement during examination.

Stand in front of the patient and hold the scope in the non-dominant hand (see Chapter 64, Otolaryngologic Procedures). Control scope maneuvers solely with the hands. The dominant hand controls the depth of scope insertion at the naris and directs the scope along the horizontal plane at the floor of the nose. This hand should rest lightly on the patient's face for comfort and to prevent abrupt changes in scope position in case of movement during examination. Flexion in the sagittal plane is achieved with the thumb lever on the scope handle. Rotation clockwise and counterclockwise is performed via simple rotation of the wrist, not the entire upper body. It is important to maintain mild tension on the two ends of the scope for wrist action to be translated to motion at the tip of the scope. Warming the tip of the scope in water and applying silicone drops helps prevent scope fogging. Manipulation against the patient's mucosa will clear the scope during endoscopy. Water-soluble lubricant aids in passing the scope but should not be applied to the distal 2 cm of the scope.

Effective examination of the oropharynx requires some practice and reference to normal anatomy. Although many patients can localize the FB, systematic examination in a caudal direction is vital.[43] Direct the patient to focus on slow, steady mouth breathing to attenuate discomfort and gagging during the procedure. Insert the scope horizontally along the floor of the nose and pass it below the inferior turbinate. Upon reaching the soft palate, deflect the scope tip inferiorly (via directing the thumb lever toward the eyepiece) and advance it into the oropharynx. Examine the laterally located palatine tonsils and palatopharyngeal arches, along with the proximal tongue and lingual tonsil. Advance the scope caudally to allow further visualization of the tongue base, epiglottis, and the interposed spaces, known as the epiglottic vallecula. Voluntary or manual protrusion of the tongue helps reveal this anatomy. Scan posteriorly to reveal the vocal cords, aryepiglottic folds, and pyriform recesses. Patients can gently exhale against a closed mouth and nose to distend the lower pharyngeal structures and improve visualization of these areas. Avoid contact with the epiglottis and vocal cords. Explore all pharyngeal walls fully and compare the structures bilaterally, even when patients localize symptoms to one side. Signs of trauma, including bleeding, mucosal hyperemia, and edema, require close investigation to differentiate retained FBs from mucosal irritation.

If an FB is visualized (Fig. 39–8), the method of extraction depends on the location and size of the retained object. Small FBs may be extracted transnasally via forceps passed through the scope side port. Large or irregular bodies may be withdrawn orally with angled forceps.[55] Alternatively, endoscopy may be used primarily for FB confirmation. Extraction can then be performed via handheld forceps under endoscopy guidance, subsequent direct laryngoscopy, or under general anesthesia. Careful attention to prevent FB dislodgment into the airway is critical with any extraction attempt.

Complications

Complications of nasopharyngoscopy are rare and typically mild. Reflex tearing, sneezing, and coughing are the most common and are self-limited. Some patients experience a residual FB sensation for several hours after manipulation. Mild bleeding, including epistaxis, is common secondary to mucosal abrasion. Extraction of an embedded FB may result in bleeding but is also generally self-limited. Vasovagal syncope has been reported in up to 3% of patients undergoing this procedure.[71] Inadvertent dislodgment of the FB farther

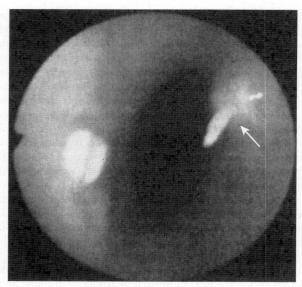

Figure 39–8 Esophageal FB seen on nasopharyngoscopy.

into the esophagus or into the airway may occur with manipulation or attempted extraction.

Esophagoscopy

Esophagoscopy is the definitive diagnostic and therapeutic procedure for impacted esophageal FBs.[9,41] Although esophagoscopy is not a procedure performed by the emergency clinician, its proper role in the ED evaluation of FBs must be understood. With esophagoscopy, the clinician can document the presence and location of the FB along with any underlying lesion. The clinician can then remove the object and reevaluate the esophagus after FB removal to rule out perforation or underlying pathology. Esophagoscopy may be necessary even if a radiologic contrast study does not reveal complete obstruction because x-ray studies are not always conclusive.[8,72] Esophagoscopy may be necessary to rule out predisposing pathology or resultant perforation, even when symptoms presumed to be due to an esophageal FB have resolved.

Esophagoscopy is the preferred method for removal of sharp or pointed objects such as bones, open safety pins, and razors. In the case of sharp objects prone to causing esophageal perforation, intravenous antibiotics should be administered before the procedure. Endoscopy is the preferred way to remove an impacted meat bolus and to evaluate for possible esophageal pathology at the same time. Esophagoscopy is also indicated for an FB retained for more than 24 to 48 hours both to remove it and to examine for esophageal wall erosion or perforation. Esophagoscopy is the only appropriate removal technique for multiple or large esophageal FBs. This technique is also indicated in the patient with an FB proved to have passed into the stomach and who has persistent symptoms possibly caused by esophageal wall injury. Flexible endoscopic procedures can usually be performed without general anesthesia, even in most children.[73] The success rate of flexible endoscopy in patients with retained esophageal FBs exceeds 96%.[41,74]

Traditionally, esophagoscopy is more expensive than other maneuvers such as Foley catheter removal or esophageal bougienage (described later),[3,7,75] largely owing to charges for the surgical suite, but it has a higher success rate than the other two techniques. The ED removal of esophageal FBs in children by experienced endoscopists, while the child is under ketamine sedation administered by the emergency clinician, has been reviewed.[76] In select cases, this approach can shorten the interval to procedural completion and expense.

ESOPHAGEAL PHARMACOLOGIC MANEUVERS

Background

Because the LES is the narrowest portion of the entire GI tract, most FBs that reach the stomach eventually move through the GI tract without further problems. Because a large number of entrapped esophageal FBs are lodged at the LES, especially in adults, several therapeutic maneuvers have been developed to assist transit into the stomach, including pharmacologic relaxation of the LES. In theory, agents that promote smooth muscle relaxation should improve mobility through the LES. Although many clinicians use pharmacologic adjuncts for all esophageal FBs, objects lodged at the LES will probably benefit most from such interventions. Nonspecific *pain relief, anxiolysis, vomiting, and spontaneous passage over time may account for the success attributed to many pharmacologic manipulations of esophageal FBs.*

Several pharmacologic agents, including diazepam, meperidine, and atropine, have been shown to be *unsuccessful* for removing or resolving esophageal FB impactions.[13] These agents, alone or in combination, have success rates below 10%, which is no better than observation alone.[2] Glucagon, nitroglycerin, nifedipine, and gas-forming agents (Table 39–3) are described later and are the most effective pharmacologic agents for treatment of distal esophageal food impactions.

Indications and Contraindications

The indication for pharmacologic relaxation of the LES is the presence of a smooth or blunt FB such as a coin or food bolus. Angulated, abrasive, or sharp FBs should not be treated with pharmacologic modalities but instead should be removed by esophagoscopy. Analgesics and sedatives are routinely indicated if pain is present or the patient is excessively anxious.

Glucagon

Pharmacology

Glucagon has been a prototype for the spasmolytic agents.[77–79] Glucagon theoretically relaxes esophageal smooth muscle and decreases the LES resting pressure. One study of normal subjects found that glucagon significantly lowers the mean LES resting pressure, but causes no significant difference in the mean amplitude of contraction in the distal esophagus.[80] Glucagon has no effect on the upper third of the esophagus, a common site of coin impaction in children, where striated muscle is present and some voluntary control is operative. It only minimally affects the middle third of the esophagus. Peristalsis is not affected by glucagon. Results with glucagon have been mixed, and the only randomized study, done in children, showed no better results than placebo.[81] Its use, however, is still advocated by some authorities and has little downside. Glucagon may cause vomiting, and this action may be responsible for some of the drug's success.[82]

TABLE 39-3 Recommended Pharmacologic Therapies for Esophageal Foreign Bodies

Class and Agents	Site of Action	Dose and Route	Adverse Effects
Spasmolytics			
Glucagon	LES	1–2 mg IV*	Nausea, vomiting, hyperglycemia, hypersensitivity
Nitroglycerin	Body and LES	0.4–0.8 mg SL†	Hypotension Tachycardia
Nifedipine	LES	5–10 mg SL‡	Bradycardia Hypotension Tachycardia *Use with caution*
Gas-Forming Agents			
Tartaric acid	Distal and proximal	15 mL tartaric acid (18–20 g/100 mL)§	Vomiting Increased intraesophageal pressure
Sodium bicarbonate	Distal and proximal	15 mL sodium bicarbonate (10 g/100 mL)§	Vomiting
Carbonated beverage	Distal and proximal	100 mL PO	Increased intraesophageal pressure

*May be repeated once or used in conjunction with nitroglycerin.
†1–2 inches of nitroglycerin paste applied under an occlusive dressing may be an alternative.
‡A capsule is punctured, chewed, held in the mouth for 3 min, and then swallowed. Owing to *hypotension*, a 5-mg dose may be used in elderly. *Do not use if the patient has cardiovascular disease, is hypotensive, or has also recently been given nitroglycerin.*
§Alternatively, dissolve 2–3 g tartaric acid and 2–3 g sodium bicarbonate in 30 mL water.
IV, intravenously; LES, lower esophageal sphincter; PO, per os (orally); SL, sublingually.

Indications and Contraindications

Glucagon is most useful for smooth FBs or food impactions at the LES that are suspected because of the patient's complaint of pain or "something stuck" in the lower chest or epigastrium. The clinical diagnosis is usually straightforward, especially if there is a complete esophageal obstruction and the patient is unable to tolerate oral secretions. Nevertheless, some clinicians recommend that the FB be localized first with radiographs (with or without contrast) to establish that the impaction is indeed there. The radiographs can then serve as the baseline study for comparison after glucagon administration. However, with a classic history and physical examination, most investigators agree that an initial contrast study can be omitted. Glucagon is not effective in upper and middle esophageal obstructions, and it is not widely recommended for use in children. Also, glucagon is usually not effective in patients with fixed fibrotic strictures or rings at the gastroesophageal junction.[78] Glucagon is contraindicated if the patient has an insulinoma, a pheochromocytoma, Zollinger-Ellison syndrome, a hypersensitivity to glucagon, or a sharp esophageal FB.

Administration of Glucagon

Some reports recommend a small test dose to check for hypersensitivity to glucagon. In practice, this is rarely done. The therapeutic dose is 0.25 to 2 mg administered intravenously over 1 to 2 minutes in the sitting patient, although one study found that in normal subjects, 1 mg provides no significant additive benefit over 0.5 mg glucagon.[80] The patient is given water orally within 1 minute after the injection of glucagon to stimulate normal esophageal peristalsis; this helps push the food through the relaxed LES into the stomach. Glucagon has a rapid onset and short duration of action. The GI smooth muscle relaxes within 45 seconds, and the duration of action is about 25 minutes. If there are no results within 10 to 20 minutes, a second administration of 0.25 to 2 mg may be tried. Success rates are higher when combining glucagon with gas-forming agents or even carbonated beverages.[83,84] It is recommended that a small volume of some oral fluid be routinely given to enhance the activity of glucagon.

Complications

Glucagon is associated with a few minor side effects. If administered too rapidly, it causes nausea and vomiting. Therefore, the adult patient must be alert and mobile enough to avoid aspiration. Occasionally, vomiting dislodges the impacted food bolus. Theoretically, there is a risk of rupture of the obstructed esophagus during induced emesis, so slow injection is preferred to minimize this side effect.

The administration of glucagon is also associated with dizziness. Mild elevation of blood glucose levels is also common but is not of clinical concern and blood glucose levels do not need to be monitored. No fatalities have been reported. Although theoretically glucagon can stimulate catecholamine release with a pheochromocytoma and induce hypoglycemia from reflex insulin release with insulinoma, these endocrine tumors are rare. Nonetheless, precipitation of either profound catecholamine or insulin reactions with glucagon use should direct a work-up for these underlying tumors.

Further Evaluation and Therapy

If the patient experiences symptomatic relief after glucagon administration, a postprocedure radiograph or contrast study may be obtained to confirm passage of a radiopaque object, but this is not mandatory. Adult patients with successful passage into the stomach may also be discharged home, but careful follow-up should be obtained to rule out coexistent esophageal pathology. This is because a significant number of patients (65%–80%) will have underlying esophageal disorders.[9,16] If glucagon fails to produce symptomatic relief or resolve radiograph findings, its use does not preclude other methods from being used.

Nitroglycerin and Nifedipine

Pharmacology

Both sublingual nitroglycerin and nifedipine have been used in a manner similar to that of glucagon to relieve LES tone and allow the passage of a distal esophageal FB.[85–87] Although these two agents have been used less than glucagon for the treatment of esophageal FBs, both are useful for the relief of chest pain associated with esophageal smooth muscle spasm[64] and may be administered concurrently with glucagon. Manometric and radiographic studies after the administration of nitroglycerin reveal abolition of repetitive high-pressure wave contractions characteristic of esophageal spasm. Nifedipine, conversely, significantly reduces LES pressure without changing contraction amplitudes in the body of the esophagus. Thus, nitroglycerin may relieve partial or complete obstruction of the middle or lower esophagus secondary either to intrinsic esophageal disease or to simple FB impaction, and nifedipine, like glucagon, is most likely to succeed when the bolus is lodged at the gastroesophageal junction.

Indications and Contraindications

Similar to the clinical indications for the use of glucagon, any patient presenting with an impacted smooth esophageal FB, especially a food bolus, may be a candidate for nitroglycerin and/or nifedipine. Also, similar to the mode of action of glucagon, neither of these agents is expected to relax a fixed fibrotic stricture or ring at the gastroesophageal junction.[78] Nevertheless, because both agents have a relatively benign side effect profile, if the patient has no contraindication to their use, they may be tried with or without previous documentation of the distal esophageal obstruction by contrast study. Contraindications to their use include a history of allergic reactions, a sharp esophageal FB, hypovolemia, and hypotension.

Use and Complications

Doses of 1 or 2 (0.4-mg) sublingual nitroglycerin tablets, 1 to 2 inches of nitroglycerin paste, or 5 to 10 mg of nifedipine have been reported.[85–87] Remember that some patients with esophageal FBs may present with some degree of dehydration due to the inability to swallow liquids or their own saliva. These patients may be prone to hypotension from the vasodilatation associated with the use of either agent. Ideally, rehydration should precede therapy with these agents. Sublingual nifedipine (5- to 10-mg capsule punctured, chewed, and swallowed) has been rarely implicated in cerebral or coronary insufficiency in patients with cardiovascular disease, so caution is warranted. *Do not use both agents simultaneously.* The smaller dose of nifedipine is suggested in the elderly or those with cardiovascular disease.

Further Evaluation and Therapy

As with the use of glucagon, if nitrate therapy fails to produce symptomatic relief or resolve radiographic findings, its use does not preclude trying another method. If a patient experiences symptomatic relief, a postprocedure radiograph may be obtained to confirm passage of a radiopaque object, but this is not mandatory. The adult patient may be discharged home, but careful follow-up should be obtained to rule out coexis-

tent esophageal pathology, because a significant number of patients will have underlying esophageal disorders.

Gas-Forming Agents

Pharmacology

The use of gas-forming agents for the treatment of distal esophageal food impactions, especially meat boluses, was first described in 1983.[88] The combination of tartaric acid solution followed immediately by a solution of sodium bicarbonate or even carbonated beverages was reported. In theory, the use of this acid-base mixture or of a carbonated beverage may produce sufficient carbon dioxide to distend the esophagus, relax the LES, and push impacted food through the gastroesophageal junction into the stomach.[89,90]

Indications and Contraindications

Gas-forming agents are indicated for the relief of smooth distal esophageal FB impactions, with or without prior FB confirmation by a radiographic study. They are often given to patients with food impaction or retained coins. Although gas-forming agents are more likely to succeed with distal esophageal impactions, they have also been successful in relieving obstructions in the proximal esophagus. Concurrent administration of spasmolytic agents may improve the effectiveness of gas-forming agents.[84]

Use and Complications

A solution of 15 mL of tartaric acid (18.7 g/100 mL), followed by 15 mL of a sodium bicarbonate solution (10 g/100 mL), or 1.5 to 3 g of tartaric acid and 2 to 3 g of sodium bicarbonate dissolved in 15 mL of water can be used.[88,89] Carbonated beverages (100 mL) have also been successful in the transit of FBs into the stomach,[89,90] and are more readily available in the ED. Many patients with esophageal FB impactions have been noted to retch after receiving gas-forming agents, which theoretically puts patients at risk for esophageal trauma including esophageal rupture. Gas-forming agents should not be given to patients with impactions of more than 6 hours duration or to patients with chest pain that might be indicative of an esophageal injury.

Further Evaluation and Therapy

As with the use of glucagon, nitroglycerin, or nifedipine, even if administration of the gas-forming agent is successful, as judged by relief of symptoms, follow-up evaluation is necessary to determine the underlying esophageal abnormality that potentially led to the FB impaction.

Papain

Papain is not recommended for treatment of an esophageal FB. It is a proteolytic enzyme that has been touted for dissolving meat impactions.[91] Papain is available commercially in a variety of meat tenderizers. This therapy has never been tested in a clinical trial. Although it is harmless when in brief contact with the normal esophagus, if it is left in the obstructed esophagus too long, papain may begin to dissolve the esophageal mucosa underlying an FB. This is likely to occur when the esophageal wall is ischemic owing to FB impaction and resultant wall pressure, when esophageal injury results from small bony spicules in the FB, or when an underlying lesion is responsible for the obstruction. The subsequent rupture and leakage of the proteolytic enzymes result in a self-perpetuating mediastinitis. Patients with esophageal FBs are at increased risk for aspiration, and pulmonary aspiration of papain results in acute hemorrhagic pulmonary edema. In general, papain is not currently recommended because of the unacceptable complication risk and the availability of safer, more effective interventions.

FOLEY CATHETER REMOVAL OF ESOPHAGEAL FOREIGN BODIES

Foley catheter removal of esophageal FBs was first described in the thoracic surgery literature in 1966[92] and in the emergency medicine literature in 1981.[93] The technique is essentially unchanged since the first reports, and is now used by emergency clinicians, radiologists, otolaryngologists, and general surgeons.[94–98] The classic patient for this technique is a small child who is brought to the hospital shortly after swallowing a coin that is documented by radiograph, but the procedure may be used for a wide variety of smooth FBs in all ages of patients. Success rates for Foley catheter removal of FBs have been cited from 85% to 100%, with complication rates of 0% to 2%.[7,74,99–103] Many of the reported complications were due to the nasal insertion of the catheter, and complication rates are lower when the catheter is inserted orally and at centers that perform the procedure frequently. Foley catheter extraction costs significantly less than endoscopy.[7,104,105] Fluoroscopic assistance may be preferable, but it is not essential. Whether the procedure is performed in the ED or the radiology department, equipment and personnel capable of emergency pediatric airway management must be present.

Indications and Contraindications

Recently ingested smooth, blunt objects that are radiographically opaque are most suitable for balloon catheter extraction. Recently ingested FBs carry little likelihood of causing pressure necrosis, perforation, or other significant injury; however, 24 to 48 hours duration of impaction should be the upper limit for consideration of this technique.[7,33,105]

Coins are particularly amenable to Foley manipulation, but food boluses and button batteries have also been extracted successfully.[95] Radiographically opaque objects are most easily located by plain radiographs. Radiolucent objects can be manipulated, but uncertainties about location mandate contrast esophagograms.

Contraindications

Contraindications to catheter removal of esophageal FBs include total esophageal obstruction, as manifested by an air-fluid level on plain radiograph or contrast esophagogram or when patients are unable to handle oral secretions. The presence of a total obstruction prevents passage of the catheter tip distal to the FB. Esophageal perforation, as recognized by the typical symptoms and signs, requires immediate surgical consultation and precludes blind esophageal manipulation, as does airway distress. The presence of multiple esophageal FBs also precludes Foley catheter use. Sharp, irregularly shaped FBs should not be removed with this technique because esophageal perforation or laceration can result, and the balloon may burst during the procedure. Finally, lack of expertise or equipment to handle an airway problem arising during the procedure is a contraindication.

Equipment

The necessary equipment is basic and present in most EDs. Although never reported, airway obstruction during the procedure is the most feared potential complication. Thus, the proper equipment and personnel capable of managing airway obstruction must also be present, including suction devices. Forceps (bayonet and Magill) of various sizes should be available to extract the FB from the pharynx. Foley catheters ranging in size from No. 8 French with 3-mL balloons to No. 26 French with 30-mL balloons may be used. In settings in which both children and adults are treated, sizes ranging from 10 to 16 French with 5- to 10-mL balloons should suffice. Child restraint devices (e.g., papoose board), topical anesthetics, or moderate sedation may be used.

Procedure

Every patient should be appropriately coached concerning the procedure. Restrain young children. Moderate sedation and nasopharyngeal topical anesthesia may be used; however, this may increase the risk of aspiration due to decreased airway protective reflexes. Place the patient in a head-down Trendelenburg, lateral decubitus, supine, or prone position. The procedure is often done under fluoroscopic guidance, although this is not mandatory if the FB has been localized on plain radiographs.

Assuming the procedure is being performed on a young child, a 12- to 16-French Foley catheter is used. After checking for symmetrical balloon inflation, insert the catheter orally (Fig. 39–9). When using fluoroscopy, visually pass the catheter distal to the FB. Intermittent inflation with 1 to 2 mL of contrast may be needed to verify the catheter tip location. If performed without fluoroscopy, estimate the distance from nose or mouth to the FB, and insert the catheter accordingly. On occasion, the operator feels the catheter tip passing the object. Fill the balloon slowly with 3 to 5 mL of saline or contrast agent (if fluoroscopy is used). Stop inflating the balloon if the patient complains of increased pain. The catheter should be repositioned before attempting inflation again. Fluid is preferable to air, because it is less compressible. Overdistention of the balloon is undesirable, and in children, no more than 5 mL of fluid should be used.

Using steady, gentle traction, withdraw the catheter with its balloon inflated beyond the FB. Contact with the object can be sensed as the friction of withdrawal increases. Terminate the attempt if there is significant impedance to traction. If the catheter slides past the object without dislodging it, deflate the balloon and reposition it. Enlarge the balloon with an additional 2 to 3 mL and make another attempt. Often, when the object reaches the hypopharynx, the balloon and gravity act in concert to fully externalize the FB. Grasp the object with the fingers, forceps, or a clamp or instruct the patient to spit it out.

A follow-up radiograph may be necessary to exclude the possibility of multiple objects. If fluoroscopy is not used and no FB is retrieved, another radiograph should be obtained, because 10% to 20% of the time, the FB will pass distally into the stomach.[106]

Multiple attempts should not be required if catheter size, placement, and balloon inflation are correct. Failed attempts are best followed by a change in one of the aforementioned parameters or repeat x-ray studies to confirm the continued presence of the esophageal FB before esophagoscopy.

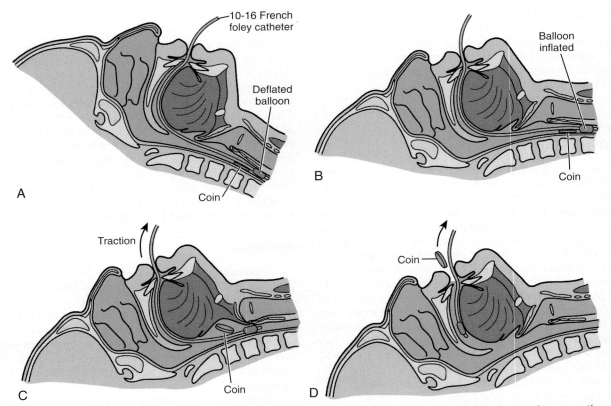

Figure 39–9 Technique of Foley catheter extraction. This can be done under fluoroscopy or blindly. Fill the balloon with contrast if fluoroscopy is used. In children, this procedure is best done with the patient restrained on a papoose board, or minimally consciously sedated (ketamine is ideal), with the head lowered. Some operators place the patient in a prone position or roll the patient to the prone position after catheter insertion to enhance oral expulsion of the foreign body. *A,* Insert a catheter (10–16 Fr size, balloon deflated) orally into the esophagus distal to the coin. Use a bite block to assist oral passage if necessary. *B,* Inflate the balloon. Apply gentle traction to move the coin proximally through the esophagus. *C,* Move the coin steadily past the glottis. *D,* Once the coin is present in the mouth either grasp it or ask the patient to expectorate it. *(A–D, Adapted from McSwain N: Esophageal foreign body. Emerg Med 21:85, 1989.)*

Complications

Complication rates of 0% to 2% have been reported.[7,74,99–103] Many complications (nosebleeds or displacement of the FB into the nose) have been related to the nasal insertion of the catheter. Complication rates are lower when the catheter is inserted orally and generally lower at centers that perform the procedure frequently. No deaths have been reported. Laryngospasm and aspiration are rare complications. Failure to either remove the object or displace it into the stomach occurs in approximately 2% to 10% of carefully selected patients,[100–103] but success rates are lower in adults or patients with underlying esophageal disorders.[102]

Disposition

Children who have an FB successfully removed by the Foley catheter need no further follow-up if they remain asymptomatic. If the FB was moved into the stomach, clinical follow-up should be adequate to verify movement of gastric FBs through the alimentary tract. Discharge instructions should include warnings about potential symptoms of GI obstruction, perforation, and hemorrhage. Parents of children who swallow coins can be instructed to watch for coins in the stool. Adults with esophageal FBs that have been removed successfully must be referred for evaluation of possible esophageal pathol-

ogy. Should a FB remain lodged in the esophagus, immediate referral for endoscopy is necessary.

ESOPHAGEAL BOUGIENAGE

Background

Displacement of esophageal FBs into the stomach can be done using naso- or orogastric tubes or esophageal bougienage. Esophageal bougienage is a technique for dislodging impacted esophageal coins by blind mechanical advancement of the coin into the stomach, a procedure first described in 1965.[107] The technique has a greater than 95% success rate with essentially no reported complications.[7,75,108,109] Rates as successful as those of endoscopy have been reported.[105] Furthermore, bougienage is unrivaled in overall cost-effectiveness, approximating 10% of the cost of endoscopic removal.[7,75,105,110]

There have traditionally been warnings against forceful advancement of esophageal FBs, but growing evidence verifies the efficacy and safety of blind esophageal bougienage as first-line therapy for coin ingestions in properly selected patients. Although early articles suggested that esophageal bougienage should be performed exclusively by pediatric surgeons, the technique is easily mastered and used by emergency clinicians.[75,109]

Indications and Contraindications

Strict patient selection is paramount for successful and uncomplicated bougienage. The criteria have changed little since initially proposed and define a group in whom a round, smooth object can be forcibly passed into the stomach with little risk.[108,111] Although many swallowed objects meet this description, only coins hold clear supportive evidence in the literature. Selection criteria are the following: a single, smooth FB, lodged less than 24 hours, in a patient with no respiratory distress or history of esophageal disease including prior FB or surgery. The procedure is contraindicated in patients who do not satisfy all criteria. It is important to ascertain time period of esophageal impaction to avoid the procedure when there may be underlying esophageal injury. For this reason, some advocate requirements for clearly witnessed ingestions less than 24 hours before presentation.[109] Plain radiographs are indicated to verify coin location and the absence of multiple esophageal bodies. Preprocedure esophagograms are not required.

Equipment

The necessary equipment should be assembled before initiating the procedure (Table 39–4). Airway equipment and drugs, topical anesthetic, suction, tongue depressor blades, bougie dilator set, water-soluble lubricant, an emesis basin, and an assistant are needed. Hurst-type esophageal dilators refer to weighted, flexible rubber bougies with a blunt, rounded tip. Nasogastric tubes and taper-tipped dilators should not be substituted. Bougie dilator size is selected based on age: 1 to 2 years, size 28 French; 2 to 3 years, 32 French; 3 to 4 years, 36 French; 4 to 5 years, 38 French; older than 5 years, 40 French.[109]

Procedure and Technique

Although not painful, bougienage may be frightening for pediatric patients and their parents. Both should have a clear understanding of the procedure, including the possible complications, before initiation. Small children may require physical restraint with bed sheets or papoose. All patients require guidance and reassurance throughout the procedure.

Topical anesthesia may be achieved with gargled 2% to 4% viscous lidocaine (Xylocaine), atomized 2% lidocaine, or topical benzocaine (20% Hurricane spray, Cetacaine). Sedation is generally not needed. Anxiolysis may be of use in some cases but must be weighed against the potential for aspiration from uncontrolled secretions or induced vomiting.

Blind esophageal bougienage is relatively straightforward and resembles placement of an orogastric tube. Patients may be positioned prone or seated upright for the procedure. The distance from nose to midepigastrium approximates the length to reach the stomach and should be noted before passage. Ask the patient to flex the head slightly forward and protrude the tongue. A tongue blade may be used to displace the tongue in uncooperative children. Pass the well-lubricated, appropriately sized bougie posteriorly along the roof of the mouth following the natural curve of the soft palate caudally to the hypopharynx. The patient will momentarily gag as the bougie meets resistance at the level of the cricopharyngeus muscle. Encourage the patient to swallow and gently pass the dilator through the cricopharyngeus muscle. Asking the patient to phonate helps exclude accidental laryngeal intubation; marked hoarseness or inability to phonate indicates airway obstruction and incorrect placement.

Once past the cricopharyngeus muscle, extend the head to enable the bougie to pass distally to the stomach with little resistance. Withdraw the bougie after a single pass. Terminate the procedure immediately for pain or resistance to advancement. A postprocedure radiograph of the chest and upper abdomen documents coin location and should be scrutinized for evidence of complications. Routine postprocedure esophagograms are not indicated unless a complication is clinically suspected. Barring a suspicion of complications, release asymptomatic patients to home with appropriate precautions including the need to return for signs of respiratory compromise, chest or abdominal pain, dysphagia, hematemesis, persistent vomiting, or other concerns. Follow-up abdominal radiographs may be performed to document passage of the coin if it is not identified in the feces within 1 week. For adult patients, follow-up is mandated owing to the 65% to 80% chance of underlying esophageal disorders.[9]

Complications

Gagging and self-limited nonbloody vomiting are not uncommon after the procedure and may reveal the dislodged coin. Patients may experience a residual FB sensation for several hours. Pulmonary aspiration and inadvertent passage into the airway are potential complications. Likewise, traumatic pharyngeal and esophageal injury, ranging from mild self-limited bleeding to frank esophageal perforation with concomitant infection, are possible but rare.

SPECIAL SITUATIONS

Childhood Coin Ingestions

Coins are among the most commonly ingested objects in preschool-aged children. In most cases, the ingestion is quickly realized by a caretaker, and in the majority of cases, the coins pass uneventfully.[112] Rarely, an esophageal coin can

TABLE 39–4 Equipment for Bougienage Manipulation of Esophageal Foreign Bodies

Tongue depressor
Topical anesthetic
Emesis basin
Yankauer suction tip and tubing connected to continuous wall suction
Water-soluble surgical lubricant
Hurst-type blunt-tipped bougie dilators (age-appropriate size)

Age (Yr)	Dilator Size (Fr)
1–2	28
2–3	32
3–4	36
4–5	38
>5	40

From Emslander HC, Bonadio W, Klatzo M: Efficacy of esophageal bougienage by emergency physicians in pediatric coin ingestion. Ann Emerg Med 27:726, 1996.

be clandestine for many weeks or months, producing a variety of vague respiratory or GI symptoms.[113] In addition, many coin ingestions are not witnessed,[39] so maintain a high index of suspicion for children presenting with dysphagia, drooling, or crying who may have esophageal FBs, most likely coins.

Most coins pass from the esophagus to the stomach with only transient symptoms. The child may be in pain for a few minutes as the coin migrates, but on arrival in the ED, the child is often asymptomatic. Coins that remain in the esophagus are likely to, but do not always, produce continued symptoms (e.g., drooling, pain, dysphagia, refusal to eat or drink). Rarely, esophageal coins can produce airway distress by external compression of the trachea, simulating an asthmatic attack. Coins below the diaphragm are asymptomatic, and the presence of pain or symptoms requires further evaluation. Coins in the trachea produce immediate and obvious respiratory distress.

The first clinical decision is whether to obtain a radiograph. Although some authors recommend that asymptomatic children not be radiographed,[34] it is important to remember that up to 44% of children with esophageal coins may be asymptomatic. Therefore, it is prudent to perform plain radiographs on all children with a suggestive history.[36] In most cases, a single film that includes the pharynx, esophagus, and stomach will suffice to prove or exclude an ingested coin. Another advantage of obtaining radiographs is to rule out multiple FB ingestions, which are not uncommon in children.[114] Only a single PA chest film is needed to prove the presence of a coin, but a lateral projection is also suggested. If the flat surface of the coin is seen (see Figs. 39–2 to 39–4), this orientation ensures an esophageal position. If the edge of the coin is seen, this orientation suggests that it traversed the vocal cords, but a coin in the airway *is not subtle and produces obvious distress*. It is advisable to also routinely obtain a lateral radiograph to determine whether multiple coins are stacked on top of each other (Fig. 39–10).

Once a coin's presence has been documented, a decision concerning removal must be made. The approach varies, and there is no agreed upon standard. *Overall, about 25% of coins will pass spontaneously, even if the coin is proximal.* Observation for 8 to 16 hours is a reasonable approach for asymptomatic children if ingestion has been within 24 hours. Coins in the upper and middle third of the esophagus are less likely to pass spontaneously, and some prefer to remove them as soon as the diagnosis is made.[18] Coins in the distal esophagus will pass spontaneously in one third to one half of patients within 24 hours.[18,35]

The decision on managing these patients depends on various factors: clinician comfort and experience with removal techniques, local protocols and procedures developed by the medical staff of each institution, and comfort level of the caretakers with various therapeutic options. Regardless of the approach, a *radiograph should be taken just before surgical removal to ensure that spontaneous passage has not occurred.*

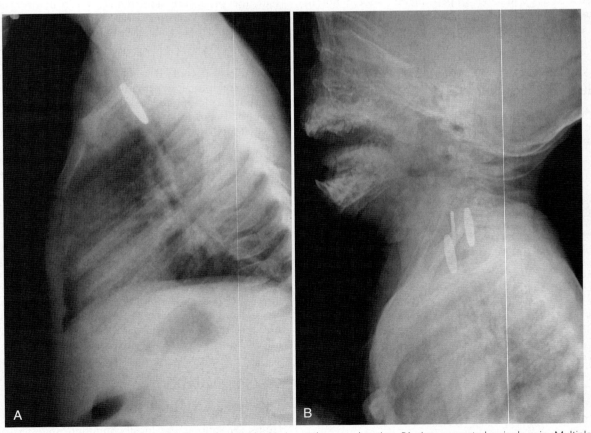

Figure 39–10 *A*, Lateral radiograph of the child shows *four stacked coins* at the same location. PA view suggested a single coin. Multiple swallowed coins are common in children. It is important to obtain both PA and lateral films to ascertain the exact number and location of swallowed coins. *B*, A single coin was seen on the PA chest film, but this lateral film suggests *three coins*. However, they do not seem to be stacked directly on top of each other. This digital radiograph was accidentally exposed three times; actually, only one coin was swallowed and x-rayed three times during minimal movement.

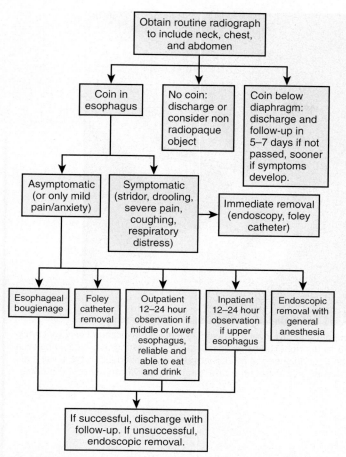

Figure 39–11 Flow diagram outlines an approach to the management of swallowed coins.

coin is not found in 1 to 2 weeks. Most coins are passed unknowingly by the patient. Any abdominal discomfort or distention warrants reevaluation in the ED. If a follow-up radiograph demonstrates a persistent coin in the intestines for more than 3 to 4 weeks, an obstructive lesion may be present, and further evaluation is warranted.

Finally, there are theoretical concerns about U.S. pennies, which contain 97.5% zinc. Theoretically, zinc can lead to mucosal ulceration from the caustic nature of zinc[116]; however, evidence to date suggests no increased risk from ingested pennies.[117]

Fish or Chicken Bones in the Throat

Patients who complain of a "bone" in their throat usually present to the ED within several hours of the onset of symptoms and usually have tried a home remedy, such as swallowing a piece of bread. These patients are typically able to pinpoint the location of their discomfort and present with an FB sensation, exacerbated with swallowing. Patients who are markedly symptomatic, vomiting, or unable to swallow require definitive therapy. Those with minor complaints may be safely evaluated over a few days, often as outpatients.

In cooperative patients, a careful examination of the oropharynx, with either direct or indirect laryngoscopy or both, should be made. If the bone is seen, it should be removed with forceps (Fig. 39–12).

If the patient feels pain in the upper throat, special attention is directed to the tonsils because bones often lodge in this area. Strands of saliva may mimic a bone, and small bones may be difficult to see. More commonly, the area of complaint is below the oropharynx. In these patients, indirect laryngoscopy or nasopharyngoscopy should be the first step, once again removing the bone if one is seen.

Most patients presenting with an oropharyngeal FB will not have an easily identified or visualized object on examination. These patients present a diagnostic dilemma for several reasons. *Only 17% to 25% of patients complaining of an FB sensation after eating chicken or fish have an endoscopically proven bone present*, and only 29% to 50% of endoscopically proven bones are seen on plain films.[64,118,119] The symptoms in those patients with an FB sensation, but no FB on endoscopy, are believed to be due to esophageal abrasions.

For these reasons, a two-tiered, but individualized, approach to managing these patients is proposed.[6,9,33,70] The patient receives a physical examination and the bone is removed if seen. Carefully examine the tonsils, posterior pharynx, and base of the tongue, *which are common places for bones to lodge*. If the bone is removed, and symptoms disappear, no further intervention is required and follow-up is as needed. *The removal of a bone usually provides immediate and complete relief of symptoms*. Persistent symptoms are cause for further evaluation based on individual circumstances.

If no bone is seen on physical examination, the bone may have passed after causing local irritation that persists, or the bone is present and not visualized due to location or consistency. Minor symptoms in the upper throat likely represent persistent local irritation. Minimally symptomatic patients can be discharged and followed up in 24 hours. Those with complaints of an FB below the visualized pharynx, or very bothersome persistent symptoms, should be evaluated with a CT scan of the neck, or possibly the chest, if symptoms are distal. Positive scans are an indication for endoscopic removal of the bone. If the CT scan reveals no FB or postbone com-

One suggested protocol (Fig. 39–11) involves radiologically localizing the coin and, if the child is *symptomatic*, immediately removing the coin. If the patient is *asymptomatic*, the coin may be removed immediately or the patient may be observed either as an inpatient or at home. If the child is asymptomatic, one common practice is to allow the child to drink a carbonated beverage and eat a small amount of soft food in the ED, wait about 1 to 2 hours, and perform another radiograph. If sent home with an asymptomatic retained FB, the patient is allowed to eat or drink but should be rechecked in 12 to 24 hours with the knowledge that up to 50% of asymptomatic coin FBs will pass into the stomach spontaneously.[18,35,115]

The techniques of esophageal bougienage and Foley catheter removal have been described earlier. Both are options for single coins in the esophagus present for less than 24 to 48 hours. Another option for coins at the LES is pharmacologic relaxation of the sphincter to aid passage into the stomach. The most common method to remove esophageal coins in use today is esophagoscopy.

About half of ingested coins are in the stomach at the time of first investigation, and such patients can be safely released home to allow for almost certain spontaneous passage with a normal diet. Spontaneous passage of a coin from the stomach to the anus usually requires 5 to 7 days. There is no need for routine cathartic. Parents should be advised to check the stool for the coin and return for repeat radiographs if the

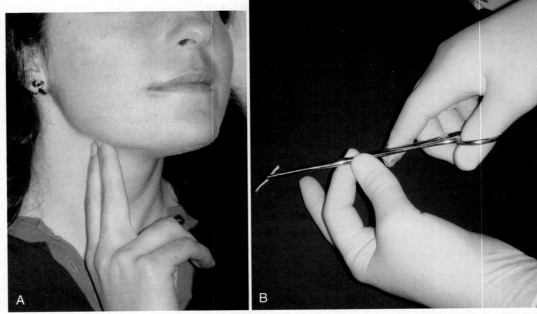

Figure 39–12 Many fish bones become impaled in the soft tissues of the upper digestive tract. This woman felt a bone catch in her throat while eating fish. As is often the case, she was able to consistently localize the FB to the right submandibular area (*A*), suggesting that it could be seen with direct visualization. With only a tongue blade, local anesthetic spray, and good lighting, a fish bone was found embedded in the tonsil and was easily removed with forceps (*B*). *Removal provided immediate and total relief*, as is usually the case. Strands of saliva can mimic a fish bone, so be careful when probing and grasping.

plication, and the patient is stable, she or he is discharged home with follow-up within 24 hours. Patients with oropharyngeal abrasions will usually be asymptomatic at that time. If still symptomatic on follow-up, endoscopy is advocated.

A small bone lodged in the esophagus for a few days is annoying and painful, but it is generally not an emergency. However, impacted bones can cause serious sequelae, often weeks later, and continued complaints cannot be ignored. Importantly, a *lodged bone will not dissolve and rarely passes spontaneously once lodged in the mucosa*. Referral, and possible endoscopy, is necessary if complaints persist for more than 2 to 3 days, even if the examination and CT scan are negative.

Sharp Objects in the Esophagus

Sharp objects cause the majority of complications seen in patients with esophageal FBs. These objects include tacks, pins, open paperclips, bobby pins, toothpicks, and razor blades (Fig. 39–13). They will usually not pass spontaneously and should be removed. The only appropriate removal technique is under direct visualization with endoscopy.

Attempts at radiographic localization are appropriate for metallic or radiopaque FBs. Most objects in the stomach, even those considered problematic, will transit the remainder of the GI tract if less than 6 cm in length or 2 cm in diameter. If larger than this, consult a gastroenterologist. If radiographs show the FB in the esophagus, endoscopic removal is indicated, and attempts to remove such objects in the ED by other methods are not indicated. Complication rates for endoscopic removal of sharp FBs range from 0% to 3%.[8,12,40]

Nonradiopaque Objects in the Esophagus

Objects such as toothpicks, aluminum tabs from beverage cans, plastic, and food boluses cannot be visualized on plain radiographs and will normally not pass spontaneously. Toothpicks cause a higher percentage of complications than any other type of esophageal FB. Localization of the FB may be accomplished by esophagogram with contrast material, although the yield is low with toothpicks. As with fish bones, toothpicks often lodge in the tonsils or posterior pharynx and can be seen on direct vision.

Impacted Food Bolus

A large bolus of food may become impacted in the esophagus, usually at the LES. This occurs most frequently in the elderly, those intoxicated while eating, or those with dentures. Often, there is underlying esophageal pathology, such as a stricture or web, even in the young (see Fig. 39–6). The diagnosis is usually straightforward, and patients may be in significant distress, gagging, and unable to swallow. A barium swallow may be used to confirm the diagnosis, but this is rarely necessary. Proceeding directly to endoscopy appears most reasonable. Food boluses may be amenable to pharmacologic relaxation of the LES, but the definitive intervention is endoscopy to both *remove the bolus and to evaluate the esophagus for pathology*. The specific approach, however, is varied and not standard.

The most logical ED approach is initial aggressive symptomatic relief (judicious narcotics, sedatives, antiemetics), followed by attempts at pharmacologic manipulation of the LES. If the bolus passes, esophageal evaluation can be performed

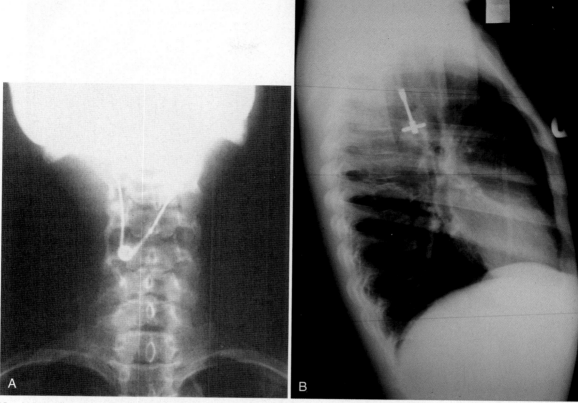

Figure 39–13   *A,* PA radiograph of an open safety pin lodged in the upper esophagus. Sharp foreign bodies in the esophagus are best removed with endoscopic visualization. *B,* This 10-year-old child came to the emergency department (ED) with severe chest pain. No history of an FB was given. Even when the radiograph demonstrated this metallic object in the esophagus, how it got there remained a mystery. Objects such as this are removed under anesthesia with an endoscope, and no ED intervention, except for pain relief, is indicated.

at follow-up. *Papain is contraindicated.* An esophagogram can be performed but seems unnecessary if the diagnosis is obvious (it usually is) and endoscopy is available or planned. A barium swallow should not be used to delay definitive treatment. Removal of impacted food is an urgent issue but need not be done immediately upon presentation, or in the middle of the night with inadequate resources. Often, pain relief and a few hours of relaxation will allow the bolus to slowly break. Vomiting occasionally dislodges the impaction.

Button Battery Ingestion

Button batteries lodged in the esophagus should be considered an emergency because of the potential for serious morbidity and mortality.[22,24,120] These batteries range in size from 7 to 25 mm and are radiopaque (Fig. 39–14). Batteries appear as round densities, similar to an impacted coin, but some demonstrate a "double-contour" configuration. It is important to distinguish between a coin and a button battery, because button batteries require immediate removal. Batteries consist of two metal plates joined by a plastic seal. Internally, they contain an electrolyte solution (usually concentrated sodium or potassium hydroxide) and a heavy metal, such as mercuric oxide, silver oxide, zinc, or lithium.

If ingested, these batteries often lodge in the esophagus. The mechanisms of injury include electrolyte leakage, injury from electrical current, heavy metal toxicity, and pressure

necrosis. Of particular concern is the development of a corrosive esophagitis or perforation as a result of caustic injury and prolonged mucosal pressure. Although essentially harmless in the stomach and intestines, batteries lodged in the esophagus should be considered an emergency situation because even new batteries demonstrate corrosion, leakage, and mucosal necrosis within a few hours of contact with the esophagus (see Fig. 39–14).[23,24]

Esophageal impaction mandates immediate removal. Options include Foley catheter removal, esophageal bougienage, or esophagoscopy. Esophagoscopy allows for direct esophageal evaluation and a more controlled extraction. In addition, the "invasive" nature of batteries may lead to rapid edema, making the catheter technique more difficult.

Once in the stomach, button batteries do not require removal. They may be followed radiographically to demonstrate passage, with little risk of GI injury or heavy metal poisoning, even if the battery opens.[121–124]

The Patient in Distress

Pharyngeal or upper esophageal FBs can cause respiratory embarrassment or respiratory arrest, usually in infants and the elderly. The Heimlich maneuver was developed for just such circumstances and can be attempted in the ED when the situation is appropriate. There are no data on the best intervention for the unknown choking patient who arrives in extremis

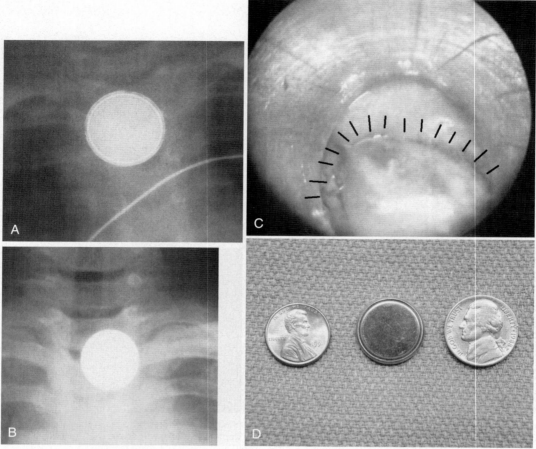

Figure 39–14 *A* and *B*, Button batteries have a wide range of sizes and can mimic coins on radiographs. Note that the battery (*upper x-ray*) has a double-density circular appearance at the border, whereas the coin has a homogeneous density with smooth borders. *C* and *D*, Endoscopic mucosal injury and size comparison of battery with coins. *(A* and B *from Kost KM, Shapior RS: Button battery ingestion. A case report and review of the literature. J Otolaryngol 16:4, 1987.)*

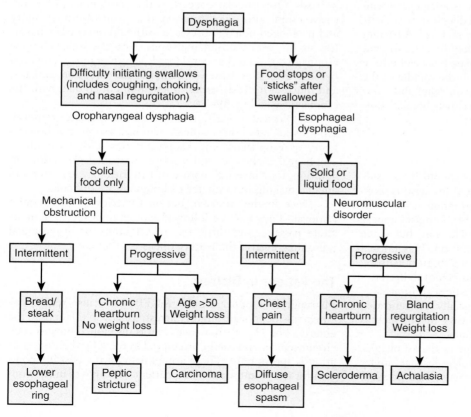

Figure 39–15 Diagnostic algorithm for the symptomatic assessment of the patient with dysphagia. *(Adapted from Saud BM, Szyjkowski RD: A diagnostic approach to dysphagia. Clin Fam Pract 6:525, 2004.)*

to the ED, often with no history. The first intervention is to ensure an adequate airway, which can be obvious by the situation or may require laryngoscopy or other means of direct visualization. For the infant who is rushed to the ED in extremis with a known FB, it seems reasonable to hold the infant by the legs, head down, and attempt a Heimlich maneuver and/or sweep the pharynx with a finger to remove an obstruction. However, blind intervention into the pharynx has the potential to change a partial obstruction into a complete obstruction. Forceps may be required to remove obstructions under direct vision. Because FBs may mimic multiple other pathologies, the approach to the acutely choking patient is indeed challenging and every situation individual.

ED Evaluation of Dysphagia/Lump in the Throat

Foreign body insult to the esophagus are usually straightforward, but patients may present to the ED with a complaint of a lump in the throat or difficulty swallowing, with no apparent reason. One common cause is acute uvulitis (see Chapter 64, Otolaryngologic Procedures). Such complaints require an examination and an investigation based on the clinical encounter and individual circumstances. The complete evaluation of these complaints is beyond the scope of this chapter, but initial modalities available to the clinician to evaluate these complaints are barium swallow, CT scan, and pharyngoscopy/

laryngoscopy. The need for consultation is based on the clinical scenario. Figure 39–15 is a suggested approach to the patient with dysphagia.

If no cause is suspected by history or examination, globus pharyngeus may be the cause. This may be associated with anxiety or a panic attack. The sensation of a painless lump in the throat is called globus pharyngeus or globus hystericus. It has many causes other than foreign bodies. Palpate, visualize, or review the anatomical structures in the area: the chin, laryngeal cartilage, cricothyroid cartilage, tracheal rings, sternum and cricopharyngeal muscle.

Foreign body sensation may be caused by infection, acid reflux, esophageal spasm, esophageal strictures, pill esophagitis, benign and malignant tumors, hiatal hernia, scleroderma, and many other causes. Globus sensation may also persist after a foreign body has been completely removed due to mucosal injury. Neurologic causes include botulism, myasthenia gravis, cerebral vascular accident, and amyotrophic lateral sclerosis. If the patient is otherwise well appearing and able to drink liquids and keep hydrated, referral to a gastroenterologist as an outpatient is standard.

 REFERENCES CAN BE FOUND ON EXPERT CONSULT

CHAPTER 40

Nasogastric and Feeding Tube Placement

Leonard E. Samuels

Nasogastric (NG) intubation is commonly used to evaluate or treat bowel obstruction, ileus, or gastric hemorrhage; pre- or postoperatively, or to administer food or medication into the gastrointestinal tract. Patients with long-term feeding tube complications and those requiring replacement or other manipulation of tubes frequently present to the emergency department (ED).

PROPERTIES OF NG AND FEEDING TUBES

Polypropylene is the most common material used for Levin and Salem sump NG tubes (Fig. 40–1), but it is too rigid for long-term use as a feeding tube. Polypropylene tubes are less likely to kink than others, but are more capable of creating a false passage during placement. Latex (rubber) tubes are moderately firm, require greater lubrication for passage, are relatively thick-walled, and induce a greater foreign body reaction than tubes of other common materials. Latex, especially in latex balloons, deteriorates more rapidly than other materials.[1] Foley catheters are primarily latex, although silicone Foley catheters are available for those patients with latex allergies. Silicone tubes are thin-walled, pliable, and nonreactive; however, the walls of silicone tubes are weaker and may rupture if fluid is introduced into a kinked tube.[2] Polyurethane tubes are nonreactive and relatively durable. Rigidity varies from manufacturer to manufacturer, depending on tube thickness. A stylet may aid in the passage of polyurethane and silicone tubes, but it increases rigidity and the potential for tissue dissection, especially in tubes that have a small distal end bulb.[3] Some feeding tubes have weights, usually made of tungsten, which are nontoxic if released into the gastrointestinal tract.

NG TUBE PLACEMENT

Indications and Contraindications

The simplest NG tube is the Levin tube, which has a single lumen and multiple distal "eyes." The advantage of the Levin tube is its relatively large internal diameter (ID) in proportion to its external diameter. The theoretical disadvantage is that a Levin tube should not be left hooked up to suction after the initial contents of the stomach have been drained because the suction will cause the stomach to invaginate into the eyes of the tube, blocking future tube function and potentially causing injury to the stomach lining. Levin tubes are, therefore, rarely used in the ED. The Salem sump tube is preferred over the Levin tube for chronic use as a drainage device because it has a separate (blue-colored) channel that vents the distal main

lumen to the atmosphere (Fig. 40–2). This vent helps to prevent excessive vacuum at the tube tip. Note that both intermittent suction and wall-unit vacuum can exceed the venting capacity of the second lumen, so the vacuum setting should be less than 120 mm Hg.[4]

The major indication for NG tube placement is to aspirate the stomach contents, particularly to differentiate upper from lower gastrointestinal bleeding. Except when frankly bloody fluid is obtained, the *sensitivity and specificity of aspiration to detect upper intestinal bleeding are not good.*[5–7] Use of Hemoccult or guaiac cards to detect bleeding in gastric aspirates is unreliable because *false-positive tests* are frequently obtained.[5] Although variceal rupture has occurred during insertion of instruments into the esophagus, several studies suggest that NG tube passage is generally safe, even in the presence of esophageal varices.[8,9] NG suction is indicated in patients in whom vomiting is likely to be recurrent or dangerous, such as with a paralytic ileus, bowel obstruction, or acute gastric dilation. The trauma patient may need an NG tube as part of the evaluation for gastrointestinal injury or to decompress the stomach before surgery or peritoneal lavage. A radiopaque NG tube may help delineate transdiaphragmatic hernia of the stomach after trauma. A deviated NG tube is a nonspecific sign of traumatic aortic rupture.

NG tubes are contraindicated in patients with special predispositions to injury from tube placement. Patients with facial fractures who have a cribriform plate injury may suffer intracranial penetration with a blindly placed nasal tube.[10] A severe coagulopathy is a relative contraindication for passage of an NG tube. For patients with a coagulopathy or significant facial or head trauma, an NG tube passed through *the mouth* may be a better alternative (Fig. 40–3). Patients who have esophageal strictures or a history of alkali ingestion may suffer esophageal perforation. Gagging will decrease venous return and increase cervical and intracranial venous pressure. Comatose patients may vomit during or after NG tube placement. Indwelling NG tubes predispose patients to pulmonary aspiration because of tube-induced hypersalivation, depressed cough reflex, or mechanical or physiologic impairment of the glottis.[11] Aspiration is also quite common with nasoenteral feedings in debilitated patients, hence the use of a gastrostomy feeding tube for this condition. An NG tube should be avoided when possible in patients with gastric bypass surgery or lap banding procedures.

Despite their traditional use, NG tubes are not routinely required in patients with mild to moderate pancreatitis,[11,12] and NG tubes may actually prolong hyperamylasemia and pain. Extended irrigation of the stomach with water in a patient with upper gastrointestinal hemorrhage can lower serum potassium levels,[14] and animal studies suggest that cold water lavage can cause, rather than control, bleeding.[15,16] No study has shown irrigation to be effective in the control of bleeding,[6,17] and vigorous lavage with cold water may lower the body temperature. An NG tube may be used to instill air into the stomach for documentation of a suspected gastric perforation by enhancing visualization of free air under the diaphragm on an upright chest film.

Equipment

Passage of standard NG tubes or feeding tubes can be messy and may be accompanied by coughing, retching, sneezing, bleeding, and spilled water or stomach fluid. For this reason, both patient and clinician should be gowned; cleanup may be

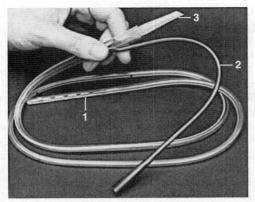

Figure 40–1 **Salem sump tube.** This tube contains a second lumen that allows venting during continuous suction. *1,* Gastric end with suction eyes. *2,* Pigtail extension (*blue*) of the air vent lumen. *3,* Connector for attachment of suction lumen to vacuum line.

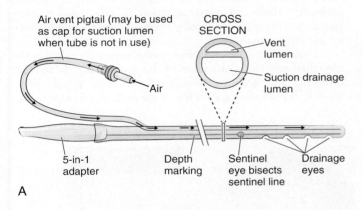

Air vent pigtail (may be used as cap for suction lumen when tube is not in use)

Air

5-in-1 adapter

Depth marking

Sentinel eye bisects sentinel line

Drainage eyes

CROSS SECTION

Vent lumen

Suction drainage lumen

A

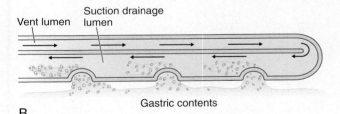

Vent lumen

Suction drainage lumen

Gastric contents

B

Figure 40–2 **Diagram of the Salem sump tube.** *A,* General design. *B,* Diagram of double-lumen principle for suction. (*A and B, Courtesy of the Argyle Division of Sherwood Medical, St. Louis.*)

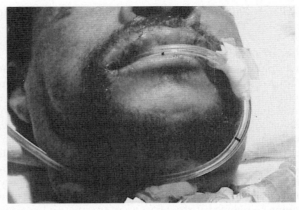

Figure 40–3 A nasogastric (NG) tube may enter the cranium or facial soft tissues in patients with severe head or facial trauma. Those with a coagulopathy may experience significant bleeding from nasal or pharyngeal trauma during passage of an NG tube. In such cases, a standard NG tube inserted *through the mouth* may be a better alternative.

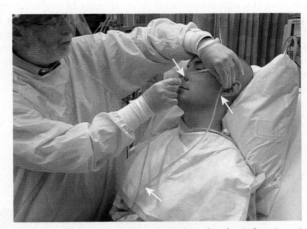

Figure 40–4 **Estimation of tube insertion depth.** Before inserting the NG tube, the clinician should estimate the length of tubing that will be required to ensure intragastric positioning without excess coiling. Holding the tube against the patient's body, measure the distance from the tip of the xiphoid to the earlobe. Add the distance from the earlobe to the tip of the nose. Then add another 15 cm. Note the total distance using markers on the tube or attach a piece of tape to the tube. (*From Thomsen T, Setnik G [eds]: Procedures Consult—Emergency Medicine Module. Copyright 2008 Elsevier Inc. All rights reserved.*)

Procedure

Explain the procedure to the patient. Written informed consent is not standard. If the patient is alert, raise the head of the bed so that the patient is upright. Place a towel over the patient's chest to protect the gown, and place an emesis basin on the patient's lap.[18] Position the tube (typically a 16- or 18-Fr sump) so that the insertion distance can be estimated, and mark the distance with tape or by noting the markers printed on the proximal tube. A simple method for measurement is to measure the tube from the xiphoid to the earlobe and then to the tip of the nose. Then add 15 cm (6 inches) to this number (Fig. 40–4).[19] *It is a common error to fail to estimate the proper length of the tube before passage,* resulting in the tip of the tube in the esophagus or the tube coiled excessively in the stomach. Check the nares for obstruction. Assess patency by direct visualization, by gentle digital nasal examination, or by having the patient sniff while first one and then the other

reduced if the bib area is covered with a towel and a supply of tissues or washcloths is available. For standard NG tube placement, a piston or bulb syringe (with a catheter slip-tip) should be available. NG feeding tubes should have a compatible 50- or 60-mL syringe (some are Luer compatible and others are slip-tip compatible).

Tape torn in 4-inch strips or a commercial NG tube holder (e.g., Suction Tube Attachment Device, Hollister, Libertyville, IL) should be handy for securing the tube after placement. Cotton-tipped applicators and tincture of benzoin may be helpful to secure the tube to the nose if the skin is greasy. Make sure the feeding tube is designed for duodenal passage if that is desired—such tubes are usually longer than regular feeding tubes.

nostril is occluded. Pass the tube down the more patent naris.

Relief of Discomfort

Ameliorate the pain and gagging associated with tube placement by using vasoconstrictors, topical anesthetics, and antiemetics. Because patients rate NG tube placement as very painful, one of the most painful procedures performed in the ED, *use these adjuncts whenever the time and clinical situation permit* (Fig. 40–5A). Spray topical vasoconstrictors, such as phenylephrine (Neo-Synephrine 0.5%) or oxymetazoline (Afrin 0.05%) into both nares at first in case one side proves to be problematic. The nares, nasopharynx, and oropharynx should all be anesthetized *at least 5 minutes before the procedure.* Gagging is reduced if the pharynx is anesthetized as well as the nose. Combinations of tetracaine, butyl aminobenzoate, and benzocaine (Cetacaine), nebulized or atomized (spray cans/bottles) lidocaine (4% or 10%), and lidocaine gels (2%) are most commonly used. Lidocaine preparations of 10% are most useful. Lidocaine may be nebulized and delivered by face mask with the equipment used to administer bronchodilators to asthmatics. This method has been found to be superior to lidocaine spray to reduce gagging and vomiting and to increase the chance of successful passage.[20,21] Cullen and coworkers[22] concluded that nebulized nasal and pharyngeal lidocaine (4 mL of 10%) reduced NG tube passage discomfort better than placebo, without lidocaine toxicity (see Fig. 40–5B).

After topical vasoconstrictor and anesthetic are administered, lubricate the tube with viscous lidocaine or lidocaine jelly.[23] Lubrication and anesthesia of the nares can be facilitated by using a syringe (without needle) filled with 5 mL of anesthetic lubricant, such as 2% lidocaine gel (see Fig. 40–5C). Simply putting anesthetic jelly *on the tube* before insertion will not provide any anesthesia. Topical anesthetics are generally quite safe, but pay attention to the total dose of administered anesthetic to avoid toxicity.[24] Note that each milliliter of a 10% lidocaine solution contains 100 mg of lidocaine and can be absorbed systemically. Topical benzocaine has been known to rarely cause methemoglobinemia in the relatively small amounts used for endoscopy.[25]

Ondansetron (Zofran 4 mg) or metoclopramide (Reglan 10 mg) given intravenously 15 minutes before NG tube passage can reduce nausea and gagging, and secondarily, it improves the pain and procedural prolongation that gagging engenders. Metoclopramide may have additional benefits on the discomfort of NG tube insertion, unrelated to its antinausea effects. Ondansetron is preferred for nausea because metoclopramide can cause agitation or facial and tongue spasm, but these can be rapidly reversed with 25 mg diphenhydramine intravenously.

Under direct vision, not blind forcing, insert the tube gently into the naris along the floor of the nose, *under the inferior turbinate,* and not upward toward the nasal bridge (Fig. 40–6A). If mild resistance is felt in the posterior nasopharynx,

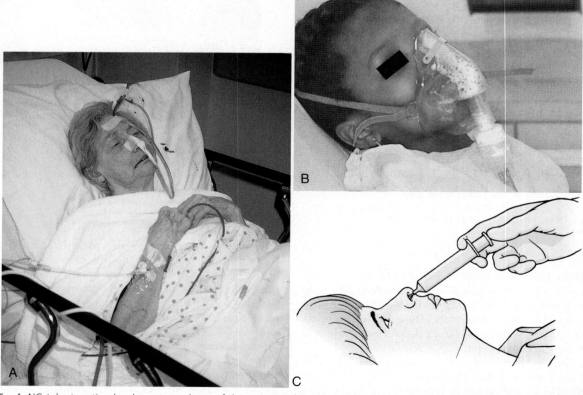

Figure 40–5 *A,* NG tube insertion has been termed one of the most painful and unpleasant procedures performed in the emergency department (ED), and it should not be used unless specifically indicated. Whenever possible, some form of topical anesthesia to *both the nose and the pharynx* should be used *at least 5 min before passing an NG tube. B,* Nebulizing 3–4 mL of 10% lidocaine (note concentration) reduces both nasal and pharyngeal discomfort. Have the patient alternately breathe through the nose and mouth. *C,* The method is effective primarily for the nasal opening, so encourage the patient to swallow. Fill a syringe barrel with 5 mL of 2% viscous lidocaine. Without using a needle, squirt the solution along the floor of the nose and allow it to drip into the nasopharynx and be swallowed. This method works best with the patient supine.

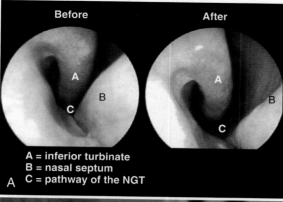

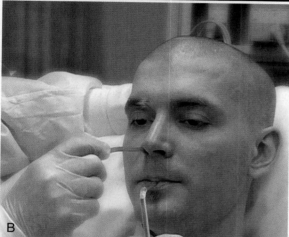

A = inferior turbinate
B = nasal septum
C = pathway of the NGT

Figure 40–6 *A,* The NG tube is passed under the inferior turbinate, made more patent after vasoconstrictors applied in the nose. The operator should actually *look into the nose during this insertion to properly guide the tube,* not force it blindly. *B,* Drinking water by straw during passage seems to help the tube go down. Once the esophagus is entered, *rapid advancement* is more tolerable and successful than slow placement. *(A and B, From Thomsen T, Setnik G [eds]: Procedures Consult—Emergency Medicine Module. Copyright 2008 Elsevier Inc. All rights reserved.)*

apply gentle pressure to overcome this resistance. If significant resistance is encountered, it is better to try the other nostril because bleeding or dissection into retropharyngeal tissue may occur if force is used. Once the tube passes into the oropharynx, pause to help the patient regain composure and enhance the chances for cooperation with the rest of the procedure.

If the patient is alert and cooperative, ask him or her to sip water from a straw and swallow while you advance the tube into and down the esophagus (see Fig. 40–6B). This often helps ease passage of the tube. Once the tube is in the nasopharynx, flex the patient's neck to direct the tube into the esophagus rather than the trachea. Withdraw the tube promptly into the oropharynx if the patient has excessive choking, gagging, coughing, a change in voice, or the appearance of condensation on the inner aspect of the tube. This indicates the possibility of passage of the tube into the trachea. Inspect the tube by way of the mouth to detect coiling or respiratory passage. If the tube is lateral to the midline, this suggests correct position in the esophagus.[26] Once the tube is in the esophagus, *advance it rapidly* to the previously determined depth. Passing the tube slowly prolongs discomfort and may precipitate more gagging.[18]

Confirmation of Tube Placement

Before the NG tube is secured, confirm successful placement by nonradiographic means or by auscultation. Use more than one method when in doubt because all confirmation methods have some possibility of error. Radiographic evaluation is the most definitive way to confirm the position of an NG tube, but it is not standard to routinely obtain x-ray confirmation.

A quick and simple method is to insufflate air into the NG tube and auscultate for a rush of air over the stomach. If increased pressure is required to instill the air or if no sounds are heard, the tube may be malpositioned or kinked. Suspect an esophageal location if the patient immediately burps upon insufflation. If the patient is awake, it will be immediately discernible if the tube is in the trachea or lungs. Unfortunately, if the patient is comatose, struggling, or demented, the tube may pass into the lungs unrecognized. Insufflation is often insufficient to detect this type of malpositioning.[3] The insufflation test is also unreliable in detecting a tube that has advanced past the stomach and into the small bowel.[27] In such patients, radiographic verification may be prudent.

Aspiration of stomach contents, especially if pH tested, is more reliable, and can be performed if positioning is in question. If the pH is less than 4, there is an approximately 95% chance that the tube is in the stomach and nonrespiratory placement is almost guaranteed.[28] Whereas aspirated fluid can occasionally be obtained from the lung or pleural space, the pH should be 6.0 or higher.[28,29] Approximately 2% of patients have an alkaline stomach pH[30] with causes including duodenal reflux, antacids, H_2 blockers, or recent instillation of formula or medications.[30,31]

If awake and cooperative, ask the patient to talk. If the patient cannot speak, suspect respiratory placement. Note that with small-bore tubes, patients may still be able to speak despite tracheal placement.[31]

Once correct tube position is tentatively confirmed, secure the tube. If the patient requires abdominal or chest radiographs for other diagnostic purposes, place the NG tube before obtaining the films. An NG tube deviated to the right may occasionally be seen in patients with traumatic rupture of the aorta, but this is not a reliable indicator.

Securing the Tube

The NG tube is generally secured to the patient with tape attached to both tube and nose (Fig. 40–7A). A butterfly bandage (or tape on each side of the nose) that then coils around the NG tube is a typical approach. The nose and the tube should both be clean and possibly prepared with tincture of benzoin. If a tape should let go or require repositioning, both the tape and the tincture of benzoin must be replaced. It is wise to also secure the tube to the patient's gown, so that a tug on the tube will encounter this resistance before pulling on the material securing the tube to the patient's nose. A rubber band tied around the tube with a slipknot (see Fig. 40–7B) and pinned to the gown near the patient's shoulder is effective. It is critical to ensure that the tube is secured in such a way that it *does not press on the medial or lateral nostril.* Necrosis or bleeding can result if a tube is not secured correctly.

When a Salem sump is used, the blue pigtail must be kept above the level of the fluid in the patient's stomach or stomach contents may leak back through the vent lumen. If a patient

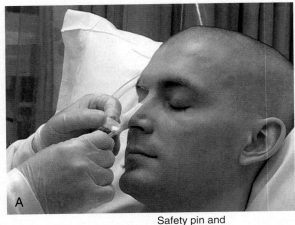

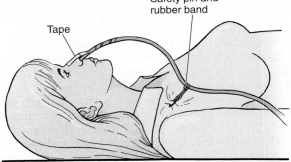

Figure 40–7 *A,* The tape on the bridge of the nose keeps the tube in the middle of the nasal opening, away from the skin, preventing irritation. *B,* Attach the NG tube to the patient's gown using a rubber band and a safety pin so that the first tug on the tube pulls the gown and not the tape holding the tube in the patient's nose. (*A, From Thomsen T, Setnik G [eds]: Procedures Consult—Emergency Medicine Module. Copyright 2008 Elsevier Inc. All rights reserved.*)

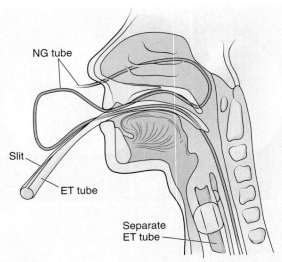

Figure 40–8 Diagrammatic representation of the separation of the NG tube from the guiding endotracheal (ET) tube through the slit in the guiding ET tube. The NG tube has first been passed through the nose and is pulled out through the mouth. The tip of the tube is then threaded into the guiding ET tube to ensure passage down the esophagus. The guiding ET tube is removed from the esophagus before being separated from the NG tube. Note the prior placement of another ET tube in the trachea (partially shown) to avert passage of the guiding ET tube into the trachea. (*Modified from Sprague DH, Carter SR: An alternate method for nasogastric tube insertion. Anesthesiology 53:436, 1980.*)

needs to ambulate with a sump tube in place, the blue pigtail can be fitted into the plastic connector at the end of the suction lumen, creating a closed loop that should not leak.

Placement Issues

If the patient is intubated, deflate the balloon of the endotracheal (ET) tube briefly to allow passage of the NG tube. In the unconscious patient, the NG tube is easily misplaced into the pulmonary tree, but misplacement is unlikely if the patient is intubated. This complication may be missed during the procedure because gag and cough reflexes may be suppressed and the patient cannot talk. In addition, the absence of swallowing may prevent successful passage of the tube. Several techniques may be used to successfully pass an NG tube in a difficult unconscious patient. If initial attempts fail, place the NG tube through a naris into the oropharynx. Visualize the tip of the tube with a laryngoscope, grasp it with Magill forceps, and pull it out of the mouth. Select an ET tube with an ID that is slightly larger than the external diameter of the NG tube. Slit it along its lesser curvature from the proximal end to a point 3 cm from its distal end. Pass the slit ET tube (generally 8 mm ID) through the mouth into the esophagus.[32] Alternatively, pass a 7-mm ID slit ET tube directly through the nose into the esophagus.[33] Passage into the esophagus is facilitated by the stiffness of the larger ET tube and does not require active swallowing. Thread the tip of the NG tube into the ET tube and advance it into the stomach (Fig. 40–8). Remove the slit ET tube from the esophagus. When the distal

part of the ET tube is visible, slit the unslit 3-cm distal part with scissors. Remove the ET tube, and the NG tube will remain in place.[34]

Advance any slack tubing with forceps or pull it back nasally, depending on the final depth required for the NG tube. The technique can also be performed by passing the slit ET tube nasally, which also saves the trouble of orally advancing or nasally retracting any slack tubing.[33,34]

In a particularly passive, sedated, unconscious, or toothless patient, guiding the NG tube with the fingers in the pharynx is occasionally successful (Fig. 40–9).[35] Displacing the larynx forward by manually gripping and lifting the thyroid cartilage can aid tube insertion,[36] as can simple jaw elevation. A soft nasopharyngeal airway, well lubricated, is at times easier to pass nasally than the NG tube, and then the lubricated NG tube can be passed through it. In addition, it affords some protection to the nasal mucosa if multiple attempts to pass the NG tube are necessary, or if it is particularly important to minimize bleeding or trauma. Cooling an NG tube increases its rigidity, and coiling it can increase the tube curvature, both of which may help pass the tube.

Ultimately, if all other methods fail, place a flexible fiberoptic bronchoscope or esophagoscope into and through the esophagus under direct visualization.[37] Thread a guidewire into the stomach. Place the NG tube over the guidewire into the stomach and then remove the guidewire.[38]

Complications

Complications of standard NG tube placement are similar to problems noted with NG feeding tube placement. The complications related to tube misplacement are discussed in that section. In addition, the clinician placing the NG tube in the patient with neck injuries should be cautious of potentiating

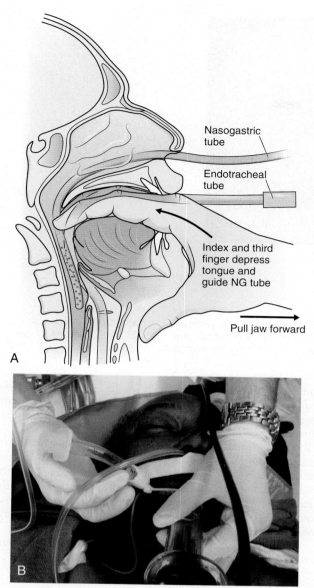

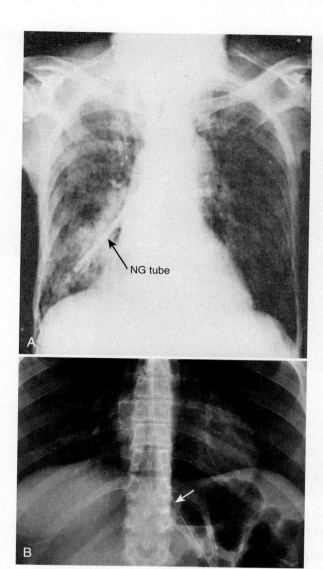

Figure 40–9 *A,* The passage of an NG tube through the nose of an intubated patient. An ET tube is in the trachea via the mouth. Place the second and third fingers in the posterior pharynx. Depress the tongue with the fingers. Guide the NG tube down the esophagus by passing it through the second and third fingers that are in the posterior pharynx. *Importantly, place the thumb under the jaw and pull the jaw forward. B,* In this intubated patient, the Video Laryngoscope (Glidescope, Verathon, Bothell, WA) can be used to manipulate the larynx to allow for visualized NE tube passage.

Figure 40–10 *A,* Levin tube inadvertently placed in the right main stem bronchus; an alveolar infiltrate consistent with early pneumonia is also shown. *B,* Proper position of the NG tube is best verified by an x-ray. (*A, From Johnson JC: Letter to the editor: Back to basics for morbidity-free nasogastric intubation. JACEP 8:289, 1979; B, from Thomsen T, Setnik G [eds]: Procedures Consult—Emergency Medicine Module. Copyright 2008 Elsevier Inc. All rights reserved.*)

cervical spine injuries with excessive motion during passage (especially in association with coughing and gagging in the awake patient). Furthermore, passage of an NG tube in the awake patient with a penetrating neck wound may exacerbate hemorrhage should coughing or gagging result. Particularly serious forms of tube misplacement are pulmonary placement (Fig. 40–10) and intracranial placement (Fig. 40–11).

A tension gastrothorax can develop in patients with an intrathoracic stomach. The tension gastrothorax can occupy much of the left hemithorax, displacing the heart and lungs and causing a clinical syndrome identical to tension pneumothorax. Whereas successful passage of an NG tube will relieve a tension gastrothorax, the high pressures of a tension gastro-

thorax often develop because torsion of the stomach in the chest prevents egress of air; that torsion may prevent ingress of the therapeutic NG tube. The condition is rare enough that further emergent therapy is based on case reports rather than substantial series. Relief of the tension gastrothorax has been accomplished with transthoracic puncture of the stomach with a 16-gauge catheter over needle. The catheter over needle was inserted in the second intercostal space in the midclavicular line, and then the needle was removed. The catheter was left in place attached to intravenous tubing with the distal end under a water seal.[39] A single 16-gauge puncture of the stomach is unlikely to leak and cause pleuritis; such punctures have long been used in percutaneous endoscopic gastrostomy (PEG) tube placement. Inserting a chest tube into the stomach is not advisable because gastric fluid may leak into the pleural space. Once the tension on the stomach is relieved, it may be possible to pass the NG tube to prevent reoccurrence of the problem. The stomach, no longer tense

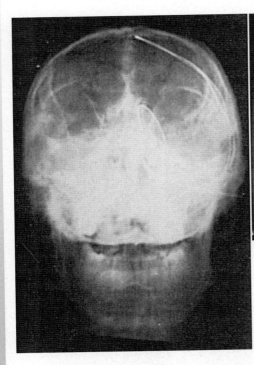
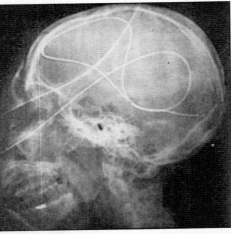

Figure 40–11 Anteroposterior and lateral skull radiographs demonstrate intracranial insertion of an NG tube in a patient with multiple skull fractures. *(From Johnson JC: Letter to the editor: Back to basics for morbidity-free nasogastric intubation. JACEP 8:289, 1979.)*

and wedged in the chest, can twist to allow the tube to pass. Surgical correction of the condition permitting intrathoracic herniation of the stomach is the definitive treatment to prevent recurrence of tension gastrothorax. NG tubes, when in place for prolonged periods, are a common cause of innocuous gastric bleeding and gastric erosions.

REPLACEMENT OF NASOENTERIC FEEDING TUBES

Indications and Contraindications

The most common indication for feeding tube replacement in the ED is unintentional removal of a preexisting feeding tube. In one prospective study, 38% of tubes were removed unintentionally. Although some of these tubes had fallen out or had been coughed out, more than half were pulled out by the patient.[40] Tube rupture, deterioration, or clogging may also necessitate replacement. Management of a clogged or nonirrigating feeding tube is discussed in the section on clogged feeding tubes.

Feeding Tube Site

Three major classes of enteral feeding tubes are in common use; classification is according to the site of insertion. Tubes can enter through the nares, a cervical ostomy, or an abdominal ostomy. Enteral tubes are often categorized by the location of the tip of the tube. Tubes may terminate primarily in the stomach, such as a gastrostomy (G) or PEG tube. They may terminate in the small intestine, a jejunosotomy (J) tube, or in both the stomach and the small intestine, a PEG-J tube. To confuse the issue, *some tubes enter the stomach and terminate in the stomach (G tube) or in the proximal small bowel (J tube), whereas some tubes enter the gastrointestinal tract directly through the small bowel wall (J tube).* Practically speaking, almost all gastric tubes are PEG tubes. They are placed endoscopically with local anesthesia and without a surgical incision. J tubes,

conversely, are placed surgically under general anesthesia, require a surgical incision, and result in a surgical scar at the insertion site. Gastric feeding results in better digestion than intestinal feeding whereas J tubes are less likely to result in reflux and aspiration. Normally about 20% of gastric antral contents pass into the duodenum, with 80% refluxing back into the body of the stomach for further mixing.[41] If the feeding tube is placed in the antrum of the stomach or in the small bowel, enteral feeding solution passing into the small bowel may not be tolerated, resulting in diarrhea and paradoxical decreased nutrition.[41,42]

The most common rationale for small intestinal feeding is to reduce regurgitation and aspiration.[43–46]

Procedure

Nasoenteric feeding tube replacement requires greater time and effort if the patient is uncooperative or has a physically obstructing lesion. Nasoenteric feeding tube migration into the duodenal bulb generally requires patient positioning in the right decubitus position for about an hour after successful intragastric passage.[47]

The clinician should explain the procedure to the patient before tube passage. It is generally advisable to restrain the hands of demented, impaired, or otherwise uncooperative patients. Prepare the nares before passage of the tube similar to the procedure for primary NG tube placement. If a feeding tube stylet is used, lubricate and insert it into the feeding tube before introducing it into the nares. Tube stylets can be lubricated with water-soluble jelly. If using Dobbhoff, Entri-Flex (Biosearch) or another tube with preapplied lubricant, you may need to activate the lubricant with a 5-mL flush of water. Never allow the stylet to protrude beyond the end of the feeding tube because these stiff, small-diameter wires have the capacity to scratch the esophagus and allow for the creation of a false passage. The stylet may lock into position on the tube at the proximal end and should be properly secured.

When the patient is uncooperative or cannot drink, introduce 5 to 15 mL of water into the mouth or into the proximal end of the feeding tube with a syringe; this may induce swallowing and facilitate tube passage. Although the patient may not swallow for several minutes, wait for her or him to swallow because this may mean the difference between a coiled or pulmonary tube placement and successful passage.

Placement Confirmation

Auscultatory confirmation of tube placement can be misleading, so confirm proper placement of the tube with a radiograph before feeding.[3] However, radiographic confirmation of tube placement may also be misleading. In viewing the radiograph, it is particularly important to study the area around the carina. An esophageal tube shows at most a mild change in course, whereas a tracheally placed tube usually deviates significantly as it travels into the right or left main stem bronchus. The end of an NG tube may appear to be in the stomach yet actually may be in the left lung behind and below the top of the diaphragm.[48] When a stylet has been used for passage, leave it in the feeding tube for the radiograph, because the tube's course is not always visible without it. The stylets of most tubes are designed to allow insufflation and aspiration while in place. Even when stomach entry is certain, the intestinal location may be misleading on radiograph. A nasoenteric tube may lie completely to the left of midline and yet have its tip in the duodenum, or it may have a position overlying the right abdomen yet not have entered the duodenum. A contrast study is necessary to ascertain duodenal position when pulmonary placement has been ruled out.[47,49]

Examine the radiograph also for the presence of mediastinal air or a pneumothorax, which may suggest pulmonary or esophageal puncture. An esophageal puncture should be evaluated with endoscopy and may require surgery, depending on the size of the rent.

The end bulb of most nasoduodenal tubes will pass into the duodenum after patient positioning in the right decubitus position for an hour. Some researchers recommend pretreatment with metoclopramide to enhance gastric emptying.[50–52] One investigator[47] found that metoclopramide enhances duodenal passage of nasogastrically placed feeding tubes in diabetic, but not in nondiabetic, patients. Gastric antral motility in diabetics is often impaired; metoclopramide helps restore normal synchronized activity in these patients but has little effect on emptying in subjects who have normal antral function. The usual dose of metoclopramide is 10 mg administered intravenously. Also, 3 mg/kg of erythromycin lactobionate given intravenously over 1 hour works similarly and may be effective even if metoclopramide fails.[53] Endoscopy or fluoroscopy may be necessary if positioning and metoclopramide are not successful.

Complications

Pulmonary intubation is an uncommon but well-known and potentially fatal complication of nasal feeding tube insertion (see Fig. 40–10). Coughing and respiratory distress are the most common symptoms of respiratory passage of an NG tube, but there may be relatively few apparent symptoms in a demented or comatose patient.[54] Decreased mentation and an absent cough reflex are predisposing factors for unrecognized nasopulmonary intubation with NG tubes.[3] A small end bulb (e.g., 2.7 mm diameter) can slip past a tracheal high-volume, low-pressure cuff and pass easily to the lung periphery.[3,54,55]

A pneumothorax may result when an NG tube dissects into or is withdrawn from the pulmonary parenchyma.[56] Bloody aspirate from a tube should heighten awareness of possible tissue damage.

A clogged or nonfunctional NG tube may be difficult to remove. Fluoroscopy may allow careful insertion of a guidewire or stylet into an in situ tube to facilitate removal. Fluoroscopy may also identify the mechanical problem interfering with the tube's removal. Bent-double segments are probably the most common cause. Knots, although uncommon, do occur. Do not use excessive force to remove an NG tube because serious injury to the patient may result.

Premature removal of the NG tube is the most frequent complication of feeding tube use. To help prevent removal by an uncooperative patient, secure the NG tube to a loop anchor passed in the same naris. The anchor works by aversive stimulation of the soft palate and nose with distraction of the NG tube, rather than by mechanical stabilization of the tube.

Sax and Bower[57] recommend a technique for creating a separate NG tube anchor. Cut a soft weighted nasoenteric tube approximately 12 inches from the top. Pass a heavy (2-0) silk suture through the tube to exit the side hole. Insert the guidewire with care, because it must not protrude from the inserted end. Sedate the patient if uncooperative. Insert the tube through the anesthetized naris into the nasopharynx, grasp it with Magill forceps and pull to remove it through the mouth (Fig. 40–12A). Trim excess tubing without cutting the silk suture. Make a closed loop by tying the silk suture in front of the nose. Leave the loop long enough that it does not apply

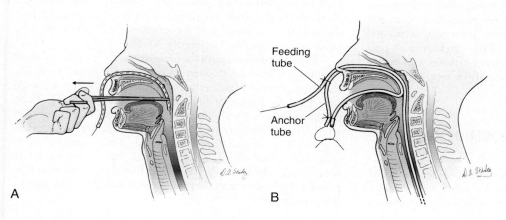

Feeding tube

Anchor tube

A   B

Figure 40–12 Placement of an NG tube anchor to secure a companion NG or feeding tube in an uncooperative patient who repeatedly pulls out the feeding tube. *A,* Using forceps, grasp the tube in the pharynx and pull it out through the mouth. This will serve as an anchor tube. *B,* Tie the ends of the short anchor tube together to form a loop, and tie the companion NG or feeding tube to the anchor loop.

continuous pressure to the nose or palate while at rest. Pass the nasal feeding tube through the same nostril and secure it to the loop (see Fig. 40–12B). This anchor is simpler to construct and more comfortable than anchors that pass through the opposite nostril.[57]

Complications of properly placed nasoenteric tubes include nasopharyngeal erosions, esophageal reflux, tracheoesophageal fistulas, gagging, rupture of esophageal varices, and otitis media.[58] One survey of nasogastrically fed patients found that the most distressing features of having an NG tube for feeding were deprivation of tasting, drinking, and chewing of food; soreness of the nose; rhinitis; esophagitis; mouth breathing; and the sight of other patients who were eating.[59]

Checking feeding tolerance is difficult with small-gauge feeding tubes. Aspiration of tubes to check for residuals is not recommended with tubes of 9 French size or smaller. Aspiration is likely to clog the tubes because they collapse under pressure and because relatively small particles can occlude the tube. For the same reasons, the residual is likely to be inaccurate.[43]

Patient Instructions

To maintain catheter patency, small tubes should be flushed with 20 to 30 mL of tap water at least two to three times daily and after administration of medication.[43,49] Water is a more effective irrigant than cranberry juice.[60] Medications should be in liquid form or be completely dissolved, or they may clog the tube. Methods of dealing with a clogged tube are discussed subsequently. The tube should be anchored to the nose and face in such a way that it is not in contact with the skin at the nasal opening. This reduces tube discomfort and prevents necrosis of the alae, nares, and distal septum. Patients who exhibit a tendency to pull on their tubes need adequate restraints. Patients receiving tube feedings should have their heads elevated to at least 30° above the horizontal.[43]

PHARYNGOSTOMY AND ESOPHAGOSTOMY FEEDING TUBES

Cervical pharyngostomy and cervical esophagostomy have both been developed relatively recently. Cervical esophagostomies are generally performed at the time of cervical or maxillofacial operations. Malignant growths of the proximal esophagus, head, or neck are the primary indications for esophagostomy. Cervical esophagostomies may eventually evolve a permanent sinus, allowing the feeding tube to be removed between meals. Such tubes will unlikely be replaced in the ED, but the concept of these feeding tubes is illustrated in Figure 40–13. Complications of pharyngostomy and esophagostomy include local soft tissue irritation, accidental extubation because of excess length of the external tube, pulmonary aspiration from vomiting, arterial erosion with exsanguination, and esophagitis or stricture of the esophagus from reflux.

G, GASTROENTEROSTOMY, DUODENOSTOMY, AND J TUBES

Since the turn of the century, more than 30 different operative techniques have been described for tube gastrostomy.[61] The "pull" technique, an endoscopic percutaneous procedure,

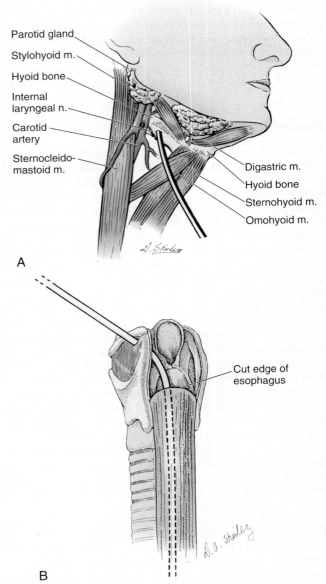

Figure 40–13 *A,* Pharyngostomy feeding tube. *B,* Pathway for an esophagostomy or pharyngostomy feeding tube.

performed under conscious sedation, is now the most common method of gastrostomy placement. This has been termed a *PEG tube.* In the "pull" technique, an endoscope is passed into the patient's stomach and the contents are aspirated. The procedure is described in Figure 40–14.

Feeding tubes may also be placed directly into the jejunum or advanced into the duodenum or jejunum via the stomach. Rarely, an operative procedure is performed to suture a jejunal tube into the lumen of the small bowel (Fig. 40–15). Tube duodenostomies are also created for duodenal decompression after partial gastrectomy with Billroth II anastomoses.[62] Permanent jejunostomies are rarely used. Tube jejunostomy is indicated when the proximal bowel has a fistula or is obstructed, when recovery of small bowel motility is anticipated long before recovery of gastric motility, and after a gastrectomy.[61,62]

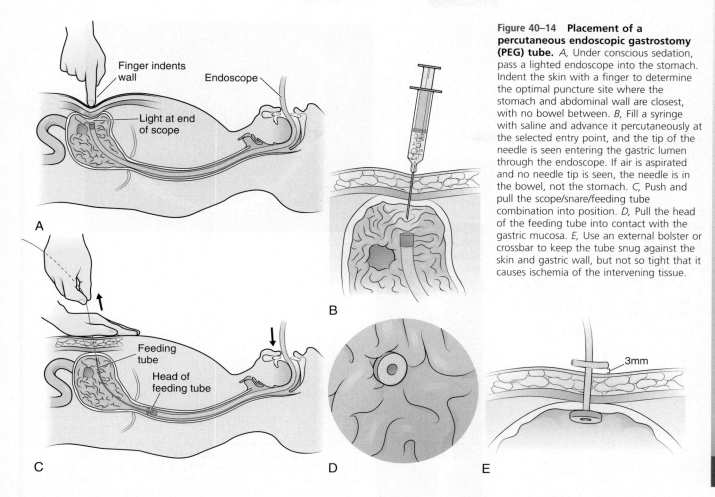

Figure 40–14 **Placement of a percutaneous endoscopic gastrostomy (PEG) tube.** *A,* Under conscious sedation, pass a lighted endoscope into the stomach. Indent the skin with a finger to determine the optimal puncture site where the stomach and abdominal wall are closest, with no bowel between. *B,* Fill a syringe with saline and advance it percutaneously at the selected entry point, and the tip of the needle is seen entering the gastric lumen through the endoscope. If air is aspirated and no needle tip is seen, the needle is in the bowel, not the stomach. *C,* Push and pull the scope/snare/feeding tube combination into position. *D,* Pull the head of the feeding tube into contact with the gastric mucosa. *E,* Use an external bolster or crossbar to keep the tube snug against the skin and gastric wall, but not so tight that it causes ischemia of the intervening tissue.

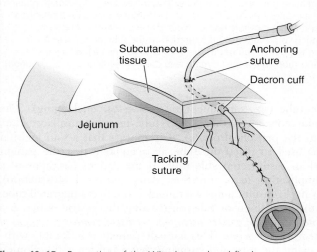

Figure 40–15 Formation of the Witzel tunnel and final permanent jejunal catheter placement. *(From Wiedeman JE, Smith VC: Use of the Hickman catheter for jejunal feedings in children. Surg Gynecol Obstet 162:69, 1986.)*

Contraindications for gastrostomy feeding include severe gastroesophageal reflux, upper gastrointestinal fistulas, repeated aspiration of gastric contents, and intestinal or gastric outlet obstruction.[61] Jejunal feeding is contraindicated if the highly osmolar feeding solutions required for jejunal feeding are poorly tolerated and cause copious diarrhea.

Indications and Contraindications for Tube Replacement

The nursing home patient with a nonfunctioning or displaced feeding tube represents a common ED presentation. The clinician cannot always determine the location of the original feeding tube by simply looking at the patient who arrives in the ED for tube replacement. Nevertheless, the emergency clinician should attempt to ensure that the terminal end of a replaced tube is in the same viscus as the original. External inspection may or may not reveal where a feeding tube should terminate (Fig. 40–16). Contrast studies and fluoroscopy usually provide such information (Fig. 40–17). A de Pezzer (mushroom) or Foley G tube is designed only for intragastric termination. Some tubes have two lumina, one terminating in the stomach for decompression and the other in the small bowel for feeding. These can be confused with tubes that have two entrances to one lumen (one for continuous feeding and the other for medications) and tubes that have a second lumen leading to an inflatable balloon.

Foley catheters are not ideal as long-term feeding tubes. They clog easily, and the balloon disintegrates in stomach acid. They may be used temporarily but should be replaced with specialized feeding tubes when feasible. A call from the nursing home indicating that a tube has been pulled out should be answered by the advice that a Foley catheter be immediately used to keep the stoma open. Always inflate the balloon with saline, and use a bolster to prevent tube migra-

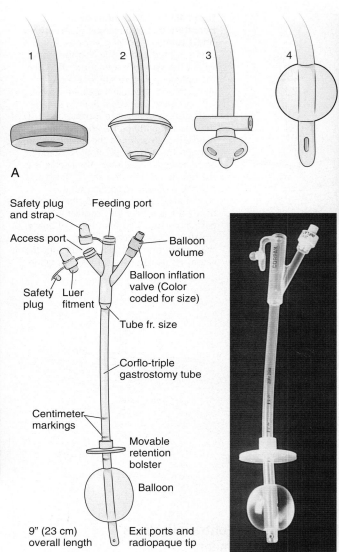

B

Safety plug and strap

Feeding port

Access port

Balloon volume

Balloon inflation valve (Color coded for size)

Safety plug

Luer fitment

Tube fr. size

Corflo-triple gastrostomy tube

Centimeter markings

Movable retention bolster

Balloon

9" (23 cm) overall length

Exit ports and radiopaque tip

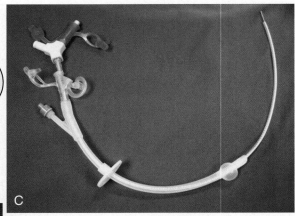

A

C

Figure 40–16 *A,* Various types of gastrostomy tubes. *1,* Silicone catheter (American Endoscopy [Bard Interventional Products, Billerica, MA]). *2,* Polyurethane catheter with collapsible foam flange (to collapse, tube should be cut) (VIASYS MedSystems, Wheeling, IL). *3,* Latex catheter with a movable external bolster and an internal mushroom or de Pezzer–type flange on the end (American Endoscopy [Bard Interventional Products, Billerica, MA]). *4,* Balloon (Foley) catheter (Wilson-Cook Co., Winston-Salem, NC). *B,* A user-friendly gastrostomy tube is supplied by VIASYS MedSystems (Wheeling, IL), the CORFLO-DUAL GT gastrostomy tube, packaged with lubricant, a prefilled syringe for inflating the balloon, and an extension set. The color-coded inflation valve indicates tube size (12–24 Fr). The silicone tube uses a retention balloon and a movable bolster. Note that the retention bolster is designed to prevent inward migration of the tube and not to be an anchoring device sutured to the skin. *C,* A gastric balloon jejunal feeding tube enters the stomach and delivers feedings into the jejunum.

tion (Fig. 40–18). An original PEG tube is pictured in Figure 40–19. This long tube has a mushroom end that is removed by traction.

The clinician has a few options when faced with the task of replacing a feeding tube. Unfortunately, old records or nursing home personnel rarely give specific information that is helpful to the emergency clinician. If only a stoma exists, one may request that the nursing home *describe or send the prior tube to the ED.* If no surgical scar is seen at the stoma site, the tube is almost certainly a G tube or a G tube that terminated in the jejunum. When in doubt, passing a Foley catheter without balloon inflation, taping it to the skin, and referring the patient to a consultant or the original referring clinician is appropriate. *Some type of tube must be placed to stent the stoma, otherwise the stoma will quickly close (in a matter of hours), and the patient might require a more complicated procedure to regain access.* The only real concern of placing a gastric tube into the jejunum is that the balloon will produce intestinal obstruction if it is fully inflated.

If the tube is nonfunctioning yet still in place, the clinician must make a judgment as to the risk versus benefit of removal and replacement versus an attempt at unclogging

the tube (see subsequent discussion on unclogging). The major concern is that a new tube may be misplaced (i.e., into the peritoneal cavity). If it appears that a skin incision was used to place the tube, it is unlikely that the patient has an easily removable tube. If the patient has signs of a complication (e.g., infection, ileus, intestinal obstruction), surgical consultation is warranted. Note that a migrated tube, with the balloon or tube obstructing the gastric outlet, *is a common cause of gastric distention, persistent vomiting, or signs of intestinal obstruction.* This is easily remedied by simply withdrawing the tube and ensuring that a bolster is functioning (Fig. 40–20).

Most PEG tubes do not have sutures joining the stomach with the abdominal wall, so there is potential for a replaced tube to end up in the peritoneal cavity. Adhesions, however, usually keep the stomach appropriately positioned, but only after the tract has matured. Nonoperative tube replacement techniques are safe only through an established tract between the skin and the bowel. *Catheter replacement should not be attempted in the immediate postoperative period.* A simple gastrostomy takes about a week to form a tract.[63] A stable tract may take 2 or 3 weeks longer to form if healing is compro-

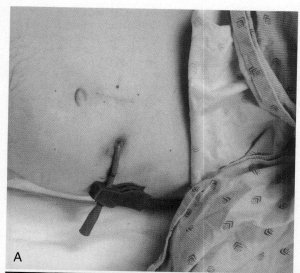

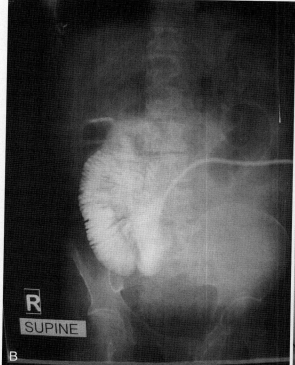

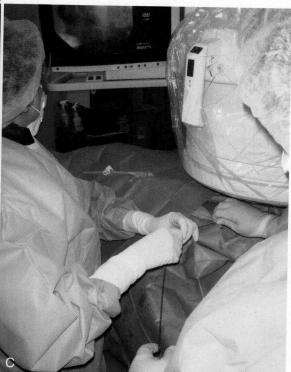

Figure 40–17 *A,* Without old records, the exact type and positioning of this nonfunctioning feeding tube are unknown. The operative scar on the abdominal wall suggests an implanted tube, not a simple gastric tube. *B,* Injection of contrast before tube removal demonstrates the tube tip ending in the small bowel, not the stomach. *C,* If the tube has been removed, and questions remain about type of tube and circumstances of placement, a new tube is best placed under fluoroscopy with guidewire assistance.

mised. Poor nutrition is the most common element compromising wound healing in patients requiring a feeding tube. A Witzel tunnel may take up to 3 weeks after the operation to mature sufficiently for safe nonoperative tube replacement.

Equipment for Replacing a Dislodged Tube

Equipment for feeding tube replacement *into a matured site* includes gloves, stethoscope, feeding tube, external bolster, lubricant, basin, and a syringe that fits the tube. Tincture of benzoin, tape, and absorbent dressing material may be used to dress the wound, although many are better left undressed.[64] Some feeding tubes require special plugs or connectors. Others need to be pinched with a clamp when not in use to prevent leakage. Some tubes are placed with the aid of accompanying guidewires or stents.

The easiest tube to replace is one that has been removed in the ED or dislodged for only a few hours. The stoma closes quite quickly, so replacement is best done as soon as possible. The stoma site can be gently probed by a cotton applicator to determine patency and direction of the tract (Fig. 40–21). In selected cases, a hemostat can gently dilate the opening to accept a replacement tube. *All such attempts should be done carefully to avoid creating a false tract.* Local anesthetic around the stoma may be used if exploration causes pain, and bleeding is common. After the tube is passed, restrain the hands to avoid tube removal by uncooperative patients.

Transabdominal Feeding Tube Removal

A feeding tube may have to be removed because it is irreversibly clogged, leaking, or broken; persistently develops kinks;

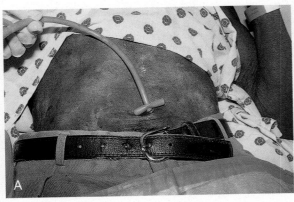

A

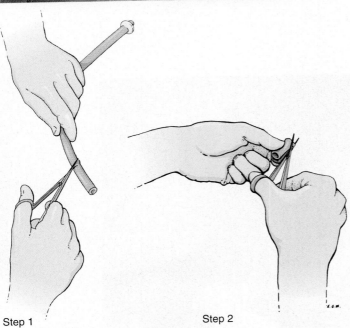

Step 1

Step 2

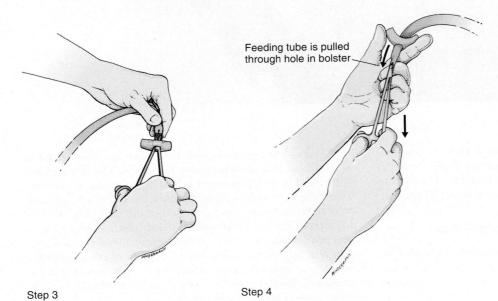

Feeding tube is pulled
through hole in bolster

Step 3

Step 4

B

Figure 40–18 *A,* Foley catheter is *not an ideal feeding tube* but can be used temporarily to maintain stoma patency, lasting only about a few months owing to disintegration of the latex. Always inflate the balloon with saline and use a bolster. *B,* To make an external bolster for a feeding tube to prevent tube migration: Step 1—Cut a 3-cm segment of tubing from the proximal segment of another Foley catheter. Step 2—Bend the tubing in half and cut to create a hole on each side of the segment. Step 3—Insert a hemostat through the holes in the completed bolster and grasp the feeding tube. Step 4—Advance the tube through the bolster to 1 cm above the skin of the external abdomen.

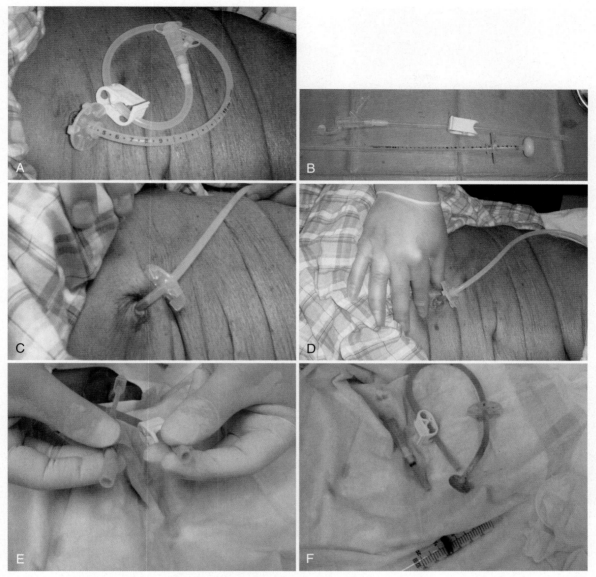

Figure 40–19 *A,* This type of tube serves as the original PEG device. It has a mushroom head, not a balloon. *B,* When replaced, a balloon-type tube is used. *C,* This original tube is leaking because the mushroom tip has been pulled out of the stomach lumen and is lodged in the soft tissue of the abdominal wall. *D,* If the tube tract has matured (at least 2 wk after placement), it may be removed by traction/countertraction. Significant force may be required, and be prepared for a pop and splattering of gastric contents. *E,* It is easy to determine if there is a balloon at the end of a PEG tube that cannot be removed. Simply cut the tube and if there is no additional port or channel to inflate the balloon (*F*), it must be the type of tube that can be removed by traction.

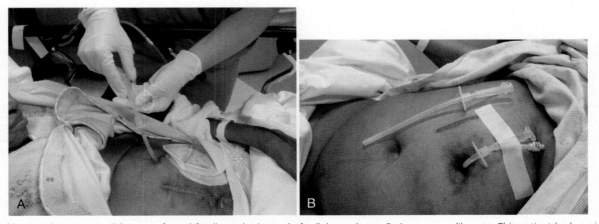

Figure 40–20 *A,* Whenever possible, use a formal feeding tube instead of a Foley catheter. *B,* A common dilemma: This patient had persistent vomiting after tube feedings, and gastric distention. The tube had simply migrated distally (note comparison of new tube and positioning of indwelling one) because the bolster was too far proximal. Withdrawing the tube and repositioning the bolster alleviated the problem.

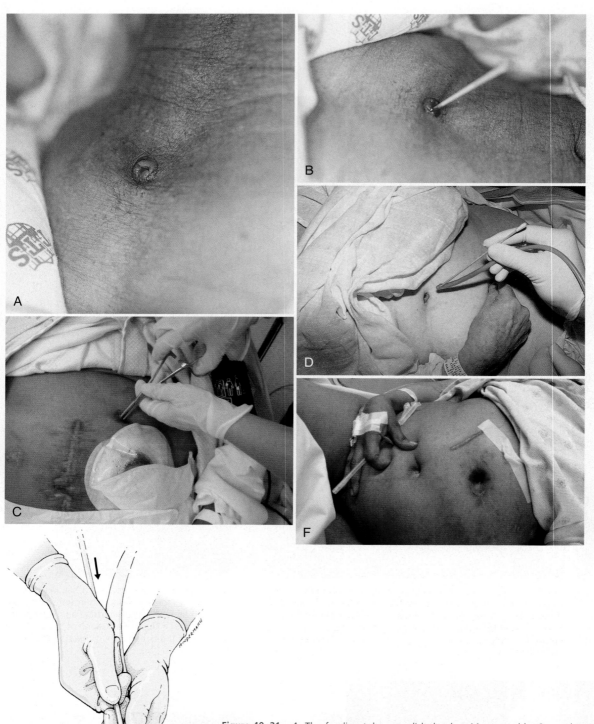

Figure 40–21 *A,* The feeding tube was dislodged at 11 PM, and by 9 AM, the stoma was too tight for easy tube replacement. It was accomplished under fluoroscopic guidance, always the best option in questionable cases. *B,* The stoma opening and direction of the tract can be investigated by gently probing the site and tract with a Q-tip; in this case, it easily entered the stomach. *C,* This tight stoma was carefully dilated under local anesthesia with a hemostat. A false passage can easily be created. This area usually readily bleeds. *D,* To give a Foley catheter rigidity to aid in passage, the end of a Q-tip was inserted in the side port of the distal catheter, and traction was applied to the catheter. *E,* If a de Pezzer catheter is used, an ET tube stylet distends the flange for passage, and the tip re-forms once in the stomach. *F,* This patient removed her recently replaced feeding tube, with balloon inflated, while still in the ED awaiting transfer. This could have been avoided if her hands were restrained.

too large or too small; causes a hypersensitivity reaction; is associated with an abscess; or is not the appropriate length for feeding into the desired viscus. Before a new transabdominal feeding tube is inserted, the old tube must be removed. Most, but not all, tubes can be removed without endoscopy. It is imperative to know whether the tube in place is safe to remove before attempting to remove it. Standard de Pezzer or mushroom catheters that have been modified with bolsters or rings at the time of endoscopic or surgical insertion may no longer be safe to remove with traction. Tubes are occasionally secured with sutures or rigid internal bumpers or stays. It is rare, however, to encounter a tube that cannot be removed with traction/countertraction. Modest force may be required; use a hand for countertraction, and be prepared for a pop and splattering of gastric contents (Fig. 40–22). This causes the tube and end mushroom to narrow, and the tube should come out easily. The inner crossbar, if present, may remain in the stomach when the rest of the feeding tube complex is removed by traction. Obstruction from the crossbar, which will pass in the stool, has yet to be reported for adults. In small children, obstruction is a possibility, and the crossbar should be removed by endoscopy.[65,66]

Recently placed feeding tubes may need to be left in until a tract has formed (1–2 wk, depending on the procedure) even if the tube is nonfunctional.

A simple Foley catheter G tube is easiest to remove. Deflate the Foley balloon and the tube should slide right out. If the Foley balloon cannot be deflated, cutting the tube may allow the balloon to deflate. Do not cut the catheter so close to the abdomen that it will be impossible to maintain a grip on it for a traction removal if the balloon still does not deflate. The balloon may also be punctured to cause it to deflate. To puncture a Foley balloon, apply traction to the catheter to draw the balloon up against the ostomy (Fig. 40–23). Using the taut feeding tube as a guide, pass a small-gauge needle along the tube to puncture the balloon. It may be necessary to try again on the other side of the catheter, because the balloon may be asymmetrically inflated, and contact with the needle may be established on one side and not the other. Be careful not to track away from the ostomy into the patient's abdominal wall or to cause separate punctures of the stomach. Allow a minute for the balloon to deflate before another attempt is made at traction removal. Large, nondeflating balloons should probably be punctured, whereas small balloons may be removed with traction.

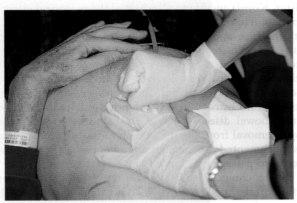

Figure 40–22 Gentle, firm traction using the flat part of the opposite hand for countertraction will remove most PEG tubes, even those with internal mushroom bumpers. Modest force may be required, and be prepared for a sudden pop and splattering of gastric contents.

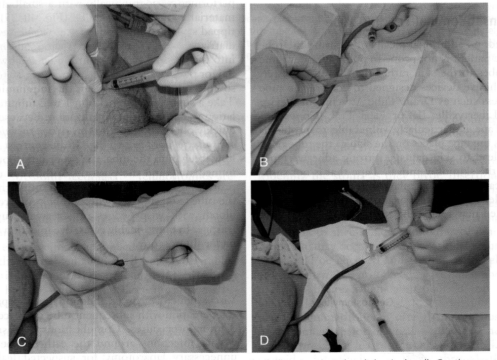

Figure 40–23 *A,* If a Foley balloon will not deflate, use traction to bring the balloon against the abdominal wall. Gently pass a small needle along the course of the catheter, puncturing as many times as necessary. Wait a few minutes for the fluid to egress. *B,* Once the balloon is deflated, it can be withdrawn. Note the encrusted condition of this longstanding Foley catheter used as a PEG tube. *C,* Occasionally the wire from a central line kit can clear the lumen and allow deflation. *D,* If the valve mechanism malfunctions, cut the catheter and attempt to drain the balloon by placing a needle in the inflation channel, by flushing and withdrawing fluid.

CHAPTER 42

Decontamination of the Poisoned Patient

Christopher P. Holstege and Pauline E. Meekins

In 2005, the Toxic Exposure Surveillance System of the American Association of Poison Control Centers reported 2,424,180 toxic exposures and 1261 resultant fatalities.[1] Of these total exposures, 22.8% were managed in a health care facility. A massive exposure to some very toxic agents (e.g., cyclic antidepressants, β-blockers, calcium channel blockers, antihistamines, chemotherapy agents, colchicine, cocaine, chloroquine, iron, cyanide, amanita mushrooms, paraquat) *will likely result in severe morbidity or fatality regardless of even the most sophisticated and timely medical intervention*. With general supportive care and the use of a few specific antidotes, however, the mortality rate of unselected overdose patients is less than 2% if the patient arrives at the hospital in time for the clinician to intervene.

The management of poisoned patients presenting to health care facilities initially focuses on confirming the diagnosis of a possible toxin exposure, providing standard cardiovascular and respiratory supportive care, and using a small cadre of specific antidotes. In selected instances, the prevention of further toxin absorption by various decontamination procedures may theoretically ameliorate morbidity or reduce mortality.

Although a better final outcome from gastric decontamination may seem intuitively reasonable, *there is no definitive evidence from prospective clinical trials proving that the use of various decontamination techniques positively alters the morbidity or mortality of the poisoned patient*.[2]

Before the availability of objective, experimental evidence addressing gastric emptying procedures, most clinicians instituted such procedures in the emergency department (ED) as a reflex response for the majority of patients suspected of drug overdose, often without much forethought and certainly without confirming data. Mounting evidence relegates *any form of gastric decontamination to selected cases and individual specific scenarios*. In fact, because of the lack of demostratable benefit and the mounting evidence for potential harm, syrup of ipecac, once a mainstay in the management of poisonings, is no longer recommended; its use is considered a class III action (may cause harm) by the American Heart Association, and parents have been instructed by the American Academy of Pediatrics to remove it from the home.[3]

Nonetheless, a selective role for other methods of gastric decontamination exists, and there will always be a role for real time clinical judgment. Because compelling circumstances may prospectively clinically support gastric decontamination, this chapter discusses specific clinical procedures. These techniques include gastric lavage, oral activated charcoal administration, and whole bowel irrigation (WBI). In addition, dermal decontamination as a result of a toxic exposure is also addressed. Before performing these techniques, the clinician responsible for the care of the poisoned patient must clearly understand that these procedures are not without hazards, and any decision on their use must consider whether the benefit of decontamination outweighs any procedure-related harm.

GASTRIC DECONTAMINATION

Gastric Lavage

Background

The use of gastric lavage in poisoned patients has decreased significantly since the late 1990s.[4] Numerous animal and human volunteer studies have been conducted examining the effectiveness of gastric lavage in removing toxins from the stomach, especially in comparison with other gastrointestinal decontamination methods.[5–15] The reported efficacy of gastric lavage in removing markers from the stomach varies significantly in these studies. The difference in these study results is due in part to the variability of the methods used (different fluid instilled markers, animal models, positioning, amount of lavage, and lavage tube sizes) and the time that elapsed from the instillation of the marker in the stomach until gastric lavage was performed. Even within individual studies, the range of effectiveness of gastric lavage to remove the marker varied considerably. For example, Tandberg and coworkers[11] performed gastric lavage 10 minutes after ingestion of the marker and reported that its effectiveness to remove the marker varied from 18.9% to 67.7%.

Many of these studies do not replicate the typical clinical scenario encountered in emergency medicine.[2,16] The efficiency of gastric lavage to remove a marker significantly decreases with increasing time after ingestion. This is due to the fact that as time increases after ingestion, the more time there is for the marker to be absorbed and for the marker to pass out of the stomach. For example, Shrestha and colleagues[17] reported that greater than 70% of the marker used in their study passed out of the stomach by 60 minutes. It is rare that gastric lavage can be performed within the first hour after toxic ingestion. Not only does it take time for these patients to present to the ED, but it also takes time for evaluation, stabilization, and for the gastric lavage to take place. For example, Watson and associates[14] reported that the mean time required by experienced emergency medicine nurses to perform lavage was 1.3 hours. Gastric lavage may also propel the marker from the stomach into the small intestine, decreasing the effectiveness of removing the toxin from the stomach and enhancing the rate of absorption.[18]

Three major studies have examined whether gastric lavage positively influences the outcome of poisoned patients.[19–21] In a study performed by Kulig and coworkers,[19] there was no difference in outcome among patients who received gastric lavage followed by charcoal versus charcoal alone when these were performed more than 1 hour after ingestion. In patients who were treated within 1 hour of ingestion, gastric lavage followed by charcoal provided a small but statistically significant advantage over activated charcoal alone. Merigian and colleagues[20] demonstrated that for symptomatic patients, the rate of intensive care admission and the need for intubation was significantly higher for those patients who received gastric lavage followed by charcoal than for those who received charcoal alone. This increased admission and intubation rate was directly attributed to the aspiration of gastric contents owing to gastric lavage. Pond and associates[21] replicated the Kulig study. They found no difference in outcome between those patients who received gastric lavage followed by charcoal versus those receiving charcoal alone,

POSITION STATEMENT: GASTRIC LAVAGE

American Academy of Clinical Toxicology; European Association of Poisons Centres and Clinical Toxicologists

Gastric lavage should not be employed routinely in the management of poisoned patients. In experimental studies, the amount of marker removed by gastric lavage was highly variable and diminished with time. There is no certain evidence that its use improves clinical outcome and it may cause significant morbidity. Gastric lavage should not be considered unless a patient has ingested a potentially life-threatening amount of a poison and the procedure can be undertaken within 60 minutes of ingestion. Even then, clinical benefit has not been confirmed in controlled studies. Unless a patient is intubated, gastric lavage is contraindicated if airway protective reflexes are lost. It is also contraindicated if a hydrocarbon with high aspiration potential or corrosive substance has been ingested.

Figure 42–1 Position statement: gastric lavage. *(From the American Academy of Clinical Toxicology; European Association of Poisons Centres and Clinical Toxicologists. Published in Clin Toxicol 35:711, 1997.)*

regardless of time of performance of gastric lavage. They concluded that "gastric emptying procedures can be omitted from the treatment regimen for adults after acute overdose, including those who present within 1 hour of overdose and those that manifest severe toxicity."

Indications

Based on the available literature, gastric lavage should not be routinely used in the management of poisoned patients[22] (Fig. 42–1). There is no universally accepted standard of care that can be applied to the use of gastric lavage in the unselected poisoned patient in the ED. Under certain circumstances, however, there may be a theoretical benefit from gastric emptying, and the local poison center should be contacted to assist in making a decision whether gastric lavage may be of benefit. Whether specific subsets of overdose patients may benefit from gastric lavage has not been clearly defined (Table 42–1).

Only patients who have ingested a potentially life-threatening amount of poison in whom the procedure can be performed within 60 minutes are the primary candidates for gastric lavage. Oral charcoal alone is considered superior to gastric lavage if a drug is adsorbed by charcoal.

Contraindications

Although generally safe, gastric lavage is not an innocuous procedure. The performance of gastric lavage is contraindicated in any person who demonstrates compromised airway protective reflexes, unless she or he is intubated. Many clinicians opt for lavage in a seriously ill patient who is intubated because airway protection is already accomplished. Tracheal intubation, however, does not ensure a totally protected airway. Paralyzing and intubating a patient merely to initiate gastric lavage is generally eschewed.

Gastric lavage is contraindicated in persons who have ingested corrosive substances (acids or alkalis), hydrocarbons (unless containing highly toxic substances such as pesticides), known esophageal strictures, or history of gastric bypass surgery.[23] Caution should be exercised in performing gastric lavage in combative patients and in those who have medical conditions such as bleeding diatheses that could be compromised by performing this procedure.

TABLE 42–1 Factors that Cumulatively Increase the Appropriateness of Gastric Emptying*

Substantial risk of consequential toxicity: e.g., ingestion of aspirin, chloroquine, colchicine, cyclic antidepressants, calcium channel blockers
Evidence of consequential toxicity: e.g., repeated seizures, hypotension, cardiac dysrhythmias, apnea, acid-base, or other metabolic disturbances
Antidotal or adjunctive therapy ineffective or nonexistent: e.g., colchicine, paraquat
Recent ingestion (<1–2 hr)
Ingestion exceeds adsorptive capacity of initial activated charcoal dosing: e.g., >100 mg/kg of pills such as aspirin, sustained-release verapamil, sustained-release theophylline
Ingested agent not adsorbed by activated charcoal: e.g., iron, lithium
Ingested agent likely to form durable mass after overdose: e.g., large amounts of aspirin, enteric-coated agents, iron, meprobamate
Ingestions of extended or sustained-release formulations: e.g., calcium channel blockers, theophylline
No antecedent vomiting
Gastric tube placement required for activated charcoal administration
No contraindications to gastric emptying

*See text for further discussion, recommendations, and caveats. *Note*: This table gives general circumstances in which the clinician may consider gastric emptying procedures (generally, gastric lavage). These recommendations are those of one textbook and are theoretical and not specifically supported by scientific data. Charcoal alone is considered superior to lavage if the toxin is adsorbed by charcoal. The table is included to give the reader a perspective that reflects the limitations of experimental gastric emptying studies and is contrary to recommendations to abandon the procedure.

From Smilkstein MJ: Techniques used to prevent gastrointestinal absorption of toxic compounds. In Flomenbaum NE, Howland MA, Goldfrank LR, et al (eds): Goldfrank's Toxicologic Emergencies, 7th ed. New York, McGraw Hill, 2002.

Equipment and Preparation

If the decision is made to perform gastric lavage, careful attention to the details of the procedure results in increased safety for the patient and more effective removal of the ingested poison. Before lavage, the patient should have intravenous access secured and should have continuous cardiac monitoring and pulse oximetry. A large, rigid suction catheter should be immediately available.

If the patient is highly anxious or agitated, give a small dose of a benzodiazepine (e.g., 1–2 mg midazolam intravenously). If the patient's level of consciousness is significantly depressed, the airway status is questionable, or the airway is likely to be compromised during the procedure, consider rapid-sequence induction and intubation with a cuffed endotracheal tube before initiating gastric lavage. If the patient is fully awake and alert, proceed to lavage without tracheal intubation. The procedure should proceed deliberately without significant patient resistance. The procedure is intended to be therapeutic, not punitive. Antiquated arguments promulgating that a noxious lavage will keep patients from overdosing again should be abandoned.

The position of the patient during gastric lavage is important. Place all patients in the left lateral decubitus position in Trendelenburg (~20° tilt on the table) (Fig. 42–2). This position diminishes the passage of gastric contents into the duo-

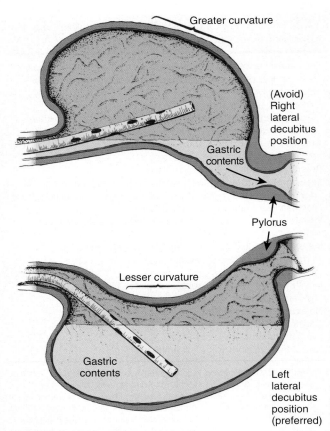

Figure 42–2 The effect of patient positioning on lavage. The left lateral decubitus position is preferred.

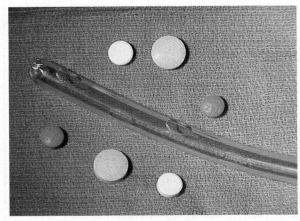

Figure 42–3 This large-diameter gastric lavage tube demonstrates the size of the holes and the size of some typical pills. Extra holes can be cut in the side of the tube to facilitate removal of large fragments.

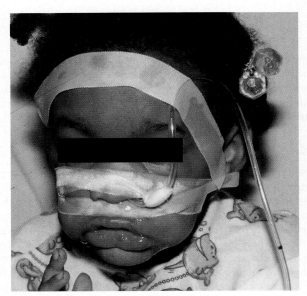

Figure 42–4 Gastric lavage in a child is always problematic. Obviously, an adult-sized large-bore oral gastric tube cannot be used, but a nasogastric (NG) tube may suffice. Some pediatric textbooks recommend a 24-Fr oral gastric tube for toddlers, and a 36-Fr tube for adolescents. In this case, a child was found with an open bottle of digoxin, and it could not be determined whether ingestion had occurred. She would not drink charcoal. The 18-Fr NG tube was used to attempt to aspirate digoxin from the stomach (none was recovered) and to instill charcoal. Some would suggest the oral route for this tube, but it was passed rather easily through the nose. An NG tube is not ideal for some ingestants (iron, sustained-release products), but most pills quickly dissolve in the stomach and the small particles can easily be removed with an NG tube. Although lavage may have been reasonable in this scenario, a potent and safe antidote for digoxin does exist. The common routine practice of passing an NG tube in a child who is unwilling to drink charcoal is controversial and while intuitively reasonable, it is of unproven value and likely done far too often for benign ingestions. *(Reprinted with permission from Seckl MJ, Rustin GJ, Newlands ES, et al. Pulmonary embolism, pulmonary hypertension, and choriocarcinoma. Lancet 338:1313, 1991.)*

denum during lavage and decreases the risk of pulmonary aspiration of gastric contents should vomiting or retching occur. Restrain the hands of an uncooperative patient to prevent removal of the gastric or endotracheal tube. Intubated patients on a ventilator may be lavaged in the supine position because of logistical reasons. Under no circumstances should the nonintubated patient undergo lavage in the restrained supine position. Such positioning invites aspiration and diminishes the patient's natural protective maneuvers, such as coughing and sitting up.

Most clinicians prefer the oral route for gastric lavage, but in selected circumstances, a standard large-bore nasogastric (NG) tube (Salem sump pump) may be used. Large-diameter gastric hoses with extra holes cut near the tip have been traditionally recommended for gastric lavage. There are no convincing data on humans to refute or support this recommendation, and one study of a small number of dogs failed to show any difference in efficacy with lavage through a 32-French tube compared with a 16-French lavage tube.[24] It is generally held that large-diameter NG or orogastric tubes (>1 cm) are more likely to retrieve particulate matter successfully, but the tube size is such that whole pills are unlikely to pass (Fig. 42–3). Smaller, more flexible tubes may kink and are significantly more difficult to pass. An NG tube may be passed through the mouth or nose, but orogastric hoses should not be passed through the nose. Because most pills disintegrate in the stomach in a few minutes, significant amounts of particulate matter may be retrieved with a large-bore NG tube such as an 18-French Salem sump tube. NG tubes are considerably easier to pass and are less traumatic for the

patient. NG tubes are preferred for liquid ingestions and in children (Fig. 42–4).

In most cases, a 36- to 40-French or 30 English-gauge tube (external diameter, 12–13.3 mm) should be used in adults and a 24- to 28-French-gauge (diameter, 7.8–9.3 mm) tube in

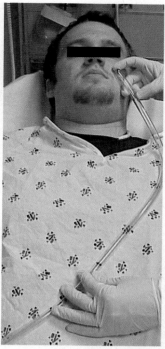

Figure 42–5 Measure and mark the appropriate depth of gastric lavage tube prior to passage. This ensures that the tip is in the stomach and that there is no excess tubing to hinder fluid egress or to allow kinking/knotting of the tube.

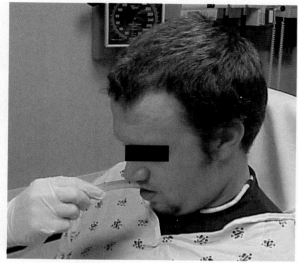

Figure 42–6 Once the pharynx has been entered, put the patient's chin on the chest to facilitate passage of the tube into the esophagus. *If the patient begins to vomit, withdraw the tube immediately to allow the patient to close the epiglottis and lessen the chance of aspiration.*

children.[22] Before passage, the length of the tube required to enter the stomach should be estimated by approximating the distance from the corner of the mouth to the midepigastrium; premeasurement avoids the curling and kinking of excess hose in the stomach (Fig. 42–5). Passage of an excessive length of hose may cause gastric distention, bruising, and perforation, whereas passage of an insufficient length of hose may result in lavage of the esophagus and the increased risk for emesis and aspiration. Commercial lavage systems are available and often use either a gravity fill-and-empty system with a Y connector or a closed irrigation syringe system. Alternatively, an irrigation syringe can be used for intermittent lavage fluid input and withdrawal.

Technique

Lubricate the gastric tube and pass it gently to avoid damage to the posterior pharynx. Use a bite block or an oral airway to avoid the patient's chewing the orogastric tube and biting the fingers of the inserter. If the patient is obtunded or paralyzed, extend the jaw to facilitate passage. Never use force to pass the tube. Once the pharynx has been entered, put the patient's chin on the chest to facilitate passage of the tube into the esophagus (Fig. 42–6). Cough, stridor, or cyanosis indicates that the tube has entered the trachea; withdraw the tube immediately and reattempt passage. Once the tube is passed, confirm that it is in the stomach. Intragastric placement is usually evident on clinical grounds and confirmed by auscultation of the stomach during injection of air with a 50-mL syringe and aspiration of gastric contents. In the intubated or obtunded patient or the young child, confirm the tube position radiographically before lavaging, although this is not routinely performed. A misplaced tube may irrigate the esophagus with a tube that has doubled back on itself during passage. The most serious complication is inadvertent passage

of the tube into the lungs. Tracheal passage of a lavage tube should be readily obvious in the awake patient before lavage, and obtunded patients are intubated, obviating this problem. If an awake patient begins to vomit during the lavage, immediately remove the tube to allow the patient to protect the airway.

Before gastric irrigation, remove the gastric contents by careful gastric aspiration with repeated repositioning of the tube tip. With the Y connector closed system, perform lavage by clamping the drainage arm of the Y adapter and infusing aliquots of fluid into the stomach from a reservoir (Fig. 42–7). Clamp the reservoir arm of the Y, and then open the drainage arm to permit gravity drainage of the stomach contents. Repeat this procedure. Some resistance is produced by the Y connector and tubing. Apply suction intermittently to the drainage tubing to enhance stomach emptying.

Lavage can be performed adequately with tap water in adults. Because electrolyte disturbance has occurred in children who were lavaged with tap water, prewarmed (45°C) normal saline is generally recommended for children.[25-27] Warmed lavage fluid increases the solubility of most substances, delays gastric emptying, and theoretically, should increase the effectiveness of the procedure.[28,29] Repeatedly introduce small aliquots of lavage solution (200–300 mL in adults and 10 mL/kg body weight in children up to a maximum of 300 mL) into the stomach and then remove them. Larger amounts of fluids create the potential for an increased risk of washing gastric contents into the duodenum or the lungs. Much smaller amounts are not clinically practical because of the dead space in the tubing (~50 mL in the 36-Fr hose) and the increase in time that is required. The amount of fluid that is returned should approximate the amount introduced. Manual agitation of the patient's stomach by gently "kneading" the stomach with a hand placed on the abdomen may increase recovery.[28] Continue lavage until the fluid becomes clear.

After gastric aspiration and lavage have been completed, administer a slurry of activated charcoal through the gastric tube. When no longer needed, clamp off the gastric tube

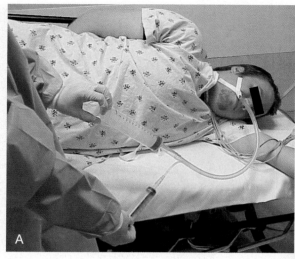
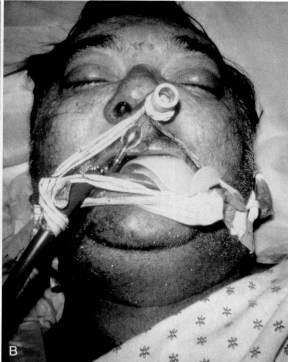

Figure 42–7 *A,* Example of a Y connector closed system with the patient in a left lateral decubitus position. *B,* Patients on a ventilator or intubated with airway protection may be lavaged in the supine position, but an awake nonintubated patient is never lavaged in the supine position.

during its removal to avoid "dribbling" fluid into the airway. With the increasing use of repetitive doses of activated charcoal, the gastric tube is often left in place after the lavage procedure is completed. Because this large tube is irritating and may predispose the patient to gagging, drooling, or aspiration, it should be removed. The alert patient should take subsequent doses orally as necessary. The patient who remains obtunded may receive additional doses via a standard NG tube.

Complications

A correctly performed procedure in the appropriate environment is generally safe but numerous complications have been associated with gastric lavage.[30] The complications can be divided into those caused by mechanical trauma and those resulting from the lavage fluid.

Depending on the route selected for tube insertion, damage to the nasal mucosa, turbinates, pharynx, esophagus, and stomach has been reported.[31–34] After tube insertion, it is imperative to confirm correct placement. Scalzo and associates[35] found radiographically that 7 of 14 children had improper tube placement (too high or too low) despite positive gastric auscultation in all cases. Radiographic confirmation of tube placement should be considered in young children and intubated patients. Instillation of lavage fluid and charcoal into the lungs through tubes inadvertently misplaced within the airways has been reported.[36]

During lavage, changes in cardiorespiratory function have been noted. Thompson and coworkers[37] reported that during lavage, 36% of patients had atrial or ventricular ectopy, 4.8% had transient ST elevation, and 29% had a fall in oxygen tension to 60 torr or less. Patients at greatest risk for these findings included the elderly, smokers, those with lung disease, or those with cyclic antidepressant overdose. Laryngospasm may also occur during gastric lavage.[22]

The lavage fluid itself is a potential source of complications. The large amount of fluid administered during lavage has been reported to cause patient fluid and electrolyte disturbances. These disturbances have been seen with the use of both hypertonic and hypotonic lavage fluids in the pediatric population.[25–27] Hypothermia is a possible complication if the lavage fluid is not prewarmed.

Pulmonary aspiration of gastric contents or lavage fluid is the primary potential risk during gastric lavage, especially in patients with compromised airway protective reflexes.[38–40] Merigian and colleagues[20] reported a 10% incidence of aspiration pneumonia in patients who received gastric lavage. This risk is reduced by using small aliquots of lavage fluid, adequately positioning the patient, and intubating patients with compromised airway protective reflexes.

If the lavage tube cannot be easily removed, do not force it. Kinking or knotting of the tube can occur, but occasionally, a tube may become stuck because of lower esophageal spasm. If fluoroscopy or a radiograph demonstrates no deformation to the lavage tube, 1 to 2 mg of intravenous glucagon can be infused in an attempt to relieve lower esophageal spasm.[41] Surgical removal may be necessary if the gastric tube is deformed by kinking or knotting.

Activated Charcoal

Background

Activated charcoal is a carbon product that is subjected to heat and oxidized to increase the surface area. It has the capacity to adsorb substances onto the porous surface of the charcoal. Activated charcoal acts both by adsorbing a wide range of toxins present in the gastrointestinal tract and by enhancing toxin elimination if systemic absorption has already occurred. It enhances elimination by creating a concentration gradient between the contents of the bowel and the circulation, but it also has the potential of interrupting enterohepatic circulation if the particular toxin is secreted in the bile and enters the gastrointestinal tract before reabsorption.[42] Oral activated charcoal is given as a single dose or in multiple doses. The adsorptive capacity of charcoal depends on the inherent properties of the toxin and the local milieu, such as pH. Adsorption begins within minutes of contact with a toxin, but may not reach equilibrium for 20 to 30 minutes. Desorption of toxins from charcoal occurs over time, although this has little clinical significance for most patients and can be overcome by administering additional charcoal.

Indications

For years, the administration of a single dose of oral activated charcoal for essentially all overdoses has been routine. Clearly, charcoal binds many toxins in the gut, thereby decreasing some systemic absorption. Despite a lack of scientific data demonstrating a decrease in morbidity and mortality, and without firm evidence to support its widespread use, charcoal is a reasonable intervention for most poisoned patients presenting to the ED if it can be easily and safely administered (Fig. 42–8). The exact indications are not established, and no universally accepted standard of care has been promulgated.[43] A single dose of activated charcoal is indicated if the clinician estimates that a clinically significant fraction of the ingested substance remains in the gastrointestinal tract, the toxin is adsorbed by charcoal, and further absorption may result in clinical deterioration. This will usually be a clinical decision, because adequate historical data may often be lacking. It may also be administered by multiple dosing if the clinician anticipates that the charcoal will result in increased clearance of an already absorbed drug. It is most effective within the first 60 minutes after oral overdose and decreases in effectiveness over time. Charcoal is generally considered to provide superior gut decontamination over gastric lavage. There is no definitive evidence that administration of activated charcoal improves outcome.

Contraindications

The administration of charcoal is contraindicated in any person who demonstrates compromised airway protective reflexes, unless he or she is intubated.[43] It is absolutely contraindicated in persons who have ingested corrosive substances (acids or alkalis). Not only does charcoal provide no benefit in a corrosive ingestion, but its administration could precipitate vomiting, obscure endoscopic visualization, and lead to complications if a perforation developed and charcoal entered the mediastinum, peritoneum, or pleural space. Charcoal should be avoided in cases of a pure aliphatic petroleum distillate ingestion. Hydrocarbons are not well adsorbed by activated charcoal, and its administration could lead to further aspiration risk. Many hydrocarbons are potential systemic toxins (e.g., carbon tetrachloride and benzene) or are mixed with other potentially significant toxins such as pesticides. In these cases, data are lacking, but charcoal administration can be considered. Caution should be exercised in using charcoal in patients with medical conditions that could be further compromised by charcoal ingestion, such as gastrointestinal perforation or bleeding. *Charcoal is not indicated for isolated ingestions of ethanol, iron, or lithium because these substances are not adsorbed.* If the airway is not secure, charcoal should be given with caution to minimally symptomatic patients who have ingested a toxin that may suddenly induce seizures. Because it is often impossible to determine the exact nature of an ingestion, a liberal use policy is advocated for potentially mixed overdoses.

Charcoal administration by paramedics and other emergency response personnel should be performed with caution.[44] The same indications and contraindications apply as for those patients who are in the hospital. The motion of the ambulance during transport may make the patient more prone to emesis. Either the spilling of charcoal or the vomiting of charcoal may result in significant contamination of the transport vehicle and subsequently place that vehicle out of commission until it can be cleaned.

Technique

There is no universally accurate dose for charcoal. A 10:1 ratio (charcoal-to-toxin) is recommended if the amount of ingestion is known. Charcoal dosing should be considered in light of the specific ingestion, but the recommended empirical doses of single-dose activated charcoal (standard aqueous products, such as Liqui-Char) are as follows:[43]

- Up to 1 year: 1 g/kg of body weight.
- 1 year to 12 years: 25 to 50 g.
- Older than 12 years: 25 to 100 g.

If the ingestion were, for example, clonidine (0.1-mg tablets) or digoxin (0.25-mg tablets), this regimen would be more than adequate for even a massive overdose to achieve the desired 10:1 ratio. If the ingestion consisted of a large number of 325-mg aspirin tablets, or 240-mg verapamil tablets, the dosing regimen could be insufficient. If toxic medications with a high milligram dosage are ingested, it would be prudent to administer more charcoal than indicated by these guidelines. There is no known benefit of mixing charcoal with a cathartic (i.e., sorbitol), and the combination is not suggested. Sorbitol increases the incidence of vomiting.

Because in many formulations the contents settle with time, shake the preparation vigorously before administering it to the patient. Follow this by rinsing the container with a small amount of tap water before administering it to the patient to allow ingestion of the full dose.[45] Aqueous activated charcoal has a gritty texture that most patients find unpleas-

---

POSITION STATEMENT: SINGLE-DOSE ACTIVATED CHARCOAL

American Academy of Clinical Toxicology; European Association of Poisons Centres and Clinical Toxicologists

Single-dose activated charcoal should not be administered routinely in the management of poisoned patients. Based on volunteer studies, the effectiveness of activated charcoal decreases with time; the greatest benefit is within 1 hour of ingestion. The administration of activated charcoal may be considered if a patient has ingested a potentially toxic amount of a poison (which is known to be adsorbed to charcoal) up to 1 hour previously; there are insufficient data to support or exclude its use after 1 hour of ingestion. There is no evidence that the administration of activated charcoal improves clinical outcome. Unless a patient has an intact or protected airway, the administration of charcoal is contraindicated.

Figure 42–8 Position statement: single-dose activated charcoal. *(From the American Academy of Clinical Toxicology; European Association of Poisons Centres and Clinical Toxicologists. Published in Clin Toxicol 35:721, 1997.)*

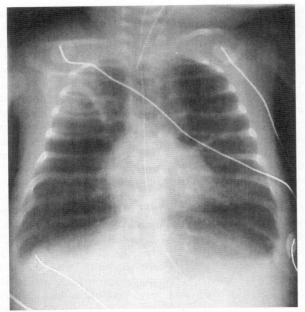

Figure 42–9 Radiographic confirmation of NG tube placement may be performed before lavage or instillation of charcoal if there is uncertainty about the position of the tube. Tracheal placement of a lavage tube is usually readily evident. Vomiting during lavage suggests that the tube has curved back into the esophagus. A confirmatory radiograph is suggested in the obtunded patient if correct gastric placement is questioned. Tracheal intubation precludes passage of a tube into the lungs, but it does not ensure proper gastric placement.

ant; attempts have been made to improve the taste and texture. Mixing activated charcoal with chocolate milk, chocolate- or cherry-flavored syrup, or ice cream may increase palatability, but mixing with these additives has been suggested, though not proved, to cause a decrease in the adsorptive capacity of activated charcoal.[46] Rangan and colleagues[47] reported no decrease in adsorption after mixing superactivated charcoal with a noncaffeinated cola. Scharman and associates[48] demonstrated that a regular, sugared cola was favored by children over a diet cola, but only 20% of the time were they able to cajole even nonpoisoned children younger than 3 years to drink a therapeutic amount of flavored charcoal.

Give activated charcoal orally if the patient is awake and cooperative and by NG tube if the patient is unconscious. If an NG tube is inserted, it is imperative to verify correct placement (Fig. 42–9). Confirm correct tube placement radiographically before administering charcoal, especially in obtunded or intubated patients. Instillation of charcoal into the lungs has been reported after inadvertent misplacement within the airways[36] and massive aspiration can be fatal[49] (Fig. 42–10). Intubation is protective but it is not uncommon to see some charcoal in the airway even if the patient has been intubated.

The common tactic of passing an NG tube in the awake but uncooperative patient merely to administer charcoal is controversial. Such a scenario is more likely to result in trauma from the tube placement, a misplaced tube, or subsequent emesis from the rapid administration of charcoal. Given the unproven efficacy of charcoal, the authors advise against the routine insertion of an NG tube simply to administer charcoal in the awake and minimally symptomatic patient. Such a decision is, however, a clinical one that must be made by the clinician and based on the entire clinical milieu (Fig. 42–11).

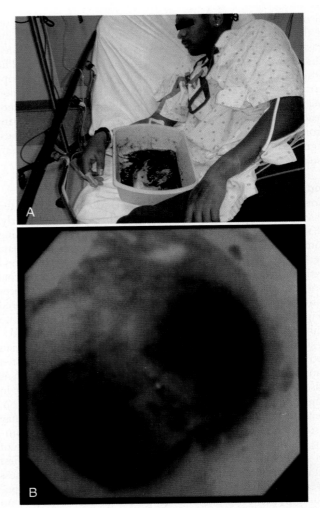

Figure 42–10 *A,* Vomiting can be expected following charcoal administration, especially if sorbitol is added (not recommended). This patient rapidly became drowsy after charcoal administration, vomited, but fortunately did not aspirate. *B,* In another patient who aspirated, the charcoal can be seen at the carina with a fiberoptic scope. Massive aspiration can be fatal. Intubation does not totally protect against minimal charcoal aspiration.

Complications

The administration of activated charcoal is not without risks and complications. Published reports have demonstrated adverse effects associated with activated charcoal therapy, including childhood deaths.[50] The most common complications of charcoal administration include constipation, diarrhea, and vomiting.[51,52] Bowel perforation has been described in a patient with diverticular disease.[53] Pulmonary aspiration of activated charcoal is a dreaded complication that can result in pneumonitis, obstruction of the respiratory tree, bronchiolitis obliterans,[33,54-56] acute lung injury, and barotrauma.[50] Risk factors for serious aspiration are large amounts of charcoal instilled over a short period of time, multiple-dose charcoal in the setting of an ileus, charcoal administration in a patient who becomes obtunded, charcoal that is inappropriately diluted, or the forced administration of charcoal via an NG tube, especially in a restrained supine patient. These complications can be prevented by prudent dosing of charcoal and associated cathartic therapy, as well as monitoring of fluid and electrolyte status, abdominal examinations, and clinical condition. Trivial aspirations of charcoal are common and usually innocuous even if the patient is intubated. Studies show a 4% to 39% incidence of aspiration pneumonia in intubated patients who received activated charcoal while intubated.[57] It has been shown that even in the face of a protected airway with a cuffed endotracheal tube, vomiting can lead to pulmonary aspiration of the charcoal.[50] This can lead to a significant increase in lung microvascular permeability, causing lung edema and pulmonary compromise.[58]

Multiple Doses of Activated Charcoal

Indications

The use of multiple-dose activated charcoal (MDAC) may be indicated in select cases[59] (Fig. 42–12). Its use has been advo-

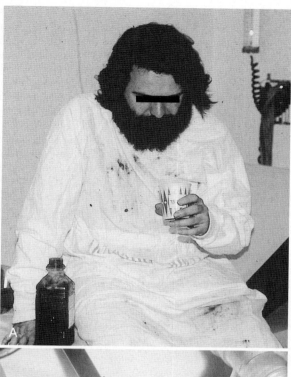

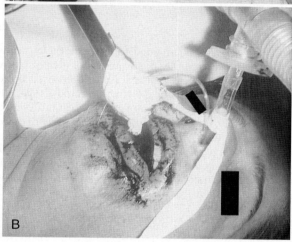

Figure 42–11 *A,* If the overdose patient will voluntarily drink charcoal, there are few reasons to withhold it, even though a definite clinical benefit in the routine case cannot be proved. If a patient will not drink charcoal, patient management becomes controversial. Passing an NG tube in a struggling patient or in a recalcitrant child merely to instill the unproven, but theoretically useful, antidote is not supported by scientific data. Nonetheless, it remains a common procedure. Although not always easy or pleasant, such an intervention is usually safe. Pulmonary aspiration, even in the awake patient, is the major downside. *Restrained supine patients are at greatest risk for aspiration,* and that position should be avoided, even in the initially awake patient. *B,* Charcoal that is voluntarily swallowed or instilled via an oral-gastric lavage tube or NG tube can induce emesis. This occurs in both the obtunded and the awake patient. In this instance, the patient was unconscious from the overdose and the airway was protected with prior tracheal intubation. Although the intubation procedure does not totally exclude pulmonary aspiration and it carries some morbidity in its own right, it is recommended prior to charcoal use in the patient who is not able to fully protect the airway. Patients who initially are asymptomatic or minimally affected but have ingested drugs that have the potential to produce rapid deterioration, seizures, or loss of airway protection make decisions on the use of charcoal difficult for the clinician. In borderline cases, some experienced clinicians avoid the use of charcoal altogether.

POSITION STATEMENT: POSITION STATEMENT AND PRACTICE GUIDELINES ON THE USE OF MULTI-DOSE ACTIVATED CHARCOAL IN THE TREATMENT OF ACUTE POISONING

American Academy of Clinical Toxicology; European Association of Poisons Centres and Clinical Toxicologists

Although many studies in animals and volunteers have demonstrated that multiple-dose activated charcoal increases drug elimination significantly, this therapy has not yet been shown in a controlled study in poisoned patients to reduce morbidity and mortality. Further studies are required to establish its role and the optimal dosage regimen of charcoal to be administered.

Based on experimental and clinical studies, multiple-dose activated charcoal should be considered only if a patient has ingested a life-threatening amount of carbamazepine, dapsone, Phenobarbital, quinine, or theophylline. With all of these drugs there are data to confirm enhanced elimination, though no controlled studies have demonstrated clinical benefit.

Although volunteer studies have demonstrated that multiple-dose activated charcoal increases the elimination of amitriptyline, dextropropoxyphene, digitoxin, digoxin, disopyramide, nadolol, phenylbutazone, phenytoin, piroxicam, and sotalol, there are insufficient clinical data to support or exclude the use of this therapy.

The use of multiple-dose charcoal in salicylate poisoning is controversial. One animal study and 2 of 4 volunteer studies did not demonstrate increased salicylate clearance with multiple-dose charcoal therapy. Data in poisoned patients are insufficient presently to recommend the use of multiple-dose charcoal therapy for salicylate poisoning. Multiple-dose activated charcoal did not increase the elimination of astemizole, chlorpropamide, doxepin, imipramine, meprobamate, methotrexate, phenytoin, sodium valproate, tobramycin, and vancomycin in experimental and/or clinical studies.

Unless a patient has an intact or protected airway, the administration of multiple-dose activated charcoal is contraindicated. It should not be used in the presence of an intestinal obstruction. The need for concurrent administration of cathartics remains unproven and is not recommended. In particular, cathartics should not be administered to young children because of the propensity of laxatives to cause fluid and electrolyte imbalance.

In conclusion, based on experimental and clinical studies, multiple-dose activated charcoal should be considered only if a patient has ingested a life-threatening amount of carbamazepine, dapsone, Phenobarbital, quinine, or theophylline.

Figure 42–12 Position statement and practice guidelines on the use of multidose activated charcoal in the treatment of acute poisoning. *(From the American Academy of Clinical Toxicology; European Association of Poisons Centres and Clinical Toxicologists. Published in Clin Toxicol 37:731, 1999.)*

TABLE 42–2 Drugs Whose Serum Clearance May Be Enhanced by Multiple Doses of Activated Charcoal

Aspirin	Phenobarbital
Caffeine	Phenytoin
Carbamazepine	Quinine
Cyclosporine	Sotalol
Dapsone	Sustained-release thallium
Digoxin	Theophylline
Disopyramide	Valproate
Nadolol	Vancomycin

cated for two purposes: first, to prevent continued absorption of a drug that may still be present within the gastrointestinal tract; second, *to increase the serum clearance of a drug that has already been absorbed* (Table 42–2).

MDAC prevents continued absorption by either binding a drug that may be present throughout the gastrointestinal tract or binding a drug that exists as extended-release or enteric-coated preparations. MDAC enhances elimination of a drug by interrupting enterobiliary recirculation or augmenting enterocapillary exsorption.[52] By interrupting enterobiliary recirculation, charcoal binds to an active drug that is secreted by the biliary system, subsequently preventing reabsorption. By augmentation of enterocapillary exsorption, charcoal produces sink conditions that drive diffusion of drug from the capillaries into the entraluminal space, where it is subsequently eliminated. This process is called *intestinal dialysis*.[60] Drug characteristics that are associated with enhanced systemic clearance with MDAC include a low intrinsic clearance, a prolonged distributive phase, low protein binding, and a small volume of distribution.[61]

MDAC has been shown to increase total body clearance of multiple drugs, including carbamazepine,[62–64] dapsone,[65,66] phenobarbital,[64,67–73] quinine,[74,75] and theophylline.[42,59,76–87] Despite the reported increase in drug clearance associated with the use of MDAC, *improved clinical outcomes have not been definitively demonstrated*. For example, Pond and coworkers[72] described 10 comatose patients following phenobarbital overdose who were randomized to receive either single-dose activated charcoal or MDAC. Despite the fact that the MDAC group had a significantly shorter phenobarbital serum half-life, no difference was found between the groups in regard to the duration of intubation or hospitalization.

Contraindications

MDAC is contraindicated if there is evidence of bowel obstruction. An ileus is a relative contraindication. Many ill patients who develop an ileus may be selected candidates for MDAC if the airway is protected. The administration of MDAC is contraindicated in any patient who does not have an intact or protected airway. MDAC should be avoided in patients who have repetitive emesis, especially when associated with decreased mental status or a decreased gag reflex. The concurrent use of cathartics with MDAC remains unproved and is not recommended.[88] MDAC with cathartics should not be administered to young children because of the propensity for laxatives to cause fluid and electrolyte imbalance. For example, MDAC with sorbitol has been associated with hypernatremia and dehydration,[89,90] and MDAC with magnesium cathartics has been associated with hypermagnesemia, neuromuscular weakness, and coma.[91,92]

Technique

Give 1 g/kg (≤100 g) for the first dose of charcoal. If a cathartic is used, administer it only with the first dose of charcoal to decrease the risk of cathartic-induced electrolyte abnormalities that can develop, especially in children.[89–92] Follow the initial dose of charcoal by 0.5 g/kg (≤50 g) every 4 hours. Stop giving MDAC if repeat examination reveals an absence of bowel sounds or a distended abdomen. In this case, consider placing an NG tube and put it on low intermittent suction. Patients receiving MDAC may be at increased risk for emesis because of the larger total dose of activated charcoal received. The use of antiemetics may help decrease the incidence of vomiting associated with MDAC.[76,93,94] Charcoal therapy should be continued until there is clinical improvement and plasma drug levels have fallen to acceptable levels.

Complications

The complications encountered in single-dose activated charcoal are also encountered in MDAC. In addition, there have been reports of gastrointestinal obstruction and perforation from MDAC therapy, especially in conjunction with the ingestion of drugs with anticholinergic properties.[95–99]

Cathartics

Background

The use of cathartics is intended to decrease the absorption of substances by accelerating the expulsion of the poison from the gastrointestinal tract. Cathartics are often used in conjunction with activated charcoal owing to charcoal's side effect of constipation. The mechanism of action of cathartics is such that, theoretically, it would minimize the possibility of desorption of drug bound to activated charcoal. There is little evidence that a single dose of aqueous activated charcoal is significantly constipating; however, cathartics are often given for this potential problem. The majority of data suggest negligible clinical benefit from cathartic use.[100,101]

Indications

The routine administration of a cathartic in combination with activated charcoal is not endorsed by the American Academy of Clinical Toxicology or the European Association of Poison Centres and Clinical Toxicologists.[102] The administration of a cathartic alone has no role in the management of the poisoned patient.

Contraindications

Cathartics are contraindicated if there is volume depletion, hypotension, significant electrolyte imbalance, corrosive ingestion, ileus, recent bowel surgery, intestinal obstruction, or perforation. The administration of cathartics is also contraindicated with patients who do not have an intact or protected airway. They should be avoided in patients who have repetitive emesis, especially when associated with decreased mental status or a decreased gag reflex. Cathartics should be used cautiously in young children and the elderly because of the propensity for laxatives to cause fluid and electrolyte imbalance.

Technique

There are two types of osmotic cathartics: saccharide cathartics (sorbitol) and saline cathartics (magnesium citrate, magnesium sulfate, and sodium sulfate). The optimal dose of sorbitol or magnesium citrate remains to be determined. The recommended dose of sorbitol is approximately 1 to 2 g/kg of body weight or 1 to 2 mL/kg of 70% sorbitol in adults and 4.3 mL/kg of 35% sorbitol in children (single administration only).[102] Many charcoal formulations come premixed with sorbitol, but the sorbitol content varies considerably. The recommended dose of magnesium citrate is 250 mL of 10% solution in an adult and 4 mL/kg body weight of 10% solution in a child. Multiple doses of cathartics should be avoided.

Complications

The administration of sorbitol has been associated with vomiting, abdominal cramps, nausea, diaphoresis, and transient hypotension.[103–105] Because the sorbitol content varies between different charcoal/sorbitol combination products, pay attention to the sorbitol content in each brand to avoid excessive sorbitol administration. Be aware that multiple doses of sorbitol have been associated with volume depletion.[89] Multiple doses of magnesium-containing cathartics have been associated with severe hypermagnesemia.[91,92] Children are particularly susceptible to the adverse effects of cathartics, and therefore, use caution or totally avoid using cathartics in children.

WBI

Background

WBI involves the enteral administration of an osmotically balanced polyethylene glycol electrolyte solution (PEG-ES) in a sufficient amount and rate to physically flush ingested substances through the gastrointestinal tract, purging the toxin before absorption can occur.[12] PEG-ES (CoLyte, GoLYTELY) is isosmotic, is not systemically absorbed, and will not cause electrolyte or fluid shifts. Available data suggest that the large volumes of this solution needed to mechanically propel pills, drug packets, or other substances through the gastrointestinal tract are safe, including in pregnant women and in young children.[106,107]

The clinical data on the efficacy of WBI remains limited. Ly and colleagues[108] found that the effect of WBI on the reduction of acetaminophen concentration versus time was not statistically significant. However, WBI did have a mechanical effect on radiopaque markers in the gastrointestinal tract with 8 of 10 subjects' markers congregating in the right hemicolon after WBI. WBI was shown to mobilize lead BB pellets in a child to the large bowel, where less absorption occurs and the foreign bodies could be removed by colonoscopic intervention.[109] In addition, PEG-ES may play a role in the pharmacologic conversion of some toxins. For example, it has been shown that the relatively high pH of PEG-ES increases the rate of spontaneous conversion of cocaine to its inactive metabolite benzoylecgonine.[110]

Indications

WBI may be considered for ingestions of exceedingly large quantities of potentially toxic substances, ingestions of toxins that are poorly adsorbed to activated charcoal (e.g., iron, lithium), ingestions of delayed-release formulations, late presentation after ingestion of a toxin, pharmacobezoars, and in body stuffers or packers[12,110–113] (Fig. 42–13). WBI remains a theoretical option for these ingestions and is often performed on body packers who have ingested many times the lethal amount of heroin or cocaine (Fig. 42–14). No definitive evidence exists that WBI improves the outcome of the poisoned

---

Position Statement: Whole Bowel Irrigation

American Academy of Clinical Toxicology; European Association of Poisons Centres and Clinical Toxicologists

Whole bowel irrigation (WBI) should not be used routinely in the management of the poisoned patient. Although some volunteer studies have shown substantial decreases in the bioavailability of ingested drugs, no controlled clinical trials have been performed and there is no conclusive evidence that WBI improves the outcome of the poisoned patient. Based on volunteer studies, WBI may be considered for potentially toxic ingestions of sustained-release or enteric-coated drugs. There are insufficient data to support or exclude the use of WBI for potentially toxic ingestions of iron, lead, zinc, or packets of illicit drugs; WBI remains a theoretical option for these ingestions. WBI is contraindicated in patients with bowel obstruction, perforation, ileus, and in patients with hemodynamic instability or compromised unprotected airways. WBI should be used cautiously in debilitated patients, or in patients with medical conditions that may be further compromised by its use. A single dose of activated charcoal administered prior to WBI does not appear to decrease the binding capacity of charcoal or to alter the osmotic properties of WBI solution. Administration of charcoal during WBI appears to decrease the binding capacity of charcoal.

Figure 42–13 Position statement: whole bowel irrigation (WBI). *(From the American Academy of Clinical Toxicology; European Association of Poisons Centres and Clinical Toxicologists. Published in Clin Toxicol 35:753, 1997.)*

---

patient.[114] Although not a proven procedure, WBI is often suggested by toxicologists, and its use in select cases is intuitively reasonable and supported by the authors. The most common indication for WBI in the ED is for the treatment of toxic sustained-release medications (such as iron, calcium channel blockers, β-blockers, theophylline, and lithium) and iron tablets (Fig. 42–15).[115]

Contraindications

WBI is contraindicated in patients with gastrointestinal obstruction, perforation, ileus, and corrosive ingestion. It should also be avoided in patients with hemodynamic instability or an unprotected airway.[115] WBI should also be avoided with patients who have repetitive emesis, especially when associated with decreased mental status or a decreased gag reflex. WBI should be used cautiously in debilitated patients.

Technique

PEG-ES is marketed in a powder form. Add tap water to make a total volume of 4 L. The recommended rate of administration is[12,115]

- 9 months to 6 years: 500 mL/hr.
- 6 years to 12 years: 1000 mL/hr.
- Older than 12 years: 1500 to 2000 mL/hr.

Cooperative patients with intact airway protective reflexes may drink the solution. The large volume and taste often limit even the most motivated patient's ability to comply. If the patient is unable or unwilling to drink this solution, administer it through a small-bore NG tube after placement is con-

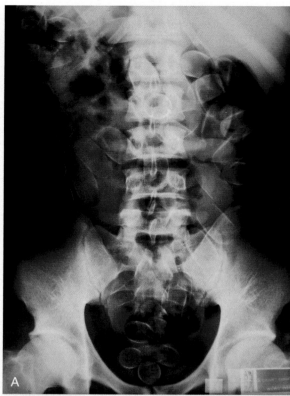

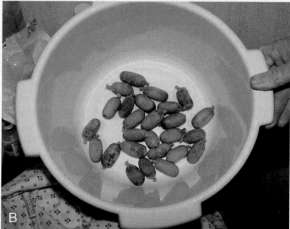

Figure 42–14 *A,* This body packer attempted to smuggle more than 50 packets of heroin. All packets were passed intact after 12 hr of whole bowel irrigation. *B,* Note the integrity of the carefully wrapped packets that were passed.

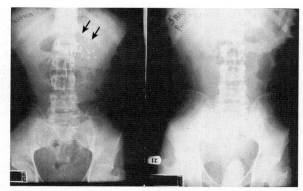

Figure 42–15 WBI is commonly recommended for the treatment of iron ingestion. These radiographs depict the effect of 5 hr of WBI. Note the marked decrease of radiopaque pills (*arrows*) in the gastrointestinal tract. Intact pills were recovered in the rectal effluent.

firmed. *Even cooperative patients have difficulty drinking adequate fluid for effective whole bowel irrigation.* Because it is common for WBI to be delayed while the patient and medical personnel attempt to administer the large volumes of oral WBI solution required to be effective, it is suggested that NG instillation be instituted early in the ED course (Fig. 42–16). Unconscious patients with protected airways may receive WBI via an NG tube. In one study, patients vomited shortly after beginning WBI infusion at a rate of 1.5 to 2L/hr. Antiemetics, such as metoclopramide, as well as gradually advancing the infusion rate over 60 minutes can help ease this side effect.[108] Prewarming the irrigant to a temperature of approximately 37°C avoids the potential complication of hypothermia. To collect the waste products, ask an awake patient to sit on a commode. In an obtunded patient, insert a rectal tube to collect the waste. Many toxicologists recommend adding two to three bottles of activated charcoal to each liter of WBI solution. The benefit is unproved, but there is little theoretical downside to this technique, and it is supported by the editors. The binding capacity of charcoal is decreased when combined with PEG-ES, but the clinical consequences of this observation are unknown. Empirically, metoclopramide may be coadministered to decrease nausea and facilitate gastrointestinal passage.

The end point of WBI is the arrival of clear rectal effluent and/or resolution of toxic effect.[115] There are rare case reports of late purging of drug packets, plant parts, and tablets after the arrival of clear effluent.[111,116] Radiographic studies may also be beneficial to determine the end point in body packers or in patients who have ingested radiopaque medications.

Complications

Few complications from WBI therapy, especially pertaining to acute poisonings, have been reported. Nausea, vomiting, abdominal cramps, and bloating have been described.[117] Nausea and vomiting may make administration of WBI difficult. Antiemetics and a 15- to 30-minute break followed by a slower rate may allow readministration. As discussed with the other methods of decontamination, attention should be directed to the airway and the potential for aspiration. Administration of a large amount of chilled or room-temperature WBI fluid to pediatric patients could potentially cause hypothermia. Consider warmed fluids in these patients. If activated charcoal is administered concurrently with WBI, there might be a desorption of toxin from charcoal.[118–120]

DERMAL DECONTAMINATION

Background

Numerous hazardous material (HAZMAT) incidents occur each year in the United States. In 2004, 7744 HAZMAT events in 15 states involving thousands of substances were reported to the Hazardous Substances Emergency Events Surveillance System (HSEESS). HAZMAT events frequently result in injuries, and the ED treatment of contaminated HAZMAT patients is not a rare event. Many of these patients, including those involved in past terrorist events, transport themselves to the ED. For example, in the Tokyo sarin gas attack, 93% of 498 patients reporting to St. Luke's Hospital

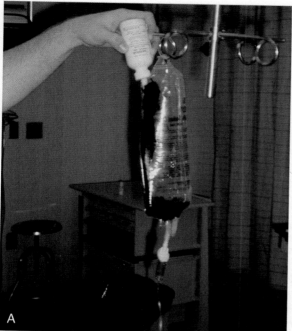

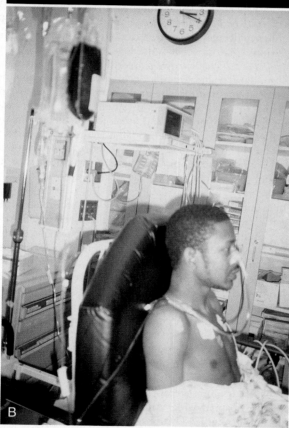

Figure 42–16 It is very difficult for even the most motivated patient to drink an effective volume of WBI solution. To enhance compliance and to decrease vomiting, polyethylene glycol electrolyte solution (PEG-ES) may be slowly and continuously administered via an NG tube. An empty bag of saline is hung on an intravenous pole, the corner of the bag is removed, and the PEG-ES is poured into the bag. Standard intravenous tubing is connected to the proximal end of an NG tube and the solution is infused continuously. In this picture, charcoal has been added to the WBI solution. Metoclopramide was coadministered to reduce nausea.

arrived by means other than ambulance.[121] The risk of injury to medical personnel incurred while treating contaminated patients is significant. Of the patients reported to HSEESS, emergency responders accounted for 10% of injuries and hospital personnel for 4.1% of injuries.[122] After the Tokyo attack, 13 of 15 clinicians (87%) reported symptoms while treating patients in the ED and 23% of involved hospital staff complained of acute poisoning symptoms.[123] Burgess and associates[124] reported that 13% of Washington state emergency care facilities had evacuated their ED or another part of the hospital for contamination during a 5-year period. Ghilarducci and coworkers[125] surveyed level 1 trauma centers in the United States and reported that only 6% had the necessary equipment required for safe decontamination. Less than 36% of emergency medicine staff had received appropriate training in handling the contaminated patient, and 5.6% had experienced injuries to their staff due to contact with contaminated patients during a 1-year period. It is imperative that EDs have plans in place to handle patients who are exposed to potential toxins, provide adequate decontamination facilities, and ensure the safety of the treating medical staff.[126]

Technique

There are a number of key components in the management of hazardous materials incidents and the care of the contaminated patients who present to the ED.[127] These components should include early recognition of a HAZMAT event, rapid activation of a plan to manage contaminated patients, initiation of primary triage, appropriate patient registration, patient decontamination, secondary triage, and final treatment.

First, the ED must be able to recognize that an event has occurred before contaminated patients gain entrance into the health care facility. Communication with local fire, police, and paramedics provides early detection of such events and allows preparation before patients arrive. Security should be arranged to prevent contaminated patients from entering the hospital, and a "lockdown" of the facility should be considered.

Second, the ED should have the authority to activate a plan expeditiously to prepare the decontamination facility and allow appropriate preselected personnel to don personal protective equipment (PPE). If necessary, the hospital disaster plan should be activated quickly at the discretion of the ED clinician who is in contact with scene operations and incoming patients. Specific data to determine the appropriate level of PPE to maintain hospital worker protection remain limited. Minimum PPE for hospital-based decontamination (level C) consists of a splash-proof, chemical-resistant suit with tape, double-layer protective gloves, and a powered air-purifying respirator per the National Institute of Occupational Safety and Health. Higher levels of protection, such as a level A Self-Contained Breathing Apparatus (SCBA) fully encapsulated chemical-resistant suit or level B SCBA chemical-resistant suit, is recommended with unknown chemical and biologic exposures and for entering hot zones, but these are not readily available in EDs.[128,129] Fortunately, most chemical exposures are known. For those that occur in the workplace, Material Safety Data Sheets can be obtained and either the local poison center or the Agency for Toxic Substances and Disease Registry (ATSDR) can be contacted for advice on what level of protection is appropriate.

Third, appropriate primary triage should occur. Contaminated patients should not enter the ED until proper decontamination has occurred to ensure that the hospital staff will not get secondary contamination. Appropriate triage should then occur, with experienced personnel performing an initial brief assessment of each patient. The triage and decontamination areas should be organized into several "zones" to prevent further contamination. The "hot" zone is the location with the highest level of contaminant, or where the incident occurred. In most cases of hospital-based decontamination, there is no hot zone because the patients have been removed from the initial chemical insult. On average, patients arrive at the ED 20 minutes after the event and have had significant off-gassing by this time; however, the majority of patients have self-transported and have received no prehospital decontamination by Emergency Medical Services/HAZMAT. Basic life-saving treatments, airway/hemorrhage control, antidote administration (e.g., for cyanide or nerve agents), and decontamination occur in the "warm" zone. The "cold" zone is safe from contaminant.[128]

Fourth, a brief sign-in process in the warm zone should capture the patient's name and date of birth, with full registration to occur after decontamination. Contaminated clothing and valuables should be placed in an impervious bag to avoid potential off-gassing.[130,131]

Fifth, decontamination should be performed. The hospital ED should have preexisting HAZMAT incident protocols that designate the decontamination area and the triage and decontamination team. Ideally, a hospital should have a permanent decontamination facility capable of handling a small number of chemically exposed patients and, in addition, a large portable unit for mass casualties. The decontamination area should meet several qualifications: (1) it should be secured to prevent spread to other areas of the hospital, (2) the ventilation system should be separate from the rest of the hospital or it should be shut off to prevent airborne spread of contaminants, and (3) provisions must be made to collect the rinsate from contaminated patients to prevent contamination of the facility and water supply. At most facilities, the best place to begin initial treatment and evaluation is outdoors (Fig. 42–17). Portable decontamination facilities are available, but their cost may be prohibitive for many institutions. A practical alternative is to have a warm shower nozzle, soap, and wading pool available outside the entrance to the ED. A tent or screen can provide privacy.

The first priority in decontaminating a patient is to remove her or his clothing while both maintaining privacy and preventing hypothermia. This step is the most important in the decontamination process and can reduce the contaminant by 75% to 90%. Cut the clothes off rather than pulling them off, if possible. Place all clothing and valuables in labeled bags, as mentioned earlier. Brush off solids with a soft brush or towel. Irrigate the skin with copious amounts of warm water and cleanse the skin with soap. Although some agents (e.g., metallic sodium, potassium, cesium, and rubidium) may react with water, irrigation is still more beneficial to immediately decontaminate the skin than to delay treatment time. Starting from head to toe, irrigate the exposed skin and hair for 10 to 15 minutes. Scrub with a soft surgical sponge, being careful not to abrade the skin. Irrigate wounds for an additional 5 to 10 minutes with water or saline. Remove contact lenses and irrigate the eyes for 10 to 15 minutes with saline. Direct irrigation away from the medial canthus to avoid

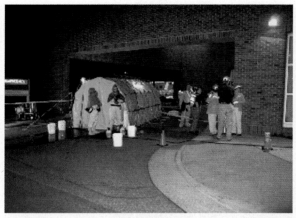

Figure 42–17 During a hazardous materials (HAZMAT) incident, a decontamination tent with personnel in protective gear is assembled outside the emergency department entrance.

forcing contaminants into the lacrimal duct. With strongly alkaline substances, irrigate for longer times. Irrigate the nares and the ear canals with frequent suctioning if contamination is suspected. Clean underneath the fingernails with a brush. Avoid using stiff brushes and abrasives because they may enhance dermal absorption of the toxin and can produce skin lesions that may be mistaken for chemical injuries. Sponges and disposable towels are effective alternatives.

Secondary triage should occur after decontamination. Transfer patients with major or moderate casualties to areas designated for such cases. Send patients with minor or no injuries to appropriate holding areas for further evaluation. Medical care at this stage depends on the toxin to which the patient has been exposed and the potential toxicity of that agent. Wounds, after copious irrigation, may need thorough exploration and possibly surgical removal of the contaminant.

In order for the ED to care for the contaminated patient, protocols should be in place and regularly rehearsed by the facility. Train staff in the procedures and protocols, establish communication between community agencies and the hospitals, regularly inspect equipment, and rehearse setups. Obtain template protocols both from peer-reviewed medical literature and in the government literature if needed.[132,133] For example, guidelines for managing HAZMAT incidents are available from the Emergency Response and Consultation Branch (E57), Division of Health Assessment and Consultation, Agency for Toxic Substances and Disease Registry, 1600 Clifton Road NE, Atlanta, GA 30333. In addition, prompted by the 2001 terrorist attacks, the U.S. Department of Veterans Affairs and several policy experts developed a "comprehensive hospital-wide emergency mass casualty decontamination program." This program has been applied at most Veterans Affairs medical centers and demonstrates a cost-effective protocol suitable for implementation at other U.S. hospitals.[134]

REFERENCES CAN BE FOUND ON EXPERT CONSULT

CHAPTER 43

Peritoneal Procedures

Michael S. Runyon and John A. Marx

Paracentesis and diagnostic peritoneal lavage (DPL) constitute the two primary intraperitoneal procedures. They are fundamentally similar in purpose and design; however, the former is generally reserved for medical concerns and the latter for traumatic pathology. There is no mandate for emergency clinicians to perform these procedures if local custom is to refer to specialists, but many emergency clinicians routinely perform these procedures.

DPL

Root and colleagues[1] introduced DPL in 1964. It has withstood the passage of more than 4 decades and remains a useful tool in the management of penetrating torso trauma. Following a blunt mechanism of injury, its greatest utility is as a triage tool in the assessment of the hemodynamically unstable multiply injured patient. The intent is to rapidly discover or exclude the presence of intraperitoneal hemorrhage (IPH). This purpose is identical with that of ultrasound (US) in the diagnostic armamentarium of the emergency clinician evaluating the blunt trauma patient.[2]

Although commonly referred to as diagnostic peritoneal *lavage*, this procedure has two distinct components: peritoneal aspiration and peritoneal lavage. Peritoneal aspiration, in which an attempt is made to retrieve free intraperitoneal blood, precedes lavage. A finding of intraperitoneal blood presages intraperitoneal organ injury and precludes the need for subsequent lavage. In the lavage portion, normal saline is introduced by catheter into the peritoneal cavity, recovered by gravity, and analyzed.

Peritoneal lavage can be used as a therapeutic tool in hypothermia and as a means of removing toxins.[3] It has also been used as a diagnostic instrument for suspected intra-abdominal infection and nontraumatic sources of hemorrhage.[4,5] However, its primary use is as a determinant for the need for laparotomy after trauma, and this chapter focuses on that use.

Indications

Blunt Trauma

Prior to the advent of computed tomography (CT) and US, DPL was the sole diagnostic option to supplement physical examination for predicting the need for operative intervention (Table 43-1). It was integral both to the reduction of unnecessary laparotomies and to the discovery of unsuspected and life-threatening intra-abdominal hemorrhage in patients with significant closed head injury.[6,7]

In a number of respected centers in the United States, DPL continues to be a focal diagnostic instrument.[8] It serves two primary functions.[9] First, it can rapidly determine or exclude the presence of IPH (Table 43-2). Thus, the patient with a critical closed head injury, the unstable motor vehicle crash victim with multiple potential sources of blood loss, or the patient with pelvic fracture and retroperitoneal hemorrhage can be appropriately routed to life-saving laparotomy.[10,11] Furthermore, given its exquisite sensitivity, a negative peritoneal aspiration allows the clinician to proceed to alternative management steps and the patient to forego unnecessary laparotomy. Second, DPL has been used in less exigent circumstances as a means of predicting solid or hollow visceral injury requiring laparotomy.[12,13] However, in this venue, its sensitivity to the presence of hemorrhage may prompt unnecessary laparotomy in patients with self-limited lacerations of the liver, spleen,[14-17] or mesentery.[17] CT scan specifically evaluates all intraperitoneal structures as well as the retroperitoneum, a region inaccessible to DPL. Because the resolution and the speed with which it can be undertaken have vastly improved, CT has become an invaluable adjunct in the management of blunt trauma[18,19] and has largely replaced DPL in the stable patient. It is most useful in the identification of injury to solid organs with accompanying IPH and greatly assists nonoperative management of those injuries. The ability of CT to discern hollow viscus and pancreatic pathology has improved but remains inconsistent.[20,21] With regard to hollow viscus injury, it is when serial clinical evaluations cannot be performed that gut perforation leads to preventable mortality. This is especially true in the patient with severe closed head injury or high spinal cord injury in whom physical assessment of the abdomen is quite compromised. It is for these express scenarios that some authorities recommend the performance of DPL. The clinician's concern should be heightened if the US or CT demonstrates minimal amounts of free intraperitoneal fluid without evidence of solid organ damage.[22,23]

Experience with US in North America is meager in comparison with that in Western Europe (notably Germany) and Asia (notably Japan). In the past, US in the United States had been used exclusively for the detection and serial examination of traumatic pancreatic pseudocysts.

Two paradigms have brought US to the forefront. First, this modality has been adopted as the primary triage instrument, in lieu of DPL, for the detection of IPH on the basis of identifying which pouches and gutters are fluid-filled.[24-27] Clinical success in this role has been mixed with reported sensitivities for IPH of 65% to 95%.[28-34] In addition, to be useful in this role, a competent technician, interpreter, and equipment must be present in real time. It has been demonstrated that emergency clinicians and surgeons can be trained in this technique to a level of competence sufficient for this need.[35] In centers that rely upon US, DPL should serve as a reliable study when US equipment is unavailable, the US is technically difficult, or when the results of the US are indeterminate, especially when the patient demonstrates hemodynamic compromise.

Second, US can determine injury to solid viscera such as the liver, spleen, kidneys, and pancreas. This requires considerably greater expertise, and in most centers, US has not supplanted CT for this purpose.[36]

DPL is a readily available procedure that can be conducted rapidly in the safe confines of the emergency department (ED). The ability to undertake CT, in particular, or to a lesser extent, US in a similar manner requires careful consideration of clinical circumstances, equipment location, and the capabilities of available personnel (Table 43-3 and Fig. 43-1).[37,38]

TABLE 43–1 Clinical Indications for Laparotomy after Blunt Trauma

Manifestation	Pitfall
Unstable vital signs with strongly suspected abdominal injury	Alternate sources shock
Unequivocal peritoneal irritation	Unreliable
Pneumoperitoneum	Insensitive; may be due to cardiopulmonary source or invasive procedures (diagnostic peritoneal lavage, laparoscopy)
Evidence of diaphragmatic injury	Nonspecific
Significant gastrointestinal bleeding	Uncommon, unknown accuracy

From Marx J, Isenhour J: Abdominal trauma. In Marx JA, Hockberger RS, Walls RM, et al [eds]: Rosen's Emergency Medicine: Concepts and Clinical Practice, 6th ed. St. Louis, CV Mosby, 2006, p 509.

TABLE 43–2 Principal Indications for Diagnostic Peritoneal Lavage in Abdominal Trauma

Indication	Clinical Scenario
Determine diaphragmatic violation	Penetrating injury to low chest, upper abdomen
Rapidly determine presence of IPH	Ultrasound unavailable, indeterminate, or negative for free-fluid in an unstable patient
Determine presence of HVI	CT nondiagnostic and SCE unreliable: • Head injury with altered mental status • Alcohol intoxication • Drug intoxication • Spinal cord injury

CT, computed tomography; HVI, hollow viscus injury; IPH, intraperitoneal hemorrhage; SCE, serial clinical evaluations.

TABLE 43–3 Diagnostic Studies in Blunt Abdominal Trauma

Scenario	Study Purpose	Primary Study	Alternate/Compensatory
Hemodynamically Unstable			
General	IPH	US	DPA
Pelvic fracture	IPH	US	DPA*
Hemodynamically Stable			
General	OI[††]	CT	SPEs, DPL
Nonoperative management[§]	OI	CT[‖]	SPEs, DPL[¶]
CHI	OI, HVI	CT,[‖] DPL[¶]	SPEs**
BAI	IPH	US, DPL	CT[††]

*Positive peritoneal aspirate mandates laparotomy, positive red blood cell count only, warrants attention to pelvic fracture.
[†]To discover fluid/blood suggesting injury.
[‡]US for OI is much less reliable than for IPH.
[§]Institutional capability should be carefully considered.
[‖]CT is less reliable for HVI than for solid visceral injury.
[¶]Complementary to CT if HVI suspected.
**SPEs are unreliable in the patient with CHI.
[††]May be more appropriate if helical CT is primary study for BAI or can be rapidly acquired.
BAI, blunt aortic injury; CHI, closed-head injury; CT, computed tomography; DPA, diagnostic peritoneal aspiration; DPL, diagnostic peritoneal lavage; HVI, hollow viscus injury; IPH, intraperitoneal hemorrhage; OI, organ injury; SPEs, serial physical examinations; US, ultrasonography.
Adapted From Marx J, Isenhour J: Abdominal trauma. In Marx JA, Hockberger RS, Walls RM, et al (eds): Rosen's Emergency Medicine: Concepts and Clinical Practice, 6th ed. St. Louis, CV Mosby, 2006, p507.

TABLE 43–4 Injury Likelihood by Entry Site

	Intraperitoneal	Retroperitoneal	Diaphragm
Anterior abdomen	++	+	+
Flank	+	++	+
Back	+	++	+
Low chest	+	+	++

From Marx JA: Diagnostic peritoneal lavage. In Ivatury RR, Cayten CG (eds): The Textbook of Penetrating Trauma. Baltimore, Williams & Wilkins, 1996, p 336.

Penetrating Trauma

The advent of DPL was seminal in the promotion of selective management for penetrating abdominal injury. Here its role is more dominant than for blunt trauma owing to the far greater likelihood of occult injury to hollow viscera and the diaphragm after a penetrating mechanism.[39,40]

Instruments and missiles may penetrate the abdominal cavity via the anterior abdominal wall, flank, back, or low chest.[41] The intraperitoneal space is vulnerable if penetration occurs as high as the fourth intercostal space anteriorly and the sixth or seventh laterally and posteriorly, because the diaphragm may rise to these levels in the expiratory phase of respiration.[42] Coincident thoracic penetration has occurred in up to 46% of abdominal injuries.[43-45] The likelihood of retroperitoneal injury increases when the entry site is over the flank or back, but the prospect of intraperitoneal pathology remains considerable with cited incidences of up to 43% for the flank and 14% for the back (Table 43–4).[46-48]

Stab Wounds. Because only one fourth to one third of patients who sustain stab wounds to the anterior abdomen

require laparotomy, diagnostic algorithms are used to decrease the rate of unnecessary operation.[39,44,49,50] An optimal approach would not sacrifice sensitivity for morbid intraperitoneal injury. A pathway using a combination of clinical mandates, local wound exploration, and DPL is well established (Fig. 43–2).[51] These clinical mandates are reasonably accurate predictors of significant intraperitoneal injury (Table 43–5). Thus, the presence of one or more mandates suggests the need for urgent laparotomy and precludes the undertaking of other diagnostic studies.

DPL fills three roles in the evaluation of patients with abdominal stab wounds (see Table 43–2): (1) rapid determination of the presence of hemoperitoneum, (2) discovery of intraperitoneal injury requiring operation in stable patients, and (3) the establishment of diaphragmatic violation. As is the

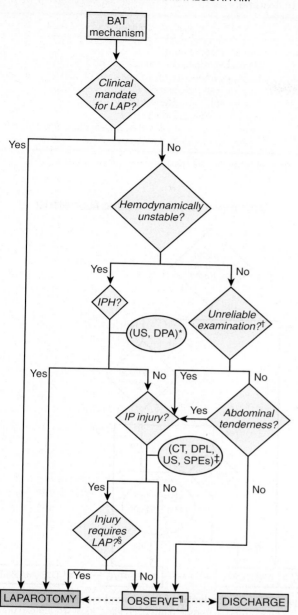

Figure 43–1   Blunt abdominal trauma (BAT) algorithm.
*Determined by unequivocal free IP fluid on US or positive peritoneal aspiration on DPA.
†Can be unreliable because of closed-head injury, intoxicants, distracting injury, or spinal cord injury.
‡One or more studies may be indicated.
§Need for LAP is based on clinical scenario, diagnostic studies, and institutional resources.
¶Duration of observation should be 6–24 hr depending on whether diagnostic tests have been performed, the results of the tests, and clinical circumstances including the absence of factors rendering the examination unreliable.
CT, computed tomography; D/C, discharge; DPA, diagnostic peritoneal aspiration; DPL, diagnostic peritoneal lavage; IP, intraperitoneal; IPH, intraperitoneal hemorrhage; LAP, laparotomy; SPE, serial physical examination; US, ultrasound. *(From Marx J, Isenhour J: Abdominal trauma. In Marx JA, Hockberger RS, Walls RM, et al [eds]: Rosen's Emergency Medicine: Concepts and Clinical Practice, 6th ed. St. Louis, CV Mosby, 2006, p 508.)*

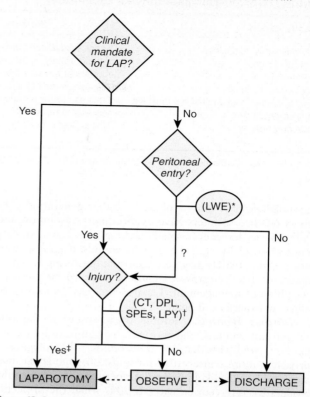

Figure 43–2   Anterior abdomen stab wound algorithm.
*Plain films, ultrasonography, LPY, and CT can also assess peritoneal entry.
†CT, DPL, SPEs, or LPY can be used in singular or complementary fashion depending on the clinical scenario.
‡Expectant management of injuries is infrequently attempted.
CT, computed tomography; D/C, discharge; DPL, diagnostic peritoneal lavage; LAP, laparotomy; LPY, laparoscopy; LWE, local wound exploration; SPE, serial physical examination. *(From Marx J, Isenhour J: Abdominal trauma. In Marx JA, Hockberger RS, Walls RM, et al [eds]: Rosen's Emergency Medicine: Concepts and Clinical Practice, 6th ed. St. Louis, CV Mosby, 2006, p 503.)*

case in blunt trauma patients, DPL can be invaluable as a rapid triage tool when the source of hemodynamic instability is not known. Pericardial tamponade, intrathoracic hemorrhage, and IPH may be contributory to hemodynamic instability or wholly causal. Again, as for blunt trauma evaluation, US is the only diagnostic modality for IPH that is competitive for this role and carries the added advantage of scanning for intrapericardial and intrathoracic hemorrhage.[45] In the determination of injury after stab wounds, DPL carries 90% accuracy.[52–54] Serial examinations,[55–57] CT, and laparoscopy[58–61] are alternative modalities in specific circumstances and centers.[62] Diaphragmatic rents created by stab wounds are generally small; thus, at the outset, they do not create apparent clinical or radiologic abnormalities.[63,64] However, morbidity due to delayed herniation of bowel is common and substantive.[65] Physical examination is notoriously insensitive and DPL is currently the most sensitive means of discerning this injury in

TABLE 43–5 Clinical Indications for Laparotomy after Penetrating Trauma

Manifestation	Premise	Pitfall
Hemodynamic instability	Major solid visceral or vascular injury	Thorax, mediastinum
Peritoneal signs	Intraperitoneal injury	Unreliable, especially immediately postinjury
Evisceration	Additional bowel, other injury	No injury in one fourth to one third of stab wound cases
Diaphragmatic injury	Diaphragmatic herniation	Rare clinical, radiographic findings
Gastrointestinal and vaginal hemorrhage	Proximal gut or uterine injury	Uncommon, unknown accuracy
Impalement in situ	Vascular impalement	High operative risk, pregnancy
Intraperitoneal air	Hollow viscus perforation	Insensitive; may be caused by intraperitoneal entry only or be due to cardiopulmonary source

Modified from Marx JA: Diagnostic peritoneal lavage. In Ivatury RR, Cayten CG (eds): The Textbook of Penetrating Trauma. Baltimore, Williams & Wilkins, 1996.

the immediate post-trauma phase.[52] Higher-generation CTs such as 64-slice scanners have extraordinary resolution and may be able to detect even small diaphragmatic tears, but data are not yet available. For these small wounds, magnetic resonance imaging (MRI) may be diagnostic, but owing to safety and accessibility concerns, it should be reserved for the non-acute phase of management. Laparoscopy has demonstrated promise in experienced hands.[58,59]

Gunshot Wounds. Multiple organ injury is the rule after gunshot wounds, and mortality is significantly greater when compared with that for stab wounds.[62] The diagnostic approach is more conservative for gunshot wounds because, in some studies, the likelihood of intraperitoneal injury requiring operative intervention exceeds 90% when the projectile has entered the intraperitoneal cavity (Fig. 43–3).[67] If clinical mandates are met (see Table 43–5) or if peritoneal violation has occurred, most centers proceed to laparotomy.[51] One series, however, cited intra-abdominal injury in 70% to 80% of cases, supporting the contention that nonoperative management could be applied to a substantial percentage of patients.[68] In a separate cohort of 152 patients sustaining solid organ injury from penetrating abdominal trauma (70% gunshot wounds and 30% stab wounds), 27% were successfully managed without laparotomy after selection by a protocol combining clinical examination and CT scanning.[69] DPL is reserved for two circumstances: (1) the wound tract is neither obviously superficial nor intraperitoneal, and (2) penetration occurred in the low chest, where diaphragmatic injury is more likely yet the possibility of intraperitoneal injury exists.

Contraindications

DPL can be undertaken in virtually any patient irrespective of age or comorbid illness. Adjustment of the technique and site of performance allows relative contraindications to be overcome. Relative contraindications include prior abdominal surgery or infections, obesity, coagulopathy, and second- or third-trimester pregnancy. The sole absolute contraindication is when clinical mandates for urgent laparotomy already exist.

Technique

Preliminary Steps
Decompress the stomach and bladder to prevent inadvertent injury. Place the patient in the supine position and administer sedation and analgesia as appropriate. Perform DPL according to compliance with standards for body fluid precautions.

ABDOMINAL GUNSHOT WOUND ALGORITHM

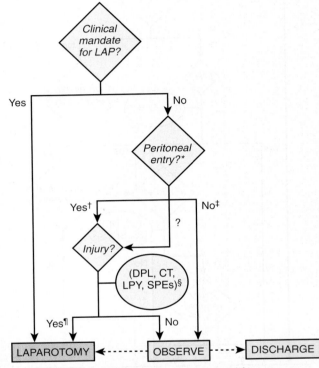

Figure 43–3 Abdominal gunshot wound algorithm.
*Can be assessed by missile path, plain films, local wound exploration, ultrasonography, and LAP.
†Most centers proceed to LAP if peritoneal entry is suspected.
‡Patients with documented superficial and low-velocity injuries can be discharged; unknown-depth or high-velocity injuries require further tests or observation.
§ DPL, CT, LPY, or SPEs can be used in singular or complementary fashion depending on the clinical scenario.
¶Expectant management of injuries caused by gunshot wounds is rarely attempted.
CT, computed tomography; D/C, discharge; DPL, diagnostic peritoneal lavage; LAP, laparotomy; LPY, laparoscopy; SPE, serial physical examination. (*From Marx J, Isenhour J: Abdominal Trauma. In Marx JA, Hockberger RS, Walls RM, et al [eds]: Rosen's Emergency Medicine: Concepts and Clinical Practice, 6th ed. St. Louis, CV Mosby, 2006, p 506.*)

Observe sterile technique throughout the procedure. Before making the skin incisions described later, prepare the site with standard skin antiseptics and drape appropriately. Prophylactic antibiotics are not indicated for routine DPL because local and systemic infections are rare.[70]

Infiltrate the area for incision and dissection with a local anesthetic such as 1% lidocaine *with* epinephrine (Fig. 43–4). Delay the incision for more than 30 seconds after local anesthetic infiltration to permit local vasospasm, which minimizes wound bleeding during the procedure. Standard equipment for an open peritoneal lavage catheter placement is shown in Figure 43–5.

DPL Catheter Placement

There are two basic methods for DPL: open and closed. The two open techniques are *semiopen* and *fully open*, and they typically require an assistant. DPL is clearly within the diagnostic armamentarium of the emergency clinician and surgeon. It may be undertaken by either or both in keeping with clinical policies established at the particular trauma center.

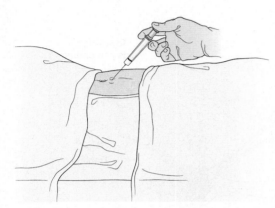

Figure 43–4   Local anesthesia is introduced at the incision or puncture site. The patient is supine with the head of the bed elevated slightly.

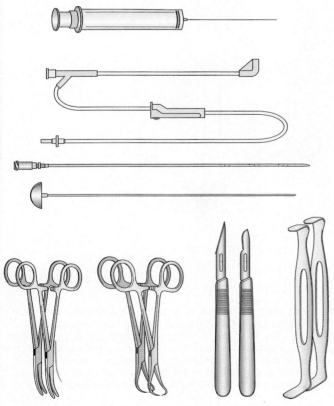

Figure 43–5   Standard equipment for open lavage technique.

Semiopen Technique. In the semiopen method, make a skin incision, 4 to 6 cm in length with a No. 11 scalpel. Using Army-Navy retractors, proceed with blunt dissection to expose the *rectus fascia* (Fig. 43–6*A* and *B*). With the infraumbilical incision in the midline, continue blunt dissection until the *linea alba* is seen. Its crossing bands of crural fibers may be apparent.[71] Make a small 2- to 3-mm opening in the linea alba with a No. 15 scalpel blade (see Fig. 43–6*C*). You may notice a tough, gritty sensation when cutting the linea alba with the scalpel. Place towel clips through this opening to grasp each side of the rectus fascia (see Fig. 43–6*D*). Ask an assistant to lift the two towel clips and carefully advance the catheter and trocar in a 45° to 60° caudad orientation. Proceed through the peritoneum into the peritoneal cavity (see Fig. 43–6*E* and *F*).[72]

One method to decrease the likelihood of penetrating underlying viscera is to hold the fingers low on the catheter-trocar instrument such that on entering the abdominal peritoneum, the fingers will prevent deep penetration. Excessive pressure during trocar penetration is a common error. Apply steady one-finger pressure to the handle sufficient to "pop" through the peritoneum. After controlled peritoneal penetration of 0.5 to 1.0 cm in the midline, retract the trocar 1.0 to 2.0 cm within the catheter, and advance the catheter carefully toward the pelvis. Some operators advance the catheter toward the right or left side of the pelvis. Use a slight twisting motion during advancement to minimize visceral or omental injury.

The *fully open* technique extends the semiopen technique by one step. Lengthen the opening in the *linea alba*, to open the peritoneum, and use direct visualization to advance the catheter placement into the peritoneal cavity. The trocar is unnecessary with the open technique.

The two open techniques can be accomplished with a single technician, but it is useful to have an assistant help with retraction and handling of instruments. The fully open method is the more technically demanding and time-consuming. Reserve this method for clinical circumstances in which neither the closed nor the semiopen technique is deemed safe or has been attempted and failed. Examples of these circumstances include pelvic fracture, pregnancy, prior abdominal surgery, infections, and obesity.

Closed Technique. For the closed techniques, introduce the catheter into the peritoneal space in a blind percutaneous fashion.[73] Utilize the simple Seldinger (guidewire) method, in which a small-gauge guide needle is inserted into the peritoneal cavity in the midline just inferior to the umbilicus (Fig. 43–7*A*). Pass a flexible wire through the needle (see Fig. 43-7*B*), and remove the needle but not the wire. Advance a soft catheter over the wire and into the peritoneal cavity. Make a small stab with a No. 11 scalpel at the entry site of the wire to allow easier passage of the catheter through the abdominal wall (see Fig. 43–7*C* and *D*). Rotate the catheter while pushing it over the guidewire to facilitate entry into the peritoneal cavity. Place the catheter into the right or left pelvic gutter.

Always control the guidewire to avert intra-abdominal migration of the wire. Withdraw the wire and aspirate for blood using a 10-cc syringe. Follow this with peritoneal lavage when necessary. Proponents of the guidewire technique promote its ease and rapidity.[74–78] Those who prefer the semiopen method argue that the time to peritoneal aspiration, the more critical interval, is minimally different and that this method may have fewer complications and thus be more accurate than the guidewire technique.[79–82] Note that for both

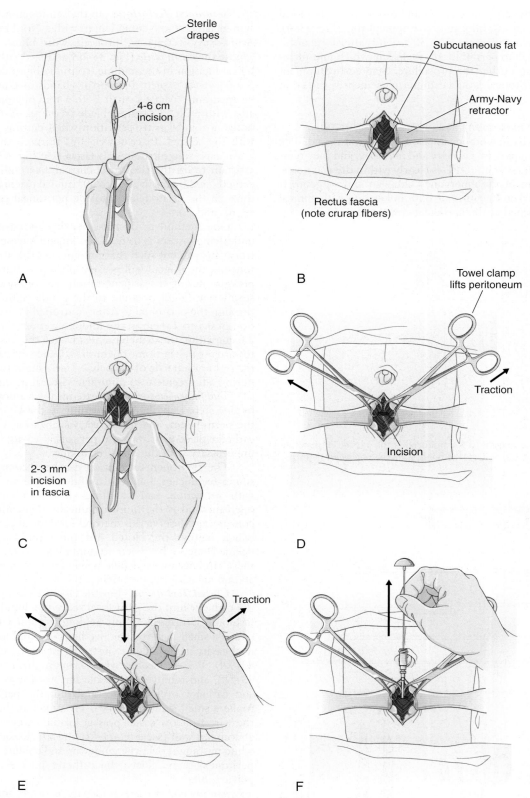

Figure 43–6   *A,* After bladder decompression (generally by Foley catheter placement), make a 4- to 6-cm long vertical infraumbilical incision with a No. 11 scalpel. *B,* Carry blunt dissection using Army-Navy retractors down to the *rectus fascia*. Crossing bands of crural fibers may be seen. *C,* Make a 2- to 3-mm incision through the *rectus fascia* in the midline (*linea alba*) with a No. 15 scalpel. *D,* Grasp each side of the *rectus fascia* with towel clips and lift it prior to insertion of the trocar and DPL catheter. *E,* Pass the trocar with DPL catheter at a 45° caudad angle into the fascial opening and through the peritoneum. In the fully open method, extend the incision in the *rectus fascia* until the peritoneum is directly visualized. Incise the peritoneum and place the catheter alone into the peritoneal cavity. *F,* As soon as the peritoneum has been entered, gently advance the catheter into the peritoneal cavity while withdrawing the trocar. It is often helpful to advance the catheter with a slight twisting motion and to direct it toward either the right or the left pelvic gutter.

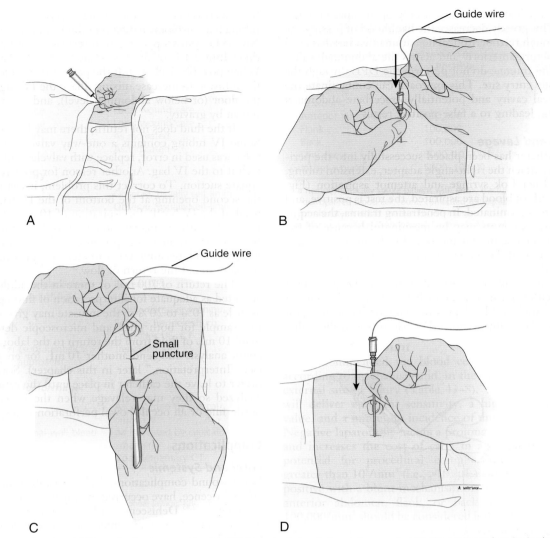

779

Figure 43–7 *A*, For the closed DPL method using a guidewire (Seldinger technique), insert the needle into the peritoneal cavity in the midline just below the umbilicus and aim it slightly caudad. *B*, Pass the flexible guidewire through the needle and into the peritoneal cavity. Ideally, direct the wire toward the right or left pelvic gutter. Withdraw the needle while stabilizing the wire with the free hand at all times. *C*, Make a stab incision with a No. 11 scalpel immediately below the wire to permit easier passage of the DPL catheter. *D*, Direct the DPL catheter over the wire and into the peritoneal cavity using a slight twisting motion. Stabilize the wire at all times and remove it after catheter placement, directing it toward the right or left pelvic gutter when advancing.

semiopen or closed approaches, the time to aspiration should be no more than 2 to 5 minutes.

Site

The optimum location for DPL is at the infraumbilical ring, at the inferior border of the umbilicus (Table 43–6). Here, between the *rectus abdominis* muscles, there is adherence of the peritoneum and relative lack of vascularity and preperitoneal fat.[71] Closed DPL should always be conducted here. In the event of second- or third-trimester pregnancy, a suprauterine approach is used. If there is midline scarring, a fully open technique at the lateral border of the *rectus abdominis* in the left lower quadrant may be necessary. The left side is preferred to avoid later confusion about whether an appendectomy has been performed. It is interesting to note that Moore and associates[83] found no increase in complications or misclassified lavages when the closed technique was used in a small series of patients with prior abdominal surgery. In the

TABLE 43–6 Preferred Site of Diagnostic Peritoneal Lavage

Clinical Circumstance	Site	Method
Standard adult	Infraumbilical midline	C or SO
Standard pediatric	Infraumbilical midline	C or SO
Second- and third-trimester pregnancy	Suprauterine	FO
Midline scarring	Left lower quadrant	FO
Pelvic fracture	Supraumbilical	FO
Penetrating trauma	Infraumbilical midline*	C or SO

*The stab wound or gunshot wound site should be avoided.
C, Closed; FO, fully open; SO, semiopen.

or more without injury. Use a smaller-gauge (20- to 22-gauge) needle for diagnostic taps, because these lessen the likelihood of postprocedural ascitic fluid leak through the wound site. However, for large-volume therapeutic paracenteses use an 18-gauge needle, because this permits expeditious outflow.[115,142]

Insert the needle directly perpendicular at the preferred site. Alternatively, use the "Z-tract" method. For this method, pull the skin approximately 2 cm caudad to the deep abdominal wall with the non–needle-bearing hand while slowly inserting the paracentesis needle (Fig. 43–13).[143] Release the skin when the needle has penetrated the peritoneum and fluid flows. This technique also holds the draining needle in place without sutures or tape. Remove the needle after the procedure, and the skin will slide to its original position and help seal the tract. In any case, insert the needle slowly in 5-mm increments to detect undesired entry of a vessel and to help prevent unnecessary puncture of small bowel. Avoid continuous suction because it may attract bowel or omentum to the end of the paracentesis needle with resultant occlusion. Once fluid is flowing, stabilize the needle to ensure a steady flow. If flow ceases, gently rotate the needle and advance it inward using 1- to 2-mm increments.

US Guidance

US-guided paracentesis may be performed by a radiologist or an experienced emergency clinician ultrasonographer. This technique clearly delineates the pocket of ascitic fluid and allows visualization of loculated collections and avoidance of bowel adhesed to the anterior abdominal peritoneum. The ultrasonographer scans the abdomen and marks the skin at the point overlying the optimal puncture site. Once the entry site is marked, the patient is kept immobile and the procedure is performed (as detailed previously) as soon as practical to avoid shifting of the fluid, which may decrease the utility of US guidance.

Complications

Complications of paracentesis can be divided into systemic, local, and intraperitoneal categories.

Systemic

An oft-cited but poorly documented concern is hemodynamic compromise caused by overzealous removal of ascitic fluid, so-called large-volume paracentesis. Because upward of 6 L has been reportedly removed in less than 15 minutes without complication, certain authorities decry this issue as folklore.[144] Others believe that rapid total paracentesis is accompanied by marked cardiovascular and humoral changes, some of which are explained by mechanical factors directly or indirectly related to relief of abdominal pressure[145,146] (Fig. 43–14). Other changes, including systemic vasodilatation and humoral deactivation, are of a nonmechanical nature. Hyponatremia, the development of the hepatorenal syndrome, and rapid reaccumulation of ascetic fluid have also been ascribed to large-volume paracentesis. Because many patients require therapeutic paracentesis on a regular basis, asking the patient about prior experience and usual volume of fluid removed may guide the clinician.

Because fluid and electrolyte shifts tend to be minimal after the removal of large amounts of fluid,[147] colloid infusion is considered strictly optional for paracentesis of more than 5 L and is not recommended for paracentesis of lesser volume.[118,148,149] When colloid is indicated, albumin has been the de facto choice. The recommended infusion is 6 to 8 g of IV albumin per liter of ascitic fluid removed.[148] However, colloid dextran 70 is favored by some authorities owing to cost and infection concerns.[150,151]

Local

Local complications include persistent ascitic fluid leak at the wound site, abdominal wall hematoma, and localized infection. Persistent fluid leak can be corrected with a single suture at the site of puncture.[142] An abdominal wall hematoma requiring transfusion is very uncommon, but careful observation in such cases is necessary.[136]

Intraperitoneal

Intraperitoneal complications include perforation of vessels and viscera.[152] In experienced hands, these are uncommon, and in most circumstances, they are self-sealing and clinically inconsequential. However, generalized peritonitis and abdominal wall abscess have been reported after paracentesis in rare

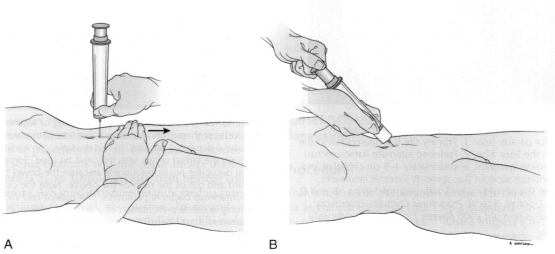

A   B

Figure 43–13 *A*, Z-tract method of needle paracentesis. Pull the skin approximately 2 cm caudad in relation to the deep abdominal wall by the non–needle-bearing hand while slowly inserting the paracentesis needle perpendicular to the skin. *B*, After penetrating the peritoneum and obtaining fluid return, release the skin. Note that the needle is now angulated caudally. See also Fig. 43–14, inset.

787

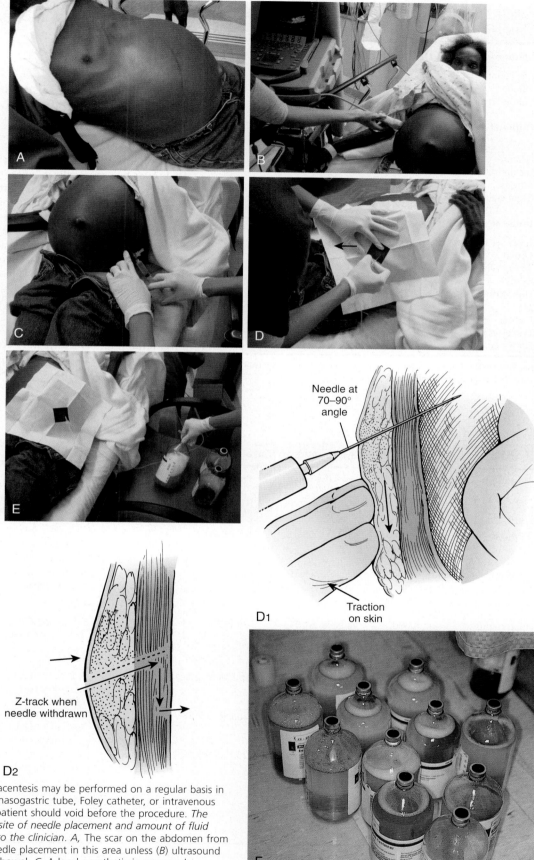

Figure 43–14 Therapeutic paracentesis may be performed on a regular basis in the emergency department. A nasogastric tube, Foley catheter, or intravenous line are not standard, but the patient should void before the procedure. *The patient's prior experience with site of needle placement and amount of fluid drained is an invaluable guide to the clinician.* A, The scar on the abdomen from a cholecystectomy prohibits needle placement in this area unless (B) ultrasound demonstrates no adherence of bowel. C, A local anesthetic is generously injected. D, Use the Z track method to insert the needle, then release the skin and the needle will stay in place without tape (inset). E, Drain fluid into vacuum bottles. F, This patient regularly tolerated a 10-L removal. A simple large needle is often used in lieu of plastic cannulas that may kink or shear, but paracentesis kits are perfectly acceptable.

TABLE 43–13 Ascitic Fluid Laboratory Data to Be Obtained on Patients with Ascites

Routine

Cell count
Albumin
Culture in blood culture bottles

Optional

Total protein
Glucose
Lactate dehydrogenase
Amylase
Gram stain

Unusual

Tuberculosis smear and culture
Cytology
Triglyceride
Bilirubin

Unhelpful

pH
Lactate
Cholesterol
Fibronectin

From Runyon BA: Ascites. In Schiff L, Schiff ER (eds): Diseases of the Liver, 7th ed. Philadelphia, Lippincott-Raven, 1993, p 997.

cases. The most common cause of postparacentesis IPH is bleeding due to a coagulopathy, rather than large-vessel injury per se.[153]

Interpretation

Ascitic fluid should undergo gross inspection. Routine laboratory testing includes a differential cell count, albumin assay, and cultures (Table 43–13).

Inspection

Ascitic fluid is typically translucent and yellow. A dark greenish-brown hue may reflect biliary perforation. Cloudy fluid generally indicates particulate matter, including neutrophils: fluid with WBC counts greater than 5,000/μL (i.e., >5,000/mm^3) are cloudy and those greater than 50,000/μL are purulent. An opaque, milky appearance may indicate elevated triglyceride levels.[154] A blood-tinged appearance requires at least 10,000/μL RBCs. This may reflect an iatrogenic complication, malignancy, hemorrhagic pancreatitis, or tuberculous peritonitis, although the last diagnosis creates hemorrhagic-appearing fluid in less than 5% of cases.[136]

Cell Count

Several milliliters of ascitic fluid are sufficient to obtain a differential cell count. Cirrhotic ascites should generally contain less than 250 WBCs/μL (Table 43–14). However, because

TABLE 43–14 Ascitic Fluid Characteristics in Various Disease States

Condition	Gross Appearance	Specific Gravity	Protein (g/dL)	Cell Count RBCs, (>10,000/μL)	Cell Count WBCs/μL (WBCs/mm^3)	Other Tests
Cirrhosis	Straw-colored or bile-stained	<1.016 (95%)*	<25 (95%)	1%	<250 (90%),* predominantly mesothelial	
Neoplasm	Straw-colored, hemorrhagic, mucinous, or chylous	Variable, >1.016 (45%)	>25 (75%)	20%	>1000 (50%); variable cell types	Cytology, cell block, peritoneal biopsy
Tuberculous peritonitis	Clear, turbid, hemorrhagic, or chylous	Variable, >1.016 (50%)	>25 (50%)	7%	>1000 (70%); usually >70% lymphocytes	Peritoneal biopsy, stain and culture for acid-fast bacilli
Pyogenic peritonitis	Turbid or purulent	If purulent, >1.016	If purulent, >2.5	Unusual	>250; mainly polymorphonuclear leukocytes	Positive Gram stain, culture
Congestive heart failure	Straw-colored	Variable, <1.016 (60%)	Variable, 15–53	10%	<1000 (90%); usually mesothelial, mononuclear	
Nephrosis	Straw-colored or chylous	<1.016	<25 (100%)	Unusual	<250; mesothelial, mononuclear	If chylous, ether extraction, Sudan staining
Pancreatic ascites (pancreatitis, pseudocyst)	Turbid, hemorrhagic, or chylous	Variable, often >1.016	Variable, often >25	Variable, may be blood-stained	Variable	Increased amylase in ascitic fluid and serum

*Because the conditions of examining fluid and selecting patients were not identical in each series, the percentage figures (in parentheses) should be taken as an indication of the order of magnitude rather than as the precise incidence of any abnormal finding.

RBC, red blood cell; WBC, white blood cell.

From Glickman RM, Isselbacher KJ: Abdominal swelling and ascites. In Isselbacher K, et al (eds): Harrison's Principles of Internal Medicine, 13th ed. New York, McGraw-Hill, 1994, p 234.

cells may exit through the peritoneal cavity more slowly than fluid does, the WBC count can rise in the ascitic fluid during the procedure.[154] Thus, an upper limit for uncomplicated cirrhotic ascites is reported as 500 cells/μL.[155] Lymphocytes should predominate, and clinical signs or symptoms of peritoneal infection should be absent.[156] In cases in which spontaneous bacterial peritonitis is a clinical consideration, the WBC criterion is 250 WBCs/μL with greater than 50% polymorphonuclear leukocytes.[133,134]

Albumin

A serum-ascites albumin gradient can be obtained by simultaneously measuring ascites and serum-ascites albumin gradient. A serum-ascites albumin gradient greater than 1.1 g/dL indicates portal hypertension with greater than 95% accuracy (see Table 43–12).[157,158]

Culture and Gram Stain

The most valuable method for determining the presence of infection is culture. The sensitivity of this test is markedly increased by the direct inoculation of blood culture bottles at the bedside in contrast to simply delivering the ascitic fluid to the laboratory.[143,159] Approximately 10 bacteria/μL of fluid is required for a positive Gram stain. Thus, the Gram stain is notoriously insensitive in spontaneous bacterial peritonitis in which the medium concentration of bacteria is 10^{-3} organisms/μL of fluid.[159] The Gram stain can be expected to be helpful only in cases of free gut perforation.

Miscellaneous

Optional tests include measurement of total protein, glucose, lactate dehydrogenase, and amylase. These will be beneficial in selected circumstances and need not be obtained on a routine basis. Immunosuppressed patients, including those with AIDS, should undergo microbiologic testing for opportunistic infections, including tuberculosis.[135] Cytologic analysis is recommended in patients with suspicious constitutional symptoms and signs.[160] Triglyceride and bilirubin studies are indicated if the gross appearance of the fluid is suggestive of increased levels.[161]

Medical Therapy and Disposition

Total paracentesis may be safely performed in the ED, even in cirrhotic patients with large volumes of ascitic fluid (>5 L). However, the immediate relief provided by the procedure is temporary and medical therapy is indicated to prevent or slow fluid reaccumulation. These measures include reduction of dietary sodium intake (<2000 mg/day) and the use of diuretics (spironolactone and lasix) to promote natriuresis. In the absence of other indications for hospital admission, these patients may be managed in the outpatient setting with close follow-up to ensure adequacy of their medical regimen.

Chronic Ambulatory Peritoneal Dialysis

Patients undergoing chronic ambulatory peritoneal dialysis are at an increased risk for peritonitis due to the presence of a chronic indwelling peritoneal catheter. Culture yield is maximized by obtaining a sample of greater than 10 mL of the peritoneal effluent under sterile conditions after a dwell time of at least 4 hours.[162] Peritonitis is defined by cloudy fluid with greater than 100 WBCs/mm² with greater than 50% polymorphonuclear cells.[163] Intraperitoneal antibiotics are indicated and catheter removal may be required for refractory or recurrent infections. Initial, empirical intraperitoneal therapy usually includes a first-generation cephalosporin along with an aminoglycoside or ceftazidime.[164] The optimal treatment strategy should be discussed with the consulting nephrologist.

 REFERENCES CAN BE FOUND ON EXPERT CONSULT

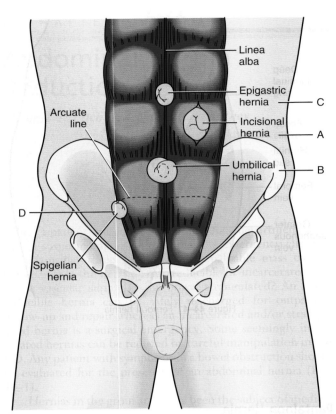

Figure 44–5. Ventral hernias. *A,* Incisional hernia. *B,* Umbilical hernia. *C,* Epigastric hernia. *D,* Spigelian hernia.

found in infants and children, is congenital in origin, and often resolves without treatment by the age of 2. If the hernia persists beyond this age, is larger than 2 cm, or becomes incarcerated or strangulated, it may be repaired surgically.[14,15] An acquired umbilical hernia may also be seen in an adult, particularly with increased abdominal pressure (such as in obesity, ascites, or pregnancy). An umbilical hernia is more prone to incarceration and strangulation in an adult than in a child.

Epigastric Hernia

This hernia occurs in the midline through the linea alba of the rectus sheath (see Fig. 44–5*C*). It is usually located in the epigastric region between the xiphoid and the umbilicus. Although previously considered rare in infants, one study found epigastric hernias in 4% of all pediatric patients seen for hernias.[16]

Spigelian Hernia

The spigelian hernia is rare and courses through a defect at the lateral edge of the rectus muscle at the level of the semilunar line (see Fig. 44–5*D*). It is caused by a partial abdominal wall defect in the transversus abdominal aponeurosis or the spigelian fascia. Patients are typically ages 40 to 70. Incarceration rates (often with omentum) have been reported as high as 20% in these uncommon hernias.[17] Some reports suggest that ultrasound may be a valuable adjunct for the diagnosis of these hernias and may be helpful during attempted reduction procedures.[18,19]

DIAGNOSIS

History and Physical Examination

A patient with a symptomatic hernia may present to the ED with swelling and/or pain in the region of the hernia or abdomen.[20] Ask whether the patient has a history of heavy lifting. Inquire about signs of infection such as fever, chills, and malaise. Determine whether the patient has signs of bowel obstruction including nausea and vomiting. Occasionally, signs and symptoms of intestinal obstruction can be so prominent that the actual hernia is unsuspected as the culprit. Document a record of previous surgeries and hernia repairs including the use of synthetic mesh.

For the physical examination, palpate the inguinal canal in males by inverting the scrotal skin and passing a finger into the external ring. Ask the patient to cough or perform the Valsalva maneuver, which increases the intra-abdominal pressure and facilitates the detection of a hernia. The palpation of the external ring is more difficult in females because it is narrower. An indirect inguinal hernia presents as a swelling in the area of the inguinal ligament or as scrotal swelling. It is often painless and may be noted as an incidental finding. On examination, this hernia can be differentiated from a direct hernia in two distinct ways. First, it starts lateral to the inferior epigastric arteries. Second, on palpation of the inguinal canal, the contents of the hernia will strike the tip of the finger instead of the pad. This occurs as the hernia protrudes down the canal to meet the finger instead of across a fascial and muscular defect. This effect can be accentuated by applying pressure over the internal ring after hernia reduction. Bulging will recur with straining if the hernia is direct, but the pressure over the internal ring should block distention of the hernia into the inguinal canal. A hernia that fills the scrotum is most likely an indirect hernia. The peritoneal contents may become incarcerated owing to swelling of the internal or external ring.

An asymptomatic hernia may present as a mass that is found incidentally on physical examination of the abdomen or groin. If a hernia is easily reducible, it requires no procedural intervention in the ED, but patients should be given instructions for appropriate outpatient surgical follow-up for potential repair. This is particularly important for inguinal hernias in which elective repair is preferred to the morbidity associated with strangulation and emergent repair.[12–14]

A child with an inguinal hernia may have a reducible inguinal or scrotal mass that occurs with straining or crying. A child may present with symptoms of vomiting, poor eating, lethargy, or irritability. Always consider incarcerated or strangulated hernias in the differential of such vague complaints.

Radiologic Imaging

When findings on physical examination are equivocal and suspicion remains for a possible occult hernia, the emergency clinician has several diagnostic options available.[4] Magnetic resonance imaging (MRI) has a high positive predictive value for patients with clinically uncertain herniations[21] and computed tomography (CT) scan can also be helpful for diagnosis of hernias and any associated complications (e.g., bowel obstruction or perforation)[22] (Figs. 44–6 and 44–7). Ultrasound examination has been shown to have good sensitivity and specificity for diagnosis of groin hernias[21,23] and may decrease the rate of emergency surgery by improving the ability to reduce hernias.[24]

Diagnosis of Incarcerated Versus Strangulated Hernias

When the patient or emergency care provider cannot manually reduce the contents of the hernia back into the abdominal cavity, the hernia is described as *incarcerated*. A patient with an incarcerated hernia often presents with a mass that is painful, discolored, enlarged, and not reducible. Associated symptoms may include nausea, vomiting, fever, scrotal pain, labial pain, or abdominal distention. Patients with incarcerated hernias do not necessarily have associated bowel obstruction, and those with a bowel obstruction are not necessarily incarcerated. Incarceration is more common with femoral hernias, small indirect inguinal hernias, and abdominal wall hernias.[25] They can be caused by the presence of a small fascial defect, by constriction of the defect by outside musculature, or by swelling of the hernia contents.

A strangulated hernia is an incarcerated hernia in which the vascular supply to the herniated bowel is compromised, thus leading to ischemia. Ischemic injury to the bowel is suggested by red, purple, or bluish discoloration of the skin over the hernia, significant abdominal tenderness with peritoneal signs, and radiographic findings of extraluminal air.[25] Patients with strangulated hernias may present with bowel obstruction, peritonitis, viscus perforation, intra-abdominal abscess, or septic shock.

It has long been suggested that strangulated hernias cannot be reduced. However, in rare instances, the hernia may inadvertently be reduced en masse to a preperitoneal location (Fig. 44–8), making the hernia sac and contents no longer palpable.[26–28] In this case, the hernia has not been

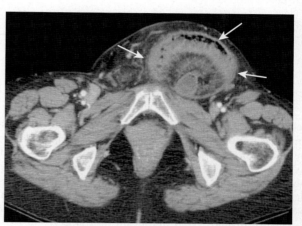

Figure 44–7 Strangulated hernia in a 56-year-old man. Axial contrast-enhanced reformatted CT image of the abdomen shows a strangulated left inguinal hernia with a C-shaped configuration (*arrows*). Note the bowel wall thickening, severe fat stranding, mesenteric engorgement, and extraluminal fluid confined to the hernia sac, findings that suggest strangulation. *(Reprinted with permission from Aguirre DA, Santosa AC, Casola G, et al: abdominal wall hernias: Imaging features, complications, and diagnostic pitfalls at multi-detector row CT. Radiographics 25:1501–1520, 2005, Figure 9a.)*

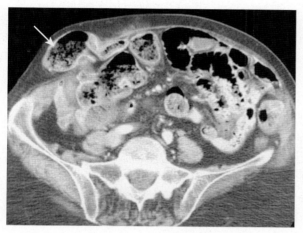

Figure 44–6 Incarcerated hernia identified on computed tomography (CT) scan in a 78-year-old man. *(Reprinted with permission from Aguirre DA, Santosa AC, Casola G, et al: Abdominal wall hernias: Imaging features, complications, and diagnostic pitfalls at multi-detector row CT. Radiographics 25:1501–1520, 2005, Figure 7a.)*

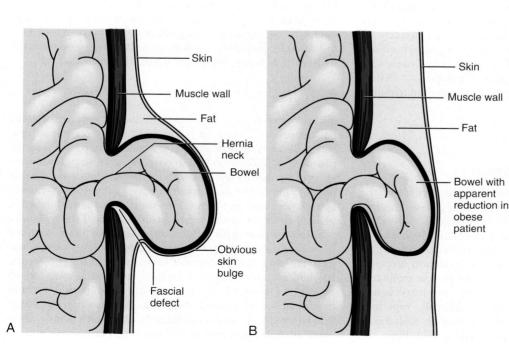

Figure 44–8 En masse reduction. *A,* When a hernia forms, it projects from the fascia into the subcutaneous fat. The object of reduction is to replace the hernia into the peritoneal cavity. *B,* If the hernia sac is partially reduced into the subcutaneous fat of an obese patient, it may appear reduced and may not be palpable owing to the patient's body habitus. However, the hernia is still susceptible to incarceration or ischemia, because it has not been returned to the peritoneal sac.

TABLE 44–1 Differential Diagnosis of Groin Masses

Hernia
Testicular torsion
Retracted or undescended testicle
Hydrocele
Spermatocele
Venous varix
Pseudoaneurysm
Lymphadenopathy
Lymphogranuloma venereum
Epididymitis
Hidradenitia suppurativa
Groin abscess
Hematoma
Lipoma
Epidermal inclusion cyst
Tumor
Tracking of intraperitoneal blood

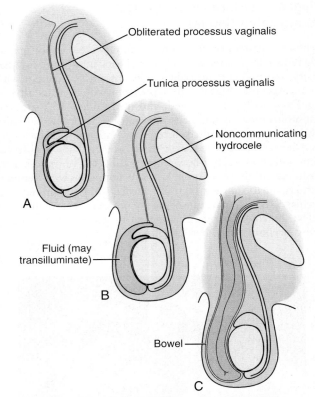

Figure 44–9   Hydrocele versus hernia. *A,* Normal anatomy. *B,* Noncommunicating hydrocele (which may transilluminate) that may be confused with hernia. *C,* Indirect hernia that can be palpated from inguinal ring to testicle.

reduced into the peritoneal cavity and the incarceration/ischemia has not been relieved. Because the clinician believes the hernia has been appropriately reduced, this can result in delay in the diagnosis of ischemic bowel. Fortunately, this is rare, occurring in less than 1% of hernias.[29] One case report described a 3-month-old patient whose gangrenous intestines were completely reduced into the peritoneal cavity, leading to delayed diagnosis and significant morbidity.[11]

Differential Diagnosis

The differential diagnosis for a groin mass is large. Table 44–1 lists a number of disease processes that may masquerade as a hernia. For example, testicular torsion can be mistaken for a hernia, especially if there is an associated reactive hydrocele. The clinician must examine the testicle for tenderness, swelling, lie, and cremasteric reflex. If there is concern for testicular torsion, urology should be notified immediately while simultaneous diagnostic studies are undertaken. A hydrocele can also be confused with a hernia because both can occupy the same anatomic space (Fig. 44–9). A hydrocele may transilluminate, whereas a hernia generally does not.[2] Differentiation can be difficult and may require ultrasound to define the contents of the scrotum.

REDUCTION

Indications and Contraindications

The indications for attempting to reduce a hernia are the presence of a hernia and the absence of strangulation. In some clinical practices, surgeons prefer consultation before an attempt at reduction by an emergency clinician. Because many patients require sedation for successful reduction, it may be helpful to have a surgeon available for reduction attempts while the patient is sedated in the ED. This may be facilitated by discussing the treatment plan with the consultant before reduction. If reduction proves to be difficult, repetitive attempts at reducing the hernia should not be undertaken because this may cause increased swelling and limit the

chances of a nonoperative reduction by the surgical consultant.

In addition to the presence of incarceration despite attempted reduction, several other clinical situations may benefit from surgical consultation. Reduction of a strangulated hernia in the ED is contraindicated and will require operative management. Surgical consultation in the ED is indicated for bowel obstruction, undescended testes or ovaries within the hernia contents, or traumatic hernias.

Procedure

The first step to successful hernia reduction is to position the patient properly, because increases in intra-abdominal pressure will work against efforts to reduce a hernia. Place the patient in a position so that gravity can work to pull the contents of the hernia sac back into the peritoneal cavity. Ensure patient comfort to decrease voluntary or involuntary muscle contraction and guarding. For ventral abdominal hernias, place the patient in the supine position. The Trendelenburg position (supine with head down) may facilitate inguinal hernia reduction. Many of these hernias spontaneously reduce if the patient is left comfortably in this position for 10 minutes. In children, spontaneous reduction has been reported in up to 80% of inguinal hernias over a 2-hour period without manipulation. If manual reduction is necessary, approach slowly with soft, ongoing dialogue and warm hands. This method encourages patient relaxation and minimizes muscu-

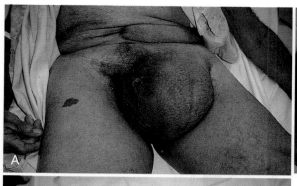
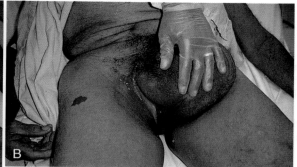
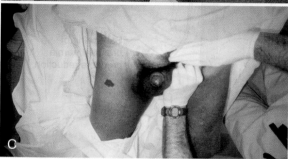

Figure 44–10 *A,* This very large hernia is challenging to reduce. *B,* Merely pushing on the distal mass will not be successful. *C,* Instead, try to first reduce the contents that are more proximal by stabilizing the neck and replacing the portion of bowel closest to the fascial defect.

lar contractions due to pain, cold, or other physical discomfort. A cool compress or ice pack may help to reduce swelling and make the hernia easier to reduce.

Before attempting reduction, consider sedation and analgesia because this will help the patient relax and minimize the pain of the procedure. Options for moderate sedation include etomidate, propofol, midazolam, and fentanyl.

Before beginning the hernia reduction, identify the components of the hernia that will be manipulated during the procedure. The hernia consists of a defect in the existing tissue (muscle and fascia) that makes up the neck of the hernia sac. If the neck is small, the hernia will have a higher incidence of incarceration and strangulation. When attempting to reduce the hernia, take care not to override the edge of the hernia orifice, because this will cause "ballooning" of the contents of the hernia sack around the hernia neck. Attempt to find the edge of the hernia defect and *position your hand or fingers opposite the reducing hand.* This will reduce ballooning and fix the fascial defect.

Begin the reduction procedure by gently guiding the hernia contents and sac back through the neck of the hernia with gentle pressure. With a small hernia, gentle steady pressure may be all that is required. If the contents of the hernia are large, *first guide the most proximal aspect of the hernia back through the neck.* Thus, reduce the hernia in the opposite order from which the contents protruded. Guiding the distal end of the hernia sac through the fascial defect may cause the proximal contents to be displaced around the opening and prevent reduction. Apply gentle, steady pressure *on the tissue at the neck of the hernia* to overcome this and then gradually reduce the hernia (Figs. 44–10 and 44–11). *Failing to perform this important procedure is a common error that precludes reduction.*

When attempting to reduce inguinal hernias in children, position the patient supine in a Trendelenburg position of about 20°, which may allow spontaneous reduction. Another option is to place the patient in the "unilateral frog-leg" position described by Fraser[30] (Fig. 44–12). Stabilize the patient by grasping the anterior superior iliac spines to prevent lateral movement of the pelvis. Abduct the ipsilateral leg, externally rotate and flex the hip to obtain the classic frog-leg position. The purpose of this position is to allow both the internal and the external rings the greatest reapproximation. After achieving this position, use the fingers of one hand to prevent the hernia contents from overriding the external ring while the other hand provides steady but gentle pressure to the contents of the hernia sac. Repeated forceful attempts are not recommended.

POTENTIAL COMPLICATIONS

Major complications may occur during the reduction of hernias. Underlying bowel may be injured due to overzealous attempts at reduction by the clinician. This may aggravate the swelling and make the hernia irreducible. This complication can be avoided with appropriate patient preparation, positioning, sedation, and careful reduction. Another complication occurs after the reduction of ischemic bowel in the setting of an undiagnosed strangulated hernia. These complications may occur when the clinician ignores or does not search for signs of ischemic tissue and inadvertently reduces ischemic bowel back into the peritoneal cavity or en masse into the preperitoneal space.

CHAPTER **45**

Anorectal Procedures

Wendy C. Coates

Patients with anorectal disorders frequently present to the emergency department (ED). In some cases, the condition is isolated, whereas in others, the anorectal complaint can be an outward manifestation of a serious underlying illness. A thorough history and physical examination must precede any procedure. Because of the nature of these complaints, extreme sensitivity and professionalism must be applied.

Patients may be anxious about an anorectal examination or associated procedure. Although sedation is rarely needed for a simple digital rectal examination (DRE), other anorectal procedures may be difficult, if not impossible, to perform without sedation, analgesia, or both. The use of a topical anesthetic on the anoscope is an effective lubricant, but does not provide adequate analgesia in a patient with severe pain or anxiety.

ANATOMY

The rectum and anus compose the most distal portion of the gastrointestinal tract. The rectum begins at the level of the third sacral vertebra and extends distally 12 to 15 cm. The blood supply to the anorectum consists of superior, middle, and inferior hemorrhoidal arteries and veins. The venous system is formed by a series of plexi that are susceptible to overdistention and thrombosis[1-3] (Fig. 45–1). The dentate or pectinate line marks the transition from the anus to the rectum, where a series of anal crypts containing submucosal anal glands lies. Infection of these glands is the likely etiology of many anorectal abscesses. Sensory innervation to the rectum is primarily visceral, whereas innervation to the anus is via cutaneous fibers. Therefore, patients are often unaware of rectal pathology because the pain associated with it may be vague or absent. By contrast, anal lesions are usually very painful and well localized.

DRE

Indications and Contraindications

Perform the physical examination in a private location and take care that the patient is completely draped and relaxed. Generally, a calm atmosphere and caring examiner are sufficient. In some cases, analgesic or anxiolytic agents may be needed to facilitate a thorough examination. In some extremely painful conditions, such as thrombosed or gangrenous hemorrhoids, postpone the examination until the patient is anesthetized. If a sharp-edged foreign body (FB; e.g., metal blade or broken glass) is suspected, performing a DRE may cause injury to the clinician as well as the patient. In these cases, defer the DRE in favor of anoscopy or sigmoidoscopy under anesthesia after radiographic evaluation.

Procedure

Place the patient in the lateral decubitus position. Wear protective gloves and lubricate the examining finger. Inspect the perianal area visually for important information regarding patient hygiene, trauma, or sexually transmitted diseases. Place the finger firmly against the anal sphincter and ask the patient to bear down. Note any prolapsing rectal mucosa or hemorrhoids. Insert the gloved finger into the anus and perform a 360° sweep to identify any irregularities. Examine the prostate. After removing the finger from the anus, examine and test adherent stool for the presence of visible or occult blood[4] (Fig. 45–2). Details of testing for blood in the stool are discussed in detail in Chapter 55.

Complications

Although DRE has been reported to cause a vasovagal response or cardiac dysrhythmias such as ventricular fibrillation, these complications are rare and do not negate the need for this examination.[5] There are essentially no clinical contraindications. As an example, this examination is standard to peform in patients with acute myocardial infarction before using heparin.

ANOSCOPY

Indications and Contraindications

When evaluating a patient for anal pathology, anoscopy may be used as an adjunct to the DRE.[3] Internal hemorrhoids, tears in the distal rectal mucosa, FBs, and distal anorectal masses may be visualized by this method. An imperforate anus is the only absolute contraindication to anoscopy; however, severe rectal pain, a common presenting complaint in the ED, may preclude awake anoscopic examination in anxious patients in pain.

Equipment and Setup

The anoscope is a clear plastic or stainless steel tube with a removable obturator. It may have an integrated light source or require an external light or head lamp. An appropriate examination table, topical anesthetics, lubricant, and gauze with forceps may also be required (Figs. 45–3 and 45–4).

Positioning

Ideally, place the patient in a prone position on a proctoscopic examination table. The prone or lateral decubitus position with knees and hips flexed may also be adequate and is sometimes better tolerated. In the lateral decubitus position, place the patient on the left side if the examiner is right-handed (Fig. 45–5).

Procedure

Although most patients do not require intravenous sedation and analgesia, administer these agents as needed to keep the patient relaxed and comfortable. Apply a topical anesthetic such as eutectic mixture of local anesthetics (EMLA) cream or 4% lidocaine ointment *for at least 30 minutes before the procedure* for painful conditions such as thrombosed hemorrhoids or anal fissures. However, complete relief of pain is not to be

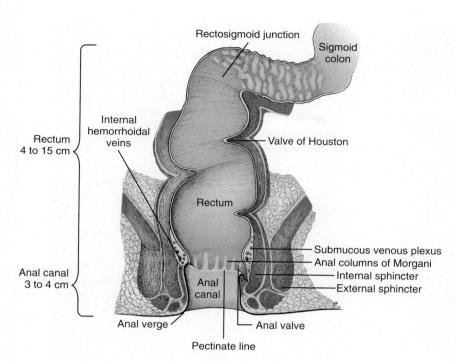

Figure 45–1 Anatomy of the terminal gastrointestinal tract. *(Redrawn from Abrahams PH, Webb PJ: Clinical Anatomy of Practical Procedures. London, Pitman, 1975.)*

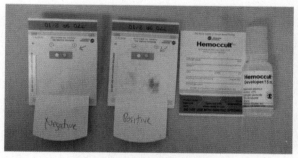

Figure 45–2 Negative (*left*) and positive (*right*) Hemoccult II test for occult blood. Evaluate both positive and negative *control areas*. (Note arrows on card indicates a positive control.) Allow stool sample to fix for 30 sec, and wait 60 sec before reading. Any blue color is positive. This is based on the following reaction:

$$\underset{\substack{\text{endogenous} \\ \text{peroxidase}}}{\text{RBC}} + H_2O_2 + \text{quaiac} \rightarrow \underset{\substack{\text{reaction} \\ \text{product}}}{\text{blue quinone}}$$

expected with this method. If patients do not tolerate anoscopy because of pain, or if they have conditions that are not limited to the anus, refer them to a specialist for a more thorough examination (e.g., sigmoidoscopy, colonoscopy, examination under anesthesia).

Before anoscopy, perform a routine DRE to identify sources of bleeding or pain and to locate any palpable masses. After the DRE and with the obturator inserted completely into the anoscope, carefully introduce the scope into the anus. Use gentle, constant pressure to overcome resistance from involuntary contraction of the external anal sphincter. Gently advance the instrument while asking the patient to bear down slightly. Pass the anoscope gently into the anorectum (Fig. 45–6). If the obturator falls back during insertion, remove the anoscope completely and replace the obturator to avoid pinching the anal mucosa. Advance the anoscope until the outer flange impinges on the anal verge. Unless the anoscope

has an internal light, use an external light source such as a penlight, otoscope, or pelvic examination light.

When the anoscope is fully inserted, remove the obturator. While gradually *withdrawing the anoscope*, visualize the anal canal. Swab away blood or debris to aid visualization, and culture any abnormal discharge that is found. Note whether there is rectal bleeding proximal to the reach of the anoscope. Look for FBs beyond the reach of the anoscope. Withdraw the anoscope slowly as the entire circumference of mucosa is inspected. Look for distal sources of pain or bleeding such as hemorrhoids, rectal fissures, ulcerations, abscesses, or tears. Near the last stage of withdrawal, be aware of the reflex spasm of the anal sphincter, which may cause the anoscope to be expelled quickly. Use firm counterpressure to prevent such a rapid expulsion, and realize that it is not uncommon to need to repeat the procedure to obtain an adequate view of the anal verge.

Complications

Anoscopy is a safe procedure and complications are rare. Patients often complain of increased pain after the examination. Local mucosal irritation with subsequent bleeding is the most common complication. To prevent transmission of infectious diseases, dispose of or sterilize instruments after each use.

MANAGEMENT OF HEMORRHOIDS

Hemorrhoids are a common affliction and have been described and treated for more than 4000 years.[2] The refined, low-fiber diet of Western nations makes hemorrhoids extremely common in the United States,[3] where 1 in 25 to 30 individuals is afflicted.[6] One million patients annually[7] seek medical attention for this condition.[2]

Hemorrhoidal tissue is composed of vascular, mucosal, and muscular tissues. Although frequently attributed to vari-

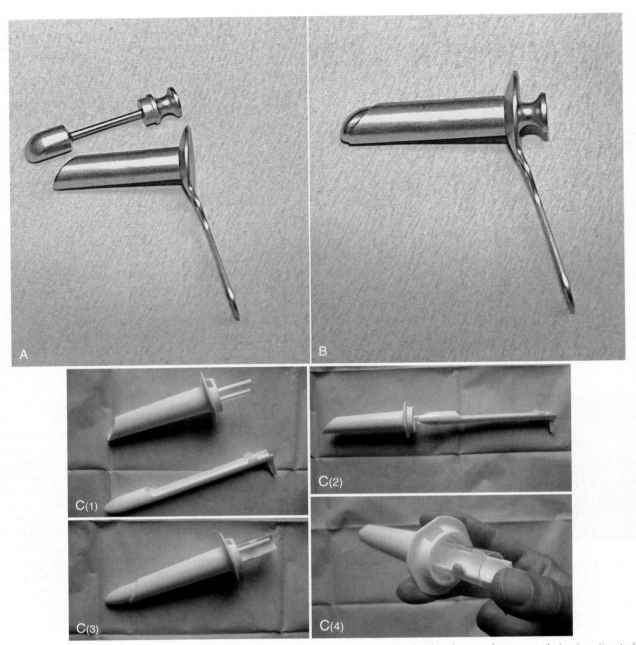

Figure 45–3 *A,* Stainless steel anoscope (reusable). *B,* Anoscope prepared for insertion. Use the thumb to apply pressure during insertion to keep the smooth round trochar protruding through the tip. *C,* Plastic disposable anoscope: parts and assembly.

cosities, all three elements compose the hemorrhoid[8] (Fig. 45–7).

There are two types of hemorrhoids: internal and external.[2,9] Internal hemorrhoids originate above the dentate line,[1,3] are covered with mucosa, and lack sensory innervation.[9] Internal hemorrhoidal prolapse may be painless.[3,9] Gangrenous, strangulated, extruded, or thrombosed internal hemorrhoids, however, may be extremely painful.

Internal hemorrhoids can be further classified as first through fourth degree. First-degree hemorrhoids do not prolapse but can be identified on anoscopic examination. Second-degree hemorrhoids prolapse upon straining, but reduce spontaneously. Third-degree internal hemorrhoids prolapse upon straining and can be reduced manually, whereas fourth-degree internal hemorrhoids prolapse and are irreducible.

Fourth-degree hemorrhoids are prone to thrombosis and strangulation (see Fig. 45–7C).[2]

External hemorrhoids originate below the dentate line[1,3] and are covered with squamous epithelium. This makes them easily recognizable because their covering matches the surrounding skin. They are innervated by the inferior rectal nerve.[2] A thrombosed external hemorrhoid appears as a bluish mass covered by epidermis.[3,4,9] Acute thrombosis occurs suddenly and is usually very painful. Many patients feel a tender mass and are unable to sit comfortably. Significant bleeding is uncommon but may occur if spontaneous rupture occurs.[3] Increased pressures from straining or trauma from constipation or diarrhea may exacerbate external hemorrhoids.[1,3] Distention and trauma predispose the hemorrhoidal venous plexus to stasis with ensuing clot formation and edema.[10,11]

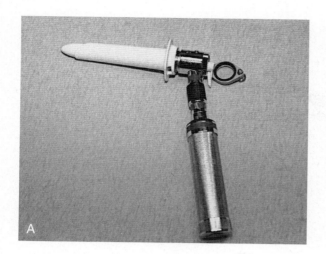

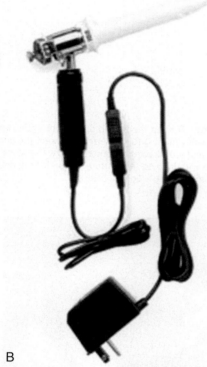

Figure 45–4 *A,* Anoscope with a light source and obturator in place (A and B). *B,* Anoscope with a light source attached. *(A and B, Courtesy of Welch Allyn Inc.)*

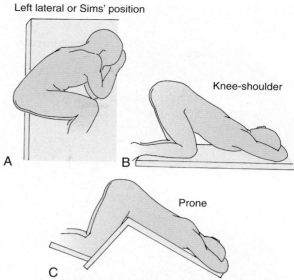

Figure 45–5 *A–C,* Positions for performing anoscopy. *(A–C, From Hill GJ II: Outpatient Surgery, 3rd ed. Philadelphia, WB Saunders, 1988.)*

Conservative Treatment

ED management of minor *internal hemorrhoids* is conservative.[7] Major prolapse is a miserable condition, will not benefit from conservative intervention, and should receive surgical consultation in the ED. A useful mnemonic for minor internal hemorrhoids is WASH: water (increase fluid intake, sitz baths in water), analgesics, stool softeners, high-fiber diet.[4] A truly adequate high-fiber diet *is almost impossible to maintain, so psyllium (Metamucil and others) is usually prescribed.* Referral for outpatient surgical consultation may be considered.[9] Banding of internal hemorrhoids is often very successful. If the patient must push the hemorrhoids back in after a bowel movement, he or she has symptomatic third-degree internal hemorrhoids and would benefit from elective surgical referral. This condition can be easily demonstrated by having the patient strain before the DRE. *Nonreducible prolapsed internal hemorrhoids*

should receive immediate surgical consultation and, often, admission.

Without treatment, thrombosed *external hemorrhoids* and those that have spontaneously ruptured, will generally resolve spontaneously over 1 to 3 weeks,[9,11] usually without complication (except for an occasional skin tag).[3] During the interim, however, they are quite painful and may bleed. Small ruptured or nonruptured hemorrhoids that present acutely with minimal discomfort may be managed conservatively with frequent sitz baths, and topical corticosteroids (Anusol HC) or Preparation H. The pain is most severe within the first 48 hours,[3] and patients presenting within this time window are most likely to benefit from *ex*cision (not incision and drainage) of the contents of their thrombosed external hemorrhoid. Patients who present after this time are usually best managed with conservative treatment[9] (see Fig. 45–7D).

Surgical Excision of Thrombosed External Hemorrhoids

Indications and Contraindications

Surgical consultation should be obtained in the ED for very distressing and painful fourth-degree internal hemorrhoids[3] and for profuse bleeding that is hemodynamically significant. Bleeding disorders, serious systemic illness, and hemodynamic instability are all relative contraindications to excision in the ED.

Procedure

Place the patient in the prone or lateral decubitus position.[3,12] Tape the buttocks apart to aid in visualization. An assistant is usually mandatory. Give parenteral analgesia and sedation as an adjunct to local anesthesia if necessary. Infiltrate with a local anesthetic (such as 0.5% bupivacaine or buffered 1% lidocaine with epinephrine at 1:100,000) just under the skin and over the dome of the hemorrhoid[9] (Fig. 45–8). The overlying skin should blanch, indicating that anesthesia has been introduced at the appropriate depth. It is usually not necessary to perform a very painful field block to anesthetize a larger

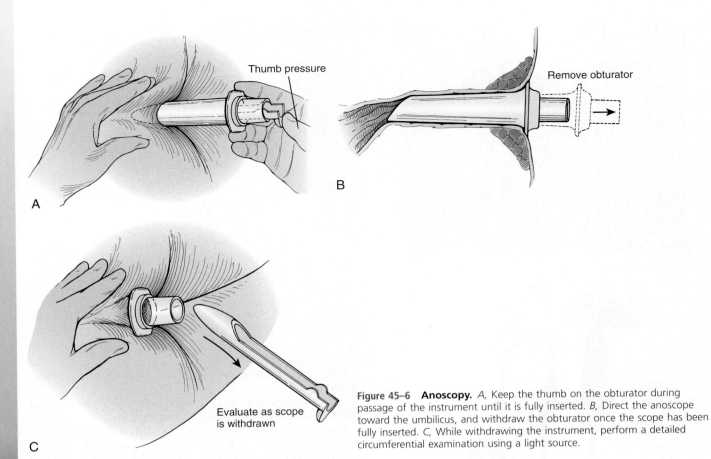

Thumb pressure

Remove obturator

A

B

Evaluate as scope
is withdrawn

C

Figure 45–6   Anoscopy. *A,* Keep the thumb on the obturator during passage of the instrument until it is fully inserted. *B,* Direct the anoscope toward the umbilicus, and withdraw the obturator once the scope has been fully inserted. *C,* While withdrawing the instrument, perform a detailed circumferential examination using a light source.

Internal
hemorrhoid

Submucous space

Ext. sphincter

Interhemorrhoidal
groove

External
hemorrhoid

A

B

C

D

Figure 45–7   *A,* Anatomic location of internal and external hemorrhoids. *B,* Thrombosed external hemorrhoid. *C,* Thrombosed prolapsed internal hemorrhoids. These hemorrhoids cannot be permanently reduced and are quite painful; occasionally, partial relief can be obtained by manual reduction. They should not be incised in the emergency department (ED); a formal hemorrhoidectomy is required if conservative measures are not successful. They are often mistaken for a partial "rectal prolapse." Sitz baths and stool softeners are often futile in such severe cases. *D,* This small external hemorrhoid ruptured and produced minor but persistent bleeding and pain. Topical corticosteroids or Preparation H and frequent sitz baths are curative in 5 to 7 days. If very symptomatic the contents can be removed under local anesthesia (see Fig. 45–10). *(A, from Hill GJ II: Outpatient Surgery, 2nd ed. Philadelphia, WB Saunders, 1980. Reproduced by permission.)*

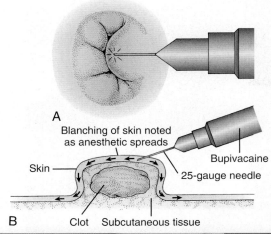

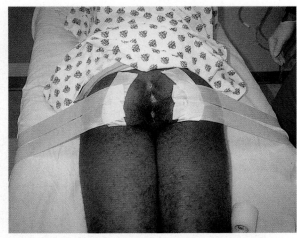

Figure 45–9 Taping the buttocks to gain exposure but an assistant will be helpful.

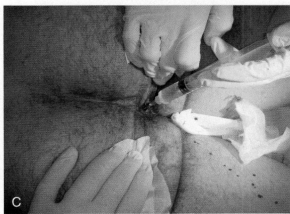

Figure 45–8 A, For surgical treatment of a thrombosed external hemorrhoid in the ED, aesthesia usually can be obtained by a *single injection* of buffered long-acting bupivacaine. In elective cases, apply eutectic mixture of local anesthetics (EMLA) cream for 1 hr before the procedure. Parenteral sedation is optional. Using a 25-gauge needle, inject an anesthetic solution in the middle of the swollen hemorrhoid just below the skin surface. B, Do not move the needle tip. With slow injection, the anesthetic will spread over the surface of the dome and into the surrounding tissue. Avoid deep field blocks at the base of the hemorrhoid because they are unnecessary and very painful. C, If pain persists, inject additional anesthetic into deeper tissues *through the cut edges, not through the intact skin.*

area or multiple hemorrhoids. *If pain persists, inject additional anesthetic through the incised tissue into the base of the hemorrhoid rather than through the intact skin* (see Fig. 45–8C).

Grasp the skin overlying the thrombosis with forceps. Make an elliptical incision around the clot and direct it radially from the anal orifice. Elevate the skin edges with forceps and excise the edges to expose the underlying thrombosis.[9] Remove the clot with forceps[1] or by applying digital pressure (Figs. 45–9 to 45–11). Often, multiple individual clots will be present. If any skin ulceration is noted over the hemorrhoid, include it in the excised portion. Pack the wound loosely with standard cotton gauze or Gelfoam to prevent the skin edges from reapproximating prematurely.[1,13]

For the trip home, place a gauze pad between the buttocks and tape the buttocks together to hold the gauze in place. Advise the patient to avoid prolonged standing or straining for the next few days. Minor bleeding may occur. Sitz baths can be started as soon as the anesthetic has worn off. If the gauze has not fallen out, instruct the patient to remove it at the first sitz bath. Gelfoam packing avoids the need for this step. After the packing has been removed, instruct the patient to apply a soothing cream to the area for a couple of days (such as Preparation H, Anusol HC, lidocaine ointment). Instruct the patient to avoid using toilet paper after a bowel movement for a few days, but to wash the area with mild soap and water in the shower. Most patients do not need a routine wound check, and they should be relatively asymptomatic in 48 hours. If pain or bleeding persists, a repeat visit is indicated. Once the clot has been removed, recurrent thrombosis is unlikely, but these patients are predisposed to future episodes. Permanent residual skin tags usually appear. Long-term therapy should be directed toward avoiding constipation by increasing dietary fiber and fluid intake.[3] Antibiotics are not indicated.

If an invasive procedure is not well tolerated by the patient, alternate nonoperative treatments include topical nitrates[4,9,14] or topical nifedipine.[11,15] Applied to the thrombosed hemorrhoid, these creams relax the anal sphincter, relieve pain, and promote healing. Systemic absorption is minimal, and the application is usually well tolerated.

Complications

Although complications are rare, bleeding and infection do occur.[9] Bleeding is usually simple skin oozing and stops with direct pressure.[1] When a simple incision and drainage is performed instead of an elliptical excision, or when the ellipse of skin is not completely removed, the skin edges can close prematurely and cause infection and a permanent perianal skin tag.[1,3,12] Premature closure can also result in incomplete evacuation of the clot.

MANAGEMENT OF ANORECTAL ABSCESS AND PILONIDAL CYST/ABSCESS

These topics are covered in detail in Chapter 37, Incision and Drainage.

MANAGEMENT OF RECTAL FOREIGN BODIES

The etiology of rectal FBs includes autoeroticism (most common),[16] iatrogenic placement (thermometer, enema tip),

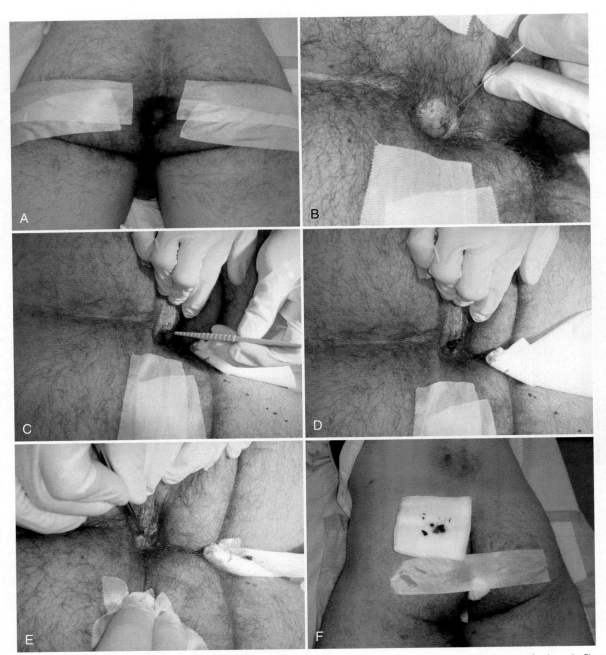

Figure 45–10 Technique to remove clot from a thrombosed external hemorrhoid. *A*, Gain proper exposure. *B*, Inject anesthesia as in Figure 45–8. *C*, Excise a triangular piece of tissue, *not merely a simple incision*. *D* and *E*, Remove all clots by manual pressure and/or forceps. *F*, Secure a piece of gauze in the buttocks with tape.

assault, self-administered treatment (enema), accidental ingestion, and concealment (body packing). The myriad of objects that have been removed include vibrators, sex toy phalluses, aerosol cans, light bulbs, glass bottles, billiard balls, fruits, vegetables, and small animals.[16–19] Most objects are cylindrical. Many of these objects can be removed successfully in the ED.[20] By following some simple guidelines, outpatient treatment can be practical and cost-effective.

Diagnosis of a rectal FB is usually made from the history. The physical examination should, therefore, concentrate on excluding anorectal or intestinal perforation and determining which objects will be accessible in the ED.[20] DRE will identify objects that are low-lying or palpable. These are most likely to be removed successfully in the outpatient setting.[16,20] Plain

radiographs can supplement the examination by delineating the shape, position, and number of the objects.[16,18] If an FB with a sharp edge is suspected from the history, omit the DRE to keep from getting cut by the object.

Indications and Contraindications

Although some objects may pass spontaneously, delayed removal may lead to obstipation, pain, infection, and perforation. For these reasons, FB removal is indicated according to the algorithm included in this chapter (Fig. 45–12). *Rectal FB removal can lead to rectal perforation. While many FBs can be removed safely in the ED, complicated or prolonged attempts may be better performed under general anesthesia.*

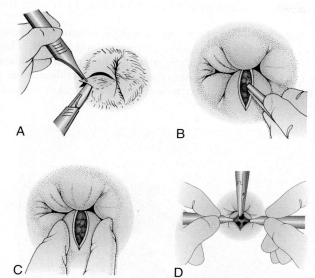

FB removal in the ED is contraindicated in patients who have severe abdominal pain or signs of perforation, a nonpalpable FB, or broken glass in the rectum. Other situations precluding ED removal include a rectal FB that is unusually difficult to remove (a set time limit has elapsed or the patient cannot tolerate removal), or when there is insufficient experience or equipment to perform the procedure.[20] Patients who present under these conditions require surgical consultation.

Equipment

The specific equipment required will often depend on the nature of the FB. In general, the clinician will need a speculum with a light source and an instrument to grasp the FB. The speculum can be an anoscope, a rigid sigmoidoscope, a vaginal speculum, or a retractor. Instruments useful for grasping the FB include ring forceps, tenaculum forceps, or obstetric forceps. In some instances, a Foley catheter or endotracheal tube will be helpful. A suction dart,[21] vacuum extractor,[16] and plaster of Paris have also been used to aid in FB retrieval. Individual situations may lead to creative use of standard medical equipment, but one must ensure safety before using a device to remove a rectal FB.

Procedure

The technique for removal depends on the size, location, orientation, and composition of the FB. Place the patient either prone in the knee-chest position or in a lateral decubitus position. Alternatively, if the patient is in the lithotomy position, pressure can be placed on the abdomen to help maneuver the FB toward the distal rectum. Parenteral analgesia is often required to relieve pain from anal stretching and manipulation. Intravenous sedation is almost always required to calm the patient and facilitate relaxation of the anal sphincter. Perform a perianal block to allow greater dilation of the sphincter. As described earlier, local infiltration with 0.5% bupivacaine or 1% lidocaine with epinephrine at 1:100,000

Figure 45–11 Schematic technique as described in Fig. 45–10. *A,* For the unroofing technique, make an elliptical or triangular incision to remove a piece of the overlying skin. To prevent skin tags, do not use a simple linear incision. *B,* Blood clots may extrude spontaneously but remove the remaining ones with forceps or express them with the fingers (*C*). *D,* Often, multiple clots are present, and they should all be removed. Ask an assistant to provide exposure with forceps if necessary.

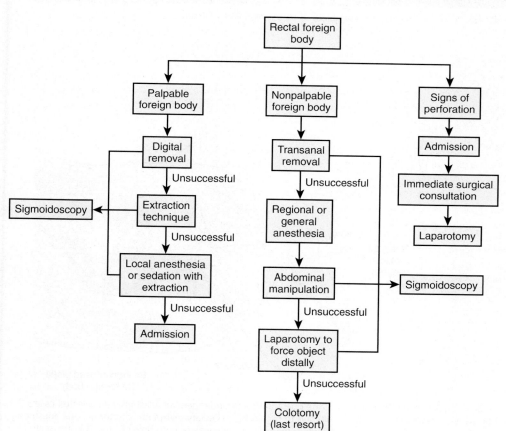

Figure 45–12 Emergency approach to the removal of rectal foreign bodies. Foreign bodies that are fragile or are associated with rectal spasm are generally managed with regional or general anesthesia. The use of supplemental analgesic, anxiolytic, and local anesthetic medications is recommended.

may be administered circumferentially around the anus in the submucosal tissue.[13,20]

After analgesia and sedation are administered, perform a DRE to gauge the position and orientation of the FB. Suprapubic pressure from above, the examiner's finger from below, and the patient performing a Valsalva maneuver may successfully deliver the object without instrumentation.[20] If the FB is lodged against the sacrum posteriorly, redirect it by cradling its posterior aspect between two fingers and directing it slightly proximally and anteriorly while the patient gently bears down.[16]

If the DRE reveals that the object has an accessible edge or lip, use an instrument to extract it under direct visualization

(Figs. 45–13 to 45–15). First, insert an anoscope, rigid sigmoidoscope, vaginal speculum, or retractor into the anus as described previously under anoscopy. If an intact object is visualized clearly, use a blunt instrument to secure it. Apply gentle traction to remove the object, the instrument, and the anoscope or speculum as a single unit. Grasp the object under direct visualization to avoid pinching or tearing the mucosa.[20]

Rigid sigmoidoscopes offer a unique advantage because air can be insufflated into the rectum around the FB. This technique can be particularly helpful when retrieving glass objects. Glass rectal FBs often create a vacuum in the segment of bowel just proximal to where they lie. This makes removal

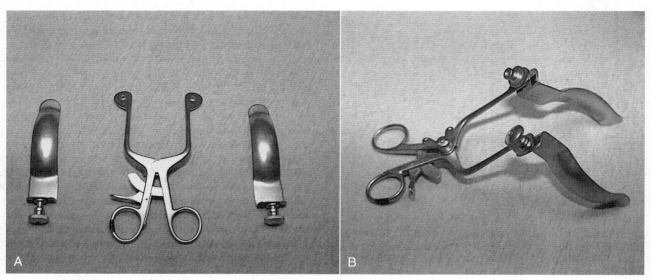

Figure 45–13 *A,* Parks retractor (unassembled). *B,* Assembled Parks retractor.

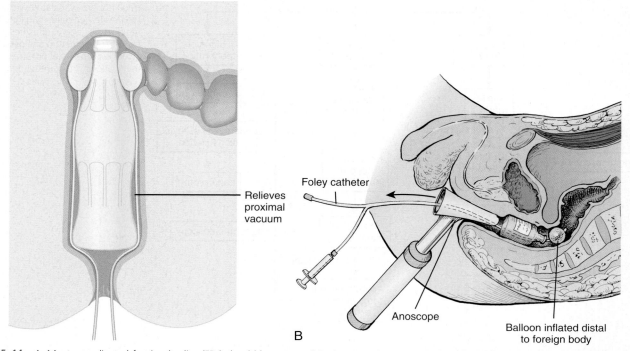

Figure 45–14 *A,* Most complicated foreign bodies (FBs) should be removed in the operating room under general anesthesia. In selected cases, removal may be attempted in the ED, but be wary of rectal perforation. It is difficult to obtain the necessary relaxation without general anesthesia. *B,* Similar procedure using an anoscope and a Foley catheter. The key to success is to remove the proximal vacuum holding the FB in the rectum.

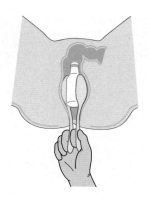

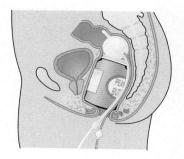

Figure 45–15 *A,* Large spoons grasp a fragile FB in the rectum. *B,* Use of an endotracheal tube or Foley catheter to remove a smooth FB made of glass. Air introduced above the obstruction overcomes the vacuum created by the FB.

with simple traction almost impossible. The vacuum can be released by distending the rectal wall around the object with air. If a sigmoidoscope cannot be used to retrieve a glass object, pass one or two Foley catheters or an endotracheal tube beyond the FB, and inflate the balloon or cuff. Then remove the object using the inflated balloons and gentle traction. Often, specific equipment is not available to remove all FBs, and the clinician must improvise based on the circumstances. Something as simple as two large spoons or an endotracheal tube may be used in lieu of complicated forceps and clamps.

Besides creating a vacuum, glass objects are especially difficult to remove because they can break and cause a tear or perforation in the rectal wall. If forceps are used for retrieval of a glass object, coat the grasping edge with rubber[22] or plastic or pad it with gauze. Plaster of Paris has been used to remove a hollow glass object if the object has an open end facing distally. Insert a hollow tube (e.g., an endotracheal tube or small chest tube) into the open end. Fill the FB with plaster using a large irrigation syringe to inject plaster through the hollow tube. Once the plaster cools around the tube, it can be used as a handle to remove the object with gentle traction. Be careful not to leak plaster onto the mucosa. In addition, heat is released as the plaster hardens and may cause the glass to crack or shatter. After removal, perform a sigmoidoscopy to evaluate for edema and possible perforation of the mucosa.[16,20] Patients with normal postextraction examinations and no evidence of perforation may be safely released home after a period of observation.

FBs that are positioned proximal to the rectum warrant surgical consultation. Management options include observation to enable passage to the rectum or surgical removal. Enemas or cathartics should not be used, because they may increase the impaction of a rectal FB or cause it to move higher into the colon.

Complications

The most common complication is the inability to remove the rectal FB, which should prompt a surgical consultation. The most serious complication of rectal FB retrieval is perforation or deep mucosal tear, which may necessitate surgery. Cracking or shattering of glass may also require surgical exploration and retrieval. Mild mucosal edema and rectal bleeding are common complications of prolonged rectal FB presence and retrieval.[18] These may not require any specific treatment. However, the presence of postprocedural abdominal pain, fever, sustained or profuse rectal bleeding, or discharge warrants a surgical consultation.[23]

MANAGEMENT OF RECTAL PROLAPSE

Rectal prolapse is the protrusion of some or all of the layers of the rectal wall through the anal orifice.[24] Prolapse is usually not an emergency, and manual reduction is often easily accomplished in the ED. The most common presenting complaint is protrusion of a rectal "mass" or tissue.[25] Patients may complain of pain on defecation, itching, incomplete evacuation, incontinence, or bloody mucosal discharge and mistake the condition for "hemorrhoids." Rectal prolapse is diagnosed by visual inspection of the anus and DRE. The differential diagnosis includes hemorrhoids, polyps, cystocele, or carcinoma.[26]

There are three types of prolapse: (1) Complete prolapse, or procidentia, involves all layers of the rectum protruding through the anal orifice (Figs. 45–16 and 45–17). (2) Incomplete, or occult prolapse, describes internal prolapse that does not reach the orifice. This type is difficult to diagnose in the ED and requires no emergency intervention. (3) Mucosal prolapse is limited to mucosal protrusion through the anal opening.[24,26,27]

Complete and partial prolapse can be distinguished from each other by digital palpation. A thick muscular layer of tissue between the examiner's thumb and forefinger suggests complete prolapse. Partial or mucosal prolapse may demonstrate radial rectal folds protruding through the rectum. This type of prolapse rarely extends more than 3 to 4 cm from the anus.[1,25] Complete prolapse can extend 10 to 15 cm outside the anal verge.[1,24]

Rectal prolapse is most common in children and older adults. Prolapse in children is typically incomplete, or mucosal. It usually affects children younger than age 3 years and is often associated with cystic fibrosis, parasitic infection, chronic diarrhea, or malnutrition or occurs as a sequelae of chronic neurologic disease. Prolapse is usually self-limited; outpatient management (after manual reduction) includes correcting constipation,[1,7] avoiding straining, and referring for testing to exclude cystic fibrosis.[26,28] Rectal prolapse in adults occurs most often in older women. Nursing home patients may have recurrent prolapses. The etiology is poorly understood but is associated with chronic constipation, chronic neurologic conditions, or pudendal neuropathies that weaken the anal sphincter.[24,27,28]

Indications for Reduction

Rectal prolapse may be reduced in the ED. If unsuccessful, outpatient surgical referral is appropriate. Definitive surgery may be attempted but occasional prolapses in debilitated

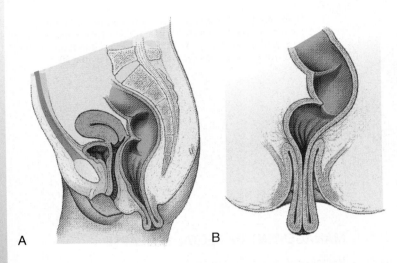

Figure 45–16 *A,* Type I procidentia (rectal prolapse). *B,* Intussusception of the sigmoid colon beyond the anus. (*A and B, From Kratzer GL, Demarest RJ: Office Management of Colon and Rectal Disease. Philadelphia, WB Saunders, 1985, pp 221–333.*)

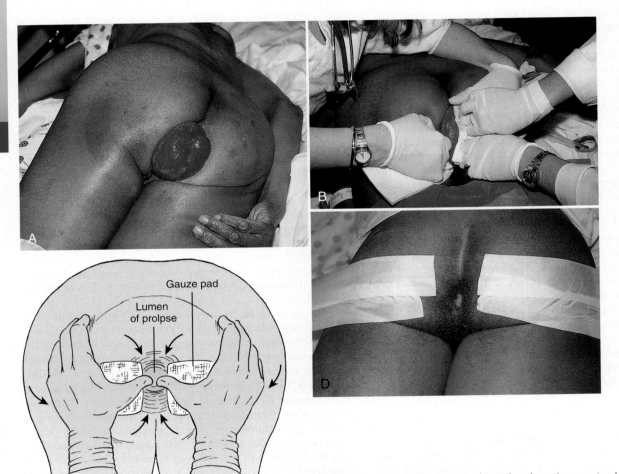

Gauze pad

Lumen
of prolpse

Figure 45–17 *A,* Complete (recurrent) rectal prolapse in a nursing home patient. *B* and *C,* To reduce the prolapse, an assistant spreads the buttocks and the clinician's hands encircle the prolapse. The key to success is adequate sedation/analgesia and a slow steady gentle pressure. *D,* Successful reduction.

patients are usually treated conservatively.[26] Referral for outpatient proctoscopy should be made to search for a polyp or malignancy that may have acted as a lead point.[28] If the prolapse is incarcerated, a surgical consultation should be obtained.[26]

Procedure

Reduce a mucosal prolapse with a few minutes of gentle, constant pressure on the mass. In children, intravenous sedation may be necessary to allow reduction. Children are often more relaxed if they are allowed to remain in the parent's lap during the procedure. After reduction, send the child home with a pressure dressing and stool softeners. Counsel the parents on the use of dietary fiber and increased fluid intake to prevent constipation and straining.[26] Refer the child for outpatient follow-up.[28–30]

For reduction of a complete prolapse, place the patient in the prone or lateral decubitus position. Parenteral sedation may be required if the patient is anxious or having difficulty relaxing the sphincteric muscles. Tape the buttocks apart to aid in reduction. Apply constant, gentle circumferential pressure to the prolapsed area, beginning with the portion closest to the lumen (the most distal segment) (see Fig. 45–17). Place the thumbs on either side of the lumen while grasping the exterior walls with the fingers. Apply pressure with the thumbs while rolling the walls inward to force the prolapse back through the anus.[26]

Complications

Complications after a successful reduction are uncommon, but may include bleeding and ulceration. Failure to reduce a prolapse requires surgical consultation. Apply saline-moistened gauze over the rectal tissue while awaiting consultation. A persistently prolapsed rectum can result in ulceration, strangulation, and perforation of the bowel wall.[25] Moreover, the possibility of anal sphincter tone loss and incontinence increases with delays in reduction of rectal prolapse.[26,28]

ANAL FISSURE

An anal fissure is a small laceration or ulcer at the anal verge. Appearing trivial on examination, it can be extremely painful, even hours after a bowel movement, owing to persistent spasm (Fig. 45–18). The condition is quite difficult to eradicate, is debilitating, and can last for months. It is occasionally associated with bright red rectal bleeding. Anal fissure is most

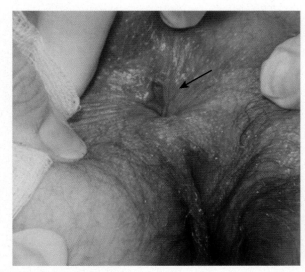

Figure 45–18 Posterior midline anal fissure is the most common type. These lesions are painful and difficult to heal. In a child, an anal fissure suggests child abuse. *(By permission of Mayo Foundation.)*

commonly found in young adults, men and women equally. In children, it can be a sign of child abuse. Usually associated with constipation, a hard or strained stool, or chronic diarrhea, the exact etiology is unknown. Multiple or recurrent fissure are associated with Crohn's disease, tuberculosis, syphilis, human immunodeficiency virus, and malignancy. Diagnosis is relatively easy, and the fissure is readily seen by spreading the buttocks. The vast majority of fissures develop in the posterior midline. Conservative therapy (high-fiber diet/Metamucil, stool softeners, sitz baths, and topical preparations [Anusol with cortisone]) may result in slow healing in 4 to 6 weeks, but in only about half of patients. Nitroglycerine gel (0.2%) and nifedipine gel (2%) relax muscles and promote blood flow as second-line therapy. Botox has been used successfully. Surgical sphincterotomy is usually curative.

Acknowledgments

Acknowledgments to Christopher M. Strear, MD, Scott M. Davis, MD, and Howard Blumstein, MD, for earlier editions of this text.

REFERENCES CAN BE FOUND ON EXPERT CONSULT

MUSCULOSKELETAL PROCEDURES

CHAPTER 46

Prehospital Immobilization

Thomas A. Brabson and Brett S. Greenfield

SPINE IMMOBILIZATION

Despite a lack of scientific data to show that it improves patient outcomes, spinal immobilization is one of the most frequently performed prehospital procedures.[1,2] Recommendations for spinal immobilization date back to 1971 when the American Academy of Orthopaedic Surgeons[3] published the first set of guidelines for spinal immobilization following blunt trauma. In these guidelines, the presence of signs (e.g., weakness, paralysis) or symptoms (e.g., neck pain, paresthesias) of spine injury was the primary indication for spine immobilization.[3] Since then, recommendations for spine immobilization have evolved considerably. Today, indications for spine immobilization are based primarily on mechanism of injury, regardless of the presence or absence of symptoms or physical findings suggestive of a spine injury.[2,4] This has resulted in routine prehospital spinal immobilization in all but the most trivial injuries.

Although spinal fracture and spinal cord injury can have devastating results, the incidence of such injuries in trauma patients is relatively small, about 2% to 5% in most reviews. Sundheim and Cruz[5] calculated that only 0.03% to 0.16% of all out-of-hospital trauma patients may be expected to have *secondary spinal cord* injury that may be helped by immobilization. The number needed to immobilize to prevent one secondary injury is between 625 and 3333 trauma patients, but the wholesale dismissal of any benefit from immobilization is not justified. It is important to note, however, *that despite zealous use of prehospital cervical spine immobilization, and countless medical legal prosecutions for worsening of injury from its absence, there is little scientific evidence quantifying the effect of spinal immobilization in trauma patients, or the possible adverse effects of its application* (Box 46–1). Simply stated, the effect of spinal immobilization on mortality, neurologic injury, spinal stability, and adverse effects in trauma patients remains uncertain by evidenced-based medicine, and no randomized prospective trials have been conducted. Because such trials are

highly unlikely, caution and clinical judgment are still prudent.

Although mechanism of injury is widely accepted as an indication for prehospital spine immobilization, focus on evidence-based medicine has led some investigators to question this practice.[4,6–8] Falls from heights and motor vehicle accidents are mechanisms most associated with spinal injury. Associated injuries, intoxication, or abnormal mental status make immediate clinical decision in the field problematic. The results of several trials support the use of clinical criteria for cervical spine clearance by prehospital care providers.[4,9–12] A few studies have found that unnecessary spine immobilization may be associated with *increased morbidity and cost.*[2,13,14] Whereas large prospective studies will be needed before prehospital spine clearance gains widespread acceptance, studies to date have prompted several emergency medical service (EMS) systems across the country to establish specific clinical criteria for prehospital spine immobilization (Table 46–1).[2,4,11,12,15]

Despite the growing controversy regarding the practice of routine prehospital spine immobilization, mechanism of injury and initial complaints or findings of neurologic dysfunction remain the primary indications for spine immobilization in the prehospital setting. This section outlines the techniques and equipment used by most prehospital care providers in the United States. All emergency care providers should be well trained in their use, limitations, and application.

CERVICAL SPINE

Trauma patients frequently sustain injuries to the cervical spine. These injuries are particularly devastating when associated with injury to the spinal cord. In the United States, approximately 10,000 to 12,000 spinal cord injuries occur each year.[1,16] Of these, more than half are in the cervical region, and most are a result of motor vehicle crashes.[16] The remainder are due to falls, recreational activities (e.g., diving, contact sports), and penetrating trauma. Therefore, it is critically important that unstable cervical spine injuries be immobilized early and effectively.

Because the minimum degree of motion required to cause spinal cord injury has not been defined, the goal of immobilization is to maintain the head in a neutral position with 0° of motion in all directions.[17] To immobilize the entire cervical spine, an orthotic device must fix the head, hold the occiput and mandible, and restrict motion at the cervicothoracic junction.[18] This approach follows the basic orthopaedic principle of immobilizing the joint above and below a

BOX 46-1 Spinal Immobilization for Trauma Patients

The current practice of immobilizing trauma patients before hospitalization to prevent more damage may not always be necessary, as the likelihood of further damage is small. Means of immobilization include holding the head in the midline, log rolling the person, the use of backboards and special mattresses, cervical collars, sandbags and straps. These can cause tissue pressure and discomfort, difficulty in swallowing and serious breathing problems.

The (Cochrane) review authors could not find any randomized controlled trials of spinal immobilization strategies in trauma patients. It is feasible to have trials comparing the different spinal immobilization strategies. From studies of healthy volunteers it has been suggested that patients who are conscious, might reposition themselves to relieve the discomfort caused by immobilization, which could theoretically worsen any existing spinal injuries.

AUTHORS' CONCLUSIONS

The effect of spinal immobilization on mortality, neurological injury, spinal stability and adverse effects in trauma patients remains uncertain. Because airway obstruction is a major cause of preventable death in trauma patients, and spinal immobilization, particularly of the cervical spine, can contribute to airway compromise, the possibility that immobilization may increase mortality and morbidity cannot be excluded. Large prospective studies are needed to validate the decision criteria for spinal immobilization in trauma patients with high risk of spinal injury. Randomized controlled trials in trauma patients are required to establish the relative effectiveness of alternative strategies for spinal immobilization.

From Kwan I, Bunn F, Roberts I, on behalf on the WHO Pre-Hospital Trauma Care Steering Committee. Spinal immobilization for trauma patients. Cochrane Database Syst Rev 2001;(2), CD002803.

TABLE 46-1 Clinical Criteria for Prehospital Spine Immobilization

Concerning mechanism of injury (such as axial loading, car rollover, fall from significant height)

Spine pain or tenderness

Focal neurologic deficit

Unreliable patient examination (not awake, alert, oriented, calm, and cooperative)

Head injury (including severe head and facial trauma)

Altered mental status:
  No available history
  Found in the setting of possible trauma (e.g., lying at the bottom of a staircase)
  Near drowning with a history or high probability of a diving injury

Distracting injury

Communication barriers

Extremes of age

suspected injury. In addition, to be useful in the prehospital setting, a cervical immobilization device must be portable and easy to apply and must allow access to the upper airway. Disposable devices have the additional advantages of not requiring cleaning or a return visit to the emergency department (ED) to pick up the device.

At present, the standard technique of spinal immobilization involves early manual stabilization of the head and neck relative to the long axis of the body. Manual stabilization is usually followed by the application of a cervical collar. Although its use is controversial, a cervical collar has value as an early adjunct in the sometimes complex process of immobilization and extrication. It is extremely important to remember, however, that even the best-supporting collars do not provide adequate immobilization when used independently. For complete cervical spine immobilization, the patient must also be secured to an intermediate spine-immobilizing device (e.g., short spine board, Kendrick extrication device [KED]), a full-length spine board (e.g., backboard, scoop stretcher, full-body splint), or both.

Complete cervical immobilization must also incorporate lateral stabilization of the head in the form of lightweight bulky objects such as foam blocks, towel rolls, blanket rolls, or cushions and tape. This can also be accomplished using factory-made devices such as the HeadBed (Laerdal Medical Corp., Wappingers Falls, NY) or the Universal Head Immobilizer (Ferno-Washington, Inc., Wilmington, OH).

Background

Since 1965, an entire industry aimed at prehospital preservation of life and limb has evolved. During the late 1960s and early 1970s, specially manufactured spinal immobilizers were developed for field use. Numerous variations of these early devices have been developed to solve specific prehospital problems and to meet the need for lightweight, durable, adaptable, and affordable equipment.

It should be stressed that although there is widespread agreement about the basic steps of spinal immobilization, prehospital care is a difficult setting for individuals who cannot easily adapt. Because of the variety of circumstances that confront prehospital care providers on a daily basis, flexibility is mandatory.

In 1965, Louis Kossuth[19] was the first clinician to support the need for extrication standards, including immobilization of the cervical spine. J. D. Farrington,[20,21] a pioneer in the use of the spine board for cervical immobilization, is credited with thrusting the concept of prehospital spinal immobilization into the venue of conventional medicine. He outlined the use of a backboard, sandbags, and tape for the prehospital extrication and care of patients with suspected spinal injuries. He fashioned extrication collars using universal dressings held in place by soft roller bandages and advocated manual traction during the extrication phase.[21]

Manual traction is no longer recommended, because it may *aggravate an underlying spinal injury*. It was replaced years ago by *in-line stabilization*.[22] In addition, although sandbags are effective devices for lateral immobilization, they may cause significant movement of the neck if the board is suddenly tilted (e.g., to decrease the risk of aspiration in a vomiting patient). As a result, sandbags have been replaced by more ergonomic and lighter-weight devices such as foam blocks, the HeadBed, or Bashaw CID. Despite these changes, the original Farrington method of splinting the head and torso to a rigid object remains the preferred technique for effective spinal immobilization.

Indications

An extrication collar should be used as a primary adjunct in cases involving trauma to the head and neck. The most common mechanism of injury involves sudden deceleration of an automobile, resulting in hyperflexion and hyperextension forces. Patients under the influence of alcohol or drugs lack the self-awareness to recognize their own spinal injury and should be immobilized routinely. Likewise, every unconscious trauma patient should be immobilized to avoid aggravating an underlying spinal injury. Any awake and alert trauma patient who complains of spine pain, paresthesia, weakness, or absent movement should be immobilized carefully to avoid secondary injury to the spinal cord. Extremes of age and the presence of communication barriers (e.g., language, hearing impairment) may affect the ability to accurately assess the patient's perception and communication of pain and should lower one's threshold for spinal immobilization.[2,4] In addition, the presence of other painful injuries or concern over other victims can easily mask the manifestations of an occult cervical spine injury.

Serious cervical cord injuries can also occur in the absence of demonstrable fractures. Spinal cord injury is common in elderly patients with cervical spondylosis, in whom an arthritic osteophyte may sever a portion of the cord as permanently as a fracture or dislocation. In such cases, there may be little subjective pain, and the mechanism of injury may appear seemingly minor.[23]

Therefore, a high index of suspicion for possible spinal injury must be maintained at all times, and the medical record should include documentation of the neurologic examination before and after spinal immobilization.

The purpose of an extrication collar is to assist in splinting the head and neck either therapeutically or prophylactically in a neutral position.[18] The collar is useful for the following reasons:

1. It provides airway protection by limiting flexion in a patient whose unsupported jaw and neck position threatens patency.
2. It helps reduce cervical spine motion, especially flexion, but also rotation, lateral bending, and extension. In this regard, however, it serves only as an adjunct.
3. If properly chosen, it can support the weight of the head while the patient is sitting and help to maintain the alignment of the cervical spine once the patient has been moved to a supine position.
4. An equally important function is to serve as a reminder to the patient and rescuers that the integrity of the basilar skull and cervical spine is suspect because of the mechanism of injury.

The cervical collar does not provide complete immobilization of the head and neck. The collar was designed as an adjunct and was never intended to provide definitive immobilization in itself. Complete immobilization is not possible until the patient is properly secured to a long backboard-type device. Nonetheless, the collar should go on first and remain in place during the entire procedure.

Contraindications

Few circumstances preclude the use of an extrication collar. The presence of a surgical airway (i.e., cricothyroidotomy or tracheotomy) may require modification of the cervical immobilization technique.

In addition, cervical dislocation with fixed angulation or a preexisting anatomic abnormality may prevent effective application of factory-made collars. This situation is rarely encountered and can be managed with an improvised cervical immobilizer, such as a collar fashioned from a towel roll or prolonged manual positioning without traction.

A third circumstance that could preclude the use of a collar is massive cervical swelling (e.g., secondary to hemorrhage or tracheal injury). In these circumstances, the compressive effect of a collar may impede air exchange, decrease cerebral perfusion, or increase intracranial pressure.[24-26] Finally, the presence of an impaled foreign body such as a knife, a piece of glass, or metal can also make cervical spine immobilization using extrication collars difficult. Fully conscious patients with isolated penetrating trauma and no neurologic deficit do not automatically require spinal immobilization.[27]

Note that improvised cervical support may work better than a manufactured collar, depending on the size and shape of the patient. This is particularly true in the pediatric population, because collars come in limited sizes and may not be well tolerated. In such circumstances, prolonged manual in-line stabilization is often necessary and allows the provider to give constant reassurance to the child.

Although not a contraindication, gunshot wounds (GSW) to the head are not considered an indication for routine cervical spine immobilization (Fig. 46–1). Cervical immobilization may raise intracranial pressure. Rhee and coworkers[28] reported that the frequency of having surgical cervical spine stabilization after a GSW in patients who were neurologically intact was 0.03% (4 in 12,559 patients). In that report, no patients required cervical neck stabilization if they were neurologically intact at presentation after a stab wound.[28] *In patients with penetrating spine injuries, neurologic deficits are essentially established and final at the time of injury.*[29]

In one study of baseball bat injuries to the head, no cervical spine injuries were identified.

Equipment

There are three types of cervical collars: cervical, head-cervical, and head-cervical-thoracic. Traditionally, cervical collars have used a four-point support structure at the bottom of the collar: namely, at the two trapezius muscles posteriorly

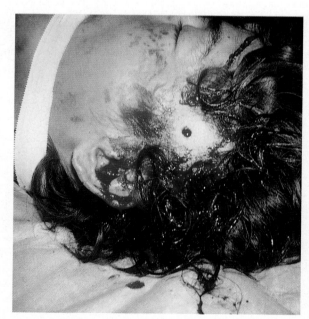

Figure 46–1 Gunshot wound (GSW) to the head is not an indication for routine cervical spine immobilization, and such intervention may lead to missed injury under the collar, airway compromise, and delay in resuscitation for fear of manipulating the spine. There is no meaningful recovery for GSW injuries to the spinal cord.

and at the two clavicles anteriorly (Fig. 46–2). Most modern collars are modified rigid head-cervical-thoracic devices that use the sternum as a fifth support structure (Fig. 46–3). Current collar designs support the head with winglike flaps on the collar's upper posterior edges. Anteriorly, the collar supports the mandible. The collar's flaring design generally prevents compression of the thyroid cartilage and cervical vessels, even when applied firmly. Semirigid collar must be comfortable to ensure patient compliance.

Soft collars, although comfortable, have no role in spinal immobilization, because they provide minimal support and do not reduce cervical motion to any significant degree.[30,31]

Investigators have attempted to evaluate cervical collars in an objective fashion. The accepted "gold standard" for comparison is the halo brace, which restricts motion to 4% flexion-extension, 1% rotation, and 4% lateral bending.[18] Unfortunately, even the best cervical collars (when used independently) restrict flexion and extension by only 70% to 75%,

and overall neck movement by less than or equal to 50%.[32] A number of studies have evaluated neck motion in volunteers immobilized supine on a backboard with various collars in place.[1,30,31,33-35] Whereas these studies demonstrated small differences among some of the collars, overall they merely confirm the fact that cervical collars alone are inadequate to immobilize the cervical spine completely. Thus, it is important to keep in mind that for effective cervical spine immobilization, differences among various types of cervical collars are less important than proper application, fit, and most importantly, use of adjunctive equipment.

Little information is available regarding the proper selection and application of spinal immobilization devices for children. Most of the available data were derived from studies of adults and might not be applicable to children. Half of the total growth in head circumference is achieved by the age of 18 months, giving children a disproportionately large head compared with the rest of the body. Prior to age 8, these anatomic and developmental differences result in a higher incidence of upper cervical spine injuries (C1–2). Because injuries in this area are frequently unstable, proper cervical immobilization in the neutral position is critically important.

In the neutral position, the pediatric cervical spine is normally lordotic or extended.[26] However, because the occiput is large, positioning the child's body on a standard backboard may force the neck into flexion or a relative kyphosis. The clinical significance of this is currently unclear, but theoretically, it may be hazardous for young children. Therefore, the standard backboard should be modified to adapt to the child's larger head size. As a rough guide, the external auditory meatus should be on the same level as the midshoulder. Suggested modifications include a cutout in the backboard that accommodates the occiput or a pad under the back at the level of the chest (Fig. 46–4). If not modified, the standard backboard in conjunction with the disproportionately large head of a child may force the neck into hyperflexion, potentially aggravating an underlying cervical spine injury. Nypaver and Treloar[36] showed that all children required elevation of the back (mean height, 25.4 ± 6.7 mm) for correct neutral posi-

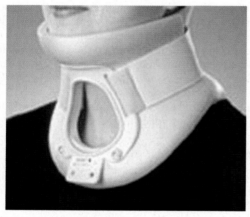

Figure 46–2 Philadelphia collar. This is a two-piece, high-type collar that comes in four sizes. The collar supports the head in a dish-shaped contour that is formed when the front and rear halves are joined by Velcro fasteners. When properly sized for a patient, this collar provides excellent support. When applied too tightly, it tends to force the mandible backward and can cause thyroid compression in some patients. It is extremely comfortable. (Courtesy of Philadelphia Cervical Collar Company, Thorofare, NJ.)

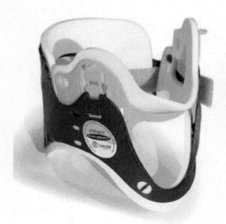

Figure 46–3 Stifneck collar. This collar is made of high-density polyethylene (a hard material) and padded with semiflexible foam margins. Note the low-reaching anterior panel, which contacts the sternum for additional support. (Courtesy of Laerdal Medical Corporation, Wappingers Falls, NY.)

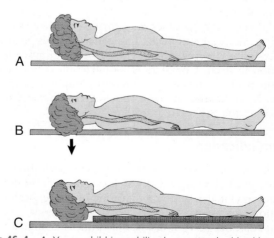

Figure 46–4 A, Young child immobilized on a standard backboard; note how the large head forces the neck into flexion. Backboards can be modified by an occiput cutout (B) or a double mattress pad (C) to raise the chest. The actual clinical consequences of this observation are unknown. (A–C, Adapted from Herzenberg JE, Hensinger RN, Dedrick DK, et al: Emergency transport and positioning of young children who have an injury of the cervical spine. J Bone Joint Surg Am 71:15, 1989.)

tion on a spine board. Children younger than 4 years required more elevation than those 4 years old or older. It must be pointed out, however, that there have been no published reports of a cord lesion resulting from the use of standard immobilization techniques and equipment in children.[26]

Procedure

Application of an extrication collar is a straightforward procedure (Fig. 46–5). A collar should be treated as a splint. The normal axiom in splinting is to immobilize the joint above and below the area of injury. Because no collar performs this function perfectly, a rescuer should be charged with maintaining manual in-line cervical stabilization in the neutral position during collar application and until the patient can be fully immobilized in an intermediate-stage corset-type device or on a full backboard. The rescuer's intentions should be thoroughly explained to the patient throughout the procedure.

Before application of the collar, the neck should be examined for swelling, ecchymosis, deformity, bony tenderness, or penetrating wounds. Once the collar is in place, a conscious patient should be cautioned repeatedly against movement of the head. Any persistent complaints of pain or dyspnea by the patient should be investigated by removal and possible replacement of the device while manual stabilization is maintained. The collar size should be determined using the manufacturer's suggested guidelines. For example, the Stifneck collar (Laerdal Medical Corp., Wappingers Falls, NY) is available

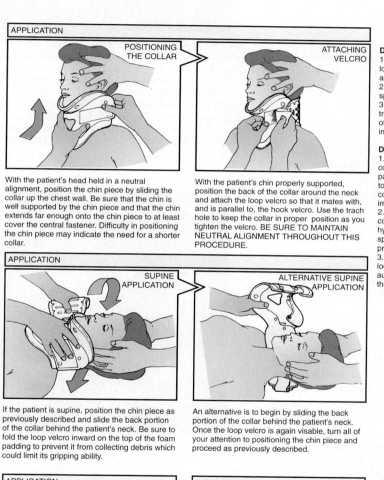

APPLICATION

POSITIONING THE COLLAR

With the patient's head held in a neutral alignment, position the chin piece by sliding the collar up the chest wall. Be sure that the chin is well supported by the chin piece and that the chin extends far enough onto the chin piece to at least cover the central fastener. Difficulty in positioning the chin piece may indicate the need for a shorter collar.

ATTACHING VELCRO

With the patient's chin properly supported, position the back of the collar around the neck and attach the loop velcro so that it mates with, and is parallel to, the hook velcro. Use the trach hole to keep the collar in proper position as you tighten the velcro. BE SURE TO MAINTAIN NEUTRAL ALIGNMENT THROUGHOUT THIS PROCEDURE.

APPLICATION

SUPINE APPLICATION

If the patient is supine, position the chin piece as previously described and slide the back portion of the collar behind the patient's neck. Be sure to fold the loop velcro inward on the top of the foam padding to prevent it from collecting debris which could limit its gripping ability.

ALTERNATIVE SUPINE APPLICATION

An alternative is to begin by sliding the back portion of the collar behind the patient's neck. Once the loop velcro is again visable, turn all of your attention to positioning the chin piece and proceed as previously described.

APPLICATION

TIGHTENING THE COLLAR

Tighten the collar gently and attach the velcro so that the two pieces are parallel. Re-check the position of the patient's head and collar for proper alignment. Tighten the collar further until proper support is obtained.

DISASSEMBLY

GRASP END OF CHIN PIECE

STIFNECK™ may be disassembled by grasping the end of the chin piece, as shown, with black fastener between the fingers and working this fastener out of its hole. Do not try to pull the white fastener apart.

DO'S
1. DO follow the directions of your local EMS authorities for the approved use of extrication collars.
2. DO use all appropriate cervical spine immobilization techniques.
3. DO refer to your EMT paramedic training manual regarding the use of extrication collars and spinal immobilization techniques.

DON'TS
1. DO NOT rely on any cervical collar to adequately immobilze a patient's cervical spine. Collars are tools to aid in immobilization, but no collar by itself provides sufficient immobilization.
2. DO NOT use an improperly sized collar. Too large a collar may hyperextend a patient's cervical spine; too small a collar may not provide appropriate stability.
3. DO NOT hesitate to contact your local EMS dealer or local EMS authority with questions regarding the use of the extrication collars.

Figure 46–5 Technique for the application of an extrication collar. *(Courtesy of Laerdal Medical Corporation, Wappingers Falls, NY.)*

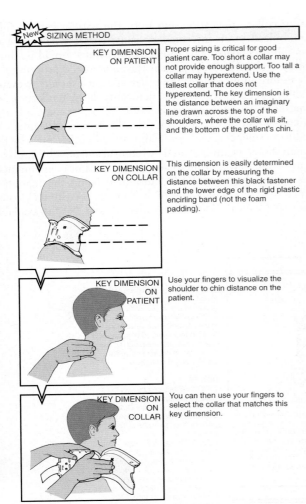

SIZING METHOD

KEY DIMENSION ON PATIENT

Proper sizing is critical for good patient care. Too short a collar may not provide enough support. Too tall a collar may hyperextend. Use the tallest collar that does not hyperextend. The key dimension is the distance between an imaginary line drawn across the top of the shoulders, where the collar will sit, and the bottom of the patient's chin.

KEY DIMENSION ON COLLAR

This dimension is easily determined on the collar by measuring the distance between this black fastener and the lower edge of the rigid plastic encircling band (not the foam padding).

KEY DIMENSION ON PATIENT

Use your fingers to visualize the shoulder to chin distance on the patient.

KEY DIMENSION ON COLLAR

You can then use your fingers to select the collar that matches this key dimension.

Figure 46–6 Method for predetermining the correct size for an extrication collar. *(Courtesy of Laerdal Medical Corporation, Wappingers Falls, NY.)*

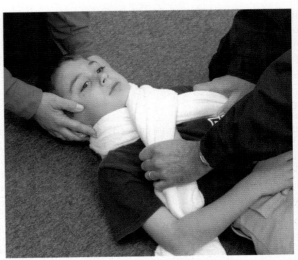

Figure 46–7 **Horse collar.** Most extrication collars are available in three to five factory sizes. If a collar is not sized properly to fit a particular patient, it performs no function. Patients with extremely long necks or especially short ones can be immobilized by means of a horse collar fashioned from a blanket or towel. The blanket (or towel) is rolled to the thickness desired and slid under the patient's neck while a bystander applies manual stabilization; the ends of the blanket (or towel) are then brought across the patient's anterior chest. *(Courtesy of AtlantiCare Regional Medical Center: Emergency Medical Services, Atlantic City, NJ.)*

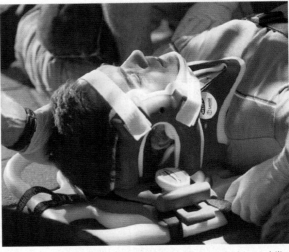

Figure 46–8 Extrication collar combined with a cervical immobilization device. *(Courtesy of Laerdal Medical Corporation, Wappingers Falls, NY.)*

in various sizes and uses the distance from the top of the shoulder to the chin to determine size (Fig. 46–6). The tallest collar that does not cause hyperextension should be used. For extremely short necks, a special extrication collar such as the No-Neck (Laerdal Medical Corp., Wappingers Falls, NY) is recommended.

In cases in which an extrication collar of the proper size is not available, an improvised device should be made from available materials (Fig. 46–7). Once the patient is in the supine position and firmly secured to a backboard, lateral stabilization should be added, using foam blocks and tape or a factory-made lateral neck stabilizer (Fig. 46–8). Because immobilization on a flat backboard has been shown to place most adult patients into relative cervical extension, it is recommended that occipital padding (mean, 3.8 cm) be added to restore neutral position in adults.[37]

It should also be remembered that application of a cervical collar should not be attempted until the patient's head has been brought into a neutral position and manual in-line stabilization has been applied.[32] If the patient experiences cervical muscle spasm, increased pain, neurologic complaints (e.g., paresthesia, weakness), or airway compromise, movement of the head and neck should be halted immediately. In these situations, patients should be immobilized in the position they are found using an alternative technique (e.g., blanket, towel roll).

Complications

Improper application of an extrication collar can occur if the wrong size is used or too little care is exercised during placement. The best means of preventing either error is strong clinician involvement in the training and continuing education of rescue crews, with vigorous feedback regarding correct and incorrect application. In addition, adherence to the manufacturer's collar-specific recommendations for size and application should be emphasized.

A collar that is too small for a patient may be either too tight for the girth of the neck (with obvious complications) or too short to provide adequate immobilization. Too large a collar commonly results in hyperextension, which can exacerbate a preexisting spinal injury.

Improper or prolonged application of an extrication collar may impede venous return and raise intracranial pressure (ICP).[38] Although the clinical significance of increased ICP produced by cervical immobilization is still unknown, two studies have confirmed that the application of a rigid cervical collar causes a statistically significant and sustained rise in ICP.[39,40] Kolb and colleagues[40] reported a 24.8–cm H_2O increase in cerebrospinal fluid pressure in 20 adult patients undergoing lumbar puncture. Hunt and associates[39] reported a 4.6–mm Hg mean rise in ICP in 30 patients with severe traumatic brain injury. The largest rise in ICP was noted in patients with a baseline ICP greater than 15 mm Hg. The authors of these studies concluded that elevation of ICP produced by cervical immobilization might have deleterious effects in patients with acute or sustained intracranial hypertension.[39,40]

The long-term use of the Philadelphia extrication collar as part of the treatment plan for an underlying cervical spine injury has been associated with pressure ulcers of the scalp.[41] Because some collars (e.g., Philadelphia [Philadelphia Cervical Collar Co., Westville, NJ] and Stifneck) have been shown to exert higher capillary closing pressures at contact points, it is suggested that collars with favorable skin pressure patterns and superior patient comfort (e.g., NECLOC [Jerome Medical, Moorestown, NJ]) be used in these settings.

One final complication should be mentioned. The patient who, for whatever reason, actively resists placement of an extrication collar or other splint *should not be forced to wear it* (Fig. 46–9). Postictal patients present such a dilemma. Immobilization of the combative patient cannot be accomplished without considerable muscular exertion not only by rescuers but also by the patient. If fractures do exist, it is

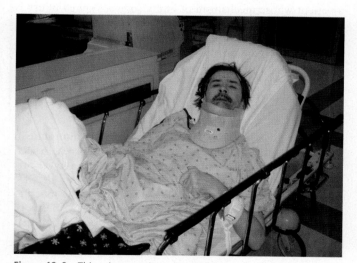

Figure 46–9 This seizure patient was initially postictal and did not allow prehospital cervical spine immobilization. Although this is a dilemma for all involved, it is best to avoid forcing such immobilization (see Box 46–1). Sedation may be an alternative if suspicion for injury exists. Despite a clear mental status, and no neck pain (and NEXUS rules negative), an unneeded collar was subsequently applied in the emergency department (ED), to the annoyance of the patient who then became very agitated and tried to elope. Note the patient *is incorrectly still upright.*

possible that struggling can cause further damage. If the patient permits manual stabilization, this should be maintained as an alternative. Sedation may be judiciously used to enhance compliance.

Conclusion

Cervical spine immobilization is an important skill for all emergency care providers; however, its true benefit has yet to be established. It may be difficult to accomplish, or counterproductive, in the combative individual. The use of a rigid cervical collar is an important first step in the immobilization of patients with potential cervical spine injuries. However, the use of a cervical collar alone does not provide complete immobilization. Proper cervical spine immobilization requires the use of a cervical collar, backboard, and lateral support device to ensure complete immobilization of the head and neck. The widespread acceptance of clinical criteria for the selective use of spine immobilization in the prehospital setting awaits the results of large prospective randomized trials.

THORACOLUMBAR SPINE

Adequate full-body thoracolumbar spine immobilization is best accomplished by means of a full-length spine board (also called a backboard). Full-body spinal immobilization includes early application of a cervical collar, lateral immobilization of the head and neck, and ample strapping of the entire body to the backboard. Proper strapping minimizes movement during transport and will help limit spinal movement associated with backboard tilting, which may be necessary in the likelihood of emesis or during transport of pregnant females in the second or third trimester.

Transferring a victim from a location and position of origin to a backboard may require the use of an intermediate-stage immobilization device such as a short spine board or a corset-type device. Corset-type devices have extensions that engage the head and neck and are equipped with weight-bearing loops that allow easier movement of the patient. Intermediate immobilizers or extrication splints should be used when a patient must be removed from a confined environment or when circumstances require movement in or from a sitting position (e.g., an automobile).

In some circumstances, a threatening environment (fire, hazardous material incident, extreme weather) or patient condition (compromised airway, shock) may necessitate rapid extrication. Rapid extrication is the process of patient removal and spinal immobilization using an abbreviated manual technique.[1] It is performed by first bringing the patient's head into the neutral position. A cervical collar is then applied and the patient is transferred to a backboard without using an intermediate-stage device. Manual in-line stabilization of the spine is maintained throughout the procedure.

When extrication is not required by a patient's location, position of origin, or route of egress, the patient is most often found lying at ground level. With an extrication collar in place and in-line manual cervical immobilization, the patient can be logrolled onto a backboard.[42] Visual inspection of the back should be carried out during the logrolling process while the body is kept in a single plane.

Although logrolling is a widely accepted method to move patients with potential spinal injuries onto a backboard, studies have shown that it may cause a small amount of anteroposterior and lateral spine displacement.[43,44] This

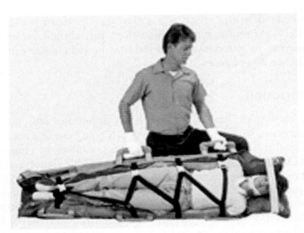

Figure 46–10 The Evac-U-Splint mattress. *(Courtesy of Hartwell Medical, Carlsbad, CA.)*

unwanted movement may be minimized by positioning subjects with the arms extended at the sides and the palms resting on the thighs.[44] It should be noted that although logrolling may cause some spinal movement, there have been no reports of neurologic deterioration after a logrolling maneuver.

An optional but effective means of moving a supine patient is provided by a type of stretcher that breaks apart longitudinally and can be slid beneath a victim without disturbing her or his position. The halves of this "scoop" stretcher are anatomically contoured to enhance comfort and limit lateral movement of the immobilized patient. Unfortunately, visual inspection of the back is not possible with the use of a scoop stretcher.

A third means of both immobilizing and moving a trauma victim consists of a specially designed full-body splint, complete with factory-made straps or harnesses. Several such immobilizers are available, most of which are highly effective and provide good lateral stability as well as anatomic conformity. One such device that is popular in European countries is the vacuum stretcher. A full-body splint marketed in the United States (Evac-U-Splint, Hartwell Medical, Carlsbad, CA) offers fast, full-body immobilization that supports the entire patient without creating pressure points (Fig. 46–10). In general, the patient must be either logrolled or lifted, using a scoop stretcher or full backboard, onto one of these devices.

Background

Until 1965, the principle of "rapid transportation above all" held widespread acceptance among rescuers, who had little or no orthopaedic training, and among clinicians whose emergency care experience, by modern standards, was just as limited. The most commonly agreed-on means of getting a sitting patient out of a wrecked automobile was to use some version of a chair-carry. If the patient originated in a position other than the sitting position, the patient was first placed into a sitting position and then moved by means of a chair-carry or simply dragged out of the vehicle.

In 1965, Col. Louis Kossuth,[19] commander of the U.S. Air Force's Medical Service School at Gunter Air Force Base in Alabama, published the first recommendations for removing victims from wrecked vehicles. Kossuth has been credited with developing the first modern-type spine board.[21] In 1967 and 1968, Farrington[20,21] authored two classic papers describ-

ing the use of an extrication collar, spinal traction, 9-ft webbing straps, and both short and long spine boards to remove people in every conceivable position from automobiles. Much of today's extrication theory is essentially identical to what was taught by Farrington.

In 1967, the Committee on Trauma of the American College of Surgeons[45] listed the minimum amount and type of equipment that should be carried in ambulances. This list included both short and long spine boards with accessories. Although the list of ambulance supplies and equipment has evolved greatly since then, the requirement for both short and long spine boards (or their equivalent) has not changed.[46]

Indications and Contraindications

Any mechanism capable of causing injury to the cervical spine should prompt rescuers to immobilize not only the head and neck but also the entire body. For complete spinal immobilization, the head, neck, and torso must be fastened into a single common plane. Extrication devices (e.g., short spine boards) will accomplish this to some extent, although movement of nonimmobilized lower extremities can lead to secondary movement of the pelvis and lumbar spine. Movement of the lumbar spine may also induce thoracic movement to some extent. Considering the fact that the most feasible position for transport is the supine position, full-body immobilization is best achieved using the long spine board with the extremities securely fastened to the board.

Mechanisms that arouse suspicion of injury to the thoracolumbar spine should also prompt full-body spinal immobilization. These include penetrating and blunt injuries to the thorax, abdomen, pelvis, and spine. Full-body immobilization should be considered whenever the mechanism for spinal injury exists, even in the absence of signs and symptoms. In such cases, the possibility of occult injury is best ruled out through clinical or radiographic examination, or both, at the hospital.

The only contraindication to full-body immobilization of a patient whose mechanism of injury suggests spinal injury is the existence of a greater threat. The threat to a patient's life may exceed the threat of possible spinal injury under the following circumstances:

- *Hazards on the scene.* Problems with traffic control, weather extremes, fire, hazardous materials, unstable structures, or unstable vehicles.
- *Ongoing gunfire at the scene.*
- *Overwhelming casualties.* Rescuers may have to improvise in cases in which casualties exceed available resources. In such cases, proper spinal immobilization may merit a lower priority than usual.
- *Patient noncompliance.* A competent rescuer can do much to make an immobilization device comfortable by means of padding and reassurance. If this fails, immobilization that is applied by force or to a combative or resistant patient may cause more harm than no immobilization at all.

Equipment

Cervical Extrication Splints

A large variety of short spine boards (Fig. 46–11) and intermediate-stage extrication devices are available for prehospital use. Generally, these devices are manufactured using rigid lightweight materials. They have a narrow board design that

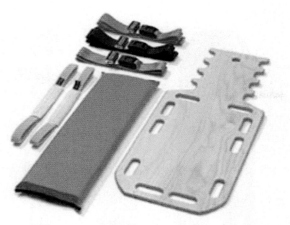

Figure 46–11 Rigid short boards. *(Courtesy of Ferno-Washington, Inc., Wilmington, OH.)*

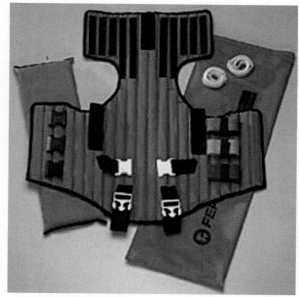

Figure 46–12 The Kendrick extrication device (KED). *(Courtesy of Ferno-Washington, Inc., Wilmington, OH.)*

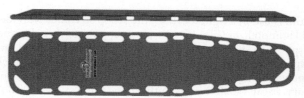

Figure 46–13 The Iron Duck long spine board. *(Courtesy of Iron Duck—A Division of Fleming Industries, Chicopee, MA.)*

permits easy application in automobiles or confined spaces and are constructed with multiple openings along the edges to allow for a variety of strapping options. Ideally, these devices should also be translucent so that radiographs can be readily obtained in the ED, and they should allow for repeated use and easy clean up.

Application of a cervical extrication splint should not produce unnecessary movement or change the position of the head, neck, shoulders, or torso. In conjunction with a good cervical collar, a properly applied cervical extrication splint should effectively limit flexion, extension, lateral, and rotational motion of the head, neck, and torso.

One commonly used device that meets all of these criteria is the KED (Fig. 46–12). This device consists of two layers of nylon mesh impregnated with plastic and sewn over plywood slats to provide rigidity. It has a nylon loop behind the patient's head that is continuous with the pelvic support straps for additional strength. Part of its anterior thoracic panels can be folded backward to fit the obese, pregnant, or pediatric patient.[47] Properly applied, the KED is a snug-fitting, highly adaptable immobilizer that can be used under even the most adverse of circumstances.

Mosesso and coworkers[48] compared six prehospital cervical immobilization devices and concluded that the devices were similar in their ability to immobilize the cervical spine.

Full-Body Spine Immobilizers

Full-Body Spine Boards (Backboards). Backboards are made from wood or plastic composites and can be either rectangular or tapered in shape (Fig. 46–13). Most rescuers prefer the tapered type because it takes up less horizontal room when angled into a narrow opening or doorway. In addition, the slight narrowing of these boards on either end enhances the effectiveness of strapping.

Most backboards have strategically placed openings along the edges that can be used to secure head-stabilizing devices, strap the patient to the board, or lift. Many also feature runners, usually about 2.5 cm thick, on their undersides that serve both as stiffeners and as spacers. These raise the board slightly off the ground so that rescuers can get their fingers under the board during lifting. The runners, however, may make it more difficult to slide a patient onto the board.

Advantages of boards over full-body splints include their ease of storage, low cost, and extreme versatility. The back-

board can be used to slide a victim out of an automobile or to protect a victim during removal of a windshield.

Backboards have a few disadvantages as immobilizers. Board splints, as a class, are the least comfortable of all immobilizers. One prospective study demonstrated that standard spinal immobilization (hard backboard, rigid cervical collar, lateral immobilization device) of healthy volunteers was associated with a variety of symptoms, including headache, backache, and jaw pain.[13] In another study using emergency medical technician (EMT) trainees, Cross and Bakerville[49] found that the occiput, lower back, and sacrum are the three most common locations for pressure pain and that pain in these areas is greater on a long backboard than on vacuum-type mattresses. Pain in these areas may become severe if patients are left immobilized on these boards for extended periods of time.[14,50,51] In addition, pain caused by the application of a backboard may be difficult to separate from other sources of pain in the trauma patient and might lead to unnecessary and costly radiographs.[4] Discomfort may be minimized by using padding at points of contact between a bony prominence and the board. This concept was reaffirmed by Hauswald and colleagues,[52] who found that increasing the amount of padding on a backboard decreased the amount of ischemic pain caused by immobilization.

Scoop Stretchers. If an injured person has to be extricated from a tight location, a smooth backboard is probably the best device to immobilize and move the victim. If the

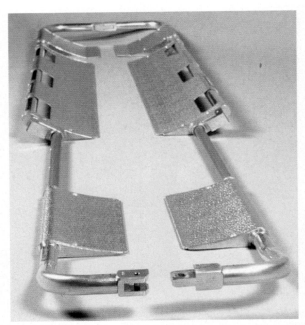

Figure 46–14 The Ferno-Washington model 65 orthopaedic (scoop) stretcher. *(Courtesy of Ferno-Washington, Inc., Wilmington, OH.)*

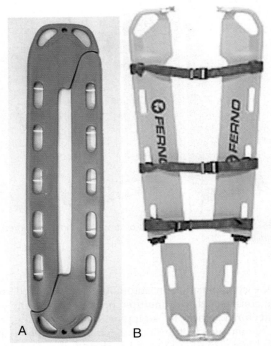

Figure 46–15 *A,* CombiCarrier. *B,* Scoop EXL. (A, *Courtesy of Hartwell Medical, Carlsbad, CA.; B, courtesy of Ferno-Washington, Inc., Wilmington, OH.)*

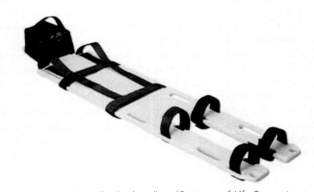

Figure 46–16 The Miller body splint. *(Courtesy of Life Support Products, Inc., Irvine, CA.)*

victim is not in a tight location, the scoop stretcher is an ideal field immobilizer (Fig. 46–14). The scoop stretcher is designed to split into two or four pieces. It is comfortable, rigid, and adaptable to patients of various lengths and provides unobstructed radiographic transparency of the entire spine. If necessary, it can be almost instantly applied or removed without disturbing the position of the victim. The scoop stretcher also provides good lateral stability owing to the troughlike shape of its top surface, and it is stable enough to be used for carrying. For optimal protection of a potential spinal injury, the spine should be completely immobilized (e.g., cervical collar, lateral supports, and secure strapping) and the scoop stretcher should be placed on a backboard before moving the patient. In addition, the scoop stretcher should be carefully reassembled to avoid trapping clothes, skin, or other objects between interlocking parts.

The scoop interferes slightly with the ischial section of a half-ring traction splint but works well with Sager-type devices. The Ferno-Washington model 65 scoop (Ferno-Washington, Inc., Wilmington, OH) is the most widely used stretcher of this type. Other devices such as the CombiCarrier (Hartwell Medical, Carlsbad, CA) and the Scoop EXL (Ferno-Washington, Inc., Wilmington, OH) offer lightweight polymer construction and additional spine support (Fig. 46–15).

Full-Body Splints. Various devices take the concept of full-body immobilization one step further than the spine board. One popular device is the Miller body splint, which consists of a polyethylene shell injected with closed-cell foam that is radiographically translucent and provides buoyancy in water (Fig. 46–16). This full-body splint features a removable head harness and a thoracic harness, as well as pelvic and lower extremity belts. The space between the lower extremities facilitates wrapping with bandage material in the event of fractures. In addition, it is shaped so that it can easily fit into a basket-type rescue stretcher. Similar spine immobilization systems are available for pediatric patients (e.g., Pedi-Pac, Ferno-Washington, Inc., Wilmington, OH).

An important innovation in the area of spine immobilization in the United States has been the vacuum mattress splint (e.g., EVAC-U-Splint Hartwell Medical, Carlsbad, CA, and Immobile-VAC MDI, Gurnee, IL) (see Fig. 46–10). It consists of a vinyl-coated polyester envelope filled with thousands of 1.1-mm-diameter polyester foam spheres. A manual or electric vacuum pump is used to evacuate the interior to a pressure of about 0.25 atm. This reduction in internal pressure causes the mattress to conform to the contours of the patient's body. Vacuum splints have been shown to produce lower sacral interface pressure and lower mean pain scores than traditional hard backboards,[49,53] and may provide better immobilization in patients with known spinal cord injuries.[54,55] It should also be pointed out, however, that vacuum splints are larger and more cumbersome than backboards, making ambulance storage more difficult.

Lateral Neck Stabilizers. Lightweight objects such as blocks (10 × 10 × 15 cm) made of medium-density foam rubber are commonly used. Foam blocks are inexpensive and disposable and do not slip on the backboard. Disposable cardboard devices that have the same advantages as foam blocks are also available (Fig. 46–17).

Another commercial device is the Universal Head Immobilizer. It is a lateral neck stabilizer designed to quickly and easily fasten the patient's head to a scoop stretcher or spine board (Fig. 46–18). The Universal Head Immobilizer is made of a Herculite nylon and polyethylene foam platform fastened to the stretcher using Velcro straps. The lateral pillows are then attached to the nylon platform by means of large Velcro interfaces.

Procedure

Despite the presence of a field cervical collar, manual in-line cervical stabilization should be continued until the patient is fully immobilized in either a cervical extrication splint or a full-body splint (e.g., a backboard or vacuum stretcher). The immobilization technique used will depend on the patient's position of origin.

Sitting Position

Patients in a sitting position are first immobilized using a short backboard or commercially available cervical extrication

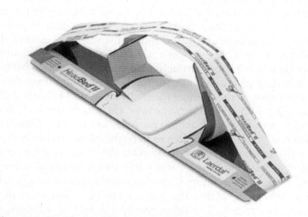

Figure 46–17 The HeadBed, a cervical immobilization device made of a water-resistant corrugated board. *(Courtesy of Laerdal Medical Corporation, Wappingers Falls, NY.)*

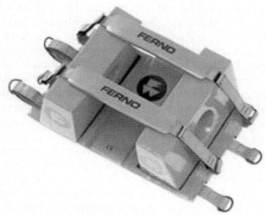

Figure 46–18 Universal Head Immobilizer. *(Courtesy of Ferno-Washington, Inc., Wilmington, OH.)*

device (e.g., KED). When using an extrication splint, it should be stored so that its straps are secured in their individual retainers to reduce their likelihood of becoming entangled during application. At least two rescuers should be present to apply an extrication splint to a sitting patient.

The device is opened, butterfly style, and gently slid behind the victim with a rocking motion. If necessary, the patient can be very carefully rocked forward a few degrees to facilitate placement of the splint.

Once behind the victim, the splint's pelvic support straps should be freed from their retainers and allowed to dangle at the patient's sides. Next, the lateral thoracic panels are brought around the chest just beneath the patient's shoulders. While grasping these panels, a rescuer slides the splint upward until the top edges of the panels firmly engage the patient's axillae.

Now the thoracic straps can be used to secure the splint, beginning with the middle strap, then the bottom strap, and finally the top strap. This procedure may need to be modified depending on injuries and preexisting conditions. For example, patients with pelvic fractures may not tolerate placement of the pelvic support and bottom straps, and the gravid abdomen of the pregnant patient may prevent placement of the middle strap. The straps should be snug, but not so tight as to interfere with respiration.

The pelvic support straps are fastened next. They can be slipped one at a time beneath the patient's lower extremities and brought directly beneath the pelvis using a back-and-forth motion. If the pelvic straps are not applied properly, considerable slippage may occur when the patient is lifted. The free end of each of these straps mates with a buckle located at the patient's hip on the outside of the splint. Once a strap is ready to be buckled, it can be either attached to the buckle on its own side or moved across the patient's lap and engaged with the opposite buckle. Most prehospital care providers prefer the latter method because it allows the patient's knees to remain together without discomfort to the patient. It is also a good idea to pad the groin area when placing the pelvic support straps because these may cause the patient considerable discomfort.

Next, the head is secured to the device. When using the KED, the head panels are wrapped snugly around the head and neck by one rescuer while another rescuer applies the diagonal head straps. It may be necessary to place padding behind the head to maintain a neutral position. The forehead can be used as a point of engagement for one strap and the cervical collar itself can be used for the other.

As the final step, all buckles should be tightened until the entire splint is firmly in place. The patient can now be moved (Fig. 46–19). If the patient is to be lifted from a vehicle, the ambulance cot, with a spine board on it, should be brought as close as possible. While one rescuer supports the patient's knees, the other rescuer uses the handholds on the splint to lift the patient. The patient should be rotated and laid in a supine position onto a backboard.

The pelvic straps should then be loosened to allow the legs to be lowered onto the backboard. The legs can then be extended and secured to the backboard or left in the flexed position with a pillow placed under the knees for support.

A lateral immobilizer should be applied to help prevent movement of the head and neck, and the body should be belted into place on the backboard. Once the patient is on the board, the thoracic straps of the cervical extrication splint may need to be readjusted.

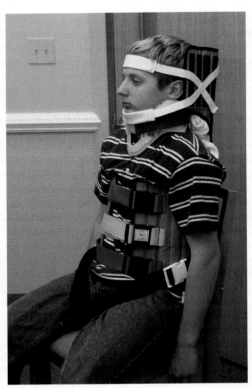

Figure 46–19 The KED. *(Courtesy of AtlantiCare Regional Medical Center: Emergency Medical Services, Atlantic City, NJ.)*

Recumbent Position

A patient who is found in a recumbent position should be placed in a supine position, if not already in one. If repositioning is necessary, the back should be examined in the process. Physical examination, spinal immobilization, airway management, and transport are easier to accomplish with the patient in the supine position.

Patients who are found supine do not require the use of a cervical extrication splint. They should, however, receive initial manual in-line cervical stabilization and an extrication collar. The patient should then be fastened to a full-body spinal immobilizer, such as a scoop stretcher, backboard, or full-body splint.

Scoop Stretcher. A patient who is in a supine position can be moved by means of a scoop stretcher. In the conscious patient, rescuers should explain that they are about to apply a scoop-type stretcher, which may be cold to the touch, beneath the patient's body. An extrication collar is applied, and manual in-line cervical stabilization is maintained until the patient is completely secured to the stretcher. Another rescuer places the scoop on the ground next to the patient and opens the latches that regulate its length. The length should be adjusted so that the scoop stretcher fits the full length of the patient's body. The latches that regulate the length of the device should then be engaged.

Next, the latches at each end should be released, allowing rescuers to separate the stretcher into two halves. Each half is then placed next to the patient. One rescuer then gently pushes half the stretcher under one side of the patient. In some cases, it may be necessary to have another rescuer rock the patient to allow proper positioning. The procedure is repeated with the opposite half of the scoop until both halves are aligned beneath the patient. The latch at the head of the device should be engaged first. The lower end of the stretcher is then brought together and the foot latch is engaged to complete the integrity of the stretcher. The patient's torso should be strapped into place and the head immobilized using a suitable lateral neck stabilizer. The patient can then be lifted onto another device for transport (e.g., Stokes stretcher or backboard). After placement on another device, the scoop stretcher can be removed without disturbing the patient's position, if necessary.

Full-Body Spine Boards (Backboards). There are several ways of placing a patient onto a spine board. The precise technique used will depend on the space available and the position of the patient within that space.

For lengthwise extrication, as from an automobile seat, the patient can be slid, either feet first or head first, onto the backboard. It is important that the patient be moved as a unit during this process.

The end of the backboard should first be placed on the seat or doorsill of the automobile. One rescuer should then stabilize and maintain the backboard level at its opposite end, while other rescuers (at least two) lift and slide the patient's body onto the board. Manual cervical in-line stabilization should be maintained throughout the procedure, and rescuers should avoid spinal compression or traction. Once the patient is completely on the board and secured, the board can be slid out and placed on a waiting stretcher.

When space permits, lateral extraction is preferred. With the patient in the recumbent position, rescuers may logroll or slide the patient onto the board. The *logroll maneuver* requires the presence of at least three rescuers. One rescuer is positioned at the patient's head and applies manual in-line cervical stabilization. It is this person's responsibility to oversee and direct body movement throughout the procedure. The backboard is then positioned next to the body. To minimize thoracolumbar movement, the patient's arms should be extended at the sides with the palms resting on the lateral thighs.[44] To keep the patient from reaching for a rescuer or object during transfer, some rescuers prefer to have the patient cross his or her arms across the thorax. However, this maneuver has not been shown to prevent or minimize thoracolumbar movement. If one arm is injured, the backboard should be placed against this side, so that the patient can be rolled onto the uninjured extremity. The other rescuers should be positioned on the side that the patient will be rolled toward, with one rescuer at the midchest and the other at the legs. The rescuer at the chest should reach across the victim, taking hold of the shoulder and hips, while the other rescuer grasps the hips and lower legs. When everyone is ready, the rescuer at the head gives the command to roll the patient. The patient's back should be examined at this point. The backboard is then slid under the patient, and when everyone is ready, the rescuer at the head gives the command to lower the patient onto the board (Fig. 46–20). The patient should then be centered and securely strapped to the board. Alternatively, during lateral extraction, a recumbent patient can be slid sideways onto the spine board. This improvised technique also requires the presence of three or four rescuers, one of whom can maintain control of the patient's head and neck.

Various techniques can be used to secure a patient to the backboard. In addition to the standard thoracic, pelvic, and lower extremity straps, the use of an abdominal strap significantly reduces lateral motion without compromising respiration.[56] In addition, proper strap placement and firm contact between the straps and the patient are also important in limiting lateral motion.[57]

After the body has been strapped to the board, the head can be secured. If necessary, padding should be placed under the occiput to maintain the head in neutral position. A lateral neck stabilizer (e.g., foam blocks, HeadBed device) is then applied and the head secured in place using tape or straps. Most taping techniques involve the use of one piece across the forehead and one piece across the cervical collar. Note that this method of securing a patient to a backboard is designed for horizontal lifting only.

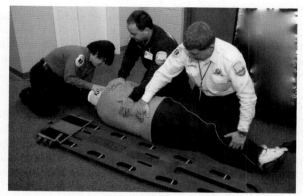

Figure 46–20 Logroll maneuver. *(Courtesy of AtlantiCare Regional Medical Center: Emergency Medical Services, Atlantic City, NJ.)*

Standing Position

The standing patient with a potential spine injury must be immobilized and placed in the supine position. One technique for placing these patients on a backboard that is quick, safe, and effective is presented here (Fig. 46–21).[58] The tallest rescuer should be positioned behind the patient to manually stabilize the head while a second rescuer applies an extrication collar. The first rescuer must maintain manual in-line cervical stabilization until the patient is completely secured to the board. The backboard should be centered behind the patient between the arms of the rescuer who is stabilizing the head and neck. Facing the patient, a rescuer on each side reaches under the patient's arms and grabs the backboard by a hand-hold at or above the patient's axillae. The patient's elbows are then brought closer to the body. If an additional rescuer is available, this rescuer should be positioned at the feet to prevent the board from sliding out. The patient should be slowly tilted back by lowering the head of the backboard. The rescuer at the head should step back during this process while maintaining the patient's head and neck in neutral alignment. When the backboard is completely horizontal, the patient can be secured to the backboard in the normal fashion.

Complications

In general, complications are more likely to occur as a result of failure to immobilize spinal injuries before movement than

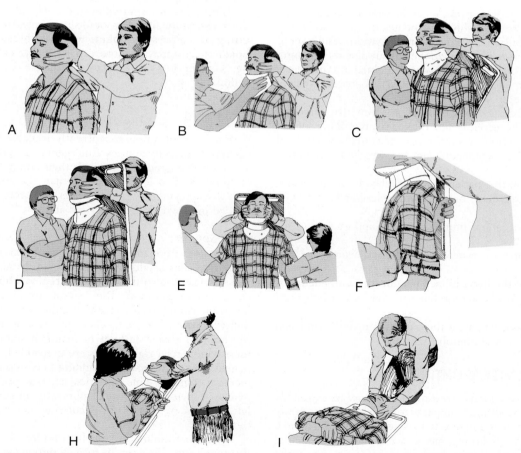

Figure 46–21 Backboarding the standing patient. *A,* Step 1: Manual stabilization. *B,* Step 2: Apply a rigid collar. *C,* Step 3: Insert a long backboard. *D,* Step 4: Center the backboard. *E,* Step 5: Emergency medical technicians grasp the board, using a handle higher than the patient's armpit (*F*). *G,* Step 6: Slowly lower the patient. *H,* Step 7: Fully immobilize the torso, then the head and neck. (*A–H, From Elling R, Politis J: Backboarding the standing patient. JEMS 12:9, 1987. Reproduced with permission.*)

from the technique of immobilization. When complications do arise, they may be related to improper choice or use of equipment.

Victims are generally strapped in place on a spine board to prevent sliding during transport. If too few straps are used or if the straps are loosely applied, motion during transport can occur. Patients who are strapped too firmly in place may complain of extreme discomfort and even panic. Excessive strapping can interfere with respiratory function in both children and adults.[59,60] Totten and Sugarman[61] evaluated the effect of two spinal immobilization methods (wooden backboard and vacuum mattress) on eight respiratory function measurements in healthy volunteers. In comparing baselines for each method, six of the eight measures (forced vital capacity [FVC], FVC%, forced expiratory volume in 1 sec [FEV_1], FEV_1%, peak expiratory flow [PEF], and forced expiratory flow [FEF_{25}%–FEF_{75}%]) showed respiratory function to be restricted an average of 15%. Whereas this may not be a problem in healthy volunteers, the effects on patients with chest trauma or preexisting respiratory disease may be significant.[61]

Once strapped into place, a patient who vomits should be protected from aspiration. The traditional means is to logroll the board and patient as a unit to the side. Although this procedure may be associated with some spinal movement, airway protection takes precedent.

Conclusion

The wide variety of circumstances in which a traumatized patient is likely to be involved mandates the need for many approaches to full-body spinal immobilization. The overall goal of rescuers is to immobilize the entire spine by fastening the victim to a boardlike full-body immobilizer. After early application of an effective cervical collar, this process involves the following steps:

1. Application of a cervical extrication splint that serves to immobilize the cervical and thoracic spine. This sort of device is often used when the patient is first encountered in a confined environment, such as a wrecked automobile or bathtub.
2. Placement of the patient on a full-body spine board, a scoop stretcher, or a factory-designed full-body immobilizer.
3. Application of lateral immobilization support devices for the head.
4. Use of straps to fasten the patient securely to the backboard.
5. Placement of the immobilized patient into a rescue litter, such as a Stokes basket stretcher, if complex terrain must be traversed.
6. Frequent reassessment of the patient's medical condition and effectiveness of immobilization.

UPPER EXTREMITY SPLINTING

Fractures and dislocations of the upper extremity are extremely common injuries. Although upper extremity injuries are rarely life-threatening, it is important to assess and manage these injuries properly. Splinting has constituted a fundamental component of orthopaedic care since 2500 BC, when the Egyptians used palm fibers and reed bundles to immobilize injured extremities.[62] In addition to decreasing pain, appropriate splinting of a minor fracture or dislocation reduces the incidence of serious complications and the risk of permanent disability.

The rescuer must not let obvious injuries to the extremities be a distraction to the care of more life-threatening injuries. In some situations, it may be necessary to rapidly secure the patient to a long backboard that supports and splints every bone and joint of the body in one efficient step.[42] Injuries to nerves or blood vessels are a frequent complication of upper extremity trauma. Circulation, motor function, and sensation distal to the injury must be assessed early and monitored continuously.

The purpose of splinting is to prevent motion of broken or dislocated bone ends. Carefully applied splints decrease pain while minimizing further damage to muscles, nerves, and blood vessels. Splinting also reduces the risk of converting a closed injury to an open one.[63]

Indications and Contraindications

Indications for splinting an extremity are usually clear. Pain with or without deformity after trauma should arouse suspicion for underlying bone or joint injury. Other signs include swelling, discoloration, deformity, crepitus, or loss of neurovascular function. However, the absence of these findings does not rule out an underlying fracture or dislocation. Whenever a musculoskeletal injury is suspected, a prophylactic splint should be applied and maintained. The old axiom, "if in doubt, splint," should be followed.

There are no contraindications to splinting suspected upper extremity fractures or dislocations. However, in the setting of multisystem trauma with life-threatening injuries, rapid transport may be more important than extremity splinting. Averting loss of life takes precedence over averting loss of limb.

Equipment

Various types of splints are currently available for immobilizing upper extremity injuries. Emergency care providers should be well trained and familiar with their equipment. The type of splint used is less important than the expertise of the provider applying the splint. Upper extremity splints can be divided into two basic types: rigid and soft.[42]

Rigid Splints

Rigid splints are made of many different materials, including cardboard, plastic, aluminum, wire, and wood. These splints must be fastened to the injured extremity using tape, gauze, cravats, or Velcro straps. Rigid splints are generally nonflexible (some commercially available splints may have some flexibility in their design) and, when applied properly, immobilize the limb in a rigid fashion to maintain stability. Although most commercial rigid splints are prepadded, many will still benefit from additional soft padding to cushion the splint and increase comfort. This is particularly true over bony prominences. When applying rigid splints, the fingertips should be left exposed so that distal circulation can be continuously monitored.

Cardboard splints are excellent for long bone fractures of the upper arm. They can be formed into many shapes and are easy to apply, inexpensive, lightweight, radiolucent, and magnetic resonance imaging (MRI) compatible. Splints made

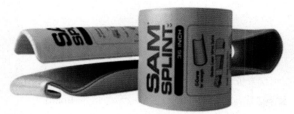

Figure 46–22 SAM splint. *(Courtesy of SAM Medical Products, Portland, OR.)*

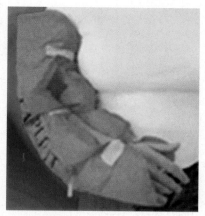

Figure 46–24 Upper extremity vacuum splint. *(Courtesy of Hartwell Medical, Carlsbad, CA.)*

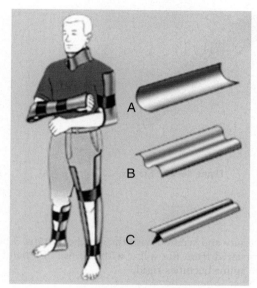

Figure 46–23 Bent into any of three simple curves (A, B, and C in the figure), the SAM splint provides support for any fractured or injured extremity. *(Courtesy of SAM Medical Products, Portland, OR.)*

from wax-impregnated cardboard are also water resistant. Plastic, aluminum, wire, and wood splints, although less malleable, are also good choices. An inexpensive aluminum splint that is popular with emergency care providers and can be found in many wilderness medical kits is the SAM SPLINT (Sam Medical Products, Portland, OR) (Fig. 46–22). The SAM SPLINT is built from a thin core of soft aluminum alloy sandwiched between two layers of closed-cell foam. The SAM SPLINT is extremely pliable. Bent into any of three simple curves, it is extremely strong and provides support for any fractured or injured extremity (Fig. 46–23). In addition, it is water resistant, lightweight, radiolucent, reusable, and not affected by extreme temperatures or altitudes. These characteristics make it an ideal tool for emergency care providers and outdoor enthusiasts.

Vacuum splints (Fig. 46–24) are a special type of rigid splint in which the air is evacuated from a closed bag containing tiny foam beads. This compresses the contents into a solid mass, resulting in a rigid splint. Injuries can be encased and immobilized in the position in which they are found, thereby reducing patient discomfort. Flexibility of the splint before removal of air allows molding of the splint to conform to the patient's position. Vacuum splints are radiolucent and do not apply external pressure, ensuring maximum circulation to the injured extremity.

Soft Splints

Soft splints include air splints, pillows, slings, and swaths. Immobilization with pillows, slings, or swaths alone is usually inadequate because these splints allow significant flexibility and motion. Therefore, they are most effective when used with some form of a rigid device.

Air splints are soft splints that become rigid when inflated. Besides providing immobilization, they help compress underlying soft tissue to reduce local hemorrhage. These devices are sensitive to differences in atmospheric pressure and temperature. Therefore, their inflation must be constantly monitored to ensure that the underlying tissue is not subject to pressure-induced ischemia and the development of a compartment syndrome. One study suggests a maximum splint pressure of 15 mm Hg to reduce the risk of ischemia.[64] With long ambulance transports, the splint should be deflated for 5 minutes every 1.5 hours.[65] Disadvantages include the inability (with most air splints) to continuously monitor pulses once the air splint is in place and the susceptibility of air splint chambers to puncture. Air splints are designed to conform to a specific shape when inflated and should not be used on angulated fractures. In addition to being radiolucent, some types can be inflated with a refrigerant to provide concurrent cooling.

Pillow splints (Fig. 46–25) can be fashioned from any soft bulky material and are excellent choices for hand or wrist injuries. These splints are extremely comfortable and can be easily applied.

Slings and swaths are usually used in combination with a rigid or a soft splint. When used alone, they can effectively immobilize injuries to the shoulder, clavicle, or humerus.

Procedures

To properly apply a splint to an injured extremity, several general rules must be followed. Communication is important to ensure that the patient understands what is being done at all times. When possible, administration of an appropriate analgesic will make splint application less painful. Any unnecessary clothing should be removed to adequately visualize the injured extremity. Manual stabilization of the fracture site helps limit unnecessary movement and prevent further injury. The neurovascular status (i.e., pulse, motor, and sensation) should be checked before and after the application of a splint.

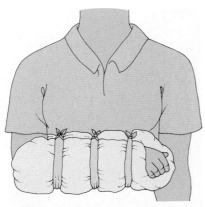

Figure 46–25 Hand/wrist pillow splint.

TABLE 46–2 Management of Specific Upper Extremity Orthopaedic Injuries

Site	Suggested Immobilization Techniques
Clavicle	Sling and swath
Shoulder	Sling and swath as it lies
Humerus	Cardboard or vacuum splint with sling and swath
Elbow	Cardboard or vacuum splint as it lies
Forearm	Cardboard, malleable metal, air, or vacuum splint with sling and swath
Wrist	Pillow, cardboard, malleable metal, or vacuum splint applied in position of presentation
Hand	Pillow, cardboard, or malleable metal splint in position of function
Finger	Tongue depressor or small malleable metal splint

A severely angulated extremity with neurovascular compromise may be reduced with gentile longitudinal traction (not exceeding 10 lb of pressure) to reduce the deformity before splinting. Only one attempt should be made at fracture reduction. If resistance or pain is encountered, the extremity should be splinted in the position found. Open wounds should be covered with a dry sterile dressing before a splint is applied. The splint (Table 46–2) should be applied using the orthopaedic principle of immobilizing the joint above and below a suspected fracture site. Cooling and elevation of the injured area may help reduce local swelling and pain. Once the splint has been applied, the distal neurovascular status should be assessed frequently. Any deterioration requires immediate evaluation of the splint to determine whether excess pressure is being applied. In addition, providers should frequently assess and treat pain.

Rigid Splints

To apply a rigid splint, an assistant should provide support and gentle traction above and below the injury. The splint is then applied on the side of the extremity away from any open wounds. The splint should be large enough to immobilize the joint above and below a fracture or the bone above and below a dislocation and be well padded to reduce the risk of pressure necrosis. The splint is then secured to the extremity using gauze, tape, cravats, or Velcro straps (Fig. 46–26).

Vacuum splints are applied in much the same manner as other rigid splints. While an assistant stabilizes the injured site and applies traction, the splint should be wrapped around

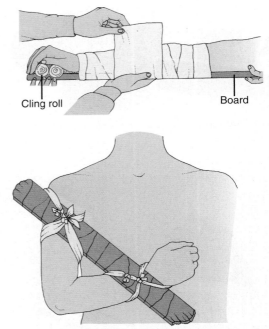

Figure 46–26 Examples of rigid splints.

the extremity and secured with the attached straps. The air is then evacuated from the splint with the use of a hand pump until the splint becomes rigid.

Soft Splints

The application procedure for an air splint depends on whether the splint is equipped with a zipper. If the splint does not have a zipper, it must first be placed on the rescuer's arm until the bottom edge lies above the wrist. Next, the rescuer grasps the hand of the patient's injured extremity while the free hand is used to provide support and gentle traction above the injury (Fig. 46–27A). An assistant should then slide the splint onto the patient's arm (see Fig. 46–27B). After making sure that the splint is not wrinkled, it should be inflated until finger pressure makes a slight dent (see Fig. 46–27C). Zippered air splints should be opened and placed around the injured area. The zipper should be closed and inflation accomplished as described previously. With air splints that completely enclose the hand, distal circulation must be continuously assessed by checking fingertip color, temperature, and capillary refill.

Pillow splints are applied by encasing the injury in the pillow and securing with tape, cravats, or gauze (see Fig. 46–25). If possible, the nailbeds should remain exposed to allow for frequent neurovascular checks.

To apply a sling, an assistant should support the injured arm in a flexed position across the patient's chest. The long edge of the triangular bandage should then be placed lengthwise along the patient's side opposite the injury, with its tip over the uninjured shoulder (Fig. 46–28). The other tip is then brought over the injured shoulder to enclose the arm in the sling. The sling should be adjusted so that the arm rests comfortably with the hand higher than the elbow. The sling is then tied together at the side of the neck, and the knot is padded for patient comfort. The point of the sling at the elbow should be drawn around to the front and pinned. With

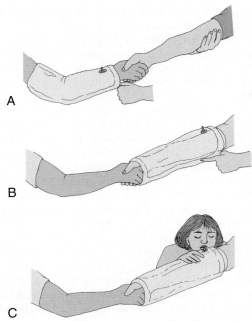

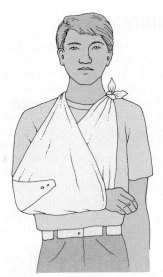

Figure 46–29 Completed triangular bandage.

Figure 46–27 **Application of an air splint.** *A,* The rescuer supports the injured extremity with one hand and places the air splint on the other arm. *B,* An assistant slides the splint onto the patient's arm. *C,* The air splint is inflated until finger pressure makes a slight dent.

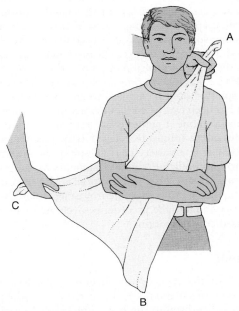

Figure 46–28 Stepwise application of a triangular bandage. *1,* Place tip A over the uninjured shoulder. *2,* Bring tip B over the injured shoulder to enclose the arm. *3,* Draw tip C around the front and pin.

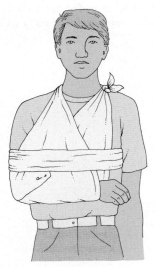

Figure 46–30 Sling with swath.

Complications

Potential complications of upper extremity splinting include pressure necrosis, conversion of a closed injury into an open one, and loss of neurovascular function. With the use of air splints, there is the additional risk of pressure-induced tissue ischemia and compartment syndrome.[66]

Conclusion

Injuries to the upper extremities, although not life-threatening, may be limb-threatening and can have significant immediate or long-term effects. A high index of suspicion for underlying neurovascular injury should always be maintained. Neurovascular status must be checked before and after application of splints and monitored frequently throughout transport. When possible, administration of an appropriate analgesia will be greatly appreciated by the patient.

the sling properly applied, the patient's arm rests comfortably against the chest with the fingertips exposed (Fig. 46–29).

To apply a swath, a cravat of sufficient length should be placed under the uninjured arm and over the injured arm at the level of the midhumerus. This should then be fastened circumferentially around the thorax so that the injured extremity is secured snugly to the chest (Fig. 46–30). In adults, two cravats may have to be tied together in an end-to-end fashion to produce a swath of sufficient length.

LOWER EXTREMITY SPLINTING

Injuries to the lower extremities, including sprains, fractures, and dislocations, are also commonly encountered by prehospital care providers. As with upper extremity injuries, the application of a splint is an essential part of the prehospital management of lower extremity injuries. Many of the principles, techniques, and complications discussed with upper extremity splinting also apply to injuries of the lower extremity; the SAM SPLINT (see Fig. 46–23) and pillow splint (Fig. 46–31) are just two examples. Table 46–3 provides recommendations for immobilizing a variety of lower extremity injuries. One fundamental difference between splinting upper extremity injuries and lower extremity injuries is the use of the traction splint in the management of femur fractures. The remainder of this section focuses on the use of traction splints.

Traction splints are a near-universal piece of equipment found on most ambulances and their application is an integral part of the prehospital care provider's skill set. The main purpose of the traction splint is to immobilize a fractured femur. In addition, application of a traction splint helps align fracture fragments, control spasm, minimize blood loss, reduce pain, prevent further damage to neurovascular structures, and lower the incidence of clinical fat embolism.[67]

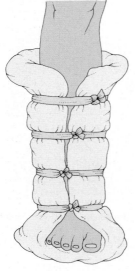

Figure 46–31 Lower leg pillow splint.

TABLE 46–3 Management of Specific Lower Extremity Orthopaedic Injuries

Site	Suggested Immobilization Techniques
Pelvis	PASG, long backboard
Hip	Traction splint and long backboard, or secure injured leg to uninjured leg
	Long backboard with limb supported by pillows
Femur	Traction splint or PASG
Knee	Cardboard or vacuum splint in position found
Tibia/fibula	Cardboard, air, or vacuum splint
Ankle	Pillow or air splint
Foot	Pillow or air splint
Toe	Tape to adjacent toe

PASG, pneumatic antishock garment.

The use of traction and countertraction for the alignment and reduction of fractures dates from the time of Hippocrates.[69] In the late 1800s, Sir Hugh Owen Thomas developed the first full-ring traction splint for the definitive management of fractured femurs.[69] Because the Thomas full-ring splint was not an emergency treatment device, it was later modified by his nephew, Sir Robert Jones, and other surgeons to a half-ring splint that made it easier to apply in the field. During World War I, the modified splint was credited with reducing the mortality rate associated with fractured femurs from 80% to 15%.[70] Since then, several additional modifications that carry the name of their inventors (e.g., Glenn Hare, Joseph Sager, Allen Klippel) have furthered the development of lower extremity traction splints.

In the setting of a fractured femur, muscle spasm and fragment overlap may cause the thigh to lose its cylindrical shape and adopt a more spherical appearance.[69] The resultant decreased tissue pressure and increased volume may allow 1 to 2 L of blood to accumulate at the fracture site. Traction splints are designed to align fracture segments and restore the cylindrical shape of the thigh. This in turn increases tissue pressure, decreases the potential space for blood loss, and inhibits further hemorrhage.

Indications and Contraindications

Application of a lower extremity traction splint is indicated whenever a fractured femur is suspected.[42,71,72] This should be clinically suspected if there is pain associated with shortening, angulation, crepitus, swelling, or ecchymosis of the thigh.

Traction splints should not be used in patients with pelvic fractures, hip injuries with gross displacement, any significant injury to the knee, or avulsion or amputation of the ankle and foot.[72] There has been some controversy over whether a traction splint should be applied to an open femur fracture. Concern has been expressed that the use of traction may allow contaminated bone fragments to retract into the wound. Should this occur, it must be relayed to the receiving clinician. As an alternative, a variety of rigid splints or the PASG can be used to immobilize the bony fragments in the position of presentation. In any case, stabilization of the fracture site to prevent further hemorrhage, neurovascular damage, or soft tissue injury should take precedence over the theoretical risk of increased contamination.

Equipment

Regardless of the type or manufacturer, the basic traction splint consists of a metal frame that extends from the proximal thigh to an area distal to the heel. The padded proximal end fits against the ischial tuberosity and serves as the anatomic fixation point. The proximal portion of the splint may be a ring that encircles the proximal thigh, a partial ring, or a padded bar. At the distal end of the splint is typically a ratchet-type device that when engaged, creates traction on the distal femur. All traction splints also have several soft elastic straps that support the thigh and leg.[72]

Currently, a variety of lower extremity traction splints are commercially available (e.g., Hare Traction Splint, Ferno-Trac, Sager Emergency Traction Splints, Kendrick Traction Device [KTD]), each with its own advantages, disadvantages, and unique method of application. For example, traction splints that utilize a half-ring design apply countertraction to the ischial tuberosity from below the shaft of the femur. This produces flexion at the hip joint of up to 30° and will not allow complete fracture alignment unless the patient is in a reclining position about 30° from horizontal or the injured extremity is elevated to create the same angle. Traction splints that do not use a half ring do not cause hip flexion.

Procedure

Application of the FernoTrac Traction Splint (Ferno-Washington, Wilmington, OH) and the Sager Emergency Traction Splint (Minto Research and Development, Redding, CA) are illustrated in Figures 46–32 and 46–33, respectively.

When possible, the splinting procedure should be explained to the patient. Pain is always associated with the application of a traction splint, and every effort should be made to provide appropriate analgesia (e.g., parenteral opiates) before splint application. In addition, the patient should be reassured that while the initial application of traction is often quite painful, stabilization of the fracture site will help reduce subsequent discomfort. The area of injury should be exposed, and the patient's shoe and sock should be removed to assess distal neurovascular status before and after splint application. Open fractures should be managed as discussed previously. If the injured leg is markedly deformed, an assistant should first attempt to straighten it using manual traction and maintain that position until a splint has been applied. The amount of traction necessary to straighten a badly deformed extremity will vary, but rarely exceeds 15 pounds. If the patient strongly resists while traction is being applied, the emergency care provider should stop and splint the injured extremity in the position it was found.

If the splint has an adjustable bar, the appropriate length should be determined by measuring the uninjured leg. The splint should extend beyond the ankle by approximately 6 inches (15 cm). With the extremity slightly elevated, the traction splint (e.g., FernoTrac Traction Splint) is placed under the injured leg and brought to rest firmly against the ischial tuberosity. The heel stand should be unfolded and locked in place to support the end of the splint. This will ensure that the injured extremity will remain elevated once manual traction has been released. Sager Emergency Traction Splints should be placed either against the symphysis pubis or positioned laterally against the greater trochanter of the femur. When the padded end of a Sager Emergency Traction Splint is placed in the groin, one should ensure that the genitalia are carefully protected. Once the splint is properly positioned, the thigh strap should be firmly secured.

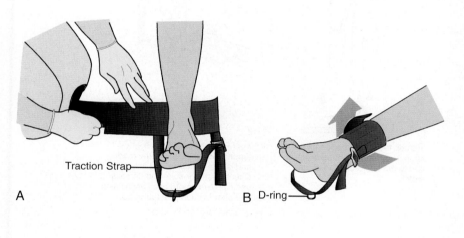

Traction Strap

A

B D-ring

Figure 46–32 Application of the Ferno traction splint. *A* and *B,* Applying the ankle wrap. *C–E,* Applying the splint. *(A–E, Reproduced and modified with permission. Ferno-Washington, Inc., Wilmington, OH.)*

C

D

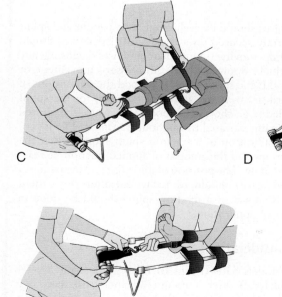

E

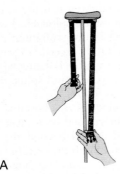

A

Before applying the splint to the leg, slide the Kydex plastic buckle so that when it is closed, it will be located on the anterior (top) surface of the thigh.

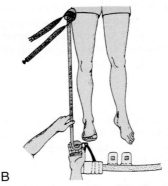

B

Prior to application of the splint, get a rough measure of length of splint needed. Extend the splint so that the wheel is at the heel. NOTE: Patients wearing tight jeans or underclothing, especially males, will find the splint uncomfortable to wear unless clothing is removed or cut open, which, of course, should be done as part of patient secondary evaluation prior to application of splint.

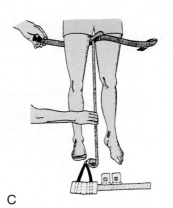

C

Grasp the Kydex buckle and slide the thigh strap up under the leg so that the perineal cushion is snug against the perineum and ischial tuberosity.

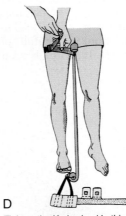

D

Tighten the Kydex buckle thigh strap, drawing the perineal-ischial pad to the lateral portion of the crotch.

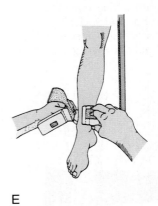

E

Apply the ankle harness tightly around the ankle above the medial and lateral maleoli of the ankle. Check posterior tibial and dorsalis pedis pulses before hitch application and after traction is established.

Figure 46–33 Application of the Sager emergency traction splint. *A–J,* Standard application.

A harness is then placed around the ankle immediately above the medial and lateral malleoli and attached to the distal end of the traction splint. FernoTrac and other similar traction splint devices use a ratchet mechanism to apply constant (static) traction to the ankle strap. For Sager-type devices, the inner shaft of the splint is gently extended until the desired amount of traction is achieved. The traction handle/scale enables providers to set and document the traction force applied. Sager Emergency Traction Splints are unique in that they provide gentile, quantifiable traction that is dynamic in nature. The dynamic function permits the traction to decrease automatically as the muscle spasm decreases and the leg length increases.[69] Regardless of which splint is being used, traction is applied gradually to approximately 10% of body weight or a maximum of 15 pounds. Only rarely will more traction be required.[71,72] The goal is to stabilize the fracture and maintain proper limb alignment; the least amount of force needed to accomplish this should be used.[73]

Before moving the patient, supportive straps are applied around the thigh, knee, and distal leg to vertically stabilize the extremity. After application of the splint, the distal neurovascular status should be rechecked. The patient and splint should be firmly secured on a backboard. Extra care should be taken while moving the patient and when closing any transport vehicle door to avoid unnecessary movement or further injury. If the splint extends beyond the dimensions of the backboard or stretcher, additional support for the splint may be needed (e.g., short spine board) to ensure the injured extremity remains elevated throughout transport. The loss of pulses with application of a traction splint requires that the position of straps and the amount of applied traction be reassessed immediately. The position of the splint and the patient's neurovascular status should be rechecked after any patient movement. Removal of a traction splint should be done in reverse order of application.

Special Considerations

The Sager Models S304 (Form III Bilateral) and the SX404 (Extreme Bilateral) offer a unique advantage in that they can be used to immobilize both legs simultaneously using only one splint (see Fig. 46–33). In addition, neither splint

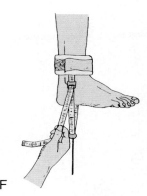

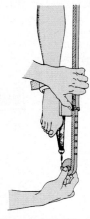

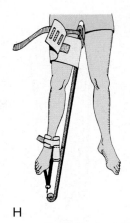

F

Shorten the loop of the harness connected to the cable ring by pulling on the strap threaded through the square "D" buckle.

G

Extend the inner shaft of the splint by opening the shaft lock and pulling the inner shaft out until the desired amount of traction is noted on the calibrated wheel. Rough guide to determine amount of traction needed: apply 10% of body weight to maximum of 22–25 pounds (10 to 12 kilograms) traction.

H

Apply the longest 6-inch wide thigh strap as high up the thigh as possible.

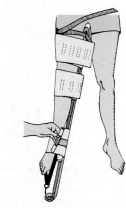

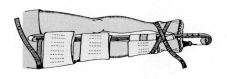

I

Apply the second longest thigh strap around the knee. Use padding as needed. Next, apply the shortest 6-inch wide strap over the ankle harness and lower the leg.

J

Apply figure-eight strap around both ankles. Patient's leg is now secured, traction is controlled, medial and lateral shift of distal fragment and internal and external rotation is prevented. Patient is ready for strapping to spine board for transport.

Figure 46–33, cont'd

Continued

831

extends beyond the patient's heels, making them ideal for use in helicopters, fixed-wing aircraft, and smaller van-type ambulances.

The use of traction splints in general is not recommended in the presence of an associated distal tibia-fibula or ankle fracture in the same extremity. In these circumstances, the amount of traction required to realign the fractured femur can distract the distal fracture site. A variety of rigid or soft splints or the PASG may be considered in these settings.

Complications

Complications are generally the result of incorrect application and include pain, ongoing hemorrhage, peroneal nerve injury, perineal injury, movement at the fracture site, or further neurovascular compromise. Once the fracture site is stabi-

lized, additional traction is unnecessary and potentially dangerous.

PELVIC SPLINTING

Pelvic fractures present a unique clinical challenge to prehospital care providers. These injuries can be immediately life-threatening and are associated with significant morbidity and mortality.[74] However, even the most experienced prehospital provider may find it extremely difficult to identify pelvic injuries in the field (the exception being an open-book fracture). Early stabilization of fracture segments and hemorrhage control are the keys to effective prehospital management of these injuries.

Several methods exist for stabilizing pelvic fractures in the prehospital setting including pelvic sheeting, pelvic cir-

APPLICATION ON THE OUTSIDE OF THE LEG

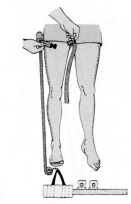 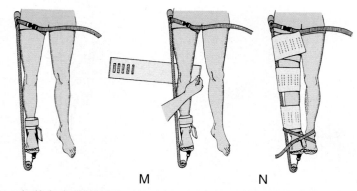

K

Application of Sager Splint on the outside of thigh is appropriate if perineal injuries or pelvic fractures are encountered. Carry out steps 1 and 2, then apply the splint on the outside of the leg as noted.

L

Leave the Kydex buckle thigh strap loose so that it makes a sling around the upper thigh and forms an angle of about 55 degrees with the shaft of the splint. Pad the strap as needed.

M

Apply the thigh straps in sequence, adding figure-eight strap as last strep prior to securing the patient on the sping board.

N

APPLICATION OF THE BILATERAL SPLINT

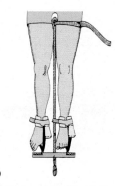 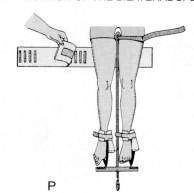 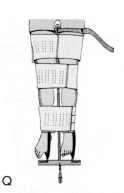

O

Application of double splint is accomplished in same manner as with the single splint. Modify step 2 by lengthening splint so that the harness bar is adjacent to the patient's heels.

P

Apply the 6-inch wide thigh straps, hooking together more than one strap to give you a proper length to wrap strap around both thighs.

Q

Apply all three sections of leg strapping to secure the legs together. A figure-eight strap may be used around ankles and feet, if needed.

Figure 46–33, cont'd

cumferential compression devices such as the SAM Sling (Fig. 46–34), vacuum "beanbag" mattress splints, and the PASG. However, with the advent of commercial pelvic binders, and its well-documented list of complications and disadvantages, application of the PASG (Table 46–4) for pelvic fracture stabilization has fallen out of favor among most prehospital care providers. Pelvic binders are designed for quick and easy application in the field or ED. They are easy to maintain, reusable, and sized to fit 95% of the adult population. The pelvic binder acts similarly to the bed sheet and, when placed properly (over the area of the greater trochanters), provides a safe and effective force to stabilize pelvic fractures.[74,75] Application of the SAM Sling is illustrated in Figure 46–35.

Conclusion

A properly applied traction splint will limit pain, hemorrhage, and movement associated with femur fractures. Careful monitoring of distal neurovascular status is imperative with the use of these splints. When contraindicated by the presence of

other injuries, most femur fractures can be adequately immobilized with a variety of rigid or soft splints, a vacuum splint/mattress, or a long spine board. For EMS systems that still carry the PASG, isolated femur fractures are one of the few remaining indications for its use. Commercially available pelvic binders (e.g., SAM Sling) are quick and easy to apply and provide safe and effective stabilization for pelvic fractures.

HELMET REMOVAL

Although originally developed for protection of the head during combat, helmets are commonly worn by motorcyclists, athletes (e.g., football, hockey, lacrosse, motor sports), and individuals participating in a host of recreational activities (e.g., cycling, rollerblading, skateboarding). Emergency care providers must therefore be equipped and trained to remove a helmet safely.

Most modern sports helmets consist of a hard polycarbonate shell lined with foam padding, adjustable air cells, or

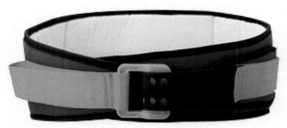

Figure 46–34 The SAM Sling. *(Courtesy of SAM Medical Products, Portland, OR.)*

TABLE 46–4 Complications and Disadvantages of Pneumatic Antishock Garment Application

Hypotension after removal
Metabolic acidosis
Respiratory compromise
Decreased renal perfusion
Other (infrequent) complications
   Pulmonary edema, congestive heart failure
   Compartment syndromes
   Increased wound bleeding
   Urination, defecation, vomiting
   Skin breakdown
   Lumbar spine movement
Mechanical problems and disadvantages
   Limitation of diagnostic and therapeutic procedures
      Physical examination
      Urinary catheterization
      Peritoneal lavage
      Vascular access
   Environmental influences
      Barometric pressure
      Temperature

both. They may be modified with additional padding so that they conform tightly to the individual's head. In addition, helmets used in contact sports (e.g., football, hockey, lacrosse) typically have some type of face mask secured to the front of helmet to provide additional protection for the athlete's eyes and face.

Motorcycle helmets may or may not have a full-face guard, but in either case, motorcycle helmet use has been shown to reduce the incidence of severe head injury and death and is associated with a shorter hospital stay and reduced hospital costs.[68] Although early studies suggested that the use of motorcycle helmets might be associated with an increased incidence of cervical spine injury,[70,76] this concern has not been substantiated.[77–79]

Most of the early research in the area of helmet removal focused on the removal of motorcycle helmets. More recently, the spotlight has turned to football helmet removal because football players commonly sustain head and neck trauma, and their care is frequently complicated by the presence of additional protective equipment.[80]

Helmet removal requires a careful, methodical approach to avoid compounding a possible injury to the spinal cord.[81,82] Fluoroscopic studies have detected spinal motion even in the best of circumstances when removing hockey and football helmets.[82–84] As with all trauma victims, the initial management of the injured athlete is to address the ABCs. However, it is important to note that a proper-fitting sports helmet holds the head securely in a neutral position of alignment,

minimizing any motion, provided that the athlete is also wearing shoulder pads. In this case, removing the face mask but leaving the helmet and shoulder pads in place will allow adequate airway control while maintaining proper alignment of the cervical spine and reducing the risk of further injury.[80,85]

Motorcycle and motor sport helmets do not usually have a removable face mask, do not always properly fit, and are worn without shoulder pads. Thus, in contrast to helmets worn by athletes, motorcycle and motor sport helmets should be routinely removed to achieve proper spinal immobilization.[80]

Indications and Contraindications

For years, the proper management of the spine-injured athlete prompted much debate and disagreement among various health care professionals. In 1998, the National Athletic Trainers' Association formed the Inter-Association Task Force (IATF) For the Appropriate Care of the Spine-Injured Athlete,[86] which in 2001 released a comprehensive set of guidelines and recommendations titled, *Prehospital Care of the Spine-Injured Athlete*. This consensus document outlines the current guidelines for helmet and shoulder pad removal, which include[86]

- If the helmet and chin strap fail to hold the head securely, such that immobilizing the helmet does not also adequately immobilize the head.
- If the helmet and chin strap design prevent adequate airway control or ventilation, even after removal of the face mask.
- If the facemask cannot be removed after a reasonable amount of time.
- If the helmet prevents proper immobilization in an appropriate position for transport.

If the athlete's helmet is not removed, cervical spine immobilization can usually be maintained with a properly fitting helmet by using tape, commercially available foam blocks, and a backboard. If it does become necessary to remove the helmet, the principle of "all or nothing" should apply. That is, the helmet and shoulder pads (if present) should be removed at the same time to avoid hyperextension of the cervical spine.[80,83]

In contrast to athletic helmets, motorcycle and motor sports helmets should be removed in the prehospital setting.[42] Motorcycle helmets with a full-face guard make it very difficult to assess and manage the airway and to evaluate injuries to the head and neck. The helmet's large size and design may cause significant neck flexion if left in place when the patient is placed on a backboard. In addition, the increasing use of head and neck restraint devices (e.g., the HANS device; Fig. 46–36) in professional motor sports has further complicated cervical spine management and helmet removal.

In the ED, stable patients typically undergo imaging studies of the cervical spine before helmet and shoulder pad removal. The National Collegiate Athletic Association and the IATF recommend that the helmet (with the face mask removed) and shoulder pads remain in place until the initial clinical and radiographic evaluation is completed.[86] However, two small studies in healthy volunteers found that the helmet and shoulder pads worn by athletes may interfere with standard cervical spine radiographic evaluation.[87,88] The authors

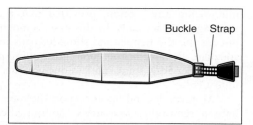

1. Remove objects from patients pocket or pelvic area. Unfold SAM Pelvic Sling with non printed side facing up. *Keep strap attached to buckle.*

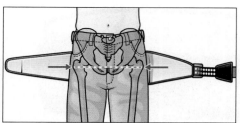

2. Place non printed side of SAM Pelvic Sling beneath patient at level of buttocks (greater trochanters).
CORRECT PLACEMENT. The correct level of application is at the greater trochanters.

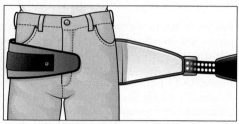

3. Wrap non buckle side of SAM Pelvic Sling around patient.

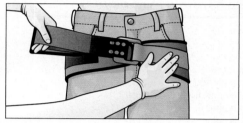

4. FIRMLY WRAP buckle side of sling around patient, positioning buckle in midline. Secure by pressing flap to sling.

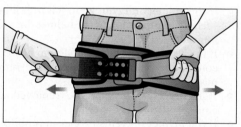

5. Lift the BLACK STRAP away from Sling by pulling upward.

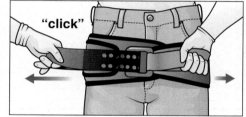

6. With or without assistance firmly pull orange and black straps in opposite directions until you hear and feel the buckle click.
MAINTAIN TENSION!

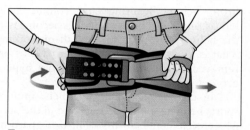

7. IMMEDIATELY press black strap on to surface of SAM Pelvic Sling to secure.
Note: do not be concerned if you hear a second "click" after sling is secured.

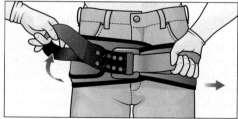

8. To remove lift black strap by pulling upward. Maintain tension and slowly allow SAM Pelvic Sling to loosen.

Figure 46–35 Application of the SAM Sling. *(Courtesy of SAM Medical Products, Portland, OR.)*

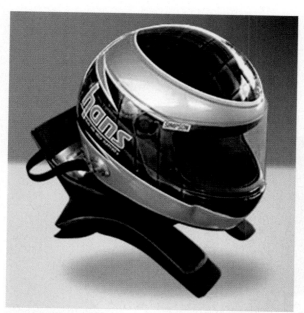

Figure 46–36 The HANS device. *(HANS Performance Products, Atlanta, GA.)*

of these studies recommend incorporating procedures for controlled and cautious removal of equipment before initial radiographic evaluation.[87,88] A study by Wanninger and associates[89] evaluated the use computed tomography (CT) as a viable alternative to cervical spine clearance in the injured helmeted athlete. Although the findings in this small study require further validation, the use of CT for initial triage and diagnosis seems promising.

The only absolute contraindication to helmet removal is neck pain or paresthesias associated with the procedure. Relative contraindications to helmet removal include unfamiliarity with the technique and lack of sufficient assistance.[90]

Procedure

Sports Helmet Removal

Whenever possible, injured athletes with a suspected cervical spine injury should be treated with their equipment (e.g., helmet, chin strap, shoulder pads) left in place to minimize any risk of further cervical spine motion.[82] However, when present, a face mask should be removed at the earliest opportunity, before transportation and despite the absence of any respiratory complaints.[86]

A variety of tools (e.g., FM Extractor, Trainer's Angel, anvil pruner, PVC pipe cutter, or power screwdriver) and techniques are used for face mask removal.[82] All emergency care providers should have tools for face mask removal readily available and be familiar with their use. The choice of equipment is less important than the skill and experience of the personnel using it.[91] The face mask of a football helmet should be completely removed (not retracted) by cutting the four plastic loop straps that secure the face mask to the helmet. Hockey and lacrosse face masks are easily removed by unscrewing the external screws holding them in place. In-line stabilization to keep the head and neck in the neutral position should be maintained during the entire procedure. With practice, the face mask of any helmet can be quickly and safely

removed with minimal risk of extraneous movement of the cervical spin.[85]

The National Athletic Trainers' Association protocol for helmet and shoulder pad removal discussed in this chapter has been shown to effectively limit motion of the cervical spine during equipment removal.[92] Proper removal of a helmet and shoulder pads requires at least two (and preferably three or four) individuals along with in-line stabilization of the cervical spine throughout the procedure.[68,90,93]

One rescuer manually stabilizes the head and neck in the neutral position by placing her or his hands on each side of the helmet, with thumbs pointing up (Fig. 46–37A). A second rescuer then removes the chin strap by cutting or snapping it (see Fig. 46–37B). Next, this rescuer removes the left or right cheek/jaw pads from the helmet by first slipping the flat blade of a screwdriver or bandage scissor between the pad snaps and the helmet's inner surface and twisting slightly. The pads are removed by sliding them out firmly and slowly. The opposite side is then removed in the same manner. Note that some helmets models (e.g., Riddell Revolution) are padded with a number of air-filled bladders that must be deflated (rather than removed) before helmet removal (Fig. 46–38).[94] In this case, the second rescuer deflates the air inflation system by releasing the air at the external ports using the inflation needle that comes with the helmet. Alternatively, an 18-gauge needle or air pump needle may be tried. If an inflation needle is not available (or an 18-gauge needle or air pump needle does not work), the bladders can be directly punctured with an 18-gauge needle.

The second rescuer then takes over in-line immobilization of the head by using one hand to grasp the patient's mandible between the thumb and the first two fingers while placing the other hand under the occiput (see Fig. 46–37C). The first rescuer then places a thumb inside each ear hole of the helmet and curls his or her fingers along the bottom edge of the helmet (see Fig. 46–37D). At this point, some experts recommend easing the helmet off by pulling laterally and longitudinally in line with the head and neck.[93] However, this maneuver may actually tighten the helmet at the occiput and the forehead.[95] The IATF recommends rotating the helmet off the head in a gentle fashion without pulling laterally.[86] The shoulder pads are removed by cutting the straps underneath the arms and the anterior straps holding the pads together (see Fig. 46–37E). If a neck roll or roll restriction pad is present, it should be unfastened from the helmet and shoulder pads before removal.

When possible, the shoulder pads and helmet should be removed simultaneously to prevent the head from falling into extension. If the shoulder pads cannot be removed simultaneously, the head must be stabilized in the neutral position during the procedure. The hands of second rescuer can be moved superiorly as the helmet is being removed so that the thumb and first fingers grasp the maxilla at each side of the nose in the maxillary notch (see Fig. 46–37F).

A cervical collar should be placed after helmet removal, and in-line stabilization maintained. It should be remembered that if the helmet cannot be removed and access to the chest area is required, the anterior half of the shoulder pads can be removed, leaving the posterior portion to maintain cervical position with the helmet in place.

Motorcycle Helmet Removal

For the reasons described earlier, motorcycle helmets should be removed in the prehospital setting. The removal method

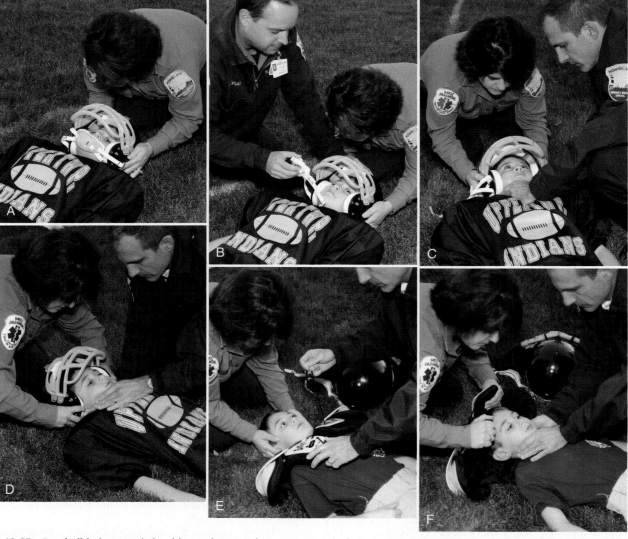

Figure 46–37   Football helmet and shoulder pad removal. Proper removal of a helmet and shoulder pads requires at least two rescuers. *A,* One rescuer manually stabilizes the patient's head and neck in the neutral position by placing his or her hands on each side of the helmet, with thumbs pointing up. *B,* A second rescuer then removes the chinstrap by cutting or snapping it. *C,* The second rescuer then takes over in-line immobilization of the head by using one hand to grasp the patient's mandible between the thumb and the first two fingers while placing the other hand under the occiput. *D,* The first rescuer then places a thumb inside each ear hole of the helmet and curls his or her fingers along the bottom edge of the helmet. Without pulling laterally, the helmet is removed by gently rotating it off the head. *E,* The shoulder pads are removed by cutting the straps underneath the arms and the anterior straps holding the pads together. *F,* The hands of the second rescuer stabilize the head as the shoulder pads are removed. When possible, the helmet (with the facemask removed) and shoulder pads should remain in place until the initial clinical and radiographic evaluation is completed in the ED. *(Note: This figure does not demonstrate removal of the facemask and cheek/jaw pads, which is recommended before helmet removal. See text for details.) (Courtesy of AtlantiCare Regional Medical Center: Emergency Medical Services, Atlantic City, NJ.)*

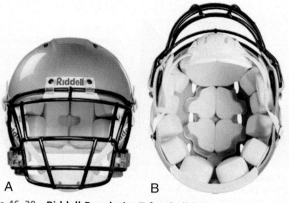

Figure 46–38 Riddell RevolutionT football helmet. These helmets are padded with a number of air-filled bladders that must be deflated (rather than removed) before helmet removal. *A,* Frontal view. *B,* Inside view. See text for details. *(A and B, Courtesy of Riddell, Elyria, OH.)*

endorsed by the American College of Surgeons in 1997 is the method most often used (Fig. 46–39).[96] Providers should be aware that unacceptable cervical motion can occur during motorcycle helmet removal if the shoulders are not properly elevated, and the addition of a folded sheet or jacket placed behind the patient's shoulders may help limit any cervical motion associated with the procedure.[97]

If attempts to remove the helmet results in pain and paresthesias, current Advanced Trauma Life Support guidelines recommend removing the helmet using a technique described by Aprhamian and coworkers.[98] This technique utilizes a cast saw to bivalve the helmet in the coronal plane. Following division of the outer rigid shell, the inner foam material is incised and removed with the head and neck maintained in neutral alignment. Although this approach does provide an alternate method of removing the helmet, the intense vibrations produced during use of the cast cutter may exacerbate an underlying spinal injury. In addition, even with the proper equipment available to the prehospital care provider, the technique may be slow and difficult with modern, well-fitting, high-quality helmets.[90]

A new and novel approach to motor sports helmet removal has recently been introduced. The HATS OFF emergency helmet removal system is a unique, low-technology and low-cost device that is rapidly becoming the preferred method for emergency helmet removal in the motor sports arena (Fig. 46–40). The HATS OFF system uses a small air bladder that is neatly folded in an accordion fashion and placed underneath the helmet liner (if removable; otherwise it fits over the lining and is covered with a supplied crown pad). A small tube runs under the padding and fastens to the bottom of the helmet rim to provide easy access. As the bladder expands, it gently pushes the helmet up and off the head. The Indycar Racing League, American Speed Association, and American Motorcycle Association have made the HATS OFF system mandatory at all of their events. In addition, the Championship Auto Racing Teams and National Association for Stock Car Auto Racing have strongly recommended its use. There are currently two versions of the HATS OFF system—the Helmet Kit, which is prefitted into the rider's helmet, and the 1st Response Kit, which consists of an insertion tool that allows the airbag to be slid up inside the top of a helmet not already equipped with the HATS OFF system. There is no scientific literature to advocate for the use of this device over the helmet removal techniques described previously. However, this novel and simple device clearly warrants further investigation and may change the approach to emergency helmet removal in the future.

Complications

Underlying cervical spine injuries may be exacerbated by failure to adhere to proper helmet removal techniques. Although this is not supported by conclusive evidence, the few related studies seem to suggest that there may be a risk to helmet removal.[82] In a cadaveric model, Donaldson and colleagues[99] demonstrated that even in the best clinical setting, there is a significant amount of motion during helmet and shoulder pad removal. Larger studies are needed to determine whether there is a real and significant risk in the clinical setting.

Conclusion

Prehospital care providers must take extreme caution when evaluating and treating an athlete with a suspected head and neck injury. Unless absolutely necessary, helmets and shoulder pads should not be removed in the prehospital setting. In contrast, motorcycle and motor sport helmets should be routinely removed to provide access to the patient's airway and allow for proper spinal immobilization. Face masks should be removed early in the management of these patients. When indicated, prehospital helmet removal can be accomplished in a safe and effective manner by well-trained prehospital care providers.

HELMET REMOVAL

The varying sizes, shapes, and configurations of motorcycle and sports helmets necessitate some understanding of their proper removal from victims of motorcycle crashes. The rescuer who removes a helmet improperly may unintentionally aggravate cervical spine injuries.

The Committee on Trauma believes that physicians who treat the injuries should be aware of helmet removal techniques. A gradual increase in the use of helmets is anticipated, because many organizations are urging voluntary wearing of helmets, and some states are reinstating their laws requiring the wearing of helmets.

Full face coverage—motorcycle, auto racer

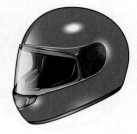

Full face coverage—motocross

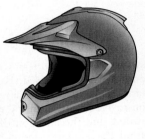

Partial face coverage—motorcycle, auto racer

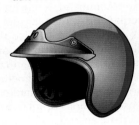

Light head protection—bicycle, kayak

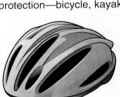

Football

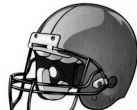

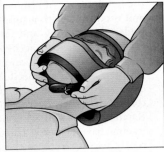

1. One rescuer maintains inline immobilization by placing her hands on each side of the helmet with the fingers on the victims mandible. This position prevents slippage if the strap is loose.

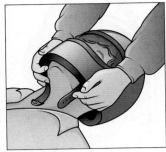

2. A second rescuer cuts or loosens the strap at the D-ring.

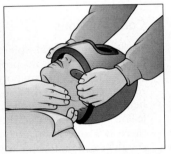

3. The second rescuer places one hand on the mandible at the angle, the thumb on one side, the long and index finger on the other. With his other hand, he applies pressure from the occipital region. This maneuver transfers the inline immobilization responsibility to the second rescuer.

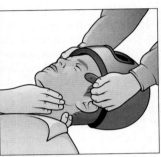

4. The rescuer at the top moves the helmet. Three factors should be kept in mind:
• The helmet is egg shaped and therefore must be expanded laterally to clear the ears.
• If the helmet provides full facial coverage, glasses must be removed first.
• If the helmet provides full facial coverage, the nose may impede removal. To clear the nose, the helmet must be tilted backward and raised over it.

5. Throughout the removal process, the second rescuer maintains inline immobilization from below to prevent unnecessary neck motion.

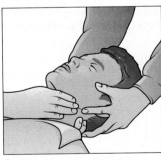

6. After the helmet has been removed, the rescuer at the top replaces her hands on either side of the victim's head with her palms over the ears.

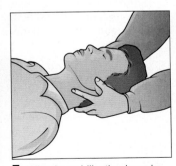

7. Inline immobilization is maintained from above until a backboard is in place and a cervical immobilization device (collar) is applied.

SUMMARY

The helmet must be maneuvered over the nose and ears while the head and neck are held rigid.
• Inline immobilization is first applied from above.
• Inline immobilization is applied from below by a second rescuer with pressure on the jaw and occiput.
• The helmet is removed.
• Inline immobilization is reestablished from above.

Figure 46–39 Motorcycle helmet removal. *(Reproduced with permission Norman E. McSwain Jr., MD, FACS, and Richard L. Garrnelli, MD, FACS— American College of Surgeons Committee on Trauma, April 1997.)*

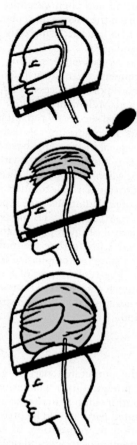

Figure 46–40 **The HATS OFF emergency helmet removal system.**
This device uses a small air bladder that is neatly folded in an accordion fashion and placed underneath the helmet liner. A small tube runs under the padding and fastens to the bottom of the helmet rim to provide easy access. The device may be prefitted into the rider's helmet or inserted at the time of removal using an insertion tool that allows the airbag to be slid up inside the top of a helmet. *(Courtesy of HATS OFF USA, Yorba Linda, CA.)*

Acknowledgments

The authors would like to thank Lynne Krider, RN, and the Mobile Intensive Care Unit staff at AtlantiCare Regional Medical Center for their contributions to this chapter.

 REFERENCES CAN BE FOUND ON **EXPERT CONSULT**

CHAPTER 47

Management of Amputations

Maria Halluska-Handy

"The first person caring for an injured hand will probably determine the ultimate stage of its usefulness."[1] Consequently, rapid and appropriate emergency care of a patient with an amputated part is crucial to the salvage and preservation of function. This chapter discusses the acute care of amputated parts before they are replanted and specifically addresses the management of distal digit amputations and dermal "slice" wounds.

Amputation may be partial or complete. Injuries with any interconnecting tissue between the distal and the proximal portions, even if it is only a small piece of bridging skin, are considered incomplete (or partial) amputations. Complete amputations are replanted, whereas partial amputations are revascularized. This distinction is arbitrary; for emergency clinicians, treatment for both injuries is very similar. The prognosis and outcome of both types of amputations are similar, although partial amputations often have better venous and lymphatic drainage, and functional recovery may be more complete if there is less anatomic damage.

The peak incidence of traumatic amputations occurs between the ages of 20 and 40 years;[2,3] men predominate over women at a ratio of 4:1. Local crush injuries are the most common mechanism of injury, and sharp guillotine amputations are the least common.[4,5] Partial amputations occur as often as total amputations.[6] Proximal amputations are less common than distal amputations.

The media have exaggerated somewhat the success of replantation and have often generated unrealistic expectations from the public. The technical limitations of successful repair of vessels that are less than 0.3 mm in diameter usually preclude replantation of digits distal to the distal interphalangeal joint.[7] Successful revascularization of amputated parts often ensures viability, but neurologic, osseous, and tendinous healing is critical for ultimate function. If there is incomplete neurologic recovery, limited range of motion, and intolerance to cold, the replanted part may have little functional value for the patient. Rehabilitation from replantation surgery may be prolonged, often requiring more than 1 year and repeated surgical procedures. The emergency clinician should be aware of the limitations of replantation surgery and *should not encourage unrealistic expectations in injured patients or their families.*

BACKGROUND

The possibility of restoring viability and function to traumatically severed parts has fascinated clinicians for centuries. Clinicians have attempted to replant parts with little more than a few sutures and secure bandaging and have occasionally had spectacular results. One of the earliest medical reports was by Fiorvanti,[8] who in 1570 reported the successful replantation of a soldier's nose, which was severed by a saber, after first cleansing it with urine and then carefully bandaging it. In 1814, Balfour[9] reported the successful replantation of a finger, which was severed by a hatchet, using only meticulous alignment and secure bandaging.

The ability to consistently replant amputated parts awaited the development of modern microvascular surgical techniques. The first reported successful upper limb replantation was by Malt and McKhann in 1962.[10] Later that year, Chen and Pao[11] reported successful replantation of a hand and arm. Developments in microsurgical techniques, advanced optics, and microsurgical instruments have created the ability to consistently replant amputated parts with a high degree of success. Since 1965, when Kleinert and Kasdan[12] reported the first successful microvascular anastomosis of a digital vessel, several large series of replantations have reported success rates ranging from 70% to 90%.[5,6,13–19] To the original pioneers in replant surgery, survival of the replanted tissue was the criterion for success, but with further technologic and surgical refinements, today's surgeons emphasize functional recovery as well as viability. The replantation of a part that is painful or useless or that interferes with function is a disservice to the patient and is less desirable than early restoration of function without replantation.

INDICATIONS

Preservation of the amputated part is generally indicated whenever there is potential for replantation or revascularization. Revascularization and reanastomosis of partially and completely amputated parts should be provided when there is hope of preservation or restoration of function. Aesthetic considerations, patient avocations, and occasional religious or social customs may also influence the decision to proceed with surgery.[20–22] In the end, the microsurgical team and the patient must reach the decision together, after a rational explanation of the potential results and successes.

Indications for replantation of fingers and hands have been proposed and are generally accepted, although they should not be applied rigidly to all circumstances. Successful functional recovery is more likely in distal than in proximal extremity amputations and more likely in multidigit amputations, single-digit thumb amputations, or transmetacarpal amputations.[23] Generally, these are indications for replantation (Table 47–1). Single digits that are both proximal to the distal interphalangeal joint and distal to the flexor digitorum superficialis may be replanted successfully, with good functional recovery (Fig. 47–1).

Successful replantations have been reported in patients from the ages of 7 months to 84 years.[24,25] There are no fixed age limits for replantation, although particularly good functional results have been reported in children, owing to their regenerative capacity and adaptability to rehabilitation.[2,26,27] The decision to replant is made on a case-by-case basis by the microsurgical team, who must weigh all the factors involved.

CONTRAINDICATIONS

There is no contraindication to managing the amputated part and stump as though replantation were going to occur, even when replantation is considered unlikely. In addition, ancillary personnel can often handle care of the amputated part and stump during resuscitation and transportation of the patient. However, it must be remembered that evaluation and

TABLE 47–1 Replantation of the Amputated Extremity

Indications

Young stable patient
Thumb
Multiple digits injured
Sharp wounds with little associated damage
Upper extremity (children)

Absolute Contraindications

Associated life threats
Severe crush injuries
Inability to withstand prolonged surgery

Relative Contraindications*

Single digit, unless thumb
Avulsion injury
Prolonged warm ischemia (≥12 hr)
Gross contamination
Prior injury or surgery to part
Emotionally unstable patients
Lower extremity

*If the victim is a child or if there are multiple losses, salvage replantations are attempted, and the relative contraindications are ignored.

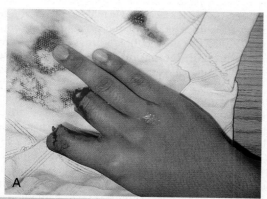

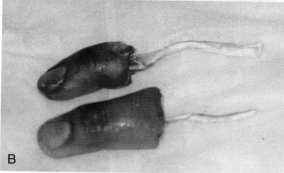

Figure 47–1 *A* and *B*, Single-digit amputations are not usually replanted unless the thumb is involved. This sharp amputation with little associated damage in a 20-year-old may qualify, but it is best to discuss this with the transplant team before giving unrealistic expectation to the patient who may expect a normal result by simply "sewing them back on." The avulsion of the tendons proximal to the amputation complicates this case.

treatment of life-threatening injuries always take precedence over that of the amputated part. Contraindications to replantation are listed in Table 47–1 and are discussed in the following sections. Note that even when replantation is contraindicated, tissue (skin, bone, tendon) from the amputated part may be useful in restoring function to other damaged parts. *Never discard amputated tissue until all possible uses of the severed parts are considered.* For example, even an amputated fingertip not suitable for replantation may be an ideal donor source for a skin graft to the stump.

GENERAL CONSIDERATIONS

Mechanism of Injury

The potential for successful replantation in terms of survival as well as useful function is directly related to the mechanism of injury. Guillotine-type injuries are the least common but have the best prognosis, owing to the limited area of destruction. Crush injuries are the most common, but produce more tissue injury and therefore have a poorer prognosis. Avulsion injuries have the worst prognosis because a significant amount of vascular, nerve, tendon, and soft tissue injury invariably occurs.[2,4–6,28]

Ischemia Time

The time that an amputated part can survive before replantation has not been determined. After 6 hours, additional delay may decrease the success rate of revascularization and lead to diminished function. Skin, bone, tendons, and ligaments tolerate ischemia much better than do muscle and connective tissue. As a general rule, the more proximal the amputation, the less ischemia time the amputated part can tolerate. Attempts to extend viability during ischemia have shown that the most important controllable factor is the *temperature* of the amputated part. Warm ischemia may be tolerated for 6 to 8 hours.[29] When the part is cooled properly to 4°C, 12 to 24 hours of ischemia may be tolerated with distal amputations.[2,4,6,13,14,30] There is a report of a successful digital replantation after 33 hours of cold ischemia.[31] Hypothermia limits the metabolic demand of tissues, preserving intracellular energy and reducing the production of toxic metabolites caused by ischemia.[31–34] It also retards the development of acidosis[35] and may prevent the no-reflow phenomenon that can follow ischemic and low-flow states.[20,31,32,36]

Delay in the replantation of proximal arm and leg amputations containing significant amounts of muscle tissue can lead to the buildup of toxic products. In such cases, when blood supply is restored, the absorbed toxins have been reported to cause respiratory failure, renal failure, cardiovascular collapse, and even death.[20,22,31,32,37–40]

Intraoperative perfusion techniques such as those used in organ transplants to extend anoxic time are being used to help cool amputated parts before replantation. However, emergency clinicians should not attempt perfusion because the risk of damaging vessels as well as the potential delay in care and in rapid transport override the theoretical benefits of emergency department (ED) cold perfusion.[20,41]

ASSESSMENT OF THE PATIENT

The initial care and treatment of the patient who has had a body part amputated are the same as those for any trauma patient. The amputated extremity or the excitement of others must not distract the clinician from assessing and stabilizing the patient's airway, breathing, and circulation. Amputations are generally not life-threatening injuries, and other potentially more serious injuries must first be assessed and treated. Hemorrhage from completely amputated limbs is often limited by the retraction and spasm of severed vessels. Partial amputations may result in more serious hemorrhage than if the vessels were totally severed. Usually, hemorrhage can be controlled adequately with direct pressure and elevation. Vascular clamps and hemostats should be avoided in the ED when possible. A proximally placed blood pressure cuff inflated 30 mm Hg above systolic pressure can be used for short periods of time (<30 min) to control severe bleeding, if necessary.

After the initial primary assessment and treatment and subsequent stabilization of the patient, care of the stump and amputated part can be initiated safely. In addition to the general history obtained from all trauma patients, particular attention should be focused on the exact mechanism of injury, the time and duration of the injury, handedness, allergies, medications, illness, prior injury to the affected part, care of the stump and amputated part before arrival in the ED, occupation, avocations, and tetanus history.

Tetanus prophylaxis and broad-spectrum systemic antibiotic therapy (e.g., cephalosporins) should be initiated. Intravenous opioids are usually required for pain; the dose should be titrated to the clinical condition. In fingertip amputations, digital or regional nerve blocks are ideal for pain relief but may make functional and neurologic evaluation by a consultant impossible (see Chapter 31, Nerve Blocks of the Thorax and Extremities). Aspirin, low-molecular-weight dextran, or both have been administered in an attempt to maintain small vessel perfusion, but have not proved beneficial in the ED management of these injuries.

Patients who have suffered an amputation often experience denial, shock, disbelief, and feelings of hopelessness about their injury; some have even become suicidal. Patients should be treated with supportive and realistic reassurance, but unrealistic medical promises should be avoided. It is important that the emergency clinician (or other non-replantation specialist) not speculate on the specifics of the ultimate prognosis.

Examination of the stump may be brief and should primarily be an assessment of the degree of damage to the surrounding tissue. Gross contamination can be removed by irrigation with normal saline. Local antiseptics, especially hydrogen peroxide or alcohol, should not be used because they may damage viable tissues. Similarly, tissues should not be manipulated, clamped, tagged, or further traumatized in any way. It is important to assess the degree of contamination, the level of the injury, and any concomitant injury. The amputated part should also be examined for the degree of tissue injury, contamination, and the presence of distal injuries. Radiographs of the amputated part and proximal stump that include at least one joint proximal to the injury site should be obtained. If not already done, preoperative laboratory studies and intravenous access in an uninjured extremity should also be initiated.

The neurologic status of the stump or distal extremity in partial amputations should be assessed by pinprick and two-point discrimination tests. The presence of sweat may indicate autonomic-neurologic functioning. Vascular competence, motor and tendon function, and neurovascular assessment

should be recorded in the medical record. The regional replantation resource center should be contacted as soon as possible to arrange transportation and provide adequate time for mobilization of the replantation team.

CARE OF THE STUMP AND AMPUTATED PART

The stump should be dealt with during the secondary assessment of the trauma victim (Table 47–2). If replantation is proposed, the goals of initial care include control of hemorrhage and prevention of further injury or contamination. All jewelry should be removed. The stump should be irrigated with normal saline to remove gross contamination; only the replantation team should perform manual débridement and dissection. Do not clamp arterial bleeders. The stump wound should then be covered with a *saline-moistened* sterile dressing to prevent further contamination and to limit damage from desiccation. The stump should be splinted for protection and to prevent further injury from concomitant fractures or compromised blood flow from a change in position. Splinting and elevation may also reduce swelling and help control bleeding.

Care of the amputated part follows the same general guidelines as for the stump. Gross contamination should be removed by irrigation with normal saline. All jewelry should be removed. The amputated part should be handled minimally to prevent further damage and should be wrapped in a saline-moistened sterile dressing. *Direct prolonged immersion in saline or hypotonic fluids should be avoided* because it may cause severe maceration of tissue and may make replantation technically more difficult. The amputated part should be cooled as soon as possible. The ideal temperature is 4°C, but care must be taken to prevent freezing of tissues. This is best accomplished by wrapping the amputated part in saline-moistened gauze, placing the gauze-wrapped part in a watertight plastic bag, and then immersing the bag in a container of ice water (Fig. 47–2). Amputated parts should not be placed directly on ice because tissue in direct contact with ice may freeze. A guideline is to use half water and half ice; excessive ice should be avoided. Cooling coils and refrigeration devices have occasionally been used but are generally not available and offer no significant advantages. The tissue containers should be labeled with the patient's name, the amputated part contained within, the time of the original injury, and the time that cooling began.

Treatment for *partial amputations* with vascular compromise is the same as that just described. Irrigate the wound with normal saline. Place a saline-moistened sponge on the

TABLE 47–2 Axioms for Care of Amputations	
Do's	**Don'ts**
Splint and elevate	Apply dry ice or freeze tissue
Apply pressure dressing	Place tags on tissue
Protect from further trauma or injury	Place sutures in tissue
Protect from further contamination	Sever skin bridges
Provide analgesia	Initiate perfusion of amputated part
Supply tetanus prophylaxis and antibiotic therapy	Place tissue in formalin or water
Obtain radiographs	

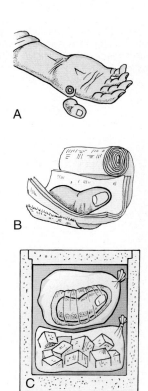

Figure 47–2 Evaluate the patient's condition to ensure that resuscitation is not necessary before transfer. *A,* The wound should be rinsed with saline solution. Do not scrub or apply antiseptic solution to the wound. Apply saline-moistened sterile dressing, wrap in Kling or Kerlix for pressure, and elevate. *B,* The amputated part should be rinsed with saline. Do not scrub or apply antiseptic solution to the amputated part. Wrap it in moist sterile gauze or a towel, depending on its size, and place it in a plastic bag or plastic container. Do not place the amputated part directly in saline. *C,* The part is then put in a container, preferably Styrofoam, and cooled by separate plastic bags containing ice or in a container of ice water. Do not pack the bagged injured part in ice, but it can be immersed in half water, half ice. *(A–C, From Hand Trauma: Emergency Care. Baltimore, MD, Emergency Services.)*

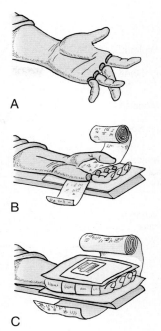

Figure 47–3 For a partial amputation, rinse with saline (*A*); then place part(s) in a functional position, apply a saline-moistened sterile dressing, and splint and elevate (*B*). Apply coolant bags to the outside of the dressing (*C*). Do not scrub or apply antiseptic solution to the wound. Control any bleeding with pressure. If a tourniquet is necessary, place it close to the amputation site. *(A–C, From Hand Trauma: Emergency Care. Baltimore, MD, Emergency Services.)*

843

open tissue, and wrap the injury in a sterile dressing, incorporating a splint to protect it from further injury. Ice packs or commercial cold packs should be applied over the dressing to cool the devascularized area (Fig. 47–3).

SPECIAL CONSIDERATIONS

Hand Function

Hand function is determined in part by pinch and grasp functions. If the index finger is removed, the pinching function of the index finger is adequately provided by the middle finger. Power in grasping and gripping is primarily an ulnar function of the fourth and fifth digits. An effective grip that provides the ability to hold a variety of objects is a central function of the ring and middle fingers. In addition to its function in pinching, the thumb is the major opposing force for successful grip and grasp. The thumb is the most important digit for adequate hand function, and its loss results in 40% to 50% disability. Such disability requires aggressive attempts to replant amputated thumbs. If this is impossible or unsuccessful, secondary alternatives are pollicization of other digits or toe transfers.[42,43]

Lower Extremity Amputations

There are few reports of successful replantation of amputated parts of the lower extremity.[44-46] Indications for replantation of lower extremity parts are different from those for replantation of amputated upper extremity parts. Isolated toe amputations are not replanted. It is generally held that if replantation does not restore function, a patient may be substantially better off with a prosthesis because lower limb prostheses, especially those used below the knee, are well tolerated and functional. Prostheses provide a secure stance and permit locomotion. Lower extremity replantation generally requires skeletal shortening, and distal nerve regeneration is often imperfect. Both deficits may produce dysfunction. A patient with a replanted lower extremity with significant shortening and without sensation would function better with a prosthesis. This is not necessarily true of someone with an upper extremity replant. For these reasons, lower limbs are not generally replanted except under ideal circumstances, usually in children. The final decision regarding replantation should be left to the replantation team.

Fingertip Amputations and Dermal "Slice" Wounds

Proper treatment of distal fingertip injuries is controversial, but good results often occur with conservative management. Fingertip amputations often heal by normal wound contracture, but occasionally this results in the loss of functional ability to palpate. The basic goals of treatment are to provide tissue coverage, an acceptable cosmetic result, and an early functional recovery. Distal amputations with a wound area

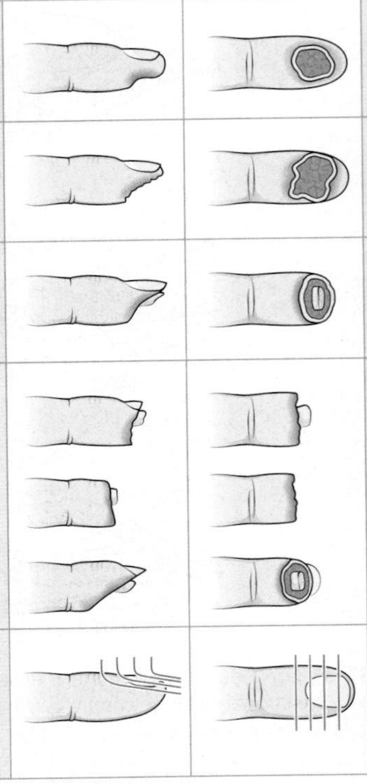

			TREATMENT
TYPE I Soft-tissue loss: Minimal Bone loss: None Nail/nail bed injury: None			Conservative management
TYPE II Soft-tissue loss: Moderate Bone loss: None Nail/nail bed injury: None			Conservative management, split-thickness skin graft
TYPE III Soft-tissue loss: Major Bone loss: Minimal Nail/nail bed injury: None			Split-thickness skin graft, operative procedure
TYPE IV Soft-tissue loss: Major Bone loss: Moderate Nail/nail bed injury: Minor to major			Operative procedure
TYPE V Soft-tissue loss: None Bone loss: Minimal Nail/nail bed injury: Minor to major			Conservative management, split-thickness skin graft

Figure 47–4 Clinical classification of fingertip injuries and treatments for each type. *(From Newmeyer WL: Managing fingertip injuries on an outpatient basis. J Musculoskel Med 2:17, 1985.)*

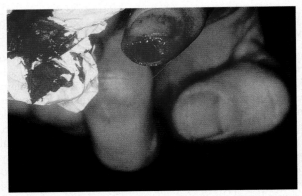

Figure 47–5 This very minimal amputation of a fat pad by a meat slicer, not involving bone or the nailbed, is a common injury and will heal well with conservative therapy (see Fig. 47–6).

less than 10 mm² are not a problem (Figs. 47–4 and 47–5). Larger dorsal wounds also heal well by secondary intention. However, when skin and soft tissue loss from the finger pad is significant, the clinician is faced with more challenging situation. Volar skin is unique in its combination of toughness and sensitivity. Wounds with significant volar tissue loss frequently require additional treatment. Children, with their regenerative capacity, often progress very well when significant volar wounds are allowed to heal primarily. For older people and for amputations that involve a more significant amount of the distal digit, a wide variety of techniques for managing the injured fingertip have been advocated. These include partial-thickness skin grafts; full-thickness skin grafts; V-Y, Kutler, Kleinert, and island advancement flaps; and various local and distal flap coverage techniques. These procedures are designed to preserve length and provide soft tissue coverage of exposed bone and sensation to the finger pad.

Each of these procedures has its own indications, complications, and limitations.[47–49] Discussion of these procedures is beyond the scope of this chapter. Most of these techniques are best performed by a specialist in the operating room at the time of injury or as delayed procedures when necessary.

In most complete fingertip amputations distal to the distal interphalangeal joint, the emergency clinician can provide adequate care initially with conservative wound management. Although thinking has changed significantly over the years, many hand surgeons still advise skin grafting to shorten the time for wound healing. Although complete transverse amputations could be handled conservatively, wound healing may take several weeks, and these patients may benefit from operative treatments. Patients with complete transactions should be referred for consultation to coordinate their initial care and subsequent follow-up. Regardless of the type of injury, definitive care is usually provided on a delayed basis, and ED intervention is conservative with subsequent consultation being considered standard.

Incomplete transections and small distal amputations without significant soft tissue loss may heal well with conservative therapy started by the emergency clinician. Nonoperative treatment in selected patients provides excellent functional and cosmetic results, minimizes recovery time, and has few complications.[48–54] Children have excellent regenerative capacity and also respond extremely well to conservative treatment. Necrotic and grossly contaminated tissue should be débrided, and the wound should be irrigated thoroughly. If bone is left exposed without soft tissue coverage, the patient will need an operative procedure; alternatively, the bone may be rongeured (shortened) to allow soft tissue coverage and primary healing with better functional recovery. The nailbed tissues should be preserved, because the presence of a nail affects the cosmetic result. After cleansing and cautious débridement, an occlusive dressing is placed directly over the wound, and the finger is bandaged and splinted for protection. If needed, tetanus prophylaxis should also be provided. Amputations that involve the distal phalanx are frequently treated as contaminated open fractures. In these cases, a recent Cochrane review supports the early use of antibiotics to reduce the incidence of infection.[55] Wounds managed conservatively must have serial dressing changes and cleansing. This helps provide superficial débridement, which may aid healing and minimize the chance of secondary infection. Wound contraction and healing usually result in acceptable cosmetic and functional recovery in 2 to 3 weeks. Patients should have appropriate follow-up to ensure adequate healing and recovery.

The emergency clinician can also manage partial fingertip amputations distal to the distal interphalangeal joint. These wounds are treated in a manner similar to that for complete amputations. However, when the amputation has substantial undamaged tissue connecting the fingertip, careful alignment and stabilization are provided by sutures or bandaging and protective splinting. Partially amputated fingertips, especially in children, may occasionally survive and regain vascularization and sensation. If the distal tissue becomes ischemic and necrotic, the amputation becomes complete.

Injury to the nailbed requires special attention to ensure proper alignment. If the nailbed tissues are not aligned properly, permanently disfigured nails may result. Complete or partial nail removal may be required for the placement of sutures.

Dermal "slice" wounds (see type 1 in Figs. 47–4 and 47–5) are managed by gentle wound cleansing and application of an antibiotic ointment and a nonadherent dressing, followed by a pressure dressing (e.g., tube gauze). The patient should return in 48 to 72 hours for a wound check and dressing change. At that time, the patient can be instructed on daily changes of nonadherent dressings for 10 to 14 days until functional epithilialization of the wound occurs. A protective finger splint or guard also minimizes the risk of further injury and pain from trauma to the sensitive wound area. Protection allows an earlier return to function and employment. Wounds larger than 10 mm² and those with deep loss of digit pulp tissue may be candidates for skin grafting.

Conservative Management of Fingertip Amputations

An amputation of the fingertip that does not involve significant bony injury or massive tissue maceration generally does well with conservative treatment. In the past, skin grafts, flaps, and advancement techniques were used for Type II and Type III injuries depicted in Figure 47–4, but currently such interventions are uncommon for simple fingertip amputations. The common transverse guillotine amputation from machinery heals with good cosmetics and adequate sensation, but it may require 6 to 8 weeks for complete healing. Such injuries may be simply cleaned and bandaged in the ED and appropriately referred. However, if ED follow-up is available, patients may be re-evaluated and selectively débrided at 1 week intervals. Figure 47–6 outlines such a conservative course.

Penis, Ear, and Nose Amputations

Replantation of the penis, ear, and nose generally results in better function and cosmesis than a prosthesis or reconstructive surgery. The amputated parts and wounds should be handled in the same manner as for digital replantations.

Penile amputations are an uncommon problem. Most cases result from self-inflicted trauma in patients who are severely psychologically disturbed. Successful replantation has been reported using microsurgical techniques. Preservation or reconstruction of the urethra to maintain a competent urinary stream is critical for success.[56,57] Ears and noses fre-

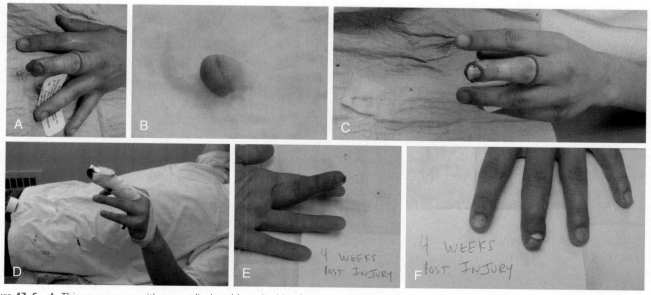

Figure 47–6 *A,* This young man with no medical problems had his fingertip cut off by a metal press. Note that the nail bed is exposed due to avulsion of the nail. The distal phalynx was not injured but was felt in the stump. *B,* The avulsed tip has skin and the avulsed nail attached. *C,* After the tip was cleaned by gentle scrubbing and minor débridement of macerated tissue, the nail was dissected from the tip and sutured back under the eponychium. The amputated tip was discarded. *D,* A protective splint and a pressure dressing was applied. Cephalexin was given for 7 days. The patient was seen weekly for dressing changes and minor débridement. *E,* At 4 weeks the finger has healed well, with good sensation and an almost normal appearance. *F,* The old nail was removed to reveal the growth of a new nail. At 8 weeks there was no deformity or problem except minor shortening of the tip.

quently are partially amputated and occasionally are totally amputated. Whenever possible, these body parts should be replanted unless they are severely traumatized and there is gross contamination. These wounds frequently heal well, and patients with such wounds have a high tissue survival rate and a low incidence of total necrosis. Replantation of these parts requires good suture technique and careful placement, but does not necessarily require skill in microsurgical techniques.[57–60]

COMPLICATIONS

The care of amputated parts should not lead to avoidable complications if the aforementioned principles are followed. Improper management of the parts or stump with subsequent additional injury of the tissue from overzealous hemostasis or cleansing should be avoided. Furthermore, desiccation, maceration, or freezing of tissue from improper storage should not occur. *Expediting the preoperative workup of the patient and immediate notification of the replantation team are crucial factors in the patient's care.*

Despite optimal initial care, replantation itself may be associated with acute or long-term complications. There is the usual risk of anesthesia and protracted surgery. Moreover, it is not unusual for second and third emergency operations to be required to reestablish adequate blood flow. Postoperative complications include vascular thrombosis, hemorrhage, infection, and reaction to accumulated toxins. Toxins accumulate in ischemic amputated parts, despite cooling. The amount of toxin is directly proportional to the amount of muscle mass and the duration of ischemia. Significant pulmonary failure, electrolyte disturbance, and even death have been reported in replantation efforts. Finally, patients are often placed on anticoagulants, which create additional risk.

Later complications include a significant percentage (60%) of patients with cold intolerance, limited function, anesthesia, pain, paresthesias, malunions, and nonunions. Repeated operative procedures may be required to obtain a functionally useful result.

Acknowledgment

The contributions by William C. Dalsey, MD, and Jeffrey Luk, MD, to earlier editions are appreciated.

 REFERENCES CAN BE FOUND ON EXPERT CONSULT

Extensor and Flexor Tendon Injuries in the Hand, Wrist, and Foot

Peter Erik Sokolove

EXTENSOR TENDONS

Extensor tendons are quite superficial, covered only by skin and a thin layer of fascia, and are thus highly susceptible to injury. Hence, they are readily injured by commonly experienced trauma. These injuries may result from lacerations, bites, or burns, but they may also be caused by closed injury with even seemingly superficial lacerations. Whereas some extensor tendon injuries must be managed by a hand surgeon, others may be treated in the emergency department (ED). The emergency clinician must understand the anatomy, principles of treatment, repair technique, and postrepair care of these injuries to ensure the best possible patient outcome.

Functional Anatomy

There are 12 extrinsic extensors of the wrist and digits, all of which are innervated by the radial nerve. The muscles that give rise to these tendons originate in the forearm and elbow (Fig. 48–1). The extrinsic extensor tendons reach the hand and digits by passing through a fibro-osseous tendon sheath (retinaculum) located at the dorsal wrist. This synovium-lined sheath provides for smooth gliding of the tendons and prevents bowstringing when the wrist is extended.[1] The dorsal retinaculum contains six compartments or subdivisions (Fig. 48–2). These compartments are numbered from the radial to the ulnar side of the wrist.

The first compartment contains two tendons, abductor pollicis longus (APL) and extensor pollicis brevis (EPB). The APL tendon, the most radial of the extensor tendons, inserts on the base of the first metacarpal. It can be palpated just distal to the radial tubercle. The APL tendon causes thumb abduction and extension and some radial wrist deviation. The EPB travels with the APL through the first compartment but inserts at the base of the proximal phalanx of the thumb. The EPB tendon can be palpated over the dorsum of the first metacarpal when the thumb is extended against resistance. Both tendons can be tested by having the patient spread the fingers apart against resistance.

The second compartment also contains two tendons: the extensor carpi radialis brevis (ECRB) and the extensor carpi radialis longus (ECRL). These two tendons arise from the lateral epicondyle of the elbow. The ECRL inserts on the base of the second metacarpal, and the ECRB inserts on the base of the third metacarpal. Both tendons are powerful wrist extensors, and the ECRL also allows some radial wrist deviation. Wrist extension plays an especially important role in the mechanics of the hand, because hand grip strength is maximal only when the wrist is extended.

The third compartment contains only one extensor tendon: the extensor pollicis longus (EPL). This tendon crosses over the ECRB and ECRL and travels along the dorsum of the thumb to insert on the distal phalanx. The EPL forms the top of the anatomic "snuffbox," and the bottom is formed by the EPB. The EPL can be visualized when the thumb is extended, and its strength can be tested by having the patient hyperextend at the interphalangeal (IP) joint against resistance. The intrinsic extensor of the thumb can provide some degree of extension at the IP joint. Therefore, if EPL injury is suspected, it is important to compare extension at the IP joint with that of the unaffected thumb.

The fourth and fifth compartments contain the six tendons that extend the index through the little fingers. Each finger has its own extensor digitorum communis (EDC) tendon. The index and little fingers have an additional independent extensor tendon—the extensor indicis proprius (EIP) for the index finger and the extensor digiti minimi (EDM) for the little finger. The fourth compartment contains the EIP and EDC tendons, and the fifth compartment contains only the EDM tendon. These six tendons can be seen over the dorsum of the hand, where they are poorly protected and prone to injury. In this region, tendinous, ligamentous, and fascial connections between these tendons are known as the *juncturae tendini.* Because of these interconnections, a patient may be able to extend a digit, albeit weakly, even when there is a complete laceration of its EDC tendon. To avoid missing a tendon injury on the dorsum of the hand, it is important that the examiner test for tendon strength and not just for active extension.

The course of the extensor tendons along the fingers is more complex, but a basic understanding of this anatomy is essential for the emergency clinician to evaluate and treat extensor tendon injuries (Fig. 48–3). The EIP tendon joins the EDC tendon at the level of the metacarpophalangeal (MCP) joint in the index finger. The EDM tendon parallels the course of the EDC tendon; the four EDC tendons eventually insert at the base of the proximal, middle, and distal phalanges. The most proximal insertion of the EDC tendon is at the level of the base of the proximal phalanx. The tendon actually inserts in two ways. First, there is a loose dorsal insertion just distal to the MCP joint. In addition, the EDC tendon inserts into the volar plate via the sagittal bands. The sagittal bands are circumferential structures at the level of the metacarpal head that serve to keep the EDC tendon centered over the metacarpal head as well as to provide a stable connection with the volar plate located on the palmar side of the hand. After its primary insertion at the level of the MCP joint, the EDC tendon then extends dorsally along the digit. The EDC trifurcates over the proximal phalanx (Fig. 48–4). Its major central slip inserts on the base of the middle phalanx (Fig. 48–5). The lateral branches of the EDC tendon join with the lateral bands from the interossei and lumbricals to form the cojoined lateral bands. The two cojoined lateral bands then fuse together over the middle phalanx to form the terminal extensor mechanism (TEM), which inserts into the base of the distal phalanx (Fig. 48–6). The triangular ligament is a connection between the two cojoined lateral bands that assists in keeping these structures on the dorsal aspect of the digit.

The sixth dorsal compartment of the wrist contains only one tendon: the extensor carpi ulnaris (ECU). This tendon originates at the lateral epicondyle of the elbow and inserts at the base of the fifth metacarpal. The ECU functions as a wrist extensor and ulnar deviator. It can be palpated just distal to the tip of the ulna, and its strength can be tested by forced ulnar deviation of the wrist.

Posterior (dorsal) view

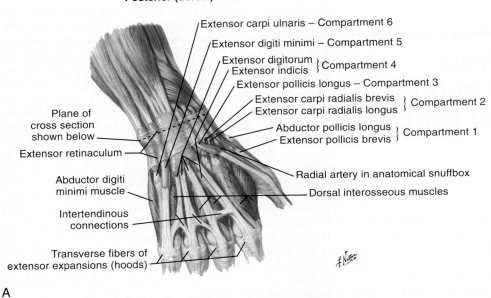

Extensor carpi ulnaris – Compartment 6

Extensor digiti minimi – Compartment 5

Extensor digitorum } Compartment 4
Extensor indicis

Extensor pollicis longus – Compartment 3

Extensor carpi radialis brevis } Compartment 2
Extensor carpi radialis longus

Abductor pollicis longus } Compartment 1
Extensor pollicis brevis

Plane of cross section shown below

Extensor retinaculum

Abductor digiti minimi muscle

Intertendinous connections

Transverse fibers of extensor expansions (hoods)

Radial artery in anatomical snuffbox

Dorsal interosseous muscles

A

Cross section of most distal portion of forearm

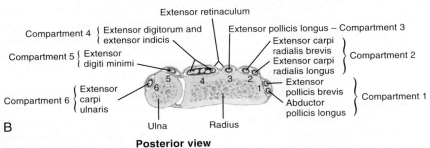

Extensor retinaculum

Compartment 4 { Extensor digitorum and extensor indicis

Extensor pollicis longus – Compartment 3

Compartment 5 { Extensor digiti minimi

Extensor carpi radialis brevis
Extensor carpi radialis longus } Compartment 2

Compartment 6 { Extensor carpi ulnaris

Extensor pollicis brevis
Abductor pollicis longus } Compartment 1

Ulna   Radius

B

Posterior view

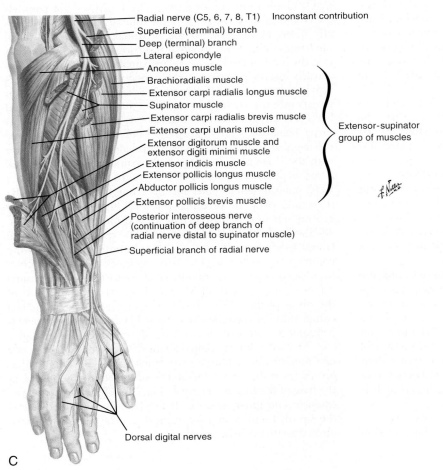

Radial nerve (C5, 6, 7, 8, T1)   Inconstant contribution

Superficial (terminal) branch

Deep (terminal) branch

Lateral epicondyle

Anconeus muscle

Brachioradialis muscle

Extensor carpi radialis longus muscle

Supinator muscle

Extensor carpi radialis brevis muscle

Extensor carpi ulnaris muscle

Extensor digitorum muscle and extensor digiti minimi muscle

Extensor indicis muscle

Extensor pollicis longus muscle

Abductor pollicis longus muscle

Extensor pollicis brevis muscle

Posterior interosseous nerve (continuation of deep branch of radial nerve distal to supinator muscle)

Superficial branch of radial nerve

Dorsal digital nerves

Extensor-supinator group of muscles

C

Figure 48–1 Extensor muscles and tendons of the right wrist and hand. *A,* Posterior (dorsal) view. *B,* Cross-section of most distal portion of forearm. *C,* Radial nerve in forearm: posterior view. *(A–C, Netter illustrations used with permission of Elsevier Inc. All rights reserved.)*

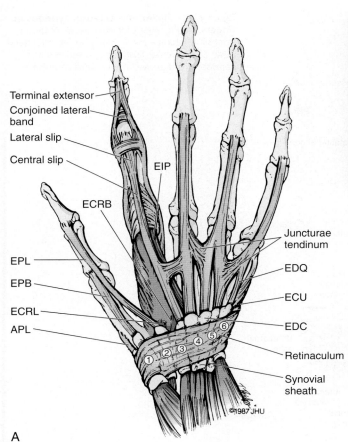

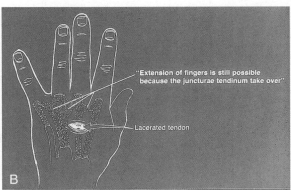

Figure 48–2 *A,* The extensor mechanism at the wrist and dorsum of the right hand. The six extensor compartments at the wrist contain (1) the abductor pollicis longus (APL) and extensor pollicis brevis (EPB); (2) the extensor carpi radialis longus (ECRL) and brevis (ECRB); (3) the extensor pollicis longus (EPL); (4) the extensor digitorum communis (EDC) II–V and extensor indicis proprius (EIP); (5) the extensor digiti quinti (EDQ); and (6) the extensor carpi ulnaris (ECU). An important anatomic detail is the presence of a synovial sheath around each tendon unit within each fibro-osseous canal. Note that the EDQ is also called the extensor digiti minimi (EDM) by some authors. *B,* Note that the juncturae tendinum allow some weak extension of the finger when the proximal extensor is completely lacerated. *(A, Adapted from Thomas JS, Peimer CA: Extensor tendon injuries: Acute repair and late reconstruction. In Chapman MW [ed]: Operative Orthopaedics, 3rd ed. Philadelphia, JB Lippincott, 2001, p 1487.)*

849

General Approach to Extensor Tendon Injuries

The key to detecting extensor tendon injuries in the ED is to perform a careful and thorough history and physical examination. Closed injuries may appear innocuous at first but may result in tendon injuries that often lead to severe deformities or dysfunction if undetected (Figs. 48–7 to 48–9). Closed injuries are also commonly associated with fractures. A hand radiograph is recommended in closed hand injuries when a fracture is suspected or in open hand injuries in which fracture or a foreign body is suspected. It is generally accepted that all open injuries that result from glass should be radiographed. Plain radiographs have a sensitivity of approximately 98% for detecting radiopaque foreign bodies (e.g., gravel, glass, metal).[2]

Injuries to extensor tendons from lacerations are quite common, especially on the dorsum of the hand, where they are superficially located. All dorsal wrist, hand, and digit lacerations should be assumed to have an underlying tendon laceration until proven otherwise. Digital extension, albeit weak, can still occur with partial tendon lacerations of up to 90%, so visualization of the tendon and careful strength testing are required to definitively rule out a partial injury. In some cases, the specific diagnosis simply cannot be made on the first examination (see later). A complete laceration of an EDC tendon on the dorsum of a hand can also still allow digital extension through the juncturae tendini.

After assessing the strength and neurovascular status of the injured hand, it is imperative that the emergency clinician visually inspect the wound thoroughly. Inspection should include an assessment of the degree of wound contamination as well as a search for foreign bodies and occult tendon lacera-

tions. It is often necessary to extend the skin laceration to aid in the visualization of a possible tendon injury. Because an extensor tendon is a mobile structure, it is imperative that if it is exposed, it is visualized in its entirety through a full range of motion. It is especially important to examine the tendon in the position of injury, because the tendon injury frequently does not lie directly under the external skin wound (see Fig. 48–8).

The definitive examination of any wound must occur under the best possible conditions—with a good light source, a bloodless field, adequate local anesthesia, and a cooperative patient. *It may be impossible to adequately assess some patients completely during the first ED visit. Final diagnosis must be delayed until the proper circumstances permit the required conditions.* Occasionally, however, patient noncompliance thwarts even the most carefully planned follow-up. Often, the patient's pain, swelling, anxiety, or degree of intoxication/altered sensorium limits the clinician's diagnostic ability; therefore, *it would not be considered standard to diagnose the presence, or the full extent, of all extensor tendon injuries immediately.* Whenever logistically possible, it is suggested that a specialist be consulted when an extensor tendon injury is suspected, by either mechanism or location of the wound, or tendon dysfunction. Under most circumstances, however, there is no value in obtaining an immediate on-site consultation with a hand surgeon/orthopaedic surgeon, because the intrinsic scenario would similarly limit any clinician's diagnostic acumen.

If the examining clinician suspects, but is unable to locate, a tendon laceration, or if a patient is uncooperative with the examination and the circumstances prohibit ideal initial care, the patient should be referred for follow-up in 1 to 3 days for a repeat examination. Interim wound care with skin closure

Posterior (dorsal) view

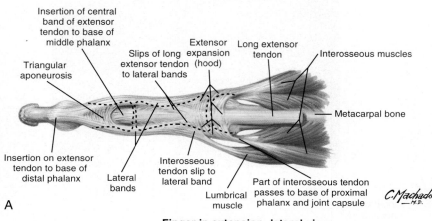

Insertion of central band of extensor tendon to base of middle phalanx

Triangular aponeurosis

Slips of long extensor tendon to lateral bands

Extensor expansion (hood)

Long extensor tendon

Interosseous muscles

Insertion on extensor tendon to base of distal phalanx

Lateral bands

Interosseous tendon slip to lateral band

Lumbrical muscle

Part of interosseous tendon passes to base of proximal phalanx and joint capsule

Metacarpal bone

C. Machado —M.D.

A

Figure 48–3   Flexor and extensor tendons in fingers. *A,* Posterior (dorsal) view. *B,* Finger in extension: lateral view. *C,* Finger in flexion: lateral view. *(A–C, Netter illustrations used with permission of Elsevier Inc. All rights reserved.)*

Finger in extension: lateral view

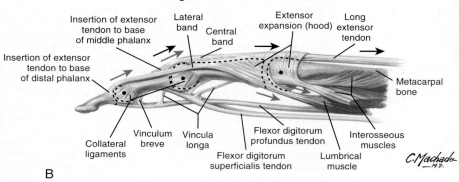

Insertion of extensor tendon to base of middle phalanx

Lateral band

Central band

Extensor expansion (hood)

Long extensor tendon

Insertion of extensor tendon to base of distal phalanx

Metacarpal bone

Collateral ligaments

Vinculum breve

Vincula longa

Flexor digitorum profundus tendon

Flexor digitorum superficialis tendon

Interosseous muscles

Lumbrical muscle

C. Machado —M.D.

B

Finger in flexion: lateral view

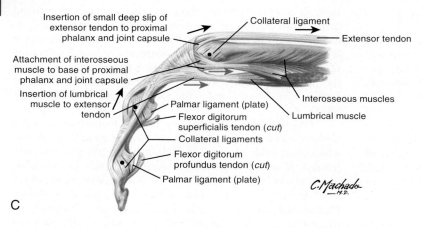

Insertion of small deep slip of extensor tendon to proximal phalanx and joint capsule

Collateral ligament

Extensor tendon

Attachment of interosseous muscle to base of proximal phalanx and joint capsule

Insertion of lumbrical muscle to extensor tendon

Palmar ligament (plate)

Flexor digitorum superficialis tendon (*cut*)

Collateral ligaments

Flexor digitorum profundus tendon (*cut*)

Palmar ligament (plate)

Interosseous muscles

Lumbrical muscle

C. Machado —M.D.

C

and splint application is advised. A delay of a few days for definitive diagnosis, surgical repair, or both does not result in any significant alteration in final outcome. Delayed primary repair, without the need for tendon grafting or tendon transfer, is a well-accepted technique. In fact, many hand surgeons are reluctant to immediately repair even a complete extensor tendon laceration in a contused, potentially contaminated, wound. The exact timeframe under which such delayed repair results in an outcome similar to immediate repair is not well defined and depends on the clinical scenario. Usually, delayed repair up to 7 to 10 days will ensure an outcome similar to that of an immediate repair, but this varies depending on the injury. Inability to rule out a tendon injury in the ED and the mandate for follow-up, with a specific following timeframe

indicated, should be clearly documented on the medical record and discharge instructions.

Antibiotic Use

There are no data to support or refute the use of prophylactic antibiotics as a routine adjunct after tendon injury. In general, prophylactic antibiotics have not been demonstrated to reduce infection rates after soft tissue injury in the setting of proper wound cleaning. Neither have they been proved to reduce infection rates in the absence of gross contamination, retained foreign material, or extensive contusion or after a delay in cleaning. Many clinicians opt for antibiotics with gram-positive (including antistaphylococcal) coverage if the tendon has been injured or sutured, but no universally accepted stan-

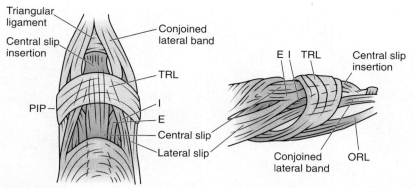

Figure 48–4 The zone of convergence of the digital extensor mechanism, which begins at about the midportion of the proximal phalanx and ends at the level of the central slip insertion into the dorsal base of the middle phalanx. Proximal to the zone of convergence, the extrinsic and intrinsic components of the extensor mechanism are separate: The central slip is extrinsic, whereas the lateral slips are intrinsic. Within the zone of convergence, there is complete reciprocal crossover of fibers from the central slip and lateral slips. The products of the completed convergence are the central slip insertion and the conjoined lateral bands, both of which have dual muscular activity. E, extrinsic contribution to conjoined lateral bands; I, intrinsic contribution to central slip insertion; ORL, oblique retinacular ligament; PIP, proximal interphalangeal joint; TRL, transverse retinacular ligament. *(From Thomas JS, Peimer CA: Extensor tendon injuries: Acute repair and late reconstruction. In Chapman MW [ed]: Operative Orthopaedics, 3rd ed. Philadelphia, JB Lippincott, 2001, p 1500.)*

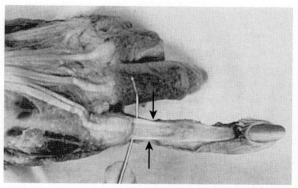

Figure 48–5 The extensor mechanism on the dorsum of a finger. *Arrows* point to the radial and ulnar lateral band portions of the extensor mechanism, and the probe lifts the entire structure up off the phalanx.

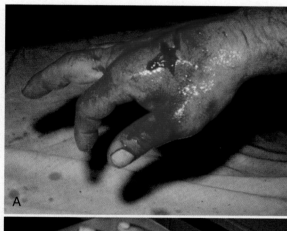

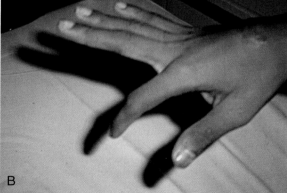

Figure 48–7 *A* and *B*, Because of their superficial location, *it is difficult to avoid at least partial injury to extensor tendons in even superficial lacerations of the dorsum of the wrist, hand, or fingers. A,* This complete extensor tendon laceration is obvious since the index finger cannot be extended. *B,* This partial tendon laceration was not appreciated on initial examination that seemingly demonstrated full tendon function. The entire tendon could not be visualized owing to an uncooperative patient. The unappreciated partial laceration progressed to complete rupture by the time of suture removal. An expeditious delayed primary repair resulted in a good outcome.

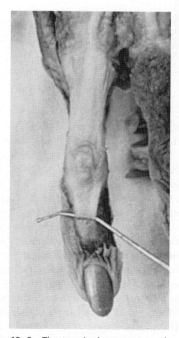

Figure 48–6 The terminal extensor mechanism.

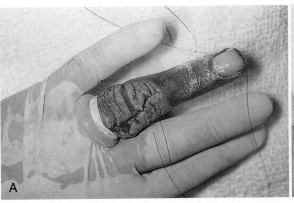
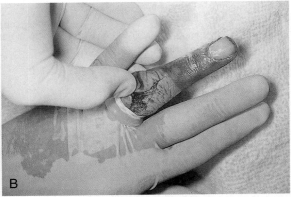

Figure 48–8 To examine for tendon injury, use a bloodless field. Note the sterile glove on the patient to maintain a clean field. *It is almost impossible to cut the dorsum on the hand/fingers and avoid at least a partial tendon injury. A,* The location and depth of this laceration suggests an extensor tendon injury. On examination, the patient had full extension. *B,* Note that no tendon injury is visualized when the laceration was examined with the fingers in extension. When the laceration was *extended and probed with the finger flexed*, a 60% laceration of the extensor tendon could be viewed in the depths of the wound.

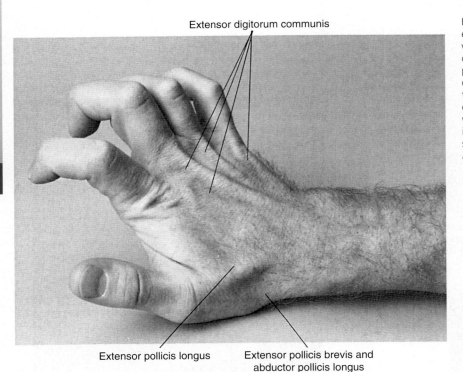

Extensor digitorum communis

Extensor pollicis longus

Extensor pollicis brevis and abductor pollicis longus

Figure 48–9 Given the superficial location of extensor tendons, suspect a tendon injury even with seemingly superficial lacerations of the dorsum of the hand and fingers. Full function is possible with a significant tendon laceration, and delayed total rupture can occur days to weeks if the injury is not repaired or splinted. Most partial extensor tendon lacerations do well with 3 to 4 weeks of splinting and no surgical repair. When in doubt, clean the laceration, suture the skin, splint, and refer for a subsequent examination in a few days.

dard of care exists. An individualized approach is advocated. Prophylaxis is generally used only for 3 to 5 days after injury unless extenuating circumstances (such as immunocompromise, human bite, unusual source of contamination, or peripheral vascular disease) exist. If there is doubt about the sterility of a wound, tendon repair should not be attempted.

Preparation for Repair

Before attempting repair of an open extensor tendon injury in the ED, it is essential that the treating clinician be prepared and has the proper equipment available. Patients should be placed supine on a gurney that ideally has an arm board attached. Bright overhead lighting is important for wound exploration so that the presence of tendon injuries and foreign bodies can be adequately assessed. Instruments should include, at a minimum, a needle holder; two skin hooks and retractors;

sharp (i.e., "iris") and blunt-nosed scissors; several small hemostats; and one pair of small, single-toothed (i.e., Adson) forceps.

The choice of suture material depends on the location of the tendon injury. For the repair of complete tendon injuries on the dorsum of the hand, nonabsorbable, synthetic, braided sutures are preferred.[3] Polyester sutures, such as Ethibond or Mersilene, are recommended. Nylon sutures are acceptable but are less ideal, because colored nylon may be visible under the skin. Chromic and plain gut should be avoided because they will dissolve before adequate tendon healing has occurred. Silk is not desirable because of its reactivity. Most extensor tendons on the dorsum of the hand will accommodate 4-0 sutures, but 5-0 suture material may be needed for smaller tendons. Small, "plastic repair," tapered needles should be used to avoid tearing the tendon. Partial tendon injuries of the digits are best repaired with fine, synthetic, absorbable sutures such as polyglactin (Vicryl).

It is imperative that the clinician use adequate anesthesia so that thorough wound exploration can occur. A field block or regional nerve block can be used on the dorsum of the hand, whereas local anesthesia or a digital nerve block can be used on the fingers. Many clinicians readily use lidocaine with epinephrine in the hand. It is important to liberally anesthetize the area around the wound, because many lacerations must be extended to afford access to the surgical field. It is a common error to neglect to extend a laceration and to attempt examination, cleaning, or repair through a small initial skin laceration.

Following the administration of anesthesia, a tourniquet may be placed on the involved limb if hemostasis is problematic. It is absolutely essential that adequate control of blood flow be obtained before attempting to repair a tendon laceration. It is very difficult to find the proximal end of a retracted tendon in a bloody field. Before application of a tourniquet, the patient's arm may be wrapped in several layers of cast padding as a comfort measure, and the arm should be elevated for at least 1 minute to allow blood to drain by gravity. A blood pressure cuff is placed on the mid- to upper arm, wrapped in several more layers of cast padding, then inflated to 260 to 280 mm Hg. Once inflated, the tubes are clamped tightly using a hemostat. The use of cast padding during inflation helps avoid inadvertent unraveling of the cuff. The use of a hemostat to clamp the blood pressure cuff tubes helps avoid a slow leak in the cuff with resultant deflation. A blood pressure cuff tourniquet is generally well tolerated by patients for approximately 15 to 20 minutes. If tendon repair cannot be accomplished in this amount of time, it is likely that the injury is too complex for repair in the ED. When necessary, the use of parenteral sedation may allow the patient to tolerate a longer tourniquet time.

Atraumatic technique is essential for minimizing adhesions and scar tissue formation. Tendons should be handled delicately, avoiding crushing forces or excessive punctures with forceps and needles. Forceps should be used only on the exposed, cut end of the tendon whenever possible.[4]

Patterns of Injury and Management

The treatment for extensor tendon injury depends primarily on whether the injury is open or closed as well as the anatomic location of the injury. The most widely accepted classification system is that developed by Verdan,[5] which divides the hand and wrist into eight anatomically based zones (Fig. 48–10). It is quite useful for emergency clinicians to become familiar with this classification, because in many instances, the zone of injury can help determine whether tendon repair should be attempted in the ED. One must keep in mind that repair of lacerated extensor tendons within 72 hours of injury is still considered primary closure. Therefore, whereas emergency clinicians may repair many extensor tendon injuries immediately, some injuries are best managed with delayed repair. In these cases, initial care in the ED should consist of sterile skin preparation, copious wound irrigation and inspection for foreign bodies, skin closure, splint application, and a referral to a hand specialist for further care in 1 to 5 days. A dorsal plaster/fiberglass splint, incorporating a metal foam finger splint, is an ideal way to totally immobilize a finger (Fig. 48–11).

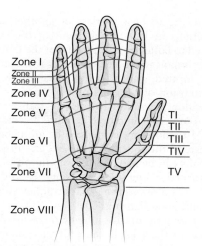

Figure 48–10 **Dorsum of left hand.** The injury classification system recommended by Verdan[5] includes eight anatomically based zones. *(From Blair WF, Steyers CM: Extensor tendon injuries. Orthop Clin North Am 23:142, 1992.)*

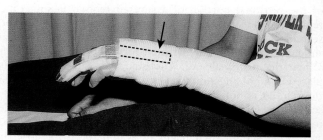

Figure 48–11 An effective way to fully immobilize a finger with a tendon laceration is to incorporate an aluminum foam splint into the middle layers *(arrow)* of a standard dorsal plaster/fiberglass short arm dorsal splint.

Zone 7 and 8 Injuries

Zones 7 and 8 consist of the area over the wrist and the dorsal forearm, respectively.[1] Extensor tendon lacerations in these regions can be quite complex and are therefore not repaired in the ED. Because of the close proximity of extensor tendons in the distal forearm, lacerations such as stab wounds may appear innocuous but often result in multiple tendon lacerations. At the wrist level, extensor tendons are covered by a retinaculum that is lined with synovium. Although this tissue allows smooth gliding of tendons during normal activity, the presence of synovium increases the risk for adhesions after tendon repair. In addition, lacerated tendons in the wrist and distal forearm may retract away from the site of initial injury. This may make tendon retrieval and repair quite difficult and may necessitate incision of the retinaculum and exploration of one or more of the compartments.

As a result of the potential complexity of these injuries, all tendon lacerations in zones 7 and 8 require formal surgical exploration and repair. ED management of these patients includes local wound care with primary repair of the skin and placement of a volar splint with 35° of extension at the wrist and 10° to 15° of flexion at the MCP joints. These patients should be promptly referred to a hand surgeon so that repair may be undertaken within 1 week of injury.

Zone 6 Injuries[1,3,6]

Zone 6 consists of the area over the dorsum of the hand. Extensor tendon injuries in this region frequently result from lacerations owing to broken glass or another sharp object. Common pitfalls in ED management of these injuries are usually related to failure to recognize that the tendon has been injured. It is important to remember that these tendons are superficially located, partial tendon lacerations may occur, and weak extension of a digit is possible in the presence of a complete tendon laceration because of transfer of extensor function through the juncturae tendini. Lacerations of the EIP or EDM tendons are evidenced by an inability to independently extend the index or little fingers, respectively. All of these pitfalls can be avoided if a careful physical examination is performed, including a thorough wound exploration under sterile conditions using a tourniquet, adequate local anesthesia, and good lighting.

Extensor tendon injuries in zone 6 are usually appropriate for repair in the ED. Because of the juncturae tendini, extensor tendons in zone 6 are less likely to retract than those in zone 7 or 8; however, the severed tendon may retract when the injury is more proximal. The distal end of a severed tendon is usually easy to find by passively extending the patient's affected digit to bring the end into view. Retrieval of the proximal portion of a severed tendon is sometimes required and usually can be accomplished in the ED. Before searching for the proximal end of the tendon, the clinician should have a 4-0 nylon suture loaded onto a needle holder. When the proximal end is located, this suture should be placed as a holding suture as far proximal as possible so that the tendon is not lost again. It is often necessary to use a scalpel to extend the wound proximally in a direction parallel to the course of the injured tendon to obtain adequate exposure. One should then begin to search for the tendon by lifting up this overlying skin with a forceps and inspecting the proximal portion of the wound. Sometimes, the blood-stained end of a tunnel can be seen; this may contain the proximal end of the tendon. By gently placing a small hemostat or toothed forceps up this tunnel, the tendon stump can often be pulled into view.

Once both ends of the injured tendon have been located, the technique used for repair depends on the size and shape of the tendon. Whereas larger, round tendons can accommodate sutures that pass through the core of the tendon, smaller or flat tendons are difficult to repair using this technique. Most of the tendons in zone 6 can be repaired with either a modified Kessler or a modified Bunnell core suture technique, using 4-0 nonabsorbable suture (Fig. 48–12). Both of these techniques involve first placing a single suture into half of the cut tendon. The suture is placed into the tendon core by inserting the suture needle into the exposed, cut end and then weaving the suture through the lateral tendon margins. Next, the same suture is placed through the core of the opposite half of the cut tendon. The suture ends are tied in a square knot in between the cut ends of the tendon, bringing the two halves together.

Smaller tendons may be repaired using a figure-of-eight or horizontal mattress suture (see Fig. 48–12). Small, tapered needles should be used to avoid tearing the tendon. In a cadaver study comparing these multiple suture techniques, it was found that the modified Bunnell technique provided the strongest extensor tendon repair.[7] In addition, this technique produced no gaping between the repaired tendon ends and minimized the post repair restriction of flexion at the MCP and proximal interphalangeal (PIP) joints. It is important to passively test the degree of flexion at the MCP joint after a zone 6 tendon repair to be certain that the tendon has not been excessively shortened.

To improve the tensile strength of the repair, a number of other suture techniques may be used.[4] One option is to increase the number of suture strands that cross the repair site (e.g., four strands rather than two). A cadaver study that compared various four-strand tendon repair techniques concluded that the Massachusetts General Hospital (MGH) technique was more resistant to gap formation than either the Krackow-Thomas or the four-strand modified Bunnell technique.[8] However, this cadaver model could not assess tendon shortening or subsequent range of motion.[9] Another way to improve tensile strength is to place a peripheral suture in addition to the core suture. A running suture can be placed circumferentially around the repair site using synthetic, absorbable material (e.g., polyglycolic acid, polyglactin, polydioxanone). Alternatively, sutures may be placed laterally along both sides

Figure 48–12 Suture techniques used in extensor tendon repair.

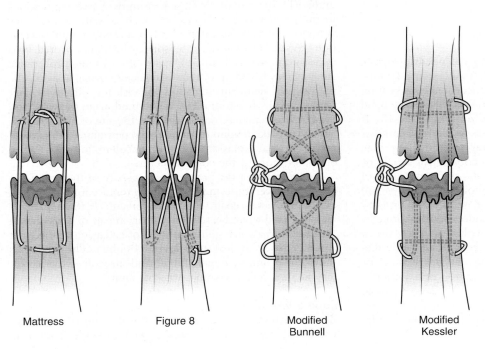

Mattress   Figure 8   Modified Bunnell   Modified Kessler

of the tendon, starting at about 1 cm on either side of the repair site. The ultimate choice of repair technique will depend largely upon the treating clinician's familiarity with extensor tendon repair as well as the size of the tendon.

The approach to partial extensor tendon lacerations is not well defined, and no definitive standard of care exists. One evidence-based analysis identified 141 papers in its literature search, but none were relevant to the question of partial extensor tendon injury repair.[10] The authors concluded that there is no direct evidence to assist in answering this question. Given the lack of literature on the subject, a reasonable approach may be to extrapolate from data on flexor tendon injuries. It has been demonstrated that many partial flexor tendon lacerations do well without repair,[11] but disagreement still remains among hand surgeons concerning the need for repair of these injuries. In a survey of hand surgeons, 30% of respondents repaired all partial flexor tendon lacerations, and 45% of respondents repaired only lacerations with greater than 50% cross-sectional area involvement.[12] Except at the wrist level, extensor tendons are not covered with synovium and are less likely than flexor tendons to develop adhesions after repair. This encourages some authors to recommend repair of most partial extensor tendon lacerations. Although the ideal approach to these injuries is not known, it is reasonable to consider repair of partial extensor tendon lacerations to be optional if less than 50% of the cross-sectional area is involved. However, such injuries must be splinted for 3 to 4 weeks to ensure that a partial laceration is not converted into a complete injury. Skin closure, splinting, and referral for follow-up is a standard approach to unsutured partial extensor tendon lacerations.

After repair of a lacerated EDC tendon in zone 6, a plaster or fiberglass volar splint should be applied so that the wrist is in 45° of extension, the affected MCP joint is in neutral (0° of flexion), and the unaffected MCP joints are in 15° of flexion. The PIP and distal interphalangeal (DIP) joints should be allowed full range of motion. After 10 days, the MCP joints are allowed 20° to 30° of flexion. If there is an isolated EIP or EDM tendon injury, then only the index or little finger must be included in this splint. Dynamic extension splinting may be used as early as 2 days after tendon repair, so close follow-up is recommended.[13]

Zone 5 Injuries[14,15]

Zone 5 consists of the area over the MCP joint. Open injuries in this region should be considered secondary to a human tooth bite until proven otherwise (Fig. 48–13). This is especially true if the injury occurs over the first or second MCP joint, because this is frequently the location of a clenched-fist ("fight-bite") injury. ED evaluation must begin with a careful and persistent history and physical examination, although patients' reluctance to admit to punching someone in the mouth is notorious. The wound should be inspected through its full range of motion, because the position of the EDC tendon changes with hand position. It is generally recommended that radiographs be obtained in all of these injuries to evaluate for metacarpal head fractures, air in the joint space, or presence of a foreign body such as a tooth fragment (Fig. 48–14).[13]

If, after a thorough evaluation, it is determined that a human bite to this region has resulted in a superficial skin laceration only, without injury to the underlying tendon or joint, outpatient management is appropriate. The wound should be copiously irrigated and left open. A volar splint is

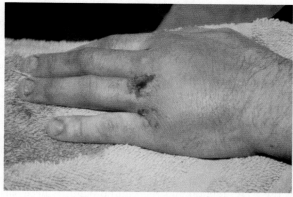

Figure 48–13 Regardless of this patient's history, this wound is highly suggestive of a human bite injury, vehemently denied by this patient. Human bites cause *extensor tendon injuries, fractures, and joint capsule injuries and can harbor foreign bodies.*

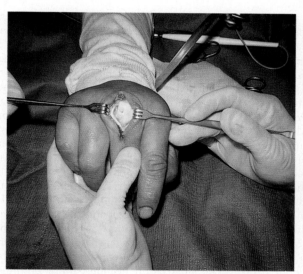

Figure 48–14 This patient stated that he sliced his hand on a piece of metal at work (expecting a Workers Compensation claim), but was unable to explain the chipped bone and *piece of tooth* that was found in the wound on exploration. Note that this puncture type wound had to be significantly extended to adequately visualize the extent of injury.

applied with the wrist in 45° of extension, the MCP joints in the neutral position (0° of flexion), and the hand dressed with a bulky dressing. Some authors recommend that 3 to 5 days of prophylactic antibiotics be given to these patients, and patients should be seen in 24 to 36 hours for a repeat examination to evaluate for wound infection. As mentioned previously, there are inadequate prospective data to prove or disprove the value of prophylactic antibiotics for extensor tendon injuries, and no universally accepted standard of care exists.

If a human bite results in tendon damage, including partial or complete laceration, some clinicians opt for admission and intravenous antibiotics. However, no specific standard of care exists. Outpatient therapy is acceptable in the reliable patient who has access to follow-up. Delayed closure with tendon evaluation/repair should be undertaken by a hand surgeon after 7 to 10 days of antibiotics.[3,13] Primary closure of even seemingly clean and well-irrigated human bites in this region is not advisable because of the increased risk of wound infection as well as the potential for septic destruction of the MCP joint if it is violated. If an open joint is noted on physical examination, a more aggressive approach is warranted. Such patients are generally admitted for intravenous antibiotics, after copious irrigation.[3,13] However, after initial ED treatment (aggressive wound care and initial intravenous antibiotics), there may be a role for outpatient therapy in selected cases. If a patient suffers a zone 5 tendon injury and it can be determined with complete certainty that it was caused by a relatively clean, sharp object rather than by a human bite, primary closure is appropriate. Referral of these injuries to a hand surgeon is a common practice, given the complexities of the injury and the sequelae. Careful repair of lacerations to both the EDC tendon and the sagittal bands is necessary to prevent subluxation of the EDC tendon away from the center of the metacarpal head. Initial ED management of non–human bite injuries is often limited to skin closure, splinting as described earlier, and referral to a hand surgeon within 1 to 5 days.

Closed extensor tendon injuries in zone 5 usually result from the acute or recurrent application of compressive forces to the MCP joint capsule. Closed injuries in this region are sometimes referred to as *boxer's knuckle*. Repetitive closed injury to the MCP joint region can produce small tears of the EDC tendon, the sagittal bands, or the joint capsule. These patients tend to present with chronic and recurrent pain and swelling at the MCP joint region and usually have normal radiographs. Acute trauma may result in the same injuries or cause more severe damage to the extensor hood. Such patients may have complete disruption of the extensor mechanism, including damage to the central tendon and the sagittal bands. The MCP joint is swollen, has decreased mobility, and may exhibit an extensor lag. Traumatic subluxation of the EDC tendon may be present, usually involving the middle finger with subluxation to the ulnar side (Fig. 48–15). Dislocation to the radial side is less common, likely due to juncturae tendinae on the ulnar side that can compensate for injuries to the ulnar sagittal band.[16] The subluxation becomes more prominent with flexion at the MCP joint. Controversy exists regarding

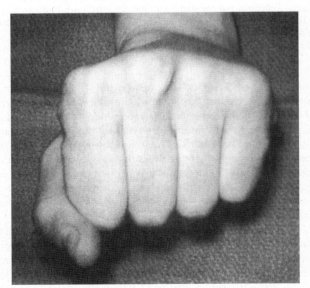

Figure 48–15 Ulnar dislocation of the extensor tendon of the metacarpophalangeal (MCP) joint of the middle finger. This is often treated with splinting with full recovery. *(From Leddy JP, Dennis TR: Tendon injuries. In Strickland JW, Rettic AC [eds]: Hand Injuries in Athletes. Philadelphia, WB Saunders, 1992, p 196.)*

the initial management of closed injuries to this region. Whereas some authors prefer initial surgical repair,[15] others use an initial trial of extension splinting in some or all cases.[3,13,14,16] Splinting the MCP joint in neutral or slight flexion for 6 weeks has been recommended for dislocations presenting within 3 weeks of injury, with operative repair reserved for more delayed presentations or patients who fail splint therapy.[13]

Zone 4 Injuries[14]

Zone 4 consists of the area over the dorsal aspect of the proximal phalanx between the MCP and the PIP joints. The extensor tendon is a broad, flat structure in this region and is relatively easy to repair. Because the extensor tendon is flat and conforms to the roundness of the proximal phalanx, tendon injuries in this area usually result from a laceration and are almost always incomplete. As a result, extension at the PIP joint is usually not impaired. It is therefore imperative that all of these wounds be explored carefully, remembering that the extensor tendon lies immediately beneath the thin overlying skin. Tendons tend not to retract in this area, so close inspection will usually result in location of the injured tendon.

A hand surgeon usually repairs central slip lacerations or any laceration that results in an extension lag at the PIP joint. The decisions of whether to repair a partial tendon laceration and whether it should be repaired by the emergency clinician in this zone are best discussed with the consulting hand surgeon. In general, because of the duality of the extensor system in this region, lacerations of a single lateral slip can either be repaired with 5-0 nonabsorbable sutures or be left unrepaired and splinted. A running suture or simple interrupted sutures with buried knots are appropriate for this area. Postrepair splinting depends on the presence of tension at the repair site. Minor lacerations in zone 4 that do not result in tension on the repair site can be treated with a finger guard for 7 to 10 days and early range of motion. Larger lacerations or those that result in tension at the repair site are usually treated in a splint that extends from the forearm to the digit for 3 to 6 weeks. The splint should be applied so that the wrist is in 30° of extension, the MCP joints at 30° of flexion, and the PIP joint in neutral position. Fingers should be grouped so that either digits 2 and 3 or digits 3 through 5 are immobilized.

It is important to recognize that complex partial tendon lacerations (e.g., a laceration of a lateral slip resulting from a saw) in zone 4 may result in damage to the gliding layer located between the tendon and the bone. If the patient is still able to actively extend the digit at the PIP joint, then these complex partial tendon lacerations are best managed by débriding the frayed tendon ends and splinting the digit in extension rather than attempting to suture the damaged tendon. The splint should be worn for 10 days, followed by active range of motion.

Zone 3 Injuries[1,13,15]

Zone 3, the area over the PIP joint, is a common site of both closed and open injury. Open injury usually results from laceration with a sharp object. It is imperative that these wounds be carefully explored in the ED to rule out penetration of the joint capsule. Patients with wounds that are suspected of penetrating the joint are generally taken to the operating room for surgical exploration, irrigation, and treatment with intravenous antibiotics, but protocols vary.

Zone 3 tendon lacerations can result in long-term deformity if not carefully repaired, and patients with such injuries are commonly referred to a hand surgeon. Partial lacerations of the central slip or lateral bands are managed variably, and it is advisable to discuss these injuries with the consulting hand surgeon. Lacerations in this area may sometimes result in a complete central slip injury. This may present as an acute boutonnière ("buttonhole") deformity, in which the PIP joint rests in 60° of flexion. The presentation may be subtler, however, and may be noticeable only by weakened extension at the PIP joint or incomplete extension by only a few degrees.

The boutonnière deformity develops when the central slip is ruptured by an open or closed mechanism, leading to unopposed action of the flexor digitorum superficialis tendon (Fig. 48–16). This results in flexion at the PIP joint, protrusion of the head of the proximal phalanx between the two lateral bands, and disruption of the triangular ligament. When this occurs, the lateral bands are displaced volar to the axis of motion of the PIP joint. The lateral bands then paradoxically become flexors of the PIP joint. In addition, the extensor hood mechanism is pulled more proximally, resulting in increased tension on the terminal extensor mechanism and hyperextension at the DIP joint. Thus, the boutonnière deformity consists of flexion of the PIP joint with hyperextension at the DIP joint.

Open central slip injuries are usually managed operatively, and complex injuries may require direct attachment of the tendon to bone or tendon reconstruction. If the consulting hand surgeon chooses not to repair the tendon injury immediately, the skin should be closed and a plaster splint applied in the same fashion as described for zone 4 injuries. Thermoplastic splints allow splinting of the hand without involvement of the wrist but are generally not available in the ED setting. These patients should be promptly referred to a hand surgeon so that repair may be undertaken within 1 week of injury.

Patients with closed injuries to zone 3 present commonly to the ED. They may complain of a direct blow to the dorsal

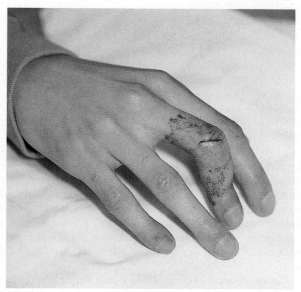

Figure 48–16   Boutonnière deformity. This can be an open or a closed injury. Note flexion of the PIP joint and extension of the distal interphalangeal (DIP) joint, from a laceration of the central slip mechanism (see Fig. 48–17).

PIP joint or of a "jammed" finger. This injury occurs when an object such as a ball delivers a sudden axial loading force with forced flexion of the PIP joint while it is extended. These patients commonly complain of a painful, swollen PIP joint, which often makes the examination difficult. Some of these injuries may represent PIP joint dislocations that were spontaneously or manually reduced before the patient's ED presentation. The tendon injury that is important to recognize in this setting is an occult isolated central slip rupture. Patients may have decreased extension at the PIP joint, but extension is usually normal because the lateral bands are the primary extenders of this joint. With forced extension against resistance, patients usually have pain and may have decreased strength. To eliminate pain as the cause of decreased mobility, it may be helpful to test PIP extension against resistance after performing a digital block. With acute central slip rupture, PIP joint extension may be particularly weak when the MCP and wrist joints are held in maximal flexion. In this position, a 15° or greater loss in active extension is highly suggestive of a central slip injury.[15] The Elson test may also help identify this injury[17] (Fig. 48–17).

The boutonnière deformity usually does not develop in patients with closed zone 3 injuries until 10 to 21 days after injury. The only way to prevent this deformity is to have a high index of suspicion for its presence and treat these patients conservatively. It is advisable that all patients with a swollen, tender PIP joint and pain with flexion or extension be splinted and referred for close follow-up. A dorsal splint should be applied overlying the PIP joint, keeping it in full extension. This can be accomplished using an aluminum foam-backed splint or a Bunnell ("safety pin") splint, although the latter may not be available in the ED.[13] The MCP and DIP joints should be left free to have full, active range of motion (Fig. 48–18). If a central slip attachment fracture is present, orthopaedic consultation is recommended because these patients may require surgical internal fixation.[18]

Zone 1 and 2 Injuries[1,3,13,15]

Zones 1 and 2 consist of the area over the DIP joint and the middle phalanx, respectively. In zone 2 the cojoined lateral bands come together to form the TEM and are held together, in part, by the triangular ligament. The TEM inserts on the base of the distal phalanx and allows extension at the DIP joint. Complete disruption of the TEM results in inability to extend at the DIP joint. Because of the unopposed action of the flexor digitorum profundus (FDP) tendon, the DIP joint rests in the flexed position. This is known as a *mallet deformity* of the finger (Fig. 48–19).

Tendon lacerations in zones 1 or 2 that result in a partial or complete mallet deformity generally warrant discussion with a hand surgeon (Fig. 48–20). Management consists of repair of the lacerated tendon and postrepair immobilization. Some surgeons will use only an external splint; others prefer placement of a K-wire through the distal phalanx into the middle phalanx to help stabilize the joint. One technique for tendon repair involves placement of a roll-type suture (dermatotenodesis), which incorporates the tendon and overlying skin into a single suture[1,13] (Fig. 48–21). The DIP joint is then splinted in full extension for at least 6 weeks. Occult partial tendon lacerations are important to recognize to prevent development of a mallet deformity. If there is a partial tendon laceration in zone 1 or 2 that does not result in any extension lag, the approach to repair is variable, and it is advisable to discuss the repair with the consulting hand surgeon. In

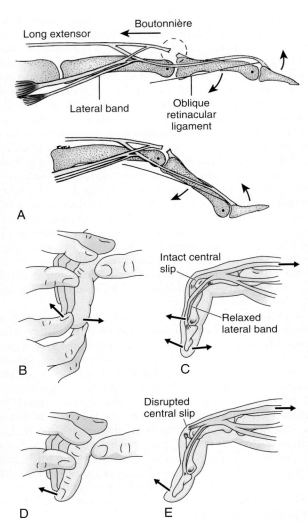

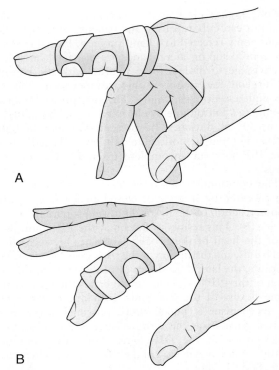

Figure 48–18 *A,* Boutonnière splint. *B,* This splint allows active flexion at the MCP and DIP joints.

Figure 48–17 *A,* Diagram of a boutonnière deformity. *B–E,* The Elson test for early diagnosis of an acute rupture of the central slip of the EDC tendon. Such rupture results in boutonnière deformity, in which the DIP joint is hyperextended, as shown. *B,* With the patient's finger flexed (over a straight edge) at the PIP joint, the examiner palpates the dorsal surface of the middle phalanx. *C,* If the central slip is intact, PIP joint flexion causes the slip to tighten distally, thereby relaxing the lateral bands and leaving distal phalanx flail (*arrows*). Thus, when the patient was asked to extend the digit, the examiner feels pressure that is necessarily being exerted by an intact central slip. *D and E,* If the central slip is disrupted, however, the examiner feels no pressure on the dorsum of the middle phalanx as the patient tries to extend the digit. It is possible for the patient to extend the injured finger successfully only by hyperextending (by action of the lateral bands) (*arrows, D and E*).

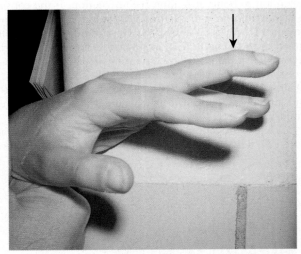

Figure 48–19 Mallet finger deformity (*arrow;* also see Fig. 49–41). *(From Leddy JP, Dennis TR: Tendon injuries. In Strickland JW, Rettic AC [eds]: Hand Injuries in Athletes. Philadelphia, WB Saunders, 1992, p 180.)*

general, partial tendon lacerations of less than 50% of the tendon area that do not result in an extension lag may be splinted in extension for 7 to 10 days with or without repair of the tendon itself.[13] Partial tendon lacerations of more than 50% that do not result in an extension lag may be repaired by a hand surgeon or an emergency clinician who is experienced in the repair of these injuries. In either case, it is advisable to discuss whether tendon repair will occur in the ED or the operating room with the consultant hand surgeon.

If the zone 1 or 2 partial tendon laceration is repaired in the ED, it can be approximated using a combination of running and cross-stitch sutures,[13] using 5-0 nonabsorbable suture material. It is important that the tendon ends be approximated but not pulled too tightly; otherwise, joint stiffness and limitation of flexion will occur. After repair of a partial tendon laceration, the DIP joint should be splinted in extension for 6 weeks, followed by 2 to 4 weeks of night splinting and active range-of-motion exercises. Patients should be warned after tendon repair that there is likely to be some residual loss of flexion at the DIP joint, even in the best case.

Closed injuries in zones 1 and 2 may result in a partial or complete mallet deformity depending on the injury pattern. These injuries are usually caused by an axial loading force with forced flexion of the DIP joint while it is being held in extension. A common ED presentation of this injury is a

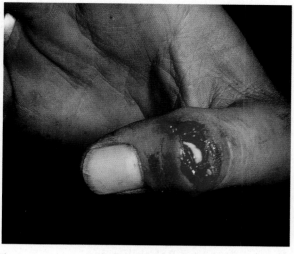

Figure 48–20 An open mallet finger can be surgically repaired.

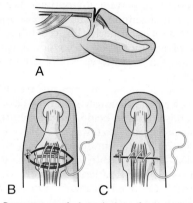

Figure 48–21 *Dermatotenodesis technique for zone 1 extensor tendon repair. A, Fresh lacerations of the extensor mechanism over the distal joint with mallet finger deformity are repaired by a running-type suture, which simultaneously approximates the skin and tendon (B and C). A small dressing is applied along with a splint, which maintains the joint in full extension. The sutures are removed at 10–12 days, but the splint is continued for a total of 6 wk. (A–C, Adapted from Baratz ME, Schmidt CC, Sugar AM, et al: Extensor tendon injuries. In Green DP [ed]: Operative Hand Surgery, 5th ed. Philadelphia, copyright 2005 by Churchill Livingstone, an imprint of Elsevier Inc., p 190.)*

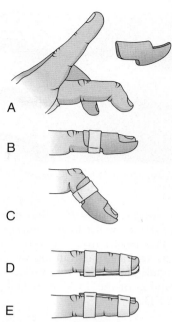

Figure 48–22 **A proper mallet finger splint.** Either a commercially available volar plastic splint (Stack mallet finger splint) (*A–C*) or a volar or dorsal aluminum foam splint (*D* and *E*) may be used. The splint should allow easy motion of the PIP joint. (*A–E, Adapted from Doyle JR: Extensor tendons—Acute injuries. In Green DP [ed]: Operative Hand Surgery, 4th ed. New York, Churchill Livingstone, 1999, p 1967.)*

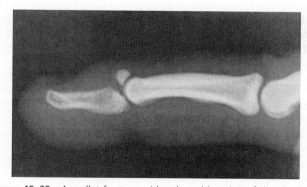

Figure 48–23 A mallet fracture with volar subluxation of the distal phalanx.

patient who complains of pain and swelling at the DIP joint after a ball strikes her or his fingertip.

Closed tendon injuries in this region can generally be classified into three types. In the first type of injury, there is a closed rupture of the TEM. The second type of injury is an avulsion fracture of the dorsal lip of the distal phalanx. This fracture is intra-articular, but there is no volar displacement of the remaining portion of the distal phalanx. Both type 1 and type 2 injuries can be treated by splinting in full extension for 6 weeks. The splint should hold the DIP joint in extension while allowing free range of motion of the PIP joint (Fig. 48–22). The splint can be constructed from an aluminum, foam-backed splint or from a prefabricated Stack splint. A Cochrane review of treatment for mallet finger injuries found inadequate data to establish the most effective type of splint.[19]

The third type of closed injury is an intra-articular avulsion fracture of the dorsal lip of the distal phalanx with volar displacement of the remaining portion of the distal phalanx (Fig. 48–23). Normally, the DIP collateral ligaments hold the distal phalanx in place; however, if there is a large-enough fracture fragment (usually > 50% of the articular surface), then the remaining distal phalanx fragment displaces in the volar direction secondary to unopposed action of the FDP tendon. When volar displacement of the distal phalanx occurs, this injury may require more aggressive treatment for an optimal outcome.[15] Unfortunately, there are not adequate published randomized, controlled trials comparing operative versus conservative treatment of these injuries.[19] Operative repair usually involves placement of a K-wire and open reduction and internal fixation of the fracture. It is important to remember that it is the presence of volar subluxation, not the size of the avulsion fracture, that is most often considered when determining the need for operative management.

Any injury, whether open or closed, that results in a complete disruption of the TEM may result in a swan-neck

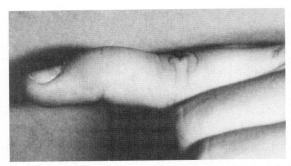

Figure 48–24 A swan-neck deformity. *(Courtesy of Raymond G. Hart and Joseph E. Kutz.)*

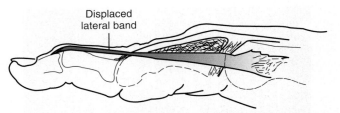

Displaced lateral band

Figure 48–25 **Diagram of the swan-neck deformity.** Lateral bands have displaced dorsal to the axis of the PIP joint, where they extend the joint and allow the DIP joint to flex. *(From Rizio L, Belsky MR: Finger deformities in rheumatoid arthritis. Hand Clin 12:531, 1996.)*

deformity (Figs. 48–24 and 48–25). This deformity consists of flexion at the DIP (a mallet finger) and hyperextension at the PIP joint. This results from a dorsal and proximal displacement of the lateral bands causing increased extension forces on the middle phalanx. This complication often can be avoided if disruption of the TEM is diagnosed and treated correctly in the ED.

Complications

All extensor tendon repairs are subject to the usual complications of wound infection and skin breakdown secondary to prolonged splinting. Tendon rupture is a rare complication after tendon repair and may result from inadequate suture technique or premature motion against resistance. It is important when extensor tendons are repaired for at least five throws to be used and a square knot to be tied. All extensor tendon repairs require some period of complete immobilization during tendon healing, and the emergency clinician must stress the necessity for patient compliance.

Extensor tendon injuries in zone 7 tend to have the worst prognosis. Because of the presence of a synovial lining, postrepair adhesions may occur. The adhesions may lead to decreased excursion of the extensor tendons with resultant decreased mobility at the wrist. There may also be limitation of finger flexion when the wrist is flexed as well as finger extension when the wrist is extended. Because of the lack of synovium, the relatively simple anatomy, and the usual lack of associated injuries, zone 6 tendon injuries tend to have fewer complications than other areas of the hand. The tendons in zone 6, however, do have a tendency to shorten if the tendon ends are approximated too tightly. This may result in a restriction of PIP and MCP joint flexion. In addition, worse outcomes may occur in complex zone 6 tendon injuries when additional soft tissue or bony injuries are present.[20]

Zone 5 injuries are particularly prone to infection, because injuries in this region commonly occur from a human bite. In addition, if the extensor hood covering the MCP joint is not carefully repaired, subluxation of the EDC tendon may occur.[6] If complex partial tendon lacerations in zone 4 are managed too aggressively, tendon shortening and stiffness may result. As discussed previously, these injuries are often best managed with splinting alone. A common complication of zone 3 extensor tendon injuries is development of a boutonnière deformity. This usually results from failure to diagnose or adequately immobilize a central slip injury. Similarly, undiagnosed or improperly treated extensor tendon injuries in zones 1 and 2 may lead to either a swan-neck or a chronic mallet deformity of the digit. DIP joint splinting itself may result in skin ulceration or tape allergy, often presenting in the 2nd week of treatment.[13] Skin breakdown may be encouraged if the DIP joint is splinted in hyperextension, because of decreased skin perfusion.

Postrepair Care and Rehabilitation

Proper care after diagnosis and repair of an extensor tendon injury is extremely important for optimal patient outcome. Even the best initial tendon repair can have a poor result if subsequently treated improperly. The rehabilitation of tendon injuries has evolved since 1980 to include dynamic splinting and active range of motion exercises to obtain maximal motion of the affected digit.

Zones 1 and 2 injuries are usually treated with static splinting, as described previously. After 6 weeks, active range of motion exercises should begin. Night splinting is recommended for an additional 2 to 6 weeks.[1,13,15] Some authors also recommend wearing the splint during the day when performing heavy tasks.[13] It is advisable to give the patient a number of extra splints so that the patient (or family) can change the splint frequently to avoid pressure injury. During splint changes, it is important that the DIP joint be held in full extension either by using the other hand or by placing the finger against a table. If an extension lag develops at any time, continuous splinting must be repeated. Closed injuries of the central slip (zone 3) are often treated with a boutonnière splint for 4 to 6 weeks, followed by 2 to 6 weeks of gradual flexion exercises and night splinting. During the initial period of immobilization, the patient should be instructed to passively flex the DIP joint every hour to maintain gliding and proper position of the lateral bands.

Lacerations in zones 3 and 4 have traditionally been treated with static splinting from the forearm to digits. An alternative approach is to splint only the DIP and PIP joints in extension and begin a "short-arc-motion" protocol within 1 to 2 days of repair.[21] This consists of active motion at the PIP joint progressing from 0° to 30° the first 2 weeks to 0° to 50° in the 4th week. When compared with static splinting, this protocol may lead to better PIP and DIP joint flexion, without resulting in tendon rupture or boutonnière deformity. Dynamic extension splints are also proving to be useful for zone 3 and 4 tendon injury rehabilitation.[13,21,22]

Early motion after extensor tendon repair has been found to be most useful in zones 5 through 7. A dynamic extension splint is commonly used in which the wrist is extended 45° and all finger joints rest in the neutral position. A volar block allows 30° to 40° of MCP joint flexion, whereas a dynamic traction mechanism passively extends the digits. Dynamic splinting is started 1 to 3 days after repair. Active motion is added at 3 to 4 weeks, and resistance is added at 7 weeks. A randomized, controlled trial of zones 5 and 6 extensor tendon repairs found superior total active motion using dynamic splinting when compared with static splinting at 4 to 8 weeks, but not at 6 months. However, grip strength in the affected hand was improved at 6 months using dynamic splinting.[23] A short-arc-motion protocol with controlled active motion at the MCP joint has also been shown to be safe and effective when started 24 to 48 hours after repair.[6] One comparative trial reported that dynamic extension splinting and controlled active mobilization worked equally well for zones 5 and 6 tendon injuries.[24] All early range of motion protocols are most beneficial when managed closely by a skilled hand therapist. Patient age, associated injuries, suture type, and repair technique all affect the choice of rehabilitation protocol.[9] Most importantly, patients must be reliable and motivated to take advantage of early range of motion techniques. It is best to refer patients to a hand surgeon or hand therapist as soon as possible after repair so that rehabilitation can begin in a timely manner.

EXTENSOR TENDON INJURIES OF THE FOOT

The extensor tendons of the foot are less commonly injured than the extensor tendons of the hand and wrist. The most important extensors of the foot and ankle that may be presented with injuries in the ED are the tibialis anterior, extensor hallucis longus (EHL), and extensor digitorum longus (EDL) tendons.

The tibialis anterior muscle originates on the shaft of the tibia and interosseous membrane and inserts on the medial cuneiform and the base of the first metatarsal. The tibialis anterior extends the foot at the ankle joint and inverts the foot at the subtalar and transverse tarsal joints. Spontaneous rupture of the tibialis anterior tendon may be seen in both elderly and young patients who have been injured during athletic activity. Injury to this tendon commonly results from forceful attempted dorsiflexion of the ankle while it is held fixed in the plantar-flexed position.[25] Patients generally present with decreased strength of foot dorsiflexion because toe extensors are used to accomplish this motion. Ruptures or lacerations of the tibialis anterior tendon should be referred promptly to an orthopaedic surgeon for consideration of formal operative repair. In some cases, closed injuries to the tibialis anterior tendon may be managed nonoperatively, depending upon the extent of the patient's symptoms and functional impairment.[25]

The EDL and EHL tendons both originate from the shaft of the fibula and interosseous membrane. The EHL tendon inserts into the base of the distal phalanx of the great toe, and the EDL tendon divides into four branches that insert on toes two through five (Fig. 48–26). Both the EHL and the EDL tendons primarily result in extension of the toes and dorsiflexion at the ankle. The extensor digitorum brevis (EDB) and extensor hallucis brevis (EHB) muscles originate from the upper part of the calcaneus. The EHB tendon joins the lateral aspect of the EHL tendon prior to inserting on the great toe. The EDB muscle gives rise to three tendons that join the lateral side of the EDL tendons going to toes two through four (see Fig. 48–26).

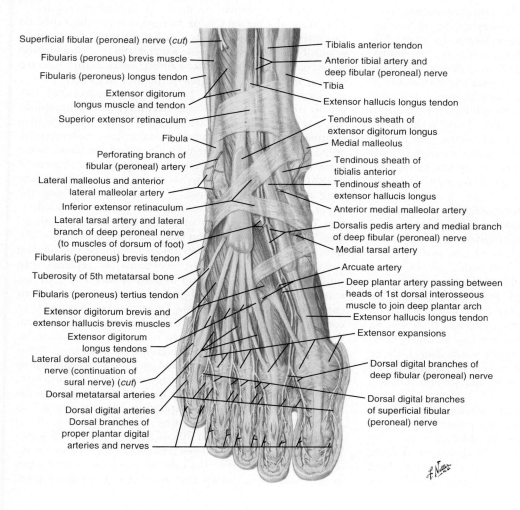

Superficial fibular (peroneal) nerve (*cut*)
Fibularis (peroneus) brevis muscle
Fibularis (peroneus) longus tendon
Extensor digitorum longus muscle and tendon
Superior extensor retinaculum
Fibula
Perforating branch of fibular (peroneal) artery
Lateral malleolus and anterior lateral malleolar artery
Inferior extensor retinaculum
Lateral tarsal artery and lateral branch of deep peroneal nerve (to muscles of dorsum of foot)
Fibularis (peroneus) brevis tendon
Tuberosity of 5th metatarsal bone
Fibularis (peroneus) tertius tendon
Extensor digitorum brevis and extensor hallucis brevis muscles
Extensor digitorum longus tendons
Lateral dorsal cutaneous nerve (continuation of sural nerve) (*cut*)
Dorsal metatarsal arteries
Dorsal digital arteries
Dorsal branches of proper plantar digital arteries and nerves

Tibialis anterior tendon
Anterior tibial artery and deep fibular (peroneal) nerve
Tibia
Extensor hallucis longus tendon
Tendinous sheath of extensor digitorum longus
Medial malleolus
Tendinous sheath of tibialis anterior
Tendinous sheath of extensor hallucis longus
Anterior medial malleolar artery
Dorsalis pedis artery and medial branch of deep fibular (peroneal) nerve
Medial tarsal artery
Arcuate artery
Deep plantar artery passing between heads of 1st dorsal interosseous muscle to join deep plantar arch
Extensor hallucis longus tendon
Extensor expansions
Dorsal digital branches of deep fibular (peroneal) nerve
Dorsal digital branches of superficial fibular (peroneal) nerve

Figure 48–26 Muscles of dorsum of foot: superficial dissection. *(Netter illustrations used with permission of Elsevier Inc. All rights reserved.)*

Injury to the EHL and EDL tendons may result from a sharp object lacerating the dorsum of the foot. Patients may present with weakness of, or an inability to extend, the involved toe. The examiner may be unable to palpate the injured tendon. Whether one should repair EHL or EDL tendon lacerations is controversial. However, many authors favor repair; failure to repair EDL tendons may result in a claw deformity of the adjacent toes.[26] Lacerations of the EHL and EDL tendons at the level of the ankle are usually repaired, whereas lacerations on the dorsum of the foot and the toe are managed variably. If the patient has significant pain or any flexion deformity of the involved toe, one should probably repair the lacerated tendon. Repair is also favored when both tendon ends are easily visualized in the wound and the patient is willing to undergo prolonged postrepair immobilization.[27] Because management of these injuries is controversial, it is advisable to discuss the care of these patients with the consulting orthopaedic surgeon. Extensor tendon repair of the foot is usually not performed in the ED setting. Superficial cutaneous nerves are easily injured on the dorsum of the foot during wound exploration, which can lead to the formation of a chronic, painful neuroma. If the injury is repaired in the ED, the technique for repair is similar to that used for the dorsum of the hand (zone 6). A posterior splint that includes the toes should be applied after tendon repair. The ankle should be splinted at 90° with the toes in the neutral position.

FLEXOR TENDON INJURIES

Flexor tendon injuries are more difficult to diagnose and more challenging to treat than extensor tendon injuries. In general, ED repair of flexor tendons is not performed by emergency clinicians. Anatomic and biomechanic issues, the physiology of flexor tendons and tendon healing, and follow-up rehabilitation/physical therapy issues are complex and formidable. A satisfactory outcome of an injured flexor tendon is more difficult to achieve than is a similar degree of injury to an extensor tendon. Unlike extensor tendons, flexor tendons are influenced by a number of pulley mechanisms. The tendon must glide through delicate tendon sheaths, so even a minor defect in tendon integrity is physiologically magnified (Fig. 48–27). In addition, flexor tendon injuries are often associated with nerve and vascular injuries.

The main clinical mandates for emergency clinicians are to diagnose, or consider, flexor tendon injuries; provide initial proper wound care; and expedite appropriate consultation and follow-up. Unlike the more superficial extensor tendons, flexor tendons are often buried deep within the hand and forearm, and it is often not possible to readily visualize the tendon in the recesses of a wound. Puncture wounds of the palm often injure flexor tendons, but deep puncture wounds prohibit visualization of the injured structures (Fig. 48–28). Therefore, a partial flexor tendon injury may be totally clinically silent until rupture occurs days or weeks later. Delayed repair of undiagnosed flexor tendons may be complicated by tendon retraction or scar formation, and tendon transfer/grafting may be necessary.

It may not be possible for the emergency clinician to diagnose the presence of all flexor tendon injuries, nor the full extent of such injuries, on the initial visit. Help may be obtained from a specialist if logistically possible, but generally, there is no mandate for such immediate on-site examination when questions about tendon integrity exist. Whereas consultation is advised before

definitive disposition, the same limitations in the examination would similarly confront a specialist. Individual scenarios and local protocols will guide the timing and degree of consultation in the ED.

Complete flexor tendon injuries are often readily apparent on physical examination, either by individual tendon testing or by the resting posture of the injured hand. Partial tendon lacerations are commonly clinically unappreciated because no functional deficit is evident. Clinical clues to a potential flexor tendon injury are weakness of flexor tendon function (difficult to evaluate in the acutely injured extremity), pain at the site of injury when performing active range of motion against resistance, or an abnormal resting posture of the hand (Fig. 48–29A and B), or by careful examination, which is always difficult in the child or uncooperative patient (see Fig. 48–29C and D). However, the clinician may not ever be able to arrive at a complete or accurate diagnosis without surgical exploration. It is counterproductive, and potentially harmful, to attempt extensive exploration of the deep recesses of the hand or forearm in the ED merely to visualize a suspected flexor tendon injury.

Completely transected flexor tendons are surgically repaired by a consultant, usually on an elective basis. Most hand surgeons are reluctant to perform a primary repair of a flexor tendon injury on ED patients and prefer to have the wound cleaned, the skin closed, and the patient schedule a subsequent definitive repair. The final outcome of flexor tendon surgery depends on multiple factors; however, surgical repair of most flexor tendons accomplished within 10 to 21 days of injury (delayed primary repair) generally manifests final outcomes similar to those of immediate repair.[28–30] Therefore, if a partial tendon laceration is not diagnosed on the initial visit and rupture is noted at the time of skin suture removal or wound check, immediate referral to a hand surgeon would be expected to produce a similar result as that expected had the injury been diagnosed at the time of injury.

Partial flexor tendon lacerations, if appreciated, are usually treated by careful wound cleaning, skin closure, splinting, and referral for reevaluation in 1 to 5 days. The definitive treatment of partial lacerations remains quite controversial. Some surgeons will explore partial tendon lacerations. Some experimental evidence suggests that surgical repair of partially lacerated tendons results in weaker tendons than if the tendons were not surgically repaired.[31] To further complicate the issues, some authors suggest no suturing and early mobilization of lacerated tendons of 25% to 95% cross-sectional area.[32] As a guideline, tendon lacerations of greater than 50% cross-sectional area are often sutured with specific surgical techniques, 25% to 50% of lacerations are repaired with simple or special sutures, and injuries of less than 25% are trimmed to promote normal gliding function.[30] All decisions concerning the type and timing of repair should be made in concert with a consultant. Some decisions concerning surgical repair of partial injuries cannot be made for weeks or months.

Following evaluation of a known or suspected flexor tendon injury, the skin is sutured and the hand splinted to protect the tendon and minimize retraction. Techniques vary, and initial splinting positions are likely inconsequential to the final outcome if the length of splinting does not exceed 7 to 14 days. As a guideline, splinting with the wrist in 30° of flexion, the MCP joints in 70° of flexion, and the IP joints flexed at 10% to 15% has been recommended.[33] There are no data to support or refute the value of prophylactic antibiotics in any soft tissue injury that has been properly cleaned.

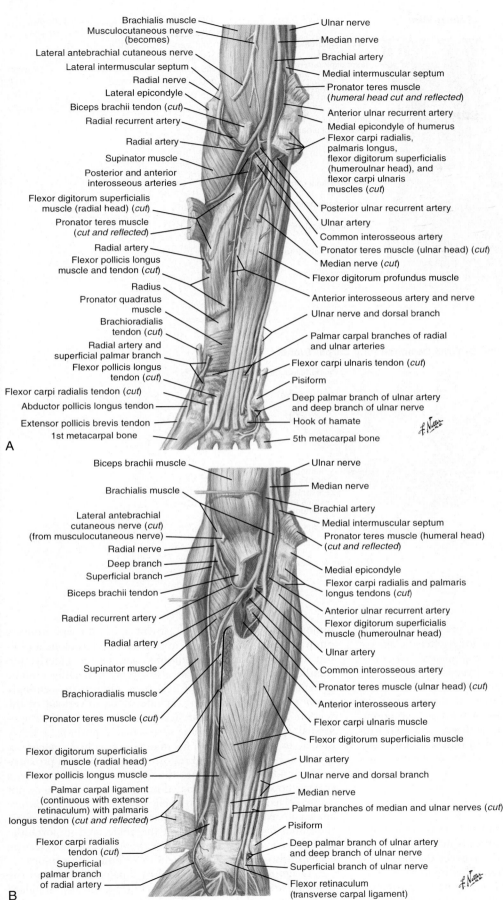

Figure 48–27 *A,* Muscles of forearm (deep layer): anterior view. *B,* Muscles of forearm (intermediate layer): anterior view.

Continued

Palmar View

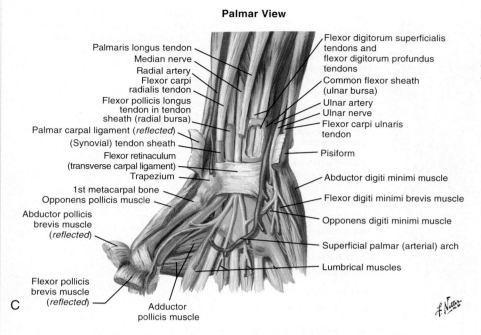

Palmaris longus tendon
Median nerve
Radial artery
Flexor carpi radialis tendon
Flexor pollicis longus tendon in tendon sheath (radial bursa)
Palmar carpal ligament (*reflected*)
(Synovial) tendon sheath
Flexor retinaculum (transverse carpal ligament)
Trapezium
1st metacarpal bone
Opponens pollicis muscle
Abductor pollicis brevis muscle (*reflected*)
Flexor pollicis brevis muscle (*reflected*)
Adductor pollicis muscle

Flexor digitorum superficialis tendons and flexor digitorum profundus tendons
Common flexor sheath (ulnar bursa)
Ulnar artery
Ulnar nerve
Flexor carpi ulnaris tendon
Pisiform
Abductor digiti minimi muscle
Flexor digiti minimi brevis muscle
Opponens digiti minimi muscle
Superficial palmar (arterial) arch
Lumbrical muscles

C

Figure 48–27, cont'd   *C,* Flexor tendons, arteries, and nerves at wrist: palmar view. *D,* Transverse cross-section of wrist demonstrates carpal tunnel. *(A–D, Netter illustrations used with permission of Elsevier Inc. All rights reserved.)*

Transverse Cross Section Of Wrist Demonstrating Carpal Tunnel

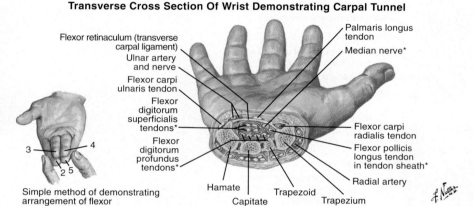

Flexor retinaculum (transverse carpal ligament)
Ulnar artery and nerve
Flexor carpi ulnaris tendon
Flexor digitorum superficialis tendons*
Flexor digitorum profundus tendons*
Palmaris longus tendon
Median nerve*
Flexor carpi radialis tendon
Flexor pollicis longus tendon in tendon sheath*
Radial artery
Hamate
Capitate
Trapezoid
Trapezium

Simple method of demonstrating arrangement of flexor digitorum superficialis tendons within carpal tunnel

D

*Contents of carpal tunnel

Although no definitive standard of care is promulgated, many clinicians prescribe 3 to 5 days of antibiotics effective against gram-positive organisms (including *Staphylococcus aureus*) if the tendon is injured. Antibiotics are recommended if the degree of contamination is significant, there has been delay in cleaning, there are unusual sources of injury, or if the patient is immunocompromised. Specific written instructions, with a definite follow-up timeframe outlined, and help with patient referral will likely improve final outcome, but *flexor tendon injuries often produce lifelong disability despite even ideal care in the ED.*

ACHILLES TENDON RUPTURE

An Achilles tendon rupture can lead to serious morbidity. Although definitive care of such injuries is not performed in the ED, it is important to make the correct diagnosis and institute proper and prompt referral. This injury is easy to miss, and it is not always diagnosed on the first visit (missed in about 25% of cases). It is usually initially considered a minor ankle sprain by both patient and clinician. Rupture often occurs in the presence of steroid use, quinolone antibiotic use, degenerative conditions, and in the elderly; but Achilles tendon rupture can also occur in healthy athletic patients, with no history of heel pain, often with seemingly *minor trauma.* Mechanisms include sudden overload of the tendon by forceful plantar flexion of the foot, as in recreational sports with jumping (basketball), pushing a heavy object, or stepping up. The injury is usually a *complete as opposed to a partial tear,* and rupture occurs 3 to 4 cm proximal to the tendon's insertion on the calcaneous. Occasionally, a snap or pop may be appreciated by the patient. Pain may not be perceived in the tendon itself, producing heel or diffuse ankle pain. Multiple structures plantar flex the foot; therefore, the initial result is weakness of the ankle, and importantly, there *is not complete loss of motion of the foot.* Characteristic ecchymosis may be evident in 48 to 72 hours after injury.

Diagnosis may be suggested by a palpable defect in the tendon, *but this can be subtle or absent* (Fig. 48–30). Standard radiographs will be normal. Magnetic resonance imaging

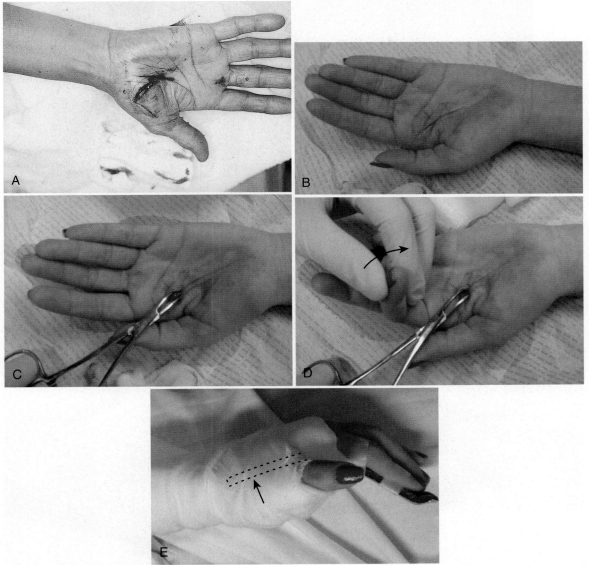

Figure 48–28 **Deep puncture wounds of the palm may injure flexor tendons.** *A,* The depth of this wound precludes extensive exploration to visualize the tendon. Partial tendon lacerations may still initially allow full function. Clues to a partial flexor tendon laceration include weakness of flexion or pain with attempts at flexion against resistance, but many partial lacerations are clinically silent. Despite full function, this wound's location and depth suggest the possibility of at least a partial tendon injury. The prudent course would include meticulous wound care, splinting, skin closure, and contact with a hand specialist to arrange reexamination in a *few days,* while cautioning the patient that a flexor tendon injury may be present and delayed repair for up to 1 to 3 weeks yields results comparable to immediate repair. Immediate repair is often eschewed due to swelling and wound contamination. Further care may be required. *B,* This palm laceration from the sharp top of a metal can seemed superficial. The function was normal. *C,* When examined with the fingers in extension, the tendon was readily visualized, a surprise to the clinician given the benign and superficial appearance of the laceration. The visualized tendon was intact. *D,* When the fingers were flexed (*arrow*), *the position of the hand when the injury occurred,* a 20–30% laceration of the tendon was demonstrated. *E,* This injury will do well with 3 weeks of splinting, and no tendon repair. Hand surgeon follow-up in a few days is prudent. Note the outrigger aluminum splint incorporated into a short arm plaster splint (*arrow;* see Fig. 48–11).

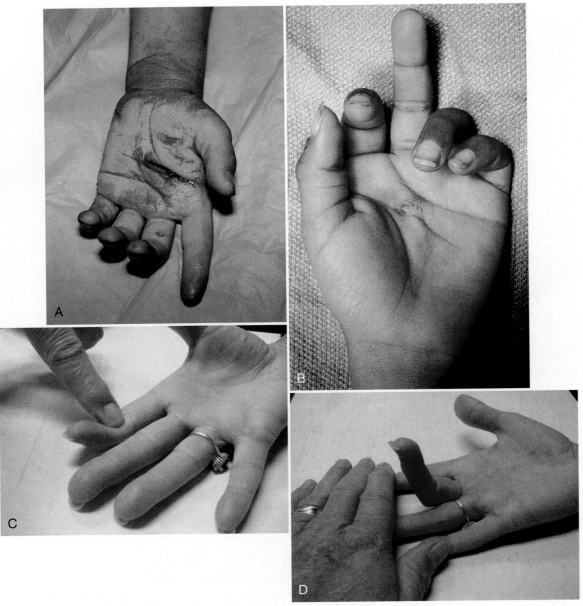

Figure 48–29 *A,* Note obvious abnormal resting posture of the hand. This boy's palm laceration involved the flexor tendons to his index finger. With his hand at rest, his index finger lies in extension, in contrast to his other fingers, which are partially flexed. *(Courtesy Robert Hickey, MD, Children's Hospital of Pittsburgh.) B,* The loss of digital cascade in the middle finger illustrated here should be indicative of a flexor tendon laceration without further exam. The small glass laceration in the palm accounts for the profundus laceration, apparent only in follow-up. Children are difficult to fully examine in the ED. Splinting and follow-up in a few days is prudent based on injury mechanism and location. *C,* The flexor digitorum profundus tendon is examined by immobilizing the digit in question and asking the patient to flex the DIP joint against resistance. *D,* The flexor digitorum superficialis tendon is examined by immobilizing the digits not being tested and asking the patient to flex the PIP joint against resistance. Pain and weakness associated with flexion against resistance may suggest a partial tendon laceration, but this is often a very subtle or inaccurate evaluation that must be repeated when pain and swelling have subsided.

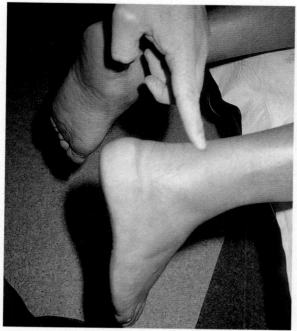

Figure 48–30 This patient complained of a sprained ankle of 3 day's duration after jumping up in a basketball game. There was moderate weakness of plantar flexion, but not complete loss. A defect in the Achilles tendon may be appreciated in some cases of Achilles tendon rupture, but not in this case. Note the characteristic bruising.

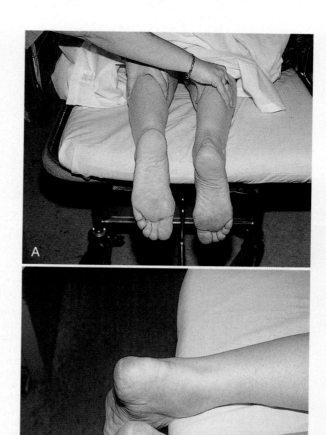

Figure 48–31 *A,* To perform the calf squeeze test (Thompson's test) place the patient prone on the stretcher with the feet overhanging the edge. *B,* Squeeze the calf and look for forceful passive plantar flexion of the foot. In this case, the left foot (note swelling and ecchymosis) did not move, confirming complete Achilles tendon rupture.

(MRI) is diagnostic. The calf squeeze test (Thompson's test) is a physical finding that is 96% to 100% sensitive. To perform this test, have the patient prone on a stretcher with the feet overhanging the edge. Squeeze the calf and observe for strong passive plantar flexion of the foot. If the foot does not move, a complete tear is diagnosed (Fig. 48–31). Treatment varies from conservative splinting to surgery and is controversial. Splinting the foot in mild plantar flexion can protect the tendon for follow-up in 1 to 5 days.

QUADRICEPS TENDON RUPTURE

Quadriceps tendon rupture is a serious injury with significant morbidity regardless of treatment. It is usually a problem for the elderly and those with systemic degenerative diseases, arthritis, or steroid use. It may be seen in younger patients, such as occurs after taking a basketball jump shot. Performance-enhancing steroid use is a risk factor. Although definitive treatment is not undertaken in the ED, early diagnosis may improve long-term outcome. As with Achilles tendon rupture, this condition is *not always initially suspected or diagnosed,* being missed by primary care providers in 20% to 30% of cases. The mechanism is a deceleration injury with the knee partially flexed, coupled with a strong quadriceps muscle contraction when the foot is fixed. The trauma can be seemingly minor, such as missing a step or jumping from a minor height. A common history is an elderly patient who is descending steps or walking off a curb, misses a step, and attempts to keep from falling. A popping or tearing sensation may be elicited. Pain may be deceptively minor. The rupture can be partial, but is more often complete. Rupture occurs just proximal to the patellar insertion, with or without an avulsion fracture of

the superior pole of the patella. Athletic patients may continue to play with a partial tear, but a complete rupture does not allow for ambulation. Bilateral complete rupture has been described, but the condition is usually unilateral.

A large hemarthrosis is usually produced, often prompting the incorrect diagnosis of a ligamentous injury (such as an anterior cruciate ligament rupture). A palpable defect superior to the patella may be appreciated, but diffuse swelling can hide this finding (Fig. 48–32). Lack of the expected defect can be misleading in the presence of a large hemarthrosis. In cases in which the history is one of only minor trauma and physical findings are subtle, malingering or noncooperation with the examination may be incorrectly contemplated by the clinician. The *supine* patient is *unable to actively extend the knee* or lift the straightened leg off the stretcher or the knee flexes when posterior thigh support is removed from the raised leg. Weak extension, especially in the sitting position, may be possible if portions of the medial and lateral retinacula are intact, even with a complete rupture of the central rectus femoris. With complete rupture, the patient cannot walk, and the knee gives way immediately. As one would intuit, however,

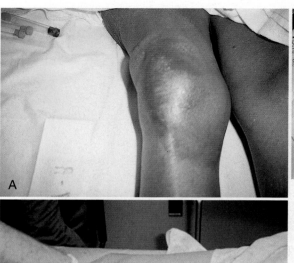
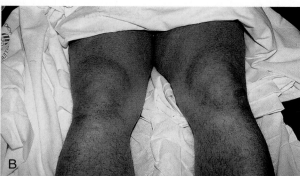
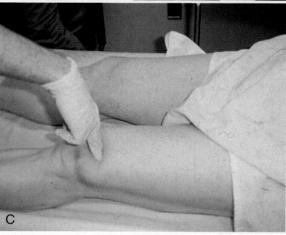

Figure 48–32 *A,* This elderly man lost his footing going down the stairs and missed *only a single step*. He felt a pop and was unable to walk. Arthrocentesis yielded a grossly bloody effusion. An obvious suprapetallar soft tissue defect, and the inability of straight leg raise while supine, made the diagnosis of a complete quadriceps tendon obvious. *B,* This man landed on both feet while jumping off a low curb and then collapsed. Pain was minimal and malingering was suspected. Diffuse soft tissue swelling, bilateral knee effusions, normal radiographs, and the ability to walk *with bilateral knee immobilizers* delayed the diagnosis of bilateral quadriceps tendon rupture until follow-up. *C,* A step off above the knee readily identified the complete quadriceps tendon rupture. The patient was unable to lift the leg off the stretcher, an activity that made the soft tissue defect obvious.

a knee immobilizer allows the patient to apparently walk normally. Partial tears may allow the patient to walk with a peculiar forward-leaning gait that helps support the knee in extension.

Plain radiographs are normal except for the occasional patellar avulsion fracture. MRI is definitive to identify nuances of the process. Partial tears may be treated conservatively; complete tears require surgical repair, usually as soon as the diagnosis is made. Delaying the diagnosis for 2 to 3 weeks makes recovery less complete and repair more problematic.

The postoperative period of recovery for the elderly is prolonged and difficult. Acute injuries diagnosed in the ED may be treated with a knee immobilizer and crutches with 1- to 2-day follow-up, but admission is often warranted to expedite definitive intervention.

 REFERENCES CAN BE FOUND ON EXPERT CONSULT

CHAPTER **49**

Management of Common Dislocations

Jacob W. Ufberg and Robert M. McNamara

Joint dislocations are frequently encountered among patients presenting to the emergency department (ED). They can range from a simple finger injury to limb- or life-threatening consequences of high-energy trauma. Although the dislocated joint is most often clinically obvious, the presentation may be obscured or masked by other injuries. Emergency clinicians must be capable of detecting and managing these injuries; appropriate timely referral to a consultant is often required for complex dislocation injuries.

This chapter addresses the diagnosis and management of joint dislocations. Keys to the clinical assessment and radiographic evaluation of these injuries are discussed along with methods of reduction. The emphasis of the chapter is on simple dislocations that should be diagnosed and initially managed in the ED. Fracture-dislocations that commonly require operative intervention and emergency orthopaedic consultation are not discussed.

PREPARATION OF THE PATIENT

Although many authors claim that their reduction method is well tolerated without premedication, they generally have not quantitatively measured the discomfort of their patients.[1-5] There are no rigid, generally accepted guidelines for the use of pharmacologic adjuncts in the management of dislocations. Each patient and presentation is unique and the treating clinician must use judgment as to whether premedication is required, which agent or agents to use, and what dose to give. In general, the editors suggest the judicious use of analgesia with or without sedation for the majority of reductions performed in the ED. The calm, cooperative patient may tolerate gentle reduction attempts of a major joint such as the shoulder, but even the most stoic of patients may be quite uncomfortable with the manipulations necessary for reduction of a dislocated finger. A radial head dislocation in a child is usually easily accomplished without analgesia; however, the reduction of a hip dislocation is unlikely to be successful without a significant amount of sedation and analgesia. Attempting any reduction technique in an extremely anxious patient without premedication will generally frustrate the operator and further upset the patient, and it may hinder a successful outcome. When multiple attempts are required, and significant force must be exerted owing to muscle spasm or an uncooperative patient, there is additional chance of producing complications during the reduction.

Verbal techniques for alleviating anxiety and discomfort are not to be discounted because they can be of great assistance during joint reduction. In field settings, simple hypnosis techniques have been successfully used for major joint dislocations.[6] In the ED, verbal reassurance and distracting conversation are useful adjuncts.

In most circumstances, analgesia or sedation of some sort, or both, will be required; generally the intravenous (IV) route for drug administration is the method of choice, because it allows for rapid relief of patient discomfort and facilitates repetitive dosing for titration to the desired effect (see Chapter 33, Systemic Analgesia and Sedation for Procedures). Alternatives to procedural sedation and analgesia include intra-articular injection of local anesthetics, hematoma blocks, peripheral nerve blocks, and regional anesthesia (see Chapters 29, Local and Topical Anesthesia; 31, Nerve Blocks of the Thorax and Extremities; and 32, Intravenous Regional Anesthesia, respectively).

GENERAL PRINCIPLES

The clinical assessment of the patient with a dislocation must include a search for other serious injuries, especially if the mechanism was of high energy. This is generally most important for hip, knee, and posterior sternoclavicular dislocations. For all dislocations, a detailed extremity neurovascular examination should be conducted before focusing attention on the injured joint.

Although many dislocations are clinically obvious, some may escape detection for some time while other injuries or issues dominate the clinical picture. A knee dislocation may be quite obvious in a 170-pound man who displays a deformity of the knee, but in a 400-pound patient, the knee may look deceivingly normal on first glance. The history and mechanism of injury can be quite helpful in certain circumstances. For example, a painful shoulder joint in a seizure patient should prompt assessment for a posterior shoulder dislocation, whereas a history of the knee striking the dashboard is a clue to the potential for a hip dislocation.

Carpal dislocations in the hand are often radiographically clandestine to the inexperienced clinician, but are clinically suggested by severe pain and swelling. Some dislocations will have been reduced prior to clinician assessment. A careful history will uncover these injuries and prompt the necessary assessment of the ligamentous integrity of the joint and the possibility of associated vascular injury and guide proper immobilization and follow-up care. *A dislocated, then spontaneously reduced, knee is a severe injury that often escapes detection by even the seasoned clinician's initial evaluation.* Other dislocations that commonly present in a reduced state include finger dislocations, patellar dislocations, and radial head subluxations.

Although the chance of a gentle reduction attempt causing a fracture or neurovascular injury is extremely low, careful evaluations before and after reduction, as well as documentation of the neurovascular status, are prudent. Often, the initial pain of the dislocation is distracting, and paresthesias or a weak pulse may not be readily apparent until the joint has been replaced. When the integrity of the pulse is in question, the *blood pressure* at the wrist or foot may be compared with that of the uninjured extremity, or a *pulse oximeter* may be applied to the distal fingers (Fig. 49–1).

Prereduction radiographs are generally recommended. Reasons for this include the difficulty in distinguishing a fracture-dislocation by clinical examination and the potential for medicolegal problems if the fracture is not identified prior to reduction attempts. More importantly, certain associated fractures predict a poor outcome from closed reduction and make orthopaedic consultation a consideration before such attempts. The obvious exceptions to this rule include suspected radial head subluxation in young children and clinical

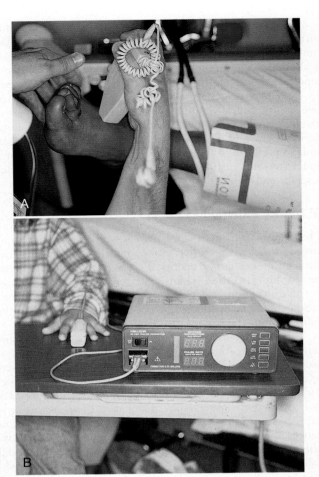

Figure 49–1 Significant vascular injuries from dislocations, such as the knee or ankle, are usually obvious, but an impaired distal circulation may be subtle or delayed owing to a slowly increasing intimal flap artery lesion. The standard techniques to assess vascular injury are the strength of the pulse and capillary refill; this should detect most arterial injuries. Taking the blood pressure distal to the injury with a cuff and Doppler (*A*) or applying a pulse oximeter distal to the injury and comparing the results with those of the uninjured extremity (*B*) may give some helpful clues to underlying vascular injuries.

films, or a previously noted minor fracture may be found to reside in an intra-articular location.[8]

The proper terminology for dislocations describes the relationship of the distal (or displaced) segment relative to the proximal bone or the normal anatomic structure. The terms *anterior* and *posterior* are used in most dislocations. Therefore, if the head of the humerus lies anterior to the glenoid fossa, the injury is an anterior shoulder dislocation. Similarly, if the olecranon lies behind the distal end of the humerus, the injury is a posterior elbow dislocation. In the hand, wrist, and foot, one uses the terms *dorsal* and *volar*. *Palmar* and *plantar* are sometimes used in place of volar to describe the position of the dislocated part. Dislocations can be *open* or *closed* and may have associated fractures requiring a separate description.

It is generally accepted that the sooner a dislocation is reduced, the better. This alleviates the patient's discomfort and corrects the distortion of surrounding soft tissue structures. In some studies, the success rate of reduction is higher when attempted closer to the time of injury.[2] However, there is no reason to forego an attempt at a closed reduction of an "old injury" in the vast majority of dislocations. Chronic dislocations of several days, weeks, or more are often difficult to reduce in a closed manner, but such presentations are infrequent.

A certain percentage of all types of dislocations are not amenable to closed reduction. Inability to complete a closed reduction is generally a result of the interposition of soft tissue structures or fracture fragments and not necessarily due to improper technique. If one has achieved sedation/analgesia adequate to permit relaxation of the patient's muscle tone, reduction should be relatively straightforward. When reduction under adequate sedation/analgesia is unsuccessful after several attempts, further attempts at closed reduction are inappropriate. Generally, orthopaedic consultation should be considered after two to three failed attempts.

Once an attempt at reduction is completed, the operator should recheck the neurovascular status that was documented before the reduction was performed. For the elbow, hand, and forefoot joints, passive range of motion is performed to assess the stability of the reduction and to ensure a smoothly gliding joint that is free of intra-articular obstruction. In addition to close monitoring of the medicated patient, proper aftercare involves adequate immobilization of the injured joint for comfort and to prevent repeat dislocation. Recommendations for follow-up care depend on the injury and its severity.

Timing of Reductions

Questions often arise concerning the necessity of immediate reduction versus delayed reduction, with the clinician fearing disastrous neurovascular consequence if a dislocation is not manipulated immediately upon arrival. In reality, there is rarely an instance in which some prereduction radiographs, even portable films, cannot be obtained before treatment. Even if the pulse is weak, or the fingers are numb, a few minutes' delay is usually acceptable in order to gain important radiographic information on the type of dislocation and the presence of an associated fracture and for documentation for the follow-up clinicians. Important clinical information may be difficult to obtain, or the specific initial injury may be impossible to reconstruct once the joint has been reduced (Fig. 49–2). Of equal importance, dislocation with concomitant neurovascular injuries should be reduced with the least amount of trauma possible, often requiring a few minutes for

circumstances in which radiographs are not readily available (e.g., in the wilderness). Obvious clinical conditions (i.e., vascular compromise or threatened skin penetration) may dictate the need for immediate reduction without x-rays; however, the few minutes required for initial radiographic evaluation rarely increase vascular/neurologic complications and provide very useful information to the consultant.

Some authors question the need for prereduction films in certain patients with obvious and/or recurrent anterior shoulder dislocations.[7,8] Although postreduction radiographs are traditionally obtained, the need for this in a clinically obvious successful shoulder joint relocation also has been questioned.[8,9] The editors strongly suggest postreduction films in virtually all patients who have had a dislocation reduced in the ED. Patients who have received sedatives and opioids may not remember the actual successful reduction or the immediate postreduction period. A reinjury after release from the ED without radiographic corroboration of a successful reduction can raise questions about the adequacy of the initial procedure. Occasionally, a fracture is detected on postreduction radiographs that was not obvious on the initial

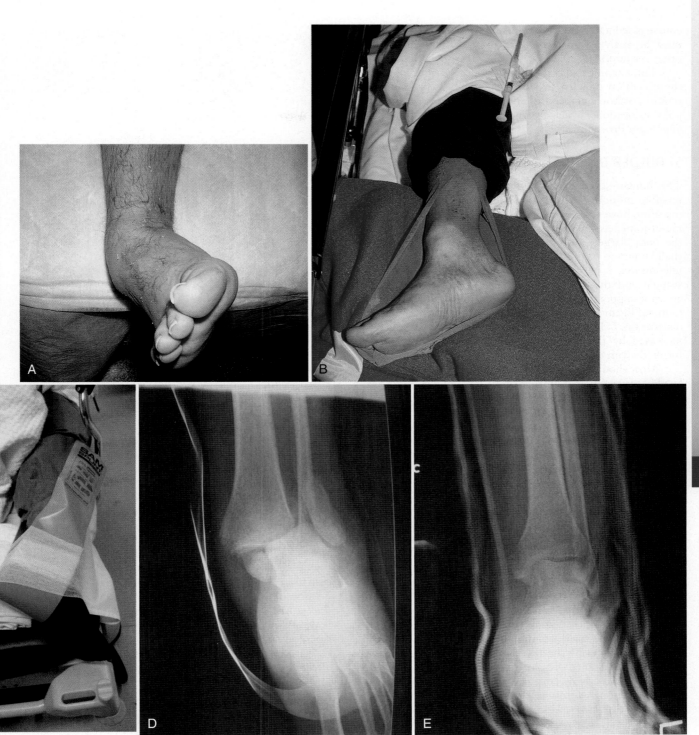

Figure 49–2 *A–C,* Because the distal pulse is weak and the toes are numb, it may be tempting, and commonly advocated and acceptable, to immediately reduce these obvious dislocations while the patient is still on the ambulance stretcher. Because proper analgesia/sedation is required, take a few minutes to also obtain at least a portable x-ray. *D,* Note the very significant fracture/dislocation on the pre-reduction x-ray. *E,* Once the reduction is accomplished, there is a remarkable difference, suggesting a minor injury. *The specific initial injury will be impossible to reconstruct from the post-reduction physical examination alone.* The few minutes required to properly prepare the patient for reduction and to document the initial injury will not result in a more serious adverse outcome than has been prognosticated by the initial injury. However, when the patient has sustained multiple trauma and extremity films are a low priority, early reduction without radiographs may be warranted.

the induction of analgesia/sedation, a time during which radiographs can be obtained. If a vascular or neurologic abnormality is documented before reduction, the joint should be reduced by the most timely and least traumatic procedure available. Each case should be handled individually, consider-

ing the specific injury, available resources, and experience of the clinician. Although multiple unsuccessful or forceful attempts at reduction in the ED should be avoided with all dislocations, this is especially important if there is vascular or neurologic compromise. Occasionally, the more prudent course is reduction under general anesthesia, but this decision must be analyzed given the availability of consultation and other resources.

This chapter covers dislocations of the various joints with the exception of wrist dislocations, which are complex and require orthopaedic consultation, and temporomandibular joint dislocations, which are discussed in Chapter 64, Otolaryngologic Procedures.

SHOULDER DISLOCATIONS

The human shoulder joint is remarkable for its degree of possible motion. The anatomic features that allow for this mobility, however, contribute to its instability. The glenohumeral joint has the greatest range of motion of any joint in the body, largely owing to the loose joint capsule and the shallow nature of the glenoid fossa.[10] Posterior dislocation is uncommon, largely owing to the anatomic support of the scapula and the thick muscular support in this area. The anterior support is less pronounced, with the inferior glenohumeral ligament serving as the primary restraint to anterior dislocation.[11] The depth of the glenoid fossa is somewhat increased by the fibrocartilaginous glenoid labrum, which forms the rim of this structure.

Most shoulder dislocations are anterior (i.e., the humeral head becomes situated in front of the glenoid fossa). Posterior dislocations are the next most common, but they generally account for less than 4% of shoulder dislocations.[12] Uncommon variations include inferior (luxatio erecta), superior, and intrathoracic dislocations. Dislocations of all types, including the shoulder, are less common in children owing to the relative weakness of the epiphyseal plate compared with that of the ligamentous support of the joint.

Anterior Shoulder Dislocations

Anterior dislocations of the shoulder are the most common major joint dislocation encountered, and reduced, in the ED. The usual mechanism of injury is indirect, with a combination of abduction, extension, and external rotation.[10,11] Only rarely is the mechanism a direct blow to the posterior aspect of the shoulder. Occasionally, *especially with recurrent dislocations*, the mechanism is surprisingly minor and can be puzzling to the clinician. Mere external rotation of the shoulder while rolling over in bed or raising the arm overhead can induce a dislocation. The occurrence of a first dislocation at a younger age is associated with a higher recurrence rate; 80% to 92% with a first dislocation before age 20 years versus 10% to 15% in patients with a first dislocation after age 40.[10] Rotator cuff injuries, however, occur more frequently in older patients with anterior shoulder dislocations.[13]

The four types of anterior dislocations are subcoracoid (accounting for >75% of anterior dislocations), subglenoid, and the uncommon subclavicular and intrathoracic.[10] These are classified according to where the humeral head comes to rest (Fig. 49–3).

Clinical Assessment

The presentation of anterior shoulder dislocation is usually obvious (Fig. 49–4). Posterior dislocations are more subtle on both clinical presentation and radiographic manifestations and can be misdiagnosed as a severe contusion (Table 49–1). The patient with an anterior shoulder dislocation supports the injured extremity and leans toward the injured side, holding

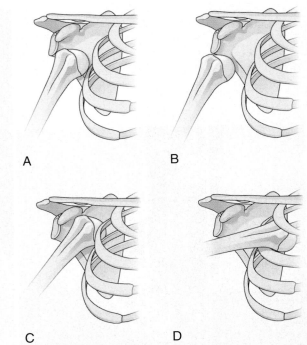

Figure 49–3 Types of anterior shoulder dislocations. *A*, Subcoracoid. *B*, Subglenoid. *C*, Subclavicular. *D*, Intrathoracic.

the arm in abduction with slight external rotation. The patient cannot adduct or internally rotate the shoulder. Visual inspection reveals loss of the rounded appearance of the shoulder due to the absence of the humeral head beneath the deltoid region. The acromion is prominent and an abrupt drop-off below the acromion can be seen or palpated. An anterior fullness in the subclavicular region is visible in thinner individuals and is easily palpable in most others. Comparison with the uninjured side is a useful aid for both visual examination and palpation. Any attempt at internal rotation is quite painful and is resisted by the patient. The inability to place the palm from the injured extremity on the uninjured shoulder is consistent with anterior shoulder dislocation; postreduction, this maneuver should be possible.

A careful assessment of the neurovascular status of the affected extremity is essential. Injury to the axillary artery is rare, usually occurring in the elderly,[13] and can be quickly assessed by palpation of the radial pulse or the presence of an expanding hematoma. It is important to assess the status of the axillary nerve, because this is the most common nerve lesion resulting from anterior dislocations.[14] The sensory component of the axillary nerve is assessed by testing for sensation over the lateral aspect of the upper arm (Fig. 49–5). The motor component of the axillary nerve would be tested by assessing the strength of the deltoid muscle, a difficult undertaking in the patient with a dislocated shoulder. Less commonly, the brachial plexus may be injured by a stretch injury, producing variable nerve deficits. The neurologic examination should include a complete assessment of all major nerves to the arm, because other nerve injuries such as to the ulnar and radial nerves may occur.[14] The presence of a neurologic deficit does not preclude closed reduction, but in the presence of a nerve injury, multiple forceful attempts at reduction should be avoided.

Brachial plexus injuries require an especially atraumatic reduction. If generous sedation/analgesia does not permit an easy reduction in the ED, reduction of the dislocation with a nerve injury may be more prudently performed in the operating room with the patient under general anesthesia. Nerve

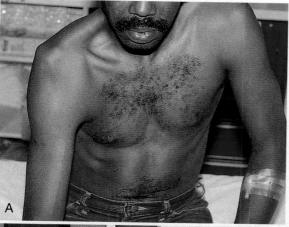

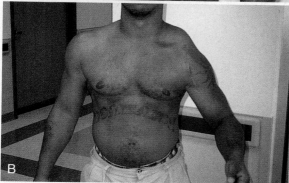

Figure 49–4 *A,* Typical presentation of an anterior right shoulder dislocation. The shoulder is very painful; thus, the patient resists movement. The outer round contour of the shoulder is obviously flattened, and the displaced humeral head may be appreciated in the subcoracoid area. Often, the patient abducts the arm slightly, bends the torso toward the injured side, and supports the flexed elbow on the injured side with the other hand. *B,* Obvious left shoulder dislocation. This chronic dislocation occurred frequently with minimal trauma, and the patient was able to dislocate it at will, feign a new injury, and score narcotics from multiple emergency departments (EDs).

injuries in this setting generally have a good prognosis, but the patient should be informed of the findings and the need for follow-up. Symptoms may require many months to resolve.

The rare vascular injuries, such as axillary artery disruption, are usually quite obvious, producing dysesthesias and coolness of the involved arm. An expanding axillary hematoma, pulse deficit, peripheral cyanosis, and pallor can be seen. Collateral circulation may produce a faint pulse in the extremity, so comparison blood pressure of the uninjured side may be helpful. Specific lesions include complete disruption, linear tears, or thrombus. Axillary artery injuries can occur in all ages, although they are more prominent in the elderly. The artery is at risk with anterior dislocations, and a dislocation–spontaneous reduction can produce the injury. Arteriography with surgical repair of the artery is required, occasionally with fasciotomy of the forearm if ischemia is long-standing.[15]

Some portion of the rotator cuff will be injured in many shoulder dislocations. Rotator cuff tears are easier to evaluate after reduction, often days later when pain and swelling have subsided.

Radiologic Examination

Associated fractures are detected in 15% to 35% of anterior shoulder dislocations, with fractures of the greater tuberosity being the most common.[10] The presence of a fracture of the greater tuberosity does not change the initial management of anterior shoulder dislocations, and these fractures usually heal well after closed reduction in the routine fashion.[10] The Hill-Sachs deformity, a sign of repeated dislocations, produces a groove in the posterolateral aspect of the humeral head and may be seen on prereduction or postreduction films (Fig. 49–6). The Hill-Sachs deformity is caused by impaction of the humeral head against the glenoid rim after dislocation. It rarely has clinical significance, but may result in a loose body within the joint.[13] Impaction of the humeral head against the glenoid during dislocation may cause a disruption of the glenoid rim, known as a *Bankart lesion*. This has been implicated as one cause of recurrent dislocations, but does not affect immediate ED management.[13]

Fractures of the humeral neck are frequently displaced with attempts at closed reduction, the result of which is often avascular necrosis of the humeral head.[16] The fact that humeral neck fractures are a known complication of shoulder relocation[10] suggests the value of prereduction radiographs in

TABLE 49–1 Comparison of Anterior and Posterior Shoulder Dislocations: Classified According to the Displacement of the Humeral Head

Type of Dislocation	Patient Presentation	Other Clinical Clues	Radiographs
Anterior 99% subcoracoid and subglenoid Humeral head is anterior to the glenoid	• Arm held in *abduction* and *slight external rotation* (abduction more prominent in subglenoid dislocation) • Patient cannot adduct or *internally* rotate shoulder	Seen from the front, shoulder appears "squared off" Distal acromion prominent from side view	*On AP view:* obvious dislocation *On lateral or "Y" view:* humeral head appears anterior to glenoid fossa
Posterior 95% subacromial 5% subglenoid and subspinous Humeral head is posterior to the glenoid	• Arm held in sling position, with adduction and internal rotation • Attempts at *abduction* and *external rotation* cause extreme pain	Coracoid process prominent, glenoid fossa empty anteriorly and humeral head bulging posteriorly	*On AP view:* vacant glenoid sign, 6-mm sign, lightbulb sign *On lateral or "Y" view:* humeral head appears posterior to glenoid fossa

AP, anteroposterior.

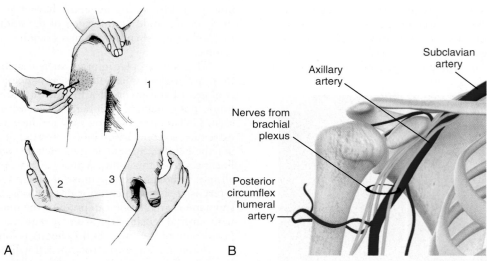

A

B

Figure 49–5 *A,* Evaluation of the upper extremity with a shoulder dislocation. Axillary (circumflex) nerve palsy is the most common neurologic complication. The axillary nerve has a sensory and motor function. Test the integrity of the nerve by assessing sensation to pin prick (*1*) in its distribution over the "regimental badge" area. (The shoulder is usually too painful to allow assessment of deltoid activity with certainty.) Look for other (rare) involvement of the radial portion of the posterior cord (*2*) and involvement of the axillary artery (*3*). *B,* Anatomy about the shoulder demonstrates the possibility of nerve and vascular damage. *(A, From McRae R: Practical Fracture Treatment. Edinburgh, Churchill Livingstone, 1981, p 84. Reproduced by permission; B, from Thomsen T, Setnik G [eds]: Procedures Consult—Emergency Medicine Module. Copyright 2008 Elsevier Inc. All rights reserved.)*

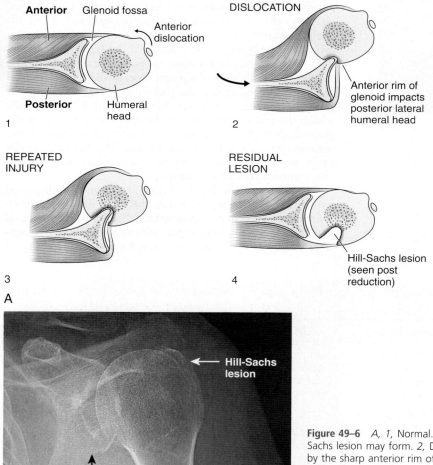

A

B

Figure 49–6 *A, 1,* Normal. With repeated anterior shoulder dislocations, a Hill-Sachs lesion may form. *2,* During the dislocation, the humeral head is damaged by the sharp anterior rim of the glenoid. *3,* With repeated dislocation, the lesion, called the "hatchet sign" develops. *4,* On the reduction film, the lesion is apparent. *B,* Radiograph demonstrates a Hill-Sachs lesion and a Bankart fracture: a fracture of the inferior glenoid rim from impaction of the dislocated humeral head. *(B, From Thomsen T, Setnik G [eds]: Procedures Consult—Emergency Medicine Module. Copyright 2008 Elsevier Inc. All rights reserved.)*

anterior shoulder dislocations. However, some argue that clinically obvious recurrent dislocations and first-time anterior dislocations without a blunt traumatic mechanism (information usually offered by the patient) can be reduced without prior radiographs, because fracture is quite unlikely in these situations.[7,8] Hendey and coworkers[17] performed a prospective validation study of an algorithm for selective radiography that incorporated the mechanism of injury, previous dislocations, and the clinician's certainty of joint position. In this study, 24 patients with recurrent atraumatic anterior shoulder dislocations who received neither pre- nor postreduction radiographs had no clinically significant fractures found on follow-up. These patients had much shorter ED lengths-of-stay than patients who received only pre- or postreduction films or both.[17]

One retrospective case-control study found that the presence of any of three risk factors (age > 40 yr, first episode of dislocation, traumatic mechanism of injury defined as fall greater than one flight of stairs, a fight or assault, or a motor vehicle crash) predicted clinically important fractures with a sensitivity of 97.7%.[18] This study has not yet been prospectively validated.

Anterior dislocations are not subtle on the routine anteroposterior (AP) radiograph, and this view detects the most important fracture to identify, that of the humeral neck. An adequate AP view, when combined with the typical clinical examination, allows for successful management of most ante-

rior shoulder dislocations. The true AP view of the shoulder is taken at a right angle to the scapula, requiring rotation of the patient to 30° to 45°, as shown in Figure 49–7A.

The typical lateral views obtained include the scapular Y view (Fig. 49–8; see also Fig. 49–7B), the transthoracic view, and the axillary view. These views rarely add to the AP view in the obvious anterior dislocation, but they are of value in posterior dislocations. The usefulness of additional views in anterior shoulder dislocations is primarily to detect fractures, and the previously mentioned lateral views (especially the transthoracic view) are quite limited in this respect.[19] The apical oblique view has been found to be more valuable than the oblique scapular projection in acute shoulder trauma.[19] This view is obtained by angling the beam 45° caudad with the patient in a 45° oblique position (see Fig. 49–7C–E).

Postreduction radiographs are obtained to document the success of the reduction. Occasionally, they will reveal a fracture not detected on the prereduction radiographs. In one series, 8% of patients with anterior shoulder dislocations had Hill-Sachs deformities noted only on postreduction films.[8]

Reduction Techniques

Hippocrates (450 bc) is generally credited with the first detailed description of reduction techniques, and it is believed that a drawing in the tomb of Upuy (1200 bc) is the earliest depiction of such a method.[10] The Hippocratic technique involves placement of the operator's foot in the axilla to effect

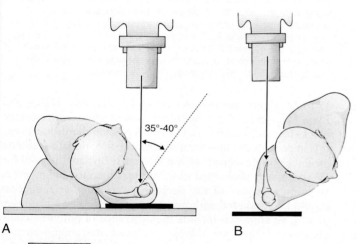

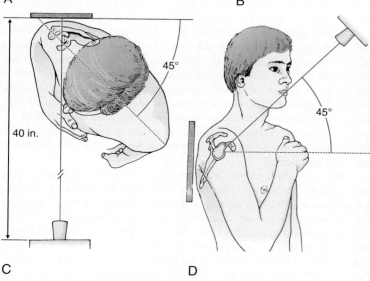

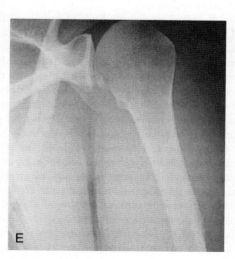

Figure 49–7 A trauma series includes two views of the shoulder made perpendicular and parallel to the scapular plane. This provides an anteroposterior (AP; *A*) and a scapular Y (*B*) view. The advantage is that roentgenograms may be obtained without moving the patient or removing the arm from the sling. *C* and *D*, Positioning for apical oblique view. The affected shoulder is placed at a 45° oblique position and the central ray is angled 45° caudad. The affected arm is adducted. *E*, Normal apical oblique view. (*A* and B, *From Heppenstall RB: Fracture Treatment and Healing. Philadelphia, WB Saunders, 1980, p 374. C to E, From Heppenstall RB: Fracture Treatment and Healing. Philadelphia, WB Saunders, 1980, p 392. Reproduced with permission.*)

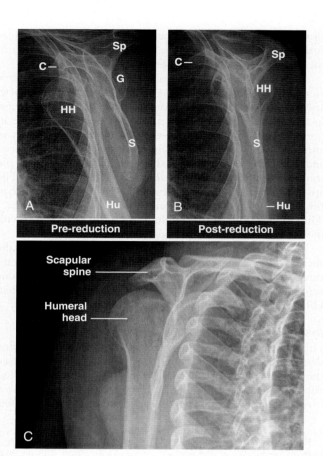

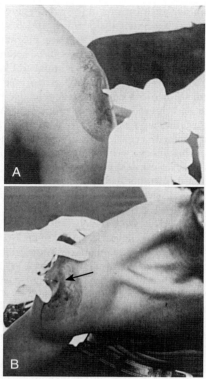

Figure 49–8 *A*, Scapular Y view demonstrates an anterior dislocation (note that the humeral head is displaced inferior and medial). *B*, Scapular Y view after dislocation is reduced. Note that the humeral head bisects the two intersecting limbs of the scapular Y. *C*, Scapular Y view of a posterior dislocation with the humeral head laterally displaced. A *posterior dislocation* may be difficult to appreciate on an AP view because it is *not inferiorly displaced and may appear to be in the glenoid fossa*. C, coracoid; G, glenoid; HH, humeral head; SP, scapular spine. (*A–C, From Thomsen T, Setnik G [eds]: Procedures Consult Emergency Medicine Module. Copyright 2008 Elsevier Inc. All rights reserved.*)

Figure 49–9 Intra-articular injection for the reduction of an acute anterior shoulder dislocation can be very effective. *A*, After aspirating blood from the joint, 10–20 mL of 1% plain lidocaine is slowly injected through the lateral sulcus, aiming slightly caudad. *B*, Anterior view. Allow 15–20 min for the lidocaine to take effect. (*A and B, From Matthews DE, Roberts T: Intra-articular lidocaine versus intravenous analgesic for reduction of acute anterior shoulder dislocations. Am J Sports Med 23:54, 1995. Reproduced by permission.*)

countertraction. This technique is problematic and is not recommended by some authors.[3,11] Likewise, the Kocher method, which involves forceful leverage of the humerus, has an increased rate of complications and is generally discouraged in favor of other techniques.[10,11]

This section discusses several methods of reduction that are well studied, proven to be safe, and easy to master. Regardless of the reduction technique used, gradual, gentle application of the technique is essential. Although all of the techniques discussed are generally acceptable and many authors state that their techniques are quite painless,[1-5] few studies have quantified the actual pain reported by patients.[20] As noted previously, intra-articular lidocaine also may be used to reduce the pain of reduction (Fig. 49–9). In studies by Matthews and Roberts[21] and Kosnick and colleagues,[22] the use of intra-articular lidocaine was found to offer significant pain relief during reduction of anterior shoulder dislocations, making it a useful alternative to procedural sedation and analgesia. When using intra-articular lidocaine, any blood should be aspirated from the glenohumeral joint before injecting anesthetic. Note that 10 to 20 mL of 1% lidocaine has been used with the intra-articular technique, and it may take as long as

15 to 20 minutes for adequate analgesia. Recently, Blaivas and Lyon[23] reported the ED use of ultrasound-guided interscalene blocks for analgesia before reduction of shoulder dislocations. It is important to note that neither local or regional anesthesia produce muscle relaxation, but these may obviate the need for IV access and prolonged observation. Operator judgment is an important part of the decision as to whether reduction should be attempted without premedication. The advantages of such an approach include the avoidance of potential complications from drug therapy, reduced staff requirements, and theoretically, a more rapid patient disposition. Certainly, the patient who is markedly intoxicated may require little, if any, supplemental sedative therapy. However, all patients who are reluctant or too anxious to cooperate with an attempt at reduction without medication and those with a high degree of muscle spasm should receive premedication. Generally, only one attempt is made; if unsuccessful, further reduction attempts are made after the administration of IV sedation. When in doubt, it is best to use pharmacologic adjuncts (see Chapter 33, Systemic Analgesia and Sedation for Procedures).

Several factors will help decide which technique is best in each situation. One factor is whether the patient will tolerate a reduction attempt without sedation, because attempts without sedation should not use forceful techniques such as traction-countertraction. The clinician's comfort level with a given technique is always a factor, because the greatest success rates will likely result from techniques with which the clinician is most familiar. The time and resources available to the clinician must be considered, because methods such as the Stimson maneuver require greater time and the availability of weights and straps. In addition, certain reduction techniques can be performed without assistance, whereas others require an additional person to apply countertraction or to help with manipulation of the scapula or humeral head. Ideally, the emergency clinician should become familiar with a number of different techniques for reducing anterior dislocations of the shoulder, because no single method has a 100% success rate nor is any technique ideal in every situation.

Stimson Maneuver. The Stimson maneuver (Fig. 49–10) is a classic technique that offers the advantage of not requiring an assistant. The patient is placed prone on an elevated stretcher and about 2.5 to 5.0 kg (5–10 lb) of weight is suspended from the wrist.[10,11] The weights can be strapped to the wrist or a commercially available Velcro wrist splint can be placed and the weights hung from this with a hook.[24] The slow, steady traction of this method often permits reduction,

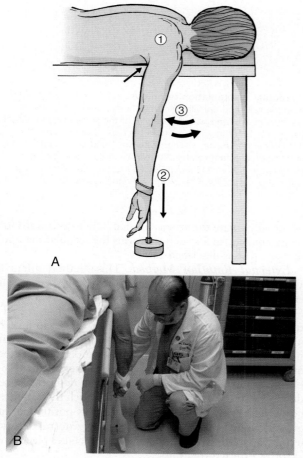

Figure 49–10 *A,* Stimson technique. This technique is often tried first, because it is the least traumatic if the patient can relax the shoulder muscles. *1,* The patient is lying prone on the edge of the table. One must be careful that the sedated or intoxicated patient does not fall off the table. Belts or sheets can be used to secure the patient to the stretcher. *2,* 5-kg weights are attached to the arm, and the patient maintains this position for 20–30 min, if necessary. *3,* Occasionally, gentle external and internal rotation of the shoulder with manual traction aids reduction. *B,* Physician applying manual traction and rotation to aid reduction. *(A, From DePalma AF: Management of Fractures and Dislocations: An Atlas. Philadelphia, WB Saunders, 1970, p 618. Reproduced by permission. B, from Thomsen T, Setnik G [eds]: Procedures Consult—Emergency Medicine Module. Copyright 2008 Elsevier Inc. All rights reserved.)*

but it may take 20 to 30 minutes. Reduction may be facilitated by gentle external rotation of the extended arm.

Variations of this method include the recommendation for flexion of the elbow to further relax the biceps tendon and the application of manual traction instead of weights.[25,26] Rollinson[27] allowed the arm to hang under its own weight after a supraclavicular block and reported a 91% success rate with usually no more than a gentle pull on the arm after 20 minutes in this position. Each variation of the Stimson method can be used in combination with the scapular manipulation technique described later. Indeed, a success rate of 96% has been reported using the combined prone position, hanging weights, IV drug therapy, and scapular manipulation.[24]

Disadvantages of the Stimson method include the time required and the danger of patients slipping off the elevated bed. A "seatbelt" strap or bedsheet may be placed around the patient and stretcher to avoid patient movement off the stretcher. In addition, a bed that elevates to a suitable height for the patient's arm length, a convenient method to hang the weights, the weights themselves, and adequate staff to monitor the patient are often difficult to locate and organize in a busy ED.

Scapular Manipulation Technique. This method is popular owing to its ease of performance, reported safety, and acceptability to patients. To date, no complications from this technique have been reported in the literature.[20,24,28] Shoulder reduction using this method focuses on repositioning the glenoid fossa rather than the humeral head, and it requires less force than many other methods.[21] The success rate is high, generally greater than 90% in experienced hands.[24,28]

The initial maneuver for scapular manipulation is traction on the arm as it is held in 90° of forward flexion. This may be performed with the patient prone and the arm hanging down, as described in the Stimson method, with or without flexion of the elbow to 90° (Fig. 49–11*A*). Alternatively, this traction may be applied by the operator placing an outstretched arm over the seated patient's midclavicle while pulling the injured extremity with the other arm (see Fig. 49–11*B* and *C*). Regardless of the means of arm traction, slight external rotation of the humerus may facilitate reduction by releasing the superior glenohumeral ligament and presenting a favorable profile of the humeral head to the glenoid fossa.[29]

The prone patient position is recommended for those not familiar with the technique, because it facilitates identification of the scapula for manipulation (medial rotation of the tip). Nonetheless, the technique can be performed with the patient supine, given that the patient's shoulder is flexed to 90° and the scapula is exposed during gentle upward traction on the humerus.[30] Although seated scapular manipulation offers the advantage of not requiring the patient to go through the awkward and potentially uncomfortable assumption of the prone position, it is a technically more difficult variation of scapular manipulation, especially if sedation is going to be necessary. When placing the patient in the prone position, it is important to place the injured shoulder over the edge of the bed to allow the arm to hang perpendicularly for the application of traction.[28]

After application of traction, the scapula is then manipulated to complete the reduction. Anderson and associates[28] recommended manipulation of the scapula after the patient's arm is relaxed; however, success is possible with no delay in the performance of this second step.[20] Manipulation of the scapula is carried out by stabilizing the superior aspect of the

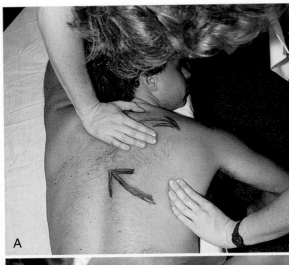

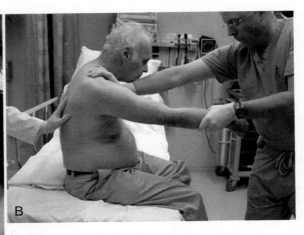

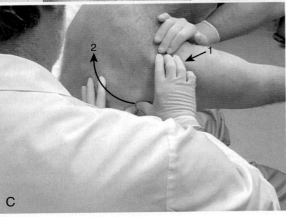

Figure 49–11 **Scapular manipulation technique.** *A*, The inferior tip of the scapula is pushed medially and dorsally with the thumbs while the superior aspect of the scapula is stabilized with the fingers of the superior hand. Weights may be attached to the hand to apply hanging traction. *B* and *C*, With the patient seated, the operator applies traction with one hand and countertraction with the other, while an assistant rotates the scapula in the same manner. (*B* and *C*, from Thomsen T, Setnik G [eds]: Procedures Consult—Emergency Medicine Module. Copyright 2008 Elsevier Inc. All rights reserved.)

scapula with one hand and pushing the inferior tip of the scapula medially toward the spine (see Fig. 49–11*A* and *B*). The thumb of the hand stabilizing the superior aspect of the scapula can be placed along the lateral border of the scapula and used to assist the pressure applied by the thumb of the other hand. A small degree of dorsal displacement of the scapular tip is recommended as it is being pushed as far as possible in the medial direction.[28]

When the patient is properly positioned, with the affected arm hanging perpendicularly, the lateral border of the scapula may be difficult to find in larger subjects. This border is generally located quite laterally with the patient in this position, and it must be properly located before any reduction attempt. The reduction itself is occasionally so subtle that it may be missed by both the patient and the operator. A minor shift of the arm may be the only clue to the successful reduction. Careful palpation of the subclavicular area in order to locate the position of the humeral head before repositioning the patient may be used to determine the success of the reduction.

A recently described variation of the seated scapular manipulation technique is the "Best of Both" (BOB) maneuver.[31] In the BOB maneuver, the patient is positioned seated sideways on the stretcher with the unaffected shoulder and hip against the fully elevated head of the stretcher. The operator stands on the foot end of the gurney at the patient's affected side and uses one hand to apply downward force on the patient's proximal forearm. The operator's other hand is used to grasp the patient's hand in order to gently internally

or externally rotate the arm as needed. Once downward force is being applied, an assistant performs the scapular manipulation maneuver as described earlier.[31]

External Rotation Method. This method offers the advantage of requiring only one person and no special equipment. The technique requires no strength or endurance on the part of the operator and is well tolerated by patients.[3] The actual pain experienced by patients with this technique has not been quantified, but Plummer and Clinton[3] stated that it can be performed with "little, if any sedation." In this technique, the basic maneuver is slow, gentle external rotation of the fully adducted arm. In 1957, Parvin[32] described a self-reduction external rotation technique in which the patient sits on a swivel-top chair and grasps a fixed post positioned waist high and slowly turns the body to enact external rotation. Parvin[32] reported that the reduction usually takes place at 70° to 110° of external rotation.

Since Parvin's initial study, this method has been described with the patient supine and the affected arm adducted tightly to the side of the patient.[1,33] The elbow is flexed to 90° and held in the adducted position with the operator's hand closest to the patient. The other hand holds the patient's wrist and guides the arm into slow and gentle external rotation (Fig. 49–12). The procedure may require several minutes, because each time the patient experiences pain, the procedure is momentarily halted. Although the report of Mirick and coworkers[1] mentioned using the forearm as "a lever," a later description clearly recommends allowing the forearm to "fall" under its own weight.[3] No additional

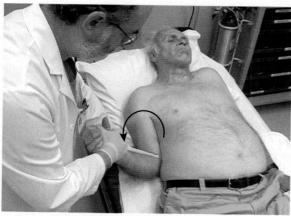

Figure 49–12 External rotation method. No traction is applied and a slow, gentle approach is essential. First, the arm is adducted to the patient's side. In one hand, the elbow is held flexed at 90° while the other hand grasps the wrist. Slowly and gently, the forearm is used as a lever to rotate the arm externally. Usually by the time the forearm has reached the coronal plane, the shoulder will have been reduced. *(From Mirick MJ, Clinton JE, Ruiz E: External rotation method of shoulder dislocation reduction. JACEP 8:528, 1979, and Thomsen T, Setnik G [eds]: Procedures Consult—Emergency Medicine Module. Copyright 2008 Elsevier Inc. All rights reserved.)*

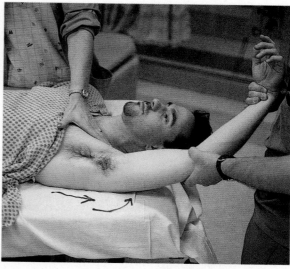

Figure 49–13 Milch technique. Slow, steady abduction with overhead traction, external rotation (not shown), and direct pressure over the humeral head are the steps of the Milch technique. The procedure may take 3–4 min to complete, and the operator should avoid sudden, jerky manipulations. It may help to ask the patient to make a motion as if he or she is reaching up and picking an apple from a tree.

force should be applied to the forearm and no traction is exerted on the arm.

The end point of the reduction may be difficult to identify, because reduction is frequently very subtle. It is therefore recommended to continue the external rotation until the forearm is near the coronal plane (lying on the bed, perpendicular to the body), a process that usually takes 5 to 10 minutes.[3] If the patient notes persistent dislocation with full external rotation, steady gentle traction at the elbow may be added at this time. Reduction may occasionally be noted when the arm is rotated back internally.[33] The success rate of this technique in three series performed by emergency clinicians was around 80%.[1,33,34]

Milch Technique. Proponents of this method praise its gentle nature, high success rate, lack of complications, and tolerance by patients.[2,5] It can be described as "reaching up to pull an apple from a tree." The basic steps of this technique are abduction, external rotation, and gentle traction of the affected arm. Finally, if needed, the humeral head is pushed into the glenoid fossa with the thumb or fingers (Fig. 49–13).

Milch,[35] in describing this technique, wrote that the fully abducted arm was in a natural position in which there was little tension on the muscles of the shoulder girdle. He postulated that this was related to our ancestral "arboreal brachiation" (swinging from trees). The primary step in this technique is to have the affected arm abducted to an overhead position. Russell and colleagues[29] had their patients raise the arm and put the hand behind the head as a first step. Although this seems odd, patients can usually do this quite readily with little assistance and be quite comfortable in this position. Alternatively, the operator may abduct the arm by grasping the patient's arm at the elbow or the wrist. Lacey and Crawford[36] found that the prone position, with the patient's shoulder close to the end of the bed, facilitated this step.

Once the arm is fully abducted, gentle longitudinal traction is applied with slight external rotation. If reduction does not occur quickly, the humeral head can be pushed upward into the glenoid fossa using the thumb or fingers of the other

hand. Beattie and associates[2] reported a success rate of 70% with the Milch technique, but others report success rates of 90% or greater.[5,29]

Traction-Countertraction. This method is commonly used in the ED, largely out of tradition, because it has a high rate of success and many emergency clinicians are most comfortable with it. Familiarity is an advantage of this technique, but it requires more than one operator, some degree of force, and occasionally, endurance. This technique is usually quite uncomfortable for the patient, and premedication is recommended before any attempt.

With the patient supine, a sheet or strap is wrapped around the upper chest and under the axilla of the affected shoulder (Fig. 49–14). An assistant holds this sheet, preferably by wrapping the sheet around the waist to take advantage of body weight rather than arm strength, to apply the countertraction. The operator's foot should not be used in the axilla to provide countertraction. Traction may then be applied to the extended arm, but this generally results in operator fatigue, especially if the operator relies on biceps strength to provide continuous traction. Preferably, the elbow of the affected side is flexed to 90° and a sheet or strap is wrapped around the proximal forearm and then around the operator's back. The bed should be elevated to a point at which the sheet can sit at the level of the operator's ischial tuberosities. This allows the operator to comfortably lean back and use the body weight to supply the force of traction, eliminating the possibility of operator fatigue. The portion of the sheet that is positioned on the patient's forearm has a tendency to ride up; flexion of the elbow beyond 90° will minimize this problem. Alternatively, the operator merely leans backward with the arms fully extended, again using the continuous weight of the body rather than the strength of the biceps to provide constant traction.

Once traction is applied, the operator must be patient, because the procedure may take a number of minutes to be successful. Inadequate premedication is noted by the patient who resists the procedure or is notably uncomfortable during

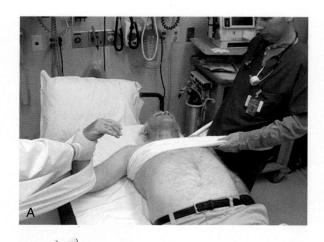

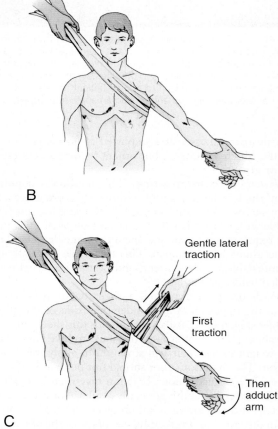

Figure 49–14 *A and B,* Traction-countertraction method. This simple technique for reducing the dislocated shoulder applies gradual and steady traction along the axis of the dislocated limb. A bedsheet, wrapped around the supine patient's upper chest wall and over the unaffected shoulder, is either tied or held by an assistant and acts as a fixed counterforce. A second bedsheet is placed around the patient's flexed forearm, just distal to the flexed elbow, and securely tied behind the operator's back. Note that a significant skin avulsion or friction burn may occur if there is excessive motion of the sheets, especially in the elderly patient with thin, delicate skin. With the patient's forearm held in a neutral rotation and the hand in a vertical position, *the operator applies traction by leaning back, rather than using the biceps to apply traction, which will soon fatigue most clinicians.* C, Gentle lateral traction on the humerus, coupled with adduction of the arm, often helps reduction. (*B and C, From Respet PB: A practical technique for reducing shoulder dislocations. J Musculoskel Med 5:29, 1988.*)

the reduction attempt. The operator should not hesitate to order supplementary medications. Gentle, limited external rotation is sometimes useful to speed reduction.[10] Applying traction to an arm that is slightly abducted from the patient's body is often successful, but some operators prefer to slowly bring the arm medial to the patient's midline while maintaining traction or to have an assistant apply a gentle lateral force to the midhumerus to direct the humeral head laterally. Successful reduction is usually presaged by slight lengthening of the arm as relaxation occurs, and a noticeable "clunk" may occur at the point of reduction. A brief fasciculation wave in the deltoid may also be seen at the time of reduction.

Spaso Technique. This technique was first reported by Spaso Miljesic as a simple, single-operator technique requiring minimal force.[37] One published series reported an 87.5% success rate among premedicated patients when performed by junior house officers.[38] The patient is placed in a supine position and the operator grasps the affected arm around the wrist or distal forearm. The affected arm is gently lifted vertically toward the ceiling, applying gentle vertical traction. While traction is continuously maintained, the arm is externally rotated (Fig. 49–15*A*). Reduction may be subtle, but is generally signaled by hearing or feeling a "clunk." Completion of this technique may require several minutes of gentle traction, allowing the muscles of the patient's shoulder to relax.[38]

Other Methods. Poulsen[39] reported a method termed the *Eskimo technique,* which may be performed in field settings. In this technique, the patient lies on the unaffected side and is lifted a short distance off the ground by grasping the abducted arm of the injured side (see Fig. 49–15*B*). The patient's body weight acts to effect the reduction. Poulsen's[39] success rate was 74% in a series of 23 patients, all of whom were premedicated. Poulsen[39] also postulated that this technique could place undue stress on the brachial plexus or axillary vessels. Use of this technique, when other options are available, should probably be reserved until a larger experience is reported.

Noordeen and coworkers[40] reported a simple method in which the patient sits sideways in a chair, with the affected arm draped over the backrest. The operator holds the arm with the wrist supinated, and the patient is instructed to stand up. The success rate was 72% in 32 patients treated in this manner. A variation of the chair technique, which was successful in 97% of 188 anterior shoulder dislocations, involves operator-applied traction to the patient's flexed elbow by means of a cloth loop or stockinette.[41] Standing beside the patient, the operator holds the involved elbow in 90° of flexion while stepping down on the cloth loop. The patient sits in the chair, and an assistant may help support the patient by applying countertraction under the involved arm.

Postreduction Care

After an attempt at reduction, the neurovascular status of the affected extremity should be rechecked and the results documented on the patient record. Indirect evidence that the reduction has been successful includes an immediate reduction in pain, restoration of the round shoulder contour, and increased passive mobility of the shoulder. No harm is done by putting the joint through a limited range of motion. If the patient can tolerate placement of the palm from the injured arm on the opposite shoulder, it is quite likely that the shoulder reduction was successful (see Fig. 49–15*C*).

Postreduction radiographs are often recommended, with a careful search for new fractures. Although most greater

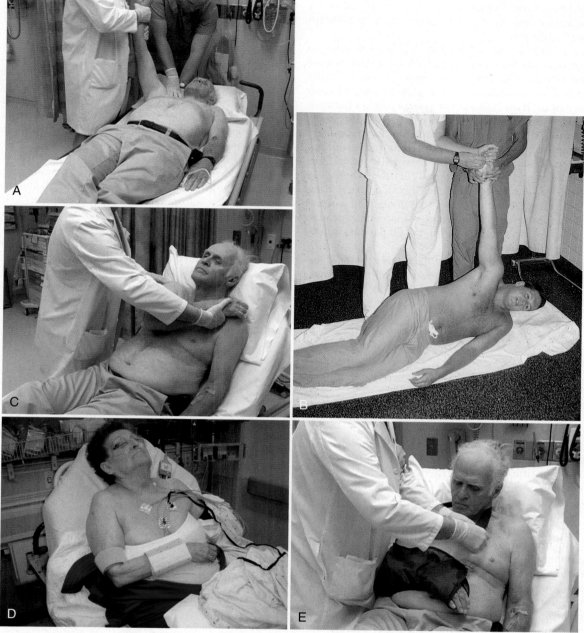

Figure 49–15 *A,* Spaso technique. While an assistant maintains gentle vertical traction-countertraction, the affected arm is externally rotated by grasping the wrist or forearm. Reduction may be subtle. *B,* Eskimo technique. The patient's body weight serves as countertraction. If the operator stands on a stool, biceps power is not needed. The operator's arms are left fully extended while grasping the patient's wrist, and the back is straightened to avoid operator arm fatigue. *C,* Regardless of the technique used, if a patient with a shoulder injury can place the palm of the injured arm on top of the contralateral shoulder, it is unlikely that a shoulder dislocation is present. Alternatively, completion of this maneuver after a reduction attempt provides strong evidence that the reduction was successful, even if the patient is still sedated. *D* and *E,* The best way to immobilize any reduced shoulder dislocation is uncertain and unlikely of consequence for a few days (see text). *D,* A typical shoulder immobilizer or a simple sling is appropriate pending referral and follow-up. *(B, D, and E, From Thomsen T, Setnik G [eds]: Procedures Consult—Emergency Medicine Module. Copyright 2008 Elsevier Inc. All rights reserved.)*

tuberosity fractures do not alter patient management, patients with greater tuberosity fractures displaced greater than 1 cm after closed reduction are almost always associated with a rotator cuff tear[42] and should receive prompt orthopaedic consultation, because they may require operative repair.

Traditional postreduction treatment has focused on the importance of preventing the shoulder from dislocating after discharge. This is best accomplished by immobilizing the joint using a commercially available shoulder immobilizer or a sling and swath, which limits external rotation and abduction (see Chapter 50, Splinting Techniques). Orthopaedic follow-up is recommended for all anterior shoulder dislocations because the incidence of rotator cuff injury is as high as 38% and might complicate restoration of normal function.[43] Younger patients are usually immobilized for approximately 3 weeks and can be instructed to follow up within 1 or 2 weeks of the event. As a general rule, the older the patient, the shorter the time of immobilization.[10] Those older than 60 years should have early follow-up (e.g., 5–7 days) to allow for early mobilization and avoidance of persistent or permanent shoulder joint stiffness.

Since the early 2000s, the wisdom of immobilization in internal rotation has been questioned. Several studies have shown that placing the arm in internal rotation actually increases labral detachment from the glenoid rim, whereas some degree of external rotation maximizes contact between the detached labrum and the glenoid rim.[44-46] In one study, cadavers were used to measure the force of contact between the labrum and the glenoid rim in different arm positions. The authors of this study found that maximal contact force was actually generated in 45° of external rotation, whereas no contact force was generated with the arm in internal rotation.[46] One prospective study showed that none of 20 patients immobilized in external rotation had recurrent dislocation after more than 1 year, compared with 6 of 20 patients immobilized in internal rotation.[45]

Despite this growing body of evidence, very little scientific data remain to guide the clinician on the most appropriate position for postreduction immobilization of anterior shoulder dislocations. In fact, a recent literature review designed to assess (1) whether traumatic anterior shoulder dislocations should be immobilized, (2) how long they should be immobilized, and (3) whether the position of immobilization affects outcomes was unable to provide any definitive answers.[47] According to the author of this study, "much of this uncertainty is due to the limited size of the evidence base, which exhibited numerous methodological weaknesses (e.g., small sample sizes, no control groups, not evaluating findings against statistical tests)."[47]

As a result, it is not unreasonable to immobilize the extremity in a manner consistent with the orthopaedic surgeons at one's institution until further evidence is presented. When in doubt, a simple sling or the traditional shoulder immobilizer will certainly suffice pending 5- to 7-day follow-up (see Fig. 49–15D and E).

It is appropriate to prescribe oral analgesics (either nonsteroidal anti-inflammatory drugs or narcotics) appropriate for the amount of patient discomfort at the time of disposition and to instruct the patient to return for any worsening of the clinical condition. Periodically, one may encounter a return visit from a successfully treated patient who is in severe pain from a hemarthrosis. Trimmings[48] reported excellent relief of pain by aspiration of the hemarthrosis 24 to 48 hours after shoulder reduction in a series of patients older than 60 years. This can be accomplished using the technique of arthrocentesis described in Chapter 53, Arthrocentesis. In addition, intra-articular instillation of 10 to 20 mL of 1% lidocaine (or longer-acting local anesthetic) as has been recommended for shoulder reduction may be helpful for further pain relief.

Posterior Shoulder Dislocations

Posterior shoulder dislocations account for less than 4% of all shoulder dislocations.[12] Because they are so uncommon, posterior dislocations are easily overlooked and the emergency clinician must be knowledgeable about these injuries to avoid a misdiagnosis. Delays in diagnosis for weeks to months have been reported with posterior dislocations.[49,50] This may lead to increased rates of dislocation arthropathy and chronic pain.[13] The mechanism of injury is almost always indirect, with a combination of internal rotation, adduction, and flexion.[10] Classic precipitating events include seizure, electrical shock, and falls. The patient may also present at a point

well past the original event.[50] Patients with seizures may not experience obvious problems in the immediate postictal period owing to their altered mental status.

Clinical Assessment

Although clinically less obvious than anterior dislocations, posterior shoulder dislocations do present in a typical, recognizable manner. Mistakes may be made if the clinician is overly reliant on the AP radiographs, which are potentially misleading,[50] and may result in misdiagnosing the injury as a soft tissue contusion or acromioclavicular (AC) strain. The principal sign of posterior dislocation is an arm that is somewhat fixed in adduction and internal rotation (Fig. 49–16). Abduction and external rotation are limited, and attempts to perform these movements generally elicit pain.[10,12] Inspection and palpation reveal a loss of the normal anterior contour of the shoulder and a prominent coracoid and acromion. The shoulder is flattened anteriorly and rounded posteriorly, whereas the humeral head may be palpable.[10,12]

Comparison with the opposite shoulder should be undertaken with the understanding that this injury may occasionally occur bilaterally. Neurovascular assessment is performed in the standard manner, although such complications are unusual with posterior dislocations.

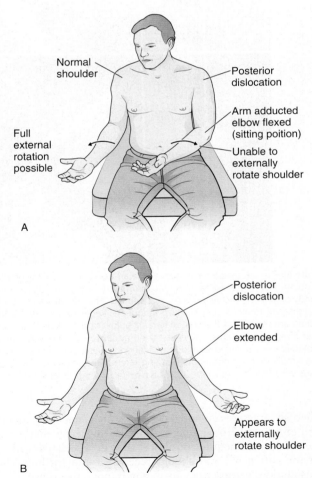

Figure 49–16 A posterior dislocation may be difficult to appreciate on x-rays. *A,* A clue to a posterior shoulder dislocation is the arm locked in adduction and internal rotation, with patient's inability to rotate the shoulder externally with the elbow flexed at 90°. *B,* Note that extension of the elbow with supination of the forearm may obscure loss of the external rotation.

Radiologic Examination

The key point regarding radiographs for posterior shoulder dislocations is the subtle nature of this dislocation on a single AP radiograph (Fig. 49–17A) and the diagnostic value of the scapular Y view (see Fig. 49–8C) or the axillary view (see Fig. 49–17B). The diagnosis of posterior shoulder dislocation using the axillary view is quite easy, whereas the routine AP and lateral views are difficult to interpret in around half of cases.[50] The axillary view is generally available in the radiology department and can be obtained with as little as 20° to 30° of abduction, with the plate placed on the shoulder.[50] In addition to easy visualization of the posteriorly situated humeral head, the axillary view often reveals an impression fracture of the humeral head (see Fig. 49–17B).

Whereas the axillary view is diagnostic, clues to posterior dislocation do exist on the AP film. The internally rotated humeral head appears symmetrical on the AP film in the shape of a lightbulb as opposed to the normal club-shaped appearance created by the greater tuberosity[51] (Figs. 49–18 and 49–19). With posterior dislocation, the space between the articular surface of the humeral head and the anterior glenoid rim is widened, and there is a decrease in the half-moon–shaped overlap of the head and the fossa (see Fig. 49–18).[49,51]

There may also be a compression fracture of the medial aspect of the humeral head, indicated by a dense line. This is known as the *trough sign*[51] (see Fig. 49–17C). A fracture of the lesser tuberosity should always prompt a search for the presence of a posterior shoulder dislocation.[49]

Reduction Technique

An acute posterior dislocation may be reduced by traction on the internally rotated and adducted arm combined with anteriorly directed pressure on the posterior aspect of the humeral head (Fig. 49–20).[10,50] Generous premedication is generally indicated, and countertraction may be applied with a sheet looped in the affected axilla much as described for anterior dislocations. Kwon and Zuckerman[10] recommend applying lateral traction on the upper humerus if the humeral head is locked on the posterior glenoid. Hawkins and colleagues[50] suggested that posterior dislocations with an impression defect of the humeral head greater than 20% of the articular surface require open reduction. Posterior dislocations that have been diagnosed late are difficult to reduce in a closed manner, but an attempt with adequate premedication is generally indicated.[50]

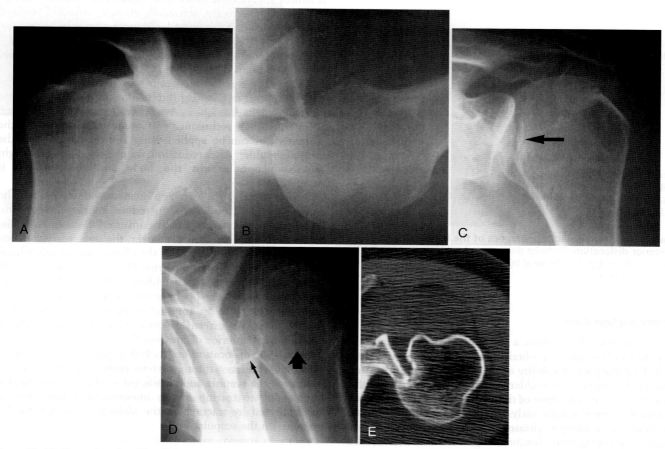

Figure 49–17 Posterior shoulder dislocation. *A,* This patient has a posterior dislocation of the humerus. Because the dislocation is directly posterior, there is no superior or inferior displacement of the humeral head. On superficial observation, the head of the humerus appears to maintain a normal relationship with the glenoid fossa and the acromion process. However, definite abnormalities exist in this film. The space between the humeral head and the glenoid fossa is abnormal, and because of the extreme internal rotation of the humerus, the head and neck are seen end on. In this projection, the humeral head resembles a lightbulb. Impaction of the humeral head on the posterior rim of the glenoid (*B*) leads to the "trough sign" (*arrow*) seen on an AP radiograph (*C*). *D,* Trans-scapular radiograph from a third patient shows posterior dislocation of the humeral head (*large arrow*) relative to the glenoid (*small arrow*). *E,* Computed tomography (CT) scan from the patient in *D* shows impaction of the anterior humeral head on the posterior glenoid. *(A, From Harris JH Jr, Harris WH: Radiology of Emergency Medicine, 2nd ed. Baltimore, Williams & Wilkins, 1981, p 629. Reproduced by permission.)*

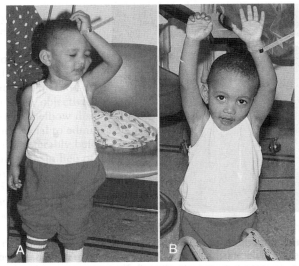

Figure 49–28 **Typical presentation of a child with a subluxation of the radial head (nursemaid's elbow).** It may be difficult to determine exactly where the pathology exists, and often the wrist is thought to be the area of injury. This child will not use the injured arm but has minimal discomfort as long as the elbow is not manipulated. *A,* The affected arm hangs down at the side, slightly flexed and pronated. *B,* Once the subluxation is reduced, full activity is generally regained in a matter of minutes.

in bed.[67] It is important to remember this and not to proceed with a child abuse investigation unless other suggestive features are present. The typical patient with a nursemaid's elbow presents in no distress with the arm held slightly flexed and pronated at the side (Fig. 49–28). This has been termed the *nursemaid's position.*[72] The exact area of pain is often difficult to locate. The child will refuse to use the arm, and this may be the chief complaint.[69] The older child will usually point to the dorsal aspect of the distal forearm when asked where it hurts. This may mislead one to suspect a buckle fracture of the distal radius.

Although tenderness about the elbow has been reported occasionally, there is often little tenderness or swelling of the elbow region.[68,69] In the cooperative child, the arm and shoulder are carefully palpated to discern any tenderness. Areas of focus on palpation should include the clavicle and the distal radius, because these are common sites of pediatric fractures. When patient anxiety interferes with a reliable assessment of tenderness in a child whose arm is in the classic nursemaid's position, the examiner can stand at a distance and have the parent or caretaker palpate the extremity to ascertain tenderness. This may also be done in the cooperative patient to reassure the doubtful parent regarding the absence of a fracture. If no tenderness is noted by palpation, it is appropriate to attempt a reduction without prior radiographs.[73]

Although resistance to or pain with supination is a frequent finding in such patients,[68] one need not test for this finding until the time of reduction.

Radiographic Examination

Radiographs are generally not needed in a child presenting with an arm in the nursemaid's position that is nontender (or minimally tender in the radial head area) on palpation, regardless of the history.[73] In these cases, radiographs are generally normal, and if obtained, the positioning of the child's arm by the x-ray technician often effects reduction.[68] However,

Frumkin[71] described three cases of nursemaid's elbow in which a line drawn through the longitudinal axis of the radius did not normally bisect the capitellum on prereduction radiographs, but did so after reduction. Radiographs are sometimes recommended if the child is not moving the arm normally 15 minutes after reduction.[72] However, this timeframe may be too short because reuse can be delayed for more than 30 minutes, particularly in children who present some time after the injury. Quan and Marcuse[69] recommended an approach in which no radiographs are obtained on the first visit, including in those children released from the ED prior to regaining full use of the arm. At the time of a 24-hour follow-up visit, radiographs are obtained only if repeat attempts at manipulation are not successful.

Whereas this condition does not generally require x-rays, they can be valuable if external signs of trauma are present (e.g., swelling, abrasions, ecchymoses), or if the child does not use the arm normally within 24 hours after the subluxation is considered reduced. Other less common conditions that can present with similar findings are fractures, joint infections, tumors, or osteomyelitis.

Reduction Techniques

Supination Method. Reduction of a nursemaid's elbow (Fig. 49–29) is generally performed without premedication. If the subluxation has been present for hours, oral or nasal midazolam can be a useful adjunct to overcome the child's anxiety related to manipulation. It is important to explain to the caretaker that the reduction will likely cause the child discomfort, but that this is transient and a clue to the diagnosis. The child is positioned seated on the lap of an assistant (often the parent) who stabilizes the arm by holding the humerus adducted to the side. The operator then grasps the elbow with one hand placing the thumb over the region of the radial head. Although it has been stated that the thumb can apply pressure to the radial head, this positioning is mainly useful for palpation of the reduction "click." The other hand grasps the wrist and is then used to supinate the extended forearm in a steady, deliberate manner. Slight traction before supination is generally recommended, but it is unclear whether this increases the likelihood of successful reduction. Once supinated, the arm can be flexed or extended; however, flexion is the most common maneuver and may actually be somewhat more successful than extension.[68] An audible or palpable click signifies successful reduction, but is not always noted. Once the reduction has been performed, the child usually cries for a few minutes. Generally, the operator should leave the room and then return in 10 to 15 minutes to do a repeat examination. Full use of the arm should be evident (see Fig. 49–28B).

Pronation Method. This technique is performed with the child positioned as in the supination method. However, the forearm is not supinated. Instead, the forearm is rapidly hyperpronated and flexed. A recent study by McDonald and colleagues[70] reported equal success rates using this technique and the supination technique.

After Attempted Reduction. If a click is detected, the child will generally regain use of the arm quickly (almost always by 30 min).[69] Therefore, if a definite click is detected, it is reasonable to observe the child for up to 30 minutes prior to further intervention. If there is still no use at 30 minutes, the operator may try to determine whether supination is still painful, which would suggest the need for a repeat attempt. In those in whom a click is not detected, the majority will not

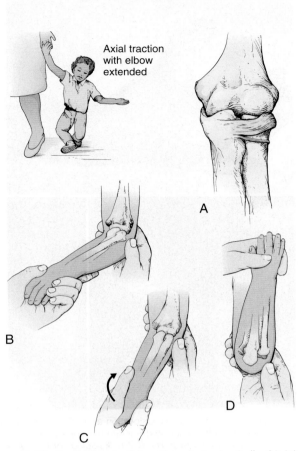

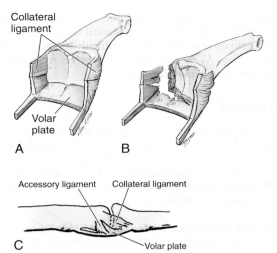

Collateral
ligament

Volar
plate

A   B

Accessory ligament   Collateral ligament

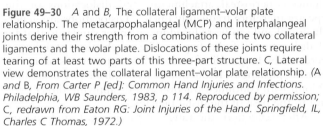

C   Volar plate

Figure 49–30 *A* and *B,* The collateral ligament–volar plate relationship. The metacarpophalangeal (MCP) and interphalangeal joints derive their strength from a combination of the two collateral ligaments and the volar plate. Dislocations of these joints require tearing of at least two parts of this three-part structure. *C,* Lateral view demonstrates the collateral ligament–volar plate relationship. *(A and B, From Carter P [ed]: Common Hand Injuries and Infections. Philadelphia, WB Saunders, 1983, p 114. Reproduced by permission; C, redrawn from Eaton RG: Joint Injuries of the Hand. Springfield, IL, Charles C Thomas, 1972.)*

Axial traction
with elbow
extended

A

B

C

D

Figure 49–29   Radial head subluxation. *A,* Anatomically, this injury represents interposition of the torn annular ligament between the radial head and the capitellum. *B,* The supination method of reduction is performed by grasping the arm about the wrist and placing the other hand about the elbow with the thumb over the radial head. The forearm is then supinated *(C)* and then the arm is flexed *(D)* in one continuous motion. *(A–D, From Fleisher GR, Ludwig S: Textbook of Pediatric Emergency Medicine. Baltimore, Williams & Wilkins, 1988, p 1322. Reproduced by permission.)*

use the arm by 30 minutes.[69] In these children, a repeat attempt at reduction is recommended after 10 to 15 minutes of nonuse. Two or more attempts are required to produce the click in up to 30% of patients.[69]

If the child has not regained the use of the arm after a few attempts and a reasonable period of time, some authors recommend that radiographs be performed.[72] X-ray films also may help relieve parental anxiety. Alternatively, instructions should be given for 24-hour follow-up if normal function is not restored, with consideration for radiographs at the time of follow-up.[69] In two series of patients with nursemaid's elbow, of 10 patients released without normal arm use, 6 had spontaneous restoration of function, and the other 4 required remanipulation, which successfully restored function.[68,69] The use of a posterior splint to protect the elbow of the child who refuses to use the arm after a presumed reduction is of uncertain value. However, some form of immobilization (e.g., splint, sling, or both) may be valuable in the child with significant residual discomfort after a prolonged period of subluxation or in whom recurrent subluxations have occurred. On occasion, a successful reduction painfully resubluxates with movement; in this case, immobilization and referral may

be necessary.[71] If reduction has been achieved clinically and maintained in the ED, analgesics or a follow-up visit is unnecessary. Because other pathology can rarely mimic this condition (e.g., occult fractures, osteomyelitis, joint infection, tumors), full, unrestricted, and painless use of the arm must be evident by 24 hours. If not, further assessment is indicated.

HAND INJURIES

The hand is an extremely common site of injury owing to the demands placed on it and the exposed nature of its location and use. Proper motion and function of the hand are intimately related to normal anatomic alignment.[74] The emergency clinician must therefore be skilled in the diagnosis and management of dislocations about the hand. An improperly managed hand injury can result in significant disability that the patient is reminded of on a daily basis.

Anatomically, the joints of the digits are quite similar and consist of a hinge joint with a tongue-in-groove–type arrangement.[74] The soft tissue support includes two collateral ligaments attached to a volar plate (Fig. 49–30). The volar plate is dense fibrous connective tissue that is thickened at its distal attachment and thinner at its proximal attachment, to allow for folding with joint flexion.[74,75] Dorsal dislocation of a digit requires failure of the volar plate, whereas lateral dislocation disrupts a collateral ligament and induces at least a partial tear in the volar plate (see Fig. 49–30).

Radiographic examination of all hand injuries is relatively straightforward, including at least two views (AP and lateral) of the injured area. The most important radiographic error in evaluating joint injuries of the hand is failing to get a true lateral view of the injured joint.[75] This may lead to missing a fracture or a loose body in the joint.

Anesthesia is generally required for the proper management of dislocations about the hand. This is most often

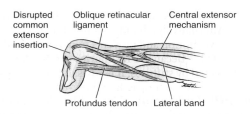

A

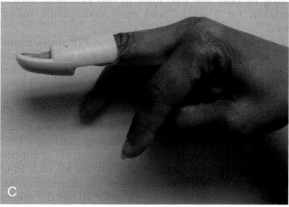

Figure 49–41 *A,* The mallet finger injury is not a dislocation; it is a rupture of the extensor tendon to the distal phalanx. It can occur with or without (demonstrated here) an avulsion fracture, *with seemingly minor trauma. B,* This mallet deformity was caused by a baseball striking the fingertip end on, producing acute flexion of the joint. *C,* A stack splint, *leaving the PIP joint free to allow for relaxation of the distal interphalangeal joint,* is kept in place for 6–8 wk. Caution the patient to avoid flexing the joint to "test it out" during splint changes. Wire fixation may be required.

48, Extensor and Flexor Tendon Injuries in the Hand, Wrist, and Foot).

MCP Dislocations

The pathology and management of finger MCP dislocations are identical to those of the thumb, as discussed earlier. The same classification of simple and complex applies; the complex type requires operative repair. Dimpling on the palmar surface suggests the presence of a complex dislocation. It is important to remember that the application of traction alone for a simple MCP dislocation may convert it to a complex dislocation. For dorsal dislocations, the wrist is flexed to relax the tendons. The next maneuver in reduction should be hyperextension as far as possible. This is followed by pressure on the base of the proximal phalanx to effect reduction. After reduction of a simple dorsal MCP dislocation, buddy taping is generally sufficient to secure the reduction.[74] Volar dislocations are rare and require orthopaedic consultation.

Carpometacarpal Dislocations

Carpometacarpal dislocations are rare injuries that are frequently misdiagnosed. The usual site of injury is the fifth carpometacarpal joint, which is dorsally dislocated.[75] The injury is usually the result of a high-energy mechanism, such as a motor vehicle crash or a fall. The diagnosis can be quite difficult because the appearance may be subtle even on the lateral radiograph. Associated fractures and other injuries are frequently present, and percutaneous fixation is usually required.[75]

HIP DISLOCATIONS

The hip is generally a stable ball-and-socket joint. The head of the femur is deeply situated in the acetabulum, and ligamentous and muscular support is very strong. Hip dislocations are therefore usually the result of significant forces, and a careful search for other limb- or life-threatening injuries must be undertaken. Common mechanisms of hip dislocation include motorcycle crashes, car crashes, and falls.[79]

Associated fractures are quite common with hip dislocations. In fact, up to 88% of hip dislocations present with an associated fracture.[80] If a fracture complicates the dislocation, orthopaedic consultation is generally indicated. However, the emergency clinician should be able to reduce simple hip dislocations, which are dislocations without an associated fracture or with a very minor fracture.[81]

Hip dislocations may occasionally be missed in the setting of severe trauma because other injuries garner more attention. A missed diagnosis can also occur when a femur fracture obscures the clinical picture of hip dislocation.[81] Common complications of hip dislocation include sciatic nerve injuries and avascular necrosis of the femoral head. Sciatic nerve injuries are seen in 10% to 14% of posterior hip dislocations.[81] Avascular necrosis of the femoral head is one of the more disabling complications associated with hip dislocation. Although it is generally stated that early reduction will reduce the frequency of this complication, evidence for this statement is hard to find. Dreinhofer and coworkers[80] noted poor outcomes despite early (i.e., <6 hr) reduction of type I hip dislocations (dislocation without significant associated fracture). Yang and colleagues[79] found that reduction beyond 24 hours was associated with a worse prognosis, but they could not find a significant time factor for those reduced in less than 24 hours. However, it is still advisable to reduce hip dislocations as soon as feasible to decrease soft tissue distortion. If evidence of nerve injury exists, the dislocation should be treated as an emergency and should be reduced as early as possible.

Radiographic Examination

Dislocation of the hip is generally obvious on the standard AP pelvic film that is often taken during trauma resuscitations. The use of a lateral or oblique view may help clarify the type of dislocation, but this can usually be deduced through clinical examination.

Analgesia and Anesthesia

Dislocation of a prosthetic hip can usually be managed with moderate amounts of IV premedication in the ED. Premedication recommendations for acute traumatic dislocations run the gamut from general anesthesia for all reductions[80] to IV

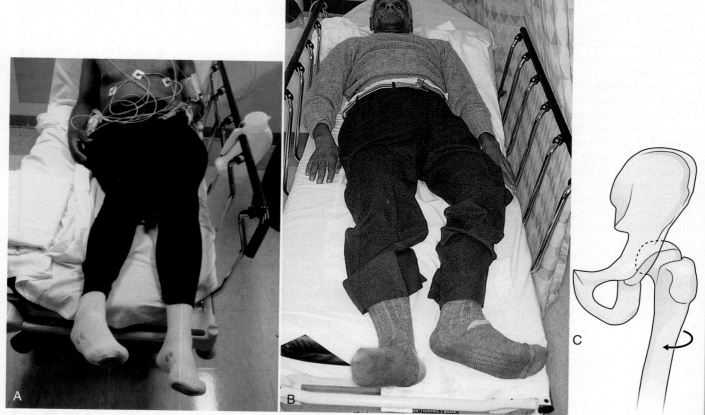

Figure 49–42 *A,* A posterior hip dislocation in a patient with a hip prosthesis: The leg is adducted, flexed at the knee, shortened, and internally rotated. *B,* The much less common anterior dislocation: The leg is shortened, abducted, flexed at the knee, and externally rotated, similar to the appearance of a hip fracture. *C,* Position of the femoral head in a posterior dislocation. *(C, From Simon R, Koenigsknecht S: Orthopedics in Emergency Medicine. New York, Appleton-Century-Crofts, 1982, p 366. Reproduced by permission.)*

sedation only.[82] Most clinicians would agree that some type of IV premedication is necessary, and patients often require deep sedation if the procedure is to be successful in the ED. One should not hesitate to opt for spinal or general anesthesia if a reasonable attempt at reduction fails in the ED.

Posterior Hip Dislocation

Posterior dislocation is the most common type of hip dislocation (Fig. 49–42). Posterior dislocations generally occur secondary to a blow to the flexed knee with the hip in varying degrees of flexion. The greater the amount of flexion of the hip at the time of the injury, the less the chance of an associated fracture.[81] The femoral head is forced out of the acetabulum and rests behind it (see Fig. 49–42*C*). The sciatic nerve is located just behind the hip joint and may be injured with posterior hip dislocation. The clinical picture includes a shortened, internally rotated, and adducted leg.

Reduction Techniques

Several basic methods for hip reduction have been reported in the literature. In the prone or gravity method described by Stimson (Fig. 49–43), the patient is placed so that the distal pelvis overhangs the edge of the stretcher. The hip, knee, and ankle are all flexed to 90° and downward pressure is applied to the proximal posterior tibia.[81] The hip can be gently internally and externally rotated to facilitate reduction, and if needed, an assistant may apply direct downward pressure to the femoral head. An alternative and more comfortable way

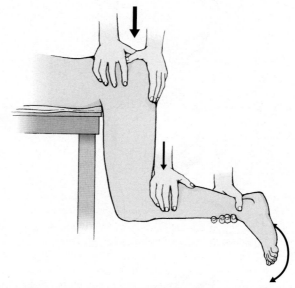

Figure 49–43 Stimson method of reduction for posterior dislocation of the hip (see text for description). *(From DeLee JC: Fractures and dislocations of the hip. In Rockwood CA, Green DP [eds]: Fractures in Adults, vol 2. Philadelphia, JB Lippincott, 1991, p 1588. Reproduced by permission.)*

to provide downward pressure on the tibia is for the operator to grasp the patient's ankle and place her or his own knee on the patient's calf, applying the body weight for pressure.[82] This method is believed to be the least traumatic; however, associated injuries or deep sedation may prevent the required prone position.[81]

Other techniques involve placing the patient in a supine position with downward stabilization of the pelvis performed by an assistant. This may be preferable in the multiply injured patient, because placing these patients in the position necessary for the Stimson technique may be difficult or impossible. In the Allis technique (Fig. 49–44), upward traction is exerted in line with the deformity, and the hip is flexed to 90°. The hip can be gently rotated internally and externally until it is reduced.[81] Some prefer to stand on the patient's stretcher to allow using body weight for leverage. Howard[83] suggested modifying this technique by applying lateral traction to the flexed upper femur to disengage the head of the femur from the outer lip of the acetabulum.

A newer method known as the Whistler technique was described by Walden and Hamer.[84] The patient is placed in the supine position with both knees flexed to 130°. While an assistant stabilizes the pelvis, the operator stands beside the

affected limb, placing an arm under the affected knee to grasp the unaffected knee. With the other hand, the operator anchors the ankle of the affected leg firmly against the stretcher (Fig. 49–45). Using the arm placed under the knee as a lever, the clinician raises the shoulder, elevating the affected knee. This allows the femoral head to move anteriorly around the acetabular rim to relocate.[84] Although there is only limited experience with this technique, it appears to be a promising, gentle reduction method.

Once reduction is achieved, the legs are immobilized in slight abduction through the placement of an abduction pillow or another object between the knees. Repeat radiographs confirm reduction, and the patient is admitted to the hospital.

Dislocations of Hip Prostheses

The dislocation of a hip prosthesis is a separate issue (Fig. 49–46A). Unlike primary dislocations that require significant trauma, a prosthetic hip may dislocate with minimal force, such as rolling over in bed or trying to get out of a chair. Most dislocations occur in the first 3 to 4 months after surgery, but recurrent dislocation may occur much later. The majority of dislocations are posterior. The emergency physician should consider consultation with the orthopaedic surgeon who placed the prosthesis.

The three major causes of prosthetic hip dislocations include (1) the patient assuming a position that exceeds the stability of the prosthesis, (2) soft tissue imbalances, and (3) component malposition.[85]

Emergency clinicians have been shown to be highly successful in reducing prosthetic hip dislocations.[86] Reduction techniques are similar to those described earlier; however, the urgency is not as paramount, because the problems with bone necrosis do not exist. Although complications are occasionally unavoidable, the clinician must be aware that forceful reduction of the dislocated hip prosthesis may dislodge the acetabular cup, fracture underlying osteoporotic bone, or loosen the prosthesis. Unlike other hip dislocations, patients with prosthetic hip dislocations often will not require hospital admis-

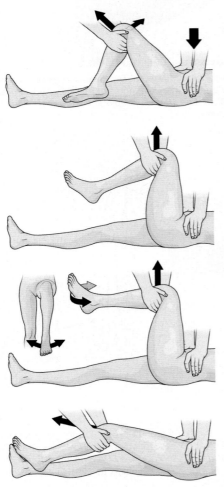

Figure 49–44 Allis method of reducing posterior dislocation of the hip (see text for description). *(From DeLee JC: Fractures and dislocations of the hip. In Rockwood CA, Green DP [eds]: Fractures in Adults, vol 2. Philadelphia, JB Lippincott, 1991, p 1594. Reproduced by permission.)*

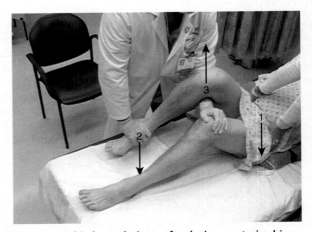

Figure 49–45 **Whistler technique of reducing posterior hip dislocation.** The operator stabilizes the affected ankle with one hand while placing the other arm under the affected knee to grasp the unaffected knee. While an assistant stabilizes the pelvis, the operator raises the shoulder, elevating the knee to reduce the dislocation. *(From Thomsen T, Setnik G [eds]: Procedures Consult—Emergency Medicine Module. Copyright 2008 Elsevier Inc. All rights reserved.)*

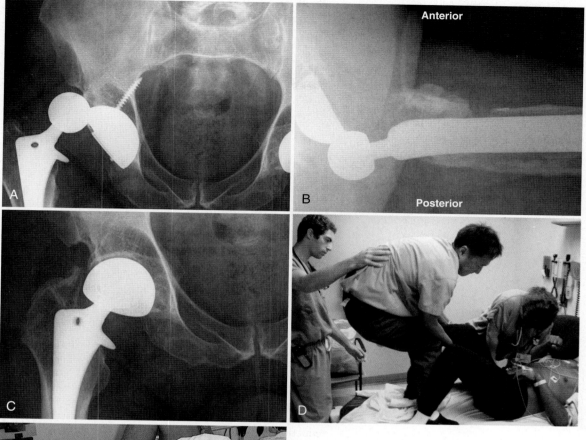

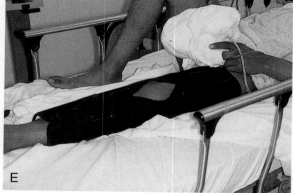

Figure 49–46 Usually a hip dislocation is the result of significant trauma, but prosthetic hips can dislocate with minimal trauma, such as rolling over in bed or a minor twisting. This method is usually successful for all hip dislocations but it is commonly used for repositioning prosthetic hip displacements. *A and B,* Posterior dislocation of a hip prosthesis. *C,* Radiograph demonstrates reduction. *D,* A common method of reducing a posterior hip dislocation is to stand on the bed as shown. Apply traction with external rotation to get the femoral head away from the metallic cup. Assistants protect the operator and provide countertraction. *E,* After reduction, a knee immobilizer prevents dislocation again since hip motion is hampered. *Note:* Care must be taken not to disrupt the prosthesis by using excessive force. Also note that osteoporotic bones can fracture during a forceful reduction. This procedure requires adequate sedation/analgesia. If reduction is not accomplished, general anesthesia may be required.

sion and may be discharged after discussion with the consulting orthopaedic surgeon. The most common way to reduce such dislocations is shown in Figure 49–46.

Anterior Hip Dislocation

Anterior hip dislocation is a less common injury than posterior dislocation, constituting 10% to 15% of all hip dislocations.[81] There are three general types of anterior hip dislocations, which are defined by where the femoral head comes to rest (Fig. 49–47): the iliac or subspinous, the pubic, and the inferior or obturator dislocation. Anterior hip dislocations generally result from a forced abduction of the thigh, which may occur in a fall or motor vehicle crash.[81] The clinical picture varies with the type of dislocation. With the obturator (inferior) type, the leg is abducted and externally rotated

with varying degrees of flexion. In the other types, the hip is usually extended and externally rotated.[81]

Reduction Techniques

The Stimson gravity method may work for anterior hip dislocation, although it is not recommended for the pubic type.[81] Alternatively, the Allis maneuver is applied in a modified fashion (Fig. 49–48). The patient is placed in a supine position and an assistant stabilizes the pelvis and applies lateral countertraction to the thigh. Traction by the operator is applied in the long axis of the femur with the hip slightly flexed. The leg is then gently adducted and internally rotated to effect reduction.[81]

In the reverse Bigelow technique, the hip is held in partial flexion and abduction. Traction is applied in the line of the deformity, and the hip is then adducted, sharply internally

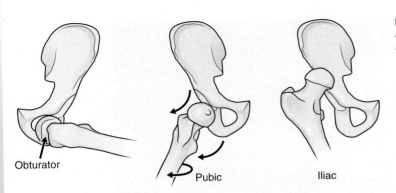

Figure 49–47 Anterior dislocations of the hip: obturator, pubic, and iliac. *(From Simon R, Koenigsknecht S: Orthopedics in Emergency Medicine. New York, Appleton-Century-Crofts, 1982, p 367. Reproduced by permission.)*

Obturator

Pubic

Iliac

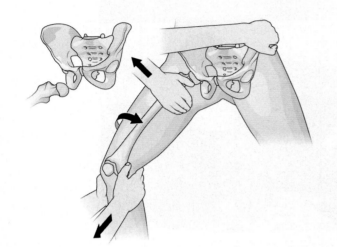

Figure 49–48 Modified Allis maneuver for reduction of anterior hip dislocation (see text for description). *(From DeLee JC: Fractures and dislocations of the hip. In Rockwood CA, Green DP [eds]: Fractures in Adults, vol 2. Philadelphia, JB Lippincott, 1991, p 1588. Reproduced by permission.)*

rotated, and extended. Caution should be exercised in using this technique because the sharp internal rotation may result in femoral neck fracture in patients with osteoporotic bone.[81] As with posterior dislocations, admission to the hospital is required for patients with these injuries.

KNEE (FEMUR/TIBIA) DISLOCATIONS

Although the knee is a simple hinge joint, dislocations are quite rare owing to its strong ligamentous support. The major ligaments include the anterior and posterior cruciate and the collateral ligaments. The usual mechanism of a knee dislocation involves a great deal of force, such as a motor vehicle crash or a sporting injury. However, knee dislocation has been reported after minor mechanisms, such as stepping off a curb or into a hole, usually associated with a twisting action.[87] Obese patients may be more likely to dislocate a knee with surprisingly minor trauma, with stepping in a hole with a twisting mechanism being a common mechanism (Fig. 49–49). There are five general types of knee dislocations, including anterior, posterior, lateral, and the less common medial and rotatory. The more common types are shown in Figure 49–50. Rotatory dislocations may be either posterolateral or posteromedial. Knee dislocations are described with respect to the position of the tibia in relation to the femur.[88]

Clinical Assessment

Knee dislocations are usually clinically obvious; however, dislocation may have been spontaneously reduced prior to ED evaluation, presenting only as severe knee pain with hemarthrosis. It is the spontaneously reduced knee dislocation, often one that is associated with other major trauma, that thwarts initial diagnosis. Obese patients may exhibit a seemingly normal appearance to the knee (see Fig. 49–49A), but an obvious deformity is often appreciated on initial examination (see Fig. 49–49B). A grossly unstable knee is probably a reduced dislocation and carries the same risk of vascular and other complications as a dislocated knee.[89] The severely unstable knee can be defined as one that has greater 30° of recurvatum (hyperextension)[89] upon lifting the leg off the stretcher by the heel or one that has gross instability after reduction.[88] Because of pain and muscle spasm that limit the physical examination for stability, a knee hemarthrosis, usually a large one with signs of posterior or calf hemorrhage, is a potential tip-off to a reduced dislocation.

An impressive effusion may not be present in knee dislocation because the joint capsule is often disrupted and extravasation occurs into the surrounding tissue, usually posteriorly. The most important part of the clinical assessment is the vascular status of the extremity (see later). Nerve injury is less common, but peroneal nerve injury is a recognized complication, particularly of a posterolateral dislocation.[88] Posterolateral dislocations may be irreducible because the medial femoral condyle buttonholes through the joint capsule.[88] A clue to this injury is the presence of a dimple sign at the medial joint line.

Vascular Injury

The most feared complication of a knee dislocation is severance or internal injury of the popliteal artery. Injury to the popliteal artery may complicate both anterior and posterior knee dislocation and occurs because the artery is relatively fixed both proximally and distally.[88] In addition, Varnell and associates[89] noted that vascular injury was as common in the severely unstable knee (e.g., field-reduced) as in an acutely dislocated knee. The incidence of popliteal artery injury in a dislocated knee is around 20% in most series.[89,90] The seriousness of this complication is largely due to the fact that collateral circulation about the knee is poor,[42] and amputation may be the end result of popliteal artery (or vein) injury. It should also be noted that nerve injuries are also more common in the patient with vascular injury.[91]

It has been previously stated that popliteal artery disruption can occur despite the presence of a normal pulse.[92] Such

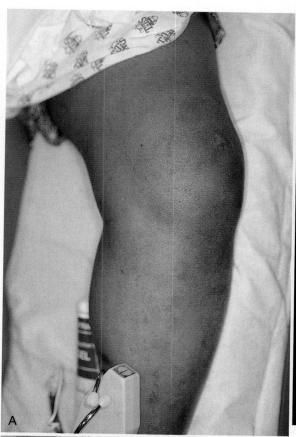

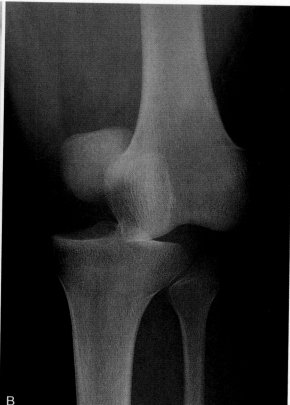

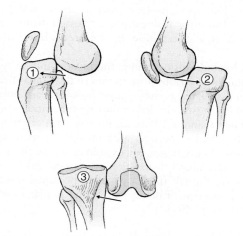

901

Figure 49–49 *A,* In an obese patient, a dislocated knee may not be obvious on initial inspection. This patient stated that she stepped into a hole and twisted the knee (a classic mechanism for dislocation), causing the clinician to suspect only a sprain. *B,* An x-ray demonstrated the seriousness of this seemingly benign injury. If a spontaneous reduction occurs before ED evaluation, this diagnosis may not even be considered. *C,* The dislocation is usually readily reduced by traction-countertraction. Tibial manipulation concurrent with traction-countertraction is often helpful. Evaluations for damage to the popliteal artery range from a careful physical examination of pulses, blood pressure determinations in the ankle, to an arteriogram. This is obviously a serious injury requiring months of rehabilitation. *Beware:* Spontaneous relocation can occur before evaluation, presenting to the clinician as only ligamentous injury and hemarthrosis.

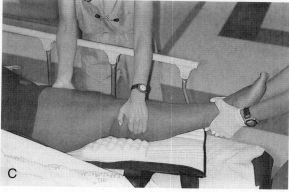

Figure 49–50 Three most common types of knee dislocations. Anterior (*1*), posterior (*2*), and lateral (*3*). *(From DePalma AF: Management of Fractures and Dislocations: An Atlas. Philadelphia, WB Saunders, 1970, p 1621. Reproduced by permission.)*

statements have led to recommendations to perform arteriography or exploration in all knee dislocations.[88] However, some studies question that perspective. Varnell and associates[89] reported a pulse deficit or absent pulse in all patients with vascular injury. Kendall and coworkers[90] also reported clear clinical evidence for all popliteal artery injuries in knee dislocations. This group recommended exploration for obvious ischemia, angiography for those patients with ischemia who have pulse restoration after relocation, and observation for all others.[90] Dennis and colleagues[93] reported that physical examination alone showed 100% accuracy in predicting the need for surgical intervention among patients with posterior knee dislocations. Miranda and associates[94] reported that popliteal artery injury can be safely and reliably predicted by a physical examination that includes specific evaluation for active posterior hemorrhage, expanding hematoma, absent pulse, or the presence of a thrill/bruit. However, it is noted that the hard physical signs of arterial injury might be delayed for 24 to 48 hours. Although the focused clinician examination may be quite accurate in the vast majority of cases, popliteal artery injury is subtle enough, or occasionally delayed, that any dislocated knee should prompt serious concern about the vascular integrity of the leg.

Simple palpation of the artery may not be sensitive enough to detect a decreased pulse, so an ankle/brachial arterial pressure index (ABI), comparison of the blood pressure at the ankle, or digit pulse oximetry of the uninjured leg should be considered (see Fig. 49–1). Mills and coworkers[91] reported a prospective study of 38 patients with knee dislocation in order to evaluate the accuracy of the ABI for identifying vascular injury. Patients with an ABI less than 0.90 underwent arteriography, and those with an ABI of 0.90 or greater underwent serial examination and delayed arterial duplex evaluation. Eleven (29%) of the patients had an ABI less than 0.90, and all had arterial injuries requiring surgical intervention. Of the remaining 27 patients with an ABI of 0.90 or greater, none had a vascular injury noted on serial examination or duplex ultrasonography. No patient in this group was found to have vascular compromise at follow-up (range, 4–36 mo).[91]

Because all knee dislocations will require orthopaedic evaluation, it is the dislocated and spontaneously reduced knee that is problematic for the emergency clinician to diagnose. Internal derangement with a knee hemarthrosis (often of the size noted with an anterior cruciate ligament tear) is a common first impression in the spontaneously reduced knee dislocation. Therefore, all knee injuries with significant swelling, hemarthrosis, or a dislocating mechanism of injury should be evaluated with a specific intent on ruling out vascular injury.

If vascular compromise is detected on clinical assessment, it is appropriate to reduce the knee dislocation without obtaining radiographs, although a few minutes to obtain portable x-rays and administer IV medication would probably be unlikely to make a difference in final outcome.[88] Use of Doppler ultrasound for pulse checks and ABIs should also be considered in these injuries (see Chapter 1, Vital Signs Monitoring). Early consultation should be sought in knee dislocations owing to the high incidence of complications and frequent need for operative intervention. The decision to pursue angiography in the patient with the dislocated knee is best made in consultation with the patient's orthopaedic surgeon.

Reduction Technique

The need for IV sedation and analgesia depends on the clinical situation, but it should be considered whenever possible (see Chapter 33, Systemic Analgesia and Sedation for Procedures). The basic initial approach for all types of knee dislocations is to apply traction to the extremity (Fig. 49–51). This alone is often all that is required for reduction owing to severe disruption of the ligamentous support of the knee.[64] For anterior dislocations, the distal femur is lifted to effect reduction. For posterior dislocations, the proximal tibia is lifted to complete the reduction.[42] For medial, lateral, and rotatory dislocations, a similar approach is acceptable, with pressure being exerted as needed in the medial or lateral direction.

After reduction, the extremity is splinted in 15° of flexion. The posterolateral dislocation may be irreducible, and operative intervention should be considered if reduction is not easily accomplished.[42]

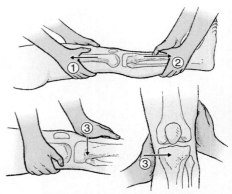

Figure 49–51 **Manipulative reduction of a knee dislocation.** *1,* An assistant fixes and provides countertraction on the thigh. *2,* Another assistant provides straight traction on the leg (this usually reduces the dislocation). *3,* The operator puts direct pressure over the displaced bones. *(From DePalma AF: Management of Fractures and Dislocations: An Atlas. Philadelphia, WB Saunders, 1970, p 1623. Reproduced by permission.)*

Postreduction Care

Appropriate aftercare for knee dislocations involves serial reassessment of the neurovascular status of the extremity. Postreduction radiographs are performed, and the patient is admitted to the hospital. The application of a knee immobilizer will provide stabilization and comfort. These injuries cause severe ligamentous and other derangements in the knee and generally require operative stabilization, with a long period of recovery and physical therapy.

DISLOCATIONS OF THE FIBULAR HEAD

The fibula can be dislocated at its proximal articulation in the knee joint. This is most commonly an anterolateral dislocation.[88] The fibular head is normally nestled in a stable manner behind the lateral tibial condyle with two supporting tibiofibular ligaments.[95] The tibiofibular joint has a separate synovial cavity, and therefore, a typical knee joint effusion will not be seen with this dislocation. When the knee is flexed, the stability of this joint is decreased owing to relaxation of the fibular collateral ligament.[95] The typical mechanism of injury is a fall on the flexed, adducted leg, often combined with ankle inversion. This mechanism is seen in sports and parachute landings.[95] Posterior dislocations can occur from a twisting mechanism or a direct blow to the area while the knee is flexed.[88]

Anterolateral dislocation is the most common type. It is accompanied by obvious prominence of the fibular head anteriorly; no associated neurovascular problems are noted. The less common posterior dislocation may be accompanied by peroneal nerve injury.[88] Patients present with varying degrees of disability, and some may walk on the leg with only mild discomfort.[95] On radiographic examination, the three cardinal signs of anterolateral dislocation are lateral displacement of the fibula on the AP film, a widened proximal interosseous space, and anterior displacement of the fibular head on the lateral view (Fig. 49–52).[95]

Reduction Technique

The position for reduction of an anterior fibular head dislocation is to place the patient supine and flex the knee to 90° in

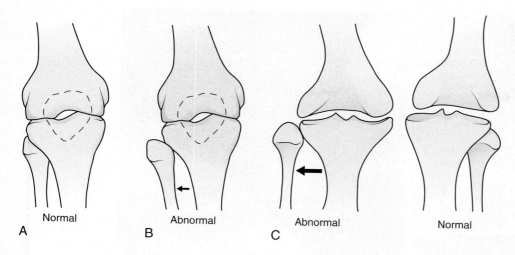

Figure 49–52 **Anterolateral fibular head dislocation compared with the normal knee.** The interosseous distance is widened and the proximal fibula is displaced laterally. *A,* Normal AP projection of knee. *B,* Lateral displacement of the proximal fibula. *C,* Use of bilateral comparison views to highlight fibular displacement.

Normal   Abnormal   Abnormal   Normal

A   B   C

order to relax the biceps femoris tendon. Direct pressure is then applied to the fibular head; reduction is usually signified by a snap.[88] The method for a posterior dislocation is the same except that direct pressure is applied in a forward direction. Patients should not bear weight for 2 weeks and should receive orthopaedic referral. Immobilization is probably unnecessary.[88]

PATELLAR DISLOCATION

Patellar dislocations are fairly common, especially among adolescents. The usual mechanism is a powerful quadriceps contraction combined with a strong valgus and external rotation component.[96] This may be seen in activities such as making a "cut" in sports or with dancing. The patella may also dislocate from a direct blow to the flexed knee.[42] Predisposing factors to patellar dislocation include chronic patellofemoral abnormalities such as genu valgum and femoral anteversion.[96] The patellar dislocation is described by the relation of the patella to the knee joint. Lateral dislocations are the most common by far. Other types include superior, medial, and intra-articular (Fig. 49–53).

Clinical Assessment

Lateral dislocation of the patella is generally clinically obvious (Fig. 49–54). The knee is held in some degree of flexion and the patella can be easily seen and palpated on the lateral side of the knee. A tenting-type action of the patella is often detectable unless significant soft tissue swelling is present.

The patella may be spontaneously reduced in the field with simple leg straightening. The patient will report that the leg "went out" and may describe actually seeing the lateral deformity caused by the displaced patella. Clinical clues to the spontaneously reduced patella include the presence of a knee effusion and tenderness along the medial edge of the patella. Fairbank's test or the patellar "apprehension" sign is elicited when the patella is pushed laterally and the patient grabs for the knee, indicating the sensation of repeat injury.[42]

Radiographs

Prereduction films are difficult to obtain because the patient is usually in flexion. Some recommend prereduction films when possible in all patients[42]; however, it is an easy matter

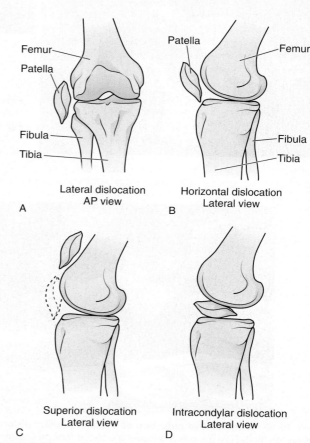

Femur   Patella   Femur
Patella

Fibula   Fibula
Tibia   Tibia

Lateral dislocation
AP view
A

Horizontal dislocation
Lateral view
B

Superior dislocation
Lateral view
C

Intracondylar dislocation
Lateral view
D

Figure 49–53 *A–D,* Various types of patellar dislocation. The lateral dislocation is the most common.

to reduce these injuries before radiography. The diagnosis is usually obvious, and there are no reports in the literature of complications from gentle reduction. Osteochondral fractures are detectable in about half of patients with patellar dislocations, but many of these are visible only on arthroscopy.[96] Postreduction radiographs are recommended, as are prereduction studies, when the diagnosis is uncertain. The clinical diagnosis of patellar dislocation in an older patient should be made with caution because these are primarily injuries of the young.

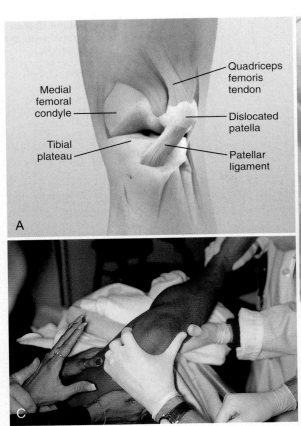

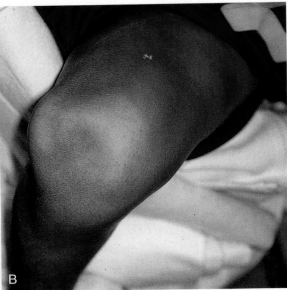

Figure 49–54 *A* and *B,* Lateral dislocation of the patella. *C,* To reduce a lateral dislocation, the knee is extended while the patella is directed medially using slight anteriorly directed elevation. *(A and B, From Thomsen T, Setnik G [eds]: Procedures Consult—Emergency Medicine Module. Copyright 2008 Elsevier Inc. All rights reserved.)*

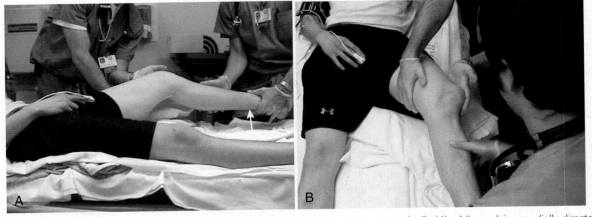

Figure 49–55 Manipulative reduction of a lateral patellar dislocation. Extend the knee gradually (*A*) while applying medially directed pressure on the patella (*B*), pushing it over the lateral femoral condyle. *(From Thomsen T, Setnik G [eds]: Procedures Consult—Emergency Medicine Module. Copyright 2008 Elsevier Inc. All rights reserved.)*

Reduction Technique and Postreduction Care

Reduction of a lateral patellar dislocation is usually quite simple. Premedication is often not required if the patient can be verbally reassured. If the patient is anxious or in great discomfort, premedication should be considered (see Chapter 33, Systemic Analgesia and Sedation for Procedures). The two basic maneuvers for patellar relocation are extension of the knee and gentle medial pressure applied to the patella, lifting the most lateral edge of the patella over the femoral condyle (Fig. 49–55; see also Fig. 49–54).[42]

The leg is then immobilized in extension. This may be done by casting or application of a commercially available knee immobilizer. Orthopaedic follow-up is necessary because of the need for physical therapy and the high rate of persistent instability.[96] However, hospitalization is not required for routine lateral dislocations of the patella. Recurrent dislocation, and those associated with an osteochondral fracture, might require operative repair.

Patellar dislocations in other locations are often irreducible, and orthopaedic consultation should be sought. Intracondylar and superior dislocations are extremely rare and

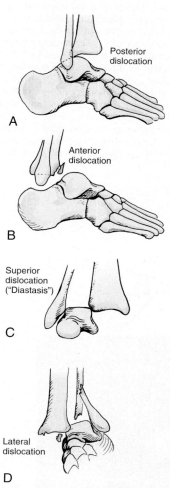

Figure 49–56 *A–D, The types of dislocations of the ankle. (From Simon R, Koenigsknecht S: Orthopedics in Emergency Medicine. New York, Appleton-Century-Crofts, 1982, p 419. Reproduced by permission.)*

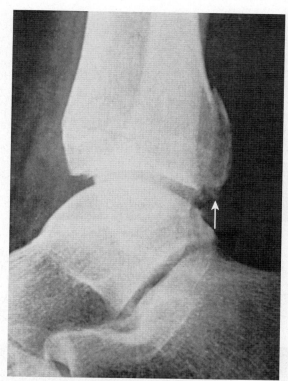

Figure 49–57 Isolated posterior tibial lip fracture (*arrow*), seen only after reduction of a posterior ankle dislocation. *(From Harris JH Jr, Harris WH: Radiology of Emergency Medicine, 2nd ed. Baltimore, Williams & Wilkins, 1981, p 629. Reproduced by permission.)*

905

require operative reduction. The rare horizontal dislocation may relocate with closed reduction but surgical reduction is often necessary.

ANKLE DISLOCATIONS

The ankle joint is a modified saddle joint in which the talus is nestled in the mortise formed by the distal tibia and fibula.[42] The ligamentous support of the ankle is quite strong, and pure dislocations are uncommon. Usually, there are associated fractures of the ankle joint (Fig. 49–56). Ankle dislocations are described by the relation of the talus to the tibia. Posterior dislocations of the ankle are more common than are anterior dislocations, and they usually result from a fall on a plantar-flexed foot. Patients with posterior dislocations often have an associated fracture of one or more of the malleoli,[42] occasionally seen only post reduction (Fig. 49–57). The clinical picture is usually one of significant deformity and disability.

Anterior dislocations generally result from forced dorsi-flexion or a blow directed posteriorly to the distal tibia while the foot is fixed. The talus is prominent anteriorly, and the dorsalis pedis pulse may be lost secondary to pressure from the talus. Superior dislocations are uncommon and result in diastasis of the tibiofibular joint. These injuries are usually the result of a significant axial force. Lateral dislocations of the ankle are always associated with fractures of the malleoli or distal fibula.

Radiographic Examination

Because of the high rate of associated fractures and the clinical difficulty in assessing for the presence or the exact nature of a dislocation, it is recommended that prereduction radiographs be obtained in all suspected ankle dislocations (see Fig. 49–2). It is acceptable to reduce the dislocation without a radiograph if severe vascular compromise is present, but for the vast majority of cases, the few minutes taken to obtain bedside radiographs and administer IV medications rarely affect final outcome. It may be impossible to accurately determine the exact type of dislocation unless prereduction films are obtained. An AP and a lateral view usually suffice for emergency management; other views can be ordered if necessary after the joint is relocated.

Reduction Techniques

Unless a strong contraindication is present, it is advisable to administer IV sedation and analgesia to patients with ankle dislocation early in their care, preferably before conducting any manipulations or radiologic studies. Reduction is always painful in the awake patient, and sufficient premedication must be administered. For posterior dislocations, the patient is placed supine and the *knee is slightly flexed* to relax the Achilles tendon (Fig. 49–58). An assistant can do this, or the patient can be positioned such that the knee hangs over the end of

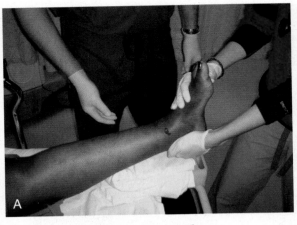

Figure 49–58 *A,* Manipulative reduction of a posterior ankle dislocation. *B,* The knee is slightly flexed (*1*), an assistant provides countertraction on the leg (*2*) while the forefoot is grasped with one hand under the heel (*3*) with the other hand over the dorsal metatarsals. The foot is first slightly plantar flexed (*4*). Apply straight downward traction on the plantar flexed foot. *C,* Pull the foot forward with longitudinal traction on the heel (*5*) and dorsiflex the foot (*6*), while a second assistant provides counterpressure on the front of the lower leg (*7*). *D,* Note that a seemingly minor laceration is evidence of the fractured bone previously protruding through the skin (compound fracture requiring antibiotics and open débridement). *E,* A sugar-tong splint is placed with the foot at 90°, so the dorsal pulse and sensation can be checked without removing the splint. (*B* and *C,* From DePalma AF: *Management of Fractures and Dislocations.* Philadelphia, WB Saunders, 1970, pp 1916 and 1917. Reproduced by permission.)

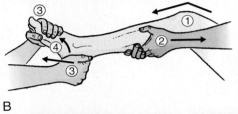
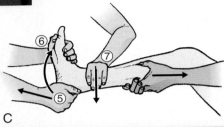

B C

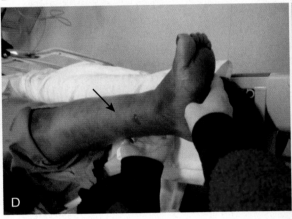

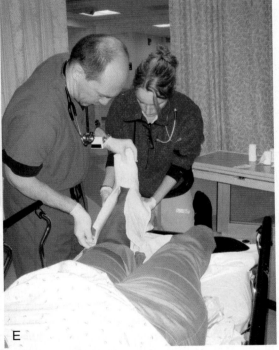

the bed. The operator then grasps the foot with both hands, placing one hand on the heel and the other on the forefoot. The foot is flexed slightly plantar, and traction is applied to the foot. A second assistant can then apply downward pressure on the distal tibia as the operator moves the heel anteriorly to effect reduction.[97]

For anterior dislocations, the initial steps and positioning are the same as those for posterior dislocation (Fig. 49–59). However, instead of plantar flexion, the foot is dorsiflexed to free the talus. The second assistant applies upward pressure to the distal tibia while the operator applies traction and pushes the foot in a posterior direction.[42]

Lateral dislocations are really fracture-dislocations, and orthopaedic consultation is generally required as part of the ED course. The emergency clinician will often need to reduce these injuries owing to the extreme lateral deformity and the occasional compromise of the dorsalis pedis artery by stretch. Open dislocations (in the absence of vascular compromise) may be better handled by cleaning in the operating room before attempting reduction. If a lateral fracture-dislocation is to be reduced in the ED, the approach is quite similar to that for posterior ankle dislocation. However, instead of pressure in the AP direction, the foot is moved medially after application of traction.[42]

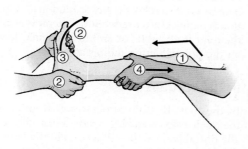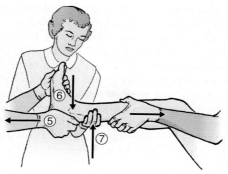

Figure 49–59 Manipulative reduction of anterior ankle dislocation. *1,* The knee is flexed. *2,* The operator grasps the forefoot with one hand and the heel with the other. *3,* Dorsiflexion of the foot is slightly increased (to disengage the talus). *4,* An assistant provides countertraction on the leg. *5,* Straight longitudinal traction is applied, then the foot is pushed directly backward (*6*) while a second assistant provides countertraction on the back of the lower leg (*7*). *(From DePalma AF: Management of Fractures and Dislocations. Philadelphia, WB Saunders, 1970, pp 1918 and 1919. Reproduced by permission.)*

Postreduction Care

The ankle is splinted at 90° with a long-leg posterior splint. The application of a stirrup splint in addition to the posterior splint may provide additional stability (see Chapter 50, Splinting Techniques). Necessity for admission to the hospital must be determined in consultation with an orthopaedic surgeon. Many patients with these injuries have associated fractures that require surgical intervention.

DISLOCATIONS OF THE FOOT

The importance of the foot is recognized by anyone who has had to spend time ambulating with an injury to this area. For the purposes of discussion, injuries to the foot can be divided into those of the hindfoot and those of the forefoot.

Hindfoot Injuries

Injuries to this area are uncommon and usually result from high-energy transfer. The major dislocations are subtalar and talar dislocations and midtarsal fracture-dislocations (Lisfranc injury). Although x-ray findings are often subtle and easily overlooked, Lisfranc injury is complex and always a fracture-dislocation because of the rigid nature of the region (Fig. 49–60). These injuries require orthopaedic management and are not discussed here.

Subtalar Dislocation

This uncommon injury generally occurs secondary to sports, falls from heights, or motor vehicle crashes. The calcaneus, navicular, and forefoot are displaced from the talus.[97] The primary mechanisms are severe inversion causing a medial dislocation or severe eversion resulting in a lateral dislocation. The medial type occurs so commonly during basketball that it has been termed *basketball foot.*[98] This injury is usually seen in young adult males. Medial dislocations constitute the majority (85%) of these injuries, with lateral dislocations making up the rest.[98]

The diagnosis is usually obvious because the talus is prominent and often tents the skin of the proximal foot. The medial type has been termed an *acquired clubfoot;* the lateral type appears as an *acquired flatfoot.*[98]

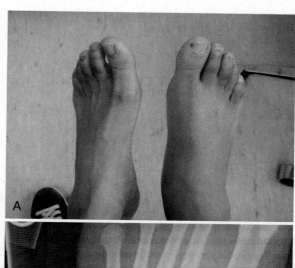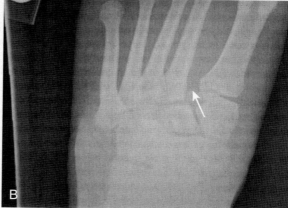

Figure 49–60 *A,* Lisfranc fracture-dislocation is a serious and debilitating injury that is easily missed. This patient complained of extremely severe pain in the foot and was unable to walk after falling down the steps while intoxicated, so the mechanism was unclear. Drug seeking was suspected, however; *note the significant soft tissue swelling,* suggesting internal injury. *B,* This x-ray was initially read as a minor avulsion fracture around base of the second metatarsal, but a closer review shows a widening of the space between the first and the second metatarsals and *lateral displacement of the rest of the metatarsals.* This injury often requires operative repair, and permanent disability is common in the best of circumstances.

Some authors recommend spinal or general anesthesia for all such injuries[98]; however, it is usually possible to reduce these injuries with IV premedication. The patient is positioned in a supine fashion and the hip and knee are flexed much as in posterior dislocation of the ankle. One hand is placed on the forefoot and the other grasps the heel. Firm longitudinal traction is required to effect reduction, and dangling the leg over the end of the bed allows the operator to use his or her body weight to assist in traction. Once traction is applied, the deformity is initially increased (inversion for medial; eversion for lateral) and then reversed to effect reduction.[98]

Dislocation of the Talus

In this extremely rare injury, the talus is essentially extruded from its normal position, coming to lie anteriorly. This injury is generally open,[98] is not amenable to closed reduction, and virtually always progresses to avascular necrosis.[99] Talectomy and arthrodesis are often required,[98] and orthopaedic referral should be emergently undertaken if vascular compromise of the foot is present.

Forefoot Dislocations

Much of what is pertinent to the diagnosis and management of forefoot dislocations has already been discussed in the management of dislocations of the fingers and hand MCP joints. Anatomically, the joints are quite similar.

Metatarsophalangeal Dislocations

These uncommon injuries are generally the result of hyperextension resulting in a dorsal dislocation of the great toe metatarsophalangeal (MTP) joint.[100] Among the lesser toe MTP joints, lateral or medial displacement of the digit on the metatarsal head is more common and usually is the result of jamming the toe on a piece of furniture.[98] As with MCP dislocations, these can be simple or complex. Complex dislocations of the first toe can be suspected by the presence of sesamoid bones in the joint space in the prereduction radiographs.[98] Complex MTP dislocations are often irreducible.

For simple MTP dislocations, reduction is accomplished by increasing the deformity through hyperextension and then applying traction while exerting thumb pressure over the base

of the dislocated proximal phalanx. Plantar flexion of the foot may be used to relax the flexor tendons.[97] Operative intervention is required after reduction if crepitus is present on motion, the joint is unstable, or an intra-articular loose body is noted on the postreduction radiographs.[98]

IP Dislocations

In the foot, IP dislocations result from an axial load to the toe, such as from kicking a wall. These dislocations are generally dorsal and can be reduced as in the hand. Dislocations of the first toe IP joint are usually buddy taped to the second toe for 2 to 3 weeks, whereas those of lesser toes can be taped for 10 to 14 days.[98] As in the hand, complex dislocations may occur and require open reduction.

CONCLUSION

The following points are important regarding the assessment and management of dislocations:

1. A search for other more serious injuries should be undertaken when there is a high-energy mechanism of injury.
2. A neurovascular assessment should be performed early in the evaluation and appropriately documented.
3. Radiographs and IV premedication are generally indicated prior to reduction attempts.
4. Reduction attempts should involve the gentle, gradual application of forces and patience on the operator's part.
5. After completing reduction, the operator should recheck the neurovascular status, request postreduction radiographs (except with radial head subluxations), and in certain circumstances, assess the stability and the range of motion of the joint.
6. A definite percentage of dislocations are irreducible, and the need for multiple attempts should halt prolonged and forceful attempts in the ED and prompt orthopaedic consultation.
7. Reductions that present with neurologic injury should be reduced by the most expeditious and least traumatic method.

 REFERENCES CAN BE FOUND ON EXPERT CONSULT

CHAPTER 50

Splinting Techniques

Carl R. Chudnofsky and Stacie E. Byers

Splints are frequently used in the emergency department (ED) for temporary immobilization of fractures and dislocations and for definitive therapy of soft tissue injuries.[1,2] Patients with a variety of nontraumatic musculoskeletal disorders (e.g., gout, infections, burns) also benefit from short-term immobilization therapy. Immobilization is the mainstay of fracture therapy, but it is difficult to find firm scientific data that support the use of splinting for soft tissue injuries.[3,4] Although the general principle of immobilizing sprains and contusions is strongly supported by custom and personal preference, its exact influence on healing, number of complications, and ultimate return to normal activity is not known. In most studies of ankle sprains, for example, the function and pain of the injured joint are similar at 6 weeks' follow-up, regardless of whether treatment consisted of ad lib walking, a simple elastic bandage, a posterior splint, or a formal cast.[5,6] A systematic review of 22 random clinical trials comparing various treatments for lateral acute ankle sprains (cast, splint, or early immobilization with support) found no favorable effect of immobilization.[7] The current data support functional management for most cases of acute ankle sprains.[7]

Similar concepts have evolved for acute cervical strain and low back strain. Although a strict standard of care cannot be promulgated, the use of short-term splinting in the ED for acutely painful conditions remains a common practice.

Most splinting techniques are handed down from house staff or experienced clinicians, but the procedure is often suboptimal and haphazard.[8] This chapter presents guidelines for the adequate immobilization of injuries commonly encountered by emergency clinicians.

Patients routinely present to the ED with injuries that are amenable to splinting to relieve pain and augment healing (Table 50–1). Emergency clinicians have virtually abandoned the use of circumferential casts in favor of premade commercial immobilizing devices or splints made from plaster of Paris or fiberglass. The impetus for this change is primarily related to the complications occasionally associated with circumferential casts, liability issues, and ease of application brought about by new technology. In most instances, properly applied splints provide short-term immobilization equal to that of casts while allowing for continued swelling, thus reducing the risk of ischemic injury. Other obvious advantages of splints are that patients can take them off when immobilization is no longer needed or can remove them temporarily to bathe, exercise the injured part, or perform wound care.

INDICATIONS

Theoretically, immobilization facilitates the healing process by decreasing pain and protecting the extremity from further injury. Other benefits of splinting are specific to the particular injury or problem being treated. For example, in the treatment of fractures, splinting helps maintain bony alignment. Splinting deep lacerations that cross joints reduces tension on the wound and helps prevent wound dehiscence. Immobilizing tendon lacerations may facilitate the healing process by relieving stress on the repaired tendon. The discomfort of inflammatory disorders such as tenosynovitis or acute gout is greatly reduced by immobilization (Fig. 50–1). Deep space infections of the hands or feet as well as cellulitis over any joint should similarly be immobilized for comfort. Limiting early motion also may reduce edema and theoretically improve the immune system's ability to combat infection. Hence, select puncture wounds and mammalian bites of the hands and feet may be immobilized until the risk of infection has passed. Splinting large abrasions that cross joint surfaces prevents movement of the injured extremity and reduces the pain produced when the injured skin is stretched. Finally, patients with multiple traumas should have fractures and reduced dislocations adequately splinted while other diagnostic and therapeutic procedures (e.g., peritoneal lavage, computed tomography scan) are completed. Immobilization decreases blood loss, minimizes the potential for further neurovascular injury, decreases the need for opioid analgesia, and may decrease the risk of fat emboli from long bone fractures.

Patients often use or request an elastic bandage for many soft tissue injuries. Although applying an elastic bandage to an injured part likely is popular, it is of minimal benefit. The downside is that the bandage may be wrapped too tightly, causing additional injury or distal swelling (Fig. 50–2).

EQUIPMENT

Support Materials

Plaster of Paris

Plaster of Paris is the most widely used material for ED splinting.[9] Its name originated from the fact that it was first prepared from the gypsum of Paris, France. When gypsum is heated to approximately 128°C, most of the water of crystallization is driven off, leaving behind a fine white powder—plaster of Paris. When water is added to plaster, the reaction is reversed, and the plaster recrystallizes or sets by incorporating water molecules into the crystalline lattice of the calcium sulfate dehydrate molecules.

Today, plaster is impregnated into strips or rolls (2-, 3-, 4-, or 6-inch widths) of a crinoline-type material. The crinoline allows for easy application, helps keep the plaster molded to the proper form during the setting process, and adds support to the finished splint. Plaster rolls and sheets are available in a variety of setting times and widths. The distinct advantage of plaster over commercially available premade splints is that plaster can be more easily molded and tailored to the individual's anatomy, negating the "one-size-fits-all" approach. Also, plaster is generally less expensive than premade splints.

Prefabricated Splint Rolls

The use of plaster splints in the form of prefabricated splint rolls (e.g., OCL) is very popular among emergency clinicians. These splint rolls have 10 to 20 sheets of plaster enclosed between a thick layer of protective foam padding on one side and a thin layer of cloth on the other. Like custom-constructed splints, they are secured to the extremity with an elastic bandage. The major advantage of prefabricated splint rolls is that significant time is saved because the splint and padding come ready to apply. In addition, prefabricated splint rolls are ideal for intermittent splinting and can be removed

TABLE 50–1 Conditions That Benefit from Immobilization
Acute arthritis, including acute gout
Severe contusions and abrasions
Skin lacerations that cross joints
Tendon lacerations
Tenosynovitis
Puncture wounds to the hands, feet, and joints
Animal bites to the hands or feet
Deep space infections of the hands and feet
Joint infections
Fractures and sprains
Reduced joint dislocations

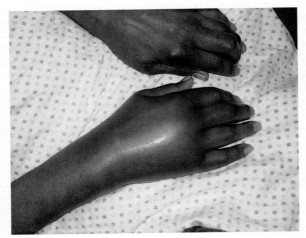

Figure 50–1 Acute gout is an indication for splinting for comfort.

and reapplied by the patient as needed. However, prefabricated plaster splint rolls are more expensive than simple plaster rolls, and they lack some of the versatility and custom-fit qualities of self-made plaster splints. The application of premade splints is shown in Figure 50–3.

Prefabricated splint rolls using layers of fiberglass between polypropylene padding (e.g., Ortho-Glass, 3M) are now commonplace in many EDs (Fig. 50–4). Fiberglass splint rolls offer the same time-saving aspect of prefabricated plaster splint rolls, but require only 3 minutes to set, making application faster. In addition, splints made from prefabricated fiberglass rolls cure more rapidly (20 min), have no messy residue (i.e., they can be hydrated using a conventional sink without a special trap), can be washed and reapplied, and are stronger and lighter than splints constructed from prefabricated plaster rolls. Another advantage is the polypropylene padding, which wicks moisture away from the skin better than polyester, nylon, or cotton padding.[10] Prefabricated fiberglass splint rolls are more expensive than both simple plaster rolls and prefabricated plaster splint rolls and, like prefabricated plaster splints, lack some of the versatility and custom-fit qualities of self-made plaster splints.

Protective and Miscellaneous Equipment

Stockinette

A single layer of stockinette is commonly used under circumferential casts and splints. It protects the skin and, when folded back over the ends of the plaster, creates a smooth,

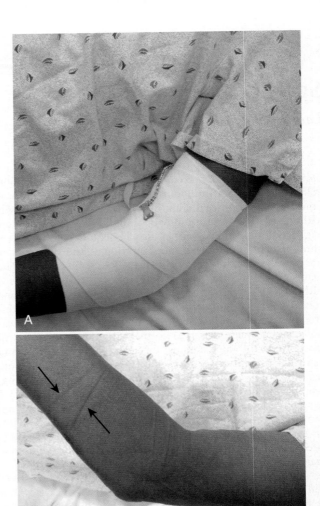

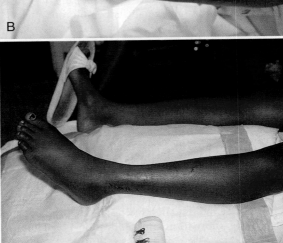

Figure 50–2 *A,* An elastic bandage is a popular home treatment for many painful conditions, such as sprains and contusions. An actual medical benefit is unproven. *B,* Wrapping an extremity too tightly may cause additional injury or distal swelling. This patient complained of a *swollen hand after an elbow injury.* Note the grooves in the skin (*arrows*) indicating that the wrap was the culprit, causing the hand swelling. *C,* Markedly swollen foot after useless elastic bandage to lower leg.

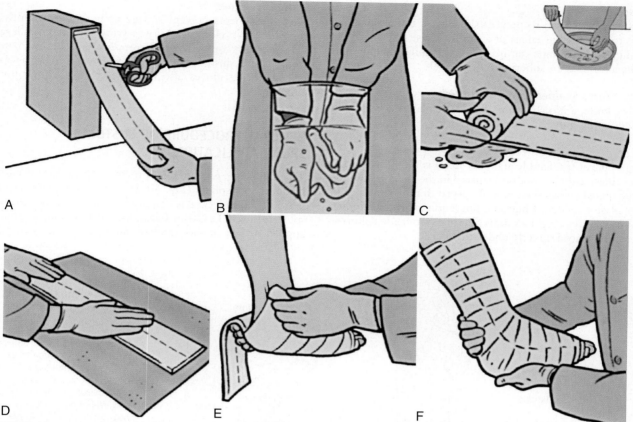

A

B

C

D

E

F

Figure 50–3 Some clinicians prefer to use premade plaster splints for temporary immobilization (e.g., OCL, J-Splint). There is less latitude for custom fitting with these products compared with the technique demonstrated in Figure 50–5. *A*, Measure the appropriate length. (Note that plain plaster slabs shrink several centimeters when wet. Cut the material slightly long, because the excess may be folded back on itself if necessary). *B*, Submerge the plaster until bubbling stops (do not oversoak). *C*, Roll and squeeze excess water from the premade splint. *Inset*, If using plain plaster slabs, allow the water to drip off. *D*, Smooth the sheets to remove wrinkles and mix the plaster throughout the layers. *E*, Apply the splint, padded site against the skin, and secure it with an elastic bandage. Some prefer to apply cotton padding (Webril) under even a padded splint for additional comfort or protection. *F*, Mold the splint to fit the contour of the extremity—an important step. *(A–F, Courtesy of Johnson & Johnson Products, Inc., New Brunswick, NJ.)*

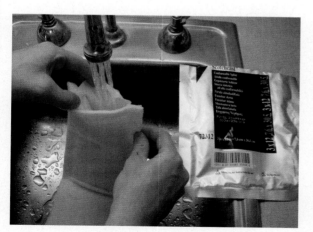

Figure 50–4 Premade fiberglass splints are also popular for temporary immobilization. Fiberglass splints set and cure more rapidly, have no messy residue (i.e., can be hydrated in a conventional sink without a special trap), can be washed and reapplied, and are lighter and stronger than plaster splints. Open the pouch and cut the splint to the desired length, stretching the padding to cover the exposed edge. A fiberglass splint requires minimal wetting. Simply run tap water through one end, and when water exits the other end, it is ready to apply. Additional Webril padding is optional. Apply the splint and secure it with an elastic bandage. When applying the splint at a right angle (e.g., posterior ankle splint), pinch and fold over any extra splinting material). See Fig. 50–6.

professional-looking, padded rim. Stockinette is available in 2-, 3-, 4-, 8-, 10-, and 12-inch widths.

Padding

Padding under the splint protects the skin and bony prominences and allows for swelling of the injured extremity. Most commercially available splints contain adequate padding in the premade product, but in some instances, additional padding is prudent. In general, the older thin cotton padding known as sheet wadding has been replaced by newer materials such as Webril (Curity) or Specialist (Johnson & Johnson) cast padding. Webril is soft cotton with a much coarser weave than sheet wadding; consequently, it has greater tensile strength, adheres better, and can be applied more evenly. Specialist padding uses micropleated cotton fibers that relax when moistened. This results in uniform, feltlike padding that conforms to the surface being wrapped. Felt (0.5-inch thick) also may be used to pad bony prominences.

Elastic Bandages

Elastic bandages are used to secure the splint in place. Elastic bandages are available in 2-, 3-, 4-, and 6-inch widths. Some bandages use metal clips; others use a Velcro-type arrangement at the end of the roll. Metal clips can be taped in place to avoid inadvertent removal.

Adhesive Tape

Adhesive tape is used to prevent slippage of the elastic bandages, to line the cut edges of a bivalved cast, and to buddy tape digits. Coban tape can be used in a similar manner and has the advantage of adhering only to itself.

Utility Knife, Scalpel, and Plaster Scissors

A utility knife, a No. 10 scalpel blade, or plaster scissors can be used to cut and shape dry plaster.

Bucket

A large bucket (preferably stainless steel) is used for wetting plaster. Plaster should not be prepared in the sink because the residue quickly clogs the drain. A special drain is required to accept plaster residue. A bucket is not required for the minimal amount of water used to soften fiberglass premade splints—they can be placed directly under the faucet.

Protective Gear

Gowns or sheets prevent soilage of both the patient's and the clinician's clothing. Gloves (vinyl or latex) and safety glasses are recommended to prevent skin or eye damage from plaster dust, wet plaster, or uncured fiberglass polymer. Wearing gloves also decreases clean-up time for the clinician.

GENERAL PROCEDURE OF CUSTOM SPLINT APPLICATION

The following section refers to the application of custom-made plaster splints (Fig. 50–5), unless otherwise stated. If periodic wound care is required, a more easily removable splint (e.g., OCL, Ortho-Glass, Velcro-type splint) should be applied in lieu of the standard splint, to be described. The

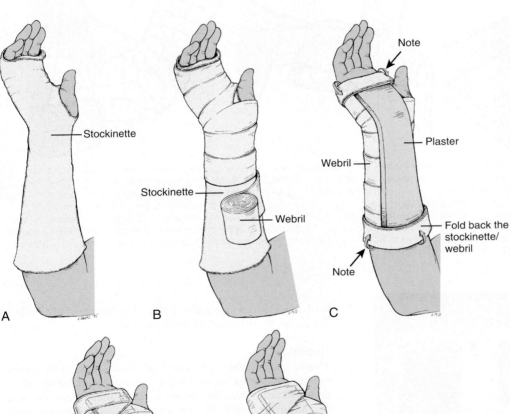

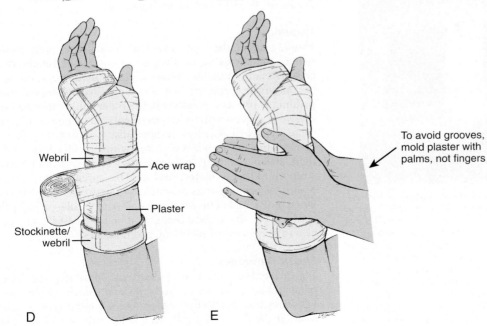

Figure 50–5 Principles of custom splint application.
A, Stockinette is applied to extend 2 or 3 inches beyond the plaster. *B,* Two or three layers of Webril are evenly and smoothly applied over the area to be splinted. *C,* The plaster slab is positioned over the area to be immobilized and the stockinette and Webril *are folded back to help secure the slab in place and to form smooth, rounded ends.* *D,* The elastic bandage is applied to secure the splint. *E,* While still wet, the plaster is molded to conform to the shape of the extremity. This is an important step that is often overlooked. See Fig. 50–6.

TABLE 50–2 Caveats for Proper Emergency Department Splinting

- Always use cool, clean water.
- Do not oversaturate the plaster splint. Minimal water is required for fiberglass splints.
- Make the splint *smooth* when placing on the patient to avoid bumps and pressure points.
- Smooth and mold the splint without squeezing. Use the palms of the hands, not the fingers, to mold the splint to fit the contour of the body part.
- Place padded side against the skin. Extra cotton padding is optimal.
- Simply roll elastic bandages over an extremity without undue tension.
- Protect or pad edges.
- Leave fingertips exposed to check for circulation and sensation.
- Keep the patient still until the splint has dried and hardened.
- Post check includes function, arterial pulse, capillary refill, temperature of skin, and sensation (FACTS).
- Emphasize and demonstrate splint elevation to the patient.
- Tape over metal clips used to fasten the elastic bandage to keep it in place and avoid ingestion by a child.

TABLE 50–3 Areas of the Upper and Lower Extremity That Require Additional Padding

Upper Extremity

Olecranon
Radial styloid
Ulnar styloid

Lower Extremity

Upper portion of the inner thigh
Patella
Fibular head
Achilles tendon
Medial and lateral malleoli

issue of removability should be addressed before the splint is applied. In addition, use of Webril (Curity) cast padding is described, but other suitable cast padding may be substituted. Caveats for proper ED splinting appear in Table 50–2.

Patient Preparation

If the clinical situation permits, the patient should be covered with a sheet or gown to protect clothing and the surrounding area from water and plaster. Nursing staff and housekeeping also appreciate this courtesy. The involved extremity should be inspected carefully before splinting. All skin lesions and soft tissue injuries should be examined and documented clearly on the ED record. All wounds should be cleaned, repaired, and dressed in the usual manner. When open fractures or joints are to be immobilized, the soft tissue defect should be covered with saline-moistened sterile gauze.

Padding

When the splint involves the digits, padding must be placed between the fingers and the toes to prevent maceration of the skin. This can be done with pieces of Webril or gauze cut to the appropriate length.

Following placement of padding between the fingers and the toes, stockinette is often used as the next protective layer in self-made splints (see Fig. 50–5A). The stockinette should extend at least 10 to 15 cm beyond the area to be splinted at both ends of the extremity. Later, after plaster has been applied, the stockinette can be folded back over the ends of the splint to create smooth, padded rims. Folding back the stockinette can also help hold the splint in place when applying elastic bandages (see Fig. 50–5C). Care is needed to avoid pressure damage from pulling the stockinette too tightly over bony prominences, such as the heel. Wrinkling over flexion creases should also be avoided by slitting and overlapping the stockinette at bony prominences. One may also use two separate pieces of stockinette (one at each end of the splint) to produce the smooth padded rims. As a general rule, 3-inch-wide stockinette is used for the upper extremity, whereas 4-inch-wide is used for the lower extremity.

After the stockinette has been properly positioned, Webril should be wrapped around the entire area that will be exposed to plaster. The Webril should be at least two or three layers thick and each turn should overlap the previous turn by 25% to 50% of its width (see Fig. 50–5B). In addition, the Webril should extend 2.5 to 5.0 cm beyond the ends of the splint so that it, too, can be folded back over the splint to help create smooth, well-padded edges (see Fig. 50–5C). Extra padding should be placed over areas of bony prominence, such as the radial condyle or the malleoli (Table 50–3). Although this can be done with Webril, the use of Mother's Cotton adds an additional measure of protection without the worry of wrinkling or ischemic injury. If significant swelling is anticipated, three or four layers of Webril should be applied as padding. Care should be taken to avoid wrinkling because it can result in significant skin pressure when a tight splint is used for a long period. Wrinkles can be eliminated by proportionately stretching or even tearing the side of the Webril that must wrap around the bigger portion of an extremity. Joints that must be immobilized in a 90° position, such as the ankle, make continuous Webril wrapping difficult. To avoid wrinkles in the area of the ankle, the joint should be placed in the proper position before padding. Webril is then wrapped around the malleolar and midtarsal regions first. The bare calcaneal region can then be covered with overlapping vertical and horizontal Webril strips until the entire heel region is evenly padded. The same approach can be used in similar areas, such as the elbow. The width of Webril that should be used varies depending on the extremity to be splinted. In general, the 2-inch width should be used for hands and feet, the 3- or 4-inch width for the upper extremity, and the 4- or 6-inch width for the lower extremity.

A final caveat when using Webril is to be aware of the potential for ischemic injury. This rare complication is most likely to occur in an extremity that continues to have significant swelling after the patient is released from the ED. Ischemia may result because the concentrically placed Webril can become a constricting band. If this situation is anticipated, it can be prevented easily by cutting through the Webril along the side of the extremity opposite to the plaster splint. The splint is then secured to the extremity in the usual manner. Alternatively, two or three layers of Webril (the same diameter as the plaster) are placed directly over the wet plaster (Fig. 50–6). The Webril-lined splint is then positioned over the area to be immobilized and secured with an elastic bandage.

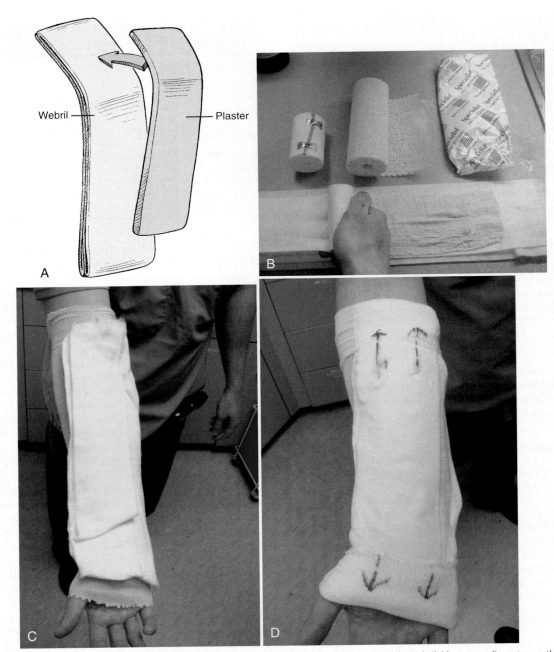

Figure 50–6 Alternative method of Webril application. *A,* If significant swelling is anticipated, Webril (the same diameter as the plaster) may be placed directly over the wet plaster, rather than wrapping it around the extremity. The Webril-lined splint is then positioned over the area to be immobilized and secured with an elastic bandage. Sandwiching the plaster strips with Webril will also minimize rigid adherence of the plaster to the elastic wrap. *B,* A personalized splint. Webril on *both sides* of a pre-measured slab of plaster provides skin protection and comfort, and the Ace bandage will not stick so the splint can be removed for wound care/exercise. *C,* Stockinette and optional additional Webril are placed on the extremity, and the splint placed over these items. Note that the padding and stockinette extend 4–5 inches past both ends of the splint. *D,* Prior to applying an Ace bandage, the Webril and stockinette ends of the splint are rolled back (*arrows*) to keep the plaster in place and provide a smooth edge.

Plaster Preparation

The choice of plaster setting time depends on the nature of the injury and the expertise of the clinician. Extra-fast-setting plaster is typically used when rapid hardening is desired to help maintain alignment of an acutely reduced fracture. However, for the majority of ED splints, plaster with slower setting times (e.g., Specialist fast-drying) is recommended.[11] Plaster that sets more slowly is easier for some clinicians to use because it affords more leeway in applying and molding the splint. Furthermore, plaster with a longer setting time produces less heat, thus reducing both patient discomfort and the risk of serious burns.[12] Table 50–4 lists the setting times for commonly used plaster. These setting times are adjusted by adding different substances to the plaster during the production process (Table 50–5). Given plaster with equal setting times, the most important variable affecting the rate of crystallization is water temperature. Warm water hardens a splint faster than cold water and should not be used when extra time is needed for splint application.

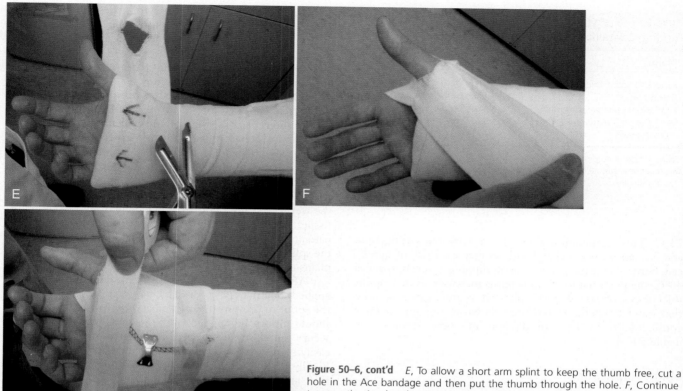

Figure 50–6, cont'd *E*, To allow a short arm splint to keep the thumb free, cut a hole in the Ace bandage and then put the thumb through the hole. *F*, Continue to wrap the Ace bandage to assure a perfect fit around the thumb. *G*, Apply tape to metal clips to avoid inadvertent loss. These clips will readily end up in the mouth of an inquisitive toddler. See Fig. 50–5.

915

TABLE 50–4 Setting Times of Fast- and Extra-Fast-Drying Plaster

Plaster	Setting Time (min)
Fast-drying	5–8
Extra-fast-drying	2–4

TABLE 50–5 Effect of Water Temperature and Different Additives on Setting Time of Plaster

Accelerates Setting Time	Slows Setting Time
Reusing dip water	Cool dip water
Higher dip water temperature	Glue
Salicylic acid	Gum
Zinc	Borax
Magnesium	
Copper	
Iron	
Aluminum	
Salt	
Alum	

The ideal length and width of plaster depends on the body part to be splinted and the amount of immobilization required. The best way to estimate length is to lay the dry splint next to the area to be splinted. It is best to use a generous length because wet plaster shrinks slightly from its dry length. Also, if the wet splint is too long, the ends can be folded back easily. The plaster width varies according to the type of splint being made and the body part that is injured, but generally, it should be slightly greater than the diameter of the limb to be splinted. Specific recommendations regarding splint length and width are discussed in the sections describing individual splints.

The thickness of a splint depends on the size of the patient, the extremity that is injured, and the desired strength of the final product. An ankle splint may crack quickly and become useless if only eight layers are used, but this thickness may be ideal for a wrist splint. In general, it is best to use the minimum number of layers necessary to achieve adequate strength. Thicker splints are heavier and more uncomfortable. It is also important to note that plaster thickness is a major determinant of the amount of heat given off during the setting process. More than 12 sheets of plaster create an increased risk of significant burns, especially when using extra-fast-drying plaster, using dipping water with a temperature greater than 24°C, or placing a pillow under or around the extremity for support during the setting process (Table 50–6). For an average-sized adult, upper extremities should be splinted with 8 sheets of plaster, whereas lower extremity injuries generally require 12 to 15 sheets. This layering usually gives the strength necessary for adequate immobilization while reducing the patient's discomfort and the risk of significant burns. In a 136-kg (300-lb) patient, however, up to 20 layers may be required to make a durable ankle splint.

The dipping water should be kept clean and fresh. Reusing water that has been used previously for wetting plaster increases the amount of heat given off during crystallization and causes plaster to set more quickly. As a rule of thumb, the temperature of the water should be kept around

TABLE 50–6 Variables That Increase Heat Production during Crystallization

Major	Minor
Increased splint thickness	High humidity
Setting time*	High ambient temperature
High dip water temperature†	Reusing dip water
Wrapping the extremity for support while drying	

*Faster setting times produce more heat.
†Dip water temperature has been a minor determinant of heat production in some studies.

24°C. This temperature allows for a workable setting time and has not been associated with an increased risk of significant burns. As the temperature of the dipping water approaches 40°C, the potential for serious burns increases, even at splint thicknesses of less than 12 plies. It is interesting to note that water temperature has been shown to be only a minor consideration in heat production in some studies (see Table 50–6).

Splint Application

The dry splint should be completely submerged in the water until bubbling stops. The splint is removed and excess water is gently squeezed out until the plaster has a wet and sloppy consistency. The splint is placed on a hard table or countertop (a protective covering is recommended to prevent water or plaster damage) and smoothed out to remove any wrinkles and to ensure uniform lamination of all layers. Lamination helps to increase the final strength of the splint. The splint is placed over the Webril and gently smoothed over the extremity. Plaster is usually somewhat adherent to Webril, but an assistant may be required to hold the splint in place. Once the splint has been properly positioned over the extremity, folding back the underlying stockinette and Webril also helps hold it in place. The splint is secured with an appropriately sized elastic bandage by wrapping in a distal to proximal direction. Finally, the extremity is placed in the desired position and the wet plaster is molded to the contour of the extremity using only the palms of the hand. Finger indentations may cause a ridge that will produce a pressure point.

Molding the wet splint to conform to the body's anatomy is probably the most important, yet the most frequently overlooked, step to ensure adequate immobilization (see Fig. 50–5E). The act of molding may cause some pain, and the patient should be forewarned. All manipulation of the wet plaster should be completed before it reaches a thick, creamy consistency. Any movement after this time, also known as the critical period, results in an imperfect crystalline network of calcium sulfate molecules and greatly weakens the ultimate strength of the splint. While the plaster is setting, a pillow or blanket should **not** be wrapped around the extremity for support. This leads to inadequate ventilation around the splint and greatly increases the amount of heat produced (see Table 50–6).

If an elastic bandage is applied directly over wet plaster, the elastic bandage may be incorporated into the drying plaster, making subsequent removal of the bandage difficult. To make it easier for patients to remove and reapply the splint, a single layer of Webril or roll gauze can be wrapped around the wet plaster loosely before application of the elastic bandage. This prevents the wet plaster from becoming stuck to the elastic bandage. Only one layer of Webril should be used over the plaster because multiple layers have been associated with high drying temperatures.

Before the patient is released from the ED, the splint should be checked for adequate immobilization and the patient should be observed for any evidence of vascular compromise or significant discomfort. If either occurs, the elastic bandage should be loosened. If the discomfort persists, additional padding should be placed over the painful areas. If this measure, too, is unsuccessful, a new splint should be made, and special attention should be paid to proper molding so that the wet plaster does not become indented. By resting tender tissue, splinting usually relieves discomfort quickly, and patients generally say that they feel better immediately after the splint has been applied. Never release a patient who complains of increased pain after a splint has been placed.

After a properly fitting, comfortable splint has been applied, one may place two strips of tape along each side of the splint to prevent the elastic bandage from slipping. Tape should always be applied over the metal fasteners used to secure the elastic bandages. Note that these objects can be easily swallowed or aspirated by infants and small children. Finally, a sling should be provided for upper extremity injuries, and if required, crutches should be dispensed (and instructions given for their proper use) for lower extremity injuries.

Patient Instructions

Patients should receive both verbal and written instructions on splint care and precautions. The importance of elevation in helping to decrease pain and swelling should be stressed and demonstrated (most patients do not understand the medical definition of elevation). At night, a pillow wrapped and secured around a hand or foot will help the patient keep the injured extremity satisfactorily elevated. If the injury is less than 24 hours old, the application of ice bags or cold packs also should be encouraged. It is useless to apply cold packs over plaster, but it can be beneficial if it is applied over Webril and an elastic bandage or directly over an injury if the splint is removed. In theory, cold therapy stiffens collagen and thus reduces the tendency for ligaments and tendons to deform. Cold therapy also decreases muscle spasm and excitability, decreases blood flow (thus limiting hemorrhage and edema), raises the pain threshold, and decreases inflammation. Because the thermal conductivity of subcutaneous tissue is poor, cold packs should be applied for at least 30 minutes at a time. This guideline is in contrast to the popular recommendation of "ice 20 minutes on, 20 minutes off," which does nothing more than cool the skin. Cold packs should not be applied for more than the first 24 to 48 hours because cold can interfere with long-term healing. The patient should be instructed not to stress the splint for at least 24 hours because plaster does not approach optimal strength until evaporation has reduced the water content of the plaster to approximately 21% of its initial hydrated level. This process of removing excess water by evaporation is called *curing* and it generally takes several days to be completed. However, by 24 hours, the water content of the plaster has usually been reduced enough to produce a strong, resilient splint. In addition, because the chemical process involved in the formation of plaster is reversible, the patient should avoid getting the splint wet. If the injury permits, the splint can be removed for showering and then reapplied. Alternatively, one or more plastic bags may be placed over a splint before showering.

Splints may crack, break, or disintegrate with wear, and such a useless splint should be removed or replaced. Patients should be given general guidelines for length of immobilization and appropriate follow-up care. Long-term immobilization, particularly in the elderly, can produce permanent disability and should be avoided. It is extremely important for the patient to continue to check for signs of vascular compromise. If the patient experiences a significant increase in pain, any numbness or tingling of the digits, pallor of the distal extremity, decreased capillary refill, or weakness, she or he should be instructed to return to the ED or to see the primary clinician without delay. As with casting, increased pain after splinting is a warning sign that should prompt a return visit— not telephone advice. Strong opioids should be avoided during the first 2 to 3 days after splinting to allow pain to prompt a follow-up visit.

UPPER EXTREMITY SPLINTS

Long Arm Splints

Long Arm Posterior Splint

Indications. The long arm posterior splint (Fig. 50–7) is used to immobilize injuries of the elbow and proximal forearm. It completely eliminates flexion and extension of the elbow, but it does not entirely prevent pronation and supination of the forearm. Therefore, it is not recommended for immobilization of complex or unstable distal forearm fractures unless used in conjunction with a long arm anterior splint. Alternatively, a double "sugar-tong" splint can be applied.

Construction. The long arm posterior splint is constructed using 8 to 10 layers of 4- or 6-inch-wide plaster. The splint starts on the posterior aspect of the proximal arm. It runs down the arm to the elbow and then continues along the ulnar aspect of the forearm and hand to the level of the metacarpophalangeal (MCP) joints. The anterior splint is constructed in the same manner. It mirrors the posterior splint by running down the anterior aspect of the arm to the antecubital fossa, where it continues along the radial aspect of the forearm to the distal radius. The anterior splint is never used alone, but rather, as an adjunct to the long arm posterior splint to improve immobilization by increasing stability and preventing pronation and supination of the forearm.

Application. Stockinette and Webril are applied as described previously. A hole should be cut in the stockinette to expose the thumb and extra padding should be placed over the olecranon to prevent pressure injury. The arm is positioned with the elbow flexed to 90°, the forearm neutral (thumb upward), and the wrist neutral or extended slightly (10°–20°). It is helpful to have an assistant hold the wet splint in place, particularly when applying both a posterior and an anterior splint. Once the splint has been properly positioned, the ends of the stockinette and Webril are folded back and the splint is secured in place using 2-, 3-, or 4-inch elastic bandages. Finally, the sides of the splint are folded up to create a gutter configuration and the splint is carefully molded using the palms of the hand. The fingers and thumb should remain free to prevent stiffness from unnecessary immobilization.

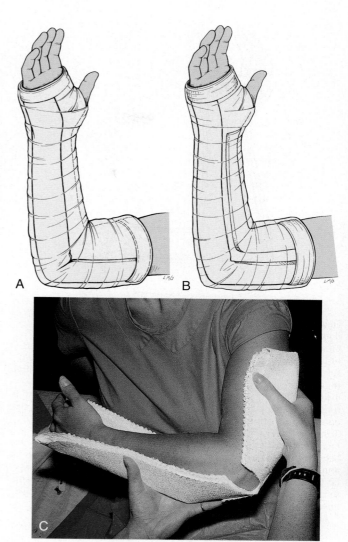

Figure 50–7 Application of a long arm posterior splint. *A,* The posterior portion of the splint begins on the posterior aspect of the proximal humerus. It runs down the arm to the elbow and then continues along the ulnar aspect of the forearm and hand to the distal metacarpals. The elbow is flexed at a 90° angle, the forearm is in the neutral (thumb-up) position, and the wrist is in a neutral position or slightly extended (10°–20°). *B,* Adding an anterior splint. The anterior splint mirrors the posterior splint by running down the anterior aspect of the arm to the antecubital fossa, where it continues along the radial aspect of the forearm and hand to the distal radius. The anterior splint is never used alone, but rather as an adjunct to the long arm posterior splint. It improves immobilization by increasing stability and preventing pronation and supination of the forearm. *C,* When measuring for a posterior splint, cut out a notch to allow for a smooth bend. Note that padding needs to be applied before splinting.

Double Sugar-Tong Splint

Indications. Like the long arm posterior splint, the double sugar-tong splint (Fig. 50–8) is used to immobilize injuries of the elbow and forearm. However, because it prevents pronation and supination of the forearm, it is preferable for some fractures of the distal forearm and elbow.

Construction. The splint consists of two separate pieces of plaster, a forearm splint and an arm splint. Each piece is constructed using eight layers of 3- or 4-inch plaster. The forearm portion of the splint runs from the metacarpal heads on the dorsum of the hand, along the dorsal surface of the forearm around the elbow. It continues along the volar surface

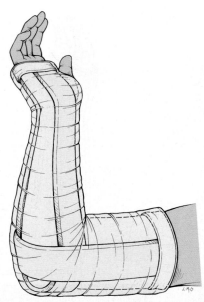

Figure 50–8 An alternative to the long arm posterior splint is a double sugar-tong splint. This splint immobilizes the elbow and prevents pronation and supination of the forearm. The splint consists of two separate pieces of 4-inch plaster, a forearm splint, and an arm splint. The elbow is flexed at a 90° angle, the forearm is in the neutral (thumb-up) position, and the wrist is in a neutral position or slightly extended (10°–20°). The forearm portion of the splint is applied first. It runs from the metacarpal heads on the dorsum of the hand, along the dorsal surface of the forearm, and around the elbow. It continues along the volar surface of the forearm, stopping at the level of the metacarpophalangeal (MCP) joints. The arm portion of this splint begins on the anterior aspect of the proximal arm. It runs down the arm over the forearm splint, and around the elbow. It then continues up the posterior aspect of the arm, once again going over the forearm splint until it reaches the starting point. The fingers and thumb should remain free to avoid stiffness.

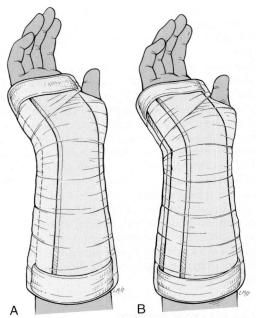

Figure 50–9 **Application of a volar splint.** *A,* The splint begins in the palm at the metacarpal heads and extends along the volar surface of the forearm to a point just proximal to the elbow. If any of the fingers are injured, the splint may be extended to incorporate the involved digits. The forearm is placed in the neutral (thumb-up) position with the wrist slightly extended (10°–20°). Wrist flexion should be avoided. *B,* For more serious injuries, an additional dorsal slab may be used to create a bivalve splint.

of the forearm to the palm of the hand, stopping at the level of the MCP joints. The arm portion of the splint begins on the anterior aspect of the proximal humerus. It runs down the arm over the forearm splint and around the elbow. It then continues up the posterior aspect of the arm, once again going over the forearm splint, until it reaches the starting point.

Application. Use of stockinette, Webril, and positioning is similar to those described for application of a long arm posterior splint. The two splints are secured in place using two 3- or 4-inch elastic bandages starting at the forearm splint at the hand. Once secure, the arm portion of the splint is wrapped beginning at the proximal end. The fingers and thumb should remain free to avoid stiffness.

Forearm and Hand Splints

Volar Splint

Indications. The volar splint (Fig. 50–9*A*) is used to immobilize a variety of soft tissue injuries of the hand and wrist. It is also used for temporary immobilization of triquetral fractures, lunate and perilunate dislocations, and second through fifth metacarpal head fractures. For these more serious injuries, some clinicians prefer to add a dorsal splint to create a more stable bivalve effect (see Fig. 50–9*B*). Because the volar splint does not completely eliminate pronation and supination of the forearm, it may not be ideal for fractures of the distal radius and ulnar, although many clinicians use this

splint for nondisplaced or minimally displaced distal ulnar and radial fractures.

Construction. The splint is constructed using 8 to 10 layers of 3- or 4-inch-wide plaster. The splint begins in the palm at the metacarpal heads and extends along the volar surface of the forearm to just proximal to the elbow. If there is an injury to any of the fingers, the splint may be extended to incorporate the involved digit.

Application. Stockinette and Webril should be applied as described previously. A hole should be cut in the stockinette to expose the thumb. In addition, Webril or gauze should be placed between any digits that are going to be immobilized. The forearm is placed in the neutral position (thumb upward) with the wrist extended slightly (10°–20°). Wrist flexion should be avoided. After the wet plaster has been properly positioned, the ends of the stockinette and Webril are folded back and a 3- or 4-inch elastic bandage is used to hold the splint in place. The sides of the splint are folded up, creating a gutter effect, and the plaster is carefully molded to conform to the contours of the palm and wrist. Some clinicians prefer to extend the splint to the fingertips and then fold the wet plaster back toward the palm, allowing the fingers to "grasp" the rounded distal end when at rest. In any event, the thumb and fingers should be free to move unless they are injured and are being intentionally immobilized by the splint.

Sugar-Tong Splint

Indications. The sugar-tong splint (Fig. 50–10) is used for fractures of the distal radius and ulna. The advantage of this splint over the volar splint is prevention of pronation and supination of the forearm. In addition, it immobilizes the

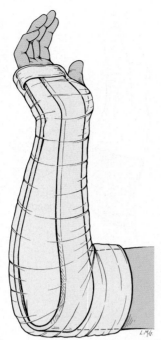

Figure 50–10 Application of a forearm sugar-tong splint. The splint runs from the metacarpal heads on the dorsum of the hand, along the dorsal surface of the forearm, and around the elbow. It continues along the volar surface of the forearm, stopping at the level of the MCP joints. The elbow is flexed at a 90° angle, the forearm is in the neutral (thumb-up) position, and the wrist is in a neutral position or slightly extended (10°–20°). The advantages of this splint over the volar splint are immobilization of the elbow and prevention of pronation and supination of the forearm.

elbow, which is desirable for the first few days after a distal forearm fracture.

Construction and Application. The splint is constructed and applied in the same way as the forearm portion of the double sugar-tong splint, described earlier.

Thumb Spica Splint

Indications. The thumb spica splint (Fig. 50–11) is used to immobilize injuries to the scaphoid, lunate, and thumb and fractures of the first metacarpal. It is also used in the treatment of de Quervain tenosynovitis. Traditionally, a thumb spica splint or cast was thought to be a requirement to properly immobilize scaphoid fractures; however, there is no totally agreed-upon standard. Clay and coworkers[13] stated that the optimal method of casting scaphoid fractures has not been definitively established. They were unable to prove a difference in patient comfort, recovery of function, or incidence of nonunion between a Colles cast and a traditional scaphoid cast that included the thumb.

The incidence of nonunion of scaphoid fractures is about 10%, regardless of the type of immobilization in the ED, but it is greatest with unstable proximal pole fractures. Because some scaphoid fractures heal poorly under the best of circumstances, it seems prudent to provide thumb immobilization in the initial splinting. Failure to do so, such as when a "sprained wrist" is suspected, should not be construed as beneath the accepted standard of care. Most volar splints will at least partly immobilize the base of the thumb, so the discussion may be moot.

Construction. The splint is constructed using eight layers of 3-inch-wide plaster. The splint extends from just distal to the interphalangeal joint of the thumb to the mid-forearm.

Application. The forearm is placed in the neutral position with the wrist extended 25° and the thumb in the wineglass position (Fig. 50–12). Stockinette and Webril are applied from the base of the palm to the mid-forearm. It may be difficult to place stockinette around the thumb. Instead, a hole can be cut in the stockinette to expose the thumb. The thumb is then padded with small vertical strips of Webril or wrapped with 2-inch Webril. The dry plaster is then placed over the radial aspect of the forearm from just beyond the thumb interphalangeal joint to the mid-forearm. Once in position, the location of the first MCP joint is marked and a small (1–2 cm) perpendicular cut is made 1 cm distal to the mark on each edge of the plaster (see Fig. 50–11 *inset*). If necessary the plaster distal to the notch may be tapered slightly. This will allow the splint to be molded around the thumb without creating a buckle in the plaster. The plaster is then dipped and secured in place with a 2- or 3-inch elastic bandage. It is important to carefully mold the wet plaster around the thumb and palm and to maintain the thumb in the wineglass position while the plaster is drying.

Ulnar Gutter Splint

Indications. The ulnar gutter splint (Fig. 50–13) is used to immobilize fractures and serious soft tissue injuries of the little and ring fingers and fractures of the neck, shaft, and base of the fourth and fifth metacarpals.

Construction. The splint is made using six to eight layers of 3- or 4-inch plaster. It incorporates both the little and the ring fingers. It runs along the ulnar aspect of the forearm from just beyond the distal interphalangeal joint of the little finger to the mid-forearm.

Application. Stockinette and Webril are applied as usual. Additional Webril or gauze should be placed between the little and the ring fingers to prevent maceration of the skin. The forearm is in the neutral position with the wrist in slight extension (10°–20°), the MCP joints in 50° of flexion, and the proximal and distal interphalangeal joints in slight flexion (10°–15°). When immobilizing a metacarpal neck fracture (i.e., boxer's fracture), the MCP joint should be flexed to 90°. Once in the proper position, the sides of the splint are folded up to form a gutter. The ends of the stockinette and Webril are then folded back to help hold the splint while it is secured in place with a 2- or 3-inch elastic bandage.

Radial Gutter Splint

Indications. The radial gutter splint (Fig. 50–14) is used to immobilize fractures and serious soft tissue injuries of the index and long fingers and fractures of the neck, shaft, and base of the second and third metacarpals.

Construction. The splint is made using six to eight layers of 3- or 4-inch plaster. It runs along the radial aspect of the forearm from just beyond the distal interphalangeal joint of the index finger to the mid-forearm.

Application. Stockinette (with a hole cut to expose the thumb) and Webril are applied as previously described. Additional Webril or gauze should be placed between the index and the long fingers to prevent maceration of the skin. The hand and fingers can be splinted in the *position of function* or in the *intrinsic plus position* (see Fig. 50–12). Neither have proven superiority for the first few weeks of splinting. Both are acceptable for initial ED splinting, for hand and finger

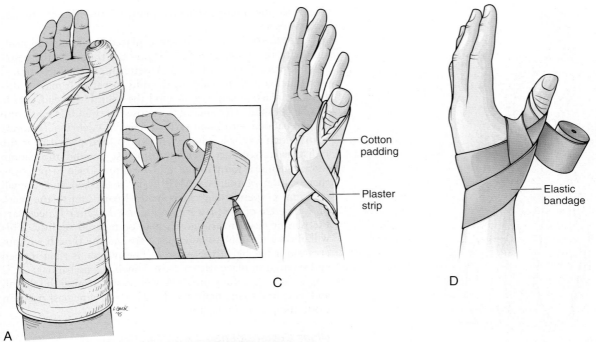

A

B

C

D

Cotton padding

Plaster strip

Elastic bandage

Figure 50–11 *A and B,* Application of a thumb spica splint. The splint extends from just distal to the interphalangeal joint of the thumb to the mid-forearm. The forearm is placed in the neutral position with the wrist extended 25° and the thumb in the wineglass position (see Fig. 50–12). *Inset,* A small (1- to 2-cm) perpendicular cut is made 1 cm distal to the first MCP joint on each edge of the plaster to allow molding of the splint around the thumb without creating a buckle in the plaster. *B,* For skier's/gamekeeper thumb, a figure-of-eight thumb splint is ideal. *C,* Cut this length of material (should be ~14″ –16″). Center the splint on the web space, crossing over the dorsal aspect of the thumb in a figure-of-eight fashion and overlapping the cut edges around the styloid process of the ulna. *D,* Wrap with a small elastic bandage, overlapping in a figure-of-eight formation. Mold and position after placement.

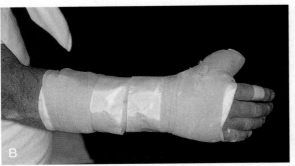

A

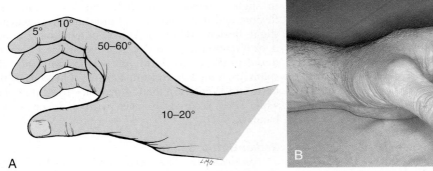

B

5° 10°
50–60°
10–20°

Figure 50–12 *A,* The wineglass position, also termed position of function, is a safe splint position for the hand and fingers for short-term splinting (7–14 days). The wrist should allow alignment of the thumb with the forearm, the MCP joint should be moderately flexed, and the interphalangeal joints should be only slightly flexed. The thumb should be abducted away from the palm. *B,* For longer splinting, fingers should be extended to prevent flexion contractions, termed the intrinsic position. The MCP joint is flexed at 90°. Either *A* or *B* are acceptable positions for initial ED splinting.

immobilization. In the position of function, the forearm is in the neutral position with the wrist in slight extension (10°–20°), the MCP joints in 50°–60° of flexion, and the proximal and distal interphalangeal joints in slight flexion (5°–10°). When immobilizing a metacarpal neck fracture, the intrinsic position is often used, with the MCP joint flexed to 90° and the fingers extended (see Fig. 50–12*B*).

The dry plaster is placed over the extremity and the location of the thumb is marked. A hole is cut in the dry plaster to expose the thumb. The plaster is then dipped and positioned over the extremity. The ends of the stockinette and Webril are folded back to help hold the splint while it is secured in place with a 2- or 3-inch elastic bandage.

Finger Splints

Fingers are splinted after sprains, fractures, tendon repair, or infection. Minor finger sprains can often be managed with dynamic splinting (e.g., buddy taping) (Fig. 50–15) or a com-

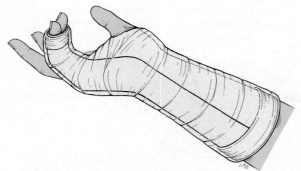

Figure 50–13 Application of an ulnar gutter splint. The ulnar gutter splint incorporates both the little and the ring fingers. Webril or gauze should be placed between the digits to prevent maceration of the skin. The splint runs along the ulnar aspect of the forearm from just beyond the distal interphalangeal joint of the little finger to the mid-forearm. The forearm is in the neutral position with the wrist in slight extension (10°–20°), the MCP joint in 50° of flexion, and the proximal and distal interphalangeal joints in slight flexion (10°–15°). When immobilizing a metacarpal neck fracture, the MCP joint should be flexed to 90°.

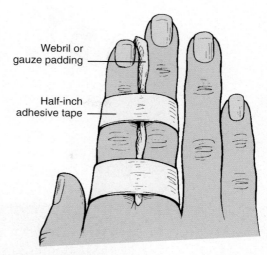

Figure 50–15 Buddy tape technique. Taping between the digital joints (toes or fingers) allows the normal adjacent finger to protect the collateral ligament of its injured neighbor. Webril should be placed between the digits to prevent maceration of the skin.

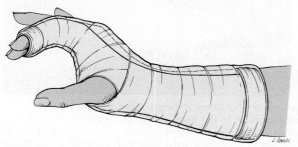

Figure 50–14 Application of a radial gutter splint. The radial gutter splint incorporates both the index and the long fingers. Webril or gauze should be placed between the digits to prevent maceration of the skin. The splint runs along the radial aspect of the forearm from just beyond the distal interphalangeal joint of the index finger to the mid-forearm. The forearm is in the neutral position with the wrist in slight extension (10°–20°), the MCP joint in 50° of flexion, and the proximal and distal interphalangeal joints in slight flexion (10°–15°). When immobilizing a metacarpal neck fracture, the MCP joint should be flexed to 90°.

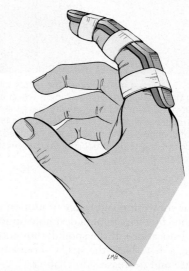

Figure 50–16 Dorsal aluminum foam splint. The bone is subcutaneous dorsally, and splints here afford better immobilization of the digit. The dorsal splint also allows preservation and use of tactile sense, which encourages function and better splint acceptance on the part of the patient.

mercially available foam splint with aluminum backing (one-surface splint) (Fig. 50–16), but fractures, tendon repairs, and some soft tissue injuries benefit from formal splinting (e.g., thumb spica, ulnar and radial gutter splints). Specific conditions, such as mallet finger, require a specialized splint (plaster or Stack splint) (Fig. 50–17). When complete immobilization of a finger is required (e.g., unstable phalangeal fractures), an "outrigger" finger splint that incorporates the wrist may be used (Fig. 50–18). Both the position of function and the intrinsic position are acceptable for initial splinting.

Sling, Swathe and Sling, Shoulder Immobilizer

Sling
The sling is used to maintain elevation and provide immobilization of the hand, forearm, and elbow. It is most often used in conjunction with a plaster splint or cast. There are a number of commercially available slings to choose from. Many of these are fairly economical and simple to use, whereas others are very expensive and do not allow the versatility of a simple,

inexpensive triangular muslin bandage. When applying a sling, it is important to have adequate support of the wrist and hand (Fig. 50–19). A sling that is too short will allow the wrist and hand to hang down (ulnar deviate) and can result in ulnar nerve injury.

Swathe and Sling, Shoulder Immobilizer
The swathe and sling is the treatment of choice for most proximal humerus fractures and shoulder injuries, such as reduced dislocations. The sling supports the weight of the arm, and the swathe immobilizes the arm against the chest wall to minimize shoulder motion. In most EDs, the swathe and sling has been replaced by the commercially available shoulder immobilizer (Fig. 50–20). Its advantage is that it may

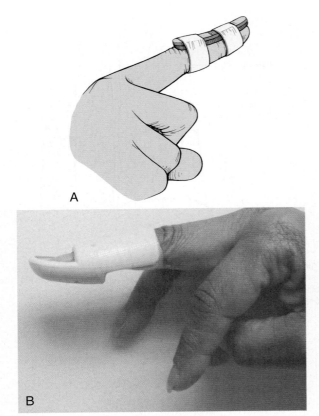

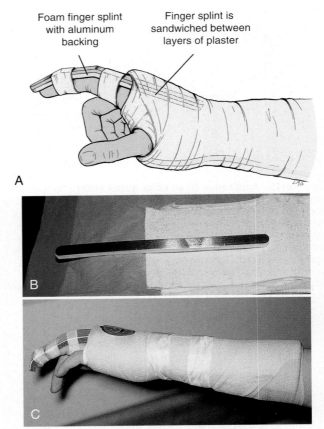

Figure 50–17   *A,* Splinting a mallet finger. The dorsal splint immobilizes only the distal interphalangeal joint, which allows use of the finger. Hyperextension of this joint predisposes to skin sloughing and should be avoided. The patient should be advised not to flex the joint during splint changes. *B,* A Stack splint is designed especially to treat a mallet finger. Long-term immobilization (8 weeks) or surgical fixation is required for this injury.

Figure 50–18   **"Outrigger" finger splint for complete immobilization of the finger.** A padded aluminum splint is incorporated into the middle of a plaster splint, forming an outrigger configuration. The plaster splint is applied to the dorsum of the hand and wrist with an elastic bandage; the finger is then taped to the aluminum splint.

be removed for showering and range of motion exercises and is easily reapplied by the patient (a desirable option in the care of a shoulder dislocation). If the shoulder immobilizer is used for more than a few days, the axilla should be padded to absorb moisture and decrease skin chafing.

The Velpeau bandage is a sling and swathe device that positions the forearm diagonally rather than horizontally across the chest with the hand elevated to the level of the shoulder. This offers no particular advantage over a standard sling and swathe, is difficult to apply, cannot be removed easily, and is not well tolerated for prolonged immobilization.

Figure-of-Eight Clavicle Strap

Clavicle fractures have been traditionally treated with an uncomfortable and complex figure-of-eight bandage. Despite its widespread use, this device has never been proved superior to a simple sling (in terms of cosmesis, functional outcome, or pain relief).[14,15] Indeed, use of the figure-of-eight dressing should be discouraged because it may actually promote nonunion or increase the deformity at the fracture site; it is very uncomfortable; prohibits bathing, often causing chafing and discomfort in the axilla; and may predispose to axillary vein thrombosis.[4] Although some orthopaedists continue to recommend the figure-of-eight bandage, a simple sling is sufficient to treat most clavicular fractures.

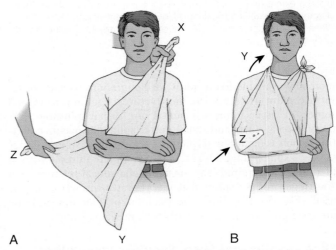

Figure 50–19   *A,* Stepwise application of a triangular muslin sling. (*1*) Place tip *X* over the uninjured shoulder. (*2*) Bring tip *Y* over the injured shoulder to enclose the arm. (*3*) Draw tip *Z* around the front and pin. *B,* Completed triangular muslin sling. (*Note:* When applying a sling, it is important to have adequate support of the wrist and hand. A sling that is too short will allow the wrist and hand to hang down [ulnar deviate] and can result in hand edema and ulnar nerve injury.)

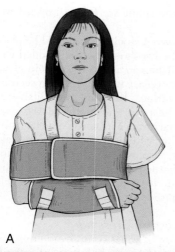

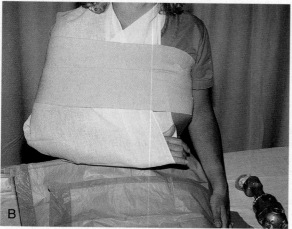

Figure 50–20 *A,* The shoulder immobilizer is used for most proximal humerus fractures and shoulder injuries. It may be removed for showering and range of motion exercises and is easily reapplied by the patient. *B,* An elastic bandage and sling provide similar shoulder immobilization. *Note that the wrist is supported by the slings.*

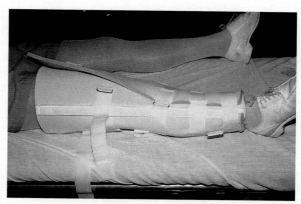

Figure 50–21 The Velcro strap bulky knee immobilizer is easily removed and readily applied by the patient. It can be worn over clothes.

TABLE 50–7 Useful Estimates of Splint Times for Various Hand Problems

Injury	Splint Type	Immobilization Time*
Mallet finger	FIN	8 wk
Boutonnière deformity	FIN	6 wk
Distal phalanx—soft tissue	FIN	1–2 wk
Extensor tendon	DHWF	3 wk
Sprain-strain†		
Interphalangeal joint	FIN	1–2 wk
Wrist	DHWF	1–2 wk
Hand burn	DHWF	5–7 wk
Infection		
Digit	DHWF	5–7 day
Hand	DHWF	5–7 day
Severe hand contusion	DHWF	5–7 day
Fracture		
Distal phalanx	FIN	2–3 wk
Middle phalanx	FIN	2–3 wk
Proximal phalanx	DHWF	2–3 wk
Metacarpal	DHWF	2–3 wk
Carpal tunnel	DHWF	Night only
de Quervain disease	DHWF	2–3 wk
Trigger finger	FIN	Night only

*These are average times only. Every patient is treated as an individual when a splint is used. Clinical judgment is critical.
†The diagnosis of a sprain should be made only after a thorough effort has been made to rule out a fracture or dislocation. This is particularly true in the wrist.
DHWF, digit-hand-wrist-forearm; FIN, finger.

Pitfalls of Hand Dressings and Splints

The two most common problems with hand dressings are putting them on too tightly and leaving them on too long (Table 50–7). One must be especially careful to avoid wrapping elastic bandages too snugly. The patient should be instructed to loosen an elastic bandage if it feels too tight. The patient should always have access to emergency follow-up care. It is often advisable to start patients on a regimen of early protected motion. This means that the patient removes the splint for a specified period, does a prescribed exercise, and then replaces the splint. A splint is not an all-or-none device, and the patient is generally weaned from it slowly before it is discarded entirely. A stiff hand is a nonfunctional one, and stiffness is often a consequence of prolonged immobilization. It is important for the patient to be made aware of his or her responsibility for the injured hand.

LOWER EXTREMITY SPLINTS

Knee Splints

Knee Immobilizer

Indications. The knee immobilizer (Fig. 50–21) is commonly used for mild to moderate ligamentous and soft tissue injuries of the knee. It is removable and extremely easy to apply, making it popular among patients and clinicians alike. In many EDs, it has almost totally replaced the more bulky plaster splint. Its use should be restricted to injuries that do not require immediate surgical intervention, traction, or casting. For these injuries, in which temporary but more complete immobilization is needed, a plaster knee splint can be used because it provides better stabilization and costs much less than a knee immobilizer. The exact scientific benefit of the knee immobilizer is poorly studied and difficult to document. However, it clearly helps relieve pain and, at least theoretically, hastens healing.

Application. The knee immobilizer is available in small, medium, large, and extra-large sizes. To choose the appropriate size, the knee immobilizer is placed next to the injured leg so that the tapered end lies distal to the patient's knee; if present, the cutout patellar area on the anterior aspect of the splint lies adjacent to the knee. In this position, the splint should extend distally to within a few inches of the malleoli and proximally to just below the buttocks crease. To apply the knee immobilizer, the open splint is slid under the injured extremity and firmly secured in place using the Velcro straps. The knee immobilizer can be applied directly over clothing, obviating the need to remove or cut the patient's pants.

Posterior Knee Splint

Indications. In many EDs, the knee immobilizer has virtually replaced the plaster knee splint for mild to moderate injuries to the knee. However, the plaster knee splint can be particularly useful in patients whose extremities are too large for the knee immobilizer, in the treatment of angulated fractures, or for temporarily immobilizing other knee injuries that require immediate operative intervention or orthopaedic referral. The posterior (gutter) knee splint (Fig. 50–22) is the type most commonly applied, but as alternatives, two parallel splints can be placed along each side of the leg and foreleg, creating a bivalve effect (see Fig. 50–22B) or a long leg U-splint can be applied (see later). The bilateral knee splint is slightly more difficult to apply than the posterior knee splint, but it may provide better immobilization of the lateral and medial collateral ligaments and can be used for injuries to these structures.

Construction. The knee splint is made with 12 to 15 layers of 6-inch plaster. It should run from just below the buttocks crease to approximately 5 to 8 cm above the malleoli.

The sides of the splint are folded upward to form a gutter configuration.

Application. A stockinette should be placed in the usual manner, and the leg should be well padded with 4- or 6-inch Webril. If available, an assistant can help elevate the leg and hold the splint in place while it is being secured with 4- or 6-inch elastic bandages. If no aide is available, the patient can be placed in the prone position and the splint laid on the posterior surface of the extremity. The leg is then wrapped in the usual manner without the need for special support of the applied plaster. Also, while in the prone position, the patient's toes can elevate the lower part of the leg off the bed, allowing sufficient room to wrap the Webril and elastic bandages around the injured extremity.

Jones Compression Dressing

Indications. A Jones compression dressing is commonly used for short-term immobilization of soft tissue injuries of the knee. It immobilizes and compresses the knee, reducing both pain and swelling. However, because it does allow slight flexion and extension of the knee, it should not be used for injuries that require strict immobilization. In addition, it is difficult to maintain the splint for more than a few days.

Construction. A Jones dressing is made using 6-inch Webril and elastic bandages.

Application. To apply a Jones dressing, the patient is placed on a stretcher, lying supine. If available, an assistant can elevate the patient's leg to facilitate wrapping. If no help is available, a pillow placed under the patient's heel should suffice. Webril is then wrapped around the extremity from the groin to a few inches above the malleoli. Two or three layers of Webril can be used, and each turn should overlap the previous turn by 25% to 50%. The elastic bandage (two are usually required) is then wrapped around the Webril. If more support is required, the process can be repeated with another two or three layers of Webril held in place by additional elastic bandages.

Ankle Splints

Posterior Splint

Indications. The posterior ankle splint (Fig. 50–23) is one of the most common splints applied in the ED. As noted in the introductory section, the entire concept of splinting an acutely sprained ankle has been questioned, with no firm evidence to support a better outcome of any type of splinting or casting versus functional management (early mobilization with an external support). Nonetheless, an acutely sprained ankle is painful, and if nothing else, splinting for a few days will alleviate pain.

The posterior splint is used primarily to immobilize severe ankle sprains, fractures of the distal fibula and tibia, and reduced ankle dislocations. It can also be used for fractures of the tarsal and metatarsal bones or for other foot conditions that require immobilization. In particularly severe or unstable injuries, an additional anterior splint may be used to provide extra immobilization resembling that of a formal cast (Fig. 50–24). For severe lateral or bilateral ligamentous injuries, a U-splint or stirrup splint (see later) may be added to the posterior splint for increased immobilization. With minor soft tissue injuries, patients may have partial weight-bearing on ankle splints after 24 hours. If the patient will be bearing weight, a cast shoe over the splint makes it easier to walk. In addition, a cast shoe increases the longevity of the

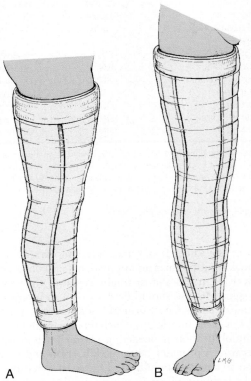

Figure 50–22 Application of a posterior knee splint. *A,* The posterior knee splint runs from just below the buttocks crease to approximately 2–3 cm above the malleoli. *B,* Alternatively, two parallel splints can be placed along each side of the leg and foreleg, creating a bivalve effect.

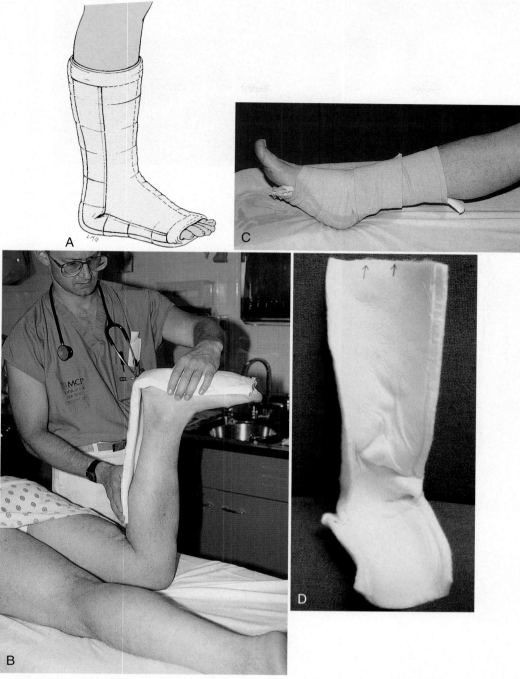

Figure 50–23 **Posterior ankle splint.** *A,* Proper application of a posterior ankle splint. This splint extends from the plantar surface of the great toe (or metatarsal heads) along the posterior surface of the foreleg to the level of the fibular head. The ankle should be at a 90° angle. *B,* The most convenient way to apply an ankle splint is to have the patient lie prone and bend the knee to a 90° angle, thereby relaxing the calf muscles. The ankle should be at a 90° angle so that the foot is flat for partial weight-bearing. *C,* Incorrect splint application. Three things are wrong with this posterior ankle splint: (1) It does not extend distally enough to support the entire foot. (2) The ankle is not maintained at a 90° angle. (3) The edges and ankle area are not molded or protected. Overall, the splint is sloppy and ineffective. *D,* This is an *unacceptable* fiberglass splint. It looked fine under the Ace wrap but the patient complained that it was uncomfortable. When removed the problems were obvious. Note the very sharp frayed fiberglass edges (*arrows*) and the multiple internal ridges and folds that will produce soft tissue trauma when worn.

Continued

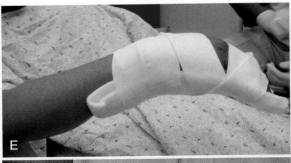

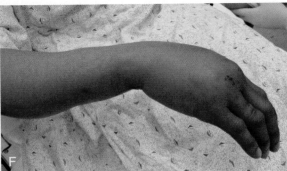

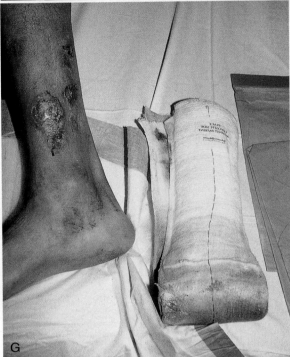

Figure 50–23, cont'd *E* and *F*, Never splint an injured wrist in flexion, even though the patient prefers this position. When immobilizing an infected human bite, this splint was not held in position until hardened, and the patient reflexively flexed the wrist. *G*, The problem with this splint is that it was intended to be used for only a few days, but the patient wore it and walked on it for 3 wk. Note the resultant full-thickness skin loss. No padding was used under the premade splint. Skin grafting was eventually required.

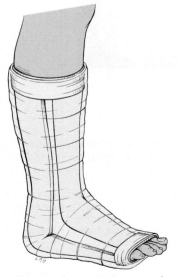

Figure 50–24 Application of an anterior-posterior ankle splint. In particularly severe or unstable injuries, an anterior splint may be added to a posterior ankle splint to provide extra immobilization resembling that of a formal cast. The anterior splint is never used by itself, but it can augment a posterior splint, creating a bivalve effect. The ankle should be at a 90° angle.

splint because walking on an unprotected splint quickly destroys the device. Generally, walking on the splint is prohibited if immobilization for more than 2 or 3 days is desired.

Construction. The posterior splint is made using 4- or 6-inch-wide plaster strips. It should extend from the plantar surface of the great toe or metatarsal heads along the posterior surface of the foreleg to the level of the fibular head. If it hurts to move the toes, they should be incorporated into the splint (after padding is placed between the digits). It is a common mistake to apply a posterior splint that does not extend far enough to support the ball of the foot. Fifteen to 20 layers should be used if partial weight-bearing is allowed because this splint frequently breaks or cracks when walked on.[16]

Application. The easiest way to apply a posterior splint is to place the patient in the prone position with the knee and ankle flexed at a 90° angle. Failure to place the ankle in a 90° angle results in a plantar-flexed splint. The supine patient may help maintain the ankle in a 90° angle by pulling up on the foot with a wide stockinette stirrup. Flexing the knee to a 90° angle relaxes the gastrocnemius muscle and facilitates ankle motion. With the knee and ankle in the proper position, stockinette may be applied and the foot and leg padded with

Webril, as described earlier. Extra padding is used over bony prominences, particularly the malleoli. Again, Webril or gauze is placed between the toes if they are to be included in the splint. The wet plaster is then laid over the plantar surface of the foot and secured in place by folding back the ends of the stockinette and wrapping with one or two 4-inch-wide elastic bandages. The wet plaster is carefully molded around the malleoli and instep to ensure maximum comfort and immobilization. The toes should be left partially exposed for later examination of color and capillary refill.

Anterior-Posterior Splint

Indications. The anterior splint is never used by itself, but it can augment a posterior splint, creating a bivalve effect (see Fig. 50–24). It is used for serious fractures and soft tissue injuries of the ankle.

Construction. A piece of plaster should be cut several centimeters shorter than the one used for the posterior splint, but because this splint does not bear weight, only 8 to 10 layers are required.

Application. The patient should be positioned and padded as for the posterior splint. After the wet posterior splint has been applied, the anterior splint is placed over the anterior aspect of the ankle and foreleg parallel to the posterior splint. The two are then held in place with elastic bandages as described earlier for the posterior splint alone. An assistant is needed to apply the anterior-posterior splint because it is extremely difficult to hold both splints in place while wrapping the elastic bandages. Once secured, both splints are carefully molded over the instep and ankle joint.

U-Splint (Stirrup Splint)

Indications. The U-splint or stirrup splint (Fig. 50–25) is used primarily for injuries to the ankle. It functions like the posterior splint, and either of the two provides satisfactory ankle immobilization. In one study that compared these splints in normal volunteers, the U-splint allowed less plantar flexion and broke less often with plantar flexion than the posterior splint.[16] Also, because it actually covers the malleoli, the U-splint may protect the medial and lateral ligamentous area from further injury better than the posterior splint.

Construction. The U-splint is made using 4- or 6-inch-wide plaster strips. The splint passes under the plantar surface of the foot from the calcaneus to the metatarsal heads and extends up the medial and lateral sides of the foreleg to just below the level of the fibular head.

Application. The patient is positioned, and the extremity is padded as described for the posterior splint. If both posterior and U-splints are used, the posterior splint is applied first. The wet plaster is laid across the plantar surface of the foot between the calcaneus and the metatarsal heads with the sides extending up the lateral and medial aspects of the foreleg. The plaster is secured in place with 4-inch elastic bandages. The elastic bandage should be wrapped around the extremity starting at the metatarsal heads and continuing around the ankle using a figure-of-eight configuration. Once the ankle has been wrapped, another 4- or 6-inch elastic bandage can be used to secure the remainder of the splint in place. The splint should be carefully molded around the malleoli. The plaster may overlap on the anterior aspect of the ankle; this overlap does not interfere with the splint's ability to accommodate further swelling.

Walking Boot (Fig. 50–26A)

Indications. A walking boot (e.g., Cam Boot, DonJoy Boot; see Fig. 50–26A, also called a sugar tong splint) can be used for the treatment of moderate to severe soft tissue injuries of the ankle, including second- and third-degree sprains.[17] In addition, many orthopaedic surgeons use it for isolated, nondisplaced lateral malleolus fractures.[18] The walking boot provides a degree of immobilization similar to that of a U-splint but is easier to remove for bathing and dressing, and the Velcro straps allow adjustment for edema.

Patients placed in a walking boot should receive follow-up with an appropriate specialist and advised on the importance of partial or non–weight-bearing as indicated by the type and degree of injury. When cleared by the follow-up physician, the walking boot allows easy transition to full weight-bearing. Studies have shown that rapid mobilization after ankle injuries improves functional outcome and reduces disability time.[7]

Application. Walking boots come in a variety of sizes from extra small to extra large, depending on the manufacturer. The boot should fit comfortably with the patient's calcaneous snugly in the heel of the boot, and the patient's toes close to, but not extending over, the front edge of the boot. Once the appropriate size has been determined, the patient places her or his bare foot and ankle into the boot, which is secured using Velcro straps.

Semirigid Orthosis

Indications. In patients with sprains of the lateral ankle associated with a stable joint, the use of a functional brace with early mobilization is frequently more comfortable, and results in an earlier return to normal function, than complete immobilization in a plaster splint or cast.[17-25] Consequently, functional bracing with early mobilization has become the standard of care. However, it should be pointed out that there is no documented difference in long-term outcome between the two methods of treatment.

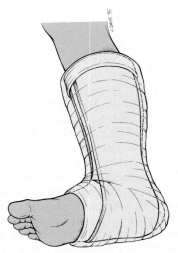

Figure 50–25 The U-splint (also called sugar-tong or stirrup splint) is also used primarily for injuries to the ankle. The splint passes under the plantar surface of the foot, extending up the medial and lateral sides of the foreleg to just below the level of the fibular head. The ankle should be at a 90° angle. For immobilization of the knee, the sides of the splint may be extended proximally to the groin, creating a long leg splint.

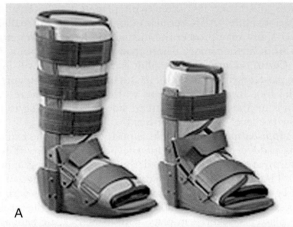

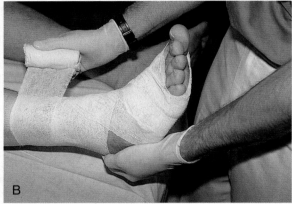

Figure 50–26 *A,* A walking boot can be used for the treatment of moderate to severe soft tissue injuries of the ankle, including second and third degree sprains, and isolated, nondisplaced lateral malleolus fractures. The walking boot provides a similar degree of immobilization as a U-splint, but is easier to remove for bathing and dressing, and the Velcro straps allow adjustment for edema. *B,* The Unna boot or an Ace wrap provide effective immobilization of an ankle soft tissue injury. The Unna boot is applied from a semisolid paste roll. The wrap is then covered with gauze or an elastic bandage. The entire dressing can be cut off by the patient at home. For similar short-term immobilization without plaster, a modified Jones dressing can be used. Copious Webril is wrapped around the ankle and foot and covered with an elastic bandage. A cast shoe can be used with this dressing.

Application. Most functional ankle braces resemble a U-splint with air bladders (Aircast, Inc., Summit, NJ) or foam padding (DeRoyal Inc., Powell, TN) for cushioning the malleoli. The braces are secured about the ankle by Velcro straps. The device is worn within the patient's shoe over a sock and appears to eliminate ankle instability.

Hard Shoe (Cast or Reese Shoe)

Indications. A hard shoe can help reduce the pain associated with ambulation in patients with fractures or soft tissue injuries to the foot. This device can also be used over a splint or cast to allow partial weight-bearing. This device is commonly used for fractured toes that have been buddy taped.

Application. If the cast shoe is going to be used by a patient with a fractured toe, the injured digit should first be buddy taped to the adjacent toe. After this is done, the patient merely slips on the hard shoe like a sandal. The shoe is then fastened with ties or Velcro straps.

Ankle Wraps and Bandages

There are no data supporting the routine use of ankle wraps for simple sprains, but some pain relief may be afforded by a proper wrap. Some type of temporary immobilization is commonly used in the ED, and usually requested and expected by patients. For minor ankle injuries, a simple elastic bandage (Ace) can be applied. A figure-of-eight configuration is preferred (see Fig. 50–26B). The wrap is applied only to give lateral support, and minimal compression. *It should not be tight enough to impair venous drainage,* a common problem when patients apply their own wraps. An Unna boot placed over Webril is an alternative. A modified Jones dressing may also be used for a variety of soft tissue injuries. To apply a Jones dressing, generously wrap the foot and ankle with large amounts of Webril (about five or seven layers) and cover it with an elastic bandage. A cast shoe can be applied over the dressing.

Soft Cast

Indications. A soft cast is basically a modified Jones compression dressing. It is useful for minor ligamentous and soft tissue injuries of the foot and ankle that do not require prolonged or complete immobilization. A soft cast can help reduce the pain and swelling often associated with mild ankle sprains and gives support for early weight-bearing (see Fig. 50–26B).

Construction. A soft cast is made using 3- or 4-inch Webril and elastic bandages.

Application. A soft cast is as simple to apply as the Jones compression dressing. To begin, the patient is placed in a supine position with the foot and ankle extending off the end of the stretcher. Alternatively, the leg can be elevated by an assistant or by placing pillows under the knee and foreleg. The ankle and foot are then wrapped with five or seven layers of Webril, starting at the metatarsal heads and continuing around the ankle in a figure-of-eight configuration. The Webril should extend 5 to 7 cm above the malleoli and, as discussed earlier, should overlap by 25% to 50% of its width. After the Webril is in place, an elastic bandage is wrapped around the foot and ankle in a similar fashion. Additional layers of Webril and elastic bandages are seldom required.

COMPLICATIONS OF SPLINTS

Ischemia

A compartment syndrome leading to ischemic injury and ultimately to a Volkmann ischemic contracture is the most worrisome complication of cylindrical casts. Although the risk of ischemia is drastically reduced with splinting, Webril or elastic bandages can cause significant constriction. To reduce the likelihood of this occurring, the elastic bandage should not be excessively tight. If the patient has a high-risk injury, the Webril may be cut lengthwise before the plaster is applied. Elevation, no weight-bearing, and application of cold packs should be stressed to each patient. Furthermore, signs and symptoms of vascular compromise should be explained carefully, and all patients whose injuries have the potential for significant swelling or loss of vascular integrity should receive follow-up in the first 24 to 48 hours. The clinician should not ignore complaints of increasing pain under a splint. Patients with splint-related discomfort should be reevaluated clinically and should not be treated with a telephone prescription for opioid analgesics.

Heat Injury

Fiberglass splints produce minimal heat when drying, but plaster generates considerable heat as it hardens. Many clinicians are unaware of the potential for drying plaster to produce second-degree burns.[26] Thermal injury can occur with both cylindrical casts and plaster splints. Some clinicians have reported a higher incidence of burns with the use of plaster splints, although the reasons for this are unclear.[26,27] Table 50–6 lists factors that can increase the amount of heat produced during plaster recrystallization. Their effects are additive, and this fact should be taken into account when applying a splint. For example, if 15 sheets of plaster are needed for strength in a particular splint, one should not increase the heat production further by using extra-fast-drying plaster or reusing warm dip water. To avoid plaster burns, use only 8 to 12 sheets of plaster when possible, use fresh dip water with a temperature near 24°C, and never wrap the extremity in a sheet or pillow during the setting process. Peak temperatures usually occur between 5 and 15 minutes after plaster wetting.

The patient should be warned that the hardening process produces warmth. The heat of drying may produce pain in patients with hemophilia-related hemarthroses. Splinting these patients may require that the plaster splint be placed only long enough to verify proper fit; the splint is then reapplied after setting (and cooling) of the plaster. If any patient complains of significant burning while the plaster is drying, *do not ignore this complaint!* Immediately remove the splint, and promptly cool the area with cold packs or cool water. Patients with vascular insufficiency or sensory deficits (e.g., diabetic neuropathy, stroke) are at high risk for plaster burns and require close observation during the drying process.

Pressure Sores

Pressure sores are an uncommon complication of short-term splinting.[28] They can result from stockinette wrinkles, irregular wadding of Webril, incorrectly padded or unpadded bony prominences, irregular splint ends, plaster ridges, or indentations produced from using the fingers rather than the palms to smooth and mold the wet plaster. Attention to detail during padding and splinting reduces the incidence of pressure sores. However, whenever a patient complains of a persistent pain or burning sensation under any part of a splint, the splint should be removed and the symptomatic area inspected closely. The padding incorporated in premade plaster and fiberglass splints is generally all that is needed for safe short-term splinting. However, the life of a splint applied in the ED may be longer than intended by the clinician; therefore, it is prudent to err on the side of additional padding when putting splints on patients who will overuse the splint, such as those who will not use crutches, or for those who may not have ready access to follow-up.

Infection

Bacterial and fungal infections can occur under a splint.[29,30] Infection is more common in the presence of an open wound but may occur with intact skin or develop in a skin lesion produced by prolonged splinting. The moist, warm, and dark environment created by the splint is an excellent nidus for infection. Toxic shock syndrome has been rarely reported from a staphylococcal skin infection that has clandestinely developed under a splint or cast. Also, it has been shown that bacteria can multiply in slowly drying plaster. To avoid infection, all wounds should be cleaned and débrided before splint application, and clean, fresh tap water should be used for plaster wetting. In some instances, it is preferable to apply a removable splint that allows for periodic wound inspection or local wound care.

Dermatitis

Occasionally, patients develop a rash under a plaster cast or splint.[31–35] Allergy to plaster is exceedingly rare, but there are several reports of contact dermatitis when formaldehyde and melamine resins are added to the plaster.[33,34] The rash is usually pruritic, with weeping papular or vesicular lesions. Because these resins are unnecessary for ED splints, their use should be avoided whenever possible. Dermatitis has also been reported with the use of fiberglass splinting materials.[36]

Joint Stiffness

Some degree of joint stiffness is an invariable consequence of immobilization. It can range in severity from mild to incapacitating and can result in transient, prolonged, or in some cases, permanent loss of function. Stiffness appears to be worse with prolonged periods of immobilization, in elderly patients, and in patients with preexisting joint diseases such as rheumatoid arthritis or osteoarthritis. Thus, splints should be left on for only that period of time necessary for adequate healing. Table 50–8 lists several injuries that commonly require splinting, along with some suggestions for length of immobilization. Fractures, dislocations, or other conditions that require prolonged immobilization (>7 days) should have orthopaedic follow-up. Patients must be told that a splint is only a short-term device and that prolonged immobilization can be detrimental. For minor injuries, the clinician can suggest that the patient use her or his own judgment about when to remove the splint, but a definite end point should be set.

CAST PAIN

Cast-related pain is a common complaint that brings patients to the ED. Because of the potential for ischemia with circum-

TABLE 50–8 Suggested Length of Immobilization for Conditions That Frequently Require Splinting

Length of Condition	Immobilization (Days)
Contusions	1–3
Abrasions	1–3
Soft tissue lacerations	5–7
Tendon lacerations	Variable*
Tendinitis	5–7
Puncture wounds and bites	3–4
Deep space infections and cellulitis	3–5
Mild sprains	5–7
Fractures and severe sprains	Variable†

*Considerable controversy surrounds the length of immobilization for tendon lacerations, and duration therefore is best left to the consultant surgeon.
†Usually requires prolonged immobilization; best determined by an orthopaedic surgeon.

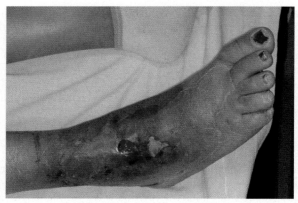

Figure 50–27 If a patient complains of a cast being too tight, it probably is. The cast must be removed to inspect the area for infection or other problems. Complaints of pain under this cast were incorrectly met with a phone call to suggest elevation and a call-in prescription for narcotics.

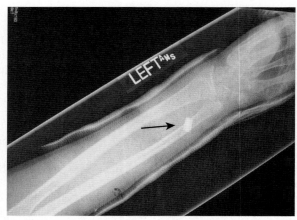

Figure 50–28 This 9-year-old tried to scratch an itch under his splint with a pencil and the eraser fell off, creating a skin irritation/infection requiring splint removal.

ferential casts, all complaints should be fully investigated, and vascular compromise must be ruled out. *If a patient states that a cast is too tight, it probably is too tight* (Fig. 50–27). Narcotics should not be prescribed for cast pain until a too-tight cast can be ruled out. A detailed history and physical examination should be performed on all such patients. The nature and onset of the pain are of particular importance. A dull, non-specific pain that has worsened gradually since the time of injury may be the only clue to an early compartment syndrome (see Chapter 54, Compartment Syndrome Evaluation). The sudden onset of throbbing pain associated with swelling and redness suggests a possible deep venous thrombosis. In both of these cases, rapid intervention is the key to decreasing morbidity and mortality. The physical examination should pay particular attention to the areas of tenderness and the effect of active and passive movement on the severity of pain.

Itching under a cast can be problematic. Patients, especially children, use various objects such as a pencil, coat hanger, or fork to get to the itch. This can cause skin maceration and possible infection, or a foreign body can be left under the cast (Fig. 50–28).

With a compartment syndrome, tenderness over the involved compartment is a common finding; stretching or contracting ischemic muscle also elicits significant pain. The examination should also evaluate the presence and quality of distal pulses, amount of edema fluid present, distal sensation, capillary refill, and color and temperature of the digits. The finding of pain, pallor, paresthesias, paralysis, and pulselessness (the five Ps) are said to be pathognomonic for ischemia. Unfortunately, they seldom occur simultaneously, and their presence together is usually a late finding that carries a poor prognosis. Hence, the emergency clinician must maintain a high index of suspicion for possible ischemia and remove the cast if any possibility of vascular compromise exists. Almost any cast can be bivalved and reapplied after inspection without significant loss of short-term immobilization.

To loosen a cast, an oscillating cast saw is used to cut along the medial and lateral aspects of the cast (Fig. 50–29). This is called *bivalving the cast*, and it allows the halves to be

spread and reapplied in a less constricting manner while still maintaining proper immobilization. To use the oscillating power saw, proceed in a series of downward cutting movements facilitated by wrist supination, removing the blade between cuts. The blade is removed between cuts to prevent it from getting hot enough to burn the skin. This is particularly important if synthetic materials have been used in the cast. Also, the blade should not be allowed to slide along the skin, and the saw should never be used on unpadded plaster. With an apprehensive patient, the clinician can demonstrate that the cast saw blade only vibrates (it does not turn) and that it does not cut the skin.

After the medial and lateral sides of the cast are completely cut through, the two halves are separated using a cast spreader, and the padding is cut lengthwise with scissors. This may be sufficient to relieve early ischemia if the problem is simple postinjury swelling, but both the padding and the cast can be totally removed to inspect the injured area if necessary. If ischemia cannot be ruled out, compartment pressures should be measured (see Chapter 54, Compartment Syndrome Evaluation), and an orthopaedic consultation should be obtained.

If vascular integrity is established and no other problems are found, the bivalved cast can be replaced. First, the extremity should be padded in the usual manner using fresh Webril. The cut ends of the bivalved cast are then lined with white adhesive tape, and the cast is replaced around the extremity. Finally, the cast is secured in place using elastic bandages.

If plaster sores are causing the patient's discomfort, the clinician who placed the cast should be consulted. In some cases, additional padding is all that is needed, but in others, a window should be cut out over the problem area. Because pressure sores can lead to significant tissue necrosis, the patient should receive follow-up care within 24 hours.

If the patient's problem is plaster (or, more likely, resin) dermatitis, treatment generally consists of topical or oral steroids and antihistamines. Therapy should be done in concert with an orthopaedic surgeon because the patient may require admission for other forms of immobilization until the cast can be replaced. With mild cases, changing the cast or splint and

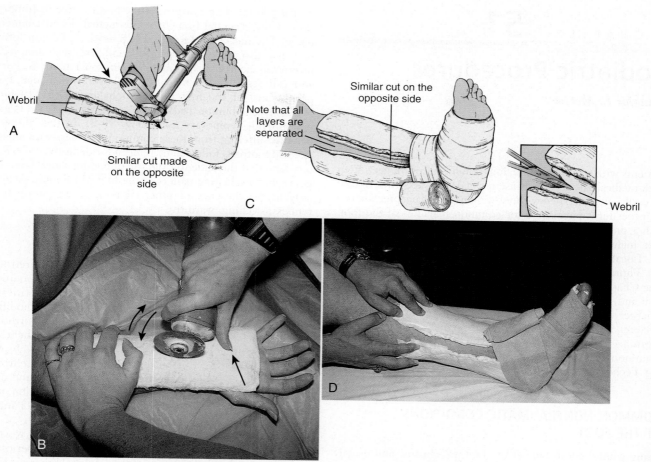

Similar cut on the
opposite side

Note that all
layers are
separated

A

Similar cut made
on the opposite
side

C

Webril

D

B

Figure 50–29 *A* and *B,* The cast saw vibrates; it does not rotate. It will not cut the patient. The blade is controlled by *placing the thumb* (*arrow*) *on the splint* and lowering the saw blade to the plaster. The blade is raised and lowered for each cut; it is not drawn across the plaster like a knife. *C* and *D,* This cast was too tight, and it was therefore bivalved from calf to forefoot with a cast saw. After separation of the edges of the cut cast, the anterior and posterior components were secured in place with an elastic bandage. Note that the underlying Webril padding was cut to relieve pressure but was not removed (*inset*). A bivalved cast provides temporary immobilization equal to that of an intact cast. Extra padding can be used to protect the skin from the cut edges.

using antihistamines for symptomatic relief may suffice. All of these patients should receive close follow-up; if the condition does not improve, the cast must be removed.

CONCLUSION

Splinting represents an important means of temporary fracture immobilization and provides protection and comfort for a variety of soft tissue injuries. The clinician should be aware of potential complications, including ischemia, thermal injury, and pressure sores, that can occur with improper splint application. Proper technique should minimize the risk of these adverse outcomes. The emergency clinician also should be facile in the release of circumferential cast and splint materials when ischemia is suspected.

REFERENCES CAN BE FOUND ON EXPERT CONSULT

CHAPTER **51**

Podiatric Procedures

Douglas L. McGee

Patients with painful or infectious conditions of the feet often seek medical attention because normal daily activities cannot be easily accomplished without walking. This chapter focuses on procedures performed for common maladies of the foot. Other procedures of the foot are described elsewhere in this text, including anesthesia of the foot and ankle (see Chapters 29, Local and Topical Anesthesia, and 31, Nerve Blocks of the Thorax and Extremities), management of nailbed injuries (see Chapters 35, Methods of Wound Closure, and 37, Incision and Drainage), incision and drainage of paronychia (see Chapter 37, Incision and Drainage), joint fluid analysis (see Chapter 53, Arthocentesis), the management of common dislocations of the foot (see Chapter 49, Management of Common Dislocations), and splinting (see Chapter 50, Splinting Techniques).

COMMON NONTRAUMATIC CONDITIONS OF THE FOOT

Many painful conditions of the foot are chronic and usually do not require definitive treatment in the emergency department (ED); however, patients often present with common conditions that require evaluation and proper referral. To accomplish this, the clinician must be cognizant of basic podiatric conditions including painful lesions over bony prominences, heel pain, foot infections, and pain on the plantar surface of the foot.

Footpad Use

Footpads redistribute pressure over an inflamed, tender area of the foot. The particular type of footpad and its placement depend on the condition being treated (Fig. 51–1). Commercially available aperture footpads are recommended for temporary relief of warts, corns, hyperkeratoses, and bunions. Verruca virus introduced into the plantar surface of the foot may produce a painful hyperkeratotic lesion, commonly referred to as a "plantar wart," on the sole of the foot. Simple callus may be painful and result in the formation of a "hard corn" when formed over the bony prominence of a digit. Once recognized, and after other conditions are ruled out, definitive care of these lesions is rarely indicated in the ED.

When tenderness is elicited over more than one metatarsal head, the diagnosis is metatarsalgia. Pain that is progressively worse while walking but relieved by rest, often beneath the second or third metatarsal heads, is typical in this case. A pad placed under the first metatarsal head to raise the second and third metatarsals may provide some relief.

A bunion develops when unbalanced forces applied to the first metatarsal cause lateral displacement of the distal hallux. Bunions typically form in women wearing heeled shoes with narrow toe boxes. The patient may complain of numbness over the distal, medial aspect of the first toe due to compression of the terminal branch of the medial dorsal cutaneous nerve. The mechanical forces that precipitate bunion formation may also cause other painful conditions including intermetatarsal neuroma, hammertoes, ingrown toenails, corns, and calluses. Bursitis may develop over the medial bony prominence of the first metatarsophalangeal (MTP) joint. Self-adherent bunion pads placed over the first MTP joint may provide temporary relief (Fig. 51–2). In the ED, treat patients suffering from these common disorders with analgesics and footpads followed by referral for definitive care. Recommend that the patient avoid the offending shoes. Consider gout when evaluating pain over the first MTP joint, particularly in the presence of other signs of inflammation (e.g., redness, swelling, warmth).

Heel Pain Syndromes

Bony spurs on the plantar surface of the calcaneus, retrocalcaneal bursitis, calcaneal apophysitis, and other conditions may cause heel pain. Treat most of these conditions with rest, nonsteroidal anti-inflammatory drugs (NSAIDs), modification of physical activities or shoewear, footpads, and orthoses. Some clinicians also include the injection of anesthetics or steroids for these conditions.

Heel spur pain can be quite bothersome and chronic. This condition is not easily remedied in the ED, and after other conditions are ruled out, minimal intervention with podiatric referral is often the best course of action. Patients typically present with pain over the medial border of the plantar aspect of the calcaneus. The pain gradually worsens over months. A bony prominence that begins as periostitis extends from the medial aspect of the calcaneal tuberosity into the central plantar fascia and may be demonstrated on radiographs. Radiographs of the calcaneus that do not demonstrate a bony spur suggest plantar fasciitis (see "Painful Conditions of the Plantar Surface of the Foot," later in this chapter), even though many patients with plantar fasciitis have plantar calcaneal and Achilles spurs. Radiographs have little value in the evaluation of nontraumatic heel pain, rarely demonstrating radiographic abnormalities that prompt additional treatment.[1]

Shoe supports using a heel pad or cup or a doughnut-shaped orthotic often help reduce the discomfort by redistributing weight. Treatment of the painful site is done with 10 to 20 mg of methylprednisolone injected from the medial aspect of the foot, avoiding the sensitive plantar surface. Few randomized, controlled trials have evaluated steroid therapy; those that have do not provide substantial evidence supporting its long-term efficacy.[2,3] Some evidence suggests that 25 mg of prednisolone acetate injected into the medial heel provides partial pain relief at 1 month compared with lidocaine only, but no advantage can be detected at 3 months.[4] A short leg-walking cast may be effective in some patients with recalcitrant heel pain.[5] There is little evidence to suggest that specific interventions aimed to reduce heel pain are superior to conservative, supportive treatment alone.

Retrocalcaneal Bursitis, Achilles Tendinitis, and Calcaneal Apophysitis

Although retrocalcaneal bursitis and Achilles tendinitis are anatomically distinct, the clinical presentation is similar. Pain at the insertion of the Achilles tendon is worsened with prolonged standing or walking and is aggravated by passive or active range of motion in both conditions. Directed palpation can distinguish one entity from the other, but both are treated similarly. Tenderness of the Achilles tendon suggests tendinitis, whereas tenderness between the tendon and the calcaneus suggests retrocalcaneal bursitis. Achilles tendinitis has been noted to develop spontaneously after quinolone antibiotic use, occasionally with rupture. Rest, elevation, ice, NSAIDs, heel pads, and an open-back shoe provide relief in the majority of patients. A corticosteroid injection is usually not performed, but it may provide some relief, although its superiority to conservative measures is unproved. Repeated steroid injection is associated with Achilles tendon rupture.[6] Osteochondrosis of the posterior calcaneal apophysis may cause pain worsened by activity in the child between 7 and 10 years old. It is thought to represent an overuse syndrome in the athletically active child with a tender posterior heel.[6,7] Treat this self-limited condition with rest, ice, and heel pads. Activity is resumed when the pain abates.

Painful Conditions of the Plantar Surface of the Foot

Plantar Fasciitis

Repeated microtrauma to the plantar aponeurosis causes pain on the plantar surface of the foot. Plantar fasciitis is typically unilateral and found in women who wear high-heeled shoes. The pain is maximally severe in the morning or after prolonged sitting and improves after walking. Some patients with plantar fasciitis may also have a calcaneal heel spur, but the presence or absence of this radiographic finding is generally immaterial (Fig. 51–3). Pain is elicited with palpation (Fig. 51–4), toe walking, or passive stretching of the plantar aponeurosis. Often, this annoying condition resolves on its own, but resolution is slow, taking as long as 6 to 18 months to resolve. Conservative therapy, including rest, elevation, ice, and NSAIDs, results in a satisfactory outcome after 6 to 8 weeks in 90% of patients.[8] Pain improves over time in most

933

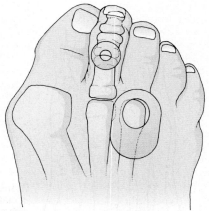

Figure 51–1 Use of aperture pads to redistribute pressure from painful areas to surrounding structures. *(Courtesy of Kenneth R. Walker, DPM.)*

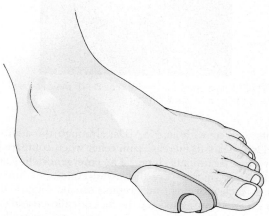

Figure 51–2 Use of a self-adherent bunion pad. *(Courtesy of Kenneth R. Walker, DPM.)*

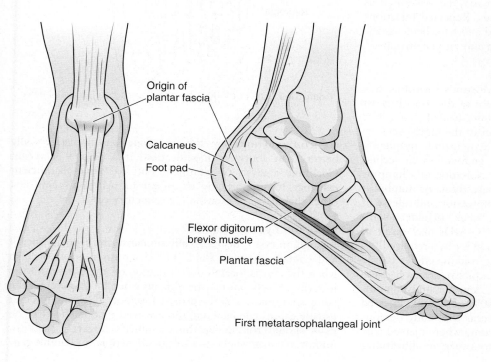

Origin of plantar fascia

Calcaneus

Foot pad

Flexor digitorum brevis muscle

Plantar fascia

First metatarsophalangeal joint

Figure 51–3 The plantar fascia spans the plantar aspect of the foot. The origin is the *medial* tubercle of the calcaneus; this is the most common site of pain. A heel spur may be seen on x-ray but inflammation of the plantar fascia, not the spur, is the source of pain.

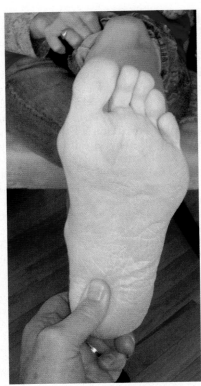

Figure 51–4 Palpation of the medial tubercle of the calcaneus reproduces the pain of plantar fasciitis.

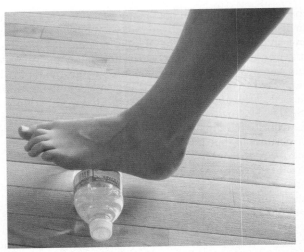

Figure 51–5 Rolling the arch of the foot back and forth over a frozen water bottle will stretch the fascia and, over time, may lessen the pain of plantar fasciitis. A tennis ball can also be used.

patients with or without NSAIDs, although the addition of NSAIDs appears to increase pain relief when compared with conservative treatments alone.[9] The emergency clinician can do little to treat this very distressful condition. Stretching exercises each morning and evening can be suggested (Fig. 51–5). Night splinting to keep the foot dorsiflexed and custom orthoses made from the patient's foot impression can be very helpful, usually requiring podiatry referral for proper fitting. Corticosteroid injection is used by some clinicians; the benefit remains unproved. A single injection may be warranted as supplemental therapy in resistant cases. Repeated injections with corticosteroids should be avoided and have been associated with rupture of the plantar fascia and fat pad atrophy.[10]

Forefoot Neuroma

A forefoot neuroma, also know as Morton's neuroma, is a painful condition of the plantar surface of the foot. It most commonly affects women who wear high-heeled shoes. The neuroma forms after chronic irritation to the digital sensory nerve between the metatarsals. The neuroma frequently occurs in the third interspace but may be found in the second space (Fig. 51–6). Patients report the sensation of a lump or cord in the interspace and describe paresthesia or numbness in the third or fourth toes. Direct compression and release of the forefoot causes pain, and often a "click" (Mulder's sign) (Fig. 51–7). Rest, elevation, ice, and NSAIDs may result in some improvement, but surgical excision is often required.[11,12] Little data support the use of corticosteroid injections. In one study, less than 50% of patients with a foot neuroma had any benefit from injected corticosteroids.[11] Another study demonstrated complete or partial relief in 80% of patients injected with corticosteroid injections.[13] Whereas this study demonstrated a trend toward improved outcome when injected corticosteroids were compared with footwear modifications,

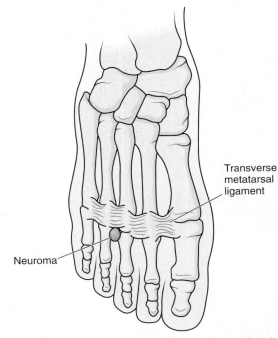

Figure 51–6 Site of Morton's neuroma, arising from a digital nerve.

corticosteroid injection therapy alone was not statistically better than footwear modification at 1 year.[13] A recent Cochrane analysis of treatment options found insufficient evidence to support any treatment for Morton's neuroma other than surgical excision for refractory cases.

Ganglion Cyst of the Foot

A ganglion cyst is histologically similar to the synovial sheath and contains synovial fluid. The diagnosis is easy to make when the cyst is located over a tendon on the dorsum of the foot (Fig. 51–8), but may be difficult when located among the compact structures of the plantar forefoot. The ganglion cyst usually causes edema along the involved tendon sheath. The mass should roll under the examiner's finger; a painless, immovable mass suggests a soft tissue neoplasm. Painful gan-

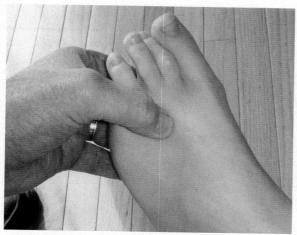

Figure 51–7 Palpation of the distal metatarsal area may reveal pain from a Morton neuroma. Squeezing and releasing this area (not shown) can elicit pain and a clinking sensation, termed *Mulder's sign*.

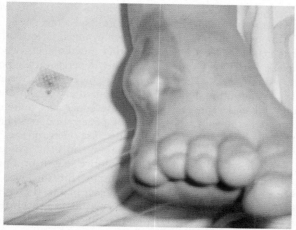

Figure 51–8 **Ganglion cysts on the dorsum of the foot.** A small amount of gel substance was aspirated with a needle, but a cyst of this size is best totally excised surgically.

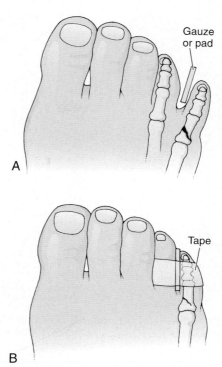

Figure 51–9 **Buddy taping of a fractured lesser toe.** *A,* A pad is placed between the injured toe and an adjacent toe. *B,* The toes are secured together with tape or self-adherent wrap. *(A and B, Courtesy of Kenneth R. Walker, DPM.)*

935

glion cysts are treated with aspiration with or without the injection of corticosteroid (see Chapter 52, Injection Therapy of Bursitis and Tendinitis). After local or regional anesthesia (see Chapters 29, Local and Topical Anesthesia, and 31, Nerve Blocks of the Thorax and Extremities), insert a 20-gauge needle into the cyst and withdraw yellow, thick, synovial fluid. Manually express any remaining synovial fluid after the needle is withdrawn. Corticosteroid injection is often advocated for ganglion cysts, but recurrence is common after aspiration and corticosteroid injection—as high as 57% in one study.[14] Recurrence, chronic pain, neuritis, stiffness, and infection are not uncommon even after surgical excision.[15]

TRAUMATIC CONDITIONS OF THE FOOT

Trauma to the feet and toes is common and covers a broad spectrum of injury. Lacerations, fractures, compartment syndromes, and nailbed injuries are described in other chapters of this text. Three specific injuries—toe fractures, sesamoid bone fractures, and puncture wounds to the plantar surface of the foot—are discussed in detail here.

Toe Fractures and Fractures of the Sesamoid Bones

Emergency clinicians often treat toe fractures and can intervene to relieve the pain and encourage healing. As with any other fracture, pay attention to the possibility of disrupted joint cartilage, hypermobility of fracture segments, and malposition or malunion of the fracture fragments. Aggressive reduction is indicated for fractures of the proximal phalanx of the great toe because it represents the main propulsive segment of the forefoot. A plaster cast alone without anatomic reduction is insufficient treatment. Displacement suggests axial rotation or abnormal biomechanical interaction between the hallux and its own interphalangeal or MTP joint.

In the acute setting, a non–weight-bearing ankle splint that extends beyond the great toe provides protection until the patient with a complicated great toe fracture obtains follow-up with a foot and ankle surgeon. Open fractures require careful cleaning, usually antibiotic therapy, and close follow-up. Fractures of the lesser toes usually result from jamming the toe into a nightstand or bedpost while barefoot. Radiographs of the lesser phalanges confirm the suspected fracture and may occasionally reveal an unsuspected interphalangeal or MTP dislocation. However, x-rays are generally not required and the injured digit is easily reduced.

Treat closed, lesser phalangeal fractures with "immobilization" for 6 weeks. After the fracture is reduced, splint the injured toe against an adjacent noninjured toe. Place a soft corn pad or other suitable material between the toes to prevent skin maceration, and hold the toes together with adhesive tape or a self-adherent wrap like Coban (Fig. 51–9). Demonstrate the procedure to the patient or family and dispense or prescribe enough material so that the splint can be changed every

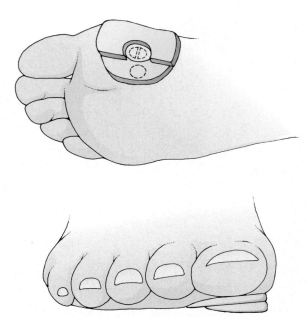

Figure 51–10 Bunion shields redistribute pressure away from fractured sesamoid bones. *(Courtesy of Kenneth R. Walker, DPM.)*

Adapted from Sanderlin BW, Raspa RF: Common stress fractures. Am Fam Physician 68:1527, 2003.

TABLE 51–1 Risk Factors for Stress Fractures
Sports involving running and jumping, especially on angled, hard, or irregular surfaces
Rapid increase in physical training program
Poor physical condition
Female gender
Hormonal or menstrual disturbances
Osteoporosis/decreased bone density
Nutritional deficiencies (including extreme dieting)
Obesity/overweight
Inappropriate footwear
Poor flexibility

2 to 3 days at home. Put the patient in a less restrictive, stiff-soled shoe. A postoperative shoe (or similar footwear) may be a comfortable alternative for the first several days.

Jumping from a height can result in a fracture of the first MTP joint sesamoid bone. The great toe sesamoid bones lie in grooves on the bottom of the metatarsal head. Each bone lies within the tendon of its respective flexor hallucis brevis muscle belly. Localized pain on the plantar aspect of the first metatarsal head accompanies a sesamoid bone fracture. Bipartite sesamoids (tibial more frequently than fibular) are common. Comparison radiographs clarify whether the radiographic abnormality represents a fracture.

For a tibial sesamoid injury, an aperture bunion-type pad, reinforced medially with 0.5- to 0.75-cm-thick felt protects the sesamoid and transfers weight-bearing to the surrounding structures (Fig. 51–10). A hard-soled shoe and NSAIDs are also helpful. Subsequent radiographs rarely show bony consolidation, but the fracture interface appears smoother.

Stress Fractures

Runners, military recruits, or those with repetitive trauma to the foot can develop a metatarsal stress fracture, commonly of the distal second and third metatarsals. Other risk factors are listed in Table 51–1.[16] There is pain on walking but minimal to no external findings. A bone scan or magnetic resonance imaging (MRI) scan may detect the subtle fracture that often eludes a plain radiograph. Women are more prone to stress fractures than men. Treatment is usually rest and alleviating the precipitant causes.

Plantar Puncture Wounds

Plantar puncture wounds present a diagnostic and therapeutic challenge for the clinician. Considerable controversy exists regarding the proper initial management of puncture wounds to the plantar surface of the foot, and no universally accepted standard of care exists. Treatment recommendations range from simple wound cleaning to aggressive débridement. No single approach has been demonstrated to be superior. The editors support a close inspection for retained foreign material and an initially conservative approach, but an aggressive one is recommended if the patient returns or presents with an infection or if pain persists for more than a few days.

Although nails produce many such wounds, various other objects may cause them including other metal objects, wood, and glass. Patient response to the injury depends on the penetrating material, location and circumstances of the wound, depth of penetration, footwear, time from injury until presentation, and underlying health. Because superficial puncture wounds generally do well, depth of penetration may be a primary determinant of outcome.[17] Because one's reflexes are not fast enough to pull back when stepping on a sharp object, the clinician should assume that the entire length of a protruding nail has entered the foot (minus the thickness of footwear). Stepping on an unknown object in a field or while walking in a stream requires a more cautious approach than does a simple puncture from a known object, such as a protruding nail.

The vast majority of patients who step on a nail suffer nothing more than transient pain and never seek medical attention. Because most minor puncture wounds are not seen in the ED, the true risk of infection, including osteomyelitis, is unknown. Consequently, reported infection rates vastly overstate the actual incidence. Probably no more than 2% to 8% of puncture wounds become infected and only a small percentage of these develop osteomyelitis.[17,18] A prospective series suggests that only the presence of symptoms (e.g., redness, tenderness, increased swelling) at 48 hours was associated with the risk of infection or potential retained foreign body (FB).[19] Retained foreign material (e.g., a portion of a tennis shoe sole) in the wound is an important factor in persistent infection. Because no single test detects all possible FBs, tailor the evaluation of a suspected FB to the suspected object.

Evaluation

The approach to the patient depends on several factors, including the time from injury to presentation, the suspicion of an FB, and the presence of infection. The extent to which an FB is pursued depends on the history and physical findings. When the patient clearly states that a needle, pin, or nail was removed intact, radiographs or local wound exploration for a retained metallic FB is not needed. Stepping on an identified

937

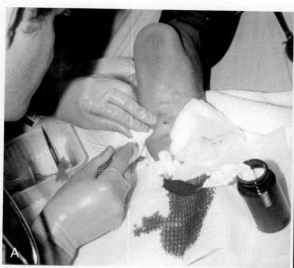

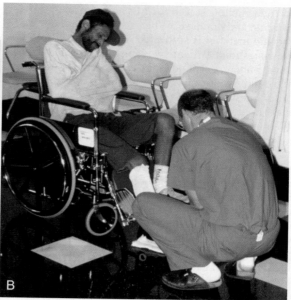

Figure 51–11 *A,* The best way to examine a puncture wound of the foot is to place the patient prone on a stretcher, have good light, and obtain a bloodless field (blood pressure cuff here). First, remove the flap of skin at the puncture site. A local anesthetic injection (lidocaine 1%) is usually required, but quite painful. *B,* An amateur move is to try to examine the bottom of the foot with the patient in a hallway chair.

intact nail does not always require a radiograph, but if there is any debate regarding a retained metallic object, plain radiographs readily demonstrate their presence. Plain radiographs also demonstrate other radiopaque objects such as glass, gravel, bone, and teeth. Rubber or pieces of a sock will not be visible on an x-ray. If the patient steps on an unknown object, a radiograph is usually indicated unless the entire depth of the wound can be ascertained and inspected. Ultrasonography is noninvasive and does not use radiation, making it potentially useful for radiolucent FBs, but soft tissue air or calcifications may suggest a retained FB when there is not one. Bedside ultrasound has been used to localize radiolucent FBs for removal.[20,21] Computed tomography (CT) can demonstrate radiopaque and radiolucent objects, but its expense and greater radiation exposure than plain films make it unsuitable as an initial screening tool. Use CT scanning when other screening tools have failed to demonstrate a suspected FB, when infection is present, or when joint penetration is suspected. Fluoroscopy may be used to help localize metallic or radiopaque FBs during exploration and removal. Fluoroscopy may be particularly useful for long metallic objects such as needles and pins. MRI provides no additional benefit and cannot be used when metallic objects are retained.

Treatment

As a general rule, the plantar surface of the foot should be *examined under good lighting and in a bloodless field.* This is best accomplished with the patient in a prone position, *not in a chair* (Fig. 51–11). Plantar puncture wounds explored for persistent infection often have contained foreign material (Figs. 51–12 and 51–13). Because most patients do not develop persistent infection, initial deep exploration in the absence of evidence or strong suspicion for retained material cannot be advocated.[17] Routine initial deep wound exploration, including coring of the wound, is not supported by scientific research and is not recommended for simple, noninfected puncture wounds.[17] However, select wounds may benefit from

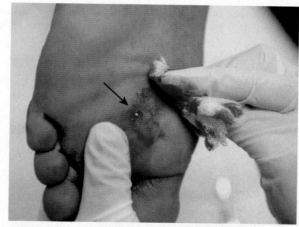

Figure 51–12 This piece of rubber (*arrow*) was introduced into a puncture when a nail went through a sneaker. It was not seen or expected until the skin flap was removed and carefully examined.

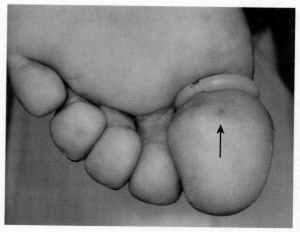

Figure 51–13 A small piece of sock is difficult to appreciate in the puncture wound of the big toe.

exploration to facilitate a search for FBs and to promote irrigation, cleansing, and drainage. When the wound is large and retained organic material is suspected, local wound exploration may be warranted. Patients wearing rubber-soled shoes during plantar puncture wounds may retain a portion of the shoe in the wound. Exploration of the wound is most productive after local anesthesia or a regional anesthetic block and excision of the epidermal flap. An incision may be required to facilitate FB removal, but extensive removal of surrounding tissue is not proven to increase successful removal of retained material.[17]

Some clinicians favor a coring technique *when an FB is found or suspected*. Although this may be aggressive for many wounds, it is the best way to remove particulate matter as a block. To accomplish coring, a No. 11 blade is advanced to the hilt and a 2- to 3-mm core is excised (Figs. 51–14 and 51–15). A hemostat may be used to grab the cutout core or may be opened in the tract to better visualize the wound. The tract can be packed with gauze for a few days or left open (Fig. 51–16). Occasionally, blunt probes may facilitate wound exploration. It is generally impossible, and likely counterproductive, to attempt to probe or visualize the entire length of the puncture tract. Patients presenting within 24 hours and without signs of infection generally require only simple topical wound care. Although irrigation of all exposed dermal tissue is recommended, high-pressure irrigation of deep tissues with distention of the soft tissues is unlikely to be helpful and not recommended. Schwab and Powers[19] described a case series of uncomplicated puncture wounds in healthy individuals who had conservative treatment with cleansing and crutches. Radiographs were obtained at the discretion of the treating clinician; antibiotics were not given. At 6-month follow-up, 88% of all patients healed without complication. The remain-

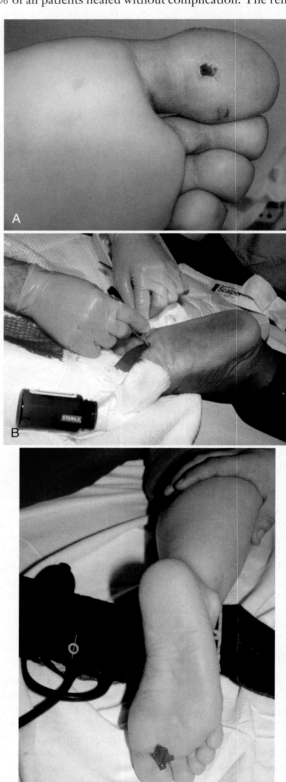

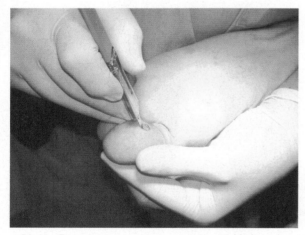

Figure 51–14 To core out a puncture, use a No. 11 blade and advance it to the hilt.

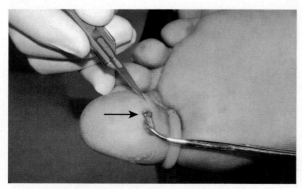

Figure 51–15 When the cored-out section is removed with a hemostat, note the present of a piece of rubber (*arrow*) deep in the wound.

Figure 51–16 After coring out a puncture tract, the wound can be left open (*A*) or packed (*B* and *C*). Packing gauze can be dry or wet with saline or iodine solution.

ing 12% developed complications including wound infection due to retained FB. *No findings on initial presentation predicted a subsequent infection.* Initial antibiotic therapy remains controversial, but there is *no evidence to suggest that prophylactic antibiotics reduce the already low rate of infection.*

Symptomatic patients who present later (≥48 hours) have an increased risk for a retained FB, because delayed presentation is often due to the development of inflammation or infection. Local wound exploration is warranted unless the patient presents without infection or with a clearly superficial cellulitis expected to respond to simple oral antibiotics. Recurrent infection, deep soft tissue tenderness, and increasing soft tissue swelling suggest a retained FB or deep space infection, such as osteomyelitis. Such patients require prompt specialty referral or additional diagnostic studies in the ED.

Patients with obvious signs of infection within a few days of a puncture wound usually have a simple cellulitis (with or without an FB) with a gram-positive organism (Fig. 51–17). In a patient with persistent pain or swelling days to weeks after a puncture wound, the presence or absence of a deep soft tissue infection or a low-grade osteomyelitis cannot be ruled in, or ruled out, by physical examination, plain radiographs, or laboratory tests (such as a sedimentation rate, complete blood count, or wound cultures). A high index of suspicion, coupled with additional investigation, is the prudent approach to the patient with minimal physical findings, normal laboratory tests, and continued pain or swelling after a seemingly simple puncture wound to the bottom of the foot. This usually entails CT, bone scan, or MRI. A study of 80 children with plantar puncture wounds presenting with signs of infection demonstrated simple cellulitis in 59, retained FBs in 11, and osteomyelitis or septic arthritis in 10 children. Because a sig-

nificant number of children in this study had retained FBs or bony infections, a cautious approach was warranted.[22]

Plantar puncture wounds complicated by *Pseudomonas* osteomyelitis and osteochondritis are clinically clandestine and particularly devastating and have been described for nearly 40 years. Some investigators have cultured *Pseudomonas* from the sole of tennis shoes, suggesting that puncture wounds made through athletic footwear may be inoculated with *Pseudomonas*[23] (Fig. 51–18). No evidence suggests that prophylactic anti-*Pseudomonas* antibiotics prescribed on an initial evaluation of an uncomplicated wound will prevent infection among patients with subsequent deep space or bone infections.[23] Some argue that prophylactic antibiotics, at the time of puncture, may select out resistant organisms.[23] Surgical débridement and prolonged intravenous antibiotics are often required for established infections.

INGROWN TOENAIL

An ingrown toenail is characterized by progressive curving or excessive widening of the lateral margin of the toenail and impingement of the nail into the periungual soft tissue (Fig. 51–19). The toenail normally grows distally in an unimpeded manner, allowing the nail to pass beyond the lateral nailfold (Fig. 51–20). Nail deformity, tight-fitting shoes, and rotational deformity of the toes increase the friction between the nail and the nailfold. Toenails that have been trimmed in a curve increase the likelihood that the lateral nail margin will impinge on the lateral nailfold. The resulting soft tissue injury may lead to hyperkeratosis, edema, and erythema of the nailfold or frank infection (Fig. 51–21). Although an ingrown toenail can be found on any toe, the majority occur in the great toe.

Evaluation

The patient presents with pain, edema, and erythema of the lateral nailfold. Pressure over the nail margins increases the pain. Because intense pain often precipitates an early visit to the ED, most inflammatory or infectious responses are confined locally. Recurrent ingrown toenails or those in patients with circulatory dysfunction, neuropathy, or diabetes may have underlying osteomyelitis. Cleanse the toe gently to facilitate visualization of periungual debris. When the free edge

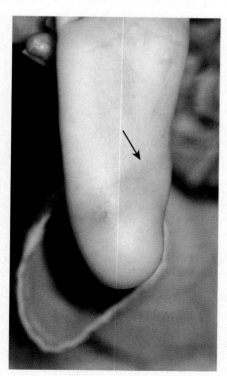

Figure 51–17 This 5-day-old inflamed and infected puncture wound tract likely harbors a foreign body. Minor lymphangitis spread (*arrow*) up the ankle, but there were no systemic complaints, adenopathy, or leukocytosis. Excision of a core of the tract found scant pus and a few pieces of the patient's sock embedded in the wound. The wound did well with oral antibiotics and warm soaks.

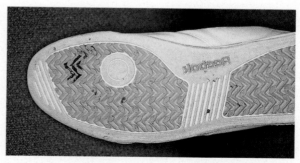

Figure 51–18 A patient stepped on a nail while wearing this shoe. An initial ED evaluation 3 weeks previous found no foreign body or infection. A week previous, the patient began taking antibiotics, but did not improve. The physical examination was quite benign, but the continued aching pain and minimal swelling suggested a deep infection. The complete blood count, sedimentation rate, and plain film were negative. A magnetic resonance imaging scan demonstrated osteomyelitis. Pseudomonas is often the offending organism in this scenario.

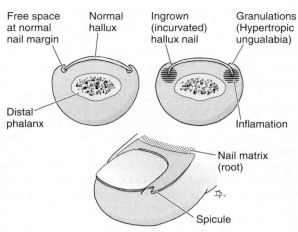

Figure 51–19 **Pathology of an ingrown toenail.** The normal free space at the nail margin is obliterated by inflammation and granulation tissue, which is caused by improper nail trimming, trauma to the matrix, and faulty footwear. *(From Hill GL II [ed]: Outpatient Surgery, 3rd ed. Philadelphia, WB Saunders, 1988. Reproduced by permission.)*

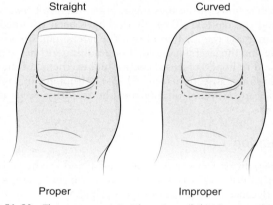

Figure 51–20 The proper way to trim a toenail that is prone to becoming ingrown is to cut the end of the nail *straight across, not at an angle.* This is counterintuitive to the patient who wants the nail to conform with the contour of the toe.

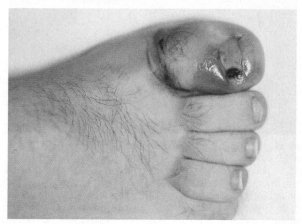

Figure 51–21 An ingrown toenail of this degree requires removal of a portion of the nail and débridement of inflamed tissue.

of the lateral nail can be easily visualized as separate from the lateral nailfold, consider other painful conditions of the toe such as trauma, gout, paronychia, and cellulitis.

Treatment

Because the toe is exquisitely tender, additional treatment will usually require digital block anesthesia. The decision to treat and what course of action to take in the ED depend on the patient's degree of discomfort. Two general courses of action are often suggested: removal of the offending nail spicule or removal of the spicule and some portion of the nail. Any degree of nail removal is usually followed with ablation of the nailbed.[24] Nail splinting techniques may also be effective and are less invasive than nail removal techniques.

Removal of the Nail Spicule and Débridement of Hyperkeratosis for Minor Ingrown Toenail

When the amount of inflammation and pain and the degree of nail deformity are both minimal, such as involving only the distal toenail area, simple removal of the impacted nail spicule is indicated and usually curative. If the condition is advanced, removal of a complete portion of the nail may be required. All procedures are best done with a tourniquet to produce a bloodless field. After a digital block and thorough cleansing, remove an oblique segment of the nail about one third to one half of the way to the proximal nailfold (Fig. 51–22). The ideal instrument is an English anvil nail splitter designed to cut the nail while minimizing trauma to the underlying nail matrix (Fig. 51–23). Sharp, pointed scissors may be substituted if care is taken to minimize nailbed injury by maintaining upward pressure while cutting the nail. Some clinicians use a dispos-

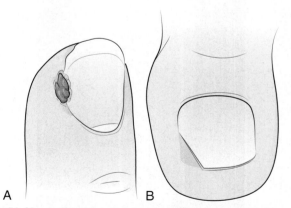

Figure 51–22 *A,* This minor ingrown toenail can be treated with removal of a portion of the distal nail. *B,* An oblique wedge of nail is trimmed from the lateral margin of the nail to free it from the hyperkeratotic area. *(A and B, Courtesy of Kenneth R. Walker, DPM.)*

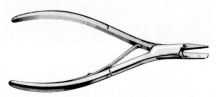

Figure 51–23 English nail anvil used to divide the nail. *(Courtesy of Gill Podiatry Supply Company, Middleburg Heights, OH.)*

able electric cautery device to cut the nail after softening it by soaking in warm soapy water.

After cutting the nail spicule free from the bulk of the nail, grasp the free edge of the nail with forceps or hemostats and remove it to expose the irritated area. The nailfold typically contains impacted debris that must be removed after the nailfold has been gently retracted away from the nail. Remove debris until the epidermis or dermis is uncovered, taking care to avoid aggressive débridement that causes bleeding. A silver nitrate stick to the débrided area may be used to control bleeding. Dress the area with antibiotic ointment and a nonadherent dressing. Soaking the toe in warm water two or three times a day, with home redressing, is explained. Harsh chemicals are avoided in the soaking regimen. The wound should be reinspected for signs of infection at 48 to 72 hours. If the problem has resolved, no further therapy is necessary. If the problem is persistent or recurrent, referral for definitive podiatric care is reasonable. Instruct patients to wear less constricting shoes and to trim the nail straight across. Like most FB reactions, removal of the nail spicule resolves the inflammation and infection. Antibiotics given without removal of the nail spicule will not ensure a satisfactory result or add benefit after spicule removal.[25] Topical antibiotics (avoid those containing neomycin) are reasonable, but systemic antibiotics are not required. Diabetics and those with peripheral vascular disease require closer follow-up. When the ingrown toenail is caused by nail deformity, a podiatrist or primary clinician can accomplish definitive removal during follow-up evaluation.

Toenail Removal for Complex/Extensive Ingrown Toenail

When irritation and/or infection are more widespread or include the entire toe, removal of a portion of the nail and débridement of the inflamed tissue may be required (Fig. 51–24). Toenail removal may be total or partial. Total nail removal is rarely needed but may be used when infection of both lateral nailfolds is present, particularly if the condition is present for more than a month. Consider partially removing the toenail when ingrown toenails are associated with chronic inflammation/infection or severe pain. Partial nail removal accomplishes two things: removal of the offending portion of nail and destruction of the underlying nail matrix to prevent nail regrowth. Phenol, the most commonly applied chemical, causes neurolysis of nerve endings and necrosis of the nail matrix in a procedure called *matricectomy*. Several studies demonstrated that 10% sodium hydroxide solution is as effec-

tive as phenol and may be associated with less postprocedure pain and faster recovery.[26–28] Considering that most EDs do not stock phenol or sodium hydroxide solution, nailbed ablation is usually not pursued on the initial visit.

After digital block, exsanguinate the toe by squeezing or wrapping, and apply a tourniquet at the base of the toe. Stabilize the toe in the nondominant hand. Separate the lateral third of the nail from the nailbed by advancing and separating scissors held parallel to the nailbed (Fig. 51–25). Split the nail lengthwise toward the cuticle. An English anvil nail splitter is desirable to begin the procedure, but sharp scissors or a No. 11 blade work. Take care to perform a controlled division along the longitudinal lines of the nail for several millimeters past the proximal nailfold (cuticle). Grasp the end of the cut toenail with a hemostat or forceps. Remove the free piece of nail by twisting it toward the remaining nail. This will pull the nail root out from under the cuticle. Inspect the remnant to be certain that the entire piece of nail has been removed as desired. Sharply remove any remaining or swollen/heaped-up skin and all hyperkeratotic debris. After nail removal, most clinicians apply a silver nitrate stick to the nailbed and to granulation tissue for 2 to 3 minutes.[29] When finished, the nailbed is open and the heaped-up tissue is now flat.

As an option, and if phenol or other ablating solutions are available, the following is suggested to permanently ablate the nailbed so a new nail will not grow. Apply a 10% sodium hydroxide solution to the nailbed with a cotton-tip applicator for 1 to 2 minutes to provide effective ablation of the nail matrix.[26–28] Alternatively, apply a 1% solution of aqueous phenol to the nail matrix beneath the involved area of the lateral nail groove and proximal nailfold using cotton-tip applicators. A 1% phenol solution can be prepared by diluting a 70% to 90% aqueous phenol solution in an 80:1 ratio (e.g., 8 mL distilled water to 0.1 mL phenol). Remove some of the cotton if the applicator is too bulky to concentrate the solution beneath the proximal nailfold and lateral nail groove. Apply thoroughly moistened (but not saturated) applicators, using three 30-second applications. Avoid forcing phenol under the remaining nail by rolling the applicator so that it rolls over the matrix and over the nail surface rather than against the split edge of the nail. Although it is necessary to cover the lateral aspect of the nailbed and lateral nailfold, do not allow excess phenol to contact the exposed nailbed or surrounding healthy tissue. After the third application, the cauterized tissue appears brown-tinged or gray. Alternatively, a 1% phenol solution can be applied for 5 minutes. Thoroughly irrigate the cauterized nailbed with water and rub the area with a gloved finger to remove traces of phenol. Snip away any remaining debris or dead skin with scissors. The technique is illustrated in Figure 51–26.

Dress the wound with antibiotic ointment (not containing neomycin) and a nonadherent dressing, followed by a dry sterile wrap. *Do not forget to remove the tourniquet after the dressing has been applied.* Instruct the patient to wash the wound twice daily followed by dry dressing changes. Systemic antibiotics do not hasten wound healing and are not necessary in most cases.[24,25] Soaking the open wound in warm water twice a day is soothing and allows the patient to view the healing process. The wound will heal in 2 to 4 weeks and may be accompanied by serous drainage for 2 weeks. The patient should be informed of this possibility. Complications include nail regrowth, infection, growth of an inclusion cyst, or delayed healing. If the condition returns, podiatric referral is recommended for more extensive nailbed ablation.

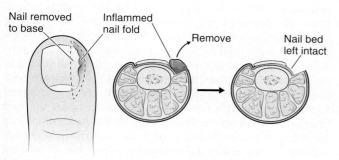

Figure 51–24 A resection of the entire length of a toenail and removal of inflamed tissue is usually a curative intervention for a complex ingrown toenail. The nailbed is left intact.

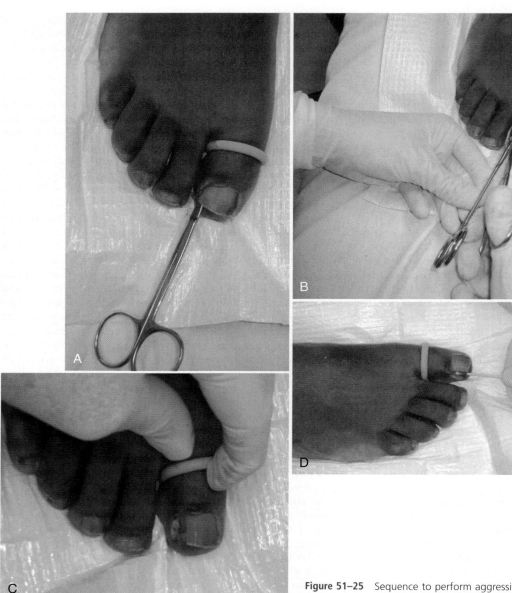

Figure 51–25 Sequence to perform aggressive treatment of a complex ingrown toenail. See text for details (see Fig. 51–26).

Nail Splinting Technique

Splinting of the nail spicule at the lateral edge of the affected nail may allow the toenail to grow out without impacting on the inflamed soft tissue. The technique provides time for the periungual tissue to heal while the nail continues to grow until it can be trimmed straight across. No portion of the nail is removed when the nail is initially splinted. When the degree of inflammation is minimal, elevation of the nail spicule is easily accomplished using forceps or a hemostat. A cotton pledget inserted under the lateral edge to maintain elevation is often sufficient in minor cases. Alternatively, a wound closure strip can be used to elevate the corner of the offending nail.[30] After cleansing the nail edge and providing draining if an abscess is present, insert a wound closure strip obliquely under the corner of the nail using a to-and-fro sawing motion until the corner is sufficiently elevated. Secure the tape closure around the toe (Fig. 51–27). Instruct the patient to soak the

toe in warm water daily, remove the tape closure, and reinsert a new tape strip. This procedure is repeated until the corner of the nail or the nail spicule has grown out and cleared the periungual soft tissue where it can be cut straight across. When the degree of inflammation is moderate, nail splinting is accomplished using the flexible tube procedure.[31,32] Obtain a surgical drain used to perform percutaneous drainage procedures that is 2 to 3 mm in diameter or the small tubing in venipuncture kits. Split a 1-cm piece of the drainage tube lengthwise. Perform a digital block and elevate the lateral edge of the nail with forceps or a hemostat. Insert the split drainage tube along the lateral edge of the nail, completely encircling the nail spicule and pushing it proximately until as much of the lateral nail and nail spicule as possible are covered (Fig. 51–28). Some authors suggest that the tube be secured with 2-0 suture passed through the nail.[31] Securing the tube with wound closure strips is more easily accomplished.[32]

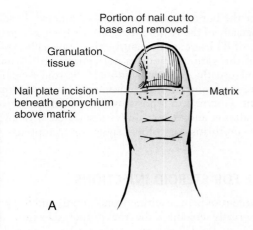

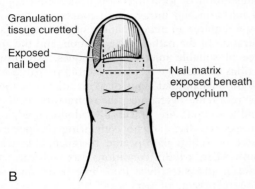

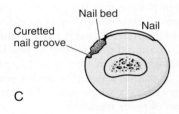

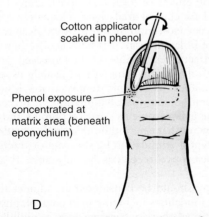

Figure 51–26 **The nail ablation technique for treatment of an ingrown toenail.** The lateral portion of the nail is cut and removed (*A*), exposing the nailbed. Granulation tissue is curetted (*B* and *C*), and the nail matrix is cauterized with hydrogen peroxide or phenol (*D*) (see text).

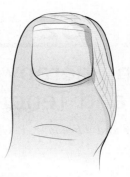

Figure 51–27 A wound closure strip is inserted under the corner of the affected nail using a sawing motion. The remaining ends of the tape strip are secured to the toe.

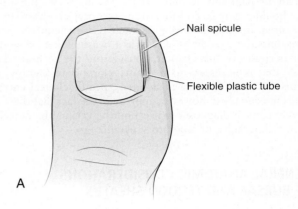

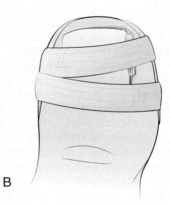

Figure 51–28 *A,* A piece of small tubing split lengthwise is inserted proximally along the lateral nail edge until the nail edge and nail spicule are encircled by the tube. *B,* The tube is secured in place with wound closure strips.

Instruct the patient to wash the affected area daily and replace loosened tape strips when needed. When the inflammation and granulation tissue have subsided, and the nail spicule has grown sufficiently so as not to impinge on the periungual soft tissue, the tube splint is removed by the patient and the nail cut is straight across.

 REFERENCES CAN BE FOUND ON EXPERT CONSULT

CHAPTER 52

Injection Therapy of Bursitis and Tendinitis

Brenda A. Foley and Theodore A. Christopher

944

Bursitis and *tendinitis* are terms frequently used to describe a variety of regional musculoskeletal conditions characterized chiefly by pain and disability at the involved site. Bursitis of the shoulder may be considered the prototypical disorder. All too often, in ill-defined regional soft tissue rheumatic problems, bursitis or tendinitis is used as a "wastebasket" diagnosis. For purposes of this chapter, considering the accurate diagnosis that is necessary to institute appropriate therapy, the terms are reserved for well-defined, specific clinical entities. The clinician must, however, appreciate the fact that these are largely clinical diagnoses that cannot be verified by objective data, radiographs, or laboratory parameters.

GENERAL ANATOMIC CONSIDERATIONS OF BURSAE AND TENDON SHEATHS

Bursae are potential spaces or sacs, subcutaneous or deep, that develop in relation to friction and facilitate the gliding motion of tendons and muscles. There are approximately 78 bursae on each side of the body. These were well described in the classic atlas of anatomy by Monro in 1788[1] and were later elaborated in greater detail in the atlas of Spalteholz.[2]

The normal bursal wall is lined with a thin layer of synovial cells that appear to be similar to those of joint synovial membrane when examined by electron microscopy.[3] When a bursa becomes subacutely or chronically inflamed, the normally thin surface of sparse cells may thicken to 1 to 2 mm. Bursitis may be caused by trauma, infection, crystal deposition, chronic friction from overuse, or a systemic inflammatory arthropathy. In addition, so-called adventitial bursae may form in response to abnormal shearing stress at sites subjected to chronic pressure; an example is a bunion over the head of the metatarsal bone of the great toe.

Involvement of the synovial lining of bursae and tendon sheaths may also result from underlying systemic diseases, including rheumatoid arthritis, ankylosing spondylitis, psoriatic arthropathy, and gout. The most common bursal lesions in these systemic inflammatory arthropathies involve the olecranon at the elbow and the trochanter region of the hip. Smaller bursae, especially those around the Achilles tendon, may also be affected. *Tendinitis* and *tenosynovitis* are useful terms that describe inflammatory reactions in tendons and tendon sheaths. Tendon sheaths are relatively long and tubular, whereas bursae are round and flat. Except for their shape, however, the structures are similar. In fact, because of the adjacent location of bursae and tendons, an inflammatory process in one may also involve the other.[4] Common sites of tendinitis in the body are depicted in Figure 52–1.

In rare cases, the etiologies of tendinitis/bursitis syndromes can be exotic, such as tendinitis caused by quinolone antibiotics or the bursitis noted in dialysis patients.[5] Tendon rupture (especially of the Achilles tendon) has been associated with the use of fluoroquinolone antibiotics (especially ciprofloxacin), but this rare condition is not appreciated by most clinicians and usually goes undiagnosed.[6] Steroid injection may facilitate tendon rupture if fluoroquinolone tendonopathy is present. Gonorrheal tenosynovitis may mimic various forms of tendinitis and is not always associated with overt vaginitis or urethritis or other signs or symptoms of bacteremia.

RATIONALE FOR STEROID INJECTIONS

The management of pain resulting from bursitis and tendinitis may be greatly enhanced by the proper selection and administration of local injections. Successful application of local injection and intrasynovial (bursa and tendon sheath) therapy requires an understanding of the diagnosis, accurate localization of the pathologic condition, and the appropriate choice of suitable injection techniques. Not infrequently, injections of lidocaine or corticosteroid preparations provide the additional aid that alone or as an adjunct to the management program, overcomes the refractory pain. Whereas steroid injections are universally administered, often with great success, there are no convincing prospective data to support or refute the specific therapeutic benefit of this therapy. Many painful conditions wax and wane; there is a significant placebo effect from injections; and there is a natural regression of pain syndromes due to a variety of factors. In fact, the primary goal of corticosteroid injection therapy is the relief of pain so that the patient is able to not only function but, more importantly, also participate in a physical rehabilitation program.[7] In many cases, a single injection may be all that is required to ameliorate a painful condition. However, injection therapy is best viewed as an adjunct in the management of painful tendinitis/bursitis syndromes. It should not be viewed as a single quick fix, but more a method of facilitation of other modalities.

The precise mechanisms of the lasting analgesia and the beneficial therapeutic effects of local injection therapy have not been clarified. Few clinical trials have adequately measured the efficacy of corticosteroid therapy. Although steroids are known to reduce inflammation, it is unclear whether the anti-inflammatory effect is responsible for the increased range of motion and relief of pain that the patient usually experiences. Histologic studies of chronic tenosynovitis lesions demonstrate degeneration, but not inflammation.[7] It is therefore possible that the pain experienced with tendinitis and/or bursitis occurs from mechanisms other than inflammation, such as mechanoreceptor stimulation by shearing or traction or activation of nociceptive receptors by substance P and chondroitin sulfate.[7]

Injection therapy should be considered an adjunct to a variety of treatment modalities including pain control, physical therapy, occupational therapy, relative rest, immobilization, and exercise. Additional pain control can be achieved with such options as nonsteroidal anti-inflammatory drugs (NSAIDs), acupuncture, ultrasound, ice, heat, and electrical nerve stimulation.[7–9] Besides pain relief, the early participation by the patient in rehabilitative activities and exercises can be an important aspect of patient recovery. Patients receiving only analgesics may have poor outcomes compared with those who also have exercise as part of their treatment.[4] Any factors that provoke the initial injury should also be identified,

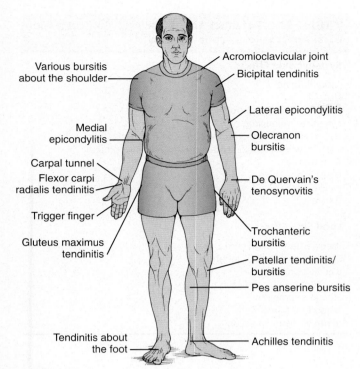

Figure 52–1 Common sites of tendinitis and bursitis. *Do not inject Achilles tendinitis or patellar tendinitis since rupture* of the weight bearing tendons can occur. Note: see Table 52–1. *(From Walker LG, Meals RM: Tendinitis: A practical approach to diagnosis and management. J Musculoskel Med 6:24, 1989. Reproduced with permission.)*

Labels (Figure 52–1): Various bursitis about the shoulder; Medial epicondylitis; Carpal tunnel; Flexor carpi radialis tendinitis; Trigger finger; Gluteus maximus tendinitis; Tendinitis about the foot; Acromioclavicular joint; Bicipital tendinitis; Lateral epicondylitis; Olecranon bursitis; De Quervain's tenosynovitis; Trochanteric bursitis; Patellar tendinitis/bursitis; Pes anserine bursitis; Achilles tendinitis

TABLE 52–1 Information for Healthcare Professionals

Fluoroquinolone Antimicrobial Drugs [ciprofloxacin (marketed as Cipro and generic ciprofloxacin), ciprofloxacin extended release (marketed as Cipro XR and Proquin XR), gemifloxacin (marketed as Factive), levofloxacin (marketed as Levaquin), moxifloxacin (marketed as Avelox), norfloxacin (marketed as Noroxin), and ofloxacin (marketed as Floxin and generic ofloxacin)]

FDA ALERT [7/8/2008].

Fluoroquinolones are associated with an increased risk of tendinitis and tendon rupture. This risk is further increased in those over age 60, in kidney, heart, and lung transplant recipients, and with use of concomitant steroid therapy. Physicians should advise patients, at the first sign of tendon pain, swelling, or inflammation, to stop taking the fluoroquinolone, to avoid exercise and use of the affected area, and to promptly contact their doctor about changing to a non-fluoroquinolone antimicrobial drug.

Selection of a fluoroquinolone for the treatment or prevention of an infection should be limited to those conditions that are proven or strongly suspected to be caused by bacteria.

This information reflects FDA's current analysis of data available to the FDA concerning fluoroquinolone antimicrobials. The FDA intends to update this sheet when additional information or analyses become available.

From MedWatch: The FDA Safety Information and Adverse Reporting Program (www.fda.gov/medwatch/safety/2008).

TABLE 52–2 Contraindications to Local Injection Therapy

Absolute

Infection (bacteremia, infectious arthritis, periarticular cellulitis/ulceration, adjacent osteomyelitis)
Uncontrolled bleeding disorder
Hypersensitivity to corticosteroid or vehicle
Osteochondral fracture

Relative

Anticoagulant therapy
Joint instability
Poorly controlled diabetes (steroids raise blood glucose)
Hemarthrosis
Decubitus ulcers
Joint prosthesis
Adjacent abraded skin
Chronic foci of infection
Internal joint derangement
Partial tendon rupture

because failure to eliminate these provoking factors can contribute to the injury becoming chronic.[7]

Although opinions in the literature differ, we recommend that corticosteroid injections should not be repeated in the same site unless there has been at least a partial clinical response. In addition, an injection should not be repeated in the same site more than once every 3 to 4 months.[7–10] Although there are little data on the outcome of repeated procedures, these recommendations are generally accepted and may limit the risk of adverse effects.

OTHER CAUSES OF TENDINITIS

It is important to realize that some forms of tendinitis may be caused by factors other than overuse, inflammation, trauma, or degenerative etiologies. Gonococcemia, for example, is one cause of tenosynovitis that should be considered. Recently, the FDA added a black box warning to fluoroquinolone antibiotics highlighting tendinopathy and potential tendon rupture (Table 52–1). Local injection therapy is best avoided under such conditions.

INDICATIONS AND CONTRAINDICATIONS

Local injection therapy with corticosteroids or local anesthetics may be effective treatment and provide relief of symptoms in a variety of acute or subacute bursitides and other painful soft tissue conditions. The indications for steroid injection are twofold: therapy and diagnosis. Injection therapy offers not only pain relief, particularly when a local anesthetic is concurrently used, but also a medium to deliver therapeutic agents.

In addition to relieving pain, injection therapy may aid with a diagnosis. When injecting a bursa, for example, bursal fluid is sometimes collected for laboratory analysis. Finally, the relief of pain helps differentiate a localized site of injury from referred or visceral pain.[9]

Absolute contraindications to local injection therapy are limited and include specific infections such as bacteremia, infectious arthritis, periarticular cellulitis or ulceration, or adjacent osteomyelitis (Table 52–2). The procedure is also contraindicated in patients with any bleeding disorders. A history of hypersensitivity, either to the corticosteroid or to the vehicle by which it is delivered, is an absolute contraindication. Finally, corticosteroid injections should not be performed in a patient who has a documented osteochondral fracture. Relative contraindications depend on both the clinician's experience and the indication for the injection. A violation of the integrity of the skin or chronic foci of infection, either locally or in the vicinity of the site of involvement, is a relative contraindication. The procedure is also relatively contraindicated in patients on anticoagulants, with poorly controlled diabetes, and with internal joint derangements or hemarthrosis. The patient with a preexisting tendon injury may be subject to tendon rupture when the corticosteroid injection removes pain and full activity is resumed. Hence, partial tendon rupture is a relative contraindication.

HAZARDS AND COMPLICATIONS

Local anesthetics are often mixed with a corticosteroid preparation to increase volume, decrease postinjection pain, and assess the accuracy of the injection. Corticosteroids used alone can be very painful. Local anesthetics may also be used alone, before injection of the corticosteroid. The major hazards in the use of local anesthetics are hypersensitivity and accidental intravenous or intra-arterial introduction. Serious or fatal hypersensitivity to procaine and other regional anesthetic compounds is encountered very rarely; the possibility is usually suggested by a history of previous reactions. Lidocaine or one of the newer amide derivatives may be used to avoid sensitivity reactions to procaine (or other ester derivatives). Bupivacaine is an excellent choice because of its safety and long duration of action. When a definite history of sensitivity is present, the use of anesthetic agents during injection therapy is absolutely contraindicated.

In the event of accidental intravenous injection of an amide drug or if symptoms of hypersensitivity arise from these compounds, such as a significant slowing of the pulse rate or a seizure, a benzodiazepine or a rapidly acting barbiturate (e.g., sodium pentobarbital) should be given promptly in accordance with the reaction and response. In addition, the patient should be placed on a cardiac monitor, oxygen should be administered, and a patent airway maintained. Severe reactions from accidental vascular injection of these drugs in the doses usually given are very rare.

Although there is evidence of allergic reactions from corticosteroids given orally and parentally, the possibility of an allergic reaction caused by corticosteroid injection is highly unlikely, and such cases are infrequent.[11] Nevertheless, the clinician should be aware that anaphylaxis after injection of methylprednisolone acetate has been reported.[12] In addition, an unusual skin rash after an intra-articular methylprednisolone injection, which appears to be consistent with a delayed type of hypersensitivity, has also been documented.[13]

Minor reactions occasionally seen after injection of amide preparations include light-headedness or dizziness, pallor, weakness, sweating, nausea, and (rarely) fainting and tachycardia. These symptoms usually disappear within a few minutes after the injection and rarely require any treatment except reassurance and a cold compress to the patient's forehead. Often, it is difficult to decide whether the symptoms are the result of sensitivity to the drug or a fright (vasovagal) reaction. *The patient should always be in a supine, prone, or reclining position during the injection to minimize the effect of any vasovagal reaction.*

The obvious ways to prevent entering a blood vessel are an awareness of the local anatomy and aspiration after every

TABLE 52–3 Potential Side Effects of Corticosteroid/Local Anesthetic Injection Therapy

Systemic Side Effects

Facial flushing
Nausea
Impaired diabetic control
Menstrual irregularity
Hypothalamic-pituitary axis suppression
Fall in erythrocyte sedimentation rate/C-reactive protein
Anaphylaxis
Dysphoria
Pancreatitis
Cataracts

Local Side Effects

Postinjection flare of pain
Skin depigmentation, fat atrophy
Bleeding/bruising
Steroid "chalk" calcification
Steroid arthropathy
Tendon rupture/atrophy
Joint/soft tissue infection

1 to 2 mL of solution is injected. Penetration into or striking a nerve may cause sharp pain or paresthesias; the patient should be warned of this possibility in advance.

Corticosteroid injections have been found to be a safe procedure with few complications[14] (Table 52–3). Although the possibility of introducing infection is one of the most serious potential complications, infections occurring as an aftermath of intrasynovial injections are extremely rare. In a study at the Mayo Clinic, no infections were reported for 3000 injections given in 1 year.[13] Others have found the infection risk to be 4.6 per 100,000 intra-articular injections.[15]

Although the problem of infection is usually avoided with meticulous attention to aseptic technique, the patient should be cautioned to report the development of any significant pain, redness, or swelling after any local injection. We do not recommend routine prophylactic antibiotic administration after corticosteroid injection.

Local undesirable reactions are usually minor and reversible. After steroid injection, about 2% of patients may experience an acute synovitis otherwise known as "postinjection" flare.[10,16] This may be more slightly common with methylprednisolone acetate (Depo-Medrol) and less common with triamcinolone acetonide (Kenalog). Characterized by an increase in pain and joint swelling, symptoms usually begin a few hours after steroid injection and can last as long as 3 days. Histologically, steroid crystals within polymorphonuclear leukocytes have been demonstrated, making it a true synovitis.[10,11] This reaction may be difficult to differentiate from an infection, and infection must be ruled out if symptoms last greater than 48 hours or are associated with fever, warmth, or other suspicious signs of infection. The incidence of postinjection flare appears to be more likely with more soluble (shorter-acting) steroid solutions and may be related to the carrier in which the steroid is manufactured.[8,13] Limiting activity of the involved area for 2 days after the injection might help reduce the incidence.[11] When it does occur, the reaction is usually mild and can be adequately controlled with application of ice or cold compresses and analgesics as needed.

Rarely, "afterpain" lasting for a few to several hours after injections may occur. Although the cause is obscure, this phenomenon may result from the trauma of needle insertion, penetration of inflamed tissue, or pressure on adjacent nerves from local swelling or bleeding. Afterpain usually is relieved by application of moist or dry heat and analgesics until the pain abates, but is best prevented by mixing a long-acting anesthetic, such as bupivacaine, with the steroid preparation.

Occasional subcutaneous bleeding at the site of injection may occur with penetration of a venule, an arteriole, or a capillary. The patient should be warned that this may occur and should be reassured that the discoloration or hematoma will disappear spontaneously. Ice packs or cold compresses applied to the involved area for the first 24 hours are commonly advised.

Another relatively minor complication is localized subcutaneous or cutaneous atrophy at the site of the injection.[10] This problem is chiefly of cosmetic concern and is recognized as a small depression in the skin frequently associated with depigmentation, transparency, and occasionally the formation of telangiectasia. These changes in the skin occur when injections are made near the surface and some of the injected steroid leaks back along the needle track. The skin depression usually recedes and the skin returns to normal with time when the crystals of the steroid have been completely absorbed. These changes are usually evident 6 weeks to 3 months after the initial injection, and usually resolve within 6 months, although these changes can be permanent.[8,10] The *two-syringe technique*, in which the anesthetic is first injected, the needle advanced to the bursa/peritendon area, and the syringe then exchanged for another in order to inject steroid, helps prevents this complication by avoiding any leaking of the steroid suspension to the skin surface.[16] A small amount of lidocaine or normal saline can be used to flush the needle of the suspension before removing it. The *Z-tract technique* is a method of creating an indirect route from skin puncture to the ultimate site of steroid injection.[16] Using this method, the needle is introduced at a site 0.5 to 1.0 cm from the actual target site and is redirected when halfway through the fat tissue to the target site of injection. This is followed by injection of both anesthetic and corticosteroid. Injection site atrophy is more likely in preparations that are less soluble and thus longer-acting.[8]

Minor skin depigmentation, especially in dark-skinned individuals, may be encountered, particularly with superficial injections. One cause is leaking of the steroid preparation back through the needle track, limited by applying pressure to the site during needle withdrawal. Hydrocortisone would be the preferable agent for superficial injections to limit depigmentation.

One of the most serious complications after local steroid injection is tendon rupture. In general, the risk is very low (<1%) and appears to be dose related.[8,10] It is believed by some that steroids injected directly into the tendon leads to a decrease in the tendon tensile strength.[10,11,17,18] However, Gray and Gottlieb[10] noted no cases of tendon rupture after more than 300 tendon sheath injections. We still advise being diligent about injection into the surrounding area of the tendon sheath and not into the tendon substance. Also, by using one size needle and syringe, the operator is more likely to appreciate the increase in resistance when injecting the needle directly into the tendon. We also suggest limiting the number of injections to no more than once every 3 to 4 months in the same site.[7–10] *Tendon rupture is especially more likely in major stress-bearing tendons, such as the Achilles tendon and the patellar tendons, in athletes. Injection of corticosteroids in these areas should generally be avoided in the ED.*[12]

There have been reports of accidental nerve injury after corticosteroid injection, particularly of the ulnar nerve (in treating medial epicondylitis) and median nerve (in treating carpal tunnel syndrome).[19] Also, up to 42% of patients undergoing local steroid therapy develop pericapsular calcifications, although these are generally asymptomatic.[10,16] Finally, within minutes to hours of injection, approximately 1% of patients may experience facial and neck flushing. This reaction may last a few days, but it is usually a benign and self-limited reaction. Facial flushing seems to be more common with triamcinolone preparations.[8,10,11]

Systemic absorption of local corticosteroid injections does occur, although at a slower rate than with oral steroids.[9] As a result, patients are at a low risk for systemic complications, but they do occur. Specifically, intrasynovial injections of steroids have been shown to suppress the hypothalamic-pituitary-adrenal axis for 2 to 7 days.[8] This complication is more likely in patients who receive repeated injections in a short period of time or multiple injections in different sites at one time.[11] Corticosteroids can also exacerbate hyperglycemia in diabetes.[9,16] Abnormal uterine bleeding has also been reported.[8,9,12]

Other potential complications of corticosteroid and local anesthetic injections are outlined in Table 52–3.

AVAILABLE PREPARATIONS AND CHOICE OF COMPOUND

Hydrocortisone and a variety of available corticosteroid repository preparations are described in Table 52–4. Local anesthetics, such as lidocaine or bupivacaine, can be mixed with the corticosteroid preparation in the same syringe. All corticosteroid suspensions, with the exception of cortisone and prednisone, can produce a significant and rapid anti-inflammatory effect (in synovial spaces). These preparations are categorized based on their solubility and relative potency. Solutions that are more soluble have a shorter duration of action, primarily because these soluble preparations are absorbed and dispersed more rapidly. The addition of tertiary butyl acetate to the solution causes decreased solubility and, therefore, a longer duration of action. For example, triamcinolone hexacetonide, the least soluble preparation, has the longest duration of action.[10] Because of the long duration of action and its greater potential for subcutaneous atrophy, some authors use this preparation only for intra-articular injections.[9,10]

Attempts have been made to incorporate steroid esters into liposomes to create an even less soluble preparation. This has been shown in both human and animal studies to offer long-lasting relief with minimal drug absorption; however, further research is necessary before this method of delivery is fully developed.[8,10,13]

There is little consensus in the literature regarding which corticosteroid should be used and what dosage is most appropriate for a given site.[7,13,16] Centeno and Moore[20] noted that the choice of injection agent seemed dependent on the institution where the clinician trained. In 1995, a survey of 172 rheumatologists found that opinions differ regarding almost every facet of soft tissue and intra-articular injection, includ-

TABLE 52–4 Injectable Corticosteroids

Intrasynovial Preparations	Potency*	Range of Usual Dosage (mg)	Solubility
Short-Acting			
Hydrocortisone acetate	1	12.5–75	High
Cortisone	0.8	15–25	High
Intermediate-Acting			
Prednisone	3.5	2.5–5	Medium
Prednisolone acetate	4	5–30	NA
Methylprednisolone acetate‡	5	5–40	Medium
Long-Acting†			
Triamcinolone acetonide‡	5	5–40	Low
Triamcinolone diacetate	5	4–40	Low
Triamcinolone hexacetonide	5	4–25	Low
Betamethasone acetate and disodium phosphatate	25	1.5–6	Low
Dexamethasone acetate	25	0.8–6	Low

*Hydrocortisone equivalents (per mg).
†Best used for intra-articular injection.
‡Preferred for emergency department use.

TABLE 52–5 A Guide for Needle Size and Dosage for Injection of Common Regional Disorders

Disorder or Injection Site	Needle Size	Usual Dosage of Methylprednisolone Acetate (mg)*
Bicipital tendinitis	1.5–2 inches, 22–25 gauge	20–40
Calcareous tendinitis / Subacromial bursitis	1.5–2 inches, 22–25 gauge	20–60
Radiohumeral bursitis / Epicondylitis	1.5 inches, 22–25 gauge	20–40
Olecranon bursitis	1–1.5 inches, 20 gauge†	15–30
Ganglia on wrist	1 inch, 22–25 gauge	10–15
de Quervain disease	⅞ inch, 22–25 gauge	10–20
Carpal tunnel syndrome	1–1.5 inches, 22–25 gauge	20–40
Digital flexor tenosynovitis	⅞ inch, 22–25 gauge	5–10
Trochanteric bursitis	1.5–2 inches, 22–25 gauge	20–40
Prepatellar bursitis	1–1.5 inches, 22–25 gauge	15–20
Anserine bursitis	1–1.5 inches, 22–25 gauge	20–40
Bunion bursitis	1 inch, 22–25 gauge	5–10
Calcaneal bursitis	1 inch, 22–25 gauge	10–20

*Empirical dose. Larger or smaller dose may be used depending on clinical scenario.
†Allows for bursa aspiration and steroid injection without removing needle.

ing patient preparation, choice of corticosteroid, and postinjection advice.[21] In general, it is recommended that for an acute or subacute diagnosis such as bursitis/tendinitis, it is prudent to use a short- or intermediate-acting agent, whereas longer-acting agents, such as triamcinolone, should be reserved for chronic and prolonged conditions, including arthritis.[8,10] Some clinicians, however, advocate mixing both shorter- and longer-acting corticosteroids in the same syringe, with little consideration for the location or category of the condition.[9,10] We recommend that longer-acting corticosteroids not be routinely used for soft tissue injections, particularly because of the increased risk of associated atrophy[7,9] including atrophy of surrounding structures, such as ligaments and fascia.[22] Triamcinolone acetonide or methylprednisolone acetate are reasonable first choices for most emergency department (ED) indications.

DOSAGE AND ADMINISTRATION

The dose of any corticosteroid suspension used for intrasynovial injection may be arbitrarily selected. Factors that influence the dosage and expected response include the size of the affected area, the presence or absence of synovial fluid or edema, the severity and extent of any synovitis, and the steroid preparation selected (Table 52–5).

A useful guideline for estimating dosage is as follows: For relatively large spaces such as subacromial, olecranon, and trochanteric bursae, 40 to 60 mg of methylprednisolone acetate or equivalent; for medium- or intermediate-sized bursae and ganglia formation at the wrists, knees, and heels, 10 to 20 mg; and for tendon sheaths, such as flexor tenosynovitis of digits and the abductor tendon of the thumb (deQuervain's disease), 5 to 15 mg. Sometimes, it may be necessary to give larger doses for optimal response. Intrabursal therapy of elbow (olecranon) or knee (prepatellar) bursae containing considerable fluid may require 30- to 40-mg doses.

Unlike intra-articular injections for synovitis in chronic joint disease, repeat infiltrations for soft tissue conditions such as bursitis and tendinitis are generally not recommended or required. However, if only a partial response occurs or if recurrence develops, a single repeat injection can be given as long as one waits at least 12 weeks between injections.[7–10]

PREPARATION OF THE SITE

Preparation of the site before injection requires meticulous adherence to aseptic technique. Anatomic landmarks may be outlined with a black or red skin pencil. Local antisepsis is applied. It is important that the injection site and needle tip remain sterile, using the "no touch" technique, although sterile drapes are not generally considered necessary.[7,16] For operator protection, universal precautions should be followed, including the use of sterile latex examination gloves.[9]

TECHNIQUES

General Considerations

Before beginning the injection, the patient should be informed of the specific indication(s) for treatment. The clinician should describe the details of the procedure, including risks and complications, and obtain informed consent. Subsequently, the details of the procedure should be documented in the medical record. Use of a written consent form is not standard and is best based on institutional and/or departmental policies.

Materials required for local injection procedures include needles, syringes, a hemostat, culture and laboratory supplies, bandages, and sterile gauze. Disposable needles and syringes are convenient and adequate for ED use. Special trays may also be stocked for this purpose. The usual sizes of needles for injection sites and corticosteroid doses are listed in Table 52–5.

Once the point of entry has been determined and the site is prepared, a superficial skin wheal is made with 1% lidocaine (Xylocaine) or 0.25% bupivacaine (Marcaine, Sensorcaine) using a 25-gauge needle. Some physicians do not use a skin wheal when the steroid is mixed with a rapid-acting local anesthetic. Ordinarily, procedural sedation and analgesia are not necessary, but occasionally, in highly nervous or agitated individuals, these may be advisable.

Local injections can be administered with corticosteroids and local anesthetics mixed together in the same syringe. This is commonly done with peritendinous injections utilizing the *Z-tract technique*, which limits the risk of a fistulous tract in the soft tissue. Because the steroid may theoretically precipitate or layer in the barrel of the syringe during the injection, the syringe should be agitated immediately before use to optimize its distribution. In addition to minimizing the pain associated with the injection, mixing the anesthetic with the corticosteroid also produces a larger volume for delivery into the soft tissue.[7]

The local anesthetic can also be given alone, before injection of the corticosteroid. This is commonly seen when injecting bursae using the two-syringe technique. After a wheal is created, a needle is introduced into the bursa and approximately half of the anesthetic is injected as the needle is inserted. Once the needle reaches the target site, the syringes are changed. Then, as much fluid as possible is aspirated before instillation of the corticosteroid suspension to reduce the dilution factor and to collect bursal fluid for laboratory analysis. Upon changing syringes again, the steroid is introduced without anesthetic. Often, syringes are changed once more, and the remaining anesthetic is used to flush out the needle, frequently causing injection and deposition of several milliliters of the local anesthetic. There is no evidence, however, that the injection of the anesthetic before the steroid provides a benefit or that there is a difference in later outcome with the use of short-acting versus long-acting steroids.[7,8]

The duration of action of lidocaine is approximately 100 minutes, whereas bupivacaine may last for a few hours. The patient should be cautioned that the local anesthetic effect may wear off within a couple of hours and that the beneficial effects of the corticosteroid may be delayed.

The accuracy of joint and soft tissue injections has not been related to outcome, and for most indications, the optimum technique is not firmly established. However, one important aspect of a successful technique is accurate positioning of the needle. Injecting an inflamed synovial space, such as a bursa containing fluid, may be as simple as puncturing a balloon. Aspiration of the fluid confirms that the needle has correctly entered the sac. Conversely, direct injection into a painful soft tissue lesion requires additional skill that can be acquired only with experience. Sometimes it is advisable to reaspirate and reinject several times within the barrel of the syringe, a procedure called *barbotage*, to obtain heterogeneous mixing and maximal dispersion of the steroid throughout the synovial cavity. Although it is desirable to inject directly into a bursa, direct injection into the tendon itself is best avoided. If the injection requires significant pressure, the needle may be in the tendon, and it should be withdrawn or advanced a few millimeters. The patient may commonly feel some myofascial radiating pain during the injection, but true paresthesias should not be elicited. "Electric shocks" felt with an injection may signal that the needle is in a nerve.

Whereas an accurate injection is desirable, using a generous volume of anesthetic (3–6 mL) to dilute and hence disperse the steroid can compensate for some less than perfect injections. As a general rule, one should allow the patient to localize the area of maximum tenderness, and the injection should begin in that area. Asking the patient to use one finger to localize the area of maximum pain and tenderness is the best way to ensure the most accurate positioning of the needle. In general, if the patient cannot localize a specific area of tenderness, the diagnosis should be reconsidered or the expectations of success lowered. Diffuse pain, such as throughout the entire shoulder or knee, is probably not tendinitis or bursitis and will not likely be cured with a local injection.

The development of ultrasound-guided therapy has led to improvement in the accuracy of corticosteroid injections. Used for musculoskeletal pathology since the 1970s, ultrasound is now steadily becoming an important tool for both diagnosis and therapy by identifying soft tissue structures such as bursae, tendons, and joint capsules.[23,24] In addition, cartilage, muscles, nerves, and blood vessels can now be easily visualized using this technique.[23] Chapter 67, Ultrasound-Guided Procedures, provides a detailed description of these procedures.

Specific Regions and Clinical Entities

Shoulder Region

Pain associated with disability may result from any of the intrinsic shoulder disorders, including bicipital tendinitis, calcareous tendinitis, and subacromial bursitis (Fig. 52–2). Because injection is easy and safe to do so, these areas are frequently injected, especially in patients who have failed more conservative therapy such as ice, rest, and oral anti-inflammatory medications. A potential long-term complication of an untreated persistent inflammation is the development of a "frozen shoulder" (adhesive capsulitis).

Bicipital Tendinitis (Tenosynovitis). This is a nonspecific low-grade inflammation of the biceps tendon and/or its sheath and is more common in those who repeatedly flex at the elbow against resistance, such as weightlifters and swimmers.[4,25] The tendon courses through the joint and along the bicipital (intertubercular) groove, which can be appreciated as the elbow is held at 90° of flexion, and the arm is internally and externally rotated.[25] Patients may have restricted or normal range of motion and normal strength; however, they usually complain of tenderness to palpation over the bicipital groove.[4] Efforts to elevate the shoulder, reach the hip pocket, or pull a back zipper all aggravate the symptoms. Tenderness over the bicipital groove does not confirm the diagnosis, however, because the supraspinatus tendon is in such close proximity to the bicipital tendon insertion.[25] Other diagnostic clues include the Lipman test, in which "rolling" the bicipital tendon produces localized tenderness; the Yergason test, which elicits pain along the bicipital groove when the patient attempts supination of the forearm against resistance, holding

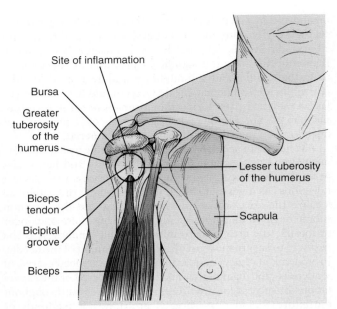

Site of inflammation

Bursa

Greater
tuberosity
of the
humerus

Lesser tuberosity
of the humerus

Biceps
tendon

Scapula

Bicipital
groove

Biceps

Figure 52–2 Pain in the shoulder may be caused by biceps tendinitis or subacromial bursitis, but this is difficult to clinically differentiate from other shoulder conditions. Sudden pain and a distinct soft tissue bulge in this area indicate rupture of the long head of the biceps. Surgical repair is usually not required. *(From Walker LG, Meals RM: Tendinitis: A practical approach to diagnosis and management. J Musculoskel Med 6:24, 1989. Reproduced with permission.)*

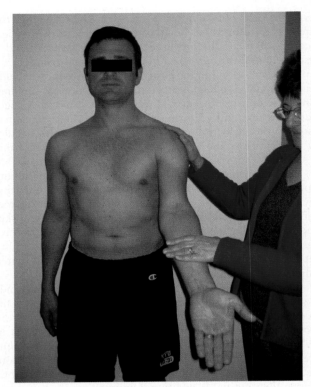

Figure 52–4 **Speed's test.** While the elbow is maintained in extension and the forearm in supination, forward flexion of the shoulder is performed against resistance. Patients with bicipital tendinitis may have pain or tenderness in the bicipital groove with this maneuver.

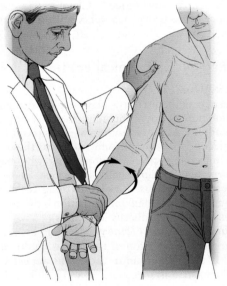

Figure 52–3 The Yergason test helps determine the stability of the long head of the biceps tendon in the bicipital groove. This test, which involves resisted supination of the forearm with the elbow flexed to 90°, may accurately reproduce symptoms of bicipital tendinitis. *(From Walker LG, Meals RM: Tendinitis: A practical approach to diagnosis and management. J Musculoskel Med 6:24, 1989. Reproduced with permission.)*

the elbow flexed at a 90° angle against the side of the body (Fig. 52–3); and Speed's test (Fig. 52–4), in which pain is reproduced on resisted forward elevation of the humerus against an extended elbow. Radiographs are normal and are not required if the clinical diagnosis is supported.

Approach. The point of maximal tenderness of the bicipital tendon is located. Entry is made with a 22- or 25-

gauge, 3.9- to 5.0-cm needle through a lidocaine skin wheal (Fig. 52–5). It is wise to *avoid an actual intratendinous injection*, which may cause weakening of the tendon and predispose the patient to tendon rupture. The needle is brought in along the side of the tendon at a 30° angle, aimed at one border of the bicipital groove to give a *peritendinous infiltration*. One third of the injection is administered at this point. The needle is then withdrawn slightly but is kept subcutaneous. It is redirected upward approximately 2.5 cm for another third of the injection, withdrawn again, and redirected downward, touching the bicipital border gently; the remainder of the drug is deposited at this point. With any of these injections, resistance to the injection suggests intratendinous needle placement, which should be avoided.[26] If the two-syringe technique is used, 1 to 1.5 mL of an intermediate-acting corticosteroid suspension, such as prednisolone tebutate, is usually instilled at the maximum area of tenderness. The anesthetic (2–4 mL of 1% lidocaine or 0.25% bupivicaine) is injected along the upper and lower borders of the tendon.

Calcareous Tendinitis, Supraspinatus Tendinitis, and Subacromial Bursitis. These inflammations are so clinically similar that their symptoms and signs are difficult to differentiate. The musculotendinous rotator cuff is composed of the supraspinatus, infraspinatus, teres minor, and subscapularis muscles, which insert as the conjoined tendon into the greater tuberosity of the humerus. The subacromial bursa lies just superior and lateral to the supraspinatus tendon (Fig. 52–6). Both the tendon and the bursa are located in the space between the acromion process and the head of the humerus and are particularly prone to impingement in this "critical zone." This can occur when the shoulder moves

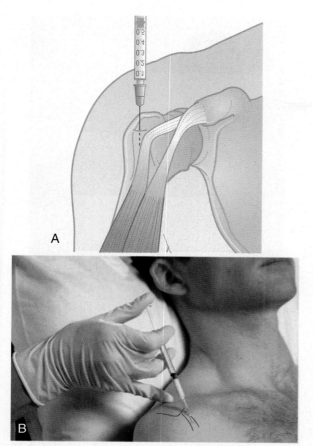

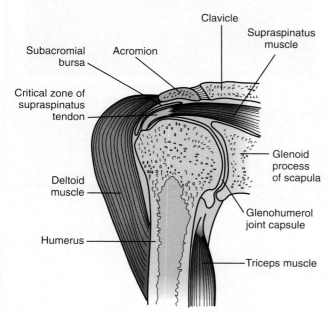

Figure 52–5 *A* and *B*, Anatomic site for injection into the bicipital groove for treating bicipital tendinitis. The anesthetic is infiltrated around the biceps tendon sheath in a fan-wise distribution, avoiding intratendinous injection. (Use 10–20 mg equivalent of Kenalog 40 [triamcinolone acetonide].)

Figure 52–6 **The "critical zone."** Note the close relationship of the supraspinatus tendon and subacromial bursa to the humeral head and acromion, making an exact clinical diagnosis very difficult.

forward, compressing the cuff and bursa under the anterior third of the coracoacromial arch. Injections into either the bursa or the tendon sheath area are commonly performed secondary to inflammation and overuse.

In *calcareous* (or calcific) tendinitis of the shoulder, a calcific deposit (hydroxyapatite) is within the substance of one or more of the rotator cuff tendons (commonly the supraspinatus).[27] These calcium crystals can occasionally rupture into the adjacent subacromial bursa, causing acute pain and tenderness in the deltoid area (Fig. 52–7*A*). The bursae in relation to the greater tuberosity and the subdeltoid (subacromial) bursa are the most common sites of calcific deposits.

During the acute or hyperacute stage, the patient holds the arm in a protective fashion against the chest wall. Pain may be incapacitating, and all ranges of motion are disturbed, with internal rotation markedly limited. Tenderness is often diffuse over the perihumeral region. The patient may also complain of pain at night when lying on the affected side and with abduction of the arm. Supraspinatus tendon impingement is most apparent with the humerus abducted and internally rotated. The Hawkins test (Fig. 52–8*A*) elicits pain with forcible internal rotation while the patient's arm is passively flexed forward at 90°, and Neer's test (see Fig. 52–8*B*) elicits pain with full forward flexion between 70° and 120° degrees. Both tests are fairly sensitive, but not specific for supraspinatus tendon impingement.[28] Constitutional symptoms are rare, but sometimes in the hyperacute form, actual swelling may be visible, and even fever and an accelerated sedimentation rate may develop. When shoulder radiographs demonstrate a calcific deposit, the shadow appears "hazy" with lightening of the periphery caused by the pressure of inflammatory edema (see Fig. 52–7*B*). Night pain may be intolerable, requiring opioids for control.

Anterior Approach. In calcific tendinitis or supraspinatus tendinitis without calcification, the injection may be given by the anterior (subcoracoid) approach. The patient is asked to rest the extremity on the lap, and the arm is rotated externally about 15°. The point of insertion is over the depression that is palpable inferior and lateral to the coracoid process and medial to the head of the humerus (Fig. 52–9).

Posterolateral Approach. With the patient sitting and the lower part of the extremity resting on the lap, a lidocaine skin wheal is made at the depression about 1 cm inferior to the posterolateral tip of the acromion, located between the head of the humerus and the acromion. A 3.9- to 5.0-cm, 22- or 25-gauge needle is then directed toward the center of the head of the humerus and upward at an angle of approximately 10°. Because the bursa does not extend posteriorly beyond the midportion of the acromion, it is important that the needle be positioned sufficiently anterior and inferior to the acromion[29] (Fig. 52–10). After the site has been penetrated 2 to 3 cm, aspiration is carried out for any fluid or calcific material. The syringe is then removed, leaving the needle in position. Another syringe containing 20 to 40 mg of methylprednisolone suspension or equivalent intermediate-acting steroid is attached, and the medication is instilled. Little resistance should be encountered when injecting the medication. If resistance is appreciated, then the needle should be repositioned, because it may be in the tendon substance of the rotator cuff. This injection can be followed with 4 to 6 mL of 1% lidocaine (or a similar volume of 0.25% bupivacaine). Alternatively, local anesthetic can be given combined with the steroid in the same syringe. One should be generous with the volume of local anesthetic to ensure adequate dispersion of

Labels in Figure 52–6: Clavicle; Supraspinatus muscle; Subacromial bursa; Acromion; Critical zone of supraspinatus tendon; Glenoid process of scapula; Deltoid muscle; Glenohumeral joint capsule; Humerus; Triceps muscle

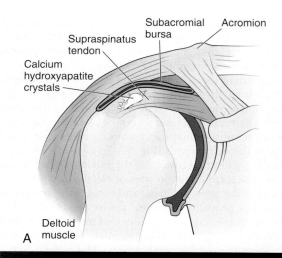

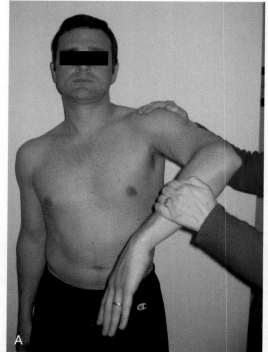

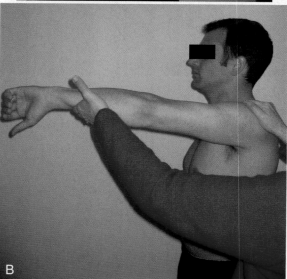

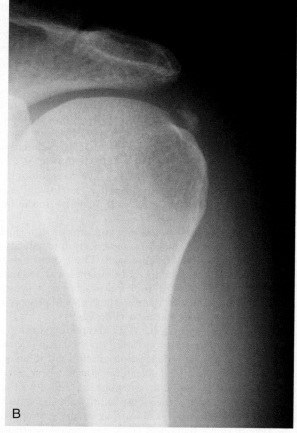

Figure 52–7 *A,* In a calcareous tendinitis of the shoulder, calcium hydroxyapatite crystals deposit in the tendons of the rotator cuff and occasionally rupture into the adjacent bursa. *B,* Abnormal calcific deposits in calcareous tendinitis of the shoulder are usually demonstrated roentgenographically in the suprahumeral region or adjacent to the greater tuberosity. When bursal calcifications appear dense (as in this x-ray film), they are frequently asymptomatic, whereas lightening at the margins of the calcium deposit is compatible with the presence of inflammatory edema in the rotator cuff, which produces pain and tenderness in the shoulder region. The location of the calcific deposit in the radiograph may be a useful guide for the point of entry of aspiration and injection. The needle is directed to the calcareous deposit, aspiration is carried out, and a portion of the steroid medication is deposited there. The calcium may subsequently disappear. Not infrequently, it does so spontaneously.

Figure 52–8 *A,* Hawkin's test. With the patient's arm and elbow flexed to 90°, the examiner rotates the forearm internally (i.e., thumb pointed down, so that the palm of the hand is directed as far posteriorly as possible). Pain is reproduced if there is impingement of the coracoacromian ligament. *B,* Neer's test. With one hand placed on the patient's scapula, the forearm is slowly forward flexed. The arm should be internally rotated such that the thumb is pointing downward. This test causes pain as the greater tuberosity of the humerus impinges on the acromion. Pain may be reproduced between 70° and 120° of forward flexion.

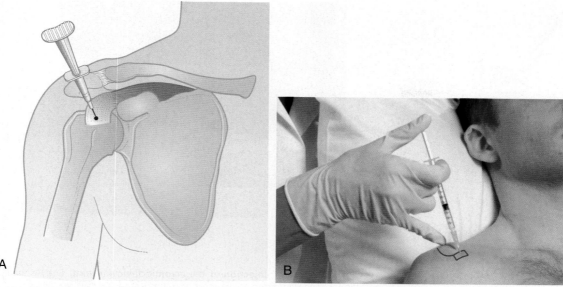

Figure 52–9 Anterior approach to the subacromial bursa or supraspinatus tendon. The needle is inserted into the depression located inferolateral to the coracoid process and medial to the humeral head. Subacromial bursitis pain is quite common and responds well to injection. Recurrent pain can be due to a rotator cuff tear, requiring magnetic resonance imaging (MRI) evaluation. Pain is felt in the deltoid area and can radiate down the arm. The bursa lies mainly under the acromion but is variable. Supraspinatus tendinopathy often occurs with subacromial bursitis.

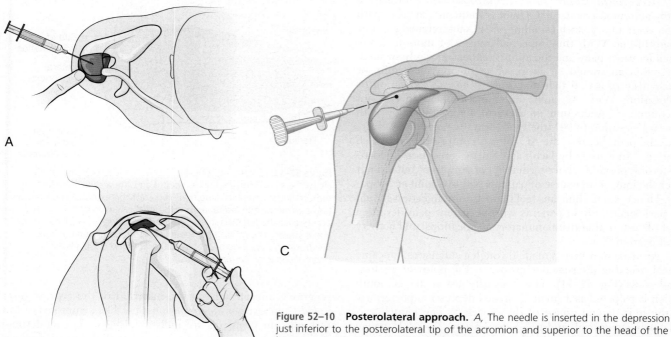

Figure 52–10 Posterolateral approach. *A,* The needle is inserted in the depression just inferior to the posterolateral tip of the acromion and superior to the head of the humerus. *B,* Injection using the posterolateral approach. The angle of entry should be approximately 10°. *C,* Lateral approach.

the steroid. A single treatment relieves the majority of acute disorders. An injection into the peritendinous space is similar to that described previously, except that the needle is advanced deeper than with a subacromial bursal injection.[30]

If calcific tendinitis is suspected, some recommend attempting to aspirate the calcium deposits. After the bursa has been anesthetized, an 18-gauge needle can be used to penetrate the calcium, often creating a "gritty" sensation.[25] In addition, the clinician may consider the technique of barbotage in order to facilitate the cleavage of calcium deposits, as well as the more diffuse dissemination of the injection.

Using this method as previously described, the steroid or anesthetic/steroid combination is aspirated and reinjected repeatedly.[27]

Sometimes, a painful reaction may follow when the analgesic has worn off. To avoid severe pain, the patient should be warned about this possibility and given appropriate analgesia. A sling may provide additional relief, and short-term use of opioids is appropriate. Whereas some authors claim that patients who do not also undergo physical therapy after corticosteroid injection have satisfactory results, some evidence supports the importance of close patient follow-up,

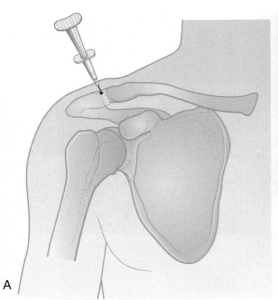

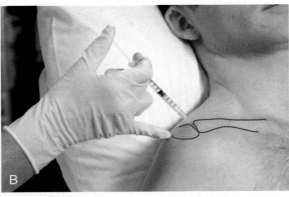

A

B

Figure 52–11   Injection of the acromioclavicular joint. Entry is made at the V-shaped depression at the most lateral aspect of the clavicle.

range of motion exercises, and physical therapy to total recovery.[25]

Acromioclavicular Joint Inflammation. Pain arising in the acromioclavicular (AC) joint is frequently an aftermath of an acute injury, such as falling on an outstretched hand or weightlifting. With this injury, all ranges of motion of the shoulder cause pain, and the joint is tender but rarely swollen. The clinician should be aware of an obvious deformity or mechanism of action that may suggest an AC separation or dislocation. With AC joint inflammation, crepitus is not uncommon.[25] Adduction of the arm across the body with forward elevation to 90° (the cross-arm test) may also exacerbate the pain, because the AC joint is compressed with such motion.[25] In a study by Jacob and Sallay,[31] injection of corticosteroids provided short-term relief of symptoms but did not alter the long-term course of patients with AC joint arthropathy. Hence, some clinicians feel that AC joint injection should be performed only in patients with persistent pain despite a trial of rest, oral anti-inflammatory medications, and activity modification.[26]

Approach. Entry is made through a cutaneous lidocaine wheal over the interosseous groove at the point of greatest tenderness (Fig. 52–11). This is usually just at the AC joint, which is palpated as a small V-shaped depression posteriorly at the most lateral aspect of the clavicle.[25] The joint line is relatively superficial, and a 2.2- to 2.5-cm, 22- or 25-gauge needle is usually advanced only approximately 5 mm. One to 2 mL of lidocaine and 5 to 10 mg of a prednisolone suspension are injected. It is not necessary to advance the needle beyond the proximal margin of the joint surface.

Elbow Region

The elbow is subject to frequently occurring characteristic extra-articular disorders. These include radiohumeral bursitis, lateral and medial epicondylitis ("tennis elbow" and "golfer's elbow"), and olecranon bursitis ("barfly's elbow").

Radiohumeral Bursitis, Lateral Epicondylitis and Medial Epicondylitis. Radiohumeral bursitis occurs at the juncture of the radial head and the lateral epicondyle of the elbow. This condition is commonly found in combination with lateral epicondylitis, which is thought to result from

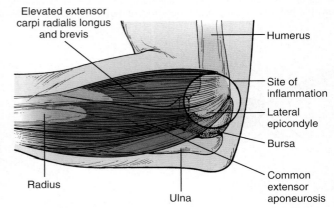

Figure 52–12   Lateral epicondylitis—commonly known as "tennis elbow"—is common and quite painful and the result of microscopic rupture and incomplete tendinous repair of the extensor carpi radialis brevis origin on the lateral epicondyle of the humerus. Pain usually occurs over the lateral humeral epicondyle during work or recreation. *(From Walker LG, Meals RM: Tendinitis. A practical approach to diagnosis and management. J Musculoskel Med 6:24, 1989. Reproduced with permission.)*

repetitive microtrauma at the insertion of the *extensor carpi radialis* and *extensor digitorum* muscles. The symptoms of the two adjacent problems are indistinguishable, but tenderness in bursitis overlies the site of the radiohumeral groove, whereas tenderness in tennis elbow occurs chiefly at the lateral epicondyle (Fig. 52–12). Although the term *epicondylitis* suggests an inflammatory cause of pain, some evidence suggests that the injury in lateral epicondylitis results from a degenerative process causing a "tendinosis."[32] Regardless of the exact pathophysiology, there is often a history of repetitive motions of the wrist (flexion, extension, supination and/or pronation) such as while golfing, gardening, or using tools.[4] A clinical sign supporting the diagnosis of tennis elbow is the provocation of pain when the patient attempts extension of the middle finger against resistance, with the wrist and the elbow held in extension. Alternatively, pain is reproduced at the elbow when the patient is asked to extend the wrist against resistance (Fig. 52–13).

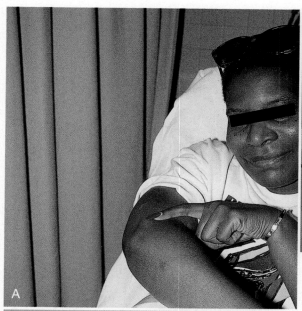

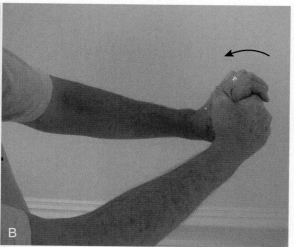

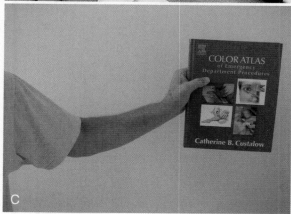

Figure 52–13 Clinical tests for lateral epicondylitis. *A,* Patients often localize the pain with one finger. *B* and *C,* Because this is an extensor tendinitis, extending the wrist against resistance or taking a book off a shelf elicits pain with lateral epicondylitis.

Medial epicondylitis (golfer's elbow) is a similar condition, although it occurs on the opposite side as that of lateral epicondylitis and is much less common[4] (Fig. 52–14*A*). This condition involves the origin of the *pronator teres* and *flexor carpi radialis* muscles. On physical examination, the patient will usually complain of pain when the wrist is *flexed* against resistance or when the forearm is pronated. Palpation of the medial epicondyle also elicits tenderness.

Some evidence supports the short-term efficacy of corticosteroid injection for these conditions.[33–35] In 1999, Hay and coworkers[34] compared local corticosteroid injection, oral NSAIDs, and other analgesics in 164 patients with lateral epicondylitis. In 4 weeks, the injection group had the highest treatment success (defined as "better") rate (82%), versus the NSAIDs (48%) and other analgesics group (50%). It should be noted, however, that after 1 year, the result was similar for all three groups (84% vs. 85% vs. 82%). Similarly, Stahl and Kaufman[36] studied 58 patients with medial epicondylitis who were first injected with methylprednisolone and then treated with both physical therapy and NSAIDs. In 6 weeks, it was noted that the patients who received steroid injections reported significantly less pain than the placebo group. However, at 3 months and 1 year after the initial injection therapy, the two groups did not differ with regard to pain.

Approach. With the forearm pronated and elbow flexed at 90°, the radial head can be palpated as a bony protrusion just distal to the epicondyle and confirmed by rotation of the patient's forearm. The entry site is the point of maximal tenderness, usually found at a point slightly distal to the lateral epicondyle (see Fig. 52–14*B*). The injection is made through a skin wheal with a 3.9-cm, 22-gauge needle, depositing 20 to 30 mg of methylprednisolone or equivalent intermediate-acting steroid mixed with anesthetic. Alternatively, the steroid is followed with 1 to 3 mL of local anesthetic. The injection should be infiltrated in a fanlike distribution, avoiding direct tendon injection. For radiohumeral bursitis, part of the repository preparation may be instilled into the radiohumeral bursa and part at the lateral epicondyle (see Fig. 52–12). In medial epicondylitis (golfer's elbow), a similar technique can be used, but it is important to remember to avoid the ulnar nerve, which lies in the ulnar groove behind the medial epicondyle. Damage to this nerve during steroid injection has been reported.[19] Subcutaneous injection should also be avoided because it can result in skin depigmentation and/or atrophy.[37]

Olecranon Bursitis (Aseptic). Olecranon bursitis is an inflammation of the olecranon bursa of the elbow, located between the skin and the olecranon process (Fig. 52–15). The

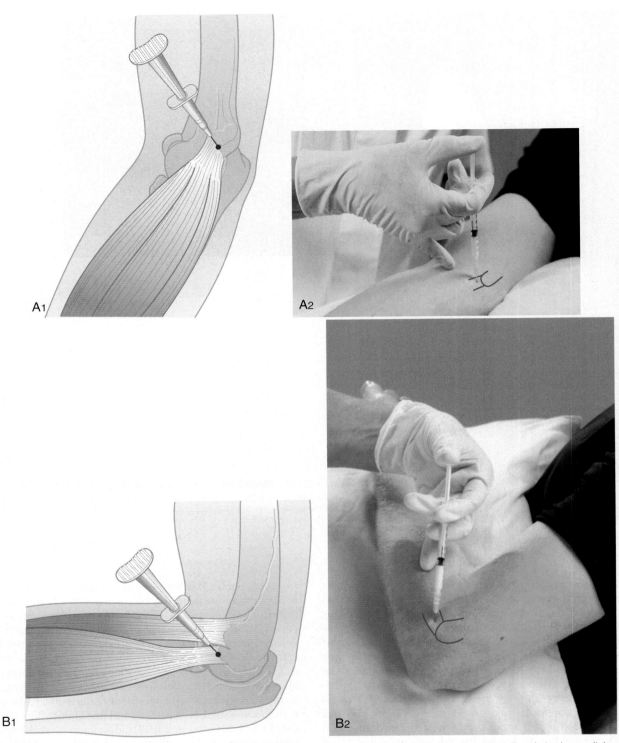

Figure 52–14 *A,* Golfer's elbow is flexor tendinitis with pain in the medial elbow, elicited by flexing the wrist. Inject directly in the medial epicondyle. *B,* Injection at the lateral epicondyle for treatment of tennis elbow is usually curative. The needle is inserted in the area of maximal tenderness, avoiding injection directly into the tendon.

most common cause of olecranon bursitis is trauma,[38] which is usually minor or results from activities that involve chronic leaning or repetitive elbow motions. As a result, olecranon bursitis is also known as "barfly elbow" or "student's elbow," so named because of prolonged leaning on the elbow leading to bursitis. Other patients at risk for olecranon bursitis include gardeners, auto mechanics, carpet layers, gymnasts, and wrestlers.[39] More significant trauma, such a direct blow to the

elbow, can also cause olecranon bursitis. In this case, hemorrhage into the bursa results in acute hemorrhagic bursitis. Other causes of olecranon bursitis include hemodialysis[40] and systemic diseases such as rheumatoid arthritis, lupus, uremia, and gout.[41]

The olecranon bursa is located superficially and, as such, is susceptible to injury. Although most cases of olecranon bursitis are sterile, the olecranon bursa is the most frequent

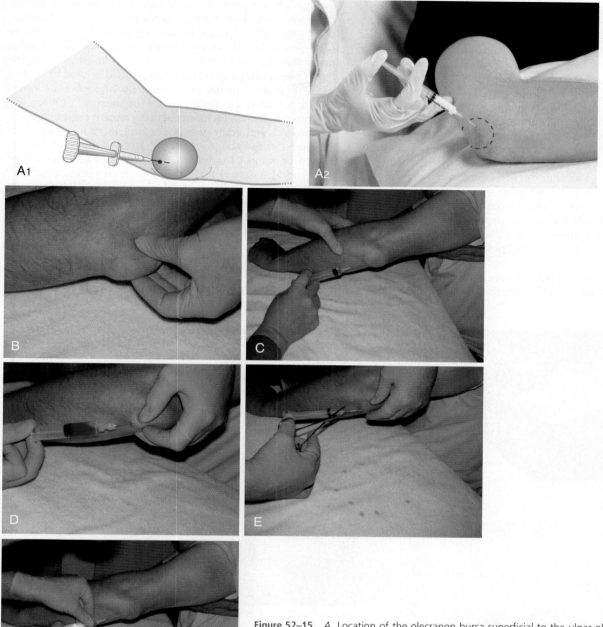

Figure 52–15 *A,* Location of the olecranon bursa superficial to the ulnar olecranon. *B,* Painless swelling over the posterior elbow is characteristic of nonseptic olecranon bursitis. The mass is soft, movable, and fluctuant. *C,* Using sterile preparation, a 20-gauge needle on a 10-mL syringe is advanced parallel to the forearm. *D,* The bursal fluid is completely aspirated. Note compression of the bursa during aspiration. Typically, slightly blood-tinged serous fluid is obtained. *E,* The aspirating syringe is changed while the needle remains in the bursal sac. *F,* A long-acting steroid preparation (such as 40 mg of methylprednisolone) is injected. An elastic bandage provides compression for 12 hr.

site of septic bursitis.[42] Therefore, it is important to accurately differentiate between the two entities. Steroid injections are absolutely contraindicated in cases of confirmed or suspected septic bursitis. Often, the diagnosis will be suggested by the history and physical examination, but it may be necessary to aspirate and analyze the fluid if septic bursitis is suspected.

In aseptic olecranon bursitis, radiographs are usually normal, but may demonstrate soft tissue swelling. Bony spurs or amorphous calcific deposits may also be seen, especially in older patients.[38] Occasionally in rheumatoid arthritis and gout, nodules or tophi may be palpated within the bursal sac.

The bursa and surrounding structures are typically nontender, and there is full and painless range of motion of the involved elbow. Signs of infection such as warmth and erythema of the overlying skin are also usually absent. It should be noted, however, that pain, warmth, tenderness, and erythema might be present in both septic and aseptic olecranon bursitis. If there is any suspicion of septic olecranon bursitis, aspiration should be performed, and corticosteroid injection deferred until an infectious etiology has been ruled out.[38]

Aseptic olecranon bursitis may be cosmetically bothersome to the patient, but usually does not cause discomfort and may resolve spontaneously. In cases of bursal swelling that is nontender and not tense, treatment is symptomatic and includes NSAIDs, compression, and avoidance of further injury.[38] In cases of acute hemorrhagic bursitis, aspiration of the bursa followed by compressive dressing and icing will decrease the incidence of chronic bursitis.[38] When the bursa is large, tense, and inflamed, provided that infection is excluded, aspiration and steroid injection have been shown to hasten the resolution of symptoms.[43] Smith and colleagues[44] demonstrated the superiority of intrabursal methylprednisolone acetate over oral naproxen or placebo at 6 months, noting faster resolution and less reaccumulation of fluid with the steroid injection. The addition of a course of an oral NSAID after steroid injection did not affect the outcome.[44] Following steroid injection, application of a compression dressing and a brief period of relative immobilization may be helpful.[38] Repetitive steroid injections for aseptic olecranon bursitis have been associated with triceps rupture and should be avoided.[45]

Septic Bursitis. Septic bursitis is most common in the olecranon, prepatellar, and superficial infrapatellar bursae owing to their superficial location and vulnerability to injury.[46] Infection of the other bursae is much less common. The infection is most likely caused by direct percutaneous inoculation of common skin organisms into the bursae caused by trauma or contiguous spread from an overlying cellulitis.[38,46,47] Septic bursitis secondary to hematogenous spread is rare.[38,46,47] Most cases of septic bursitis are caused by *Staphylococcus aureus* (80%) followed by streptococcal organisms.[48] Other less common organisms include coagulase-negative staphylococci, enterococci, and gram-negative organisms such as *Escherichia coli* and *Pseudomonas aeruginosa*.[46] Isolated cases of bursitis caused by fungi (*Aspergillus terreus*, *Candida lusitaniae*), *Brucella*, and *Mycobacterium tuberculosis* have also been reported.[38] Such unusual organisms should be considered in cases of septic bursitis that are subacute or chronic and those discovered in an immunocompromised host.[38]

The most common cause of olecranon septic bursitis is trauma (Fig. 52–16). It has been estimated that as many as 70% of cases of septic bursitis are related to trauma, either chronic, caused by repetitive injury, or acute, often associated with occupational or recreational activities.[46] Other risk

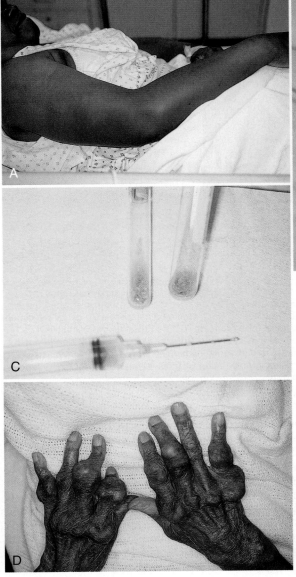

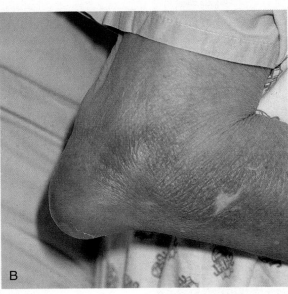

Figure 52–16 *A,* Fully developed septic bursitis is usually distinguished from nonseptic bursitis by clinical parameters. In the septic variety, there is diffuse swelling (as opposed to a discrete mass), and the area is red, warm, and quite tender. In addition, bursal fluid leukocytosis is present. *B,* Acute gout can cause painful olecranon bursitis resembling septic bursitis. *C,* Aspiration can yield urate paste. *D,* Tophi in a patient with advanced gout.

factors for developing septic bursitis include chronic illnesses (e.g., diabetes mellitus, alcoholism) and prior inflammation of the bursa, as occurs in gout, rheumatoid arthritis, or uremia.[46] Infection may follow an injection of corticosteroids into the bursae in up to 10% of cases.[49]

At times, the diagnosis of septic bursitis can be challenging. Acute gouty olecranon bursitis may present with a very similar clinical picture, and often can be accurately differentiated from septic arthritis only by fluid analysis. Other conditions that may mimic bacterial septic olecranon bursitis include acute rheumatoid bursitis, aseptic bursitis secondary to oxalosis induced by dialysis, or infectious bursitis caused by unusual organisms such as *Mycobacterium*, *Serratia marcescens*, or fungal organisms. About one third of all cases of olecranon bursitis are septic.[38]

In some cases, the diagnosis of septic bursitis is obvious. The onset of pain and swelling may be quite rapid (over 8–24 hr) compared with the more gradual onset of aseptic bursitis. The bursa is erythematous, tense, swollen, warm, and very painful (see Fig. 52–16). Flexion of the elbow is limited by pain; however, some joint mobility may be present because the bursa usually does not extend into the joint.[46] The patient may report a history of trauma to the area, which may be evident on physical examination. Some patients will also have a fever. Smith and associates' study[50] found that the infected bursa was generally 2.2°C or greater warmer than the unaffected elbow.

Aspirating infected bursal fluid and culturing bacteria from the aspirate confirm the diagnosis of septic bursitis. Fluid is usually easily obtained from the tense bursa and (in the case of established infection) may be cloudy or grossly purulent. The white blood cell count of the fluid in septic bursitis is usually 5000 to 100,000 cells/mm[3] or greater, and polymorphonuclear cells usually exceed 90%. Neither fever nor systemic leukocytosis is considered sensitive or specific for the disease. However, in immunocompromised patients (e.g., those with diabetes mellitus, alcoholism), the white blood cell count in the bursal fluid tends to be higher.[51] Because of some overlap in the leukocyte count of bursal fluid in septic versus nonseptic bursitis, it is important to remember that a low bursal white blood cell count does not exclude a septic etiology. Moreover, the sensitivity of the Gram stain may be 50% or less.[52] In a large study of 200 patients with septic olecranon bursitis, cell count and Gram stain were not always helpful in the acute evaluation and treatment of new cases of septic bursitis.[53] Therefore, if there is high clinical suspicion for septic olecranon bursitis, even in the presence of a normal or equivocal fluid cell count and/or Gram stain, *steroid injection should be delayed* and empirical antibiotic therapy started until culture results are available.[38]

Treatment of septic bursitis includes the use of antibiotics directed against penicillinase-producing *Staphylococcus*, splinting, warm soaks, and drainage of the bursa. Drainage may be adequately performed with needle aspiration performed daily until the fluid is sterile.[47] However, open incision and drainage might be required, particularly if the infection is recurrent or refractory.[54] In addition to daily drainage of the bursa as necessary, antibiotics are administered for at least 2 weeks.[47] Additional antibiotic coverage against methicillin-resistant *S. aureus* (MRSA) should be considered based on the patient's risk factors and epidemiology.[46] Outpatient therapy with oral antibiotics is generally acceptable, although this approach has been challenged for immunocompromised patients.[51] This decision is generally guided by the clinical appearance of the bursa as well as associated comorbidities, compliance, and other factors regarding patient care. Response to antibiotic therapy might be slow. Thus, it is important to initiate antimicrobial treatment once clinical suspicion for septic bursitis exists. Additional treatment with oral NSAIDs also may be effective. Standard gout medications will generally resolve acute gouty bursitis.

Approach. A 2.5- to 3.9-cm, 20-gauge needle is introduced at a dependent aspect of the bursal sac through a lidocaine skin wheal or the skin may remain unanesthetized (see Fig. 52–15B–F). To minimize the risk of persistent drainage after aspiration and contamination of the overlying skin, skin penetration should occur 2 to 3 cm from the bursa.[38,39] If infected or inspissated fluid is anticipated, a 16- to 18-gauge needle may be necessary for aspiration of the viscous contents. After as much fluid as possible is aspirated, 15 to 30 mg of methyprednisolone or an equivalent intermediate-acting preparation is injected. In aseptic bursitis, the aspirated fluid may be yellow and clear, but often, it is mildly serosanguineous in appearance. There are no compelling reasons to routinely send aspirated fluid for laboratory analysis or culture. The leukocyte count of aspirated fluid of aseptic bursitis should be less than 1000/mm[3]. Counts of about 2000 to 10,000/mm[3] are associated with a higher incidence of infection or acute gout. The elbow is wrapped with an elastic compression bandage for 5 to 7 days after aspiration and injection. *Again, if septic olecranon bursitis is suspected, corticosteroid injections should not be performed.*

Wrist and Hand Region

Ganglion Cysts of Wrist or Hand. These are cystic swellings occurring frequently on the hands, especially on the dorsal aspect of the wrist. Ganglion cysts are common and make up approximately 60% of all soft tissue tumors affecting the wrist and hand. They usually develop spontaneously in adults between 20 and 50 years old, with a female-to-male ratio of 3:1. Ganglion cysts may also be seen on the foot and ankle, generally on the extensor surface.

The etiology of ganglia remains obscure; there is usually no history of trauma.[55] The word *ganglion* is derived from the Greek word meaning "cystic tumor." The mesothelium- or synovium-lined cystic structures are attached to or may arise from tendon sheaths or near the joint capsule and do not extend into the joint itself.[56] Attachment is often by a pedicle. The wall of the ganglia is smooth, fibrous, and of variable thickness. The cyst is filled with a clear, gelatinous, sticky, or mucoid fluid of great density. The viscous fluid in the cyst may sometimes represent almost pure hyaluronic acid.

The types of ganglia vary with their location. The most common ganglion is the dorsal wrist variety, which arises from the scapholunate joint and constitutes approximately 65% of ganglia. The volar wrist ganglion, which arises over the distal aspect of the radius, constitutes another approximately 20% to 25% of ganglia. Dorsal ganglion cysts also occur relatively frequently (Fig. 52–17). Flexor tendon sheath ganglia make up the remaining 10% to 15% found on the hand and wrist.

Most ganglia are of no great clinical significance and most do not require treatment. Spontaneous regression is common. However, if the appearance of the cyst is disturbing to the patient or if the ganglion is painful or tender (from soft tissue or nerve compression or bone erosion), then simple aspiration with or without injection of a corticosteroid suspension is usually an effective approach. Up to three aspira-

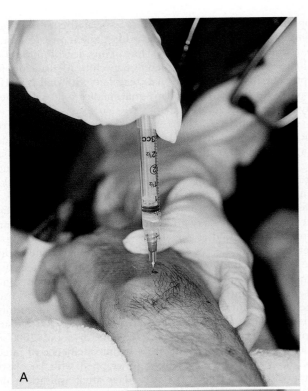

A

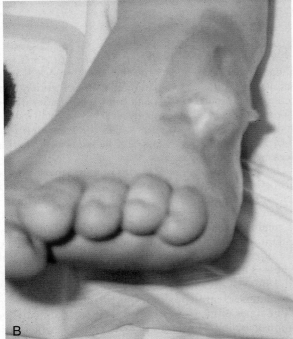

B

Figure 52–17 A typical dorsal ganglion cyst of the wrist (*A*) and dorsum of the foot (*B*).

injection is associated with considerable cost savings[44] and shorter recovery times compared with surgery, and because there is no difference in recurrence rates, aspiration appears to be the initial treatment of choice.[58] In the event that non-surgical treatment fails, surgical excision may be indicated. The "old" treatment of attempting to rupture the ganglion with a heavy book is not advised owing to the potential for local injury.

Approach. Following instillation of 1% lidocaine for local anesthesia, a 2.5-cm, relatively large-bore needle (17- to 18-gauge) is inserted into the center of the ganglion. The cyst is aspirated, with an attempt to achieve maximum evacuation of the contents. Usually 1 to 2 mL of mucinous fluid can be aspirated. Milking the contents of the cyst toward the aspiration needle can maximize the volume removed.[59] After the cyst is localized by aspiration, another smaller needle is used to simultaneously administer 10 to 15 mg of methylprednisolone (or equivalent intermediate-acting steroid). The use of steroids instilled into the cyst is a common procedure that has been proved to significantly augment the success of simple aspiration.[60] Following aspiration, a splint is usually not required, and activity need not be restricted. There is no proven role for routine NSAIDs or oral steroid therapy.

de Quervain Disease and Intersection Syndrome. de Quervain disease, a relatively common disorder, is a stenosing tenovaginitis of the short extensor tendon (extensor pollicis brevis [EPB]) and long abductor tendon (abductor pollicis longus [APL]) of the thumb. Although commonly referred to as a tenosynovitis, denoting inflammation of synovial sheaths of the tendons of the EPB and APL, this condition is more accurately described as a tenovaginitis.[61] *Tenovaginitis* refers to thickening of the fibrous sheath of the first extensor compartment. In 1912, de Quervain described "thickening of the dense fibrous connective tissues without any fresh sign of inflammation, neither round cell inflammation nor increase in numbers of cells."[61] Histologically, the thickening is caused by accumulation of mucopolysaccharide within the tendon sheath.[62,63]

It is commonly thought that the disorder more often occurs after repetitive use of the wrists, especially with a wringing motion. The syndrome has been called "washerwoman's sprain," and often no specific etiology is apparent. Women during pregnancy or within 12 months of childbirth are also frequently affected.[41] However, a study by Kay[61] challenges the association between repetitive motion and de Quervain disease. In a retrospective study of 100 cases, there was not a strong correlation with occupation and/or history of repetitive activities in patients diagnosed with de Quervain disease. Thus, it may be possible that repetitive activities exacerbate the pain associated with a condition for which the etiology is unclear.

Tenderness and occasionally palpable crepitation are elicited just distal to the radial styloid process, where both tendons come together in an osseofibrous tunnel. Patients usually present with wrist pain and often mistakenly attribute the discomfort to some distant, albeit irrelevant, trauma. The condition may be confused with first carpometacarpal arthrosis (osteoarthritis of the thumb) and intersection syndrome. Radiographs will be normal in de Quervain disease but might be appropriate to rule out other pathologic abnormalities. Ultrasound may demonstrate thickening and edema of the synovial sheath[64] but has not yet been routinely used to make or confirm the diagnosis. Rarely, gonococcal tenosynovitis might simulate this inflammatory condition.

tions may be required before the technique is considered a failure. In one study, 69% of 116 patients required only a single aspiration for successful treatment.[57] Two or three aspirations were required for 19%, and only 12% of patients ultimately needed surgical excision.[57] It should be noted, however, that ganglia might recur after aspiration or surgery. In a study by Dias,[58] 42% of palmar wrist ganglions treated with surgical excision and 47% treated with aspiration recurred within 5 years. Because aspiration with or without steroid

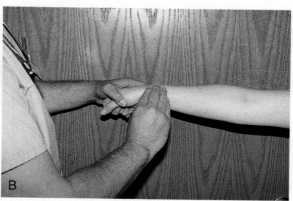

Abductor pollicis longus

Extensor pollicis brevis

Positive Finkelstein test

A

B

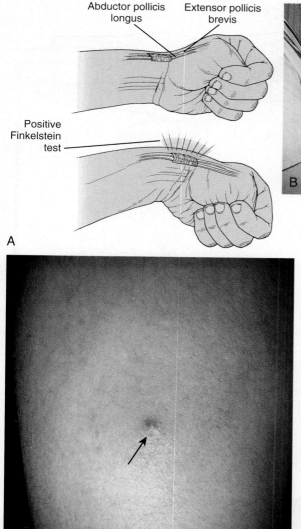

C

Figure 52–18 *A,* de Quervain tenosynovitis occurs in the first dorsal compartment of the wrist secondary to tenosynovitis of the abductor pollicis longus and extensor pollicis brevis tendons. Symptoms, which include pain over the radial styloid, are generally caused by overuse. The Finkelstein test is positive when pain is reproduced by ulnar deviation of the wrist while the patient grasps the thumb with the fingers. *B,* Occasionally, crepitus may be palpated over the involved area. To elicit this sign, the examiner's fingers are placed over the painful area and the patient's wrist is placed in ulnar deviation, which produces the characteristic sensation. *C,* Signs and symptoms of tenosynovitis of the wrist in a 25-year-old woman, which were initially thought to be de Quervain disease. The single hemorrhagic papule (*arrow*) demonstrating a septic embolus was found on the forearm, and is a subtle but classic lesion of gonococcal bacteremia. One aspect of this sexually transmitted disease is tenosynovitis. Cervical cultures were positive for *Neisseria gonorrhoeae*, despite the absence of vaginal symptoms. *(A, From Walker LG, Meals RM: Tendinitis: A practical approach to diagnosis and management. J Musculoskel Med 6:24, 1989.)*

A useful specific clinical maneuver that indicates de Quervain disease is the Finkelstein test (Fig. 52–18*A*), performed by abducting the patient's thumb into the palm of the hand and folding the fingers over the thumb. Forcible ulnar deviation at the wrist is then carried out, with severe pain at the site of the affected tendon sheaths indicating a positive test. When examining for the Finkelstein test, one should also evaluate the tender area for palpable crepitus (see Fig. 52–18*B*). If axial traction or compression (the carpometacarpal grind test) and rotation of the thumb produce pain, the condition is most likely due to degenerative changes of the carpometacarpal joint of the thumb rather than from de Quervain disease. It should be noted that gonococcal tenosynovitis of the wrist may mimic de Quervain disease, and one should inquire about other symptoms (e.g., sore throat, penile or vaginal discharge, or fever) and carefully look for the characteristic rash of this sexually transmitted disease (see Fig. 52–18*C*).

In a study comparing steroid injection of de Quervain disease with a splint and oral NSAID therapy alone, the latter traditionally accepted initial treatment was effective only in a small group of patients with minimal symptoms.[65] Steroid injection therapy was recommended as the initial treatment once the disease began to interfere with activities of daily living or if symptoms were more severe. Overall, increasing evidence supports the effectiveness of local corticosteroid injection as the therapeutic preference for de Quervain tenovaginitis. In a retrospective study, 84% of 58 cases were effectively managed either with a single injection (60%) or with repeat injections (24%), with only 12% requiring surgical treatment.[66] These data support a meta-analysis that found an 83% cure rate with injection alone among 495 subjects, in comparison with 61% for injection and splint, 14% for splint alone, and 0% for rest or NSAIDs.[67] The strikingly favorable response to local injection therapy suggests that surgery to release the tendon sheaths is seldom needed. Interestingly, some evidence suggests that failure of steroid injections may be due to an anatomic variant, in which the EPB is located in a separate synovial compartment.[67,68] This is supported by a study in which steroids selectively injected into the EPB tenosynovium resulted in resolution of symptoms in all 50 patients.[69] Clinical suspicion for this anatomic variant should be raised when previous steroid injections have failed and in patients who have pain with firm resistance to thumb metacarpophalangeal joint extension (the EPB entrapment test).[68] In these patients, selective injection into the EPB tenosynovium should be considered.

Accurate injection of the corticosteroid has been found to be an important aspect of the patients' response to treatment.[70] Using radiographic dye to verify correct corticosteroid placement, researchers have found that when the corticosteroid and anesthetic injection did not successfully reach either the EPB or the APL compartment, the patient did not experience a relief of pain. Conversely, when the medication was accurately injected, most patients reported an improvement of symptoms. If available, ultrasound may help guide the injection. In 2002, Kamel and coworkers[71] used ultrasound to guide steroid injection in 21 patients with the clinical diagnosis of de Quervain disease. No complications were reported, and all patients had decreased edema and thickening of the tendons at 6 and 12 weeks. Larger studies will be needed to confirm the benefits of ultrasound.

Intersection syndrome is a condition that may be easily confused with de Quervain disease. Because the treatment approach and clinical course of intersection syndrome differ from that of de Quervain tenovaginitis, it is important that the clinician is also familiar with this entity. First described in 1841 by Velpea, intersection syndrome describes a clinical entity approximately 4 to 8 cm proximal to the location of de Quervain disease.[72] Although the etiology is not yet clear, intersection syndrome is thought to result from inflammation of the second dorsal compartment of the wrist, which houses the extensor carpi radialis longus (ECRL) and extensor carpi radialis brevis (ECRB) tendons.[73] Other possible causes include inflammation of a bursa that develops between the APL and the ECRB tendons[55] and inflammation of the ECRL and ECRB tenosynovia where they cross the muscle bellies of the APL and EPB[74] (Fig. 52–19).

Intersection syndrome presents with pain, tenderness, edema, and occasional crepitus 4 to 8 cm proximal to the radial styloid and may be mistaken for de Quervain disease. This condition is seen in athletes who play sports requiring forceful repetitive wrist flexion and extension, such as rowing, weightlifting, gymnastics, and tennis.[55] Treatment includes rest, NSAIDs, and immobilization with a thumb spica splint in 15° wrist extension. Corticosteroid injection therapy is recommended only after a 2- to 3-week trial of splinting. In contrast, steroid injection therapy is recommended earlier in the course of de Quervain disease. Some authors, in fact, recommend corticosteroid injection therapy on initial presentation of de Quervain disease.[75] Surgery is generally reserved for refractory cases of intersection syndrome because most patients respond well to nonoperative treatment.[74]

Approach. For de Quervain disease, the hand is positioned with the ulnar side of the wrist on the table and the radial side facing upward. A 2.2-cm, 25-gauge needle is introduced at the most tender point (about 1 cm distal to the radial styloid) through a skin wheal, and 10 to 20 mg of prednisolone or equivalent intermediate-acting steroid suspension mixed with 4 to 5 mL of lidocaine 1% is deposited adjacent and parallel to the tendon sheath (peritendinous infiltration) (see Fig. 52–19). The injection should be under the edge of the first dorsal compartment retinaculum, within the first extensor compartment. If firm resistance is appreciated or if needle movement is noted when the patient abducts and extends the thumb, the needle should be redirected to prevent

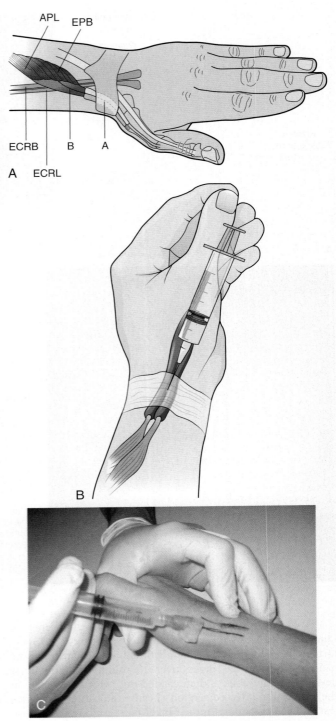

Figure 52–19 *A,* Site of de Quervain disease at the extensor pollicus brevis (EPB) and abductor pollicus longus (APL) tendons. *B,* Site of intersection syndrome at the extensor carpi radialis longus (ECRL) and extensor carpi radialis brevis (ECRB) tendons. *C,* Injection for de Quervain tenosynovitis usually produces a good result.

intratendinous injection.[75] Because there are many superficial vessels in this area, it is important to aspirate before injecting to verify that the needle is not in a blood vessel.[70] One should be generous with the injection volume, because a common reason for failure is the inability to get medication into both tendon sheaths. This may be partially overcome by increasing the volume of steroid-lidocaine injected in a more diffuse area. Often, there is visible edema at the radial aspect of the first metacarpal base and at the thumb metacarpophalangeal joint dorsally after successful injection.[70] A lightweight thumb or wrist splint for wrist support and protection may be used at night for several weeks after the injection, but routine splinting after injection is not required.[72] Oral NSAIDs may be prescribed for analgesia but will likely not affect a cure by themselves. There is no proven role for oral corticosteroids.

Injection for intersection syndrome is similar to that of de Quervain disease, except that the target site is at the point of maximal tenderness, which is usually 4 to 8 cm proximal to the radial styloid.

Carpal Tunnel Syndrome.
Carpal tunnel syndrome is the most common nerve entrapment neuropathy of the wrist.[76] Caused by median nerve compression in the fibro-osseous tunnel of the wrist, carpal tunnel is characterized by pain at the wrist that sometimes radiates proximally into the forearm and is associated with tingling and paresthesias of the medial aspect of the thumb, palmar side of the index and middle fingers, and the radial half of the ring finger. Typically, the patient wakes during the night with burning or aching pain, numbness, and tingling. Occasionally, the discomfort is extremely severe, causing the patient to seek emergency care. Clinical signs supporting the diagnosis include a positive Tinel sign, elicited by reproducing the tingling and paresthesias by tapping (with a reflex hammer) over the median nerve at the volar crease of the wrist.[77] In addition, one can perform Phalen's test, described as flexed wrists held against each other for several minutes in an effort to provoke the symptoms in the median nerve distribution.[77] Phalen's test is more sensitive than Tinel's sign and is more specific for carpal tunnel syndrome.[76] Severe muscle atrophy of the thenar eminence may develop in advanced or neglected cases. In many cases, the disturbance is idiopathic, without a recognizable underlying cause. However, people who participate in repetitive activities of the wrist, such as typing, driving, assembly-line work, and racquet sports are at risk for developing carpal tunnel syndrome.[41] Other conditions associated with carpal tunnel syndrome include rheumatoid arthritis (sometimes as the presenting manifestation), pregnancy, hypothyroidism, diabetes, and acromegaly.

The initial therapy of carpal tunnel syndrome consists of activity modification and splinting; the latter is particularly helpful at night.[41] Of the medications sometimes used to treat carpal tunnel syndrome, diuretics, NSAIDs, and pyridoxine have been shown to offer little to no relief.[78] In contrast, the benefits, at least in the short term (e.g., 4–6 wk), of local steroid injections for carpal tunnel syndrome have been well proved.[79] In a Cochrane review of randomized trials by Marshall and colleagues,[80] local steroid injection provided greater clinical improvement 1 month after injection compared with placebo and up to 3 months after injection compared with oral steroid treatment. However, symptoms after local corticosteroid injection were no different than either NSAIDs or splinting at 8 weeks. The benefits of initial steroid injection compared with surgical intervention for carpal tunnel syndrome are controversial because there is little scientifically valid information on which to draw any conclusions. In one small study, Hui and associates[81] found that surgery resulted in better symptomatic outcome (but not grip strength) when compared with local steroid injection over a 20-week period. It appears that local steroid injection for carpal tunnel syndrome offers improvement in symptoms, but this improvement may not be permanent or long term. Current recommendations include a trial of conservative treatment (including possible steroid injection) for those patients that have mild to moderate symptoms and lack thenar wasting.[82] Surgery is indicated for those patients with persistent symptoms after conservative treatment and for those with severe weakness of the thumb abductors.[76] Nerve compression should be confirmed by nerve conduction studies before surgery.[70]

Approach. When injecting the carpal canal, one should insert the needle through a skin wheal at a site just ulnar to the palmaris longus tendon about 1 cm proximal to the distal crease at the wrist. The palmaris longus tendon can be appreciated by having the patient pinch all the fingertips together while holding the wrist in a neutral position[83] (Fig. 52–20). Injecting medial (ulnar) to the palmaris longus is preferred because it avoids direct injection of the median nerve and superficial veins. A 2.5- to 3.9-cm, 25-gauge needle is directed at an angle of approximately 45° to the skin surface, pointing toward the tip of the middle finger. The needle is advanced 1 to 2 cm, and 20 to 40 mg of methyprednisolone (or other intermediate-acting steroid equivalent) with or without lidocaine is injected along the track and into the tissue space. If the patient complains of paresthesias or the needle meets resistance during injection, the needle should be redirected to avoid injecting directly into a nerve or tendon, respectively.[83] Up to 2 weeks may be required for paresthesias to abate significantly, although it usually takes only a few days for an improvement in nocturnal pain.[84] A lightweight wrist splint may hasten recovery. Repeat injections may be given, but if a response is not elicited or permanent after two or three injections, decompressive surgery should be considered.

Digital Flexor Tenosynovitis ("Trigger Finger").
A "trigger" or "snapping" finger is one of the most common problems of the hand and is characterized by a stenosed tendon sheath at the level of the first annular pulley (A1), which is located on the palmar surface over the base of the metacarpal head.[85] In this condition, the A1 pulley becomes inflamed, causing a nodule to develop on the tendon as it gets "pinched" under the constricted sheath.[85] Locking occurs when the involved digit is in flexion and is especially troublesome when the patient awakens in the morning. This can occur in any finger but is seen most frequently in the ring and middle fingers.

Besides a thickening and stenosing of the tendon sheath, trigger finger may also be characterized by flexor tendon synovitis. The tendon sheaths are long and tubular, and the walls are lined with a thin layer of synovial cells. Symptoms develop when the tendon becomes trapped and is unable to glide within the tendon sheath (Fig. 52–21). A nodule or fibrinous deposit may form at a site in the tendon sheath, usually over or just distal to the metacarpal head in trigger finger. When the digit is flexed, the nodule moves with the tendon proximally and, on extension, gets "stuck" on the pulley, leading to intermittent catching of the tendon.[85] The nodule may be palpable on physical examination, but this is not necessary for diagnosis.[41] Carpal tunnel syndrome commonly coexists with trigger finger and may be caused by tenosynovitis. The common causes of tenosynovitis include trauma, diabetes mellitus, and rheumatoid arthritis, although it may also be a primary and idiopathic disorder.[73]

Conservative treatment, including local rest or splinting, application of moist heat, and NSAID therapy, is the usual initial approach for symptomatic tenosynovitis. If these simple measures fail to control symptoms, then corticosteroid injection, appropriately administered to the involved tendon

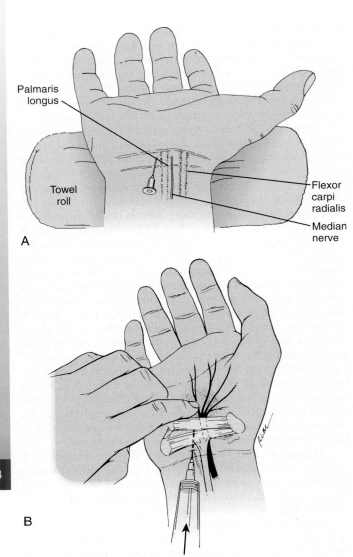

Palmaris
longus

Towel
roll

A

Flexor
carpi
radialis

Median
nerve

B

Figure 52–20 *A,* Injection of the median carpal tunnel with the wrist dorsiflexed over a rolled towel. To avoid direct injection of the median nerve, the needle is introduced just medial (ulnar) to the palmaris longus tendon, which can be appreciated by having the patient pinch all the fingertips together with the wrist in a neutral position. *B,* A palpable bulge at the distal edge of this ligament indicates correct placement of the injection. Direct injection into the median or ulnar nerve is to be avoided. *(A, Redrawn from Steinbrocker O, Neustadt DH: Aspiration and Injection Therapy in Arthritis and Musculoskeletal Disorders: A Handbook on Technique and Management. Hagerstown, MD, Harper & Row, 1972; B, from Dehaan MR, Wilson RL: Diagnosis and management of carpal tunnel syndrome. J Musculoskel Med 6:47, 1989. Reproduced with permission.)*

sheath, is indicated. One double-blind, placebo-controlled, randomized study of trigger finger demonstrated that steroid injection was significantly more effective than placebo.[86] At follow-up 3 weeks after treatment, 9 of the 14 patients receiving a combination lidocaine and steroid injection were asymptomatic versus 2 of the 10 patients receiving lidocaine injections alone. A similar study showed complete resolution of symptoms in 52% of patients receiving a corticosteroid injection, whereas 47% had improvement of symptoms.[85] Steroid injections are more successful when performed in patients with a palpable nodule or symptoms for less than 6 months.[87] Alternatively, some evidence suggests that the efficacy of steroid injections for trigger finger diminishes with

each subsequent injection in the same site.[88] As a guideline, if treatment fails after three injections (separated by several weeks/months), the patient should be considered for surgery.[41] In addition, patients with diabetes mellitus more often require surgical release for trigger finger than non–insulin-dependent diabetics.[85] Division of the first annular pulley, digital nerve injury, scarring, and recurrence are well-known complications of surgical release.[88]

Approach. Preparation of the site before the injection requires meticulous adherence to aseptic technique. The technique for injecting flexor tenosynovitis includes placing the palm in an upward direction and locating the tendon point at the base of the finger flexion crease, which is located between the A1 and the A2 tendon pulleys. Subcutaneously inject 0.25 to 0.35 mL of an intermediate-acting corticosteroid suspension mixed with 1.5–3 mL of anesthetic using a 2.2-cm, 25-gauge needle angled slightly proximally into the involved tendon sheath (see Fig. 52–21). The needle enters the skin at an angle of approximately 30° and is inserted into the tendon sheath, parallel to the tendon fibers. If resistance is felt on needle insertion, this suggests an intratendinous location, and the needle should be slightly withdrawn before injection. Similar injections can be administered to the base of the thumb metacarpal for a "snapping" thumb. Whereas injecting into the tendon sheath is the goal, Taras and coworkers[89] showed that steroid injection into the subcutaneous tissue surrounding the tendon sheath provided similar improvement to intrasheath injections. If relapses are frequent or the clinical response is not satisfactory, surgical release is indicated.

Carpal/Metacarpal Inflammation. Overuse and aging can lead to pain at the base of the thumb and fingers. This can be quite painful, especially common in elderly women. The first metacarpal articulates with the trapezium, a common site for this condition. Injection therapy is usually quite successful (Fig. 52–22).

Hip Region

Trochanteric Bursitis. Trochanteric bursitis is the second leading cause of lateral hip pain after osteoarthritis.[90] However, the condition can be confused with other conditions at or about the hip, such as sacrolumbar disease, hip/femur pathology, and metastases.[91–93] Patients with trochanteric bursitis, however, usually demonstrate discrete tenderness to deep palpation at or adjacent to the greater trochanter, and relief of symptoms with a proper corticosteroid injection can help confirm the diagnosis.[91]

The principal bursae associated with this condition are the subgluteus maximus bursa, the subgluteus minimus bursa, and the gluteus minimus bursa, although other bursae of the hip may be affected (Fig. 52–23). Pain may be acute but is more often subacute or chronic; frequently, patients have tried NSAIDs without success and have been given a number of incorrect diagnoses. The chief locus of the pathologic condition is in the abductor mechanism of the hip. Pain occurs near the greater trochanter and may radiate down the lateral or posterolateral aspect of the thigh and, rarely, into the knee.[94] Pain is described as "deep," "dull," and "aching," and it often interferes with sleep.

Lying on the affected hip, stepping from curbs, and descending steps provoke pain. Tenderness may be elicited over and adjacent to the greater trochanter. In contrast with true hip involvement, the Patrick FABERE sign (*f*lexion, *ab*duction, *e*xternal *r*otation, and *e*xtension) may be negative,

Figure 52–21 *A,* Trigger finger (stenosing tenosynovitis) can affect any digit, including the thumb, but it is most common in the ring and middle fingers. *Injection is often very effective,* but the nodule may persist. *B,* In advanced cases, inflammation at the proximal (A-1) pulley of the flexor tendon sheath overlying the metacarpophalangeal joint may hold the digit in either a flexed or an extended position. Generally, the tendon becomes thickened either proximal or distal to the pulley, causing a snapping or a locking phenomenon with finger flexion or extension. Palpation of the flexor tendon sheath over the metacarpophalangeal joint often reproduces symptoms. *C,* Injection technique for trigger finger, note use of small needle. *(B, From Walker LG, Meals RA: Tendinitis: A practical approach to diagnosis and management. J Musculoskel Med 6:41, 1989. Reproduced with permission.)*

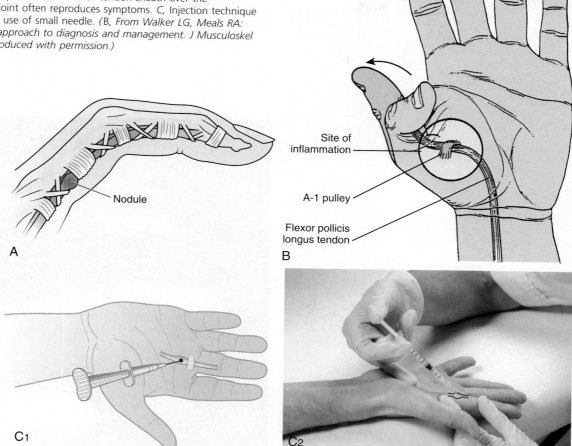

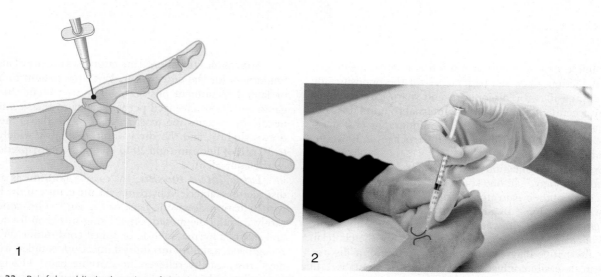

Figure 52–22 Painful and limited motion of the thumb is often caused by inflammation at the first carpal/metacarpal joint. Inject at the apex of the snuffbox, avoiding the radial artery. This is usually quite successful therapy for a very painful condition (common in elderly women).

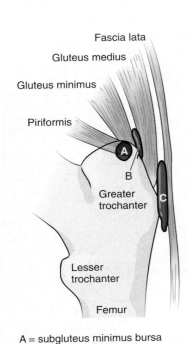

Fascia lata
Gluteus medius
Gluteus minimus
Piriformis
Greater trochanter
Lesser trochanter
Femur

A = subgluteus minimus bursa
B = subgluteus medius bursa
C = subgluteus maximus bursa

A

Figure 52–23 **Trochanteric bursitis** *A,* The principal bursa lies between the gluteus maximus and the greater trochanter, although other bursae may also be involved. *B,* Injection of the trochanteric bursa. The injection is made at the area of maximal tenderness.

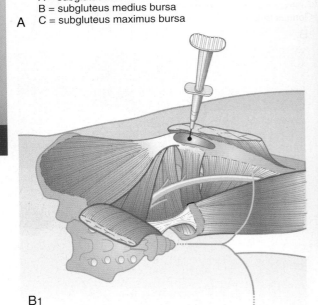

B1

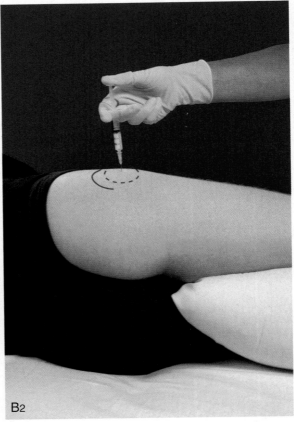

B2

and complete passive range of motion is relatively painless. Active abduction when the patient lies on the opposite side typically intensifies the discomfort, and sharp external rotation may accentuate the symptoms. Internal rotation does not usually affect the level of pain.[91] Hip radiographs may demonstrate a calcific deposit adjacent to the trochanter; however, the incidence of this is low.[92]

Corticosteroid injection for trochanteric bursitis is often an effective therapy.[92] In one study, 77% of patients reported improvement of their pain after an injection of betamethasone mixed with lidocaine.[95] In addition, 61% of patients reported improvement of pain 26 weeks after receiving the injection. Failure of corticosteroid therapy should prompt the clinician to seek alternative diagnoses, such as true hip joint disease, which can be easily confused with trochanteric bursitis.[96] In addition, although rare, there have been case reports of septic trochanteric bursitis caused by tuberculosis.[97]

Approach. Intrabursal injection uses the site of maximum tenderness for the entry point. With the patient in a supine or lateral recumbent position, a 3.9- to 5.0-cm, 20- or 21-gauge needle is advanced perpendicular to the skin until the needle tip reaches the trochanter. The needle is then withdrawn slightly, and the site is infiltrated fairly widely with 3 to 10 mL of lidocaine and 20 to 40 mg of methylprednisolone or the equivalent.

Ischiogluteal Bursitis. "Weaver's bottom" is a painful disorder characterized by pain over the center of the buttocks with radiation down the back of the leg.[92] This condition is rarely initially diagnosed, often being mistaken for lumbosacral strain, a herniated disk, or spinal cord tumor. When it is recognized, a skillful intrabursal injection, coupled with a few days' rest, usually relieves the extreme pain. The ischial or ischiogluteal bursa is adjacent to the ischial tuberosity and overlies the sciatic and posterior femoral cutaneous nerves.

Sitting on hard surfaces, bending forward, and standing on tiptoe provoke pain. Tenderness is present over the ischial tuberosity. At times, a soft tissue mass may also be felt in this area.[98]

Approach. The usual technique for injection requires that the patient lie in a prone position. A 5.0-cm, 20- to 22-gauge needle is inserted through a skin wheal and is advanced cautiously in an effort to avoid the sciatic nerve, which lies at a depth of approximately 6.5 to 7.5 cm. Paresthesias occur on striking the nerve, and if this occurs, the needle should be withdrawn from the nerve. Generally, 5 to 10 mL of lidocaine and 20 to 40 mg of methylprednisolone are introduced into the bursa.

Knee Region

Prepatellar Bursitis. "Housemaid's knee" or "nun's knee" is characterized by swelling with effusion of the superficial bursa overlying the lower pole of the patella (Fig. 52–24). In contrast to intra-articular pathology, passive motion of the knee is fully preserved, and pain is generally mild, except during extreme knee flexion or direct pressure. Although the disorder is usually caused by pressure from repetitive kneeling on a firm surface ("rug cutter's knee"), rarely it can develop after direct trauma, and occasionally, it is a manifestation of rheumatoid arthritis or gout.[99] Although uncommon, the prepatellar bursa is one of the most common sites of septic bursitis.[4] Moreover, patients with septic prepatellar bursitis may not present with the classic signs of infection such as erythema, warmth, or fever, making it difficult to differentiate from aseptic bursitis.[100] The bursal aspirate should therefore always be sent for laboratory analysis, particularly if infection is suspected.[4]

Approach. The patient should be in a supine position with the leg extended. The bursa is located superficially, between the skin and the patella, and can often be "milked" during the procedure to facilitate aspiration. This aspiration often yields a surprisingly scant amount of clear, serous fluid because the prepatellar bursa is a multilocular structure rather than the usual single cavity. Once aspiration is complete, the instillation of 1 to 2 mL of lidocaine with 15 to 20 mg of a prednisolone (or equivalent) suspension with a 2.5-cm, 20- to 21-gauge needle is usually sufficient to cause the swelling to abate. In some cases, the procedure may need to be repeated more than once (in 6- to 8-wk intervals) to obtain a lasting result. The provocative activity should be discontinued.

Suprapatellar Bursitis. Suprapatellar bursitis usually is associated with synovitis of the knees. On occasion, the bursa is largely separated from the synovial cavity with only a very minor communication, and the swelling and effusion are chiefly confined to the suprapatellar area. This may be traumatic in origin or an associated manifestation of an inflammatory arthropathy.

Approach. The procedure for aspiration and injection of the suprapatellar area is similar to that for the knee.

Anserine Bursitis. "Cavalryman's disease" now mainly occurs in heavy women with disproportionately large thighs in association with osteoarthritis of the knee, although this entity is also seen in athletes who are involved with running, baseball, and racquet sports.[92] The bursa is on the anteromedial side of the knee, inferior to the joint line at the site of the insertion of the conjoined tendons of the sartorius, semitendinous, and gracilis muscles and superficial to the medial collateral ligament (Fig. 52–25; see also Fig. 52–24). The entity is characterized by a relatively abrupt onset of knee pain, with localized tenderness and a sense of fullness in the vicinity of the anserine bursa about 4 to 5 cm below the anteromedial aspect of the tibial plateau. Pain is exacerbated by flexion of the knee. Corticosteroid injection for anserine bursitis has been shown in clinical trials to be an effective treatment.[101]

Approach. The patient is positioned with the knee flexed at 90°. An injection of 2 to 4 mL of lidocaine, with or followed by approximately 20 to 40 mg of a corticosteroid suspension, is given using an anterior or medial approach with a 2.5- to 3.9-cm, 22-gauge needle (see Fig. 52–25). At the point of greatest tenderness, the needle is gently advanced until the tibia is reached, the needle is withdrawn 2 to 3 mm, and the steroid is then injected. Prompt symptomatic relief is frequently obtained, but the duration of benefit is variable and probably correlates with the patient's weight-bearing activities. It is important to avoid direct injection of the corticosteroid suspension into the nearby tendons.

Medial Collateral Ligament Bursa. This bursa is located anterior to the tibia and posterior to the medial collateral ligament. Injury to this bursa often occurs when the patient undergoes a twisting motion, with concurrent external rotation of the tibia. Tenderness may be appreciated along the anteroinferior aspect of the medial collateral ligament, and the pain is exacerbated with extension of the knee. This condition may sometimes be confused with a medial meniscus tear, and MRI might be necessary in order to differentiate the two conditions. Treatment is usually successful with conservative measures, including relative rest, compression, and NSAIDs.[92]

Popliteal Cyst. "Baker's cysts" are herniated fluid-filled sacs of the articular synovial membrane that extend into the popliteal fossa, sometimes through the natural communication between the bursa of the posterior knee and the joint itself. These cysts may also be due to swelling of the medial gastrocnemius or semimembranosus bursae alone. Baker's cysts can occur secondary to trauma, although they are also seen in patients with rheumatoid arthritis, gout, and osteoarthritis.[92] The patient will often complain of *popliteal fossa* tenderness and swelling that may extend into the calf. Activities that involve active flexion of the knee, such as walking or jumping, will exacerbate the symptoms.

The clinical presentation of Baker's cysts can mimic that of a deep venous thrombosis (DVT), and it is important to take great care in differentiating the two. For this reason, symptomatic Baker's cysts are also known as the pseudothrombophlebitis syndrome.[102] In most studies, 2% to 6% of patients suspected of having a DVT actually have a popliteal cyst as the cause of their knee/calf pain. Ultrasound is an important tool in this diagnosis.

Many cases of Baker's cysts resolve spontaneously over a few weeks. However, treatment of Baker's cysts may require surgery to correct any articular injury or to remove the cyst. Steroid injections are not usually performed because of the risk of neurovascular injury.

Ankle, Foot, and Heel Region

Ankle Tendinitis. This is a relatively uncommon condition. It may result from unusual repetitive activity or, rarely, from acute trauma. The disorder is differentiated from ankle joint involvement by the lack of pain or restricted motion during passive flexion and extension of the ankle. Active flexion and extension of the toes does produce pain. Local tenderness is elicited along the involved tendons. Initial treat-

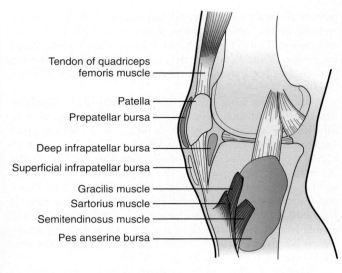

Tendon of quadriceps femoris muscle

Patella

Prepatellar bursa

Deep infrapatellar bursa

Superficial infrapatellar bursa

Gracilis muscle

Sartorius muscle

Semitendinosus muscle

Pes anserine bursa

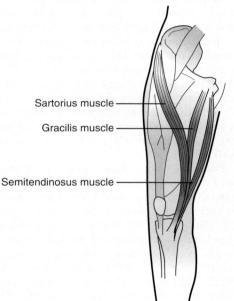

Sartorius muscle

Gracilis muscle

Semitendinosus muscle

Figure 52–24 *A,* Prepatellar bursitis and pes anserine bursitis. The prepatellar bursa lies superior to the patella, and the pes anserine bursa lies deep to the insertion of the sartorius, gracilis, and semitendinosus tendons. Prepatellar bursitis is common in carpet layers, and pes anserine bursitis is seen in dancers and runners. *B,* Infrapatellar bursitis is common in long-distance runners and can be mistaken for patellar tendinitis. Pain is below the patella at the midpoint of the patellar tendon and is elicited by knee extension. Note that there are two infrapatellar bursae. Osgood-Schlatter disease is similar in adolescents, a condition that *should not be injected.*

A

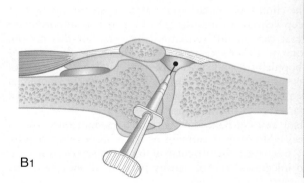

B1

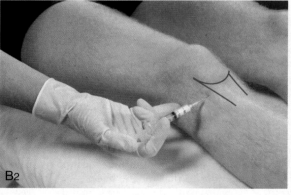

B2

ment consists of rest, NSAIDs, and immobilization, sometimes for several weeks. Some patients may eventually need operative intervention for prolonged symptoms.[103] Local steroid injections have been used successfully in patients who do not respond to conservative measures; however, the risk of tendon rupture is well documented. As a result, tendon sheath injections should be reserved for those patients with persistent symptoms despite an adequate trial of conservative therapy and should be done in consultation with a foot and ankle specialist.

Approach. A 2.5- to 3.9-cm, 22- or 25-gauge needle is used. One makes a tangential entry to the enlarged tendon

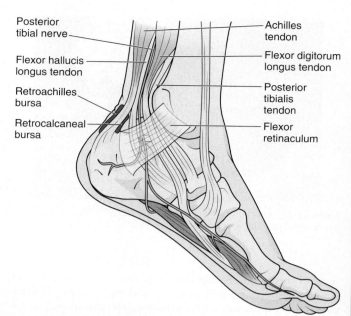

Posterior
tibial nerve

Flexor hallucis
longus tendon

Retroachilles
bursa

Retrocalcaneal
bursa

Achilles
tendon

Flexor digitorum
longus tendon

Posterior
tibialis
tendon

Flexor
retinaculum

Figure 52–26   Heel pain. Talalgia may involve the tendons, bursa, or fascia around the heel. Do not inject Achilles tendinitis since tendon rupture may occur. *Fluoroquinolones can cause significant Achilles tendinopathy* (see Table 52–1).

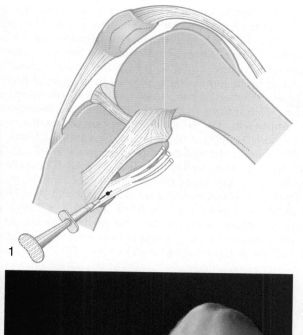

Figure 52–25   Injection of the anserine bursa of the knee. Note that the point of entry, which is the point of maximal tenderness, is inferior to the patella and medial to the tibial tuberosity.

sheath, distending the sheath with approximately 2 to 4 mL of a mixture of corticosteroid (20–40 mg of methylprednisolone) and lidocaine.

Bunion Bursitis. It is common for bunion bursitis to overlie the first metatarsophalangeal joint at its medial surface on the great toe. On occasion, tense swelling occurs, and decompression is required. Aspiration with culture of the fluid should be performed.

Approach. If no infection is present, the bursa is injected with 5 to 10 mg of methylprednisolone with a 2.5-cm, 20-gauge needle. Special shoes or an orthopaedic correction will be needed if the swelling recurs.

Heel Pain. Talalgia may be caused by many different etiologies, including Achilles tendinitis, retrocalcaneal bursitis, or plantar fasciitis (Fig. 52–26). An additional discussion is found in Chapter 51 (Podiatric Procedures). The bursae of clinical significance around the heel include the space between the skin and the Achilles tendon (known as the retroachilles bursa), the retrocalcaneal bursa (located between the Achilles tendon and the calcaneus), and the subcalcaneal bursa. Achilles tendinitis or bursitis may be traumatic in origin but is more apt to be part of a systemic disease, such as rheumatoid or gouty arthritis. Although the normal Achilles tendon is thick and strong, when affected by an inflammatory arthropathy, it is predisposed to degeneration, and because the Achilles tendon is not invested by a full synovial sheath, it is more vulnerable to intratendon instillation. Because of the potential

hazard of tendon rupture after local steroid injection, it is wise to avoid infiltration of steroids into this area. In a double-blind, randomized, controlled trial, it was shown that the injection of methylprednisolone and bupivacaine (Marcaine) had no benefit over injecting bupivacaine alone.[7] It is preferable to treat Achilles tendinitis with rest, splinting, and oral NSAIDs and to avoid injection therapy.

Retrocalcaneal bursitis is often seen in association with Haglund's deformity, a bony ridge on the posterosuperior aspect of the calcaneus. The bursa lies anterior to the Achilles tendon, and posterior to the calcaneus. Local swelling and tenderness at the posterior heel, proximal (and sometimes lateral) to the insertion of the Achilles tendon, characterize this bursitis. Treatment is focused on minimizing pressure on the bony ridge, which includes wearing open-heeled shoes (clogs), bare feet, sandals, or a heel lift. Conservative measures such as ice, oral NSAIDs, and rest are other common treatment modalities. Corticosteroid injections are not recommended owing to the risk of Achilles tendon rupture.[104,105]

The condition in this region most amenable to injection therapy is plantar fasciitis, also the most common cause of heel pain in adults.[106] The plantar fascia is located deep to the fat layer of the foot and extends from the calcaneus to the base of the digits. It is responsible for the support of the medial longitudinal arch of the foot.[107] Signs of this condition include pain on the plantar medial aspect of the heel, which is often worse in the morning, after long periods of rest, and with passive dorsiflexion of the toes.[106] The pain may be relieved with activity. Although patients may have a heel spur, many symptomatic patients do not, and the presence of a heel spur should not be considered pathognomonic of the condition. Although still debated, the pathology is generally thought to originate from microtears in the fascia, often due to overuse.[104,105] Obesity may also increase the risk of plantar fasciitis owing to the excessive load on the fascia.[106]

Most cases of plantar fasciitis eventually resolve with nonsurgical management.[108] Treatment begins with elimina-

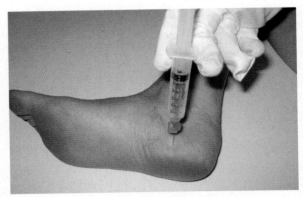

Figure 52–27 Injection of the calcaneal bursitis with heel spur. A lateral injection is preferred (see Chapter 51).

tion of precipitating activity, relative rest, strength and stretching exercises, arch supports, and night splints. If these conservative measures are not effective, injection of the painful heel will usually provide short-term improvement. In a recent Cochrane review, steroid injections for plantar fasciitis resulted in significant improvement at 1 month but not at 3 or 6 months when compared with control groups.[109] In addition, there is a risk of plantar fascia rupture and fat pad atrophy with corticosteroid injections.[104] One study found a rupture rate of close to 10%.[110] Therefore, caution should be exercised when administering steroids to the painful heel. In addition, because this tends to be a chronic or recurring condition, referral to an appropriate specialist is recommended.

Approach. The needle is inserted on the medial aspect of the heel. At the spot of maximal tenderness, a 2.5-cm, 22- to 24-gauge needle enters the plantar surface at 90°, sliding into the space at the midpoint of the calcaneus. The tip of the needle lies in the aponeurosis of the attachment to the os calcis (Fig. 52–27). One milliliter of lidocaine and 10 to 20 mg of methylprednisolone are instilled. Injection through the more superficial aspect of the base of the foot should be avoided, because this may result in dispersion of medications into the fat pad, producing fat pad atrophy.[107]

REFERENCES CAN BE FOUND ON EXPERT CONSULT

CHAPTER 53

Arthrocentesis

Steven J. Parrillo, Daniel S. Morrison,
and Edward A. Panacek

Arthrocentesis, the puncture and aspiration of a joint, is an acknowledged, useful procedure that is easily performed in the emergency department (ED). It has been established as both a diagnostic and a therapeutic tool for various clinical situations. Many clinicians are wary of joint fluid aspiration owing to a lack of experience and the fear of introducing infection. When performed properly, however, the procedure offers a wealth of clinical information and is associated with few complications. In the ED, it is difficult, if not impossible, to make an accurate assessment of an acutely painful, hot, and swollen joint without performing arthrocentesis.

INDICATIONS AND CONTRAINDICATIONS

The indications for arthrocentesis include[1]:
1. Diagnosis of nontraumatic joint disease by synovial fluid analysis (septic joint or crystal-induced arthritis).
2. Diagnosis of ligamentous or bony injury by confirmation of the presence of blood in the joint. Arthrocentesis may be needed to differentiate a traumatic joint effusion from an inflammatory process.
3. Establishment of the existence of an intra-articular fracture by the presence of blood with fat globules in the joint.
4. Relief of the pain of an acute hemarthrosis or a tense effusion. Although a minor hemarthrosis need not be drained, arthrocentesis can reduce the pain associated with large effusions and examination of an injured joint.
5. Local instillation of medications in acute and chronic inflammatory arthritides. Instillation of lidocaine into an injured joint also makes the initial examination of a traumatic injury less painful.
6. Obtaining fluid for culture, Gram staining, immunologic studies, and cell count in cases of suspected joint infection.
7. Determining whether a laceration communicates with the joint space.

Infection in the tissues overlying the site to be punctured is generally considered an absolute contraindication to arthrocentesis. However, inflammation with warmth, swelling, and tenderness may overlie an acutely arthritic joint, and this condition may mimic a soft tissue infection. Once convinced that cellulitis does not exist, the clinician should not hesitate to obtain the necessary diagnostic joint fluid. Known bacteremia is a relative contraindication because infection can spread to the joint.

Bleeding diatheses are rarely a relative contraindication, and arthrocentesis to relieve a tense hemarthrosis in bleeding disorders, such as hemophilia, is an accepted practice after infusion of the appropriate clotting factors. There are little data regarding the safety or dangers of arthrocentesis in a patient receiving anticoagulants or platelet inhibitors. Studies have demonstrated that the risk of iatrogenic hemarthrosis in patients on oral anticoagulation therapy is quite low, even in those who have International Normalized Ratios as high as 4.5.[2] One prospective trial of 32 patients on warfarin found no complications after arthrocentesis.[3] Hence, when necessary, arthrocentesis should be performed in patients on anticoagulants. The value of reversing a coagulopathy with blood components before the procedure is not proved, and clinical judgment should prevail. Prosthetic joints are at high risk for infection, and arthrocentesis should be avoided whenever possible. However, if an infected prosthesis is suspected, arthrocentesis should be performed.

Articular versus Periarticular Disease

Periarticular diseases such as trauma, tendinitis, bursitis, contusion, cellulitis, or phlebitis may mimic articular disease and suggest the need for arthrocentesis. Therefore, evaluation of acute joint disease requires that the clinician first determine whether the patient's constellation of signs and symptoms derives from the joint itself or from some other musculoskeletal or periarticular structure. Such a distinction, however, may be difficult, if not impossible, to make without synovial fluid analysis. No specific test or physical finding has high specificity for solving this dilemma; however, some physical findings may prove helpful.

If swelling is secondary to joint effusion or inflammation, the entire articular capsule will be inflamed and distended and fluid can often be palpated within the joint. In the knee, this condition must be differentiated from effusion into the prepatellar bursa, where swelling distends the bursa that lies mainly over the lower portion of the patella, between it and the skin. Effusion into the joint occurs posterior to the patella, whereas bursal swelling occurs anterior to it (Fig. 53–1). When considerable articular effusion of the knee is present, the capsule of the joint is distended and an inverted U-shaped swelling of the joint occurs. This characteristic shape occurs because the dense patellar ligament prevents distention of the capsule along its inferior border. Also, with the knee extended, a large effusion causes the patella to "float" or lift away from the femoral condyles. Complete extension and flexion are often impossible because of the joint tension produced by the effusion.

Joint effusion causes limited movement of the joint in all directions, with active and passive motion producing pain. The pain arising from a pathologic condition involving a joint may be diffuse or clearly localized to the joint or it may radiate. Hip pain, for example, frequently radiates into the groin or down the front of the thigh into the knee. Shoulder joint pain commonly radiates into the elbow or the neck. Therefore, complete examination of contiguous structures is essential for adequate diagnosis.

In contrast, pain from a periarticular process is often more localized and tenderness can be elicited only with certain specific movements or at specific points around the joint. In periarticular inflammation, one can often passively lead a joint through a range of motion with minimal discomfort, yet pain is significant when the patient attempts active motion. Crepitus may be elicited in tendinitis or the pain may be traced along the course of a specific tendon.

Septic Arthritis

Acute monoarticular arthritis is a common problem in emergency medicine. Although acute monoarticular arthritis has many causes, septic arthritis is the one requiring most urgent diagnosis and treatment. Infectious arthritis is still relatively frequent, and suspicion of a septic process in the joint is the first step in appropriate management; confirmation requires arthrocentesis and synovial fluid culture. In the ED, synovial fluid analysis is the diagnostic test most heavily relied upon in making the diagnosis of an acute intra-articular infection. Culture remains the most definitive study, although it is not

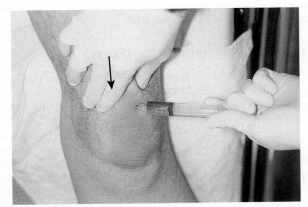

Figure 53–1 **Periarticular problems may mimic an intra-articular process.** This patient had trauma to the knee and presented with anterior soft tissue swelling and fluctuance, representing a hematoma of the prepatellar bursa, *not a hemarthrosis.* Pressure applied to the edge of the swelling aids the aspiration of all blood from the bursa (*arrow*).

100% sensitive.[4] Repeated arthrocentesis might be needed when treating a septic joint. Such therapy is usually performed on an inpatient basis and may be facilitated with ultrasound guidance.[5]

Infection of a joint occurs by one of these mechanisms: (1) hematogenous spread, the most common scenario, (2) spread from a contiguous source of infection, (3) direct implantation, (4) postoperative contamination, or (5) trauma.[4] The joint distribution of septic arthritis is typically monoarticular with a swollen, erythematous, and painful joint. The noninfectious differential diagnosis includes crystal-induced arthritis, fracture, hemarthrosis, foreign body, osteoarthritis, ischemic necrosis, and monoarticular rheumatoid arthritis.[4] In addition, osteomyelitis may mimic septic arthritis because of the close proximity of the infected metaphysis and joint space.[6] In many instances, an acutely inflamed joint from gout or other arthritides simply cannot be clinically distinguished from infection. Early diagnosis is essential to prevent complications such as growth impairment, articular destruction with ankylosis, osteomyelitis, or soft tissue extension.[7]

Because an acutely swollen joint may be indicative of a number of disease entities, a thorough history and physical examination are the cornerstones of evaluation, followed by arthrocentesis (Fig. 53–2). Laboratory findings can be useful in diagnosis, as can response to therapy (e.g., response to penicillin in gonococcal arthritis is often the only criterion for diagnosis because the organism is difficult to culture). Patients with malignancy (especially leukemia) or who are immuno-

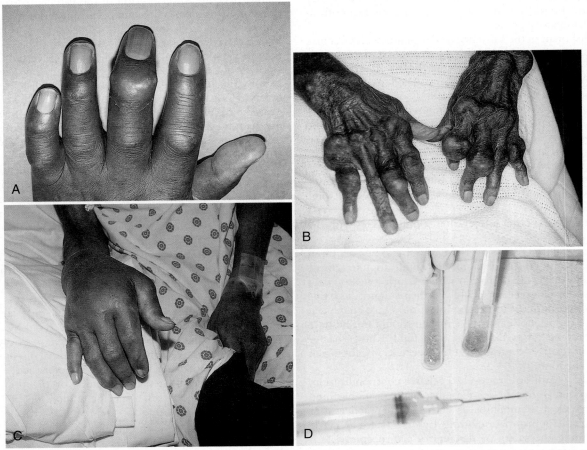

Figure 53–2 *A* and *B,* Tophaceous gout. These nodules are painless and full of uric acid crystals. *C,* An acutely swollen and painful joint in this patient is most likely acute gouty arthritis and can produce fever and leukocytosis. In some cases, joint fluid analysis is the only way to differentiate gout from a septic joint. *D,* Aspiration of a tophus yields precipitated/waxy/soft uric acid conglomeration.

suppressed or otherwise debilitated are at particular risk for a septic etiology. Infectious arthritis should be primarily considered in these patients as well as in those with such preexisting joint diseases as rheumatoid arthritis. In general, a swollen joint is usually not injected with corticosteroids until the possibility of infection has been eliminated.[8]

Neisseria gonorrhoeae, *Staphylococcus*, and *Streptococcus* are the most frequently identified etiologic agents. *N. gonorrhoeae* is the most common organism causing septic arthritis among adolescents and young adults. Patients older than 40 years and those with other medical illnesses are more likely to have *Staphylococcus* joint infections. In children, *Staphylococcus*, *Streptococcus*, and *Escherichia coli* predominate. *Haemophilus influenzae* was a common cause of septic arthritis in the past, but widespread use of the conjugate vaccine has reduced *H. influenzae* infection rates to near zero.[9,10] In neonates, staphylococci, enterobacteriaceae, group B *Streptococcus*, and *N. gonorrhoeae* are the most likely organisms. Injection drug abusers commonly develop staphylococcal or pseudomonal infections. Salmonella arthritis is more prevalent in patients with sickle cell disease than in the general population; however, more common organisms still predominate. Prosthetic joints or postoperative infections have high rates of *Staphylococcus aureus*, *Streptococcus epidermidis*, enterobacteriaceae, and pseudomonas.[11]

Although precise incidences for nongonococcal septic arthritis have not been established, predisposing factors have been described. These include age 80 years or older, diabetes mellitus, rheumatoid arthritis, hip and/or knee prosthesis, joint surgery, and skin infection.[12] The simultaneous occurrence of gout and septic arthritis is possible, and one should not allow the establishment of a diagnosis of crystal-induced disease to stop a thorough search for infection.[9,13]

Because *N. gonorrhoeae* is the most common organism causing septic arthritis, gonococcal arthritis deserves special mention. Disseminated gonococcal infection occurs in 0.5% to 3% of cases of mucosal infection. Gonococcal septic arthritis is more common in women, especially during pregnancy or after menstruation, because infected women are more likely to be asymptomatic. Time for local infection to disseminate can vary from several days to weeks. Patients will often experience systemic symptoms including fevers, chills, and malaise as well as migratory polyarthralgias. Tenosynovitis occurs in two thirds of patients. A dermatitis is also present in two thirds of patients (Fig. 53–3). The most common rash is scattered painless, nonpruritic 0.5- to 0.75-cm macules or papules with necrotic or pustular centers distributed on the extremities and trunk. Overt urethritis and vaginitis may be absent. Eventually, the infection settles into one or two large joints, yielding a purulent arthritis.[9,14]

Whereas *N. gonorrhoeae*–infected joint fluid is usually "septic" in character, the yield of positive synovial fluid cultures has ranged from 25% to 50%. Blood cultures appear to be less helpful, being positive in only 20% to 30% of cases. However, the organism can often be identified in genitourinary tract cultures,[9] and cultures from the primary mucosal site are positive in up to 80% of infected patients.[14] A positive Gram stain is immediately diagnostic of septic arthritis. Gram staining is positive in only 65% of cases of septic arthritis; therefore, a negative Gram stain does not rule out an infectious process. An elevated synovial white blood cell (WBC) count and a synovial fluid glucose reduction may give confirmatory data. However, the synovial fluid WBC count in gonococcal arthritis is often between 10,000 and 20,000 cells/

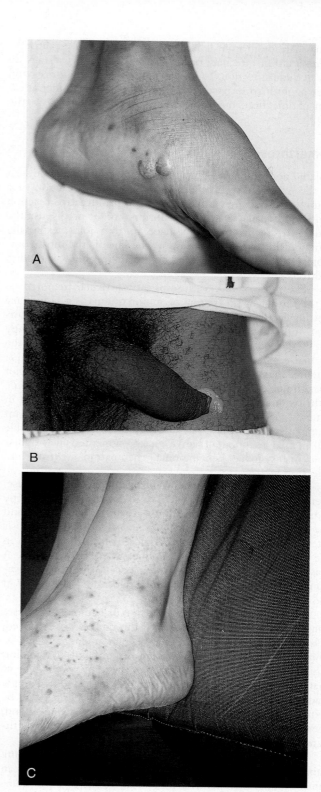

Figure 53–3 *A*, Often mistaken for insect/spider bites, these multiple embolic skin lesions, ranging from single or multiple petechiae to pustules, may be seen in patients with acutely swollen joints infected with *Neisseria gonorrhoeae*. Skin lesions are usually found on the extremities, especially the feet and hands, and may be present before a large joint effusion accumulates or with gonococcal tenosynovitis. *B*, Genital manifestation of urethritis/vaginitis may be seen, but can be rather clinically silent. *C*, Maculopapular rash of *N. gonorrhoeae*.

mm.[3,4] Although mild leukocytosis and elevated erythrocyte sedimentation rate may occur, normal laboratory values do not exclude infection.[14] Counterimmunoelectrophoresis and latex agglutination have shown promise for early identification of infection, but these have limited availability in the ED.[15]

Hemarthrosis

Isolated nontraumatic hemarthrosis may occasionally be seen by the emergency clinician. An inflammatory reaction may follow an intracapsular bleed, and the proliferative reaction and the hyperplastic synovium formed might predispose the patient to recurrent hemorrhage in that joint, especially patients with bleeding diatheses. The knee is the most commonly affected joint, followed by the ankle, elbow, shoulder, and hip.[1]

The most common cause of intra-articular hemorrhage in the setting of no trauma or minor trauma is a hereditary clotting factor deficiency such as hemophilia. Hemarthrosis is an infrequent complication of oral anticoagulant therapy but might occur even with prothrombin times within the normal range.[16] Cessation of anticoagulant therapy in these patients must be weighed against the risks of adverse clot formation (e.g., acute cerebrovascular accident). Chronic arthritis does not appear to be a long-term complication in patients with intra-articular bleeding from oral anticoagulant therapy. Hemarthrosis may also be a complication of sickle cell anemia, pseudogout, amyloidosis, pigmented villonodular synovitis, synovial hemangioma, rheumatoid arthritis, and infection.[17,18]

Management of acute hemarthrosis depends on the cause. Hemarthrosis associated with oral anticoagulant therapy improves only after the oral anticoagulant is discontinued and the prothrombin time returns to normal.[16,19] Hemarthrosis after trauma is a frequent occurrence. It is most common in the knee and often denotes significant internal damage. A massively swollen knee after trauma is seen with knee dislocation (occasionally with spontaneous relocation) and a tear of the anterior cruciate ligament.

Distension of the joint by effusion or hemorrhage causes considerable pain and disability. If the fluid is not removed, it is partially absorbed but part of it may undergo organization, resulting in formation of adhesions or bands in the joint. This is one argument for drainage of the joint.[2] Some believe that in an otherwise healthy joint that is subjected to a single traumatic event, even a relatively large hemarthrosis will be spontaneously reabsorbed without significant sequelae and, therefore, presents no pressing need to drain.[16,19] Unfortunately, little literature exists to guide the best approach.

Nonetheless, a large, tense, traumatic effusion is quite painful, and its presence precludes proper evaluation of an injured joint. Therapeutic arthrocentesis to drain a symptomatic traumatic effusion is a well-accepted practice.[2,20] The source of blood after trauma is frequently (1) a tear in a ligamentous structure, capsule, or synovium or (2) a fracture. Cruciate (especially anterior) ligament injury is the most common cause of significant hemarthrosis after trauma to the knee.[21] A joint effusion that develops 1 to 5 days after trauma may be secondary to a slow hemorrhage or reinjury, but the swelling is often caused by a nonhemorrhagic irritative synovial effusion.

Occasionally, one will diagnose an occult fracture by the presence of fat globules in the arthrocentesis specimen (see Fig. 53–17 later). This may be appreciated when the bloody effusion is placed in a clear container (e.g., test tube or specimen jar) and held to the light. If the history of trauma is vague, arthrocentesis may be required to differentiate hemorrhage from other causes of joint effusion. Following therapeutic arthrocentesis for a hemarthrosis, it may be desirable to inject 2 to 15 mL of a local anesthetic, depending on joint size, into the joint to facilitate examination or provide temporary symptomatic relief.[20]

Intra-articular Corticosteroid Injections

In 1951, Hollander and coworkers[22] first demonstrated that intra-articular corticosteroid injections are useful for symptomatic relief in patients with severe rheumatoid arthritis. The use of steroids has proved to be a dependable method for providing rapid relief from pain and swelling of inflamed joints, although it is strictly local, usually temporary, and rarely curative.[2,23,24] It is not commonly performed in the emergency setting. Acute gout responds well to joint injection, and this may be preferable in the patient who cannot tolerate indomethacin or colchicine.

Corticosteroid injections are most helpful when only a small number of joints are actively inflamed. The most frequently used corticosteroids for intra-articular injection are shown in Table 53–1.[2] Diminution of joint pain, swelling, effusion, and warmth is usually evident within 6 to 12 hours after injection.

Although very rare, the most serious complication of this practice is intra-articular infection.[2] Therefore, steroids should not be injected into a joint if there is suspicion of a joint space infection. Repeated injections into one joint carry the risk of necrosis of juxta-articular bone with subsequent joint destruction and instability and suppression of the hypothalamic-pituitary axis from systemic absorption. Other complications include local soft tissue atrophy and calcification, tendon rupture, intra-articular bleeding, and transient nerve palsy.[2,24] Transient elevations of blood glucose as well as erythema, warmth, and diaphoresis of the face and torso may also occur after intra-articular steroid injections. Deposition of steroid crystals on the synovium might give rise to a transient, self-limited flare-up of a synovitis.[2,25]

It is always important to determine whether local corticosteroid therapy has been used previously, not only to consider the array of clinical conditions associated with steroid

Preparation	Large-Joint Dose (mg)	Small-Joint Dose (mg)†
Triamcinolone hexacetonide	20	2–6
Triamcinolone acetonide	20	2–6
Prednisolone tebutate	25	2.5–7.5
Methylprednisolone acetate	40	3.5–10.5
Triamcinolone diacetate	20	2–6
Prednisolone acetate	30	3–9
Dexamethasone acetate	5	0.5–1.5

TABLE 53–1 Intrasynovial Corticosteroid Preparations*

*Listed in approximate descending order of duration of action.
†Dose will depend on joint size, capsular distensibility, and degree of inflammation.
From Gray RG, Gottlieb NL: Corticosteroid injections in RA: Appraisal of a neglected therapy. J Musculoskel Med 7:53, 1990. Reproduced by permission.

use but also because crystalline corticosteroid material can hinder proper interpretation of crystals found in synovial fluid.[25]

EQUIPMENT

Necessary materials for arthrocentesis include skin preparation solutions, sterile gloves and drapes, local or topical anesthetics, a syringe, and various-sized needles.

Depending upon the size of the effusion to be drained, a 10-, 20-, or 30 mL Luer-Lok syringe can be used. If a large effusion is suspected, a three-way stopcock between the needle and the syringe allows for complete drainage with a single joint penetration. Recently, a one-handed reciprocating syringe has been introduced for performing joint aspiration and injection (Fig. 53–4).[26] This syringe allows the index and middle fingers to remain in one position while the thumb moves to an alternating plunger to control the direction of aspiration or injection. Studies have shown that this syringe reduces unintended forward penetration and retraction and pain during the procedure.[27] It was also associated with increased clinician satisfaction, a decrease in the procedure duration, and a greater return of synovial fluid with fewer red blood cells.[26,27]

Fluid for cell count should be collected in a lavender-topped tube; however viscosity, protein, and glucose determinations do not require anticoagulants and should be placed in a red-topped tube. Although still common practice in many institutions, recent evidence suggests that synovial fluid protein and glucose levels are poor differentiators of noninflammatory versus inflammatory effusions and are no longer recommended (see "Synovial Fluid Interpretation," later).[2,28] Immediately examine fresh synovial fluid in its unadulterated form for crystals. Calcium oxalate and lithium heparin anticoagulants have been reported to introduce artifactual crystals into the fluid. Joint fluid to be analyzed for crystals should be collected in a green-topped tube containing sodium heparin. If culturing for *N. gonorrhoeae*, the fluid should be immediately placed on proper medium and stored in a low-oxygen environment in the ED.

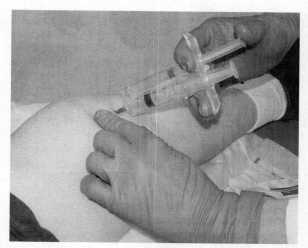

Figure 53–4 **Reciprocating syringe being used to aspirate the knee.** With this syringe, the operator depresses the smaller plunger (shown) to aspirate. If one wishes to inject the joint, the larger plunger would be depressed. *(With permission from Wilmer L. Sibbitt Jr., MD.)*

RADIOGRAPHIC APPLICATIONS

Conventional plain film radiography should be considered if there is suspicion of a fracture, dislocation or foreign body.[29] In addition, in patients with severe degenerative joint disease or ankylosis, plain films may improve the chances of successful arthrocentesis by better defining joint anatomy.[29]

Plain radiographs as well as computed tomography (CT) and magnetic resonance imaging (MRI) have been used to evaluate joint spaces for fluid accumulation.[29] Ultrasound is also an effective modality for identifying joint effusions.[30,31] In addition, ultrasound has been shown to facilitate proper needle placement for joint aspiration and may be more reliable than traditional palpation-guided technique[5,32,33] (see Chapter 67, Ultrasound-Guided Procedures).

GENERAL ARTHROCENTESIS TECHNIQUE

Joint fluid may be obtained even when there is little clinical evidence of an effusion. Although one may successfully aspirate where the joint bulges maximally, certain landmarks are important. The most crucial part of arthrocentesis is defining the joint anatomy by palpating the bony landmarks as a guide. A puncture site and an approach to the joint should be selected; tendons, major vessels, and major nerve branches should be avoided. In most instances, the approach is via the extensor surfaces of joints because most major vessels and nerves are found beneath flexor surfaces. Also, the synovial pouch is usually more superficial on the extensor side of a joint. Ultrasound may be particularly helpful in locating small effusions.

Aseptic technique, including the use of sterile gloves and instruments, is essential to avoid infection. Arthrocentesis should not be attempted if there is a definite or suspected infection overlying the joint. Antiseptic preparation solution should be allowed to dry for several minutes because the bactericidal effects of iodine are both concentration and time dependent. Iodine solution is then removed with an alcohol sponge to prevent transference of iodine into the joint space with a resultant inflammatory process. Although the utility of draping is unproved and may obscure the site, a sterile perforated drape may be placed over the joint.

With appropriate local anesthesia, arthrocentesis should be a relatively painless procedure; without anesthesia, it may be quite painful and distressing to the patient. The synovial membrane itself has pain fibers associated with blood vessels, and the articular capsule and periosteum are richly supplied with nerve fibers and are very sensitive. The articular cartilage has no intrinsic pain fibers. It is important to have the patient relax during the procedure. Tense muscles narrow the joint space and make the procedure more difficult, requiring repeated attempts at aspiration, or result in inadequate drainage. Distraction of the joint may enhance the target area, especially in areas such as the wrist and finger joints. Traction not only increases the chance of entering the joint but also lessens the chance of scoring the articular cartilage with the needle.

Anesthesia is best accomplished by infiltrating the skin *down to the area of the joint capsule along the entire route of needle penetration*, using a local anesthetic agent such as 1% or 2% lidocaine (Xylocaine) with a 25- to 27-gauge needle. For extremely painful joints, a regional nerve block is appropriate.

The landmarks described in "Specific Arthrocentesis Techniques," later in this chapter, should be used and care should be taken not to bounce the needle off bony structures as a means of finding the joint space because this may cause unnecessary pain. However, in contrast to earlier beliefs, striking bone with the arthrocentesis needle is unlikely to damage articular cartilage.[2] An 18- to 22-gauge needle or intravenous catheter and needle set of appropriate length attached to a syringe is inserted at the desired anatomic point through the skin and subcutaneous tissue into the joint space. The largest needle that is practical is used to avoid obstructing the lumen with debris or clot. In large joints such as the knee, which can accommodate large effusions, it is suggested that one use a 30- to 60-mL syringe because it may be difficult to change a syringe when the needle is within the joint cavity (Fig. 53–5). A three-way stopcock placed between the needle and the syringe is an option for draining large effusions. If the syringe must be changed during the procedure, the hub of the needle should be grasped with a hemostat and held tightly while the syringe is removed. If an intravenous catheter and needle set is used, the needle is removed, leaving the outer atraumatic plastic catheter in the joint space. The syringe is then attached to the catheter for aspiration. Now manipulation of the joint or catheter can occur with little threat of tissue injury.

Aspiration of synovial fluid and the easy injection and return of fluid indicate intra-articular placement of the needle tip. As a general rule, *one should try to remove as much fluid or blood as possible*. If the fluid stops flowing, it indicates that the joint has been drained completely, the needle tip has become dislodged, or debris or clot is obstructing the needle. One should slightly advance or retract the tip of the needle, rotate the bevel, or lessen the force of aspiration. One should never *reintroduce* a needle through a plastic catheter that has been left in the joint. Occasionally, reinjecting a small amount of fluid into the joint space confirms the needle placement and may clear the needle. If fluid flows freely back into the joint and is easily reaspirated, one has probably removed all the fluid. If resistance is met, the needle has probably been jarred from the joint space and is lodged in the soft tissue. In some instances, minor position changes produced by flexion or extension of the joint may allow the fluid to flow more freely. Scraping or shearing the articular cartilage with the needle should be avoided. One should enter the joint in a straight line and avoid unnecessary side-to-side motion of the needle.

Synovial fluid should be sent for studies as indicated by the clinical situation. Studies usually obtained include cell count with differential, crystal analysis, Gram staining, and bacterial culture and sensitivity analysis. Synovial protein,

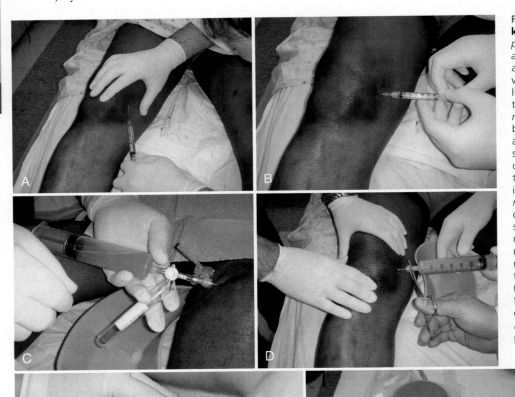

Figure 53–5 Arthrocentesis of the knee. Note that an assistant *applies palm pressure on the suprapatellar areas* to milk fluid into the joint to assist entry and aspiration. *A,* Raise a wheal with local anesthetic (1% lidocaine). *B,* Inject anesthetic along the *entire tract of the aspiration needle*. *C,* Always use a large syringe but if the syringe is too small to accommodate all of the fluid, a stopcock will negate the need to change the syringe. Turn the stopcock to collect and then expel fluid, or inject lidocaine or steroid *without moving the needle*. *D,* An assistant continually applies *pressure*. If the syringe needs to be changed to collect more fluid or inject steroid, grasp the needle hub with a hemostat and remove the syringe without disturbing the correct position of the needle (inset). *E,* Cloudy fluid such as this is from an inflammatory source; in this case, it was acute gouty arthritis. Always remove as much fluid as possible.

glucose, and lactate dehydrogenase determinations have been shown to be unreliable in distinguishing noninflammatory from inflammatory and infectious etiologies and are no longer recommended.[2,28] Less frequently obtained studies include rheumatoid factor analysis, lupus erythematosus cell preparation, viscosity analysis, mucin clot, fibrin clot, fungal and acid-fast stains, Lyme titer, fungal and tuberculous culture, and synovial fluid complement analysis. If the arthrocentesis is performed for the relief of a hemarthrosis, the fluid need not be sent for analysis. One should be selective in ordering tests. There is no need to order a large battery of tests routinely on all fluids. If the volume of fluid collected is low, Gram stain, culture, and examination of the "wet preparation" under regular and polarizing microscopy have the highest priority. Prompt examination of specimens should be performed to avoid misdiagnosing borderline inflammatory fluids, missing crystals that dissolve with time, or overinterpreting the findings because of new artifactual crystals that appear over a prolonged time.[34]

COMPLICATIONS

Significant complications are rare with arthrocentesis and include:

1. *Infection.* Skin bacteria may be introduced into the joint space during needle puncture. Nevertheless, infection rarely occurs because the bacteria are either quickly cleared or not viable.[2] One can further limit this complication by maintaining rigorous sterile technique and avoiding inserting the needle through obviously (or possibly) infected skin or subcutaneous tissue. Various studies report the incidence of infection after routine arthrocentesis to be in the range of 1/10,000.[35] However, in immunocompromised patients, particularly those with rheumatoid arthritis, the incidence is higher (1/2000 to 1/10,000 aspirations).[36] Joint aspiration in the presence of bacteremia was discussed previously.

2. *Bleeding.* Bleeding with subsequent hemarthrosis is rarely a complication, except in the patient with a bleeding diathesis. In patients with a bleeding diathesis, such as hemophilia, arthrocentesis should be delayed until clotting competence has been enhanced by infusing specific clotting factors. In general, spontaneous bleeding into a hemophiliac's joint is an indication for replacement of clotting factors. Occasionally, a small quantity of blood may be aspirated along with the synovial fluid. This happens most often when the joint is nearly emptied. A small amount of blood-tinged fluid is generally the result of nicking a small synovial blood vessel; this is usually inconsequential.

3. *Allergic reaction.* Hypersensitivity to the local anesthetic can usually be prevented by thorough history taking. Facial and torso flushing associated with corticosteroid injection may represent and idiosyncratic reaction to preservatives in the steroid preparation.[2] Fainting during the procedure is not uncommon and most often the result of vasovagal influences.

4. *Corticosteroid-induced complications.* See "Intra-articular Corticosteroid Injections," earlier.

SPECIFIC ARTHROCENTESIS TECHNIQUES

Arthrocentesis of the hip is generally performed by an orthopedic surgeon under fluoroscopic, ultrasound, MRI, or CT guidance and is not discussed here. If available, fluoroscopy

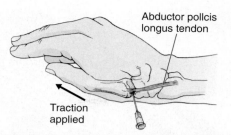

Figure 53–6 Landmarks for arthrocentesis of the first carpometacarpal joint (see text). *(From Akins CM: Aspiration and injection of joints, bursae, and tendons. In Vander Salm TJ, Cutler BS, Wheeler HB [eds]: Atlas of Bedside Procedures. Boston, Little, Brown, 1979. Reproduced by permission.)*

or ultrasound can also be used to guide aspiration of other joints, but these imaging adjuncts are generally not required. For small joints, *applying traction* is often very helpful in obtaining fluid.

First Carpometacarpal Joint (Fig. 53–6)

Landmarks. The radial aspect of the proximal end of the first metacarpal is the arthrocentesis landmark for this joint. The abductor pollicis longus (APL) tendon is located by active extension of the tendon.

Position. Oppose the thumb against the little finger so that the proximal end of the first metacarpal is palpable. *Apply traction to the thumb* in order to widen the joint space between the first metacarpal and the greater multangular bone.

Needle Insertion. Insert a 22- to 23-gauge needle at a point proximal to the prominence at the base of the first metacarpal, on the palmar side of the APL tendon.

Comments. Degenerative joint disease commonly affects this joint. Arthrocentesis is moderately difficult. The anatomic "snuffbox" (located more proximally and on the dorsal side of the APL tendon) should be avoided, because it contains the radial artery and superficial radial nerve. A more dorsal approach may also be used.

Interphalangeal and Metacarpophalangeal Joints (Fig. 53–7)

Landmarks. The landmarks are on the dorsal surface. For the metacarpophalangeal joints, palpate for the prominence at the proximal end of the proximal phalanx. For the interphalangeal joints, palpate for the prominence at the proximal end of the middle or distal phalanx. The extensor tendon runs down the midline.

Position. Flex the fingers to approximately 15° to 20° and *apply traction.*

Needle Insertion. Insert a 22- to 25-gauge needle into the joint space dorsally, just medial or lateral to the central slip of the extensor tendon.

Comments. Synovitis causes these joints to bulge dorsally. Normally, it is unusual to obtain fluid in the absence of a significant pathologic condition.

Radiocarpal Joint (Wrist) (Fig. 53–8)

Landmarks. The dorsal radial tubercle (Lister's tubercle) is an elevation found in the center of the dorsal aspect of the distal end of the radius. The extensor pollicis longus

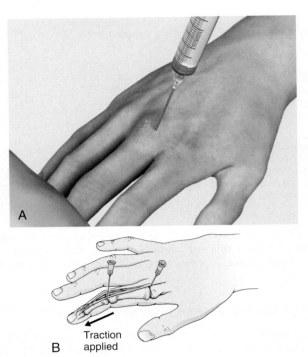

Figure 53–7 *A and B,* Landmarks for arthrocentesis of the interphalangeal and metacarpophalangeal joints (see text). *(A, From Thomsen T, Setnik G [eds]: Procedures Consult—Emergency Medicine Module. Copyright 2008 Elsevier Inc. All rights reserved; B, from Akins CM: Aspiration and injection of joints, bursae, and tendons. In Vander Salm TJ, Cutler BS, Wheeler HB [eds]: Atlas of Bedside Procedures. Boston, Little, Brown, 1979. Reproduced by permission.)*

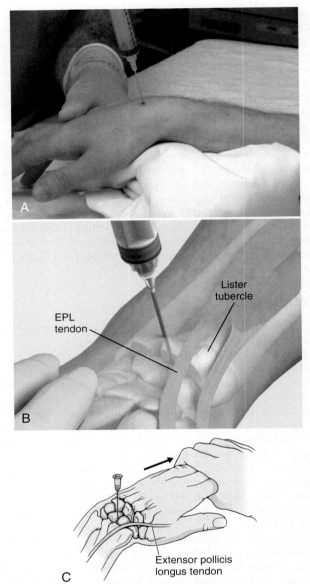

Figure 53–8 *A and B,* Landmarks for arthrocentesis of the radiocarpal (wrist) joint. C, Traction is applied with slight flexion. Minimal to *no* radial deviation is applied. *(A and B, From Thomsen T, Setnik G [eds]: Procedures Consult—Emergency Medicine Module. Copyright 2008 Elsevier Inc. All rights reserved.)*

tendon runs in a groove on the radial side of the tubercle. The tendon can be palpated by active extension of the wrist and thumb.

Position. Position the wrist in approximately 20° to 30° of flexion with accompanying ulnar deviation. *Apply traction to the hand.*

Needle Insertion. Insert a 22-gauge needle dorsally, just distal to the dorsal tubercle on the ulnar side of the extensor pollicis longus tendon. The anatomic snuffbox, located more radially, should be avoided to prevent injury to the radial artery or superficial radial nerve.

Radiohumeral Joint (Elbow) (Fig. 53–9)

Landmarks. The lateral epicondyle of the humerus and the head of the radius are the arthrocentesis landmarks for the radiohumeral joint. With the elbow extended, palpate the depression between the radial head and the lateral epicondyle of the humerus.

Position. With the palpating finger still touching the radial head, flex the elbow to 90°. Pronate the forearm, and place the palm flat on a table.

Needle Insertion. Insert a 20-gauge needle from the lateral aspect just distal to the lateral epicondyle and directed medially.

Comments. Elevation of the anterior fat pad, or the presence of a posterior fat pad, on a lateral soft tissue elbow radiograph signifies blood, pus, or fluid in the elbow joint (see Fig. 53–9*A*). Effusions in the elbow joint may bulge and be readily palpated (see Fig. 53–9*B* and *C*). Often, the effusion appears inferior to the lateral epicondyle. The bulge can then

be aspirated from a posterior approach on the lateral side (see Fig. 53–9*D*). A medial approach is not recommended because the ulnar nerve and the superior ulnar collateral artery may be damaged. Gout and septic arthritis commonly affect this joint. The most common cause of an elbow hemarthrosis after trauma with no obvious fracture is a nondisplaced radial head fracture. A small hemarthrosis need not be aspirated, but removal of blood from a tense elbow joint will significantly hasten recovery and facilitate range of motion in patients with a radial head fracture.

Glenohumeral Joint (Shoulder), Anterior Approach (Fig. 53–10)

Landmarks. Anteriorly palpate the coracoid process medially and the proximal humerus laterally.

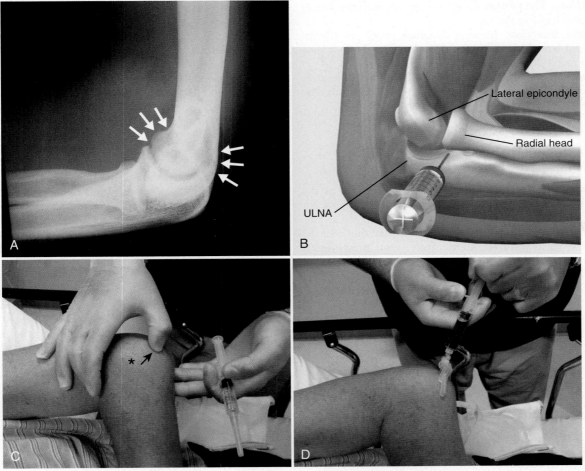

Figure 53–9 *A,* On a lateral elbow radiograph, displacement of the anterior fat pad (*arrows*) or the presence of a posterior fat pad (*arrows*) indicate blood, pus, or fluid in the joint. *B,* Landmarks for arthrocentesis of the radiohumeral joint. *C,* An effusion in the elbow joint can usually be readily palpated. A palpating finger is placed over the lateral epicondyle (*) and slid posteriorly/inferiorly toward the olecranon (*arrow*). Usually, a depression is felt as the finger leaves the epicondyle, but a bulge is appreciated if there is a joint effusion. *D,* Removal of only a few milliliters of blood will reduce pain and hasten recovery of the range of motion. The most common pathology after trauma with an x-ray negative for fracture, but positive for a hemarthosis, is a nondisplaced radial head fracture. (*A, From Akins CM: Aspiration and injection of joints, bursae, and tendons. In Vander Salm TJ, Cutler BS, Wheeler HB [eds]: Atlas of Bedside Procedures. Boston, Little, Brown, 1979. Reproduced by permission; B, from Thomsen T, Setnik G [eds]: Procedures Consult—Emergency Medicine Module.Copyright 2008 Elsevier Inc. All rights reserved.*)

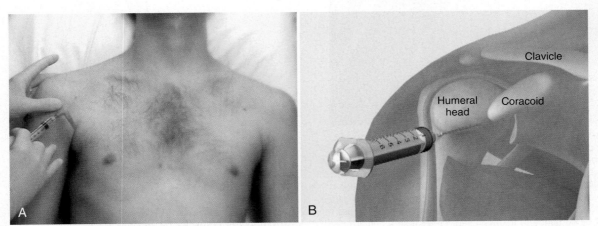

Figure 53–10 *A and B,* Landmarks for arthrocentesis of the glenohumeral (shoulder) joint *(A and B, From Thomsen T, Setnik G [eds]: Procedures Consult—Emergency Medicine Module.Copyright 2008 Elsevier Inc. All rights reserved.)*

Position. The patient should sit upright with the arm at the side and hand in the lap.

Needle Insertion. Insert a 20-gauge needle at a point inferior and lateral to the coracoid process and direct it posteriorly toward the glenoid rim.

Comments. Arthrocentesis of this joint is moderately difficult. Other approaches have been suggested but are less well accepted.

Knee Joint, Anteromedial Approach (Fig. 53–11*A*)

Landmarks. The medial surface of the patella at the middle or superior portion of the patella is the landmark for the knee joint.

Position. It is usually recommended that the knee be extended as far as possible. Alternatively, some practitioners prefer to flex the knee 15° to 20° by placing a towel under the popliteal region in order to open up the joint space. Relaxation of the quadriceps muscle greatly facilitates needle placement. Keep the foot perpendicular to the floor.

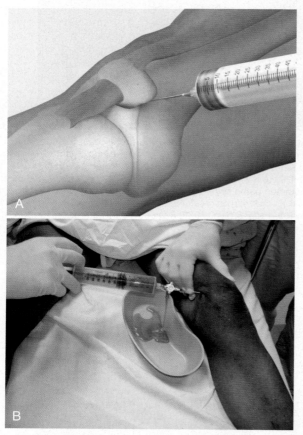

Figure 53–11 *A,* Landmarks for arthrocentesis of the knee joint, medial approach. *B,* Note the use of a stopcock on the syringe to allow complete drainage without repositioning the needle. Note that the syringe is held parallel to the table. *Compression of the suprapatellar region by the operator or an assistant will facilitate complete aspiration.* For the knee, a 60-mL syringe and an 18-gauge needle should be used to drain large effusions. Note that the red streaks of blood denote a traumatic tap, rather than a hemarthrosis. The blood streaks started after clear fluid had been withdrawn. (*A, From Thomsen T, Setnik G [eds]: Procedures Consult—Emergency Medicine Module. Copyright 2008 Elsevier Inc. All rights reserved.*)

Needle Insertion. Insert an 18-gauge needle or catheter and needle set at the midpoint or superior portion of the patella approximately 1 cm medial to the anteromedial patellar edge. Direct the needle between the posterior surface of the patella and the intercondylar femoral notch. The patella may be grasped with the hand and elevated to aid needle entry into the joint. *Keeping the needle/syringe parallel to the bed limits internal injury.*

Comments. If the patient is tense, contraction of the quadriceps will greatly hinder entering the joint. However, the knee is probably the easiest joint to enter and removal of a tense hemarthrosis will relieve pain and facilitate examination for ligamentous injury. If fluid stops flowing, the operator or assistant should squeeze the soft tissue area of the suprapatellar region to "milk" the suprapatellar pouch of fluid (see Fig. 53–11*B*). Alternatively, wrap the patient's thigh with a 6-inch elastic bandage from the groin to the suprapatellar area before beginning the procedure. The knee can easily accommodate 50 to 70 mL of fluid, and the clinician should therefore use a large syringe. Holding/securing the hub of the needle with a hemostat allows the clinician to remove the syringe without changing the position of the intra-articular needle. Alternatively, a stopcock on the needle will allow for complete removal of fluid without changing the position of the needle. The knee is a common site for septic arthritis (especially gonococcal) and various inflammatory or degenerative diseases. An anterolateral approach can be accomplished in a similar manner.

Tibiotalar Joint (Ankle) (Fig. 53–12)

Landmarks. The medial malleolar sulcus is bordered medially by the medial malleolus and laterally by the anterior tibial tendon. The tendon can be easily identified by active dorsiflexion of the foot.

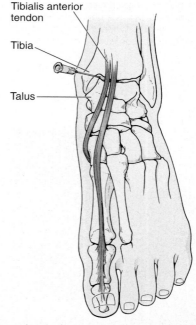

Tibialis anterior tendon

Tibia

Talus

Figure 53–12 Landmarks for arthrocentesis of the tibiotalar joint. (*From Akins CM: Aspiration and injection of joints, bursae, and tendons. In Vander Salm TJ, Cutler BS, Wheeler HB [eds]: Atlas of Bedside Procedures. Boston, Little, Brown, 1979. Reproduced by permission.*)

Position. With the patient lying supine, plantar flex the foot.

Needle Insertion. Insert a 20- to 22-gauge needle at a point just medial to the anterior tibial tendon and directed into the hollow at the anterior edge of the medial malleolus. The needle must be inserted 2 to 3 cm to penetrate the joint space.

Comments. If the joint bulges medially, one may use an approach that is more medial than anterior, entering at a point just anterior to the medial malleolus. The needle may have to be advanced 2 to 4 cm with this approach.

Metatarsophalangeal and Interphalangeal Joints (Fig. 53–13)

Landmarks. For the first digit, landmarks are the distal metatarsal head and the proximal base of the first phalanx. For the other toes, the landmarks are the prominences at the proximal interphalangeal and distal interphalangeal joints. The extensor tendon of the great toe can be located by active extension of the toe.

Position. With the patient supine, flex the toes 15° to 20°. *Then apply traction.*

Needle Insertion. Insert a 22-gauge needle on the dorsal surface at a point just medial or lateral to the central slip of the extensor tendon.

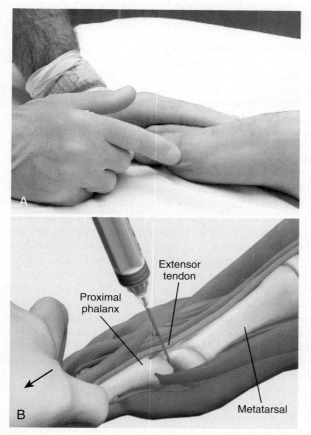

Figure 53–13 *A* and *B*, Landmarks for metatarsophalangeal and interphalangeal joints. Note that traction on the first toe aids aspiration. *(From Thomsen, Todd & Gary Setnik. [eds.] Procedures Consult – Emergency Medicine Module.*Copyright 2008 Elsevier Inc. All rights reserved.)*

SYNOVIAL FLUID INTERPRETATION

Synovial fluid examination is essential for the diagnosis of septic arthritis, gout, and pseudogout. Inflammatory joint disease of previously unknown etiology can often be diagnosed precisely by synovial fluid analysis. Joint fluid is a dialysate of plasma that contains protein and hyaluronic acid. Normal fluid is clear enough to read newsprint through and will not clot. It is straw-colored and flows freely, with the consistency of machine oil. Normal fluid produces a good mucin clot and gives a positive "string sign" (see next section). The uric acid level of joint fluid approaches that of serum, and the glucose concentration is normally at least 80% that of serum. Clarity of fluid reflects the leukocyte count. High leukocyte counts result in opacity, the degree of which generally correlates with the degree of elevated synovial fluid leukocytes. However, the degree of opacity cannot be used to reliably determine the synovial fluid leukocyte count and should not be used as a surrogate for laboratory cell count measurements.

String Sign

Viscosity correlates with the concentration of hyaluronate in the synovial fluid. Any inflammation degrades hyaluronate, characteristically resulting in low-viscosity synovial fluid. The string sign is a simple test for assessing viscosity. The practitioner measures the length of the "string" formed by a falling drop extruded from a syringe of synovial fluid or stretched between the thumb and the index finger of a gloved hand. Normal joint fluid produces a string of 5 to 10 cm (Fig. 53–14). If viscosity is reduced, as in inflammatory conditions, the synovial fluid forms a shorter string or falls in drops.

Mucin Clot Test

The mucin clot test also corresponds to viscosity and inflammation. The greater the inflammatory response, the poorer the mucin clot and the lower the viscosity. This test may be useful to define the degree of polymerization of hyaluronate. Mucin clots are produced by mixing 1 part joint fluid with 4 parts 2% acetic acid. A good clot indicates a high degree of polymerization and correlates with normal high viscosity. In inflammatory synovial fluid, such as that seen in osteoarthritis and rheumatoid arthritis–related effusions, the mucin clot is poor. This test is rarely performed.

Cell Count

A leukocytosis consisting predominantly of neutrophils is usually seen with inflammatory arthritides; a WBC count greater than 50,000/mm³ (i.e., >50,000/μL) is highly suggestive of a septic joint. Shmerling and colleagues[37] found a WBC count of greater than 2000/mm³ to be 84% sensitive and 84% specific for *all* inflammatory arthritides. Of their septic arthritis patients, 37% had a synovial WBC count less than 50,000/mm³. However, 89% of their patients with a synovial WBC count greater than 50,000/mm³ had a septic joint.[37]

Glucose and Protein

Recent literature suggests that synovial protein and glucose are highly inaccurate markers of inflammation.[2,28] In one

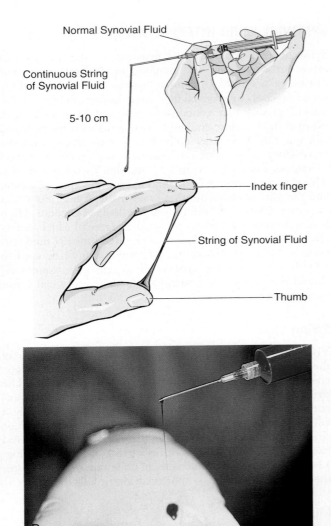

Normal Synovial Fluid

Continuous String
of Synovial Fluid

5-10 cm

Index finger

String of Synovial Fluid

Thumb

B

Figure 53–14 *A*, Ability of normal synovial fluid to form a long tenacious string. (*Note*: Gloves should be worn during the procedure.) *B*, Bloody joint fluid from recent trauma forms a normal string sign.

study of 100 consecutive patients undergoing diagnostic arthrocentesis, the sensitivity of synovial protein and glucose were found to be 0.52 and 0.20, respectively.[37] The authors of this study recommended that ordering chemistry studies on synovial fluid should be discouraged because these are likely to provide misleading or redundant informatuion.

Serology

Although available, most of the serologic tests are not likely to be useful in the emergency setting. Polymerase chain reaction (PCR) is an effective means of identifying septic arthritis, even in the setting of a negative fluid culture or when antibiotics have been administered previously.[28] PCR can also help isolate slow-growing microorganisms. Gas-liquid chromatography, a rapid and sensitive method for detection of short-chain fatty acids, may complement the currently available methods used to diagnose septic arthritis.[38]

Counterimmunoelectrophoresis and latex agglutination are also useful and available in some centers on an emergency

basis. Other immunologic markers such as complement, rheumatoid factor, and antinuclear antibodies have little diagnostic value in the acute setting but may be useful to the clinician providing follow-up care when compared to serum levels.

Fluid Processing

Proper collection of the joint fluid is essential for examination and testing. Tests for viscosity, serology, and chemistries are done on fluid collected in a red-topped (clot) tube, whereas cytology samples are collected in tubes with an anticoagulant (purple top). One should always transfer the fluid for crystal examination into a tube with liquid heparin (green top) because undissolved heparin crystals from powdered anticoagulant tubes can be seen on microscopy. Early transfer of synovial fluid to this green-topped tube is essential to prevent clotting. Culture requirements for transport and processing should be accessed before the procedure to ensure appropriate processing or plating of specimens.

Polarizing Microscope

No synovial fluid analysis is complete until the fluid has been examined under a polarizing light microscope for crystals. The polarizing microscope used for crystal identification differs from the ordinary light microscope because it contains two identical polarizing prisms or filters. One filter, called the *polarizer*, is positioned below the condenser. The other filter is called the *analyzer* and is inserted at some point above the objective. Examination for crystals is performed by most hospital laboratories.

Polarization Physics
The polarizer allows passage of light in only one specific orientation. The analyzer acts as a crossed filter, removing all light in the light path unless the material being examined rotates the beam from the polarizer into the plane of the analyzer. The compensator functions by imparting color of a certain wavelength (red at about 550 nm). Birefringent materials change the wavelength to blue or yellow, depending on the direction (negative or positive) of refringence.

Microscopic Analysis
When examining crystals under polarized microscopy, the technician orients crystals on a stage according to two axes, referred to as X and Z. If the long axis of the crystals is blue when parallel to the Z-axis and yellow when perpendicular to it, it is calcium pyrophosphate and termed *positively birefringent*. If the long axis of the crystal is yellow when parallel to the Z-axis and blue when perpendicular to it, it is monosodium urate and termed *negatively birefringent*. Urate crystals are 2 to 10 μm and usually needle-shaped. Calcium pyrophosphate crystals range from 10 μm down to tiny crystals that have to be examined with the oil objective; they appear as rods, rhomboids, plates, or needle-like forms and are weakly birefringent. Cholesterol crystals are sometimes seen and are large, very bright, square, or rectangular plates with broken corners.[39]

Items found in synovial fluid that can be confused with sodium urate (Fig. 53–15) or calcium pyrophosphate crystals (Fig. 53–16) include collagen fibrils, cartilage fragments, cholesterol crystals, metallic fragments from prosthetic arthroplasty, and corticosteroid esters.[38] One may also identify fat globules (Fig. 53–17). Note that rare cases of uric acid spheru-

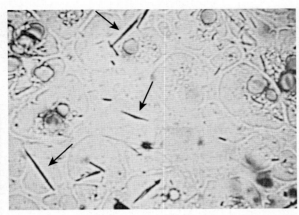

Figure 53–15 Synovial fluid with needle-shaped uric acid crystals (*arrows*). Many crystals are characteristically engulfed by leukocytes. (*From Schumacher HR, Finkinson CA, Weiss JJ: Guidelines for obtaining and analyzing synovial fluid. ER Reports 4:40, 1983. Reproduced by permission.*)

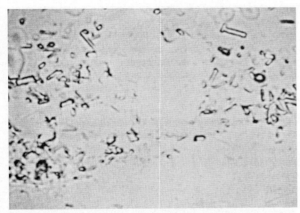

Figure 53–16 Synovial fluid with calcium pyrophosphate crystals. (*From Schumacher HR, Finkinson CA, Weiss JJ: Guidelines for obtaining and analyzing synovial fluid. ER Reports 4:40, 1983. Reproduced by permission.*)

lites in gouty synovia have been reported.[40] The spherulites are birefringent and do not take up fat stains.

Table 53–2 summarizes synovial fluid features for the joint diseases commonly encountered and studies commonly performed in the ED.

JOINT ARTHROGRAMS

Background

Wounds near joints raise concerns regarding joint penetration. Treatment and interventions may be significantly altered if a joint space has been traumatically violated. Plain radiographs may demonstrate air in the joint, clinching the diagnosis, but for questionable cases, the diagnostic approach includes injection arthrograms. Historically, these were performed by injecting methylene blue into the joint in question and assessing leakage from the joint. However, the dye can interfere with arthroscopic evaluation and produce an inflammatory reaction, so a saline arthrogram is now preferred. Saline arthrograms (SAs) or a "saline load test," were first described in 1975, but became more popular in the 1990s.

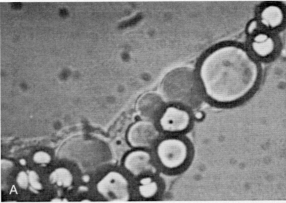

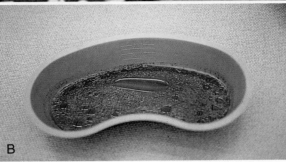

Figure 53–17 Microscopic (*A*) and gross (*B*) appearance of fat globules in synovial fluid. This finding suggests a fracture extending into the joint. (*A, From Schumacher HR, Finkinson CA, Weiss JJ: Guidelines for obtaining and analyzing synovial fluid. ER Reports 4:40, 1983. Reproduced by permission.*)

983

Indications and Contraindications

SA should be performed in patients with penetrating injuries near a joint in which violation of the joint itself is unclear (Fig. 53–18). Smaller joints such as those of the hand are visually inspected. However, for larger joints, an SA is the preferred test.

Contraindications to performing an SA are essentially the same as for performing arthrocentesis. When indicated, underlying fracture of the joint should first be ruled out. An obvious open fracture would preclude the need to perform an SA.

Equipment and Procedure

Aseptic technique is essential, but the equipment and procedure are essentially the same as for performing an arthrocentesis, with minor differences. First, a source of sterile saline is required (e.g., a small bag of intravenous fluid). Second, larger joints require more saline infusion, and this is most easily performed if a stopcock is used to allow refill of the syringe (Fig. 53–19).

Because saline is not as viscous as joint fluid, a 20-gauge needle is sufficient. Once the joint space has been reliably entered, a variable amount of saline, to "load" that joint, is slowly injected. The amount of saline injected varies with the size of the joint. In general, a *sufficient volume should be injected to visibly distend the joint or create injection resistance and cause patient discomfort*. The sensitivity of the test to detect small traumatic joint injuries is proportional to the volume injected. Specifically, for knee injuries, injecting 50 mL of saline was

TABLE 53–2 Characteristics of Synovial Fluid

	Appearance	Viscosity	Cells per mm³	PMN (%)	Crystals
Normal	Transparent	High	<180	<10	Negative
Osteoarthritis	Transparent	High	200–2000	<10	Occasional calcium pyrophospate and hydroxyapatite crystals
Rheumatoid arthritis	Translucent	Low	2000–50,000	Variable	Negative
Psoriatic arthritis	Translucent	Low	2000–50,000	Variable	Negative
Reactive arthritis	Translucent	Low	2000–50,000	Variable	Negative
Spondyloarthropathy	Translucent	Low	2000–50,000	Variable	Negative
Gout	Translucent to cloudy	Low	200 to >50,000	>90	Needle-shaped, positive birefringent monosodium urate monohydrate crystals
Pseudogout	Translucent to cloudy	Low	200–50,000	>90	Rhomboid, negative birefringent calcium pyrophosphate crystals
Bacterial arthritis	Cloudy	Variable	2000 to >50,000	>90	Negative
PVNS	Hemorrhagic or brown	Low			Negative
Hemarthrosis	Hemorrhagic	Low			Negative

PMN, polymorphic nuclear cell; PVNS, pigmented villonodular synovitis.
Adapted from Harris ED, Budd RC, Genovese MC, et al (eds): Kelley's Textbook of Rheumatology, 7th ed., Section VI, Table 46–1. Philadelphia, Elsevier, 2005.

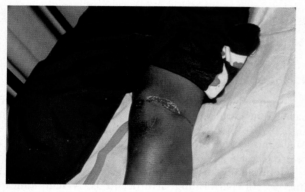

Figure 53–18 This periarticular laceration raises the question of knee joint penetration. A plain radiograph may demonstrate air in the joint space, but a saline arthrogram may also be used. Methylene blue alone is not generally required and it can cause an inflammatory reaction and obscure arthroscopy. A small amount of methylene blue may be added to color saline.

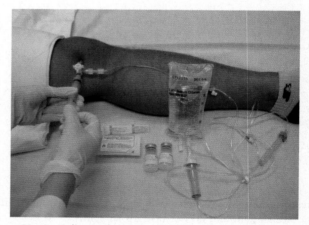

Figure 53–19 Saline arthrogram. Using a stopcock and a 18-gauge needle, enter the joint in a manner identical to that for arthrocentesis. Note that a bag of intravenous saline, or additional vials of saline, introduced into the syringe may be required to provide enough saline to distend the joint properly. Unless the joint is markedly distended, a false-negative test may result. When completed, drain the injected saline via the original needle. A positive test is saline egress into the original wound or a slow loss of saline from the joint. A small amount of methylene blue may be added to the saline.

46% sensitive; injecting 100 mL, 75% sensitive; to achieve 95% sensitivity required an average of 194 mL of saline.[41,42]

The recommended volume of injection per joint is

- Knee—100–200 mL
- Elbow—20–30 mL
- Ankle—20–30 mL
- Wrist—5 mL
- Shoulder—40–60 mL

Once the injection is complete, do not remove the needle, but close the stopcock to avoid backflow. Examine the joint for evidence for leakage of fluid from the wound. This is performed in a static position, but if negative, also with some gentle passive movement of the joint. Visible leakage of fluid into the laceration confirms the diagnosis of joint space violation. A negative test is defined as absence of evidence of leakage after an appropriate amount of saline has been injected. A slow loss of fluid may indicate a small insult to the joint, and saline can be left in the joint for a few minutes to observe for this. After completion, the fluid should be evacuated for patient comfort. This is generally performed by leaving the original needle in place with a closed stopcock attached, which is then used to aspirate joint saline.

Complications

Complications associated with performing SAs are essentially the same as those for performing arthrocentesis. In addition, some temporary patient discomfort should be assumed, due to joint distention.

Conclusion

Small traumatic joint penetration can be difficult to diagnose clinically. The SA test can help confirm the diagnosis. To be a sensitive test, it must be performed using an adequate amount of saline infusion to truly "load" the joint. If the test is positive, orthopedic consultation is indicated.

 REFERENCES CAN BE FOUND ON EXPERT CONSULT

CHAPTER 54

Compartment Syndrome Evaluation

Merle A. Carter

Open fractures, dislocations, and exposed joints are true orthopaedic emergencies that must be managed aggressively to prevent morbidity and mortality. Even when managed appropriately, these injuries may be further complicated by compartment syndrome, a condition of increased pressure within a limited space resulting in compromised tissue perfusion and, ultimately, dysfunction of neural and muscular structures contained within that space.[1] The magnitude of the trauma is usually significant, but compartment syndrome may also develop after seemingly minor injuries, prolonged proximal arterial occlusion, or prolonged external pressure in the absence of acute injury.

Causes of compartment syndrome are categorized into those that decrease compartment volume capacity, those that increase compartment contents, and those that create externally applied pressure[1] (Table 54–1). Subtleties in the early presentation of compartment syndrome or other clinical priorities render some cases *simply impossible to recognize and treat early enough to thwart ultimate disability*. This is particularly true in uncooperative, comatose, or critically injured patients. Unfortunately, the vagaries of the clinical scenario result in failure to recognize the early signs and symptoms of compartment syndrome might have severe and irreversible limb- or life-threatening consequences.

Numerous drugs and toxins have been reported to cause rhabdomyolysis, possibly owing to a direct effect or secondary to agitation and exertion, with *the theoretical potential* for the development of compartment syndrome (Fig. 54–1). This list is exhaustive but includes heroin, various hydrocarbons, cocaine, amphetamines, antidepressants, antipsychotics, salicylates, propoxyphene, nonsteroidal anti-inflammatory drugs (NSAIDs), succinylcholine, human immunodeficiency virus (HIV) medications, antimetabolites/cancer drugs, antimalarials, diphenhydramine, baclofen, ecstasy, ethanol, anticoagulants/thrombolytics, strychnine, statins, and phenothiazines.[2,3]

Although compartment syndrome is essentially a clinical diagnosis, objective measurement of compartment tissue pressure may help confirm the diagnosis and determine whether operative treatment is required. This chapter discusses the indications, complications, and interpretation of compartment pressure monitoring. The equipment and techniques required to perform compartment pressure monitoring are described.

BACKGROUND

Although recognized as a clinical syndrome in the mid-19th century, the pathophysiology of extremity ischemia was not fully described until more than a century later. Postischemic myoneural dysfunction and its associated contractures were first described in the 1870s by German surgeon Richard von Volkmann[4] who recognized the effects of increased pressure causing vascular compromise of the limb.

In 1935, Henderson and coworkers[5] developed a simple technique for measuring muscle "tonus" involving a syringe, a three-way connection, a mercury manometer, and a straight large-bore needle placed directly into the muscle. Forty years later, Whitesides and colleagues[6] refined this technique to accurately reflect muscle compartment pressures and delineated the threshold at which fasciotomy is indicated. To improve the accuracy and reproducibility of intermittent pressure measurement, Matsen[7] refined Whitesides' simple needle technique by adding a constant-infusion pump, which permitted continuous pressure monitoring. Whereas this appeared to provide more accurate measurements, concerns were raised over the injection of fluid into an already compromised compartment. The wick catheter[8,9] and the slit catheter[10,11] were later introduced to reduce the risk of increasing compartment contents while providing a mechanism for continuous pressure monitoring.

Various needles and equipment have been developed to measure compartment pressure (Fig. 54–2). The wick catheter, originally developed to measure subcutaneous and brain tissue pressures, was modified during the mid-1970s to provide continuous compartment pressure measurements. This catheter is rarely used today because of fears of catheter breakdown leading to measurement errors and retained foreign bodies, prompting the development of the slit catheter in 1980[10,11] (see Fig. 54–2C). This catheter has slits at the end being inserted into the tissue. The proximal end of the catheter is connected to a transducer and infusion system permitting continuous monitoring. The slits help prevent catheter clogging. Early reports found both methods to have similar accuracy and reproducibility as long as the patency of the catheter was ensured.[11,12]

In emergency medicine, the Stryker 295-2 Intracompartmental Compartment Pressure Monitoring System (Kalamazoo, MI) has become the most commonly used commercially available handheld device to measure compartment pressures. This device uses a fluid-filled pressure measurement catheter, a pressure monitor, and a fluid infusion mechanism that maintains catheter patency ensuring measurement accuracy. In contrast to earlier devices that utilized fluid injection to measure compartment pressures, the Stryker system uses a minimal amount of saline (>0.3 mL). This helps ensure accurate measurements and reduces the chance of causing a further increase in compartment pressure. The Stryker system also has the ability to record a single measurement or provide continuous compartment pressure recordings when required (Fig. 54–3).

Noninfusion systems like the transducer-tipped fiberoptic system offer a distinct advantage over the conventional fluid-filled systems because they do not produce hydrostatic pressure artifacts or require injections of fluid for long-term or continuous measurements. However, the fiberoptic transducer is relatively large and must be attached to a sheath 2.1 mm in diameter likely to cause pain during measurements.[13] In recent years, noninvasive, less painful methods for measuring compartment pressures have been studied in both acute and chronic exertional compartment syndromes. Investigations of magnetic resonance imaging (MRI), single-photon emission computed tomography (SPECT), myotonometry, electromyography, near-infrared spectroscopy, and ultrasound have provided encouraging results in the evaluation of

TABLE 54–1 Etiologies of Compartment Syndrome

Decreased Compartmental Volume

Closure of fascial defects
Application of excessive traction to fractured limbs

Increased Compartmental Content

Bleeding
Major vascular injury
Coagulation defect
  Bleeding disorder
  Anticoagulation therapy
  Thrombolytic therapy
Postarterial line placement

Increased Capillary Filtration

Reperfusion after ischemia
  Arterial bypass grafting
  Embolectomy
  Ergotamine ingestion
  Cardiac catheterization
  Lying on limb
Trauma
  Fracture
  Contusion
Intensive use of muscles
  Exercise
  Seizures
  Eclampsia
  Tetany
Burns
  Thermal
  Electric
Intra-arterial drug injection
Cold
Orthopaedic surgery
  Tibial osteotomy
  Hauser procedure
  Reduction and internal fixation of fractures
Snakebite

Increased Capillary Pressure

Intensive use of muscles
Venous obstruction
  Phlegmasia cerullea dolens
  Ill-fitting leg brace
  Venous ligation

Diminished Serum Osmolarity, Nephrotic Syndrome

Other Causes of Increased Compartmental Contents

Infiltrated infusion
Pressure transfusion
Leaky dialysis cannula
Muscle hypertrophy
Popliteal cyst
Carbon monoxide poisoning

Externally Applied Pressure

Tight casts, dressings, or air splints
Lying on limb
Pneumatic antishock garment
Congenital bands

Modified from Matsen FA: Compartmental Syndromes. New York, Grune & Stratton, 1980.

compartment syndrome.[14–22] In addition, externally applied devices, which measure muscle tissue "hardness," are under investigation as an economic alternative to these modalities, although support of their use has been mixed.[23–25]

Although promising, these evolving noninvasive methods have not yet replaced the needle-driven techniques as the standard for measuring intracompartmental pressures. The remainder of this chapter describes the most commonly employed measurement techniques used in the acute setting in which compartment syndrome of an extremity is suspected. Each method described provides rapid measurements with reasonable accuracy. The method chosen will depend upon the availability of the supplies and equipment necessary for the procedure and the experience of the operator.

PATHOPHYSIOLOGY

Several theories have been proposed to account for the tissue ischemia associated with compartment syndrome. These include the "arteriovenous (AV) gradient" theory, which suggests that reduced AV pressure or perfusion gradients prevents adequate blood supply;[26] the "critical closure" theory, in which blood flow arrests well before the AV perfusion gradient declines to zero;[27,28] and the "venous occlusion" theory,[29] which states that externally applied pressure, thrombotic events, and reperfusion contribute to increased compartment pressures and, ultimately, tissue ischemia. Although the exact mechanism has not been agreed upon, inherent in each of these theories is a decrease in blood supply insufficient to meet the metabolic demands of the involved tissues.

Adequate blood flow to tissues is a function of AV gradients across capillary beds. Once reduced below a critical level, oxygen delivery to these structures is impaired and aerobic cellular metabolism is no longer possible. Anaerobic metabolism then ensues until these energy stores become depleted. Muscles then become ischemic, and reduction in venous and lymphatic drainage creates increased pressure within this confined space. Note that ischemia and necrosis of the musculature can occur despite an arterial pressure *high enough to produce pulses* so merely assessing distal pulses is insufficient.[30]

A drop in blood pressure, an increase in compartment pressure, or a combination of the two can reduce AV gradients and lead to insufficient blood flow to tissues. Hypotension can occur from a variety of problems including hypovolemia, acute blood loss, cardiac disease states (e.g., ischemia), and sepsis. An increase in the contents of a compartment, a decrease in its volume capacity, or an increase in the external pressure applied to the compartment will increase the pressure within it, also reducing the AV gradient. Thus, the relationship between the intracompartmental pressure and the circulatory status of the extremity is an important factor in the development of compartment syndrome.[31] Compartment syndrome may develop in an extremity in the absence of direct trauma from prolonged ischemia associated with acute arterial occlusion by thrombus or proximal arterial injury.

The pressure of normal skeletal muscle at rest is typically below 10 mm Hg. However, deviations of 2 to 6 mm Hg have been reported.[1,8–10,12] The *perfusion pressure* of a compartment is defined as the difference between the diastolic blood pressure and the intracompartmental pressure.[32] A model using legs of normal volunteers has shown that a progression of neuromuscular deficits occurs when intracompartmental

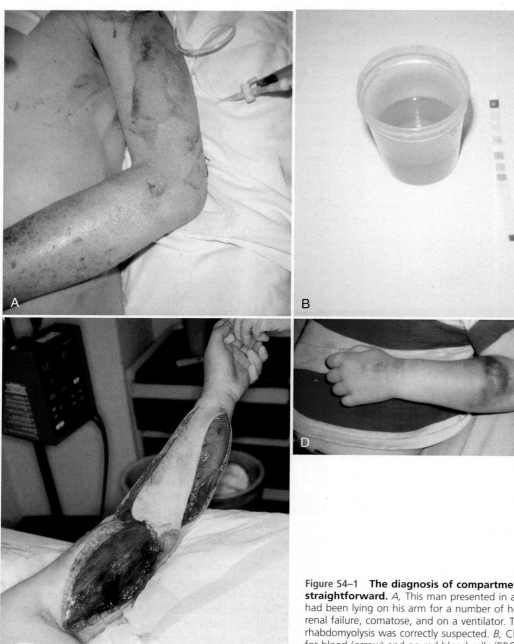

Figure 54–1 The diagnosis of compartment syndrome is not always straightforward. *A,* This man presented in a coma from a heroin overdose and had been lying on his arm for a number of hours. He was hypotensive, in renal failure, comatose, and on a ventilator. The entire arm was swollen and rhabdomyolysis was correctly suspected. *B,* Clear urine strongly positive dipstick for blood (*arrow*) and no red blood cells (RBCs) by microscopy equates to myoglobinuria. Because of the coma, he was unable to voice any complaint of pain. *C,* When he awakened 20 hr later, the pain was severe, and compartment pressures demonstrated the need for fasciotomy. Heroin can cause rhabdomyolysis, and hypotension/reperfusion, and certainly prolonged pressure on the muscles may have exacerbated the condition. *D,* The classic wringer washer injury predisposes to compartment syndrome, but industrial rollers are now usually the culprit.

pressure rises to within 35 to 40 mm Hg of the diastolic blood pressure.[33] Above this level, tissue perfusion is interrupted. Studies of neuromuscular tissue ischemia have demonstrated that inflammatory necrosis can occur at pressures between 40 and 60 mm Hg.[34]

Whitesides and colleagues[6] demonstrated that when tissue pressure within a closed compartment rises to within 10 to 30 mm Hg of the patient's diastolic blood pressure, inadequate perfusion ensues resulting in relative ischemia of the involved limb. Heppenstall and associates[35] further clarified this relationship demonstrating that the difference (ΔP)

between the mean arterial pressure (MAP) and the measured compartment pressure is directly related to blood flow to the tissue. They noted that as compartment pressure increases to approach the MAP, the ΔP decreases. Once ΔP falls below 30 mm Hg, tissue ischemia becomes more likely. In normal musculature, a ΔP of less than 30 mm Hg results in the loss of normal aerobic cellular metabolism.[35] In traumatized muscle, a ΔP of less than 40 mm Hg was associated with abnormal cellular function, highlighting the importance of maintaining an adequate systemic blood pressure in the setting of neuromuscular injury.[35]

Transducer tips

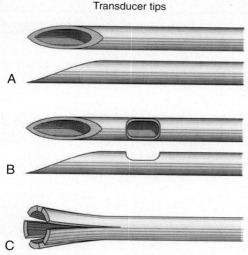

Figure 54–2 *A,* An 18-gauge straight needle. *B,* An 18-gauge side-port needle. *C,* A slit catheter. *(A–C, Boody AR, Wongworawat MD: Accuracy in the measurement of compartment pressures: A comparison of three commonly used devices. J Bone Joint Surg Am 87:2415, 2005.)*

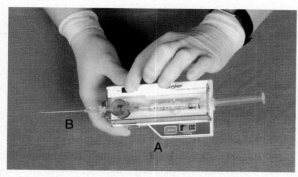

Figure 54–3 The Stryker 295 intracompartmental pressure monitor system. *(From Custalow CB. Color Atlas of Emergency Department Procedures. Philadelphia: Elsevier Saunders, 2005; p. 28.)*

For years, conventional wisdom maintained that immediate reperfusion of traumatized tissue would provide improved motor and neurologic function after injury. In the last decade, research suggests that muscle tissue may remain viable even after prolonged periods of ischemia and that a substantial percentage of the injury is generated upon reperfusion.[36] Tissue acidosis, intra- and extracellular edema, free radical–mediated injury, loss of adenine nucleotide precursors, and interruption of mitochondrial oxidative rephosphorylation by increased intracellular calcium have been implicated in the development of reperfusion-associated compartment syndromes.[36–39] Even in the absence of local trauma, ischemia followed by reperfusion has been shown to increase compartment pressures in canine models of hypovolemic shock.[40]

Evidence also suggests that elevated compartment pressure itself (in addition to causing ischemia) plays a role in the cellular deterioration seen with compartment syndrome.[41] In a study comparing muscle ischemia caused by tourniquet placement with an experimentally derived high-pressure compartment syndrome, there was no difference in the degree to which phosphocreatine levels fell between groups. However, levels of adenosine triphosphate (ATP) diminished rapidly in the compartment syndrome group compared with the tourniquet group. Moreover, phosphocreatine levels, ATP, and tissue pH normalized within 15 minutes of releasing the tourniquet. In the compartment syndrome group, these levels remained low even after fasciotomy. These results suggest that elevated tissue pressure plays a synergistic role with ischemia in cellular deterioration.[41]

CLINICAL PRESENTATION

Any compartment limited by fascial planes is potentially at risk for compartment syndrome. However, because of their propensity for injury and the presence of several low-volume compartments, the lower extremities are most commonly affected. In the leg, the anterior compartment is involved most often,[42] whereas the posterior compartment is a site frequently missed. The hands, feet, forearms, upper arms, thighs, abdomen, gluteal musculature, and back are other locations where compartment syndrome is known to occur.[1]

Increased compartment pressures may be caused by a variety of conditions (see Table 54–1). Risk factors for developing a compartment syndrome include recent extremity trauma (including acupuncture,[43] venipuncture, intravenous infusions, or intravenous drug use), bleeding within an extremity, a restrictive cast or splint, a crush or compression injury, prolonged lithotomy position,[44–47] tourniquet placement during an operative procedure, or a circumferential burn. In addition, some evidence suggests that compartment syndrome may occur in the setting of chronic exertion and overuse.[48,49] Although the exact etiology remains elusive, studies have demonstrated elevated lactate concentration and water levels in the tibialis anterior muscle after exercise with a reduction in these after fasciotomy.[50,51] Increases in muscle mass (related to a rise in blood volume during exertion) and hypertrophy of muscle and fascia with chronic use have also been reported.[52–56]

Clinical hallmarks of compartment syndrome include *pallor* of the extremity, a *pulse deficit* compared with that in the opposite limb, *paresis or paralysis* of the involved extremity, *paresthesias* in the distribution of the involved nerves, and *pain on passive stretch* of the involved musculature (*note:* the 5 Ps). These signs and symptoms may be unreliable in pediatric populations.[57] In addition, although commonly seen, pain and paralysis are late findings. Early, more subtle, signs of compartment syndrome include a burning sensation over the involved compartment, nonspecific sensory deficits, or poorly localized deep muscular pain that seems out of proportion to clinical examination and that intensifies when the musculature is passively stretched.

The period between the injury and the onset of symptoms can be as short as 2 hours and as long as 6 days.[58] The peak interval appears to be 15 to 30 hours. Often, the first symptom described by patients is pain greater than expected given the clinical scenario. Although pain out of proportion to the visible injury may raise the question of drug-seeking behavior, a focused evaluation for the possibility of limb-threatening disorders must precede this diagnosis of exclusion. Physical examination may reveal muscles that are weak and tense, with hypesthesia in the distribution of the nerves involved. Sensory deficits are often an indicator of the involved compartment, including loss of two-point discrimination and decreased vibratory sensation.[59–61] The presence or absence of a palpable arterial pulse is not an accurate indicator of relative tissue pressure or the relative risk of developing compartment syndrome. Pulses may be present in a severely compromised

TABLE 54–2 Compartment Syndromes and Associated Physical Signs

Compartment	Sensory Loss	Muscles Weakened	Painful Passive Motion	Tenseness Location
Forearm				
Dorsal	—	Digital extensors	Digital flexion	Dorsal forearm
Volar	Ulnar/median nerves	Digital flexors	Digital extension	Volar forearm
Hand				
Interosseus	—	Interosseus	Abduct/adduct (metacarpophalangeal joints)	Dorsum of hand between metacarpals
Leg				
Anterior	Deep peroneal nerve	Toe extensors Tibialis anterior	Toe flexion	Anterior aspect leg
Superficial posterior	—	Soleus and gastrocnemius	Foot dorsiflexion	Calf
Deep posterior	Posterior tibial nerve	Toe flexors Tibialis posterior	Toe extension	Distal medial leg, between Achilles tendon and tibia
Gluteal	(Rarely sciatic)	Gluteals, piriformis, or tensor fascia lata	Hip flexion	Buttock
Upper Arm				
Flexor	Ulnar/median nerves	Biceps and distal flexors	Elbow extension	Anterior upper arm
Extensor	Radial nerves	Triceps and forearm extensors	Elbow flexion	Posterior upper arm
Foot	Digital nerves	Foot intrinsics	Toe flexion/extension	Dorsal/plantar foot
Lumbar	—	Erector spinae	Lumbar flexion	Paraspinous

extremity.[62] Table 54–2 lists the signs and symptoms of compartment syndrome specific to each compartment.

DIAGNOSIS

Even experienced clinicians find it difficult to evaluate a potential compartment syndrome, and no specific standard of care exists with regard to a time interval from injury to definitive treatment. In the unconscious patient or for those with other life-threatening conditions that mandate other priorities, the clinical scenario simply does not allow for a diagnosis to be made in a timely fashion. In the nontrauma case or for the patient unable to voice pain or cooperate with an examination, this diagnosis is often not considered or the diagnosis is delayed. Regional nerve blocks or epidural anesthesia might obscure signs or symptoms of increased compartment pressure, causing further delays in diagnosis.

The difficulty in diagnosing an acute compartment syndrome was highlighted in a report by Vaillancourt and coworkers.[63] In a retrospective review of 76 patients who underwent fasciotomy at major university trauma centers/teaching hospitals, the interval from initial patient assessment to diagnosis of a compartment syndrome was up to 8 hours. As one would intuit, delay was most common in nontraumatic cases. The interval from the precipitating event to definitive surgery was up to 35 hours, reflecting the difficulty in suspecting this diagnosis and instituting definitive therapy in clinical practice. Such statistics describe actual care that may be less than ideal with regard to theoretical benchmarks.

Not withstanding the difficulty described previously, the diagnosis of compartment syndrome is primarily a clinical one, supplemented by direct measurement of compartment pressures. In a study evaluating of the utility of clinical findings in the diagnosis of compartment syndrome, Ulmer[64] noted that the sensitivity and positive predictive value of clinical findings (see later) are low, whereas the specificity and negative predictive value of these findings are high. Nevertheless, the study found that whereas the sensitivity of an individual clinical finding may be low, the probability of compartment syndrome rises considerably when more than one clinical hallmark is present.[64]

The differential diagnosis of compartment syndrome is extensive and includes primary vascular, nerve, or muscle injuries that produce similar findings. Acute arterial occlusion, cellulitis, osteomyelitis, neuropraxia, reflex sympathetic dystrophy, synovitis, tenosynovitis, stress fractures, envenomations, necrotizing fasciitis, deep vein thrombosis, and thrombophlebitis are additional diseases that should be considered. Differentiating compartment syndrome from these and other orthopaedic disorders requires a detailed history and thorough physical examination with a high index of suspicion (Table 54–3).

ANCILLARY STUDIES

In general, laboratory and radiographic studies are not helpful in confirming the diagnosis of compartment syndrome. However, they might be useful in identifying other diagnoses, associated conditions, and complications. Table 54–4 lists useful studies for patients with the possibility of a compartment syndrome.

INVASIVE COMPARTMENT PRESSURE MONITORING

Indications and Contraindications

The earliest objective manifestation of acute compartment syndrome is an elevation in the tissue pressure of one or more compartments. However, signs and symptoms generally do

TABLE 54–3 Clinical Findings of Compartment Syndrome, Arterial Occlusion, and Neuropraxia

	Compartmental Syndrome	Arterial Occlusion	Neuropraxia
Pressure increased in the compartment	+	−	−
Pain with stretch	+	+	−
Paresthesia or anesthesia	+	+	−
Paresis or paralysis	+	+	+
Pulses intact	+	−	+

From Mubarak S, Carroll N: Volkman's contracture in children: Etiology and prevention. J Bone Joint Surg Br 61:290, 1979.

TABLE 54–4 Ancillary Studies That May Be Helpful in Identifying Other Diagnoses, Associated Conditions, and Complications in Patients Suspected of Having a Compartment Syndrome

Laboratory Studies

- Complete metabolic profile (including electrolytes and renal function testing)
- Complete blood count with differential
- Serum and urine myoglobin
- Creatine phosphokinase
- Urinalysis to evaluate for concurrent rhabdomyolysis
- Coagulation studies

Imaging Studies

- Radiography of the affected limb to evaluate for fracture or foreign body
- Ultrasonography to rule out deep vein thrombosis or Doppler ultrasonography to evaluate blood flow to the extremity

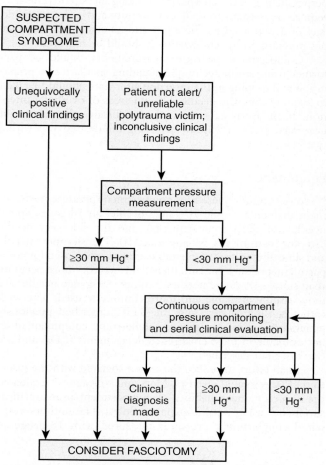

Figure 54–4 Algorithm for management of a patient with suspected compartment syndrome. Pressure thresholds (*) are based on published case series. Clinical correlation is paramount to proper interpretation of compartment pressure measurements. *(From Rorabeck CH: Compartment syndromes. In Browner BD, Jupiter JB, Levine AM, Trafton PG [eds]: Skeletal Trauma: Fractures, Dislocations, Ligamentous Injuries, vol 1, 2nd ed. Philadelphia, WB Saunders, 1992, p 290.)*

not occur until the tissue pressure has reached a critical level (see "Pathophysiology"). In some patients, the diagnosis of compartment syndrome is clinically obvious, and one can proceed directly to fasciotomy. However, when clinical findings are equivocal or difficult to interpret, tissue pressure measurement may help guide treatment (Fig. 54–4). It is important to remember that whereas tissue pressure measurements may suggest a compartment syndrome, *equivocal measurements will still require clinical judgment.*

There are several groups of patients in whom clinical findings are difficult to interpret and would benefit from compartment pressure measurement. These include unresponsive patients, uncooperative patients, children, patients with multiple or distracting injuries, those with peripheral nerve deficits attributable to other causes (e.g., fracture-associated nerve injuries, diabetic peripheral neuropathies), and those whose clinical findings are equivocal.

There are no absolute contraindications to performing compartment pressure measurements or continuous pressure monitoring. Caution should be taken when performing these procedures on patients with platelet dysfunction or other coagulation disorders. If possible, avoid needle insertion through areas of cellulitis, infection, or burns.

Patient Preparation and Positioning

Explain the procedure to the patient or surrogate. Written informed consent is not a universal standard, but is suggested when possible. Patient and extremity positioning for compartment pressure measurement depends upon the extremity and

compartment being studied, coexisting injuries, and the clinical status of the patient. Whereas the effect of positioning of the extremity on intracompartmental pressures has been studied,[65] generally, patients should be in the supine position. The exceptions to supine positioning are discussed in subsequent sections related to the extremity of interest.

For most patients, compartment pressure measurement is a painful procedure requiring adequate local anesthesia, systemic analgesia, procedural sedation (see Chapter 29 for a discussion of local anesthetics and Chapter 33 for a discussion of procedural sedation and analgeon). The skin should be anesthetized with a small amount of anesthetic, avoiding the underlying muscle and fascia. Inadvertent injection into the underlying structures may falsely elevate the compartment pressure. Movement (owing to inadequate analgesia or improper positioning) may also falsely elevate compartment pressures, particularly if the patient requires limb restraint. To minimize the discomfort of multiple attempts at localizing the correct compartment, some have advocated the use of ultrasound guidance to improve needle accuracy.[66]

The extremity being studied should be at the level of the heart and in a position that permits insertion of the needle perpendicular to the compartment being measured. This may require an assistant to hold an extremity above the stretcher. Any obstruction to needle entry and all structures that may put pressure on the compartment should be removed.

Compartment pressure measurements should be performed using sterile technique including standard skin preparation and draping at the insertion site. Care should be taken to avoid placing the needle through areas of overlying infection. If an overlying cast is present, bivalve the cast or, if necessary, create a window overlying the desired area with a cast saw.

Equipment

Needles commonly used for compartment pressure measurement include a simple 18-gauge needle, an 18-gauge spinal needle (for deep compartments), and the side-port needle (Stryker Instruments, Kalamazoo, MI). The side-port needle and slit catheter have comparable efficacy when used for compartment pressure measurement and may be more accurate than simple 18-gauge needles.[31] Simple 18-gauge needles are more readily available and more commonly used. The wick catheter, slit catheter, and the STIC described previously generally require specialized, cumbersome equipment often not available in most emergency departments (EDs) and are therefore not described.

In an effort to reduce the pain associated with the insertion of larger gauge needles, Mars and colleagues[67] evaluated the accuracy and reliability of compartment pressure measurements using smaller-gauge needles. The authors compared compartment pressures measured with 18-gauge to 25-gauge needles and found that smaller-gauged needles provided results similar to or better than the more traditional 18-gauge needles. Furthermore, the addition of a side port did not improve accuracy.[67] Unfortunately, no additional studies have been done to corroborate these findings. As a result, most clinicians continue to use 18-gauge needles.

Pressure Measurement Systems

Mercury Manometer System (Fig. 54–5)
Equipment
- Two 18-gauge simple or spinal needles
- Two plastic extension tubes
- One 20-mL syringe
- One three-way stopcock
- One vial of sterile normal saline
- One mercury manometer

Setup and Procedure
1. Prepare and anesthetize the patient and extremity according to the guidelines described earlier.
2. Assemble the syringe, tubing, extension tubing, and needle as shown in Figure 54–5A.
3. Insert the needle into a vented vial of sterile saline. Aspirate a column of saline into the tubing halfway to the stopcock; care should be taken to avoid bubble formation. Close the three-way stopcock to the tube to avoid losing saline during needle insertion.
4. Insert the needle into the muscle of the compartment being measured (see "Needle Placement Techniques," later in this chapter).
5. Attach the second extension tubing to the monitor and to the third port of the three-way stopcock. Turn the stopcock so that the syringe is open to both extension tubes (see Fig. 54–5B). This closed system has equal pressure in both extension tubes.
6. Increase the pressure in the system gradually by *slowly* depressing the syringe plunger while simultaneously watching the column of saline. The mercury manometer will rise as the pressure in the system rises. When the pressure in the system exceeds that of the tissue, inject saline into the compartment, causing the saline column to move. Read the manometer at the moment the saline is noted to

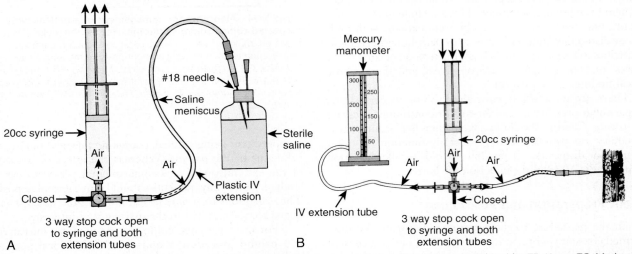

Figure 54–5 A and B, Mercury monitor technique for compartmental pressure monitoring. (A and B, From Whitesides TE, Haney TC, Morimoto K, et al: Tissue pressure measurements as a determinant for the need of fasciotomy. Clin Orthop 113:43, 1975.)

move. This reading corresponds to the tissue pressure in millimeters of mercury.

7. To obtain a second reading, completely remove the needle and repeat steps 4 through 6. A third measurement might be necessary to achieve two readings in agreement. Check the needle for tissue plugs and blood clots between readings.

Procedural Caveats. The most common error with this system is depressing the syringe plunger too quickly. Only when the saline is slowly injected into the compartment will the mercury column (which has greater inertia) accurately reflect the compartment pressure. Another source of error is obstruction of the needle with a plug of tissue (or blood clot) if the plunger of the syringe is pulled back. Finally, aneroid manometers are prone to inaccuracy, are not well calibrated at lower pressure ranges, and should not be substituted for the more accurate mercury manometers for this procedure.

Arterial Line System (Fig. 54–6)
Equipment
- One 18-gauge simple or spinal needle
- High-pressure tubing
- Pressure transducer with cable
- Pressure monitor
- Sterile saline
- Transducer stand that allows for variable height adjustments
- Two three-way stopcocks
- One 20-mL syringe

Setup and Procedure
1. Prepare and anesthetize the patient and extremity according to the guidelines described earlier.
2. Connect the transducer cable to the pressure monitor.
3. Assemble the stopcocks, transducer, transducer cable, syringe, high-pressure tubing, and needle as shown in Figure 54–6.

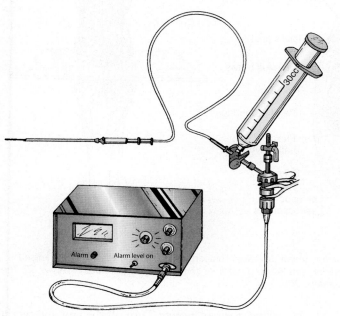

Figure 54–6 The arterial line system for compartmental pressure measurement. (From Rorabeck CH: Compartment syndromes. In Browner BD, Jupiter JB, Levine AM, Trafton PG [eds]: Skeletal Trauma: Fractures, Dislocations, Ligamentous Injuries, vol 1, 2nd ed. Philadelphia, WB Saunders, 1992, p 290.)

4. Fill the syringe with 15 mL of sterile saline and place one of the stopcocks on the syringe. Turn the stopcocks to allow filling of the transducer, high-pressure tubing, and needle. Once these are filled, close the stopcock to the high-pressure tubing.
5. Open the top stopcock to air and place the transducer at the height of the compartment being measured. Calibrate the transducer to zero and then close the top stopcock.
6. Open the lower stopcock that is attached to the high-pressure tubing.
7. Insert the needle into the desired muscle compartment (see "Needle Placement Techniques," later in this chapter for details). If the needle is in the proper location, applying slight external pressure to the compartment or passively moving the muscles within the compartment should cause a pressure spike on the monitor. Allow the compartment to equilibrate for several seconds after this maneuver, and then measure the mean compartment pressure.
8. To obtain a second reading, completely remove the needle and repeat steps 4 through 7. A third measurement might be necessary to achieve two readings in agreement. Check the needle for tissue plugs and blood clots between readings.

Stryker 295-2 Intracompartmental Pressure Measurement (Fig. 54–7)
Equipment
- Stryker 295-2 Quick Pressure Monitor Set (disposable pouch)
- Stryker handheld pressure monitoring unit (included)
- One 3-mL prefilled syringe with saline (included)
- One side-port needle (included)
- One diaphragm chamber (included)

Setup and Procedure (see Fig. 54–7, steps 1–8)
1. Prepare and anesthetize the patient and extremity according to the guidelines described earlier.
2. Open the 295-2 Quick Pressure Monitor Set and remove the contents while maintaining sterile conditions.
3. Place the needle firmly on the tapered chamber stem .
4. Remove the cap on the prefilled syringe and screw the syringe onto the remaining chamber stem. Take care to avoid contaminating the fluid pathway.
5. Open the monitor cover and inspect the device for damage or contamination. Place the chamber into the device well (black surface down) and push gently until it seats.
6. Snap the cover closed—DO NOT FORCE. The latch must have "snapped" in place.
7. Hold the needle at approximately 45° up from horizontal and slowly force fluid through the disposable system to purge it of air. Caution: DO NOT allow saline to roll down the needle into the transducer well.
8. Turn on the unit; it should read between 0 and 9 mm Hg.
9. Hold the device at the intended angle of insertion and press the "ZERO" button to calibrate. After a few seconds, the display should read "00." It is important to note that failure to calibrate the device while in the intended angle of insertion may result in inaccurate readings. Note: The display must read "00" before continuing. If it does not, follow the troubleshooting instructions provided by the manufacturer before proceeding.
10. Now insert the needle into the compartment to be measured (see "Needle Placement Techniques," later in this

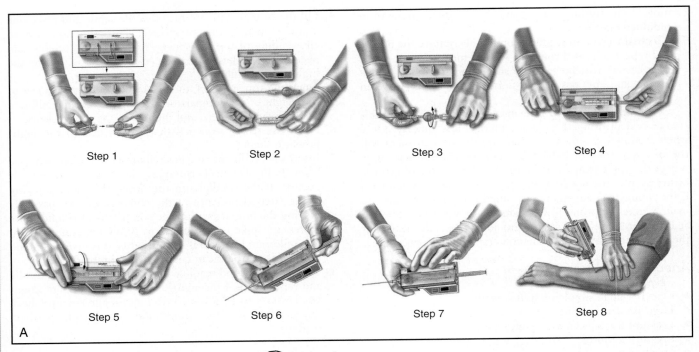

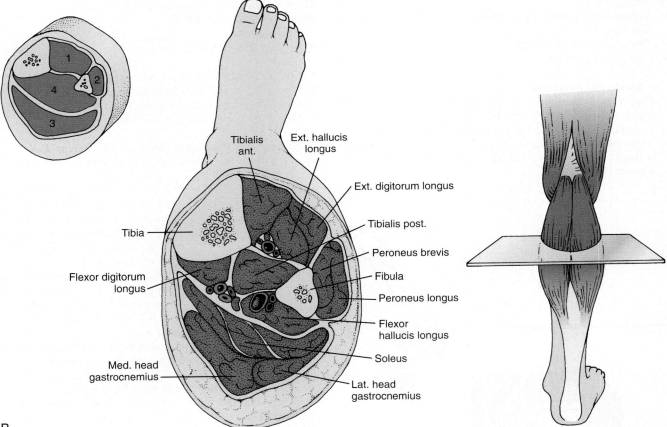

Figure 54–7 *A,* Setup of the Stryker 295 intracompartmental pressure monitor system. *B,* Fascial compartments of the lower leg with enclosed muscle groups (insert upper left): (1) anterior; (2) lateral; (3) superficial posterior; and (4) deep posterior compartments. *(A, From Custalow CB: The Color Atlas of Emergency Department Procedures. Philadelphia, Elsevier Saunders, 2005.)*

chapter for details). Slowly inject no more than 0.3 mL of saline into the compartment to equilibrate with interstitial fluids.

11. Wait for the display to reach equilibrium and record the resulting pressure.

12. *For additional measurements:* Turn off the unit and repeat steps 8 through 11. Recalibrate the unit to zero before each measurement.

13. For continuous monitoring using an indwelling slit catheter, refer to the instructions accompanying the system.

NEEDLE PLACEMENT TECHNIQUES FOR SPECIFIC COMPARTMENTS

General Principles

Accurate pressure measurements depend on careful needle insertion and confirmation of correct placement. The requirements of proper technique include (1) reliable placement into the compartment being measured; (2) avoidance of important neurovascular structures; (3) simplicity and reproducibility; and (4) minimal patient discomfort.[68] Most compartments are superficial and easily accessible. Only the deep posterior compartment of the lower leg and the gluteal compartment might require a spinal needle to reach the required depth. Most approaches require that the needle enter the tissue perpendicular to the skin. In conjunction with the text, provide landmarks for proper needle placement and passage to ensure proper compartment placement and avoidance of neurovascular structures.

Lower Extremity

Because of its high vulnerability to injury and limited fascial compliance, the lower leg, especially the anterior compartment, is predisposed to compartment syndrome. The anterior compartment is the most frequent site of compartment syndrome associated with injury to the lower extremity.[33] The lower leg traditionally has four compartments: anterior, lateral, deep posterior, and superficial posterior.[1] In addition, in some patients, the tibialis posterior muscle may occupy its own compartment, separate from the rest of the deep posterior compartment.[69-71] Keep this possibility in mind when measuring compartment pressures in this area.

The easiest cross-sectional level for needle placement for any compartment is approximately 3 cm on either side of a transverse line drawn at the junction of the proximal and middle thirds of the lower leg. When measuring the compartment pressure of the leg, place the patient in the supine position with the leg at the level of the heart. An exception to this is when measuring the superficial posterior compartment. In this case, place the patient in the prone position. Otherwise, patient preparation should be performed as described previously in this chapter.

Anterior Compartment

With the patient supine, palpate the anterior border of the tibia at the level of the junction between the proximal and the middle third of the lower leg (Fig. 54-8). The entry point for needle insertion is 1 cm *lateral* to the anterior border of the tibia. Direct the needle perpendicular to the skin to a depth of approximately 1 to 3 cm. Observing a severalfold rise in pressure during (1) external compression of the anterior compartment just proximal or distal to the needle insertion site, (2) plantar flexion of the foot, or (3) dorsiflexion of the foot confirms proper needle depth.

Lateral Compartment

With the patient supine and the leg at heart level, an assistant should elevate the leg slightly off the stretcher (if the clinical situation permits). Palpate the posterior border of the fibula at the level of the junction between the proximal and the middle thirds of the lower leg. Insert the needle into the skin just anterior to the posterior border of the fibula and direct it toward the fibula to a depth of 1 to 1.5 cm (Fig. 54-9A). If

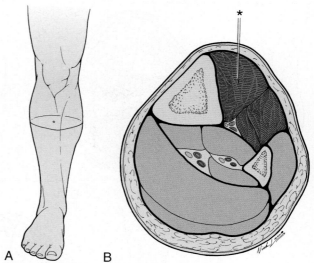

Figure 54–8 Anterior compartment syndrome of the lower leg. Suggested needle entry point is indicated by the small circle (A). The needle should be inserted (*) to a depth of 1 to 3 cm (B). (*Modified with permission from Matsen FA (ed): Compartmental Syndromes. New York, Grune & Stratton, 1980, p 91.*)

the needle contacts bone, retract it approximately 0.5 cm. Confirm proper needle depth by observing a rise in the pressure during (1) external compression of the lateral compartment just inferior or superior to the needle's entrance or (2) inversion of the foot and ankle.

Deep Posterior Compartment

With the patient supine, an assistant should elevate the leg slightly off the stretcher (if the clinical situation permits). Palpate the medial border of the tibia at the level of the junction of the proximal and middle thirds of the lower leg while simultaneously palpating the posterior border of the fibula on the lateral aspect of the leg at the same level. Insert the needle perpendicular to the skin just posterior to the medial border of the tibia and direct it toward the palpated posterior border of the fibula to a depth of 2 to 4 cm (final depth depends on the amount of subcutaneous adipose tissue; see Fig. 54-9B). Confirm proper needle depth by observing a rise in pressure during (1) toe extension or (2) ankle eversion.

Superficial Posterior Compartment

With the patient in the prone position and the leg at heart level, identify an imaginary transverse line (or draw one with a marking pen) at the level of the junction between the proximal and the middle thirds of the lower leg. Insert the needle at this level, 3 to 5 cm on either side of a vertical line drawn down the middle of the calf (see Fig. 54-9C). The needle's path should be perpendicular to the skin and directed toward the center of the lower leg to a depth of 2 to 4 cm. Confirm proper needle depth by observing a rise in pressure during (1) digital external compression of the posterior compartment just inferior or superior to the needle insertion point or (2) dorsiflexion of the foot.

Forearm

Traditionally, the forearm has been considered a two-compartment limb.[1] However, some authors place the

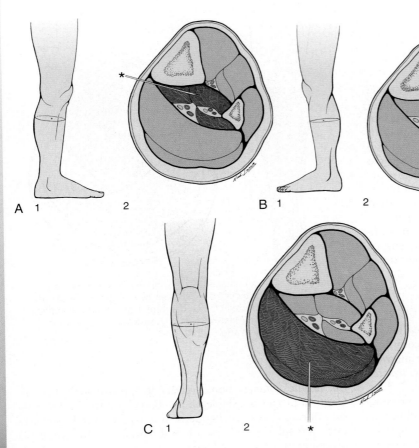

Figure 54–9 *A*, Deep posterior compartment syndrome of the lower leg. Suggested needle entry point indicated by the small circle (*1*). The needle should be inserted (***) to a depth of 2 to 4 cm (*2*). *B*, Lateral compartment syndrome of the lower leg. Suggested needle entry point indicated by the small circle (*1*). The needle should be inserted (***) to a depth of 1 to 1.5 cm (*2*). *C*, Superficial posterior compartment syndrome of the lower leg. Suggested needle entry point indicated by the small circle (*1*). The needle should be inserted (***) to a depth of 2 to 4 cm (*2*). (*A–C*, Modified with permission from Matsen FA (ed): *Compartmental Syndromes.* New York, Grune & Stratton, 1980, p 92.)

extensor carpi radialis brevis, the *extensor carpi radialis longus*, and the *brachioradialis* musculature in a third compartment called the "mobile wad."[72,73] The forearm compartments (particularly the volar compartment) are predisposed to compartment syndrome because of their use during vigorous exercise, accessibility for drug injection, and vulnerability to injury and burns.[1]

The junction of the proximal and middle thirds of the forearm is the cross-sectional level for needle insertion.[73] When measuring forearm compartment pressures, place the patient in the supine position with the arm at the level of the heart. Prepare the patient as previously described.

Volar Compartment (see Fig. 54–13A)

Hold the forearm in supination. Identify the *palmaris longus* tendon by having the patient oppose the thumb and small finger with the wrist flexed against resistance. Trace the tendon to the junction between the proximal and the middle thirds of the forearm. Palpate the posterior border of the ulna and insert the needle perpendicular to the skin just medial to the *palmaris longus* tendon. Direct the needle toward the palpated posterior border of the ulna to a depth of 1 to 2 cm. Confirm proper needle depth by observing a rise in pressure during (1) external compression of the volar compartment just proximal or distal to the needle insertion or (2) extension of the fingers or wrist.

Dorsal Compartment (see Fig. 54–13B)

Hold the forearm in supination with the elbow flexed and the dorsum of the forearm facing down. Palpate the posterior aspect of the ulna at the level of the junction between the proximal and the middle thirds of the forearm. Insert the needle perpendicular to the skin 1 to 2 cm lateral to the posterior aspect of the ulna to a depth of 1 to 2 cm. Confirm proper needle placement by observing a rise in pressure during (1) digital external compression of the dorsal compartment just proximal or distal to needle insertion or (2) flexion of the wrist or fingers.

Mobile Wad (see Fig. 54–13C)

Hold the forearm in supination. Identify the most lateral (radial) portion of the forearm at the level of the junction between its proximal and its middle thirds. Insert the needle into the muscle tissue lateral to the radius perpendicular to the skin to a depth of 1 to 1.5 cm. Confirm proper needle placement by observing a rise in pressure during (1) digital external compression of the mobile wad just proximal or distal to needle entry or (2) deviation of the wrist.

Gluteal Musculature

A two-layer fascia encases the muscle bellies of the tensor fascia lata anteriorly and the gluteus maximus posteriorly. This fascia divides the musculature into three distinct compartments: maximus, tensor, and medius/minimus (Fig. 54–10). The sciatic nerve is deep to the fascia but lies between the pelvis-external rotator complex and the gluteus maximus, making it vulnerable to injury when compartment syndrome occurs here. Gluteal compartment syndrome is very rare and unknown to many clinicians. Most reported cases of gluteal compartment syndrome result from prolonged immobilization and local compression in association with drug or alcohol intoxication.[74] Prolonged pressure from a toilet seat or significant soft tissue contusions (whipping, paddling) may predis-

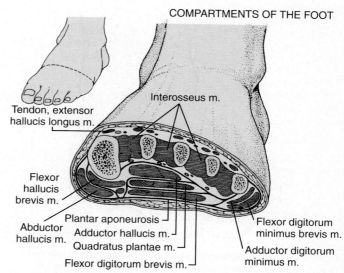

Figure 54–11 The compartments of the foot. (*From Mubarak SJ, Hargens AR: Compartment Syndromes and Volkmann's Contracture. Philadelphia, WB Saunders, 1981.*)

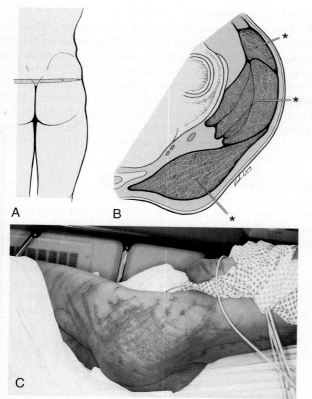

Figure 54–10 Gluteal compartment syndrome. *A,* Suggested entry points are indicated along the blue line. The needle should be inserted to a depth of 4 to 8 cm depending on which compartment is being measured. *B,* Needle tips (*) are shown entering the muscle compartments. *C,* This patient suffered extensive soft tissue trauma to the buttocks from repeated blows from a stick (domestic abuse), and is at risk for rhabdomyolysis and gluteal compartment syndrome. (*A and B, Modified with permission from Owen CA, Moody PR, Mubarak SJ, et al: Gluteal compartment syndromes. Clin Orthop 132:57, 1978.*)

pose to this condition. Patients typically present with gluteal tenderness that is often attributed to contusion or hematoma; this, combined with the rarity of a compartment syndrome in this area, frequently results in a delayed or missed diagnosis. Rhabdomyolysis should be considered in patients with gluteal compartment syndrome, given the large muscle mass involved.

Gluteal Compartments
To measure gluteal compartment pressures, place the patient in the prone position with the gluteal structures at the level of the heart. Prepare the patient as described previously. Cutaneous landmarks for the three compartments are not consistent from patient to patient. Therefore, in cases of suspected gluteal compartment syndrome, needle insertion at the point of maximal tenderness is considered sufficient to provide adequate pressure measurements.[74] Insert an 18-gauge spinal needle perpendicular and direct it toward the point of maximal tenderness to a depth of 4 to 8 cm. Confirm proper needle placement by observing a rise in pressure during external compression of the gluteal musculature.

Foot

Crush injuries account for the majority of the reported cases of compartment syndrome in the foot, but may also be seen

after vascular injuries, fractures, and other high-energy injuries. Although compartment syndrome of the foot is rare, it is being reported with increasing frequency as clinicians become more aware of this entity. Although there is no universal agreement on the number or exact location of the anatomic compartments in the foot,[75,76] it is generally accepted that there are at least nine compartments separated into four groups: the central/calcaneal, intrinsic/interosseous, medial, and lateral (Fig. 54–11).

For pressure measurements in any of the foot compartments, place the patient in the supine position with the foot at the level of the heart and prepare the patient as described previously. Note that pedal edema has been shown to increase the resting tissue pressure of the foot.[77]

Medial Compartment
The medial compartment contains the *abductor hallucis* and the *flexor hallucis brevis*. The compartment is bounded medially and inferiorly by an extension of the plantar aponeurosis, laterally by an intramuscular septum, and dorsally by the first metatarsal (Fig. 54–12A). To measure the pressure in this compartment, insert the needle at the medial aspect of the foot just inferior to the base of the first metatarsal into the *abductor hallucis* muscle, which is approximately 1 to 1.5 cm deep.[78] Confirm proper needle depth by observing a rise in pressure during external compression of the medial compartment of the foot.

Central (Calcaneal) Compartment
The central compartment contains the *flexor digitorum brevis*, the *quadratus plantae*, the *lumbricals*, and the *abductor hallucis* muscles. Its boundaries are the plantar aponeurosis inferiorly, the osseofascial tarsometatarsal structures dorsally, and the intermuscular septa medially and laterally. To measure the pressure in this compartment, insert the needle at the medial aspect of the foot just inferior to the base of the first metatarsal. Advance the needle through the *abductor hallucis* muscle to a depth of 3 cm.[78] Confirm proper needle depth by observing a rise in pressure during external compression of the central compartment of the foot.

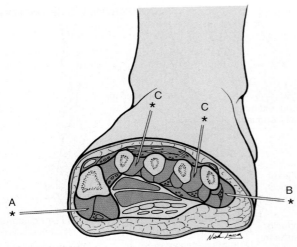

Figure 54–12   Compartment syndromes of the foot. Suggested needle pathways (*) to measure intracompartmental pressures: *A,* Medial. *B,* Lateral. *C,* Interosseous. The central compartment is surrounded by these compartments. *(A–C, Modified from Myerson M: Acute compartment syndromes of the foot. Bull Hosp Jt Dis 47:251, 1987.)*

Lateral Compartment

The lateral compartment contains the *abductor, flexor,* and *opponens* muscles of the fifth toe. The boundaries are the fifth metatarsal dorsally, the plantar aponeurosis inferiorly and laterally, and an intermuscular septum medially.[79] To measure the pressure in this compartment, insert the needle parallel to the plantar aspect of the foot just inferior to the base of the fifth metatarsal (see Fig. 54–12*B*). Advance the needle to a depth of 1 to 1.5 cm. Confirm proper needle depth by observing a rise in pressure during external compression of the lateral compartment of the foot.

Intrinsic (Interosseous) Compartment

The intrinsic compartment contains the seven interossei muscles and is bounded by the metatarsals and the interosseous fascia. Pressure in this compartment is measured in two areas, the second and fourth web spaces. Avoid the first web space to prevent inadvertent puncture or disruption of the *dorsalis pedis* artery or the *deep peroneal* nerve.[78] Insert the needle perpendicular to the skin at the dorsum of the second and fourth web spaces at the base of the metatarsals, and advance the needle to a depth of 1 cm[78] (see Fig. 54–12*C*).

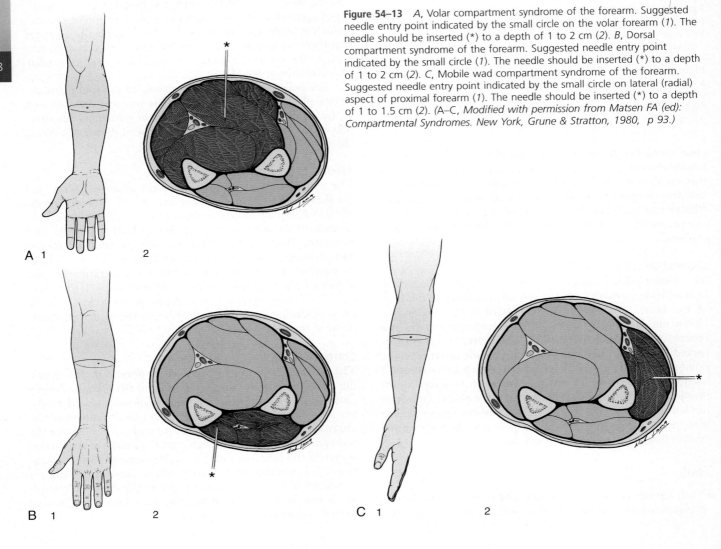

Figure 54–13   *A,* Volar compartment syndrome of the forearm. Suggested needle entry point indicated by the small circle on the volar forearm (*1*). The needle should be inserted (*) to a depth of 1 to 2 cm (*2*). *B,* Dorsal compartment syndrome of the forearm. Suggested needle entry point indicated by the small circle (*1*). The needle should be inserted (*) to a depth of 1 to 2 cm (*2*). *C,* Mobile wad compartment syndrome of the forearm. Suggested needle entry point indicated by the small circle on lateral (radial) aspect of proximal forearm (*1*). The needle should be inserted (*) to a depth of 1 to 1.5 cm (*2*). *(A–C, Modified with permission from Matsen FA (ed): Compartmental Syndromes. New York, Grune & Stratton, 1980, p 93.)*

Confirm proper needle depth by observing a rise in pressure during external compression of the intrinsic compartment adjacent to the needle insertion site.

INTERPRETATION

Compartment pressures must be interpreted within the context of the clinical picture. Inaccurate measurements are far worse than no measurement at all, and a *clinical evaluation is more telling than pressure measurements alone.* To be most accurate, compartment pressures should be measured in the area of highest pressure and greatest tissue damage.[62] Inaccurate measurements may result from needle placement into tendon or fascia, plugged needles, defective or poorly calibrated devices, injection of fluid into the compartment, and movement during the procedure. Whitesides and colleagues[6] found an increase in compartment pressure of 1 mm Hg for every 1 mL of saline infused into the anterior compartment of the lower extremity. It is difficult to assess the relevance of this finding, but recognition of the potential for its occurrence is important.

Reports of normal human compartment pressures vary in the literature. In comparing several techniques, Shakespeare and associates[12] found an average pressure of 8.5 mm Hg with slightly higher pressures in individuals who were physically fit. Wiley and coworkers[13] found a mean of 15 mm Hg (±8 mm Hg) using the electronic transducer-tipped probe in healthy volunteers. Although the generally accepted range of normal is between 0 and 10 mm Hg, others have noted pressures in normal subjects ranging from 0 to as high as 18 mm Hg.[1,8,61,80]

When properly performed, each method has acceptable accuracy in the clinical setting. Studies have found standard deviations between 2 and 6 mm Hg with all of the techniques described earlier.[1,8-10,12] It is generally agreed that the mercury manometer method of compartment pressure measurement is the least accurate. The arterial line system used with a simple (straight) or side-port needle provides a higher degree of accuracy for simple, episodic readings. The Stryker 295-2 Intracompartmental Pressure Monitoring System provides consistent, accurate readings for episodic and continuous monitoring situations. Development of miniature transducer-tipped devices is ongoing. Noninvasive modalities, including MRI, SPECT, myotonometry, electromyography, near-infrared spectroscopy, and ultrasound continue to be investigated as painless alternatives to needle-driven compartment measurements, and although early results are promising, they are not in widespread use.[14-22]

Mubarak and coworkers[9,81] and Hargens and colleagues[82] suggested that an absolute compartment pressure of 30 mm Hg is the "critical pressure" requiring fasciotomy. Despite the fact that this tissue pressure is abnormal and corresponds to the onset of pain and paresthesias,[9] it does not necessarily precipitate a compartment syndrome in the absence of other factors and must be interpreted within the context of the clinical scenario. Whereas some patients may develop compartment syndrome at this pressure others will not because tolerance to increasing pressures appears to be variable.[1,8,12,61]

Despite a body of literature addressing compartment pressure measurement, *no consensus exists on the threshold at which a fasciotomy should be performed.* Some argue that an absolute compartment pressure of 30 mg Hg or greater should be the threshold for fasciotomy.[9,81,82] Matsen[1] found that no patients with pressures of less than 45 mm Hg had symptoms of compartment syndrome, whereas all patients with pressures greater than 60 mm Hg had symptoms. Whitesides and colleagues[6] found that fasciotomy was required when the intracompartmental pressure approaches 20 mm Hg below the diastolic pressure, whereas McQueen and associates[83] recommended using a differential pressure (diastolic minus the compartment pressure) of less than 30 mm Hg as a criterion for fasciotomy. Heppenstall and associates[35,41] concluded that using either the Whitesides or McQueen criteria would produce similar results and recommended using a ΔP (MAP minus the measured compartment pressure) of 30 mm Hg or less in nontraumatized muscle and a ΔP of 40 mm Hg or less in traumatized muscle as a guide for fasciotomy.

Factors other than compartment pressure alone are important in the development of compartment syndrome and the need for fasciotomy. Situations in which the MAP is low (e.g., hypovolemia) might interfere with the patient's ability to tolerate even mildly elevated compartment pressures. The duration of increased compartment pressures is also an important factor in the development and severity of a compartment syndrome.

COMPLICATIONS

The risk of both local and systemic infection is similar for all of the measurement procedures described in this chapter. Strict adherence to aseptic techniques and universal precautions is mandatory. This includes sterilization of catheters and use of sterile solutions in addition to use of sterile gloves and supplies whenever possible.

All of the invasive monitoring systems have some degree of pain associated with needle or catheter insertion. Adequate analgesia and, when necessary, procedural sedation are often necessary to gain the patient's cooperation and prevent patient movement during pressure measurements. When using local anesthetics, avoid injections into the compartment, because this can increase pain and result in inaccurate (higher) readings.

Acknowledgments

The author recognizes the contribution of Neal R. Frankel, DO, and L. Albert Villarin, Jr., MD, to the previous edition of this text.

 REFERENCES CAN BE FOUND ON EXPERT CONSULT

GENITOURINARY, OBSTETRIC, AND GYNECOLOGIC PROCEDURES

CHAPTER **55**

Urologic Procedures

Michael A. Silverman and Robert E. Schneider

This chapter addresses urologic conditions that are either initially or eventually associated with an emergency procedure or may need to be performed in the absence of a urologic surgeon.

Testicular torsion is an emergency that can be difficult to diagnose under the best clinical conditions. Although some argue that surgical exploration, rather than radionuclide scanning or color Doppler ultrasonography, is the diagnostic and therapeutic procedure of choice, most urologists prefer some study before surgical exploration. This chapter addresses bedside maneuvers including testicular detorsion for this entity in the setting of scrotal pain.

Access to and the subsequent evaluation of bladder urine are clinically important to every practicing clinician. Various approaches to urine sampling, including the techniques and complications of male and female urethral catheterization in various clinical situations, are addressed.

Finally, a discussion of radiographic imaging of the genitourinary system is provided, with an emphasis on assessing lower urinary tract injury. Although the timing of genitourinary radiologic examinations within the work-up of the critically ill multiple trauma patient must be individualized, general guidelines are provided.

PHIMOSIS AND DORSAL SLIT

Phimosis, the inability to retract the penile foreskin, is not by itself an emergency unless it results in complete obstruction of the preputial opening (rare) or is transposed into paraphimosis. *Paraphimosis*, the inability to replace the foreskin back over the glands penis, is a urologic emergency, or an emergency if it inhibits urinary flow. Phimosis has been recognized since ancient times. Models of phimotic foreskin have been found near the altars of Hygeia and Aesendopius in ancient Greece. Orikosius (AD 325–403) was the first to describe the dorsal slit as definitive treatment for phimosis.

Circumcision, removal of the foreskin that renders phimosis and paraphimosis anatomically impossible, is common-place in America; but circumcision rates vary among socioeconomic status, religious affiliation, and racial and ethnic groups. In the mid-1990s, several medical societies published statements that did not recommend routine circumcision.[1-3] Between the mid-1960s and 2003, circumcision rates declined by approximately 20%, thus making the potential for complications such as phimosis more common. Congenital phimosis is common in young patients, but typically declines with age and pediatric patients rarely require treatment.[4]

After any injury or inflammatory event, the foreskin (prepuce) reacts by forming scar tissue. The normally soft pliable foreskin can develop sufficient distal scarring to make routine retraction of the tissue over the glans penis difficult or impossible. This is especially true if the end of the foreskin is injured, such as in zipper injuries, toilet seat trauma, or other crush injuries (known as the Tristram Shandy syndrome, after the well-known literary character who had a window sash fall on his penis while he was urinating out the window). A chronically irritated and infected foreskin often occurs in diabetic patients.[5] Rarely, a tight phimosis and accompanying poor hygiene may lead to abscesses of the foreskin, which can result in further contracture.

Asymptomatic phimosis does not ordinarily require any treatment. It may prevent or make easy urethral catheterization more difficult. In such situations, the phimotic opening may need to be dilated. An alternative strategy is to crush a portion of the foreskin followed by an incision (dorsal slit), using light sedation and local anesthesia to allow access to the urethral meatus. This minor operative procedure can be easily performed in the emergency department (ED).

Dorsal Slit: Indications and Contraindications

Dorsal slit of the foreskin is performed in any emergent situation either to gain access to the urethral meatus for urethral catheterization or as definitive treatment after simple foreskin reduction or phimotic ring incision and foreskin reduction in a patient with paraphimosis. Elective circumcision rather than dorsal slit of the foreskin is the definitive procedure of choice in nonemergent situations. Medical management for patients in the ED who will be discharged can include the application of steroid creams (0.1% triamcinolone) once or twice daily. Topical antibiotics or antifungals may be required to treat concomitant balanitis (inflammation of the glans or head of the penis) or balanoposthitis (inflammation of the foreskin and the glans).

TABLE 55–1 Equipment Needed to Perform Dorsal Slit for the Emergency Treatment of Phimosis

1% lidocaine (Xylocaine) without epinephrine
5-mL syringe
27-gauge needle
1 straight Crile clamp
1 straight scissors
1 needle holder
4-0 absorbable suture

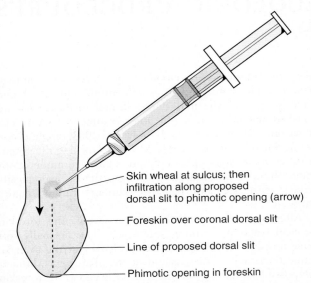

Skin wheal at sulcus; then infiltration along proposed dorsal slit to phimotic opening (arrow)

Foreskin over coronal dorsal slit

Line of proposed dorsal slit

Phimotic opening in foreskin

Figure 55–1 Technique for obtaining anesthesia before performing a dorsal slit. See also Figure 55–7 for anesthesia for paraphimosis.

Procedure

Table 55–1 lists the equipment needed to perform dorsal slit of the foreskin. With the patient in the supine position, clean and drape the penis with sterile towels. Clipping of the pubic hair is unnecessary. Then infiltrate 1% *plain lidocaine without epinephrine* into the dorsal midline of the foreskin just beneath the superficial fascia throughout the course of the proposed incision, starting proximally at the level of the coronal sulcus and proceeding distally to the tip of the foreskin (Fig. 55–1; see Fig. 55–7 later). Consider mixing equal volumes of 1% lidocaine with 0.5% bupivicaine. After 3 to 5 minutes, grasp the foreskin with toothed forceps to test for anesthesia. The operator must be certain that the inner surface of the foreskin is also anesthetized. If this area is not numb, use a dorsal nerve block or "ring block" at the base of the penis (Fig. 55–2).[6]

After achieving both adequate local anesthesia and light sedation, the operator takes a straight hemostat and carefully advances both jaws of the hemostat proximally to the area of the coronal sulcus between the inner layer of the foreskin and the smooth glans penis, carefully separating any existing preputial adhesions. Take care that the meatus and urethra are visualized or palpated at all times to avoid inadvertent injury during this maneuver. Once release of adhesions is complete, open the hemostat, and place one jaw of the hemostat in the recently developed plane between the glans penis, opened to tent the skin to ensure proper placement, and the superior overlying inner layer of foreskin. Advance the hemostat to the level of the coronal sulcus and then close it, effectively crushing the interposed anesthetized foreskin (Fig. 55–3). Leave

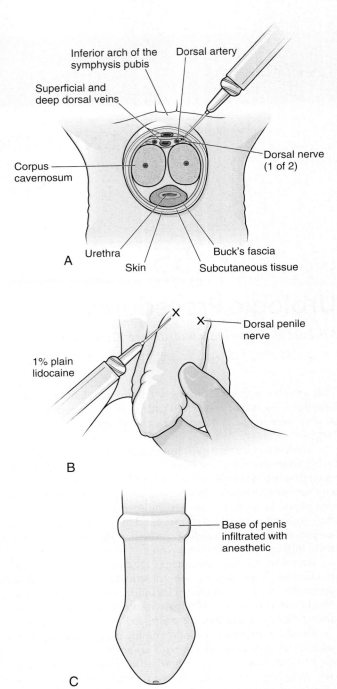

Figure 55–2 *A,* The penis has two dorsal penile arteries and two nerves (running together) and one dorsal penile vein (in the midline). To block the dorsum of the penis, infiltrate both nerves at the base of the penis. Dorsal nerve block at the base of the penis will provide anesthesia of *only the dorsum of the penis. B,* Landmarks for penile block: Inject at the base of the penis lateral to the midline at approximately the 10 and 2 o'clock positions. *C,* Circumferential subcutaneous lidocaine (without epinephrine) infiltration for a ("ring") field block at the base of the penis can provide anesthesia to the entire distal penis. *(A, From Soliman MG, Tremblay NA: Nerve block of the penis for postoperative pain relief in children. Anesth Analg 57:495, 1978. Reproduced by permission.)*

the closed hemostat in place for 3 to 5 minutes, then remove it and cut the resultant serrated crushed foreskin longitudinally with straight scissors throughout the extent of the crushed tissue. Normally, the incised, anatomically approximated skin edges bleed and ooze. Not infrequently, these skin

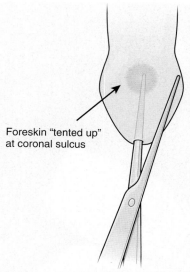

Figure 55–3 **Placement of a hemostat for treatment of phimosis.** The "tenting up" of the foreskin (*arrow*) in this manner proves that the tip of the hemostat is not in the urethra or under the glans. Once the hemostat is properly placed between the glans and the overlying foreskin, close it to crush the area of the foreskin to be cut.

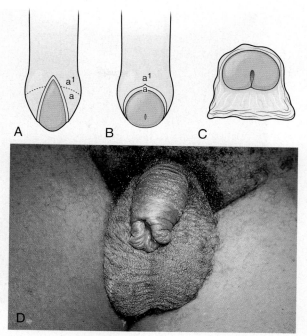

Figure 55–4 **Treatment of phimosis.** *A,* Dorsal slit in the phimotic foreskin. The exposed glans is *shaded.* A single (dorsal) lengthwise incision has been made through crushed tissue (a^1, outer layer of foreskin; *a,* inner layer of foreskin). *B,* Cut edges of the foreskin drawn back around glans penis. First, suture a^1 to *a,* then sew the remainder of the cut edges together for hemostasis. *C,* Final "beagle-ear" deformity of the ventral transposed foreskin after the dorsal slit procedure has been completed. *D,* Postoperative appearance of the dorsal slit showing "beagle-ear".

edges of the foreskin separate into two layers, the outer foreskin and the inner foreskin (Fig. 55–4*A* and *B*). Two absorbable chromic or Vicryl (4.0–5.0 for children and 3.0–4.0 for adults) running hemostatic sutures may be placed, each beginning proximally at the apex of the dorsal slit and carried distally, reapproximating the two leaves of foreskin. Bacitracin ointment may be used to lubricate the suture material to facilitate passage of the suture through the delicate skin tissues.

After successful dorsal slit of the foreskin, the prepuce is easily retracted for cleansing of the glans penis or exposure of the urethral meatus. Postprocedural conscientious foreskin reduction to its normal anatomic position must be ensured after any distal penile procedure to avoid iatrogenic paraphimosis.

Ideally, a definitive elective circumcision is recommended after a dorsal slit. Some patients complain about the appearance of their incised foreskin ("dog ears") and the relative inconvenience during urination, whereas others are pleased they no longer have their phimosis and refuse further treatment (see Fig. 55–4*C* and *D*).

Complications

Injury to the urethral meatus and the glans penis may occur if the hemostat or straight scissors are blindly and unknowingly introduced into the urethra. Bleeding may occur if the hemostat has not adequately crushed the foreskin or the scissor incision is made lateral to the serrated crushed tissue. The latter two problems are easily resolved with the previously described running hemostatic suture.

PARAPHIMOSIS AND FORESKIN REDUCTION

Background

Paraphimosis is a urologic emergency. By definition, it is the *inability to reduce the proximally positioned uncircumsized foreskin*

over the glans penis to its normal anatomic position (Fig. 55–5*A*). As with phimosis, a decline in circumcision rates has the potential to increase complications such as paraphimosis in the uncircumcised male. In the obtunded or demented patient, subjective pain may not be perceived or communicated. Today, the most common cause of paraphimosis is iatrogenic: The catheterist or examining health care provider forgets to reduce the foreskin after penile examination or urethral instrumentation. Other causes include failure to return the foreskin to its normal position after intercourse, exotic dancing, and genital piercing.[7,8] Paraphimosis can be quite subtle and may be either unrecognized or misdiagnosed as an allergic reaction, penile trauma, or an infection by those unfamiliar with the condition (see Fig. 55–5). This cannot occur if the patient has been circumcised, so this information is sought.

The coexisting phimotic ring initially interferes with venous and lymphatic drainage, precipitating foreskin swelling. Over time, the degree of swelling prevents manual reduction of the retracted foreskin. When left untreated, eventual arterial embarrassment leads to tissue anoxia, skin ulceration, and ultimately, infection or penile gangrene, or both.[9]

Emergent manual or surgical reduction of the edematous foreskin is mandatory to restore proper circulation, relieve discomfort, and permit resolution of potential serious sequelae: skin ulceration and gangrene. It must be done as soon as a paraphimosis is recognized. Once the foreskin is successfully reduced, dorsal slit as previously described is advised in those cases of potential patient noncompliance until definitive circumcision can be performed.

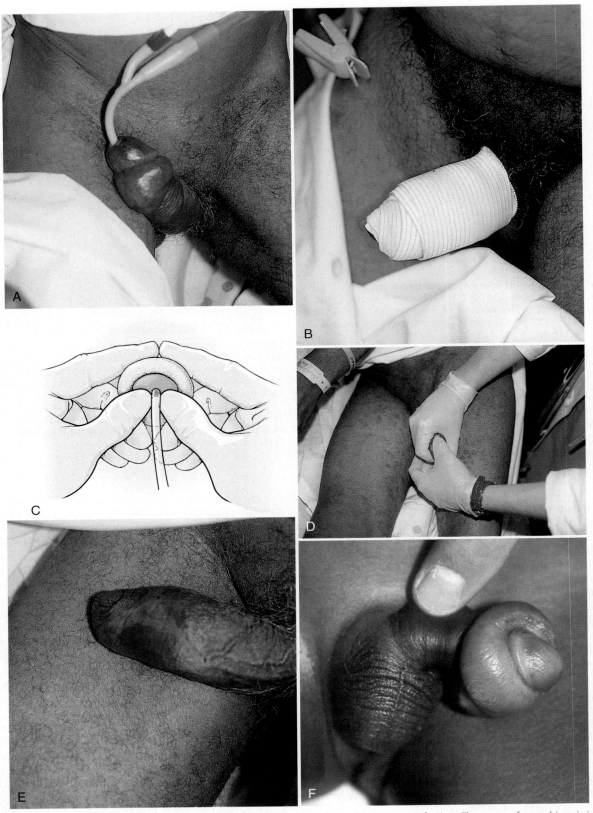

Figure 55–5 *A,* Paraphimosis, pictured here, may be mistaken for penile trauma, angioedema, or infection. The cause of paraphimosis in this case was failure to replace the foreskin in an uncircumsized man after a catheter change in a demented nursing home patient. Before reduction, *the catheter is usually removed.* When the edema is minimal, the catheter may be left in place during reduction. *B,* Compression of the foreskin by wrapping the penis with an elastic bandage for a few minutes may reduce edema before attempting a reduction of the paraphimosis. *C,* Technique for reduction of paraphimosis. Place gentle, steady pressure on the glans with the tips of the thumbs while applying gentle traction to the foreskin. In this line drawing, the catheter is left in place during reduction but removal may be required. *D,* In a manner reminiscent of removing a rubber glove, the thumb forces the glans through the foreskin that is encircled by the entire palm to achieve final reduction (*E*). The catheter may be replaced, ensuring that the foreskin is properly replaced afterward. *F,* Uncircumcised boy with paraphimosis. This may be mistaken for infection or localized trauma especially if it is unclear whether or not a circumcision has been performed. Always seek this history. (*C, from Neuwirth H, Frasier B, Cochran ST: Genitourinary imaging and procedures by the emergency clinician. Emerg Med Clin North Am 7:1, 1989.*)

Indications and Contraindications

Emergent reduction of a paraphimotic foreskin is indicated whenever the condition exists. There are no contraindications.

Procedure

Manual Reduction[9]

The current standard for reducing paraphimosis is manual reduction. This can be accomplished by using a nonirritating topical anesthetic lubricant applied to the inner surface of the foreskin (not to the shaft of the penis) and the glans to reduce friction and decrease the discomfort of the procedure. A previously described penile block may be performed if required. Light sedation is an excellent adjunct. Then compress the foreskin for several minutes to reduce as much edema fluid as possible (see Fig. 55–5B). Several authors have suggested ways to reduce the edema before attempting manual reduction or if manual reduction fails. Snugly wrapping the distal penis from the glans to the base in a 5-cm piece of Elastoplast (or elastic bandage) for 10 minutes has also been described.[10] Osmotic methods are used to produce a high solute concentration on the surface of the edematous area to draw water from the engorged tissue along the osmotic gradient. Granulated sugar has been studied, but a better alternative for the ED patient is to soak a swab in 50 mL of 50% dextrose solution and leave it wrapped around the paraphimosis for 1 hour.[11] This is obviously time consuming and does not provide immediate reduction of the foreskin. Another alternative is to inject 1 mL of hyaluronidase (150 U/mL Wydase) by tuberculin syringe into one or two sites in the edematous prepuce to reduce edema fluid immediately, thus allowing the foreskin to be retracted over the glans with minimal patient discomfort.[12,13] If the patient is catheterized, the catheter may be removed and replaced later, but that is not generally recommended or necessary. Most often, reduction of minor paraphimosis can be completed with the catheter in place.

The index and long fingers of both hands are placed in apposition just proximal to the phimotic ring. Both thumbs are aligned on the urethral meatus. Constant force is applied as the thumbs try to invert the glans penis proximally while the index and long fingers attempt to reduce the phimotic ring distally over the glans penis into its normal anatomic position (see Fig. 55–5C). Successful reduction results in the appearance of an uncircumcised penis with a phimotic foreskin. Alternatively, the thumb may be used to push the glans through the foreskin that has been encircled by the entire palm—in a maneuver similar to taking off a rubber glove (see Fig. 55–5D and E). The key to success in both of these maneuvers is the application of slow, steady pressure.

The Puncture Method

The puncture method was originally described in the early 1990s as a way to facilitate manual reduction of paraphimosis.[14,15] A penile block is used to provide anesthesia. Approximately 20 puncture holes are made in the edematous tissue with a 26-gauge needle. Then compress the prepuce manually to express edema fluid out of the puncture sites. Manual reduction can then be more easily accomplished. A key point to remember is that the edema fluid is not under pressure and the manual compression might not decrease the swelling as much as the operator will need to successfully accomplish this technique.

Assisted Manual Reduction ("Iced-Glove" Method or Babcock Clamp Method)

If the constricting phimotic ring cannot be brought down over the glans easily, additional measures may be used. In the "iced-glove" method,[16] cold compression is used to reduce foreskin swelling and induce vasoconstriction in the glans penis. Half fill a large glove with crushed ice and water, and tie the cuff end securely. Invaginate the thumb of the glove and then draw it over the lubricated paraphimotic penis. Hold the thumb of the glove securely in place over the penis for 5 to 10 minutes. The combination of cooling and compression usually decreases the edema sufficiently to permit manual reduction of the foreskin. If the constricting ring cannot be brought down over the glans after this maneuver, it may be necessary to use Babcock clamps. Use from six to eight Babcock clamps (not Allis clamps, which are serrated and intolerably painful for the patient) to grasp the phimotic ring circumferentially.[17] Then slowly pull the clamps distally over the glans. With gentle, slow traction, the phimotic ring can hopefully be reduced over the glans penis (Fig. 55–6).

Complications

Penile shaft laceration or simple tearing of compromised penile skin may occur during manual or surgical paraphimotic reduction. Simple suturing will resolve most injuries.

If reduction of a paraphimosis cannot be achieved with other means, then surgical interventions should be considered. Figure 55–7 describes the dorsal slit procedure which involves carefully sterilizing the field, anesthetizing the penis on the dorsal aspect followed by a linear incision.

PRIAPISM AND PENILE INJECTION/ASPIRATION

Priapism is manifested by a persistent, usually painful, penile erection, unrelated to sexual stimulation and not relieved by ejaculation. Most often, priapism is a urologic emergency associated with a high incidence of impotence, regardless of treatment. It is characterized clinically by a soft glans penis and spongy urethra in the presence of two erect penile bodies or corpora cavernosa. Although reported in most age groups, the condition is most common between the ages of 30 and 50 years.

The pathophysiology of priapism is complex. The pharmacologic basis for treatment is based on manipulating blood flow via the α- and β-receptors. Priapsm is believed to result from increased arterial inflow of blood into the corpora cav-

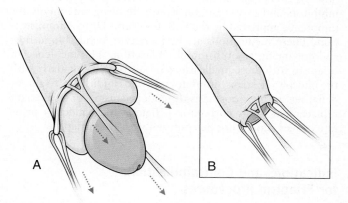

Figure 55–6 *A,* Application of Babcock clamps to reduce paraphimosis. *B,* Foreskin reduced.

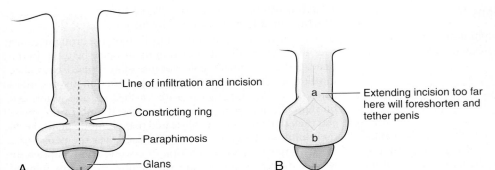

Figure 55–7 *A,* Anesthetizing the penis for surgical treatment of paraphimosis that cannot be manually reduced. Line of infiltration of local anesthesia used before performing the dorsal slit. *B,* Incision for paraphimosis. Diamond-shaped defect results from linear incision of foreskin. Approximate the two apices of the dorsal slit (*a* and *b*) after the foreskin is reduced.

ernosa secondary to dilatation of the cavernosal arteries. Relaxation of the cavernosal tissue occurs and secondary compression of the emissary veins leads to engorgement of both corpora cavernosa during an erection. When the cavernosal pressure approaches the arterial pressure, blood flow is markedly reduced. Ischemic or low-flow priapism results after several hours of continuous painful erection, leading to intracavernosal acidosis and sludging of blood with subsequent thrombosis of the cavernosal arteries, fibrosis of the corporal tissue, and irreversible impotence. This urologic emergency is frequently treated by the emergency clinician, often with urologic input and arranged follow-up.

High-flow priapism is less common than low-flow priapism and usually results from traumatic production of an arteriocavernosal fistula. It is not associated with intracavernosal ischemia or acidosis and is, therefore, painless and may be treated electively rather than emergently.

In the past, priapism was most often encountered as a complication of a number of medical (e.g., hematologic, neoplastic, and drug-related) conditions (Table 55–2). Today, many cases are idiopathic or iatrogenic, resulting from the current practice of using vasoactive substances (e.g., papaverine and phentolamine) and newer erectile dysfunction medicines to induce penile erections in impotent men. Sickle cell disease continues to be a leading cause of priapism. Sickle cell patients may experience such a high rate of recurrence that home self-injection of vasoactive drugs into the penis has been advocated. Cocaine use is one etiology that is likely underreported.[18] A drug screen may unravel some discrepancies between clinical findings and history. As an end result, vasoactive drugs promote engorgement of the corpora cavernosa and reduction in venous outflow, which may result in low-flow or ischemic priapism.[19–21] Several phosphodiesterase inhibitors and prostaglandin E_1 are the drug treatments for impotence approved by the U.S. Food and Drug Administration. These medications act by increasing penile blood flow and enhancing smooth muscle relaxation. The incidence of priapism with these medications is quite low, particularly with the phosphodiesterase inhibitors. Penile rigidity due to a nondeflating penile prosthesis (pseudopriapism) or malignant replacement of the corpora in patients with bladder or prostate cancer should not be confused with true priapism.

Indications and Contraindications for Priapism Procedures

The emergency clinician should attempt to identify reversible causes for low-flow priapism and, in conjunction with a urolo-

gist to provide follow-up, initiate specific corrective therapy as soon as possible. Almost 66% of cases of low-flow priapism in children and young adults are due to sickle cell disease, and such cases may respond to noninvasive standard antisickling measures (including exchange transfusion).

TABLE 55–2 Etiologies of Priapism	
Intracavernosal Agents	Hydroxyzine
Papaverine	Total parenteral nutrition
Phentolamine	**Hematologic**
Prostaglandin E_1	Anemia
Antihypertensive Agents	Fat emboli
Ganglion-blocking agents	Leukemia
Arterial vasodilators	Multiple myeloma
α-Antagonist agents	Sickle cell disease
Calcium-channel blocking agents	Thalassemias
Psychotropic Drugs	**Metabolic**
Phenothiazines	Amyloidosis
Butyrophenones	Fabry disease
Hypnotics	Gout
Trazodone	**Miscellaneous**
Selective serotonin-reuptake inhibitors	Carbon monoxide
Anticoagulants	Malaria
Heparin	Black widow spider venom
Warfarin	Scorpion sting
Recreational Drugs	Asplenism
Cocaine	**Neurogenic**
Marijuana	Spinal cord lesions
Ethanol	Cauda equina compression
Performance-enhancing drugs	Autonomic neuropathy
Hormones	Spinal stenosis
Gonadotropin-releasing hormone	Anesthesia
Tamoxifen	**Trauma**
Testosterone	Genital
Medications	Pelvic
Metoclopramide	Perineal
Omeprazole	

Adapted from Mulhall JP, Honig SC: Priapism: Etiology and management. *Acad Emerg Med* 3:810, 1996. Reproduced with permission.

Regardless of the etiology, this distressing condition is *first treated with adequate analgesia, often consisting of parenteral opiates and benzodiazepines.* Empirical terbutaline, 0.25 to 0.5 mg, given subcutaneously, is recommended for every patient presenting with low-flow priapism as soon as the diagnosis is suspected. This treatment may be repeated, when needed, in 15 to 20 minutes.[22] If a patient with previous low-flow priapism calls from home with a recurrence and has the appropriate supplies, he should be instructed to inject himself with terbutaline (as described earlier) or take a 5-mg terbutaline tablet by mouth, if available, before coming to the ED. The pharmacotherapeutic action of terbutaline for priapism is not well elucidated. Oral pseudoephedrine (60–120 mg) also has been suggested as a noninvasive initial therapy for low-flow priapism secondary to intracavernosal agents, but its efficacy has not been well studied.[23] Although terbutaline and other oral or parenteral medications have been advocated for the treatment of priapism, such interventions might not be successful, and many cases will require more aggressive procedures. Table 55–3 lists the reversible causes of low-flow priapism with their respective therapies.

In the majority of patients, no reversible cause will be identified. When detumescence does not occur with subcutaneous terbutaline, the condition necessitates corporal aspiration/injection alone or corporal aspiration and irrigation with an α-agonist (epinephrine or phenylephrine [Neo-Synephrine]). Conservative measures, such as sedation and analgesia, oral estrogens, ice-water enemas, transurethral diathermy, spinal/epidural/general anesthesia, and local anesthetic injections have not proved to be of value and should not be used in lieu of definitive intracavernosal therapy.[23] Should initial medical and corporal aspiration and irrigation fail, Lue and coworkers[24] recommended that further therapy be guided by cavernosal blood gas and pressure measurements. If one elects to use blood gas analysis of aspirated corporal blood to help guide therapy, the initial results will reflect the degree of ischemia present in the priapismic penis. Sequential blood gas analyses that fail to show an improvement in the initial acidosis (pH remaining at ≤7.10) despite corporal aspiration or irrigation, or both, suggest that a more aggressive definitive corpus cavernosum-spongiosum shunt may be indicated, and more urgent urologic intervention should be sought. Although not usually performed, the aspirating or irrigating corporal needle may also be used for measurement of intracorporal pressures similar to the approach outlined for muscular compartmental pressures.[25] A variety of regimens and protocols have been suggested for the treatment of priapism. No single intervention has shown superior efficacy.

The mainstay of therapy for advanced priapism is aspiration of the corpora cavernosa combined with saline irrigation, usually coupled with the intracavernosal injection of α-adrenergic agents. When urologic consultation is unavailable or delayed, the emergency clinician can initiate therapeutic corporal aspiration. Because prolonged priapism increases the risk of subsequent erectile dysfunction, an aggressive management strategy is advised. Impotence rates of up to 35% to 60% have been reported when priapism persists for 5 to 10 days, respectively.[23] If present for more than 24 hours, priapism often does not respond to aspiration techniques. Recurrence is not uncommon, and some patients require multiple procedures on a frequent basis. Shunting procedures might be required if the measures described earlier are not successful.

Procedure

Simple Intracorporal Injection

Table 55–4 lists the equipment needed for aspiration and irrigation of corpus cavernosum. Whereas the aspiration/irrigation technique is often recommended, some clinicians have had success with the simple injection of vasoactive solutions into the corpus cavernosum. This negates the more complicated irrigation procedure, and the minimally invasive procedure may be attempted as an initial approach. This procedure is used by outpatients as a self-injection technique for recurrent priapism. With this technique, a 25- to 27-gauge needle

---

TABLE 55–3 Treatment of Low-Flow Priapism Based on Etiology

A. Terbutaline 0.25–0.5 mg subcutaneously in the deltoid muscle area or thigh for all patients with priapism (may be repeated in 15–20 min); alternatively, 5 mg terbutaline per os may be used (1 dose). Note: this is often not successful.

B. Reversible causes
   1. Sickle cell anemia
      a. Packed red blood cell transfusion
      b. Hyperbaric oxygenation (investigational)
   2. Iatrogenic injection of prostaglandin E₁, papaverine, or phentolamine for impotence
      a. Corporal aspiration of 30–60 mL of blood, followed by observation
         (1) Detumescence: no further treatment
         (2) Persistent erection: Inject an equal volume of an α-agonist (e.g., phenylephrine, 10 mg in 500 mL of normal saline)
   3. Leukemic infiltration
      a. Specific chemotherapy
   4. Medication (phenothiazines, trazodone)
      a. Corporeal aspiration, observation
      b. α-Agonist instillation, observation
      c. Heparin irrigation of corporeal bodies, observation
      d. Corpus cavernosum-spongiosum shunt

C. Nonreversible causes
   1. Idiopathic
   2. High spinal cord lesion

TABLE 55–4 Equipment Needed for Aspiration of Corpus Cavernosum for Low-Flow Priapism

27-gauge needle (for penile block)
1-mL syringe (for local anesthetic)
1% lidocaine without epinephrine (for penile block)
Sterile drapes
Gauze sponges
Chlorhexidine preparation solution
19-gauge butterfly needles (for aspiration)
2 30-mL syringes (for aspiration and injection)
Sterile basin for aspirated blood
Blood gas syringe with cap
Irrigation fluid (one of the following vasoactive agents* is diluted with 500 mL of normal saline and up to 20–30 mL is administered in small aliquots; 5000 units of heparin added to solution is optional; see text)
Phenylephrine, 10 mg/500 mL of saline
Norepinephrine, 1 mg/500 mL of saline
Epinephrine, 0.5 mg/500 mL of saline

*Systemic absorption of vasoactive agents may occur with adverse cardiovascular effects.

is used to inject vasoactive substances into the corpus at the base of the penis, with the goal of pharmacologically reversing the priapismic process. Often, this can be done without anesthesia. Specific protocols are not established, but one option is to draw up 0.5 mg of phenylephrine into a 3-mL syringe and add 2 mL of saline diluent. Puncture the corpus with the needle at the 10 o'clock or 2 o'clock position at the base of the penis, aspirate blood to confirm position, and inject the solution. If not successful in 30 minutes, give a repeat injection, up to a total of three injections (Fig. 55–8). In one small study, successful detumescence was achieved in eight of nine patients by simple intracorporal injection of phenylephrine with this regimen, with three or fewer injections being required.[26] Alternatively, 0.1 mg of epinephrine (0.1 mL of 1:1000) diluted with 1 mL of saline may be used. Anecdotal success has been noted by injecting the corpus cavernosum with 2 to 3 mL of the local anesthetic lidocaine (2% with epinephrine 1:100,000) in a similar manner. Only one side need be injected, and two or three injections might be necessary. Wait at least 20 minutes before additional interventions after each injection. *Note that this is essentially an intravenous injection and systemic effects may be produced.* Proceed with caution in patients with cardiovascular disease. Additional injections with partial detumescence are more likely to introduce medication as a bolus into the general circulation.[27,28]

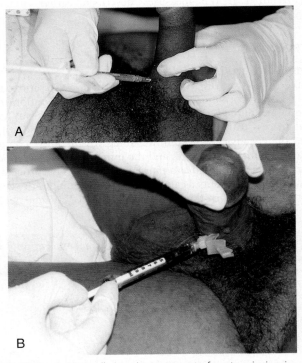

Figure 55–8 *A,* Minimally invasive treatment of acute priapism is often successful and can be used at home by the motivated patient with recurrent problems (such as sickle cell disease). As an initial approach to priapism and as an alternative to aspiration/irrigation, the intracorporeal injection of vasoactive drugs such as epinephrine or phenylephrine may be used. Use a small-gauge needle to inject the corpus at 10 o'clock or 2 o'clock, at the base or proximal shaft of the penis. *B,* Aspiration of blood confirms proper needle placement prior to injection. Only one side need be injected. Repeat injection might be required if unsuccessful after 20 min. Injections with 0.1 mg of epinephrine (0.1 mL of 1:1000 concentration) plus 1 mL saline is often used. *Note that this procedure is akin to an intravenous injection and systemic effects may be precipitated, especially if repeat doses or injections during partial detumescence are given.*

Aspiration and/or Irrigation (see Table 55–4)

This procedure entails drainage of blood from the erect penis and the instillation of a vasoactive medication. Alternatively, irrigation (aspirate, infuse, aspirate) with aliquots of a dilute vasoactive solution is also effective. Place the patient in the supine position (Fig. 55–9A–D). Parenteral analgesia and sedation are suggested. Local anesthesia at the puncture site is recommended for this procedure. An injection of 1% plain lidocaine placed at the base of the penis for a dorsal penile nerve block or placement of a circumferential penile block can be performed, but are usually not necessary (see Fig. 55–2). Sterilely prepare and drape the penis. The clinician grasps the shaft of the penis with the left hand using the thumb and index finger. Palpate an engorged corpus cavernosum laterally (2 and 10 o'clock) and insert a 21- to 19-gauge butterfly needle into one of the corpus cavernosum.[25] Alternatively, a 20-gauge intravenous catheter may be used, but the butterfly needle catheter is preferred. If palpation fails to demonstrate the corpus, blindly inserting the needle at either 10 o'clock or 2 o'clock will usually gain access to this large vascular structure. Because there is communication of blood flow between both sides, the operator needs access to only one of the corpora. Either side may be punctured. The site of needle placement is one of personal preference, and locations from the base to the proximal shaft of the penis have been suggested. The editors suggest using the proximal shaft, 3 to 4 cm from the base, for irrigation, and the base for simple injection. *The glans should not be used as a puncture site.*

The needle is advanced in a 45° angle, using constant suction. *Blood is usually readily aspirated;* once it is obtained, the needle is not advanced further and is stabilized. Deep penetration is to be avoided to minimize the risk of injury to the cavernosal artery during this procedure.

An initial 20 to 30 mL of corporal blood is aspirated while the operator milks the corpus with the left hand. *Excessive suction should not be applied because this often halts the aspiration. A common error is to use too much suction with a 60-mL syringe.* Using a 10-mL syringe, and changing it if it fills with blood, is preferable. Use of a butterfly reduces the danger of dislodging the needle when changing syringes. Continue this initial aspiration until the original egress of dark blood ceases and bright red arterial blood returns or complete detumescence is obtained and persists. Because multiple anastomoses exist between the two corpora cavernosa, bilateral aspiration is not required.

If detumescence is achieved after initial aspiration, no further treatment may be required. However, if this is successful, some advise injecting an aliquot of vasoactive substance, such as 0.1 mg epinephrine (0.1 mL of 1:1000 or 1 mL of 1:10,000). *If the irrigating solution contained epinephrine/phenylephrine, additional medication is not suggested.*

A number of irrigating solutions have been suggested, but none has proved superiority. Some suggest 20 to 30 mL of a phenylephrine/normal saline solution (10 mg of phenylephrine in 500 mL of normal saline) as the exchange for 20 to 30 mL of aspirated corporal blood. Some clinicians add 2500 to 5000 units of heparin to the solution, but the value of heparin is unproved. Alternatively, 1 mg of epinephrine can be added to 1 L of saline, with irrigation performed using 20 to 30 mL aliquots. A norepinephrine solution also may be used. Note that the corpus cavernosum has ready access to systemic circulation, and injecting a drug into it is essentially the same as an intravenous injection. When detumescence occurs, the unmetabolized drug enters the venous system;

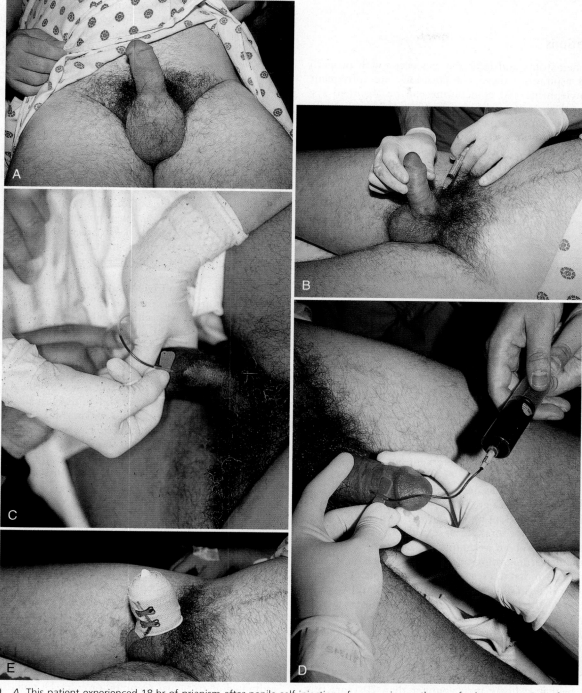

Figure 55–9 *A,* This patient experienced 18 hr of priapism after penile self-injection of papaverine as therapy for impotence. *B,* Perform a penile dorsal nerve block. *C,* Insert a 19-gauge butterfly needle into the corpus via the proximal penile shaft at either the 2 o'clock or the 10 o'clock position and aspirate. Only one side need be punctured. *D, Slow steady suction will be most successful,* whereas excessive suction may halt the aspiration. Do not puncture the corpus via the glans (see text). After initial aspiration, irrigate (slowly inject and withdraw) 10- to 20-mL aliquots of vasoactive solution until detumescence persists. *E,* After detumescence with the first aspiration or with aspiration-irrigation-aspiration of a vasoactive medication (see text), wrap the penis with an elastic bandage to discourage re-engorgement and to compress the puncture site. *Note:* Acceptable procedures include aspiration alone followed by instillation of a small aliquot of epinephrine (0.1 mg) and combined multiple aspiration and irrigations with a vasoactive solution. The end point is the appearance of bright red arterial blood and/or persistent detumescence.

therefore, vasoactive drug dosages should be monitored. Some clinicians wrap the penis snugly in an elastic wrap with the needle securely in place after aspiration to discourage retumescence and decrease hematoma formation of the penile shaft.

Complications

Although hematoma and infection can occur with properly performed aspiration, these complications are infrequent. Both phenylephrine and epinephrine can be absorbed systemically, with the potential for toxic effects.[24] Therefore, the intracavernosal use of vasoactive agents is contraindicated in patients with conditions sensitive to these agents (e.g., severe hypertension, dysrhythmias, monoamine oxidase inhibitor use). Blood pressure and cardiac rhythm should be monitored throughout the procedure if the patient is at risk. Supplemental oxygen should be considered in any patient undergoing conscious sedation. Failure to aspirate blood is a potential complication, usually because of a misplaced needle, applying excessive suction, or if blood has clotted. Because impotence is a well-recognized complication after priapism, regardless of the cause or the promptness of therapeutic intervention, the patient must be advised both verbally and in writing of this potential complication.

ADJUNCTIVE TESTING IN ACUTE SCROTAL PAIN

Establishing a diagnosis in the patient with acute scrotal pain creates significant clinician anxiety. The condition most easily confused with torsion of the testicle is acute epididymitis. The prompt diagnosis of testicular torsion and differentiation of this condition from epididymitis can be quite difficult, but it is obviously crucial to the patient's care. The treatment of acute epididymitis requires appropriate antimicrobial and supportive therapy. The treatment of testicular torsion requires emergent operative intervention, not excessive adjunctive testing.[29]

Testicular salvage rates decrease with time. Some studies suggest that salvage rates are 80% to 100% when detorsion occurs within 6 hours but are near 0% at 12 hours. It is recognized that testis may torse, detorse, and retorse so clinicians should be cautious about assigning an exact time as the time of onset and deferring urologic consultation based on an erroneous assumption that the testis is not salvageable. The "gold standard" for determining testicular viability is intraoperative visualization of the affected testis, which dictates early urologic involvement. Although all clinicians recognize the need for expedient surgery in the setting of known torsion, not all consultants will agree on surgical exploration without some adjunctive testing.

Torsion of the testicle is the most frequent cause of acute testicular pain in celibate men younger than 20 years (Fig. 55–10). One pediatric series of patients presenting with a painful scrotum reported a 6% incidence of epididymitis versus a 42% incidence of testicular torsion and a 32% incidence of torsion of the appendix testis and epididymis.[30] It is interesting to note that pyuria was seen in 10% of the patients with testicular torsion and in 80% of the children with epididymitis. In men 20 years or older, testicular torsion is less common, but it must always be considered in the differential diagnosis because it may occur well into the 7th decade of life.[31]

In contrast, epididymitis is an uncommon condition in young celibate boys unless a congenital lower urinary tract abnormality is present, promoting urinary tract infection (UTI) with subsequent epididymitis.

As with all difficult diagnostic dilemmas, the patient's history is of paramount importance in establishing the correct diagnosis. The evaluation of acute scrotal pain is no different. In considering epididymitis, detailed and often probing questions must be asked regarding the patient's work habits and his sexual experiences. The pathophysiology of epididymitis is believed to be related to the generation of increased pressure in the prostatic urethra as a result of either heavy lifting (e.g., in roofers or construction workers), detrusor external sphincter dyssynergia (e.g., in patients with neurogenic bladder dysfunction), or iatrogenic promotion of a Valsalva maneuver for whatever reason. These mechanisms force sterile or infected urine out through the ejaculatory ducts into the vas deferens (urethrovasal reflux), then retrograde down the vas into the tail of the epididymis (globus minor). Initially, this may cause nonspecific lower quadrant abdominal pain or inguinal canal pain (vasitis) before it causes scrotal or testicular pain, and vasitis should be included in the initial differential diagnosis in any male presenting with lower abdominal pain.

Sexually transmitted diseases (STDs) with subsequent epididymitis are quite common in sexually active young men, usually associated with chlamydial or gonococcal urethritis. Signs and symptoms of infection may be minimal when the patient is first examined.[32] The presence of genitourinary infection, a history of previous STDs, or a history of multiple sexual partners and the absence of penile protection during intercourse may all be important clues to the diagnosis of epididymitis. In older men, epididymitis is usually due to UTI secondary to outlet obstruction or urethral stricture disease. In such cases, Enterobacteriaceae, *Entercocci*, and *Pseudomonas* species are the predominant organisms. If one cannot be certain after taking a careful history and examining the patient that epididymitis or torsion of the appendix testis or epididymis is the correct diagnosis, then urologic consultation to exclude testicular torsion is required. A clinical diagnosis of epididymitis should be based on the focal finding of epididymal induration and tenderness (the vas deferens also might be involved) in the proper patient population. The site of tenderness is best discerned when examining the patient in the relaxed supine position. Although testicular tenderness can develop with advanced epididymo-orchitis, the time course is generally gradual and on the order of days. However, marked testicular tenderness in a patient with advanced epididymo-orchitis may reflect secondary testicular ischemia and also warrants urologic consultation.[33]

The gold standard for the diagnosis of testicular torsion is scrotal exploration.[34] However, some clinicians incorporate radionuclide testicular scanning or color Doppler ultrasound examination in their diagnostic work-up.[35] Radionuclide scans have a sensitivity of 90% to 100% and specificity of 90% for detecting testicular blood flow.[36] Color Doppler ultrasound has a sensitivity of 70% to 89%, a specificity of 97% to 100% and an accuracy of 91% to 97% in diagnosing testicular torsion when the presence or absence of intratesticular blood flow is the single criterion for diagnosis.[36-38] Whereas these studies may complement each other for indeterminate cases, they are unfortunately time-, technician-, and reader-dependent examinations in a clinical situation in which time is

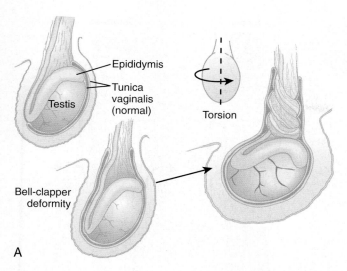

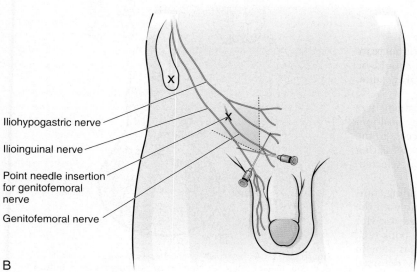

Figure 55–10 *A,* Anatomy of testicular torsion. *B,* Achieve anesthesia of the spermatic cord by injecting lidocaine at the superficial inguinal ring. *(A, From Snyder HM III, et al: In Fleisher GR, Ludwig S [eds]: Textbook of Pediatric Emergency Medicine, 4th ed. Philadelphia, Lippincott Williams & Wilkins, 2000.)*

A labels: Epididymis, Tunica vaginalis (normal), Testis, Torsion, Bell-clapper deformity

B labels: Iliohypogastric nerve, Ilioinguinal nerve, Point needle insertion for genitofemoral nerve, Genitofemoral nerve

essential. The quintessential point in testicular torsion is that no markers, signs, or symptoms will distinguish incomplete from complete testicular ischemia. One minute there may be total absence of blood flow to the involved testis; the next minute sufficient spontaneous detorsion may have occurred to provide temporary testicular perfusion. This is the dilemma. Scrotal exploration, detorsion, and orchiopexy or orchiectomy of the involved testis and orchiopexy of the contralateral testis is a relatively benign, straightforward operative procedure.

Intravaginal testicular torsion is a congenital bilateral abnormality. The ischemic testis must be detorsed and pexed with nonabsorbable (e.g., nylon, polypropylene), rather than absorbable (e.g., chromic, Vicryl), suture. The torsed testis that is pexed with absorbable suture remains at risk for subsequent postoperative torsion. Orchiopexy of the nonischemic contralateral testis is mandatory to ensure prevention of future torsion.

Once the diagnosis of testicular torsion is suspected, immediately place a call to notify a urologist of the suspected diagnosis, the perceived need for surgical exploration, and the fact that you will be attempting testicular detorsion while awaiting patient transport to the operating room. At some point before the patient leaves the ED, meticulous charting to document time, suspected diagnosis, notification of the urologist, and any manipulation of the affected testis must be done. All efforts are then focused on attempting testicular detorsion.

Manual Detorsion and Spermatic Cord Anesthesia

Manual detorsion is performed in the following manner. Advise the patient that the procedure will be uncomfortable and painful and offer light sedation if it seems appropriate. The rationale for not using spermatic cord anesthesia with attempted detorsion is that the anesthesia takes away an important subjective end point (i.e., relief of the patient's pain after manipulation of the testis). However, many authors do advocate spermatic cord anesthesia before detorsion, and if anesthesia of the spermatic cord is elected, it can be done in the following manner.

Spermatic Cord Anesthesia

Local anesthesia of the spermatic cord using 1% plain lidocaine is usually done at the external inguinal ring[39] (see Fig. 55–10). First prepare the skin with an antiseptic solution. The cord can usually be grasped between the thumb and the index finger, and 10 mL of 1% plain lidocaine can be directly injected into the cord. If the cord is swollen, as it often is in testicular torsion, or if the testicle is lying very high in the hemiscrotum as a result of spermatic cord torsion (so as to preclude grasping), the cord may be palpated at the pubic tubercle as it passes over the pubis and the lidocaine injected at this landmark. Lee and colleagues[40] were able to perform manual detorsion with local spermatic cord anesthesia in 70% of their adult cases of torsion. Kresling and associates[41] had success in 15 of 16 patients and noted a fair amount of associated cremasteric muscle spasm, which must also be relieved. In their experience, torsion usually resulted from an initial lateral-to-medial rotation (Fig. 55–11), with an occasional caudal-to-cranial component.

Manual Detorsion

The goal of manual detorsion is to reestablish or increase blood flow to a previously ischemic testis. This should be done in conjunction with preparation of the operating suite. It should never delay operative intervention.

Before initiating detorsion, ensure that the patient is as comfortable as possible in a reclining or supine position. Lithotomy position gives the examiner the most access to the patient's genitalia and prevents the patient from retreating during the procedure. If light analgesia/sedation is selected, implement them at this time.

Manual detorsion begins with the clinician standing comfortably at the side of the bed or stretcher, preferably on the patient's right side if the clinician is right handed, or vice versa. Detorsion is begun just as one would open a book (i.e., an initial 180° detorsion of the patient's right testis is done in a counterclockwise fashion). The patient's left testis is detorsed 180° in a clockwise fashion (see Fig. 55–11). Pain relief is an objective end point. If one rotation relieves some but not all of the pain, continue with another rotation. The degree of torsion may range from 180° to 1080° with medians of 360° to 540° that correlated to salvage rate.[42] Therefore, many patients may require two or three rotations to alleviate pain. If the initial detorsion is mechanically difficult (which it will be if one is detorsing in the wrong direction) or makes the pain worse, detorse the testis in the opposite direction and observe the result. Approximately one third of testicular torsions occur in the lateral, or unexpected, direction.[42] The objective success or failure of any testicular manipulation can be substantiated by an increase in Doppler signal and the patient's relief of pain.

With successful detorsion, the testicle returns to its normal anatomic position. Resolution of induration and swelling of the spermatic cord, testis, and epididymis will depend on the degree and duration of ischemia. Thus, the more severe the torsion and the longer it has been present, the longer it will take for the edema and induration to resolve. With significant ischemia, the entire epididymis often becomes enlarged like a link sausage (uncommon in epididymitis except in severe cases or those that are initially misdiagnosed or seen late in their clinical course), and the testis becomes quite firm, simulating a testicular tumor. In the author's experience (RES), both of these reversible changes usually resolve over 3 to 4 hours. Occasionally, the testis will torse in the opposite

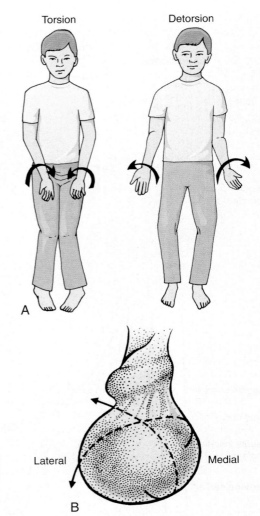

Figure 55–11 *A,* Testicular torsion usually occurs in a medial direction. Initially attempt detorsion by rotating the testis outward toward the thigh. This is most successful if attempted within the first few hours of torsion, before the onset of significant scrotal swelling. Intravenous narcotics (such as fentanyl) or a cord block can be administered before attempting detorsion. *B,* Detorsion of the testicle may require testicular rotation through two planes. To release the cremasteric muscle, rotate the testis in a caudal-to-cranial direction simultaneously with medial-to-lateral rotation. The right testis is shown. *(B, from Freeman S, Chapman J: Urologic procedures. Emerg Med Clin North Am 4:543, 1986.)*

direction (medial to lateral) or have multiple twists. This may become apparent as the clinician assesses the results of the detorsion procedure by palpation, relief of edema, and return or increase of the Doppler signal. Even though manual detorsion will save an ischemic testicle, it should not be substituted for definitive scrotal exploration.

URETHRAL CATHETERIZATION

Alternatives to Catheterization

The merits of alternative approaches to urine specimen collection over patient catheterization depend on the patient's age and clinical setting.

In children, the collection technique reported by Amir and coworkers[43] consists of placing the young child on his or her back. In very young children, collection and analysis of spontaneously voided urine specimens after penile cleansing or suprapubic "finger tap" showed urine culture results identical to those specimens obtained by suprapubic aspiration.[43] The applicability of this to a busy ED is questionable. Often, it is possible to collect a spontaneously voided midstream specimen in a child if ED personnel are prepared in advance. The problem is that the voiding events tend to occur as the child is undergoing venipuncture, spinal tap, or attempted urethral catheterization. Even more important, if the first specimen is missed or inadequate, how long are we willing to wait for another chance? Urethral catheterization is quick, definitive, and routinely used.

In adult circumcised men without anatomic lesions, first-voided midstream specimens can define the presence or absence of culture-proven bacteriuria.[44] This certainly represents a user-friendly approach to urine collection in a busy ED and needs to be carefully considered.

In adult women, properly collected clean-catch midstream specimens has been found to be as bacteriologically reliable as catheterized specimens.[45] A few caveats are worth mentioning: Patients must sit backward on the toilet when collecting the specimen (i.e., facing the wall, which theoretically promotes labial spreading). Of more concern is the fact that these studies excluded patients with vaginitis, urologic abnormalities, pregnancy, and vaginal bleeding. These diagnoses represent the clinical circumstances for which urine is commonly examined in young women visiting the ED. In this at-risk population, catheterized urine specimens are preferred.

Urethral catheterization seems a simple task—insertion of one tube into a larger tube. Nonetheless, many difficulties might arise. Patients often remember catheterization as either painful or uneventful depending on the operator's expertise, confidence, and gentleness.

Patients are often apprehensive about catheterization. If the clinician shows concern regarding positioning and exposure, the patient will be reassured. Although adequate exposure may be obtained in the frog-legged position, the use of an examination table with stirrups (lithotomy position) is ideal, especially for female catheterization.

Anticipation and preparation of all materials necessary for urethral catheterization beforehand are reassuring to the patient. It is frustrating for the health care provider and upsetting to the patient when the patient is told "not to move or touch anything" while a search is made for additional equipment. Most catheterizations are performed using a standard catheterization tray. Often, these trays contain more equipment than is truly needed. This necessitates opening the tray and establishing a sterile field at the bedside, selecting those items that will be needed, and discarding the rest of the equipment. Once the penis or labia has been touched in preparation for the procedure, the touching hand (usually nondominant) is contaminated and ideally should not be handling any of the sterile equipment. When a standard catheterization tray is not used or is not available, catheterists should go through the anticipated procedure mentally to secure all of the appropriate equipment before actually starting the procedure.

Indications and Contraindications

Urinary catheterization and instrumentation are rarely a primary cause of urinary infection in otherwise healthy patients who urinate normally and carry small amounts of postvoid residual urine. As with any procedure, catheteriza-

tion needs to be limited to those clinical situations in which the benefits outweigh the risks. The following are considered to be indications for urethral catheterization:

1. Acute urinary retention.
2. Urethral or prostatic obstruction leading to compromised renal function.
3. Urine output monitoring in any critically ill or injured patient.
4. Collection of a sterile urine specimen for diagnostic purposes.
5. Intermittent bladder catheterization in patients with neurogenic bladder dysfunction.
6. Urologic study of the lower urinary tract.

Urethral catheterization should be avoided when other less invasive procedures will be as informative. A traditional, albeit currently relative, contraindication to urethral catheterization (see following discussion on alternate views) is the trauma patient with suspected urethral injury as evidenced by blood at the urethral meatus, an abnormal-feeling or high-riding prostate on rectal examination, penile, scrotal, perineal hematoma, or radiographic evidence of urethral/bladder trauma. In the setting of a severely fractured pelvis or diastasis of the pubic symphysis, urethrogram should always precede attempts at catheterization.[27] Although some authors, and more liberal clinical protocols, allow for gentle attempts at catheter passage in the presence of the previously discussed traditional contraindications, these findings dictate a selective approach, and/or the need for retrograde urethrography to define the integrity of the urethra before any attempted urethral catheterization.[46]

Equipment

The equipment listed in Figure 55–12B is included in most standard catheterization trays and must be at hand before attempting urethral catheterization. The catheterist should check the list of contents before opening the tray because some trays do not include certain items. For most routine adult in-and-out catheterizations, a 14-French red rubber catheter or Foley balloon catheter is adequate. In infants or neonates, a 2- or 5-French feeding tube taped in place produces the least amount of urethral trauma. In older boys, a 5- to 12-French red rubber catheter or Foley balloon catheter may be used. Table 55–5 lists appropriate-sized catheters and feeding tubes for all ages. A 14- to 18-French coudé catheter should be considered after unsuccessful passage of a straight Foley balloon catheter or in any male patient with known enlargement of the prostatic median lobe. If a coudé catheter is not available, a larger 18- to 22-French Foley balloon catheter can be tried. In a male patient with a urethral stricture in whom attempts at catheterization with a straight Foley or

TABLE 55–5 Pediatric Urethral Catheter Size

Age Group	Pediatric Catheter Size*
Infants	8 Fr feeding tube
1–3 yr	10 Fr feeding tube
4–6 yr	10–12 Fr red rubber catheter (Robinson)
7–12 yr	5–8 Fr feeding tube
>12 yr	14 Fr red rubber catheter (Robinson)

*6 Fr is the smallest balloon catheter and is quite flimsy; would recommend 8 Fr in most cases; 12 Fr is the smallest coudé catheter.

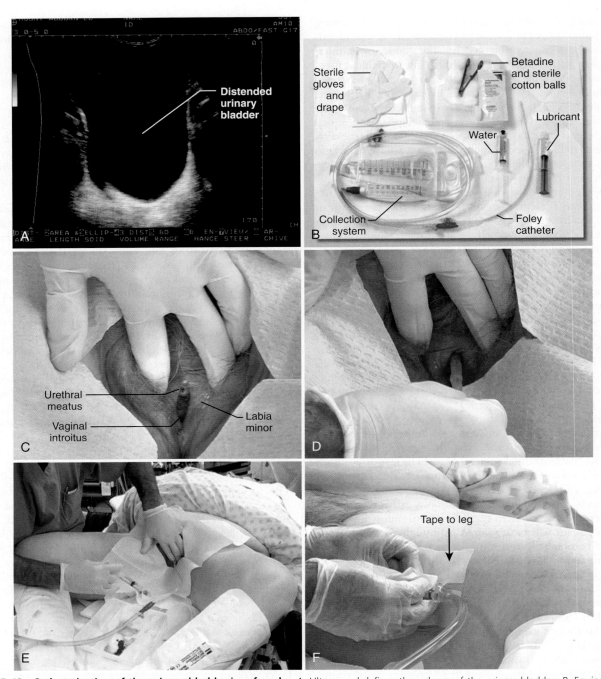

Figure 55–12 **Catheterization of the urinary bladder in a female.** *A,* Ultrasound defines the volume of the urinary bladder. *B,* Equipment for Foley catheterization. *C,* Anatomy of the female urethra. *D,* After a sterile preparation, spread the labia and advance the catheter. *D,* Uncomplicated catheterization in the female. *E,* Fill the balloon with water, not air. *F,* Sterile connection to the drainage bag with catheter taped to the leg. *(A–F, From Thomsen T, Setnik G [eds]: Procedures Consult—Emergency Medicine Module. Copyright 2008 Elsevier Inc. All rights reserved.)*

coudé catheter have failed, passage of filiforms and followers is the next logical step. This requires special expertise that can be learned quickly. If immediate bladder access is required in this circumstance or in any emergency, suprapubic placement of a peel-away sheath and Foley balloon catheter using the Seldinger technique will be needed.[47]

Anatomic Considerations

Female Catheterization

The female urethra is a short (~4 cm) straight tube, usually of wide caliber, lying on top of the vagina. It must be approached between double labia, and the urethral meatus is occasionally hidden and not obvious (in contrast to most males, except those with hypospadias). If the female patient nervously adducts her legs, successful catheterization will be very difficult if not impossible.

The female urethral meatus is oval but may appear as an anteroposterior slit with rather prominent margins situated directly superior to the opening of the vagina and approximately 2.5 cm inferior to the glans clitoris (see Fig. 55–12).[48] It is the first of three orifices encountered when examining any female genitalia cephalad to caudad in the lithotomy position. The urethral meatus might be especially difficult to find in the very young infant and the older, postmenopausal woman. Anticipation of this and knowledge of the anatomic variances will help to modify any patient discomfort associated with needless catheter tip probing, which is an unsettling experience for both the patient and the catheterist.

Occasionally, the urethral meatus recedes superiorly into the vagina and is not immediately visible because of either prior surgical procedures or atrophic postmenopausal changes. Anticipation of such cases will allow the examiner to gently advance a nondominant index finger into the vagina in the superior midline. The urethral meatus can usually be palpated then visualized as a soft mound surrounded by a firmer ring of supporting periurethral tissue. Rarely, the meatus will have receded so far superiorly and intravaginally that it cannot be visualized at all, and catheterization must be carried out by palpation alone. From the meatus (if the patient assumes a supine position), the urethra proceeds straight back to slightly downward as it advances into the bladder just behind the symphysis pubis (Fig. 55–13A).

In women with a urethrocele or cystourethrocele, in whom the urethra or the bladder falls into the vagina, the "normal" urethral course might be more significantly posterior .The normal anatomic relationships in these situations may be re-created by spreading the index and long fingers and placing them along the superior vaginal wall and gently applying upward support (see Fig. 55–13B). This reconstitutes the normal anatomic relationships and permits straight, rapid

urethral catheterization. Because the female urethra is so short, only half the total length of the catheter has to be inserted before it is safe to inflate the Foley balloon.

Male Catheterization

Because the urethral meatus is usually evident in most males, it might seem a simple matter to insert a urethral catheter.[49] Yet catheterization can be quite difficult. The normal male urethra is approximately 20 cm long from the external urethral meatus to the bladder neck (Fig. 55–14). The posterior prostatic urethra is approximately 3.5 cm long, and the contiguous external sphincter or urogenital diaphragm that encompasses the membranous urethra is 4 cm from the bladder neck. In males, *any catheter must be fully inserted to the balloon-inflating side-arm channel before it is safe to inflate the balloon* (Fig. 55–15). At the first egress of urine from the catheter, the balloon is just passing through the membranous urethra. *The catheter balloon still has about 3 cm to go before clearing the bladder neck.* Inflation of the Foley balloon at any point before full insertion of the catheter might result in iatrogenic urethral injury.

The male urethra is relatively fixed at the level of the urogenital diaphragm and symphysis pubis; traction downward on the penis kinks and promotes urethral folding at the level of the penile suspensory ligament (Fig. 55–16A), which creates a level of spurious obstruction. For this reason, the penis should always be held taut and upright during any urethral instrumentation including catheterization (see Fig. 55–16B). The catheter then needs to make only a single curve rather than a complex S curve as it traverses into the bladder.

General Procedure

As stated previously, urethral catheterization must be done using sterile technique. Both male and female patients have special urethral meatal considerations. In the uncircumcised or partially circumcised male, absolute total control of the penile foreskin is paramount to ensuring success. Before establishing a sterile field, retract the available foreskin to its fullest extent proximal to the glans penis (Fig. 55–17A). Unfold a standard 4 × 4 gauze pad, then refolded in its longest dimension, and carefully wrap it around the retracted foreskin at the level of the coronal sulcus (see Fig. 55–17B). This will

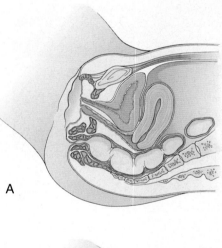

A

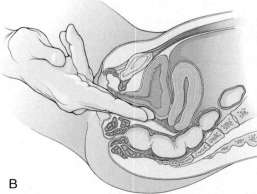

B

Figure 55–13 *A,* Normal sagittal anatomy of the female urethra. *B,* In a patient with a cystocele/urethrocele or prolapsed bladder, the normal anatomy may have to be re-created for catheter passage. Insert two fingers into the vagina and lift upward while passing the catheter.

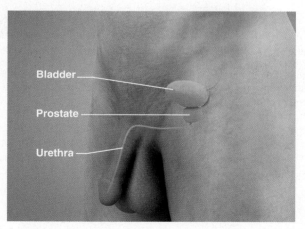

Bladder

Prostate

Urethra

Figure 55–14 Anatomy of the male urethra. *(From Thomsen T, Setnik G [eds]: Procedures Consult—Emergency Medicine Module. Copyright 2008 Elsevier Inc. All rights reserved.)*

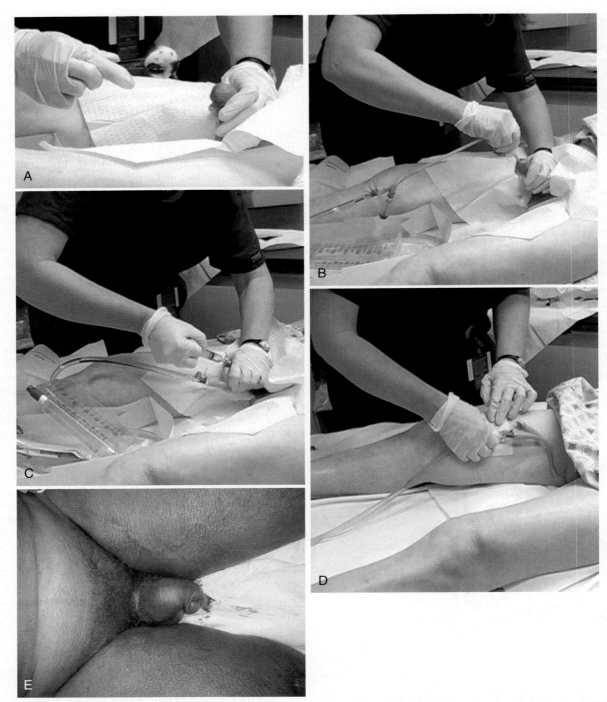

Figure 55–15   Foley catheter placement in a male. *A,* Use sterile technique. *B,* Holding the penis taut and upright prevents urethral folding, lessens external sphincter spasm, and promotes unobstructed catheterization. *C,* Advance the catheter *fully to the hilt* before inserting the balloon with water. *D,* Then withdraw the catheter until the balloon stops the egress. Tape the drainage tube to the leg. *E,* The urethral meatus cannot be found in the markedly edematous penis in this patient with massive anasarca.

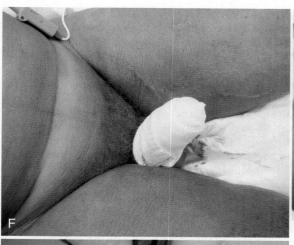

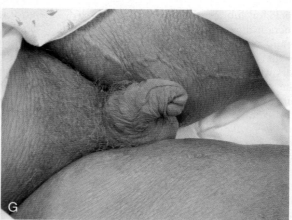

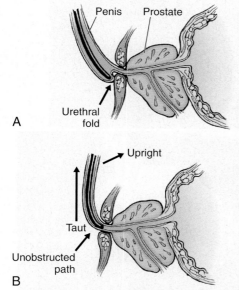

Figure 55–15, cont'd *F,* Wrap the penis in an elastic bandage for 8–10 minutes. *G,* The edema is reduced with compression alone. *H,* An assistant stabilizes the penis shaft with the thumb and index finger (*arrow*) while the operator (***) spreads the redundant tissue with forceps to visualize the meatus deep within the swollen tissue, and advances the catheter. *(A–D, From Thomsen T, Setnik G [eds]: Procedures Consult—Emergency Medicine Module. Copyright 2008 Elsevier Inc. All rights reserved.)*

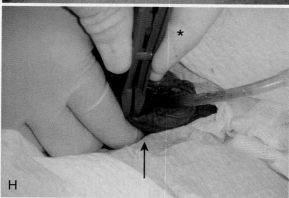

Figure 55–16 *A,* The urethra may fold and kink if the penis is not held taut and upright. *B,* The taut and upright position allows for an unobstructed path for the catheter.

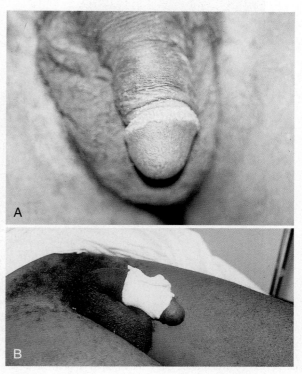

Figure 55–17 *A,* In this uncircumsized male, the foreskin has been fully retracted for catheter placement. *B,* A gauze pad allows for a firm grasp on the foreskin to prevent movement during catheterization. *Reduce the foreskin to its original position once the catheter is in place.*

prevent the tendency for lubricant-associated normal anatomic foreskin reduction during catheterization and provide a continuously dry and sterile field. Secure the folded 4 × 4 gauze surrounding the foreskin between the nondominant long and ring fingers when beginning the procedure and do not release until the procedure is completed. This position leaves the nondominant index finger and thumb available for manipulating the catheter. After catheterization, remove the 4 × 4 pad and *reduce the penile foreskin to its normal anatomic position to prevent the development of iatrogenic paraphimosis.*

After exposing the urethral meatus in the female and the glans penis and urethral meatus in the male, use an antiseptic solution (e.g., povidone-iodine) soaked into cotton balls or oversized cotton-tipped applicators to cleanse the exposed meatus and surrounding tissues. This is best done by hand but can also be done using the plastic forceps in the catheterization tray. Begin the cleansing circular motion on the urethral meatus and proceed outward, intentionally moving any debris toward the periphery and thus creating a sterile field.

An appropriately sized catheter (10 Fr is adequate for small children, whereas 14–16 Fr is commonly used in adults) that has been lubricated with viscous rather than inspissated

lubricating jelly is gently passed by hand, or with the aid of a hemostat or plastic forceps, into the urethra and upward into the bladder. Injection of the male urethra with 5 mL of 2% viscous lidocaine (Anestacon) or a similar syringe filled with anesthetic lubricant can be helpful for urethral distention and topical anesthesia. Regardless, advise the patient of mild urethral discomfort and the potential urge to void. During slow, gentle passage of the catheter, be aware of the anatomic considerations discussed previously. A catheter that inadvertently enters the vagina should be discarded.

After passing the catheter "to the hilt" in all male patients (Fig. 55–18A), slowly inflate the balloon with 10 mL of air or tap water. Sterile water or saline is not required. Most 5-mL balloons will easily accommodate up to 30 to 50 mL of air or water without bursting. Obvious resistance or patient discomfort on balloon inflation should signal potential erroneous urethral positioning and mandates reevaluation. If this occurs,

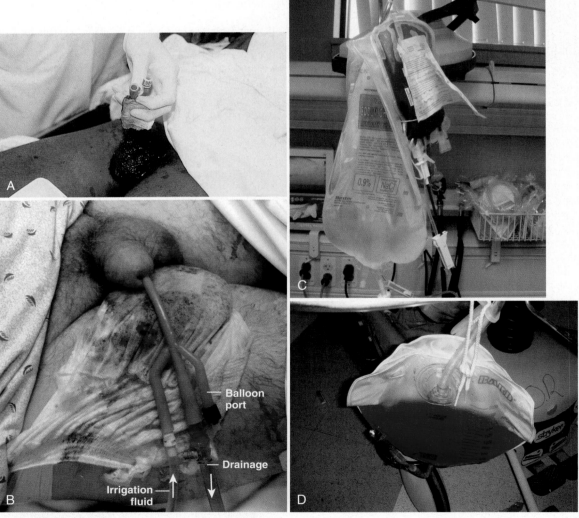

Figure 55–18 *A,* When urine is returned from a catheter (in a male), the balloon might not be within the bladder and could be inflated in the urethra unless the catheter is passed to the hilt before balloon inflation. Note bleeding when balloon was inflated in the urethra (see Fig. 55–38). *B,* Large three-way Bardex® 22-26F Foley catheter for bladder irrigation to remove blood clots after prostate surgery. *C,* Continuously irrigate the bladder with irrigation fluid to remove clots. Blood loss can be substantial (note transfusion requirement). *D,* Irrigate the bladder until bleeding stops. This procedure may require sedation or parenteral analgesia. Use only saline infused under gravity, using 500 to 1000 mL/hr to begin. Overdistension may occur if the egress is blocked by clots.

immediately deflate the Foley balloon and reposition or slightly withdraw the catheter, then pass it to the hilt again before balloon reinflation (see Fig. 55–18*A*). If this is unsuccessful a second time, catheter removal and urethral evaluation for a potential obstructive problem or false passage using retrograde urethrography is recommended (see "Retrograde Urethrography," later in this chapter). It may be difficult or impossible to pass a Foley catheter in a male with a markedly edematous penis (see Fig. 55–15*E–H*). If this cannot be accomplished, a suprapubic catheter may be required.

After successful catheter passage and Foley balloon inflation, slowly withdraw the catheter until the approximation of the balloon with the bladder neck precludes further withdrawal. Then connect the catheter to either a sterile leg bag or a closed-system bedside drainage bag. If the patient will be released with an indwelling Foley catheter, it can be initially connected to a leg bag, which is then comfortably fastened to the lower thigh and upper calf. The patient and family must be instructed regarding proper care of the catheter and drainage device. In most other cases, the catheter may be secured to either the thigh or the lower abdomen (preferred with males) with adhesive tape or simply placed under the knee and left to drain dependently into the bedside drainage bag.

It is a foregone conclusion that the urine in any catheter will eventually become colonized with bacteria; it simply cannot be prevented. Therefore, prophylactic antibiotics for the duration of catheterization is useless and selects out resistant organisms. The use of antibiotics before simple catheterization is not warranted. However, patients with known valvular heart disease, suspected urinary tract bacteremia, chronic UTI, urethral stricture disease, or outlet obstruction associated with infection are considered to be at theoretical risk for procedure-induced bacteremia. In these patients, any urinary instrumentation, especially urethral dilation, can be given prophylactic parenteral gram-negative antibiotic coverage before beginning any instrumentation. These patients may be released with appropriate antibiotic coverage and be scheduled for early urologic follow-up within 1 to 2 days.[50] The need for prophylactic antibiotics in the ED for initial catheter placement in this subset of patients at theoretical risk is unknown, and no standard presently exists. Most clinicians do not provide routine prophylactic antibiotics prior to simple Foley catheter passage, even in patients at theoretical risk for transient bacteremia.

Bladder Irrigation

After prostate surgery (transurethral resection), blood clots may form in the bladder and cause acute urinary retention. Blood loss can be significant. This condition is usually easily relieved by the use of a large three-way irrigation catheter. A Bardex 22-26F Foley catheter is preferred. Saline irrigation fluid is continuously infused into the bladder, while allowing the egress of fluid and blood clots. Continue the procedure until the bladder remains decompressed and/or bleeding stops (see Fig. 55–18*B–D*). Gravity alone usually provides adequate ingress-egress of fluid, but gentle syringe irrigation with 60 mL aliquots of saline may be used. Irrigation can be brisk, 1 to 2 L/hr or more, as long as the *volume of drained saline is equal to the volume infused.* Only saline (supplied in 2 or 4 L bags) is used and infused only *via gravity.* Syringe irrigation of a Foley catheter with 60 to 100 mL aliquots is an alternative. The goal is to obtain clear urine.

Difficulties in Male Catheterization

Phimosis

Physiologic adhesions between the foreskin (prepuce) and the glans penis with associated inability to retract the foreskin are normal in children. This condition must be distinguished from phimosis, which is the inability to retract the foreskin proximally over the glans penis due to recurrent inflammation or trauma, which results in gradual scarring of the preputial opening.[51] It is not essential to retract the foreskin in uncircumcised boys at the time of catheterization if the urethral meatus can be visualized. At birth, the foreskin is fully retractable in only 4% of boys. Sufficient foreskin retraction to visualize the urethral meatus is possible in only half of newborn boys. Although the foreskin can be retracted completely in only 20% of 6-month-old boys, 90% of 3-year-old boys have a fully retractable foreskin. By 17 years of age, the foreskin should be physiologically separated and fully retractable in all males unless they have experienced secondary infections or repeated preputial trauma.[52]

The foreskin, especially in diabetics, is susceptible to recurrent infections and inflammation. A scarred, contracted, difficult-to-retract preputial opening might result, leading to phimosis. Phimosis precludes optimal hygiene of the glans penis and coronal sulcus, resulting in an increased risk of bacterial infection, transmission of STDs (especially human immunodeficiency virus), and the development of penile malignancies. Occasionally, the phimotic opening becomes so tight that the meatus cannot be visualized or palpated. If the patient requires catheterization, it will be necessary either to perform a dorsal slit of the foreskin to expose the glans and urethral meatus sufficiently for cleansing and catheterization or to dilate the phimotic opening sufficiently to identify the urethral meatus and blindly pass the catheter. These procedures are discussed at the beginning of the chapter.

Edema of the Foreskin

Patients with penile trauma, paraphimosis, anasarca, or significant lymphatic obstruction from irradiation or cancer may have marked edema of the foreskin, subsequently burying the urethral meatus and glans penis in several centimeters of boggy foreskin (see Figs. 55–15 and 55–19). Because the latter group of patients often requires careful fluid monitoring, they might need an indwelling catheter. The clinician's first responsibility is to determine the proper etiology for the foreskin edema. This will require enough foreskin manipulation to identify the glans penis, coronal sulcus, and urethral meatus, as well as the relationship of the prepuce and preputial opening to these structures, to ensure the absence of foreign body strangulation or paraphimosis.

Two separate methods of visualizing the glans penis and urethral meatus are available to the clinician.[53] The simplest method is to manually compress the swollen foreskin by hand or between opposing cold packs in an attempt to reduce the edema fluid (see Fig. 55–5*C* and *D*). Snugly wrapping the distal penis with Elastoplast for 10 minutes may also be helpful. In most mild cases, manual compression is often successful, and no further maneuvers are required. Often, close inspection is the only way to fully evaluate an edematous foreskin (see Fig. 55–19).

Meatal Stenosis

The urethral meatus may be either congenitally or secondarily narrowed by scarring, resulting in meatal stenosis. The

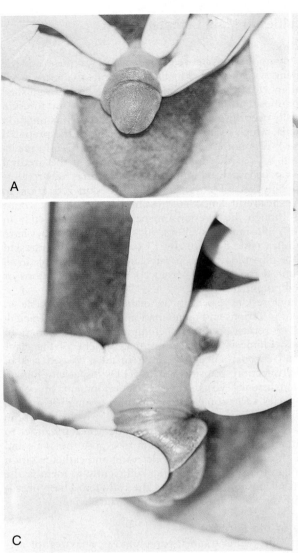
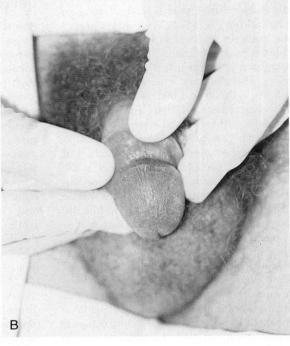

Figure 55–19 *A,* This edematous foreskin may have numerous etiologies, from benign edema to paraphimosis, and at first glance, the cause might not be obvious. This patient has paraphimosis that is appreciated by careful inspection to identify the normal coronal sulcus (*B*) and a phimotic foreskin band proximal to the glans (*C*).

stenosis may prevent admission of a normal-sized catheter. If the meatus admits a small-caliber tube (i.e., 5-Fr or larger pediatric feeding tube), this may be all that is required for the short term. Remember that the inner diameter of the feeding tube or catheter is the important diameter for urinary drainage. A smaller, single-lumen tube may provide better drainage than a larger, double-lumen Foley balloon catheter.

If a larger-caliber catheter or a Foley balloon catheter is required, meatal dilation or meatotomy might be necessary. Meatal dilation is accomplished by repeatedly inserting larger meatal dilators to a certain end point. This procedure is painful and should be performed with topical meatal anesthesia in conjunction with light intravenous sedation. On occasion, a ventral meatotomy might be required in men in whom repeated instrumentation or long-term catheterization has resulted in severe meatal stenosis. This procedure is best performed by a urologist.

Urethral Stricture

Urethral obstruction encountered in the anterior or bulbous urethra during catheterization is usually the result of urethral stricture disease.[54] Urethral strictures develop as a result of trauma, infection (especially STDs), lower urinary tract instrumentation, or long-term indwelling catheter drainage.

Strictures might remain asymptomatic for a period of time, but eventually, most become symptomatic and cause urethral voiding symptoms, hematuria, or bloody urethral discharge that might or might not be associated with infection. Manual force should not be used to negotiate or to dilate urethral strictures. Force merely promotes a vicious circle of false passages, bleeding, and eventual increased scarring, which makes catheterization more difficult. Inability to negotiate a urethral stricture with a simple straight Foley catheter or coudé catheter leads to consideration of urethral dilation using filiforms and followers as well as urologic consultation.

Although usually not performed by the emergency clinicians, filiforms and followers have been a longstanding technique to pass a catheter in the presence of a urethral stricture. The procedure is included for completeness and for occasions when urologic consultation is unavailable and a suprapubic drainage catheter is not possible.

Filiforms are very narrow, flexible, solid catheters, usually not exceeding 4 French in caliber. They are not dilators. Their sole function is to locate and successfully navigate a strictured urethral segment. Each filiform has a straight or pigtailed (curved) distal end and a proximal female-threaded coupling into which the distal male end of a follower may be threaded. After generous topical anesthesia with 2% lidocaine

(Anestacon), grasp the previously prepared penis between the nondominant long and ring fingers and stretch upward. The filiform is slowly passed down the urethra in an attempt to negotiate the strictured iris or narrowed segment of involved urethra (Fig. 55–20*A*). This is all done by "feel" and experience and might require several attempts. Always advance the filiform with the gentlest of pressure.

Filiforms should never be forced through the urethra. Any encountered resistance represents the potential edge of the strictured urethra or fold of urethral mucosa. Undue force applied to the filiform at this point might result in perforation of the urethral mucosa and creation of a false passage along the urethral body or inferiorly into the perineum. If the fili-

form meets resistance, it should be partially withdrawn, rotated 90° to 180°, then gently reinserted. If resistance is met again at the same location, leave the first filiform in place (to occupy that particular obstructing site) and advance a second filiform alongside it. A third and fourth filiform might be necessary before one of them successfully navigates the narrowed aperture of the stricture and advances upward through the normal proximal urethra and into the bladder (see Fig. 55–20*B–D*). The sine qua non of success is the effortless passage of the filiform through the strictured area without spontaneous discharge of the filiform when it is released. Any amount of filiform return should alert the catheterist that the filiform has not negotiated the stricture and requires replace-

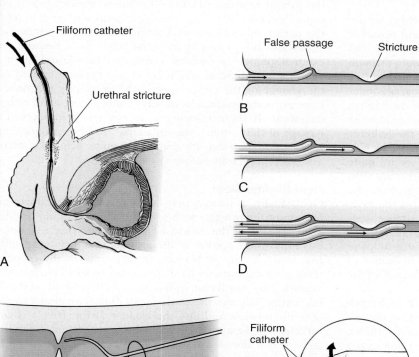

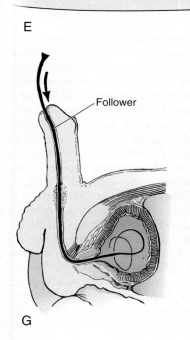

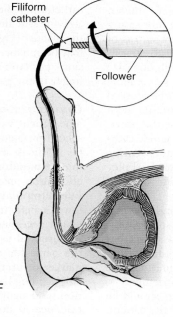

Figure 55–20 *A,* Passage of the filiform past the urethral stricture. *B,* Sequential passage of filiforms, with entry of the first catheter into the false passage. *C,* Advancement of the second filiform to the stricture site. *D,* Passage of the third filiform past the stricture. After passing the filiform into the bladder, remove redundant catheters. *E,* Pigtail filiform passing through the stricture. *F,* Attachment of a follower to the filiform. *G,* Dilation of the stricture with a follower. (B–D, *From Hill GJ: Outpatient Surgery. Philadelphia, WB Saunders, 1973. Reproduced by permission; E, from Blandy J: Operative Urology. Oxford, Blackwell Scientific Publications, 1978, p 204.)*

ment. Pigtail filiforms (with a corkscrew-shaped tip) (see Fig. 55–20E), rather than straight-tipped filiforms, are often easier to advance over an abrupt urethral edge and through the smallest of strictured openings. Once through the stricture, advance the filiform until the threaded coupling is near the urethral meatus (see Fig. 55–20F).

Because filiforms are very pliable, they must be grasped securely. This is ensured by stabilizing the retracted foreskin and penis just proximal to the glans between the long and the ring fingers of the nondominant hand as described previously and holding the filiform between the nondominant index finger and thumb. This allows controlled attachment and subsequent detachment of graduated followers while performing serial dilation (see Fig. 55–20G).

A follower of the smallest caliber (usually 8 Fr) should always be selected first; lubricate it copiously and thread it onto the filiform. When it has been threaded completely (no threads showing), gently advance it without pressure through the upwardly stretched penis and urethra into the bladder (see Fig. 55–20G). Stretching the penis upward discourages telescoping of the urethra and subsequent kinking of the filiform and follower (see Fig. 55–16B). Advance the follower into the bladder until spontaneous egress of urine from the follower occurs, guaranteeing successful passage. Note that the side drainage holes of the 8- and 10-French followers are quite small and frequently become occluded with lubricating jelly. This might prevent spontaneous urinary drainage from the follower even though it has successfully negotiated the stricture and passed into the bladder. In this circumstance, easy passage of the 8-French follower into the bladder and the lack of gross blood or bloody drainage at the filiform-follower coupling site when changing follower sizes are indicative of successful passage and dilation rather than creation of a false passage.

Absolute certainty of location of the 8- or 10-French follower can be established at any time by irrigating the follower with sterile saline, much like irrigating a Foley catheter. The irrigating fluid will dislodge any obstructing lubricating jelly from the side holes of the follower and allow egress of urine from the follower. The entire dilating procedure is repeated with sequentially larger followers until one size larger than the proposed retention catheter is successfully introduced. Following completed dilation, remove the coupled filiform and follower intact, relubricate the urethra with topical lidocaine (Anestacon) anesthesia, and pass the previously selected 14- to 16-French balloon Foley or coudé catheter to its fullest extent into the bladder. When return of urine from the Foley ensures proper placement, inflate the Foley balloon and withdraw the catheter and leave it to drain as described previously.

Occasionally, a urethral stricture is so dense and irregular that a filiform and 8-French follower may pass successfully, but the density and length of the stricture prevent further dilation. In this circumstance, tape the indwelling filiform and follower to the penile shaft for 1 to 2 days to provide adequate bladder drainage and probable softening of the stricture.

Urethral dilation with filiforms and followers should be neither bloody nor excessively uncomfortable for the patient. If the procedure is bloody or uncomfortable or if no urine is returned despite advancement of the follower for at least 24 cm, the clinician should consider that the filiform may not be in the urethra, but instead has created a false passage. In such a situation, retrograde urethrography will define the urethral anatomy. In cases in which urethral instrumentation

is unsuccessful for whatever reason, it may be necessary to place a suprapubic cystostomy tube rather than persist with unsuccessful urethral dilation.

Spasm of the External Urethral Sphincter

The male patient may voluntarily or involuntarily contract the urogenital diaphragm (external sphincter), the striated urethral sphincter at the apex of the prostate. (This is especially true of trauma patients and men with neurogenic bladder dysfunction and pelvic floor spasms.) This produces spurious urethral resistance at approximately 16 cm from the meatus. Because increased abdominal pressure or voluntary perineal contraction causes reflex contraction of the external sphincter, the patient in these situations should be encouraged to lay supine and take slow, deep breaths, consciously trying to relax the perineum and rectum. Plantar flexion of the toes and ankles also aids in relaxation of the pelvic floor. Because the external sphincter is composed of striated muscle and fatigues within a few minutes, gentle but steady pressure exerted on the syringe or the catheter while the previously mentioned maneuvers are undertaken usually results in successful catheterization. If these maneuvers do not result in successful passage of the catheter, the catheterist may be encountering an anatomic abnormality that will require definitive retrograde urethrography before instrumentation.

High Bladder Neck

Occasionally, a patient may have an enlarged intravesical portion of the prostate with a secondary high-riding bladder neck. The tip of the standard Foley catheter may encounter this intravesical portion of the prostate and may not readily pass above it into the bladder. Resistance is usually encountered after the catheter has been passed 16 to 20 cm into the urethra. Slow instillation or injection of 20 to 30 mL of sterile lubricating jelly into the urethra may allow the catheter to slip over the prostate and into the bladder. If this fails, a coudé catheter may be inserted. This catheter has a bend in the tip, and one will almost always be able to maneuver it gently into the bladder (Fig. 55–21A). Passage of the coudé catheter often may be enhanced by having an assistant exert digital compression and flattening of the elongated prostate using a gloved finger in the patient's rectum (see Fig. 55–21B).

Catheterization in the Patient with Pelvic Trauma

The patient with pelvic trauma or a straddle injury presents special problems in urinary management. The patient might be in shock from associated injuries. Accurate minute-to-minute monitoring of urinary output requiring bladder catheterization may be necessary in the initial resuscitation. Furthermore, radiographic evaluation to define the extent of lower urinary tract injury may require a retrograde cystogram, which necessitates urethral catheterization. Before performing urethral catheterization in all trauma patients, examine the penis for evidence of blood at the urethral meatus, a marker of urethral injury.[46] Blood at the urethral meatus; a "high-riding" or abnormal-feeling prostate on rectal examination; and penile, scrotal, or perineal ecchymoses might be evidence of potential urethral or bladder injury. However, such clinical findings have a low sensitivity for such injuries despite being in Advanced Cardiac Life Support guidelines. Shlamivotz and McCullough[27] noted that grossly bloody urine had excellent sensitivity for bladder or urethral injuries; however, blood at the meatus had only a 6% sensitivity for bladder injury and a 60% sensitivity for urethral injury. In

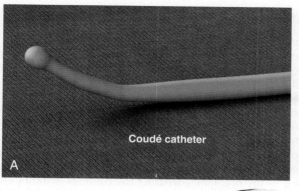

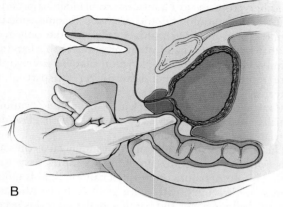

Figure 55–21 *A,* Coudé catheter, available in a self-retaining model, shown here, or with a balloon. *B,* Superior pressure on the prostate may facilitate catheter passage. (*A, From Thomsen T, Setnik G [eds]: Procedures Consult—Emergency Medicine Module. Copyright 2008 Elsevier Inc. All rights reserved.*)

addition, this author found that digital rectal examination in trauma patients had only a 23% sensitivity, but a 95% specificity, for pelvic fracture and urethral disruption.[28] Traditionally, blood at the meatus was considered a contraindication to empirical urethral catheterization without an antecedent normal retrograde urethrogram (RUG).[46] Despite this admonition in the literature, clinical practice has found no firm evidence that attempted urethral catheterization produces additional harm in patients with bladder or urethral injury, some authors have advocated gentle attempts at catheterization in the presence of suspected urethral injury.[27] Caution is still advised, and the approach to this scenario varies among institutions and is undergoing evolution. Patients with severe pelvic fracture and diastasis of the pubic symphysis are generally ideal candidates for an RUG before attempting catheter passage.

The theoretical hazard of injudicious urethral catheterization in the pelvic trauma patient is the potential worsening of an already existing, less serious urethral injury that is often associated with such trauma. Pelvic fractures most often impart injury to the prostatomembranous urethra just above the urogenital diaphragm. The shearing pelvic fracture fragments transect the urethra and puboprostatic ligaments, thereby displacing the prostate superiorly from its normal anatomic attachment to the posterior surface of the pubic bone. A partial or complete urethral injury might occur. An appropriately recognized and treated partial urethral disruption may heal with little or no scarring. However, a complete urethral disruption requires surgical repair and usually results

in some degree of postoperative urethral stricture and, occasionally, urinary incontinence and impotence, all of which portend significant morbidity.

The prognosticated danger of injudicious urethral catheterization in this situation is the potential conversion of a partial injury into a complete urethral injury, with its associated complications. Retrograde urethrography is the diagnostic procedure of choice to clarify urethral injury (see "Retrograde Urethrography," later in this chapter).

In the event that contrast material flows easily from the urethra into the bladder without extravasation, complete urethral integrity is ensured, and an attempt to pass a 14- or 16-French Foley catheter should be made. If any urethral resistance is encountered other than that normally expected at the voluntary external sphincter (urogenital diaphragm) in a conscious, anxious patient, immediately abort the catheterization and consult a urologist. If passage is successful, inflate the catheter balloon and withdraw the catheter until it approximates the bladder neck. At this point, leave it to dependent drainage, and pay very careful attention to the initial bladder effluent. Any colored urine other than clear or yellow is considered gross hematuria and mandates evaluation of the bladder and upper urinary tract to disclose the source.

If the RUG shows urethral extravasation AND passage of contrast into the bladder, a partial urethral injury has been identified. One gentle attempt at passage of a 12- to 14-Fench Foley or coudé catheter may be attempted, depending on the experience and confidence of the catheterist. Once again, any degree of resistance dictates termination of the procedure and urologic consultation.

In the patient without external sphincter spasm in whom the RUG shows evidence of urethral extravasation without any contrast filling the bladder, a complete urethral injury has been identified. Upon identification, immediate urologic consultation is indicated for placement of a suprapubic catheter and subsequent surgical repair of the complete urethral injury. One caveat: If more than 50 to 60 mL of contrast is used at any time for urethrography and more than gentle pressure is exerted during urethral contrast instillation, it is possible to create objective penile venous intravasation of contrast, which is benign. This intravasation of contrast may simulate urethral extravasation and produce a spurious examination result similar to urethral injury. The distinguishing feature with intravasation is that any subsequent film (i.e., postvoid film) will disclose immediate clearing of the iatrogenic penile venogram, whereas urethral extravasation will persist indefinitely.

Suprapubic placement of a catheter as an alternative to urethral catheterization for the trauma patient is covered elsewhere in this chapter.

Complications of Urethral Catheterization

Although urethral catheterization performed by skilled personnel in appropriate circumstances has an acceptable complication rate, untoward sequelae of catheterization are not unusual.

The frequency of bacteriuria after a single catheterization in a healthy outpatient population is probably less than 1%.[50] However, in hospitalized, elderly, debilitated, or postpartum patients, the rate might be considerably higher. Urinary catheterization is the leading cause of nosocomial UTIs. The mortality in patients with nosocomial UTI is approximately three times that in patients not acquiring infection.[55] Of patients catheterized with a closed system for 2 to 7 days, 8% to 10% will have significant bacteriuria once the catheter is removed.[56] Patients with catheters indwelling more than 10 days almost always acquire an infection. Infection from the urethra and the bladder might disseminate to cause epididymitis, pyelonephritis, and bacteremia. Although the use of a povidone-iodine lubricating gel has been shown to reduce the inoculation of bacteria into the bladder at the time of catheterization,[57] further study is needed to determine whether this antiseptic lubricant actually reduces infectious sequelae.

With long-term catheterization, bacteriuria is inevitable. Although episodes of high temperature (≥38.8°C) due to UTI in patients with long-term catheterizations are rare (2/1000 patient-days), these episodes can be associated with bacteremia and death.[58] Use of a condom catheter, adult diapers, and intermittent self-catheterization[59] represents noninvasive alternatives to long-term Foley catheterization in nonambulatory incontinent men and women. Other rare complications of long-term indwelling urethral catheterization include bladder stones, recurring bladder spasm, periurethral abscesses, bladder perforation,[60] and urethral erosion.[61]

In addition, complications might occur during the act of catheterization. False passages might be established in any area of the urethra when force is exerted on the catheter. In an uncircumcised patient, negligence in reducing the retracted foreskin to its normal anatomic position after urethral catheterization or instrumentation might lead to painful paraphimosis and associated complications.

Leaving a catheter indwelling too long or using a larger catheter than is needed promotes poor drainage of the periurethral glands, urethritis and might contribute to the formation of periurethral abscesses, all of which may lead to urethral stricture disease. Likewise, concretions might form around the catheter balloon and lead to the formation of bladder stones, many of which require operative removal.

The use of silicone rather than latex catheters for postoperative urinary drainage in adult males undergoing cardiac surgery has been shown to reduce the incidence of subsequent urethral stricture formation.[62] Although patients with indwelling latex catheters were catheterized less than 48 hours, a 2% incidence of urethral stricture was still noted at 1 year and a 5% incidence at 2 years. None of the patients with indwelling silicone catheters developed a stricture.

Hematuria has long been considered to be common immediately after even atraumatic catheterization. Although Sklar and colleagues[63] found a small increase in urinary red blood cell (RBC) count with catheterization, only 1 in 47 patients had an increase of greater than 4 RBCs per high-power field (HPF) attributable to the procedure. They suggest that greater than 4 RBCs/HPF after catheterization is unlikely to be due to the procedure and is, in fact, evidence of preexisting hematuria, which must be explained.

Undesirably retained urethral catheters are an uncommon but frustrating problem. Catheters may be retained because of balloons that do not deflate (see the next section) or, very rarely, because of a knot that has spontaneously developed in the catheter (very rare). Catheter knotting has been associated with the insertion of a highly flexible catheter far into the bladder.[64] A guidewire passed up the catheter may be successful in reducing an infrequent knot, but urethral dilation with progressively larger catheters adjacent to the retained catheter might be needed to permit subsequent urethral passage of the knot.

REMOVING THE NON-DEFLATING CATHETER

The self-retaining Foley balloon-type catheter obviates the need for cumbersome taping or suturing of the catheter to keep it in place. Occasionally, however, an indwelling catheter balloon does not deflate. Needless to say, this problem has challenged and frustrated many clinicians and has produced a number of ingenious solutions. A common cause of the non-deflating catheter balloon is the malfunction of the flap-type valve in the balloon lumen of the catheter, which normally allows fluid to fill the balloon of the catheter but prevents passive egress (Fig. 55–22).[65] The ideal solution is one that resolves the problem—deflating the balloon—without creating another problem (i.e., unnecessary bladder irritation or balloon fragmentation). Of the methods recommended to decompress non-deflating catheter balloons, the only technique that approaches the ideal directly attacks this flap valve deformity. Other methods of deflation may be effective but require more creativity and dexterity on the part of the catheterist.

A variation on the non-deflating balloon is "cuffing," essentially an *asymmetrical deflation* in which the balloon does not deflate flush with the catheter.

The irregularity becomes more pronounced as the catheter is withdrawn into the urethra, preventing easy withdrawal. This occurs more often when balloon fluid is quickly aspirated and less often with more gradual fluid withdrawal. Inflate the balloon again and try slow deflation if this occurs. Reinflating the balloon to a smooth surface with 0.5 to 1 mL of saline during withdrawal may also obviate this. An example of cuffing is shown in Figure 55–23D and this is more common in suprapubic tubes.

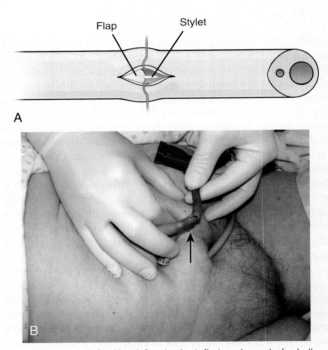

Figure 55–22 *A,* A flaplike defect in the inflating channel of a balloon catheter that is being raised by a wire stylet (from a central venous pressure [CVP] kit) passed down the inflating channel to deflate the balloon. *B,* Note that the entire inflation channel is filled with debris *(arrow),* preventing egress of fluid from the retaining balloon *(A, From Eichenberg HA, Amin M, Clark J: Nondeflating Foley catheters. Int Urol Nephrol 8:171, 1976. Reproduced by permission.)*

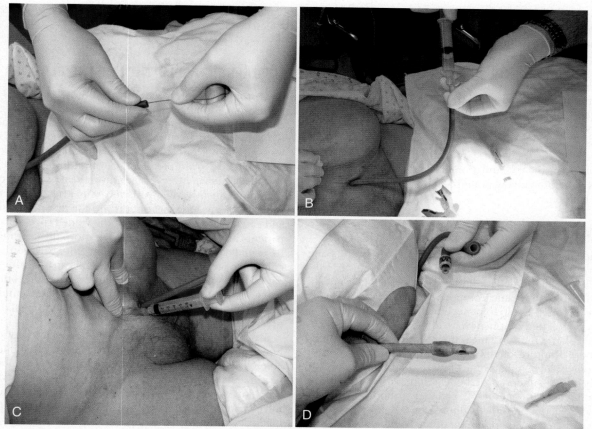

Figure 55–23 A, The inflation port has been removed and the catheter is cut so the inflation channel can be cannulated with the firm end of a CVP guidewire. The wire may puncture the balloon or simply clear the channel so fluid escapes. B, Insert a 20-gauge needle gently into the inflation channel to suck out balloon fluid once the path has been cleared. C, This nondeflating suprapubic balloon was filled with 50 mL of saline and a 25-gauge spinal needle was inserted parallel to the catheter to puncture the balloon while maintaining *traction on the catheter to stabilize the balloon.* D, This balloon demonstrates "cuffing" where the balloon deflated asymmetrically, getting caught up during withdrawal.

Techniques

The first way to deflate a non-deflating balloon is to attack the inflate-deflate channel that normally prevents the passive egress of inflating fluid or air (see Fig. 55–23A). Occasionally, cutting off the inflation port will deflate the balloon, but usually, this is not the problematic area. Once the port has been removed, use a needle/syringe in the inflation channel to suck out balloon fluid (see Fig. 55–23B). Cutting the catheter closer to the bladder may fortuitously cut off the offending area, but do not cut off excessive catheter because additional techniques may be used. More often, the inflation channel may have a valve defect or be filled with debris (see Fig. 55–22B). When presented with this situation, it is best to insert a thin, rigid wire into the balloon-port lumen in an attempt to deflate the valve-flap defect sufficiently and promote the escape of fluid from the balloon. Occasionally, the balloon itself may be punctured by this wire. A stainless steel wire suture of 3-0 or 4-0 gauge is the thinnest suitable material. The wire stylet from an angiographic or central venous pressure catheter, guidewires from ureteral catheters, and very small, well-lubricated ureteral catheters themselves have all been reported to be successful. When a ureteral catheter guidewire was used in one series, 34 of 39 balloons were deflated without fragmentation.[66] In the 5 unsuccessful cases, needle puncture of the balloon was required and was successful.

A common method of deflating the balloon is to puncture it with a needle. This may be accomplished by overinflating the balloon (with 50–100 mL saline) and puncturing it via a suprapubic needle under bedside ultrasound guidance.

With gentle traction, inflate the balloon with additional fluid, draw against the bladder neck, and puncture with a thin 25- or 27-gauge *spinal needle* (see Fig. 55–23C). With gentle traction on the catheter to stabilize the balloon, the thin needle may be directed suprapubically (transvesically), transvaginally, transperineally, or transrectally. The procedure may be done either blindly[66,67] or with the aid of ultrasound. In women, a spinal needle may be gently introduced transurethrally alongside the catheter. It may take a few minutes for all of the balloon fluid to drain. Fragmentation during puncture can occur, but it is much more rare than in the two techniques described previously.

One approach is to use a stepwise series of maneuvers. If the balloon does not deflate, remove the syringe adapter plug from the balloon-inflating channel. This rules out a malfunction of the adapter. If the balloon water does not escape, next insert an angiographic catheter stylet into the balloon-inflating channel and rotate it. Usually, the water from the balloon flows out along the wire. If it does not, place the catheter on traction and attempt to locate the balloon by palpation either perineally, transvaginally, or transrectally. If this is successful, use a 25- to 27-gauge spinal needle with or without local anesthesia to blindly puncture the balloon and then remove the catheter. If localization is unsuccessful, multiple blind passes with the 27-gauge needle can be attempted; this is usually successful in decompressing the balloon and removing the catheter.[68] If the patient requires a permanent indwelling catheter, it may be replaced immediately after removal by any of these techniques. Concomitant inadvertent needle punctures of the rectum are usually of no clinical significance.

Once a malfunctioning balloon has been deflated, inspect the balloon itself for missing fragments. If a piece of the balloon is missing, arrange for subsequent cystoscopy to look for and remove the fragment. Unfortunately, pretesting Foley catheter balloons by trial inflation and deflation before insertion does not eliminate the potential for a non-deflating Foley catheter balloon.

Other Methods

A traditional method of balloon deflation involves injecting an erosive substance into the balloon port. The caustic substance allows balloon deflation after part of the balloon wall has been eroded. Organic compounds that attack the latex polymers are often used. Toluene, ether, acetone, mineral oil, and even petrolatum ointment have all been used. In general, the more volatile the substance, the more rapidly it ruptures the balloon. Rupture of the balloon may be partly a result of the rapid expansion that some of these volatile substances—especially ether—undergo at body temperature. Ether was reported to rupture 58 of 60 catheter balloons within 2 minutes of injection into the balloon port.[65] Unfortunately, in 55 of the catheters, a free fragment of the balloon was created. Mineral oil, which works more slowly, was associated with fragment production in 95 of 100 catheters tested.[65] When released into the bladder, organic substances often produce a symptomatic chemical cystitis. Toluene is less likely to cause fragmentation. If mineral oil is used, instill 10 mL into the balloon, and an additional 10 mL if rupture does not occur in 10 minutes. Regardless of substance used, inspect the balloon for possible retained fragments. If fragmentation is noted, cystoscopy and, occasionally, irrigation can be used. After withdrawal, insert a new catheter and irrigate the bladder copiously with saline to remove small particles and to mitigate chemical cystitis. For obvious reasons, use of these substances has fallen out of favor.

Another prior method, although effective, is not in favor because it almost always results in balloon fragments that must be retrieved cystoscopically. This consists of simply overfilling the balloon with air or water to the point of rupture. If the in port is still functioning, add 50 to 100 mL of saline into the bladder to cushion the effects of a ruptured balloon. Up to 200 mL of fluid or air can be injected before a 5-mL balloon will rupture.[65,69] Adding volume to an empty bladder might not be a problem. Unfortunately, this same technique might produce unacceptably painful bladder distention in a patient whose catheter is blocked and whose bladder is either secondarily contracted due to chronic infection or neurogenic bladder dysfunction or distended to the point of maximum filling. As stated, the main reason not to use this technique is the disconcerting frequency of balloon fragmentation with subsequent foreign body bladder stone formation. In an experimental study of 100 catheters (50 of which were overdistended with water and 50 of which were overdistended with air), all 100 catheter balloons ruptured, producing bladder fragments.[65] Cystoscopic inspection of the bladder with removal of any fragments will be required to prevent bladder stone formation if this method of balloon deflation is selected.

SUPRAPUBIC ASPIRATION OF THE BLADDER

One problem of interpreting voided urine samples is that the urine from the bladder passes through a progressively more contaminated urethral conduit. In the female, the perineum is a culture medium in which bacteria are seemingly eager to be swept along into the sterile collection cup and onto the agar plate. To avoid the dilemma of interpretation, clinicians have devised maneuvers to minimize the presence of contaminating organisms. Male patients are instructed to retract the foreskin, cleanse the meatus, discard the first portion of urine, and catch the midstream part of the voided specimen. Female patients are asked to perform even more difficult maneuvers to avoid bacterial contamination: Sit backward on the commode facing the wall, hold the labia apart with one hand, cleanse the periurethral skin blindly with the other, then reach for the cup, initiate voiding, and catch the midstream urine—all while holding the labia apart and maintaining the precarious position on the commode.

In standard transurethral bladder catheterization, even under ideal circumstances, the procedure is often uncomfortable. The catheter must traverse the distal contaminated urethra and might infrequently introduce contaminating bacteria into the specimen and into the bladder, resulting in infrequent infections, in patients who do not empty their bladder with normal voiding.

Suprapubic aspiration of the bladder, first reported as a method of collecting urine for bacteriologic study in 1956,[70] offers the clinician a relatively simple means of obtaining uncontaminated bladder urine. Urethral contamination is successfully avoided, and positive results always represent true bacteriuria. The one caveat is that the bladder must be full to avoid multiple painful needle sticks, a clinical situation that may be difficult to discern in a sick child.

Indications

In the neonate or the young child, suprapubic aspiration or urethral catheterization can provide the clinician with a sample that is reliable for bacteriologic interpretation.[70–72] Although disconcerting to some parents (they may wish to leave the room or look away during the procedure), suprapubic aspiration is not a dangerous procedure, and the sensitivity of urinalysis of this urine for bacteriuria approaches 100%. However, for children age 2 years or older, urine can generally be more easily collected by urethral catheterization.

For adult patients, the indications for suprapubic aspiration are more limited because these patients usually can cooperate with the clinician. Men with condom catheters or phimosis, however, may require suprapubic aspiration to minimize urethral contamination. Aspirated cultures, rather than catheterized specimens, may help rule out contamination in patients with asymptomatic bacteriuria on routine urine collection. In infections caused by organisms that in other circumstances are often discounted as contaminants (e.g., *Staphylococcus epidermidis* or *Candida albicans*), suprapubic aspiration or a catheterized specimen is required to confirm the presence of such pathogens.

In patients in whom the possibility of infravesical infection is a concern (e.g., patients with chronic infections of the

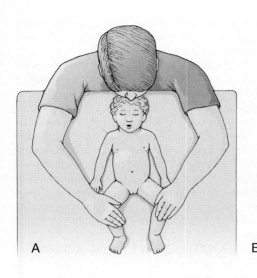

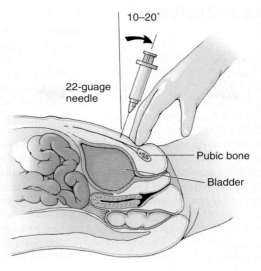

Figure 55–24 *A*, For a suprapubic bladder tap, restrain the infant and place it in a frog-legged position. *B*, A 22-gauge needle punctures the abdominal wall in the midline approximately 1 to 2 cm cephalad to the superior border of the pubic bone. The syringe is perpendicular to the plane of the abdominal wall (usually 10°–20° from the true vertical). The bladder is an abdominal organ in infants, and placing the needle too close to the pubic bone or angling toward the feet might cause the needle to miss the bladder. Localizing the bladder with bedside ultrasound facilitates this procedure.

10–20°

22-guage needle

Pubic bone

Bladder

urethra or the periurethral glands), suprapubic aspiration may help localize a bladder from a urethral source.

Procedure

The clinician must first locate the bladder. A full, palpable, or percussible bladder should be readily apparent, but this can be difficult to discern in all but the thinnest patients. If there is any question about the location or the amount of bladder urine, a quick ultrasound examination is informative. The point of entry in the skin should be 1 to 2 cm above the superior edge of the symphysis pubis. The syringe and needle are passed perpendicular to the abdominal wall toward the bladder, usually a 10° to 20° angle from the true vertical, somewhat *cephalad* in children (Fig. 55–24) and somewhat *caudad* in adults (Fig. 55–25). Note that the bladder of a newborn is an abdominal organ and that it will be missed if the needle is inserted too close to the pubis or angled toward the feet.

Place the child supine and restrain with the legs in a frog-legged position. After draping the prepared skin and choosing the point of entry, raise a skin wheal of local anesthesia to reduce discomfort. After anesthetizing the skin, advance a longer, larger-caliber needle (usually 22-ga, 3.75 to 8.75 cm in length) in the midline through the skin and quickly into the bladder. The authors prefer to advance the needle attached to a syringe, with active aspiration during advancement. As soon as the bladder is entered, urine appears in the syringe. A short needle is adequate for virtually all pediatric patients. After collecting the urine, withdraw the syringe and needle. Microscopic hematuria always follows the procedure but gross hematuria is uncommon. A bandage may be placed over the puncture site. If urine is not obtained, do not remove the needle but withdraw it to a subcutaneous position and redirect it at a different angle. Often, a child may spontaneously start to void after any type of invasive stimulus (e.g., bladder irritation by a probing needle, venipuncture, or lumbar puncture). Hence, preparation to collect a spontaneously voided specimen is recommended, should that option arise. Anticipate this before beginning blood or spinal fluid collection during the bacteremic work-up of the febrile neonate.

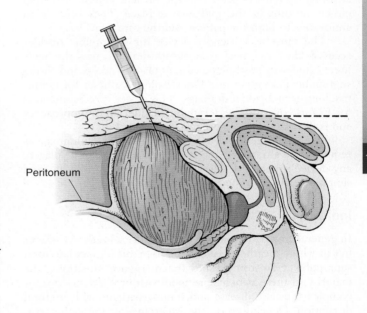

Peritoneum

Figure 55–25 The peritoneum is pushed cephalad by the filled bladder during suprapubic aspiration in an adult. Direct the needle slightly caudad.

In most patients, an acceptable urine sample can be obtained with the first needle pass. If the needle points too caudad in an effort to avoid entering the peritoneum, it is possible to enter the retropubic space, skimming the bladder muscle and never penetrating the bladder mucosa.

Complications

Bacteremia does not result from this procedure.[73] Bowel penetration has occurred in children with distended abdomens from gastrointestinal disturbances.[74] The combination of gaseous bowel distention and relative hypovolemia might displace and flatten the relatively empty bladder against the pelvic floor. Even when the large bowel has been penetrated, patients recover uneventfully. Simple penetration of the bowel with a needle is considered an innocuous event and requires no specific treatment.

PERCUTANEOUS SUPRAPUBIC CYSTOSTOMY

Background

Although suprapubic cystostomy was described as early as 4 centuries ago, the safety of the procedure was first demonstrated by Garson and Peterson in 1888. The first modern method was the Campbell trocar set, described in 1951.[75,76]

Perhaps the most widely known and frequently used trocar-type cystostomy tube is the Cystocath.[77] It is available in 8- and 12-French sizes. The latter is more commonly used for adult patients. The Cystocath is packaged as a self-contained set supplying virtually everything needed for insertion. The device is easy to insert and may be satisfactory for relatively long periods of trouble-free use if the patient is given conscientious nursing care.

The major difficulty with cystostomy tubes of all designs has been securing them to the patient's skin. Those with retention balloons, such as the standard Foley urethral catheter or the Ingram catheter, are most secure and need only tape to secure them to the anterior abdominal wall. Virtually all other systems depend on tape or skin adhesive to hold either the tube or the appliance in place. They become an annoyance to both the patient and the care provider.

The most user-friendly device for suprapubic bladder access is the Cook peel-away sheath unit.[47] It uses the Seldinger (guidewire) technique to gain bladder access and allows suprapubic placement of a Foley balloon catheter for definitive long-term bladder drainage. This device is recommended for ED use over other suprapubic bladder access approaches and is discussed in the next section.

In an emergency, when emergent bladder drainage is required and a transurethral Foley catheter cannot be placed, any device suitable for central venous access can be inserted suprapubically with the Seldinger technique.

Indications

In general, any patient who would require a urethral catheter but in whom a catheter cannot be passed is a candidate for a suprapubic cystostomy tube. In emergency situations, the majority of these patients are men with urethral stricture or complex prostatic disease and trauma patients with urethral disruption. Depending on the experience of the catheterist, dilation can usually be performed in patients with urethral strictures using filiforms and followers. If there is any difficulty with urethral instrumentation, a suprapubic cystostomy tube is prudent and prevents further urethral injury. Complete urethral transection associated with a pelvic fracture is an absolute indication for emergent suprapubic cystostomy. Many affected patients need laparotomy because of associated injuries, and a large suprapubic catheter can be placed intraoperatively. However, if the patient does not require laparotomy, a percutaneously placed Foley catheter allows urologic surgery to be done electively after the patient's condition has stabilized clinically.

Patients with lower genitourinary infection deserve special care before instituting any type of urethral instrumentation. The risk of inciting an episode of gram-negative bacteremia with urethral dilation must be considered, and appropriate intravenous gram-negative antibiotic coverage started before the patient is instrumented. Foley catheter drainage is the first choice, and suprapubic drainage is an option in patients with acute prostatitis or epididymitis who require bladder drainage. Ideally, a suprapubic catheter allows both bladder drainage and unobstructed drainage of prostatic, seminal vesicle, and urethral secretions but requires an invasive procedure with its associated risks.

Neurologically disabled patients (e.g., quadriplegics or paraplegics) or those with any type of neurogenic bladder dysfunction who have been successfully maintained on a program of intermittent self-catheterization occasionally have difficulty with urethral catheterization. In these patients, especially those with high spinal cord lesions, suprapubic needle aspiration or suprapubic cystostomy can be a rapidly effective method of relieving autonomic hyperreflexia associated with acute bladder distention. Bladder decompression in the dysreflexic, profusely perspiring, hypertensive quadriplegic in sympathetic crisis provides dramatic symptom resolution, whether by suprapubic bladder decompression or Foley catheter placement.

Suprapubic catheterization is not recommended as first-line treatment for the patient who is voiding poorly from lower urinary tract prostatic obstruction. Such patients, although symptomatic, are better off with intermittent self-catheterization or an indwelling Foley catheter if they are in retention or have chronically infected urine. Young women with psychosocial or emotional neurogenic bladder dysfunction are best managed by intermittent self-catheterization. In all such cases, clinical judgment will dictate the most appropriate form of treatment and whether concomitant antibiotic therapy is required.

Contraindications

Because placement of a suprapubic tube involves some risk, patient selection is important. The procedure should not be performed in a patient whose bladder is not definable. Although no absolute reported minimum bladder volume has ever been established, there must be enough urine in the bladder to allow the needle to fully penetrate the bladder dome without immediately exiting through the base. There must also be enough urine in the bladder to displace the bowel away from the anterosuperior surface of the bladder and the entrance of the needle. Ultrasound may be helpful in defining bladder anatomy.

Individuals who have a history of previous lower abdominal surgery, intraperitoneal surgery, or irradiation may have developed adhesions or adherence of the bowel to the anterior bladder wall. They are potentially at greater risk for bowel injury during percutaneous suprapubic cystostomy tube placement than those without previous abdominal surgery. Blind suprapubic cystostomy tube placement should be avoided in these patients. The absence of any of these risk factors does not totally exclude the risks of bowel or intraperitoneal injury, but it reduces them significantly.

Patients with bleeding diatheses are at greater risk for postinsertion bleeding, either into the bladder or into the retropubic space, than their normal counterparts.

Procedure

The following comments describe the placement of the Cook peel-away sheath. With modifications, these guidelines are adaptable for any type of suprapubic catheter placement.

Preparing the Patient

If necessary, the lower abdomen is shaved and antiseptic topically applied. Fill a 6-mL syringe with 1% lidocaine, and attach a 22-gauge, 7.75-cm spinal needle. Raise a skin wheal in the proposed site (~2–3 cm above the pubic symphysis), and infiltrate the subcutaneous tissue and rectus abdominis muscle fascia at a 10° to 20° angle toward the pelvis.

Locate the bladder by advancing the needle in the prescribed direction while aspirating the syringe. Urine is easily aspirated when the bladder is entered (Fig. 55–26*A*).

Placing the Tube

Once the bladder has been located, remove the syringe from the needle and advance a guidewire through the needle into the bladder (see Fig. 55–26*B*). Withdraw the needle, leaving only the guidewire traversing the anterior abdominal wall and positioned inside the bladder. Use a No. 15 scalpel blade to make a stab incision directly posterior to the wire through the skin, subcutaneous tissue, and superficial anterior abdominal wall fascia. Then pass the peel-away sheath and indwelling fascial dilator together over the wire into the bladder (see Fig. 55–26*C*). Remove the guidewire and fascial dilator, leaving only the peel-away sheath inside the bladder (see Fig. 55–26*D*). Then pass a preselected Foley balloon catheter through the indwelling intravesical sheath into the bladder (see Fig. 55–26*E*). Aspirate urine to confirm proper placement. Inflate the Foley balloon with a minimum of 10 mL of air, water, or saline (see Fig. 55–26*F*). Withdraw the peel-away sheath from the bladder and anterior abdominal wall and literally peel it away from the catheter, leaving only the indwelling suprapubic Foley catheter (see Fig. 55–26*G*). Withdraw the catheter slowly until the inflated balloon approximates the cystostomy site (see Fig. 55–26*H* and *I*). Connect the catheter to a drainage bag, and then dress the wound with 4 × 4 gauze pads to complete the procedure.

Complications

A wide variety of complications specific to each procedure have been reported, which serve as reminders that suprapubic cystostomy is not innocuous. Occasionally, despite the best intentions, the suprapubic tube or catheter cannot be positioned or maintained successfully without untoward sequelae (Table 55–6).

The most serious complications involve perforation of the peritoneum or the intraperitoneal contents. Any condition that might fix the anterior peritoneum so that the filled bladder cannot lift the peritoneum cephalad might result in either transperitoneal bladder puncture or possible perforation of small or large bowel.[78] Although finding the bladder using a small-gauge scout needle may help reduce bowel injury, even in the most apparently successful of bladder punctures, a complication might result.

TABLE 55–6 Reported Complications of Suprapubic Cystostomy

Bowel perforation
Intraperitoneal extravasation (without a prior history of surgery)
Extraperitoneal extravasation
Infection of space of Retzius
Ureteral catheterization
Obstruction of tubing by blood, mucus, or kinking
Tubing comes out
Hematuria

The cystostomy tube or catheter that merely traverses the peritoneum might produce a mild ileus, serve as a route for peritoneal infection, or drain the bladder contents into the peritoneal cavity. The last situation would be expected if a Cystocath, rather than a peel-away sheath, was used and one of the extra holes of the Cystocath tubing opened into the peritoneal cavity. Through-and-through bladder penetration with associated rectal, vaginal, or uterine injury has been reported, although the consistent use of small-gauge bladder locator needles and the judicious advancement of fascial dilators should reduce the incidence.

Occasionally, the clinician is tempted to proceed with suprapubic cystostomy when the bladder is not palpable and has not been located with a syringe and needle. Injury of adjacent organs is much more frequent in these circumstances. If clinicians remind themselves that the bladder eventually refills, they will find waiting much more tolerable. If faced with an emergency, ultrasound guidance may be helpful for determining bladder size and location.

Infection may occur at the suprapubic cystostomy skin site or anywhere along the course of the catheter.[79] Use of antimicrobial ointment daily after cleaning the catheter entry site may reduce purulence around the tube. However, topical care does not prevent eventual deep space or bladder infection from the presence of a foreign body. Deeper tissue infections may result from extravasated infected urine or from a superficial infection spreading along the tube to a hematoma at the bladder or fascial level. Parenteral antibiotics might be required. Open drainage is rarely needed unless a loculated abscess has formed.

Hematuria is rarely more than a transient problem.[80] After suprapubic Foley catheter insertion, bladder irrigation may occasionally be required to clear the hematuria. Transient Toomey syringe aspiration may be needed to evacuate clots.

EMERGENCY LOWER GENITOURINARY RADIOLOGIC PROCEDURES

Trauma to the urinary tract accounts for about 10% of all injuries seen in EDs. Although the signs of genitourinary trauma in general can be quite subtle, lower urinary tract injury can often be quickly identified and thoroughly evaluated radiographically in the ED. Radiologic imaging of the upper urinary tract is generally a less urgent matter and can usually be done in the radiology suite or, when important for emergency operative decision-making, as a single shot intravenous pyelogram (IVP) in the operating room. Hence, this section does not discuss the role or technique of IVP in detail. Note that the timing of any radiologic evaluation can be challenging to the emergency clinician, especially when faced with a critically ill multiple trauma patient. The trauma team of clinicians involved in each resuscitation must determine the priority and extent of such an evaluation.

Indications for Evaluation

The urinary tract includes the kidneys, ureters, bladder, urethra, and external genitalia. Approximately 8% to 10% of blunt abdominal trauma is associated with injuries to the urinary tract.[81] In one large series,[82] 7% of gunshot wounds and 6% of stab wounds to the abdomen resulted in penetrating wounds to the kidney. For injury identification purposes,

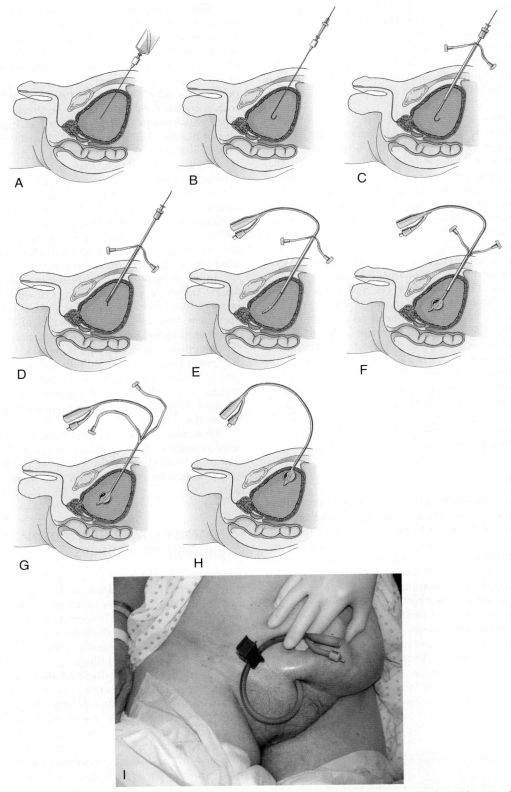

Figure 55–26 Any catheter that can be used as a central venous catheter can be inserted suprapubically with the Seldinger technique. The more traditional, and more permanent, suprapubic cystostomy with the Cook peel-away sheath introducer is demonstrated here. *A,* Enter the bladder with a syringe and needle. Confirm location by aspirating urine. *B,* Remove the syringe and pass the guidewire through the needle into the bladder. *C,* Remove the needle, then pass the dilator and peel-away sheath over the wire into the bladder. A small stab wound in the anterior abdominal fascia may be required to accommodate the dilator and sheath. *D,* Remove the dilator and wire, leaving only the sheath inside the bladder. *E,* Pass the preselected Foley balloon catheter through the sheath into the bladder. Aspirate urine to confirm location. *F,* Inflate the balloon with a minimum of 10 mL of air, saline, or water. A 5-mL balloon will accommodate 10 mL easily and make accidental catheter distraction less likely. *G,* Remove the sheath from the bladder, anterior abdominal wall, and cutaneous entry site, and then literally peel it away from the indwelling catheter. *H,* Withdraw the catheter until a snug fit is ensured at the cystostomy site. *I,* A suprapubic Foley catheter in place.

the genitourinary system is best divided into lower urinary tract (i.e., urethra and bladder), upper urinary tract (i.e., kidneys and ureter), and external genitalia (i.e., penis, scrotum, and testes or vagina, labia majora, and labia minora). Each of these subdivisions has its own markers for potential injury. These markers are addressed during the resuscitation phase of trauma care and during secondary injury survey when the abdomen, pelvis, external genitalia, vaginal vault, and rectum are systematically examined.

The markers for lower urinary tract injury are blood at the urethral meatus, abnormal position of the prostate on rectal examination (in men), and gross hematuria.[83] Perineal ecchymosis and scrotal hematoma also represent potential lower urinary tract injury, but these findings are usually seen later in the patient's course rather than acutely in the ED.

Gross hematuria or microscopic hematuria (≥3–5 RBCs/ HPF-spun specimen) in conjunction with any history of shock (systolic blood pressure ≤ 90 mm Hg) in the field or in the ED after blunt trauma are markers of potential upper urinary tract injury in any adult.[84] Research has suggested that pediatric patients can be managed similarly to adults; a meta-analysis defined 50 RBCs/HPF as the quantity below which imaging may be omitted and no significant injuries missed.[85,86] This can be particularly justified if there are no other associated injuries and the mechanism of injury was not severe (e.g., high speed motor vehicle collision).[87,88] In genitourinary trauma, always evaluate the lower urinary tract before the upper urinary tract. Retrograde urethrography and retrograde cystography are the diagnostic procedures of choice to evaluate potential injury to the lower urinary tract. These studies must be carried out in the proper sequence and in a retrograde fashion to avoid missing potential injuries. *Retrograde* refers to the technique of instilling contrast retrograde through the urethra or by gravity filling of the bladder. It must be distinguished from antegrade filling, in which intravenous contrast for IVP or abdominal computed tomography (CT) is excreted from the kidneys and allowed to fill the bladder passively over time.

Contrast-enhanced CT is the diagnostic examination of choice for suspected renal trauma. It provides greater resolution and sensitivity than bolus infusion IVP with nephrotomography and has the advantage of evaluating other intra-abdominal structures as well.[89] Contrast-enhanced CT should also be performed initially if thoracic or intra-abdominal injuries are present or suspected, or if there is concern about renal pedicle injury.

Gross Hematuria

Gross hematuria is indicated by any color of urine other than clear or yellow. It is an absolute marker for urinary tract injury and an indication for diagnostic evaluation. The resuscitating clinician must be responsible for observing the initial bladder effluent after Foley catheter insertion. Vigorous fluid resuscitation may quickly clear initial gross hematuria and eliminate the only marker for potential injury. When gross hematuria is encountered after injury, the bladder and kidneys are thought of as potential sources for the hematuria. In most cases, gross hematuria in association with a pelvic fracture will implicate the bladder as the most likely source of injury. In the absence of a pelvic fracture and with a history of upper abdominal or chest trauma, the kidneys are the most likely source of the hematuria. In urologic trauma, the lower urinary

tract must always be studied before the upper urinary tract (e.g., study the urethra before the bladder, study the bladder before the kidneys). Always perform the specific diagnostic studies in a retrograde fashion. This allows the responsible clinician to directly control the amount of contrast used to investigate potential urethral or bladder injuries. Whenever any doubt exists about the mechanism of injury, the patient's physical examination, or the source of gross hematuria, the resuscitating clinician is always advised to begin with an evaluation of the lower urinary tract before evaluating the upper urinary tract.

Evidence of Lower Urinary Tract Injury

In the resuscitation of any trauma patient, placement of a Foley catheter has become the standard method of monitoring urinary output. Blood at the urethral meatus, however, indicates a potential partial or complete urethral disruption and dictates the need for an RUG to delineate urethral integrity. This study can be done by the resuscitating clinician in the ED or on the operating room table by the trauma surgeon or urologist if the patient requires immediate surgical intervention for life-threatening injuries. The approach to gentle catheter insertion in the setting of possible bladder or urethral injury has been discussed previously. The traditional approach is outlined later, using contraindications previously stated to be absolute, now thought, by many, to be relative.[27,28]

The male posterior urethra, which includes the membranous and prostatic urethra, is injured more frequently than the anterior urethra. The urogenital diaphragm encloses and fixes the membranous urethra; the prostate and prostatic urethra are firmly attached to the posterior surface of the symphysis pubis by the puboprostatic ligaments. Blunt trauma and pelvic fractures, especially in the presence of a full bladder, may result in shearing forces that partially or completely avulse portions of the firmly attached posterior urethra. Usually, the bladder and prostate gland are sheared from the membranous urethra, resulting in a complete urethral disruption (Fig. 55–27). The female urethra, in contrast, is short and relatively mobile and generally escapes injury in blunt trauma. Occasionally, a significant pelvic fracture will result in a laceration or avulsion of the female urethra at the bladder neck. Direct injuries to the female urethra may also occur secondary to penetrating trauma to the vagina or perineum. These injuries often are disclosed by blood at the introitus or an abnormal vaginal examination in the female pelvic fracture patient.[90]

Contusions or lacerations of the male anterior urethra occur when the bulbous urethra is compressed against the inferior surface of the symphysis pubis. This happens most commonly as a result of straddle injuries in males but may result from any blunt perineal trauma. Significant trauma to the penile urethra is rare without penetrating injuries or urethral instrumentation. Anterior urethral injuries may result in extravasation of blood or urine into the penis, scrotum, or perineum or along the anterior abdominal wall, depending on whether or not Buck's fascia has been violated (Fig. 55–28).[46] This is in contrast to posterior urethral injuries, in which blood and urine extravasate into the pelvis.

The rectal examination is highly specific, although not as sensitive, in the evaluation of a posterior urethral disruption. If the prostate is not clearly defined (it should have the consistency of the examiner's thenar eminence), is high-riding rather than in its normal anatomic location, or if a pelvic

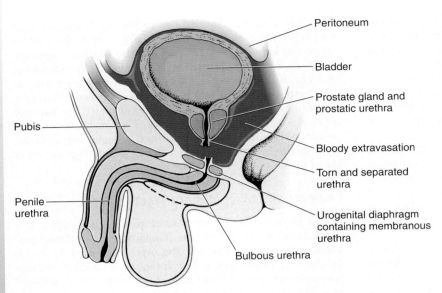

Peritoneum

Bladder

Prostate gland and prostatic urethra

Pubis

Bloody extravasation

Torn and separated urethra

Penile urethra

Urogenital diaphragm containing membranous urethra

Bulbous urethra

Figure 55–27 A common posterior urethral injury is a disruption of the membranous urethra. In this case, a distended bladder and attached prostate gland are sheared from the fixed membranous urethra. Note the development of a perivesical hematoma and the presence of a "high-riding" prostate gland.

hematoma can be palpated (see Fig. 55–27), one should be suspicious of a posterior urethral injury and an RUG should be performed before attempting urethral catheterization. However, a normal rectal examination, by itself, should not be considered definitive evidence of an intact urethra if other clinical signs raise suspicion for urethral injury. Retrograde urethrography is a quick, technically easy study to perform and should be part of every emergency clinician's armamentarium.

Pelvic Fracture

Pelvic fractures commonly occur in patients with urethral or bladder injury. The incidence of lower tract injuries in males with pelvic fractures ranges from 7% to 25%. Conversely, approximately 80% of all posterior urethral and bladder injuries are associated with pelvic fractures.[83] Because of the severity of late complications, especially urethral strictures, which most often require difficult surgical repair, it is paramount that these injuries not be missed. Again, in any female patient with a pelvic fracture, it is most important to examine the introitus and vaginal vault for blood, which may be indicative of urethral, bladder neck, or vaginal wall lacerations. In male patients, rectal examination of the prostate to assess its position will be most helpful in assessing the posterior urethra. A pelvic fracture in association with gross hematuria is an absolute indication for retrograde cystography. In a review of 234 patients with traumatic pelvic fractures, no major lower urinary tract injuries were found in the absence of gross hematuria.[83]

Radiographic Contrast Material

To evaluate the urethra and bladder, inject or instill contrast into these structures in a retrograde manner. To evaluate the kidneys and ureters, CT scan or a bolus of contrast material is injected into the venous system, opacifying the renal parenchyma and collecting system as it is excreted unchanged in the urine. Three types of contrast material are currently available (Table 55–7). All contain iodine, and all are hyperosmolar with respect to blood. Conventional agents, such as Hypaque and Renografin (diatrizoate), are triiodinated water-

soluble agents (ionic monoacetic monomers) that completely dissociate into anion and cation moieties on intravascular injection. Osmolality is quite high, ranging from 1200 to 2000 mOsm/kg. Many of the side effects of contrast agents have been attributed to their osmolarity. Although iodine concentrations do determine the quality of the radiographic image, iodine itself is not thought to play a major role in the typical anaphylactoid side effects.[91]

Two new classes of contrast agents are ioxaglate (Hexabrix), an ionic monoacetic dimer, and nonionic (nondissociating) agents, such as iopamidol (Isovue), iohexol (Omnipaque), and iodixanol (Visipaque). The newer agents have twice as many iodine atoms per particle in solution as conventional agents and, therefore, provide a significantly higher urinary iodine concentration, offering better diagnostic imaging. The osmolality of the newer agents is markedly lower, ranging from 600 to 700 mOsm/kg. The lower osmolality and improved chemical structure may be associated with fewer adverse side effects.[92,93] Although these new agents are promising for intravascular use, there is still some skepticism that they will truly limit major or clinically significant contrast reactions.[94] The lower-osmolarity nonionic agents have not been associated with a lower incidence of contrast-induced nephropathy. Furthermore, there is no indication for using these more expensive products in the retrograde evaluation of the injured lower urinary tract.

Contrast-induced nephropathy is a common cause of acute renal failure. Emergency clinicians can perform several interventions to minimize the patient's risk of developing this. One newer intervention is the use of sodium bicarbonate 154 mEq/L in dextrose and water given at 3 ml/kg starting 1 hour before the contrast procedure and then continued at 1 ml/kg/hr for 6 hours after the procedure. This can be used as preventive hydration for procedures involving intravenous contrast and has been shown to reduce the risk of patients developing contrast-induced nephropathy.

Radiographic Techniques

Kidneys, Ureters, and Bladder

A CT scan is the best intervention to fully evaluate pelvic trauma. The plain film, scout film, or KUB (kidneys, ureters,

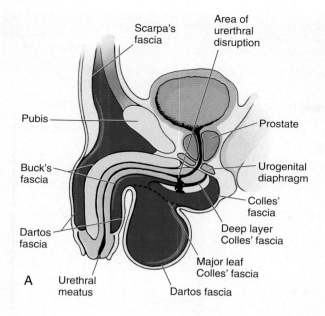

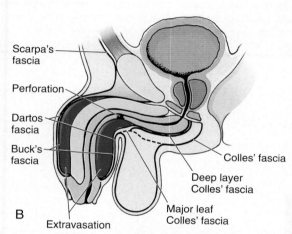

Figure 55–28 *A,* Disruption of the anterior urethra (bulbous urethra) occurs with straddle-type injuries in the male. Extravasation of urine and blood may occur in the perineum or scrotum or along the anterior abdominal wall. Note that in this diagram, Buck's fascia has been penetrated. *B,* Anterior urethral injury in which Buck's fascia remains intact. In this situation, extravasation is confined and results in a swollen and ecchymotic penis. Such an injury usually results from instrumentation of the anterior urethra.

and bladder) film of the abdomen, is used in conjunction with the following radiographic techniques. Incidental nondiagnostic findings on initial KUB that may alert the clinician to the possibility of urinary tract injury include:

1. Loss of one or both psoas shadows secondary to blood in the retroperitoneum.
2. Spinal curvature secondary to splinting—usually concave to the side of the injury.
3. Lower rib or transverse process fractures, both of which may be associated with upper urinary tract injury.
4. Pelvic fracture.

The KUB must always precede the injection or instillation of contrast material because radiopaque shadows seen on the plain film must be differentiated from extravasation on the postevacuation film.

Retrograde Urethrography

Retrograde urethrography is indicated whenever uncertainty exists about the integrity of the urethra. In cases associated with pelvic fracture, the patient should remain supine throughout the entire radiographic examination. This is important to ensure stability of any possible retropubic hematoma that may result from extensive venous bleeding associated with the initial pelvic fracture. In cases of suspected urethral injury not associated with pelvic fracture, it is acceptable to obtain oblique films during the study that may complement the examination findings. Perpendicular stretching of the penis across the thigh or oblique films may be needed to ensure urethral unfolding and a high-quality RUG.

Although several techniques have been promoted for retrograde urethrography, this section emphasizes one. The choice of technique is not as important as attention to detail. Solutions of either full-strength Hypaque (50%), Cystografin, or Renografin-60, or the same agents diluted to a less than 10% solution using sterile saline as the diluent, are frequently used (see Table 55–7). First, take a plain film (KUB) of reference before injecting any contrast material.[85] Retract and secure the penile foreskin with a folded 4 × 4 gauze sponge. Second, hold the penis between the long and the ring fingers of the nondominant hand (Fig. 55–29*A*) to allow a snug fit of the contrast-filled syringe or catheter inside the urethra (see Fig. 55–29*B*).

After sterile penile preparation, inject dye. A small Foley catheter may be used (Fig. 55–30). Alternatively, gently advance a catheter-tipped Toomey irrigating syringe or a regular 60-mL syringe with an attached Christmas-tree adapter or a non–Luer-Lok syringe inside the urethral meatus until a snug fit is ensured. Always gently squeeze the meatus over the injecting device to prevent leaking. If a Foley catheter is placed just inside the urethral meatus, inflate the balloon to ensure a snug fit in the fossa navicularis and then inject contrast through the catheter (see Fig. 55–30). If not done carefully, this technique often results in the spillage and deposition of contrast outside the urethra and onto the patient and the examination table, yielding a spurious result.

Then *slowly* inject approximately 50 to 60 mL of full- or half-strength contrast material under constant pressure into the urethra. Before injecting contrast, *stretch the penis perpendicularly across the patient's thigh to prevent urethral folding* (i.e., the double image of the proximal penile and bulbous urethra superimposed on one another) (Fig. 55–31). Overly forceful injection of contrast material may cause intravasation of contrast material into the venous plexus of the urethra, simulating an injury (Fig. 55–32). Finally, during the injection of the last 10 mL of contrast, a film (the urethrogram) is taken.

The extravasation of contrast material from a urethral disruption usually appears as a flamelike density outside the urethral contour (Fig. 55–33*A* and *B*). If any contrast material is seen within the bladder in conjunction with urethral extravasation, a partial rather than complete urethral disruption is more likely. In a complete urethral disruption, urethral extravasation will be present without evidence of contrast within the bladder. The examiner needs to be certain that the lack of bladder contrast is not secondary to voluntary contraction of the external sphincter. Occasionally, as mentioned previously, intravasated contrast material is seen in the periurethral penile venous plexus (see Fig. 55–32). It is of no clinical significance and should not be mistaken for urethral extravasation. As expected, penile venous intravasation (venous plexus opacification) is seen to clear spontaneously on any

TABLE 55–7 Clinical Use of Radiographic Contrast Material for Intravenous Pyelogram and Retrograde Studies

Use of RCM for IVP	Iodine Content (mg/mL of Solution)	Osmolality (mOsm/kg) (H₂O)	Average Volume for IVP
Conventional Ionic RMC			
Renografin-60 (diatrizoate sodium)	288	1511	Adult: 100 mL over 30–60 sec* Child: 1.5 mL/kg†
Hypaque (50%) (diatrizoate sodium)	300	1500	Adult: 100 mL over 30–60 sec* Child: 1.5 mL/kg†
Conray (methyl glucamine iothalamate)	282	1217	Adult: 100 mL over 30–60 sec* Child: 1.5 mL/kg†
New Nonionic RMC			
Isovue (iopamidol)	300	616	Adult: 50 mL over 30–60 sec‡ Child: 1–1.5 mL/kg†
Omnipaque 300 (iohexol)	300	672	Adult: 50 mL over 30–60 sec‡ Child: 1–1.5 mL/kg†
Visapaque 320 (iodixanol)	320	652	Adult: 100 mL over 30–60 sec Child: 1–2 mL/kg§

Use of RCM for Retrograde Studies	Use	Procedure
Renografin-60 or Hypaque (50%)	Dilute stock solutions with saline 1:10 (10% solution)	Urethrogram: 10–15 mL of dilute solution injected slowly through the urethral meatus. Children: 0.2 mL/kg Cystogram: after plain film and with Foley catheter in place, fill bladder of adult with 400 mL of dilute contrast material, introduced under gravity. Children: 5 mL/kg

*Average dose of iodine for IVP with ionic RCM: 350–400 mg/kg or 1.5 mL/kg.
Adult: Low dose: 10 g
      Intermediate dose: 30 g
      High dose: 60 g
†Do not exceed 3 mL/kg total dose.
‡Because the ratio of iodine atoms to dissolved particles is 1.5 with conventional ionic agents and 3.0 with the nonionic agents, less volume is required with the new agents. Average dose is 200–350 mg/kg.
§Do not exceed 4 mL/kg per dose.
IVP, intravenous pyelogram; RCM, radiographic contrast material.

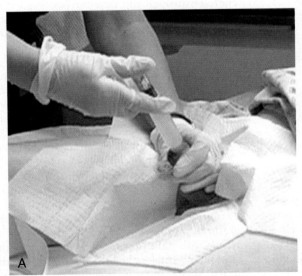

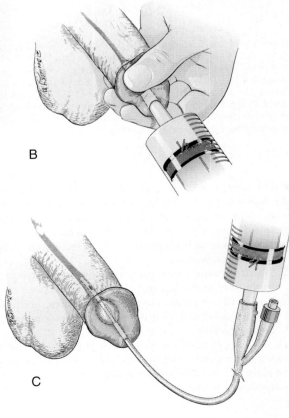

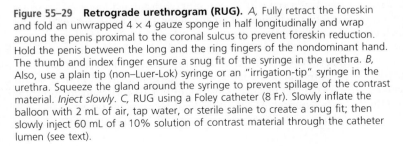

Figure 55–29 Retrograde urethrogram (RUG). *A,* Fully retract the foreskin and fold an unwrapped 4 × 4 gauze sponge in half longitudinally and wrap around the penis proximal to the coronal sulcus to prevent foreskin reduction. Hold the penis between the long and the ring fingers of the nondominant hand. The thumb and index finger ensure a snug fit of the syringe in the urethra. *B,* Also, use a plain tip (non–Luer-Lok) syringe or an "irrigation-tip" syringe in the urethra. Squeeze the gland around the syringe to prevent spillage of the contrast material. *Inject slowly. C,* RUG using a Foley catheter (8 Fr). Slowly inflate the balloon with 2 mL of air, tap water, or sterile saline to create a snug fit; then slowly inject 60 mL of a 10% solution of contrast material through the catheter lumen (see text).

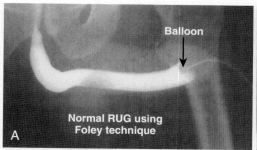

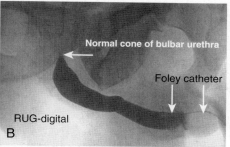

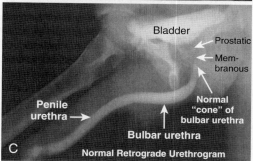

Figure 55–30 *A,* Normal RUG using a Foley catheter technique with the Foley balloon in the fossa navicularis. Note the air bubble in the penile urethra (conventional radiographic technique). *B,* Digital RUG using the Foley catheter technique. *C,* Labeled normal RUG. *(Reprinted from Older RA, Hertz M: Cystourethrography. In Pollack HM, McClennan BL, Dyer R, Kenney PJ [eds]: Clinical Urography, 2nd ed. Philadelphia, WB Saunders, 2000.)*

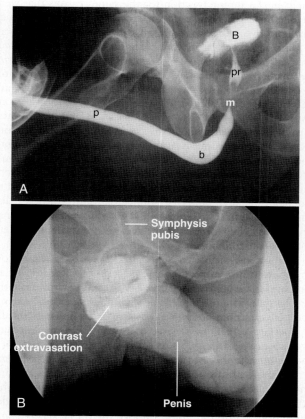

Figure 55–31 *A,* Normal RUG. Place the patient supine on the examination table. Stretch the penis perpendicularly across the patient's right thigh to allow urethral unfolding and complete urethral visualization. B, bladder; b, bulbar urethra; m, membranous urethra; p, penile urethra; pr, prostatic urethra. *B,* Obvious abnormal urethrogram. *(B, From Thomsen T, Setnik G [eds]: Procedures Consult—Emergency Medicine Module. Copyright 2008 Elsevier Inc. All rights reserved.)*

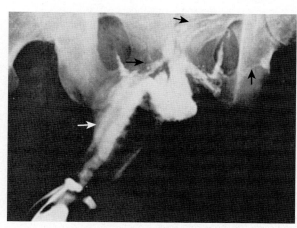

Figure 55–32 Always inject contrast material slowly. A too-fast injection causes venous intravasation *(arrows)* during a forceful RUG. This may mimic urethral extravasation but it clears immediately, as opposed to actual extravasation, which remains indefinitely. If unsure, take another film in 10 min. The presence of intravasation is benign but can confuse the clinician. *(From Richter MW, Lytton B, Myerson D, Grnja V: Radiology of genitourinary trauma. Radiol Clin North Am 11:626, 1973.)*

postvoid films, unlike urethral extravasation, which remains indefinitely.

If a Foley catheter has been successfully placed into the bladder and a partial urethral injury is suspected later, such an injury can be easily demonstrated without removing the catheter. Place the lubricated end of a pediatric feeding tube into the penile urethra alongside the existing Foley catheter (Fig. 55–34). Obtain a seal by compressing the glans penis with the nondominant thumb and index finger and gently inject contrast material via a Luer-Lok syringe with the dominant hand. In this way, extravasation can be demonstrated. It should be noted, however, that successful placement of the Foley catheter obviates the need for further treatment of a partial urethral tear in the emergency setting because an indwelling catheter alone is appropriate initial management for this type of injury. The finding of an associated urethral

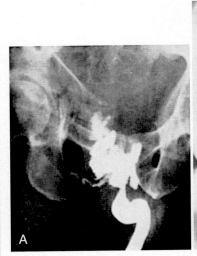
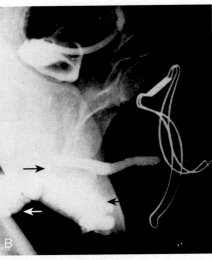

Figure 55–33 *A*, RUG. Urethrogram in a case of supramembranous urethral rupture. Contrast extravasation is typical of that seen with this type of injury. *B*, A rupture at the proximal bulbous urethra into the scrotum (*arrows*). (A, *From Morehouse DD, MacKinnon KJ: Posterior urethral injury: Etiology, diagnosis, initial management. Urol Clin North Am 4:74, 1977.*)

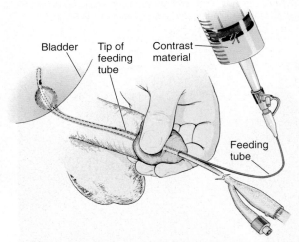

Figure 55–34 Evaluation of a urethral injury with a Foley catheter in place. A lubricated pediatric feeding tube has been advanced into the urethra beside the indwelling Foley catheter.

injury must be conveyed to a urologist because it will dictate the duration of definitive Foley catheter drainage.

Retrograde Cystogram

Perform a retrograde cystogram any time a bladder injury is suspected. It assumes that the urethra is normal before passing the Foley catheter. Obtain a preliminary KUB that will serve as the reference film for the entire examination. Next, fill the bladder under direct operator supervision by gravity instillation of contrast material. After removing the central piston from a 60-mL catheter-tip syringe, attach the catheter-tipped end of the syringe to the Foley catheter and hold it above the level of the patient's bladder. Pour the contrast material into the syringe and allow it to fill the bladder by gravity instillation to one of three end points: (1) 100 mL with evidence of gross extravasation on fluoroscopy or on plain film (if the examiner elects to check at this point); (2) 400 mL in an adult or any child age 11 years or older. In children younger than 11 years, bladder capacity, and therefore appropriate contrast volumes, are estimated based on the formula "(age in years +2) × 30"; or (3) the point of initiating a bladder contraction (see later), then add an additional 50 mL by hand injection under pressure.

Obtain anteroposterior (AP) and complementary oblique projections so long as there is no evidence of a pelvic fracture. In the presence of a pelvic fracture, obtain all films with the patient in the supine position for the same reasons that were elucidated for retrograde urethrography. A lateral film may be informative when oblique films are not possible. Obtain an AP *postevacuation film in all cases after bladder drainage to disclose posterior perforation in select cases, especially those associated with penetrating trauma.* Again, a dilute solution of contrast material (see Table 55–7) may be used, rather than full-strength contrast. Some authors recommend a dilute solution of contrast material (≤10%) because extravasation into periurethral or perivesical tissues may cause considerable inflammatory reaction at higher concentrations. The dilute solutions do not appear to compromise the quality of the study, but this must be a consideration. Retrograde cystography done by any technique other than hand-poured gravity instillation is subject to inadequate bladder filling or connector tubing-catheter disconnection. Both conditions will result in spurious examination results, which may adversely affect important patient management decisions.

It must be stressed that in the absence of initial gross extravasation, the bladder must be filled to 400 mL in an adult, and to an appropriate capacity in a child, and the catheter clamped with a Kelly clamp. Volumes less than 400 mL have been associated with false-negative findings, especially in penetrating bladder injuries.[95] At times, the patient may have difficulty cooperating with bladder filling because of a head injury or associated pain; and in the case of severe injury, the patient may have involuntary bladder contractions, causing contrast material to back up into the Toomey syringe. If this occurs, refill the bladder to the point of initiating a bladder contraction, clamp the Foley, remove the initial syringe, and replace it with a 60-mL contrast-filled syringe, unclamp the catheter, hand-inject the additional 50 mL under pressure, and reclamp the catheter. The goal is to overdistend the bladder. Once the filled-bladder films have been obtained and reviewed, unclamp the Foley catheter and allow the contrast material to drain into a bedside drainage bag. Then obtain the AP postevacuation film to visualize any posterior extravasation that may have been hidden by the distended bladder during the AP filled-bladder film (Fig. 55–35). Once again, take care to ensure that contrast material is not spilled onto the patient or the examination table during the procedure. Spilled contrast can lead to spurious examination results.

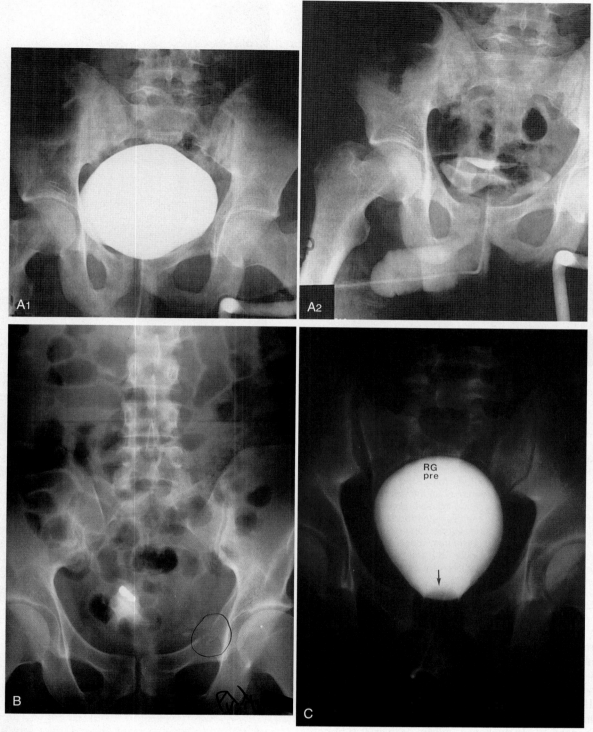

Figure 55–35   Retrograde cystogram. *A,* In patients with pelvic fractures, retrograde cystography should be done with the patient supine throughout the examination. This is a normal study. Note that a film must be taken after voiding/drainage to search for a posterior bladder injury. A lateral film may help define the extent of any extravasation. *B,* Note the subtle collection of contrast material on this postevacuation film, signifying a bladder tear from a gunshot wound (note the bullet and ramus fracture [circle]). This would be missed unless a postvoid film was taken and carefully examined. This bladder appears intact (Foley balloon seen by *arrows;* C) but the evacuation film demonstrates significant posterior extravasation.

Continued

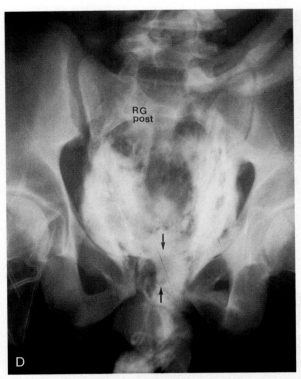

Figure 55–35, cont'd (D). A lateral film would have shown this while the bladder was still full of contrast material.

Figure 55–36 Pathology demonstrated by retrograde cystogram. *A,* Bladder rupture. A cystogram done in a patient after a motor vehicle accident shows extravasation of contrast (*arrows*) into the tissues surrounding the bladder, an extraperitoneal bladder rupture. With an intraperitoneal bladder rupture, contrast would be seen outlining loops of bowel. *B,* Cystogram of an intraperitoneal bladder rupture. Conventional cystogram shows injected contrast material outlining the paravesical space in the dependent portion of the pelvis, tracking up the right paracolic gutter (*arrows*) and surrounding bowel loops. *C,* Grade IV urethral injury. Cystogram shows extravasated contrast from the region of the bladder neck and proximal posterior urethra (*arrows*). There is vertical displacement of the left hemipelvis. The urogenital diaphragm is disrupted.

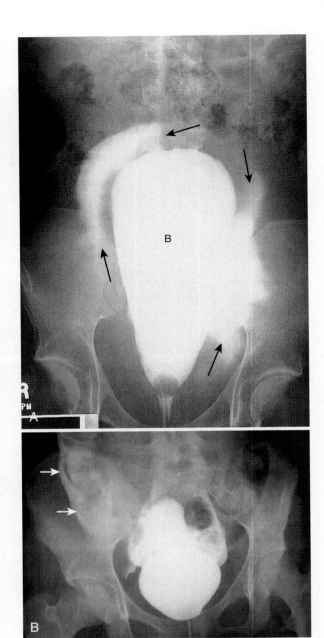

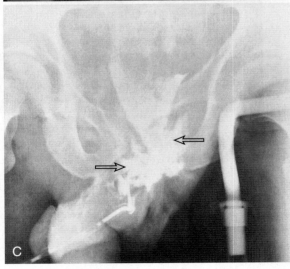

Extravasation from an injured bladder may be intraperitoneal, extraperitoneal, or both. Extraperitoneal extravasation is usually seen as flamelike areas of contrast material confined to the pelvis and projecting laterally to the bladder (Fig. 55–36). If the contrast material extravasates intraperitoneally, it tends to fill the paracolic gutters and outline intraperitoneal structures, particularly the bowel, spleen, or liver. It is important to distinguish extraperitoneal from intraperitoneal injury because the treatment options are totally different (i.e., surgical repair for all intraperitoneal injuries and for extraperitoneal injuries that extend into or primarily involve the bladder neck, especially in women). Most other extraperitoneal injuries can be managed confidently by Foley catheter drainage alone.

Retrograde cystography may be done in conjunction with contrast-enhanced abdominal CT scanning (Fig. 55–37). The bladder must be filled just as if a conventional retrograde cystogram were being obtained. Clamp the catheter, and seek evidence for contrast ascites on the CT scan. When this is

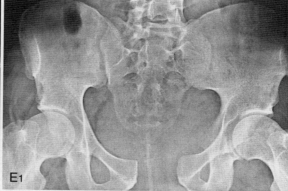

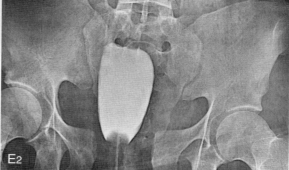

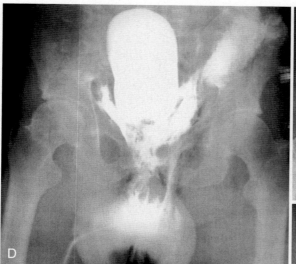

Figure 55–36, cont'd *D,* Plain film cystogram reveals extraperitoneal bladder rupture with extravasation into the scrotum. Surgical exploration revealed anterior bladder neck and prostatic urethral laceration. *E,* (*1*) "Open-book" injury with pubic symphysis diastasis and sacroiliac joint widening. The increase in soft tissue density in the pelvis is compatible with hematoma. (*2*) Cystogram demonstrates a pear-shaped bladder secondary to pelvic hematoma.

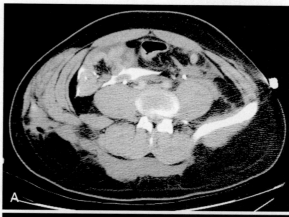

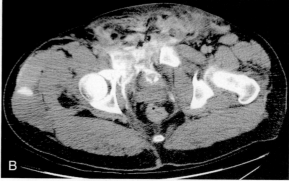

Figure 55–37 **Retrograde cystogram and abdominal computed tomography (CT) scan.** These two procedures can be done concomitantly. *A,* Intraperitoneal rupture shows contrast material extravasated from the bladder outlining loops of bowel in the lower abdomen. *B,* Extraperitoneal rupture shows contrast material extravasating into the disrupted soft tissue plains of the anterior and left pelvic side wall. Fill the bladder in the standard retrograde fashion and clamp the catheter. Intravenous and oral contrast can then be administered and CT scanning performed. This film demonstrates contrast ascites, which is consistent with intraperitoneal bladder rupture and extravasation. (*A and* B, *Courtesy of Charlotte Radiology, Emergency Radiology Section, Charlotte, NC.*)

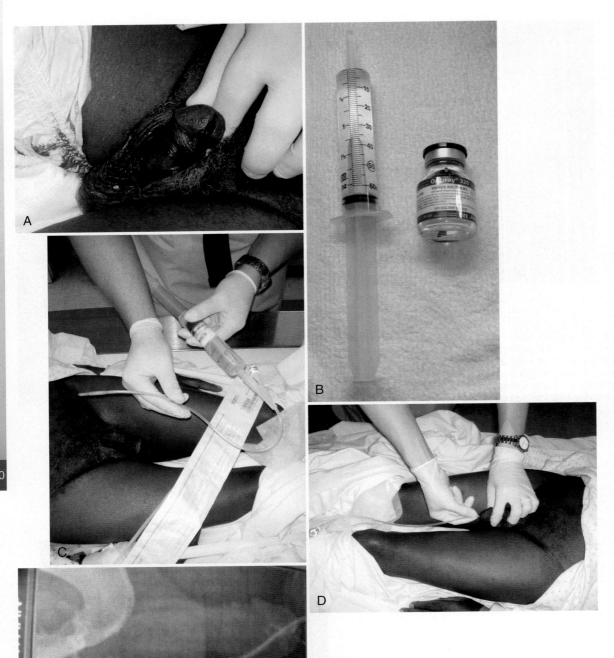

Figure 55–38 *A,* This patient pulled out his Foley catheter with the balloon inflated. Blood appeared at the meatus. His mental status prevented assessment of his ability to void spontaneously. *B,* Given the large volume of the inflated balloon and gross blood, it was decided to perform a retrograde urethrogram, although some would simply try to gently pass a new catheter. Place a balloon-tipped catheter into the meatus (*C*) and squeeze the gland while an assistant slowly injects contrast material (*D*). *E,* Overzealous injection resulted in venous uptake of the dye and spillage on the patient's leg. The urethra is intact. A new catheter was easily passed.

encountered, bladder injury with extravasation must be looked for with selective images of the pelvis.

Contrast Medium Reactions and Toxic Effects

In the lower genitourinary tract radiologic procedures described in this section, administer the contrast material within the urinary collecting and drainage system. Hence, the patient is at low risk for systemic absorption and allergic reaction. Even with intravenous infusion, contrast medium reactions are rare; the incidence of significant reactions (i.e., of sufficient severity to require medical intervention) with intravenous administration is between 1 in 1000 and 1 in 10,000 uses.

The ED use of contrast agents is often necessary and justified despite the small possibility of untoward reactions. At times, the patient's past history may not be known, underlying renal function cannot be rapidly assessed, or alternative imaging techniques (e.g., ultrasonography) are unavailable. In such circumstances, carefully weigh the risks versus the benefits of emergent imaging using intravenous contrast. Often the potential information gain from contrast-enhanced imaging in the unstable patient far outweighs the small associated additional risk.

Traumatic Foley Catheter Removal

Occasionally, uncooperative or demented patients will pull out their Foley catheter with the balloon still inflated (Fig. 55–38). One would intuit that urethral injury is possible; however, there are no prospective data on the incidence or type of injury from this maneuver or how to deal with this situation. Usually, there is blood at the meatus, and it may de

difficult to know whether the patient can spontaneously urinate. If the patient can spontaneously urinate, it would seem reasonable to gently pass another Foley catheter to avoid urethral obstruction by tears or clots and allow healing of urethral trauma with a new catheter in place. Most of the time, however, the clinician has minimal data yet is faced with the decision on how to approach this conundrum. Surprisingly, this incident does not usually result in massive urethral injury. It is assumed that a new catheter will be required, either to continue the original catheter indication or to provide a stent while any urethral injury heals. In the absence of available urologic consultation, gentle attempts to pass another Foley catheter are reasonable, without a routine RUG. If the catheter does not pass easily, stop and perform an RUG to assess the extent of the pathology. Most of the time, simply replacing the catheter will be the most prudent approach. Prophylactic antibiotics are reasonable under these circumstances. Complete eversion and prolapse of the bladder have been rarely associated with this misadventure.[96]

Acknowledgments

The authors and editors acknowledge the contributions made to previous editions by Ivan Zbaraschuk, MD, Richard E. Berger, MD, Jerris R. Hedges, MD, Martin Schiff, Jr., MD, Morton G. Glickman, MD, and Geoffrey E. Herter, MD.

 REFERENCES CAN BE FOUND ON EXPERT CONSULT

CHAPTER 56

Emergency Childbirth

Beatrice D. Probst

The emergent delivery of an infant is one of the most challenging procedures facing emergency clinicians. The actual number of infants born or delivered emergently in the ambulance bay or emergency department (ED) is unknown. Of the over 4.1 million births in 2003, 4.05 million were delivered in the hospital, which included those en route to or on arrival at the hospital.[1] Few situations create more stress for the emergency health care team than ensuring the safe delivery of a healthy infant. One must quickly assess both mother and fetus, prepare for a normal delivery, and anticipate potential difficulties or complications.

Some of the procedures discussed in this chapter may be out of the area of expertise of emergency clinicians, but they are included to aid the clinician should such emergency interventions be required. The degree to which the emergency clinician interacts in the process of labor and delivery varies among institutions, depending on the availability of on-site obstetric services. The duties of the emergency physician may be only to determine that labor is active and delivery imminent or, alternatively, be responsible to manage a complicated delivery and neonatal resuscitation. The emergency clinician should be familiar with the stages and timing of labor, assist the mother in delivery of the infant and placenta, as well as provide initial stabilization of the newborn.

LABOR

Labor is the coordinated sequence of involuntary uterine contractions that result in progressive effacement and dilatation of the cervix. Labor is normally divided into three stages. The first stage begins when uterine contractions are of sufficient force to cause cervical effacement and dilatation and ends when the cervix is completed dilated. In parous women, this stage of labor is about 4 hours compared with 7 hours in nulliparous women, but with much individual variation in these times.[2] The second stage of labor begins when dilatation of the cervix is complete and ends with delivery of the infant. The duration of this stage is also variable, with a median of 50 minutes in nulliparas and 20 minutes in multiparas.[2] The third stage of labor begins after delivery of the infant and ends after delivery of the placenta. Infrequently, a fourth stage of labor is described as the hour immediately after delivery, the period in which postpartum hemorrhage is most likely to occur.[2]

IDENTIFICATION OF LABOR

Contractions late in pregnancy of parous women are not uncommon, although not all are true or effective labor contractions. Irregular, brief *Braxton-Hicks* contractions of the uterus, usually with discomfort confined to the lower abdomen and groin, are typically irregular in timing and strength. These pains do not change the contour of the cervix nor result in descent of the fetus. Although these pains usually stop spontaneously, they may convert rapidly to effective contractions of true labor. Therefore, a period of observation may be necessary.

True labor is characterized by a regular sequence of uterine contractions, with progressively increasing intensity and decreasing intervals between contractions. The interval between contractions gradually diminishes from 10 minutes at the onset of labor to as short as 1 minute or less in the second stage of labor. True labor begins in the fundal region of the uterus and radiates into the lower back. It is accompanied by effacement and dilatation of the cervix, with descent of the presenting part of the uterus.

Show or *bloody show* is a rather dependable sign of the approach of labor. Show consists of a small amount of blood-tinged mucus discharged from the vagina, indicating that labor is already in progress or will likely occur during the next several hours to a few days. Extrusion of the mucus plug that filled the cervical canal during pregnancy is evidence of cervical effacement and dilatation. If more than a few drops of blood escape with the mucus plug, an abnormal cause such as abruption of the placenta or placenta previa should be suspected. Vaginal examination under these circumstances is generally contraindicated.[2]

Spontaneous rupture of membranes usually occurs during the course of active labor, typically evident by a sudden gush of a variable amount of clear or slightly turbid fluid. Rupture of membranes before the onset of labor, at any stage of gestation, is referred to as *premature rupture of membranes* (PROM). Term PROM, occurring before the onset of labor, complicates approximately 8% of pregnancies.[3] In the majority of cases, it is followed by the onset of labor and delivery within 5 hours.[3] The most significant maternal risk of term PROM is intrauterine infection. Fetal risks associated with PROM include umbilical cord compression and ascending infection.[3]

Membrane rupture occurring before 37 weeks of gestation is called *preterm premature rupture of membranes* (pPROM). In 75% of patients, delivery occurs regardless of the management or clinical presentation.[3] The most significant maternal risk of pPROM is intrauterine infection. The most significant risks to the fetus are complications related to prematurity.[3]

Whereas membrane rupture during labor typically manifests by a sudden gush of fluid, presentation of PROM may be more subtle. Because accurate diagnosis is crucial to management, suspected PROM should be confirmed by examination that minimizes the risk of introducing infection. Avoid digital cervical examinations unless prompt labor and delivery is anticipated. A sterile speculum examination can be performed, looking for amniotic fluid extruding from the cervical os or pooling in the posterior fornix.[2,3]

Differentiation of amniotic fluid from vaginal fluid may be made by testing the pH of the fluid with nitrazine paper or similar swab devices (Fig. 56–1). Amniotic fluid has a pH of 7.0 to 7.5 and turns the paper blue-green to deep blue. In the presence of vaginal secretions, with a pH of 4.5 to 5.5, nitrazine paper remains yellow.[2,3] In cases of questionable rupture in which the amniotic fluid is small and more subject to pH changes from admixed blood and vaginal secretions, the result is less reliable. False-positive results may occur with blood, semen, or bacterial vaginosis.

If rupture of the membranes is documented in the ED, notify the patient's obstetrician and consider hospital admission.

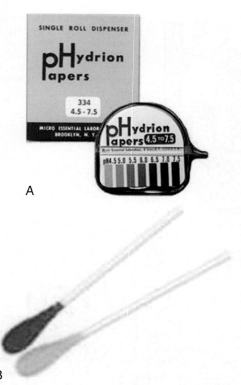

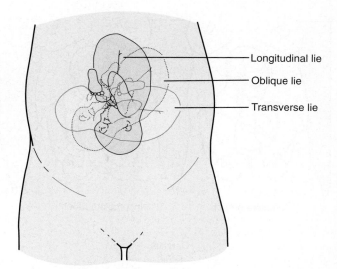

Longitudinal lie
Oblique lie
Transverse lie

Figure 56–2 Examples of different fetal lie. *(From Gabbe SG: Obstetrics: Normal and Problem Pregnancies. Philadelphia, Elsevier Churchill Livingstone, 2007.)*

Figure 56–1 Amniotic fluid has an alkaline pH, whereas normal vaginal secretions are acidic. Both nitrazine or pH paper (*A*) or a indicator swab (*B*) (Amnicator device/Amnicator.com) will turn yellow in the absence of amniotic fluid and *dark blue in a few seconds in contact with amniotic fluid.*

EVALUATION OF LABOR

When a woman presents in labor, quickly ascertain the general condition of the fetus and mother by means of the patient history and physical examination. Inquire as to the onset and frequency of contractions, the presence or absence of bleeding, the possible loss of amniotic fluid, and the prenatal care and condition of the mother and fetus. In the absence of active vaginal bleeding, determine the position, presentation, and lie of the fetus by abdominal palpation and sterile vaginal examination. Assess the staging of labor by vaginal examination. Monitor fetal well-being by auscultation of fetal heart tones, particularly immediately after a uterine contraction.

Lie refers to the relation of the long axis of the fetus to that of the mother. Lie is longitudinal, oblique, or transverse (Fig. 56–2). Longitudinal lies occur in greater than 99% of pregnancies at term.[2]

The *presentation*, or presenting part, refers to that portion of the body of the fetus nearest to or foremost in the birth canal. Feel the presenting part through the cervix on sterile vaginal examination. In longitudinal lies, the presenting part is the fetal head, the buttocks, or the feet. In *transverse lie*, the presenting part is the shoulder.

Cephalic presentations are classified by the relation of the fetal head to the body of the fetus Ordinarily, the head is sharply flexed so that the occipital fontanel is the presenting part. This is referred to as the *vertex* or *occiput presentation*. Less commonly, the neck is fully extended and the face is foremost in the birth canal; this is termed *face presentation*. Occasionally, the fetal head assumes a partially flexed or partially extended position, resulting in *sinciput* and *brow presentations*, respectively. Sinciput and brow presentations, asso-

ciated with preterm infants, are almost always unstable and convert to either the occiput or the face presentation as labor progresses.

Breech presentations are classified as frank, complete, or incomplete (Fig. 56–3). When the fetus presents with the hips flexed and the legs extended over the anterior surfaces of the body, this is termed *frank breech*. Flexion of the fetal hips and knees results in *complete breech* presentation. When one or both of the feet or knees are lowermost in the canal, an *incomplete breech* results.

At or near term, the incidence of the various presentations is approximately 97% for vertex and 3.5% for breech.[2]

Position refers to the relation of the presenting part to the birth canal and may be either left or right. The occiput, chin, and sacrum are the determining parts in vertex, face, and breech presentations, respectively. The presentation and position of the fetus are best determined by ultrasound examination.

Vaginal Examination

Unless there has been bleeding in excess of a bloody show, perform a vaginal examination (not speculum) to identify the fetal presentation and position and assess the progress of labor. Cleanse the perineum with an antiseptic and use a sterile lubricant to decrease potential contamination. Introduce the gloved index and middle fingers into the vagina while avoiding the anal region. Do not withdraw the fingers from the vagina until the examination is complete. Assess cervical effacement and dilatation as well as fetal station. Confirm fetal presentation and position.[2] The number of vaginal examinations during labor correlates with infectious morbidity, especially in cases of early membrane rupture.[2]

Cervical effacement refers to the process of cervical thinning that occurs before and during the first stage of labor as the cervical canal shortens from a length of about 2 cm to a circular opening with almost paper-thin edges (Fig. 56–4). Assess the degree of cervical effacement by palpation and determine the palpated length of the cervical canal compared with that of the uneffaced, or normal, cervical canal. Express effacement as a percentage from 0%, or totally uneffaced, to 100%, or completely effaced.

1043

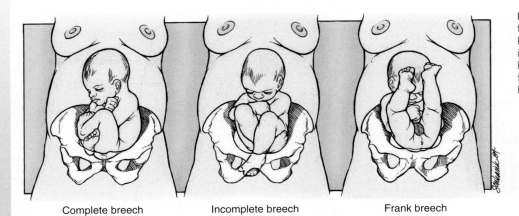

Figure 56–3 The complete breech is flexed at the hips and flexed at the knees. The incomplete breech shows incomplete deflexion of one or both knees or hips. The frank breech is flexed at the hips and extended at the knees.

Complete breech   Incomplete breech   Frank breech

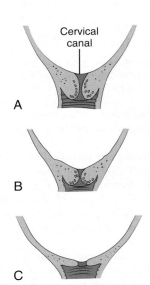

Figure 56–4 Effacement of the cervix. *A,* None. *B,* Partial. *C,* Complete. *(A–C, From Romney S, Gray MK, Little AB, et al [eds]: Gynecology and Obstetrics: The Health Care of Women. New York, McGraw-Hill, 1975.)*

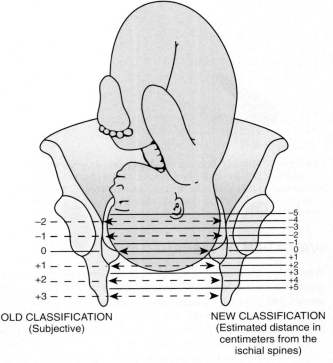

OLD CLASSIFICATION (Subjective)   NEW CLASSIFICATION (Estimated distance in centimeters from the ischial spines)

Figure 56–5 The relationship of the leading edge of the presenting part of the fetus to the plane of the maternal ischial spines determines the station. Old and new classification are included. *(From Gabbe SG: Obstetrics: Normal and Problem Pregnancies. Philadelphia, Elsevier Churchill Livingstone, 2007.)*

Determine *cervical dilatation* by estimating the average diameter of the cervical os. Sweep the examining finger from the cervical margin on one side across the cervical os to the opposite margin. Express the transverse diameter in centimeters. Ten centimeters constitutes full cervical dilatation. A diameter of less than 6 cm can be measured directly. For a diameter greater than 6 cm, it is frequently easier to determine the width of the remaining cervical rim and subtract twice that measurement from 10 cm. For example, if a 1-cm rim is felt, dilatation is 8 cm.

Station refers to the level of the presenting fetal part in the birth canal relative to the ischial spines, which lie halfway between the pelvic inlet and the pelvic outlet (Fig. 56–5). Zero station is used to denote that the presenting part is at the level of the ischial spines. The new classification (−5 to +5) is an attempt to quantitate in centimeters the distance of the leading bony edge from the ischial spines. When the presenting part lies above the spines, the distances are stated in negative figures (−5, −4, −3, −2, −1). Below the ischial spines, the presenting fetal part passes +1, +2, +3, +4, and +5 stations to delivery. Make this determination by simple palpation.[2] Three maneuvers are used to determine fetal presentation and position. In the first maneuver, introduce two fingers into the vagina and advance them to the presenting part, differentiat-

ing face, vertex, and breech presentations. In vertex presentations, move your fingers up behind the symphysis pubis and then sweep posteriorly over the fetal head toward the maternal sacrum, identifying the course of the sagittal suture. Define the positions of the two fontanels, located at opposite ends of the sagittal sutures, by palpation. The anterior fontanel is diamond shaped; the posterior fontanel is triangular.

In face and breech presentations, the various parts are more readily distinguished. In breech presentations, the fetal sacrum is the point of reference; in face presentations, the easily identifiable fetal chin is used.

FETAL WELL-BEING

Auscultation

Make the initial determination of fetal well-being by assessing fetal heart rate with a stethoscope, a fetoscope, or preferably, a Doppler ultrasound device placed firmly on the maternal abdominal wall overlying the fetal thorax and repositioned until fetal heart tones are heard. When a Doppler device is used, apply a conducting gel to the abdominal wall, interfacing with the Doppler receiver. To avoid confusion of maternal and fetal heart sounds, palpate the maternal pulse as the fetal heart rate is auscultated.

The normal baseline fetal heart rate is 120 to 160 beats/min, varying considerably from beat to beat.[2,4] Rates above or below this range may indicate fetal distress. Brief accelerations in fetal heart rate, that is, those lasting less than 20 seconds, occur commonly during labor and are probably a physiologic response to fetal movement.[2,4,5] Persistent fetal tachycardia occurs most commonly in response to maternal fever or amnionitis but may also indicate fetal compromise.[2,4]

As with brief accelerations in fetal heart rate, decreases in rate that reach their nadir with the peak of a contraction and end with or slightly after the end of a contraction (early decelerations) are physiologic and probably the result of vagal nerve stimulation due to compression of the fetal head. Decelerations that occur independently of uterine contractions (variable decelerations) and those that persist significantly after a contraction (late decelerations) are ominous and may represent cord compression and uteroplacental insufficiency, respectively.[2,4,5]

Changes in the fetal heart rate indicating fetal distress are usually evident immediately after a uterine contraction, and therefore, fetal heart rate is optimally assessed at this time. If prolonged monitoring of labor is necessary in the ED, fetal heart sounds should be assessed at 15-minute intervals during the first stage of labor and at 5-minute intervals during the second stage in the pregnancies at risk. In the absence of risk factors, intervals of 30 minutes and 15 minutes, respectively, are probably sufficient.[2,4] If trained personnel and equipment are available, external tocography provides a noninvasive method for continuous assessment of fetal heart rate and maternal uterine contractions.

Management of Fetal Distress

Perform the definitive evaluation of fetal distress in the obstetric unit by the delivery team. There is no role nor standards for sophisticated fetal monitoring in the ED. In the absence of a dedicated obstetric unit, transfer to another hospital is the only option, albeit a less than ideal circumstance. The emergency clinician working in an ED without adequate obstetric backup can do little to effect a positive outcome in high-risk situations. Eclampsia, bleeding, and abnormal fetal presentation may be identified, but the emergency clinician needs to focus attention on maternal well-being while expediting transfer and/or referral. Some emergency interventions, however, can be undertaken, as described later.

If fetal distress is suspected on the basis of resting fetal heart rate or changes after contractions, change the maternal position, typically into the *left lateral decubitus position*, and reevaluate. Administer *supplemental oxygen* to the mother in order to optimize fetal oxygenation. In the absence of bleeding, perform a vaginal examination to rule out the possibility of umbilical cord prolapse.[4,6] *Cord prolapse* usually occurs at the same time as rupture of the membranes and is diagnosed by palpation of the umbilical cord on vaginal examination or by visualization of the cord protruding through the introitus.

Cord prolapse is frequently encountered with breech presentation, multiple pregnancies, and prematurity.[7–9]

The management of cord prolapse is directed at sustaining fetal life until delivery is accomplished. Unless immediate delivery is feasible or the fetus is known to be dead, prepare for an emergency cesarean section. If immediate obstetric services are not available, administer tocolytic therapy to decrease uterine contractions and improve fetoplacental perfusion.[10,11] Minimize compression of the umbilical cord by exerting manual pressure through the vagina *to lift and maintain the presenting part away from the prolapsed cord*. Place the patient in the knee-chest or deep Trendelenburg position, and maintain this position until delivery is accomplished.[6,9,11] After manual elevation of the presenting part, some clinicians recommend instilling 500 to 700 mL of saline into the bladder to maintain cord decompression. Once the bladder is filled, the vaginal hand may be removed.[10,11] Unfortunately, and realistically speaking, outcomes of true obstetric emergencies are often bleak and essentially out of the hands of the emergency clinician.

Tocolytic Therapy

Before instituting pharmacologic tocolytic therapy for either preterm labor or fetal distress, initiate basic maneuvers to improve uterine and fetal status. Because uterine hypoxia may induce uterine contractions, administer supplemental oxygen, intravenously infuse 500 mL of crystalloid, and place the mother in the left lateral decubitus position to improve uterine perfusion.[2,6,12] Because uterine, cervical, or urinary tract infections account for 20% to 40% of cases of preterm labor, search for a specific cause and treat infections appropriately.[6,13,14] If contractions persist and cervical changes are documented despite these basic interventions, consider pharmacologic therapy.[2,6,12] Although tocolytic agents are commonly used and have been shown to prolong pregnancy by several days, there are little data to suggest that tocolysis improves long-term perinatal or neonatal outcome.[2,12,15,16] The principal benefit of pharmacologic therapy may be only to prolong pregnancy to allow maternal transfer to a tertiary care facility or to delay delivery sufficiently to improve fetal maturation with corticosteroids.[2,12–14,17] General contraindications to tocolytic therapy include severe preeclampsia, placental abruption, intrauterine infection, advanced cervical dilatation, and evidence of fetal compromise or placental insufficiency.[18]

There are no clear "first-line" tocolytic agents to manage preterm labor (Table 56–1). Clinical circumstances and preferences should dictate treatment. The most commonly used tocolytic agents in the United States are magnesium sulfate and the β_2-receptor agonists ritodrine and terbutaline. Other agents such as calcium channel blockers, the prostaglandin inhibitor indomethacin, and most recently, the oxytocin receptor antagonist atosiban have shown varying efficacy in clinical trials.[2,12,13,15–17]

β_2-Receptor Agonists

The traditional mainstays of pharmacologic tocolytic agents are the selective β_2-adrenergic agents ritodrine and terbutaline. The β-mimetic agents prevent contraction of the myometrium through activation of the enzyme adenyl cyclase. Adenyl cyclase enhances the conversion of adenosine triphosphate to cyclic adenosine monophosphate that in turn initiates

TABLE 56–1 Drugs for the Emergency Management of Preterm Labor

β₂-Receptor Agonists

Ritodrine

Dose	50–100 μg/min IV infusion ↑ 50 μg/min q 10–20 min
End point	Cessation of uterine contractions
	Intolerable maternal side effects
	Maximum dose, 350 μg/min

Terbutaline

Dose	0.25 mg SC
End point	May repeat q 20–60 min
	Cessation of uterine contractions
	Intolerable maternal side effects

Magnesium Sulfate

Dose	4–6 g IV over 20 min → 2–4 g/hr IV infusion
End point	Cessation of uterine contractions
	Signs of magnesium toxicity (e.g., respiratory depression, hypotension, somnolence)

Nifedipine*

Dose	10 mg PO
End point	May repeat q 15–20 min
	Cessation of uterine contractions
	Harmful maternal side effects, e.g., hypotension
	Maximum dose, 40 mg

*Variable doses have been used. Data on effects, particularly uteroplacental blood flow, are limited.
IV, intravenously; PO, by mouth; SC, subcutaneously. Sublinqual dose may cause excessive hypotension. It is best to avoid SL route.

a number of reactions that reduce the intracellular concentration of ionized calcium, thereby preventing activation of contractile proteins.[2] Although both ritodrine and terbutaline stimulate β₂-receptors primarily, both have some β₁-activity, which is responsible for their cardiovascular side effects.

Ritodrine is the only agent approved for tocolysis in the United States. Prepare an intravenous infusion by mixing 150 mg ritodrine in 500 mL fluid, preferably with 5% dextrose solution, yielding a final concentration of 0.3 mg/mL (i.e., 300 μg/mL). Begin initially at an infusion rate of 50 μg/min (i.e., 10 mL/hr) and increase it by 50 μg/min (i.e., by 10 mL/hr) every 10 to 20 minutes until uterine contractions cease, intolerable maternal side effects develop, or a maximum dose of 350 μg/min (i.e., 70 mL/hr) is reached.[13,19,20] Ritodrine is contraindicated in patients with cardiac disease, pulmonary hypertension, hyperthyroidism, and uncontrolled diabetes. It should be used cautiously in patients on other sympathomimetic amines.[20]

The usual clinical side effects of ritodrine are related to its inherent activity as a β-mimetic drug. Whereas side effects are usually self-limited and resolve with dosage reduction or discontinuation of the drug, infusions have resulted in serious and sometimes fatal side effects including arrhythmias, myocardial ischemia, and pulmonary edema.[2] Treatment of the majority of side effects is supportive; severe cardiovascular effects may be treated with β-blocking agents.[19,20]

Although not approved for use by the U.S. Food and Drug Administration as a tocolytic agent, terbutaline is commonly used in the treatment of preterm labor.[2,13,21] When given subcutaneously, administer terbutaline as a 0.25-mg dose, and repeat every 20 to 60 minutes until contractions cease or intolerable maternal side effects occur.[6,18,19,22] Use terbutaline with caution in patients with cardiovascular disease, hypertension, hyperthyroidism, diabetes, and seizures and those taking other sympathomimetic amines.[20] Side effects associated with the parenteral use of terbutaline are similar to those of ritodrine.[18–20]

Magnesium Sulfate

Magnesium sulfate ($MgSO_4$) is not approved in the United States for use as a tocolytic agent. Nevertheless, some perinatal centers prefer $MgSO_4$ over the β-mimetic agents because of its lower incidence of side effects.[6,23,24] Although its mechanism of action is not fully understood, magnesium probably decreases myometrial contractility through its role as a calcium antagonist.[2]

When used as a tocolytic agent, administer 4 to 6 g of $MgSO_4$ intravenously over 20 to 30 minutes, followed by a maintenance intravenous infusion beginning at 2 to 4 g/hr.[6,19,24] Infusion of $MgSO_4$ typically produces sweating, warmth, and flushing. Rapid parenteral administration may cause transient nausea, vomiting, headache, or palpitations.[13,24] The major side effect of magnesium therapy is related to impairment of the muscles of respiration with subsequent respiratory arrest, an effect usually not seen until the serum magnesium level exceeds 10 mEq/L. At levels of 12 mEq/L or greater, respiratory arrest may occur.[20]

The first sign of magnesium toxicity, decrease of the patellar reflex, typically occurs as serum magnesium levels exceed 4 mEq/L, with loss of the reflex as levels approach 10 mEq/L. Monitor the patellar reflex throughout therapy. Because magnesium is almost totally excreted by the kidney, it is contraindicated in the presence of renal failure. Monitor urinary output and renal function throughout therapy. If respiratory depression develops, inject 10 mL of a 10% solution of calcium gluconate or calcium chloride over 3 minutes as an effective antidote. For severe respiratory depression and arrest, prompt endotracheal intubation may be life saving.[2]

Calcium Channel Blockers

Calcium antagonists inhibit the influx of calcium ions through the muscle cell membrane and reduce uterine vascular resistance. The decreased intracellular calcium also results in decreased myometrial activity. Although dosing regimes vary, nifedipine is frequently given as an initial loading dose of 30 mg orally, then 10 to 20 mg every 4 to 6 hours.[19] When oral nicardipine (Cardene) was compared with magnesium sulfate, it required less time to achieve tocolysis, 3.3 versus 5.3 hours, respectively; less recurrence of preterm labor was noted with nicardipine.[25] The calcium channel blocker–induced decreased vascular resistance can lead to maternal hypotension and thus decreased uteroplacental perfusion.

Prostaglandin Inhibitors

A number of prostaglandin synthesis inhibitors have been evaluated for their efficacy as tocolytic agents. Prostaglandin synthetase inhibitors inhibit cyclooxygenae that decrease prostaglandin synthetase and block conversion of free arachidonic acid to prostaglandin. Because prostaglandin E and F series are mediators of uterine contractions, a decrease in production results in decreased contractile activity.[19] Indomethacin is administered as an initial oral or rectal dose of 50 to 100 mg followed by a total 24-hour dose of not greater than 200 mg.[2]

VAGINAL BLEEDING DURING THE THIRD TRIMESTER

Bleeding during the third trimester should always be considered an emergency because shock may occur within minutes. Prepare for the most typical causes of bleeding in late gestation, placenta previa and placental abruption. *Placenta previa* refers to implantation of the placenta in the lower uterine segment with varying degrees of encroachment on the cervical os. Placenta previa is classically characterized by vaginal bleeding with little or no abdominal or pelvic pain. Premature separation of the placenta, or *abruptio placentae*, refers to separation of the placenta from its site of implantation in the uterus before delivery of the fetus. Although the clinical signs and symptoms with placental abruption can vary considerably, abruptio placentae is typically associated with varying degrees of abdominal pain and uterine irritability.[2]

Stabilization of a patient with third trimester bleeding should be initiated with large-bore intravenous access. Blood should be drawn for a complete blood count with platelets and a type and cross-match. If abruption is suspected, clotting studies including a fibrinogen level and a toxicology screen for cocaine may be indicated owing to the association of abruption with disseminated intravascular coagulation and cocaine abuse, respectively. Until the diagnosis of placenta previa is excluded, digital vaginal examination is *contraindicated* because of the possibility of tearing or dislodging a placenta previa, which may result in profuse, potentially fatal hemorrhage.[2] The simplest and most precise method of placental localization is by transabdominal ultrasound, which has an accuracy of locating a placenta previa of about 96%. In contrast, ultrasonography has limited sensitivity in detecting abruptio placenta, with a reported negative predictive value of between 63% and 88%.[2] Therefore, negative findings on ultrasound should not be used to exclude placental abruption. Immediately transfer the patient to the care of her obstetrician for further evaluation.

LABOR MOVEMENTS: VERTEX

Full dilatation of the cervix signifies the second stage of labor, heralding delivery of the infant. Typically, the patient begins to bear down with descent of the presenting part. Uterine contractions may last 1.5 minutes and recur after a resting phase of less than 1 minute.

The mechanism of labor in vertex and breech presentations consists of engagement of the presenting part, flexion, descent, internal rotation, extension, external rotation or restitution, and expulsion (Fig. 56–6). The mechanism of labor is determined by the pelvic dimensions and configuration, the size of the fetus, and the strength of uterine contractions. Essentially, the fetus will follow the path of least resistance by adaptation of the smallest achievable diameters of the presenting part to the most favorable dimensions and contours of the birth canal.

The sequence of movements in vertex presentations is:

1. *Engagement* refers to the mechanism by which the greatest transverse diameter of the head, the biparietal diameter in occiput presentations, passes through the pelvic inlet. In the primiparous patient, it usually occurs in the last 2 weeks of pregnancy; in the multiparous patient, it occurs at the onset of labor.
2. *Flexion* of the head is necessary to minimize the presenting cross-sectional diameter of the head during passage through the smallest diameter of the bony pelvis. In most cases, flexion is necessary for both engagement and descent.
3. *Descent* is gradually progressive and is affected by uterine and abdominal contractions as well as by straightening and extension of the fetal body.
4. *Internal rotation* occurs with descent and is necessary for the head or presenting part to traverse the ischial spines. This movement essentially turns the head such that the occiput gradually moves from its original, more transverse position, anteriorly toward the symphysis pubis or, less commonly, posteriorly toward the hollow of the sacrum.
5. *Extension* occurs as the flexed head reaches the anteriorly directed vulvar outlet. With increasing distention of the perineum and vaginal opening, an increasingly larger portion of the occiput appears gradually. The head is born by further extensions as the occiput, bregma, forehead, nose, mouth, and finally, chin pass successively over the anterior margin of the perineum. Immediately after its birth, the head drops downward such that the chin lies over the maternal anal region.
6. *External rotation* or restitution follows delivery of the head as it rotates to the transverse position that it occupied at engagement. After this movement, the shoulders descend in a path similar to that traced by the head, rotating anteroposteriorly for delivery. First, the anterior shoulder is delivered beneath the symphysis pubis followed by the posterior shoulder across the perineum.
7. *Expulsion* of the remainder of the fetal body occurs with ease. Delivery of the vertex-presenting infant usually occurs spontaneously. The role of the clinician or attendant is principally to provide control of the birth process, preventing forceful, sudden expulsion or extraction of the infant with resultant fetal and maternal injury.

LABOR MOVEMENTS: BREECH

The mechanism of labor for breech presentations varies. Usually, the hips engage in one of the oblique diameters of the pelvic inlet. As descent occurs, the anterior hip generally descends more rapidly than the posterior hip. Internal rotation occurs as the bitrochanteric diameter assumes the anteroposterior (AP) position. Lateral flexion occurs as the anterior hip catches beneath the symphysis pubis, allowing the posterior hip to be born first. The infant's body then rotates, allowing engagement of the shoulders in an oblique orientation. Gradual descent occurs, with the anterior shoulder rotating to bring the shoulders into the AP diameter of the outlet. The anterior shoulder follows lateral flexion to appear beneath the symphysis, with the posterior shoulder delivered first as the body is supported. The head tends to engage in the same diameter as the shoulders. Subsequent flexion, descent, and rotation of the head occur to bring the posterior portion of the neck under the symphysis pubis. The head is then born in flexion.

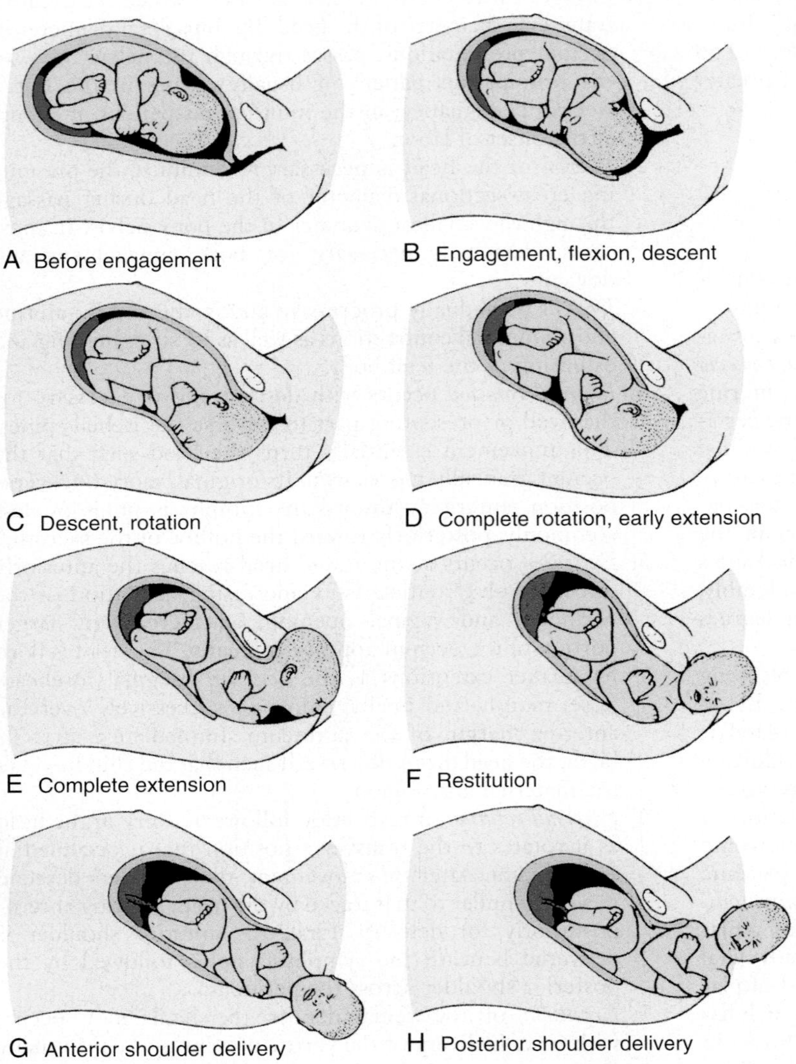

A Before engagement

B Engagement, flexion, descent

C Descent, rotation

D Complete rotation, early extension

E Complete extension

F Restitution

G Anterior shoulder delivery

H Posterior shoulder delivery

Figure 56–6 Cardinal movements of labor. (From Gabbe SG, Niebyl JR, Simpson JL [eds]: Obstetrics: Normal and Problem Pregnancies, 5th ed. Philadelphia, Elsevier Churchill Livingstone, 2007.)

Technique for Uncomplicated Delivery

Although complete sterility is not a priority, when time permits, use sterile technique. Equipment in the obstetric pack should be sterile. Wear sterile gloves, a gown, mask, and eye protection for protection of both the mother and the health care providers. Clean the perineum and vulva as for a vaginal examination and drape with sterile towels so that only the immediate area about the vulva is exposed. Be careful to avoid fecal contamination of the infant.

Ideally, place the patient on a delivery table in the dorsal lithotomy position to increase the diameter of the pelvic outlet. Alternatively, position the patient on a stretcher with her hips and knees partially flexed, her thighs abducted, and the soles of her feet placed firmly on the stretcher. If the foot of the bed cannot be removed, enhance the delivery position by placing the underside of a bedpan under the patient's buttocks, which will provide additional space between the bed and the perineum.

SPONTANEOUS VERTEX DELIVERY

Spontaneous delivery of the vertex-presenting infant is divided into three phases: delivery of the head, delivery of the shoulders, and delivery of the body and legs.

Delivery of the Head

Anticipate delivery when the presenting part reaches the pelvic floor. With each contraction, the perineum bulges increasingly and the vulvovaginal opening becomes more and more dilated by the fetal head. Just before delivery, *crowning* occurs, which is when the head is visible at the vaginal introitus and the widest portion, or the biparietal diameter of the head, distends the vulva.

Gentle, gradual, controlled delivery is desirable. Avoid explosive delivery of the head. Once the fetal head distends the vaginal introitus to 5 cm or more during a contraction, place the palm of one hand over the occipital area and provide

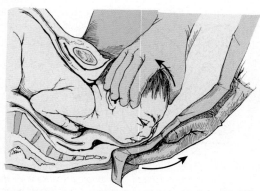

Figure 56–7 For a controlled and gentle delivery of the head, use the modified Ritgen maneuver. *(From Seils A, et al [eds]: Williams Obstetrics, 22nd ed. New York, McGraw-Hill Medical Publishing Division, 2005.)*

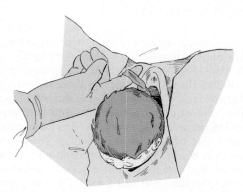

Figure 56–8 Check for the cord around the infant's neck.

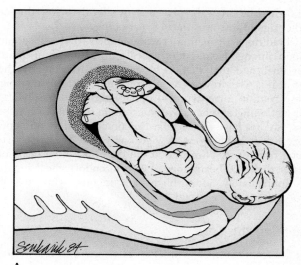

A

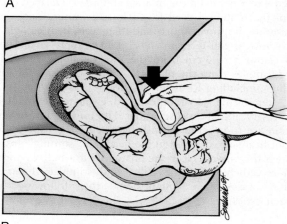

B

Figure 56–9 *A,* When delivery of the fetal head is not followed by delivery of the shoulders, the anterior shoulder has often become caught behind the symphysis. The head may retract toward the perineum. *Desperate traction on the fetal head is not likely to facilitate delivery and might lead to trauma.* Delivery of shoulder dystocia often results in fracture of the clavicle or humerus to accomplish delivery. *B,* Moderate suprapubic pressure will often disimpact the anterior shoulder.

gentle pressure to control delivery of the head. With the other hand, preferably draped with a sterile towel to protect it from the anus, exert forward pressure on the chin of the fetus through the perineum just in front of the coccyx in a modified Ritgen maneuver (Fig. 56–7). This maneuver extends the neck at the proper time, such that the smallest diameter of the head passes through the introitus and over the perineum, to protect the maternal perineal musculature.

Gently support the head during subsequent delivery of the forehead, face, chin, and neck. With delivery of the neck, pass a finger around the infant's neck to determine whether it is encircled by one or more coils of the umbilical cord. If a loop of cord is felt, loosen it carefully and gently slip it over the infant's head (Fig. 56–8). If this cannot be done easily, clamp the cord doubly, cut the cord between the clamps and promptly deliver the infant.

Delivery of the Shoulders

Just before external rotation, the head usually falls posteriorly, bringing it almost into contact with the mother's anus. As rotation occurs, the head assumes a transverse position and the transverse diameter of the thorax rotates into the AP diameter of the pelvis. In most cases, the shoulders are born spontaneously. Aid delivery by grasping the sides of the head and exerting *gentle* downward (posterior) traction until the anterior shoulder appears beneath the symphysis pubis (Fig. 56–9). Gently lift the head upward to aid delivery of the posterior shoulder. The remainder of the body usually follows without difficulty. Some practitioners prefer to deliver the

anterior shoulder before suctioning the nasopharynx or checking for nuchal cord to avoid shoulder dystocia.

If delivery of the body is delayed after the shoulders have been freed, assist by providing *moderate* traction on the fetal head along with *moderate* pressure on the uterine fundus. In order to avoid brachial plexus injury, do not hook the fingers in the axilla during delivery. Always exert traction in the direction of the long axis of the infant. If traction is applied obliquely, it may cause bending of the neck and excessive stretching of the brachial plexus.[2,26]

Clearing the Airway

Once the head has been delivered, quickly wipe the infant's face and mouth. Gently suction the nose and oral cavity with a bulb syringe. This minimizes the chance of aspiration of amniotic fluid, debris, and blood, which may occur with inspiration during delivery of the thorax. Some controversy exists as to the optimal timing and position of the infant in relation to the mother during this stage, but most authorities recommend that the infant be placed at or slightly below the level of the vaginal introitus during suctioning.[26]

Traditional teaching recommended that meconium-stained infants have endotracheal intubation immediately after birth and that suction be applied to the endotracheal tube as it is withdrawn. Current recommendations no longer advise routine intrapartum oropharyngeal and nasopharyngeal suctioning of infants with meconium staining of amniotic fluid. Studies have shown that this practice offers no benefit if the infant is vigorous. A vigorous infant is one who has strong respiratory effort, good muscle tone, and a heart rate greater than 100 beats/min.[27] Perform endotracheal suctioning immediately after birth for infants who are not vigorous.[27]

Clamping the Cord

Cut the umbilical cord with scissors between two Kelly clamps placed 4 to 5 cm from the infant's abdomen. Delayed clamping of the umbilical cord for at least 2 minutes after birth consistently improves short- and long-term hematologic and iron status of full-term infants.[28] Later, apply an umbilical cord clamp 2 to 3 cm from the infant's abdomen. Collect blood samples from the placental end of the cord for infant serology, including Rh determination.[26]

After cutting the umbilical cord, evaluate the infant, and if necessary, initiate resuscitation. The initial steps of resuscitation are to provide warmth by placing the baby under a radiant heat source, position the head in a "sniffing" position to open the airway, clear the airway with a bulb syringe or suction catheter, dry the baby, and stimulate breathing. Rapidly assess the infant for the following four characteristics:

- Was the baby born after a full-term gestation?
- Is the amniotic fluid clear of meconium and without evidence of infection?
- Is the baby breathing or crying?
- Does the baby have good muscle tone?

If the answer to these questions is "yes," the baby does not need resuscitation.

If the answer to any of these questions is "no," there is general agreement that the infant should receive one or more of the following: (1) initial stabilization (provide warmth, position, clear airway, dry, stimulate, reposition), (2) ventilation, (3) chest compressions, and (4) administration of epinephrine and/or volume expansion.[27]

Delivery of the Placenta

Placental separation usually occurs within about 5 minutes after delivery of the infant and may be recognized by the following signs:

1. The uterus becomes globular and firmer as it contracts.
2. There is a sudden gush of blood as the placenta separates from the uterine wall.
3. The umbilical cord lengthens and protrudes further out of the vagina.

Ask the mother to bear down; the increased intra-abdominal pressure produced by this maneuver may be enough to effect complete expulsion of the placenta. If maternal force alone is insufficient, aid in the delivery of the placenta. After ensuring that the uterus is firmly contracted and placental separation has occurred, use one hand to exert gentle

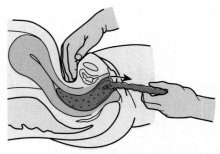

Figure 56–10 Delivery of the placenta and fetal membranes using controlled *traction on the cord and suprapubic pressure with the abdominal hand to prevent uterine inversion.* Care should be taken to avoid avulsion of the cord. Active management with uterotonic agents such as oxytocin administered at delivery hastens delivery of the placenta and may reduce the incidence of postpartum hemorrhage and total blood loss. *(From Gabbe SG, Niebyl JR, Simpson JL [eds]: Obstetrics: Normal and Problem Pregnancies, 5th ed. Philadelphia, Elsevier Churchill Livingstone, 2007.)*

pressure through the abdominal wall to lift the uterine fundus cephalad while keeping the umbilical cord slightly taut with the other hand (Fig. 56–10). Repeat this maneuver until the placenta reaches the introitus. At this time, stop uterine pressure and gently lift the placenta upward and out of the vagina. Never force the expulsion of the placenta before placental separation has occurred and never use forceful traction to pull the placenta out of the uterus. Both of these premature maneuvers may result in uterine inversion with catastrophic hemodynamic consequences. The placenta should be examined for completeness and saved for later evaluation by the obstetrician.[2,6,26]

Examine the vulva, vagina, and cervix for traumatic lacerations. Cervical lacerations most typically occur at the 9 or 3 o'clock position; vaginal lacerations typically occur at the point of the ischial spines. If found, note the extent of the lacerations and repair them using adequate analgesia.

After delivery of the placenta, the primary mechanism by which hemostasis is achieved at the placental site is through myometrial contraction. Agents such as oxytocin, methylergonovine, and ergonovine may be used to stimulate myometrial contraction. Oxytocin (Pitocin, Syntocinon) is the most commonly used oxytocic drug and is usually given by intravenous infusion. Add 20 units of oxytocin to 1 L of normal saline and administer at a rate of 10 mL/min for several minutes until the uterus remains firmly contracted and bleeding is controlled. At this point, reduce the infusion rate to 1 to 2 mL/min.[2,6,26] Alternatively, ergot derivatives such as methylergonovine maleate (Methergine), 0.2 mg, or ergonovine maleate (Ergotrate), 0.2 mg, may be given intramuscularly.[2,6] Because of their vasoconstrictive properties, ergot preparations are relatively contraindicated in patients with hypertension, including pregnancy-associated hypertension or preeclampsia.[2] Do not use oxytocic agents before delivery of the placenta because the resultant uterine contraction may entrap the placenta or an undiagnosed twin within the uterus.[2,26] Even when oxytocics are administered, the hour after delivery of the placenta is the time during which postpartum hemorrhage due to uterine atony is the most likely to occur. For this reason, palpate the uterus frequently to ensure that it is well contracted. A normally contracted uterus will feel firm with its upper margin just below the maternal umbilicus. If the uterus is flaccid and bleeding, gently massage the uterus through the abdominal wall. Occasionally, the placenta may fail to separate completely, resulting in a retained placenta or placental fragments, with persistent uterine bleeding. Support the patient with intravenous fluids and blood transfusions as indicated until definitive therapy is available. Constant firm uterine massage can lessen hemorrhage and may be life saving.

Complex Deliveries

Shoulder Dystocia

Shoulder dystocia refers to impaction of the fetal shoulders in the pelvic outlet occurring after delivery of the head which occurs in 0.15% to 1.7% of vertex presentations.[29] Shoulder dystocia is associated with several risk factors in 50% of cases, including fetal macrosomia, maternal diabetes, obesity, multiparity, and post-term pregnancy (see Fig. 56–9).

Impaction of the fetal shoulders and thorax in the maternal pelvis prohibits adequate respiration, and compression of the umbilical cord frequently compromises fetal circulation. For these reasons, shoulder dystocia is a serious, and potentially fatal, complication of delivery.[26,30] Fetal complications include brachial plexus injuries, clavicular fractures, humeral fractures, and infrequently, death.[30–32]

Management. The techniques used to treat shoulder dystocia frequently require an assistant and delivery can result in fetal injury or hypoxia. Call for assistance emergently from a pediatrician, an obstetrician, and an anesthesiologist. A wide episiotomy may be used to reduce the incidence of major perineal lacerations and provide additional space for manipulation. It should be noted that a fetal fracture or nerve injury is not unusual with shoulder dystocia with any delivery technique, occurring in about 25% of cases (clavicle or humerus fracture). The clavicle may be fractured by intent to accomplish delivery.

Although a variety of techniques have been described to free the anterior shoulder from its impacted position beneath the symphysis pubis, some cases of shoulder dystocia can be resolved with one of two simple maneuvers. In the McRoberts maneuver, place the mother in the extreme lithotomy position with her hips completely flexed, thereby allowing her knees to rest on her chest. This causes a flattening of the lumbar lordosis and rotation of the maternal pelvis cephalad and frequently frees the impacted anterior fetal shoulder (Fig. 56–11).[2,30,32–34] If the McRoberts maneuver fails to effect delivery, ask an assistant to apply moderate suprapubic pressure to the maternal abdomen while providing gentle downward traction on the fetal head (see Fig. 56–9B).[30,31]

If these simple maneuvers fail to effect delivery, several other techniques exist, the choice of which will depend on clinician preference and experience (Figs. 56–12 and 56–13). In the first maneuver, place two fingers in the vagina and exert pressure on the fetal scapula, rotating the posterior shoulder 180° in a corkscrew fashion ("reverse Wood's screw" or Rubin maneuver). This may cause the impacted anterior shoulder to be released and delivery to progress.[30,35] Alternatively, attempt to deliver the posterior arm. In this maneuver, insert the hand along the hollow of the maternal sacrum to the level of the fetus' posterior elbow. Exert pressure at the antecubital fossa, flex the fetus' posterior forearm. and grasp the hand or forearm. Next, carefully sweep the posterior arm of the fetus across its chest to effect delivery of the posterior arm and shoulder. Rotate the shoulder girdle into one of the oblique diameters of the pelvis and subsequently deliver the anterior

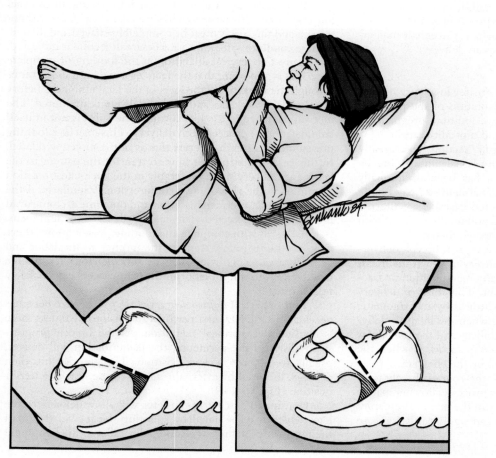

Figure 56–11 The least invasive maneuver to *disimpact the shoulders in shoulder dystocia* is the McRoberts maneuver. Position: extreme lithotomy position with hips completely flexed (knee-chest position) may free the anterior fetal shoulder. *(From Gabbe SG, Niebyl JR, Simpson JL [eds]: Obstetrics: Normal and Problem Pregnancies, 5th ed. Philadelphia, Elsevier Churchill Livingstone, 2007.)*

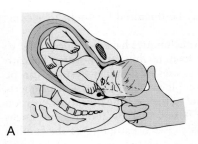

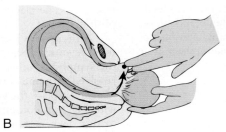

Figure 56–12 **Rubin or reverse Wood's screw maneuver for shoulder dystocia.** *A,* Rotate the posterior shoulder. *B,* Deliver the rotated shoulder.

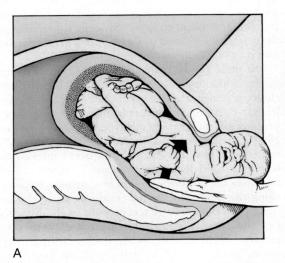

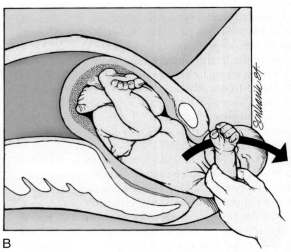

Figure 56–13 *A* and *B,* For shoulder dystocia, insert a hand and sweep the posterior arm across the chest and over the perineum. Take care to distribute the pressure evenly across the humerus to avoid unnecessary fracture. *(From Gabbe SG, Niebyl JR, Simpson JL [eds]: Obstetrics: Normal and Problem Pregnancies, 5th ed. Philadelphia, Elsevier Churchill Livingstone, 2007.)*

shoulder.[2,30] If all of these strategies fail, it may be necessary to perform a controlled destructive procedure, such as fracture of the fetal clavicle, or the cephalic replacement maneuver (Zavanelli) with subsequent cesarean delivery.[2,26]

Breech Delivery

Breech delivery is associated with a greater incidence of prematurity, prolapsed cord, low implantation of the placenta, uterine and congenital abnormalities, multiple pregnancies, and increased perinatal morbidity and mortality rates.[2,36–38]

The increased use of cesarean section has greatly decreased the morbidity and mortality associated with breech delivery. Although cesarean section has been traditionally considered the standard of care, vaginal delivery may be the method of choice in carefully selected cases.[36,39,40] Alternatively, the emergency clinician could potentially be faced with the imminent vaginal delivery of a breech infant.

Types. There are three types of vaginal breech deliveries. *Spontaneous breech* is a breech delivery in which the infant is delivered spontaneously without any manipulation or traction other than supporting the infant. This form of delivery is rare with term infants, and there is little associated traumatic morbidity. *Partial breech extraction* is when the infant is delivered spontaneously as far as the umbilicus and the remainder of the body is extracted. *Total breech extraction* is when the entire body of the infant is extracted by the clinician.

Similar to vertex presentations, the role of the clinician is to assist the mother in the birthing process, allowing maternal expulsive efforts to effect delivery of the infant. Premature or aggressive assistance or traction can significantly increase fetal and maternal morbidity.

To perform any vaginal breech delivery, the birth canal must be sufficiently large to allow passage of the fetus without trauma and the cervix must be completely effaced and dilated. If these conditions do not exist, a cesarean section is indicated. To ensure full cervical dilatation in the footling or complete breech, it is important that the feet, legs, and buttocks advance through the introitus to the level of the fetal umbilicus before the clinician intervenes and further delivery is attempted. The mere appearance of the feet through the vulva is not in itself an indication to proceed with delivery. This may be a footling presentation through a cervix that is not completely dilated. In this case, there may be time to transfer the patient to the labor and delivery suite, preferably in the knee-chest position to minimize the risk of cord compression.[26] Similarly, if the breech is frank, cervical dilatation and outcome are improved if the infant is allowed to deliver to the level of the umbilicus. Before this, as with complete and footling presentations, there may be time to safely transfer the mother to the labor and delivery area. Tocolytics such as subcutaneous terbutaline may be used to inhibit labor until such patients can be safely transferred.[26]

Technique. If *assisted delivery of the frank breech* becomes necessary in the ED, first perform an episiotomy unless there is considerable perineal relaxation. As the breech progressively distends the perineum, the posterior hip will deliver, usually from the 6 o'clock position. The anterior hip then delivers, followed by external rotation to the sacrum anterior position (Fig. 56–14*A*).

Continued descent of the fetus will allow delivery of the legs, which may be aided by splinting the medial thighs of the fetus with the fingers positioned parallel to the femur and

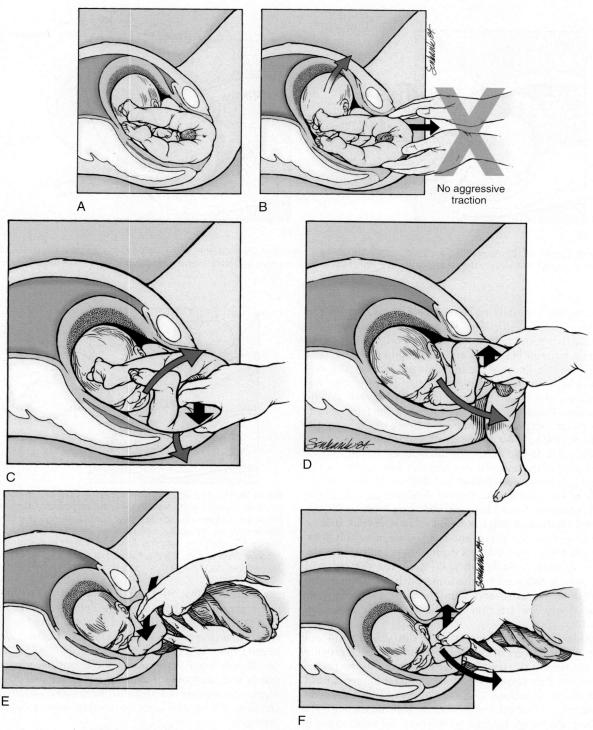

Figure 56–14 The fetus emerges spontaneously (*A*), while uterine contractions maintain cephalic flexion. Avoid premature aggressive traction (*B*) which encourages deflexion of the fetal vertex and increases the risk of head entrapment or nuchal arm entrapment. After spontaneous expulsion of the umbilicus, rotate each thigh externally (*C*) combined with opposite rotation of the fetal pelvis which will result in flexion of the knee and delivery of each leg (*D*). When the scapulae appear under the symphisis, reach over the left shoulder, sweep the arm across the chest (*E*), and deliver the arm (*F*). *(From Gabbe SG, Niebyl JR, Simpson JL [eds]: Obstetrics: Normal and Problem Pregnancies, 5th ed. Philadelphia, Elsevier Churchill Livingstone, 2007.)*

Continued

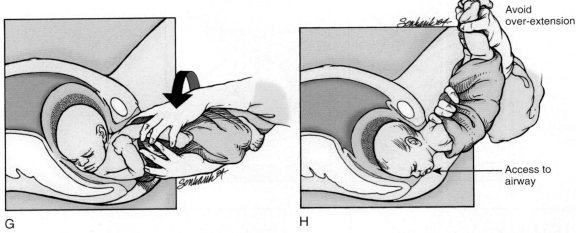

G   H

Figure 56–14, cont'd *G,* Gently rotate the shoulder girdle to facilitate delivery of the right arm. *H,* Following delivery of the arms, wrap the fetus in a towel for control and elevate the fetus slightly. The fetal face and airway may be visible over the perineum. Avoid excessive elevation of the trunk.

exerting pressure laterally to sweep the legs away from the midline (see Fig. 56–14*B*). After delivery of the legs, grasp the fetal bony pelvis using both hands with the fingers resting on the anterior superior iliac crests and the thumbs on the sacrum (see Fig. 56–14*C*). Because the fetal body is slippery and difficult to hold, wrap it in a towel to assist delivery. Use the maternal expulsive efforts in conjunction with gentle downward traction. Rotate the fetal pelvis to bring the fetal sacrum into the transverse position to effect delivery of the scapulae (see Fig. 56–14*D*). Two methods of shoulder delivery are commonly used. In the first, with the scapulae visible, rotate the trunk so that the anterior arm and shoulder appear at the vulva and can be easily released and delivered. Next, rotate the body of the fetus in the reverse direction to deliver the other shoulder and arm beneath the symphysis pubis. In the second method, if trunk rotation is unsuccessful, deliver the posterior shoulder. Grasp the feet in one hand and draw them upward over the mother's groin. Exert leverage on the posterior shoulder, which will slide out over the perineal margin, usually followed by the arm and hand. Deliver the anterior shoulder, arm, and hand beneath the symphysis pubis by downward traction on the fetal body (see Fig. 56–14*E–G*).

Occasionally, spontaneous delivery of the arm and hand does not follow delivery of the shoulder. If this occurs, provide upward traction of the fetal body after delivery of the posterior shoulder. Pass two fingers along the fetal humerus until the fetal elbow is reached. Use the fingers to splint the fetal arm, sweep it downward and deliver it. Deliver the anterior arm by depression of the fetal body alone. In some cases, it may be necessary to sweep the anterior arm down over the thorax using two fingers as a splint.

After the shoulders appear, the head usually occupies one of the oblique diameters of the pelvis, with the chin directed posteriorly. Extract the head using the Mauriceau maneuver. With the fetal body resting on the clinician's palm and forearm, place the index and middle finger of the hand over the infant's maxilla, flexing the fetal head. Hook two fingers of the other hand over the fetal neck and, grasping the shoulders, apply downward traction until the suboccipital region appears under the symphysis pubis. Elevate the body of the fetus toward the mother's abdomen and the fetal mouth, nose, brow, and eventually, occiput successively emerge over the

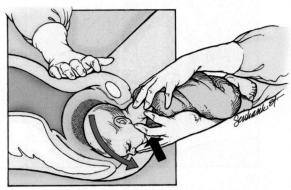

Figure 56–15 In a breech delivery, maintain cephalic flexion by pressure (*arrow*) on the fetal maxilla (not mandible). Often, delivery of the head is easily accomplished with continued expulsive forces from above with the abdominal hand and gentle downward traction. *(From Gabbe SG, Niebyl JR, Simpson JL [eds]: Obstetrics: Normal and Problem Pregnancies, 5th ed. Philadelphia, Elsevier Churchill Livingstone, 2007.)*

perineum (see Fig. 56–14*H*). Ask an assistant to apply suprapubic pressure to help with the delivery of the head (Fig. 56–15). If delivery of the head is not effected by the Mauriceau maneuver, forceps delivery may be necessary but is beyond the scope of this text.

Rarely *breech extraction* of the infant becomes necessary and is indicated only if there is a definite diagnosis of fetal distress unresponsive to routine maneuvers, obstetric services are unavailable, and cesarean section cannot be performed promptly.

If extraction of the incomplete or complete breech is deemed necessary, introduce the hand into the vagina and grasp both feet of the fetus, with the index finger placed between the fetal ankles. Apply gentle traction until the feet are pulled through the vulva. Continue gentle downward traction as successively higher portions of both legs and thighs are grasped. When the breech appears at the vulva, apply gentle traction until the hips are delivered. As the buttocks emerge, the fetal back usually rotates anteriorly. Place the thumbs over the sacrum and the fingers over the hips and deliver the remainder of the breech as described earlier. At times, delivery of a frank breech may be necessary. Facilitated by an episiotomy, the breech should be allowed to deliver spontaneously as far as possible. Place a finger in each fetal groin and then exert moderate traction. Once the knees appear outside the birth canal, flex the legs slowly to assist delivery, and proceed with delivery as described earlier.

EPISIOTOMY

Routine use of episiotomy has been abandoned. Contrary to prior thinking, episiotomy actually increases the risk of third- and fourth-degree tears. Selected indications include breech delivery, shoulder dystocia, occiput posterior presentations, and imminent perineal tear (Table 56–2). Two types of episiotomy have been used: the median or midline episiotomy and the mediolateral episiotomy. The median approach is the easiest type to perform and repair, results in the least amount of blood loss, heals rapidly with minimal discomfort, and is generally preferred in the United States. The median episiotomy should be avoided[26] because the major disadvantage is inadvertent extension of the incision into the anal sphincter or rectum, resulting in third- and fourth-degree lacerations,

respectively.[2,26,41,42] The mediolateral episiotomy seldom results in extension into the anal sphincter, but blood loss is greater, repair is more difficult, and healing is more painful.[2,26]

Technique

Time the episiotomy so that it precedes trauma to the maternal tissues and fetus but avoids excessive maternal blood loss before delivery. With vertex presentations, the episiotomy should be performed when the fetal head begins to distend the perineum and the caput becomes visible to a diameter of 3 to 4 cm during a contraction.[2] Anesthesia for the episiotomy in the ED is usually limited to local infiltration of the perineum with 1% or 2% lidocaine (Fig. 56–16).

Extend the incision through the skin and subcutaneous tissues, the vaginal mucosa, the urogenital septum, and the superior fascia of the pelvic diaphragm. If the incision is mediolateral, extend the incision through the lowermost fibers of the puborectalis portion of the levator ani muscles. As the head crowns, place the index and middle fingers inside the vaginal introitus to expose the mucosa, posterior forchette, and perineal body. Use tissue scissors to incise the median raphe of the perineum almost to the anal sphincter. For the mediolateral episiotomy (see Fig. 56–16), direct the incision downward and outward in the direction of the lateral margin of the anal sphincter either to the right or to the left. After delivery of the infant and placenta, repair the episiotomy. The goals of episiotomy repair are to restore both anatomy and hemostasis with minimal amount of suture material. Perform the closure after delivery of the placenta and after inspection and repair of the cervix and upper vaginal

TABLE 56–2 Traditional Indications for Episiotomy

Fetal macrosomatia
Shoulder dystocia
Breech delivery
Operative vaginal delivery
Occiput posterior position
Risk of major perineal laceration
Non-reassuring fetal heart rate tracing

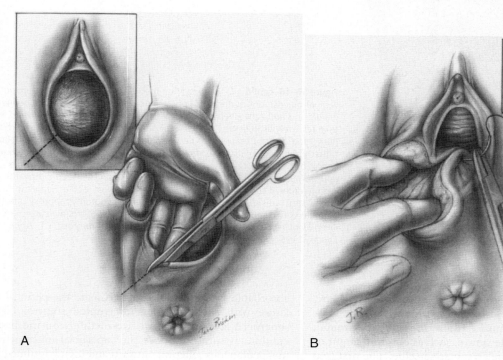

Figure 56–16 In normal deliveries, routine episotomy should be avoided. If one is performed (see text), the mediolateral approach is preferred. In general, the midline episiotomy should be avoided because it leads to excessive perineal trauma. *A,* Perform a right mediolateral episiotomy when approximately 3 to 4 cm of the fetal head is seen distending the perineum during a uterine contraction. Be careful to make the incision at 5 or 7 o'clock to avoid extension into the rectal sphincter muscle. *B,* To repair the mediolateral episiotomy, expose the full extent of the episiotomy with the left hand. Place the first suture at the vaginal apex approximately 1 cm cephalad to the most superior margin of the episiotomy or laceration. It is important to place the initial suture above the apex to ensure hemostasis of the repair. *Inset,* The correct position of the needle at the tip of the needle holder.

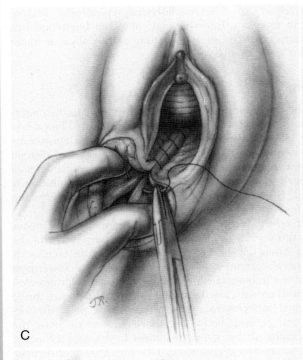

C

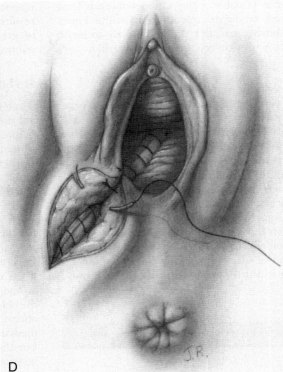

D

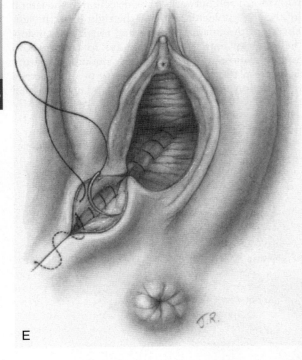

E

Figure 56–16, cont'd *C,* To repair the mediolateral episiotomy, approximate the vaginal mucosa not quite to the posterior commissure. Spread the perineum widely and unite the deep perineal tissues to avoid leaving dead space. Medially, take relatively little tissue on the needle to ensure that the rectum will not be punctured. Do not reapproximate the wound surfaces in a horizontal plane but rather at an angle with lower medial tissues joined to higher lateral tissues. *D,* Repair of the mediolateral episiotomy. Suture the vaginal wound to the approximate level of the posterior commissure. Join the deep perineal tissues with additional sutures, taking care to join the lower medial tissues to higher lateral structures. *E,* To repair the mediolateral episiotomy, approximate the perineal skin edges using a subcuticular stitch of reabsorbable suture. *(A–G, From Hankins GD, et al [eds]: Operative Obstetrics. Stamford, CT, Appleton & Lange, 1995.)*

canal if indicated. The principles of repair are the same, regardless of the type of episiotomy location.

Because there is minimal tension on the closed wound, use a 2-0 or 3-0 absorbable suture, such as chromic catgut or polyglycolic acid, on a large atraumatic needle. The first step is to close the vaginal mucosa using a continuous suture from just above the apex of the incision to the mucocutaneous junction, reapproximating the margins of the hymenal ring. Burying the closing knot in the incision minimizes the amount of scar tissue and prevents tenderness and dyspaurenia. Ligate large actively bleeding vessels during closure with separate

absorbable suture. Next, reapproximate the perineal musculature with three or four interrupted sutures. Close the superficial layers by one of two methods. In the first, use a continuous suture to close the superficial mucosa from the mucocutaneous junction outward and then continued upward as a subcuticular skin closure, returning to and ending at the mucocutaneous junction. Alternatively, place several interrupted sutures through the skin and subcutaneous fascia and tie them loosely. This last method of skin closure avoids burying two layers of suture in the more superficial layers of the perineum.[2,26]

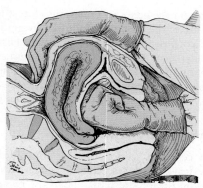

Figure 56–17 Use uterine massage to control postpartum bleeding. Insert one hand into the vagina to compress the anterior uterine wall, while massaging the posterior aspect of the uterus through the abdominal wall with the other hand.

TABLE 56–3 Drugs for the Management of Immediate Postpartum Hemorrhage

Oxytocin*	
Dose	20–40 units in 1 L crystalloid initially infused at 200–500 mL/hr → titrate to sustain uterine contractions and control hemorrhage
Comments	Do not administer as IV bolus
	If IV access unavailable, may use 10 U IM

Methylergonovine Maleate or Ergonovine Maleate	
Dose	0.2 mg IM
Comments	Avoid in patients with hypertensive disease including preeclampsia

Carboprost Tromethamine	
Dose	0.25 mg IM → repeat q 15 min until uterine hemorrhage controlled or maximum dose of 2 mg
Comments	Concurrent use of antiemetics and antidiarrheals recommended to control side effects

*Note increased concentration of oxytocin infusion when used for the treatment of postpartum hemorrhage compared with that given to stimulate uterine contractions after uncomplicated delivery.

IM, intramuscularly; IV, intravenously.

The most common complication of episiotomy is hematoma formation that requires evacuation and drainage. Infection is an infrequent complication that usually responds to sitz baths, good hygiene, and antibiotic therapy.

IMMEDIATE POSTPARTUM HEMORRHAGE

Maternal blood loss greater than 500 mL or bleeding that exceeds the clinician's estimate of "normal" defines postpartum hemorrhage. Postpartum hemorrhage is divided into immediate hemorrhage occurring, within 24 hours of delivery, and delayed hemorrhage, occurring more than 24 hours after delivery.

Postpartum hemorrhage is frequently characterized by steady, moderate bleeding that persists until serious hypovolemia develops rather than by sudden massive hemorrhage. Careful observation for blood loss, including evaluation of uterine size and consistency, is therefore needed during the early postpartum period. The most common cause of immediate postpartum hemorrhage is uterine atony. Less common causes include lacerations of the vagina and cervix, retained placenta or placental fragments, coagulation disorders, uterine rupture, and uterine inversion.[2,43–45]

Management

Management of postpartum hemorrhage consists of replacement of intravascular volume with crystalloid and blood products as needed as well as correction of the underlying cause of hemorrhage. The diagnosis of uterine atony, the most common cause of bleeding, is made when uterine palpation reveals a soft boggy uterus. Diagnosis may be suspected on the basis or abdominal examination with confirmation made on bimanual examination (Fig. 56–17).

Uterine atony is initially managed with firm manual massage of the uterine fundus through the abdominal wall in conjunction with the administration of oxytocic agents (Table 56–3). If bleeding persists, bimanual uterine compression is indicated. One hand of the clinician is used to compress and massage the posterior aspect of the uterus through the abdominal wall while the fist of the other hand is used to gently massage the anterior aspect of the uterus through the vaginal wall. Avoid vigorous downward massage, which can result in acute uterine inversion.

Oxytocics

Administer oxytocin as an intravenous infusion. Prepare it by adding 20 to 40 units of oxytocin to 1 L of crystalloid and infuse at a rate of 200 to 500 mL/hr. Titrate to sustain uterine contractions and control uterine hemorrhage. Slowing of hemorrhage should be observed within minutes of administration. If an intravenous line is unavailable, administer 10 units of oxytocin intramuscularly.[20] Profound hypotension and arrhythmias may occur if oxytocin is administered as an intravenous bolus.[2]

If bleeding persists and the uterus remains boggy despite oxytocin therapy, consider giving an ergot derivative such as methylergonovine or a prostaglandin. Give methylergonovine (Methergine) as a 0.2-mg dose intramuscularly with uterine contractions occurring within 2 to 5 minutes of administration and lasting for several hours.[20] Owing to their tendency to cause vasoconstriction and severe hypertension, avoid giving ergot preparations in women with hypertensive disease, including preeclampsia.[20,43] Alternatively, give 15-methyl prostaglandin $F_{2\alpha}$ (carboprost tromethamine [Hemabate]) to stimulate uterine contractions.[43,45] Administer carboprost at a dose of 0.25 mg intramuscularly repeated at 15-minute intervals as determined by clinical course, not to exceed 2 mg.[20,44]

Procedures

If vaginal bleeding persists despite uterine massage and a firmly contracted uterus, search for another cause. Inspect the labia, vagina, and cervix for lacerations. Control bleeding by direct pressure or by gentle application of ring forceps to bleeding cervical lacerations. Use absorbable sutures to control bleeding from accessible lacerations. Adequate visualization of the upper vagina and cervix can be difficult, and repair of lacerations may require general anesthesia and obstetric intervention.

Although rare, uterine inversion is frequently thought to be the result of traction on the umbilical cord during the third stage of labor.[2,44,46] The principal signs and symptoms of uterine inversion are lancinating and often violent pelvic pain and excessive postpartum hemorrhage. Up to 40% of patients develop shock.[43,46–48] Diagnosis is made by visualization or palpation of the soft purplish-red mass of the uterus filling the vaginal vault or protruding through the introitus. On abdominal examination, no mass representing the uterus may be palpated, or when palpated, the uterus may have a cuplike dimpling of the fundus.[43,44,47,48] Treat with crystalloid intravenous fluids to maintain cardiovascular stability. Reposition the uterus immediately (Fig. 56–18). Conscious sedation and general anesthesia might be necessary. Use tocolytic agents such as terbutaline or magnesium sulfate for uterine relaxation and repositioning.[2,43,48]

To reposition the uterus, insert one hand into the vagina with the tips of the fingers at the uterocervical junction and the uterine fundus firmly held in the palm of the hand. Gently

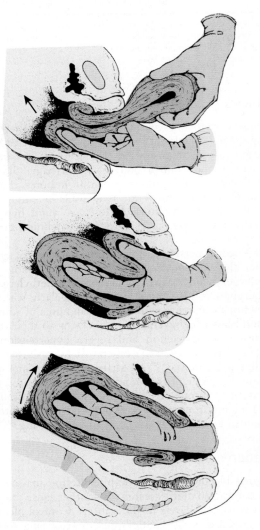

Figure 56–18 Manual replacement of an inverted uterus. Uterine inversion should be suspected with the sudden onset of brisk vaginal bleeding in association with an absent palpable fundus abdominally and maternal hemodynamic instability. It may occur before or after placental detachment. The diagnosis is made clinically with bimanual examination, during which the uterine fundus is palpated in the lower uterine segment or within the vagina. Use sonography to confirm the diagnosis if the clinical examination is unclear.

exert pressure on the edges of the uterus closest to the cervix in the direction of the umbilicus followed by gradual replacement of the corpus. Do not exert pressure centrally on the fundus initially because this will cause the uterus to be compressed, forcing more "layers" of the uterus to lie within the relatively tight cervical ring.[46–48] General anesthesia and laparotomy might be necessary for uterine positioning.

PERIMORTEM CESAREAN SECTION

Perimortem cesarean section, one of the oldest and most dramatic surgical procedures, has long been used as an attempt to preserve the life of the fetus.[49] Earliest records trace its origin back to 715 BC, when the legendary king of Rome, Numa Pompilious, decreed that the child be excised from the womb of any woman who died late in pregnancy. Under the emperors of Rome, the *caesars*, this law became known as the "lex caesare"; hence, the name cesarean operation.[50]

From 1879 until 1986, there were 188 reports of perimortem cesarean section resulting in the delivery of a live infant.[51] Since that time, only isolated cases of long-term fetal survival have been reported.[52,53] Because most of the literature on perimortem cesarean section involves only small numbers of cases with emphasis on those that are successful, accurate survival statistics are unknown. When reported, infant survival rates range from 11% to 70%.[50,51,54] Because the rare potential for survival of a normal infant exists, cesarean delivery may be considered in any woman who suffers a cardiac arrest after 24 weeks' gestation and is unresponsive to brief resuscitation.[51,52] Although the procedure is rare, the decision and its performance may fall to the emergency clinician. However, no standard of care is promulgated with regard to the procedure in the ED or the mandate of the emergency clinician to perform a perimortem cesarean section.

Indications

Survival of the infant is directly related to the elapsed time from death of the mother to delivery, the maturity of the fetus, the performance of cardiopulmonary resuscitation (CPR) on the mother, and in certain circumstances, the availability of neonatal intensive care facilities.[50–52] Although the lower limit of fetal viability varies among institutions, in general, performance of the procedure before the point of fetal viability at approximately 24 weeks is not indicated.[6] If the duration of gestation is not known from the history, fetal maturity may be quickly estimated by calculating gestational age on the basis of the date of the patient's last normal menstrual period or by measuring the height of the uterine fundus. Between 18 and 30 weeks' gestation, the age of the fetus in weeks will correspond to the distance in centimeters from the uterine fundus to the symphysis pubis (e.g., at 28 weeks' gestation the fundus is approximately 28 cm above the symphysis pubis or halfway between the umbilicus and the costal margin).[55] Criteria for intervention should be established prospectively at each institution and be in accordance with the institution's general neonatal policies.[6,55]

The potential for infant survival decreases and the chance of neurologic damage increases as the time from maternal death (cessation of circulation) to cesarean section rises (Table 56–4). When cesarean section is performed within 5 minutes of death of the mother, neonatal outcome is best, but not guaranteed; from 5 to 10 minutes, good; from 10 to 15 minutes, fair; and from 15 to 20 minutes, poor. Because, even

TABLE 56–4 Outcome of 61 Infants Who Survived Post-mortem Cesarean Section from 1900 to 1985 as a Function of Time from Maternal Death to Delivery

Time (min)	No. of Patients (%)	Normal	Neurologic Sequelae
0–5	42 (69)	42	0
6–10	8 (13)	7	1 (mild)
11–15	7 (11)	6	1 (severe)
16–20	1 (2)	0	1 (severe)
21–25	3 (5)	1	2 (severe)

From Katz VL, Dotters DJ, Droegemueller W: Perimortem cesarean delivery. Obstet Gynecol 68:571, 1986.

under optimal conditions, CPR results in a cardiac output of 30% to 40% of normal and placental perfusion may be severely compromised, make every attempt to begin cesarean delivery within 4 minutes of the cardiopulmonary arrest, completing the procedure within 5 minutes of arrest.[6,51,52,55] Fetal prognosis is generally better after the sudden death of a previously healthy mother than after the death of a mother with a prolonged and debilitating illness.[50,51,55]

CPR should, of course, be initiated immediately on cardiac arrest of the mother and be continued until after delivery of the infant. The pregnant state produces certain physiologic changes that adversely affect the adequacy of standard CPR. Vena caval occlusion by the gravid uterus hampers venous return and thus compromises maternal cardiac output. A decreased functional residual capacity of the lungs may impede ventilation. An assistant may attempt manual displacement of the uterus away from the inferior vena cava. However, perimortem cesarean delivery in itself may represent the most important variable for a successful maternal resuscitation.[50,51,56]

Legal and Ethical Considerations

To the editors' knowledge, no clinician has been found liable for performing, or not performing, a perimortem cesarean section. Whereas some believe this is a futile procedure, with the best outcome being a brain-damaged baby, others consider that the clinician has the right and responsibility to provide the fetus with every possible chance of survival when there is no hope of survival of the mother.[51,55] *This is an unsettled issue at the current time and likely will remain so.* Verbal permission for the operation should be obtained from the family when possible but not at the expense of delaying the procedure. Failure to obtain permission should not preclude cesarean section.[51,55]

Because there is no standard of care relating to emergency clinicians performing a perimortem cesarean delivery, each case must be individualized. Limited resources often place the clinician in the difficult situation of deciding whether to continue efforts to resuscitate the mother or to attempt to deliver the fetus in a difficult situation under less than ideal conditions. In the absence of obstetric backup immediately at hand, it is reasonable for the emergency clinician to proceed with delivery of the child if the mother cannot be resuscitated. Prolonged attempts to resuscitate the mother are unlikely to benefit either the mother or the fetus.

Technique

Perimortem cesarean section should be performed by the most experienced person present, preferably an obstetrician. When possible, a neonatologist should be in attendance. Their arrival, however, should not delay onset of the procedure. CPR should be initiated for the mother at the time of cardiac arrest and continued throughout the procedure. Although it is helpful if fetal heart tones are present premortem, time should not be wasted searching for them or attempting to evaluate fetal viability with abdominal ultrasonography.

Because neonatal survival is enhanced as the time from maternal death to delivery decreases (whereas the irreversible nature of maternal cardiac arrest becomes more apparent as resuscitative efforts progress), the decision to perform this procedure may be one of the most difficult that the emergency clinician makes.

Rapid extraction of the infant while avoiding fetal and maternal injury is the goal of the procedure (Fig. 56–19). Hence, time should not be wasted preparing a sterile operating field or transporting the patient to an operating suite outside the ED. Using a large (e.g., No. 10) scalpel, make a midline vertical incision through the abdominal wall extending from the symphysis pubis to the umbilicus and carried through all abdominal layers to the peritoneal cavity. In most gravid women, the hyperpigmented "linea nigra" is apparent and may serve as a guide for the incision. If available, place retractors in the abdominal wound and draw them laterally to expose the anterior surface of the uterus. Reflect the bladder inferiorly; if it is full, it may be aspirated to evacuate it and permit better access to the uterus. While avoiding injury to fetal parts, make a small (~5 cm) vertical incision through the lower uterine segment until amniotic fluid is obtained or until the uterine cavity is clearly entered. Then insert the index and long fingers into the incision and use them to lift the uterine wall away from the fetus. Use bandage scissors to extend the incision vertically to the fundus until a wide exposure is obtained. Then gently deliver the infant, suction the mouth and nose, and clamp and cut the cord. Because the incision is relatively high in the uterus, the infant's head may not be readily accessible to the clinician, in which case grasp the infant's feet and deliver the infant through maneuvers similar to those for a breech delivery. Carry out neonatal resuscitation as necessary.

Because, in rare instances, relief of vena caval compression by the uterus improves maternal hemodynamics such that survival of the mother is possible, check maternal pulses and continue CPR after delivery of the infant.

THE NEWBORN

Approximately 5% to 10% of newborns require some degree of active resuscitation at birth (e.g., stimulation to breathe), and approximately 1% to 10% of those born in hospitals require assisted ventilation.[57] Evaluation of the newborn begins before delivery with assessment of maternal well-being and gestational age and with the recognition of fetal distress, as evidenced by meconium staining of the amniotic fluid, fetal bradycardia, or evidence of cord prolapse. Care of the newborn begins with delivery of the head when the nose and mouth are suctioned.

Newborn resuscitation can be divided into four categories of action: (1) basic steps including assessment and initial

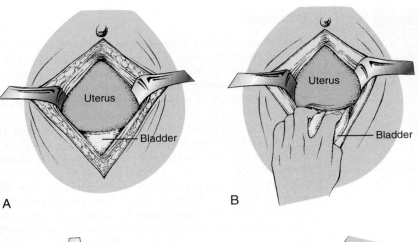

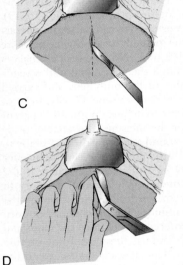

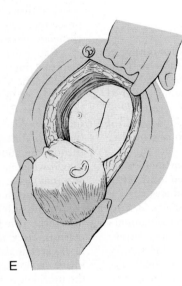

Figure 56–19 **Cesarean delivery.** *A,* Make a vertical incision through the abdominal wall from the level of the uterine fundus to the symphysis pubis. *B,* If available, use retractors to expose the anterior surface of the uterus and retract the bladder inferiorly. *C,* Use a scalpel to make a small vertical incision through the lower uterine segment. *D,* Use bandage scissors to extend the incision vertically to the fundus. *E,* Deliver the infant, suction the nose and mouth, and clamp and cut the cord.

stabilization, (2) ventilation including bag-valve-mask or bag-tube ventilation, (3) chest compressions, and (4) administration of medications or fluids. Although most newborns require only basic steps such as suctioning, drying, stimulation, and perhaps supplemental oxygen, some require further intervention, the most crucial action of which is the establishment of adequate ventilation.[57]

Evaluation

Traditionally, the Apgar scoring system, applied at 1 and 5 minutes after birth, has been the standard of newborn evaluation (Table 56–5).[2,58] In general, the higher the score, the better the condition of the infant. Although traditionally the 1-minute Apgar score has been used to indicate the need for immediate resuscitation, the decision to begin resuscitation should not be delayed until an Apgar score is obtained. Rather, resuscitation decisions are based on the clinical triad of respiration, heart rate, and color.[57,58]

Respiration. Normally, the newborn begins to breath and cry almost immediately after birth.[2] After initial respiratory efforts, the newborn should be able to establish regular respirations sufficient to improve color and maintain a heart rate of more than 100 beats/min. Gasping and apnea are signs

indicating the need for assisted ventilation.[57] If initial respirations are shallow or slow, a brief period of stimulation may be attempted while 100% oxygen is administered.[57,58] Establishing adequate ventilation and oxygenation will restore vital signs in the vast majority of newborns.[57]

Heart Rate. Heart rate may be determined by auscultation or by palpation of the pulse at the base of the umbilical cord. Heart rate should be consistently greater than 100

TABLE 56–5 Apgar Scoring System			
Sign	**0**	**1**	**2**
Heart rate	Absent	Slow (<100)	>100
Respiratory effort	Absent	Slow, irregular	Good, crying
Muscle tone	Flaccid	Some flexion of extremities	Active motion
Reflex irritability	No response	Grimace	Vigorous cry
Color	Blue, pale	Body pink, extremities blue	Completely pink

beats/min in an uncompromised newborn. If heart rate is less than 100 beats/min, initiate positive-pressure ventilation (PPV) with 100% oxygen. If the heart rate is less than 60 beats/min, despite adequate ventilation with 100% oxygen for 30 seconds, initiate chest compressions.[57] Because chest compressions may diminish the effectiveness of ventilation, do not initiate them until lung inflation and ventilation have been established.[57]

Color. An uncompromised newborn will be able to maintain a pink color of the mucous membranes without supplemental oxygenation. Central cyanosis is determined by examining the face, trunk, and mucous membranes and, if present, should be treated with supplemental oxygen. Acrocyanosis is usually a normal finding in the newborn and not a reliable indicator of hypoxemia. It may, however, indicate other conditions such as cold stress.[57,58]

Stabilization Technique

Following delivery of the infant and cutting the umbilical cord, place the newborn on her or his side with the neck in a neutral or slightly extended position.[57] A rolled blanket or towel placed under the back and shoulders of the supine infant, thus elevating the torso 2 to 2.5 cm, may help in maintaining head position.[57,58] Preventing heat loss in the newborn is vital because cold stress can increase oxygen consumption and impede effective resuscitation.[57] Hyperthermia, however, should be avoided because it is associated with perinatal respiratory depression.[57,59] Placing the infant under a radiant warmer, rapidly drying the skin, and wrapping the infant in warmed blankets will reduce heat loss.[57,58] Alternatively, the mother's body may be used as a heat source. If initial evaluation indicates the infant is stable, the infant may be dried and placed skin to skin on the mother's chest or abdomen and both covered with blankets.[57,58]

Healthy vigorous newborns generally do not require suctioning after delivery. If suctioning is necessary, secretions should be cleared first from the mouth and then the nose with a bulb syringe or suction catheter (8 or 10 Fr). Because aggressive pharyngeal suctioning can cause laryngeal spasm and vagal bradycardia, mechanical suctioning should be limited in

depth and duration, and negative pressures should not exceed 100 mm Hg.[57] Generally, drying and suctioning are enough to stimulate effective respirations in the newborn. If effective spontaneous respirations are not established after drying with a towel or gentle rubbing of the back, flicking the soles of the feet may initiate spontaneous respiration.[57] If these maneuvers do not initiate spontaneous respirations, PPV will be required.[57,58]

Meconium aspiration is a significant cause of morbidity and mortality in newborns. Careful suctioning of the nose and mouth should be performed in all infants born through meconium-stained amniotic fluid. Intubation and tracheal suctioning are indicated for depressed infants, as discussed earlier.[57,59,60]

Most newborns who require PPV can be adequately ventilated with a bag and mask. Indications for PPV include apnea or gasping respirations, heart rate less than 100 beats/min, and persistent central cyanosis despite 100% oxygen.[57,58] Assisted ventilations are performed at a rate of 40 to 60 per minute (30 breaths/min if mechanical compressions are being performed). Typically, higher inflation pressures ($\geq$30–40 cm H_2O) and longer inflation times are required for the first several breaths than for subsequent breaths. Visible chest expansion is probably a more reliable indicator of appropriate inflation pressures than any specific manometer reading.[57,58] Because bag-valve-mask ventilation can produce gastric distention, which impedes respiration, insert an orogastric tube (8 Fr) in infants undergoing prolonged PPV.[57]

Endotracheal intubation may be indicated when bag-valve-mask ventilation is ineffective, when tracheal suctioning for meconium is required, when chest compressions are performed, or when prolonged PPV is required.[57,58] Alternatively, the neonatal laryngeal mask airway may provide effective airway management, especially in the case of ineffective bag-valve-mask ventilation or failed endotracheal intubation.[57] Use of the laryngeal mask airway, however, has not been adequately studied in preterm infants and those with deliveries complicated by meconium-stained fluid. Its use, therefore, cannot be recommended in these situations.[57]

Monitor the heart rate during the course of neonatal evaluation and stabilization with either direct auscultation

---

TABLE 56–6 Medications Commonly Used in Neonatal Resuscitations

Drug	Dose	Indications	Comments
Epinephrine*	0.01–0.03 mg/kg (0.1–0.3 mL/kg of 1:10,000 solution)	Bradycardia, asystole	May be repeated every 3–5 min as indicated Data regarding high-dose epinephrine in newborns inadequate to support routine use
Naloxone*	0.1 mg/kg (0.25 mL/kg of a 0.4-mg/mL solution or 0.1 mL/kg of a 1-mg/mL solution)	Respiratory depression induced by maternal narcotics during delivery	May be repeated every 2–3 min as needed May be given IM or SC if perfusion adequate May induce narcotic withdrawal in the newborn chronically exposed to narcotics; therefore, relatively contraindicated
Volume expanders (normal saline or Ringer's solution)	10 mL/kg IV over 5–10 min	Suspected hypovolemia, shock, or blood loss	May be repeated after determination of clinical response Higher initial dose not recommended and may result in volume overload
Bicarbonate	1–2 mEq/kg of a 0.5-mEq/mL solution given over at least 2 min	Prolonged arrests unresponsive to other therapy	Not indicated during brief periods of CPR Should be used only after adequate ventilation and perfusion established

*May also be given via endotracheal tube.
CPR, cardiopulmonary resuscitation; IV, intravenously; IM, intramuscularly; SC, subcutaneously.
From Pediatric Working Group of the International Liaison Committee on Resuscitation: Neonatal resuscitation. Circulation 102:343, 2000.

over the chest or palpation of the pulse at the base of the umbilical cord. A readily discernible heartbeat of 100 beats/min or greater is acceptable. If the heart rate is less than 60 beats/min, despite adequate ventilation with 100% oxygen for 30 seconds, institute chest compressions while ventilation is continued.[57] Deliver chest compressions on the lower third of the sternum and not over the xiphoid to avoid damage to the liver.[58] There are two techniques for performing chest compression in the newborn. In the preferred method, two thumbs of the resuscitator's hands are positioned side by side over the lower third of the sternum just below the nipple line. If the infant is large or the resuscitator's hands are too small to encircle the chest, two finger compressions using the ring and middle fingers may be used.[57,58] The depth of compression should be approximately one third to one half of the anterior-posterior diameter of the newborn's chest, such that a

palpable pulse is generated.[57] Coordinate compressions and ventilations to avoid simultaneous delivery, which may compromise the efficacy of ventilation. The compression to ventilation ratio should be 3:1 with 90 compressions and 30 breaths to achieve approximately 120 respirations/min.[57] If the heart rate remains less than 60 beats/min, despite these interventions,[57] establish an umbilical or intravenous line and initiate appropriate drug therapy. Alternatively, intraosseous access can be used but may not be as effective in the preterm infant.[57] The medications most commonly used in neonatal resuscitation are listed in Table 56–6.

 REFERENCES CAN BE FOUND ON EXPERT CONSULT

CHAPTER 57

Culdocentesis

G. Richard Braen and David Lee Pierce

Culdocentesis is a procedure in which a hollow needle is inserted through the posterior vaginal wall into the peritoneal space to obtain peritoneal fluid for analysis and culture. This procedure is simple, rapid, and safe. The technique is used primarily to diagnose ruptured ectopic pregnancies and ruptured ovarian cysts and, rarely, to obtain cultures to aid in the diagnosis of pelvic inflammatory disease (PID). The availability of high-resolution transvaginal ultrasound and highly sensitive β subunit human chorionic gonadotropin (β-hCG) quantatative assays have led to a decline in the use of the procedure. Despite this change; however, culdocentesis is still valuable in patients in whom a ruptured ectopic pregnancy is suspected but a sonographic examination cannot be obtained.[1]

ANATOMY

Before attempting culdocentesis, the clinician must be familiar with the anatomy of the vagina and rectouterine pouch (pouch of Douglas). In the adult female, the vagina is approximately 9 cm long. From its inferior to its superior aspect, the posterior wall of the vagina is related to the anal canal by way of the perineal body, the rectum, and the peritoneum of the rectouterine pouch.[2] The uterus lies nearly at a right angle to the vagina. The rectouterine pouch and the posterior wall of the vagina are adjacent only at the upper quarter (~2 cm) of the posterior vaginal wall. The vaginal wall in this area is less than 5 mm thick.

The blood supply of the upper vagina comes from the uterine and vaginal arteries, which are branches of the internal iliac artery. The area is drained by a vaginal venous plexus that communicates with the uterine and vesical plexuses. The vagina has its greatest sensation near the introitus and little sensation in the area adjacent to the rectouterine pouch.

The rectouterine pouch is formed by reflections of the peritoneum, and it is the most dependent intraperitoneal space in both the upright and the supine positions. Blood, pus, and other free fluids in the peritoneal cavity pool in the pouch because of its dependent location. This pouch separates the upper portion of the rectum from the uterus and the upper part of the vagina. The pouch often contains small intestine and, normally, a small amount of peritoneal fluid.

INDICATIONS

Culdocentesis is indicated in any adult female when fluid aspirated from the rectouterine pouch will help to confirm a clinical diagnosis. If ultrasound examination is not readily available in the emergency department (ED), or if the patient is too hemodynamically unstable to be transported to an off-site location for ultrasound, culdocentesis may be the fastest and most accurate diagnostic technique available to the emergency clinician.[3] Analysis of peritoneal fluid is also a reliable method of differentiating inflammatory from hemorrhagic pelvic pathologic conditions. Conditions in which culdocentesis may be of diagnostic value include a ruptured viscus (particularly an ectopic pregnancy or a corpus luteum cyst), PID, and other intra-abdominal infections (particularly appendicitis with rupture or diverticulitis with perforation), intra-abdominal injuries to the liver or the spleen, and ruptured aortic aneurysms.[4]

Ectopic Pregnancy

Ectopic pregnancy is often one of the most difficult gynecologic lesions to diagnose.[5] The incidence of ectopic pregnancy is on the rise, accounting for 1.6% of all pregnancies. Ectopic pregnancy is the most common obstetric cause of maternal death in the first trimester.[5] In a series of 300 consecutive cases of ectopic pregnancy, 50% of patients received medical evaluation at least twice before the correct diagnosis was made.[6] In 11% of the patients in this series, the diagnosis was not made until the third medical visit.

The clinical picture of ectopic pregnancy may include vascular collapse, pelvic pain, isolated rectal or back pain, amenorrhea, abnormal menses, shoulder pain, syncope, cervical or adnexal tenderness, adnexal mass, anemia, and leukocytosis. It is important to note that blood in the peritoneal cavity does not consistently correlate with peritoneal irritation, blood pressure, or pulse rate.[7] In fact, bradycardia in the presence of significant intraperitoneal bleeding from a ruptured ectopic pregnancy is not unusual (Tables 57–1 and 57–2).

There is often a history of salpingitis, use of an intrauterine contraceptive device, or tubal ligation; however, no combination of these signs, symptoms, or historical data is diagnostic for an ectopic pregnancy. To confuse the diagnosis further, a normal menstrual history is reported in approximately 50% of patients with ectopic pregnancy. A urine pregnancy test is occasionally negative.[8] Although rarely seen, the combination of a uterine decidual cast (Fig. 57–1) and a positive pregnancy test is virtually pathognomonic of an ectopic pregnancy. A uterine cast is decidua that has been hormonally stimulated by the ectopic pregnancy but is passed vaginally when the tissue can no longer be supported. The cast is an outline of the uterine cavity, but it can be mistaken for products of conception if not inspected carefully. Therefore, all tissue passed vaginally should be carefully inspected before it is sent to the laboratory for analysis for products of conception. Ectopic pregnancy can rarely occur with an intrauterine pregnancy. Patients who have had a therapeutic abortion may actually have had an unrecognized ectopic pregnancy; hence, the need for pathologic evaluation of any tissue obtained by uterine evacuation procedures.

The greater sensitivity of the serum and urine β-hCG radioreceptor assay, coupled with the proliferation of transvaginal ultrasound and laparoscopy, has greatly increased the chances for early diagnosis of unruptured and ruptured ectopic pregnancy.[9] Urinary β-hCG tests (enzyme-linked or solid-phase immunoassay) provide sensitivity to 20 to 50 mIU/mL, being positive in the first few weeks of pregnancy. However, ectopic pregnancy is often associated with very low production of this hormone.

Quantification of the serum test adds additional information being sensitive to 5 mIU/mL. Therefore, a negative *urine* β-hCG test rules out pregnancy in greater than 98% of cases, and pregnancy in any site can be ruled out in virtually all patients with a negative *serum* β-hCG test.[10] A single

TABLE 57–1 Correlation between the Results of Culdocenteses Performed on 77 Patients with Ectopic Gestation and Various Clinical Parameters

	Classic Triad			Peritoneal Signs	Pulse ≥ 100/min	Blood Pressure < 90/40 mm Hg	Mean Hematocrit (%)	Hemoperitoneum ≥ 100 mL	Ruptured Tube	Total
	Bleeding	Pain	Adnexal Mass							
Positive	37	54	10	26	19	9	35	52	30	54
Negative	8	8	3	1	1	0	39	0	0	8
Inadequate	13	15	6	5	4	1	38	13	7	15
Total patients	58	77	19	32	24	10	65	37	77	

Note: There is a lack of correlation between positive culdocentesis and peritoneal signs and changes in vital signs. Patients are grouped by culdocentesis result (i.e., positive, negative, or inadequate). Note that only 10 patients were hypotensive and only 24 experienced tachycardia.
From Cartwright PS, Vaughn B, Tuttle D: Culdocentesis and ectopic pregnancy. J Reprod Med 29:88, 1984. Reproduced by permission.

TABLE 57–2 Correlation between Tubal Status and Hypotension, Tachycardia, Hematocrit, Signs of Peritoneal Irritation, and Hemoperitoneum in 77 Patients with Ectopic Gestation

Culdocentesis	Culdocentesis Positive	Peritoneal Signs	Blood Pressure < 90/40 mm Hg	Pulse ≥ 100/min	Hemoperitoneum ≥ 100 mL	Average Hematocrit (%)
Ruptured (n = 37)	30	25	8	19	37	33.6
Intact (n = 40)	24	7	2	5	28	37.3
Total patients	54	32	10	24	65	

Note: Culdocentesis is frequently positive in the absence of rupture. Patients are grouped by the presence (i.e., "ruptured") or absence (i.e., "intact") of hemoperitoneum. Note that only about half of patients with "ruptured" status had tachycardia.
From Cartwright PS, Vaughn B, Tuttle D: Culdocentesis and ectopic pregnancy. J Reprod Med 29:88, 1984. Reproduced by permission.

quantitative β-hCG is a poor predictor of size of the pregnancy or the risk of ectopic pregnancy, but serial testing is quite helpful. It is expected that the quantitative serum β-hCG level should double approximately every 2 days in the first trimester.

Serum progesterone determinations are not standardly used in the ED, but these may also help to identify a normal or abnormal pregnancy. Although not infallible, a serum progesterone level of less than 10 ng/mL is usually associated with a nonviable intrauterine pregnancy or ectopic pregnancy and a level greater than 25 ng/mL is usually associated with a viable intrauterine pregnancy.

To increase the accuracy of diagnosis, it is helpful to combine quantitative β-hCG testing with ultrasound examination. An empty uterus by transvaginal or abdominal ultrasound combined with certain quantitative serum β-hCG results can be quite helpful to the clinician. The quantitative range in which the ultrasonographer should detect an intrauterine pregnancy varies, but an intrauterine pregnancy should be detected if the serum β-hCG level is in the range of 1200 to 1500 mIU/mL when using a *transvaginal probe*, and greater than 6500 mIU/mL when using a *transabdominal probe*. Endovaginal ultrasonic scanning consistently identifies a 4-week gestational sac if the β-hCG level is 2000 mIU/mL or greater. The presence of a fetal pole and cardiac activity are detectable with endovaginal ultrasound scanning at approximately 6 and 7 weeks, respectively.[11] It is important to note that the absence of an intrauterine pregnancy by ultrasound, when the β-hCG level is *below the discriminatory zone* associated with positive ultrasound findings, is *nondiagnostic* and could represent an early viable normal pregnancy, a nonviable intrauterine pregnancy, a completed abortion, or an ectopic pregnancy. When no intrauterine pregnancy is detected by

ultrasound and the serum β-hCG *exceeds the discriminatory zone*, the chance of an ectopic pregnancy ranges from 86% to 100%.[12]

Culdocentesis, for some patients, may play an important role in the diagnosis of ectopic pregnancy. The test has an accuracy rate of 85% to 95%.[3,13,14] Romero and coworkers[15] reported that an ectopic pregnancy was found in 99% of patients when a positive pregnancy test and a positive culdocentesis were present. Although culdocentesis is most often positive in the presence of a frankly ruptured ectopic pregnancy, it may be diagnostic even in the nonruptured case when bleeding has been slow or intermittent. Note that many ectopic pregnancies leak varying amounts of blood for days or weeks before rupture. Hemoperitoneum has been found in 45% to 60% of cases of *unruptured* ectopic pregnancy proven at surgery.[7,16]

Hence, culdocentesis may be helpful in the stable patient whose ultrasound examination does not demonstrate an intrauterine pregnancy despite a quantitative serum β-hCG level in the appropriate range. Although some clinicians opt for outpatient monitoring of serial β-hCG levels in this setting, patients for whom the clinician has a high suspicion for ectopic pregnancy (e.g., the patient who has or had significant discomfort) or for whom close follow-up cannot be ensured may be candidates for culdocentesis.[3] Although a negative culdocentesis does not rule out an early ectopic pregnancy, patients with a nondiagnostic ultrasound and a negative culdocentesis generally represent patients at lower risk for "rupture" of an ectopic pregnancy during outpatient serum β-hCG monitoring. Patients with a nondiagnostic ultrasound examination and a serum β-hCG level below the threshold at which an intrauterine pregnancy should be visible on the ultrasound examination also must be individualized. Those patients with

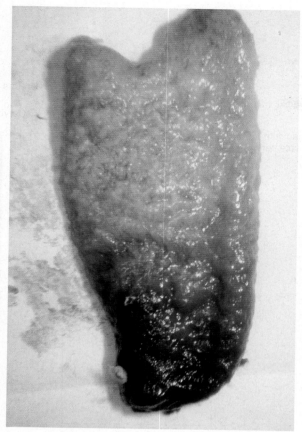

Figure 57–1 This decidual cast, a perfect outline of the uterine cavity, was initially thought to be a product of conception when found in the vaginal vault of a pregnant woman treated for abdominal pain and vaginal bleeding. The initial diagnosis was a spontaneous abortion, but this cast is *virtually diagnostic of an ectopic pregnancy.* The woman later developed hypotension and was found to have a ruptured tubal pregnancy.

TABLE 57–3 Equipment for Culdocentesis

Adjustable examination table with stirrups
Bivalve vaginal speculum
Uterine cervical tenaculum
19-gauge butterfly needle or 18-gauge spinal needle
27- or 25-gauge needle (for local anesthetic infiltration)
Ring sponge forceps
Syringes (20 mL)
Surgical preparation (iodinated, such as povidone-iodine)
Sterile water, cotton balls, 4 × 4 gauze sponges
Cocaine (10% solution) or benzocaine (20% solution)
Lidocaine (1%) with epinephrine
Culture media or test tube without anticoagulant

CONTRAINDICATIONS

The contraindications to culdocentesis are relatively few and include an uncooperative patient, a pelvic mass detected on bimanual pelvic examination, a nonmobile retroverted uterus, and coagulopathies. Pelvic masses may include tubo-ovarian abscesses, appendiceal abscesses, ovarian masses, and pelvic kidneys. It has been suggested that the only major risk with the procedure is that of rupturing an unsuspected tubo-ovarian abscess into the peritoneal cavity. This can be avoided by careful bimanual pelvic examination to exclude patients with large masses in the cul-de-sac.[19] Although there are no data to guide the age at which culdocentesis may be safely performed, the procedure is generally limited to patients who are beyond puberty. This limitation is suggested on the basis of anatomy and with the consideration that the procedure is difficult to perform through a small prepubertal vagina.

EQUIPMENT

The equipment required for culdocentesis is listed in Table 57–3. Either an 18-gauge spinal needle or a 19-gauge butterfly needle held by ring forceps is acceptable. It may be helpful to anesthetize the posterior vaginal wall at the site of the puncture with 1% to 2% lidocaine with epinephrine administered through a 27- or 25-gauge needle. Some physicians use a topical anesthetic (eutectic mixture of local anesthetics [EMLA], benzocaine) or a cocaine-soaked cotton ball to anesthetize the mucosa before infiltration with a local anesthetic. Although local anesthesia is often unnecessary (because *puncture of the posterior vaginal wall at the upper fourth of the vagina is generally no more painful than a venipuncture*), there is some advantage to use of a local anesthetic if multiple attempts at culdocentesis are required, as is sometimes the case. In addition, the epinephrine may produce vasoconstriction and may reduce bleeding associated with the needle puncture. Culdocentesis is often stressful to the patient, and all attempts should be made to render the procedure as painless as possible. Consideration of parenteral analgesia and sedation should also be made when the patient is uncomfortable or anxious.

TECHNIQUE

Preparation

Culdocentesis is an invasive procedure that in some hospitals requires a written, witnessed, and signed consent form from the patient, parent, or guardian when the patient's condition

significant pain, an unexplained low hematocrit reading, or postural vital sign changes (or near syncope) might be candidates for culdocentesis.

Blunt Abdominal Trauma

Historically, the diagnostic peritoneal lavage (DPL) and computed tomography (CT) have been used to identify hemoperitoneum in blunt trauma patients. The use of culdocentesis has also been advocated to aid in this diagnosis.[4,17] In the ED, two factors have largely obviated the need to perform invasive procedures to diagnose hemoperitoneum: (1) the increasing availability of high-resolution CT and (2) emergency clinicians trained to perform the bedside ultrasound FAST. (focused assessment with sonography for trauma). However, because small amounts of blood tend to collect in the recto-uterine pouch, the aspiration of clear peritoneal fluid is of great potential value in excluding a diagnosis of hemoperitoneum. This is especially helpful in situations in which ultrasound is unavailable or the patient is too unstable to leave the ED for a CT scan. In fact, culdocentesis may be more advantageous than DPL in some instances because there is less risk of urinary bladder perforation or bowel injury. In addition, previous abdominal surgery is not a relative contraindication to culdocentesis, as it is with DPL.[18]

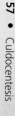

permits. If verbal consent is obtained, this action should be witnessed and a notation made in the medical record documenting that the procedure was described, complications were discussed, and any alternatives (e.g., CT, sonography, immediate laparoscopy) were offered when appropriate.

Once written or verbal consent is obtained, place the patient in a lithotomy position with the head of the table slightly elevated (reverse Trendelenburg position) so that intraperitoneal fluid gravitates into the rectouterine pouch. Place the patient's feet in stirrups. Premedicate with intravenous opioids or sedatives if appropriate. The administration of nitrous oxide analgesia also is an accepted practice. *When nitrous oxide is used during the procedure, make sure that there is a chaperone in the room (and documented) because some patients develop sexual delusions under this agent.* Although pain associated with culdocentesis needle passage is generally minor, the judicious use of analgesia and sedation makes the procedure easier for both clinician and patient.

If radiographs are indicated, take them before culdocentesis, to avoid confusion of a procedure-induced pneumoperitoneum.

Exposure

Perform a bimanual pelvic examination before culdocentesis to rule out a fixed pelvic mass and to assess the position of the uterus. It is possible to palpate an adnexal mass if the mass exceeds 3 cm in diameter. Insert the bivalve vaginal speculum and open it widely by adjusting both the height and the angle thumbscrews. Grasp the posterior lip of the cervix with the toothed uterine cervical tenaculum and elevate the cervix (Fig. 57–2). Warn the patient in advance that she may feel a sharp pain when the cervix is grasped with the tenaculum. Inform the patient also that bleeding from the tenaculum puncture site or culdocentesis site, or both, may produce postprocedure spotting.

Use the tenaculum to elevate a retroverted uterus from the pouch, exposing the puncture site, and stabilizing the posterior wall during the needle puncture. Some clinicians prefer to use longitudinal traction on the cervix to produce the same result. The vaginal wall adjacent to the rectouterine pouch will be tightened somewhat between the inferior blade of the bivalve speculum and the elevated posterior lip of the cervix. This tightening of the vaginal wall exposes the puncture site and keeps it from moving away from the needle when the wall is punctured.

After the tenaculum is applied and the posterior lip of the cervix is elevated or traction is applied, swab the vaginal wall in the area of the rectouterine pouch with surgical preparation followed by a small amount of sterile water. Administer local anesthesia (1% lidocaine with epinephrine) at this point. Anesthesia may be injected with a separate 27- or 25-gauge needle or by the spinal needle to be used for the culdocentesis. Use a cotton ball soaked in cocaine or benzocaine solution for topical anesthesia of the posterior vaginal wall before infiltration with a local anesthetic. Attach the needle to a 20 mL syringe. *A smaller syringe might not be long enough to allow adequate control of the needle*, and the clinician's hand may block the view of the puncture site if a smaller syringe is used.

Aspiration

Following local anesthesia, advance the syringe and the spinal needle parallel to the lower blade of the speculum. Fill the

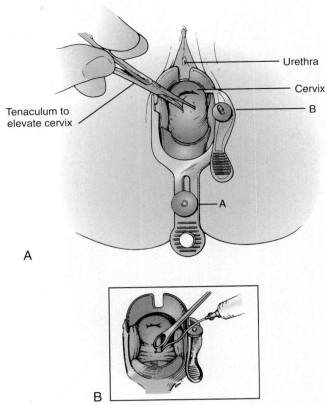

Figure 57–2 *A,* Preparation for culdocentesis. Note that one opens the speculum widely by using both the height (*A*) and the angle (*B*) adjustments. The cervix is grasped on the posterior lip with a toothed tenaculum. X marks the site for puncture of the vaginal wall. *B,* The use of a butterfly needle for culdocentesis. The needle is inserted 1 cm posterior to the point at which the vaginal wall joins the cervix. (*A, From Vander Salm TJ, Cutler BS, Wheeler HB: Atlas of Bedside Procedures. Boston, Little, Brown, 1979; B, from Webb MJ: Culdocentesis. JACEP 7:452, 1978.*)

syringe with 2 to 3 mL of saline (nonbacteriostatic) before puncture. Following needle puncture, the free flow of the fluid from the syringe expels tissue that may have clogged the needle and confirms that the needle tip is in the proper position and is not lodged in the uterine wall or the intestinal wall. Use saline rather than air, because if air is used, it is difficult to interpret the presence of free peritoneal air on subsequent radiographs. To avoid the need to change the syringe during the procedure, 1% lidocaine may be used for both anesthesia and confirmation of proper needle placement; however, the bacteriostatic property of this agent precludes its use if the procedure is performed to obtain fluid for culture.

Penetrate the vaginal wall in the midline 1 to 1.5 cm posteriorly (inferiorly) to the point at which the vaginal wall joins the cervix (Fig. 57–3).[20] Pass the needle a total of 2 to 2.5 cm.[20,21] Apply gentle suction with the syringe while slowly withdrawing the needle. Avoid aspirating any blood that has accumulated in the vagina from previous needle punctures or from cervical bleeding because this may give the false impression of a positive tap. Minimize bleeding from the puncture site in the vaginal wall by adding epinephrine to the local anesthetic.

Blood or fluid may be obtained immediately but may also be obtained as the needle is withdrawn from the peritoneal

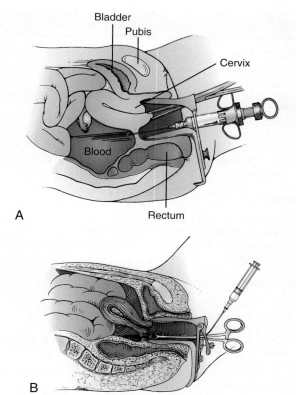

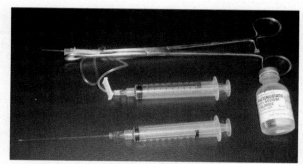

Figure 57–4 Culdocentesis may be performed with a 19-gauge butterfly needle held with ring forceps, or with a spinal needle on a 10-mL syringe. Fill the syringe with saline and confirm intraperitoneal penetration with the free flow of fluid into the cavity, avoiding creation of a pneumoperitoneum. The ringed forceps grasp the wings of the butterfly needle to direct its placement under direct vision. An assistant aspirates for fluid through the proximal end of the tubing. With the spinal needle, the operator applies suction and continues suction during slow withdrawal. (*From Webb MJ: Culdocentesis. JACEP 7:451, 1978.*)

Figure 57–3 The needle is advanced parallel to the lower blade of the speculum. Aspiration is continued throughout the gradual withdrawal of the needle. *A*, The use of a spinal needle. *B*, The use of a butterfly needle and ringed forceps. (*A, from Vander Salm TJ, Cutler BS, Wheeler HB: Atlas of Bedside Procedures. Boston, Little, Brown, 1979; B, from Webb MJ: Culdocentesis. JACEP 7:452, 1978.*)

cavity. Therefore, it is important to aspirate throughout the *gradual withdrawal* procedure. If no fluid is aspirated, reintroduce the needle and direct it only slightly to the left or right of the midline. Directing the needle too far laterally may result in puncture of mesenteric or pelvic vessels. If no fluid is obtained on the first attempt, *repeat the procedure.*

Some physicians prefer the use of a 19-gauge butterfly needle held with a ring forceps (Fig. 57–4).[20] This technique offers a built-in guide to needle depth and allows for good control of the needle during puncture. An assistant must aspirate the tubing while the physician controls positioning and withdrawal of the needle.

Fluid that is aspirated may be old nonclotting blood, bright red blood, pus, exudate, or a straw-colored serous liquid. Any fluid that is not blood should be submitted for Gram staining, aerobic and anaerobic culture, and cell counts. Blood should be observed for clotting. Blood should also be sent for a hematocrit determination.

INTERPRETATION OF RESULTS

An interpretation of the results of culdocentesis depends primarily on whether any fluid was obtained. In the absence of a pathologic condition, one will often aspirate 2 to 3 mL of clear yellowish peritoneal fluid. When there is no return of fluid of any type (a so-called dry tap), the procedure has *no diagnostic value.* Because a dry tap is nondiagnostic, it should not be equated with normal peritoneal fluid. In addition,

when less than 2 mL of clotting blood is obtained, this is also considered to be a nondiagnostic tap because the source of this small amount of blood may be the puncture site on the vaginal wall. Such blood will usually clot. More than 2 mL of *nonclotting blood* is certainly suggestive of hemoperitoneum. However, some researchers interpret as little as 0.3 mL of *nonclotting* blood as a positive tap.[7] There is no particular significance to larger amounts of blood, because absolute volume may be related to the needle position or the rate of bleeding. Brenner and colleagues[6] reported no blood from culdocentesis in 5% of patients with proven ectopic pregnancies even when rupture had occurred. In the series of 61 patients with surgically proven ectopic pregnancy reported by Cartwright and associates,[7] culdocentesis performed within 4 hours of surgery was positive in 70%, negative in 10%, and inadequate in 20%. "Positive" in their series was defined as obtaining at least 0.3 mL of nonclotting blood with a hematocrit of greater than 3%. "Negative" was defined as obtaining 0.3 mL of fluid with a hematocrit of less than 3%. An "inadequate" tap was one in which no fluid was obtained. In the 252 surgically proven ectopic pregnancy patients having culdocentesis reported by Vermesh and coworkers,[16] 83% had a positive tap. They defined a positive tap as nonclotting blood with a hematocrit of greater than 15%.

Because culdocentesis is usually used to diagnose an ectopic pregnancy, a "negative tap" is one that yields pus or clear, straw-colored peritoneal or cystic fluid. A large amount of clear fluid (>10 mL) indicates a probable ruptured ovarian cyst, aspiration of an intact corpus luteal cyst, ascites, or possibly, carcinoma. The significance of these fluids and the interpretation of results are outlined in Tables 57–4 and 57–5. Elliot and colleagues[22] cautioned that obtaining greater than 10 mL of clear fluid should not automatically rule out an ectopic pregnancy because the latter may coexist with other pathologic conditions.

A "positive tap" is one in which nonclotting blood is obtained, although the presence of nonclotted blood does not confirm a tubal pregnancy. Intraperitoneal blood from any source (ectopic pregnancy, ovarian cyst, ruptured spleen) may remain unclotted after aspiration for days in the syringe as

TABLE 57–4 Interpretation of Culdocentesis Fluid

Aspirated Fluid	Condition and Suggested Differential Diagnosis
Clear, serous, straw-colored (usually only a few milliliters)	Normal peritoneal fluid
Large amount of clear fluid	Ruptured or large ovarian cyst (fluid may be serosanguineous); pregnancy may be coexistent
	Ascites
	Carcinoma
Exudate with polymorphonuclear leukocytes	Pelvic inflammatory disease
	Gonococcal salpingitis
	Chronic salpingitis
Purulent fluid	Bacterial infection
	Tubo-ovarian abscess with rupture
	Appendicitis with rupture
	Diverticulitis with perforation
Bright red blood*	Ruptured viscus or vascular injury
	Recently bleeding ectopic pregnancy* (ruptured or unruptured)
	Bleeding corpus luteum
	Intra-abdominal injury
	Liver
	Spleen
	Other organs
	Ruptured aortic aneurysm
Old, brown, nonclotting blood	Ruptured viscus
	Ectopic pregnancy with intraperitoneal bleeding over a few days or weeks
	Old (days) intra-abdominal injury (e.g., delayed splenic rupture)

*Note: The hematocrit of blood from a ruptured ectopic pregnancy is usually 15% or greater (97.5% of cases), but some authors use greater than 3% as positive.

TABLE 57–5 Interpretation of Culdocentesis

Positive

>0.5 mL nonclotting, bloody fluid (hematocrit > 12%)
Indicates hemoperitoneum
    When β-hCG also positive, ectopic pregnancy found in greater than 95%
    Nonspecific—can occur in intrauterine pregnancies and nonpregnant women (e.g., ruptured cyst, retrograde bleeding)
Does not necessarily indicate tubal rupture
    50%–62% of ectopic pregnancies with peritoneal blood may be unruptured

Negative

Serous fluid
    Excludes hemoperitoneum and tubal rupture
    False negative in 10%–15% of ectopic pregnancies (generally unruptured)

Nondiagnostic

Dry tap or clotting blood
    Excludes neither ectopic pregnancy nor hemoperitoneum
    15% of procedures are nondiagnostic
    16% of ectopic pregnancies have nondiagnostic study results

β-hCG, β subunit human chorionic gonadotropin.
From Brennan DF: Ectopic pregnancy: II. Diagnostic procedures and imaging. Acad Emerg Med 2:1090, 1995.

COMPLICATIONS

Culdocentesis is one of the safest procedures performed in the emergency setting, and there are probably fewer complications with this technique than with peripheral venous cannulation. Complications have been reported, the most serious being rupture of an unsuspected tubo-ovarian abscess.[20] Other complications include perforation of the bowel, perforation of a pelvic kidney, and bleeding from the puncture site in patients with clotting disorders. Because the most common complications result from the puncture of a pelvic mass, careful bimanual examination of the patient should help prevent this problem. Puncture of the bowel and the uterine wall occurs relatively frequently, but this does not generally result in serious morbidity. Obviously, penetration of the gravid uterus has greater potential for harm. Occasionally, one will aspirate air or fecal matter, confirming inadvertent puncture of the rectum. Although this may be disconcerting, it is seldom of serious clinical concern and requires no immediate change in therapy.

 REFERENCES CAN BE FOUND ON EXPERT CONSULT

a result of the defibrination activity of the peritoneum. The return of a serosanguineous fluid also suggests a ruptured ovarian cyst. The hematocrit of blood from active intraperitoneal bleeding is greater than 10%. In one series, the hematocrit of blood from a ruptured ectopic pregnancy was 15% or greater in 97% of cases.[6]

It should be emphasized that a positive culdocentesis in the presence of a positive pregnancy test does not always prove an ectopic pregnancy.[16] A ruptured corpus luteum cyst in the presence of an intrauterine pregnancy test is probably the most common cause of a false-positive scenario. When possible, ultrasound may help corroborate the culdocentesis findings.

CHAPTER **58**

Examination of the Sexual Assault Victim

Carolyn Sachs and Malinda Wheeler

Despite a decrease in violent crime overall, sexual assault remains a significant societal problem that affects hundreds of thousands of American men and women yearly, and millions worldwide. Approximately 18% of U.S. women and 3% of U.S. men experience attempted or completed rape sometime in their lives. This correlates to a 1-year incidence of rape of 876,100 for women/yr and 111,300 men/yr.[1] The majority of victims do not report the assault to anyone. Victims reported an average of one third of sexual assaults to law enforcement. After reporting to law enforcement, sexual assault victims may be transported to the emergency department (ED) for evaluation, examination, and treatment. Sexual assault victims may also present to the ED for treatment without prior contact with law enforcement. Victims are usually willing to cooperate with police investigation; others are not. Many states have laws that require medical personnel treating sexual assault victims to report the assault to local law enforcement. Clinicians must know their own state laws regarding this.

DEFINITIONS

Although many use the term synonymously with rape, *sexual assault* more accurately refers to any sexual contact of one person with another without appropriate legal consent.[2] Physical force may be used to overcome the victim's lack of consent, but this is not mandatory to prove assault. Lack of consent for sexual contact by intimidation, threats, or fear equals sexual assault. State law differs slightly on the definition of exact acts that constitute sexual contact and on which populations are unable to give legal consent. In general, persons under the influence of drugs or alcohol, minors, and persons who are mentally incapacitated are deemed unable to give consent for sexual contact.

Clinicians who treat sexual assault victims have a professional, ethical, and moral responsibility to provide the best medical and psychological care possible. At the same time, they must collect and preserve the proper medicolegal evidence that is unique to the evaluation of sexual assault cases.

Many hospitals and jurisdictions are affiliated with designated sexual assault examination teams that provide specialized evaluation and treatment for victims. These sexual assault response teams (SARTs) provide clear advantages, which are outlined toward the end of the chapter. However, victims may be brought to an ED that does not routinely provide specialized care for sexual assault. This chapter is designed to aid clinicians in such a general care location. Prepared emergency personnel can help attenuate the psychological and physical impact of sexual assault. Through proper care of the victim and careful acquisition of evidence, ED staff can help the victim to recover from the assault and can aid society in improving the prosecution and conviction of sexual predators.

EVALUATION AND TREATMENT OF PATIENTS SUFFERING FROM SEXUAL ASSAULT

Preparation

In most places, local jurisdictions or hospitals provide clinicians with detailed forms and instructions for the examination and documentation of sexual assault. This chapter is meant to supplement these instructions and forms. Clinicians should familiarize themselves with such local documents before performing a sexual assault examination. Careful step-by-step planning, using written protocols to guide the way in which a victim is handled in the ED and in follow-up, helps both to ensure the best care for the victim and to aid in the prosecution and conviction of assailants.

The ED must secure patient privacy and designate a separate area for the care of sexually assaulted patients. If medically and logistically possible, interview the victim in a private room separate from the examination room. EDs often have such an area frequently called the "grieving room" or the "family room." Many legal jurisdictions provide examination kits for the collection of forensic evidence from the victims. These kits should be available in the ED, and the staff should be familiar with them. If such kits are not provided by local jurisdiction, hospital staff may need to assemble their own kits from materials found in most EDs. Alternatively, private companies assemble and sell such kits (www.lynnpeavey.com or The Lynn Peavey Company, PO Box 14100, Lenexa, KS 66285-4100). Prepared kits save a tremendous amount of nursing and clinician time when a victim comes to the ED. A checklist for local requirements for sexual assault examinations should be included in the kits and serves as a reminder for all of the medicolegal procedures to be completed.

Although this chapter is primarily devoted to the evaluation of the adult female sexual assault victim, guidelines for the evaluation of the adult male sexual assault victim, the female child victim, the male child victim, and the accused assailant are provided in separate sections of this chapter. The same examiners designated to perform adult female examinations may easily perform male victim and assailant examinations; however, the examination of the child sexual assault victim often requires considerable expertise and training. When possible, medical staff with extra training in the examination of the child sexual assault victim should perform these examinations. If this is not possible, the special section of this chapter should provide emergency medical personnel with a framework to perform an initial examination.

Consent

Consent for the treatment of a sexual assault victim is mandatory. The victim has undergone an experience in which her right to grant or deny consent was taken from her, and obtaining consent for medical treatment and for the gathering of evidence has important psychological and legal implications. The victim has the right to decline medicolegal examination and even medical treatment. Before beginning evaluation and treatment, obtain witnessed, written, informed consent. If there are no local forensic examination forms, use the standard ED "consent to treat" forms, but make sure that the

1069

patient is well informed and gives her verbal consent to each step of the examination. Although some states mandate that medical personnel report sexual assaults to law enforcement, victims may decline to discuss the event with police. If the victim cannot give consent for a forensic examination owing to a reversible process (e.g., intoxication, an acute psychological reaction), wait several hours for the victim's mental status to improve to a reasonable level for consent to be obtained. When victims cannot give consent owing to minor status or developmental disability, the person authorized to give medical consent for the patient may consent for the examination unless he or she is a suspect in the assault. Many states allow an adolescent victim of a certain age (e.g., >12–14 yr) to consent to an examination for conditions related to sexually transmitted diseases (STDs), sexual assault, and pregnancy. State laws also differ in examiners' requirements to make an attempt to contact the legal guardian (unless he or she is a suspected perpetrator). Clearly, emergency personnel must be informed regarding their local laws concerning these requirements. In the rare case that a victim cannot give consent owing to a potentially irreversible medical condition, such as severe head trauma and coma, seek the advice of institutional legal council before proceeding with a forensic examination. In some cases, the next of kin may provide the needed consent, whereas in others, it may be necessary to obtain a court order to proceed.

History

The history of the event should include only those elements necessary to complete required forms, to perform a focused physical examination, and to collect evidence. Questions beyond this, such as the details leading up to the assault, should be left to the police investigators. Avoid the urge to "help" the alleged victim by unduly embellishing or detailing uncorroborated or nonmedical information supplied during the examination. Limiting the history not only shortens the evaluation in the ED but also helps to prevent discrepancies between the ED history and the official police investigation report, which could weaken the victim's case in court. Document pertinent medical history including last menstrual period, current contraception, recent anal-genital injuries or surgeries, and preexisting injuries.

The history of the event required by legal forms and/or protocol usually includes the time, date, and place of the alleged assault and a description of the use of force, threats of force, and the type of assault. Elements of force may include the type of violence used (e.g., grabbing, hitting, kicking, strangling, weapon use), threats of violence, the use of restraints, the number of assailants, the use of alcohol or drugs (forcibly or willingly) by the victim, and any loss of consciousness experienced by the victim. Sexually assaultive acts may include fondling (of breasts and/or genitalia); vaginal, oral, or anal penetration or attempted penetration (with fingers, penis, and/or objects); ejaculation on or in the body; and the use of a condom. The use of physical force or violence is partly a police matter, but from a medical standpoint, it is desirable to correlate positive findings on the physical examination (e.g., abrasions, ecchymosis, scratches) with a description of any force, restraint, or violence.

Document postassault activity commonly requested by forms including douching, bathing, urinating, defecating, gargling, or brushing teeth. These can alter the recovery of seminal specimens and other sexual assault evidence. In

TABLE 58–1 Maximal Reported Time Intervals for Sperm Recovery

Body Cavity	Motile Sperm	Nonmotile Sperm
Vagina	6–28 hr	14 hr–10 days
Cervix	3–7 days	7.5–19 days
Mouth	—	2–31 hr
Rectum	—	4–113 hr
Anus	—	2–44 hr

From Marx J (ed): Rosen's Emergency Medicine: Concepts and Clinical Practice, 6th ed. Philadelphia, Elsevier, 2006.

addition, question victims about potential injuries from any preassault bodily trauma.

Elements of the victim's history should help in deciding which potential samples to collect. For example, sperm may be recovered after intercourse from the cervix for up to 12 days and from the vagina for 5 days (Table 58–1).[3] If the victim had voluntary intercourse 48 hours before the examination and was sexually assaulted 3 hours before the examination, obtain samples from both the vagina and the cervix, and keep the two specimens separate. Taking a careful history makes it possible to perform an appropriate examination given these two separate events. In general, cervical swabs should be collected in addition to the usual vaginal swabs if the time between assault and examination is greater than 48 hours or if intercourse with a different person took place within a few days of the assault.

Obtain a gynecologic history in preparation for injury documentation and treatment plans. From a medicolegal standpoint, question victims about any recent gynecologic surgical procedures or unintentional genital trauma that might alter the expected normal genital appearance. The history should also include the use of any method of birth control before the attack (with information regarding any missed birth control pills), last normal menstrual period, last voluntary intercourse, gravidity and parity, and recent STDs. As with all assaulted patients, the medical history should include current medications, tetanus immunization status, and allergies.

While taking the history, observe the patient's ability to understand and respond appropriately to questions. Victims of sexual assault may not possess the capacity to consent to intercourse because of developmental disability, young age, or intoxication with drugs or alcohol. Consider obtaining blood, urine, or both, and testing for drugs or alcohol when the history suggests lapses of (or impaired) consciousness. Most often, victims who lack consenting capacity owing to developmental disability will have sufficient prior documentation of the condition. In the rare instance in which an examiner suspects previously undocumented developmental disability, formal examination of the patient's mental capacity can be assessed at a later time by request of the district attorney.

Physical Examination

The physical examination of the sexual assault victim differs from most other ED examinations because examiners are not only caring for a patient's physical and mental well being but also investigating a crime scene and collecting specific evidence. Remember to explain every step of the examination to the victim. Remind the victim to communicate any discomfort or questions during the examination and to ask for a break from the examination if needed. In addition, remind the victim of her right to decline any portion of the examination and the ability to stop at any point. Each victim should have the opportunity to have a family member, friend, victim advocate, or a combination of these, in the room during all parts of the examination. In some jurisdictions, state law mandates that victims be informed of this right.

Collection of Clothing

If not already collected by law enforcement, collect the clothes that the victim wore during the assault for potential evidence. The victim should disrobe by dropping clothes onto a clean sheet or a large clean piece of paper. Using gloved hands, place each item of clothing in a separate paper bag. Label all collected material meticulously and describe it in the chart. Bundle the sheet or paper and any material that might have fallen during the victim's disrobing and place it in a separate paper bag. When a victim's clothing must be collected, be sure to provide suitable dress for the victim to wear home after release from the ED.

General Body Examination

After the patient disrobes and is placed in a gown or other suitable covering, examine her body for signs of trauma and foreign material. Uncover one part of the body at a time to examine and then carefully re-cover it. This allows the victim to retain some modesty during the examination. Important areas for evaluation are the back, the thighs, the breasts, the wrists, and the ankles (particularly if restraints were used). Even in the absence of ecchymosis, note tender areas during the examination. Leaves, grass, sand, and other materials can occasionally be found in the hair or on the skin. Retain these materials as evidence. Document areas of trauma and evaluate further (e.g., with radiographs) as indicated by the type and extent of injury. Approximately 10% to 67% of sexual assault victims display bodily injuries.[4] Document these bodily injuries because they correlate significantly with successful perpetrator prosecution.[5] Bodily evidence may range from abrasions to major blunt and penetrating trauma. If the victim has not bathed, bodily evidence in the form of dried semen stains may be visible on the hair or the skin of the victim. In a darkened room, dried semen (and, unfortunately, many other substances) on skin may fluoresce under examination with short-wave light, such as that produced by a Wood's lamp or an alternative light source (ALS)[6] but may be noticed equally well by its reflective appearance under regular room lighting.[7] Use moistened swabs to collect potential dried secretions; then air-dry them thoroughly and preserve as evidence. The underside of fingernails can also contain evidence. Rape victims may have fragments of the assailant's skin, blood, facial hair, or other foreign material from the rape site beneath their fingernails. Obtain fingernail scrapings by cleaning under a victim's nails with a toothpick or small swab or by cutting the nails closely over a clean paper. Fold the toothpick and debris into the paper, place it in an envelope, and package it with the other specimens.

Imaging

Photographs can be a valuable addition to the documentation of bodily injury. Medical institutions may employ professional-quality photographic teams; others must rely on law enforcement for photo documentation. Most institutions require patient consent for photographs taken by hospital personnel. Optimally, institutions should arrange a prior plan to handle film or digital media according to a written "chain of custody." Alternatively, self-developing film (Polaroid) that can be permanently labeled (e.g., subject, date, details of pictured injury) may be used. The photographs should be labeled immediately and may be added to the legal evidence. In some jurisdictions, photographs of physical injuries will be taken and retained by an accompanying law officer. These photographs may serve as evidence or may simply refresh the examiner's memory at the time of the trial.

Oral Evaluation

If indicated by the history, inspect the oral cavity closely for signs of trauma and collect evidence if indicated. Mouth injuries from forced oral copulation include lacerations of the labial or lingual frenulum, mucosal lacerations, and abrasions. Injury to the lips is often produced by the victim's own teeth as her lips are forced inward with the perpetrator's penis. Potential injuries to the posterior pharyngeal wall and soft palate include petechiae, contusions, and lacerations. Document these injuries at the time of initial examination because mucosal injuries heal quickly and may not be present hours or days later. Collect potential evidence with swabs rubbed between the teeth and the buccal mucosa on both upper and lower gingival surfaces bilaterally. Spermatozoa have been identified in oral smears for hours after the attack despite toothbrushing, using mouthwash, or drinking various fluids and may show valuable evidence up to 12 hours after examination.[8] Collect any foreign material (e.g., hair) to include as potential evidence. During oral inspection, local law enforcement may request that examiners collect buccal cell swabs to provide the crime laboratory with a sample for victim DNA reference.

Genital Examination

Once the victim is in the lithotomy position, inspect the thighs and perineum for signs of trauma and for foreign materials, such as seminal stains. Use an ultraviolet light again to look at suspicious dried secretions. Many jurisdictions recommend routine collection of swabs from the external genital area owing to the high likelihood of evidence being present and the inconsistent fluorescence of seminal fluid with the Wood's lamp.

Pubic Hair Samples

Before the pelvic examination, comb the victim's pubic hair for foreign material (particularly pubic hair belonging to the assailant). Place a clean paper below the victim's buttocks with the victim in the lithotomy position and comb the pubic hair onto the paper. Fold these hairs and the comb into the paper and place them directly into a large paper envelope to be given to law enforcement. Foreign pubic hairs can often provide enough cellular DNA material from the root to enable the crime laboratory to perform DNA analysis. In addition, specialized laboratories possess the capability of performing mitochondrial DNA analysis from the hair shaft in many cases.

Significant hair transfer occurs in less than 5% of assaults.[9] In the small minority of cases in which foreign suspect hairs must be compared with victim hairs, a pulled victim sample may be desired. Although the routine pulling of the patient's hair from the roots may provide the best sample, the act of pulling the victim's hair may be considered insensitive and

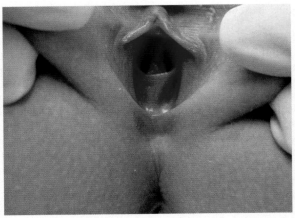

Figure 58–1 The hymen in a pre-pubertal female as seen with inferior labial traction.

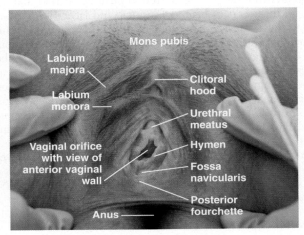

Figure 58–2 Female anatomy.

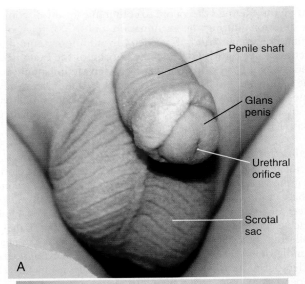

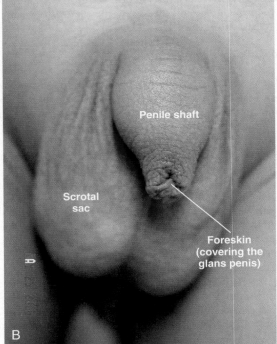

Figure 58–3 Male anatomy. *A,* Circumcised male. *B,* Uncircumcised male.

unnecessary during the initial evaluation. In addition, these hairs will rarely be needed because the vast majority of cases are never adjudicated, and those that are rarely concern this type of evidence. A victim can provide the hairs at a later time, if needed; often, the victim is willing to pluck the hairs herself at that time.

The genital examination of the sexual assault victim differs considerably from most ED pelvic examinations. First, perform a careful evaluation of the vulva and the vaginal introitus for signs of trauma. The techniques of separation and traction move the tissues most likely to suffer injury into view. In performing separation, use both hands to separate the labia laterally in each direction and inspect the posterior fourchette and vaginal introitus. Similarly, in performing tractions, use both hands to grab each labia majora and apply gentle inferior labial traction (i.e., toward the examiner); this gives a much-improved view of the hymen, especially in pre-pubertal females (Fig. 58–1). If the examiner fails to perform these maneuvers, traumatic genital injuries may be missed.

Be familiar with female (Fig. 58–2) and male (Fig. 58–3) genital anatomy, including all terms used to describe these areas. Although most novice examiners concern themselves with detecting injuries to the hymen, the majority of *sexual assault–related vaginal injuries occur to the posterior fourchette*[10] (Fig. 58–4). In fact, hymenal injuries are rare in sexually active adult women and are more commonly observed in sexually inexperienced adolescents[11,12] (Fig. 58–5). More uncommon injuries to the vaginal walls and cervix may be discovered during the speculum examination. Reported rates of genital injury among forensically examined victims range from 6% to 20% without colposcopy to 53% to 87% with colposcopy.[10,12] Most importantly, examiners must be cognizant of the fact that a completely normal genital examination can still be consistent with forced sexual assault. In fact, a study of more than 1000 sexual assault victims found that almost half of all victims with forensic evidence positive for sperm had no genital injury.[4]

Colposcopy

Teixeira[13] first described the use of colposcopy for documentation in sexual assault in 1981. Although it is not readily available in most EDs, the use of colposcopy has revolutionized the documentation of injury. The colposcope provides magnification, a bright light source, and usually permanent documentation of injuries in the form of traditional film or digital pictures or video. In one small study, the colposcope increased the rate of genital injury detection from 6% to 53%.[14] Colposcopes with photo or video attachments provide excellent photographic documentation for court and allow for expert practitioner review for court testimony without subjecting the victim to reexamination (Fig. 58–6). Experienced sexual assault examiners programs are increasingly using

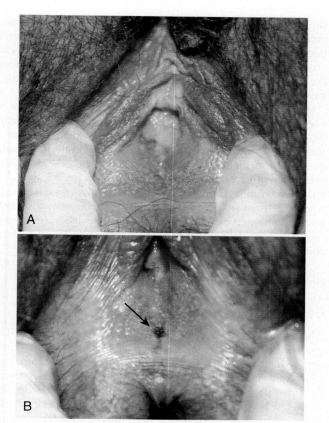

Figure 58–4 Posterior fourchette injuries are the most common site in the adult victim of sexual assault. *A,* Before toluidine blue application. *B,* After toluidine blue application.

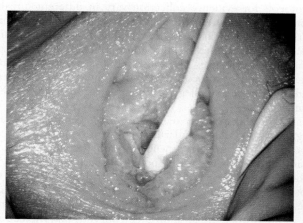

Figure 58–5 Hymenal injury at the 6 o'clock position (*arrow*), usually found in the adolescent female. Such injuries are uncommon in adults.

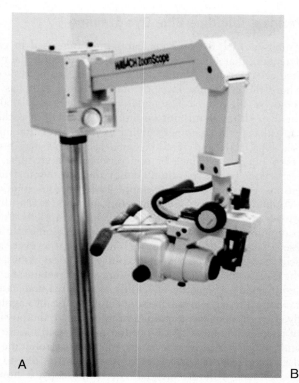

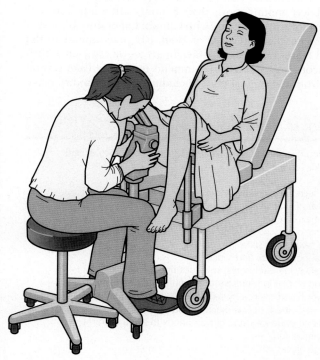

Figure 58–6 Colposcope (*A*) and method of examination (*B*). This technique is not a standard intervention by an emergency physician.

high-quality digital cameras mounted on a tripod to obtain excellent images that are indistinguishable from those obtained with colposcopy. ED practitioners often have access to such equipment. Colposcopically visible injuries have also been described in adolescent women after first consensual intercourse; hence, genital injury does not always correlate with nonconsensual vaginal penetration.[15] Conversely, a totally normal genital examination by colposcopy is often found after sexual assault. Even in sexually inexperienced adolescents, forced penetration can occur without leaving discernible genital injury.[16] Although prior victim sexual experience decreases the likelihood of finding genital injury, experts cannot fully explain the reasons why some rape victims sustain measurable genital injury when others do not.

Forensic Evidence Collection

Protocols for evidence collection vary in different jurisdictions. Many rape evaluation centers have abandoned the cumbersome rape kits that have been used in the past, substituting simple collection methods that concentrate on important and usable legal evidence. The following discussion is patterned after the model protocol suggested by the state of California and the American College of Emergency Physicians (ACEP) manual.[2]

During inspection of the external genitalia, rectum, vagina, and cervix, standard forensic specimens should be obtained. Lubricate the speculum with warm water rather than lubricant owing to the potential spermicidal activity of lubricants. However, if lubricants are inadvertently used, the potential for corruption of DNA evidence should be negligible.[17] Generally, the specimens collected will be determined by victim history and local protocol, but they may include any of the items listed in Table 58–2. Some protocols recommend that examiners make a wet mount of one swab from the vaginal pool and look at it under the microscope for the presence of motile sperm. Because of rapid cell death, studies have shown a negligible chance of finding motile sperm from a vaginal wet mount more than 8 hours after intercourse.[18] Furthermore, in complying with Clinical Laboratory Improvement Amendments (CLIA) of 1988, ED practitioners in the United States rarely have sufficient access or experience with microscopy to routinely recommend this step. Take several swabs from the vaginal pool (including the one used to make

TABLE 58–2 Potential Evidence Collected

Clothing (list and describe all clothing collected on chart and checklist form)
Debris
Dried secretions, swabs, and slides
External genital swabs and slides
Pubic hair combings
Oral mucosal swabs and slides
Rectal swabs and slides
Vaginal pool swabs and slides
Vaginal lavage fluid in test tube or urine container
Tampon or condom present in vagina (dried or frozen)
Urine or blood toxicology sample (timed collection)
Reference blood, buccal mucosa, and/or hair sample
Collect all evidence using gloved hands to avoid DNA contamination
Change gloves when necessary to avoid interlocation contamination

the wet mount, if done) and the external genitalia and run them over clean slides for a dry mount. Air-dry, label, and package all swabs and slides in paper envelopes for the local crime laboratory. Some EDs maintain specific equipment (i.e., a Dry Box) to aid the drying of specimens; in others, the swabs and slides must be left out until completely dried.

Many crime laboratories also request collection of a vaginal washing. For this procedure, insert 5 mL of sterile (but not bacteriostatic) water or saline into the vagina and then remove it. Place the washing in a sealed container (such as those for urine collection or a red-top blood tube) for later examination for evidence. In addition, collect cervical swabs if the time from assault to examination (the postcoital interval) is greater than 48 hours or if there is a history of recent consensual intercourse as well. The crime laboratory may recover sperm from cervical specimens up to 12 days after coitus.[3]

Label each sample separately. Record the area from which the specimen was collected in the chart.

Genital Testing for STDs

The Centers for Disease Control and Prevention (CDC) guidelines suggest obtaining a (cervical, rectal, or oral) culture or polymerase chain reaction (PCR) specimen, or both, for *Chlamydia trachomatis* and for *Neisseria gonorrheae*. However, the majority of SART programs in the United States do not routinely perform these tests.[19] STD testing during sexual assault examination can detect only preassault infection and provides no meaningful information for the crime laboratory. In addition, the routine prophylactic treatment with antibiotics effective against *N. gonorrheae* and *C. trachomatis* makes detection of these preexisting infections superfluous; however, clinicians might want to consider obtaining cultures on child victims in whom the presence of an STD would be indicative of previous abuse.

Perineal Toluidine Blue Dye Staining

Toluidine blue dye is a nuclear stain, often used in cancer detection, that adheres to areas of injury (subepithelial nucleated cells) but not to intact epithelial cells. It adheres to skin where the epidermal layer of non-nucleated cells has been removed (Fig. 58–7). The underlying nucleated cells take up the dye. Although it is not a uniform standard of care, the dye can enhance the examiner's ability to visualize genital injuries (see Figs. 58–4 and 58–5). Genital lacerations may provide corroborating evidence of nonconsensual intercourse. The test is done before speculum examination or other instrumentation. To outline injuries, apply a 1% aqueous solution of toluidine blue dye to the perineum and wipe excess dye off with a cotton ball moistened with lubricating jelly. A swab containing the dye is commercially available. Some examiners use 1% acetic acid to remove the excess; however, acetic acid may produce pain when it contacts injured tissues. After the excess dye is removed, any areas that retain the stain signify injury. Separate any folds of the area and carefully examine them to avoid missing injuries. Ideally, apply the dye before speculum examination to eliminate the possibility of iatrogenic injury. The procedure is shown in Figure 58–7 and Table 58–3. In one study, the use of toluidine blue dye increased the injury detection rate from 16% to 40% in women without the use of colposcopy;[20] however, injuries detected with the aid of toluidine blue dye are not

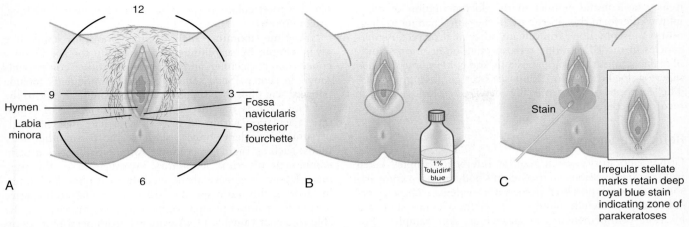

Figure 58–7 *A*, During a sexual assault, injuries are often multiple and typically occur between the 3, 6, and 9 o'clock positions. *B* and *C*, Traumatic skin injury can be highlighted by applying toluidine blue to the perineum and vaginal area, then wipe it off to show the lesions. (*A, From Marx: Rosen's Emergency Medicine: Concepts and Clinical Practice, 6th ed. Philadelphia, Elsevier, 2006.*)

TABLE 58–3 Toluidine Blue* Staining of the Perineum to Detect Microabrasion
1. Collect all external genital specimens as indicated by examination before dye application.[†]
2. Before speculum examination or instrumentation, apply 1% toluidine blue to the entire vulva (labia majora, labia minora, posterior fourchette, perineal body, and perianal area). The anus may also be stained. Do not use dye in the vaginal vault or mucous membranes.
3. Allow to dry for approximately 1 min.
4. Remove excess dye with a spray of 1% acetic acid, irrigating the area until excess dye is removed. A water-soluble lubricant can also remove excess stain.
5. Gently blot the area with 4 × 4 gauze pads. DO NOT rub the area.
6. Photograph the area if indicated.
7. The dye will fade in 1–2 days.

*A prefilled swab (T-Blue Swab/TBS, Tri-Tech, Inc.) is available through The National Forensic Nursing Institute).

[†]This does not interfere with DNA or semen testing.

Modified from The National Forensic Nursing Institute (NFNI.org/t-blueswab.html).

100% specific for sexual assault because such injuries have also been found after consensual intercourse, especially in adolescents.[21]

If seminal stains are noted on the perineum, collect samples before toluidine blue application. Contrary to earlier thinking, the use of toluidine blue dye does not interfere with recovery of DNA evidence[22] and has proved safe for mucosal application.[23]

Anal Evaluation

The anal examination follows the genital examination in most cases (Fig. 58–8). Because of a reluctance of some victims to admit to anal penetration, some clinicians recommend an anal examination in all cases. Documentation of anal penetration holds significant value because it is a separate crime in addition to vaginal penetration and can add years to the sentence of the alleged perpetrator. Insert anal swabs approximately 2 cm into the anus. Gently move them in a circular motion and then remove them. Use the swabs to make slides, air-dry

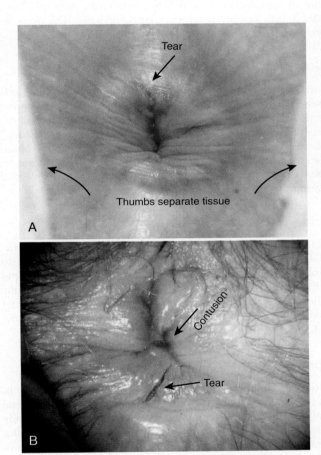

Figure 58–8 Anal injury is best seen with separation of perianal tissues. *A*, Anal tear in a 13-year-old boy after forced penile-anal penetration. *B*, Anal contusion and tear (*arrows*) in an adult male after forced penile-anal penetration.

them, and include them in evidence sent to the crime laboratory. In some jurisdictions, rectal washings may also be requested. To do this, inject 5 to 10 mL of normal saline into the rectum with a syringe and a small plastic intravenous catheter. Then aspirate and preserve the fluid as evidence. Use toluidine blue dye, as described earlier, to better visualize injury. Anoscopy is not a routine part of the examination, but it may be a useful adjunct in the documentation of rectal injuries. Perform this procedure in the same manner as diagnostic anoscopy done to evaluate other anal or rectal emergencies in the ED. In one retrospective observational study of male victims, the use of anoscopy and colposcopy provided superior documentation of injuries over colposcopy alone.[24] The location of anoscopically detected injuries may be recorded geographically.

Reference Samples

Crime laboratories often request reference samples taken from various locations on the victim's body to use in comparison testing with potential perpetrator evidence. These reference samples include blind swabs on the victim's skin in a location complementary to suspicious skin samples. For example, if a suspicious discharge is swabbed from the victim's right shoulder, take a control swab from the victim's left shoulder as well. Crime laboratories may also request other control samples for victim DNA reference, such as blood, buccal mucosa cells, head hairs, or pubic hairs. The need for such samples will be determined by local protocol.

Blood Tests

Some crime laboratories request blood samples for DNA reference or toxicology analysis or both. Include these samples in the materials sent to law enforcement and not to the hospital laboratory unless a firm procedural "chain of custody" has been established for this purpose. When collecting blood for toxicology testing, record the exact time of collection on the specimen so that the criminologist may estimate dose and timing of substances used to perpetrate the assault.

Urine Tests

Perform bedside urine β–human chorionic gonadotropin (β-hCG) testing in all women victims of childbearing age to exclude preexisting pregnancy before giving pregnancy and STD prophylaxis. Collect urine as requested by local crime laboratories for toxicology testing. Collect the victim's first available voided urine to optimize recovery of potential toxicologic evidence.

Spermatozoa, Semen, and DNA Testing

Motile and immotile sperm may be found microscopically in wet mounts of vaginal aspirates and in vaginal, oral, and rectal swabs. If the examiner is formally trained, evaluate the slide microscopically immediately after the physical examination. Examiners find sperm in 13% to 26% of vaginal wet mount specimens.[4,25] Early discovery of sperm may be helpful to law enforcement investigation. However, most ED examiners lack formal training in this process, and crime laboratories possess much higher sensitivity for sperm detection, making a negative initial wet mount unhelpful. For these reasons, many examiners do not routinely perform the wet mount examination.[4] After consensual intercourse with normal ejaculate, laboratory testing of vaginal secretions will likely be able to detect sperm after 3 days and in 50% of cases at 4 days.[26] However, despite penile penetration during sexual assault, the crime laboratories may fail to detect sperm. Reasons for this failure include inadequate specimen collection, degradation of ejaculate, azoospermia, failure of the per-

petrator to ejaculate, perpetrator vasectomy, victim washing, or condom use.

A crime laboratory analyst initially looks for semen in a given sample by searching microscopically for sperm on a concentrated specimen and by testing for other components found in semen. Such seminal plasma components include p30 and acid phosphatase. p30 is a glycoprotein specific to the prostate[27] and is regarded as conclusive evidence of semen (i.e., ejaculation within 48 hr), whereas acid phosphatase is presumptive evidence only because it can occur in other body fluids, such as vaginal secretions. Although this was a main component of crime laboratory investigation in the past, many laboratories have abandoned the acid phosphatase test in favor of the more specific p30 test.[27,28] Despite negative testing for seminal plasma components, laboratories may be able to detect valuable DNA evidence from persistent sperm cells or perpetrator epithelial cells.[29,30] As DNA testing technology rapidly changes, crime laboratory ability to perform a specific forensic test varies by location and over time. Most crime laboratories use PCR testing, which requires minimal material.

Chain of Custody

Give samples and other evidence to the police, a crime laboratory, or a forensic pathologist. Label each sample with the patient's name, hospital number, date, time of collection, area from which the specimen was collected, and collector's name. Package these specimens according to local crime laboratory specifications and transfer them to the next appropriate official (police officer, pathologist, or other individual) along with a written chain of custody, including a list of the specimens, the signature of each person who provided them, and the signature of each person who received them. If this chain is broken, important evidence might be deemed inadmissible in court.

TREATMENT

STD Prophylaxis

Address the issues of STD, pregnancy, psychological distress, and follow-up in the treatment of a sexual assault victim. Because preassault infection rates are not known, the risk of contracting an STD as a consequence of a sexual assault has been difficult to determine, and estimates vary widely (Table 58–4). Jenny and colleagues[31] found the postassault incidence of STDs to be 2% for chlamydia and 4% for gonorrhea. The reported rates of 12% for *Trichomonas* and 19% for bacterial vaginosis may reflect a preexposure infection because male

TABLE 58–4 Risk of Sexually Transmitted Disease after Sexual Assault	
Disease	**Risk (%)**
Gonorrhea	6–18
Chlamydia	4–17
Syphilis	0.5–3
HIV	<1

HIV, human immunodeficiency virus.
From Marx J. (ed): Rosen's Emergency Medicine: Concepts and Clinical Practice, 6th ed. Philadelphia, Elsevier, 2006.

transmission of these organisms is rare. The risk of developing herpes, hepatitis B, or human immunodeficiency virus (HIV) infection from being sexually assaulted has not been determined. However, HIV transmission has been noted.[32]

Although the chance of contracting an STD is small, examiners may choose to treat a victim prophylactically for gonorrhea, syphilis, and chlamydia; alternatively, examiners may choose to rely on follow-up cultures. Although most often termed *prophylaxis*, technically this antibiotic administration is considered "treatment" given so early that the disease is subclinical. The need for routine administration of medication to combat *Trichomonas* is unclear and many clinicians do not recommend it as a routine intervention. Gonorrhea resulting from a sexual assault may possibly be culturable within hours of the attack but is almost always culturable at a 2-week follow-up visit. Because of the omnipresent fear of contracting an STD from a sexual assault, it is reasonable to routinely offer some medication to all victims. Because victims tend to have a relatively low compliance with keeping follow-up visits, most examiners offer, at the least, gonorrhea and chlamydia treatment at the time of the initial examination.[19]

With the increasing prevalence of *N. gonorrheae* strains resistant to penicillin, tetracycline, and fluroquinolones, ceftriaxone and cefixime have become the CDC's recommended antibiotics of choice in targeting gonorrhea after sexual assault. In 2007 the recommendation for fluoroquinolone prophylaxis was withdrawn due to increased resistance patterns. Ceftriaxone also treats incubating syphilis. (The World Health Organization also considers the 1-g dose of azithromycin to be effective against incubating syphilis.) Spectinomycin (2 g intramuscularly) is a single-dose alternative for penicillin- and cephalosporin-allergic patients, but is not effective against incubating syphilis. No single-dose regimen for gonorrhea is effective against coexisting *C. trachomatis* infection. Therefore, give patients either a single dose of azithromycin (1 g orally) or a 7-day course of doxycycline (100 mg orally twice a day) or tetracycline (500 mg orally four times a day). A negative pregnancy test is a prerequisite for using either of the latter two antibiotics. Erythromycin may be used as a second alternative for chlamydia prophylaxis in the pregnant patient. Some examiners administer prophylaxis for *Trichomonas* with a single 2-g oral dose of metronidazole; although effective and recommended by the CDC,[33] this dose of metronidazole may cause significant nausea, vomiting, and/or diarrhea, which can interfere with the efficacy of pregnancy prophylaxis. Table 58–5 provides several options for STD prophylaxis.

Hepatitis B Prevention

Most sexual assaults involve perpetrators whose hepatitis B status is unknown by the victim. In these cases, the CDC recommends hepatitis B vaccination at the time of examination, followed by two more vaccines at the age-appropriate vaccine dose and schedule.[34] Give the vaccine to victims as soon as possible after the assault. The CDC recommends that it be given within 24 hours, but this may not be possible in all cases. When a perpetrator is known to be hepatitis B antigen–positive and the victim is known to be hepatitis B antigen–negative and has not been adequately vaccinated, the CDC recommends the administration of hepatitis B immunoglobulin (HBIG) in addition to vaccination. HBIG is not recommended if the patient is first seen by medical providers 14 days or more after the sexual exposure. Hepatitis B vaccine

TABLE 58–5 Centers for Disease Control and Prevention Recommended Regimens for Sexually Transmitted Disease Prevention after Sexual Assault[‡]

Ceftriaxone 125 mg IM in a single dose (for gonorrhea prevention)

or

Cefixime 400 mg orally in a single dose[ǁ]

plus

Metronidazole 2 g orally in a single dose (for trichomonas and bacterial vaginosis prevention)

plus

Azithromycin 1 g orally in a single dose (for chlamydia prevention)

or

Doxycycline 100 mg orally twice a day for 7 days

Alternative Oral Single-Dose Therapy for Preventing Sexually Transmitted Disease after Sexual Assault

Single-Dose Therapy for the Prevention of Gonorrhea (GC) in areas lacking GC quinolone resistance[‡]

Ofloxacin[†]	400 mg PO
or	
Ciprofloxacin*	500 mg PO
or	
Cefixime	400 mg PO

*Not for use in pregnancy. In pregnant cephalosporin-allergic patients, use spectinomycin 2 mg IM for prevention of GC.

[†]Also treats incubating syphilis.

[‡]Due to widespread resistance, fluoroquinolones are no longer recommended. Prophylaxis for hepatitis B (vaccination without HBIG) is also suggested.

[ǁ]Current recommendations for treatment of uncomplicated infection that may intuitively substitute for prophylaxis.

IM, intramuscularly; PO, by mouth.

should be administered simultaneously with HBIG in a separate injection site and the vaccine series should be completed. Complete CDC recommendations for hepatitis B treatment in sexual assault can be found at http://www.cdc.gov/mmwr/preview/mmwrhtml/rr5416a4.htm

HIV Prevention

In the nonassault scenario, the risk of transmission of HIV from one episode of unprotected consensual receptive vaginal intercourse with an infected individual is approximately 1 in 1000. The incidence with unprotected receptive anal intercourse is significantly higher, at 8 to 32 in 1000.[35] However, sexual assault victims often sustain tissue injury owing to the violent nature of the act, which may increase the transmission rate of the virus. Although treatment of parenteral occupational exposure to infected body fluids (i.e., needle stick) is believed to be effective based upon case-control studies, there is no proof that treatment of human sexual exposure prevents the transmission of the virus.[36] Furthermore, victims of sexual assault frequently present for treatment much later than those patients who have occupational exposures.

However, 40% of sexual assault victims fear contracting HIV after assault and should, at a minimum, receive counseling and, some argue, the option of taking anti-HIV medicines because they may be effective.[37,38] Unfortunately, immediate testing of the perpetrator remains a remote option. The majority of cases lack a perpetrator in custody for testing, and few state laws provide for legal preconviction HIV testing of alleged perpetrators.[39] In 2005, the U.S. Department of Health and Human Services (DHHS) Working Group on

Nonoccupational Postexposure Prophylaxis (nPEP) recommended administering postexposure prophylaxis (PEP) to sexual assault victims only in cases in which the perpetrator is known to be HIV-positive. This recommendation specifies a 28-day medication course for sexual assault victims who present for care less then 72 hours after the event with an HIV-positive perpetrator when that exposure represents a substantial risk for transmission (i.e., mucosal contact with genital secretions). As with occupational exposure, antiretroviral medications should be initiated as soon as possible after exposure. For sexual assault exposures with a perpetrator of unknown HIV status, the working group declined to offer a recommendation concerning antiretroviral administration; this must be addressed by practitioners on an individual case-by-case basis (http://www.cdc.gov/mmwR/preview/mmwrhtml/rr5402a1.htm). Given extreme negative outcome, the relative safety of treatment, and the lack of conclusive scientific evidence, at least two states have written policies to guide examiners with this complex issue. One such policy is shown in Table 58–6.

TABLE 58–6 Empirical Guide to Offering Human Immunodeficiency Virus Postexposure Prophylaxis

Has less than 72 hr passed since the assault occurred?
If no, do not offer PEP but recommend or refer for baseline and follow-up HIV antibody testing.
If yes, continue risk analysis.

Is survivor 12 yr of age or older?
If yes, continue risk analysis.
If no, consult pediatric HIV specialist.

What is the risk of HIV transmission from the assault?
Was the assault one with measurable risk of HIV transmission, such as an assault with anal penetration, vaginal penetration, or injection?
Was the assault one with possible risk of HIV transmission, such as oral penetration with ejaculation, an assault involving other mucous membranes (e.g., eyes), an unknown assault, an assault in which the victim bit the assailant or the assailant (with a bloody mouth) bit the victim?
Was the assault one with no risk of HIV transmission, such as kissing, object or digital penetration, ejaculation on intact skin, or an assault in which a condom was used?
What other risk factors were present in the assault, including presence of blood, survivor or perpetrator with STD, significant trauma to survivor; ejaculation by assailant, or multiple penetrations of the survivor?

Is the assailant's HIV status known?
If known HIV negative, do not offer PEP.
If known HIV positive:
  Recommend PEP if assault with measurable risk of HIV transmission has occurred.
  Recommend PEP if assault with possible risk of HIV transmission has occurred and at least one additional risk cofactor was present in assault.
  Offer PEP if assault with possible risk of HIV transmission has occurred with no additional risk cofactors present.
  Do not offer PEP for exposures carrying no risk.

Does the assailant engage in behaviors that put him or her at risk for contracting HIV?
High-risk groups include men who have sex with men, past or present injection drug users, commercial sex workers, individuals with multiple sex partners, individuals with prior convictions for sexual assault, and individuals with a history of prison incarceration.
If known or suspected risk factors exist:
  Recommend PEP if assault with measurable risk of HIV transmission has occurred.
  Recommend PEP if assault with possible risk of HIV transmission has occurred and more than one additional risk cofactor was present in assault.
  Recommend or offer PEP if assault with possible risk of HIV has occurred and only one additional risk cofactor was present in assault.
  Offer PEP if assault with possible risk of HIV transmission has occurred with no additional risk cofactors present.
  Do not offer PEP for exposures carrying no risk.
If assailant is not known and/or if assailant's risk factors are unknown:
  Offer PEP if assault with measurable risk of HIV transmission has occurred.
  Offer PEP if assault with possible risk of HIV transmission has occurred and more than one additional risk cofactor was present in assault.
  Offer PEP if assault with possible risk of HIV transmission has occurred and only one additional risk cofactor was present in assault.
  Offer or do not offer PEP if assault with possible risk of HIV transmission has occurred with no additional risk cofactors present.
  Do not offer PEP for exposures carrying no risk.

Offering PEP after sexual assault

Exposure Risk	Source		
	Known HIV[†]	Known or Suspected Risk Factors	Unknown Risk Factors or Unknown Assailant
Measurable risk*	R	R	O
Possible risk + more than 1 cofactor[†]	R	R	O
Possible risk + 1 cofactor[†]	R	R/O	O
Possible risk + 0 cofactors	O	O	O/N
No risk[‡]	N	N	N

*Acts with measurable risk of HIV transmission, including anal penetration, vaginal penetration, and injection with a contaminated needle.
[†]Acts with possible risk of HIV transmission, including oral penetration with ejaculation, unknown act, contact with other mucous membrane, victim biting assailant, and assailant with bloody mouth biting victim.
[‡]Acts with no risk of HIV transmission, including kissing, digital or object penetration of vagina, mouth, or anus, and ejaculation on intact skin.
HIV, human immunodeficiency virus; N, do not offer; O, offer; PEP, postexposure prophylaxis; R, recommend; STD, sexually transmitted disease.

Pregnancy Prophylaxis

Pregnancy occurs in up to 4.7% of sexual assault victims.[40] An estimated 22,000 annual rape-related pregnancies could be avoided if all victims received pregnancy prophylaxis within 72 hours.[41] Obtain a urine pregnancy test before administering postcoital contraception (PCC). Modern urine pregnancy tests possess a detection threshold approaching 20 to 25 mIU/mL and usually will be positive 1 to 2 weeks after conception, often before a menstrual period is missed.

Offer pregnancy prevention, using available oral PCC, to all sexual assault victims. The drug of choice for PCC is levonorgestrel, available in the United States in a commercial kit called "Plan B." In 2006, the U.S. Food and Drug Administration (FDA) approved the sale of Plan B without a prescription for individuals age 18 or older. Although the kit includes two pills containing 0.75 mg of levonorgestrel, each approved for administration 12 hours apart, a large World Health Organization (WHO) trial demonstrated that both pills may be taken at once with the same efficacy as the divided dose and the potential for increased compliance.[39] In the rare instance in which Plan B is unavailable, there are several combined oral contraceptive pills, known as the *Yuzpe regimen*, that may be used for PCC (Table 58–7).[42] The Yuzpe method prevents approximately 75% of pregnancies that would have otherwise occurred.[43] Plan B prevents 89% of pregnancies that would have otherwise occurred and causes fewer side effects. Potential adverse side effects of both methods include nausea, vomiting, and breast tenderness. If the patient vomits within 1 hour of taking a dose, repeat the dose. Some practitioners routinely offer prophylactic antiemetic therapy; others reserve such treatment for patients who vomit. All available evidence demonstrates no untoward effects on the fetus should pregnancy occur despite PCC.[44] The common practice of obtaining written patient consent for these medications seems unwarranted.

Unfortunately, religious preferences may deter some hospital EDs from providing PCC.[45] In these instances, the website and number listed in this paragraph provide practitioners information to give referral for easy access to PCC for patients who cannot obtain Plan B (i.e., those under 18 or those lacking funds to pay for the medication). In addition, given the ever-increasing availability of new methods and drugs for PCC, examiners may want to obtain up-to-date information from this site (www.not-2-late.com; telephone: 1-800-not-2-late).

Psychological Support

Sexual assault precipitates a psychological crisis for the patient, and psychological care should begin when the patient first arrives in the ED.[46,47] Reassure the victim that she will be in control of the examination, that she may ask questions at any point, and that she should notify the examiner whether anything hurts or whether she needs a break. Giving the victim control over her body and the examination is the first step toward psychological support. Unfortunately, if this is not made a priority, full recovery may be impaired. Sexual assault victims often develop post-traumatic stress disorder (PTSD), manifested by numbed responsiveness to the external world, sleep disturbances, guilt feelings, memory impairment, avoidance of activities, and other symptoms.[46] *Rape trauma syndrome* is the specific label for PTSD in this population.[46] The victim is particularly vulnerable to this stress disorder because of the following characteristics of sexual assault: (1) it is sudden and the victim is unable to develop adequate defenses; (2) it involves intentional cruelty or inhumanity; (3) it makes the victim feel trapped and unable to fight back; and (4) it often involves physical injury. Attention to the initial psychological care of the rape victim in the ED is fundamental and can reduce distress during forensic examination.[48]

Many areas have a local sexual assault crisis agency that can dispatch an advocate to be with victims during the interview and examination. This same agency may then provide the follow-up psychological support that must be offered to all victims. It is critical that all examiners maintain current contact information with these agencies and use their services when at all possible. The importance of this contact is emphasized in some areas by the fact that state law dictates that medical personnel contact a local sexual assault crisis agency when a victim presents for examination (California penal code 264.2, Notification of a Counseling Center). In the absence of immediate local crisis services, a hospital social worker may fill this role.

Postexamination Follow-Up

Medical and psychological follow-up for sexual assault victims is essential. Unfortunately, fewer than one third of the victims complete follow-up medical care.[49] Many protocols recommend a 2-week follow-up to reexamine any injuries and to repeat testing for STDs and pregnancy. The timing of this

---

TABLE 58–7 Emergency Contraception		
Brand	**Manufacturer**	**Pills**
Progestin Only Emergency Contraception Oral Therapy: Recommended		
Plan B	WCC	2 white pills immediately
Combined Emergency Contraception Oral Therapy Alternative When Plan B Unavailable		
Ovral	Wyeth-Ayerst	2 white pills immediately and in 12 hr
Ogestrel	Watson	2 white pills immediately and in 12 hr
Alesse	Wyeth-Ayerst	5 pink pills immediately and in 12 hr
Levlite	Berlex	5 pink pills immediately and in 12 hr
Nordette	Wyeth-Ayerst	4 light orange pills immediately and in 12 hr
Levlen	Berlex	4 light orange pills immediately and in 12 hr
Levora	Watson	4 white pills immediately and in 12 hr
Lo/Ovral	Wyeth-Ayerst	4 white pills immediately and in 12 hr
Low-Ogestrel	Watson	4 white pills immediately and in 12 hr
Triphasil	Wyeth-Ayerst	4 yellow pills immediately and in 12 hr
Tri-Levlen	Berlex	4 yellow pills immediately and in 12 hr
Trivora	Watson	4 pink pills immediately and in 12 hr

Note: Some regimens cause nausea and an antiemetic may be used. If vomiting occurs, repeat the dose of antiemetic.

follow-up seems less important, given the widespread use of prophylactic medication to prevent STDs and pregnancy. However, given the measurable failure rate of PCC, repeat pregnancy testing is critical for a victim who does not experience an expected menses. Further follow-up evaluations may be performed at 4 or 6 weeks and 4 to 6 months to repeat serologic tests for HIV, hepatitis B, hepatitis C, and syphilis. In addition, local volunteer support groups can be of immense assistance to a sexual assault victim; contact with such a group should be offered to each victim.

SPECIFIC POPULATIONS

Male Evidentiary Examinations

Male evidentiary examinations include all of the same forensic evidence collection as female victims except vaginal specimens. The forensic examination is guided by the history of events related by the victim. Most male victims suffer from anal penetration, or sodomy, by their perpetrator. In addition to rape trauma syndrome, heterosexual male victims may suffer psychological trauma, wondering whether the assault dictates a change in their sexual orientation. Examiners should inform such victims that the act of forced sodomy in and of itself does not indicate homosexuality. The increased risk of HIV transmission with anal intercourse is noted (see "HIV Prevention," earlier in this chapter). Because of the extreme emotional reaction men often feel after a sexual assault, they report the crime even more infrequently than do female victims.[50,51] The male victim deserves the same unhurried, nonjudgmental manner that the female victim deserves. Penile samples from the shaft, glans, corona, and scrotum may be obtained if there is oral or anal contact with the perpetrator.

Child Sexual Assault Examinations

In general, the care and treatment of the pediatric sexual assault patient requires expert knowledge and experience. Often, ED practitioners are the first professionals to examine a child victim and the presence of obvious genital injury and trauma may speak for itself, based on the history provided. However, in less obvious cases, the subtle variations of developmental changes and congenital anomalies may leave many clinicians ill-equipped to render an opinion concerning the findings indicative of sexual assault. The lives of children and families may be disrupted or severely affected, depending on the practitioner's opinion on the presence of genital penetration–type findings.

A well-known study by Adams and associates[52] demonstrates that the majority of children reporting sexual abuse have normal or nonspecific genital findings. As these authors succinctly stated with child sexual assault, it is "normal to be normal." In spite of expert physical examination, the vast majority of sexually abused children cannot be differentiated from nonabused children.[53] The discovery of one of the rare examination markers of injury should be confirmed with experts, and a discussion of these findings, although beyond the scope of this chapter, is covered extensively in other resources.[54] The potential sexual assault history provided by the child or caretaker should, therefore, remain the primary indicator that inappropriate genital contact has occurred. At the very least, the history warrants an investigation of the possibility of sexual abuse.

It cannot be emphasized enough that the examiners' responsibility to the care of the child victim of sexual abuse remains within the realm of experts. However, in EDs lacking timely availability of local experts, inspect the genitalia carefully in a nonhurried, child-friendly manner and, if indicated, collect forensic specimens. For the very young child with small genital orifices, the aid of a magnification source may be extremely helpful. Ask a parent to assist in the calming, reassurance, and positioning of the child for careful inspection. However, when the parent is a suspect, the practitioner must exclude that parent from the examination. Whereas the basic lithotomy position may be used for the older, more mature child or adolescent patient, using alternative positioning of the pediatric female patient is essential to inspection. The frog-leg position (with feet together and knees spread apart widely) using labial and/or gluteal separation and traction is often most beneficial in children (Fig. 58–9). Take care to gently separate the labia to avoid superficial examiner-induced injuries. In addition, to get a better look at the hymenal perimeter in prepubertal girls and the anus in girls and boys, ask them to turn over into the knee-chest position (Fig. 58–10). Genital findings that are deemed definitive of sexual abuse or penetration or are nonspecific are included in Table 58–8. However, many normal hymenal differences exist from one child to the next, and the definitive diagnosis of "abnormal" is often difficult for experts. When any doubt exists in the ED, describe the findings and refer the child for a later examination by experts. The availability of a colposcope or alternative photographic equipment with magnification clearly aids in documentation of any injuries that may heal before a time when an expert examination can be performed.

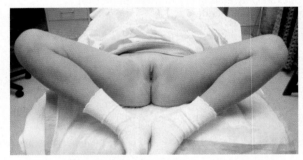

Figure 58–9 "Frog-leg" position to examine children.

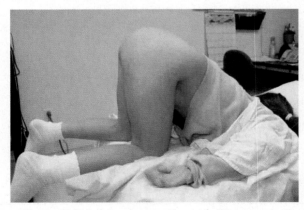

Figure 58–10 Child in knee-chest position to facilitate examination of the hymen.

TABLE 58–8 Genital Findings Possibly Related to Sexual Assault in Prepubertal Children*

Clear Evidence

Local areas of hymenal absence in knee-chest position
Hymenal transection
Anal laceration

Suspicious or Suggestive

Extremely narrow hymen (<1 mm)
Acute abrasions or lacerations of labia or vagina external to hymen
Excessive anal dilatation (<15 mm without stool in rectum)

Nonspecific

Redness
Increased vascularity
Labial adhesions

*Adapted from Adams JA, Harper K, Knudson S, et al: Examination findings in legally confirmed child sexual abuse cases: It's normal to be normal. Pediatrics 94:310, 1994.

When disclosure or genital injuries confirm possible penetration of the child, collect specimens for potential evidence. On all conscious prepubertal children, collect the specimens without inserting a pediatric speculum. If there is no bleeding or significant trauma, procedural sedation is rarely indicated in the majority of cases. If a child proves too uncooperative for an ED examination, refer the patient to a child sexual assault expert for examination the next day. For cases involving severe vaginal trauma or suspected internal genital injury (presenting with bleeding) that will possibly require surgical repair, conduct the examination under deep procedural sedation or general anesthesia. External anal and vulvar swabs are usually collected without difficulty on a child of any age. Owing to a lack of estrogen, contact with the prepubertal hymen generates much pain, making vaginal samples difficult to obtain. The samples should remain the very last evidence collected. Make every effort possible to avoid swab contact with hymenal tissues during collection. Vaginal aspirates using a feeding tube or plastic angiocatheter may provide an alternative to vaginal swabs.

Genital specimens to screen for STDs remain a controversial issue in the realm of child abuse experts. For *N. gonorrheae*, at least, the literature supports the notion that all infected children will display an abnormal discharge.[55] With very young children, the practitioner may have only one opportunity to collect vaginal specimens without causing agitation that prohibits further examination. Forcing specimen collection using physical restraint is considered a second assault on the child. Because the child presents for possible sexual abuse, the primary specimens collected should be for forensic DNA analysis. STD detection and treatment can be performed at a later time. Clinicians should consult local child abuse centers for protocols regarding immediate STD specimen collection, referrals, and follow-up services.

Suspect Examinations

As forensic evidence collection in the form of DNA retrieval continues to evolve, EDs may see more requests from local law enforcement for evidence collection from suspects. EDs should be familiar with local and state protocols, especially regarding consent. Some jurisdictions permit suspect examination without consent, given imminent degradation of potential biologic evidence. Other jurisdictions require that suspects give consent or, at the very least, that police obtain a search warrant from the court. The sooner a suspect is apprehended and brought in for a medical-forensic examination, the better the quality of forensic biologic evidence.

Performing a medical-forensic examination on a suspect can give important corroborating information for the investigation of a crime. It can also help to exonerate the innocent. Law enforcement should always be in attendance during any suspect examination to address safety issues for the examiner. Furthermore, the suspect and victim should never encounter one another in the hospital setting during the examination period, and care should be taken to examine the victim and suspect in separate locations within the ED. It is extremely beneficial to conduct the victim examination and history before the suspect's examination to search for physical findings on the suspect that may be indicated by the victim's history. For example, if, during the victim's history, she relates that she scratched the suspect's left shoulder in defense, the examiner can be certain to examine, document, and preferably photograph the presence (or absence) of the injury on the suspect's left shoulder.

The physical and evidentiary examination for the alleged suspect is similar to the victim examination. The primary differences lie in history taking, reference samples, and more "blind" samples. During suspect examinations, law enforcement officers, rather than the suspect, provide the history of the event. Collect reference samples of head and pubic hairs as well as blood, saliva, and urine, if possible. Apply special attention not only to nail scrapings but also to swabbing all of the fingers for possible vaginal epithelial cells from digital penetration. Penile swabs include collecting from the shaft and corona of the glans, then separately collecting swabs from the scrotum for vaginal secretions. From an unwashed penis, swabs almost uniformly show evidence of female cells up to 24 hours after coitus.[29]

Suspect examinations require the same amount of professional sensitivity and respect that any patient receives within the ED. It is not within the realm of the clinician's expertise to determine whether or not the suspect is guilty or innocent.

The Unconscious Victim and "Date Rape"

Alcohol and other drugs play an important role in many sexual assaults. Half of all sexual assaults involve drug or alcohol ingestion.[56] In many cases, it is unclear whether a drug was taken voluntarily or whether it was surreptitiously given to the assaulted victim.

Popular media has raised public awareness of drugs used to facilitate sexual assault under the term *date-rape drugs* (Table 58–9).[57] *Whereas date-rape drugs are of significant concern, extensive forensic testing in the United States shows that a minority of SA cases involve the scenario in which a victim's drink is covertly spiked with a tablet, capsule, or powder or liquid containing mind-altering drugs.*[58]

The drugs most commonly associated with drug-facilitated sexual assault are ethanol, marijuana, cocaine, and benzodiazepines. Often, more than one drug is found. Although *any type of sedative or hypnotic drug, or combination of both, may be used to facilitate sexual assault,* the most publicized drugs include flunitrazepam (Rohypnol) and γ-hydroxybutyr-

TABLE 58–9 Date Rape Drugs*

Alprazolam
Amphetamines
Barbiturates
1,4 Butanediol (BD)[†]
γ-Butyrolactone (GBL)[†]
Cannabis
Cocaine
Chloral hydrate[†]
Clonazepam[†]
Clonidine[†]
Diazepam
Ethanol
Flunitrazepam (Rohypnol)[†]
γ-Hydroxybutyrate (GHB)[†]
Ketamine[†]
Lorazepam
Meprobamate[†]
Methamphetamine
Midazolam (Versed)[†]
Oxazepam
Phencyclidine (PCP)
Propoxyphene[†]
Scopolamine[†]
Secobarbital
Temazepam
Triazolam
Zolpidem[†]

*Often, more than one drug is found. Most common are alcohol, marijuana, cocaine, and benzodiazepines, others account for <5% of positive tests.
[†]Will not be detected on a routine immunoassay drug screen. A more detailed analysis will be required.
After Slaughter L: Involvement of drugs in sexual assault. J Reprod Med 45:425, 2000; and Schwartz RH, Milteer R, LeBeau M: Drug-facilitated sexual assault ("date rape"). South Med J 93:558, 2000.

ate (GHB).[59] Despite their reputation in the lay press, flunitrazepam and GHB are associated with drug-facilitated sexual assault in *fewer than 3% to 5% of cases*.[59] Flunitrazepam is a benzodiazepine unavailable in the United States but available in Mexico. It can be detected in the urine up to 3 weeks after ingestion.[60] In the United States, GHB is a Schedule 1, federally banned central nervous system depressant. Legally, it is available only by prescription as the drug Xyrem for narcolepsy with a Schedule 3 exception, but it can easily be manufactured illegally by users. It can be detected in drinking material residue by crime laboratories as well in the victim's urine up to 4 hours after ingestion.

Drugs similar to GHB are 1,4 butanediol (BD) and γ-butyrolactone (GBL). Often, the victim's last memory is of using drugs or alcohol and then passing out. Some remember short segments of activity that may indicate some type of sexual acts. Some victims have no memory at all but desire to be "checked" for intercourse. A comprehensive medical-forensic examination should be conducted on these individuals. Collect standard sexual assault evidence from all orifices (oral, vaginal, and anal) and evaluate for injuries. Without a history from the victim, collect samples from every potential oral or genital contact including neck, breasts, and vulva. Obtain toxicology samples (including ethanol) from both blood and urine, if possible, with exact times of collection documented. Many of the touted date-rape drugs are not found on routine hospital laboratory testing. Some forensic laboratories offer a "date-rape panel" that tests for a variety

of commonly used substances. Obviously, a positive drug test does not prove date rape, and it may be impossible to distinguish self-administration to clandestine ingestion.

Extreme sensitivity must be used for discussing positive genital findings with a victim who has no memory of any sexual activity. Many times, the imagined sexual acts can create just as severe a traumatic response as an actual remembered sexual assault. For the unconscious victim, there is no memory of events to fill in the blanks, only her terrifying imagination of what could have happened.

LEGAL ISSUES

When the local government decides to proceed with a sex crime case against an alleged perpetrator, the district attorney will commonly contact the examiner to give legal testimony. A well-documented chart often negates the need for a clinician's appearance in court. When required for this task, it is best for the examiner to work with the prosecuting attorney to prepare testimony. As is the case for all ED patients, chart notes should be carefully written with the expectation that the ED evaluation and evidence collection may be presented in court. In some jurisdictions, it is possible to minimize the time spent away from work by arranging to be called to the courtroom just before the time of testimony or by giving a deposition before the court date. Once on the witness stand, the examining clinician is most often considered a percipient witness, and not necessarily an expert in the area of sexual assault. The law requires that one testify only to one's best recollection and to what is indicated in the chart. Factual information in answer to questions should be given only if one knows the facts; assumptions should be avoided. One should not be afraid to acknowledge the limits of one's knowledge or expertise. Statements such as "there were marks on the body that were consistent with bite marks" are preferable to statements such as "there were bite marks." It is the court's decision whether or not a person was sexually assaulted, and the clinician is there to give information about the patient's presentation, statements, what was found, and what was done for treatment.

SARTs

Prior to the 1990s, sexual assault examinations mostly fell to the responsibility of emergency clinicians. However, since the early 1990s, nurses or nurse clinicians have been performing an increasing number of sexual assault examinations. Called SANE (sexual assault nurse examiners), these nurses are the core members of the SARTs. Other members of the SARTs include law enforcement individuals, victim advocates, prosecutors, and forensic laboratory personnel.

Most examinations still take place in the ED but may be done in a space near the ED or an affiliated clinic. To establish SARTs, extra funding by government or charitable organization is often needed, because many local police jurisdictions do not reimburse adequately for the evidentiary examination to support a program. However, law enforcement is increasingly willing to pay more for a SANE-performed forensic examination because they feel it provides superior documentation for legal proceedings. Nurse examiners have formed The International Association of Forensic Nurses (IAFN). This group has drafted standards of practice for sexual assault examiners' education and the examinations themselves. Advantages of SARTs using SANEs include:

1. The practitioner performing the examination is specifically dedicated to treating the victim, not tending to multiple patients in a busy ED.
2. The clinician has usually completed more extensive training on sexual assault examination (mean, 80 hr)[19] and evidence collection and, as such, may perform a more comprehensive examination with better evidence collection.[61]
3. Many involved feel that designated clinicians consider more fully the emotional needs of the victim because of their extra time in training.

Useful guidelines and resources for establishing SANE programs are currently available.[2,62]

Acknowledgment

The editors and author wish to acknowledge the contributions of G. Richard Braen to this chapter in previous editions, Mary Hong of the Orange County Crime Laboratory and Elizabeth Swanson of the LAPD crime laboratory for their technical advice.

 REFERENCES CAN BE FOUND ON EXPERT CONSULT

CHAPTER **59**

Radiation in Pregnancy and Clinical Issues of Radiocontrast Agents

Denis J. Dollard

Pregnant women are frequently evaluated in emergency departments (EDs) with varied complaints that may require diagnostic imaging. Their chief complaint may be pregnancy-related, an acute illness/injury, or related to a chronic condition diagnosed before pregnancy. Potential teratogenic effects to the developing fetus from diagnostic radiation and radionuclide procedures are more perceived than real. Because fetal safety is a major concern, it is important for clinicians to have a clear understanding of the actual risk and benefits associated with radiographic imaging during pregnancy.

Radiologic tests are ordered every day in a busy ED. The current actual number is unknown, but approximately 40 million x-ray examinations were done on female patients in the childbearing age group, 15 to 44 years old, in 1980.[1] With such a high volume of imaging studies, there is a high likelihood of caring for a patient who requires an imaging study and has an early unknown or known pregnancy.

In utero radiation exposure of the embryo or fetus generally causes great, but largely unnecessary, anxiety among the parents, their families, and the clinician. Much of this anxiety is secondary to a general misconception that any radiation exposure is harmful and will result in an anomalous fetus. More often than not, clinicians themselves add to the confusion and fear by providing exposed women with erroneous information. Many clinicians, nurses, and even radiologists are ignorant of the qualitative and quantitative effects of ionizing radiation.[2] Multiple surveys in the literature reveal clinicians' dearth of knowledge about radiation exposure. This misinformation could lead to inappropriate abortions and litigation. For example, in Greece, after the Chernobyl disaster, 23% of pregnancies were terminated owing to unsubstantiated fears of teratogenicity.[3] A better understanding of the true risk estimates will help alleviate this fear.

It is widely held and published that concerns about possible effects of ionizing radiation exposure should not prevent medically indicated diagnostic procedures from being performed on the mother. It is not standard of care to withold necessary radiologic studies because of fear of fetal injury from diagnostic studies. According to the American College of Radiology, "No single diagnostic x-ray procedure results in radiation exposure to the degree that would threaten the well being of the preembryo, embryo, or fetus."[4-6] This remarkable statement helps put into perspective the effects of diagnostic radiation exposure on pregnancy. Standard diagnostic radiologic procedures performed in the ED are not associated with significant proven fetal risks. A clear understanding of these risks enables the clinician to make an informed decision and knowingly counsel patients in order to provide more benefit than harm.

Evaluation of radiation exposure on a pregnant patient should involve consideration of the type of radiation, types of examinations performed, gestational age, and radiation dose in order to determine risk estimation. The radiation dose of interest is the dose absorbed by the embryo or fetus, and not by the mother. However, recent articles[7,8] have raised concern about radiation exposure to maternal breast tissue and postulate a relation to breast cancer decades later. The main goal of this chapter is to review the basic issues of pregnancy and radiation exposure and provide a practical approach for clinicians in choosing a technique that entails the least risk and to counsel the patient who has or will receive an emergent diagnostic procedure.

TYPES OF RADIATION

All imaging techniques involve radiation or transmission of energy from one body or source to another. Imaging modalities used for diagnosis during pregnancy can be subdivided into ionization techniques (x-rays, computed tomography [CT] scans, nuclear imaging) and nonionization techniques (magnetic resonance imaging [MRI] and ultrasonography [US]). The nonionization techniques have insufficient energy to ionize target cells. It is the ionization process and its sequelae that induce health-related fetal effects.

Ionizing Radiation

Ionization is the transfer of energy to a medium by either electromagnetic or particulate radiation that is sufficient to overcome the binding energy of an electron. The electron may be ejected from the atom. Both electromagnetic waves consisting of uncharged particles (x-rays and γ-rays) and charged particles (α and β) can produce radiation. Indirect ionization modalities such as x-rays release an electron from a source that interacts with the target. Direct ionization refers to charged particles, α and β, that strike the target directly.

UNITS OF RADIATION

The units used to measure the effects of x-rays can be confusing. Descriptive terms include the rad and rem, along with the modern International System of Units (SI) of Gray and Sievert. In terms of radiation protection, the significant radiation quantity is the absorbed dose. The unit of absorbed radiation is the rad or the Gray (Gy) (1 Gy = 100 rad). Any risk associated with radiation is related to the amount of energy absorbed.

The dose equivalent expressed in rem or Sievert (Sv) is used to quantify the degree of biologic effect (1 Sv = 100 rem). This unit reflects the biologic response and can be used to compare effects of different types of radiation. The dose equivalent is the product of the absorbed dose times a quality factor. The quality factor depends on the mass and charge of the radiated particle. The quality factor is approximately 20 for an α particle, and equal to 1 for x-rays and γ-rays. Therefore, for diagnostic x-rays, CT scans, and ^{99}Tc nuclear studies, the absorbed dose is equal to the dose equivalent; that is, an absorbed dose of 1 rad yields a dose equivalent of 1 rem (1 Gy = 1 Sv) (Table 59–1). All reference data were converted into rads for uniformity and comparison throughout the chapter.

TIMING OF RADIATION DURING PREGNANCY AND ITS EFFECTS

The effects of exposure to radiation on the conceptus depend on the gestational age and the amount of absorbed dose. The relationship between radiation-induced effects and stage of pregnancy is shown in Figure 59–1.[1] The harmful effects of ionizing radiation have the following principal biologic effects: intrauterine death, organ malformations, mental impairment, fetal growth retardation, cancer, and genetic mutation.[2]

Radiation-induced health effects are divided into two broad categories, stochastic and nonstochastic (Table 59–2). Stochastic effects, such as cancer or genetic mutation, can result from alterations produced in a single cell and are presumed to exist even at low exposure.[2] The probability of such an effect occurring increases with dose and there is no identifiable threshold dose below which the chance is known to be zero. It is important to recognize that at low doses of radiation, the risks are far below the spontaneous incidence of carcinogenesis[9] or mutagenesis.[10]

The remaining harmful biologic effects mentioned earlier are nonstochastic effects. Nonstochastic effects require multicellular injury and have a threshold dose below which deleterious effects do not occur.[2] It is important to emphasize that the vast majority of embryopathologic effects are believed to be threshold phenomenon; therefore, a dose of ionizing radiation below the threshold will not produce these effects.

Stages of Fetal Development

Development of the unborn child is expressed as postconception age and can be divided approximately into three major phases. These include (1) the preimplantation/implantation phase (0–2 wk), from conception to implantation, (2) the phase of major organogenesis, which extends from the 3rd to approximately the 8th week after conception, and (3) the phase of fetal development, lasting from 9 weeks until birth.

Preimplantation/Implantation

During the preimplantation and implantation phase, the principal radiation-induced health effect is abortion.[11] When the number of cells in the conceptus is small and their nature not yet specialized, the effect of damage to these cells is most likely to take the form of failure to implant or an undeterminable death of the conceptus.[9] The no-effect threshold of absorbed dose is quite high, estimated at 10 to 15 rad,[11] and not likely to be approached by diagnostic ED radiographs or radionuclide testing. By the time the pregnancy is at term, the threshold to cause intrauterine mortality has risen to about 100 rad.[11] These estimates have been extrapolated from animal data. This period has been referred to as the "all or none period" because radiation is more likely to kill the embryo than result in a live malformed newborn.

Few human epidemiologic data are available for this period of gestation. Because many women are certainly unknowingly exposed to diagnostic radiation during this period, the lack of such data suggests a nonassociation between diagnostic radiation exposure and embryo death. Data from the Japanese atomic bomb experience have been cited for reference, but such a correlation is difficult to justify scientifically. Nonetheless, these data show a decrease in the number

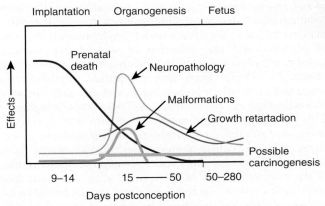

Figure 59–1 Schematic presentation of the various adverse effects associated with radiation and their relative incidence at different stages of gestation. (*Adapted from Mettler FA Jr, Upton A [eds]: Medical Effects of Ionizing Radiation, 2nd ed. Chapter 8. Philadelphia, WB Saunders, 1995.*)

TABLE 59–1 Units of Radiation			
Quantity	**Unit**	**SI Unit**	**Relationship between Units**
Absorbed dose	rad	Gray (Gy)	1 Gy = 100 rad 100 mGy = 10 rad 10 mGy = 1 rad 1 mGy = 100 mrad
Equivalent dose	rem	Sievert (Sv)	1 Sv = 100 rem 100 mSv = 10 rem 10 mSv = 1 rem 1 mSv = 100 mrem

Absorbed dose (Gy) × quality factor = equivalent dose (Sv). The quality factor for x-rays = 1. Therefore, 1 rad = 1 rem, 1 Gy = 1 Sv.

TABLE 59–2 Stochastic and Nonstochastic (Threshold) Comparison				
Phenomenon	**Pathology**	**Diseases**	**Risk**	**Definition**
Stochastic	Damage to a single cell may result in disease	Cancer, germ cell mutation	Some risk exists at all dosages; at low doses, risk may be less than spontaneous risk.	The incidence of the disease increases, but the severity and nature of the disease remain the same.
Nonstochastic (threshold)	Multicellular injury	Intrauterine death, organ malformations, mental impairment, growth retardation	No increased risk below the threshold dose.	Both the severity and the incidence of the disease increase with dose.

Modified from Brent RL: Utilization of developmental basic science principles: The evaluation of reproductive risks from pre- and postconception environmental radiation exposures. Teratology 54:182, 1999.

of offspring who retrospectively would have been 0 to 3 weeks postconception at the time of this significant radiation exposure, suggesting increased fetal loss caused by irradiation during preimplantation.[12] This decrease in birth rate is likely multifactorial because stress, disease, and malnutrition were coexistent during this traumatic time. Importantly, fetal loss from exposure to an atomic bomb cannot be scientifically extrapolated to exposure to diagnostic radiation.

Any discussion concerning the potential adverse effects from diagnostic radiation must consider the natural incidence of spontaneous abortion. Because the main effect of radiation exposure during the first few weeks postfertilization is abortion due to embryo death, it is paramount to note that the normal incidence of spontaneous abortion in humans not exposed to radiation is in the 30% to 50% range.[2] Exposure to less than 10 rad yields no statistical change in the rate of preimplantation/early postimplantation spontaneous abortion from the expected baseline (Table 59–3).

Organogenesis

Very high dose radiation exposure, far greater than could be delivered by even aggressive diagnostic radiographs/radionuclide procedures, has been reported to result in teratogenesis. Such information is gleaned from women who received therapeutic radiation (in the range of 250 rad) during early pregnancy for conditions such as pelvic malignancies. Organ malformations are the main consequence of radiation exposure during the organogenesis period (3–8 wk). Abnormalities result from cell killing during the active phase of proliferation and differentiation. Because the embryo is unable to completely replace damaged cells, malformations occur. The most common effects of exposure during organogenesis are malformations caused in the organs under development at the time of exposure and the reduction of skeletal development. Growth retardation and microcephaly are the predominant effects.[9,11,12] These effects have a reported threshold dose range of 5 to 20 rads or higher, but are not generally observed unless the exposure is several orders of magnitude or higher.[9,11] This dose range is significantly higher than what is reached in diagnostic radiology or diagnostic nuclear medicine procedures. Whereas ocular abnormalities, developmental facial abnormalities, genital abnormalities, and physical deformities of the extremities have been reported after very high dose embryonic exposure, such abnormalities are not linked to the amount of radiation that would be delivered from even multiple diagnostic radiographic procedures. Importantly, there are no reports of external radiation inducing morphologic malformations in humans unless offspring also exhibited either growth retardation or a central nervous system abnor-

mality. Simply stated, a fetus exposed to radiation will not develop isolated structural abnormalities. The fear of extra toes, cleft palate, or heart or kidney malformations from diagnostic radiation during pregnancy is simply unfounded, yet often believed by the general public.

Temporary growth retardation is likely with doses in the range of 10 to 25 rad.[12] Infants with low birth weights and lengths may recover fully, attaining normal adult stature. The natural incidence of a live birth having a developmental anomaly is 2% to 4%[1] and intrauterine growth retardation is 2% to 3%.[1] Again, it is important to emphasize that exposure to less than 5 rad yields no change in the risk of occurrence of organ malformations or growth retardation[12] (see Table 59–3).

Fetal Period

The predominant observable effects of radiation exposure during this period are growth retardation, microencephaly, and severe mental retardation (SMR). The fetal stage has been subdivided into early fetal (8–15 wk), mid-fetal (16–25 wk), and late fetal (26 wk–term) because of identifiable periods of risk to the developing central nervous system.

Mental Impairment. From the 8th to the 15th week, there is a rapid increase in the number of neurons that migrate to their ultimate sites and lose their capacity to divide. At 15 to 25 weeks, there is more differentiation and architectural definition.[1] These embryologic changes make the fetus susceptible to CNS damage during the early and mid-fetal periods.

The in utero atomic bomb survivor data indicate that the risk of SMR per rad was higher if exposed during the early fetal versus the mid-fetal period.[12] In children receiving greater than 50 rad between 8 and 15 weeks postconception, a drop in IQ score of 0.3 points per rad was estimated.[12] There is no documented increased risk of mental retardation in humans at gestation age less than 8 weeks or greater than 25 weeks evaluated with doses of less than 50 rads.[13] The highest risk for SMR occurs during the early fetal period with fetal doses in the range of 100 rad. All the clinical observations on significant IQ reductions and SMR relate to fetal doses of about 50 rad and higher.[9] This dose range greatly exceeds the dosages utilized for diagnostic imaging.

It is important to relate the magnitude of radiation effects to those abnormalities that occur spontaneously in the population. Multiple causes of mental retardation have been identified, including malnutrition, lead poisoning, rubella infections during pregnancy, and maternal alcoholism. Current prevalence figures indicate that the normal incidence of a person with an IQ below 70 is approximately 3%.[9] At fetal doses of

TABLE 59–3 Risks and Threshold Doses of the Main Effects of Prenatal Irradiation

Gestational Age	Stage	Potential Biologic Effect	Threshold	Risk
0–2 wk	Preimplantation/implantation	Abortion	$>10^{2.8}$ rad	
		Organ malformation	$>5^8$; $>10^{2.9}$ rad	
3–7 wk	Organogenesis	Growth retardation	$>10^{2.9}$ rad	
8–25 wk	Fetal	Growth retardation	$>10^{2.9}$ rad	
		Mental impairment	$>10^{9.8}$ rad	
Whole pregnancy		Carcinogenesis	None	6×10^{-4} per rad
		Mutagenesis	None	1×10^{-2} per rad

Modified from Fattibene P, Mazzei F, Nuccetelli C, Risica S: Prenatal exposure to ionizing radiation: Sources, effects, and regulatory aspects. Acta Paediatr 88:693, 1999.

10 rad, the spontaneous incidence of mental retardation is much larger than any potential radiation effect on IQ reduction.[9] Regardless of the time of gestation, IQ reduction cannot be clinically identified at fetal doses of less than 10 rad (see Table 59–3).[9]

Growth Retardation. The human data for Hiroshima and Nagasaki reveal that the major congenital anomaly observed was microencephaly.[12] Studies have demonstrated no increased risk for microencephaly in the population exposed to less than 150 rad in Nagasaki; however, an increased risk in the Hiroshima population exposed to doses as low as 10 to 19 rad has been reported.[14] It is possible that the difference between the two cities is secondary to other causes (e.g., trauma, stress, malnutrition) than radiation. In experimental animal data, a dose of 10 to 20 rad does not increase the incidence of microencephaly.[14] A dose threshold for microencephaly, as well as other congenital anomalies, is generally accepted to be in the range of a few rad. Permanent growth retardation is not typically seen unless doses exceed 50 rad.[12] Irradiation of the human fetus at doses below 10 rad has not been observed to cause congenital malformations or growth retardation (see Table 59–3).[1,2,4]

Carcinogenesis

The magnitude of risk for carcinogenesis after low-dose radiation exposure and whether the risk changes throughout gestation have been the subject of many publications,[15–17] yet interpretation of the data remains open to date. Numerous studies[18–21] indicate a 1.3- to 3.0-fold higher incidence of leukemia in children exposed to diagnostic radiation in utero, although some studies fail to substantiate the association.[14,22] Excess cancer as a result of in utero exposure has not been clearly demonstrated among Japanese atomic bomb survivor studies even though the population has been followed for about 50 years, but the number exposed is not large.[9] Identification and control of confounding factors make interpretation of radiation carcinogenesis studies difficult, if not impossible, to interpret. Brent and coworkers[14] noted that most investigators agree that low doses of radiation present a carcinogenic risk to the embryo; however, findings of an increased cancer risk among children exposed in utero to low-dose diagnostic radiation must be reconciled with the fact that high-dose animal and human studies have not found a marked increase in cancer incidence.

Risk can be expressed in several ways, including as relative risk or absolute risk. Relative risk indicates the risk as a function of the "background" cancer risk. A relative risk of 1.0 indicates that there is no effect of irradiation, whereas a relative risk of 1.5 for a given dose indicates that the radiation is associated with a 50% increase in cancer above background rates. The absolute risk estimate simply indicates the excess number of cancer cases expected in a population due to a certain radiation dose.[9]

The International Commission on Radiological Protection Publication 84[9] noted that a recent analysis of many of the epidemiologic studies conducted on prenatal x-ray and childhood cancer are consistent with a relative risk of 1.4 (a 40% increase over the background risk) following a fetal dose of about 1 rad. The best methodological studies, however, suggest that the risk is probably lower than this. Even if the relative risk were as high as 1.4, the individual probability of childhood cancer after in utero irradiation would be very low (~0.3%–0.4%) because the background incidence of child-

hood cancer is so low (~0.2%–0.3%). Absolute risk estimates for cancer risk from ages 0 to 15 after in utero irradiation have been estimated to be in the range of 600/10,000 persons each exposed to 100 rad, or 0.06%/rad.[9,11] If a fetus is exposed to 0.1 rad, the increased risk for carcinogenesis is 0.006% or 3/50,000, compared with the background incidence of 0.2% to 0.3% or 100 to 150/50,000. The increased carcinogenic risk from 0.1 rad exposure is approximately 50 times smaller than the already low natural incidence of cancer.

Mutagenesis

Investigating possible radiation-induced alteration to the human genome is exceedingly difficult. The geneticists who studied the radiated populations in Japan are convinced that there were radiation-induced mutations. However, the calculated and demonstrated risks were so small that the investigators were unable to demonstrate statistically significant genetic effects.[23]

The risk of radiation-induced hereditary disease in humans is reported to be around 1%/100 rad.[12,14] If a fetus is exposed to 0.1 rad, then the increased risk is approximately 0.001% or 1/100,000. The natural frequency of genetic disease manifesting at birth is approximately 3%[10] or 3000/100,000. For 0.1 rad, the increased genetic risk is minute compared with the natural incidence of genetic disease.

In order to put all risks into proper perspective, the range of fetal absorbed doses for diagnostic imaging must be reviewed. The vast majority of diagnostic radiographic studies are markedly less than 5 rad. A comparison of fetal absorbed doses for the more common ED radiographic procedures follows.

Radiation Exposure from Diagnostic Radiographs

Table 59–4 lists estimated fetal exposure for various diagnostic imaging modalities.[25] The number of examinations required to reach a cumulative dose of 5 rads is calculated in the second column to underscore the order-of-magnitude difference between the dose considered to have negligible risk (5 rad) and the actual exposed fetal dose. For example, one would require 5000 x-rays of an upper or lower extremity, 125 pelvic x-rays, or an impressive 70,000 two-view chest x-rays before the 5-rad limit is reached.

Radiation Exposure from CT Scans

Many variables affect the calculation of fetal radiation dose from CT scans, especially slice thickness, number of cuts, distance of target organ from fetus, and gestational age. Table 59–4 summarizes estimated maximal fetal doses from CT scans. It should be noted that a CT of the lumbar spine delivers radiation to the fetus that approaches the safe cutoff range. A CT scan of the abdomen exposes the fetus to less radiation than the 5-rad cutoff, but alternative methods of investigation such as US or MRI should be considered in early pregnancy if the clinical condition warrants.

The head CT is the most commonly requested CT scan in pregnancy. The expected fetal absorbed dose is less than 50 millirad (mrad), which is 100 times less than the dose with negligible risk. The estimated radiation dose to the fetus for CT of the chest is less than 0.100 rad. Spiral CT is common-

TABLE 59–4 Estimated Fetal Exposure for Various Diagnostic Imaging Methods

Examination Type	Estimated Fetal Dose per Examination (rad)	Number of Examinations Required for Cumulative 5-rad Dose
Plain Films		
Skull	0.004	1,250
Dental	0.0001	50,000
Cervical spine	0.002	2,500
Upper or lower extremity	0.001	5,000
Chest (2 views)	0.00007	71,429
Mammogram	0.020	250
Abdominal (multiple views)	0.245	20
Thoracic spine	0.009	555
Lumbosacral spine	0.359	13
Intravenous pyelogram	1.398	3
Pelvis	0.040	125
Hip (single view)	0.213	23
CT Scans (Slice Thickness: 10 mm)		
Head (10 slices)	<0.050	>100
Chest (10 slices)	<0.100	>50
Abdomen (10 slices)	2.600	1–2
Lumbar spine (multiple views)	3.500	1–2
Pelvimetry (1 slice with scout film)	0.250	20
Fluoroscopic Studies		
Upper gastrointestinal series	0.056	89
Barium swallow	0.006	833
Barium enema	3.986	1
Nuclear Medicine Studies		
Most studies using technetium (^{99m}Tc)	<0.500	>10
Hepatobiliary technetium HIDA scan	0.150	33
Ventilation-perfusion scan (total)	0.215	23
Perfusion portion: technetium	0.175	28
Ventilation portion: xenon (^{133}Xe)	0.040	125
Iodine (^{131}I), at fetal thyroid tissue	590.000	
Environmental Sources (for Comparison)		
Environmental background radiation (cumulative dose over 9 mo)	0.100	N/A

CT, computed tomography; HIDA, hepatobiliary iminodiacetic acid; rad, the unit of absorbed radiation.

Reproduced from Toppenberg KS, Hill DA, Miller DP: Safety of radiographic imaging during pregnancy. Am Fam Physician 59:1813, 1999.

Ordering CT scans of the head, chest, abdomen, and pelvis is a daily occurrence for emergency medicine clinicians. With that in mind, it is sobering to realize that the seventh National Academy of Science report on Biological Effects of Ionizing Radiation (BEIR VI) indicated that a 10-rad dose is associated with a lifetime attributable risk for developing a solid cancer or leukemia in 1:1000.[28,29] As data on the effects of ionized radiation accumulate, and the technology of non-ionizing techniques improves, our utilization of ionization based modalities will diminish.

The American College of Radiology notes that iodinated low-osmolality contrast media (LOCM), most of which are nonionic agents, have been shown to be associated with less discomfort and have a lower incidence of minor (1% vs. 5% for high-osmolality contrast media [HOCM]) and severe reactions (0.015% vs. 0.1% for HOCM). Many Radiology departments routinely use LOCM.[30] Although authors have expressed concern over the possibility that iodinated contrast may suppress fetal or neonatal thyroid function for a short period of time,[7] the added benefit of a nonionic contrast material is that the intravascular use of nonionic contrast media has been reported to have no effect on neonatal thyroid function.[31] To note, routine postnatal screening in the United States includes thyroid function tests.

Iodinated contrast material that is injected intravenously for CT scans does not emit radiation and is classified as pregnancy category B. The product insert for barium sulfate suspension used as oral contrast for an abdominal CT scan (e.g., Redicat) notes no adverse fetal reactions under the heading "Usage in Pregnancy." Barium preparations do not emit radiation.

NUCLEAR MEDICINE STUDIES

A common nuclear medicine procedure ordered from the ED is the ventilation perfusion ($\dot{V}/\dot{Q}$) scan. The perfusion portion of the scan is performed by injecting a radioisotope intravenously. The isotope emits radiation and is detected by sensitive cameras. This requires that a radioisotope (e.g., ^{99}Tc) be tagged to a substrate, most commonly albumin. The albumin-technetium aggregate is temporarily trapped in the arterioles and capillaries in the lung and its distribution can be identified. The principal photon that is useful for detection and imaging with technetium studies is the γ-ray.[32] When the radio-tagged substrate is excreted into the maternal bladder, the fetus will receive additional radiation exposure based on the proximity of the maternal bladder. Patient hydration and frequent voiding or bladder catheterization after a $\dot{V}/\dot{Q}$ scan will lessen the radiation exposure to the fetus.

The measurement of radioactive substances is based on its decay, and the units are the Curie (Ci) or the Becquerel (Bq). Doses are usually expressed in milliCurie (mCi). The usual dose of technetium for the lung perfusion portion of the scan is 1 to 5 mCi of ^{99}Tc. Reduced doses, as low as 1 mCi, are often used in pregnancy.

Depending on the radioisotope and substrate employed, the average fetal exposures can be calculated. Commonly used radiopharmaceuticals and estimated fetal doses for $\dot{V}/\dot{Q}$ scans and other radionuclide studies are given in Table 59–5.[13] A 5-mCi ^{99}Tc albumin scan results in 175 mrad fetal exposure. Reducing the dose to 2 mCi results in a 70-mrad fetal exposure. ^{99}Tc albumin is contraindicated in patients with severe pulmonary hypertension and is pregnancy category C.

place in radiology departments and is a popular diagnostic tool used for suspected pulmonary embolism (PE) in the pregnant patient. The dose for a spiral CT of the chest is less because the duration of the procedure is much shorter.[26] Van der Molen[27] reported that using 16-slice versus 4-slice CT can equate to a radiation dose reduction of 20% to 30%.

TABLE 59–5 Radiopharmaceuticals Used in Nuclear Medicine Studies

Examination	Estimated Activity Administered per Examination (mCi)	Dose to Uterus/ Embryo per Pharmaceutical (mrad)
Brain	20 mCi ^{99m}Tc DTPA	700
	20 mCi ^{99m}Tc O$_4$	960
Hepatobiliary	5 mCi ^{99m}Tc sulfur colloid	55
	5 mCi ^{99m}Tc HIDA	150
Bone	20 mCi ^{99m}Tc phosphate	500
Respiratory		
Perfusion	5 mCi ^{99m}Tc-macroaggregated albumin	175
Ventilation	10 mCi ^{133}xenon gas	40
Renal	20 mCi ^{99m}Tc DTPA	700
Abscess or tumor	3 mCi ^{67}Ga citrate	840
Cardiovascular	20 mCi ^{99m}Tc-labeled red blood cells	120

DTPA, diethylenetriamine penta-acetic acid; HIDA, hepatobiliary iminodiacetic acid; mCi, millicurie; mrad, millirad.

Reproduced from Cunningham GF [ed]: Williams Obstetrics, 21st ed. New York, McGraw-Hill, 2001.

Ten mCi of ^{133}Xe is used for the ventilation portion of the $\dot{V}/\dot{Q}$ scan. ^{133}Xe has a short half-life and results in 40 mrad fetal exposure. Normal findings on the perfusion scan may obviate the need for the ventilation scan, and some centers routinely perform only the perfusion portion because most pregnant women have normal ventilation.

PE DIAGNOSIS

The reported incidence of PE associated with pregnancy is equivalent to roughly 1 in every 2000 pregnancies.[7] The mortality rate of untreated acute PE is about 30% compared with 3% in treated patients.[33] Therefore, the potential morbidity of PE and the attendant risk of anticoagulant therapy in pregnant patients necessitate definitive diagnosis.

The radiologic modalities of choice for definitive diagnosis are $\dot{V}/\dot{Q}$ scan versus CT pulmonary angiography. Although conventional pulmonary angiography was long considered the "gold standard" against which other imaging techniques were compared, it is now thought to be no more accurate than well-performed CT pulmonary angiography.[7]

The calculated radiation exposure to the fetus from both $\dot{V}/\dot{Q}$ scanning and CT of the chest confers minimal, and essentially only theoretical, fetal risk.[26] Fetal exposure from CT of the chest is less than 0.100 rad. Fetal exposure from CT has been reported as low as 0.026 rad using a single-detector row helical CT and 0.013 rad for a multidetector row helical machine.[7] A 5-mCi ^{99}Tc perfusion scan and 10 mCi ^{133}Xe ventilation scan summates to 0.225 rad.[25] The dose of fetal radiation from the perfusion scan can be altered and is often lowered in the evaluation of pregnant patients (Table 59–6). Lowering the dose by 60%, a level that will usually produce a suitable study, results in lowering fetal exposure to 0.110 mrad. Pulmonary angiography results in an estimated fetal exposure of 0.22 to 0.37 rad when done via the femoral route but can be lowered to less than 0.05 rad using the brachial route.[26]

TABLE 59–6 The Technique of Ventilation/Perfusion ($\dot{V}/\dot{Q}$) Scanning

This test uses both intravenous (perfusion) and aerosolized (ventilation) agents.

Perfusion

1. Before injection, prepare the IV technetium. Mix sodium pertechnetate ^{99m}Tc with macroaggregated human albumin (MAA), forming ^{99m}Tc-MAA, the substance that is injected intravenously to investigate blood flow in the lungs. If the preparation is not used within 8 hr, discard it.
2. The usual dose is 1–5 (mCi. Doses as low as 1 mCi are used in pregnancy.
3. Within 5 min of injection, more than 90% of the Tc albumin aggregate is trapped in the arterioles and capillaries of the lung. The particle size determines where the ^{99m}Tc will be localized in the body.
4. The accumulation in the lung is temporary, and fragile albumin aggregate quickly breaks down, allowing the Tc to enter the general circulation.
5. Once in the body, the half-life of ^{99m}Tc is 6 hr.
6. The majority of the ^{99m}Tc is excreted in the urine. If it remains in the urinary bladder, it is in close proximity to the fetus.
7. Tc in the bladder also exposes the fetus to small amounts of radiation.
8. Frequent voiding or bladder catheterization after the study will lessen radiation exposure to the fetus.
9. Tc is relatively contraindicated in patients with severe pulmonary hypertension (because the ^{99m}Tc-MAA temporarily blocks blood flow in the lungs).
10. Allergic reactions to Tc and human serum albumin are extremely rare.
11. The radiation exposure to the total body from 2.5 mCi is extremely low: <0.1 rad.

Ventilation

1. Some radiologists forgo the ventilation portion of the $\dot{V}/\dot{Q}$ scan in pregnancy to limit the total radiation exposure.
2. Most hospitals use ^{133}Xe for the ventilation portion of the $\dot{V}/\dot{Q}$ scan.
3. The fetal radiation from xenon is extremely low, and the 5-rad cutoff is not reached until >125 scans have been performed.
4. The estimated dose to the fetus of a standard 10 mCi of xenon used in a $\dot{V}/\dot{Q}$ scan is 0.04 rad.
5. If Tc-based aerosol is the marker used for the ventilation portion, fetal exposure is higher than with xenon aerosol.

CT scan has supplanted $\dot{V}/\dot{Q}$ as the standard diagnostic test in ruling out PE. Because perfusion scan is being done on a relatively young healthy subset of the population, one would suspect that the percentage of nondiagnostic studies (low or intermediate probability) would be less. However, Chan and colleagues[34] published that ventilation perfusion scintigraphy is nondiagnostic in 25% of patients, with 73.5% read as normal, and only 1.8% read as high probability (113 patients in the study). Interestingly, 86% (24/28 patients) that received the nondiagnostic finding were not anticoagulated and were found to be free of a thromboembolism event for the following 20.6 months.

Recognizably, the utility of a test that does not answer your question 25% of the time is concerning but should be tempered with the fact that there is a 75% chance of getting a definitive diagnosis, along with published concerns that the higher level of radiation exposure to childbearing women's breasts via CT may cause cancer decades later.[7,8] Remy-Jardin and associates[35] and Scarsbrook and coworkers[7] reported that an exposure of 10 rads to the breasts of a woman aged 35 years increases the risk of breast cancer by approximately 14% over the background rate for the general population.

So which study does one order? Both modalities expose a fetus to low levels of radiation of similar magnitude (CT less than $\dot{V}/\dot{Q}$) with very low theoretical fetal risk. Scarsbrook and coworkers[7] presented an algorithm mindful of the radiation exposure to both fetus and mother and provided convincing evidence for the recommendation (Fig. 59–2). Scarsbrook and coworkers[7] suggested that an echocardiogram is a good first step in critically ill pregnant patients in which one considers PE. All others should start with a chest x-ray with shielding of the fetus. If the x-ray is normal, then do an US of the lower extremities to evaluate for deep venous thrombosis. Although this will have low diagnostic yield, it exposes the mother and fetus to no risk. If deep venous thrombosis is present, then treat. If US is negative, then move onto a half-dose lung perfusion scan if there is no patient history of obstructive lung disease. The literature reports that up to 75% of these scans are normal in the pregnant population. An important stipulation for using this algorithm is that one's hospital radiologist needs to be comfortable reporting a normal scan as opposed to low probability because all nondiagnostic tests would then go on for a CT pulmonary angiogram. The authors note that utilizing this algorithm allows a definitive diagnosis in the vast majority of cases while minimizing risk to both mother and fetus.

Scarsbrook and coworkers[7] recommended several dose reduction methods when using CT pulmonary angiography on pregnant patients. Although these do not fall into the realm of emergency medicine, it is worthwhile to raise these points with the radiologists when developing a protocol to lower the radiation exposure to your patients (Table 59–7).

The role of D-dimer levels in the diagnosis of PE is evolving.[36,37] During pregnancy, D-dimer levels increase and should be considered physiologic. D-Dimer levels are similar to those in nonpregnant patients up to around 20 weeks, then are noted to increase throughout pregnancy to three times higher than the mean of a healthy nonpregnant patient.[38]

Recently, attempts have been made to establish a range of normal D-dimer values throughout pregnancy, which may be of great value, but as of yet, have not been tested in clinical practice.[7]

DIAGNOSIS OF PREGNANCY AND CONSENT

If exposure of less than 5 rad does not measurably affect the exposed embryo, then why should the clinician determine the pregnancy status of the patient? Brent[2] reported sound reasoning for diagnosis of pregnancy before radiographic study. First, the diagnosis of pregnancy may be in the differential diagnosis for the patient's presenting problem and may change or obviate any further need for imaging. Second, it is beneficial to have the patient informed of pregnancy status before the imaging, if possible. An informative discussion about the risk/benefit aspects of the test before the study conveys a concern for the patient and fetus. Discussing the risk/benefit aspects of imaging after the study may be misconstrued as "back-stepping" and make the patient upset. Many lawsuits are stimulated by the factor of surprise. A frank discussion before the imaging may prevent misguided litigation.

Amenorrhea and physical changes in size and shape of the uterus may be consistent with pregnancy. However, menstrual history by itself may not be totally reliable in the determination of pregnancy. A history of recent menstruation, intrauterine device, tubal ligation, no coitus, or the proper use of birth control pills will result in the suggestion of pregnancy

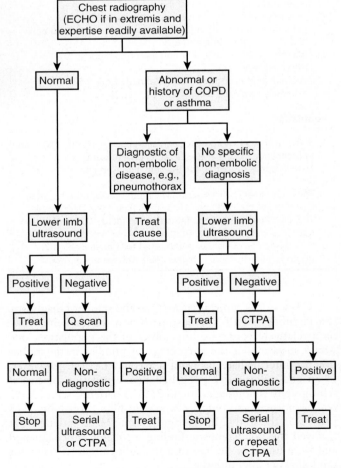

Figure 59–2 Suggested imaging algorithm for investigation of suspected pulmonary embolism in pregnancy. COPD, chronic obstructive pulmonary disease; CTPA, computed tomography pulmonary angiography. *(Modified from Scarsbrook AF, Evans AL, Owen AR, et al: Diagnosis of suspected venous thromboembolic disease in pregnancy. Clin Radiol 61:1, 2006.)*

TABLE 59–7 Dose Reduction Methods When Using Computed Tomography Pulmonary Angiography to Image Suspected Pulmonary Embolic Disease in Pregnancy
Reduce milliampere-second (mAs)
Reduce kilovoltage (kVp)
Increase pitch
Increase detector and beam collimation
Reduce field of view
Reduce z-axis scan volume (caudal extent limited to top of diaphragm)
Eliminate frontal and lateral scout views
Circumferential shielding of the abdomen and pelvis

From Scarsbrook AF, Evans AL, Owen AR, et al: Diagnosis of suspected venous thromboembolic disease in pregnancy. Clin Radiol 61:1, 2006.

more than 90% of the time, but these parameters are not 100% accurate. If the diagnosis of pregnancy is in the differential or imaging is ordered, or both, the definitive determination of the patient's pregnancy status should be strongly considered if the clinical scenario is reasonable. It is not standard of care to order a pregnancy test on all women of childbearing age before obtaining routine diagnostic radiographs. However, a menstrual history and other information should be obtained whenever possible. Urine pregnancy tests to detect early pregnancy are quite sensitive and reliable, and it is not necessary to routinely order a quantitative serum test. Theoretically, there will be a few days' window between fertilization and implantation when no method will exist to confirm the presence or absence of early pregnancy.

The pregnant patient has the right to know the magnitude and type of risks that might result from in utero exposure. The Annals of the International Commission on Radiological Protection Publication 84[9] summarized the need for informed consent as follows: "The need and degree of disclosure is usually measured by what a reasonable person believes is material to the mother's decision to be exposed to radiation. The level and degree of disclosure should be related to the level of risk. For low-dose procedures, such as chest x-rays, <100 mrad, the only information that may be needed is a verbal assurance that the risk is judged to be extremely low. When fetal doses are >100 mrad, usually a more detailed explanation is given. The information should include potential radiation risks and potential alternative modalities as well as the risk of harm from not having the medical procedure. The degree of documentation of such explanations and consent is variable but many clinicians will include a note of any such counseling or consent in the record of the patient."

PATIENT COUNSELING

When a pregnant patient requires an imaging study, be prepared to discuss the risk associated with the test. Counseling can be accomplished after attempting to estimate the dose to the conceptus from the procedure and comparing the radiation risk with other risks of pregnancy. It is important to use terminology that is easily understood by the patient. Figure 59–3 depicts three different strategies to inform the patient about the level of exposure from her study compared with established limits. Table 59–8 compares the level of exposure to established background risks.

The main bar graph (A) in Figure 59–3 compares the fetal exposure level for various radiographic studies with the maximum accepted fetal dose during pregnancy (5 rad). A patient's particular study may be plotted on this graph, showing the clear margin of safety that exists for all single diagnostic tests.

The middle graph (B) equates the exposure from the low-level diagnostic studies to the number of hours needed to accumulate a similar exposure dose from background terrestrial radiation. One of the most commonly ordered studies in pregnancy is a chest x-ray. The potential risk to the fetus can be put into perspective for the patient by comparing the absorbed dose for the chest x-ray with the natural background radiation exposure. The environmental background radiation over 9 months has a cumulative dose of 100 mrad,[39] or 0.015 mrad/hr. The fetal dose exposure for a chest x-ray (two views) is estimated at 0.07 mrad. Therefore, the exposure dose to the fetus from a chest x-ray is equivalent to the same

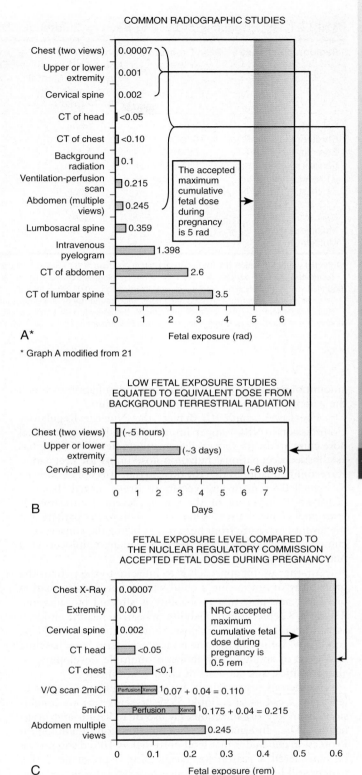

Figure 59–3 *A,* Comparison of common radiographic studies with the accepted 5-rad cumulative fetal exposure limit. *B,* Low fetal exposure studies equated to equivalent dose from background terrestrial radiation. *C,* Fetal exposure level compared to the Nuclear Regulatory Commission's accepted fetal dose during pregnancy.

TABLE 59–8 Probability of Bearing Healthy Children as a Function of Radiation Dose

Radiographic Study	Fetal Exposure (rad)	Increased Risk of Abortion, Growth Retardation, Mental Impairment, and Malformation	Probability That Child Will Have No Malformation (%)	Probability That Child Will Have No Genetic Disease Present at Birth* (%)	Probability That Child Will Not Develop Cancer (Age 0–19 yr)† (%)
No study	0	None	97	97	99.7
Chest x-ray (2 views)	0.0007	None	97	97	99.7
Extremity	0.001	None	97	97	99.7
Cervical spine	0.002	None	97	97	99.7
CT head	<0.05	None	97	97	99.7
CT chest	<0.10	None	97	97	99.7
$\dot{V}/\dot{Q}$ scan 3 mCi	0.145	None	97	97	99.7
$\dot{V}/\dot{Q}$ scan 5 mCi	0.215	None	97	97	99.6
Multiple studies	1	None	97	97	99.4
Multiple studies	5	None	97	97	99.4

*Rounded values. Radiation risk for genetic mutation assumed at 0.01%/rad fetal dose and a linear dose-response relationship. Background rate for genetic mutation estimated at 3%. From Osie IK: Fetal doses from radiological examinations. Br J Radiol 72:773, 1999.
†Rounded values. Radiation risk for fatal cancer assumed to be 0.06%/rad fetal dose and a linear dose-response relationship. Many epidemiologic studies suggest that the risk may be lower than that assumed here. Background risk of childhood cancer calculated from NCI-SEER: Surveillance, Epidemiology and End Results Cancer Statistics Review 1973–1991: Tables and Graphs. Bethesda, MD, National Cancer Institute, 1994.
Modified from International Commission on Radiological Protection. Publication 84: Pregnancy and medical radiation. Ann ICRP 30:iii, 1, 2000.

amount of naturally occurring background radiation to which the patient was exposed in the previous 5 hours.

The lower graph (C) depicts the Nuclear Regulatory Commission's (NRC) upper limit for cumulative gestational dose compared with various diagnostic studies. The NRC has established occupational radiation dose limits for pregnancy. Its recommendation is that the dose to the fetus not be allowed to exceed 0.5 rem during gestation. Brent[2] noted that this factor-of-10 lowering of the widely accepted threshold is "extremely conservative." One can explain to the patient that the level of exposure from her x-ray is below the conservative cumulative acceptable dose for a pregnant employee at a nuclear facility in the United States.

Another useful approach is to indicate to the patient the probability of not having a child with either a malformation or cancer and how that probability is affected by radiation. Table 59–8 depicts the probability of bearing healthy children as a function of radiation dose. This discussion should be coupled with the fact that the nonexposed fetus has a baseline incidence of spontaneous abortion, multiple developmental abnormalities, and subsequent childhood cancer.

Numerous organizations have declared fetal exposure to less than 5 rad as safe. Table 59–9 presents various conclusions from key organizations on use of radiation and pregnancy. The International Commission on Radiological Protection concludes that fetal doses below 10 rad should not be considered a reason for terminating a pregnancy.[9] If a patient still has considerable concern or has possibly received greater than 5 rad, referral of the patient to a radiation physicist or genetic specialist for further counseling is reasonable.

NONIONIZING RADIATION: MRI AND US

The term *radiation* describes the transmission of energy from one body or source to another. Nonionizing radiation includes the portion of the electromagnetic spectrum in which the energy of emitted photons is insufficient to ionize atoms and molecules. MRI and US are forms of nonionizing radiation.

MRI

MRI is currently not approved by the U.S. Food and Drug Administration (FDA) for use in pregnant patients.[40] However, a body of data in this population is developing. MRI is becoming a valuable complement to US when additional information is needed to make treatment decisions during pregnancy.[41,42] Recent advances in fast MRI techniques have helped to eliminate prior obstacles of slow imaging times and fetal movement. Possible indications for MRI use in a pregnant patient include further evaluation of adnexal masses, placental evaluation, hydronephrosis, pelvic vein thrombosis, appendicitis, and small bowel obstruction.[43]

Magnetic resonance direct thrombus imaging (MR-DTI) is a technique that allows direct visualization of PEs and simultaneous imaging of the legs without the need for intravenous contrast. Early data suggest it is highly accurate in the detection of PE.[7] As more studies become available and availability to MRIs improve, MRI may replace ionizing techniques for diagnosis of thromboembolism.

One of the most common reasons for emergent MRI scans from the ED is evaluation of neurologic emergencies (e.g., spinal cord compression). In light of the serious sequelae of spinal cord compression along with a lack of data supporting adverse fetal effects, a pregnant patient exhibiting symptoms of a cord compression should have an MRI scan taken to establish a diagnosis.

The Safety Committee of the Society for Magnetic Resonance Imaging states that MRI procedures are indicated for use in pregnant women when other nonionizing diagnostic imaging methods are inadequate or when the examination will provide important information that would otherwise require exposure to ionizing radiation.[44] It is required to inform pregnant patients that although to date, there is *no indication that the use of clinical MRI procedures during pregnancy produces deleterious effects*, according to the FDA, the safety of MRI procedures during pregnancy has not been definitively proved. It is advisable to obtain informed consent for MRI of a pregnant patient. Also, because of limited data, most facilities avoid

TABLE 59–9 Key Statements on Diagnostic Imaging Modalities during Pregnancy

X-Ray Imaging

"No single diagnostic procedure results in a radiation dose that threatens the well-being of the developing embryo and fetus." (American College of Radiology; From Hall EJ: Scientific view of low-level radiation risks. Radiographics 11:509, 1991.)

"[Fetal] risk is considered to be negligible at 5 rad or less when compared to the other risks of pregnancy, and the risk of malformations is significantly increased above control levels only at doses above 15 rad." (National Council on Radiation Protection and Measurements; From NCRPM: Medical Radiation Exposure of Pregnant and Potentially Pregnant Women. NCRPM Report No. 54. Bethesda, MD, NCRPM, 1977.)

"Women should be counseled that x-ray exposure from a single diagnostic procedure does not result in harmful fetal effects. Specifically, exposure to less than 5 rad has not been associated with an increase in fetal anomalies or pregnancy loss." (American College of Obstetricians and Gynecologists [ACOG], Committee on Obstetric Practice; From ACOG: Guidelines for Diagnostic Imaging During Pregnancy. ACOG Committee Opinion No. 299. Washington, DC, ACOG, September 2004.)

Magnetic Resonance Imaging

"Although there have been no documented adverse fetal effects reported, the National Radiological Protection Board arbitrarily advises against its use in the first trimester." (American College of Obstetricians and Gynecologists [ACOG], Committee on Obstetric Practice; From ACOG: Guidelines for Diagnostic Imaging During Pregnancy. ACOG Committee Opinion No. 158. Washington, DC, ACOG, 1995.)

Ultrasound Imaging

"There have been no reports of documented adverse fetal effects for diagnostic ultrasound procedures, including duplex Doppler imaging." "There are no contraindications to ultrasound procedures during pregnancy, and this modality has largely replaced x-ray as the primary method of fetal imaging during pregnancy." (American College of Obstetricians and Gynecologists [ACOG], Committee on Obstetric Practice; From ACOG: Guidelines for Diagnostic Imaging During Pregnancy. ACOG Committee Opinion No. 299. Washington, DC, ACOG, September, 2004.)

TABLE 59–10 Summary of Magnetic Resonance Imaging during Pregnancy

1. MRI involves no ionizing radiation.
2. There are no known biologic risks associated with MRI and no specific fetal abnormalities have been linked with standard low-intensity MRI scanning.
3. Most obstetric problems can be adequately evaluated with ultrasound.
4. Contrast material is often avoided in conjunction with MRI scanning during pregnancy.
5. Both maternal and fetal anatomy, including the fetal central nervous system, can be evaluated with MRI.
6. The FDA requires documented informed consent and cautions that the full effects of MRI during pregnancy have not yet been determined.
7. MRI is usually eschewed during the first trimester unless there is a clear risk-to-benefit indication, such as possible spinal cord compression.
8. Claustrophobia and the pregnant woman's inability to tolerate prolonged lying on the back can occasionally be problematic.
9. Fetal movement limits information on the fetus unless sedation is provided or ultrafast scans are available.

FDA, U.S. Food and Drug Administration; MRI, magnetic resonance imaging.

TABLE 59–11 Guidelines for Emergency Department Diagnostic Imaging during Pregnancy

1. Women should be counseled that x-ray exposure from a single diagnostic procedure does not result in harmful fetal effects. Specifically, exposure to <5 rad has not been associated with an increase in fetal anomalies or pregnancy loss.
2. Concern about possible effects of high-dose ionizing radiation exposure should not prevent medically indicated diagnostic x-ray procedures from being performed on a pregnant woman. During pregnancy, other imaging procedures not associated with ionizing radiation (ultrasonography and MRI) should be considered instead of x-rays when appropriate.
3. Ultrasonography and MRI are not associated with known adverse fetal effects.
4. Consultation with an expert in dosimetry calculations may be helpful in calculating estimated fetal dose when multiple diagnostic x-rays are performed on a pregnant patient.
5. The use of radioactive isotopes of iodine is contraindicated for therapeutic use during pregnancy.
6. Radiopaque and paramagnetic contrast agents are unlikely to cause harm and may be of diagnostic benefit, but these agents should be used during pregnancy only if the potential benefit justifies the potential risk to the fetus.

MRI, magnetic resonance imaging.
Reproduced from American College of Obstetricians and Gynecologists (ACOG), Committee on Obstetric Practice: Guidelines for Diagnostic Imaging During Pregnancy. ACOG Committee Opinion No. 299. Washington, DC, ACOG, September 2004.

imaging patients in their first trimester. With an inadvertent exposure in a wanted pregnancy, however, the present accumulated data would not warrant an interruption of the pregnancy (Table 59–10).

Although no direct adverse effects on the fetus have been documented, gadolinium-based contrast material *is not recommended for use in pregnant patients.*[43] Gadolinium-based contrast material has been shown to cross the placenta and appear within the fetal bladder moments after intravenous administration.[45] It is then excreted into the amniotic fluid and potentially reabsorbed from the gastrointestinal tract.[45] Because of this reabsorption, the half-life of gadolinium-based contrast material in the fetal circulation is not known.

There is concern about the use of gadolinium in any patient with renal insufficiency owing to the development of a very rare gadoliniun-related syndrome, nephrogenic systemic fibrosis.

US

US continues to be the screening modality of choice for the evaluation of the maternal pelvis and the fetus because of its safety profile, relatively low cost, and real-time capability. Obstetric and gynecologic US account for more than half of the US imaging volume in the United States.[46] Human data accumulated over 25 years has revealed no consistent adverse effects from prenatal diagnostic US examinations.[47,48] US in pregnancy is considered a safe procedure.

The American College of Obstetricians and Gynecologists has reviewed the effects of x-rays, US, and MRI exposure during pregnancy and suggested guidelines for radiographic examination during pregnancy (Table 59–11).[6]

TABLE 59–12 Prevention of Contrast-Induced Nephropathy

Renal Failure: Radiocontrast Agents

Radiocontrast acute renal failure is more likely to occur in the presence of advanced age, renal insufficiency, diabetes mellitus, severe congestive heart failure, multiple myeloma, volume depletion, low cardiac output states, and high-dose contrast studies (>125 mL). The incidence of nephrotoxicity varies depending on the underlying risk factors and the sensitivity of the measure used to determine nephrotoxicity. Using a rather sensitive index of renal dysfunction (an increase in the level of serum creatinine > 0.3 mg/dL and > 20% on day 1, 2, or 3 and day 5, 6, or 7), the incidence of nephrotoxicity is about 2% in nondiabetic, nonazotemic patients and 16% in diabetic, nonazotemic patients. Diabetic patients with azotemia had about a 38% incidence of nephrotoxicity. In a study of 59 diabetic patients with advanced azotemia (mean serum creatinine, 5.9 mg/dL) undergoing coronary angiography, 30 (51%) developed contrast nephrotoxicity as defined by a serum creatinine that was 25% above baseline 48 hr after angiography. Nine patients (15%) required hemodialysis.

Risk Factors for Radiocontrast Nephrotoxicity

Advanced age
Renal insufficiency
Decreased absolute and effective circulatory volume
Diabetes mellitus
Multiple myeloma
Coadministration of other nephrotoxic agents

Note: Renal failure may be oliguric or nonoliguric, with nonoliguric renal failure being more common in patients with near-normal prior renal function. Most episodes of contrast nephrotoxicity are mild, characterized by a reversible 1–3 mg/dL rise in serum creatinine; dialysis therapy is rarely needed and usually only in those patients whose baseline serum creatinine is high, for example, >3 mg/dL

From Brenner and Rector's The Kidneys, 7th ed. Philadelphia, Saunders, 2004, Table 34–3; from MD Consult.

Prevention of Radiocontrast Nephropathy

The development of acute renal failure significantly complicates intravascular contrast medium (CM) use and is linked with high morbidity and mortality. The increasing use of CM, an aging population, and an increase in chronic kidney disease (CKD) will result in an increased incidence of contrast-induced nephropathy (CIN)—unless preventive measures are used. The Canadian Association of Radiologists has developed these guidelines as a practical approach to risk stratification and prevention of CIN. The major risk factor predicting CIN is preexisting CKD, which can be predicted from the glomerular filtration rate (GFR). In terms of being an absolute measure, serum creatinine (SCr) is an unreliable measure of renal function. Patients with GFR >60 mL/min have a very low risk of CIN, and preventive measures are generally unnecessary. When GFR <60 mL/min, preventive measures should be instituted. The risk of CIN is greatest in patients with GFR <30 mL/min. Preventive measures: Alternative imaging that does not require CM should be considered. Fluid volume loading is the single most important protective measure. Nephrotoxic medications should be discontinued 48 hr prior to the study. CM volume and frequency of administration should be minimized, but satisfactory image quality should still be maintained. High-osmolar contrast should be avoided in patients with renal impairment. There is some evidence to suggest that iso-osmolar contrast reduces the risk of CIN among patients with renal impairment, but further study is necessary to determine whether iso-osmolar contrast is superior to low-osmolar contrast. N-acetylcysteine (NAC) has been advocated to reduce the incidence of CIN; however, not all studies have shown a benefit, and it is difficult to formulate evidence-based recommendations at this time. Its use may be considered in high-risk patients but is not considered mandatory.

From Benko A: Canadian Association of radiologists: Consensus guidelines for the prevention of contract-induced nephropathy. Can Assoc Radiol J 58:79, 2007.

Prevention of Radiocontrast Nephropathy—cont'd

Additional Caveats

1. Metformin use is not a contraindication to CM, but metformin should be withheld for 48 hr after CM, and after evaluation of renal function.
2. Whereas GFR is the best way to predict renal dysfunction after CM, patients with normal creatinine are at minimal risk.

Potential Prevention of Contrast-Induced Nephropathy*

NAC (N-acetylcysteine)

Suggested regimen for **oral NAC:** 600 mg (3 mL of 20% solution in liquid) twice a day for 24 hr before and 24 hr after procedure.
Suggested **IV NAC:** 150 mg/kg IV bolus over 30 min, followed by 50 mg/kg infusion over 4 hr.[†]
Example in 80-kg patient: 12,000 mg NAC in 500 ml normal saline over 30 min, followed by 4000 mg NAC in 500 ml normal saline over 4 hr.

Hydration

Suggested regimen for fluid therapy in elective cases: normal saline, at least 1 ml/kg/hr 12 hr before and 12 hr after procedure.
Alternate if emergency procedure required: A 5-mL/kg bolus normal saline 1 hr before and 1 mL/kg/hr for 12 hr after procedure.
Alternative fluid regimen with bicarbonate: add 154 mL of 1000 mEq/L sodium bicarbonate to 850 mL of 5% dextrose in water (or add 3 ampules of standard bicarbonate to 1 L D$_5$W). Initial bolus 3 mL/kg for 1 hr before contrast injection, followed by 1 mL/kg/hr for 6 hr after procedure.

*Suggested but unproven, minimal downside.
[†]From Baker CS, Wragg A, Kumar S, et al: A rapid protocol for the prevention of contrast-induced renal dysfunction: The RAPPID study. J Am Coll Cardiol 41:2114, 2003.
From Merten GJ, Burgess P, Gray LV, et al: Prevention of contrast-induced nephropathology with sodium bicarbonate: A randomized controlled trial JAMA 291:2328, 2004.

Dispensing and Administration Guidelines for CIN (Contrast-Induced Nephropathy)

NAC (N-acetylcysteine) + Hydration

Oral NAC dosing	Hydration
Give NAC 600 mg liquid (3 mL of 20% solution) in 9 mL ginger ale or cola	0.9% sodium chloride IV fluid at 1 mL/kg/hr 12 hr pre- and postcatheterization (normal saline preferred, but 0.45% has also been used with success)

IV Sodium Bicarbonate (154 mEq/L) mixed in 1 L of D$_5$W

	3 mL/kg IV Bolus over 1 Hr	1 mL/kg/hr × 6 Hr IV infusion	Total mL Infused
60 kg	180 ml	360 mL (60 mL/hr)	**540**
70 kg	210 ml	420 mL (70 mL/hr)	**630**
80 kg	240 ml	480 mL (80 mL/hr)	**720**
90 kg	270 ml	540 mL (90 mL/hr)	**810**
100 kg	300 ml	600 mL (100 mL/hr)	**900**
≥110 kg	330 ml	660 mL (110 mL/hr)	**990**

From Merten GJ, Burgess WP, Gray LV, et al: Prevention of contrast-induced nephropathy with sodium bicarbonate: A randomized controlled trial. JAMA 291:2328, 2004.

TABLE 59–12 Prevention of Contrast-Induced Nephropathy—cont'd

Potential Prevention of Contrast-Induced Nephropathy*—cont'd

IV N-Acetylcysteine

	150 mg/kg IV bolus over 30 minutes	50 mg/kg IV infusion over 4 hours
60 kg	9,000 mg/500 ml NS	3,000 mg/500 ml NS
70 kg	10,500 mg/500 ml NS	3,500 mg/500 ml NS
80 kg	12,000 mg/500 ml NS	4,000 mg/500 ml NS
90 kg	13,500 mg/500 ml NS	4,500 mg/500 ml NS
≥100 kg	15,000 mg/500 ml NS	5,000 mg/500 ml NS

From Baker CS, Wragg A, Kumar S, et al: A rapid protocol for the prevention of contrast-induced renal dysfunction. The RAPPID study. J Am Coll Cardiol 41:2114, 2003.

Potential Prevention of Contrast-Induced Nephropathy*—cont'd

UMMC Pharmacy Cost Comparisons with treatment regimens for CIN

Regimens	Cost
600 mg NAC × 8 doses (oral)	$5.82
2 L NS	$1.60
Sodium bicarbonate 154 mEq/L D_5W	$1.32 (drug only)
70-kg patient: 10,500 mg/500 mL NS bolus IV NAC	$183.00 (drug only)
70-kg patient: 3500 mg/500 mL NS infusion IV NAC	$61.00 (drug only)

TABLE 59–13 Magnetic Resonance Imaging Contrast Agent Concerns and Contraindications

Information for Health Care Professionals Gadolinium-based Contrast Agents for Magnetic Resonance Imaging (marketed as Magnevist, MultiHance, Omniscan, OptiMARK, ProHance)

FDA ALERT [6/2006, updated 12/2006 and 5/23/2007]: This updated Alert highlights FDA's request for addition of a boxed warning and new warnings about risk of nephrogenic systemic fibrosis (NSF) to the full prescribing information for all gadolinium-based contrast agents (GBCAs) (Magnevist, MultiHance, Omniscan, OptiMARK, ProHance). This new labeling highlights and describes the risk for NSF following exposure to a GBCA in patients with acute or chronic severe renal insufficiency (a glomerular filtration rate < 30 mL/min/1.73 m²) and patients with acute renal insufficiency of any severity due to the hepatorenal syndrome or in the perioperative liver transplantation period. In these patients, avoid the use of a GBCA unless the diagnostic information is essential and not available with non–contrast-enhanced MRI. NSF may result in fatal or debilitating systemic fibrosis. Requested changes to GBCA product labeling are summarized below.

- Evaluate renal function in all patients before administering a gadolinium-based contrast agent.
- Whenever possible, avoid gadolinium-containing contrast media for MRI and MRA in patients with moderate to end-stage renal failure. Contrast agents that contain gadolinium include Magnevist, MultiHance, Omniscan, OptiMARK, and ProHance.
- If gadolinium-containing agents must be used, consider prompt dialysis after the procedure to eliminate circulating gadolinium. However, it is unknown whether dialysis can prevent or treat NSF/NFD.
- Encourage patients to contact their health care provider if they have signs of NSF/NFD.
- Report cases of NSF/NFD to the FDA's MedWatch program at www.fda.gov/medwatch/index.html or by calling 1-800-332-1088 (1-800-FDA-1088).

FDA, U.S Food and Drug Administration; MRA, magnetic resonance angiography; MRI, magnetic resonance imaging; NFD, nephrogenic fibrosing deformity.

Contraindications for Magnetic Resonance Imaging

(Because this is an area of continuing change, and there are rapid advancements in the technology to produce magnetic resonance imaging (MRI)–safe materials, consultation with the radiology department is suggested if any questions arise concerning the safety of MRI scanning.)

Overview

There are few contraindications to MRI. Overall, no biologic adverse effects are associated with conventional MRI. Most contraindications to MRI are relative and essentially precautions related to the effect of MRI on devices and material within the body that may be affected by the MRI magnetic field.

Implanted Devices and Foreign Bodies

Electronic devices and magnetizable materials represent potential hazards to the patient. Titanium objects are safe for MRI.

- **Intracoronary stents**: It is considered safe to perform an MRI at any time after placement of coronary artery stents of any type.
- **Sternal wires after sternotomy**: Sternal wires sutures are considered safe for MRI imaging.
- **Mechanical cardiac valves**: It is safe to scan most prosthetic cardiac valves because, at most, they experience only a mild torque. An exception involves the pre-6000 series Starr-Edwards caged ball valves, devices rarely used now.
- **Pacemakers, implantable defibrillators, and implanted electronic devices**: The risks of scanning patients with cardiac pacemakers are related to possible movement of the device, magnetically induced programming changes, electromagnetic interference, and induced currents in lead wires leading to heating and/or cardiac stimulation. It is currently considered inadvisable for patients with pacemakers or other intracardiac wires to undergo MRI. Nerve stimulators, insulin pumps, cochlear implants, and other implanted electronic devices also may be affected by MRI and are considered unsafe.

Continued

TABLE 59–13 Magnetic Resonance Imaging Contrast Agent Concerns and Contraindications—cont'd

○ **Implanted vagal nerve stimulator**: A brain MRI performed at < 2 Tesla, with a send and receive head coil and the stimulator turned off, appears to be safe under guidelines published by the manufacturer. Other MRI studies are not known to be safe.

○ **Aneurysm clips and magnetizable materials**: Any ferromagnetic object within the body represents a potential hazard when exposed to the large magnetic field of an MRI system. The hazard primarily reflects the possibility of deflecting the foreign body sufficiently to injure vital structures. For example, certain older-model vascular clips used in cerebral aneurysms are ferromagnetic and could be moved by the magnetic field, with obviously dire consequences.

○ **Intraorbital or intraocular metallic fragments**, such as might be acquired from machining, are a potential risk, and generally contraindicate MRI.

• **Cutaneous metal objects**: Although most metallic biomaterials are now nonferrous and nonmagnetizable, any metallic device within or connected to the patient needs to be evaluated for safety. The presence of dental alloys, wires, splints, dental braces, and prostheses does not appear to pose a risk to the patient,

although these materials may result in artifactual changes. Cutaneous burns can result from skin contact with metal objects, including neurosurgical halo pins, pulse oximetry probes, and drug-eluting medical patches that contain metal foil (e.g., nicotine patch), although the mechanism of this injury is unclear.

○ **Orthopaedic/neurosurgical hardware**: It is safe to perform MRI in patients with titanium implants, screws, rods, and artificial joints.

○ **Bullets/shrapnel**: These foreign objects within the body are relative contraindications to MRI scanning. Many bullets are safe but those with metal (specialized bullets, such as metal jackets) may pose a risk.

○ **Tattoos**: The majority of professionally obtained tattoos are safe for MRI; however, tattoos containing lead, such as those obtained in prison, can burn the skin if exposed to MRI.

• **Oxygen cylinders**: Standard metal oxygen cylinders should not be used in the MRI suite. Oxygen cylinders that are safe are available.

• **Credit cards**: Credit card and other information containing strips may be destroyed in the MRI scanner.

SUMMARY

In summary, the threshold dose for the nonstochastic effects throughout the gestational period is less than 5 rad. Prenatal doses of greater than 5 rad present no measurable increased risk of prenatal death, malformations, growth retardation, or impairment of mental development over the background incidence of these entities. The risk for stochastic effects, carcinogenesis or mutagenesis, is related to the fetal absorbed dose and is very small compared with the natural background incidence of childhood cancer and genetic disease for most diagnostic procedures.

The vast majority of radiographic imaging obtained in the ED exposes the fetus to 100 times less than the threshold for adverse effects. The 5-rad threshold for onset of concern for adverse fetal effects is quite conservative, and any statistically significant change in fetal outcome probably requires at least several times this dose. Utilization of one of the methods put forth in this chapter to counsel pregnant patients in need

of diagnostic imaging, and for women inadvertently exposed to radiation prior to the recognition of pregnancy, should help to educate patients and alleviate their fear.

CLINICAL USE OF RADIOCONTRAST MATERIAL

Emergency clinicians must frequently initiate studies with the use of radiocontrast material. A full discussion of these procedures is not within the scope of this chapter, but basic issues of contrast material–induced nephropathy, the possible prevention thereof, and recent concern over the use of gadolinium for MRI studies have been included for completeness and ready reference (Tables 59–12 and 59–13).

 REFERENCES CAN BE FOUND ON EXPERT CONSULT

CHAPTER 60

Management of Increased Intracranial Pressure and Intracranial Shunts

Frederick K. Korley

Headache and head injury are commonly encountered in emergency departments (EDs). If either of them is accompanied by vomiting, decreased level of consciousness, and abnormal vital signs, the possibility of increased intracranial pressure (ICP) must be considered. Accompanying clinical symptoms may be vague or subtle, making the diagnosis of increased ICP difficult. The clinician must rely on the physical examination, diagnostic studies, and a high index of suspicion to diagnose increased ICP. *Many cases are subtle and escape initial detection despite a conscientious evaluation by competent clinicians.* Increased ICP is a neurologic emergency that must be managed quickly before further brain damage ensues. Familiarity with the pathophysiology of increased ICP facilitates the understanding of the diagnosis and management of increased ICP.

PATHOPHYSIOLOGY OF ICP

Alexander Monro, an anatomist in the 18th century, defined the intracranial contents as a fixed volume. The fixed-volume theory was supported by George Kellie a few years later and became known as the Monro-Kellie doctrine. This doctrine has guided our understanding of intracranial dynamics and the principles of autoregulation.

The components of the calvaria are the brain, the cerebrospinal fluid (CSF), the venous blood supply, and the arterial blood supply (Fig. 60–1). The CSF and the venous blood supply have the greatest ability to change their volume to compensate for increases due to other reasons.

These dynamic changes in relative cranial content proportions may not affect the patient if the ICP is not excessive. If a pathologic process overwhelms the compensating mechanisms, the result will be an increase in ICP. Unfortunately, ICP increases nearly exponentially as the brain volume increases, despite compensating mechanisms (Fig. 60–2).

Normal supine ICP usually ranges from 5 to 15 mm Hg relative to the foramen of Monro. Transient increases of ICP as high as 80 to 100 mm Hg can be noted with coughing or straining. Other factors that can transiently increase ICP are movement, pain, and fever. A space-occupying lesion such as a tumor, hematoma, pus, or foreign body can also raise ICP. Figure 60–3 demonstrates that the area and the etiology of increased ICP will determine where the brain shift occurs to produce herniation.

Brain

The brain volume can be increased by edema, benign intracranial hypertension, tumor, or bleeding. The three types of edema are vasogenic, cytotoxic, and interstitial. Vasogenic edema is due to increased permeability of the capillaries leading to the passage of excess fluid into the extracellular space. Cytotoxic edema is due to brain tissue (neurons and glia) accumulation of intracellular fluid due to dysfunction of the adenosine triphosphatase (ATPase) pump. Interstitial edema is increased brain fluid due to a block in the absorption of CSF.

Benign (idiopathic) intracranial hypertension (BIH) is also known as pseudotumor cerebri. It is increased CSF pressure not due to a tumor, edema, or hydrocephalus. Its exact pathophysiology remains a mystery. Common associated conditions are listed in Table 60–1. BIH is a diagnosis of exclusion. Owing to its subtle presentation, and normal computed tomography (CT) findings, *it is often not suspected or diagnosed on initial clinical evaluations*. It is seen more frequently in obese women. Presenting symptoms may include headache, nausea, and blurry vision. Occasionally, the headache is worse upon awakening or with exertion. In general, patients with BIH have a normal neurologic examination except for the occasional papilledema. Severe cases can lead to permanent vision loss.

Brain tumors encompass neoplasms that originate in the brain itself (primary brain tumors) or involve the brain as a metastatic site (secondary brain tumors). *Primary brain tumors* include tumors of the brain parenchyma, meninges, cranial nerves, and other intracranial structures (the pituitary and pineal glands). Primary central nervous system (CNS) lymphoma refers to non-Hodgkin's lymphoma confined to the CNS. The site of origin of this type of tumor remains unknown. *Secondary brain tumors* originate elsewhere in the body and metastasize to the intracranial compartment. They are the most common types of brain tumors.

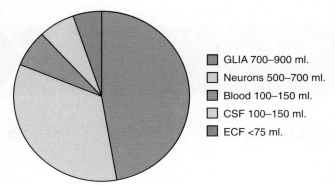

GLIA 700–900 ml.

Neurons 500–700 ml.

Blood 100–150 ml.

CSF 100–150 ml.

ECF <75 ml.

Figure 60–1 Intracranial contents and their volumes for healthy adults.

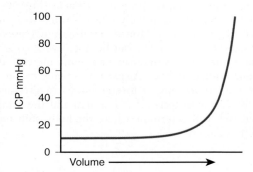

Figure 60–2 Intracranial volume-pressure relationship demonstrates the limits of compensatory mechanisms.

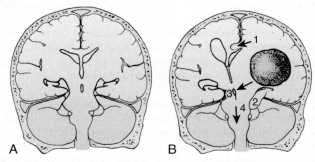

Figure 60–3 Intracranial shifts from supratentorial lesions. *A,* Relationships of the various supratentorial compartments as seen in a coronal section. *B,* Herniation of the cingulate gyrus under the falx (*1*); herniation of the temporal lobe into the tentorial notch (*2*); compression of the opposite cerebral peduncle against the unyielding tentorium, producing Kernohan's notch (*3*); and downward displacement of the brainstem through the tentorial notch (*4*). *(A and B, From Plum F, Posner JB: The Diagnosis of Stupor and Coma, 2nd ed. Philadelphia, FA Davis, 1972. Reproduced by permission.)*

TABLE 60–1 Clinical Conditions and Factors Associated with Idiopathic or Benign Intracranial Hypertension (Pseudotumor Cerebri)

Hematologic Disorders

Iron deficiency anemia
Pernicious anemia
Polycythemia vera
Thrombocytopenia
Lupus
Cushing disease
Hypoparathyroidism
Hypothyroidism

Endocrine Conditions and Disorders

Addison disease
Menstrual irregularities, menstrual cycle
Pregnancy

Medical/Surgical Conditions with Impaired Cerebral Venous Drainage

Otitis media, mastoiditis
Idiopathic dural sinus thrombosis
Radical neck surgery
Chronic pulmonary disease with venous hypertension
Heart failure with venous hypertension
Congenital heart disease
Renal failure
High-flow arteriovenous malformation
Chronic obstructive pulmonary disease
Sleep apnea
Growth hormone
Cimetidine

Dietary Considerations

Hypervitaminosis A
Hypovitaminosis A
Obesity
Malnutrition

Common Drugs

Systemic steroid withdrawal
Topical steroid withdrawal (infants)
Oral contraceptives
Tetracycline/minocycline
Nitrofurantoin
Sulfamethoxazole
Vitamin A excess
Glucocorticoids
Nalidixic acid
Levothyroxine
Lithium
Isotretinoin (Accutane)
Nonsteroidal anti-inflammatory drugs
Tamoxifen
Cyclosporine

Bleeding in the brain can occur spontaneously (as in the case of subarachnoid hemorrhage [SAH]) or can be a result of trauma. Spontaneous SAH is often the result of a ruptured berry aneurysm. Traumatic injury to the brain can often result in increased ICP by causing either epidural hematomas, subdural hematomas, or intraparenchymal hemorrhage. Diffuse axonal injury (DAI) may occur in isolation or conjunction with intracerebral bleeding. With DAI, it is believed that the axons are not actually torn, but instead suffer significant injury that may lead to swelling (shearing effect).[1]

CSF

The CSF is produced by the choroid plexus at a daily rate of 500 mL. It flows freely from the lateral ventricles into the cisterns and the subarachnoid space and is drained by the arachnoid villi of the dural sinuses to maintain a volume of 100 to 150 mL. Blockage of this flow at any point can cause hydrocephalus proximal to the obstruction. The two types of hydrocephalus are obstructive and communicating. *Obstruc-*

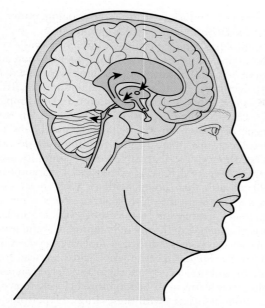

Figure 60–4 Cerebrospinal fluid production and flow. *(From Rengachary, Wilkins [eds]: Principles of Neurosurgery. Philadelphia, Mosby, 1994.)*

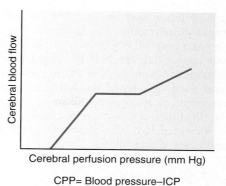

CPP= Blood pressure–ICP

Figure 60–5 Cerebral autoregulation.

tive hydrocephalus happens when the blockage occurs at the ventricular system by a tumor, colloid cyst, or primary stenosis. *Communicating hydrocephalus* is due to blockage outside of the ventricular system by either impedance of flow through the basal cisterns or lack of absorption by the arachnoid villi. Communicating hydrocephalus is often due to infection or SAH (Fig. 60–4).

Blood

Up to a certain range, cerebral blood flow (CBF) is maintained by an autoregulatory mechanism despite fluctuations in cerebral perfusion pressure (CPP) (Fig. 60–5). This autoregulatory zone is CPP of 60 to 160 mm Hg.

Once the CPP is out of the autoregulatory zone, CBF is linearly related to CPP. CPP less than 60 mm Hg can lead to ischemia whereas that above 160 mm Hg can cause hypertensive encephalopathy.

CLINICAL PRESENTATION

The neurologic examination can be normal in someone with a mild increase in ICP owing to the brain's compensatory mechanisms. Patients who present with a complaint of headache or head injury may not initially manifest the more dramatic and worrisome symptoms of increased ICP such as vomiting, syncope, altered mentation, or Cushing's triad (bradycardia, increased blood pressure with wide pulse pressure, and irregular respirations). ICP correlates poorly with clinical symptomatology. One of the earliest clinical signs is decreased venous pulsation on funduscopic examination. This may be difficult to detect in the uncooperative individual. Initially, head CT scan findings might not correlate well with the patient's neurologic insult. However, as compensatory mechanisms fail, head CT findings as well as clinical symptoms will become more obvious.

Signs and symptoms of severe ICP increases include Glasgow coma scale (GCS) score of 8 or less, decreased level of consciousness, papilledema, cranial nerve findings, or CT scans showing compression of the third ventricle or midline shift. When any of these findings are noted, urgent intervention is warranted, including neurosurgical consultation, because invasive ICP reduction and monitoring may be warranted. The risk of such invasive intervention should be weighed carefully and should be performed by a neurosurgeon. The emergency clinician may initiate medical management of increased ICP pending definitive neurosurgical intervention.

MEDICAL TREATMENT OF INCREASED ICP

Oxygenation

In any trauma or medical patient, managing the airway deserves primary attention. If the patient is hypoxic, supportive oxygenation is necessary to prevent further ischemia. Once the patient's GCS is 9 or lower or if any impending sign of inadequate respiratory status is observed, rapid-sequence intubation should be considered to protect the airway, control the carbon dioxide partial pressure (Pco_2) level, and optimize the oxygen partial pressure (Po_2) level based on the entire clinical scenario.

Sedation and Paralytics

The sequence and types of medications administered have been discussed with regard to limiting further increases in ICP while facilitating rapid intubation. *The value of such interventions once thought to be helpful is questionable and debatable.* Rapid assessment of the patient's neurologic examination must be done before giving sedation and paralytics in order to determine any changes in the patient's status. If time allows, the patient may be premedicated 3 minutes before intubation with lidocaine at 1 to 1.5 mg/kg while preoxygenating the patient. Lidocaine has been reported to blunt the rise in ICP associated with laryngoscopy, and may protect against some hypoxia-related dysrhythmias. A defasciculating dose (1/10 of the intubating dose) of a non-depolarizing neuromuscular blocking agent may be administered. This theoretically counteracts the transient fasciculation and increase in ICP that occurs when succinylcholine is initially administered. Atropine (0.02 mg/kg) may be included in this premedication if the patient is younger than 10 years old because succinylcholine can be associated with bradycardia in that age group. However, the value of atropine is quite questionable, even in infants. This regimen is followed by sedation with drugs that may block the rise in ICP, such as etomidate (at 0.3 mg/kg) or thiopental (50–100 mg intravenously or 3–5 mg/kg).

Etomidate is preferred over thiopental if the patient has an unstable hemodynamic status. Etomidate has two significant benefits—it has a minimal effect on systemic blood pressure and does not appear to increase ICP.[2,3] A paralytic of choice is succinylcholine at 1.5 mg/kg (2 mg/kg in pediatric patients). Sedation and paralytics should be short-acting in order to follow the patient's neurologic examination. Fentanyl (3 μg/kg) is an excellent drug for pain control, which, if untreated, can lead to increased ICP. This should be given during the pretreatment phase if time allows.

Hyperventilation

Once the patient's airway has been secured, he or she should be maintained on adequate oxygenation, starting at 100%, and titrating to lower levels after transport to intensive care unit settings.[1] In the past, aggressive hyperventilation was widely used to maintain the arterial carbon dioxide pressure (Pa_{CO_2}) at 25 mm Hg in order to reduce ICP. However, aggressive hyperventilation is no longer recommended because Pco_2 levels of 25 mm Hg can cause cerebral vasoconstriction resulting in decreased CBF.[1] The most recent recommendations state that in the short term, the target goal for ventilation is now 35 to 40 mm Hg.[4] The long-term recommendation is to avoid hyperventilation because it may cause prolonged vasoconstriction leading to ischemia and worse long-term outcome.[5] The role of hyperventilation in the rapidly deteriorating patient with elevated ICP remains controversial.

Head Position

If shock is not present, some literature supports head elevation to about 30° in order to decrease ICP. According to Feldman and Kanter and coworkers,[6] elevation of the head to 30° significantly reduces ICP in a majority of patients without impairing CBF, CPP, and cerebral metabolic rate of oxygenation. This position allows drainage of cerebral veins. Raising the head in a patient with hypotension would further decrease the patient's mean arterial pressure (MAP) and hence lower CPP. If head elevation is to be used, MAP must be maintained above 90 mm Hg.[7] It is also important to avoid neck rotation, flexion, or any intervention that could result in jugular compression. If jugular veins are compressed, venous outflow from the head can be further compromised.

Fluid Management

The goal in fluid management is to maintain euvolemia. Patients with increased ICP are often dehydrated due to profuse vomiting or are in shock due to loss of vasomotor sympathetic tone. The traditional practice of fluid restriction for patients with increased ICP is no longer in favor. Head-injured patients with hypotension have twice the mortality risk. Cardiac pressors, in addition to fluids, are often used to maintain CPP greater than 70 mm Hg and MAP greater than 90 mm Hg.

Diuresis

Mannitol has been shown to be effective in reducing ICP. If increased ICP causes further deterioration in the patient's status, mannitol can be given at 0.5 to 1.0 g/kg infused every 2 to 6 hours. Current recommendations suggest bolus therapy over continuous infusion. This is a bridging effort while awaiting definitive therapy such as craniotomy.

Mannitol has two properties—it initially acts as a volume expander and then serves as an osmotic agent. Upon administration of mannitol, intravascular volume expands and blood viscosity decreases, resulting in augmentation of CBF. This is the reason the bolus should be administered as rapidly as possible. Once volume expansion has occurred, an osmotic movement of fluid from the cellular compartment to the intravascular compartment begins, resulting in a decrease in ICP. The osmotic effect usually occurs within 15 minutes, resulting in decreased ICP. The half-life of mannitol ranges from 90 minutes to 6 hours. Patients with intact cerebral autoregulation benefit the most from the effects of mannitol.[8] If the patient's serum osmolality is above 320 mOsm/L, little benefit is obtained with the use of mannitol. Careful monitoring is necessary to maintain the osmolarity between 310 to 320 mOsm/L.[7] Higher levels of osmolality can lead to renal damage. In addition to serum osmolality, electrolytes, pH, and pulmonary status must be monitored closely to avoid the complications associated with these drugs. Hypertonic saline has been suggested as an alternative to mannitol.[9] Mannitol should not be used prophylactically, but instead, reserved for those patients with impending transtentorial herniation.

Seizure Prophylaxis

Controlling seizure activity is important to avoid elevation of ICP and possible herniation. Rapid-acting benzodiazepines such as lorazepam and diazepam are first-line therapy, followed by antiepileptic agents such as pentobarbital or phenytoin. Fosphenytoin has the advantage of rapid administration compared with that of phenytoin, which can be given only at a maximum rate of 50 mg/min. Phenytoin can induce hypotension and lower CPP, even at rates below 50 mg/min. Some clinicians give patients with severe head injury prophylactic phenytoin or fosphenytoin. The value of this practice for reducing seizure risk is unknown.

Patients who are paralyzed, either chemically or by their neurologic disease, are hard to monitor for seizure unless electroencephalogram (EEG) monitoring is available. These patients manifest seizures by elevation in their heart rate or blood pressure or spikes in their ICP monitor. If seizure control is not obtained with benzodiazepines or phenytoin, or both, paralysis and the inducement of a pentobarbital coma should follow. Pentobarbital has been used to treat uncontrolled increased ICP if medical and surgical management have failed. It decreases cerebral blood flow, metabolism, oxygen consumption, and cerebral edema and also scavenges free radicals.[10] Pentobarbital is given at a loading dose of 10 mg/kg over 30 minutes followed by infusion of 3 mg/kg/hr with an EEG monitor available for burst suppression. Intensive monitoring of the patient's hemodynamic status is necessary owing to pentobarbital's hypotensive effect. Similarly, intubation and controlled ventilation are needed for patients receiving this much barbiturate.

Steroids

Steroids have been shown to be beneficial in patients with vasogenic edema—edema associated with brain tumors. Its benefit has been noted to decrease CSF production, stabilize membranes, and restore normal membrane permeability.[11-13] Dexamethasone is usually given at 10 to 20 mg intravenous loading dose, followed by 4 to 10 mg every 6 hours. No studies support the use of steroids in head-injured patients.

Glucose Control

Head-injured patients tend to be hyperglycemic as a response to stress or steroid administration. Optimization of blood glucose levels is desirable in order to avoid cellular edema of brain tissue. Hypoglycemic states should be avoided. However, the long-term value of tight glycemic control is unclear.

Hypothermia

Lower body temperatures have been associated with a decrease in blood flow, ICP, and metabolism. The prior method of keeping core temperatures to less than 30°C has been abandoned. It fell out of favor owing to complications of cardiac arrhythmias and difficulty maintaining this level. One study has shown a statistically significant benefit in terms of survival and decreased ICP with mild hypothermia (32°C–34°C).[14] It is important to avoid hyperthermia. A 1° rise in body temperature results in several millimeters of mercury rise in ICP. Acetaminophen is effective in fever control.

Operative Management

Operative management is the definitive treatment if ICP cannot be adequately managed by the previously discussed measures. This entails craniotomy to relieve the compressive edema, hematoma, or tumor or ventriculostomy with drainage of the increased blood or CSF fluid.

INTRACRANIAL SHUNTS

Intracranial shunts are used for the long-term management of increased ICP. A recurrent elevation in ICP due to shunt malfunction can occur days to years after shunt placement.

Intracranial shunt malfunctions are often diagnosed in the ED. In many cases, the patient's significant other or caretaker provides the subtle clues to diagnose a shunt malfunction. Depending on the age of the patient, recurrent symptoms of increased ICP include changes in behavior, headache, nausea, vomiting, or visual disturbances. In children, lethargy, poor feeding, vomiting, ataxia, decreased or increased activity level, fever, diaphoresis, and fussiness can be indications of shunt malfunction. In children, lethargy and shunt site swelling are the most predictive of shunt malfunction.[15] Failure to gaze upward is another sensitive sign of nonacute shunt malfunction (sunset eyes). Cranial nerves and visual field examination should be routine in the assessment of older, cooperative patients with intracranial shunts.

The essential elements of any shunt system include the proximal and distal catheters, a valve, and a reservoir. A wide array of valves, catheters, and other devices is available for use in shunt systems. Most of them are more or less satisfactory and the selection of a particular one is more subjective than scientific. The valve allows unidirectional flow, incorporates a pumping chamber, and regulates the pressure at which flow will occur by responding to the pressure difference across it. The reservoir is usually located between two valves. The proximal valve allows flow from the ventricles to the reservoir, whereas the distal valve allows flow from the reservoir to the distal portion of the catheter (Fig. 60–6). Many different types of shunt systems are available incorporating a variety of

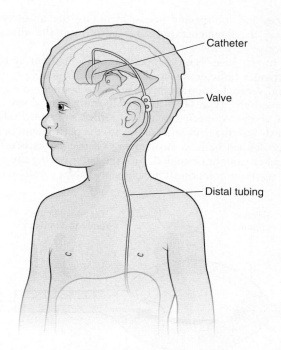

Figure 60–6 The basic tripartite ventricular shunt system is composed of a ventricular catheter, valve mechanism, and distal tubing. A slit valve may be used in the far end of the distal tubing instead of a more proximally placed valve, as shown.

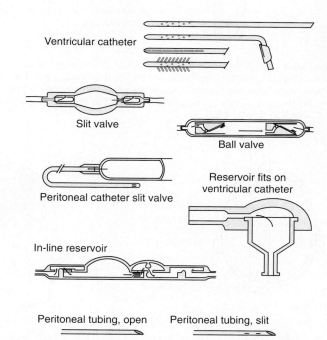

Figure 60–7 Shunt components. *(From Rengachary, Wilkins [eds]: Principles of Neurosurgery. Philadelphia, Mosby, 1994.)*

designs (Fig. 60–7). Some have one valve or unique characteristics such as a double dome or an absence of valves altogether.

In most cases, the reservoir gives successful access to the system for pressure measurement, patency testing, fluid sampling, and injection of medication or contrast material. In more rare cases, other equipment is available that can be incorporated into the shunt system under special circumstances and for specific needs, including the on-off switch device, the telemetric pressure sensor, and the antisiphon device.

In the basic ventriculoperitoneal (VP) shunt system, a ventricular catheter is placed in the right frontal horn of the lateral ventricle (nondominant brain) to connect to a subcutaneous valve (Fig. 60–8) traversing the temporal side. This valve is then connected to a distal catheter threaded subcutaneously into the neck and finally into the peritoneum or some other defined body compartment. Ventricular catheters can be either straight or angled, with the latter having the option of a reservoir component attachment. Valves usually come in four different types (ball, diaphragm, miter, slit), each with unique flow characteristics. The distal catheter is either a closed or an open end. Identifying the type of shunt in place is often difficult unless the patient has that information available. The skin overlying the subcutaneous part at the temples can often scar, thus rendering palpation of the shunt type impossible.

The principle of any extracranial shunting technique is to divert CSF into a body cavity from which it can readily be eliminated and drained. VP shunts are at present the mainstay of hydrocephalus treatment in infants and children because of their ease of insertion and reliable long-term function (Fig. 60–9). Other types of extracranial shunts include ventriculovenous (VV), ventriculoatrial (VA), ventriculopleural (VPl), and lumboperitoneal. These other shunts are usually reserved for circumstances in which VP shunting has failed because of complications or if there is a history of multiple abdominal surgeries or peritoneal infections.

Shunt Assessment

The usual cause of shunt malfunction is catheter obstruction. Proximal blockage may be due to tissue debris or choroid plexus within the ventricular catheter. Distal obstruction of venous shunts may result from thrombus or venous occlusion (such as in the VA shunt). Peritoneal shunts may be associated with infection (peritonitis) or mechanical obstruction (e.g., omentum blockade). Some evidence suggests that delayed hypersensitivity to shunt material is an occasional cause of obstruction. Symptoms of shunt malfunction may be difficult to interpret, particularly if the symptoms are atypical or nonspecific or if they occur in young children. Likewise, asymptomatic shunt obstruction can take place in children who have developed shunt independence. The clinical evaluation of a child may not always be diagnostic of a shunt malfunction.

The characteristics of valve pumping may be useful in shunt malfunction diagnosis in only about 5% of cases.[16]

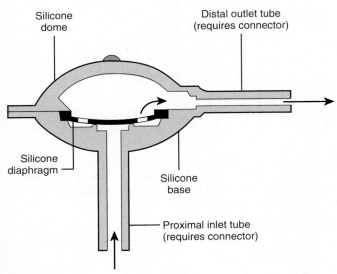

Figure 60–8 Cross-section of a Pudenz flushing valve (American Heyer-Schulte, Santa Barbara, CA) illustrates the diaphragm valve. The proximal inlet tube and silicone base are placed in the bur hole so that only the reservoir (silicon dome) protrudes above the skull. *(Courtesy of PS Medical, Goleta, CA.)*

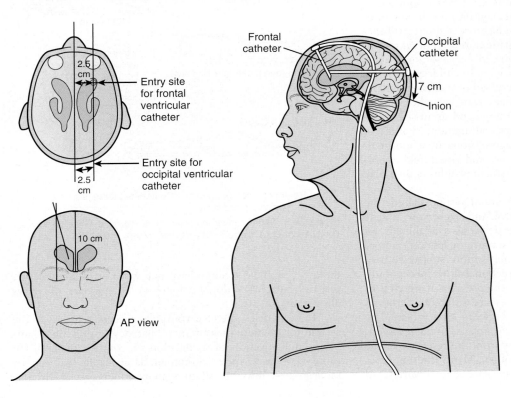

Figure 60–9 Ventriculoperitoneal shunt and alternative occipital placement. *(From Rengachary, Wilkins [eds]: Principles of Neurosurgery. Philadelphia, Mosby, 1994, Fig. 7–6.)*

Partial shunt valve compression should be done because full depression and release may lead to choroid plexus suction. If the CT scan shows narrow (slit) ventricles, indicating overdrainage, further valve compression may cause blockage of the shunt by suction of the choroid plexus. When palpating the shunt, a normal refill time of 15 to 30 seconds should be seen. If the valve fills slowly but can be compressed easily, the obstruction is proximal to the valve. If the valve is not compressible, blockage is either at the valve or distal to it. Proximal obstruction is more common than distal. Other sources of proximal blockage are blood clots or debris related to the surgical procedure. Sources of distal occlusion include malposition, infection, shunt disconnection, and pseudocyst formation. The entire shunt tract and surgical incisions should be examined for signs of wound infection, disruption of the tubing, or CSF leakage around the tract. Definitive treatment usually requires shunt revision.

Infection is often due to skin organisms overlying the valve that may ulcerate and colonize the shunt.[17] The typical organisms are *Staphylococcus epidermidis* or *aureus*. Approximately 70% of these infections are seen within 2 months of shunt placement. Other risk factors associated with shunt infection include perioperative infection or any subsequent dental or urologic instrumentation. The VA shunt has been largely avoided because of chronic bacteremia associated with it. Two studies have shown that approximately 8% of neurosurgical patients with implanted shunts acquire infections.[18,19] Treatment often involves replacement of the system.

Radiographic evaluation of shunt function in the ED begins with both a noncontrast head CT scan and shunt series x-rays. Shunt series x-rays consist of anteroposterior (AP) and lateral skull, AP chest, and AP abdominal x-rays (Figs. 60–10 to 60–18). They may reveal kinking, breakage, or disconnection of the catheter. Head CT scan has a sensitivity of 83% in detecting shunt obstruction and a negative predictive value of 93% (Figs. 60–19 and 60–20). Shunt series x-rays have a sensitivity of 20% and a negative predictive value of 22%. When combined, the two tests have a sensitivity of 88% and a negative predictive value of 95%. Because they are complementary, it is important to obtain both studies.[20–22] It should be noted, however, that the finding of large ventricles on CT reveals little about shunt function unless it can be compared with a baseline or serial scans show progressive ventricular expansion.

If the distal catheter is in the peritoneum and a distal obstruction is suspected or the patient complains of abdominal pain, an abdominal ultrasound should be obtained. The ultrasound may reveal a pseudocyst at the distal portion of the catheter or an abnormal fluid collection.

Finally, CSF analysis is important whenever an assessment of infection or shunt function is undertaken. Shunt

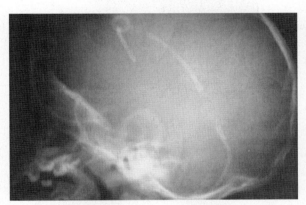

Figure 60–11 Lateral skull radiograph of patient in Figure 60–10. This view better reveals a cylindrical Holter valve situated a few centimeters distal to the Rickham reservoir.

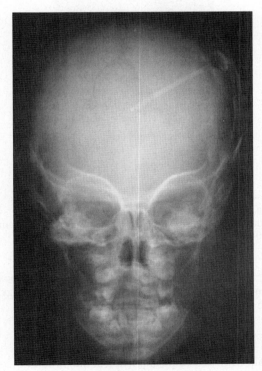

Figure 60–10 A standard shunt series includes an anteroposterior (AP) skull, lateral skull, chest radiograph and kidney, ureters, bladder (KUB) series. This intact shunt is a Rickham reservoir over the bur hole, with a cylindrical Holter valve a few centimeters distal. This AP skull radiograph reveals the proximal intracranial portion of the shunt and a Rickham reservoir over the burr hole. A non-contrast CT scan of the head is usually performed to further evaluate complaints in patients with shunts.

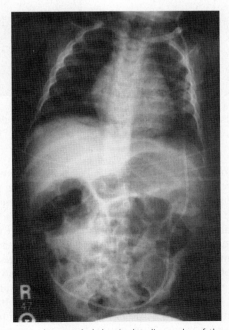

Figure 60–12 AP chest and abdominal radiographs of the patient in Figure 60–10. This radiograph reveals the distal portion of the shunt. Note the length of the catheter to allow for patient growth.

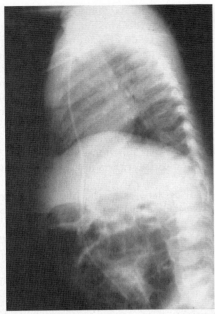

Figure 60–13 Lateral chest radiograph of the patient in Figure 60–10.

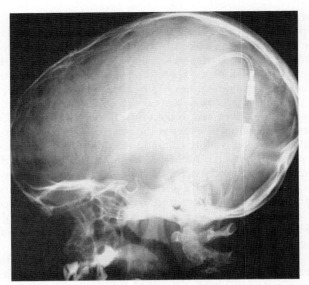

Figure 60–15 Normal lateral skull radiograph demonstrates an intact ventricular peritoneal shunt in a young patient with a Holter valve. This shunt later became disconnected (see Figs. 60–17 and 60–18).

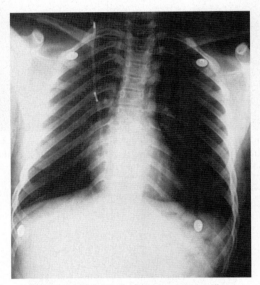

Figure 60–14 Chest radiograph from a shunt series illustrates connector discontinuity of a ventricular peritoneal shunt at the level of the clavicle.

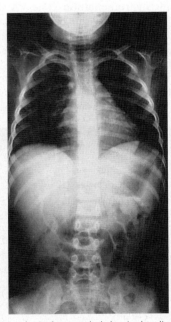

Figure 60–16 Normal AP chest and abdominal radiographs demonstrates an intact ventricular peritoneal shunt in the patient in Figure 60–15.

devices should include tapping the reservoir proximal to the distal valve to allow percutaneous testing of the proximal shunt patency. Although this is useful in most instances, it can be difficult to assess the rate of inflow or runoff adequately with a small-bore needle, particularly if the patient is a child or uncooperative. The potential for infection is a disadvantage of percutaneous tapping. Other invasive techniques include injection of either radionuclide or contrast material into the shunt as a marker of flow. If ventricular fluid pressure is low, there may be little evidence of flow, giving a false indication of shunt malfunction. Various noninvasive techniques have been devised for assessing shunt function. Visual evoked potential (VEP) changes associated with elevated ICP have been suggested as a means of determining function. Thermo-graphic and Doppler detection of shunt flow is also possible. Using magnetic resonance imaging (MRI) technology, it is possible to assess CSF flow and shunt patency.

Shunt Tapping

The scalp hairs should be clipped over and around the reservoir, then prepared with a surgical scrub brush for 10 minutes, followed by povidone-iodine solution, which is allowed to fully dry. After appropriate draping, the skin is infiltrated using 1% plain lidocaine to a level of adequate local anesthesia. Use a 25-gauge butterfly needle with tubing and enter the reservoir percutaneously at a 20° to 30° angle. Lack of CSF flow from the reservoir would indicate a proximal obstruction

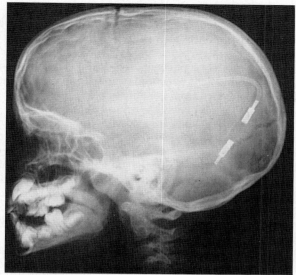

Figure 60–17 Repeat films from the patient in Figures 60–15 and 60–16 illustrate shunt disconnection at the level of the valve and subsequent migration of the distal catheter into the pelvis. This lateral skull radiograph demonstrates the disconnection from the valve.

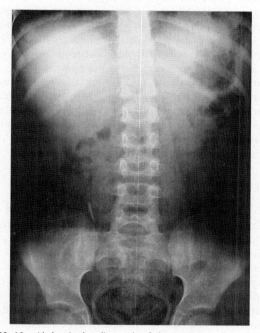

Figure 60–18 Abdominal radiograph of the patient in Figure 60–17 demonstrates migration of the catheter into the pelvis.

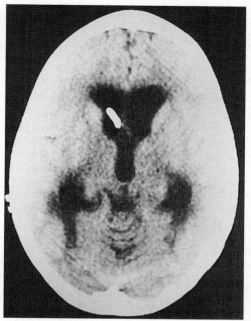

Figure 60–19 Cranial computed tomography (CT) scan of the patient with shunt disconnection shown in Figure 60–17. This CT scan at presentation reveals ventriculomegaly. After revision, the ventricles returned to normal size (see Fig. 60–20).

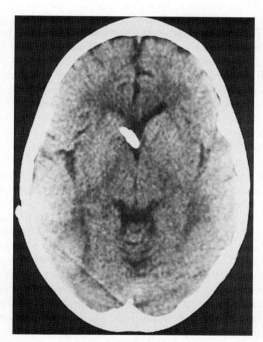

Figure 60–20 Cranial CT scan of the patient in Figure 60–19 after shunt revision. The ventricles have returned to normal size.

unless the ventricles are completely deflated (slit ventricles syndrome). Even so, a small amount of CSF should be obtained within the tubing, thus ensuring that entry into the lumen of the reservoir has been accomplished. If the ventricles are deflated and only a small amount of CSF is aspirated, the end of the tubing can be held 5 to 10 cm below the level of the reservoir to see whether CSF will fill the tubing and eventually begin to drip at the rate of 2 to 3 drops/min. If the CSF readily aspirates from the reservoir, the tubing is held vertically to give an indication of the intraventricular pressure (Fig. 60–21). This pressure reading, as well as the ease with which CSF is aspirated, will give some indication of proximal

obstruction. To assess the runoff or distal end patency, apply pressure to the tubing proximal to the reservoir and then deflate the reservoir without any resistance. If any resistance is encountered when deflating the reservoir, suspect a distal obstruction.

It is imperative to send any aspirated CSF for the relevant studies including cells, differentials, protein, and most of all, Gram stains and cultures for evaluation of possible infection.

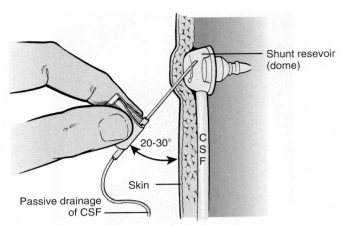

Figure 60–21 A 25-gauge butterfly needle puncture of a reservoir. To avoid damage to the reservoir, the angle should be approximately 20° to 30°. Note that the dome reservoir is under the skin. Before passing the butterfly needle, the skin is anesthetized, sterilized with povidone-iodine, and nicked with a No. 11 scalpel or a larger needle. Fluid is not aspirated but is allowed to drain passively.

Shunt reservoir (dome)

20-30°

Skin

CSF

Passive drainage of CSF

Special Consideration—Postoperative Complications of Shunts

Major complications after shunting include hemorrhage, overdrainage, migration, obstruction, malpositioning, fractured tubing, infection, radiculopathy, and seizures.

Hemorrhage. Bleeding can also occur after the placement of the shunt. Both intracerebral and subdural hemorrhages have been noted. Intracerebral hemorrhage is due to trauma to the brain parenchyma as the catheter is passed through the ventricles. Subdural hematoma is due to sudden decompression of the ventricles that leads to tearing of the bridging veins as the brain pulls away from the dura. An acute or chronic subdural bleed is also encountered in shunts with overdrainage problems.

Shunt Malfunction. If shunt malfunction is suspected, the first step is to perform a head CT scan and shunt series imaging to visualize ventricular size and anatomic alignment of the tubes and devices. The ventricles usually begin to diminish in size within a week after shunt placement in high-pressure hydrocephalus, so continued enlargement suggests shunt malfunction. The shunt series images confirm the continuity of a drainage system from the insertion site through the proximal catheter, reservoir, and distal catheter to the receiving draining cavity, most commonly the peritoneum. It is important to know that in normal-pressure hydrocephalus, the ventricles may remain large despite good functional shunting. The timing and indications of shunt placement are imperative to know when assessing the urgency of the management, especially when consulting a neurosurgeon.

Seizures. These are an infrequent complication of the shunt placement and occur in about 5% of patients. Technically, occipital catheter placement may lessen the incidence of seizures because their location is far from the motor cortex. In patients thought to be at risk for a seizure, antiepileptic medication may be indicated.

Shunt Infection—Treatment and Prevention. Of all the potential complications associated with shunting proce-

dures, infection is the most notorious, occurring in 2% to 10% of the operated cases.[16] Most shunt infections appear within the first 2 months after surgery. The diagnosis may be obvious with variable systematic signs, wound infection, meningitis, peritonitis, or septicemia. It is also possible the shunt may harbor an indolent infection without symptoms or signs. CSF culture obtained from a shunt tap may be negative, even when the shunt is ultimately shown to be infected.[23,24]

Most shunt infections are caused by otherwise nonvirulent bacteria such as *S. epidermidis*. In the presence of the shunt, these organisms exhibit unusual virulence. This reflects a variety of factors, including the ability to adhere to shunt surfaces, as well as production of mucoid substances that protect the bacteria from host defenses. The Silastic shunt material itself has an adverse effect on the immune system. Specifically, leukocytes cannot adhere to such surfaces as well as bacteria. This situation allows phagocyted bacteria to remain viable within the cell. Controversy exists over the need for shunt removal in the context of treatment of infection. Although the systemic antibiotics alone are of unpredictable benefit, the addition of intraventricular drugs has allowed more success in treating without removal of a functioning shunt. Having said this, many neurosurgeons still recommend ultimately replacing the entire shunt after the infection is eradicated. The most important single factor in preventing shunt infection is obviously aseptic operative technique and postoperative shunt handling for diagnostic procedures. The role of prophylactic preoperative antibiotic treatment remains equivocal. Consultation with neurosurgeons and infectious disease specialists is recommended when deciding to administer antibiotics directly into the CSF via either the shunt or a lumbar puncture. Among the antibiotic options, oxacillin, nafcillin, and vancomycin are good empirical choices. If a shunt infection is suspected, systemic antibiotics may be given; as with any serious infectious process, the earlier the administration, the better for the patient.

CONCLUSION

ICP is difficult to assess without obvious clinical and radiologic findings. Because of compensatory mechanisms, the degree of increased ICP does not correlate with the degree of clinical and radiologic abnormalities. Therefore, it is important to recognize by history, examination, and other ancillary tests how to detect early neurologic findings that may indicate elevations of ICP before further damage occurs. Understanding intracranial shunts and their complications is also necessary to assess patients with possible shunt malfunction.

Acknowledgments

The authors thank Khosrow Tabassi, MD, and Cecile G. Silvestre, MD, for their contributions to this chapter in previous editions.

 REFERENCES CAN BE FOUND ON EXPERT CONSULT

CHAPTER 61

Spinal Puncture and Cerebrospinal Fluid Examination

Brian D. Euerle

Cerebrospinal fluid (CSF) examination is performed in an emergency department (ED) to obtain information relevant to the diagnosis and treatment of specific disease entities. Many urgent and life-threatening conditions require immediate and accurate knowledge of the nature of the CSF. However, on rare occasions, certain harmful consequences may result from a spinal puncture. The procedure should follow a careful neurologic examination, with thought given to the risks and merits of the procedure in each situation.

In 1885, Corning[1] punctured the subarachnoid space to introduce cocaine anesthesia into a living patient. In 1891, Quincke[2] first removed CSF in a diagnostic study and introduced the use of a stylet. He studied cellular contents and measured protein and glucose levels. Quincke[2] was also the first to record pressure with a manometer. Subsequently, increasingly sophisticated bacteriologic, biochemical, cytologic, and serologic techniques were introduced. In 1918, Dandy[3] replaced CSF with air to determine normal brain anatomy and identify changes that indicate disease. Water-soluble contrast media have been used to delineate the spinal subarachnoid space and cerebral cisterns. Other uses of spinal puncture include drainage of fluids and injection of anesthetic agents, chemotherapeutic agents, and antibiotics.

CSF FORMATION AND CIRCULATION

In the adult, CSF occupies approximately 140 mL of the spinal and cranial cavities, with approximately 30 mL in the spinal canal. This volume is the result of a balance between continuous secretion (primarily by the ventricular choroid plexus) and absorption into the venous system (mainly by way of the arachnoid villi). After formation, the fluid passes out of the ventricles by way of the midline dorsal foramen of Luschka and the lateral ventral foramina of Magendie. The fluid then flows into the spinal subarachnoid space, the basilar cisterns, and the cerebral subarachnoid space. The rate of production is approximately 0.35 mL/min, and CSF ventricular production is such that there is a net flow out of the ventricles of 50 to 100 mL/day. The usual volume of CSF (15–20 mL) removed at lumbar puncture is commonly regenerated in about 1 hour.

CSF may have an embryologic nutritive function; at maturity, the CSF most likely acts as a mechanical barrier between the soft brain and the rigid fibro-osseous dura, skull, and vertebral column. It also appears to support the weight of the brain.[4] When buoyed by CSF, the functional brain weight is reduced from 1400 to 50 g. Contraction and expansion of the CSF may accommodate changes in brain volume.

INDICATIONS FOR SPINAL PUNCTURE
General Indications

The indications for spinal puncture have been reduced with the introduction of noninvasive diagnostic procedures—magnetic resonance imaging (MRI) and computed tomography (CT). A few clinical situations require early, or even emergent, spinal puncture. The primary indication for an emergent spinal tap is the possibility of central nervous system (CNS) infection (meningitis), with the exception of suspected brain abscess or a parameningeal process. The need for early detection of meningitis results in the performance of many more lumbar punctures than ultimate diagnoses of infection.[5] No other method can be used to completely exclude meningitis.

The mere presence of a fever does not mandate lumbar puncture. However, CSF generally should be examined for evidence of infection in patients with a fever of unknown origin, especially if consciousness is altered or the immune system is impaired, even in the absence of meningeal irritation. Meningeal signs may not be present in patients who are old, debilitated, immunosuppressed, or receiving anti-inflammatory drugs or who have had partial treatment with antibiotics.[6,7] In a newborn, even a fever is not a dependable sign; temperatures may be normal or even subnormal. For infants younger than 1 year, a high index of suspicion is required to make the diagnosis of meningitis. Approximately 25% of infants with meningitis will not have nuchal rigidity, but most will usually appear toxic or moribund. A tense and bulging fontanel is somewhat more reliable, although this sign may be absent in a dehydrated child. Neonatal meningitis occurs in 25% of sepsis cases. In addition, 15% to 20% of infants with meningitis have negative blood cultures.[8,9]

In a child between the ages of 1 month and 3 years, fever, irritability, and vomiting are the most common symptoms of meningitis. Typically, handling is painful for the child, and the child cannot be comforted. In addition, an older child may complain of a headache. In all ages, the patient generally looks unusually ill and appears drowsy with a dulled sensorium.

Physical signs become more useful in diagnosing meningitis in children older than 3 years.[10] These include nuchal rigidity, Kernig's sign (efforts to extend the knee are resisted), and Brudzinski's sign (passive flexion of one hip causes the other leg to rise, and efforts to flex the neck make the knees come up). A useful aid in distinguishing neck rigidity of meningeal origin from that caused by primary pain in the cervical muscles and the soft tissues is the preservation of lateral movement (indicative of meningeal irritation). A petechial rash in a febrile child should also raise the possibility of *Neisseria* meningitis.[11] Prior use of antimicrobial agents may modify the clinical presentation and alter CSF findings; partially treated children are less likely to be febrile or exhibit an altered mental status. In addition, patients in the early stages of meningitis may lack the classic features associated with advanced disease.

The second indication for emergent spinal puncture is suspected spontaneous subarachnoid hemorrhage (SAH). The diagnosis is usually made by head CT scan or the finding of blood in the CSF.[12,13] CT sensitivity is 95% soon after hemorrhage, but it drops in patients presenting later than 24 hours after the event to 76% after 48 hours and to about 50% at 1 week. Before a major hemorrhage, 20% to 60% of patients with aneurysmal SAH have had a "sentinel thunderclap" or "warning leak" headache (i.e., an unusual sudden headache without nuchal rigidity, caused by a "minor" leak of blood from the aneurysm). The headache may precede major rupture by days to months. The goal of early clinical recognition is surgical treatment before a major hemorrhage. After a warning leak, the head CT scan is usually negative, giving added importance to the performance of a lumbar puncture. Migraine or "vascular" headache is a common misdiagnosis in patients with an SAH who have an initially negative head CT scan.

The usual clinical picture of SAH is a severe and instantaneous excruciating headache. Patients usually recall the exact moment the headache occurred. The location of the headache is variable and does not give a clue as to the site of hemorrhage. Nausea, vomiting, and prostration are common symptoms, with approximately one third of patients becoming unconscious at the onset. Examination shows an acutely ill patient with irritability or overt altered mental status. Meningeal signs are commonly present at the time of the initial examination and usually develop in all cases within 2 to 3 days. Meningeal signs may become more severe during the 1st week after hemorrhage and correspond to the breakdown of blood in the CSF. During the 1st week, many patients are febrile, reflecting a chemical hemic meningitis.[14] Failure to detect blood radiographically in an awake patient may indicate a small hemorrhage or a predominant basal accumulation of blood. If a patient is seen several days after the hemorrhage, the blood may have become isodense with brain and may no longer be visible on a CT scan. The proper diagnosis would then require spinal puncture.

Newer CT scanners detect *recent* SAH quite accurately, close to 100% with fifth-generation scanners.[15] However, because acute SAHs are not detected by the initial CT scan in 2% to 5% of all patients, lumbar puncture is appropriate to rule out the diagnosis with certainty.[16–18] In theory, blood from a small SAH may take several hours to reach the lumbar region. Thus, it is possible that CSF from the lumbar region will remain normal soon after rupture. A second, delayed lumbar puncture may be required for diagnosis. If the neurologic picture demonstrates localizing findings, the presence of a large intracranial hematoma should be suspected, and spinal puncture is contraindicated until CT (or arteriography) delineates the nature of the lesion.

The emergency clinician also may be called on to perform a therapeutic lumbar puncture in a patient with known pseudotumor cerebri (also known as benign intracranial hypertension or idiopathic intracranial hypertension). The patient has elevated intracranial pressure (ICP) for unknown reasons and often has headaches, vision changes, and papilledema. The headache worsens with maneuvers that increase the ICP (e.g., Valsalva, squatting, bending, coughing). See the following section for details.

Other nonemergent reasons for CSF examination include evaluation of CNS syphilis, unexplained seizures, instillation of chemotherapy and contrast agents, a suspected demyelinating or inflammatory CNS process, and treatment of headache from SAH. Carcinomatous meningitis and suspected spinal cord compression from metastatic disease may require spinal puncture for myelography and cytologic examination. MRI is a suitable alternative for identifying compressive myelopathies.

Idiopathic Intracranial Hypertension (Pseudotumor Cerebri)

Pseudotumor cerebri, more commonly known as idiopathic or benign intracranial hypertension (IIH), is a rare condition that may be seen in the ED.[19] IIH is an elevation of intracranial pressure (usually to 250–450 cm H_2O) without hydrocephalus or mass lesions, in the setting of normal CSF composition. This is a diagnosis of exclusion. Most patients have headache, papilledema, occasionally vision changes, and minimal or absent focal findings, *with a normal CT or MRI scan*. Most patients appear otherwise well, but some complain of tinnitus, nausea, or blurred vision. IIH has been related to hypervitaminosis A, tetracycline, estrogen therapy, and a plethora of other conditions, such as sarcoidosis, tuberculosis, and carcinomatosis. Most cases are idiopathic. Because of the nonspecific presentation, *many cases initially escape detection by clinicians*. IIH is most common in obese adolescent girls and young women, but it can occur in childhood and in men. The mechanism by which CSF pressure increases is unclear; the brain appears normal. One proposed mechanism is decreased CSF outflow.

IIH may regress spontaneously after a few months. The major concern is visual loss, which may be permanent. The diagnosis can be made only by lumbar puncture, performed after neuroimaging. *This condition underscores the need to measure opening pressure during lumbar puncture whenever possible*. Many cases can be controlled with medication, but occasionally, lumbar puncture is required to lower ICP, measured in the lateral decubitus position, to 200 mm H_2O. One way to lower ICP in the ED is to drain CSF via lumbar puncture by removing 5- to 10-mL aliquots of CSF and checking ICP after each removal. Herniation does not occur despite elevated pressures. Because spinal fluid is regenerated rapidly, the procedure may need to be performed every few days to keep CSF pressure at this level. Analysis of the CSF is normal in all parameters. Drug therapy, in the form of acetazolamide, glycerol, diuretics, corticosteroids, and others, has been advocated and may negate the need for repeated lumbar puncture. Resistant cases may require shunting procedures.

CONTRAINDICATIONS FOR SPINAL PUNCTURE

Spinal puncture is absolutely contraindicated in the presence of infection in the tissues near the puncture site.[4,20] Acute meningitis, in a clinical scenario that does not suggest severe increased ICP, is not a contraindication for spinal puncture. Spinal puncture is relatively contraindicated in the presence of *increased ICP caused by a space-occupying lesion*. Caution is particularly advised when lateralizing signs (hemiparesis) or signs of uncal herniation (unilateral third nerve palsy with altered level of consciousness) are present. In such cases, a tentorial or cerebellar pressure cone may be precipitated or aggravated by the spinal puncture. Cardiorespiratory collapse, stupor, seizures, and sudden death may occur when pressure is reduced in the spinal canal.[21]

The risk of herniation seems to be particularly pronounced in patients with brain abscess.[22,23] Brain abscesses frequently occur as expanding intracranial lesions that induce headache, mental disturbances, and focal neurologic signs rather than as infectious processes with signs of meningeal irritation. In 75% of cases, a primary source of chronic suppuration is present. Common predisposing factors for brain abscess include craniofacial trauma; craniocerebral trauma;

penetrating injuries that push bone fragments into the brain; large animal bites of infants' skulls; neurosurgical procedures; cardiovascular disorders treated with right-to-left shunts; bacterial endocarditis, gram-negative sepsis in neonates, dental infections, chronic sinusitis, otitis, mastoiditis, chronic abdominal, pulmonary, or pelvic infections; bacterial meningitis; and immunosuppression. Abscesses may develop in infarcted brain tissue in septic patients if the blood-brain barrier is compromised.[24] Although the CSF is usually abnormal (elevated pressure, elevated white blood cell (WBC) count, and elevated protein concentration), spinal puncture in patients with a known, or highly probable, abscess is contraindicated in most cases. Herniation markedly reduces the patient's likelihood of survival.

A brain abscess may rupture spontaneously into the ventricular system, producing ventriculitis and meningitis. If the history suggests brain abscess, CT can rapidly diagnose and localize the lesion.[25] *Because the appearance of brain abscesses on a CT scan is similar to that of neoplastic and vascular lesions, false-positive reports of brain abscess are possible.*[26]

Spinal epidural hematomas may occur in some subpopulations of patients undergoing lumbar puncture. Individuals most at risk are patients with some sort of bleeding diathesis, including those on anticoagulant therapy or those with abnormal clotting mechanisms, especially thrombocytopenia. Spinal subdural hematomas after lumbar puncture are even more rare than epidural hematomas.[27,28] Lumbar puncture can injure the dural or arachnoid vessels, which may result in minor hemorrhage into the CSF. This generally is of little consequence. However, the number of patients with hemophilia and human immunodeficiency virus (HIV) infection who require lumbar puncture has increased since the late 1990s.

When a patient is anticoagulated or has a coagulopathy, attempts should be made to correct the clotting deficiency if clinically feasible and time permitting. Also, the tap should be performed by experienced clinicians, who are less likely to traumatize the dura. After the procedure, the patient should be followed carefully for progressive back pain, lower extremity motor and sensory deficits, and sphincter impairment. Complaints of motor weakness, sensory loss, or incontinence after lumbar puncture should be investigated thoroughly. Lumbar puncture may be performed in the presence of a coagulation defect if the procedure is expected to provide essential information, such as in the diagnosis of meningitis. In cases of severe thrombocytopenia, the infusion of platelets before the puncture may be desirable. Coumadin-induced coagulopathy is corrected with fresh frozen plasma and vitamin K.

The infusion of clotting factors into the hemophiliac patient and normalization of the prothrombin time with fresh frozen plasma in the anticoagulated patient before a puncture are desirable if the clinical situation permits such delay. Lumbar puncture can be performed safely in patients with hemophilia A or B whose deficit clotting factor is replenished before the procedure.[29] The use of additional factor replacement after lumbar puncture is of unknown value.

The performance of lumbar puncture in patients with leukemia and low platelet counts has been studied. Howard and coworkers[30] reported on 5223 lumbar punctures done in 958 children with newly diagnosed acute lymphoblastic leukemia. The platelet count was 10×10^9/L or less in 29 children, 11 to 20×10^9/L in 170 children, and 21 to 50×10^9/L in 742 children. *No serious complications were reported.* The overall rate of traumatic taps was 10.5%, but these were not associated with adverse sequelae. The authors concluded that in children with acute lymphoblastic leukemia, prophylactic platelet transfusion for lumbar puncture is not required if the platelet count is higher than 10×10^9/L. The number of patients with platelet counts lower than 10×10^9/L was too small to allow any conclusion about this group.

If the history and physical examination suggest a treatable illness, such as meningitis or SAH, the clinician may perform a spinal puncture after careful consideration of the entire clinical picture. In all cases, the study should be undertaken after careful thought regarding how the results will contribute to patient evaluation and treatment. It is unlikely that the spinal puncture will beneficially alter management in patients with a neoplasm, a cranial hematoma, an abscess, a completed nonembolic infarction, or cranial trauma.

EQUIPMENT

The standard equipment for a spinal puncture should be assembled before beginning the procedure, and it should be placed where the operator can easily access it. The standard-point Quincke cutting needle is most often used and supplied with the kit. Some operators prefer to use an "atraumatic Sprotte spinal needle" (Havel's, Inc, Cincinnati, OH) or Whitacre needle (Becton Dickinson and Company, Rutherford, NJ) to minimize the dural injury associated with needle passage (Fig. 61–1). These styletted needles have a side port for fluid withdrawal and, theoretically, are more likely to separate rather than cut the dural tissue.

Although commercial kits provide most of the items needed for lumbar puncture, the operator should bring additional supplies, including supplemental spinal needles and specimen tubes, gauze and antiseptic solution, additional local anesthesia, needles/syringes, and extra sterile gloves of the appropriate size (Fig. 61–2).

TECHNIQUE

Lumbar puncture is commonly carried out with the patient in the lateral recumbent position. A line connecting the posterior-superior iliac crests intersects the midline at approximately the L4 spinous process (Fig. 61–3). Spinal needles entering the subarachnoid space at this point are well below the termination of the spinal cord, and the only important neurologic structure is the cauda equina. Generally, the needle pushes isolated nerves to the side during advancement. The adjacent interspace above or below may be used, depending on which area appears to be most open to palpation. The space between the lumbar vertebrae is relatively wide. In the thoracic region, the spinous processes overlap and are directed caudad; therefore, there is no midline area free of overlying bone. In the adult, the spinal cord extends to the lower level of L1 or the body of L2 in 31% of persons, eliminating higher levels as sites for puncture. The puncture in adults and in older children may be performed from the L2 to L3 interspace to the L5 to S1 interspace.

Developmentally, the spinal canal and the spinal cord are of equal length in the fetus. Growth of the cord does not keep pace with longitudinal growth of the spinal canal. At birth, the cord ends at the level of the L3 vertebra. In infants, the needle should be placed at the L4 to L5 or L5 to S1 interspace. The subarachnoid space extends to an S2 vertebral level; however, the overlying bony mass prevents entry into this lowermost portion of the subarachnoid space.

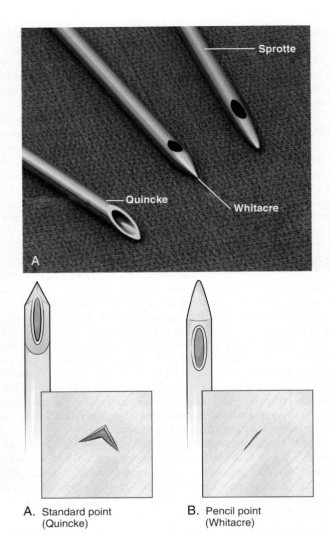

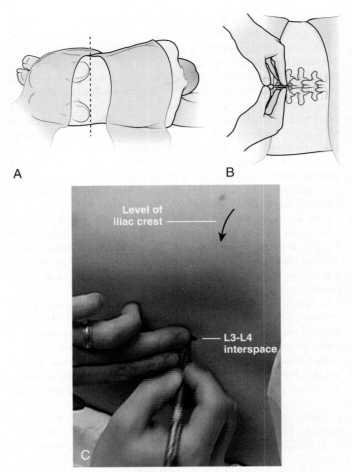

Figure 61–3 *A,* When the patient has been correctly positioned for the lumbar tap, an imaginary line connecting the iliac crests will be exactly perpendicular to the bed. Insertion sites are marked by *x*; the operative field is draped. *B,* The needle should be inserted perpendicular (or nearly so) to the plane of the back, with the forefingers of both hands guiding it in. *C,* Landmarks on the patient. *(A and B, From Cole M: Pitfalls in cerebrospinal fluid examination. Hosp Pract 4:47, 1969. Illustration by Carol Donner. Reproduced by permission; C, from Thomsen T, Setnik G [eds]: Procedures Consult—Emergency Medicine Module. Copyright 2008 Elsevier Inc. All rights reserved.)*

Figure 61–1 *A,* Various spinal needles. *B,* Penetration of the dura by Whitacre (pencil-point) and Quincke (cutting) needles. The Quincke needle cuts the fibers of the dura, whereas the Whitacre needle separates the fibers without cutting them. The Quincke needle leaves a hole in the dura through which CSF can leak until it heals several days or weeks later. *(A, From Thomsen T, Setnik G [eds]: Procedures Consult—Emergency Medicine Module. Copyright 2008 Elsevier Inc. All rights reserved.)*

When performed with parenteral sedation and proper local anesthesia, a spinal tap is neither overly distressing nor very painful to most patients. Almost all patients are likely to have some anxiety about a spinal puncture for several reasons including the stories commonly told of severe complications. Explaining the procedure in advance and discussing each step during the course of the test reduces the patient's anxiety. The clinician should inquire about history of allergies to local anesthetic agents and topical antiseptics. Use of a written informed consent is recommended whenever possible. In all cases, a detailed procedural note should be included that documents the process of patient/guardian education regarding the indications, procedural techniques, risks/benefits and alternatives to the procedure, and the patient's/guardian's assent to the procedure. This step may need to be abridged when the patient is critically ill or eliminated when the patient is mentally incapacitated and no guardian is present. In anxious patients, a benzodiazepine agent given parenterally (e.g., midazolam, 0.05–0.075 mg/kg intravenously) will facilitate the procedure and is recommended.

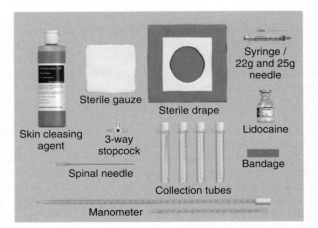

Figure 61–2 Commercial kit with equipment for lumbar puncture. *(From Thomsen T, Setnik G [eds]: Procedures Consult—Emergency Medicine Module. Copyright 2008 Elsevier Inc. All rights reserved.)*

The next important step is positioning the patient. Generally, place older children and adults in the lateral decubitus position for this procedure. Give the patient a pillow to keep the head in the same plane as the vertebral axis. Position the shoulders and the hips perpendicular to the table. A firm table or bed is desirable. Contrary to common belief, *flexion of the neck does not facilitate the procedure to any great extent*; and because severe flexion may add to the patient's discomfort, this step may be omitted. *Severe flexion of the neck in an infant may cause airway compromise.* Arch the patient's lower back toward the clinician by having the patient's knees drawn toward the chest.

Some clinicians place the patient in an upright sitting position because the midline is more easily identified. This position can be used in both adults and infants (Fig. 61–4). The higher CSF hydrostatic pressure while sitting may aid CSF flow in a dehydrated patient. Observe caution regarding orthostatic blood pressure changes and airway maintenance. Generally, allow the sitting patient to lean onto a bedside stand using a pillow to rest the head and arms. Have an assistant support the patient during the procedure. Radiographic studies by Fisher and colleagues[31] have shown the advantages of hip flexion when the sitting position is used. Accomplish this by using a stool to support the patient's feet and effectively pulling the knees up toward the chest, as is generally done when the lateral decubitus position is used. This will increase the lumbar interspinous width, which may increase the success or ease of needle passage.

Iatrogenic infection after lumbar puncture is extremely rare. The use of sterile gloves during the procedure is customary, but the need for face masks is debatable.[32-34] It seems reasonable to apply the same guidelines for central line infection control (caps, gowns, gloves, and masks) to lumbar puncture.[35] Wash the patient's back with an antiseptic solution applied in a circular motion, increasing the circumference of the cleansed area with each motion. Place a sterile towel or drape between the patient's hip and the bed. Commercial trays have a second sterile drape with a hole that may be centered over the site selected for the tap.

Infiltrate the skin and deeper subcutaneous tissue *generously* with local anesthetic (1% lidocaine). Buffered or warmed lidocaine is preferred. Warn the patient about transient discomfort from the anesthetic. Anesthetizing the deeper subcutaneous tissue significantly reduces the procedural discomfort. Merely raising a skin wheal is insufficient anesthesia. Some operators not only anesthetize the interspinous ligament but also apply local anesthesia in a vertically fanning distribution on both sides of the spinous processes near the lamina. This field block on each side of the spinous processes anesthetizes the recurrent spinal nerves that innervate the interspinous ligaments and muscles.

While waiting for the anesthetic to take effect, attach the stopcock and manometer and ensure that the valve is working. Commonly, a 3.5-inch, 20-gauge needle is used in adults, and a 2.5-inch, 22-gauge needle is used in children (a 1.5-inch, 22-gauge needle is available for infants). Needles of these sizes have enough rigidity to allow the procedure to be accomplished easily but make less of a dural tear than do larger needles. The patient should be told to report any pain and should be informed that she or he will feel some pressure.

With the patient in the lateral decubitus position, place the needle into the skin in the midline, parallel to the bed. Hold the needle between both thumbs and index fingers (Fig. 61–5). After the subcutaneous tissue has been penetrated, angle the needle toward the umbilicus. The bevel of the needle should be facing straight up toward the ceiling. Pointing the bevel parallel to the longitudinal axis of the spine may allow the needle to separate the fibers of the dura rather than cut through them, causing less CSF leakage after the needle has been withdrawn.

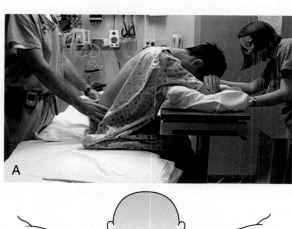

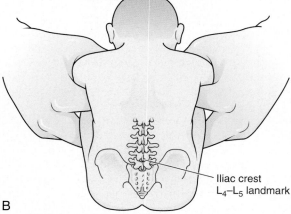

Figure 61–4 *A,* Many clinicians prefer the sitting position for lumbar puncture because of the ease of entering the dural space. Opening pressure in this position is not accurate. If possible, the patient can be placed in the lateral decubitis position for measurement of pressure, usually after fluid has been collected. *B,* Upright positioning in an infant. *(A, From Thomsen T, Setnik G [eds]: Procedures Consult—Emergency Medicine Module. Copyright 2008 Elsevier Inc. All rights reserved; B, from Dieckmann R, Selbst S [eds]: Pediatric Emergency and Critical Care Procedures. St. Louis, Mosby, 1997.)*

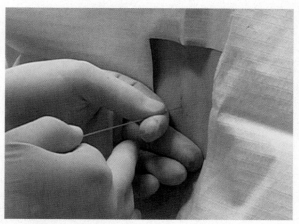

Figure 61–5 Hold the spinal needle between the thumb and the index finger to facilitate the entrance into the dural space.

The supraspinal ligament connects the spinous process; the interspinal ligaments join the inferior and superior borders of adjacent spinous processes. The ligamentum flavum is a strong, elastic, yellow membrane that may reach a thickness of 1 cm in the lumbar region. The ligamentum flavum covers the interlaminar space between the vertebrae and assists the paraspinous muscles in maintaining an upright posture (Fig. 61–6). The ligaments are stretched in a flexed position and are more easily crossed by the needle. The ligaments offer resistance to the needle, and a "pop" is often felt as they are penetrated. Remove the stylet frequently to see whether the subarachnoid space has been reached (Fig. 61–7). The pop may not be felt with the very sharp needles contained in disposable trays.

If bone is encountered, partially withdraw the needle to the subcutaneous tissue. Repalpate the back and ascertain that the needle is in the midline. Directing the needle tip toward the navel often enhances navigation of the interspinal space. If bone is encountered again, slightly withdraw and reangle the needle, with the point placed so that it angles more sharply cephalad. This approach should avoid the inferior spinous process.

Normal CSF is a clear fluid and will flow from the needle when the subarachnoid space has been penetrated. In normal patients, the dura will be penetrated when the needle is advanced about one half to three fourths of its length. In obese patients, the entire needle length may be required to reach the subdural space (Fig. 61–8).

If feasible, attach the manometer and record the opening pressure (Fig. 61–9). This step is commonly omitted in critically ill patients. Pressure readings from a struggling patient may be inaccurate. Pressure readings are valid only if taken with the patient in the lateral decubitus position (not the sitting position). A three-way stopcock, supplied in disposable trays, allows both collection and pressure to be measured by a single needle. Positioning of the manometer is often more convenient if an extension tube (provided with most disposable trays) connects the needle hub to the stopcock, which is

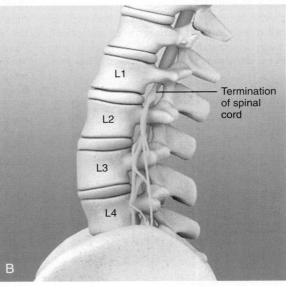

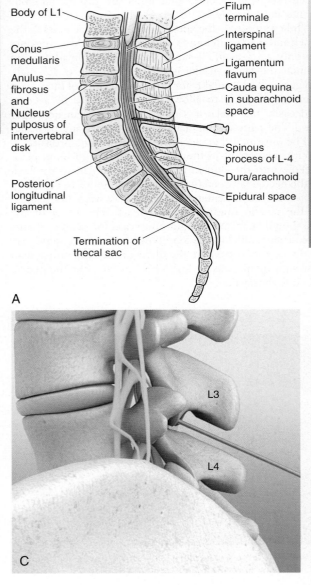

Figure 61–6 *A,* Midsagittal section through the lumbar spinal column with a spinal puncture needle in place between the spinous processes of L3 and L4. Note the slightly ascending direction of the needle. The needle has pierced three ligaments and the dura/arachnoid and is in the subarachnoid space. *B and C,* Spinal cord termination and angle of needle entrance. *(A, From Lachman E. Anatomy as applied to clinical medicine. New Physician 17:145, 1968; B and C, From Thomsen T, Setnik G [eds]: Procedures Consult—Emergency Medicine Module. Copyright 2008 Elsevier Inc. All rights reserved.)*

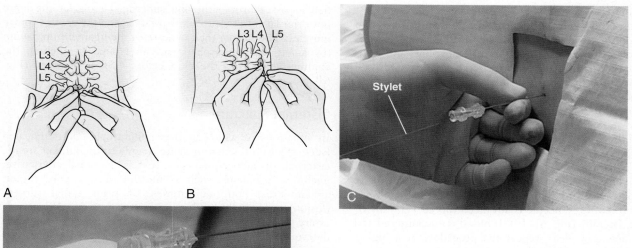

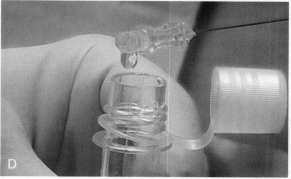

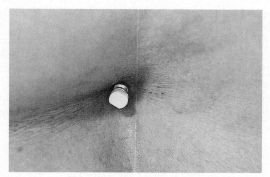

Figure 61–7 *A,* Various ways to stabilize and advance the needle. *B,* Advance the needle with the stylet in place, and remove it when a pop is felt, or to check for dural puncture. *C* and *D,* A drop of fluid from the needle hub signifies dural puncture. A syringe may be used to withdraw fluid if a very small spinal needle is used; otherwise, it should flow spontaneously. *(A–D, From Thomsen T, Setnik G [eds]: Procedures Consult—Emergency Medicine Module. Copyright 2008 Elsevier Inc. All rights reserved.)*

1113

Figure 61–8 The spinal needle is usually advanced one half to three fourths of its length before the spinal canal is reached. In this obese patient, the needle was advanced all the way to the hub of the needle before spinal fluid was returned.

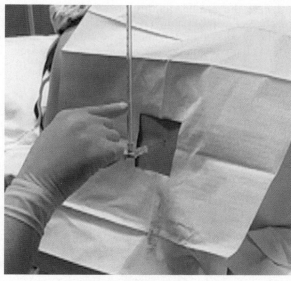

Figure 61–9 Opening pressure is measured, whenever possible, in the lateral position. An assistant holds the manometer while the operator works the stopcock. The first specimen collected is the fluid that has filled the manometer, obtained by manipulating the stopcock to flow into the collection tube. *(From Thomsen T, Setnik G [eds]: Procedures Consult—Emergency Medicine Module. Copyright 2008 Elsevier Inc. All rights reserved.)*

in turn attached to the manometer. Position the manometer so that the "zero" mark is at the level of the spinal needle. Then, ask the patient to relax. Extending the legs after needle placement does not meaningfully decrease the opening CSF pressure.[36] The observation of phasic changes in the fluid column with respirations and arterial pulsations confirms needle placement in the subarachnoid space. If the needle is against a nerve root or is only partially within the dura, the pressure may be falsely low, and respiratory excursions will not be seen in the manometer. Minor rotation of the needle may solve these problems. Hyperventilation will reduce the pressure readings, owing to hypocapnia and resultant cerebral vasoconstriction.

After measuring the pressure, turn the stopcock and collect enough fluid to perform all desired studies. The first sample of fluid exits from the manometer if pressure has been

measured, then additional fluid flows from the spinal canal. Even if the pressure is elevated, remove sufficient fluid for performance of all indicated studies, because the risk of the procedure involves the dural rent, not the amount of fluid initially removed. Presumably, more fluid will be lost subsequently through the hole in the dura. Replace the stylet into the needle before withdrawing it.

Commercial trays supply four specimen tubes. Generally, tube 1 is used for determining protein and glucose levels and for electrophoretic studies; tube 2 is used for microbiologic and cytologic studies; and tube 3 is for cell counts and serologic tests for syphilis. In the presence of bloody CSF, cell counts should be performed in tubes 1 and 3 to help differentiate traumatic taps. Tube 4 can be stored under refrigeration in the laboratory for subsequent studies.

Traumatic taps are common and usually clinically inconsequential, but they can be minimized by proper patient and needle positioning. A traumatic tap most commonly occurs when the subarachnoid space is transfixed at the entrance of the ventral epidural space, where the venous plexus is heavier. A plexus of veins forms a ring around the cord, and these veins may be entered if the needle is advanced too far ventrally or is directed laterally (Fig. 61–10). If blood is encountered and the fluid does not clear, repeat the procedure at a higher interspace with a fresh needle. A traumatic tap, per se, is not a particularly dangerous problem in the patient with normal coagulation, and no specific precautions are needed if blood-tinged fluid is obtained. However, observation for signs of cord or spinal nerve compression from a developing hematoma within the first several hours should be routine in patients with a coagulopathy.

Lateral Approach in Lumbar Puncture

The supraspinal ligament might be calcified in older persons, making a midline perforation difficult. A calcified ligament may deflect the needle. In this case, use a slightly lateral approach. As the lower lamina rises upward from the midline, direct the needle slightly cephalad to miss the lamina and slightly medially to compensate for the lateral approach. The needle passes through the skin, superficial fascia, fat, the dense posterior layer of thoracolumbar fascia, and the erector spinae muscles. The needle then penetrates the ligamentum flavum (bypassing the supraspinal and interspinal ligaments), the epidural space, and the dura before CSF is obtained (Fig. 61–11).

Cisternal Puncture

In situations in which lumbar puncture is contraindicated (such as local infection or acute trauma to the lumbar spine), cisternal, or suboccipital, puncture is the usual alternative. Technical problems, such as morbid obesity, cord tumor, arachnoiditis, bony deformities, or prior spinal surgery (fusion), might make lumbar puncture impossible. When necessary inject contrast material into the cisterna magna to determine the rostral extent of an obstructing lesion identified by lumbar myelography.

Shave the patient's neck from the external occipital protuberance to the mastoid process laterally. Clean the skin and anesthetize the patient in a manner similar to that for a lumbar puncture. The lateral decubitus position is preferable, but a sitting position can be used. Place a pillow under the patient's head to keep the neck and the vertebral axis in the same plane. Flex the patient's neck by moving the head toward the chest. Place the spinal needle in the midline halfway between the spinous process of C2 and the inferior occiput. Angle the needle cephalad through the subcutaneous tissue until it comes in contact with the bony occiput. Then withdraw the needle and subsequently advance it at a less-acute angle with the horizontal plane of the cervical spine. Repeat this action until the dural pop is felt. As in the lumbar region, remove the stylet frequently so that the dura is not punctured unknowingly. Remove fluid in the usual manner. Dural veins are less extensive in this area, and bloody taps are less common. Low-pressure headaches are less common, presumably because the subarachnoid pressure is lower and the dural tear can heal faster.

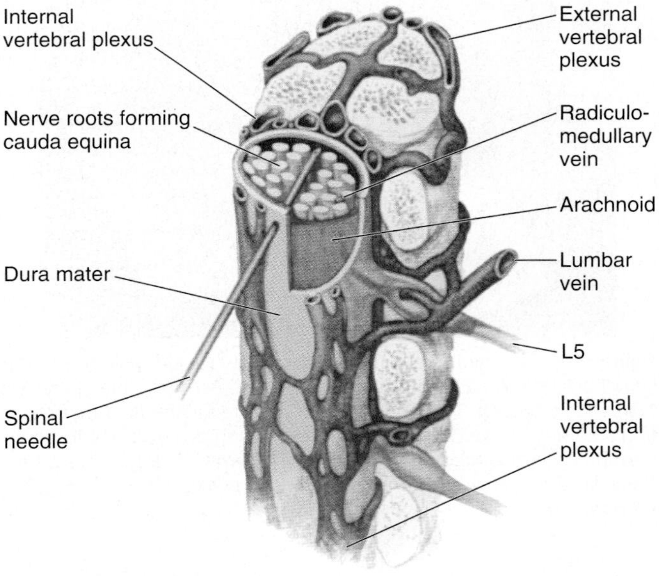

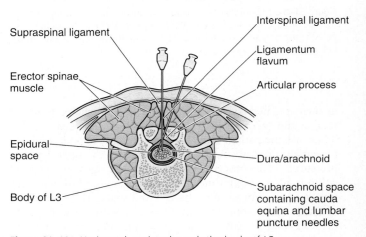

Figure 61–10 Spinal contents at L4 and L5 show the relationship of a lumbar puncture needle to the major vessels at this level. The major radiculomedullary vein, shown accompanying the L5 nerve root, is situated far laterally to a needle correctly positioned in the midline of the dural sac. Note the avascular subdural space. *(From Edelson RN, Chernik IVL, Rosner JB: Spinal subdural hematomas. Arch Neurol 31:134, 1974. Illustration by Lynn McDowell. Reproduced by permission. Copyright 1974, American Medical Association.)*

Figure 61–11 Horizontal section through the body of L3. Note the two puncture needles in the subarachnoid space. The medial needle is in the midline, corresponding to the position in Figure 62–3. The lateral exemplifies the lateral approach, which avoids the occasionally calcified supraspinal ligament. Note the lateral needle piercing the intrinsic musculature of the back and only one ligament, the ligamentum flavum. *(From Lachman E: Anatomy as applied to clinical medicine. New Physician 17:145, 1968.)*

Lateral Cervical Puncture

Place the patient in a supine position, fully sterilized and anesthetized. Insert a 20-gauge lumbar puncture needle perpendicular to the neck and parallel to the bed. The landmark for insertion is a point 1 cm inferior and 1 cm dorsal to the mastoid process. Remove the stylet frequently to check for fluid return and, as at other sites, advance the needle slowly. If the needle goes too deeply and encounters paraspinous muscles, it is probably too deep posteriorly and should be repositioned more anteriorly. If bone is encountered, more dorsal placement is needed. Measure pressure and collect fluid samples, as in other sites.[37]

The contraindications to cisternal and cervical punctures are the same as those to lumbar puncture. Both techniques are easily mastered, but observation of a demonstration of the procedure by an experienced operator is advised.

Lumbar Puncture in Infants

Lumbar puncture in infants is usually performed to exclude meningitis. The sitting position may allow the midline to be more easily identified. The use of a nonstyletted needle in small infants has been suggested because this device allows the pressure to be estimated as the needle punctures the dura.[38] However, failure to use a stylet may be the cause of the subsequent development of an intraspinal epidermoid tumor.[39] The use of a butterfly infusion set needle simplifies the procedure, which is helpful when managing a squirming or hyperactive patient.[38] In general, a stylet is recommended primarily at the time of skin penetration and on needle withdrawal. Although many operators use the stylet during any advancement of the needle, frequent placement and withdrawal after skin penetration is optional.

If the child's neck is very tightly flexed, CSF might not be obtained. However, if the head is held in midflexion, CSF usually flows briskly. If CSF fails to flow, gentle suction with a 1.0-mL syringe may be used to exclude a low-pressure syndrome. Because pressure readings are inaccurate in the struggling child, pressure measurement is not commonly attempted in infants and young children.[40]

Prolonged severe flexion of the neck in an infant should be avoided because it may produce dangerous airway obstruction. If the infant suddenly stops crying, check the airway immediately.[41] Proper positioning is best accomplished by an assistant, who maintains the spine maximally flexed by partially overlying the child using the holder's chest and body weight to immobilize the thorax and hips while holding the child behind the shoulders and the knees. Infants have poor neck control; therefore, the assistant must also ensure that the child maintains an open airway. Give particular attention to avoiding marked neck and trunk flexion. Incorrect positioning usually results in multiple punctures and a bloody tap.

Newborn and preterm infants may experience significant hypoxia during lumbar puncture, with clinical deterioration; a sitting position appears preferable.[42] Lumbar puncture in infants with respiratory distress syndrome may cause greater risk than benefit.[43] This is a problem primarily in neonates but may occur in younger infants with sepsis. Closely monitor all infants with serious cardiopulmonary disease during the procedure. Preoxygenation with or without oxygen saturation monitoring may be used as a precaution.

Although local anesthesia or sedation has not been a routine practice during lumbar puncture in the infant or child,

it is being reconsidered. Neonates perceive pain, and local anesthesia neither produces physiologic instability nor makes the procedure more difficult.[44,45] The use of topically applied EMLA (eutectic mixture of local anesthetics; Astrazeneca) reduces the pain of needle insertion in newborns.[46] Sedation of the anxious child may be considered, but sedatives are relatively contraindicated in the obtunded infant, in a child without a protected airway, and in the setting of hemodynamic instability.

Coley and associates[47] advocate ultrasound evaluation in cases of failed lumbar puncture in neonates and infants. Ultrasound provides information concerning the presence or absence of CSF and the cause of the failed lumbar puncture and thus indicates whether to proceed with further attempts.

COMPLICATIONS

Headache after Lumbar Puncture

A number of complications from lumbar puncture have been reported. One of the most common is headache, which occurs after 1% to 70% of spinal taps.[48-52] In general, the development of post-puncture headache *cannot be prognosticated nor prevented*. The syndrome starts up to 48 hours after the procedure and usually lasts for 1 to 2 days (occasionally as long as 14 days). Cases lasting months have been described. *The headache usually begins within minutes after the patient arises and characteristically ceases as soon as he or she assumes a recumbent position*. The pain is mild to incapacitating and is usually cervical and suboccipital but might involve the shoulders and the entire cranium. Exceptional cases include nausea, vomiting, vertigo, blurred vision, ear pressure, tinnitus, and stiff neck. The headache may change to a positional backache or neckache.

The technique of spinal puncture has little to do with the development of a post-procedure headache. The syndrome is thought to be caused by leakage of fluid through the dural puncture site. This results in a reduction of CSF volume below the cisterna magna and a downward movement of brain tissue, with displacement and stretching of pain-sensitive structures, such as meninges and vessels, causing a traction headache. The recumbent position brings relief because the weight of the brain is shifted cephalad. Another proposed mechanism is cerebral vasodilatation. A more recent hypothesis suggests that the headache is caused by an altered distribution of craniospinal elasticity and acute intracranial venous dilatation.[53] Some authors have commented on the incidence and severity of post–dural puncture headache as related to spinal needle bevel orientation[54,55] and type/size.[56-64] It is clear that the incidence of post–dural puncture headache is lower when the bevel of the needle is oriented parallel to the longitudinal axis of the spine. Until relatively recently, the explanation for this was that the parallel bevel would separate rather than cut the longitudinal dural fibers and thus produce a smaller dural hole and less CSF leakage. However, it is now known that the dural fibers are not oriented longitudinally but rather randomly.[65] Even with random fiber orientation, it is more likely that a longitudinal dural hole will be pulled closed during back flexion than a horizontal dural hole.

Two basic types of spinal needles are cutting (Quincke) and noncutting or pencil-point (Sprotte and Whitacre). Noncutting needles cause a lower incidence of headache after dural puncture, perhaps because the tip of the needle tends to separate rather than cut dural fibers. It has traditionally been thought that the dural hole resulting from noncutting needle puncture is smaller than that created by cutting needle puncture; however, this may not be true. The important difference may be that the cutting needle causes a clean-cut opening in the dura while the noncutting needle produces a jagged opening with rough edges.[66] The jagged opening may produce a more intense inflammatory response, resulting in edema and more complete hole closure. The use of atraumatic spinal needles is not routine. As more spinal kit manufacturers include them in kits, their use might increase.[67] In thick-skinned individuals, passage of a thin, noncutting needle may be technically difficult. The initial pass of a thicker cutting needle to the level of the interspinal ligament, followed by removal and advancement of the noncutting needle in the same soft tissue tract, can be helpful.

A smaller-diameter needle is one intervention that likely will cause a smaller incidence of postpuncture headache because it causes a smaller dural hole. If diameter were the only consideration, as small a needle as possible would be used. However, a needle must have adequate CSF flow rates in order to allow timely CSF collection and pressure measurement. With a very small needle, a syringe may be needed to withdraw fluid, and pressure cannot be easily recorded. In addition, technically, a small needle such as a 26-gauge is difficult to place and manipulate into a position in which it does not become intermittently obstructed by nerve roots. When these characteristics are considered, the 20-gauge atraumatic needle seems the best overall choice for diagnostic lumbar puncture.[57]

Despite common beliefs about techniques and postprocedure interventions, *lumbar puncture headaches likely cannot be prevented.* Studies of the influence of activity, such as strict bedrest, on postpuncture headache have yielded contradictory results: worsening of, improvement in, and no effect on the incidence. Brocker[68] reported a reduction in the incidence of headache from 36.5% to 0.5% when patients lay prone instead of supine for 3 hours after puncture with an 18-gauge needle. He postulated that the prone position caused hyperextension of the spine and disrupted alignment of the holes in the dura and the arachnoid, making leakage less likely. Thoennissen and coworkers[69] concluded that there was no evidence that longer bedrest after lumbar puncture was better than immediate mobilization or short bedrest in reducing the incidence of headache.

Other factors that might influence the incidence of post–spinal puncture headache were reviewed by Fishman[20] and Lin and Giederman.[70] The incidence is higher in young patients than in older patients and is also increased in females and individuals with a history of headache. Many medications have been advocated for treatment of headache after lumbar puncture: barbiturates, codeine, neostigmine, ergots, diphenhydramine (Benadryl), dimenhydrinate (Dramamine), caffeine amphetamine sulfate (Benzedrine), ephedrine, intravenous fluids (normal saline, Ringer's lactate), magnesium sulfate, and vitamins.[20,71,72]

Most postpuncture headaches can be managed with bedrest, with the head in the horizontal position. Avoid dehydration because it lowers CSF pressure and might aggravate the headache. Although dehydration should be avoided, the role of fluid supplementation in the prevention of post–dural puncture headache remains uncertain.

Simple analgesics are commonly prescribed, but they have no apparent advantage over bedrest and fluid intake.

A patient with a prolonged headache after spinal puncture should be reassessed to rule out structural causes. Because a spinal headache has a rather classic presentation, if the headache is not postural, while being relieved by lying flat, consider other causes.

For patients with prolonged low-pressure headache, placement of an epidural blood patch by experienced operators is highly successful[73–75] and often provides dramatic relief.[75] Consider a blood patch in all cases of seriously symptomatic spinal headaches. Perform an epidural tap at the level of the previous lumbar puncture. Use the loss-of-resistance technique with sterile saline to locate the epidural space.[76] Ten to 20 mL of autologous blood is then drawn aseptically into a syringe and slowly injected (1–2 mL every 10 sec) into the epidural space at the site of the dural puncture. Slow or discontinue the injection if back pain or paresthesias develop. Keep the patient supine for 1 hour while intravenous hydration is administered. Relief usually occurs within 20 to 30 minutes after the procedure. Epidural patches are less likely to be effective if symptoms have been present for more than 2 weeks. Pain is relieved when the blood patch forms a gelatinous tamponade, stopping the CSF leak and immediately elevating CSF pressure. Patch failures (15%–20%) are believed to be caused by improper needle placement, injection of an inadequate quantity of blood, or an incorrect diagnosis. A second patch is often successful.

Complications reported after placement of an epidural patch include back stiffness, paresthesias, radicular pain, subdural hematoma, adhesive arachnoiditis, and bacterial meningitis.[74] The procedure should be used in patients with refractory headaches who fail to respond to conservative therapy and should be performed by clinicians trained in it.

Infection

Spinal puncture is contraindicated in the presence of local infection at the puncture site (cellulitis, suspected epidural abscess, or furunculosis) because of the danger of inducing meningitis. A large concentration of bacteria in the bloodstream at the time of CSF examination is associated with meningitis. The meningitis could be coincidental ("spontaneous") or could result from leakage of blood containing bacteria into the subarachnoid space after lumbar puncture ("induced"). It is likely that many cases of puncture-induced meningitis occur when the cautious clinician performs a lumbar puncture early in the course of meningitis, before the infection has had time to be reflected in the CSF. A recent review concluded that the majority of cases of postpuncture meningitis are probably caused by contamination of the site by aerosolized bacteria from medical personnel, contamination from skin flora, or least commonly, direct or hematogenous spread from an endogenous infectious site.[35] Suspected bacteremia is not a contraindication to lumbar puncture; delay in diagnosis because of concern regarding the risks of a lumbar puncture is more serious than the risk of causing meningitis with the procedure.[77,78]

Herniation Syndromes after Lumbar Puncture

Lumbar puncture is of value in confirming a diagnosis of meningitis, encephalitis, and SAH. Generally, when the patient has symptoms consistent with bacterial meningitis, it is safe to perform lumbar puncture before a head CT scan. Lumbar puncture may be the best initial procedure to diagnose SAH, thus reducing the need for routine CT scanning in certain low-risk patients with acute sudden headache.[79] However, in patients with a suspected intracranial mass lesion, generally perform a CT scan before the lumbar puncture. When meningitis remains on the differential diagnosis list, antibiotics are best administered after blood cultures are obtained and before the CT scan.

Particularly with supratentorial mass lesions, there may be a large pressure gradient between the cranial and the lumbar compartments. When brain volume is increased because of a mass lesion or edema, rostrocaudal displacement may occur after lumbar puncture if the skull is intact. Techniques for management of increased ICP are discussed in Chapter 60, Management of Increased Intracranial Pressure and Intracranial Shunts.

The specific question whether or not lumbar puncture causes brain herniation, when herniation would not have occurred spontaneously, cannot be answered with certainty. Controversy still exists regarding the risk of cerebral herniation caused by lumbar puncture in acute bacterial meningitis, and clinicians are caught in a huge clinical bind, much pontification, and little scientific data, with this issue.[80] Obviously, herniation has occurred in the absence of lumbar puncture in the setting of acute bacterial meningitis and also has been temporally related to the procedure. Brain herniation occurs in about 5% of patients with acute bacterial meningitis and accounts for about 30% of the mortality with this process.[80] A CT scan may find causes to contraindicate lumbar puncture, but a normal CT scan does not mean that a lumbar puncture is always safe.

Lowering the lumbar spinal canal pressure by removing CSF might increase the gradient between the cranial and the lumbar compartments, theoretically promoting both transtentorial and foramen magnum herniation. The frequency with which a lumbar puncture causes or accelerates transtentorial herniation is unknown because a seriously ill patient might have developed herniation spontaneously without the procedure. With the current use of small-caliber spinal needles and aggressive concurrent use of ICP-lowering agents, herniation appears extremely rare and is not fully predictable by CT scan or opening CSF pressure readings.

A careful neurologic examination should precede all spinal punctures. When there is a history of headache and fever with progressive mental status deterioration and the development of localizing neurologic signs, spinal puncture should not be performed as the initial diagnostic procedure. Gopal and colleagues[81] identified three statistically significant predictors of new intracranial masses: papilledema, focal abnormalities on neurologic examination, and altered mental status. Greig and Goroszeniuk[82] made similar recommendations. Hasbun and associates[83] demonstrated that in adults with suspected meningitis, the presence of any of 13 clinical features portends abnormal CT findings (Table 61–1). Theoretically, the presence of an abnormal CT portends potential herniation, with or without lumbar puncture. The absence of the findings suggests the patient is a good candidate for immediate lumbar puncture because the risk of brain herniation as a result of the procedure is low (see Table 61–1). Joffe[80] contended that *clinical signs of impending herniation* are the best predictors to delay lumbar puncture in acute bacterial meningitis. Findings that may mitigate against lumbar puncture prior to CT scan include a significantly decreased level of

TABLE 61–1 Clinical Characteristics Associated with Abnormal Findings on Head Computed Tomography in Adults with Suspected Meningitis

Age ≥ 60 yr
Immunocompromised state*
History of central nervous system disease†
Seizure within 1 wk before presentation
Neurologic findings
Abnormal level of consciousness
Inability to answer two questions correctly
Inability to follow two commands correctly
Gaze palsy
Abnormal visual fields
Facial palsy
Arm drift
Leg drift
Abnormal language‡

*Includes patients with human immunodeficiency virus infection or acquired immunodeficiency syndrome, those receiving immunosuppressive therapy, and those who had undergone transplantation.
†Mass lesion, stroke, or focal infection.
‡Aphasia, dysarthria, or extinction.
From Hasbun R, Abrahams J, Jekel J, Quagliarello VJ: Computed tomography of the head before lumbar puncture in adults with suspected meningitis. N Engl J Med 345:1727, 2001.

consciousness (Glasgow coma scale ≤ 11), brainstem findings (papillary changes, posturing, irregular respirations), and a very recent seizure.[80] These individuals would obviously appear quite ill. When these findings are present, empirically administer an initial dose of antibiotic while awaiting results of CT or MRI, which will help the clinician assess the safety of a subsequent lumbar puncture. Obtain appropriate cultures of blood and other body fluid before antibiotic administration. Blood cultures are positive in 80% of infants with meningitis. Measures to lower ICP before spinal puncture can also be instituted.

In summary, *patients critically ill with acute bacterial meningitis often deteriorate rapidly and experience fatal brain herniation, both shortly after lumbar puncture and in the absence of the procedure.* A direct cause-effect relationship between lumbar puncture and brain herniation in the setting of suspected meningitis is obscure and likely cannot be prospectively defined in the ED when clinical decisions must be made. A recent review identified only 22 case reports in the medical literature of rapid deterioration and herniation after lumbar puncture in adults and children with acute bacterial meningitis.[80] This risk of not doing a diagnostic lumbar puncture in critically ill patients is small because all should be aggressively and empirically treated with meningitis doses of antibiotics. The general consensus is that less ill patients (clearly a clinical judgment subject to clinician variability) with a clinical scenario *possible for meningitis* can safely be evaluated with lumbar puncture.

A CT scan should identify hemorrhagic lesions and most neoplasms. Its results should contribute to the decision regarding the need for and the risk involved with spinal puncture. Head CT may identify patients with unequal pressures between intracranial compartments who are at greater risk for cerebral herniation. CT findings that suggest unequal pressure between intracranial compartments include (1) lateral shift of midline structures, (2) loss of suprachiasmatic and circum-mesencephalic cisterns, (3) shift or obliteration of the fourth ventricle, and (4) failure to visualize the superior cerebellar and quadrigeminal plate cisterns, with sparing of the ambient cisterns.[84] The presence of a posterior fossa mass is a strong contraindication to lumbar puncture. Because of bone and motion artifact, the posterior fossa unfortunately may be a difficult area to visualize on CT scan.

In summary, with regard to CT scan before lumbar puncture, there is no totally agreed-upon standard of care that mandates when a lumber puncture should or should not be performed. A reasonable and logical approach is to avoid initial lumbar puncture, and first perform a CT scan when a mass lesion is suspected or if the patient has signs and symptoms of increased ICP (see Table 61–1). This approach correlates with the clinical policy promulgated by the American College of Emergency Physicians in 2002.[85]

Epidermoid Tumor

An epidermoid tumor or cyst is a mass of desquamated cells containing keratin within a capsule of well-differentiated stratified squamous epithelium. Congenital lesions arise from epithelial tissue that becomes sequestered at the time of closure of the neural groove between the 3rd and the 5th weeks of embryonic life; these lesions are rare. Acquired intraspinal epidermoid tumors result from implantation of epidermoid tissue into the spinal canal at the time of lumbar puncture performed with needles without stylets or with ill-fitting stylets. The clinical syndrome consists of pain in the back and the lower extremities, developing years after spinal puncture. Failure to use a stylet upon needle withdrawal might also result in aspiration of a nerve root into the epidural space.

Backache and Radicular Symptoms

Minor backache from the trauma of the spinal needle occurs with a frequency of 90%. Frank disk herniation has been reported from the passing of the needle beyond the subarachnoid space into the annulus fibrosis. Transient sensory symptoms from irritation of the cauda equina are also common.

Other reported complications include transient unilateral or bilateral sixth nerve palsies caused by stretching or displacement of the abducens nerve as it crosses the petrous ridge of the temporal bone, SAH, subdural and epidural hematoma, anaphylactoid reactions to local anesthetics, settling of cord tumors, and retroperitoneal abscess produced by dural laceration in patients with meningitis.[86,87] Most of these are rare and seldom encountered.

The complications associated with lateral cervical and cisternal puncture are similar to those encountered with lumbar puncture. In addition, perforation of a large vessel with resultant cisterna magna hematoma or obstruction of vertebral artery flow has been described. Puncture of the medulla oblongata may cause vomiting or apnea, and puncture of the cord may be associated with pain. Long-lasting side effects of cord puncture seem to be rare. Traumatic tap and postpuncture headache may occur.

INTERPRETATION

Pressure

The pressure of the CSF is of great clinical importance. Measure it accurately whenever feasible. Unfortunately, in some cases, it will be logistically impossible to obtain. If the lumbar puncture is being performed with the patient in a seated position, place the patient in the lateral decubitus position before a measurement is obtained. This may be done initially, before fluid is collected, or after fluid collection, in which case a closing pressure is obtained. By repositioning the patient and measuring the pressure after the fluid is collected, the impact of needle displacement due to repositioning is minimized.[12,16] Accurate measurement depends on patient cooperation. Measurements from struggling or agitated patients will probably be inaccurate; in such cases, sedation may allow more accurate readings to be obtained.

Elevated pressures are abnormal. Opening pressure is taken promptly, avoiding falsely low values caused by leakage through and around the needle. Normal pressure is between 70 and 180 mm H_2O. Herniating cerebellar tonsils may occlude the foramen magnum and prevent increased ICP from being reflected in the lumbar pressure reading. Increased ICP can result from expansion of the brain (edema, hemorrhage, or neoplasm), overproduction of CSF (choroid plexus papilloma), a defect in absorption, or obstruction of flow of CSF through the ventricles. Cerebral edema may be associated with meningitis, CO_2 retention, SAH, anoxia, congestive heart failure, or superior vena cava obstruction. Pressure may be falsely elevated in a tense patient, when the head is elevated above the plane of the needle, and possibly, with marked obesity or muscle contraction.[20] Pressure is not usually measured in the neonate because a struggling or crying child will have a falsely elevated pressure. In children, the manometer reading is falsely elevated in the sitting position, but the level should not rise above the foramen magnum.

Low pressure suggests obstruction of the needle by the meninges. Low pressure can also be seen with spinal block. Rarely, a primary low-pressure syndrome occurs in a setting of trauma, after neurosurgical procedures, secondary to subdural hematomas in elderly patients, with barbiturate intoxication, and in cases of CSF leakage through holes in the arachnoid.[88,89]

The Queckenstedt test is useful for demonstrating obstruction in the spinal subarachnoid space.[4,20] The test is seldom performed today because myelographic techniques have been refined and the availability of MRI has reduced the number of myelograms and associated lumbar puncture studies. However, because situations might arise when the timeliness of this simple and reliable test is important diagnostically, the technique is described here. With the patient in the lateral recumbent position, jugular vein compression causes decreased venous return to the heart. This distends cerebral veins and causes a rise of ICP, which is transmitted throughout the system and is measured in the manometer. After 10 seconds of bilateral compression, CSF pressure usually rises to 150 mm H_2O over the initial reading and returns to baseline 10 to 20 seconds after release. If there is no change in the lumbar pressure or if the rise and fall are delayed, conclude that the spinal subarachnoid space does not communicate with the cranial subarachnoid space. In this situation, injecting Pantopaque before needle removal facilitates subsequent performance of a myelogram. This is necessary because the lumbar dural sac may collapse, making it impossible to reenter the canal. If cervical cord disease is suspected, repeat the test with the neck in the neutral position, hyperextended, and flexed. When lateral sinus obstruction is suspected, use unilateral jugular venous compression (Tobey-Ayer test).

Appearance

If the CSF is not crystal clear, a pathologic condition of the CNS should be suspected. The examiner should compare the fluid with water, viewing down the long axis of the tube or holding both tubes against a white background. A glass tube is preferred, because plastic tubes are frequently not clear. Note that the fluid *may appear clear with as many as 400 red blood cells (RBCs)/μL and 200 WBCs/μL.*[20]

Xanthochromia, a yellow-orange discoloration of the supernate of centrifuged CSF, is generally considered to be the result of SAH of at least a few hours' duration and has been used to differentiate prior bleeding from a traumatic tap. A traumatic tap usually does not exhibit xanthochromia (see "The Traumatic Tap," later). Xanthochromia is produced by red cell lysis and is caused by one or more of the following pigments: oxyhemoglobin, bilirubin, or methemoglobin.

Xanthochromia has traditionally been evaluated by visual inspection by a laboratory technician after centrifugation of a sample of CSF. Most hospitals currently use this method. Recently, spectrophotometry, designed to demonstrate both oxyhemoglobin and bilirubin, has been advocated as a more precise way of determining xanthochromia. Oxyhemoglobin alone, *without bilirubin*, in a CSF sample is thought to be artifactual (traumatic). Visually, bilirubin and oxyhemoglobin cannot be differentiated. Therefore, *the presence of bilirubin by spectrophotometry should define xanthochromia and prompt additional investigation for SAH.* Relying on spectrophotometry to identify xanthochromia, without pigment differentiation, will cause a high false-positive interpretation. The *absence* of both oxyhemoglobin and bilirubin by spectrophotometry does not support SAH. Visual inspection still appears to be a reliable method to identify xanthochromia, and the need for routine spectrophotometry is unclear.

Oxyhemoglobin causes red coloration; bilirubin, yellow; and methemoglobin, brown. Oxyhemoglobin is seen within 2 hours after subarachnoid bleeding and red cell lysis, but may be immediate if bleeding is profuse. Formation peaks 24 to 48 hours after hemorrhage, and the discoloration disappears in 3 to 30 days.[4]

Blood must be within the CSF (in vivo) for a number of hours for bilirubin to appear; it will not appear spontaneously once CSF is in the collection tube. The appearance of bilirubin in the CSF involves the conversion of oxyhemoglobin by the enzyme heme oxygenase. The enzyme is found in the choroid plexus, the arachnoid, and the meninges. Enzyme activity appears approximately 12 hours after the hemorrhage.[4] Bilirubin may persist in CSF for 2 to 4 weeks. Bilirubin in CSF caused by hepatic or hemolytic disease does not appear until a serum level of 10 to 15 mg total bilirubin per 100 mL is reached, unless underlying disease associated with a high CSF protein is present. Xanthochromia may be seen with CSF protein values above 150 mg/dL. CSF may clot in patients with complete spinal block and very high CSF protein.

Graves and Sidman[90] noted that an RBC concentration of 5000/μL created by addition of RBCs to a cellular CSF fluid will produce spectrophotometrically evident xanthochromia by 2 hours. The addition of RBCs to produce RBC concentrations of 20,000/μL and 30,000/μL will produce xanthochromia by 1 hour or immediately, respectively. Therefore, xanthochromia may occur with a traumatic tap and does not always diagnose SAH.

Methemoglobin is a reduction product of oxyhemoglobin characteristically found in encapsulated subdural hematomas and in old intracerebral hematomas.

Cells

In adults, WBC counts over 5 cells/μL indicate the presence of a pathologic condition. Conversely, normal neonatal CSF may show up to 32 WBCs/μL with prominent neutrophils, whereas infants 4 to 8 weeks old may have 22 WBCs/μL.[91] Polymorphonuclear leukocytes are never seen in normal adults. However, with the use of the cytocentrifuge, an occasional specimen may show a neutrophil in an otherwise normal individual.[92] Such a finding should routinely prompt culture of the CSF because the presence of neutrophilic pleocytosis is commonly associated with bacterial infections or the early stages of viral infections, tuberculosis, meningitis, hematogenous meningitis, and chemical meningitis caused by foreign bodies.

As many as 30% of patients may exhibit CSF pleocytosis after a generalized or focal seizure. This finding should prompt a search for infection and assessment of the seizure as being possibly secondary to a serious intracranial pathologic processes (subdural hematoma, SAH, or stroke).

Small lymphocytes may be seen in normal individuals. Small and large immunocompetent cells are found with a variety of bacterial, fungal, viral, granulomatous, and spirochetal diseases.

Eosinophils always indicate an abnormal condition, most commonly a parasitic infestation of the CNS. They may also be seen after myelography and pneumoencephalography and, to a minor degree, in other inflammatory diseases, including tuberculous meningitis and neurosyphilis. Normal CSF RBC counts are less than 10/μL. Herpes simplex virus encephalitis may elevate the CSF RBC count. Myeloid and RBC precursors may contaminate CSF with bone marrow cells from an adjacent vertebral body.[93]

Glucose

Glucose enters the CSF by way of the choroid plexus as well as by transcapillary movement into the extracellular space of the brain and the cord via carrier-mediated transport. It then equilibrates freely within the CSF subarachnoid space. Once in the CSF, glucose undergoes glycolysis and there is an invariable rise in CSF lactate levels. Glucose levels remain subnormal for 1 to 2 weeks after the effective treatment of meningitis.

The normal range of CSF glucose is 50 to 80 mg/dL, which is 60% to 70% of the glucose concentration in the blood. Ventricular fluid glucose levels are 6 to 8 mg/dL higher than in lumbar fluid. A ratio of CSF glucose–to–blood glucose of less than 0.5 or a CSF glucose level below 40 mg/dL is invariably abnormal. The ratio is higher in infants, for whom a ratio of less than 0.6 is considered abnormal. Hyperglycemia may mask a depressed CSF glucose level; when present, the CSF glucose–to–blood glucose ratio should be measured routinely. With extreme hyperglycemia, a ratio of 0.3 is abnormal.[94] Between 90 and 120 minutes is required before the CSF glucose reaches a steady state with blood glucose changes (e.g., after an intravenous injection of glucose). When CSF glucose is of diagnostic importance, obtain CSF and blood samples ideally after a 4-hour fast.

TABLE 61–2 Low Cerebrospinal Fluid Glucose Syndromes

Bacterial meningitis	Syphilis
Tuberculous meningitis	Chemical meningitis
Fungal meningitis	Subarachnoid hemorrhage
Sarcoidosis	Mumps meningitis
Meningeal carcinomatosis	Herpes simplex encephalitis
Amebic meningitis	Hypoglycemia
Cysticercosis	
Trichinosis	

Low CSF glucose levels may be associated with several diseases of the nervous system (Table 61–2). Only low concentrations of glucose are of diagnostic value; elevated CSF glucose levels generally have no significance, usually reflecting hyperglycemia. A rapid estimate of the CSF glucose level can be obtained by using bedside reagent strip testing with a commercial autoanalyzer. Formal laboratory testing is recommended for confirmation of bedside levels.

Protein

The normal range of the lumbar CSF protein level is 15 to 45 mg/dL. Infants normally have a lower level than adults, and protein levels may drop after a lumbar puncture. The concentration is lower in the ventricles (5–15 mg/dL) and the basilar cisterns (10–25 mg/dL), reflecting a gradient in the permeability of capillary endothelial cells to proteins in the blood. Levels of CSF protein in premature infants and full-term neonates are higher than in adults, with a mean of 90 mg/dL; protein levels decline by age 8 weeks, reflecting maturation of the blood-brain barrier.

Most of the proteins in CSF normally come from the blood, which normally has a protein concentration of up to 8000 mg/dL. Protein entry is determined by its molecular size and the relative impermeability of the blood-CSF barrier. A full range of serum proteins is found in CSF at several hundred-fold dilution.

An increase in the CSF total protein level is a nonspecific abnormality associated with many disease states. Levels higher than 500 mg/dL are uncommon and are seen mainly in meningitis, in subarachnoid bleeding, and with spinal tumors. The high levels seen with cord tumors result from an increase in local capillary permeability. With high levels (generally 1000 mg/dL), CSF may clot (Froin syndrome).

Hemorrhage into the CSF or the introduction of blood by a traumatic tap increases CSF protein levels. If the serum protein concentration is normal, the CSF protein should theoretically rise by 1 mg/dL for every 1000 RBCs, but this relationship varies. The inflammatory effect of hemolyzed RBCs may also significantly increase CSF protein.

Selective measurement of immunoglobulin fractions in CSF has proved to be of diagnostic value in suspected cases of multiple sclerosis. Elevated CSF immunoglobulin levels may reflect blood-brain barrier disruption or local antibody response to a CNS immune response.[95] Stimuli may be infectious or antigenic, producing an inflammatory response. Immunoglobulin elevation has been found in many conditions, including syphilis, viral encephalitis, subacute sclerosing panencephalitis, progressive rubella encephalitis, tuberculous meningitis, sarcoidosis, cysticercosis, and acute inflammatory demyelinating polyneuropathy (Guillain-Barré syndrome).

The Traumatic Tap

The incidence of a traumatic tap is 10% to 30%, depending on the criteria used to define the condition.[96] *Currently, there is no consensus as to what constitutes a traumatic tap.* Traditionally, the number of RBCs in the CSF, the rate of clearance of RBCs from tube 1 to tube 4, and the presence or absence of xanthochromia have guided the clinician in attempts to define the need for further investigation for SAH when blood is detected during the lumbar puncture.

The Absolute Number of RBCs. The current literature makes no firm recommendations regarding the absolute CSF RBC count that can be used as a cutoff to differentiate SAH from a traumatic tap. However, SAH consistently produces more RBCs in CSF than does a traumatic tap. In tube 3 or 4, an absolute RBC value of 400 to 500 RBCs/μL or less is very suggestive of a traumatic tap, and this value has been traditionally used by clinicians.[12] In a retrospective study of 300 patients, Gorchynski and coworkers[97] reported a 100% *negative predictive value for SAH* with an RBC count, in tube 4, of 500 RBCs/μL or less, with a *sensitivity for SAH* in this range of 100%. In this study, no radiographically normal subject had an RBC count of more than 10,000 RBCs/μL, suggesting that results above this number are suspicious for a radiographically detectable SAH. In this study when the RBC count in tube 4 ranged between 500 and 10,000 RBCs/μL, SAH could not be ruled out without further study.

RBC Clearance from Tube 1 to Tube 3/4. In traumatic punctures, the fluid generally clears of RBCs between tubes 1 and tubes 3/4 as the needle is washed by CSF. Theoretically, the RBC count *should not decrease* between tubes if there is actual blood in the CSF (SAH). Therefore, a decrease in the RBC count between the first and the third tubes has traditionally been considered as strong evidence of a traumatic tap.[2] However, after a recent hemorrhage, some declining cell count may also be seen, representing layering of cells in a recumbent patient. A decrease in RBC count of more than 30% between the first and the last tube has been a longstanding guideline to suggest a traumatic tap.[98] Others have reported a more dramatic decrease in CSF RBC count in subsequent tubes with traumatic taps. Gorchynski and coworkers[97] reported an 82% RBC clearance from tube 1 to tube 4 in traumatic taps and a 9% clearance in the SAH group. These authors suggested that a decrease in RBC count from tube 1 to tube 4 of at least 70%, coupled with a total RBC count of less than 500 RBCs/μL could exclude patients with a radiographically detectable SAH.

Xanthochromia. RBCs undergo hemolysis in the CSF after a few hours to produce xanthochromia. Xanthochromia persists for up to 4 weeks, depending on the number of RBCs originally present. Xanthochromia is suggestive of, but not pathognomonic for, SAH. An early CSF examination may show clear fluid before the development of hemolysis, even after spontaneous subarachnoid bleeding. However, xanthochromia may be detected immediately after a traumatic tap if the RBC count exceeds 30,000/μL.[90] The presence of a clot in one of the tubes strongly favors a traumatic tap. In SAH, clotting does not occur because blood is defibrinated at the site of the hemorrhage. Lumbar puncture performed several days after a traumatic tap may yield stained fluid. The collection of clear CSF from an immediate repeat puncture done at a higher interspace also indicates a traumatic tap. The fluid from a traumatic tap should contain about 1 WBC/700 RBCs if the complete blood cell count is normal, but this ratio is highly variable. All blood-contaminated CSF should be cultured, especially samples from uncooperative infants and children being evaluated for sepsis.

A D-dimer test on CSF can be used to determine SAH by identifying local fibrinolysis. Other conditions such as disseminated intravascular coagulation, a previous traumatic tap, or prior thrombolytic therapy may produce false-positive results. Eskey and Ogilvy[99] suggested that the routine use of fluoroscopy-guided lumbar puncture in patients with suspected SAH and negative CT scan would reduce the frequency of traumatic punctures.

CSF Analysis with Infections

Bacterial Infections

The CSF findings are essential to establishing a provisional diagnosis of acute bacterial meningitis. CSF analysis establishes not only the diagnosis but also the causative organism and therefore the choice of antibiotics (Table 61-3). CSF must be transported to the laboratory immediately and examined at once. CSF cells begin to lyse within 1 hour of collection; this process can be slowed by refrigeration. In cases of meningococcal infection, a delay in processing may cause the diagnosis to be missed because the organism tends to autolyze rapidly. For other organisms, speed is slightly less important but still warranted because early initiation of antibiotic therapy is crucial.

The Gram stain is of great importance because the results dictate the initial choice of antibiotic therapy. Gram-negative intracellular or extracellular diplococci are indicative of *Neisseria meningitidis*. Small gram-negative bacilli may indicate *Haemophilus influenzae*, especially in children. The presence of gram-positive cocci indicates *Streptococcus pneumoniae*, other *Streptococcus* species, or *Staphylococcus*. Twenty percent of Gram stains may be falsely negative because too few organisms are present. The Gram stain smear is more likely to be positive in patients who have not received prior antibiotic therapy. Acridine orange stain may improve the yield in stains of Gram-negative organisms.[100]

For culture, blood and chocolate agar are required. *N. meningitidis* and *H. influenzae* grow best on chocolate agar. The plates are incubated under 10% CO_2. Thioglycolate medium is used for possible anaerobic organisms. Cultures are examined at 24 and 48 hours, but plates should be kept for at least 7 days. Large volumes of CSF may improve yields.

While the culture results are pending, bacterial infection should be suspected in patients with an elevated opening pressure and marked pleocytosis, ranging between 500 and 20,000 WBCs/μL.[3] The differential count with bacterial infections is usually chiefly neutrophils. A count of more than 1000 cells/μL seldom occurs in viral infections. Occasionally, acellular fluid may be collected from a severely immunosuppressed patient or others with appropriate presentations. Repeat lumbar puncture may be required in febrile patients in whom the clinical features remain compatible with meningitis.[94,101,102]

CSF glucose levels of 40 mg/dL or less or less than 50% of a simultaneous blood glucose level should raise the question of bacterial meningitis, even in the presence of a negative Gram stain and a low cell count. Glucose levels with bacterial meningitis are occasionally below 10 mg/dL; levels are normal in a small percentage of patients with bacterial meningitis.[94] The CSF protein content in bacterial meningitis ranges from 500 to 1500 mg/dL and usually returns to normal by the end of therapy. Of note, previous antibiotic therapy may adversely affect the sensitivity of cultures and Gram stains for bacterial meningitis but does not significantly affect WBC counts, CSF glucose–to–blood glucose ratios, or CSF protein values.[103] Spanos and colleagues[104] developed a useful nomogram to help distinguish bacterial from viral infections.

Microbial Antigens and Polymerase Chain Reaction

Several tests other than CSF culture and Gram stain are available to establish a bacterial cause of meningitis. These include blood cultures, CSF counterimmunoelectrophoresis (CIE), CSF latex agglutination (LA), and coagglutination CIE.[6] These ancillary tests have a low sensitivity for bacterial meningitis, thus limiting their use. In 50% to 80% of bacterial meningitis cases, blood cultures are positive for the etiologic agent.[105]

CIE uses wells in two rows of agarose gel. A different antiserum is placed in each well. A current is passed through the gel, causing the reactants to move toward each other by electrophoretic mobilization of the antigen. A line of precipitation visualized in 1 to 4 hours represents a positive reaction between antiserum and antigen.[106] Commercial kits are available to detect *S. pneumoniae*; *Listeria monocytogenes*; *H. influenzae*; *N. meningitidis* A, B, and C and W135; group B streptococci; K1 strains of *Escherichia coli*; *Klebsiella*; and *Pseudomonas* species.[107]

Particle agglutination involves staphylococcal coagglutination and latex agglutination. Antibody on the surface of a colloid combines with antigen-binding sites to cross-link the colloid-forming antigen bridges. A matrix forms and appears as a macroscopic agglutination. Agglutination tests can detect approximately 10 times less antigen than CIE. False-positive tests can occur in the presence of rheumatoid factor, serum complement components, and possibly other serum proteins. The technique may be used in infections with *H. influenzae*, *S. pneumoniae*, *N. meningitidis*, and group B streptococci.

Another technique having some potential use for identification of bacterial meningitis is the enzyme-linked immunosorbent assay. This technique may detect 100 to 1000 times less antigen than agglutination tests but is technically more difficult and requires 4 hours to perform.

TABLE 61–3 Cerebrospinal Fluid Analysis in Bacterial and Viral Meningitis*

	Bacterial Meningitis	Viral Meningitis
Opening pressure	Usually elevated	Usually normal
WBC count/mm³	Elevated, 500–10,000+	Elevated, 6–1000
Differential count	Polymorphonuclear predominance	Lymphocytic predominance
Glucose level	Decreased, 0–40 mg/dL	Usually normal
Protein level	Elevated, >50 mg/dL	Normal or slightly elevated

*This is only a guide and care must be taken when interpreting these parameters, especially early in the clinical course.

Adapted from Fong B, Van Bendegem J: Lumbar puncture. In Reichman E, Simon R (eds): Emergency Medical Procedures. New York: McGraw-Hill, 2004, p 875.

A positive CSF antigen test may be expected in 70% to 90% of patients with *Neisseria* meningitis. This compares with a positive Gram stain in approximately 70% of patients. Positive latex antigen tests have been reported in approximately 60% of *S. pneumoniae* meningitis cases, with a positive Gram stain in 80%. A positive latex test and Gram stain are reported in approximately 85% of *H. influenzae* meningitis cases.[105,106] Group B streptococci can be detected with 60% to 90% sensitivity. The Gram stain may be difficult to assess after antibiotic therapy has been initiated. Bacterial antigens may persist in the CSF for several days after antibiotic therapy. With appropriate antimicrobial therapy, 25% to 33% of positive tests are lost per day. A negative test, however, does not rule out bacterial meningitis.[107] In addition, blood and urine should be examined for antigen. Often, antigen may be found only in the urine. Urine needs to be concentrated and may have the disadvantage of reflecting urinary tract infections. The particle agglutination test for *H. influenzae* type B may be positive up to 10 days after children have received *H. influenzae* polysaccharide vaccine. Antigen tests are not useful in diagnosing gram-negative bacillary, staphylococcal, and *Listeria* meningitis. In addition, although antigen tests may identify the bacterial pathogen, they do not provide information about the antibiotic susceptibility of the organism.

Future use of polymerase chain reaction (PCR) will aid the rapid diagnosis of CNS infection when results of current techniques are suboptimal. PCR amplifies target nucleic acid in CSF by use of repeated cycles of DNA synthesis. PCR requires use of flanking DNA sequences at the opposite ends of the target DNA. Synthetic primers anneal to their respective recognition sequences at the opposite end of the target sequence; they serve as primers for new DNA synthesis. PCR allows detection and quantification of organisms whose genetic material is DNA or messenger RNA. PCR permits the diagnosis of infectious disease with a high degree of sensitivity and specificity and allows rapid reliable detection of microbes present in small numbers. False-negative and false-positive laboratory results may occur.

Empirical Antibiotic Use before Lumbar Puncture

Many patients are transported within a facility or to a referral center for a CT scan to rule out an intracranial mass after clinical concern for meningitis is raised. In such instances, CSF examination might not be performed before transport because of technical problems (an uncooperative or a large patient) or concerns regarding the safety of lumbar puncture in an obtunded patient with possible increased ICP.[94,108] The initial clinician may have to decide whether to initiate empirical antibiotic therapy. Antibiotic administration could obscure the bacterial source, whereas a delay in initiating therapy might increase morbidity and mortality. It may be difficult to identify individuals at risk for a fulminant course, and bacterial meningitis cannot always be diagnosed with confidence; some cases may be misdiagnosed as SAH or metabolic encephalopathy.

After administration of parenteral antibiotics, a window of 2 to 3 hours exists when CSF cultures are not adversely affected. Twenty-four hours after treatment, as many as 38% of meningitis patients may still have positive CSF cultures. Kanegaye and associates[109] demonstrated that CSF sterilization may depend on the infecting organism. They reported CSF sterilization after antibiotic administration within the following timeframes: meningococcal, less than 2 hours; pneumococcal, less than 4.3 hoursr; and group B streptococcal, longer than 8 hours.

When CSF is cultured more than several hours after parenteral antibiotics are administered, antigen tests may be helpful. Of course, blood cultures should be obtained immediately before antibiotic administration whenever possible. Occasionally, patients may develop lymphocytic pleocytosis in response to antibiotic therapy, but in most cases, cell count, differential, glucose, and protein concentrations are not changed in the first 2 to 3 days of antibiotic therapy.[94] Although there are no data to confidently address the advantages or disadvantages of antibiotic therapy before lumbar puncture, it is reasonable to initiate therapy on the premise that a delay might be deleterious. If a lumbar puncture cannot be done, consultation with clinicians at the referral center seems appropriate. If a lumbar puncture is performed before a transfer, a portion of the CSF (chilled on ice) should be sent with the patient or held in the referring hospital laboratory.

Bacterial meningitis occurring in children younger than 10 years of age historically has been caused by *H. influenzae*. Fortunately, this organism appears to be easier to grow from early postantibiotic cultures and is more likely to be associated with positive blood cultures and antigen tests. In the pediatric population, a single dose of an antibiotic before transport is unlikely to prevent bacterial identification. In neonates, adults, and immunosuppressed patients, the sensitivity of blood cultures and immunologic tests is less reliable. CSF examination before antibiotic administration or early in the course of treatment is preferred.

For suspected or confirmed cases of acute bacterial meningitis, antimicrobial therapy can be started based on the most likely causative organism based on age of the subject, associated diseases, and renal function.

For immunocompromised patients and after neurosurgery, a third-generation cephalosporin (cefotaxime, ceftizoxime, ceftazidime, or ceftriaxone) plus ampicillin and vancomycin should be used for coverage against staphylococci, *Listeria monocytogenes*, and gram-negative organisms.[6] Tables 61–4 through 61–6 offer guidelines for emergency antibiotic therapy. The third-generation cephalosporins are efficacious in many empirical regimens or situations in which the organism is known. Reliance on third-generation cephalosporins alone for all cases of bacterial meningitis would result in treatment failures for all *Listeria* species and increasing numbers of *Enterobacter*, *Serratia*, and *Pseudomonas* groups.

Dexamethasone Therapy in Bacterial Meningitis

In acute bacterial meningitis, bacterial cell wall components including lipopolysaccharides and teichoic acid initiate and exacerbate the host response. These stimulate the production of cytokines, including interleukin-1 and tumor necrosis factor, from macrophages and monocytes. Cytokines may injure vessels, diminish cerebral perfusion, and stimulate cerebral swelling.[108] The outcome of acute bacterial meningitis has been related to the severity of the inflammatory process in the subarachnoid space.

Studies have suggested benefit from adjunctive dexamethasone therapy in reducing neurologic sequelae, especially hearing loss, in children with *H. influenzae* meningitis and for a lower mortality and a better overall outcome in adults with community-acquired acute bacterial meningitis due to *S. pneumoniae*.[110] There appear to be no adverse sequelae from steroid therapy. The adjunctive benefit of corticosteroids during treatment of meningitis caused by other organisms (viral, fungal, parasitic) is unknown. *A recent Cochrane review concluded that "the corticosteroid dexamethasone leads to a major reduction in hearing loss and death in both children and adults with bacterial meningitis, without major adverse effects."*[111] Interestingly, and somewhat puzzling, for children in low-income countries, the use of corticosteroids was associated with neither benefit nor harmful effects.

The dosage of dexamethasone is 0.15 mg/kg (10 mg intravenously in adults) every 6 hours for 4 days. It is recommended that the corticosteroid be given *before antibiotic use*, but the exact timing and specific benefits are unclear. It has been suggested that caution should be exercised in immunocompromised and leukopenic patients when administering corticosteroids in the presence of bacterial meningitis, but currently no specific recommendations are forthcoming.

A moderate inflammatory response in the meninges is required for penetration of the CNS by many antibiotics. Reducing meningeal inflammation reduces the concentration of antibiotics in the CSF. Corticosteroids should be discontinued after approximately 4 days of treatment, at which time meningeal inflammation should have been reduced by antibiotics.[112,113]

Neurosyphilis

The true incidence of neurosyphilis is unknown. Approximately 5000 new cases of this disease are estimated to occur in the United States each year.[114] The natural history and clinical manifestations have been modified in the antibiotic era. The widespread use of oral antibiotics has changed neurosyphilis into chronic, partially treated meningitis. Partial therapy may clear peripheral infection and attenuate the immune response. Therapy may be sufficient to minimize symptoms but insufficient to eradicate organisms in the CNS and eye, which may then multiply.

CSF findings suggestive of neurosyphilis include greater than 5 WBCs/μL, elevated protein concentration, elevated γ-globulin concentration, and a positive serologic test for syphilis. The glucose concentration is usually normal. Higher cell and protein values are seen in early as opposed to late neurosyphilis.

Diagnostic certainty remains difficult. The diagnostic criterion standard is darkfield microscopy to identify morphology and flexing "corkscrew" motility of spirochetes. Serologic tests for syphilis are either treponemal or nontrepo-

---

TABLE 61–4 Empirical Therapy for Purulent Meningitis*

Predisposing Factor	Antimicrobial Therapy[†]
Age	
0–4 wk	Ampicillin plus cefotaxime; or ampicillin plus an aminoglycoside
4–12 wk	Ampicillin plus a third-generation cephalosporin[‡]
3 mo–18 yr	Third-generation cephalosporin[‡] or ampicillin plus chloramphenicol
18–50 yr	Third-generation cephalosporin[‡§]
>50 yr	Ampicillin plus a third-generation cephalosporin[‡]
Immunocompromised state	Vancomycin plus ampicillin plus ceftazidime
Basilar skull fracture	Third-generation cephalosporin[‡]
Head trauma	Vancomycin plus ceftazidime postneurosurgery
Cerebrospinal fluid	Vancomycin plus ceftazidime shunt

*Consider corticosteroids before antibiotic administration (see text).
[†]Vancomycin should be added to all empirical therapeutic regimens when highly penicillin- or cephalosporin-resistant strains of *Streptococcus pneumoniae* are suspected.
[‡]Cefotaxime or ceftriaxone.
[§]Add ampicillin if meningitis caused by *Listeria monocytogenes* is suspected.

TABLE 61–5 Recommended Dosages of Antimicrobial Agents for Meningitis in Adults with Normal Renal and Hepatic Function*

Antimicrobial Agent	Total Daily Dose (IV)	Dosing Interval (hr)
Ampicillin	12 g	4
Cefotaxime	8–12 g	4–6
Ceftazidime	6 g	8
Ceftriaxone	4 g	12–24
Chloramphenicol[†]	4–6 g	6
Gentamicin[‡]	3–5 mg/kg	8
Tobramycin[‡]	3–5 mg/kg	8
Vancomycin[‡]	2–3 g	8–12

*Consider corticosteroids before antibiotic administration (see text).
[†]High dose recommended for pneumococcal meningitis.
[‡]Peak and trough serum concentrations must be monitored.

TABLE 61–6 Recommended Total Daily Dosages (With Dosing Intervals in Hr) of Antimicrobial Agents for Meningitis in Neonates, Infants, and Children with Normal Renal and Hepatic Function

Antimicrobial Agent*	Neonates (0–7 days)[†]	Neonates (8–28 days)[†]	Infants and Children
Amikacin[‡]	15–20 mg/kg (12)	20–30 mg/kg (8)	20–30 mg/kg (8)
Ampicillin	100–150 mg/kg (8–12)	150–200 mg/kg (6–8)	200–300 mg/kg (6)
Cefotaxime	100 mg/kg (12)	150–200 mg/kg (6–8)	200 mg/kg (6)
Ceftazidime	60 mg/kg (12)	90 mg/kg (8)	125–150 mg/kg (8)
Ceftriaxone	—	—	80–100 mg/kg (12–24)
Chloramphenicol	25 mg/kg (24)	50 mg/kg (12–24)	75–100 mg/kg (6)
Gentamicin[‡]	5 mg/kg (12)	7.5 mg/kg (8)	7.5 mg/kg (8)
Tobramycin[‡]	5 mg/kg (12)	7.5 mg/kg (8)	7.5 mg/kg (8)

*Consider corticosteroids before antibiotic administration (see text).
[†]Smaller dosages and longer intervals of administration may be advisable for very low birth weight neonates (<2000 g).
[‡]Peak and trough serum concentrations must be monitored.

nemal. Nontreponemal tests detect a nonspecific globulin complex called reagin. Reagin tests, such as the Venereal Disease Research Laboratory (VDRL) flocculation test, lack sensitivity and should not be used to exclude the diagnosis of neurosyphilis. One third to one half of patients with neurosyphilis have a negative VDRL test in the serum, and more than one third have a negative VDRL test in the CSF.[114] CSF VDRL is quite specific, with false-positive results seen primarily with traumatic taps.

Treponemal tests provide evidence of a specific immune response to *Treponema pallidum*. These include serum fluorescent treponemal antibody absorption (FTA-ABS), microhemagglutination tests for *T. pallidum* (MHA-TP), and the *T. pallidum* hemagglutination assay (TPHA). A positive serum treponemal test indicates past infection with syphilis and may be reactive indefinitely, even after treatment. Therefore, CSF is used as a guide to the presence and activity of neurosyphilis. The VDRL test is the test of choice in CSF and, when positive, is strong evidence for neurosyphilis. False-positive CSF VDRL tests are rare. The FTA-ABS test is not used in CSF; the false-positive rate is between 4% and 6% and is believed to represent antibodies that have passively entered from serum.[115] The FTA-ABS test measures immunoglobulin G (IgG) antibody and cannot differentiate active from past infection. The CSF VDRL may be reactive by contamination with seropositive blood (traumatic tap, SAH) or may occur with entry of serum reagin into CSF during meningitis.

There is some concern that many patients with parenchymal neurosyphilis have normal CSF. This finding leads to the recommendation that a patient with signs of progressive neurosyphilis and a positive treponemal serologic test be treated with antibiotics regardless of the CSF findings. CSF pleocytosis may be provoked after 1 week of therapy and may supply supportive evidence for a diagnosis of neurosyphilis. PCR may have future applications for diagnosis of neurosyphilis (see "Neurosyphilis in Patients with HIV Infection," later in this chapter).

Viral Meningitis

The organisms most commonly isolated in viral meningitis are the enteroviruses (coxsackieviruses, echoviruses) and mumps virus. Enteroviruses are most commonly seen in the summer and fall, and mumps appears most frequently in the winter and spring. Viral cultures in most hospitals are not available and play little role in acute decisions regarding diagnosis and treatment. A serial rise in CSF antibody titers may be helpful but difficult to obtain in patients who have clinically recovered. Intrathecal production of organ-specific antibodies (IgM, IgG, and IgA isotopes) may be diagnostic of neurologic infection if there is no history of infections. Serum and CSF antibody titers must be measured in a specialized laboratory. Viral meningitis is diagnosed when bacterial culture and Gram stain are negative. A tentative diagnosis may be based on analysis of the CSF.

The WBC count in viral meningitis and encephalitis characteristically shows 10 to 1000 cells/μL. The differential cell count is predominantly lymphocytic and mononuclear in type. In the early stages of meningoencephalitis, however, polymorphonuclear cells may predominate, making the distinction between viral and bacterial infections difficult. In such cases, a repeat tap in 12 to 24 hours will assist in clarifying the diagnosis. Protein levels are usually mildly elevated, but normal levels may be seen. Antibiotic coverage pending culture results may be reasonably initiated if the diagnosis of viral meningitis is in doubt.[94] The CSF glucose concentration is characteristically normal; however, notable exceptions include some cases of mumps meningoencephalitis and herpes simplex encephalitis. CSF pleocytosis and elevated protein levels have also been found in asymptomatic HIV-seropositive individuals.[116]

If the CSF cannot be delivered to the viral laboratory in 24 to 48 hours, it should be refrigerated at 4°C. Members of the enterovirus group are occasionally isolated from CSF. Herpes viruses and arboviruses are rarely found in CSF. The PCR is the diagnostic test of choice for herpes simplex meningoencephalitis and will be increasingly applied to the diagnosis of other CNS viral infections.

CSF Analysis in Immunocompromised Patients

The number of immunocompromised individuals is increasing because of the HIV epidemic and the increased survival of patients with cancer and autoimmune disorders. The nervous system is a major target of the HIV virus: 40% to 60% of infected individuals develop neurologic disease during their lifetime. One third of HIV-infected patients present with neurologic complaints as the initial manifestations of the acquired immunodeficiency syndrome (AIDS), and an even higher incidence of nervous system involvement is found at autopsy.[117] Risk of CNS infection depends on the underlying disease, treatment, duration, and type of immune abnormality. Abnormalities include defects in T-lymphocyte and macrophage cellular immune function, defects in humoral immunity, defects in number and function of neutrophils, and loss of splenic function with inability to remove encapsulated bacteria.[118] The major neurologic manifestations of HIV infection, including clinical characteristics, are summarized in Table 61–7.

Patients with defects of cell-mediated immunity include those with lymphoma, organ transplant recipients, those taking daily corticosteroid therapy, and patients with AIDS. These individuals are vulnerable to infections with microorganisms that are intracellular parasites. The most common source of acute bacterial meningitis in such patients is *L. monocytogenes*. The clinical presentation includes fever, headache, seizures, focal neurologic deficits, and brainstem encephalitis.

Patients with defective humoral immunity include those with chronic lymphocytic leukemia, multiple myeloma, and Hodgkin's disease after radiotherapy or chemotherapy. These patients have difficulty controlling infection by encapsulated bacteria. They may develop a fulminant meningitis due to *S. pneumoniae*, *H. influenzae* type B, and *N. meningitidis*. After splenectomy, patients are at risk for the development of meningitis for the same reason. Neutropenic patients are at risk for meningitis due to *P. aeruginosa* and the Enterobacteriaceae.

Establishing a specific diagnosis in HIV and organ transplant patients may be difficult or impossible because of overlapping clinical and radiographic presentations, the presence of simultaneous infections with more than one organism, and CSF changes that may be nonspecific. The immune response may be altered with the absence of signs of meningeal irritation; patients may present with a diffuse encephalopathy or

TABLE 61–7 Major Neurologic Manifestations of Human Immunodeficiency Virus Infection

	CD4+ Count (cells/mm³)	Presenting Symptoms	Neurologic Signs	Diagnostic Studies	Therapy
HIV dementia	<200	Memory loss, gait disorder, behavioral change	Dementia, spasticity, psychosis	CT/MRI: brain atrophy, white matter abnormalities; CSF: increased β₂-microglobulin	High-dose zidovudine, clinical trial
Toxoplasma encephalitis	<200	Headache, fever, confusion, lethargy, seizures	Dementia, ataxia, hemiparesis	Serum *Toxoplasma* antibodies; CT/MRI: multiple enhancing lesions, edema	Pyrimethamine, sulfadiazine, clindamycin
CNS lymphoma	<100	Headache, confusion, lethargy, memory loss, seizures	Dementia, hemiparesis, aphasia	CT/MRI: enhancing lesions (especially if single); stereotactic biopsy	Radiotherapy
Progressive multifocal leukoencephalopathy	<100	Lethargy, confusion, weakness	Hemiparesis, ataxia, visual disturbance	CT/MRI: multiple hypodense, nonenhancing white matter lesions, stereotactic biopsy	High-dose zidovudine, Ara-C (IV, IT); clinical trial
CMV encephalitis	<50	Rapidly progressive confusion, apathy, weakness	Dementia, cranial neuropathies, spasticity	CT/MRI: periventricular and meningeal abnormalities; CSF: CMV culture, PCR; electrolyte abnormalities	Ganciclovir, foscarnet
Vacuolar myelopathy	<200	Gait dysfunction, lower extremity weakness and stiffness, urinary dysfunction	Spastic paraparesis, Babinski signs, sensory abnormalities	MRI/CSF: normal or nonspecific abnormalities	Baclofen, physical therapy
Cryptococcus neoformans meningitis	<200	Fever, headache, neck stiffness, memory loss	Lethargy, confusion, meningeal signs, cranial nerve palsies	CSF India ink, serum and CSF *Cryptococcus neoformans* antigen and culture	Amphotericin B (plus or minus flucytosine), fluconazole
Neurosyphilis	Any	Headache, memory loss, visual disturbances	Dementia, stroke, meningeal or myelopathic signs, cranial nerve palsies	CSF: increased leukocyte count, increased protein, serum and CSF VDRL	IV penicillin (plus probenecid)
Distal symmetrical polyneuropathy	<200	Distal numbness, paresthesias, pain	Stocking-glove sensory loss, decreased ankle reflexes	EMG: distal axonopathy	Neurotoxin withdrawal, analgesics, tricyclic antidepressants, anticonvulsants, capsaicin
Inflammatory demyelinating polyneuropathy	>500, ≥50	Progressive weakness, paresthesias	Weakness, areflexia, mild sensory loss	CSF: increased leukocyte count, elevated protein; EMG: demyelination	Early (increased CD4 count): plasmapheresis, IV Ig, steroids. Late (decreased CD4 count): Ganciclovir
Manoneuropathy multiplex	>500, ≥50	Facial weakness, footdrop, wristdrop	Multifocal cranial and peripheral neuropathies	EMG: multifocal axonal neuropathy; nerve biopsy: inflammation, vasculitis, CMV inclusions	Early: none Late: ganciclovir
Progressive polyradiculopathy	<50	Lower extremity weakness, paresthesias, urinary dysfunction	Flaccid paraparesis, saddle anesthesia, decreased reflexes, urinary retention	CSF: increased leukocytes (PMNs), CMV culture, PCR; EMG: polyradiculopathy	Ganciclovir, foscarnet
Myopathy	Any	Muscle weakness, myalgia, weight loss	Proximal muscle weakness	Increased creatine kinase; EMG: irritative myopathy; muscle biopsy: myofiber degeneration, inflammation, inclusions	Zidovudine reduction or withdrawal, corticosteroids

CMV, cytomegalovirus; CNS, central nervous system; CSF, cerebrospinal fluid; CT, computed tomography; EMG, electromyography; HIV, human immunodeficiency virus; IT, intrathecal; IV, intravenous; IV Ig, intravenous immunoglobulin; MRI, magnetic resonance imaging; PCR, polymerase chain reaction; PMNs, polymorphonuclear leukocytes; VDRL, Venereal Disease Research Laboratory.
From Simpson DM, Tagliati M: Neurologic manifestations of HIV infection. Ann Intern Med 121:770, 1994.

with focal neurologic deficits. CSF is abnormal in 60% of asymptomatic HIV-infected individuals, complicating CSF/clinical correlation.[117]

Neurosyphilis in Patients with HIV Infection

Syphilis and HIV infection are sexually transmitted diseases, and patients with syphilis are at increased risk of HIV infection. CNS invasion is probably no more common in patients with HIV than in those not infected with the virus.[119] Both diseases may cause elevation in CSF WBC counts, protein levels, and γ-globulin levels. The incidence of syphilitic meningitis, meningovascular syphilis, and ocular syphilis seems to be increasing. HIV-infected patients treated for syphilis may have viable organisms in the CSF after therapy or have persistent CSF VDRL titers. Treatment failures are more likely to occur with single-dose benzathine penicillin therapy.

Neurosyphilis may be more difficult to diagnose in HIV-infected patients. A small number of patients with secondary or ocular syphilis have negative serum reagin tests. Positive treponemal tests may revert to nonreactivity after treatment, particularly in individuals with advanced symptomatic HIV disease and a low VDRL titer at the time of diagnosis. CSF pleocytosis and increased γ-globulin levels may not help distinguish between HIV infection and CNS syphilis.

HIV-infected patients should undergo serum treponemal and nontreponemal tests early in their illness to minimize the likelihood of false-negative results.[119] Infected patients should undergo a CSF examination. Previously treated patients without a CSF examination at the time of initial syphilis treatment should have a lumbar puncture because of a probable increased risk of neurosyphilis even with a decline in serum nontreponemal titers. Asymptomatic patients with neurosyphilis should be treated to prevent CNS relapse.

Cryptococcal Meningitis

The most common CNS fungal infection is caused by *Cryptococcus neoformans*. Infection with this common fungus develops in approximately 5% of AIDS patients. Clinical presentation in AIDS and non-AIDS patients includes nonspecific symptoms of headache and altered mental status with or without meningeal signs. Most patients have increased ICP. Immunocompetent patients show a lymphocytic pleocytosis with CSF WBC counts less than 500/μL. Glucose levels are depressed, with elevation of CSF protein. India ink preparations are positive in 50% of cases. The CSF is less likely to have abnormal cell counts and chemistries in HIV infection. However, CSF cultures and cryptococcal polysaccharide capsular antigens are almost always positive. False-positive antigen tests are rare but may be seen in the presence of rheumatoid factor. Blood cultures are frequently positive in AIDS patients. Cisternal puncture for fluid analysis may be helpful in undiagnosed cases of lymphocytic meningitis in which multiple lumbar punctures have not established a diagnosis.[117]

Toxoplasmosis

Toxoplasma gondii, an intracellular protozoan, is associated with CNS infection in up to 30% of AIDS patients who have antibodies to this organism. Most adults have antibodies against this organism; infection is believed to represent reactivation of latent primary infection. *Toxoplasma* encephalitis usually develops within the first 2 years after the diagnosis of AIDS. Cerebral toxoplasmosis usually presents with the acute/subacute appearance of focal disease, including seizures.

MRI or CT scanning often reveals multiple abscesses that may represent multiple pathogens. The distinction between toxoplasmosis and lymphoma may be difficult to make clinically. Less commonly, the presentation is chronic meningitis with confusion, memory loss, and lethargy similar to the AIDS-dementia complex. CSF in these patients is nonspecific with increased protein, mononuclear pleocytosis (<100 cells/μL), and rarely, reduced glucose concentration. Serum and CSF serologies may be either positive or negative and do not help make a diagnosis, although most patients with encephalitis have detectable IgG antibodies. Diagnosis is usually based on clinical and imaging responses to antibiotics (pyrimethamine or sulfadiazine) or brain biopsy. Treatment failures with relapse occur in 50% of AIDS patients and 15% to 25% of non-AIDS patients, necessitating life-long treatment.

Mycobacterial Tuberculosis

CNS mycobacteria infection is almost always the result of infection with *Mycobacterium tuberculosis*. Infection occurs in the setting of disseminated tuberculosis. Atypical *Mycobacterium* infection occurring in HIV-infected individuals uncommonly affects the CNS. Clinical presentation is meningitis (particularly involving the basal cistern), encephalitis, or abscess formation. If tuberculosis is suspected, a large volume of CSF (10 mL) is required for adequate culture. The cell count varies from 100 to 400 cells/μL, with a lymphocytic predominance; 30% may show predominantly neutrophils early in the course of infection. Protein levels are elevated (100–500 mg/dL); the CSF glucose level may be depressed. Acid-fast stains should be examined by experienced technicians. Fluid is inoculated onto Löwenstein-Jensen medium, and the absence of visible growth on the medium should not be considered negative for 8 weeks. CSF cultures are more sensitive than stains.

Primary CNS Lymphoma

The risk of developing CNS lymphoma in an AIDS patient is 2%. Presentation is diffuse encephalopathy, although occasionally focal neurologic deficits occur. Leptomeningeal spread of malignancy is reflected in a modest lymphocytic pleocytosis with slightly elevated protein and decreased glucose levels. Cytologic yield is improved by repeat lumbar punctures and submitting large quantities of CSF or sampling fluid obtained by cisternal puncture.[117]

Progressive Multifocal Leukoencephalopathy

Progressive multifocal leukoencephalopathy is an uncommon disorder in individuals with impaired cell-mediated immunity and is caused by reactivation of the JC papovavirus in the kidney. Progressive demyelination presents as combinations of dementia, blindness, aphasia, hemiparesis, and seizures that progress until death. MRI and CT demonstrate nonenhancing white matter lesions without mass effect. Definitive diagnosis is made by brain biopsy, but CSF may show the presence of myelin basic protein, increased IgG, with acellular or a mild CSF pleocytosis (<50 WBCs/μL). Average survival is 4 months.[118]

Cytomegalovirus Infection

Cytomegalovirus may be detected in 30% of brains of HIV-infected persons at autopsy. A distinct CNS disorder has not been defined. CSF pleocytosis may be minimal. Retinitis and painful polyradiculopathies are recognized, with a prominent CSF pleocytosis in the latter condition.[117]

CONCLUSION

A spinal tap should be performed only when the treating clinician believes the CSF specimen(s) will be of diagnostic or therapeutic value, as in the case of patients with symptomatic pseudotumor cerebri. The procedure is often indicated in the diagnosis of meningitis or SAH. Complications are uncommon, and risks are usually outweighed by the benefit of the procedure. Most contraindications are relative and not absolute, particularly if CNS infection is an overriding consideration.

Acknowledgments

The editors and author acknowledge the contributions of Jon Kooiker to this chapter in previous editions. The author would like to thank Linda J. Kesselring, MS, ELS, for copyediting the manuscript and incorporating his revisions into the final document.

 REFERENCES CAN BE FOUND ON EXPERT CONSULT

CHAPTER 62

Special Neurologic Tests and Procedures

J. Stephen Huff

Neuro-otologic tests and procedures are used in a variety of clinical scenarios ranging from evaluation of the dizzy patient to diagnosing brain death. Some of these procedures have been replaced by neuroimaging, electrophysiologic, or other tests, but in selected patients, there is still utility in bedside testing.[1] In this chapter, caloric testing for oculovestibular responses, the Dix-Hallpike maneuver for diagnosing benign paroxysmal positional vertigo (BPPV), and techniques of canalith repositioning are summarized. A discussion of brain death directed at the emergency clinician follows, and a brief synopsis of emergency department (ED) testing for myasthenia gravis completes the section.

CALORIC TESTING

An accurate assessment of the comatose patient requires a thorough neurologic examination including careful evaluation of the patient's responses to a variety of external stimuli. In a comatose individual with normal brainstem and cranial nerve function, stimulation of the vestibular labyrinth results in well-described and reproducible extraocular movements. This response is known as the *vestibulo-ocular reflex* and forms the physiologic basis for caloric testing. Caloric testing (*calor* from Latin, meaning *heat*) involves delivering a thermal stimulus to the external auditory canal to activate the labyrinth. Pathologic conditions involving either the vestibular or the oculomotor reflex pathways will alter or abolish the usual response to caloric stimulation.

Caloric tests may be performed in either conscious or unconscious patients, depending on the diagnostic circumstances. Quantitative caloric examination is conducted in the awake ambulatory patient for evaluation of possible vestibular dysfunction. This type of testing requires precisely controlled irrigation temperatures and specialized recording devices and is best undertaken in a properly equipped laboratory under the supervision of an experienced neuro-otologist. However, the neurologist, neurosurgeon, or emergency clinician may perform *qualitative* caloric testing in the comatose patient to detect gross disruption of vestibulo-ocular reflex pathways that may indicate structural lesions or metabolic abnormalities affecting the labyrinth, vestibulocochlear nerve, or brainstem. In this clinical setting, ice water is used to provide stimulation of the vestibular system. Such testing needs no special expertise and can be done at the bedside using equipment readily available in the ED. This simple procedure can provide valuable diagnostic and prognostic information necessary for management of the comatose patient.

Background

Brown-Séquard[2] first described the effects of introducing cold water into the ear canal in the mid-19th century. The clinical importance of the phenomenon was first realized in 1906 by Bárány,[3] who developed a caloric procedure using an ice water stimulus. He postulated, correctly, that caloric stimulation of the auditory canal induced the formation of convection currents within the semicircular canals of the vestibular labyrinth.

Standardization of the procedure awaited the introduction of the Fitzgerald-Hallpike technique in 1942.[4] This technique used both warm and cool water stimuli under rigidly specified conditions, permitting quantification of normal and abnormal caloric responses. Today, most formal caloric testing of conscious patients is based on variations of the original Fitzgerald-Hallpike procedure.[4]

The value of caloric testing in the assessment of the comatose patient was emphasized by the work of Klingon[5] and Bender and associates.[6] More recent advances include the development of electronystagmography (ENG), which provides a graphic record of reflex eye movements and permits precise determination of the intensity of the caloric response.[7]

Physiology and Functional Anatomy

Proper performance and interpretation of the caloric test require a basic understanding of the structure and function of both the vestibular and the oculomotor systems. The anatomic pathways underlying the vestibulo-ocular reflex begin in the posterior portion of the labyrinth of the inner ear. The peripheral vestibular apparatus is located within the temporal bone and consists of the utricle, the saccule, and the lateral, anterior, and posterior semicircular canals. Because of its proximity to the external ear canal, the lateral or horizontal canal is of principal interest in caloric testing. The lateral canal is oriented at a 30° angle to the horizontal plane. Deflections of the cupola due to movement of end lymphatic fluid within the canal result in polarization changes in the underlying hair cells, which in turn are relayed to the afferent limb of the primary vestibular neuron.

Impulses of the primary neuron travel via Scarpa's ganglion and cranial nerve (CN) VIII to the brainstem to synapse with secondary vestibular neurons in the superior and medial vestibular nuclei of the upper medulla and lower pons (Fig. 62–1). Although the connections between the vestibular and the oculomotor nuclei in the brainstem are quite complex, two main pathways exist. The direct projection runs from the vestibular complex to the nuclei of CNs III and VI via the medial longitudinal fasciculus (MLF) and involves only three neurons: (1) primary vestibular, (2) secondary vestibular, and (3) oculomotor.[8] The indirect projection between these nuclei occurs over multisynaptic circuits in the tegmental reticular formation.[9] Another brainstem structure that contributes to the vestibulo-ocular interaction is the parapontine reticular formation (PPRF), a poorly characterized group of pontine neurons that coordinates both voluntary and involuntary lateral gaze. The PPRF receives multiple inputs, including projections from the vestibular system and the contralateral frontal cortex, and sends output to oculomotor neurons through both the direct and the indirect pathways. Excitatory impulses originating in the lateral canal finally travel via the oculomotor and abducens nerves to the ipsilateral medial rectus and contralateral lateral rectus muscles.[10]

Rotation of the head generates flow of endolymphatic fluid within the semicircular canals. The firing rate of the primary vestibular neuron is dependent on the direction of flow. For example, in the lateral canal, flow toward the ampulla

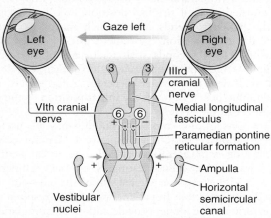

Figure 62–1 Vestibulo-ocular reflex and its contribution to horizontal eye movements. The semicircular canals respond to rotational acceleration of the head by driving the vestibulo-ocular reflex to maintain the eyes in the same direction in space during head movement. Fibers from the horizontal semicircular canal travel first to the vestibular nuclei and then to each paramedian pontine reticular formation. Excitatory projections that travel to the contralateral sixth cranial nerve nucleus and, via the medial longitudinal fasciculus, to the ipsilateral medial rectus subnucleus cause gaze to the left. In a similar manner, inhibitory projections are sent to the antagonist ipsilateral lateral rectus and contralateral medial rectus. *(Modified from Lavin PJ, Donahue SP: Disorders of supranuclear control of ocular motility. In Yanoff M, Duker JS (eds): Ophthalmology, 3rd ed. St. Louis, Mosby, 2008.)*

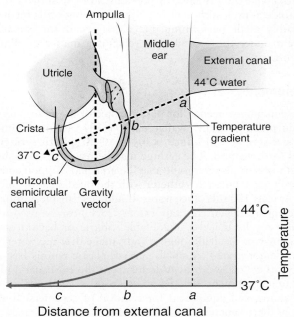

Figure 62–2 Convective flow mechanism of the caloric response. Irrigation with warm or cold water (or air) results in a temperature gradient across the horizontal semicircular canal. With the horizontal canal oriented in the earth-vertical plane, gravity induces the convective flow of endolymph from the cooler area of the canal in which endolymph is more dense into the warmer area of the canal in which endolymph is less dense. For the warm caloric irrigation shown in this diagram, an ampullopetal deflection of the cupula results from this flow of endolymph. Vestibular-nerve afferents innervating the horizontal semicircular are excited, and a horizontal nystagmus with slow-phase components directed toward the opposite ear is produced. A cold caloric stimulus results in an oppositely directed response with ampullofugal deflection to the cupula, inhibition of horizontal canal afferents, and a nystagmus with slow-phase components directed toward the ear to which the cold caloric is applied. *(Modified from Baloh RW, Honorubia V [eds]: Clinical Neurophysiology of the Vestibular System, 3rd ed. Philadelphia, FA Davis, 2001.)*

(ampullopetal) increases the firing rate, whereas flow away from the ampulla (ampullofugal) decreases the firing rate. Increased firing on one side results in conjugate deviation of the eyes toward the opposite side, whereas decreased firing causes deviation to the same side. This principle forms the physiologic basis of caloric testing. When the lateral canal is placed in the vertical position (patient placed supine) and ice water is infused into the ear, the endolymph nearest the canal cools and sinks, resulting in ampullofugal flow (Fig. 62–2). As the firing rate decreases, the eyes deviate conjugately toward the side of irrigation. When warm water is used in the same position or when the canal is inverted 180°, the opposite occurs.

Eye movements induced by caloric stimulation in conscious, neurologically normal individuals are more complex. Ice water infusions induce a rhythmic jerking of the eyes that includes a slow deviation toward the irrigated side followed by a quick compensatory saccade toward the midline. This is known as *caloric nystagmus.* By convention, *caloric nystagmus is named for the fast component,* thus the popular mnemonic "fast COWS" (Cold irrigation—Opposite beating nystagmus; Warm irrigation—Same-sided beating nystagmus). Most sources attribute the slow phase of nystagmus to vestibular activity transmitted over the direct pathway, whereas the fast phase is believed to be generated by the PPRF in conjunction with cortical activity and carried over indirect pathways within the reticular formation. Numerous factors, including physiologic, pharmacologic, and pathologic factors, can alter caloric-induced eye movements.

Indications and Contraindications

Caloric testing of the comatose patient is indicated when the clinician needs information regarding the functional integrity of the brainstem. When the cause of the coma is initially unknown, qualitative caloric testing at the bedside may assist in differentiation among structural, metabolic, or psychogenic causes of unresponsiveness. Even when the cause of coma is clear, caloric testing may provide an indication of the depth of coma and possibly the prognosis for eventual recovery.

In conscious patients who complain of vertigo, quantitative caloric testing may rarely be indicated for the nonemergency evaluation of possible vestibular disorders. These patients are best referred to a qualified neuro-otologist or audiologist, who may conduct more accurate testing in the audiology laboratory.

Few contraindications exist to caloric testing in the unresponsive patient. An absolute contraindication is the presence of a basilar skull fracture, either documented radiologically or suspected by clinical signs, because of the risk of introducing infection into the central nervous system (CNS) through an associated dural tear. If a basilar skull fracture is discovered to be unilateral, testing of the intact ear with warm then cold water will yield results similar to those of the standard bilateral examination with cold water stimulation.

Relative contraindications to caloric testing using water include perforations of the tympanic membrane (including those not due to temporal fractures), otitis media and externa, and the presence of previous otologic surgery (e.g., mastoidectomy). Although the risk of causing otitis media is probably small, performing the caloric test in the comatose patient under these conditions remains a matter of clinical judgment.

Equipment

The equipment needed for performance of the caloric test is minimal and is readily available in the ED. Although almost any size syringe will suffice, a 30- or 50-mL plastic syringe is ideal for irrigation. The syringe may be used as is or a short length of soft plastic tubing may be attached. A good source of tubing is a butterfly catheter with the needle cut or pulled off. At least 100 mL of ice water should be available, although larger quantities of cool tap water (<25°C) can be used with similar results if ice is unavailable. Sterile or bacteriostatic saline may be used, although no advantage over tap water has been demonstrated. A small, curved, plastic emesis basin is useful to collect water as it drains from the ear canal. Other required equipment includes an otoscope, several sizes of ear speculums, and equipment for removal of cerumen. Towels and a thermometer that reads from 0° to 50°C may be helpful.

Procedure

Defer vestibulo-ocular reflex testing until the patient's condition has been stabilized, with attention to the airway and the evaluation of the cervical spine in trauma patients. Perform a thorough neurologic assessment before caloric testing, with special attention given to the ocular examination. Observe pupillary responses, spontaneous ocular movements, and resting eye position. Inspect the ears before inserting the otoscope. If active bleeding or cerebrospinal fluid otorrhea or rhinorrhea is noted in the trauma victim, defer caloric testing and evaluate the patient for a probable basilar skull fracture. If the external ear canal appears normal, complete the otoscopic examination. Signs of active ear infection or perforation of the tympanic membrane are contraindications to caloric testing. Tympanic rupture, hemotympanum and stepoff deformities of the canal may indicate fracture of the temporal bone; caloric testing is contraindicated in this situation. Remove excess cerumen and foreign material. The tympanic membrane should be clearly visualized. The ear speculum may be left in the canal as a guide for irrigation.

Perform the test with the patient in the supine position, with the head and upper body raised to 30° if possible (two pillows will provide the appropriate angle). This amount of elevation places the lateral canal in the vertical plane and ensures a maximal response. Drape the patient with a towel and position a small emesis basin below the ear to collect the water outflow. Fill a container with ice water and place it near the bedside.

Fill a syringe and catheter system (*minus the needle*) with 10 mL of ice water, and direct the irrigation stream at the tympanic membrane. Because the goal of qualitative caloric test is to induce a maximum response, the amount and rate of infusion are not critical. As a general guide, infuse 5 to 10 mL of ice water initially and infuse over a period of 5 to 10 seconds. Amounts less than 5 mL may be advisable in suspected cases of light coma or psychogenic unresponsiveness. If no response is noted within a moment, infuse at least

100 mL before declaring that there is no response. Begin testing the contralateral ear 5 or 10 minutes after the eyes have returned to their original position. Ask an assistant to hold the patient's eyelids open, which makes it easier to observe for eye deviation. Movement usually occurs after a latency of 10 to 40 seconds, with persistence of the response for as long as 4 to 5 minutes. Focusing on a small scleral vessel makes small deviations easier to detect. Alternatively, use a dermographic pencil to mark the initial position of the pupil with respect to the eyelid.

Variations of the caloric technique may be useful in certain situations. If there is no response to bilateral ice water caloric testing or in cases in which only one ear can be tested, perform warm water caloric testing. Keep water temperature below 50°C. The response elicited will be the opposite of that obtained with ice water. In patients who fail to respond to ice water caloric testing alone, provide additional stimulation by combining irrigation with repeated head turning away from the irrigated side (*doll's-eye maneuver*). In trauma patients, *exclude cervical injury before using this technique*. This combination of techniques may produce eye movements in patients who do not respond to caloric testing alone.[11] Eviatar and Goodhill[12] described a technique for caloric testing in tympanic perforations using a small latex finger cot placed in the ear canal to prevent water from entering the middle ear.

Complications

The few complications that are possible with caloric testing can be avoided by carefully selecting both the patients to be tested and the equipment and technique to be used. Using needles or other sharp objects to irrigate the ear may result in laceration or perforation of the tympanic membrane or canal wall if the patient moves unexpectedly. The use of plastic syringes and soft catheter tubing aids in reducing such occurrences.

Other potential complications of caloric testing include otitis media, meningitis, and the induction of vomiting and subsequent aspiration. Although meningitis may follow basilar skull fractures with meningeal tears, the additional risk of calorics in such situations is not known. Therefore, caloric testing should be omitted in the head-injured patient if there is any suspicion of temporal bone fracture. Although ice water irrigation might produce nausea and even emesis in awake patients, vomiting with aspiration has not been reported as a complication of caloric testing in the comatose patient. Nevertheless, some operators may prefer to delay testing until the patient's airway is protected.

Interpretation

First Phase of Interpretation. Analyze initial eye position and spontaneous movements before irrigation. A description of eye movement abnormalities of the comatose patient is beyond the scope of this chapter and is only briefly summarized here. The eyes of comatose patients with intact oculomotor pathways are usually directed straight ahead or are slightly divergent. Unilateral destructive lesions of the cerebral hemisphere can cause conjugate deviation of the eyes toward the side of the lesion, whereas irritative foci, as might be seen in status epilepticus, can cause conjugate deviation away from the affected side. Deviations of this type can usually be overcome by caloric stimulation, although combined irrigation with head turning may be required in the first hours after the insult. Lesions in or near the PPRF in the brainstem cause conjugate deviation away from the side of the lesion. This finding usually cannot be overcome by calorics. Conjugate downward deviation can be seen with structural lesions of the brainstem or in the deeper phases of metabolic coma. Dysconjugate gaze might indicate damage at the level of the oculomotor nuclei or below or might reflect disruption of the ocular muscles themselves.[13] Dysconjugate gaze may also be seen in drug-induced coma in the presence of a structurally intact brainstem pathway. In the very late stages of brainstem dysfunction, the eyes usually return to the central position. Spontaneous roving movements of the eyes, either conjugate or dysconjugate, may be seen in supratentorial insults, but these, too, disappear with brainstem involvement.[11] Ocular "bobbing" is an intermittent, spontaneous downward jerking of the eyes that may occur with massive pontine lesions. Ocular "dipping" is a more prolonged, downward conjugate deviation of the eyes and has been reported in cases of severe anoxic encephalopathy (e.g., carbon monoxide poisoning).[14] The pathophysiologic basis of these eye movements is poorly understood.[15]

Second Phase of Interpretation. After irrigation, the ocular movements should be observed for any response to the stimulus. Again, typically there is a latency of response of 10 to 40 seconds. Reactions to ice water irrigation may be divided into four categories: (1) caloric nystagmus, (2) conjugate deviation, (3) dysconjugate deviation, and (4) absent responses (Fig. 62–3). The first reaction, caloric nystagmus with the fast component beating away from the side of ice water irrigation, is seen in normal, alert individuals; in cases of psychogenic unresponsiveness; and in those who have very mild organic disturbances of consciousness. The intensity of nystagmus is highly variable in conscious subjects and depends on the degree of visual fixation and the level of mental alertness. The response is present in more than 90% of children by age 6 months and declines in magnitude only after the 7th decade of life.[16]

Caloric-induced nystagmus after cold water irritation in the apparently comatose individual usually results from testing individuals with psychogenic unresponsiveness due to catatonia, conversion reactions, schizophrenia, or feigned coma. Hyperactive caloric responses may result from testing in the presence of tympanic perforation or mastoid disease. Hypoactive caloric responses are recorded in a wide variety of vestibular and neurologic disorders.

Hypoactive or abnormal caloric responses may be further evaluated with quantitative caloric testing, ENG, or other techniques such as auditory evoked responses. Caloric-induced nystagmus may be *inverted* (beating to the wrong side) or *perverted* (beating in the wrong plane); both responses may be seen in brainstem lesions. *Pseudocaloric nystagmus* is a preexisting latent nystagmus that is brought out by the general arousal of ice water irrigation; it can be distinguished from true nystagmus by its failure to reverse direction with warm water irrigation.

As the level of coma deepens, the fast phase of nystagmus becomes intermittent and then disappears, probably as a result of decreased activity in the cerebral cortex.

In the second type of response to cold caloric stimulation, the eyes deviate conjugately toward the side of ice water stimulation (they "look" toward the source of irritation). When present, this reaction indicates intact brainstem function as well as intact afferent and efferent limbs of the reflex. This is seen during general anesthesia, in supratentorial

lesions *without brainstem compression*, and in many metabolic and drug-induced comas. In such situations, bilateral simultaneous irrigation with ice water might result in conjugate downward deviation, implying that brainstem centers for vertical gaze are functional.

Dysconjugate reactions constitute the third type of caloric response to ice water stimuli. The most common dysconjugate reaction is internuclear ophthalmoplegia, in which a lesion of the MLF causes weakness or paralysis of the *adducting* eye after caloric irrigation. Internuclear ophthalmoplegia might be due to acute damage to the rostral pons or might be seen as a manifestation of multiple sclerosis or stroke.

In acute supratentorial lesions, the development of dysconjugate caloric responses is a significant sign that may indicate compression of the brainstem and impending herniation. Caloric responses of this type are less common with metabolic and drug-induced coma; when present in metabolic coma, their significance is less ominous. Reversible internuclear ophthalmoplegia has been reported in hepatic coma and may occur during toxic response to phenytoin, barbiturate, or amitriptyline. Forced downward deviation of the eyes, either conjugate or dysconjugate, may be seen in sedative-hypnotic drug–induced coma when unilateral caloric testing is performed.[17]

Palsies of the oculomotor nerves are another cause of dysconjugate reactions, although most should be apparent before irrigation. Causes include diabetic neuropathy, increased intracranial pressure, and Wernicke's encephalopathy. Finally, Plum and Posner[13] reported that unusual and poorly characterized caloric responses may be obtained from the testing of comatose patients with longstanding severe brain injury.

Absent caloric response is the fourth category of reactions to ice water stimuli. As a general rule, the oculovestibular response is preserved more than other brainstem reflexes; however, the oculocephalic or doll's eye response may persist in the absence of caloric responses owing to bilateral labyrinthine disease because of additional input from proprioceptive receptors in the neck. Loss of caloric responses in comatose patients with structural lesions is usually a sign of brainstem damage. In supratentorial lesions, progressive loss of caloric responses may be seen in the final stages of transtentorial herniation. The oculovestibular reflex may also be transiently absent or decreased on the side opposite massive supratentorial damage during the first hours after injury.[18] Absent caloric responses may occur in any subtentorial lesion that affects vestibular reflex pathways, including pontine hemorrhage, basilar artery occlusion, cerebellar hemorrhage, or infarction with encroachment on the brainstem, and in any expanding mass lesion within the posterior fossa. Calorics may disappear in deep coma resulting from subarachnoid hemorrhage, perhaps owing to pressure on the brainstem.

The vestibulo-ocular reflex is usually retained until the late stages of metabolic coma. Nevertheless, caloric responses may be transiently absent in certain types of drug-induced coma, with the *eventual complete recovery of the patient*. The vestibulo-ocular reflex seems particularly sensitive to the effects of sedative-hypnotic drugs (e.g., barbiturates, glutethimide), antidepressants (e.g., amitriptyline, doxepin), and anticonvulsants (e.g., phenytoin, carbamazepine).[19,20] As one would expect, neuromuscular blocking agents (e.g., succinylcholine) will abolish caloric-induced ocular movements.

Finally, the caloric response may be absent for reasons other than the neurologic causes responsible for the coma.

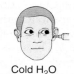

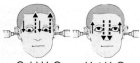
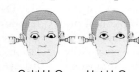

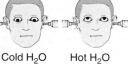

1. Normal nystagmus
----► Fast component
  → Slow component

Cold H₂O Cold H₂O   Cold H₂O Hot H₂O

2. Conjugate deviation

Cold H₂O Cold H₂O   Cold H₂O Hot H₂O

3. Dysconjugate deviation (with MLF lesion)

Cold H₂O Cold H₂O   Cold H₂O Hot H₂O

4. Absent responses

Cold H₂O Cold H₂O   Cold H₂O Hot H₂O

A

Figure 62–3 *A,* The four types of caloric responses seen with unilateral and bilateral irrigations: *1,* Normal nystagmus; *2,* Conjugate deviation; *3,* Dysconjugate deviation. The most common type, internuclear ophthalmoplegia, is shown here. Vertical eye movements usually remain intact in this lesion; *4,* Absent caloric responses. MLF, medial longitudinal fasciculus. *B,* Oculocephalic and oculovestibular testing in selected clinical conditions. (A, *Modified from Plum F, Posner JB [eds]: The Diagnosis of Stupor and Coma, 3rd ed. Philadelphia, FA Davis, 1980, p 55; B, from Smith M, Bleck T: Techniques for evaluating the cause of coma. J Crit Illn 2:51, 1987.)*

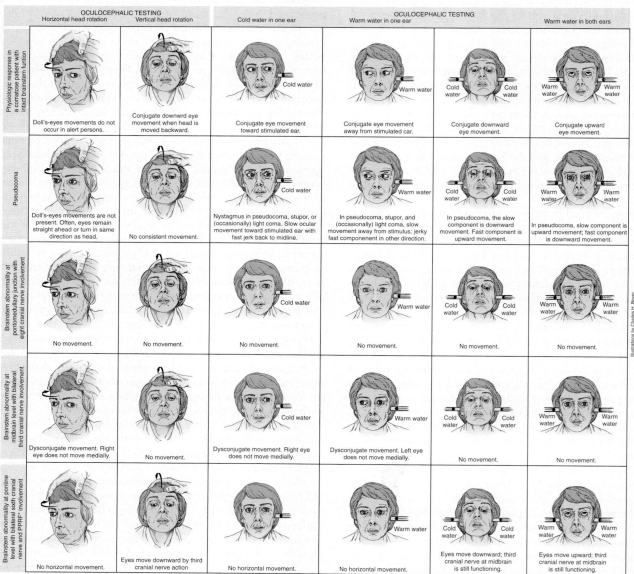

B

TABLE 62–1 Possible Causes of Absent Vestibulo-ocular Reflex in Conscious Patients

Inadequate irrigation	Traumatic
Cerumen impaction	Previous temporal fracture
Postinfection	Previous head injury
Meningitis	Postlabyrinthectomy
Encephalitis	Labyrinthine
Syphilis	Vestibular neuronitis
Neoplastic	Suppurative labyrinthitis
Acoustic neuroma	Congenital
Other cerebellopontine angle	Congenital hydrocephalus
tumors	Hereditary spinocerebellar
Posterior fossa tumors	degeneration
Inflammatory	Idiopathic
Systemic lupus	Drugs
erythematosus	Aminoglycoside antibiotics
Cogan syndrome	Neuromuscular blocking
	agents
	Anticonvulsants*

*Reported rarely in conscious patients who have taken more than the normal therapeutic dosage.

Inadequate irrigation owing to excess cerumen or poor technique and unilateral or bilateral dysfunction of the peripheral vestibular apparatus must be considered. Bilateral loss of caloric response (areflexia vestibularis) is uncommon in conscious patients, constituting 1.7% and 0.2%, respectively, of the ENG clinical population in two large series of patients.[21,22] Some of the causes of unilateral and bilateral loss of oculovestibular reflexes in conscious patients are listed in Table 62–1.

The vestibulo-ocular reflex has prognostic as well as diagnostic significance in the comatose patient. In a study of 100 patients who were comatose from head trauma, absence of calorics at 1 to 3 days after injury was associated with extremely high mortality.[23] Testing in the immediate post-traumatic period may yield inconsistent responses and is of considerably less prognostic value. Levy and coworkers[24] studied 500 cases of nontraumatic, non–drug-induced coma in a large multicenter effort. Absence of the vestibulo-ocular reflex correlated with less than a 5% chance of achieving functional recovery within 1 year when tested within 6 to 24 hours of coma onset. In one study of comatose patients, the combination of absent vestibulo-ocular reflex and absent pupillary light reflex at 24 hours was associated with 100% mortality.[25] Complete loss of caloric responses is part of the criteria for the diagnosis of brain death and correlates with the irreversible cessation of cerebral function at least as well as an isoelectric electroencephalogram (EEG).[26] Excessive reliance on a single clinical sign must be avoided in the consideration of brain death, and decisions regarding neurologic prognosis and future therapy should be based on complete consideration of all evidence available. The topic of clinical diagnosis of brain death is discussed in detail subsequently.

Summary

Caloric testing is a simple, easily performed bedside procedure that may enhance the neurologic assessment of the comatose patient. When reliably interpreted, caloric testing may furnish valuable diagnostic and prognostic information. Even if the cause of the coma is known, the test may provide a baseline for the evaluation of changes in the patient's status.

In the emergency patient, this test should be reserved for the stable patient undergoing secondary assessment. The examination requires minimal equipment and can be conducted in a few minutes while awaiting laboratory results or during preparation for computed tomographic scanning. Complications are few if patients are properly selected and correct technique is used.

DIX-HALLPIKE TEST IN DIAGNOSIS OF POSITIONAL VERTIGO

Vertigo occurring only and repeatedly with position change is probably BPPV; the head-hanging positioning maneuver (Dix-Hallpike test, sometimes referred to as the Nylen-Bárány maneuver) is useful in confirming the clinical suspicion of BPPV because the provoked abnormal nystagmus is characteristic of the disorder.[27,28] Evolving pathophysiologic theory is that calcium crystal material displaced from the vestibule floats within the endolymph of the posterior semicircular canal and head movement induces bidirectional forces in the fluid acting on the cupula, triggering the BPPV attack.[29–32] The posterior semicircular canal is most commonly affected,[24,31] but at times, the horizontal canal is thought to be involved, leading to variants of typical BPPV.[33–35]

Background

BPPV is a common mechanical disorder of the inner ear in which vertigo is precipitated by certain head movements; nystagmus and autonomic symptoms such as nausea commonly accompany the vertigo. Syndromes of positional vertigo and provocative maneuvers have been described by clinicians for more than 100 years; the description of BPPV has been attributed to Adler, Bárány, Nylèn, Bruns, Borries, Dix, and Hallpike.[36] Current consensus is that Dix and Hallpike most fully defined the disorder and that the provocative technique they described is superior and most accurately should bear the eponymic *Dix-Hallpike positioning test* or the *Dix-Hallpike test*.[28,36]

Indications and Contraindications

The Dix-Hallpike test may be a useful diagnostic test in confirming BPPV by provoking a specific type of nystagmus and in selecting patients suitable for positional therapy (discussed later). The maneuver should not be performed in patients with severe cervical spine disease, unstable spinal injury, high-grade carotid stenosis, or unstable heart disease.[28] Patient discomfort or physical infirmity are relative contraindications; some elderly patients or patients with ongoing nausea or vertigo may not tolerate the body position changes necessary for performance of the procedure. If nystagmus is present at rest without any provocation or if associated neurologic signs or symptoms exist, the diagnosis of BPPV is likely excluded and the maneuver is not clinically indicated.

Procedure

Perform the Dix-Hallpike maneuver as illustrated in Figure 62–4. In summary, place the patient initially in the seated position on the stretcher with the head turned 45° to one side. Quickly lay the patient down flat with the head hanging over the edge of the bed and observe the eyes for induced

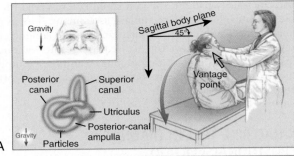

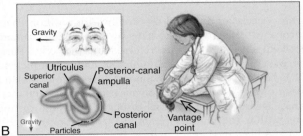

Figure 62–4 The Dix-Hallpike test of a patient with benign paroxysmal positional vertigo (BPPV) affecting the right ear. *A,* The examiner stands at the patient's head 45° to the right to align the right posterior semicircular canal with the sagittal plane of the body. *B,* The examiner moves the patient, whose eyes are open, from the seated to the supine right ear–down position and then extends the patient's neck slightly so that the chin is pointed slightly upward. The latency, duration, and direction of the nystagmus, if present, and the latency and duration of vertigo, if present, should be noted. Inset, The *arrows* over the eyes depict the direction of nystagmus in patients with typical BPPV. The presumed location in the labyrinth of the free-floating debris thought to cause the disorder is also shown. (*A and* B, *From Furman C: Benign paroxysmal positional vertigo. New Engl J Med 341:1590, 1999.)*

nystagmus.[28] Repeat the entire maneuver with the head turned 45° toward the opposite side.[28]

Interpretation

The Dix-Hallpike head-hanging positioning maneuver produces vertigo only in patients with positional vertigo that is most commonly characterized as BPPV. The stereotypic positive response in BPPV is provoked vertigo developing after a brief delay (1–10 sec), lasting less than a minute, and with direction-fixed rotary or vertical nystagmus. Nausea or other systemic symptoms are often present.[27,28] The eye movements are mixed torsional and vertical nystagmus of both eyes with the upper pole of the eye beating toward the dependent ear and the vertical nystagmus beating toward the forehead. The side of the ear in the downward position during the Dix-Hallpike test that elicits the greater nystagmus likely identifies the affected ear. After the patient is returned to the sitting position, the nystagmus may again be transiently observed in a reversed direction. If the positional nystagmus is atypical or if the maneuver fails to elicit nystagmus in a patient with ongoing symptoms of vertigo, another diagnostic possibility should be considered.[28,37]

Complications

The maneuver may precipitate brief vertigo and nausea in patients with BPPV.

Summary

The Dix-Hallpike test may be useful in confirming the diagnosis of BPPV in patients when there is doubt in localizing the abnormality to one ear. Accurate identification of BPPV is of interest because of the possibility of interventional therapies, as described subsequently.

CANALITH-REPOSITIONING MANEUVERS

If the clinical evaluation of the patient with vertigo is consistent with the diagnosis of BPPV and the Dix-Hallpike test is supportive of the diagnosis and lateralizes to one ear, the patient may be a candidate for attempted canalith-repositioning maneuvers. These techniques have largely been described in the otologic and neurologic literature and have been only little studied in the emergency patient population. Success rates of 44% to 100% are reported.[28] One small ED-based study concluded that the Epley maneuver was more efficacious than a placebo maneuver.[38]

Background

With theory suggesting that stray material in the posterior semicircular canal is causative of the symptoms of BPPV, maneuvers were designed using sequential head movements to reposition the debris to the vestibule.[28,32,39,40] The manipulation of head position theoretically allows the debris ("canaliths") to sequentially fall from the problematic location in the semicircular canal to the vestibule of the labyrinth where they presumably adhere. The currently recommended maneuver was introduced by Epley.[32] Other maneuvers are described but require repeated trials or are more difficult to perform and perhaps more uncomfortable for the patient.[28,39–41] The Semont maneuver is also described because it may be performed at the bedside. In theory, the Semont maneuver would be effective primarily in patients in whom the displaced canaliths were adhering to the cupola of the posterior semicircular canal (Schuknecht cupolith theory), although it might be effective as well when the debris are free floating in the long arm of the semicircular canal; the Epley maneuver would be effective only in patients with debris floating in the long arm of the posterior semicircular canal (canalith theory).[42] In one small trial comparing the efficacy of either the Semont or the Epley maneuver in a carefully selected outpatient otolaryngology population, the maneuvers were found to be of roughly the same effectiveness (90%) in relieving or improving symptoms of BPPV.[42]

Indications and Contraindications

The indication for any canal-clearing or "liberatory" procedure is the clinical diagnosis of BPPV as confirmed by history and physical examination including the Dix-Hallpike maneuver. Careful patient selection is likely a key point in success of any of these maneuvers as well as correct identification of the impaired ear, which will govern the initial position and movement of the patient. Contraindications are the same as for the Dix-Hallpike maneuver, as noted earlier.

Procedure

The Epley procedure is illustrated in Figure 62–5. Briefly, as in the Dix-Hallpike maneuver, place the patient initially in

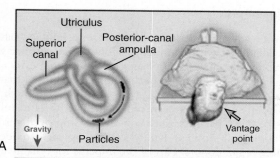

A

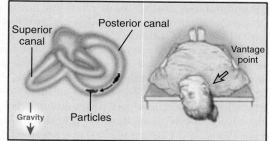

B

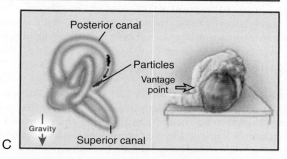

C

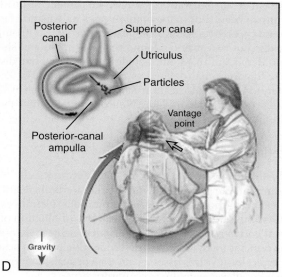

D

Figure 62–5 Bedside maneuver for the treatment of a patient with BPPV affecting the right ear. The presumed position of the debris within the labyrinth during the maneuver is shown in each panel. The maneuver is a three-step procedure. *A,* First, a Dix-Hallpike test is performed with the patient's head rotated 45° toward the right ear and the neck slightly extended with the chin pointed slightly upward. This position results in the patient's head hanging to the right. *B,* Once the vertigo and nystagmus provoked by the Dix-Hallpike test cease, the patient's head is rotated about the rostral-caudal body axis until the left ear is down. *C,* Then the head and body are further rotated until the head is face down. The vertex of the head is kept tilted downward throughout rotation. The maneuver usually provokes brief vertigo. The patient should be kept in the final, face-down position for about 10 to 15 sec. *D,* With the head kept turned toward the left shoulder, the patient is brought into the seated position. Once the patient is upright, the head is tilted so that the chin is pointed slightly downward. (*A–D, From Furman C: Benign paroxysmal positional vertigo. New Engl J Med 341:1590, 1999.*)

symptoms of nystagmus or vertigo to resolve.[28] Others suggest a period of 4 minutes after the head is placed in the hanging position and again after rotation of the head ("modified Epley maneuver").[42] The maneuver may be repeated a few times until some improvement in symptoms occurs, although this is not typically described in the literature.[42] After a successful procedure, advise the patient to remain in a head-upright position for 24 hours.

The Semont maneuver involves larger and more abrupt body movements. Identify the affected ear by the Dix-Hallpike maneuver. With the patient seated on the side of an examination table or bed, turn the patient's head toward the unaffected side. Quickly lay the patient down into a side-lying position (Fig. 62–6) and keep there until symptoms subside. Move the patient abruptly through the sitting position to the opposite side-lying position and keep there until symptoms subside. Return the patient to the upright position.[41,42] As in the Dix-Hallpike maneuver, advise the patient to remain in a head-upright position for 24 hours after a successful procedure.

Complications

Exacerbation of vertigo occurs occasionally and is thought to result from displacement or the dislodgment of the canal debris. Repeating the procedure is recommended for relief. Similar symptoms may occur in up to 50% of patients with up to 20% in the first 2 weeks.[29]

Summary

In most patients with correctly identified BPPV, canalith-repositioning techniques may be useful and may bring immediate relief or improvement of symptoms. Experience in an emergency patient population with treatment by emergency clinicians is limited,[38] although with careful patient selection, some success should be achieved.

BRAIN DEATH TESTING

In a textbook of emergency medicine from 1988, the author wrote that because emergency medicine was a life-supporting–oriented specialty, the determination of brain death was outside the practice of the emergency clinician.[43] The date of

the seated position on the stretcher with the head turned 45° toward the affected side. Lay the patient down flat with the head hanging over the edge of the bed. After 20 seconds or after symptoms subside, rotate the patient's head to face the opposite shoulder while maintaining the head-hanging orientation. Roll the patient further onto his or her side and rotate the head further into a face-down position. Again, after 20 seconds or after any symptoms subside, return the patient to a seated position.[29,37,41] Some authors suggest keeping the patient's head in each position long enough for any provoked

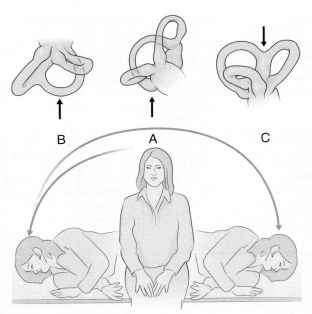

Figure 62–6   Semont's maneuver. The patient is moved quickly into the position that provokes the vertigo and remains in that position for 4 min. The patient is then turned rapidly to the opposite side, ear down, and remains in this second position for 4 min before slowly sitting up (for detailed description of the technique, see text). *Insets,* The right labyrinth as it would be viewed from the front of the patient. The orientation of the labyrinth is shown for when the patient is sitting (*A*), lying on the affected side (*B*), and lying on the opposite side (*C*). The *solid black arrow* indicates the location of the relative position of free-floating debris within the canal during the different stages of this maneuver.

publication reflects practice at that time; neuroimaging was not often performed while patients were in the ED and delays for inpatient bed availability were unusual. With increased use of neuroimaging in the ED and general trends to increased ED length of stay, the occasion may arise for emergency clinicians to be involved in assessment of brain death. The duty to identify potential organ and tissue donors is another consideration in identifying patients with irreversible loss of brain function. Local practices, policies, regulations, and laws differ and these remarks are general; the clinician is urged to be familiar with local practices and administrative policies regarding the issue of brain death.

For purposes of this discussion, *brain death* is defined as irreversible loss of functioning of the cerebral hemispheres and brainstem consistent with definitions in the literature.[44-47] The cause of the brain injury should be known or identified because some toxicologic syndromes, notably barbiturate toxicity, exactly duplicate the clinical syndrome of brain death. In keeping with the theme of this book, this chapter focuses on clinical procedures commonly used to delineate brain death. Radiologic, electrophysiologic, and other tests are mentioned only in passing. This chapter is not a historical summary of the complex legal and ethical issues surrounding this topic or a guide to approaching the family of a severely injured or impaired patient. Frequently in current practice, if a cause for coma or neurologic injury is identified and prognosis is shared with family, the option of withholding or withdrawing advanced life support is considered. This is entirely within the realm of patient, family, and clinician interactions, and the discussion of brain death does not surface in these circumstances.

Background

With the advancement of intensive care techniques, patients were identified with continuing spontaneous cardiovascular function while on ventilatory support but without evidence of CNS activity. Observation of these patients showed that cardiovascular function would eventually fail, although rare prolonged survival has been reported.[48,49] Efforts to reliably identify these patients were sought for improved resource allocation and optimal family counseling and to identify possible organ donors. Part of the impetus for reliably establishing clinical brain death was to allow the medical and legal pronouncement of death and allow discontinuation of advanced life support without fear of legal consequences. Death had long been defined as cessation of cardiac function; these deeply comatose patients with persistent cardiac activity but without demonstrable brain function challenged the traditional definition of death. The concept of brain death has been entangled in ethical, legal, and policy discussions roughly since the advent of clinical application of mechanical ventilation in the 1960s.[44,50,51] Current medical practice in the United States allows withdrawal of life-sustaining therapies when they are considered futile. In most patients, formal declaration of brain death is not necessary before withdrawing support.

Indications and Contraindications

Assessment of brain function is part of the ongoing care of every patient. Evaluation for brain death implies that severe CNS dysfunction has been identified, that the cause of CNS dysfunction is known, and that reversible causes of profound coma have been confidently excluded.[45,47] Formal brain death assessment is in preparation for pronouncement of death to allow organ harvest or in uncommon cases of disparate family or caregiver convictions regarding patient prognosis. Complex medical issues that may confound the assessment and should be considered and ruled out include severe electrolyte disturbances, hypothermia (defined as core temperature < 32°C), hypotension, drug intoxication or poisoning, and pharmacologic neuromuscular blockade.[47] Neuroimaging studies should be carefully reviewed.

Procedure

Establishment of Coma and Cortical Assessment

By definition, the patient under evaluation for brain death will be in a coma without spontaneous respirations. Certain examination techniques are used to establish loss of function of the cerebral cortex and brainstem; the clinical neurologic examination remains the standard for determination of brain death.[47] This typically involves assessment for cortical function and brainstem reflexes including respiratory drive.

While holding the patient's eyes open, give loud verbal commands such as "Look up!" and assess for voluntary eye movements, particularly important for patients with the locked-in syndrome. Additionally deliver a strong painful stimulus by forcefully pressing on brow, sternum, or nailbed. Should any cerebral or brainstem function be discovered, the patient is not brain dead by definition in spite of what may be severe brain injury. Some institutions require evaluation by two clinicians of particular specialty training. The clinician must be familiar with local practices and policies, which may also require ancillary testing with EEG, nuclear angiography, or other techniques. Brain death in the pediatric population is more complex with varying recommendations of repeat examinations and ancillary tests; that discussion is outside the scope of this chapter but is summarized elsewhere.[47]

Brainstem Reflex Testing

Pupillary Response. The pupils in brain-dead patients are unreactive and midposition to dilated. Shine a bright light into the pupil and observe for a reaction; there will be none in the brain-dead patient. Should any reactivity be noted, the patient is not brain dead.

Auditory Reflex. Deliver a loud handclap into each ear. Observe for eye blink or other reaction. Any reaction establishes that some brainstem function remains and excludes brain death.

Caloric Testing. Perform cold water irrigation of the external auditory canals with large volumes (≥100 mL) to elicit any eye movements through the oculovestibular reflexes (described in detail earlier in this chapter). In the brain-dead patient, there will be no movement of the eyes in response to irrigation. Any eye movement excludes brain death.

Corneal Reflex. Stimulate the cornea with a cotton wisp or applicator. Observe for any eye closure, which indicates that the CN V to VII reflex arc remains intact and excludes the diagnosis of brain death.

Cough Reflex. Stimulate the trachea or mainstem bronchi by deep suctioning and observe for coughing. A cough excludes brain death.

Apneic Oxygenation Test. CNS control of respiratory drive resides in the medulla. Establishing apnea is necessary to confirm medullary failure. Mechanical hyperventilation may artificially depress respiratory effort. Recall that it is hypercapnia, not hypoxia, that triggers respiratory effort. Simply disconnecting the ventilator to allow development of hypercapnia for apnea testing may lead to hypoxia.[52] A variety of techniques have been described that allow adequate hypercapnia for medullary stimulation to develop but ensure that oxygenation is adequate during the test. The most commonly described technique is to disconnect the patient from the ventilator and deliver oxygen at 10 to 15 L/min through a catheter inserted into the trachea and then observe for respiratory efforts for 8 minutes. Any observed excursion of the abdomen or chest sufficient to produce a tidal volume suggests that brain death is not present. If there are no observed respiratory excursions, arterial blood gas analysis is obtained and the patient is reconnected to the ventilator pending results. An arterial partial carbon dioxide pressure (Pco_2) of 60 mm Hg or higher and the absence of respiratory excursions are the criteria for a positive apnea test.[46] Others suggest that a possibly safer technique is to simply set the ventilator rate to zero while allowing continuous oxygen flow to continue and maintaining any necessary continuous positive pressure through the ventilator.[53]

Declaration of Death

If the criteria for brain death are satisfied, the family and all clinicians involved in patient care should be informed to allow further management decisions. At some institutions, the patient is declared dead at the time criteria are met and further care is assumed by transplant services if that is the anticipated course. Per institutional protocol, confirmation of brain death by two clinicians may be required. Families are generally given the option of being present at the bedside while mechanical ventilation is discontinued, although some advise against this because spontaneous reflex movements such as the Lazarus sign (discussed later) may occur and disturb the family.[14] Again, for patients age 18 years or younger, particularly infants, repeated examinations and confirmatory tests are generally recommended.[47,51] A model for direct family conversation in this sensitive interaction has been described and includes a sample script and procedure.[54]

Complications

Carefully following the physical examination protocol reliably identifies the majority of patients with irreversible loss of brain function. Two basic areas of error are possible: either erroneously declaring a patient brain dead when in fact some CNS function is retained or failing to correctly identify brain death.

Profound barbiturate intoxication may simulate the picture of brain death at times. To guard against the error of failing to detect surreptitious pharmacologic coma, some protocols include toxicologic screening tests for barbiturates as part of the process of assessment for brain death. Ancillary techniques for assessing intracranial blood flow would also prevent this error. Two examinations both confirming brain death performed several hours apart have been part of some protocols with the idea that toxicologic coma might improve during this period of observation. Again, familiarity with local policies and practices is necessary.

A variety of movements have been observed in brain-dead patients; at times these spinal-level–mediated reflexes may be dramatic and erroneously lead observers to believe that the brain-dead patient is demonstrating voluntary movements or brain-mediated reflex movements. Finger jerks and facial myokymia (spontaneous, fine fascicular muscular contractions) have been reported to be spontaneously present in brain-dead patients. Decerebrate-like extensor posturing, the Lazarus sign (flexion of the arms at the elbow, shoulder adduction, lifting arms, dystonic posturing of the hands with crossing of the hands), undulating toe flexion, triple flexion response in the lower extremities, and flexion of the trunk (giving the appearance of sitting up) are among the signs described during apnea testing and after the termination of ventilation or triggered by tactile stimuli.[14,55-59]

Summary

The emergency clinician may become involved in assessment of patients for brain death in the course of current practice. The screening physical examination for assessing brain death is described earlier. Again, the cause of irreversible coma should be known. The clinician is urged to be familiar with local practices and regulations in this sometimes-complex medicolegal process.

MYASTHENIA GRAVIS TESTING

Background

Myasthenia gravis is the most common disease of neuromuscular transmission, but still, the incidence is only 1 in 20,000 in the general population. Patients with myasthenia may be grouped into two major categories. The first group shows weakness in proximal muscles, which increases with activity and improves with rest. The other group presents with ocular complaints of diplopia or ptosis. Patients in the ocular weakness group may or may not have generalized symptoms as well. Fatigue is the hallmark of the disease; symptoms typically wax and wane. Patients often see a number of clinicians before a correct diagnosis is made.[60,61]

Myasthenia gravis results from an immune-mediated destruction of postsynaptic acetylcholine (ACh) receptors, with variable failure of neuromuscular transmission.[60,61] ACh is the transmitter at the neuromuscular junction. When the nerve terminal is stimulated, ACh is released in a quantity far in excess of that needed for effective activation of the ACh receptor. ACh diffuses across the synaptic cleft to transiently interact with the ACh receptor, and an electrical potential is generated at the myoneural end plate. If it is of sufficient magnitude, the end plate potential initiates an action potential that is propagated along the muscle membrane and muscle fiber contraction follows. The ACh is rapidly hydrolized by acetylcholinesterase in the synaptic cleft. Figure 62–7 summarizes neurotransmitter action at the neuromuscular junction. Of the millions of receptors at each myoneural junction, only a fraction must depolarize to stimulate muscle fiber contraction. Any factor that decreases interactions of ACh with ACh receptors decreases the probability of an action potential being generated and may lead to failure of neuromuscular transmission with resulting weakness. Acetylcholinesterase inhibitors (anticholinesterases) have been the mainstay of therapy for myasthenia gravis for years, but they have been supplemented by immunosuppressive regimens and thymectomy. Failure of neuromuscular transmission may also occur with excessive acetylcholinesterase inhibition; the persistence of ACh in the synaptic cleft leads to continuous depolarization of the receptor.

Bedside diagnostic testing for myasthenia gravis has been described in patients presenting to the ED with two different clinical pictures. The first presentation involves a known patient with myasthenia gravis on cholinesterase inhibitor therapy with increased weakness; pharmacologic testing in this setting is controversial. The second presentation involves a previously undiagnosed patient in whom the diagnosis of myasthenia gravis is suspected with ptosis, diplopia, or fluctuating muscular weakness; bedside testing may be helpful in select patients in this group.

A battery of tests can be used in the assessment of the patient with suspected myasthenia gravis, but only a few are available to the emergency clinician.[62] ACh receptor antibody assay is positive in more than 80% of patients with myasthenia but has a turnaround time of several days.[63,64] Repetitive nerve stimulation and single-fiber electromyography tests are available in the electrophysiology laboratory.[65] Several pharmacologic tests have been used to aid in the diagnosis of suspected myasthenia gravis including parenteral administration of edrophonium chloride (Tensilon), neostigmine, or curare. Edrophonium chloride administration for diagnosis of myasthenia gravis (Tensilon test) is described in detail because of the drug's rapid onset, short duration of action, and widespread acceptance for this diagnostic challenge; the emergency clinician may find occasion to use this test. The ice pack test is discussed because of favorable reports of its utility and its noninvasive nature.[66,67] The use of curare has been described to aid in diagnosis of myasthenia gravis by both systemic and regional administration. A technique is described for administration into an ischemic arm; this modification is known as the *regional curare test*.[65] The use of curare in this setting is outside the realm of practice of the emergency clinician.

Edrophonium (Tensilon) Test

Background

Edrophonium chloride (Tensilon) is an acetylcholinesterase inhibitor that has been used in the diagnosis of myasthenia gravis since the 1960s. The short duration of action of edrophonium that made it unsatisfactory as a therapeutic agent for myasthenia gravis makes it useful as a diagnostic agent. The drug's onset of action is rapid, and the duration of maximal effect is short, usually less than 2 minutes. Any effect resolves within 5 to 10 minutes.[68]

Edrophonium administration has also been recommended in the past to monitor acetylcholinesterase inhibitor therapy.[69,70] However, edrophonium administration is not sufficiently reliable for titrating the effect of anticholinesterase medication.[71] The use of the Tensilon test in a patient with known myasthenia gravis is controversial and should be done only in consultation with or in the presence of the treating neurologist, if at all.

Myasthenic crisis may be loosely defined as respiratory distress in a patient with myasthenia gravis. Earlier concepts included "myasthenic" crisis from insufficient drug administration, "cholinergic" crisis from cholinesterase inhibitor overdosage, and the "brittle" patient with rapidly changing drug requirements,[72,73] but terminology in this setting remains controversial.[74] Even the clinical existence of the different types of crisis has been debated.[71] Certainly, in the myasthenic patient with respiratory distress, airway management and assisted ventilation are top priorities. Edrophonium administration should not be viewed as a possible alternative to intubation and mechanical ventilation. Several authorities advocate withdrawing all cholinesterase inhibitors in this setting because most patients show increased responsiveness to cholinesterase inhibitors after several days without taking the drug.[71,74] Others advocate a trial of edrophonium chloride at reduced dosage (1–2 mg) only after respiratory support is achieved.[72,75]

Indications and Contraindications

The bedside Tensilon test is indicated for diagnosis of patients with suspected myasthenia gravis when there is clinical need to make that diagnosis immediately. If other bedside tests

NEUROMUSCULAR JUNCTIONS

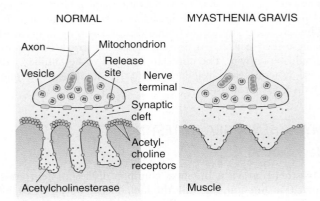

NORMAL   MYASTHENIA GRAVIS

Axon
Mitochondrion
Release site
Vesicle
Nerve terminal
Synaptic cleft
Acetylcholine receptors
Acetylcholinesterase
Muscle

Figure 62–7 Neuromuscular junctions. In myasthenia gravis, acetylcholine is released from presynaptic vesicles and diffuses across the synaptic cleft to the postsynaptic receptors. Acetylcholinesterase, located deep within the synaptic folds, hydrolyzes acetylcholine. There is also a simplification of the postsynaptic site with a reduced number of receptors.

such as the ice pack test (discussed later) are conclusive, or if eyelid fatigue on prolonged upgaze can be demonstrated, there is no need to administer edrophonium.[76] If the tempo of the clinical scenario is such that consultation or admission and obtaining specialized electromyelograms or serologies is feasible, then deferring the Tensilon test in the ED may be the preferred strategy, realizing that serologies and neurophysiologic testing will not be completed for some days.

Administration of edrophonium is commonly performed in office settings by neuro-ophthalmologists with occasional complications of bradycardia that at times may be symptomatic with hypotension and loss of consciousness.[77,78] One study reports the complication rate in office settings as 0.16%.[77] A history of asthma or cardiac dysrhythmias is a relative contraindication to administration of cholinesterase inhibitors. Complications reported in the literature from Tensilon testing largely date from the era when it was used in cardiology to differentiate supraventricular rhythms.[76] Reported complications include cardiac rhythm disturbances and even death; several of these patients were taking digoxin or β-blockers.[79–82] One report noted transient asystole after edrophonium administration in a patient with suspected myasthenia; the patient was critically ill and had been receiving intravenous labetalol.[76] Hence, caution is advised in edrophonium administration in patients receiving β-blocking agents, digoxin, or other drugs with atrioventricular-blocking properties.

Administration of edrophonium to a patient with myasthenia gravis being treated with cholinesterase inhibitors is controversial. Many investigators consider myasthenic crisis to be a contraindication to edrophonium administration, although in a series of patients with myasthenic crisis, its use continues to be reported.[72,75]

A muscle that is clearly weak must be identified to monitor during Tensilon testing; ptosis is a commonly monitored sign. If a specific muscle cannot be isolated for objective testing, edrophonium administration should be deferred and other approaches to diagnosis pursued.

Equipment

The following materials are needed for testing an adult. Intravenous access should be secured with D_5W at a keep-open rate or with a saline lock. Ten milligrams of edrophonium chloride should be drawn up in a tuberculin syringe. Edrophonium chloride is supplied in 1- and 10-mL vials at a concentration of 10 mg/mL. A second syringe of normal saline should be available to administer as a placebo, although some clinicians have recommended nicotine, calcium chloride, or atropine for this purpose.[70] Atropine and other cardiovascular drugs and resuscitative equipment should be readily available. Cardiac monitoring is generally recommended. Photographic recording equipment is desirable to objectively document any improvement in motor function.

Procedure

Identify a muscle that is clearly weak. A clinically evident extraocular muscle weakness or the presence of ptosis allows direct observation of a single weak muscle becoming stronger in response to the drug. Simple grip dynamometry does not aid in evaluation; a repetitive measure of grip strength (ergogram) is necessary. Ideally, one person is available to administer the edrophonium or placebo and a second person is free to observe the effect of medication on the patient. It is best if both the observer and the patient do not know which syringe contains edrophonium and which contains saline, thus creating a double-blind testing situation.

Again, ptosis is an easily testable sign and is generally used if present. The principles involved with assessing the effect of edrophonium on ptosis may be extended to testing other muscles. Ask the patient to look upward for several moments to fatigue the levator muscles. Note the degree of ptosis and document by measurements or photographs. After a moment's rest, ask the patient to look straight ahead. Inject 0.2 mL of the test substance in one syringe (2 mg of edrophonium or saline). If there is no response within 1 minute, inject 0.3 mL (3 mg of edrophonium or saline); if no response, inject the remainder. Note any increase in strength as reflected by an increase in palpebral fissure size. Repeat the procedure with the other test substance.

Complications

A small percentage of individuals are hypersensitive to even the initial small dose of edrophonium and show cholinergic side effects of salivation, lacrimation, and miosis. These effects are transient. Atropine, 0.5 mg, may be given intravenously if necessary to counteract these symptoms. A smaller number of patients may experience symptomatic bradycardia that responds to atropine. As described earlier, rare cardiac arrhythmias and death have been reported, usually in patients taking digoxin or β-blockers.

Interpretation

The key to the procedure is its interpretation. If a clearly paretic muscle has been identified, objective signs of improvement in the strength of that muscle within a moment of administration of edrophonium and the fading of that improvement over the next 5 minutes are criteria for a positive test result. Up to 90% of patients with myasthenia have a positive test result under ideal circumstances.[69,70] False-negative results do occur consistently.

For evaluating the effect of edrophonium on ptosis, a positive test consists of the patient having increased ability to elevate the eyelids after administration of 5 to 10 mg of edrophonium. The ptosis returns within 5 minutes. Subjective increases in general strength or relief of fatigue do not constitute a positive test. Fasciculations, brief twitches of muscles, are not usually observed in the patient with myasthenia who has received edrophonium, in contrast to normal subjects. The Tensilon test may be repeated in 30 minutes if desired.

Normal subjects have no change in muscle strength. They may transiently experience the side effects of salivation, lacrimation, and diaphoresis. Perioral, periocular, or lingual fasciculations are almost always noted in the normal patient after edrophonium administration.

The reproducible and unequivocal reversal of weakness in a specific muscle is extremely specific for myasthenia.[83,84] False-positive test results have been reported in patients with Eaton-Lambert syndrome and rarely in patients with intracranial lesions.[85–87] Other rare reports of positive test results involve patients with amyotrophic lateral sclerosis. A "perverse" reaction has been noted rarely, in which a paretic extraocular muscle, weak from other causes, becomes even weaker with edrophonium administration.[88]

Ice Pack Test

Background

It has been observed clinically that myasthenic patients have exacerbations of weakness with environmental heat and improvement in strength with cold temperatures. A simple bedside test uses these observations to evaluate ptosis.[66,67] Ice placed in a surgical glove or wrapped in a towel is placed lightly over the eyelid of a patient. Cooling of the eyelid below 29°C is accomplished within 2 minutes. The ptosis has been noted to improve in 80% or more of patients tested and may be more sensitive than the edrophonium test in detecting ocular myasthenia gravis. Although the reported number of patients evaluated by this method continues to be small, the test is included here because of its potential application in the ED, its lack of side effects, and its noninvasive nature.

Indications

Unilateral or bilateral ptosis of uncertain etiology in which myasthenia is a diagnostic possibility is the sole indication for this test.

Procedure

Ice and a surgical glove or towel are the only materials required. A camera to record any response is optional. Measure or photograph the degree of the patient's ptosis. Ask the patient to look upward, which often provokes the ptosis. If bilateral ptosis is present, use the more affected eye for evaluation. Cool the eyelid by lightly holding the wrapped ice to the patient's eyelid for 2 minutes or until patient discomfort limits the application. Compare the width of the palpebral fissure with the pretest width (Fig. 62–8).

Complications

Patient discomfort from the ice pack application may limit the cold exposure time to less than 2 minutes but may still allow a successful test.

Interpretation

A clear improvement of ptosis in the cooled eye is the criterion for a positive test. The effect should be reproducible. In small clinical studies, the ice pack test is at least as sensitive as edrophonium administration in improving ptosis in patients with ocular myasthenia. False-negative results do occur, probably at about the same frequency as those in Tensilon testing. One individual has been reported to have had a negative ice pack test result with a positive Tensilon test result. Negative or equivocal Tensilon tests have been reported in other individuals who had clearly positive ice pack test results. Normal individuals showed no change in palpebral fissure width after the cold exposure. False-positive results are rare.[66,67,89]

Summary

The bedside Tensilon test has a long history of utility in diagnosing myasthenia gravis, but it has been largely replaced by acetylcholinesterase receptor assay and electrodiagnostic studies in the ambulatory setting.[63,65,76,84] On occasion when rapid diagnosis is desired or myasthenia gravis is suspected in the presence of a normal ACh receptor titer, a carefully performed Tensilon test is still clinically valuable. The use of the Tensilon test in the setting of myasthenic crisis is controversial and is discouraged.

The ice pack test is so simple and noninvasive that it should become the initial procedure of choice in the ED for evaluating the possibility of ocular myasthenia. A positive ice pack test result strongly suggests ocular myasthenia gravis and alleviates any need for the Tensilon test. False-negative results do occur, and additional testing should be performed if the clinical suspicion of myasthenia gravis is strong.

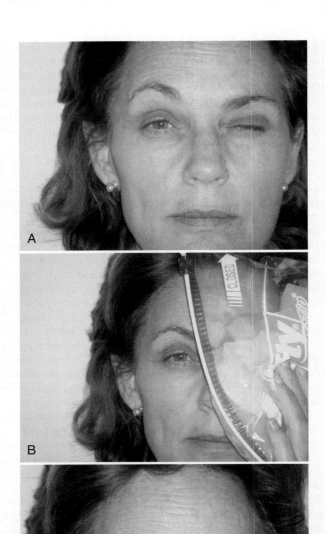

Figure 62–8 *A,* Before ice pack placement. *B,* Ice pack is placed over the eyelid for about 2 min. *C,* After ice pack placement, improvement is noted in ptosis of the right eye. *(For details, see Sethi KD, Rivner MH, Swift TR: Ice pack test for myasthenia gravis. Neurology 37:1383, 1987.)*

It is often the case with neuromuscular diseases, given the broad diagnostic possibilities, that the emergency clinician is unable to establish a confident diagnosis at a single patient encounter.[90] Appropriate consultation and referral are necessary.

Acknowledgments

The author would like to thank Paul B. Baker, MD, for his contributions to this chapter in earlier editions of this work.

 REFERENCES CAN BE FOUND ON **EXPERT CONSULT**

OPHTHALMOLOGIC, OTOLARYNGOLOGIC, AND DENTAL PROCEDURES

CHAPTER 63

Ophthalmologic Procedures

Kevin J. Knoop, William R. Dennis, and Jerris R. Hedges*

The following discussion focuses on procedures performed by emergency clinicians during the evaluation and treatment of injuries and diseases of the eye. The emphasis is on the practical application of the techniques; cautions to be heeded by the emergency clinician are included.

VISUAL ACUITY ASSESSMENT

Visual acuity may initially be deferred in simple, obvious, or straightforward cases, such as a stye, periorbital laceration, or minor eye irritation; however, visual acuity assessment should be the first procedure performed in the majority of patients who present to the emergency department (ED) with an eye complaint. Whereas it may be initially deferred in the triage or trauma room setting, or under other relevant scenarios, it is incumbent upon the emergency clinician to ensure that visual acuity or function is ultimately adequately assessed.

Indications

Visual acuity should be done as soon as practicable and before the patient is examined with bright lights. In the event of blepharospasm from an injury (e.g., abrasion, chemical exposure), a topical anesthetic may facilitate the examination. Patients often present in the context of an eye complaint saying that they "can't see." In these instances, emergent visual acuity assessment should first be performed beginning with the assessment of light perception, then hand motion, and finally counting fingers at 3 feet (Fig. 63–1). If the patient

*This article represents the views of the authors and is not to be interpreted as official, representing the U.S. Navy or the Bureau of Medicine.

succeeds in performing these assessments, a near vision card may then be used or distant visual acuity assessed. Under emergent circumstances, detailed formal vision testing is not essential; however, some form of visual acuity assessment is needed. In this situation, the ability to count fingers or read newsprint gives some indication of gross visual function. Formal visual acuity testing should never delay important therapeutic interventions such as eye irrigation.[1]

Distant Visual Acuity Procedure

For formal vision testing, ask the patient to face a well-lit standard Snellen or similar eye chart from a premeasured distance of 20 feet. Use a card or the palm of the hand to occlude one eye at a time. If possible, all patients should be examined while wearing their current lens correction in order to obtain the best corrected distant visual acuity. If this is not available, measure visual acuity first without correction, then with a pinhole device, and note any improvement in visual acuity. This device functions as a corrective lens by reducing corneal refractive error. In general, visual acuity is improved with the pinhole device. Decreased visual acuity that is not improved with this device suggests that corneal refractive error is not the cause. Construct a pinhole device by punching several holes in the center of a card (3- × 5-inch index card) with an 18-gauge needle. Devices with one or more pinholes drilled into an eye cover are available commercially (Fig. 63–2A and B). Figure 63–2C presents a chart for visual acuity testing while the patient is on a stretcher or in a chair. The chart can be used directly from this text if it is held 14 inches from the eye. Begin by testing the affected eye or the one presumed to have the worst visual acuity. First, instruct the patient to read the smallest letters on the chart that can easily be seen. Then, ask the patient to read letters that can just barely be made out (i.e., they do not have to be clear). If the patient is unable to read the largest letter on the chart, move the patient to one half the distance from the chart (10 ft) or move the figure 7 inches closer to the edge and repeat the procedure. Record the results reflecting the change in distance (e.g., 10/200). The numerator in the vision ratio is the distance of the patient from the chart and the denominator is the distance at which a patient with normal vision can read the line of letters. For the patient who still cannot read the letters on the chart, test vision progressively as follows: ability to count fingers, detect hand motion, perceive light (with or without projection and ability to perceive the direction of light), and finally inability to perceive light.[2]

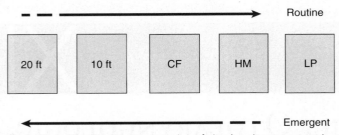

Figure 63–1 The "routine" progression of visual acuity assessment is reversed in the emergent presentation. Assessing an intact visual pathway begins with quickly discerning whether the patient has light perception (LP), can see hand motion (HM), and can count fingers at 3 ft (CF). Subsequent progression to assess vision at 10, then 20, feet from a standard eye chart ensues.

Near Visual Acuity Procedure

Perform near visual acuity in the ED at the bedside or at triage. Hold a pocket near vision card (see Fig. 63–2C) or any printed material at a distance of approximately 14 inches in good light in front of the patient and occlude each eye alternately as described earlier. When using available printed material in lieu of a near vision card, measure the size of the letters that are discerned by the patient. At a later time, compare these with the letter size on the near vision card to deduce the actual visual acuity. When near vision is decreased, it is usually either from loss of visual function or as a result of poor accommodation from advancing age (presbyopia). Less commonly, it is caused by traumatic mydriasis. Thus, examine patients with presbyopia with their reading correction in place to obtain the best corrected near visual acuity.

For patients who cannot communicate or in whom factitious blindness or malingering is suspected, check for optokinetic nystagmus (OKN) to determine whether there is an intact visual pathway. To test for OKN, pass a regularly sequenced pattern in front of the eyes. If an optokinetic drum is available, rotate the drum in front of the patient (Fig. 63–3). This is not available in many EDs, however. In place of the drum, substitute a printed piece of paper such as newsprint (without photographs or large areas with no print) or a standard tape measure. Pass it in front of the patient's eye at reading distance while instructing the patient to look at it as it rapidly moves by. Evaluate for tracking as demonstrated by nystagmus-like eye movements seen when the test object is moved from side to side in front of the patient. This movement indicates an intact visual pathway. Finally, another effective method is to hold a mirror in front of the patient and slowly rotate the mirror to either side of the patient. The patient with an intact visual pathway will maintain eye contact with herself or himself as demonstrated by eye movement as the mirror is moved. A large mirror that reflects the patient's entire face is most effective for this purpose.

All patients with decreased visual acuity from their baseline require routine referral for further ophthalmologic follow-up; however, those patients with moderately or severely decreased visual acuity not explained by refractive error require ophthalmologic consultation in the ED.

DILATING THE EYE

Dilating the eye is useful for both diagnostic and therapeutic purposes. Be advised, however, that an attack of narrow-angle (angle-closure) glaucoma may be precipitated by dilating the pupil. The most common form of glaucoma, however, is open-angle glaucoma and this type is not precipitated by dilating the pupil. Some patients may have a "mixed-mechanism" glaucoma with both open-angle and narrow-angle components. Systemic reactions, such as bradycardia from β-blocker eye drops, can be produced by mucosal absorption of dilating medications.

There are two types of dilators: sympathomimetic agents, which stimulate the dilator muscle of the iris, and cycloplegic agents, which block the parasympathetic stimulus that constricts the iris sphincter. Cycloplegic agents also block the contraction of the ciliary muscles, which control the focusing of the lens of the eye. This second effect of cycloplegic agents is of great importance in the therapeutic use of dilators for iritis.

Cycloplegic agents were used cosmetically as early as Galen's time. Beginning in the early 1800s, extracts from the plants Hyoscyamus and belladonna were used in ophthalmology. Atropine was first isolated in 1833. Epinephrine was used on eyes in 1900 as the first sympathomimetic agent.[3]

Indications and Contraindications

There are diagnostic and therapeutic indications for dilating the pupil. Dilation is indicated for diagnosis when the fundus cannot be examined adequately through an undilated pupil. The elderly patient with miotic pupils and cataracts is an example of a patient in whom dilation may facilitate funduscopic examination. Dilation is therapeutically useful for many ophthalmic conditions, including inflammation in the eye. In the emergency setting, corneal injury with a secondary traumatic iritis is a common example. Dilation helps the inflamed eye in two ways. First, it may hinder adhesions (synechiae) from forming between the iris and other ocular structures. Such adhesions eventually limit the movement of the pupil and may precipitate glaucoma. Second, cycloplegic dilating agents relax the ciliary muscle spasm that often accompanies an inflamed eye and thus may reduce the pain associated with inflammation. Although traditionally used for these purposes, both benefits are largely theoretical with little formal evidence to support or refute their use in the ED.

Dilation is discouraged in the patient with head injury at risk for herniation, when it is necessary to monitor pupil findings. Dilation is contraindicated in the presence of narrow anterior chamber angles. Patients who are predisposed to having narrow angles may be unaware of this condition. Evaluate the depth of the anterior chamber before this procedure and do not dilate the eye if there is any question of a narrow angle. To estimate the depth of the anterior chamber, shine a penlight in tangentially from the lateral side of the eye. When the depth of the anterior chamber is normal, a uniform illumination of the iris is seen. However, when there is a forward convexity of the iris in the case of a narrow anterior chamber, only a sector of iris is illuminated and there will be a shadow on the medial (nasal) side of the iris (Fig. 63–4). With a slit lamp, the depth of the anterior chamber angle can be assessed directly. The definitive test for assessing the anterior chamber angle is gonioscopy, in which the anterior chamber angle structures are viewed directly by means of a special mirrored contact lens and the slit lamp. Gonioscopy is not a technique normally performed by emergency clinicians.

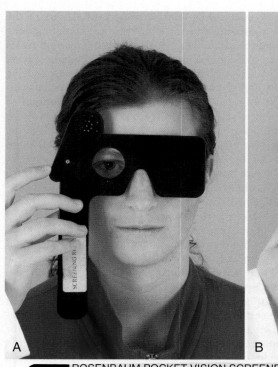

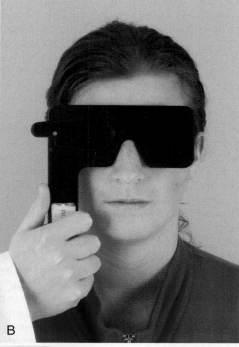

ROSENBAUM POCKET VISION SCREENER

Card is held in good light 14 inchest from eye. Record vision for each eye separately with and without glasses. Presbyopic patients should read thru bifocal segment. Check myopes with glasses only.

		Point	Jaeger	Distant equivaletn
95				$\frac{20}{800}$
874				$\frac{20}{400}$
2843		26	16	$\frac{20}{200}$
6 3 8 E Ш Э	X O O	14	10	$\frac{20}{100}$
8 7 4 5 Э M Ш	O X O	10	7	$\frac{20}{70}$
6 3 9 2 5 M E Э	X O X	8	5	$\frac{20}{50}$
4 2 8 3 6 5 Ш E M	O X O	6	3	$\frac{20}{40}$
3 7 4 2 5 8 Э Ш Э	x x o	5	2	$\frac{20}{30}$
9 3 7 8 2 6 Ш m E	x o o	4	1	$\frac{20}{25}$
4 2 8 7 3 9 E ш m	o o x	3	1+	$\frac{20}{20}$

PUPIL GAUGE (mm.)

2 3 4 5 6 7 8 9

DESIGN COURTESY J.G. ROSENBAUM, M.D., CLEVELAND, OHIO

Figure 63–2 A commercial pinhole device reveals refractive error caused by corneal aberration (excess tearing or nearsightedness). *A,* First measure visual acuity without the device. *B,* Then measure with the pinhole cover lowered. Document the acuity with and without the pinhole device. *C,* If the patient cannot stand or a formal eye chart is not available, ask the patient to read this "distance equivalent" chart by holding this Figure 14 inches away from the patient.

Systemic effects can develop after the application of eyedrops.[4-10] Review the following sections on agents and complications before using these drugs in patients with compromised cardiovascular function.

Agents

Only two dilating agents are really needed in the ED. Phenylephrine (Neo-Synephrine) 2.5% is used for diagnostic dilation of the pupil for visualization of the fundus. The drug is short-acting, and because accommodation is not affected, the patient's vision is not altered. Phenylephrine 10% should not be used routinely because it can be absorbed systemically and, in rare cases, has caused hypertensive crisis, myocardial infarction, and death.[8,9]

For therapeutic cycloplegia in iritis, homatropine 5% works well. Although Table 63-1 indicates a maximum duration of 3 days, 24 hours is more common. Therefore, homatropine 5% is a useful therapeutic agent for traumatic iritis. Atropine should not be used for traumatic iritis because the undesirable effects of pupillary dilation and blurred vision persist for a week or longer after healing of associated corneal

abrasions. Atropine drops may be prescribed as part of the therapy for nontraumatic iritis after appropriate ophthalmologic consultation. Individuals with lightly pigmented irides tend to have a greater sensitivity to the cycloplegic agents than do individuals with greater pigmentation; the cycloplegic effect might, therefore, be more prolonged in people with light eyes. It might be difficult to dilate some patients with deeply pigmented irides, and numerous applications of drops might be required.

Malingerers may use mydriatic agents to dilate a pupil unilaterally for the purpose of feigning neurologic disease. Normally, a pupillary dilation caused by intracranial third cranial nerve compression will constrict with 2% pilocarpine eye drops. The mydriatic-treated eye can be identified by full motor function of the third cranial nerve and the absence of miosis after pilocarpine instillation. A fixed and dilated pupil in an awake and alert patient cannot be secondary to brain herniation. Although other neurologic problems may be present, in the normal-appearing patient with a fixed and dilated pupil, a pharmacologic cause is highly likely. It should be noted that legitimate patients may not recall the name of an eye medicine that they used but will usually recall whether the bottle had a red cap, as is found on all cycloplegic solutions. An unexpected mydriasis in a trusted patient may be the result of such an agent. Medications that constrict the pupil, such as pilocarpine, have a green cap. Pressure-lowering drops for glaucoma may be yellow- or blue-topped (β-blockers), purple-topped (adrenergic agents) or orange-topped (topical carbonic anhydrase inhibitors).

A fixed and dilated pupil from a pharmacologic cause may be encountered after both nasotracheal and orotracheal intubation (Fig. 63-5). In such ill or injured patients, cerebral herniation must be considered. When phenylephrine is used to constrict the nasal mucosa prior to nasal intubation (endotracheal tube, nasogastric tube), the inadvertent contamination of the eye will cause a fixed and dilated pupil. The same scenario may occur after endotracheal epinephrine has been instilled into the lungs during resuscitation, and cardiopulmonary resuscitation has expelled epinephrine into the eye. Under such scenarios, the affected pupil will not constrict after intraocular pilocarpine administration. Finally, a fixed and dilated pupil might occur from inadvertent contamination of the eye with scopolamine after application of a scopolamine patch.

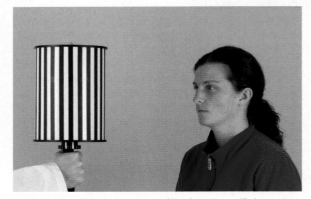

Figure 63–3 Optokinetic nystagmus (OKN) testing will determine whether there is an intact visual pathway. Induce OKN by passing a regularly sequenced pattern in front of the eye such as this commercially available drum. Hold the drum in front of the patient. Direct the patient to look at the drum as you rotate it slowly. Alternatively, draw a tape measure across the line of sight while asking the patient to look directly at it as it passes.

TABLE 63–1 Mydriatic Agents

Agent	Maximum Mydriasis	Duration of Mydriasis[§]	Common Trade Name
Sympathomimetics			
Phenylephrine*, 2.5%[†]	20 min	3 hr	Neo-Synephrine
Cocaine, 5% or 4%	20 min	2 hr	—
Parasympatholytics (Cycloplegics)			
Atropine, 1%	40 min	12 days	—
Scopolamine, 0.25%	30 min	7 days	—
Homatropine, 5%[‡]	30 min	1–3 days	—
Cyclopentolate, 1%	30 min	6–24 hr	Cyclogyl
Tropicamide, 1%	30 min	4 hr	Mydriacyl

*Preferred for funduscopic examination.
[†]A 10% solution may produce cardiovascular reaction and hence should not be used.
[‡]Preferred for iritis or corneal abrasion therapy.
[§]The duration of effect shows considerable individual variation. These are general estimates.

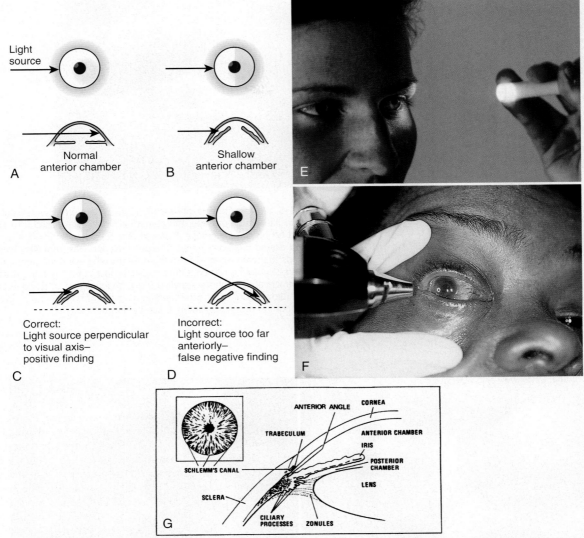

Figure 63–4 **Anterior chamber depth and transillumination test.** *A,* Normal anterior chamber with negative transillumination test. Note that the entire iris is illuminated. *B,* Shallow anterior chamber with positive transillumination test. Note the shadow on the outer half of the iris. *C,* Shallow anterior chamber with correctly placed light source yielding a true-positive test result in the presence of a shallow anterior chamber. *D,* Shallow anterior chamber with incorrectly placed light source giving a false-negative test result. *E,* Clinical use of the penlight examination to assess the depth of the anterior chamber. The examiner sits face-to-face with the patient to ensure that the light source is perfectly perpendicular to the line of vision. *F,* Note the shadow cast on the nasal portion of the iris, indicating a very narrow anterior chamber in this patient with acute angle-closure glaucoma. *G,* Diagram of the eye to explain the etiology of acute angle-closure glaucoma. When the pupil is dilated, the egress of fluid is hindered by the narrow angle at the canal of Schlemm, causing a sudden increase in intraocular pressure. *(A–D, From Bresler MJ, Hoffman RS: Prevention of iatrogenic acute narrow-angle glaucoma. Ann Emerg Med 10:535, 1981. Reproduced by permission.)*

Procedure

The instillation of mydriatic agents is similar to the administration of other eye solutions. For medicolegal purposes, note the visual acuity before the instillation of the medicine. This documents that any decreased vision is not the result of the mydriatic agent. Whenever dilation is performed, note on the patient's chart the dose and time that agents have been given to avoid confusion during subsequent neurologic evaluation.

Place the patient in a supine or a comfortable semi-recumbent position. Instruct the patient to gaze at an object in the upper visual field, such as a fixture on the ceiling. Gently depress the lower lid using a finger on the epidermis (Fig. 63–6). Instill a single drop of the solution into the lower lid fornix, and ask the patient to blink to spread the medication. Do not use more than a single drop because it produces reflex tearing and reduces the concentration in contact with the conjunctiva. Forewarn the patient that the medication is uncomfortable when it goes into the eyes. After the medication is in, the patient may blot the eye when it is closed but should not rub it with a tissue. If the desired effect is not noted in 15 to 20 minutes, repeat the dose, but this is seldom required.

Complications

As mentioned in the section on "Indications and Contraindications," any dilator can precipitate an attack of angle-closure glaucoma in susceptible patients.[10] In a case of angle-closure glaucoma, it may take several hours before symptoms become evident. The patient often complains of smoky vision with "halos" around lights as well as an aching pain that is some-

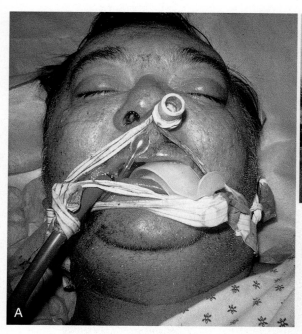

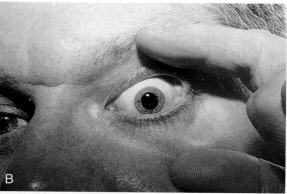

Figure 63–5 *A,* After phenylephrine (Neo-Synephrine) drops were instilled in the nose to facilitate tube passage, this comatose patient was nasotracheally intubated for his drug overdose. *B,* On a subsequent examination, a unilateral fixed and dilated pupil was noted. The pupil dilation was from Neo-Synephrine nose drops that were snorted from the nose into the eye during intubation, simulating cerebral herniation. Other unusual causes of a fixed and dilated pupil are endotracheal epinephrine expelled from the lungs and splashed in the eye during cardiopulmonary resuscitation and inadvertent contamination of the eye after application of a scopolamine patch behind the ear.

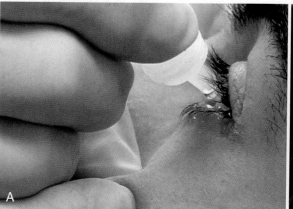

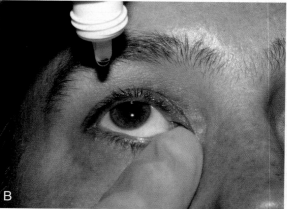

Figure 63–6 *A,* Administration of eye drops. The patient should lie in a supine position or with the head tilted back. The patient's gaze should be directed upward. Pull the lower lid downward and instill a single drop of medicine in the lower conjunctival fornix. Instruct he patient to close the eyelids for 1 minute to increase the contact of the medicine with the globe and to decrease the medication outflow down the tear duct and over the lid margin. *B,* If administering large amounts of eye drops that have systemic effects, such as β-blocker drops, the operator's index finger is placed under the inferior eyelid along the nasal borders of the eye, firmly compressing the nasolacrimal duct against the globe for a few minutes, thereby preventing migration of the drops into the nose and reducing systemic absorption. *(A, From Thomsen T, Setnik G [eds]: Procedures Consult—Emergency Medicine Module. Copyright 2008 Elsevier Inc. All rights reserved.)*

times severe. There may be nausea and vomiting. If the affected eye becomes injected in association with a hazy cornea, elevated pressure on tonometry, and an oval, fixed pupil, consult an ophthalmologist immediately. The treatment usually includes osmotic agents, carbonic anhydrase inhibitors, β-blocker drugs, pilocarpine, and later, definitive laser or surgical procedures (Table 63–2).

Be aware that using an eye medication might introduce infection. Most solutions contain bactericidal ingredients, but contamination of the tips of the droppers can still occur.[11] Use only newly opened bottles of eye medication, particularly if there is a deep corneal injury or if the patient has recently had eye surgery. Promptly discard out-of-date drops and drops in which crust or other material is found around the nozzle.

TABLE 63–2 Treatment Options for Acute Angle-Closure Glaucoma

1. Pilocarpine 4%: 2 drops every 15 min for 1–2 hr*
2. Glycerol: 1 mL/kg by mouth (as 50% solution in citrus juice)
3. Mannitol: 1.5–3 g/kg intravenously over 20 min (as 20% solution)*
4. Acetazolamide: 500 mg intravenously*
5. β-Blocker drugs (e.g., timolol 0.5%) 1 drop every 30 min for 2 doses*†
6. α₂-Agonist (apraclonidine [Iopidine] 0.5%) 1 drop†

*First-line therapy.
†May cause cardiovascular effects.

Forewarn the patient that any cycloplegic (in contrast to a sympathomimetic) will blur a patient's near vision. Vision will be less blurred in adults older than 45 years of age, who generally have a reduced ability to focus for near vision. Although most adults will be able to drive safely, even with both eyes affected, it is advisable to have someone else drive whenever feasible. Light sensitivity caused by pupillary dilation may also be bothersome; sunglasses are sufficient for this problem.

Systemic reactions can rarely be produced by sympathomimetic and cycloplegic eyedrops.[4-10] In one report of 33 cases of adverse reactions associated with 10% phenylephrine, there were 15 myocardial infarctions (11 deaths), 7 cases of precipitation of angle-closure glaucoma, and a variety of systemic cardiovascular or neurologic reactions.[9]

After instillation of eye drops into the conjunctival sac, systemic absorption can occur through the conjunctival capillaries as well as by way of the nasal mucosa, the oral pharynx, and the gastrointestinal tract after passage through the lacrimal drainage system. Mucosal hyperemia enhances absorption. Symptoms can often be avoided by maintaining digital pressure on the nasal canthus, thus occluding the puncta, for several minutes after administration.[4]

THE FLUORESCEIN EXAMINATION

Perform fluorescein staining of the eye as part of the evaluation of all cases of eye trauma and infection. It is a quick and easy technique that is crucial for the proper diagnosis and management of common eye emergencies. View the fluorescein-stained cornea and conjunctiva under a "blue" light and ideally in conjunction with slit lamp magnification (see "Slit Lamp Examination," later in this chapter).

Sodium fluorescein is a water-soluble chemical that fluoresces. It absorbs light in the blue wavelengths and emits the energy in the longer green wavelengths. It fluoresces in an alkaline environment (such as in the Bowman membrane, which is located below the corneal epithelium), but not in an acidic environment (such as in the tear film over an intact corneal epithelium).[12] Thus, it is useful in revealing even minute abrasions on the cornea (Fig. 63–7).

Fluorescein was first used in ophthalmology in the 1880s.[13] It was first used as a drop, but when the danger of contamination by bacteria (especially *Pseudomonas*) was recognized in the 1950s,[14] paper strips impregnated with fluorescein were developed. These are now supplied in individual sterile wrappers and should be used instead of the premixed solution.

Indications and Contraindications

Fluorescein staining is indicated for evaluation of suspected abrasions, foreign bodies (FBs), and infections of the eye.[15] This includes "simple" cases of conjunctivitis, which may actually be herpetic keratitis. Pepper spray exposure to the face has been associated with corneal abrasions, and these patients should be stained with fluorescein and evaluated with a slit lamp or Wood's lamp.[16] Corneal defects may be seen after unprotected viewing of a welder's arc flame.

Fluorescein permanently stains soft contact lenses. Therefore, when fluorescein is used, remove soft contact lenses before instilling the fluorescein and caution the patient not to put the lenses back into the eye for several hours. Topically administered fluorescein is considered nontoxic, although

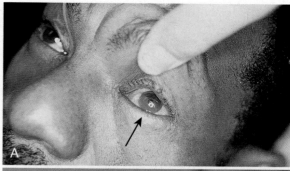

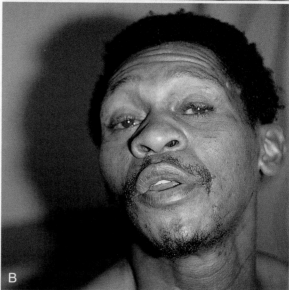

Figure 63–7 *A,* This large corneal abrasion (*arrow*) is readily seen without the slit lamp when fluorescein is instilled into the eye. Smaller abrasions, or corneal injuries produced by keratitis or welder's arc flash injuries, require slit lamp evaluation to identify minor corneal defects. Even minor traumatic abrasions will escape detection with only a blue light examination by the naked eye. *B,* This patient had severe eye pain, diffuse scleral injection, and tearing. A slit lamp was needed to discover multiple corneal defects due to keratitis from welding without eye protection.

reactions to a fluorescein-containing solution (not impregnated strips) have been described.[17] These reports consisting of vagal reactions[18] and generalized convulsions[19] are rare, not rigorously supported, and believed to be caused by agents other than fluorescein in the solution. If using one of these fluorescein-containing solutions rather than the fluorescein-impregnated strips, be aware of these potential, yet scientifically suspect, idiosyncratic reactions.

Be aware also that fluorescein dye may enter the anterior chamber of the eye in the presence of deep corneal defects. This form of intraocular fluorescein accumulation is nontoxic. When the anterior chamber is viewed under the blue filter of the slit lamp, a fluorescein "flare" is visible and should not be confused with the flare reaction noted with iritis.

Procedure

Theoretically, one should not use topical anesthetics before fluorescein staining, because some patients may develop a superficial punctate keratitis from the anesthetic,[12] which can confuse the diagnosis. However, with patients who are tearing

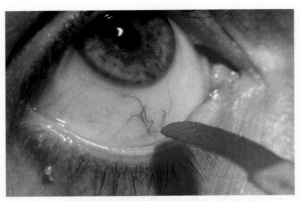

Figure 63–8 The fluorescein strip has been moistened with 1 drop of saline or topical anesthetic. Depress the lower lid and gently place a wetted strip onto the inside of the patient's lower lid so that only the smallest amount is instilled. Excess fluorescein may obscure subtle findings and thus should be avoided. Fluorescein will permanently stain contact lenses not removed (as seen in this model).

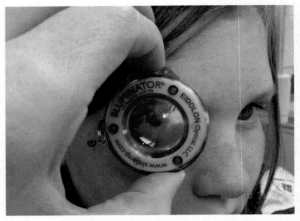

Figure 63–9 The Eidolon BLUMINATOR ophthalmic illuminator provides an intense blue LED light with 7× magnification. *(Courtesy Michael W. Ohlson, OD, FAAO, and Victor J. Doherty, Eidolon Optical, LLC.)*

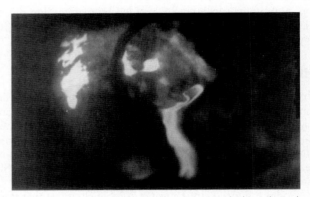

Figure 63–10 Positive Seidel's test shows aqueous leaking through a full-thickness corneal wound. Aqueous will turn fluorescein lime-green under cobalt-blue light as it oozes through the wound while being observed at the slit lamp. *(From Mitchell JD: Ocular Emergencies. In Tintinalli JE, Kelen GD, Stapcynski JS [eds]: Emergency Medicine—A Comprehensive Study Guide, 5th ed. New York, McGraw-Hill, 2000. Reproduced by permission.)*

profusely and who are squeezing their eyes shut from an abrasion or an FB, the examination often is impossible if a topical anesthetic is not first used. Theoretical downsides notwithstanding, it is common practice to apply a local anesthetic before instilling fluorescein.

Grasp the fluorescein strip by the non-orange end and wet the orange end with 1 drop of saline. There are several conveniently available forms including a small bottle of artificial tears, or a 5-mL "bullet" or "fish" of normal saline commonly used for nebulizer treatments. Alternatively, wet the strip with tap water or the recently used local anesthetic drops. Once the strip is moistened, place it gently into the inside of the patient's lower lid (Fig. 63–8). Withdraw the strip, and ask the patient to blink, which spreads the fluorescein over the surface of the eye. The key to a good examination is to have a thin layer of fluorescein over the corneal and conjunctival surfaces. If the strip is too heavily moistened before placing it in the lower fornix, the eye may become flooded with the solution, which makes the evaluation difficult. If too much dye accumulates, the patient can remove the excess by blotting the closed eye with a tissue. Conversely, placing a dry strip in the unanesthetized eye may be irritating. Next, use a Wood's lamp (4× magnification), the blue filter of a slit lamp, or simply a penlight with a blue filter to examine the eye in a darkened room. Check for areas of bright green fluorescence on the corneal and conjunctival surfaces. The naked eye may not be able to see small defects. Ideally, use a slit lamp, with 10× or 25× magnification, to examine the stained cornea before ruling out a pathologic process. A new handheld magnification device, the Eidolon BLUMINATOR ophthalmic illuminator, provides an intense blue light-emitting diode (LED) light with 7× magnification (Fig. 63–9). After completion of the fluorescein examination, irrigate excess dye from the eye to minimize damage to the patient's clothing from dye-stained tears.

The Seidel test uses fluorescein to detect perforation of the eye.[20] To perform this test, instill a large amount of fluorescein onto the eye by profusely wetting the strip. Examine the eye for a small stream of fluid leaking from the globe (Fig. 63–10). This stream will fluoresce blue or green in contrast to the orange appearance of the rest of the globe flooded with fluorescein.[12]

Interpretation

Fluorescein is mainly used for evaluation of corneal injuries. Although conjunctival abrasions pick up the stain, most of the staining on the conjunctiva represents patches of mucus rather than a real pathologic condition. Corneal staining is more specific for injury and the pattern of injury often reflects the original insult.

Corneal staining patterns are illustrated in Figure 63–11. Abrasions usually occur in the central cornea because of the limited protection of the patient's closing eyelids. The margins of the abrasions are usually sharp and linear if seen in the first 24 hours. Circular defects are seen about embedded FBs and may persist for up to 48 hours after removal of a superficial foreign object. Deeply embedded objects may be associated with defects persisting for longer than 48 hours. Objects under the upper lid (including some chalazia) often produce vertical linear lesions on the upper surface of the cornea. *When vertical lesions are noted, search diligently for a retained FB under the upper lid.* Hard contact lens overuse diminishes the nutrient supply to the cornea. The central cornea receives the most injury and thus fluoresces brightly when stained. Ultraviolet light exposure from sunlamp abuse, snow blindness, or

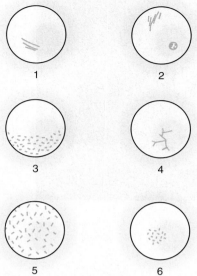

Figure 63–11 **Patterns of acute corneal injury.** *1,* Traumatic abrasion: usually with linear features and sharp borders when seen early (<24 hr). Occurs more in the central cornea. *2,* Abrasion from foreign body (FB): vertical abrasions on the upper cornea seen when an FB is embedded in the upper lid. Also shown is a rust ring with a metallic FB. *3,* Exposure pattern: seen with prolonged exposure to ultraviolet (e.g., welding flash, sunlamp exposure); produces bandlike keratitis over lower half of the cornea. Squinting in the setting of the bright light protected the upper corneal surface. *4,* Herpes simplex keratitis: classic dendritic pattern. *5,* Adenovirus keratitis: diffuse minute corneal staining seen in epidemic keratoconjunctivitis about 7 days after symptoms. *6,* Contact lens overuse: central punctate staining. *(From Knoop K, Trott A: Ophthalmologic procedures in the emergency department—Part III: Slit lamp use and foreign bodies. Acad Emerg Med 2:227, 1995. Reproduced by permission.)*

welding flash produces a superficial punctate keratitis, which in its mildest form may not be visible without a slit lamp. The central cornea is the least protected by the lids, and a central horizontal band–like keratitis can result. Herpetic lesions may develop anywhere on the cornea. Classically, these lesions are dendritic, although ulcers may also be punctate or stellate.[21,22]

Any area of corneal staining with an infiltrate or opacification beneath or around the lesion should alert the practitioner to the possibility of a viral,[21,22] bacterial,[23] or fungal[24] keratitis. Obtain urgent ophthalmologic consultation so that cultures of the possible etiologic agents can be procured and appropriate treatment initiated.

Many *Pseudomonas* organisms fluoresce when exposed to ultraviolet light;[25] therefore, presence of fluorescence before the instillation of fluorescein in the red eye should suggest the possibility of a pseudomonal infection.

Summary

Fluorescein staining is a quick, easy diagnostic procedure that should be part of every eye evaluation. The extra minute that the examination takes provides a wealth of diagnostic information for patients with eye trauma or infection. With the exception of the reactions noted with fluorescein solution, the potential discoloration of soft contact lenses, and the potential for infection when premixed solutions rather than fluorescein-impregnated paper strips are used, no complications are associated with the procedure.

EYE IRRIGATION

The crucial first step in the treatment of chemical injuries to the eye is eye irrigation. Irrigate as clinically appropriate to the exposure and severity of the injury. Serious chemical injury to the eye requires irrigation at the site of injury, before the patient is brought to the ED.[15] Corneal injury can occur within seconds of contact with an alkaline substance. Eye irrigation must often be continued in the ED.

This section discusses methods of irrigation. Although it is best to irrigate liberally, copious irrigation is not needed when the patient has gotten a small amount of a noncaustic, nonalkaline compound in the eye.

Indications and Contraindications

Irrigation is indicated for all acute chemical injuries to the eyes. Irrigation may also be therapeutic for patients having an FB sensation with no visible FB. Small, unseen foreign material in the conjunctival tissues may be flushed out with irrigation. There is no contraindication to eye irrigation, but if there is the possibility of a perforating injury to the eye, perform the irrigation especially gently and carefully.

Equipment

The following equipment is necessary for eye irrigation:
Topical anesthetic, such as proparacaine 0.5%
Sterile irrigating solution (warmed intravenous saline or lactated Ringer's [LR] solution in a bag with tubing)*
A basin to catch the fluid
Cotton-tipped applicators
Gauze pads to help hold the patient's lids open
Lid retractors
Irrigating device (e.g., Morgan Therapeutic Lens, modified central venous catheter, or Eye Irrigator) for prolonged irrigation
Optimal: 10 ml of 1% lidocaine added to a liter of irrigating fluid

Procedure

Basic Technique

First, instill a topical anesthetic in the eye. Evert the eyelid and sweep out any particulate matter in the conjunctival fornices with a moistened, cotton-tipped applicator[15] (see Ocular FB Removal," later in this chapter, and Fig. 63–12). Hold the eyelids open during irrigation. The easiest method is to use gauze pads to grasp the wet, slippery lids and hold them open. If the patient has severe blepharospasm, however, consider using lid retractors (Desmarres or paper clip retractors; Figs. 63–13 and 63–14). When lid retractors are used, be certain that the eye is well anesthetized, that the retractors do not injure the globe or the lids, and that chemicals are not harbored under the retractors. Be aware that simple retractors fashioned from metal paper clips (especially those that are nickel-plated and shiny) may have surface chipping, which can create an ocular FB.[26] Use caution to avoid ocular injury when using such a makeshift retractor.

---

*A balanced salt solution designed for eye irrigation is preferred by some (when available) and may produce less corneal edema with chemical injuries. Readily available normal saline and lactated Ringer's solution are equally well tolerated.

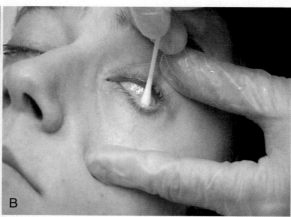

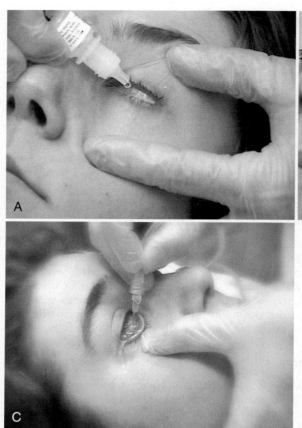

Figure 63–12 Eye irrigation. Note the severe blepharospasm from a chemical irritation. If this prohibits eye opening, circumferentially inject lidocaine anesthetic into the obicularis oris muscle to paralyze eye closure (see Fig. 63–15). *A,* First apply anesthesic drops. *B,* Sweep the eye with a wet cotton swab to remove particulate matter from under the lids. *C,* Begin irrigation by streaming saline or Ringer's solution directly from an intravenous bag. *(A and B, From Thomsen T, Setnik G [eds]: Procedures Consult—Emergency Medicine Module. Copyright 2008 Elsevier Inc. All rights reserved.)*

Deutsch and Feller[15] recommended an ipsilateral facial nerve block for severe blepharospasm (Fig. 63–15). To avoid swelling of the periorbital tissue, block the facial nerve just anterior to the condyloid process of the ipsilateral mandible. Place a subcutaneous line of anesthesia (2% lidocaine) to temporarily paralyze the orbicularis muscle.

Irrigate with normal saline or LR solution directed over the globe and into the upper and lower fornices. The choice of fluid initially is less important than initiating irrigation as rapidly as possible. If tap water is available at the scene of the injury, begin irrigation immediately with copious amounts of fluid before transporting the patient to the hospital. Teach out-of-hospital care providers to irrigate all acid injuries of the eye for at least 5 minutes at the scene and to irrigate all alkali injuries for at least 15 minutes.[27,28] LR solution or normal saline is preferred over tap water or D5W for eye irrigation, because these are isotonic and do not contain dextrose. Dextrose can be quite sticky if spilled and might serve as a nutrient for an opportunistic bacterial infection. Although one clinical trial found a balanced salt solution less painful in patients with a chemical eye injury,[29] another volunteer study on uninjured eyes found that LR solution is better tolerated than normal saline and balanced saline solution when used with a Morgan lens.[30] Warmed fluids are also better tolerated than fluids at room temperature.[31] Warmed LR solution should be considered when both it and normal saline are available for eye irrigation.

Be careful to direct the irrigating stream onto the conjunctiva and then across the cornea without letting the stream splash directly onto the cornea, because the mechanical injury of the solution striking the eye can in itself be harmful. Direct irrigation of the cornea can result in the development of a superficial punctate epithelial keratopathy.

Prior to irrigation, instill anesthetic eye drops, such as 0.5% tetracaine. Adding 10 ml of 1% lidocaine to a liter of saline irrigating fluid can decrease patient discomfort during prolonged irrigation.

Duration of Irrigation

Although Deutsch and Feller[15] recommended that a full liter of irrigating solution be used in every case of caustic injury, the duration of the irrigation is best determined by the extent of exposure and the causative agent. Acids are quickly neutralized by the proteins of the eye surface tissues and, once irrigated out, cause no further damage. The only exceptions are hydrofluoric and heavy metal acids, which can penetrate through the cornea. Alkalis can penetrate rapidly and, if not removed (because of the slow dissociation of the cation from combination with proteins), will continue to produce damage for days.[15] Therefore, prolonged irrigation is indicated; at least 2 L of solution should be used. Although rapid flushing with the first 500 mL is prudent, slow continuous irrigation as discussed later at a rate sufficient to generate a continuous trickle is often more effective and better tolerated than continued high-volume flushing. If the nature of the offending agent is in doubt, use prolonged irrigation.

Consult ophthalmology for all alkaline, hydrofluoric acid, and heavy metal acid injuries. Irrigation on an inpatient basis may be required for a period of 24 hours or more. This is especially likely when the cornea is hazy or obviously thickened. Note that the magnesium contained in sparklers combines with water from tears to produce magnesium hydroxide.[32]

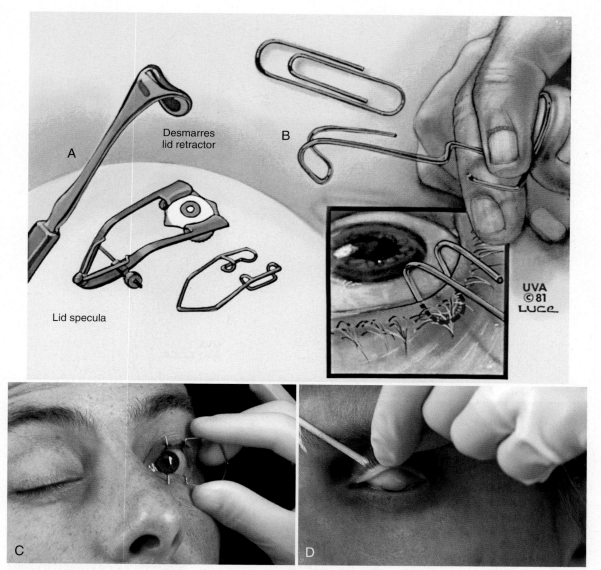

Figure 63–13   Devices for separating eyelids. Desmarres retractor (A) and a retractor improvised from a paper clip (B) allow active manipulation of lids. Free-standing specula may require a seventh nerve block to reduce blepharospasm. C, A lid retractor in place. D, Lid eversion is easily accomplished with a cotton applicator. Have the patient look down, grasp the eyelash, pull out the lid and turn it over the swab that has been placed over the upper lid. (A and B, From Fogle JA, Spyker DA: Management of chemical and drug injury to the eye. In Haddad LM, Winchester JF [eds]: Clinical Management of Poisoning and Drug Overdose, 2nd ed. Philadelphia, WB Saunders, 1990. Reproduced by permission.)

Treat such fireworks injuries as alkaline injuries rather than thermal injuries. Treat eye damage from hair straighteners,[33] phosphate-free detergents,[34] and automobile airbags[35] as alkaline injuries also.

Measure the pH of the conjunctival fornices with a pH paper strip to check the effectiveness of irrigation. In addition to litmus paper, the pH indicator on urine multi-indicator sticks can be used. The pH indicator on urine dipsticks is conveniently closest to the handle; all the distal indicator squares can be cut off with scissors. The normal tear film pH is 7.4. Use the noninjured eye as a control if the results are equivocal. If the pH measured in the conjunctival fornices after the initial irrigation is still abnormal, continue irrigation. If the pH is normal after irrigation, wait 20 minutes and check it again to make sure that it remains normal, especially in the presence of an alkaline contamination. Delayed pH changes are usually the result of incomplete irrigation and inadequate swabbing of the fornices. In anticipation of this deficiency,

measure the pH deep in the fornices. Consider double-lid eversion with a lid elevator to expose the upper fornix for swabbing, irrigation, and pH testing (see Fig. 63–12).

Prolonged Irrigation

Alkaline burns may require prolonged irrigation and it is essential to consult ophthalmology in these cases. The Morgan therapeutic lens is a contact lens-type irrigation device, that can provide slow, continuous irrigation once the more vigorous initial irrigation has been done. First, anesthetize the eye with topical anesthetic drops. Then, place the device carefully on the surface of the eye with the lids closed around the intravenous tubing adaptor (Fig. 63–16). Attach the intravenous tubing to the adaptor and provide continuous flow through the device onto the cornea and into the fornices. As the local anesthetic agents wash out during the irrigation process, the device can become uncomfortable, so reapply the anesthetic drops frequently during irrigation for patient

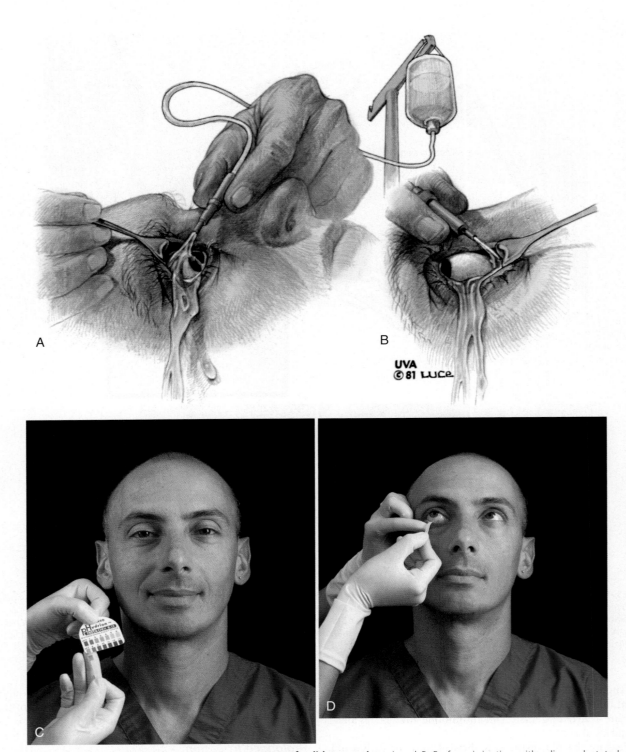

Figure 63–14 Irrigation technique using a Desmarres retractor for lid separation. *A* and *B*, Perform irrigation with saline or lactated Ringer's solution. *C*, For alkaline injuries, check the pH of the eye with pH paper to assess the adequacy of irrigation (normal pH = 7.4). *D*, Because a rebound may occur with alkaline products, *recheck the pH 20–30 min after irrigation to ensure complete removal. (A and B, From Fogle JA, Spyker DA: Management of chemical and drug injury to the eye. In Haddad LM, Winchester JF [eds]: Clinical Management of Poisoning and Drug Overdose, 2nd ed. Philadelphia, WB Saunders, 1990. Reproduced by permission.)*

comfort. Such short-term use of local anesthetics will not inhibit healing of the cornea.

Complications

The only significant complication from irrigation is abrasion of the cornea or the conjunctiva. This can be a mechanical injury from trying to keep the lids open in an uncooperative patient, a small corneal epithelial defect from a Morgan irrigating lens, or a fine punctate keratitis from the irrigation itself.[36] For this reason, do not direct the stream directly onto the cornea. If a superficial corneal defect occurs, treat it in the usual manner. Deep or penetrating corneal injuries are likely to be the result of the caustic chemical and require emergency

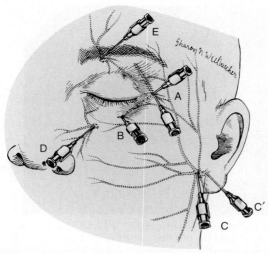

Figure 63–15 Injection points for facial and orbital anesthesia and akinesia. *A,* Van Lint technique of orbicularis infiltration. *B,* Retrobulbar injection site. *C,* O'Brien facial nerve block. *C′,* Alternative facial nerve block by tympanomastoid fissure injection. *D,* Infraorbital sensory block. *E,* Supraorbital sensory block. *Injection of orbicularis (A) or facial nerve (C or C′) permits examination and treatment of the eye in the setting of severe blepharospasm. Anesthesia is placed within several millimeters of the nerves.* (A–D, From Deutsch TA, Feller DB [eds]: Paton and Goldberg's Management of Ocular Injuries, 2nd ed. Philadelphia, WB Saunders, 1985, p 17.)

ophthalmologic consultation. Continue to provide slow continuous irrigation pending the arrival of the ophthalmologist. Some experimental evidence suggests that massive parenteral or oral ascorbic acid supplementation may prevent the development of deep corneal injury,[37] but this treatment has not gained universal acceptance.

Summary

Eye irrigation is easy, and complications associated with the technique are usually minimal. At times, the clinician may be unsure whether a chemical injury is toxic enough to warrant irrigation. If any doubt exists, err on the side of irrigating the eye, rather than omitting this vital procedure and permitting the progression of eye injury.

OCULAR FB REMOVAL

Patients with an external FB in the eye are frequently seen in EDs. They are often in pain and desperate for help. Maintain a high degree of suspicion for FB injuries and perforation of the eye because such injuries might be occult and not readily detected. Not all FB injuries are associated with pain. Glass embedded in the cornea may be particularly difficult to detect. This section is a review of the procedures for locating and removing extraocular FBs and appropriate postprocedural care. Finally, a brief discussion covers evaluating the eye for a potential perforation of the globe and to detect the presence of an intraocular FB.

1153

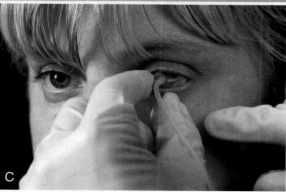
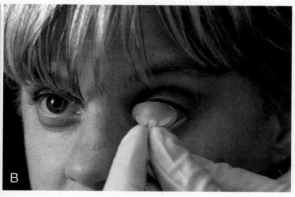
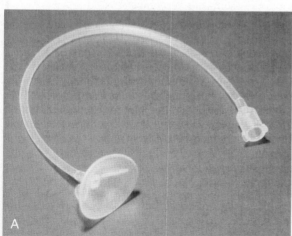

Figure 63–16 *A,* Morgan therapeutic lens: Instill anesthetic drops. Attach the lens to intravenous solution (Ringer's lactate or saline) and start the flow wide open so the Morgan lens floats on the fluid (it does not rest on the cornea). *B,* Insertion: Have the patient look down, insert the lens under the upper lid. Have the patient look up, retract the lower lid, drop the lens in place. *C,* Release the lower lid over the lens and adjust the flow.

Continued

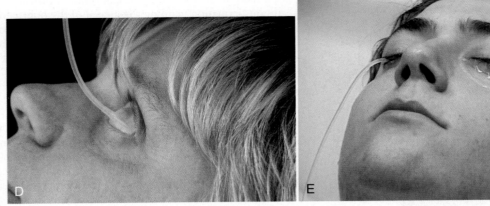

Figure 63–16, cont'd *D,* Tape tubing to the patient's forehead to prevent accidental lens removal. Absorb outflow. DO NOT RUN DRY. To remove, continue the flow, have the patient look up, retract the lower lid—hold position. Slide the lens out; terminate the flow. *E,* Bilateral irrigations. Place the patient's head over a sink. Note: adding 10 ml of 1% lidocaine to a liter of saline irrigating fluid can lessen patient discomfort from prolonged irrigation. *(D, Courtesy of Mortan, Inc., Missoula, MT; E, from Thomsen T, Setnik G [eds]: Procedures Consult—Emergency Medicine Module. Copyright 2008 Elsevier Inc. All rights reserved.)*

Indications and Contraindications

Extraocular FBs must always be removed. The timing of removal and the technique required vary according to the patient's clinical status and the type of injury. For the most part, the emergency clinician can proceed directly to removal of the object using the techniques described in this section. When the patient is extremely uncooperative (e.g., an intoxicated patient, a mentally deficient patient, or a young child) or when the injury is complicated (e.g., deeply embedded object, multiple foreign objects from a blast injury, or possible globe penetration), consult ophthalmology immediately. A patient who presents with a suspected FB or abrasion after exposure to a projectile (e.g., grinding wheel, hammering, metal objects colliding) should be rigorously evaluated for the presence of a deep intraocular FB. See further discussion later in this chapter. A penetrating injury to the cornea is of particular concern because the iris tissue may prolapse and look like a corneal FB (Fig. 63–17). Hence, in addition to the history of projectile exposure, an irregular pupil, especially a pear-shaped pupil, should alert the clinician that a penetrating injury might have occurred.

Globe Protection

In the evaluation of a patient in whom a penetrating injury to the globe is suspected, perform a careful expeditious examination of the eye, preferably with a slit lamp. Avoid any pressure on the eye or rapid eye movements. If perforation is obvious (e.g., teardrop pupil, flaccid globe, flat anterior chamber, prolapsed iris) or confirmed by slit lamp (Seidel's test positive; see Fig. 63–10), do not perform any procedures (save perhaps irrigation) and consult ophthalmology early for definitive diagnosis and care. Until the ophthalmologist has arrived, protect the eye from further harm by keeping the patient quiet, elevating the head of the bed, and placing a protective shield over the eye. Commercial shields are available for this purpose. When a metal shield is not available, construct a makeshift protective shield with available materials (e.g., paper, plastic, or Styrofoam cups; Fig. 63–18). The protective shield functions to avoid pressure on the globe and overlying tissues to prevent extrusion of vitreous and other ocular con-

tents. Extend the shield edges up to or beyond the bony orbital rim for this purpose. Apply adhesive tape over the shield from forehead to cheek to secure the shield in position.

If a patient has a globe perforation, treat with systemic antibiotics (a combination of cefazolin and gentamycin is a good initial choice), tetanus toxoid, and antiemetics in doses aggressive enough to halt vomiting.

Equipment

The following equipment is necessary for extraocular FB removal:

Topical anesthetic, such as proparacaine 0.5%
Sterile cotton-tipped applicators
Fluorescein strips
Magnification: loupes plus a Wood's lamp, Eidolon BLUMINATOR ophthalmic illuminator or a slit lamp
Eye spud or 25-gauge needle attached to a 1- or 3-mL syringe or to the tip of a cotton-tipped applicator
Dilator drops, such as homatropine 5%
Antibiotic ointment, such as erythromycin

Consideration of Intraocular FB

When examining a patient with an ocular "FB" sensation, always remain cognizant of the potential for an intraorbital or intraocular FB. Penetrating injuries represent a greater threat of visual loss than an extraocular FB and can be disastrous if overlooked. Note that an intraocular FB can be deceptively subtle on initial presentation.

The clinical presentation is most helpful in determining which patients are at risk for a penetrating injury to the globe. An individual who complains of an FB sensation in the absence of trauma or one whose history is simply that something "fell" or "blew" into the eye is at low risk for a globe perforation. Conversely, there is a greater probability of globe penetration in the individual who has sustained a high-velocity wound to the eye (e.g., drilling, hammering, grinding metal, blasting rock). The presence of any of the following physical findings should alert the clinician to a probable intraocular FB: irregular pupil, shallow anterior chamber on slit lamp examination,

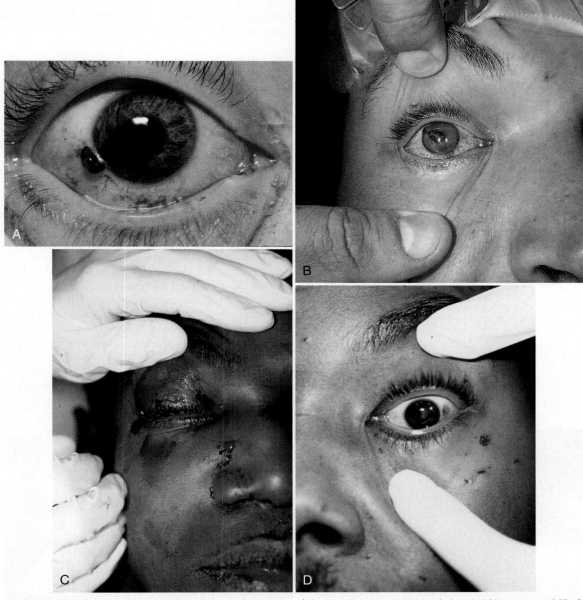

Figure 63–17　Serious eye injuries. *A,* Corneal laceration with prolapse of the iris. The extruded iris is dark, mimicking a corneal FB. Often, the only clue is an abnormal pupil, and the extruded iris may not be appreciated as intraocular tissue. The pupil is irregular (often pear- or teardrop-shaped), pointing toward the laceration. *B,* A pear-shaped pupil without protrusion of the lens is a more subtle, yet characteristic, indication of a perforated globe. *C,* Another indication of a penetrating globe injury is periorbital fat protruding from an upper eyelid laceration. This patient was stabbed by a knife. *D,* This patient has an obviously cloudy lens soon after trauma. A projectile entered the temporal portion of the globe and produced a seemingly minor scleral hemorrhage. Patients with penetrating injuries to the globe should be treated with systemic antibiotics (such as cefazolin/gentamycin combination), tetanus toxoid if indicated, and antiemetics to control vomiting (which raises intraocular pressure). (A, *Courtesy of Lawrence B. Stack, MD.*)

prolapsed iris, positive Seidel's test (see "The Fluorescein Examination," earlier in this chapter), focal conjunctival swelling, hemorrhage, hyphema, lens opacification, and reduced intraocular pressure (IOP). Do not perform tonometry if penetrating injury to the globe is suspected. Be aware that a penetrating injury may not be associated with eye pain. If there is strong historical evidence and physical findings to support a diagnosis of globe penetration, obtain emergent ophthalmologic consultation.

An intraocular FB is often not visible on direct ophthalmoscopy. Although orbital radiography for radiopaque objects and ultrasonography of the globe have been used for indirect FB localization,[15] computed tomography of the orbit is now considered the most useful technique.[38,39] When plain orbital radiography is performed looking for an intraocular FB, be aware that an eyelid FB may mimic an intraocular FB.[40] Patients with a suspected metallic FB should not undergo magnetic resonance imaging if the FB may be intraocular. Therapy for intraocular and intraorbital FBs must be individualized. Often, an ophthalmologist can localize an intraocular FB (if the vitreous is clear) using indirect ophthalmoscopy. The role of the emergency clinician is to suspect

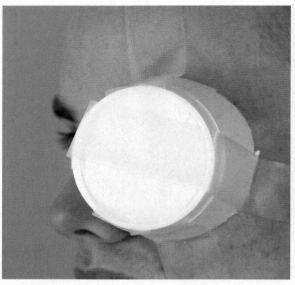

Figure 63–18 When a penetrating globe injury is suspected and a metal shield is not available in the emergency department or prehospital setting, a makeshift shield can be fashioned with available materials. A paper cup was used to fashion this shield.

the diagnosis, to protect the eye from further harm, and to obtain ophthalmologic consultation. The remainder of this section addresses the problem of extraocular FBs.

Procedure

FB Location

The first step is to locate the FB. Apply a drop of topical anesthetic to the inside of the lower lid (see Fig. 63–6*A*). Vertical corneal abrasions from FBs under the lids are helpful for localizing these hidden foreign objects (see Fig. 63–11, *2*). Use a penlight and loupes or a slit lamp to examine the bulbar conjunctiva by having the patient look in all directions. Examine the inside of the lower lid by pulling it down with the thumb while asking the patient to look up. Evert the upper lid by asking the patient to look down as the end of an applicator stick is pressed against the superior edge of the tarsal plate of the upper lid. Meanwhile, grasp the lashes and pull down, out, and then up to flip the eyelid over (Fig. 63–19).

Minute FBs under the lid may be missed with simple visual inspection. Ideally, examine the everted lid under magnification with loupes or a slit lamp. With simple lid eversion, it is still not possible to see the far recesses of the upper conjunctival fornix. Although double eversion of the upper lid (see Fig. 63–12) is helpful, the best way to rule out an FB in the upper fornix is to sweep the anesthetized fornix with a moistened applicator as the upper lid is held everted. Examine the applicator tip for removed foreign material. Small con-

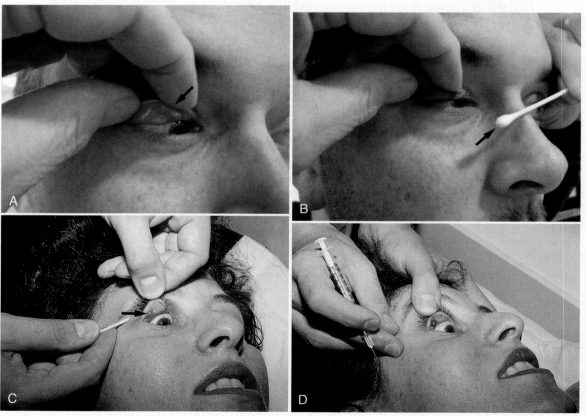

Figure 63–19 This patient complained of an FB in the eye, despite irrigation. *A*, Lid eversion (technique described in Fig. 63–13*D*) revealed a small speck (*arrow*) under the upper lid. This could cause a cornea abrasion characterized by vertical striations. *B*, It was easily removed (*arrow*) by touching it with a moistened cotton-tipped applicator. *C*, This patient presented with a swollen and tender upper eyelid thought to be secondary to a stye. With lid eversion, a small pustule (*arrow*) was found under the upper eyelid. *D*, With a 27-gauge needle, the pustule was incised and a drop of pus was expressed; she made a rapid and uneventful recovery.

junctival FBs not hidden by the lids are often best removed with a moistened nasopharyngeal swab (e.g., nasopharyngeal Calgiswab).

Reexamine the cornea. Most corneal FBs have an area of fluorescein staining around them. Use a slit lamp or other magnification device such as the BLUMINATOR to make the examination easier. If the clinician is limited to loupes and a penlight, shine the light diagonally on the cornea to locate the FB. With a history of a high-speed projectile hitting the eye, rule out an intraocular FB. In the case of a blast injury, multiple FBs may penetrate the eye. If an FB cannot be found on the surface despite a suggestive history, examine the eye for physical evidence of penetration, as discussed earlier. Dilate the pupil, and examine the fundus. Although not fool-proof, bedside ultrasonography may identify the presence of a metallic FB (sensitivity of 87.5%, specificity 95.8%, with positive predictive value and negative predictive value of 96.5% and 85.2%, respectively).[41] If in doubt regarding an intraocular FB, consider computed tomography and ophthalmologic consultation.

FB Removal

Once an extraocular FB is located, the technique of removal depends on whether it is embedded. If the FB is lying on the surface, eject a stream of water from a syringe through a plastic catheter, which will usually wash the object onto the bulbar conjunctiva. Once the FB is on the inner lid or bulbar conjunctiva, gently touch a wetted cotton-tipped applicator to the conjunctiva and the object will adhere to the applicator tip. Be aware that overzealous use of an applicator for corneal FB removal can lead to extensive corneal epithelial injury. A spud device is required for removal of objects that cannot be irrigated off the cornea.

To remove embedded corneal FBs (Fig. 63–20), use a commercial spud device, a bur drill, a short 25- or 27-gauge needle on a small-diameter syringe (e.g., insulin or tuberculin syringe), or a cotton-tipped applicator (Fig. 63–21A and B). Use the applicator or syringe as a handle for the attached needle. Contrary to what one might expect, it is difficult to penetrate the sclera or the cornea with a needle, especially

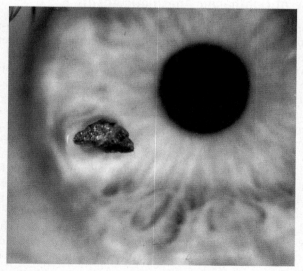

Figure 63–20 This embedded corneal FB is readily seen under slit lamp examination. A removal device (needle, spud, or bur drill) should be used for careful removal. A rust ring will remain if the FB has been there for only a few hours.

when it is applied tangentially to the cornea.[31] As with removal of conjunctival FBs, anesthetize the eye. Position the patient so that the head is well secured (preferably in a slit lamp frame). At this point, provide a simple explanation of the procedure, which usually ensures excellent compliance on the part of the patient. *Rest your hand on the patient's cheek so that unexpected movements on the part of the patient will not result in large movements of the removal device.* Instruct the patient to gaze at an object in the distance (e.g., the practitioner's ear when a slit lamp is used) to further stabilize the eye. Bring the removal device close to the eye under direct vision; then, while it is in focus, manipulate it under the magnification device [e.g., Wood's Lamp, Eidolon BLUMINATOR ophthalmic illuminator (see Fig. 63–9), or slit lamp] to remove the FB. Hold the device tangentially to the globe, and pick up or scoop out the foreign object. If a bur drill is used, press the side of the drill against the FB until removal is accomplished (see Fig. 63–21C).

During removal, rest your hand against the patient's face. It may be also helpful to brace the elbow with a pad or half-full tissue box to provide further support to the arm as the FB is removed. If right-handed, place your lower hand against the left maxillary bone when removing a foreign object from the patient's left eye and against the bridge of the patient's nose or infranasal area when removing an object from the right eye. If left-handed, reverse these positions. Using loupes or a slit lamp for magnification is highly recommended to minimize further injury during removal. In particular, corneal contact with the spud device is more readily discerned when magnification is used. Only topical anesthesia is required to remove FBs from the cornea. Although the patient may feel pressure during FB removal, pain should not be felt after the eye is anesthetized.

Rust Rings

A common problem with metallic FBs is that they develop rust rings (Fig. 63–22). *These can develop within hours* because of oxidation of the iron in the FB. There are two preferred techniques for removal of a rust ring. The most direct is to remove it at the same time as the FB, either with repeated picking away with a spud device or with a rotating bur. The second approach is to let the iron of the rust ring oxidize and kill the surrounding epithelial cells during a 24- to 48-hour period. After that, the rust ring will be soft and often comes out in one solid plug.[42] Generally, a small rust ring produces little visual difficulty unless it is directly in the line of sight. The rust ring, if large, may delay corneal healing. Close follow-up is important to ensure healing of the cornea and total removal of the rust ring and FB.

Multiple FBs

If a patient has multiple FBs in the eye, such as from an explosion, refer him or her to an ophthalmologist. One technique that may be chosen by the ophthalmologist is to denude the entire epithelium with alcohol and remove the superficial FBs. The deeper ones gradually work their way to the surface, sometimes years later.

Aftercare

After removing the FB, an antibiotic ointment is frequently instilled. Although commonly used, the value of the ointment

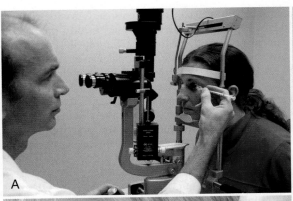

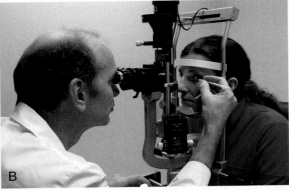

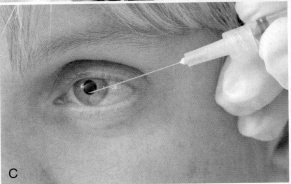

Figure 63–21 It is preferable to remove the corneal FB under the slit lamp. Apply a topical anesthetic and use a small syringe with a short 25- to 27-gauge needle (such as a tuberculin syringe). *Be certain that the needle is firmly attached to the syringe.* A, Under direct vision (not looking through the slit lamp), bring the syringe close to the eye while resting the hand on the patient's cheek. Be sure that the patient's forehead maintains continual contact with the crossbar on the slit lamp. B, While looking through the slit lamp, bring the needle to the cornea and remove the FB. C, Hold the side of the instrument (drill bit or beveled edge of the needle) *tangential to the cornea.* (A and B, From Knoop K, Trott A: Ophthalmologic procedures in the emergency department—Part III: Slit lamp use and foreign bodies. Acad Emerg Med 2:224, 1995. Reproduced by permission.)

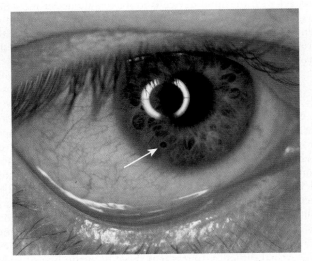

Figure 63–22 A typical rust ring is seen at 8 o'clock on the cornea (*arrow*). Essentially, these are retained FBs, and are removed in a similar manner. Rust rings can form in only a few hours. Most rust rings should be removed, but there is no urgency. Small ones out of the line of sight may remain. A bur drill can be used for attempted removal, which if unsuccessful, can be reattempted in 24 hr. Alternatively, a small needle can be used to loosen the edges, then scoop out the ring. Both procedures will leave a corneal abrasion. *(From Knoop KJ, Stack LB, Storrow AB [eds]: Atlas of Emergency Medicine, 2nd ed. New York, McGraw-Hill, 2002. Reproduced by permission.)*

for superficial corneal defects after FB removal is unproved, and no specific standard of care is supported by scientific evidence. Conjunctival and corneal abrasions do not need patching. Data suggest that eye patching offers no benefit in healing corneal abrasions secondary to FBs.[43] If the patient sustains a superficial injury from the FB, instruct her or him

to return only if the eye does not feel completely normal or if there is any blurred vision. The majority of superficial injuries heal without difficulty. The patient should be warned that the FB sensation might return temporarily when the anesthetic agent has worn off. One animal study with direct ocular exposure to *Clostridium tetani* organisms suggested that nonpenetrating ocular injuries are unlikely to lead to tetanus.[44] Tetanus prophylaxis after a corneal FB removal is not standard, but it may be considered. However, tetanus prophylaxis appears essential for injuries that penetrate through the cornea or sclera.

Use of Ophthalmic Anesthetic Agents

Application of topical anesthetic agents can be both diagnostic and therapeutic. Relief of discomfort with topical anesthetic use often suggests, but does not ensure, a conjunctival or corneal injury. An ocular irritant may also be masked by the use of these agents. Classic teaching is that patients should not self-administer the anesthetic preparations. It is thought that they delay wound healing by disrupting surface microvilli causing a decrease in the tear film layer and tear break-up time.[45] Although self-administered topical anesthetic agents are now routinely used after photorefractive keratectomy (PRK) surgery for the first 3 or 4 postoperative days, this has not become a part of the ED practice.[46] The absence of protective reflexes while the patient is under the effect of the medicine may encourage the patient to use the eye while an FB or a corneal infection inflicts further corneal injury. While not advised for outpatient use, topical anesthetic drops can be used safely for a few days without documented adverse effects.

Bartfield and coworkers[47] found that the pain of instillation of 0.5% proparacaine was significantly less than that of 0.5% tetracaine. As evident from Table 63–3, the anesthetic

TABLE 63–3 Ophthalmic Anesthetic Agents

Generic Name	Trade Name	Concentration (%)	Onset of Anesthesia	Duration of Anesthesia (min)	Comments
Tetracaine	Pontocaine	0.5–1.0	<1 min	15–20	Marked stinging; also available in ointment
Proparacaine	Ophthaine, Ophthetic	0.5	<20 sec	10–15	Least irritating; no cross-sensitization with other agents
Benoxinate	Dorsacaine	0.4	1–2 min	10–15	Only anesthetic compatible with fluorescein in solution

solutions commonly used have a duration of action of less than 20 minutes. The patient with a large corneal lesion may need a more extended period of pain relief. The discomfort associated with a large healing corneal lesion is usually made tolerable by bedrest, opioid analgesics, and appropriate sedatives. Even in the absence of infection or a retained FB, the long-term repeated use of ophthalmic anesthetic ointments might be detrimental to corneal healing.[48]

A final word of caution should be added regarding the use of ophthalmic solutions. Guaiac solutions are commonly supplied in dropper bottles similar in size and appearance to those containing ophthalmic solutions. Well-intentioned ED personnel may store the guaiac reagent bottles with the ophthalmic bottles. One should encourage both color-coding of the bottles and examination of them and their labels before each use to avoid corneal injury from inadvertently instilling guaiac reagent in the eye.

Complications

Complications associated with ocular FB removal are rare. The most frequent problem is incomplete removal of the FB. In such cases, the epithelium has difficulty healing over the affected area, and thus the eye stays inflamed. Eventually, the diseased epithelium either sloughs off and heals or heals over the FB remnants, which are gradually absorbed. In either case, the adverse effects on the eye are minimal; a minute scar on the cornea, even directly in the center, will rarely affect the vision. Nonetheless, incomplete removal of a corneal foreign object warrants ophthalmologic follow-up.

Conjunctivitis may develop after removal of an extraocular FB. In most cases, the bacteria producing the infection are introduced by the patient through rubbing of the irritated eye.

Although perforation of the globe by the clinician's spud device is theoretically possible, this complication is exceedingly rare. Treatment of this type of corneal puncture wound consists of antibiotics, eye shield placement, and ophthalmologic consultation. In the absence of resultant endophthalmitis, permanent sequelae are unlikely to develop.

Epithelial injury can occur when cotton-tipped applicators are vigorously used to remove corneal FBs. Indeed, the use of cotton-tipped applicators for embedded corneal FB removal is condemned.

Summary

Ocular FBs are one of the most common eye emergencies. Searching for and removing the FB is usually straightforward. The only real trap is missing an intraocular FB. This must be ruled out if there is a history of a high-speed projectile hitting the eye or if physical findings suggest globe penetration.

Use of Ophthalmic Nonsteroidal Anti-Inflammatory Drugs

Ophthalmic nonsteroidal anti-inflammatory drugs (NSAIDs) have been evaluated for their effectiveness in the treatment of traumatic corneal abrasions. Examples include ketorolac tromethamine, diclofenac, and flurbiprofen. These agents are safe to use and effective for the relief of pain associated with corneal abrasions.[49-52]

EYE PATCHING

Patching the lids shut has traditionally been the last step in treatment of a number of common eye emergencies; however, multiple studies have shown that eye patching offers no benefit in pain relief or healing rates with conjunctival or corneal abrasions.[43,53-55] A meta-analysis of studies on eye patching and corneal abrasions or ulcers showed that patching might actually slow healing rates and patients might actually have worsening of pain. This was found to be true in children as well.[56-58] Patching is also contraindicated in contact lens wearers and in situations in which the abrasion or ulcer may be infected.[54] In summary, eye patching is no longer indicated and might actually worsen the ophthalmologic process that it once was thought to help. The use of a therapeutic bandage contact lens applied directly to the cornea has been recommended as a possible treatment for corneal epithelial defects. Evidence from several small studies suggests that a bandage contact lens is safe, effective, and well tolerated and allows a significant number of patients to immediately resume their regular activities while maintaining baseline visual acuity. Further study for the application of this modality in the ED setting is needed.[59-62]

CONTACT LENS PROCEDURES

An estimated 24 million Americans wear a form of contact lenses.[63] Removal of these lenses in the ED may be required to permit further evaluation of the eye or to prevent injury from prolonged wear. Emergency clinicians also evaluate patients for "lost" contact lenses, which may be trapped under the upper lid. At times, the patient may request that the clinician remove a lens that he or she has failed to extract from the cornea. Corneal ulcers may occur in patients who wear contact lenses and may require prompt treatment. This section on contact lens procedures addresses these concerns and discusses injuries associated with removal attempts, the mechanism of injury from prolonged wear, and instructions to be given to patients at discharge.

The first contact lenses were scleral lenses made of glass. These lenses, covering the cornea as well as much of the surrounding sclera, are reported to have been in use from 1888 to 1948.[64] Glass corneal lenses (sitting entirely on the cornea) made by the Carl Zeiss Optical Works of Jena were first described in 1912. A practical synthetic scleral lens using methyl methacrylate rather than glass was discussed by Obrig and Mullen in 1938.[65,66] In 1947, Tuohy redeveloped the corneal lens using methyl methacrylate.[67] This was the forerunner of the current hard contact lens.[67] The development in Czechoslovakia of lenses made of soft gas-permeable polymers was reported in 1960.[68] These hydrogel (hydrophilic gelatinous–like) lenses have evolved into today's soft contact lenses. Soft contact lenses now come in a variety of types including extended and daily wear. The majority of soft contact lenses in use are now disposable.

Mechanism of Corneal Injury from Contact Lens Wear

Hard Contact Lenses

The oxygenation of the cornea is dependent on movement of oxygen-rich tears under the hard contact lens during blinking. During the "adaptation" phase of early wear, the wearer of hard contact lenses produces hypotonic tears as a result of mechanical irritation from the lens.[64] This results in corneal edema, which reduces subsequent tear flow under the lens during blinking. Overwearing a lens at this time leads to corneal ischemia, with superficial epithelial defects predominantly in the central corneal area (see Fig. 63–11), where the least tear flow occurs. With adaptation, the tears become isotonic and the blinking rate normalizes, permitting increased wear time. During early adaptation, blinking is more rapid than normal and then slows to a subnormal rate during late adaptation. Mucus delivery to the cornea in the tear film may also play an important role in maintaining corneal lubrication. Tight-fitting contact lenses may never permit good tear flow despite an adaptation phase; individuals with tightly fitted lenses may never be able to wear their original contact lenses for longer than 6 to 8 hours. Lenses that are excessively loose can also cause irritation by moving during blinking. Rough or cracked edges can cause corneal abrasions.

In the ED, the patient who presents with irritation caused by prolonged wear may be either a new or an adapted wearer. The adapted wearer may have been exposed to chemical irritants (e.g., smoke), which reduce the tonicity of tears and lead to corneal edema and decreased tear flow. Alternatively, the adapted wearer with irritation may have ingested sedatives (e.g., alcohol) or may have fallen asleep wearing the contact lenses, thus decreasing blinking and tear flow. Another possibility is that the patient may actually be wearing tight-fitting contact lenses that have never allowed true adaptation despite many months of wear.

The patient with the overwear syndrome usually awakens a few hours after removing the lenses. The patient experiences intense pain and tearing similar to that caused by an FB. The delay in the onset of symptoms until after removal of the lenses is caused by a temporary corneal anesthesia produced by the anoxic metabolic byproducts that build up during extended lens wear.[69] A second factor is the slow passage of microcysts of edema, which are pushed up to the corneal surface by mitosis of the underlying cells. When the cysts break open on the surface, the corneal nerve endings are exposed.[70]

Most patients with the overwear syndrome can be managed with reassurance, frequent administration of artifi-cial tears, oral analgesics, and advice to "wait it out" in a darkened room. Some patients require patching for comfort. A patient who has experienced no problems with contact lenses before an overwear episode can return to using the lenses after 2 or 3 days of wearing glasses but should be advised to build up wearing time gradually. A patient who was having chronic problems with lens comfort before the episode should check with an ophthalmologist before using the contact lenses again.

Soft Contact Lenses

Although there is also oxygenation of the cornea by way of the tear film with soft contact lenses, only approximately one tenth of the flow behind the lens that occurs with a hard lens is present during soft contact wear.[64] The high degree of lens gas permeability permits the majority of oxygenation to occur directly through the lens. The hydrogel lens is more comfortable than the hard contact lens because lid motion over the lens is smooth. The minimization of lid and corneal irritation allows a more rapid adaptation phase because the initial reflex-induced tearing and blinking changes are reduced. Nonetheless, the lenses may still lead to corneal edema and secondary hypoxic epithelial changes if worn for an excessive period when blinking is inhibited. Some individuals can tolerate the lenses for extended periods and may on occasion sleep with the contact lenses in place, although this practice is not encouraged. Newer extended-wear hydrogel lenses (e.g., Permalens) permit wear for several days without injury. These lenses are not discernible from standard soft lenses on examination.

Although the acute overwear syndrome that occurs with hard contact lenses can also occur with soft lenses, it is infrequent. More commonly, ocular damage from soft contact lenses falls into one of three categories:

1. Corneal neovascularization. Often, the patient is asymptomatic, but on slit lamp examination, fine vessels are seen invading the peripheral cornea. Refer the patient to an ophthalmologist to refit with looser or thinner lenses or with contact lenses that are more gas permeable.
2. Giant papillary conjunctivitis.[71] The patient notes decreased lens tolerance and increased mucus production. On examination of the tarsal conjunctiva (best seen on eversion of the upper lid), large papillae are seen. These grossly appear as a cobblestoned surface. Instruct the patient to discontinue wearing the lenses until the process reverses and to see an ophthalmologist to have the lenses refitted.
3. A sensitivity reaction to the contact lens solutions (usually thimerosol or chlorhexidine).[72,73] There is diffuse conjunctival injection and sometimes a superficial keratitis. Advise the patient to switch to preservative-free saline with the use of heat sterilization. Often, the contact lenses will need to be replaced before lens wear can be resumed.

All of these problems with soft lenses have bilateral, sub-acute onsets and do not require emergency treatment. The only form of ocular damage associated with soft contact lenses that is a true emergency is a bacterial (often *Pseudomonas* or *Acanthamoeba* with soft contact lenses) or fungal corneal ulcer.[74–76] Because the nature of soft contact lenses is to absorb water, they can also absorb pathogens, which then can invade the cornea. This is especially true if the soft lens is worn continuously for extended periods of time. The patient presents with a painful, red eye with associated discharge and a white infiltrate on the cornea. Immediately consult an ophthalmologist for appropriate culturing and antimicrobial treatment. These infections can permanently affect the patient's visual acuity.

Indications for Removal

Remove a contact lens in the following situations:

1. Contact lens wearer with an altered state of consciousness. The emergency clinician should always be aware that the patient with a depressed or acutely agitated sensorium might be unable to express the need to have her or his contact lenses removed. Furthermore, it is likely that patients with a depressed sensorium will have decreased lid motion. During the secondary survey of these patients, identify the presence of the lenses and arrange for their removal and storage to prevent harm from excessive wear or possible accidental dislodgment at a later time. Without magnification, soft contact lenses may be difficult to see. Examine the eye with an obliquely directed penlight to reveal the edge of the soft lens 1 to 2 mm from the limbus on the bulbar conjunctiva.

2. Eye trauma with lens in place. After measurement of visual acuity with the patient's lenses in place, remove them and perform a more detailed examination of the cornea. Fluorescein may discolor hydrogel lenses; when possible, remove extended-wear lenses before using this chemical. After the dye is instilled, flush the eyes with normal saline. Advise the patient to wait at least 1 hour before reinserting the lenses.[64] The availability of single-use droppers of 0.35% fluorexon (Fluresoft) has permitted the safe staining of eyes when soft lenses are to be worn immediately after the examination. A limited eye irrigation after the use of fluorexon drops is still recommended before the reinsertion of soft contact lenses.

3. Inability of the patient to remove the contact lens. A patient may present with a hard contact lens that cannot be removed because of corneal edema from prolonged wear. Alternatively, the patient may present with a "lost" contact lens believed to be behind the upper lid. There is no urgency for contact removal in the out-of-hospital setting; hence, removal can wait until the patient has been evaluated by a clinician.

Contraindication to Removal

The only major problem with contact lens removal occurs when the cornea may be perforated. In this case, the suction cup technique of removal, described later, is preferred.

Procedure

Hard Contact Lens Removal

A number of maneuvers have been devised for removal of the corneal lens. One technique is to first lean the patient's face over a table or a collecting cloth. Pull the lids temporally from the lateral palpebral margin to lock the lids against the contact lens edges. Ask the patient to look toward the nose and then downward toward the chin. This movement works the lower eyelid under the lower lens edge and flips the lens off the eye. The technique requires a cooperative patient because the clinician must pull the patient's lids tightly against the edge of the contact lens. The movement of the patient's eye then flips the contact free.

In the unresponsive patient in the supine position, modify the technique. Take a more active role in lid movement using

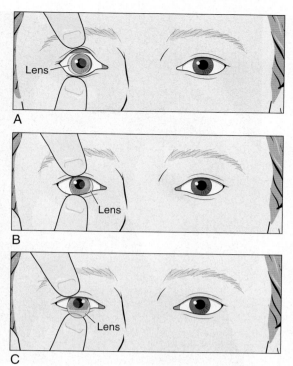

Figure 63–23 Manual technique for removing a hard contact lens. *A,* Separate the eyelids. *B,* Entrap the lens edges with the eyelids. *C,* Expel the lens by forcing the lower lid under the inferior edge of the lens. (*A–C, From Grant HD, Murray RH, Bergeron JF [eds]: Brady Emergency Care, 5th ed. Englewood Cliffs, NJ, Prentice Hall, 1990, p 338. Reproduced by permission.*)

the following procedure: Place one thumb on the upper eyelid and the other on the lower eyelid near the margin of each lid. With the lens centered over the cornea, open the eyelids until the lid margins are beyond the edges of the lens (Fig. 63–23*A*). Then press both eyelids gently but firmly on the globe of the eye and move the lids so that they are barely touching the edges of the lens (see Fig. 63–23*B*). Press slightly harder on the lower lid to move it under the bottom edge of the lens. As the lower edge of the lens begins to tip away from the eye, move the lids together, allowing the lens to slide out to where it can be grasped (see Fig. 63–23*C*). Remember to use clean hands (and preferably wear examination gloves that have been rinsed in tap water or saline) when removing the lens.

Alternatively, move the lens gently off the cornea using a cotton-tipped applicator to guide the lens onto the sclera. Force the applicator tip under an edge of the lens and flip the contact loose. Use topical anesthesia when using an applicator and the patient is awake. Take care with this technique to avoid contact of the applicator with the cornea when the lens is moved off the eye. Perhaps the easiest technique is to use a moistened suction-tipped device and simply lift the lens off the cornea (Fig. 63–24).

Several lenses (those hard contact lenses that cover both the cornea and an amount of the sclera) can be removed by an exaggeration of the manual technique described earlier (Fig. 63–25). Elevation of the lens with a cotton-tipped applicator or a suction-tipped device is also an effective technique. Soft contact lenses should not be removed with a suction-tipped device because tearing or splitting of the lens might occur.

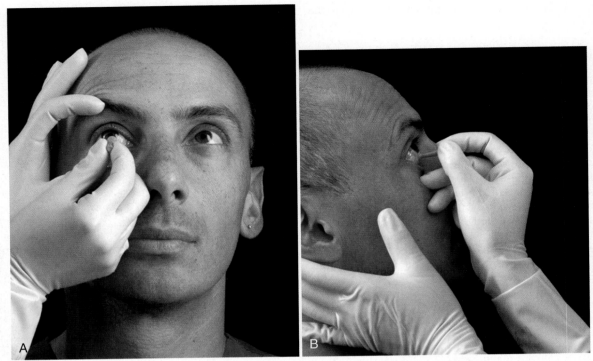

Figure 63–24 *A* and *B*, Use of a moistened suction cup to remove a hard contact lens.

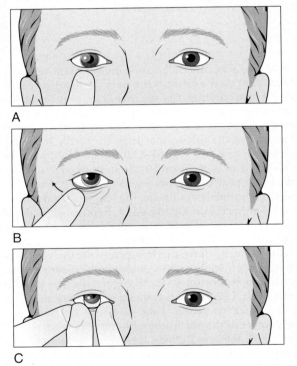

Figure 63–25 **Removal of a hard scleral lens.** *A,* Separate the eyelids. *B,* Force the lower lid beneath the edge of the scleral lens by temporal traction on the lower lid. *C,* Lift the lens off the eye. *(A–C, From Grant HD, Murray RH, Bergeron JF [eds]: Brady Emergency Care, 5th ed. Englewood Cliffs, NJ, Prentice Hall, 1990, p 338. Reproduced by permission.)*

Soft Contact Lens Removal

With clean hands (preferably using gloves rinsed in saline or tap water), pull down the lower eyelid using the middle finger. Place the tip of the index finger on the lower edge of the lens. Slide the lens down onto the sclera and compress it slightly between the thumb and the index finger. This pinching motion folds the lens so it can be removed from the eye (Fig. 63–26). Alternatively, use a cotton-tipped applicator (e.g., Q-Tip) instead of a gloved hand. Occasionally, a tight-fitting lens will be difficult to remove. One potential method is the use of topical anesthetic drops, lubricating eye drops (e.g., Refresh Celluvisc lubricant eye drops) and a cotton-tipped applicator to lift the edge of the lens from the limbus. This breaks the seal of the lens on the cornea and allows removal.

Lens Storage

After a contact lens is removed, store it in sterile normal saline solution. Use the patient's own storage container and lens solution if available. A variety of alternative sterile containers are available for use in the ED. Be certain to keep right and left lenses separate and in appropriately labeled containers. The containers should be kept with the patient until a friend or family member can procure them, or they should be locked with the patient's valuables.

Evaluation of the "Lost" Contact

A patient may present with a request to be examined for a "lost" contact lens. The patient may be unsure whether the lens is hidden under a lid, remains on the cornea, or is truly outside the eye. The evaluation of the patient with a "lost" contact should begin, as should all eye examinations, with the

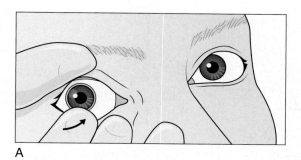

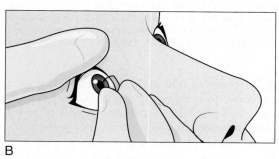

Figure 63–26 **Removal of a soft contact lens.** *A,* Separate the eyelids and then move the contact onto the sclera with the index finger. *B,* Pinch the lens between the thumb and index finger. (*A and B, From Grant HD, Murray RH, Bergeron JF [eds]: Brady Emergency Care, 5th ed. Englewood Cliffs, NJ, Prentice Hall, 1990, p 338. Reproduced by permission.)*

measurement of visual acuity. Measure visual acuity preferably using a 20-foot eye chart. Diminished visual acuity in the eye with the lost contact is convincing evidence that the lens is missing, although transparent, soft contact lenses in proper position are usually seen when viewed closely with loupes or a slit lamp. The lens forms a fine line where it ends on the sclera several millimeters peripherally to the limbus. Hard contact lenses are even more evident as they change in position on the cornea.

If the contact is not evident on initial inspection, evert the lids as discussed in the section on "Ocular FB Removal" (double eversion of the upper lid). If the lens is still not visible, place a drop of topical anesthetic in the eye. Gently sweep the upper fornix with a moistened cotton-tipped applicator while the patient looks toward the chin. If the lens is still not evident even though the patient remains insistent that it is in the eye, perform a fluorescein examination after explaining that the dye will color the lens (permanently). Evert the upper lid again and examine with an ultraviolet light source.

If the lens remains elusive, reassure the patient that a thorough examination was performed and that no object was located under the eyelids or on the cornea. Next, examine the cornea for defects that warrant antibiotic ointment and a pressure patch placed over the eye (as discussed in "Eye Patching"). Follow-up with the patient's eye specialist for a replacement lens and provide further reassurance. Ask the patient to retrace movements at the time the contact began to give trouble or was missed. Check the clothing being worn at that time and look for the lens there. A final possibility is that the patient may have accidentally placed the two lenses together in the same side of the carrying case, causing them to stick together. Hence, take a methodical approach, as outlined earlier, to ensure that no lens remains hidden in the eye.

Complications of Lens Removal

A corneal abrasion can occur during lens removal. It is difficult at times to determine whether the injury was produced by the patient or was a result of the removal by the clinician. Fortunately, the corneal injury is usually of a superficial nature and responds well to eye patching or other symptomatic care.

Summary

Contact lens removal is usually simple. Challenging situations include identifying patients at risk for corneal injury due to overuse, helping patients who have lost a contact lens in the eye, and providing aftercare instructions for patients with contact lens–related problems.

INFECTIOUS KERATITIS

Infectious keratitis with corneal ulceration can have a variety of causes, including the overwear of contact lenses. Diagnosis of a corneal ulcer requires the use of a slit lamp and an accurate determination of the patient's history. Infectious keratitis is a frequent problem in ophthalmic practice. Herpes simplex is a common corneal pathogen. *Acanthamoeba* is another pathogen particularly associated with contact lens use and exposure to organism-tainted environments. When a patient presents to the ED with a corneal ulcer, promptly refer the patient to an ophthalmologist. When immediate referral is not possible, obtain telephone guidance from the ophthalmologist in order to initiate therapy and arrange for ophthalmology follow-up within 24 hours.

Patients with herpes simplex keratitis often give a history of prior episodes of the disease. Patients who undergo almost any form of corneal stress may sustain an activation of preexisting corneal disease. Herpes simplex keratitis is classically recognized by its dendritic pattern on fluorescein staining.

Acanthamoeba keratitis is a disease with potentially devastating consequences. Its frequency seems to be increasing, particularly in contact lens wearers, and its pathophysiology is not completely understood. Patients often present with a red eye in which initial bacterial culture results are negative.

Bacterial keratitis occurs in a variety of settings. Organisms range from the relatively common *Staphylococcus* (including methicillin-resistant *Staphylococcus aureus*) or *Streptococcus* to *Mycobacterium*, which can be difficult to identify. A variety of antibiotics are used against bacterial agents. Ciprofloxacin is a quinolone that has demonstrated efficacy against most of the common causative agents. Bacterial organisms in the cornea can develop resistance to any antibiotic, and resistance to fluoroquinolones has also been observed.[77] Ideally, treatment follows culturing of the ulcer.

In instances in which a cellular infiltrate is seen on slit lamp examination and in which there will be a delay of hours before an ophthalmologic consultant can culture the patient, it is prudent to initiate therapy with topical ciprofloxacin. In such circumstances, under the telephone guidance of the consultant, obtain corneal cultures before starting the antibiotic. One approach is to lightly touch a culture-moistened cotton-tipped swab against the ulcer and then streak standard culture media. If the ulcer is chronic or the patient is immunocompromised, a fungal organism may be the causative agent.

Finally, a saline-moistened cotton-tipped swab may be used to obtain a Gram stain of the ulcer. Initiation of therapy before obtaining specimens for culture makes the subsequent identification of an organism difficult. For this reason, consider the circumstances of the individual case before initiating treatment.

TONOMETRY

Tonometry is the estimation of IOP. It is obtained by measuring the resistance of the eyeball to indentation by an applied force. Prolonged elevated IOP is associated with visual field loss and blindness. Sudden elevation of IOP can result from trauma or primary angle-closure glaucoma. Patients with primary angle-closure glaucoma often come to the ED with systemic complaints including nausea, vomiting, and headache. Occasionally, these patients are surprisingly free of pain in or about the eye. The emergency clinician must determine the IOP and its relationship to the systemic symptoms.

Ophthalmologists depended on tactile estimation of eye pressure until the 1860s when von Graefe developed the first mechanical tonometer.[3,13] Applanation tonometry was introduced in 1885 by Maklakoff[78] but was not popularized until Goldmann[79] improved the instrument in the 1930s. Schiøtz[80] developed an impression tonometer in 1905 and modified it in the 1920s; this form is still in use today. Aside from modifications in configuration, current tonometers closely resemble the devices popularized by Schiøtz[80] and Goldmann.[79] The most dramatic variations are the Mackay-Marg tonometer,[81] which permits a continuous tonographic recording, and the noncontact tonometer, a pneumatic applanation tonometer.[82] Pocket-sized tonometers using the MacKay-Marg tonometer principle are available. One such device is the Tono-Pen XL (Reichert, Inc, Depew, NY).[83] These devices are portable, lightweight, and relatively accurate, with built-in provisions for calibration. They have the advantage of a one-time-use replaceable cover that eliminates concern about the possible transmission of an infectious agent. Whereas numerous devices are available, the Schiøtz tonometer is the standard way for emergency clinicians to measure IOP.

Tonometric Techniques

Three tonometric techniques are reliable and clinically useful for estimating IOP:
1. The impression method uses a plunger (3 mm in diameter) to deform the cornea and the "indentation" is then measured. This technique was popularized by Schiøtz[80] and commonly bears his name.
2. The MacKay-Marg method[81] is a refined version of the impression technique in which smaller amounts of cornea are indented.
3. In the applanation method, a planar surface is pressed against the cornea.

The Schiøtz tonometer (Fig. 63–27) actually measures the total IOP (initial pressure plus the pressure added by the weight of the tonometer and the plunger). Friedenwald[84] empirically found that a "rigidity coefficient" could be introduced to allow an estimation of the true IOP. One must be aware, however, that calculated conversion tables for Schiøtz tonometers use an average estimate of the rigidity coefficient and, hence, are not accurate when eye rigidity is altered (e.g., after scleral buckle procedures for retinal detachment or with extreme myopia).

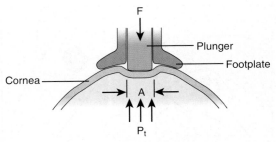

Figure 63–27 Principle of impression tonometry in the Schiøtz tonometer. In reality, P_t is increased slightly by the weight of the instrument. *(From Draeger J, Jessen K: Tonometry and tonography. In Bellows JG [ed]: Glaucoma: Contemporary International Concepts. New York, Masson Publishing USA, 1979. Reproduced by permission.)*

Measurement of IOP in the ED by tonometry is a technique available to most emergency clinicians. Tonometry is not a standard procedure for many eye-related complaints, but special situations in which tonometry may be particularly helpful are

- Confirmation of a clinical diagnosis of acute angle-closure glaucoma. The middle-aged or elderly patient who presents with acute aching pain in one eye, blurred vision (including "halos" around lights), and a red eye with a smoky cornea and a fixed midposition pupil obviously needs a pressure reading. Sometimes, the findings are less dramatic, and sometimes, the patient complains mostly of nausea and vomiting that suggest a "flu" rather than an eye disorder.
- Determination of a baseline ocular pressure after blunt ocular injury. Patients with hyphema often have acute rises in IOP because of blood obstructing the trabecular meshwork.[85] Later, angle recession can cause a permanent form of open-angle glaucoma. Arts and colleagues[86] suggested that an IOP greater than 22 mm Hg or a difference of 3 mm Hg or greater between eyes is a good marker for "ocular injury" in the setting of an orbital fracture.

Tonometry may also be considered under the following scenarios:

- Determination of a baseline ocular pressure in a patient with iritis. Patients with iritis can develop both open- and closed-angle glaucoma as well as corticosteroid-induced glaucoma. Because most cases of iritis are referred, tonometry may also be deferred unless there are signs of increased IOP.
- Documentation of ocular pressure in the patient at risk for open-angle glaucoma. All patients older than 40 years with a familial history of open-angle glaucoma, optic disk changes, visual field defects, and pressures of 21 mm Hg or higher should be referred to an ophthalmologist for further workup. Referral should also be made for those patients with suspiciously cupped disks who have normal pressures; some of these patients may have "low-pressure" glaucoma associated with visual field defects. This is usually part of an ophthalmologist's examination.

Contraindications to Tonometry

Tonometry is relatively contraindicated in eyes that are infected unless one is using a device such as the Tono-Pen

XL, which uses a sterilized cover.[2] Sterilize a tonometer before and after applying it to a potentially infected eye. Measure infected eyes with either a noncontact tonometer or a device with a covered tip (e.g., Tono-Pen). Swab the contact portions of any device with alcohol and allow it to dry before using on another eye. Not all viruses are destroyed by alcohol cleansing. Hydrogen peroxide is effective for deactivating the human immunodeficiency virus responsible for the acquired immunodeficiency syndrome (AIDS). Ultraviolet sterilization, cold-sterilizer bathing of the footplate and plunger, and ethylene oxide sterilization have all been advocated as alternatives to sterilizing the Schiøtz tonometer tip. The Schiøtz tonometer may also be used with sterile disposable coverings (marketed as Tonofilm). Nonetheless, defer the measurement of IOP in an obviously infected eye until a subsequent visit to the ED or private clinician unless the red eye demands an immediate determination of IOP.

Examples of indications for immediate tonometry in the setting of a red eye are suspected angle-closure glaucoma (acute onset of redness and pain in the eye with smoky vision, a cloudy cornea, and a fixed pupil in mid-dilation, often with headache and nausea) and iritis (ciliary injection with photophobia), in which secondary angle-closure or corticosteroid-induced pressure changes may occur (Fig. 63–28). Reported cases of conjunctivitis spread by tonometry predominantly tend to be viral infections. Particular efforts should be made to avoid use of the instrument on patients with active facial or ocular herpetic lesions or who may have AIDS.

The presence of corneal defects also represents a relative contraindication to tonometry.[3,13] The use of a tonometer on

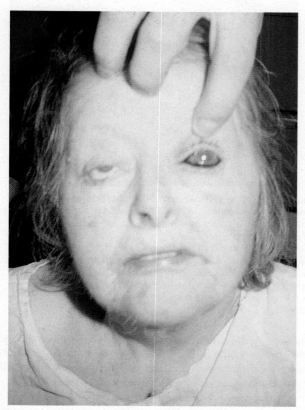

Figure 63–28 This woman complained of severe headache, nausea and blurry vision. The eye was obviously red, the pupil was dilated and minimally reactive, and the cornea was slightly cloudy. This is acute angle-closure glaucoma.

an abraded cornea may lead to further injury and is commonly deferred until a subsequent visit. Patients who cannot maintain a relaxed position (e.g., because of significant apprehension, blepharospasm, uncontrolled coughing, nystagmus, or uncontrolled hiccups) are unlikely to permit an adequate examination and can receive corneal injury when sudden movements occur during an examination. Furthermore, tonometric examination, with the exception of the palpation technique (through the lids) and the noncontact method, should not be performed on a cornea without complete anesthesia.

Tonometry should not be performed with a suspected penetrating ocular injury.[2] Globe perforation may be exacerbated by pressure on the globe with resultant extrusion of intraocular contents. Slit lamp examination can be used for detection of a possible perforation.

Procedure

Palpation Technique

All forms of tonometry are essentially ways of determining the ease of deforming the eye; an eye that is easily deformed has a low pressure. The most direct way to do this is simply to press on the sclera through the lids and grossly compare one eye with the other. One can easily distinguish the rock-hard eye of acute glaucoma from the normal opposite eye by this method. Direct the patient to look down without closing the lids. Rest both hands upon the patient's forehead and apply just enough digital pressure on the involved eye to indent it slightly with one index finger. With the other index finger, alternately feel and compare the compliance of the other eye (Fig. 63–29). An experienced examiner is able to estimate the IOP within 3 to 5 mm Hg of the actual IOP with the palpation technique, but most emergency clinicians do not have enough experience to trust this method.[31]

Another method is to anesthetize the eyes topically and press a wetted applicator on the sclera of each eye. Again, eye deformation is inversely related to ocular pressure. Rigidity of the globe also is a factor in this crude method of tonometry.

Impression (Schiøtz) Technique

Use of the Schiøtz tonometer requires relaxation on the part of the patient and steadiness on the part of the clinician. Place the patient in either a supine or a semi-recumbent position and instruct him or her to gaze at a spot directly above the eyes. A spot on the ceiling should suffice; alternatively, the patient can stretch the arm up over the head and gaze at the thumb. Place a drop of topical anesthetic in each eye. After the irritation of the drop passes, allow the patient to blink while blotting the tears away with a tissue. Rubbing the eyes lowers IOP. Reassure the patient that further discomfort will not occur during the procedure.

Ask the patient to keep both eyes wide open and fixed on an object. Separate the eyelids on the side you are standing on. Test the tonometer on a flat surface to confirm smooth movement of the device (Fig. 63–30). Take care to direct pressure onto the orbital rims rather than into the orbit, because pressure directed into the orbit falsely raises the reading. Hold the tonometer momentarily over the open eye, and inform the patient that the instrument will block vision in the one eye. Instruct the patient to continue to gaze at the fixation point as though the instrument were not there. After the patient relaxes the involuntary muscle contraction that occurs when the instrument is first placed in the line of sight,

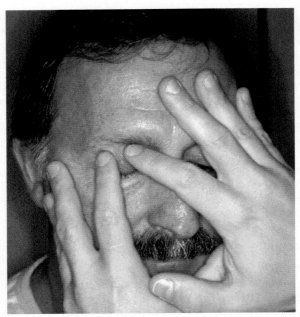

Figure 63–29 The relatively unskilled examiner can detect very high intraocular pressure of acute angle-closure glaucoma with tactile tonometry. The examiner rests both hands on the patient's forehead and alternately applies just enough digital pressure on the globe to indent it slightly with one index finger while feeling the compliance of the globe with the other.

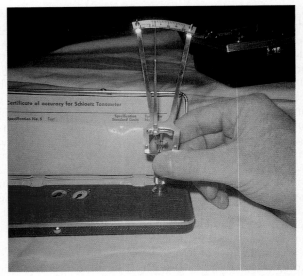

Figure 63–30 Before using the Schiøtz tonometer, test it on a flat surface to ensure smooth motion of the device and that the zero line is achieved.

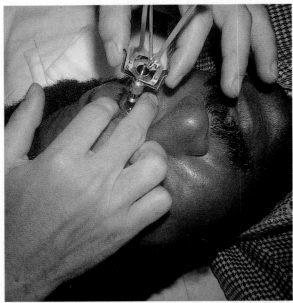

Figure 63–31 One technique of lid separation and Schiøtz tonometer placement. Lid separation pressure is applied to the bony orbital rims. An assistant may separate the lids while the operator concentrates on proper placement of the tonometer. The tonometer is held vertically during use, and the clinician's hand is established against the patient's facial bones. After anesthetic drops are instilled, the patient will not experience any pain from this procedure. It is important to have a relaxed patient, because squinting and blepharospasm may interfere with the reading. Note: gloves should be worn.

gently lower the instrument onto the middle portion of the cornea (Fig. 63–31). This is a painless experience for the patient with an anesthetized cornea. Vertically align the instrument with the footplate resting on the cornea; the reading should be in midscale. Should the reading be on the low end of the scale (<5 units), place additional weight onto the plunger after the instrument has been removed. Repeat the process as before with the additional weight.

Measure the opposite eye in the same fashion. Use the chart provided to determine the converted reading based on the reading and the amount of weight on the scale. Refer to ophthalmology if the converted scale reading is higher than 21 mm Hg (Table 63–4). Patients with elevations of IOP ≥ 30 mm Hg require more urgent consultation and initiation of therapy. Associated symptoms or signs of angle-closure glaucoma (primary or secondary) represent an ophthalmologic emergency.[87]

Errors with Impression Tonometry. Inaccurate readings occur with the Schiøtz tonometer for a variety of reasons. Falsely low readings may occur if the plunger is sticky. Check the plunger motion and the zero point of the tonometer on a firm test button before use. If the plunger is sticky, clean it with isopropyl alcohol and dry it with a tissue. Inadvertently directing pressure onto the orbit when the lids are held open may elevate the IOP and provide a falsely elevated reading. The following eye movements have been found to elevate the IOP: closing the lids (increase by 5 mm Hg), blinking (increase by 5–10 mm Hg), accommodation (increase by 2 mm Hg), and looking toward the nose (increase by 5–10 mm Hg).[88] Repeated or prolonged measurements have been found to lower the IOP approximately 2 mm Hg and may also lower the pressure in the opposite eye.[89] As mentioned in the introduction to this section, the calibration of the Schiøtz tonometer is based on a mean rigidity coefficient. Factors that

produce a reduction in ocular rigidity falsely lower the measured pressure. These factors include high myopia, anticholinesterase drugs, overhydration (e.g., four large cups of coffee or six cans of beer), and scleral buckle operations.[88,90]

Ocular pressure measurements can vary with ocular perfusion. When measured after a premature ventricular contraction, the IOP may be reduced as much as 8 mm Hg.[91] Similarly, decreased venous return as produced by breath holding, the Valsalva maneuver, or a tight collar can increase the IOP.[88]

TABLE 63–4 Schiøtz Tonometry*

Tonometer Scale Reading (Units)	Tonometer Weights (g)		
	5.5 (mm Hg)	7.5 (mm Hg)	10 (mm Hg)
2.50	27	39	55
3.00	24	36	51
3.50	22	33	47
4.00	21	30	43
4.50	19	28	40
5.00	17	26	37
5.50	16	24	34
6.00	15	22	32
6.50	13	20	29
7.00	12	18	27
7.50	11	17	25
8.00	10	16	23
8.50	9	14	21
9.00	8	13	20
9.50	8	12	18
10.00	7	11	16

*The table provides estimates of the intraocular pressure to the nearest mm Hg for the different weight of the Schiøtz tonometer. Accuracy is most dependable with scale readings greater than 5. If the scale reading is less than 5, use the next highest weight that will give a reading of 5 or more.

Impression (Tono-Pen XL) Technique

When using this device (Fig. 63–32), the preparations for testing are similar to those for the Schiøtz device. Encourage the patient to relax, and apply a topical anesthetic to numb the cornea (Fig. 63–33). Ask the patient to stare with both eyes at a distant object during testing. As noted previously, help to separate the eyelids but do not apply direct pressure on the globe. One major advantage to using the Tono-Pen XL is that the patient may be evaluated in any position as long as the device is applied perpendicular to the corneal surface. Another advantage is that the device can be used in cases of irregular or high corneal astigmatism.

Ideally, the complete instructions provided with the device should be consulted before each use; however, the following synopsis is provided to help in circumstances in which instructions are unavailable (Table 63–5).

First, spray the probe tip with compressed gas to clean the mechanism and ensure its free movement. Place an Ocu-Film (latex) cover snugly (but without tension) over the probe tip.

Perform calibration before use at least once each day (see Table 63–5). Depress and release the activation switch momentarily. The liquid crystal display (LCD) should show "—." If the device beeps and "= = = =" appears on the LCD, push the activation switch again so that the "—" reappears. If the prior calibration shows "bAd" (on LCD), a long beep sounds, followed by "CAL" (on LCD). A short beep follows and then the desired "—" is displayed. Once the "—" is displayed, hold the probe vertically with the tip pointing straight down. Press and release the activation switch twice in rapid succession. Two beeps will then sound, and "CAL" will appear (on LCD). Hold the probe in this position (up to 20 sec) until a beep sounds and "-UP-" appears (on LCD). Immediately turn the probe 180° so that the tip points straight up. In a few seconds, another beep occurs, and the LCD changes. If the LCD reads "Good," the calibration was successful. If the LCD reads "bAd," the calibration was unsuccessful.

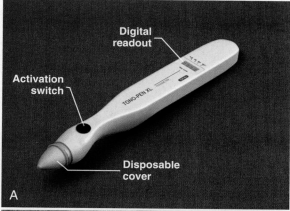

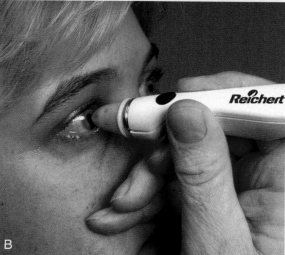

Figure 63–32 *A*, Bedside tonometry is easily accomplished with the Tono-Pen XL. The battery-powered device averages four consecutive readings and reports statistical reliability. *B*, Note the disposable sterile cover used to cover the Tono-Pen to ensure sterility. (*A, Courtesy of Reichert, Inc., from Thomsen T, Setnik G [eds]: Procedures Consult—Emergency Medicine Module. Copyright 2008 Elsevier Inc. All rights reserved.*)

With an unsuccessful calibration, repeat the calibration steps described earlier until two consecutive "Good" readings are obtained. If further attempts are unsuccessful, loosen the Ocu-Film tip cover and repeat the calibration process. If attempts are still unsuccessful, press the RESET button and repeat the process. If still unsuccessful, use compressed air to clean the probe tip and repeat the process. If still unsuccessful, the battery should be replaced and the process repeated. Continued failure warrants a call to the Reichert Technical Support (http://www.reichertonopen.com/ss.html) at 1-888-849-8955.

Proceed to measurement once the device is calibrated and the patient is prepared as outlined earlier. Depress and release the activation switch to obtain "= = = =" (on LCD). A beep will occur when ready. If the switch is not depressed long enough, the LCD will be blank. If a blank screen is seen, press and release the activation switch again to obtain "= = = =" (on LCD). Hold the probe like a pen and touch it to the cornea briefly and lightly (see Fig. 63–32*B*). Touch the cornea four times. A click will sound and a reading will appear on the LCD each time a valid reading is obtained. After four valid readings, a final beep will sound and the averaged measurement will appear on the LCD. The number represents the

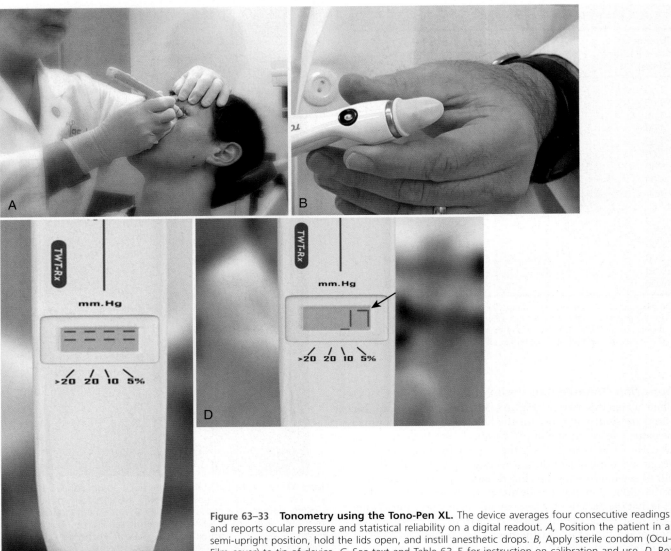

Figure 63–33 **Tonometry using the Tono-Pen XL.** The device averages four consecutive readings and reports ocular pressure and statistical reliability on a digital readout. *A,* Position the patient in a semi-upright position, hold the lids open, and instill anesthetic drops. *B,* Apply sterile condom (Ocu-Film cover) to tip of device. *C,* See text and Table 63–5 for instruction on calibration and use. *D,* Read out of ocular pressure. *(A–D, From Thomsen T, Setnik G [eds]: Procedures Consult—Emergency Medicine Module. Copyright 2008 Elsevier Inc. All rights reserved.)*

IOP in millimeters of mercury. The associated bar reflects the statistical reliability (a reading > 20% reflects an unreliable measurement, and should be repeated).

If four dashes ("----") appear on the LCD after the final beep, too few valid readings were obtained. In such a case, reactivate the probe (without recalibration) and repeat the measurement procedure. If the probe is not reactivated within 20 seconds, the LCD will clear, but the device can be activated as noted previously without recalibration.

The values are interpreted as outlined earlier for the Schiøtz device. Readings may be affected by the same features noted as causes of errors with impression tonometry via the Schiøtz device. Store the device with an unused Ocu-Film cover protecting the probe tip.

Complications

When tonometric instruments are used properly and reasonable precautions are taken, complications are unusual. The eye with preexisting corneal injury should be spared the additional trauma of tonometer placement. Corneal abrasions can be produced by ocular movement during testing. In particular, patients with uncontrollable nystagmus, hiccups, or coughing or those who are extremely apprehensive should not be subjected to tonometry. Infection can be transmitted by the use of the instrument. Careful cleansing of the device and avoidance of tonometry in patients with obvious conjunctivitis, corneal ulcers, or active herpetic lesions should minimize the risk of spreading the infection to the unaffected eye or to subsequent patients. Although protective coverings can be placed over the tonometer contact, tonometry can usually be postponed in the aforementioned individuals until the risk of infection is minimal. Extrusion of ocular contents with penetrating injuries is a potential, but rare, complication.

SLIT LAMP EXAMINATION

The slit lamp is an extremely useful instrument for examination of the anterior segment of the eye. The instrument can reveal pathologic conditions that would otherwise be invisible, such as minor corneal defects, anterior chamber hemorrhage, and inflammation.

TABLE 63–5 Tono-Pen Instructions

Steps in Setting up Tono-Pen:

1. Remove the Ocu-Film tip cover from the probe.
2. To help prevent buildup of debris around the probe post, spray the probe tip with compressed gas before the first use of the day.
3. Cover the Tono-Pen XL probe tip with a new Ocu-Film tip cover.
4. Check calibration only before the first use of each day.
   a. Depress the activation switch momentarily, then release.
   b. If the previous calibration check was good, the LCD will briefly display "—" followed by "====," accompanied by a beep.
   c. If the previous calibration was bad, a long beep sounds, after which "CAL" appears and a short beep sounds. The display then changes to "—" and another short beep sounds.
5. Hold the Tono-Pen vertically with the probe tip pointing straight down.
6. Press and release the activation switch twice in rapid succession. Two beeps will sound and "CAL" appears.
7. Wait (up to 20 sec) until a beep sounds and "-up-" appears.
8. Quickly turn the probe straight up.
9. Wait a few seconds. A second beep will sound, indicating the end of the calibration check.
10. Instill a drop of topical anesthetic (proparacaine) into both eyes.
11. Instruct the patient to look straight ahead at the fixation target with his or her eyes fully open.
12. Brace the heel of your hand on the patient's cheek for stability
13. Activate the Tono-Pen by pressing the activation switch.
14. The LCD will display "=====" and a beep will sound.
15. Once activated, touch the Tono-Pen probe against the patient's cornea lightly and briefly. **Repeat several times.**
16. A click will sound and a digital intraocular pressure measurement is displayed.
17. Proceed to the other eye. Repeat steps 12 through 15.

LCD, liquid crystal display.
Adapted from Auerbach PA: Wilderness Medicine, 5th ed. St. Louis: Elsevier Mosby, 2007. Copyright © 2007 Mosby, An Imprint of Elsevier.

Indications and Contraindications

The slit lamp can be used in the majority of eye examinations. It is especially useful in the ED for the diagnosis of corneal abrasions, FBs, and iritis.[31] The slit lamp facilitates FB removal and is also used in conjunction with most applanation tonometers. Although portable slit lamp instruments exist, emergency clinicians generally have access only to a stationary, upright device. Therefore, in the absence of a portable device, a slit lamp examination is contraindicated in patients who cannot tolerate an upright sitting position (e.g., those with orthostatic syncope).

Equipment

The slit lamp has three essential components: a binocular microscope mounted horizontally, a light source that can create a beam of variable width, and a mechanical assembly to immobilize the patient's head and manipulate the microscope and the light source. The location and arrangement of the knobs that control these components vary in devices made by different manufacturers. Usually, by simply turning each knob and watching the results, one can quickly master a new machine. Figure 63–34 illustrates the location of the functional controls on one particular instrument.

First, locate the on/off switch for the instrument. Often, this switch incorporates or is adjacent to a rheostat that provides two or three different power settings. The lowest setting is adequate for routine examination and will preserve bulb life. One can use a high-intensity setting when examining the anterior chamber with a narrow slit beam. Often, these controls are located on a transformer placed beneath the table to which the slit lamp has been attached. The second knob that one should find is the locking nut for the mechanical assembly. Loosen the nut so the assembly can be moved.

Make adjustments so the patient is comfortable while sitting with the head in the device. Ask the patient to press her or his forehead firmly against the headrest with the chin in the chinrest. By varying the table height and height of the chinrest, one should be able to maximize the comfort of the patient's neck and back. Adjust the chinrest to align the patient's eye level with the mark on the headrest support rods.

The binocular microscope has a control for varying the magnification. Usually low powers, such as 10× or 16×, are the most useful. Use a higher power to examine the anterior chamber for cells and flare and when the cornea is examined in minute detail. Adjust the binocular interpupillary distance to match that of the examiner. Focus the eyepieces by moving the instrument forward and backward until the narrowed vertical beam is sharpest on the patient's cornea when viewed with the unaided eye. Then, while viewing through each eyepiece individually, adjust the focus of each to produce a sharp image of the anterior cornea.

Notice that the light source is mounted on a swinging arm. Find the knobs that adjust the width and the height of the light beam. Click various filters in as needed, usually white and blue filters for standard examination. Alter the angle of the slit lamp beam from vertical to horizontal. The vertical alignment is preferred for routine examinations in the ED.

Both the microscope and the light source are mounted on swivel arms, linked at their base to a movable table. Change the position of this table by pushing on any part of it. Find the joystick on the table that can be used for finer movements. Vary the height of the microscope and the light source by twisting either the joystick or a separate knob at the base, depending on the design of the instrument.

Procedure

There are three setups that every slit lamp operator must know.[92] The first is for an overall screening of the anterior segment of the eye. *For examination of the patient's right eye, swing the light source to your left at a 45° angle while the microscope is directly in front of the patient's eye.* Set the slit beam to the maximum height and the minimum width using the white light. To scan across the patient's cornea, first focus the beam on the cornea by moving the entire base of the slit lamp forward and backward. Then, move the whole base left and right to scan across the cornea. The 45° angle between the microscope and the light source is the default position. The most common mistake is to try to scan by swinging the arm of the light source in an arc; this does not work because the light beam will remain centered on the same point of the patient's eye. Scan across at the level of the conjunctiva and the cornea and then push slightly forward on the base or joystick and scan at the level of the iris. The depth of the anterior

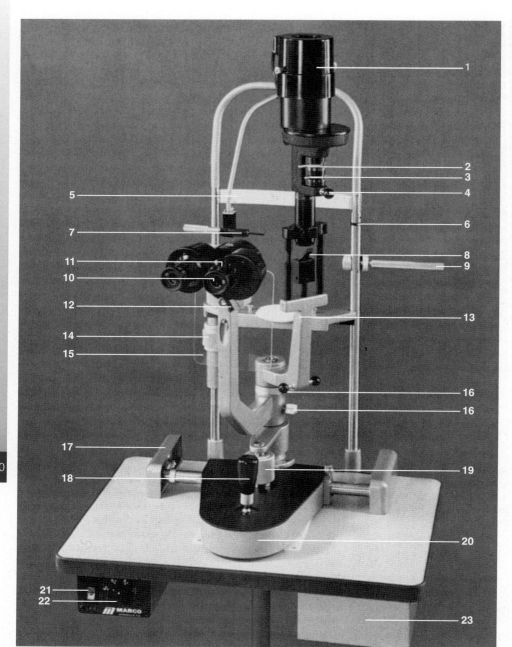

Figure 63–34 Typical slit lamp controls.
1. Cover for Lamp Bulb
2. Slit Width Controls (Red-Free Filter)
3. Slit Height Control (Cobalt Blue Filter)
4. Control of the Rotation of Slit
5. Headrest
6. Eye Level Marker
7. Fixation Lighthead
8. Mirror
9. Examiner's Handrest
10. Eyepieces
11. Knurled Rings for Refractive Error Adjustment
12. High-Low Magnification Lever
13. Patient's Chinrest
14. Headrest Elevation Control
15. Breath Shield
16. Fixing Screws for Arm
17. Rail Covers
18. Joystick
19. Elevation Control
20. Slit Lamp Base
21. On-Off Switch
22. Intensity Control
23. Accessory Storage Drawer

chamber is easily appreciated with this low-magnification setup (Fig. 63–35). When the depth of the anterior chamber is reduced, suspect a corneal perforation or a predisposition to angle-closure glaucoma.

Use this basic setup to examine the conjunctiva for traumatic lesions, inflammation, and FBs. Examine the eyelids for hordeolum, blepharitis, or trichiasis. Completely evert the lids (as described earlier in the section on "Ocular FB Removal") in conjunction with the slit lamp examination to permit evaluation of the undersurface of the upper lid for FB retention.

Corneal FB removal can be enhanced by use of the slit lamp. In particular, the instrument allows stabilization of the patient's head. Magnification also minimizes corneal injury during FB or rust ring removal. The upper eyelid may be immobilized by a cotton-tipped applicator, as discussed previ-

ously. The clinician's hand can be steadied against the patient's nose, cheek, or forehead or against the support rods of the headrest. The patient should be instructed to stare straight ahead at a fixed light or at the clinician's ear during removal of the FB.

The second setup is essentially the same as the first but uses the blue filter. The purpose is to identify any areas of fluorescein staining. After fluorescein is applied, "click" the blue filter into position and widen the beam to 3 or 4 mm. A patient can tolerate a wider beam without photophobia if it is blue. Search for corneal defects (as discussed earlier in "The Fluorescein Examination") with this setup. The blue filter may also be used with applanation tonometry, as discussed earlier in "Tonometry."

The purpose of the third setup is to search for cells in the anterior chamber—either the white cells of iritis or the

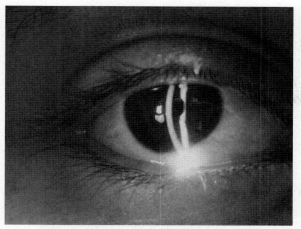

Figure 63–35 Slit lamp photograph of a normal right eye under low power. The curved slit of light on the left is reflected off the cornea and the slit on the right is reflected off the iris. The depth of the anterior chamber can easily be appreciated under this low-magnification setup. *Note that the light source is on the patient's right side to examine the right eye, with the path of the light going in a temporal-to-nasal direction. (Courtesy of D. Price.)*

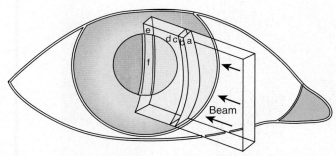

Figure 63–36 Appearance of the left eye during anterior chamber examination under low power: *a*, corneal epithelium; *b*, corneal stroma; *c*, corneal endothelium; *d*, anterior chamber (potential location of cells or flare); *e*, iris; *f*, lens reflection. The slit of light shines in the temporal-to-nasal direction at 45° to the anterior surface of the cornea. The depth of the cornea and anterior chamber examinations are best done under high power in a dark room.

red cells of a microscopic hyphema. Shorten the height of the beam to 3 or 4 mm and make it as narrow as possible. Switch the microscope to high power. Focus the beam on the center of the cornea and then push forward slightly so that it is focused on the anterior surface of the lens. Pull back the joystick again to a focus point midway between the cornea and the lens where it will be focused on the anterior chamber (Fig. 63–36). Keep the beam centered over the pupil so that there is a black background. Normally, the aqueous humor of the anterior chamber is totally clear. Small particles visible floating up or down through the beam are usually circulating cells. If the beam lights up the aqueous like a searchlight in the fog, then the examiner has found the protein flare that accompanies iritis. Note that fluorescein can penetrate an abraded cornea, producing a fluorescein flare on slit lamp evaluation. To avoid confusion, some clinicians prefer to examine for anterior chamber flare before the stain is used. A variety of conditions evaluated by the slit lamp are pictured in Figure 63–37.

UNILATERAL LOSS OF VISION

There are a variety of reasons that an individual may sustain a complete loss of vision in one eye, but most commonly, such loss is caused by occlusion of the central retinal vein, occlusion of the central retinal artery, or optic nerve damage. Less commonly, pressure in the orbit from a retro-orbital hemorrhage may compromise the ophthalmic artery.

Although discussion of all the potential causes of unilateral loss of vision is beyond the scope of this text, amaurosis fugax deserves special mention. Amaurosis fugax is a transient loss of vision most commonly due to cholesterol or platelet emboli from atherosclerotic carotid occlusive disease. When plaques are visualized in the retinal vasculature, auscultate the neck for carotid bruits and refer the patient for ultrasound examination of the carotid artery.[93,94]

Central Retinal Artery Occlusion

The patient with central retinal artery occlusion generally presents with a recent sudden (complete or nearly complete) unilateral vision loss. On examination, there is an afferent pupillary defect (i.e., sluggish or nonreactive pupil in the affected eye with direct illumination with a normal consensual response) and reduced visual acuity. Immediately after the event, the fundus may appear nearly normal; however, it soon becomes pale and a classic "cherry-red spot" in the macula may be evident as a result of patent choroidal vessels showing through the transparent fovea.

Therapy

Visual recovery has been noted to occur up to 3 days after central retinal arterial obstruction. Start treatment if the patient is seen within 24 hours after onset of symptoms.[95] Consult ophthalmology while initiating therapy.

Most of the emergency techniques suggested to treat vascular insults to the eye in the ED are theoretically sound but are not supported nor refuted by rigorous scientific data. No specific standard of care has been promulgated for these interventions by emergency clinicians. Techniques discussed later are likely safe and possibly useful, and may be attempted in an emergency situation. It is unknown whether or not these interventions will be vision saving.

Slow rebreathing into a paper bag is believed to increase the arterial carbon dioxide level, thus aiding vasodilation and permitting the occlusion to move more peripherally, possibly reducing the ischemic area. At the same time, initiate digital globe massage. With the patient lying supine, apply firm steady pressure with the thumbs to the affected globe through the patient's closed lids. Apply pressure for 5 seconds and then abruptly release it (Fig. 63–38). Immediately repeat this maneuver several more times for up to 20 minutes. The object of this technique is to help break up the occlusion and to encourage its movement more peripherally.

A more aggressive therapy, generally performed only by ophthalmologists, is anterior chamber paracentesis. In the absence of available consultation, consider this technique when central retinal occlusion is recent and unresponsive to the previously described therapeutic approaches. For this procedure, keep the patient supine with the head and eyelids secured. Anesthetize the cornea with topical anesthetic drops (e.g., 0.5% proparacaine drops). Inject the conjunctiva adjacent to the limbus using a 27- or 30-gauge needle until the entire perilimbal area is infiltrated, giving the appearance of

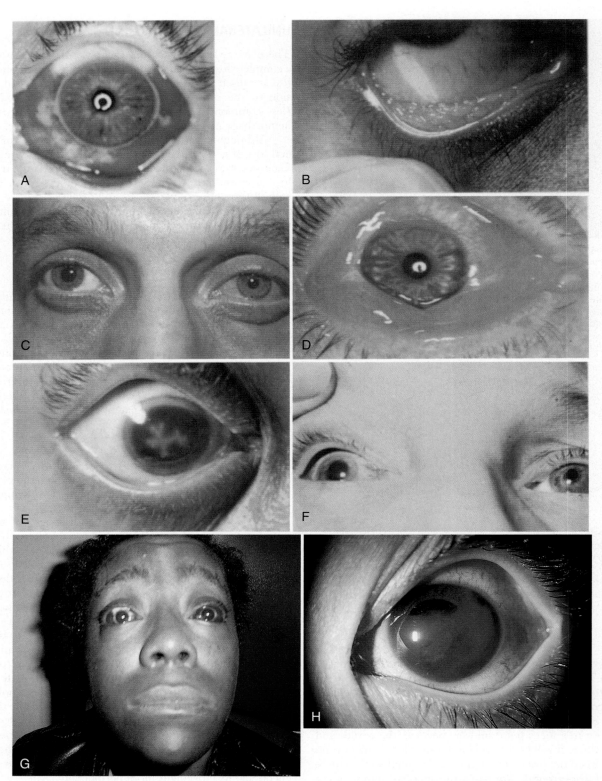

Figure 63–37 **External signs of eye pathology.** *A,* Subconjunctival hemorrhage. *B,* Ocular allergy, enlarged lid follicles. *C,* Acute iritis. *D,* Acute epidemic keratoconjunctivitis shows corneal infiltrates and chemosis. *E,* Herpes simplex (dendritic keratitis). *F,* Narrow angle-closure glaucoma shows dilated pupil, loss of corneal luster, and red eye. *G,* Bilateral subconjunctival hematoma. *H,* Large hyphema.

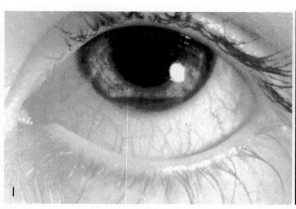

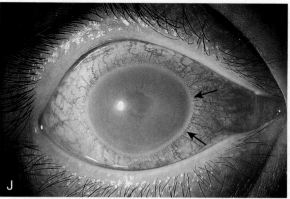

Figure 63–37, cont'd *I*, Small hyphema layering out in the inferior portion of the anterior chamber may be missed in the supine position and without a slit lamp examination. *J*, Nontraumatic iritis. Note that the conjunctival injection goes right up to the cornea (*arrows* demonstrate "perilimbal flush"), whereas with conjunctivitis, the peripheral conjunctiva is predominantly involved. These patients will have photophobia and eye pain. *(A–F, From Scheie HG, Albert DM [eds]: Textbook of Ophthalmology, 9th ed. Philadelphia, WB Saunders, 1977; J, courtesy Steve Chalfin, MD, University of Texas Health Science Center, San Antonio, TX.)*

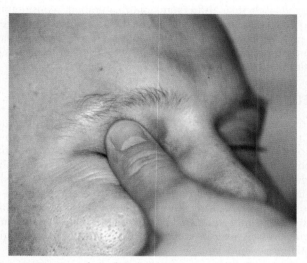

Figure 63–38 To perform digital globe massage, apply firm steady pressure with the thumb on the globe for approximately 5 sec, then abruptly release the pressure for 5–10 sec. Repeat the process for up to 20 min or until improvement of vision is observed.

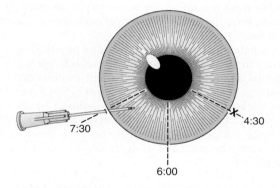

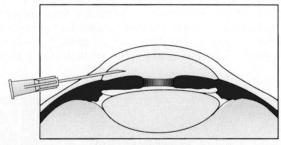

Figure 63–39 Anterior chamber paracentesis. After topical and subconjunctival anesthesia (see text), a 30-gauge needle is directed obliquely from the 4:30 or 7:30 o'clock position toward the 6 o'clock position to avoid the lens. An assistant stabilizes the globe with forceps, grasping the conjunctiva (see text). *Top,* Anteroposterior projection. *Bottom,* Tangential projection. *(Top and bottom, From Knoop K, Trott A: Ophthalmologic procedures in the emergency department: I. Immediate sight-saving procedures. Acad Emerg Med 1:408, 1994.)*

chemosis in all quadrants. During the remainder of the procedure, ask an assistant to firmly grasp the conjunctiva with toothless forceps at the 3 and 9 o'clock positions to stabilize the eye. Insert a 30-gauge needle on a tuberculin syringe obliquely just adjacent to the limbus, at either the 4:30 or the 7:30 o'clock position and direct it toward the 6 o'clock position to avoid the lens (Fig. 63–39). Apply gentle pressure on the globe and, after 1 to 2 drops of aqueous are expressed, withdraw the needle.[96,97]

One study describes a systematic approach in which ocular massage, sublingual isosorbide dinitrate 10 mg, acetazolamide 500 mg intravenously, mannitol 20% (1 mg/kg,) or oral glycerol 50% (1 mg/kg), anterior chamber paracentesis, methylprednisolone 500 mg intravenously, streptokinase 750 kIU, and retrobulbar tolazoline 50 mg were given until visual symptoms improved or until all steps were complete.[98] Of the 11 patients in this arm of the study, 8 had improved visual acuity. In those who improved, all had symptoms in 12 hours or less. The presumed cause was either platelet-derived

or cholesterol embolus from atheroma or glaucoma.[97] Although this study is small, it supports emergent ophthalmology consultation and aggressive treatment of patients who present within 12 to 24 hours of symptom onset.

Complications

Overzealous globe massage has the potential to produce intraocular trauma including retinal detachment and intraocular hemorrhage. Anterior chamber paracentesis may produce hemorrhage, infection, or mechanical injury to the cornea, iris, or lens.[99] Although these complications are rare, ophthalmologic consultation for assistance with the underlying central retinal artery occlusion and surveillance for these potential complications should be initiated on an emergent basis.

Orbital Compartment Syndrome

Acute facial trauma or recent retrobulbar anesthesia may produce retrobulbar hemorrhage with sufficient pressure to compromise the ophthalmic artery, resulting in an orbital compartment syndrome. A form of post-traumatic glaucoma may also occur when the retrobulbar hematoma forces the globe against the eyelids. In this case, IOP rises precipitously because the globe is in a relatively closed space owing to the firm attachment of the eyelids to the orbital rim by the medial and lateral canthal ligaments. The optic nerve and its vascular supply and the central retinal artery are compressed, resulting in ischemia and subsequent visual loss. In this situation, an emergency lateral canthotomy may be considered for relief of the pressure on the eye. It would not be considered a standard of care for most emergency clinicians to possess the skills for this procedure, but under the proper scenario, it may be a prudent intervention.

Ophthalmoscopic evaluation reveals a blanched ophthalmic artery in the presence of obvious retrobulbar pressure and ecchymosis around the eye. The patient exhibits decreased visual acuity, and an afferent pupil defect is often seen. The IOP is markedly elevated but may be relieved by an emergency lateral canthotomy and cantholysis. Such a procedure needs to be performed quickly because the ischemic retina will not retain function if it is deprived of blood for a long period of time.

Technique: Lateral Canthotomy and Cantholysis

The goals of the procedure are to release pressure on the globe and to decrease IOP enough to reinstitute retinal artery blood flow. Because retinal recovery is unlikely to occur if rapid relief of ischemia is not accomplished, taking time to clean the eye beyond simple saline cleansing of the lids and lateral canthus is ill advised. Stabilize the patient's head and lids and anesthetize the lateral canthus by injecting 1% to 2% lidocaine with epinephrine. Before incising, crush the lateral canthus with a small hemostat for 1 to 2 minutes to minimize bleeding. Incise the canthus by using iris or Steven's scissors. Take precautions to avoid injury to the protruding globe (Fig. 63–40). Begin the incision at the lateral canthus and extend it toward the orbital rim. Find the superior and inferior crus of the lateral canthal tendon and release them from the orbital rim (Fig. 63–41). Some operators prefer to release the inferior crus and reassess the IOP before considering release of the superior crus. An instructional video of the procedure can be found at www.brown.edu/Administration/Emergency_Medicine/eye.htm.[100]

Complications

Although hemorrhage, infection, and mechanical injury might result from the procedure, these complications generally respond to therapy better than does retinal injury from prolonged ischemia. Emergent ophthalmologic consultation should be obtained, although when the procedure is indicated, it may be considered by the emergency clinician. Lateral canthotomy incisions generally heal without suturing or significant scarring.

REDUCTION OF GLOBE LUXATION

Although luxation of the globe is uncommon, the emergency clinician should be aware of the condition and its mechanisms, know how to reduce the globe, and know when to prioritize ophthalmologic consultation. With luxation of the globe, there is extreme proptosis, which permits the lids to slip behind the globe equator (Fig. 63–42). Subsequent spasm of the orbicularis oculi muscles sustains the luxation and limits extraocular movements. Traction on the optic nerve and retinal vessels may produce direct or indirect injury to the optic nerve and retina.

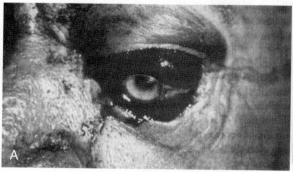
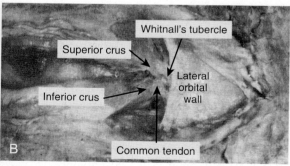

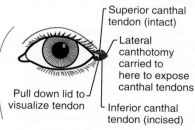

Figure 63–40 Indications for lateral canthotomy and cantholysis include decreased visual acuity, ocular pressure greater than 40 mm Hg, proptosis, afferent papillary defect (Marcus Gunn pupil), cherry-red macula, ophthalmoplegia, optic nerve pallor, and severe eye pain. A ruptured globe is a contraindication. *A,* Severe proptosis secondary to acute traumatic retrobulbar hemorrhage. *B,* Anatomy of orbital structures demonstrates the inferior and superior crura of the lateral canthal tendon beneath the lateral canthus. The crura join and as a common tendon are attached to the inner aspect of the lateral orbital wall, forming Whitnall's tubercle. The lateral canthus, formed by the upper and lower eyelid, has been removed. *C,* Lateral canthotomy. Only the inferior crus need be incised initially. (*A and B, From Vassallo S, Hartstein M, Howard D, Stetz J: Traumatic retrotubular hemorrhage: Emergent decompression by lateral canthotomy and cantholysis. J Emerg Med 22:251, 2002.*)

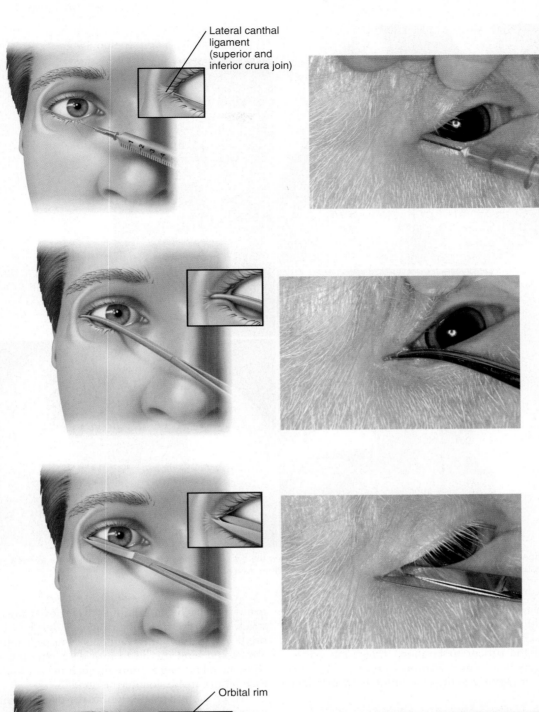

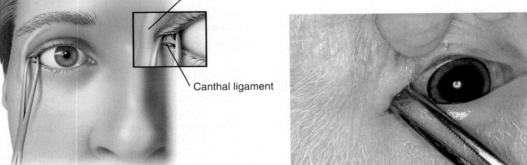

Figure 63–41 Procedure for lateral cathotomy. Step 1: Local anesthesia of the lateral canthus. Step 2: Crush the lateral canthus with a clamp to reduce bleeding when it is incised. Step 3: Lateral canthus incised to allow the inferior crus to be exposed. Step 4: To decompress the eyeball, cut the canthal ligament with scissors pointed inferoposteriorly toward the lateral rim. Pull the lower lid down and away from the lateral orbital rim, separating the skin and conjunctiva. If bleeding hinders identification of the inferior crus, it may be palpated. Only the inferior crus need be lysed initially. If intraocular pressure is not reduced, the superior crus is lysed. *(From Custalow CB: The Color Atlas of Emergency Department Procedures. Philadelphia, Elsevier Saunders, 2005.)*

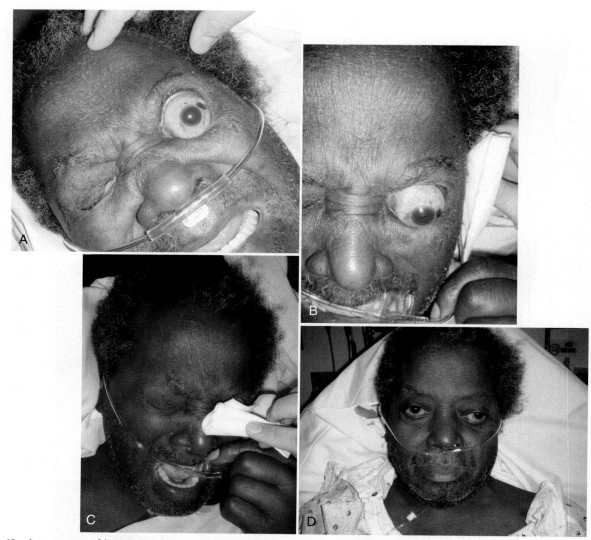

Figure 63–42 Appearance of luxated globe. This globe protruded when the eye was opened for pupil examination. It was easily reduced with slight manual pressure on the closed upper lid. Afterward, the patient had no eye or vision complaints.

Luxation may be spontaneous, voluntary, or traumatic. A variety of conditions (e.g., orbital neoplasms, Graves disease, histiocytosis X, cerebral gumma, and craniofacial dysostoses) may predispose the patient to luxation. Triggering events include maneuvers increasing intraorbital pressure (e.g., the Valsalva maneuver), trauma to the orbit or forehead, or eyelid manipulation.

Indications and Contraindications

Early globe reduction is indicated to relieve symptoms and to minimize visual impairment. Attempts at reduction in the ED are relatively contraindicated when there is obvious rupture of the globe.

Technique

Before globe reduction, perform a rapid eye examination to document visual acuity, range of eye motion, pupillary reactivity, and any evidence of globe rupture (see earlier discussion).[101] Place the patient in a recumbent position, and administer a topical ocular anesthetic agent (e.g., 0.5% proparacaine). When the lashes are visible, ask an assistant to apply steady outward and upward traction while the globe is

gently pushed behind the lids. Use gloved fingers to apply steady scleral pressure and manipulate the globe back into the orbit. When the lashes cannot be grasped, introduce a lid retractor behind the lid to provide countertraction. Others recommend placing a suture through the anesthetized skin of each lid to provide countertraction.

After the procedure, repeat the eye examination documenting visual acuity and extraocular movement. It is not uncommon for return of full visual function to be delayed for several days, or occasionally longer.

Complications

It is common with this procedure for lashes to be retained in the conjunctival fornices. Evaluate for and remove any free lashes to prevent corneal injury. Edema, retrobulbar hemorrhage, or orbital deformity may prevent outpatient reduction. When reduction is not possible in the ED, saline drops should be applied to the globe and a noncontact eye shield applied.

Aftercare

Patients with spontaneous luxation and no visual impairment in whom the globe is easily reduced warrant follow-up within alternate wet washcloths for 15 to 20 minutes. Topical ophthalmic antibiotics (drops q2h or ointment five to six times a day) are usually prescribed. Erythromycin ointment is often suggested. Topical treatment is usually sufficient, but antistaphylococcal oral antibiotics (dicloxacillin, cephalosporins) might occasionally be needed, especially if there is significant surrounding lid cellulitis. More formal incision and drainage may be necessary if the infection is unresponsive to conservative therapy.[102] Spread of the infection can lead to preseptal cellulitis.

AFFERENT PUPILLARY DEFECT OR MARCUS-GUNN PUPIL

An afferent papillary defect (APD), or Marcus-Gunn pupil, is caused by a variety of diseases of the afferent, or "in-going," pathways of the eye. It is produced by a *unilateral* lesion of the retina or optic nerve. Causes include optic neuritis (as seen with multiple sclerosis), ischemic optic neuropathy, optic tumor, and retrobulbar hematoma (an indication for lateral canthotomy). To evaluate for an afferent pupillary defect, the swinging flashlight test may be used.[103] *Normally, shining a light in either eye causes bilateral pupil constriction.* To evaluate for an APD (no light reaching the brain via the optic nerve on the affected side), record the pupil size at baseline. Shine a light into the affected eye. Record the direct response (constriction of the illuminated pupil in response to light) and the indirect or consensual response (constriction of the opposite pupil in response to light). Next, shine the light into the other eye and record the direct and indirect responses. Repeat this procedure back and forth until the pattern of response to light is identified. In the APD, there is a *decreased direct response to light along the afferent or "in-going" pathways,* whereas the efferent or "out-going" pathways to the opposite eye are preserved. Thus, light shined into the affected eye will cause neither a direct nor a consensual response, but light shined into the unaffected eye will cause bilateral pupillary constriction.

SUBCONJUNCTIVAL HEMORRHAGE

Subconjunctival hemorrhage may occur spontaneously (often noticed on awakening) or after straining, vomiting, or serve coughing. The patient notices a painless bright red hemorrhage of the eye (sclera). It may be bilateral (see Fig. 63–37). Vision is not affected. Although this is concerning to the patient, it is benign. No laboratory evaluation is required unless that patient is anticoagulated; then, clotting studies should be performed. The hemorrhage will disappear spontaneously over a few weeks, turning various colors as it recedes. No treatment will hasten resolution.

Acknowledgment

The authors recognize the many contributions by John R. Samples, MD, and David Barr, MD, to this chapter through the first four editions of the textbook.

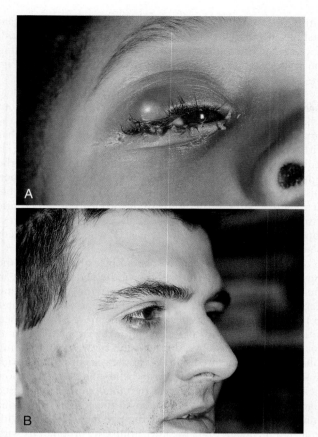

Figure 63–43 Stye (hordeolum). *A,* External hordeolum. An erythematous, tender swelling at the lid margin points externally. *B,* Internal stye. This may form a pustule on the inner surface of the lid that may be incised and pus expressed (see also Fig. 63–19C).

24 to 48 hours. Instructions to avoid potential triggering maneuvers should be given. Recurrent luxation may warrant lateral tarsorrhaphy. Further evaluation of potential precipitating illness can be pursued on an outpatient basis.

Patients with traumatic luxation are at greater risk for underlying ophthalmic injury and warrant emergent consultation. A computed tomography scan of the orbit is helpful for evaluating both the soft tissue and the bony structures about the globe.

STYE

A stye, or hordeolum, is an acute purulent inflammation (bacterial infection) of the eyelid characterized by pain, swelling, and redness. They can be quite annoying and painful to the touch. A small nodule or abscess first develops in an eyelid hair follicle or a modified sebaceous gland at the eyelid margin. This may be external (pointing at the lid margin) or internal (pointing under the conjunctival lid; Fig. 63–43). An obvious pustule may be seen, and if so, incising it with a small needle and expressing pus produces a faster cure. The lid may be inverted to find a small pustule on the inner lid that can be nicked with a 25-gauge needle (see Fig. 63–19C). *S. aureus* is the organism most frequently isolated from the infection.[1] Treat with warm compresses on the eyelid as frequently as possible. One method is to fill a sink with very hot water and

 REFERENCES CAN BE FOUND ON EXPERT CONSULT

CHAPTER 64

Otolaryngologic Procedures

Ralph J. Riviello and N. Adam Brown

The procedures presented in this section are most effectively performed using special equipment and techniques. Some are within the realm of general emergency medicine clinical expertise; others are not. They are reviewed from the perspective of the emergency clinician who must decide whether the patient needs treatment acutely in the ED, can be managed with timely referral, or requires urgent consultant expertise.

PHARYNX/LARYNX

Examination of the Larynx

Laryngoscopy has traditionally been discouraged in the patient with a high potential for epiglottitis because oropharyngeal manipulation may, in rare cases, precipitate laryngospasm and acute respiratory arrest. However, careful laryngoscopy may be performed in stridulous patients with the presumed diagnosis of croup to rule out epiglottitis when the suspicion for the latter condition is low.[1] When impending airway obstruction from epiglottitis is suspected, quickly assemble a predesignated team (usually consisting of an anesthesiologist and an otolaryngologist) in the operating room. Prepare fully for a surgical airway or rigid bronchoscopy before attempting laryngoscopy. Approach patients with severe laryngeal trauma or partially obstructing hypopharyngeal foreign bodies (FBs) in a similar manner. When examining the mouth and larynx, follow guidelines for "universal precautions" to protect patients and yourself from infection transmitted by blood and body fluids. The relevant anatomy of these structures is depicted in Figure 64–1.

Illumination

Illumination is key in evaluating pathology of the mouth and larynx. Use the reflected light from direct illumination from a head lamp or overhead light source not only for indirect laryngoscopy but also for inspection of, and procedures in, the oropharynx, nares, and auditory canal. For example, a peritonsillar abscess (PTA) is afforded excellent illumination for drainage with such devices. The advantages of a head mirror are the high degree of brightness it provides into deep recesses and its simplicity of design. Generally, the beam of light from an electric head lamp is easier to focus than the head mirror.

Procedure

Head Lamp. Attach the electric head lamp to your head with the forehead strap and place the light equidistant between your eyes to be maximally effective. The intensity of light in this position is nearly as bright as that from the head mirror. After securing the head lamp, hold your hands in front of you at a distance comfortable for working. Focus the beam of light at this point by adjusting the head lamp into position

without moving your head or eyes. This allows for the beam to shine on and follow the area on which your eyes are focused. An assistant often greatly aids in visualization by retracting the cheek and helping position the patient's head (Fig. 64–2A).

Indirect (Mirror) Laryngoscopy. This traditional method is most commonly used by the otolaryngologist, but it has some application in the emergency setting if the necessary equipment is readily available. The clinician unfamiliar with this method should practice frequently, because it requires significant eye-to-hand coordination to reflect the light beam off the angulated mirror onto the larynx. When this procedure is properly performed, most patients are able to tolerate it without anesthesia of the oropharynx. Fiberoptic nasopharyngoscopy has largely replaced indirect laryngoscopy in the emergency department (ED) when the equipment is available.

Establish rapport with the patient by explaining how the examination will be performed. Have the patient sit erect in the "sniffing position," with the feet flat on the floor and leaning slightly forward. Warm the mirror with warm water to prevent fogging, but check the temperature of the mirror with your hand before placing it into the oropharynx so as not to burn the patient. Alternatively, apply an antifogging solution to the mirrored side. Wrap the patient's tongue with gauze to prevent it from slipping or being injured by the lower incisors and then grasp it with the nondominant hand (see Fig. 64–2B). Apply gentle traction to the tongue with your thumb and index finger and lift the patient's upper lip with your middle finger. Slide the mirror into the oropharynx with the glass surface parallel to the tongue but not touching it. Place the back of the mirror against the uvula and soft palate, smoothly lifting until the larynx is visualized. Although this should not induce gagging, try to make only slight changes in mirror position to inspect the appropriate structures.

In patients who cannot tolerate this procedure without gagging, apply topical anesthetic to aid in the examination. Benzocaine (Hurricaine spray or Cetacaine gargle) or aerosolized tetracaine or lidocaine may be used. One or two quick sprays of benzocaine into the posterior oropharynx is sufficient. Prolonged or repeated spraying may rarely result in methemoglobinemia. Reassure the patient beforehand that, although this may make the throat feel as if it is swelling or paralyzed, in actuality, it is just the numbness that accounts for the sensation. The tendency to gag can also be minimized by having the patient concentrate on his or her breathing efforts and keep the eyes open, with the eyes fixed on an object in the distance.

Once the patient is anesthetized, repeat the steps described earlier and position the mirror against the soft palate. Rotate the angle of the mirror and systematically inspect the base of the tongue, valleculae, epiglottis, pyriform recess, arytenoids, false and true vocal cords, and if possible, the superior aspect of the trachea (Fig. 64–3). Observe for masses, evidence of infection, asymmetry, or FBs. Further evaluate the anterior structure of the larynx and function of the vocal cords by having the patient say "eeee" in a high-pitched voice. This should move the epiglottis away from blocking the view of the larynx and bring the true cords together at the midline.

Flexible Fiberoptic Laryngoscopy

Fiberoptic examination of the nasopharynx and larynx can be accomplished with either a flexible nasopharyngoscope or a

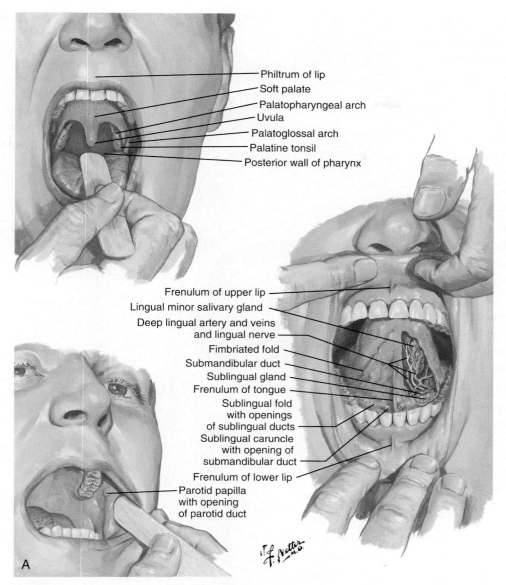

Philtrum of lip
Soft palate
Palatopharyngeal arch
Uvula
Palatoglossal arch
Palatine tonsil
Posterior wall of pharynx

Frenulum of upper lip
Lingual minor salivary gland
Deep lingual artery and veins
and lingual nerve
Fimbriated fold
Submandibular duct
Sublingual gland
Frenulum of tongue
Sublingual fold
with openings
of sublingual ducts
Sublingual caruncle
with opening of
submandibular duct
Frenulum of lower lip
Parotid papilla
with opening
of parotid duct

A

Figure 64–1 *A,* Anatomy of the oropharynx. *B,* Sagittal section of the neck. (*A and B, Netter illustrations used with permission of Elsevier Inc. All rights reserved.*)   *Continued*

bronchoscope. The nasopharyngoscope is thinner, shorter, and easier to manipulate (Fig. 64–4). Fiberoptic visualization is especially useful in patients who are difficult to examine because of persistent gagging or unusual anatomy. This scope used in the ED is for examination purposes only because most EDs do not have suction or equipment to extract objects or perform biopsies.

Attach the endoscope to its light source and the suction tubing to its port (if available). Ensure that both are functioning properly before beginning. Before inserting the scope, adjust the eyepiece to your visual acuity; it is helpful to check the focus on newsprint or a small object. Review the scope's directional controls. Examine both nares and choose the more patent one to enter. Anesthetize and vasoconstrict the naris with lidocaine and epinephrine. You may also anesthetize the pharynx to minimize gagging. Warm the end of the scope in warm water to help prevent fogging. Place the patient in the seated position, with the head placed against a headrest, in the sniffing position. Insert the tip of the lubricated scope just inside the naris. Some use a series of soft nasal trumpets to gradually dilate the nasal cavity, allowing easier passage of the scope. The movement of the scope against the inside of the nasal passage may be irritating to the patient. *Minimize this sensation by resting the fourth and fifth fingers on the bridge of the patient's nose while stabilizing and guiding the scope between the thumb and the index finger* (Fig. 64–5).

While looking through the eyepiece, slowly advance the endoscope past the inferior turbinate into the nasopharynx or through the lumen of a nasal trumpet. To clear fogging or mucus off the lens, ask the patient to swallow, wipe the lens against the pharyngeal mucosa, or use the suction. Once the scope is in the nasopharynx, direct the tip inferiorly by using the thumb control near the eyepiece. Use the thumb control to accomplish up-and-down movements of the scope. Rotate the scope about its axis and then apply thumb control to provide for lateral movement and visualization. At this point, the base of the tongue and tonsils will come into view. Slide the scope farther caudad to bring the larynx into focus. Once

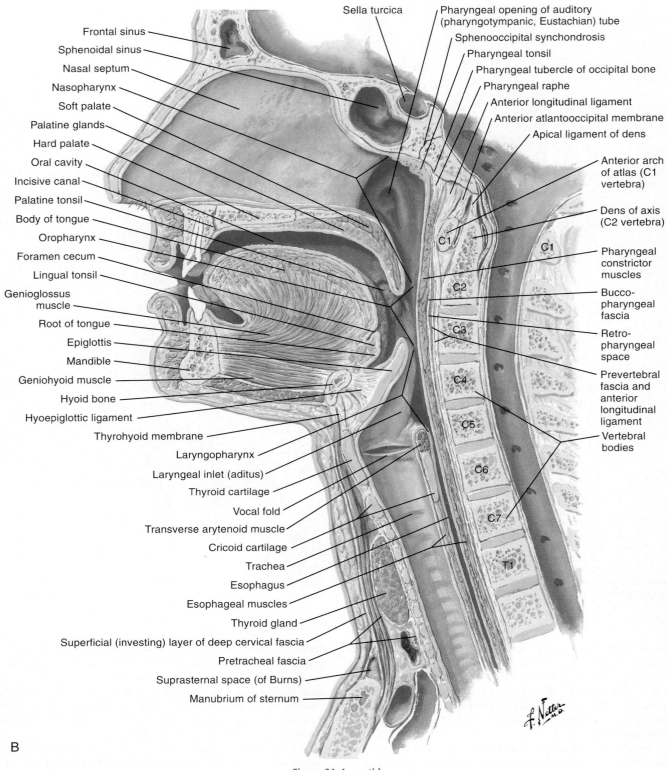

Frontal sinus
Sphenoidal sinus
Nasal septum
Nasopharynx
Soft palate
Palatine glands
Hard palate
Oral cavity
Incisive canal
Palatine tonsil
Body of tongue
Oropharynx
Foramen cecum
Lingual tonsil
Genioglossus muscle
Root of tongue
Epiglottis
Mandible
Geniohyoid muscle
Hyoid bone
Hyoepiglottic ligament
Thyrohyoid membrane
Laryngopharynx
Laryngeal inlet (aditus)
Thyroid cartilage
Vocal fold
Transverse arytenoid muscle
Cricoid cartilage
Trachea
Esophagus
Esophageal muscles
Thyroid gland
Superficial (investing) layer of deep cervical fascia
Pretracheal fascia
Suprasternal space (of Burns)
Manubrium of sternum

Sella turcica
Pharyngeal opening of auditory (pharyngotympanic, Eustachian) tube
Sphenooccipital synchondrosis
Pharyngeal tonsil
Pharyngeal tubercle of occipital bone
Pharyngeal raphe
Anterior longitudinal ligament
Anterior atlantooccipital membrane
Apical ligament of dens
Anterior arch of atlas (C1 vertebra)
Dens of axis (C2 vertebra)
Pharyngeal constrictor muscles
Bucco-pharyngeal fascia
Retro-pharyngeal space
Prevertebral fascia and anterior longitudinal ligament
Vertebral bodies

C1
C2
C3
C4
C5
C6
C7
T1

B

Figure 64–1, cont'd

again, systematically view the anatomy and function during both respiration and phonation.

If the nasopharyngeal scope will not pass through either naris, pass it through the oropharynx. Properly anesthetize the oropharynx and avoid contacting the posterior tongue to prevent gagging. A plastic bite block can be used. Alternatively, cut a 10-mL syringe (without the plunger) in half and

ask the patient to hold this in the mouth between the incisors. Pass the fragile endoscope through this tube to prevent accidental biting of the scope.

Complications include traumatic abrasions and bleeding anywhere along the path of the laryngoscope. In patients with head injury, there is always the slight risk of passing the scope intracranially if a basilar skull fracture exists; use of a soft nasal

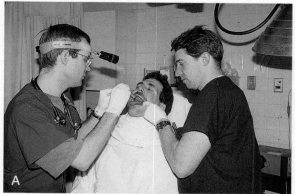

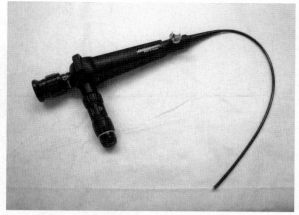

Figure 64–4 Fiberoptic nasopharyngoscope. This is for examination only and does not have suction or extraction apparatus.

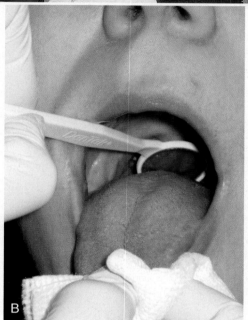

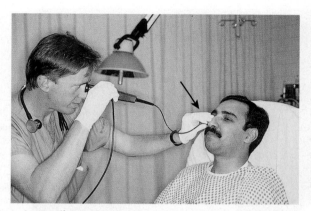

Figure 64–5 Fiberoptic nasopharyngoscope in use. Prepare the patient's throat and nares with topical anesthetic. Topical vasoconstrictors may also be used in the nares. The use of a nasal trumpet to dilate the passage for a few minutes before examination is optional. Advance the scope slowly into the naris with your hand *stabilized on the bridge of the patient's nose* (*arrow*); guide the scope using the thumb and index finger. Visualize the passage of the scope through the naris into the posterior nasopharynx. Always use universal precautions.

Figure 64–2 *A,* A good light source (head lamp) and an assistant facilitate any ear, nose, and throat examination or procedure. *B,* Indirect mirror evaluation of the oropharynx. Grasp the patient's tongue between the thumb and the first finger, using a gauze pad to provide traction. Elevate the upper lip with the middle finger. Advance the warmed (prevents fogging) laryngeal mirror into the posterior oropharynx, taking care not to stimulate the posterior tongue or pharynx. Remember that the structures in the mirror will be reversed. Always use universal precautions.

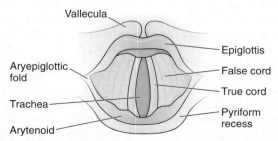

Figure 64–3 View of the larynx from above. The true and false vocal cords are sketched, with the arytenoid eminences behind them on each side. The epiglottis, piriform fossae, and valleculae are also identified.

trumpet significantly reduces this risk. Laryngospasm and acute airway compromise can be induced in patients with paraglottic infections.

TONSIL: PERITONSILLAR ABSCESS (PTA)

Anatomy

PTA, also known as quinsy, is most common during the 2nd and 3rd decades. It is rarely seen in children younger than 6 years of age, making it diagnostically challenging in younger children and infants. It remains the most common head and neck abscess in children and adults. Understand the relative anatomy before attempting to treat a PTA (Fig. 64–6). The palatine tonsils are located between the anterior and the posterior pillars of the throat, bound in a capsule and covered by mucosa. The lateral wall of the tonsil is defined by the superior pharyngeal constrictor muscle. Of great importance is the internal carotid artery, which lies approximately 2.5 cm posterolateral to the tonsil.

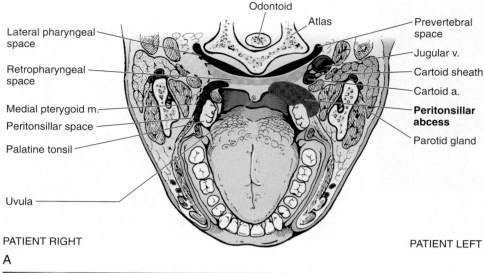

Odontoid
Atlas
Lateral pharyngeal space
Retropharyngeal space
Medial pterygoid m.
Peritonsillar space
Palatine tonsil
Uvula
Prevertebral space
Jugular v.
Cartoid sheath
Cartoid a.
Peritonsillar abcess
Parotid gland

PATIENT RIGHT

A

PATIENT LEFT

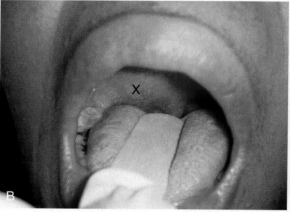

B

Figure 64–6 *A,* Anatomy of a peritonsillar abscess. The palatine tonsil and peritonsillar space are identified on the patient's left. A peritonsillar abscess (x) is shown on the patient's right. Note that the abscess can extend medially, displacing the uvula. *The carotid artery and jugular vein are posterior and lateral to the abscess.* Avoid lateral angulation of the aspirating needle and use a needle guard to prevent injury. *B,* An obvious bulging of the peritonsillar space can be either a true abscess or cellulitis, and needle aspiration (or ultrasound, if available) may be required to differentiate the two.

Pathophysiology and Presentation

PTAs can occur in patients with inadequately treated tonsillitis and in those with recurrent tonsillitis. The abscess is usually unilateral and is defined as a collection of pus between the tonsillar capsule, the superior constrictor muscle, and the palatopharyngeus muscle. It is believed to arise from the spread of infection from the tonsil or from the mucous glands of Weber located in the superior tonsillar pole.[2] The abscess is most commonly initiated from the upper pole of the tonsil. However, it can also spread from the middle or inferior poles. Complications may include pharyngeal obstruction or extension into the closely approximated neurovascular bundles and parapharyngeal space.

Most patients present primarily with a PTA, but some are already undergoing antibiotic therapy for tonsillitis. There are no data proving that antibiotics, even the correct ones in proper doses, invariably prevent the progression of tonsillitis to abscess formation. Inadequately treated tonsillitis can progress to abscess when a patient fails to follow the prescribed regimen or when the regimen is inadequate. The latter may occur as the result of an improperly chosen antibiotic or because of increasing antibiotic resistance. Although group A Streptococcus remains the leading cause of peritonsillar abscess, *Staphylococcus aureus, Haemophilus influenzae, Bacteroides, Peptostreptococcus,* and mixed anaerobic infections are also common. β-Lactamase–producing organisms are present in about 50% of cases.[3] Fine-needle aspiration of PTAs may allow identification of organisms and appropriate modification in antibiotic therapy, thus avoiding the need for tonsillectomy.

Patients with PTAs present with sore throat, odynophagia, low-grade fever, and a variable degree of trismus. The trismus develops secondary to pterygoid muscle irritation. The patient may also complain of ipsilateral otalgia. As the abscess expands, the patient may experience dysphagia with drooling. Patients may be dehydrated secondary to poor oral intake. Voice changes are common (hot-potato voice) and are caused by transient velopharyngeal insufficiency and muffled oral resonance. Rancid breath is also common. Tender ipsilateral anterior cervical lymphadenopathy is usually present. Examination of the oropharynx may be difficult because of associated trismus. Ask the patient to sit up with the head in the sniffing position. Encourage the patient to open the mouth as wide as possible, and depress the tongue to obtain a better view of the oropharynx. Use a head lamp or head mirror/light source to ensure adequate illumination. Digital palpation for a fluctuant site can be useful and may be the best way to differentiate abscess from cellulitis. The clinician places the gloved index finger into the mouth and feels for hardness or fluctuance in the peritonsillar region (Fig. 64–7). If no abscess or fluctuance can be appreciated, the diagnosis is unlikely. This technique is usually well tolerated but the patient may gag or bite the examiner by reflex. Physical findings are often diagnostic of a PTA; however, in some cases, *the diagnosis is in doubt until needle aspiration is performed.*

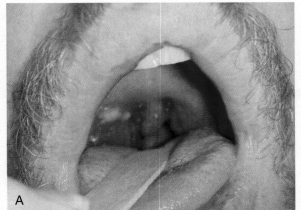
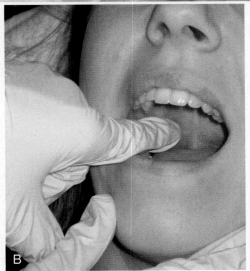

Figure 64–7 *A,* Severe tonsillitis/peritonsillar cellulitis may present with symptoms suggestive of an abscess. This may progress to an abscess. *B,* Clinical symptoms and visual inspection may not be sufficient to differentiate peritonsillar abscess from cellulitis. The clinician's gloved index finger is used to palpate the peritonsillar area to search for fluctuance and localized swelling.

Inferior and medial displacement of the tonsil and uvula are noted along with a fluctuant mass involving the tonsillar pillar. Swelling obliterates the normally sharply delineated pillar-like structure. The tonsil looks edematous and erythematous and may be covered with a whitish exudate.

The differential diagnosis for this acute process includes unilateral tonsillitis, peritonsillar cellulitis, retropharyngeal abscess, infectious mononucleosis, herpes simplex tonsillitis, retromolar abscess, neoplasm, FB, and internal carotid artery aneurysm. Chronic conditions include leukemia, carcinoma, and parapharyngeal space tumor. Differentiation of a PTA from peritonsillar cellulitis may be difficult, especially in the early stages of an abscess. The history and time course for the two disease processes are quite similar. Trismus and uvular deviation are uncommon in peritonsillar cellulitis.[4] Needle aspiration will be diagnostic if purulent material is removed. However, a negative test does not rule out an abscess. The abscess may be located posteriorly and not accessible by the aspiration needle.

Intraoral sonography may augment diagnostic accuracy. Blaivis and coworkers[5] found ED ultrasound was effective in diagnosing and aiding drainage of five cases of PTA. Ultrasound excluded the diagnosis in one case. If there is still a question as to the diagnosis or actual location of the abscess, computed tomography (CT) scanning may be helpful but is not usually performed.

General Treatment

The treatment of PTA has undergone significant change in the past 100 years and continues to do so at this writing. A myriad of opinions exist on the appropriate treatment method, although most agree that some form of drainage procedure should be performed in conjunction with antibiotics and pain control. Three options for surgical drainage include needle aspiration (most common), incision and drainage, and immediate (quinsy) tonsillectomy. Each method is discussed.

Needle aspiration is relatively simple, can be performed by clinicians who are not head and neck specialists, does not require special equipment, and is relatively inexpensive. Other benefits of needle aspiration over incision and drainage include decreased pain and trauma. Many feel that this should be the initial surgical drainage procedure for adults and children. The recurrence rate after aspiration is 10%,[6] and its cure rate is about 94%.[2] About 4% to 10% of patients require repeat aspiration.[2,6,7] One drawback is that needle aspiration may miss the PTA and, therefore, allow misdiagnosis as peritonsillar cellulitis. Therefore, some authors propose admission of patients with negative aspirations with the presumed diagnosis of peritonsillar cellulitis for intravenous antibiotics and observation to prevent further morbidity. Although most studies were performed with hospitalization and intravenous antibiotics, selected outpatient treatment with oral antibiotics has also been successful and is usually the option chosen unless the patient appears septic.[7]

Incision and drainage is commonly done as an outpatient procedure under local anesthesia. This procedure is usually performed after pus is obtained by needle aspiration, but occasionally, it is the primary procedure. It seems most logical to first attempt aspiration and follow with incision and drainage only if additional pus is suspected or there are other extenuating circumstances. The recurrence rate after incision and drainage is similar or less than aspiration alone.[2] Despite these shortcomings, incision and drainage is the initial surgical treatment used by an estimated 54% of U.S. otolaryngologists.[2]

Immediate (quinsy) tonsillectomy is thought by some to be the only way to completely drain the abscess and completely eliminate the risk of recurrence. They also feel that hospital time and the patient's disability are shortened. Arguments against this rationale include:

1. An initial PTA is no longer an indication for tonsillectomy.
2. Needle aspiration/incision and drainage have high success rates.
3. Studies have shown longer recovery times for patients after immediate tonsillectomy compared with the other drainage procedures.
4. There is a time delay (6–70 hr) in assembling equipment and personnel for the tonsillectomy.

Treatment guidelines based on a review of the literature[2,6–8] suggest that patients with PTA should be initially treated with needle aspiration. Incision and drainage and immediate tonsillectomy should be reserved for treatment failures or recurrences. Adult patients with recurrent tonsillitis/PTA should be treated either with needle aspiration followed by delayed tonsillectomy or with abscess tonsillectomy

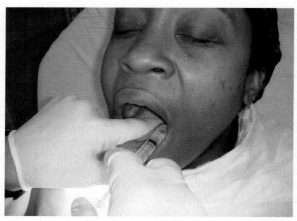

Figure 64–8 Prior to needle aspiration of a peritonsillar abscess, inject the mucosa with 1–2 ml of lidocaine with epinephrine, and observe an area of blanching. Use a small-gauge needle (25- to 27-gauge) but a larger syringe so the view of the operative area is not blocked. Often, the tongue is best displaced with the finger rather than a tongue blade. Wait a few minutes and the puncture will be painless.

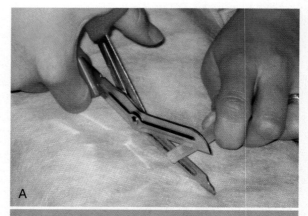

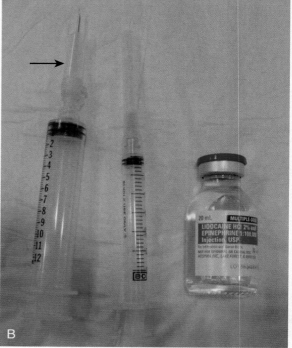

Figure 64–9 *A*, As a safeguard to prevent deep penetration of a needle used to drain a peritonsillar abscess, select a long 18- to 20-gauge needle. Remove the plastic needle guard and cut off the distal 1 cm. *B*, Then, replace the cut off guard on the needle (*arrow*) and secure it to the hub.

alone. These procedures can be done in combination with hospital admission and administration of intravenous antibiotics or as an outpatient treatment with oral antibiotics. One evidence-based review analyzed 42 articles, 5 of which were clinical studies on surgical technique.[9] They found all three techniques are effective to treat PTA and the recurrence rate is low (grade C recommendation). The approach depends on the patient's clinical status and medical history. Decisions about the treatment of a PTA in the ED are often made by the emergency clinician, but as local protocols dictate, consultation with an otolaryngologist is also appropriate.

Needle Aspiration/Incision and Drainage

The two procedures described here include needle aspiration and incision and drainage. They should be performed only in the cooperative patient without severe trismus. With the carotid artery located 2.5 cm behind and lateral to the tonsil, there is minimal room for error, patient movement, or poor anesthesia.

Have the patient sit upright with a support behind the head. This is best done as a two-person procedure. Ask an assistant to retract the cheek laterally to maximize visibility. A head lamp provides optimal lighting; a double tongue-blade setup aids visualization of the operative area (see Fig. 64–2*A*). Administer parenteral narcotic analgesia, mild sedation, or both, before attempting aspiration. Fentanyl, 2 to 3 µg/kg administered intravenously a few minutes before the procedure, is often ideal. Midazolam may be judiciously used, but the patient should not be overly sedated. The combination of midazolam, ketamine, and glycopyrrolate has been reported as being safe and effective for the outpatient peritonsillar drainage in children.[10]

Some opt to anesthetize the area topically with Cetacaine spray or 4% to 10% lidocaine. Use manual palpation to locate the fluctuant area of the abscess. Additionally, or primarily, anesthetize this area with local infiltration of 1 to 2 mL of 1% lidocaine with epinephrine via a 27-gauge needle. Use a 5-mL syringe with a long needle to visualize the area to be injected (Fig. 64–8). A small needle or syringe can cause your hand to block the view. Displacing the tongue with a finger, rather

than a tongue blade, may provide a better view. Infiltrate the lidocaine intramucosally for the best results but be careful not to increase the abscess size by direct injection into the abscess cavity. The area should blanch. With proper local infiltration, the patient will not feel the penetration of the aspirating needle. If the trismus is so pronounced as to prevent adequate anesthesia administration, it will probably be too difficult to aspirate or incise the abscess properly.

For aspiration, prepare a long 18- to 20-gauge needle on a 10- to 20-mL syringe. Fashion a needle guard by cutting off the distal 1 cm of the plastic needle cover, replace the cover on the needle, and securely attach this guard to the needle and syringe with tape to prevent inadvertent displacement (Fig. 64–9). Ensure that the needle protrudes only 1 cm beyond the cover. This procedure will limit the depth of needle penetration and lessen the risk of entering any major vascular structures. If pus is not obtained at a 1-cm depth, deeper penetration is discouraged. Insert the needle into the

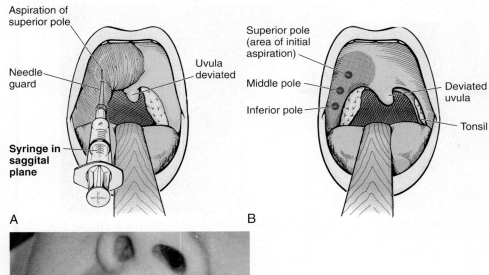

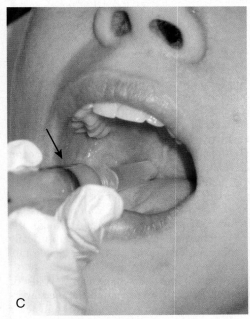

Figure 64–10 *A,* Needle aspiration of a peritonsillar abscess. Anesthetize the posterior pharynx with topical lidocaine spray. Blanch the mucosa with lidocaine/epinephrine with a 27-gauge needle on a long syringe (to allow visualization of the site) in the area to be aspirated. Advance an 18- or 20-gauge needle with needle guard into the area of greatest fluctuance, usually the superior pole. Aspirate as you advance the needle. Advance the needle in the sagittal plane. *Do not direct the needle laterally toward the carotid artery or jugular vein. B,* The superior pole is aspirated first, but the middle and inferior poles should be aspirated if pus is not obtained initially. Note that the tonsil itself is not aspirated. *C,* The peritonsillar space contains the actual abscess. Note pus in syringe *(arrow).*

most fluctuant (or prominent) area as previously determined, which is most commonly the superior pole of the tonsil (Fig. 64–10). Importantly, *advance the syringe/needle in the sagittal plane only, do not angle it to the side toward the carotid artery.* Do not aspirate the tonsil itself because the abscess develops in the peritonsillar space surrounding the tonsil. Advance the needle in the sagittal plane and do not direct it laterally where it could injure the carotid artery. If the aspirate is positive for pus, remove as much purulent material as possible. If the aspirate is negative, attempt aspiration again in the middle pole of the peritonsillar space, approximately 1 cm caudal to the first aspiration. Perform a third and final attempt at the inferior pole. Up to 30% of abscesses will be missed if only the superior pole is aspirated. It must be stressed that a negative aspirate does NOT rule out a PTA.

Usually, 2 to 6 mL of pus is obtained. It is unusual to recover more than 8 to 10 mL (Fig. 64–11). There is no specific advantage of sending the aspirate to the laboratory for culture. When significant amounts of pus are aspirated, the patient usually feels immediate improvement in pain and dysphagia. After the needle is removed, some bleeding will be noted. A slight ooze may be noted for a few hours, especially if warm water rinses are used. Drainage of pus may continue, often sensed as a foul taste by the patient. Significant addi-

tional drainage of pus may be an indication for a repeat aspiration, incision and drainage, or hospital admission.

Some clinicians advise a formal incision and drainage if frank pus is obtained; whereas others now accept needle aspiration (with close follow-up) as the definitive initial treatment. Combined aspiration and formal drainage in the same visit may be indicated if large amounts of pus are obtained (>5–6 mL) or if pus continues to drain from the aspiration site. There are no agreed-upon standards regarding the best practice for this issue.

To incise a PTA, anesthetize the area as described earlier. Prepare a No. 11 or 15 scalpel blade by taping over all but the distal 0.5 cm of the blade to prevent deeper penetration (Fig. 64–12). Incise the area of maximal fluctuance or the area where a preceding aspiration (if one was performed) located pus. Incise the mucosa in an area 0.5 cm long in a posterior to anterior direction. A stab incision with a No. 11 blade usually suffices. Warn the patient that the pus will flow posteriorly and she or he must expectorate this. Expect bleeding, because this is a vascular area. Suction the incised area with a No. 9 or 10 Frazier suction tip or a tonsil suction tip to aid in removal of the purulent material. Place a closed Kelly clamp into the opening and gently open it to break up the loculations. Allow the patient to rinse and gargle with a saline

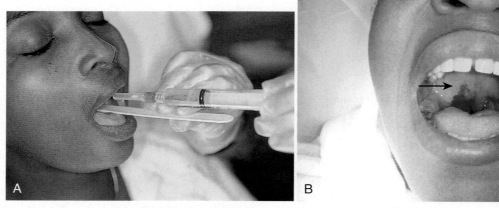

Figure 64–11 *A*, Needle aspiration usually yields 2–6 mL of thick pus. Greater volumes are unusual. Aspirate as much pus as possible, but removing only a small amount will produce a marked reduction in symptoms. *B*, After aspiration, minimal bleeding is expected (*arrow*).

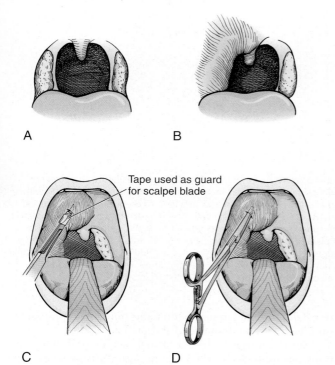

Tape used as guard for scalpel blade

Figure 64–12 Aspiration is often the only procedure required to successfully treat a peritonsillar abscess, but it has a 10% failure rate. In some instances, the clinician will opt for incision and drainage of a peritonsillar abscess. This procedure may be used initially, or after aspiration if copious pus is aspirated or if pus continues to drain or reaccumulate. *A*, Normal-appearing oropharynx. *B*, Peritonsillar abscess on the right side of the throat. *C*, Incision of the abscess at the area of greatest fluctuance. Notice that the scalpel is taped to prevent deep penetration. *D*, Remove loculations by gentle probing with hemostats.

prolonged observation. Frequent rinses with warm saline are quite helpful in relieving postaspiration symptoms.

After either needle aspiration or incision and drainage, prescribe antibiotics to eradicate the offending organisms. Penicillin, clindamycin, or cephalosporins are reasonable first choices. Resistance rates to penicillin range from 0% to 56%, but laboratory sensitivity testing is not always reflective of a clinical response.[6] Alternatives include ampicillin/sulbactam and amoxicillin/clavulanate. Reasonable cure rates have been obtained with oral penicillin in modest doses (500 mg PO four times a day). Many clinicians prefer to administer an intravenous loading dose of penicillin (5 million units) or cefazolin (1 g) before releasing the patient. Although the benefit is not well established, many clinicians empirically administer parenteral steroids as well to further ameliorate symptoms. A randomized trial by Ozbeck and colleagues[11] compared needle aspiration plus intramuscular steroids or placebo. They found a statistically significant difference favoring the use of steroids, especially for pain control and fever resolution. There were no complications in the steroid group.

Any patient who appears to have a toxic response, whose immune system is compromised, who is unable to take oral antibiotics, or who is dehydrated should be admitted for intravenous fluid hydration and antibiotic administration. Others may be discharged if no other issues are involved. Reevaluate all patients treated with needle aspiration in 24 to 36 hours to assess the need for repeat aspirations or formal incision and drainage. At 24 hours, most patients are markedly improved; failure to see this response requires further evaluation. Recommend that the patient use warm saline gargles and mild opioid analgesics. Advise all patients to return immediately for recurrence of symptoms, fevers, or continued bleeding from the incision.

Complications

Needle aspiration is an accepted, safe, and effective technique for the ED treatment of PTA. Most patients can be discharged after a short period of ED observation with 24- to 36-hour follow-up. There is an approximate 10% failure rate and need for subsequent drainage.[7] Aspiration or incision of the carotid artery or a misdiagnosed carotid artery aneurysm may have devastating results, but this complication is not documented in the recent literature. If the patient has cellu-

or dilute peroxide/saline solution. Packing is not used in the drainage of this abscess. After aspiration or incision, it is prudent to observe the patient for about an hour to watch for complications (e.g., bleeding) and to ensure the ability to tolerate oral fluids. Most patients can be discharged with 24-hour follow-up. Toxic patients, those with excessive volumes of aspirate, those with persistent bleeding, and those unable to take oral antibiotics are candidates for admission or more litis, the aspiration will be of no help, but it will not worsen morbidity. Failure to obtain pus should prompt high-dose antibiotics and a recheck in 24 hours. Many clinicians will opt for admission in such instances. A too-large or too-small incision may lead to poor healing or inability to completely evacuate the abscess, respectively.

EAR

Anatomy of the External Auditory Canal

The external auditory canal (EAC) extends from the tympanic membrane (TM) to the concha and measures approximately 2.5 cm in the adult. It is relatively short and straight in early infancy but begins to take on its adult S-shape and overall anterocaudal orientation beginning at age 2 years. Initially, the EAC is almost entirely cartilaginous, but by adulthood, its medial two thirds is composed of bony support with an overlying thin, stratified, squamous epithelium. The lateral third has a less sensitive, thicker, hairy epithelium that produces cerumen and retains its cartilage as support. The arterial supply to the EAC originates from the external carotid artery via the posterior auricular, maxillary, and superficial temporal branches. The mandibular branch of the fifth cranial nerve (V3) and the vagus nerve innervate the ear.

Other important anatomic considerations include (1) Two natural narrowings of the EAC exist, which are important when considering FBs. One is located at the junction of bone and cartilage and the other lies just lateral to the TM. (2) A blind spot may occur in the tympanic sulcus (inferior and anterior to the TM) owing to the oblique orientation of the TM. An examiner using a simple otoscope may not visualize an FB in this sulcus.

Anesthesia of the Ear

External Ear/Auricle

Indications for local anesthesia of the auricle include closure of extensive lacerations or other painful procedures such as hematoma incision and drainage. Four nerve branches supply the external ear; knowledge of their anatomy is required to understand the location for anesthesia injection (Fig. 64–13). The greater auricular nerve (branch of the cervical plexus) innervates most of the posteromedial, posterolateral, and infe-

rior auricle. A few branches of the lesser occipital nerve may contribute to this area. The auricular branch of the vagus supplies the concha and most of the area around the auditory meatus. The auriculotemporal nerve (from the mandibular branch of the trigeminal nerve) supplies the anterosuperior and anteromedial aspects of the auricle.

Procedure. Fill a 10-mL syringe with either 1% lidocaine or 0.25% bupivacaine. Mix with epinephrine if a regional block is planned in an area without evidence of traumatized vascularity. Attach the syringe to a 25- or 27-gauge needle (5–7 cm in length). One of several methods may be used to accomplish partial or complete anesthesia, depending on the area of concern. To anesthetize the nerve branches of the greater auricular and lesser occipital nerve branches, inject between 3 and 4 mL of anesthetic in the posterior sulcus (Fig. 64–14A). Insert the needle behind the inferior pole of the auricle and gradually aspirate and inject toward the superior pole, following the crescent-shaped contour of the posterior auricle. Anesthetize the auriculotemporal nerve anteriorly by placing 3 to 4 mL of anesthetic just superior and anterior to the cartilaginous tragus. Provide anesthesia to the auricular branch of the vagus nerve and the more central areas of the auricle using the technique shown in Figures 64–15 and 64–16.

Another and possibly more effective option is the regional block shown in Figure 64–14B. Insert the needle subcutaneously at a point approximately 1 cm above the superior pole of the auricle and direct it to a point just anterior to the tragus. Be sure to inject the skin of the scalp while avoiding the auricular cartilage. Aspirate, then slowly withdraw the needle, injecting anesthetic until the needle is almost to the puncture site. Redirect the needle posteriorly and repeat the process while aiming at the skin just behind the midauricle. Remove the needle and perform the same procedure, but insert the needle just inferior to the insertion of the ear lobule and anesthetize in a superior direction. Again, block the auricular branch of the vagus as described in Figure 64–17 if additional anesthesia of the concha is required.

Use caution if adding epinephrine to the anesthetic solution when placing regional blocks of the ear, especially if the blood supply has already been traumatically reduced. Do not include epinephrine when directly infiltrating wounds of the auricle, because restriction of blood flow through end arteries here may result in tissue necrosis. Other complications related

Figure 64–13 *A* and *B,* External anatomy of the ear and innervation of the auricle.

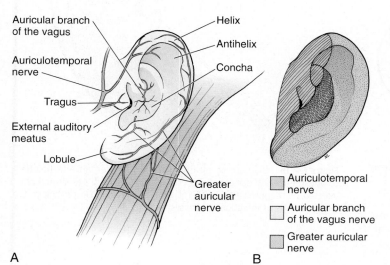

Auricular branch of the vagus

Auriculotemporal nerve

Tragus

External auditory meatus

Lobule

Helix

Antihelix

Concha

Greater auricular nerve

A

B

Auriculotemporal nerve

Auricular branch of the vagus nerve

Greater auricular nerve

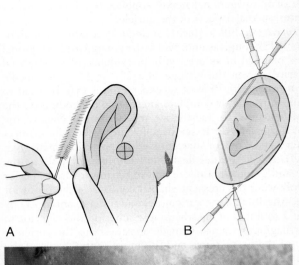

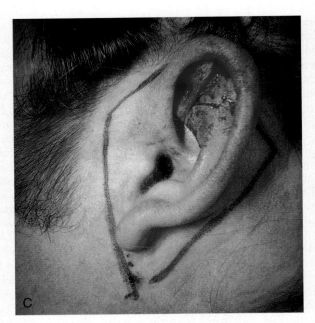

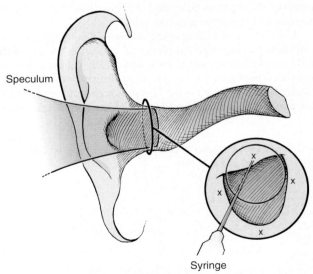

Figure 64–14   Field blocks of the auricle. *A,* One method uses approximately 3–4 mL of anesthetic, both in the posterior sulcus and at a point just anterior to the tragus. *B,* Alternative field block technique that deposits 2–3 mL of anesthetic for each needle pass. *C* and *D,* Location of anesthetic injections.

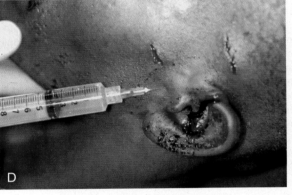

Speculum

Syringe

Figure 64–15   Four-quadrant field block anesthesia of the external auditory canal. Local anesthetic is injected subcutaneously in the four quadrants of the lateral portion of the ear canal. The largest speculum that will fit is used to guide the injections. The speculum is withdrawn slightly, tilted toward each of the four quadrants, and the needle is inserted subcutaneously (*x*). Inject a very small amount of anesthetic (0.25–0.50 mL) to produce a slight bulge in the soft tissue. A total of 1.5–2.0 mL of anesthetic is usually sufficient to anesthetize the ear canal and permit painless removal of a foreign body (FB). Ketamine procedural sedation may be a better option.

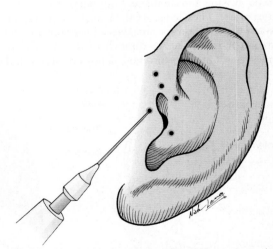

Figure 64–16   Diagram of injection sites for an alternative technique to anesthetize the ear canal and central concha. Each site should be injected with approximately 0.5 mL of 1% lidocaine. Do not inject if external signs of infection are present.

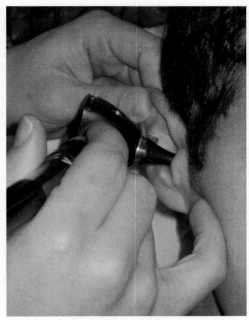

Figure 64–17 Examination of ear canal. Retract the pinna in a superior and posterior direction to straighten out the ear canal. Hold the scope in the other hand and stabilize it against the patient's head. This prevents inadvertent injury if the patient moves unexpectedly.

to local anesthetics and regional blocks of the head and neck are reviewed elsewhere in the text.

External Auditory Canal and Tympanic Membrane

The EAC is innervated by the auricular branch of the vagus (inferiorly and posteriorly) and by the auriculotemporal nerve (superiorly, anteriorly, and inferiorly). The primary indication for local anesthesia of the auditory canal is for FB removal, including débridement of otitis externa or removal of significant cerumen impaction. *It is very difficult to obtain adequate anesthesia of the inner ear and TM for painful procedures.* Simply stated, no easy and completely effective procedure consistently works well. If total anesthesia is required, general anesthesia, especially in children, is often the only alternative. *Ketamine is an ideal agent for short procedures, especially for children with foreign objects in the ear.* Topical anesthetics are inadequate owing to their poor absorption through the rather impermeable and keratinized epithelial surface of the EAC. Although effective for some procedures, injecting local anesthetics in and around the auditory meatus is quite painful and is often difficult to perform in a struggling and uncooperative patient. Certain instances warrant adjunctive use of procedural sedation Auralgan, a combination of benzocaine and other ingredients, may provide analgesia for painful earaches due to otitis, but it does little to benefit painful procedures.

Procedure. Local anesthesia is performed with a 25- or 27-gauge needle (3–5 cm in length) attached to a syringe of 1% lidocaine with epinephrine. A 1:10 mixture of 8.4% sodium bicarbonate to lidocaine helps to reduce pain during injection in this sensitive area. Place a speculum just inside the auditory meatus and inject 0.3 to 0.5 mL of the anesthetic into the subcutaneous tissue, stopping after a small bulge in the skin is raised. Inject all four quadrants in this manner by moving the speculum after each injection (see Fig. 64–15). If additional anesthesia is necessary, give two more small injec-

tions. Inject the same amount slightly farther into the canal, once along the anterior wall and again at the posterior wall at the bone-cartilage junction.

Another similar technique involves depositing the anesthetic just lateral, or exterior, to the external auditory meatus. Using the same size needle and type of anesthetic solution as just described, inject approximately 0.5 to 1.0 mL into each of five points around the auditory meatus and tragus (see Fig. 64–16).

Examination

Several methods are available to examine the EAC and TM. In all methods, grasp the superior pinna and pull cephalad and posterior to straighten the slightly tortuous EAC. The most common manner of examination is with a fiberoptic otoscope (see Fig. 64–17). Insufflate the TM and examine the EAC with the diagnostic head. Use the operating head to pass instruments into the EAC and to maneuver them more easily. Place a plastic or metal speculum into the auditory meatus for examination, using a head lamp or head mirror/light bulb as a light source. Although this provides excellent illumination, use magnifying loupes for adequate visualization during procedures. The ideal setup for cerumen or FB removal consists of an operating microscope and a speculum. This provides binocular vision and frees the examiner's hands for instrumentation. Unfortunately, this equipment is seldom found outside of the otolaryngology clinic setting. Stabilize the hand holding the otoscope against the patient's temporal skull to prevent inadvertent canal injury if there is unexpected patient movement.

Cerumen Impaction

The excretion of the ceruminous or apocrine and sebaceous glands together with cells exfoliated from the EAC combine to form cerumen. One study found that cerumen is composed of lipids, complex proteins, and simple sugars.[12] Cerumen repels water, has documented antimicrobial activity, and forms a protective barrier against infection. Cerumen often becomes impacted, causing complaints of a "blocked" ear, hearing impairment, or dizziness. Symptomatic impaction is an indication for removal, although symptoms are rare until complete obstruction is present. Sudden loss of hearing is a common complaint in patients with totally occluding impacted cerumen. Cerumen obstructs visualization of the TM and can be evacuated as a part of the evaluation of a febrile child or the patient complaining of ear pain. However, cerumen removal in a child is rarely indicated in the ED simply to visualize the TM.

Cerumen is usually impacted for prolonged periods, and vigorous attempts to remove it may precipitate otitis externa. It is reasonable to instill antiseptics (Vol Sol and others) or antibiotic ear drops for a few days after cerumen removal to prevent this. Neomycin-containing ear drops are best avoided owing to the precipitation of a contact dermatitis. Diabetics, for example, commonly experience otitis externa after seemingly minor manipulation of the ear canal. No standard exists, however, and practices vary widely.

Cerumen Removal

Irrigation is an effective approach for cerumen removal and has the advantage of being painless and simple to perform. The patient does not have to remain completely still; thus, it is ideal for the pediatric population. It is estimated that 150,000 ears are irrigated in the United States each week.[13] Although usually more time-consuming and messy than manual extraction, irrigation is an appropriate initial method to attempt and can be performed by technicians with guidance from the clinician. One contraindication is known or suspected TM perforation. Use irrigation judiciously in elderly and immunocompromised patients, because malignant otitis externa can be preceded by irrigation of the EAC.[14] Such patients may benefit from antibiotics for a few days after cerumen removal if the skin has been abraded. Generally, the procedures used to remove cerumen are safe; however, otologic injury has resulted from this "minor" procedure and has even resulted in litigation.[13]

A recent evidence-based review concluded that current evidence suggests little difference in the efficacy of water-based and oil-based preparations for the treatment of cerumen removal.[15] Non–water-, non–oil-based preparations appear most effective for clearing cerumen and improving syringing, but further research is needed.[15] Whichever of the following techniques are used, some tips for successful cerumen removal include use proper lighting, pay attention to patient comfort, and never continue beyond the patient's comfort level.

Ceruminolytics

These products may soften obviously hardened or impacted cerumen. They are used as adjuncts to other procedures—simply instilling ceruminolytics into the canal will not remove enough cerumen to aid the emergency clinician. If irrigation fails, the continued outpatient use of ceruminolytics is often prescribed, usually combined with home irrigation using a bulb syringe or a repeat visit in a few days. Although many products are available as ceruminolytics, a 5% or 10% solution of sodium bicarbonate disintegrates cerumen much more quickly and efficiently than commercially prepared ceruminolytics and other products.[16] Cerumenex, Cerumol, Auralgan, Buro-Sol, alcohol, and oils were all tested and took more than 18 hours to disintegrate cerumen versus approximately 90 minutes for the sodium bicarbonate solutions.[16] Hydrogen peroxide is another commonly used ceruminolytic, but its use has not been systematically studied. One study found the liquid preparation of the stool softener docusate sodium (Colace) was much more effective as a ceruminolytic than Cerumenex.[17] One evidence-based review of agents found docusate sodium given 15 minutes before irrigation was most effective for facilitating cerumen removal.[18] Triethanolamine (Cerumenex) and olive oil were the next most effective treatments.

Place the patient in the supine position with the affected ear up and instill the solution at least 15 minutes before attempts at removal. Repeat instillation between attempts at manual extraction or irrigation.

Irrigation (Ear Syringing)

Ask the patient to sit upright and hold an emesis or ear irrigation basin flush tightly against the skin just below the earlobe. Insert the irrigation tip into the EAC only as far as the cartilage-bone junction, and direct the stream of water superiorly to wash the impacted cerumen away from the TM. Warm water to nearly body temperature to prevent caloric stimulation. Multiple attempts may be necessary, and intermittent attempts at manual removal of loosened cerumen may help hasten the process. During the irrigation, *ask an assistant to apply traction to the pinna to straighten the canal for more efficient*

irrigation. Patients usually feel some discomfort with forceful irrigation, but not severe pain.

Attach a 30- to 60-mL syringe to a 19-gauge or larger butterfly device, cut off the needle and wings, leaving the resultant tubing for irrigation. A plastic or Teflon intravenous catheter (16 or 18 gauge with the needle removed) can similarly be affixed to a syringe. Contraindications to ear syringing include[19]:

Patient aversion to or history of injury from syringing.
History of middle ear disease.
History of ear surgery.
Perforated TM.
Severe otitis externa.
Narrow ear canals.
FBs, especially sharp objects and vegetable matter.
Uncooperative patient.
Occluding aural exostoses.
Known inner ear disturbance, especially if the patient has severe vertigo.
History of radiation therapy to the external or middle ear, skull base, or mastoid.

The most common way to irrigate an ear is with a syringe and catheter (Fig. 64–18). The use of oral jet irrigators (Water Pik) is another accepted method but a syringe/catheter is readily found in the ED and unlikely to generate enough pressure to cause injury. After irrigating the EAC, apply several drops of isopropanol in the EAC to facilitate evaporation of residual moisture. Do not use isopropanol if the TM is ruptured. Furthermore, topical steroid-containing suspension drops (ciprofloxacin/hydrocortisone) may be soothing after prolonged irrigation. Because diabetics can develop severe otitis externa after irrigation, some clinicians routinely prescribe antibiotic ear drops (e.g., fluoroquinolones) for a few days after irrigation in high-risk patients.

Although complications are more common with jet irrigators, they may occur with any method of ear irrigation. These include otitis externa, TM perforation, or middle ear injury from a preexisting defect in the TM. Stop the irrigation and examine the TM if the patient is experiencing sudden pain, tinnitus, hearing loss, nausea, or vertigo. If the membrane is ruptured, give prophylactic oral antibiotics for otitis media, keep the ear canal perfectly dry with cotton, and refer the patient to an otolaryngologist. This complication is usually intimately benign.

Manual Instrumentation

Manual instrumentation is more advantageous because it is usually quicker, and the examiner may more easily remove hardened or larger concretions of cerumen under direct visualization. However, it is difficult to manually remove cerumen without causing significant pain, so irrigation is preferred. *Manual removal may be the initial procedure in some cases, followed by irrigation when the cerumen is partially disrupted.* Place the diagnostic or operating head of the fiberoptic otoscope or a speculum to serve as a protective port through which instruments are passed and manipulated (Fig. 64–19). An operating microscope works best in this situation but, again, is usually not available. To prevent startling or agitating an already anxious patient, allow the patient to experience the sensation of an instrument in the canal by first placing the instrument softly against the ear canal wall.

Instruments used for cerumen removal include flexible plastic or wire loops, right-angle hooks, suction-tip catheters, or plastic scoops (Fig. 64–20). The spoonlike instruments and

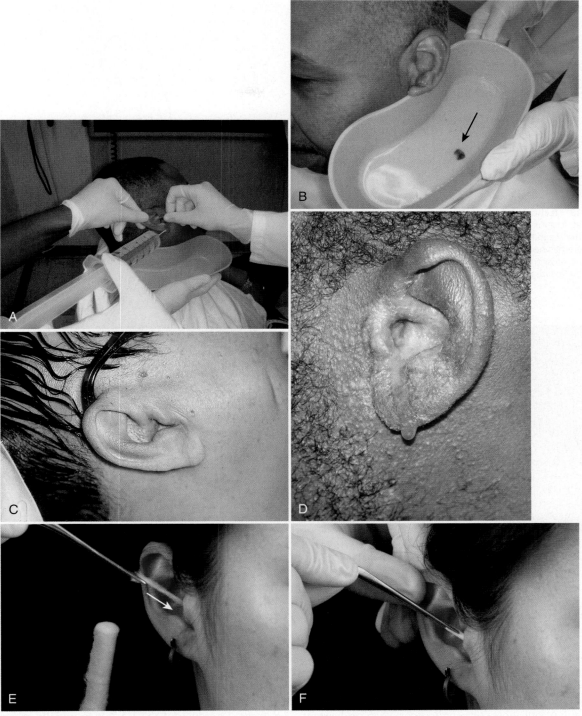

Figure 64–18 *A,* Irrigation, although time consuming and potentially messy, is usually successful in removing impacted cerumen and much less traumatic than manual removal. Irrigate with an 18-gauge flexible catheter attached to a 60-mL syringe. Because multiple irrigations may be required, small syringes are counterproductive. Use only *warm* water. Cerumenolytics, such as liquid colace, may be used for 15–20 min before irrigation. Note that an assistant *retracts the pinna* to open the canal. *B,* Often, repeated irrigations are required, followed by a sudden successful flush. If irrigation is aggressive or extensive, some will instill antibiotic/antiseptic drops for a few days in an attempt to prevent otitis external. *C,* Malignant otitis externa in a diabetic patient followed her manual removal of cerumen with cotton swab and a pencil, but it may develop without canal manipulation. *D,* Extensive contact dermatitis from the use of neomycin-containing ear drops. *E* and *F,* An ear wick can be used to draw antibiotic drops into an inflamed ear canal. Keep it wet with antibiotic solution. Either cotton (*E*) or an expandable sponge (*F;* Merocel) may be used.

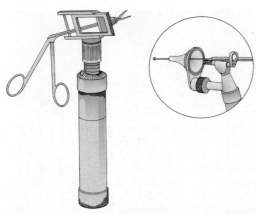

Figure 64–19 **Technique for direct visualization and mechanical FB removal.** Use of alligator forceps through a diagnostic otoscope. Note that the magnification device has been slid laterally and that no ear speculum has been attached. *Inset,* Use of ear curettage through an operating otoscope. *(From Fritz S, Kelen GD, Sivertson KT: Foreign bodies of the external auditory canal. Emerg Med Clin North Am 5:184, 1987.)*

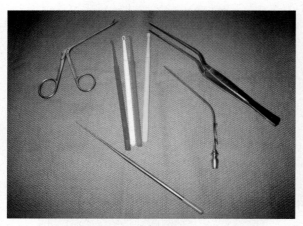

Figure 64–20 **Instruments used for FB extraction.** *Left to right,* Alligator forceps, various plastic loops and scoops, bayonet forceps, Frazier suction, right-angle hook.

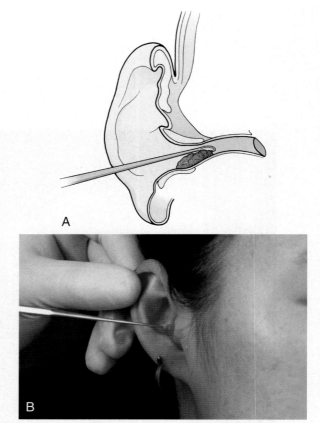

A

B

Figure 64–21 *A,* Removal of impacted cerumen. Pass the tip of the wire loop beyond the wax and gently tease the wax off the ear canal wall. Extract the wax slowly from the canal. Under direct visualization, avoid contact with the skin of the ear canal to prevent pain and excoriation. *B,* Only a very delicate touch and a cooperative patient allow cerumen removal with a spoon. Distract the pinna for better exposure and try to avoid touching the canal itself. Once cerumen is broken up, irrigation may finalize removal.

irrigation are both more effective in removing softer cerumen. Firm cerumen ordinarily is more easily withdrawn with loops or right-angle hooks. Gently tease the cerumen off of the canal wall using loops and then pass hooks or loops around the cerumen and withdraw it slowly (Fig. 64–21). Take care to keep both hands in contact with the patient's head, because any sudden movement may cause trauma to the canal or the TM. Complications most commonly occur when inadvertent contact is made with the thin, friable skin of the bony canal. Trauma may cause EAC laceration, hecatombs, otitis externa, or TM perforations.

Otitis Externa

Otitis externa, or "swimmer's ear," is an inflammation of the skin of the EAC. This is essentially a cellulitis of the ear canal. Otitis externa can be disabling enough to cause 36% of patients to interrupt their daily activities for a median duration of 4 days.[20] Precipitants of otitis externa include water exposure and trauma. Excessive moisture in the canal raises the pH and removes the cerumen. Keratin can not absorb

water, creating a medium for bacterial growth. Trauma, especially self-manipulation with FBs (e.g., cotton swabs, fingernails), causes abrasions to the ear canal and introduces infection. Removal of cerumen by water irrigation is a well-recognized risk factor for the development of otitis externa.[20]

The disease process involves a continuum of gradually worsening inflammatory changes. The patient may present with symptoms ranging from slight itching and discomfort to severe pain, purulent discharge, or systemic toxicity. Pain with manipulation of the pinna is the hallmark for otitis externa. Otoscopy of the EAC may initially reveal minimal debris and erythema, but as the infection progresses, more edema, exudate, erythema, and possibly, even a surrounding cellulitis may become apparent. In severe stages, the edema may obstruct the canal, preventing instillation of ear drops.

Common bacteria cultured from patients with otitis externa include *Pseudomonas aeruginosa* and *S. aureus*. Other bacteria include *Acinetobacter*, *Proteus*, *Enterococcus*, and *Bacteroides*. Approximately 50% of patients have polymicrobial infection and 8% have anaerobic isolates.[21] One study found that 6% of staphylococcus isolates were methicillin resistant.[22] Fungi are identified in about 10% of otitis externa cases and are often coexistent with bacterial infections. *Aspergillus* is responsible for 80% to 90% of cases followed by *Candida*. It characteristically presents as a furry lining of the ear canal with a fluffy white discharge. Herpes zoster affecting the geniculate ganglion may appear as grouped vesicles on an erythematous base within the canal. This condition, known as *Ramsay Hunt syndrome*, is associated with facial nerve palsies, hearing loss, and other cranial nerve impairment.

Diabetics and other immunocompromised patients, especially human immunodeficiency virus–positive patients, are susceptible to malignant (necrotizing) otitis externa, a life-threatening form of otitis externa caused by *Pseudomonas*. Deep tissue necrosis, osteomyelitis, intracranial extension, and systemic toxicity are hallmark features. Malignant otitis externa is difficult to treat and the mortality rate can be as high as 53%.[20] The diagnosis of malignant otitis externa should be considered in the diabetic or immunocompromised patient with significant symptoms who fails to respond to initial outpatient treatment.

Canal Débridement/Wick Placement

It has been touted that the key to successful treatment is adequate removal of canal debris. However, vigorous attempts to remove debris on the first visit are frequently painful, of unproven value, and often eschewed. Use small swabs (e.g., urethral swabs) to gently remove debris. Gently irrigate the canal, but realize that *many patients will be cured without extensive débridement*. Because the inflamed canal is susceptible to trauma, remove debris by suctioning under direct visualization using the open or operating otoscope head and a 5- or 7-French Frazier tip suction. Irrigate the canal only if you are sure that there is no TM perforation, which may be difficult to confirm owing to edema and patient discomfort.[20,21] For more advanced cases presenting with significant exudate and edema, debris removal is necessary but intensely painful. One approach is to use a local block of the EACl (see Fig. 64–16) as long as the cellulitis has not extended out to the tragus or concha. Administer parenteral analgesics if additional pain control is required.

When edema, debris, and exudate are marked enough to impede antibiotic drops from contacting the canal skin, use an ear wick. The wick works as a conduit to deliver the antibiotic solutions to the ear canal. The true benefit of wick implantation is unknown and often is not performed because it is painful. One approach is to place a 0.25-inch strip of Nu-Gauze dressing covered with an antibiotic and steroid cream (Cortisporin Otic cream) into the external acoustic canal in a fashion similar to the technique used for anterior nasal packing. Using an otoscope and alligator forceps, place the leading edge of the gauze deeply in the canal until it is fully packed. Withdraw the otoscope and finish by packing the lateral aspect of the canal as well.

Another choice is to use commercially available ear wicks, such as the Pope Merocel ear wick. Place this dehydrated and trimmed wick into an edematous canal and apply antibiotic/hydrocortisone drops onto it. The wick swells and helps to reduce edema by the antimicrobial and anti-inflammatory effects of the solution and through pressure exerted against the walls as it expands. Keep the wick moist with drops and leave it in place until the patient is followed up in 24 to 48 hours for removal and further evaluation. Although relatively safe to use, the ear wick is designed for short-term use. Generally, these wicks will fall out of the canal as edema subsides. However, the unusual retention of these wicks can harbor bacteria and cause tissue ingrowth, resulting in long-term problems for the patient.[23]

Antibiotic Therapy and Follow-up

Most cases of otitis externa can be effectively treated with débridement and topical antibiotic drops. A study by Halpern and associates[24] showed that fewer than 20% of patients have a concomitant diagnosis treatable by oral medications, yet 40% of patients receive topical and oral medications, and many of the oral antibiotics prescribed are not active against *Pseudomonas* and *Staphylococcus*. They also found that only 7% of adult doctor visits and 2% of pediatric clinician visits reported ear irrigation. Antibiotic ear drops most frequently consist of some combination of neomycin and polymyxin, but an acetic acid solution is another acceptable first-line therapy. Ear drops are instilled as 2 to 4 drops four times a day for 7 to 10 days. Hydrocortisone may be added to either the antibiotics (Cortisporin suspension or solution) or the acetic acid (VoSol HC). Cortisporin Otic solution (clear-appearing) is harmful to the middle ear if it passes through the TM, but the cloudy suspension appears safe. At times, it is difficult to distinguish between a ruptured TM secondary to otitis media and severe otitis externa in a child. Therefore, the cloudy-appearing Cortisporin suspension is recommended in any case of suspected or known TM perforation. Topical antibiotic preparations are recommended for chronic suppurative otitis media, tympanostomy tube otorrhea, and acute otitis media.[25] Antibiotic preparations entering the middle ear are rarely problematic. There is no compelling reason to withhold drops if the TM has been ruptured, but in that circumstance, do not use gentamycin preparation or corticosporin *solution*—use the Cortisporin Otic *suspension* instead.

Fluoroquinolones have good activity against *Pseudomonas* and *Staphylococcus*. Two topical fluoroquinolone preparations are available, ofloxacin 0.3% (Floxin Otic) and Ciprofloxacin 0.2% with hydrocortisone 1% (Cipro HC Otic). Ofloxacin solution is approved for treatment of otitis externa and otitis media with perforated or ventilated TM. Ciprofloxacin suspension, approved for the treatment of otitis externa only, may be used in patients 1 year of age and older. The topical fluoroquinolones show equal efficacy when compared with polymyxin B–neomycin–hydrocortisone suspension. Side effects are minimal and there is no reported ototoxicity.[26] Some practitioners consider these agents first-line therapy.

Holten and Gick[27] provided an evidence-based review of otitis externa treatment. The best evidence demonstrated equivalent results with ear cleaning, ear wick, and topical agents. Treatment with one of three regimens for 4 days was recommended. The regimens are (1) ear cleaning + ear wick + acidifying agent dosed four times a day, or (2) ear cleaning + ear wick + topical antibiotic dosed four times a day (twice daily if fluoroquinolone), or (3) ear cleaning + ear wick + topical antibiotic/steroid combination dosed four times a day (twice if fluoroquinolone). There was less evidence for the use of single topical treatment or oral antibiotics. This paper also provided evidence-based treatment options for malignant otitis externa.

Inform patients to avoid getting water in the ear for the full course of treatment and to apply ear drops immediately if water does contact the ear canal. Follow-up severe cases in 24 to 36 hours and repeat débridement if needed. Administer oral opioids generously for the first 24 to 48 hours because this condition can be quite painful. Use nonsteroidal anti-inflammatory drugs also because they are effective for pain control. To prevent the recurrence of otitis externa, advise patients to avoid its many precipitants. Precipitants include excessive perspiration, regular participation in water sports, unusually viscous cerumen, a narrowed EAC, or exposure to systemic allergies. Preventive measures include drying the EAC with a hair dryer on the lowest heat setting after bathing or swimming, using prophylactic acidifying drops with alcohol (Swim Ear) or without alcohol (Burow's solution, Star-Otic), avoiding scratching or overzealous cleaning, and using protective barriers while swimming (tight-fitting bathing cap or well-fitting ear plugs).

Use broad-spectrum oral antibiotics in cases of persistent otitis externa, concomitant otitis media, systemic symptoms, and local cellulitis. Add criprofloxacin for greater coverage of *Pseudomonas* when treating the mild to moderate case of otitis externa in an immunocompromised patient without toxic reaction. Promptly admit suspected cases of malignant otitis externa and begin an intravenous antipseudomonal antibiotic. In addition, immediately consult an otolaryngologist for possible surgical débridement.

Treat patients with Ramsay Hunt syndrome with antivirals. Some clinicians suggest admission for administration of intravenous acyclovir. Treat otomycosis by swabbing the canal with a cotton-tipped applicator saturated with an antifungal solution (such as clotrimazole or boric acid/alcohol) in an effort to remove debris. Repeat this if necessary on follow-up in 3 to 7 days. If the infection is not responding, add over-the-counter clotrimazole 1% solution (Lotrimin). If the TM is perforated, use tolnaftate 1% solution (Tinactin). Topical solutions of thimerosol and M- cresyl acetate are also effective. All of these topical agents are prescribed as 3 or 4 drops twice daily for 7 days. Because *Aspergillus* may be resistant to clotrimazole, oral itraconazole (Sporanox) can be used.[20] Do not administer corticosteroids in cases of known fungal otitis externa.

FBs of the Ear Canal

Despite its small size, the EAC may play host to numerous types of FBs.[28,29] Living insects account for most FBs found in adults. Children frequently place food (e.g., peas, beans), organic matter (e.g., grass, leaves, flowers), and inorganic objects (e.g., beads, rocks, dirt) into the ear canals during play, and they often fail to admit this to parents. Button batteries may cause significant tissue destruction in a matter of hours, and it is vital to immediately obtain otolaryngologic consultation for removal if the button battery is not easily extracted. Symptoms of FB retention are usually ear pain, fullness, or impaired hearing in the adult; the pediatric patient may not present until an associated otitis externa with a purulent discharge has developed. Tinnitus, vertigo, significant hearing loss, or bleeding from behind the object should raise a high suspicion for an associated TM rupture.

As previously described, the anatomy of the EAC predisposes to the entrapment of FBs in either a lateral or a deeper position. Removal of more medial objects can be much more painful and anesthesia is usually required. *Even the most cooperative patient may become difficult after feeling pain during manipulation of the ear canal. It is probably impossible to adequately immobilize the head of an uncooperative awake child to delicately extract an FB.* Some authorities claim local anesthesia makes extracting FBs even more difficult because of soft tissue distortion, although swelling should be minimal if proper amounts of anesthetic are used. Anesthesia of the EAC may be difficult to achieve. Topical anesthetics have a partial effect, and a four-quadrant technique may not produce complete anesthesia, especially of the TM.[30] If the FB is deeply

or firmly embedded, the patient should be referred early for removal under an operating microscope, before canal trauma and swelling mandate admission for removal under general anesthesia. Procedural sedation (preferably an analgesic-sedative combination or dissociative anesthetic) can aid in the removal of FBs in the distraught child by preventing further struggling and potential canal trauma. *Ketamine is an excellent anesthetic for simple FB removal in the outpatient setting.* The care provider must weigh the inherent risks of procedural sedation against those of general anesthesia and the cost of hospital admission.

Before initiating removal, the clinician should set realistic limits on the number of attempts to be made. Even the best clinician can become too aggressive as frustration builds with failed attempts to extract the object. Early consultation with an otolaryngologist should not be considered a failure in cases of difficult FBs. Indeed, with the proper equipment and experience, most objects can be removed atraumatically.

Adequate visualization of the object is needed for successful removal. One study showed that canal lacerations occurred in 48% of patients in whom removal was attempted without a microscope and 4% when it was used.[30] The otoscope is the traditional ED instrument for viewing FBs of the ear canal. The otoscope is less likely to be useful in retrieval because it is difficult to insert the instrument through or around the small speculum end. A specialized ear, nose, and throat (ENT) speculum allows more space for instrumentation. A head lamp provides a good light source and leaves both hands free. Magnifying loupes also provide hands-free magnification.

Procedures

Make a judicious effort to remove an ear FB in the ED setting. Avoid prolonged traumatic attempts because this often terrifies the patient, complicates subsequent attempts, and can cause bleeding and swelling, thus making subsequent efforts more difficult. Most approaches to FB removal are anecdotal and are found in the literature as case reports or case series rather than as prospective clinical trials. Familiarize yourself with several techniques, because the most appropriate choice varies depending on the size, shape, consistency, and depth of impaction of the object.

Irrigation is the least invasive method; the techniques and related complications are explained in detail earlier in this chapter (see "Cerumen Removal"). Deeply embedded vegetable matter (e.g., beans, peas, or seeds) should not be irrigated because swelling may occur, making extraction more difficult. Irrigation works particularly well with small rocks, dirt, or sand that lie deep in the canal next to the TM.

Suction-Tip Catheters. This technique works well with objects that are round and difficult to grasp. Suction is readily available in the ED and needs to provide 100 to 140 mm Hg of negative pressure to be useful. To prevent iatrogenic injury, inform the patient of the impending noise to prevent sudden movements from a startle reflex. Place either the blunt or the soft plastic tip against the object and slowly withdraw. If using a suction instrument with a thumb-controlled release valve (as with the Frazier suction), remember to cover the port to activate the suction.

The Hognose (IQDr, Inc.), a commercially available device designed by an emergency clinician, aids in the removal of auditory canal FBs. It is used in combination with an otoscope and suction setup. It is essentially an otoscope speculum with suction attachment and a soft self-molding tip that can attach to objects. The flange comes in three color-coded sizes:

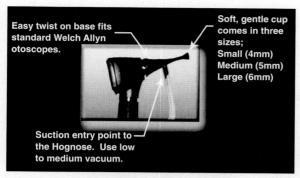

Easy twist on base fits standard Welch Allyn otoscopes.

Soft, gentle cup comes in three sizes; Small (4mm) Medium (5mm) Large (6mm)

Suction entry point to the Hognose. Use low to medium vacuum.

Figure 64–22 The Hognose device for FB removal. *A,* The Hognose attached to the otoscope and to wall suction. Occlusion of the open insufflation port to engage suction and remove the FB. Device available through IQDr, Inc (iqdr.com).

4, 5, and 6 mm. To use, first attach the Hognose to the otoscope and standard wall suction set at low to medium vacuum setting (Fig. 64–22). Next, under direct visualization, approach the FB with the otoscope. Finally, engage suction by applying finger pressure to the open insufflation port and withdraw.

Manual Instrumentation. This approach may be attempted with various instruments (Fig. 64–23). Use the diagnostic or operating head of a fiberoptic otoscope for illumination and magnification. Ask an assistant to hold the pinna back and out so that you may hold the otoscope with one hand and manipulate the instrument with the other. A speculum and either a head lamp or a head mirror/light source can also provide illumination; magnifying loupes are usually required for adequate visualization. Use small alligator forceps to remove objects with edges that can be grasped, but avoid trying to encircle an impacted round FB because this may cause trauma to the canal wall. A small right-angle hook is another choice. Place the tip past the object, rotate it 90°, and then pull the object from the canal. Fine-tissue or Adson forceps, curets, and skin hooks are other instruments used occasionally. Use of these instruments is commonly associated with abrasions and bleeding of the ear canal.[30] They should be used only on compliant, cooperative patients. Direct visualization of the object is essential.

Fogarty Catheters. Small Fogarty catheters (biliary or vascular) may be used in a manner similar to that described later in the chapter under "Nasal FB removal." Attach the catheter tip to a 3-mL syringe. Pass the catheter beyond the FB. Once the tip is past the object, gradually inflate the balloon and drag the FB out along with the balloon. Immediately deflate the balloon if sudden pain occurs because TM rupture is a potential complication.

Cyanoacrylate (Superglue). The use of glue in FB removal was first reported in India in 1977.[30,31] Glue is most effective in removing smooth, round objects that are difficult to grasp (see Fig. 64–23E and F). The FB should be dry and easily visualized. Apply a small amount of glue to the tip of a thin paintbrush, a straightened paper clip, or the blunt end of a wooden cotton-tipped applicator. Allow the glue to become tacky. Place the tip against the object, allow it to dry, and then carefully withdraw the FB. Minor complications are possible if the tip dries against the canal wall (abrasion, excoriation) or if the glue spills or drips onto the wall (creating a new FB). This technique may be more useful in adults because cooperation is required.[31]

Removal of Insects. Cockroaches are the most commonly found live insect in the ears. Treatment is to instill various substances into the ear canal to immobilize or kill the bug before removing it. This helps retrieval by allowing for a stationary target and also halts the disturbing and painful movement of the insect. Controversy exists about which agent most effectively accomplishes this. Mineral oil has traditionally been used, but lidocaine has been reported to paralyze insects and allow for easier extraction than the more viscous mineral oil. An in vitro comparative study showed that immersion in mineral oil and 2% or 4% lidocaine solution killed roaches in less than 60 seconds (~27 and 41 sec, respectively).[32] The roaches struggled less in the viscous oil than in the lidocaine, which did not appear to cause paralysis. Other substances (Auralgan, isopropanol, water, succinylcholine, hydrogen peroxide) were shown to be ineffective in killing the roaches in a reasonable amount of time. Once disabled, insects are removed with mechanical extraction as previously described; pieces can be suctioned out if fragmentation occurs (see Fig. 64–23G and *H*).

Follow-up/Complications

Evaluate hearing before and after FB removal, especially in patients with suspected TM or middle ear injuries. Examine also the opposite ear and nose of children to search for the rare but possible second FB. Minor lacerations or excoriations of the canal usually heal quickly with or without antibiotic ear drops, as long as the canal is kept clean and dry. Document preexisting canal trauma or suspected TM rupture before attempts at removal; otherwise, this may falsely be attributed to iatrogenic causes at a later date. Indications for otolaryngologic referral include failed removal in the ED, existent injury to the EAC or TM, TM rupture, EAC infection, object wedged in the medial EAC or up against the TM, glass or other sharp-edged FB, and special circumstances (disk batteries and putty).[33] Generally, no routine follow-up is necessary except in cases of infection, severe trauma, or TM perforation. Parents should be educated to reduce the exposure of children to potential FBs.

Auricular Hematoma

Auricular hematomas occur after a shearing force to the ear, most commonly in wrestlers, boxers, rugby players and after fights. A subperichondrial hematoma forms, separating the perichondrium from the cartilage. The hematoma may also arise from the cartilage itself. Recurrent or untreated injuries allow the development of new cartilage, which subsequently deforms the auricle (cauliflower ear).

Procedure

The treatment of an auricular hematoma is to completely evacuate the subperichondrial hematoma and reapproximate the perichondrium to the cartilage.

Needle Aspiration. Aspiration of an auricular hematoma is performed by perforating the hematoma with a 20-gauge needle (Fig. 64–24). "Milk" the hematoma between the thumb and the forefinger until the entire hematoma is evacuated. Apply a pressure dressing. Reexamine the ear frequently for reaccumulation of the hematoma. Reaccumulation of blood requires reaspiration. For small hematomas that are acute, needle aspiration alone with a bolster dressing is adequate therapy.[34]

Incision. An auricular hematoma, if less than 7 to 10 days old, may be incised along the natural skin folds. Anesthetize the pinna using local infiltration of 1% lidocaine

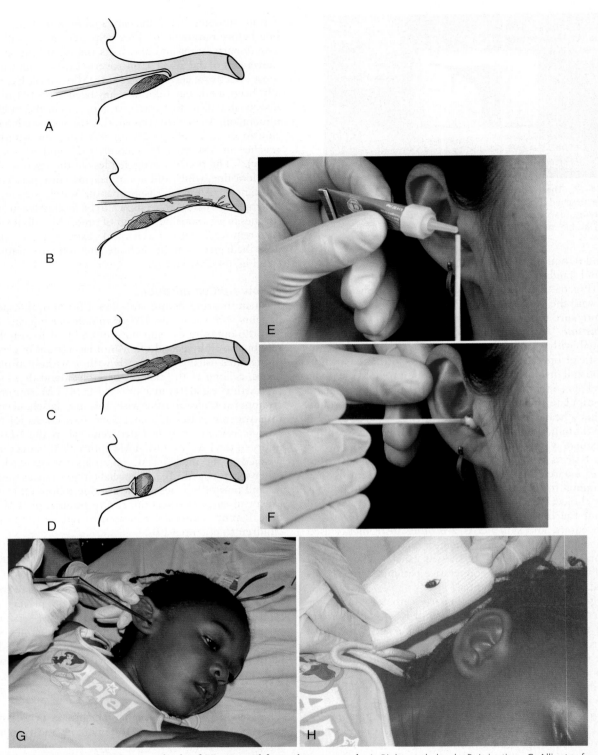

Figure 64–23 **Application of various methods of FB removal from the ear canal.** *A,* Right-angle hook. *B,* Irrigation. *C,* Alligator forceps. *D,* Soft-tipped suction. *E* and *F,* Putting Superglue on a stick and allowing it to attach to an FB may be successful. *G* and *H,* Removal of an insect can be a disaster or relatively easy. The easy way is to use ketamine anesthesia with careful direct extraction. No patients can cooperate with more than minimal inner ear canal manipulation.

(without epinephrine) or by an auricular block (described earlier). Incise the skin with a No. 15 blade at the edge of the hematoma, following the curvature of the pinna (Fig. 64–25). Gently peel the skin and perichondrium off the hematoma and underlying cartilage. Completely evacuate the hematoma and irrigate the remaining pocket with normal saline.

After removing the hematoma, apply antibiotic ointment and reapproximate the perichondrium to the cartilage with a pressure dressing. Apply a compression dressing to the ear as shown in Figure 64–26. An alternative technique is to suture dental rolls over the area (see Fig. 64–25).[35] To accomplish this, pass a 4-0 nylon suture through the entire thickness of

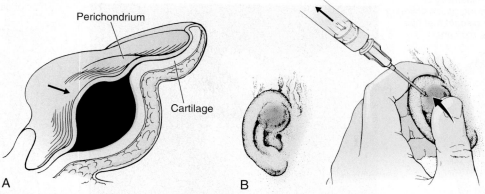

Figure 64–24 *A,* Subperichondrial hematoma within the concha of the ear. *B,* Needle aspiration of an auricular hematoma. A topical antiseptic is used to clean the ear, but local anesthesia is seldom required. While stabilizing the pinna with the thumb and fingers, puncture the most fluctuant part of the hematoma with a 20-gauge needle. Use the thumb to "milk" the hematoma into the syringe until the entire hematoma has been evacuated. Be very careful not to puncture your thumb with the needle. The thumb maintains continued pressure on the ear for 3 min after the needle has been withdrawn. A pressure dressing is then applied, and the ear is checked for reaccumulation of blood in 24 hr. Reaspiration may be required, and persistent accumulations require incision and drainage. *(B, Redrawn with permission from Ruddy RM: Aspiration of an auricular hematoma. In Fleisher GR, Ludwig S, Henretig FM, et al [eds]: Textbook of Pediatric Emergency Medicine, 5th ed. Philadelphia, Lippincott, Williams & Wilkins, 2006, p 1889.)*

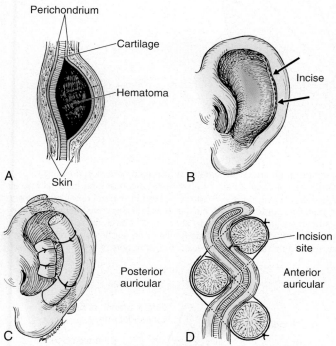

Figure 64–25 Auricular hematoma. *A,* Hematoma separates the perichondrium from the cartilage. *B,* Incision (*arrows*) made along the skin curvature at the posterior edge of the hematoma. The hematoma is evacuated and the area irrigated. *C,* Two anterior dental rolls are secured with sutures to a posterior dental roll to maintain normal anatomy of the pinna. *D,* Side view illustrates the position of sutures and dental rolls in relation to the incision site. Note that the perichondrium is apposed to the cartilage. *(A–D, From Clemons JE, Seveneid LR: Otohematoma. In Cummings CW [ed]: Otolaryngology—Head and Neck Surgery, 2nd ed. St. Louis, Mosby–Year Book, 1993, p 2866.)*

the ear over the hematoma. Wrap the suture around a dental roll on the posterior aspect of the ear and then pass the needle back through the pinna. Wrap and tie the suture around a second dental roll on the anterior aspect of the pinna. A second suture may be placed to secure a third dental roll. The dressing should firmly reapproximate the perichondrium to

the cartilage without vasculature compromise. Remove the dressing in 1 week.

Prescribe antistaphylococcal antibiotics and instruct the patient to inspect the wound frequently for evidence of vascular compromise, infection, or both. Reevaluate the wound in 24 hours for recurrence of the hematoma. Treat infection with removal of the bandage, surgical drainage, and intravenous antibiotics. Refer patients with auricular hematomas of longer than 7 days' duration to a surgeon, because the new perichondrial growth must be débrided to prevent deformity of the ear.

1197

NOSE

Anatomy

The nose consists of the vestibule, nasal septum, lateral wall, and nasopharynx. The vestibule is the anteriormost portion of the nares, which is composed of skin and contains the hair follicles. The nasal septum is the midline structure, which is composed of cartilage anteriorly and bone posteriorly. The lateral wall of the nose contains the superior, middle, and inferior turbinates as well as the auditory tube opening.

Three major arteries supply the nose and conjoin via anastomoses. The sphenopalatine artery emerges from the sphenopalatine foramen, which is located at the posterior aspect of the middle turbinate (Fig. 64–27). This is the most common source of posterior epistaxis. This artery supplies the lateral turbinates and the posterior septum. The anterior and posterior ethmoidal arteries branch off the ophthalmic artery and penetrate the cribriform plate to supply the superior nasal mucosa. The superior labial branch of the facial artery completes the triad, supplying the nasal septum and vestibule. The watershed area on the anterior septum, also known as Kiesselbach's plexus, is the most common source of anterior epistaxis (Fig. 64–28).

Anesthesia

Have the patient first blow the nose to expel all clots. Apply local anesthetic and vasoconstrictors on cotton swabs (Fig. 64–29). If a larger area of anesthetic is required, use cotton

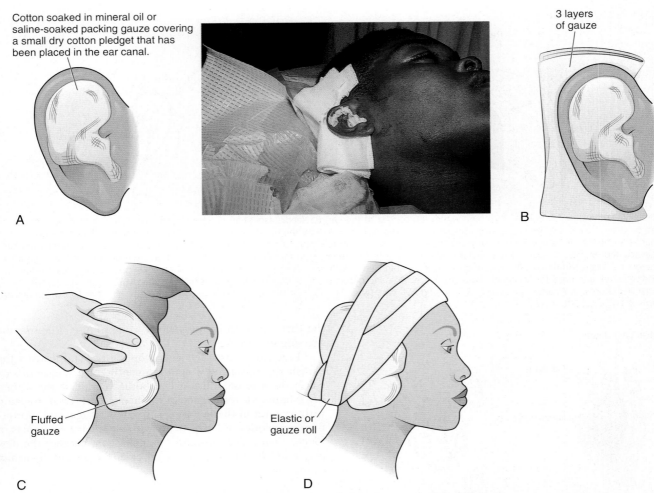

Cotton soaked in mineral oil or saline-soaked packing gauze covering a small dry cotton pledget that has been placed in the ear canal.

A

3 layers of gauze

B

Fluffed gauze

C

Elastic or gauze roll

D

Figure 64–26 Compression dressing of the ear. Following successful aspiration of an auricular hematoma, use a compression dressing to prevent reaccumulation of the hematoma or fluid. *A,* First, place dry cotton into the ear canal. Then, carefully mold a conforming material into all the convolutions of the auricle. One may use Vaseline gauze, saline-soaked ¼-inch packing gauze, or cotton soaked in mineral oil or saline. *Inset,* Note the gauze pack behind the pinna and the use of saline-soaked packing gauze to conform to the auricle. *B,* When the convolutions are fully packed, place a posterior gauze pack behind the ear. A V-shaped section has been cut from the gauze to allow it to fit easily behind the ear. *C,* Place multiple layers of fluffed gauze over the packed ear, and hold the entire dressing in place with Kling gauze or an elastic gauze roll. *Do not wrap this too tight. D,* The ear is thus compressed between two layers of gauze, and the packing ensures even distribution of pressure to all parts of the auricle.

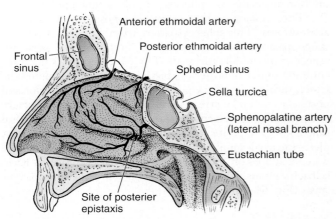

Frontal sinus

Anterior ethmoidal artery

Posterior ethmoidal artery

Sphenoid sinus

Sella turcica

Sphenopalatine artery (lateral nasal branch)

Eustachian tube

Site of posterier epistaxis

Figure 64–27 Vascular supply to the lateral wall. The most common site of posterior epistaxis is the sphenopalatine artery as it emerges posterior to the middle turbinate. *(From Maceri DR: Epistaxis and nasal trauma. In Cummings CW [ed]: Otolaryngology—Head and Neck Surgery, 2nd ed. St. Louis, Mosby–Year Book, 1993, p 728.)*

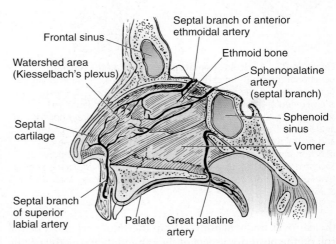

Frontal sinus

Septal branch of anterior ethmoidal artery

Ethmoid bone

Sphenopalatine artery (septal branch)

Watershed area (Kiesselbach's plexus)

Septal cartilage

Sphenoid sinus

Vomer

Septal branch of superior labial artery

Palate

Great palatine artery

Figure 64–28 Vascular supply to the septum. The most common site of anterior epistaxis is within the area labeled Kiesselbach's plexus. *(From Maceri DR: Epistaxis and nasal trauma. In Cummings CW [ed]: Otolaryngology—Head and Neck Surgery, 2nd ed. St. Louis, Mosby–Year Book, 1993, p 728.)*

pledgets. Figure 64–30 describes the procedure of making pledgets. Soak each pledget in anesthetic or a vasoconstricting substance and then squeeze the excess fluid out of the pledget. *Cocaine is the preferred agent for both vasoconstriction and anesthesia.* Alternatively, lidocaine 2% with epinephrine (local anesthetic solution) may be used but is less effective. Be aware of the total amount of cocaine being administered and stay within recommendations for the maximum safe dosage. This is an issue only with elderly patients with cardiovascular disease. Place each pledget horizontally on the floor of the

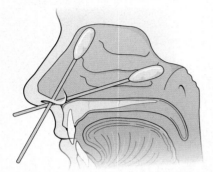

Figure 64–29 Placement of local anesthetic in the nose for anesthesia before reduction of nasal fracture by blockage of the anterior ethmoidal nerve superiorly and the sphenopalatine ganglion at the posterior end of the middle turbinate. Cocaine is the preferred agent. *(From Schuller DE, Schleuning AJ, DeMaria TF, et al [eds]: DeWeese and Saunders Otolaryngology: Head and Neck Surgery, 8th ed. St. Louis, CV Mosby, 1994, p 152.)*

nasal cavity, stacking the next pledget on top. Three pledgets are usually required to pack the nasal cavity. These can be replaced with new pledgets in 5 minutes if the desired anesthetic effect is not achieved. Benzocaine (Hurricaine) spray may also be used as a topical anesthetic. Remind the patient that excess anesthetic may numb the throat but will not inhibit swallowing.

Examination

Examination of the nares is relatively straightforward, albeit *often quite stressful to the patient.* When using a nasal speculum, insert it into the naris with the handle parallel to the floor and slowly open the blades in the *superior to inferior direction.* Stabilize your hand on the patient's nose to prevent damage to the mucosa due to unexpected movement (Fig. 64–31). When attempting to visualize the nasal passageway, remember to have the patient keep the floor of the nose parallel to the ground. Tilting of the head allows for a view only of the anterosuperior area. A nasopharyngoscope may be used to view the nasal passageways as well, and its use is described in the previous section on examination of the pharynx.

Epistaxis

Nasal hemorrhage commonly presents to the ED and accounts for about 1 in 200 ED visits.[36] Epistaxis is more common in the young (<10 yr) and old (70–79 yr). Most cases are traumatic and occur in winter months. Approximately 6% require hospitalization.[36]

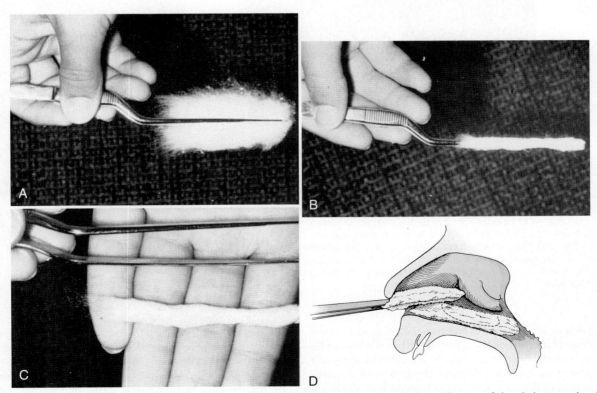

Figure 64–30 Topical anesthetic and vasoconstrictors are applied on individually made cotton pledgets. The size of the pledget may be changed according to the extent of the nasal cavity to be anesthetized and the size of the patient. *A,* Grasp an appropriately sized cotton pledget with bayonet forceps. *B,* Then grasp the cotton with the opposite hand and rotate the forceps. *C,* The pledget is removed and is ready for insertion. *D,* To completely anesthetize the nasal cavity, three pledgets are necessary. The first is placed on the floor of the nose, the second in the middle meatus between the inferior and the middle turbinates, and the third in the roof of the nasal cavity and the anterior nasal vestibule. *Note:* This pledget technique can be used to make a cotton wick for the treatment of otitis externa.

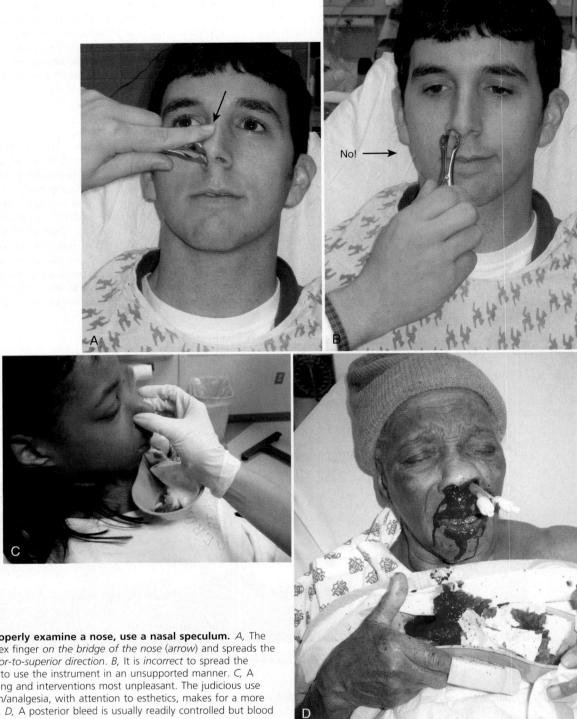

Figure 64–31 **To properly examine a nose, use a nasal speculum.** *A,* The clinician rests the index finger *on the bridge of the nose (arrow)* and spreads the speculum in an *inferior-to-superior direction. B,* It is *incorrect* to spread the speculum laterally or to use the instrument in an unsupported manner. *C,* A nosebleed is frightening and interventions most unpleasant. The judicious use of parenteral sedation/analgesia, with attention to esthetics, makes for a more rewarding encounter. *D,* A posterior bleed is usually readily controlled but blood loss can be significant.

Identification of the source of bleeding and subsequent control are paramount to the treatment of epistaxis. Although this can be frightening to both clinician and patient, a systematic approach with the proper equipment will lessen the anxiety of the situation. The goal of the procedure is to tamponade or cauterize the bleeding site. If the source is anterior, this may be the final treatment. For posterior bleeds, these are generally temporizing maneuvers until the process stops or a consultant can complete a definitive hemostatic procedure. The procedures can be performed in the ED with proper lighting and the

equipment listed later in this section. Controlling epistaxis may be a time-consuming process without proper equipment or patient cooperation.

In preparation for any procedure to treat epistaxis, evaluate the patient's hemodynamic status by assessing vital signs and orthostatic symptoms and by quantifying blood loss. Also determine whether the patient has any underlying medical problems, such as angina or chronic obstructive lung disease, which may be exacerbated owing to hypovolemia or anemia. If the patient is symptomatic in any of these areas, or if the blood loss is deemed significant, start a large-bore intravenous line and administer fluid boluses. Hematologic testing is rarely useful and not required for most patients, but if there are extenuating circumstances, obtain a complete blood count and consider a type and screen. Coagulation studies are not routinely indicated but should be undertaken in patients taking anticoagulant therapy, those with underlying hematologic abnormalities, or those with recurrent or prolonged epistaxis.[37]

Many patients with epistaxis are hypertensive as well, often transiently secondary to stress. No direct causal correlation between hypertension and overt epistaxis has been proved. Hypertension is probably a stress response instead of an inciting event.[38] Therefore, hypertension does not require treatment until the bleeding is controlled and the anxiety of the situation has resolved. However, any patient exhibiting other signs of a hypertensive emergency needs immediate treatment in addition to control of the epistaxis.

Indications/Contraindications

Any continuing episode of epistaxis can be treated with the following techniques. Massive facial trauma with the possibility of a basilar skull fracture would preclude the use of an intranasal balloon, because it may travel into the skull cavity.

Equipment

Preparation is the key to successful management of a patient with epistaxis. The following list of equipment should be readily available to the emergency clinician:

Chair with headrest or gurney with inclinable back.
Headlight with light source, head mirror.
Wall suction with multiple suction catheters.
Gloves, mask, and gown for the clinician.
Gown or drapes for the patient.
Topical anesthetic.
Topical vasoconstrictor.
Nasal speculum.
Tongue depressors.
Small red rubber catheters.
Bayonet forceps.
Scissors.
Kidney basin.
Gauze (4 × 4 inch, 2 × 2 inch).
Dental rolls or cotton.
No. 2 surgical silk ties.
1.2-cm wide Vaseline gauze or 0.5-inch wide Nu-Gauze packing.
Antibiotic ointment.
Silver nitrate sticks or electrocautery.
Pediatric Foley catheters (12 Fr).
Nasal tampons.
Dual-balloon pack.

Epistaxis Examination

Because most patients are frightened by continued epistaxis, and nasal instrumentation is quite annoying or painful, reassure the patient that you will control the bleeding with minimal discomfort. *The judicious use of parenteral sedation or narcotic analgesia is well supported*, making the entire interaction more palatable to the patient and ultimately more successful (see Fig. 64–31C). Drape the patient with a gown to protect his or her clothing from the bleeding. Have the patient hold an emesis basin to collect any continued bleeding and as a precaution to emesis of swallowed blood. Minor anterior bleeds are usually easily controlled with minimal techniques.

Ask the patient to sit upright in the sniffing position with the neck flexed and head extended. The base of the nose should remain parallel with the floor. After putting on a face shield, gown, and protective gloves, position yourself in front of the patient, level with the patient's nose. Have the patient blow the nose to remove clots or suction the nasal passageway carefully. Suction from front to back along the nasal septum, then laterally. If the bleeding is minimal, *attempt to locate the specific bleeding source.* If the bleeding is too profuse for visualization, administer a topical anesthetic and vasoconstrictor. Numerous preparations are available. A 4% cocaine solution would be ideal, but it is not commonly stocked. Lidocaine 4% is quite effective for anesthesia of the nose. A solution of 1% tetracaine and 0.05% oxymetazoline (Afrin) is an effective topical anesthetic and vasoconstrictor.[39] To administer the solution, soak a cotton pledget in it and place it in the nose for 4 to 5 minutes. Ask the patient to clamp the nostrils to limit bleeding and promote contact with the mucosa. If a discrete bleeding site is initially identified, an effective way to provide hemostasis and anesthesia before cautery is to inject the mucosa at the base of the bleeder with 2% lidocaine with epinephrine via a tuberculin syringe (Fig. 64–32A).

Insert the nasal speculum into the naris and use the suction catheter to evacuate any blood. Reapply anesthetic or vasoconstrictor if necessary. As most cases of anterior epistaxis occur in the Kiesselbach's plexus, inspect this area closely for areas of bleeding, ulceration, or erosion. After vasoconstriction, the only evidence of the former bleeding site may be a small prominent vessel. Many clinicians will gently stroke the septum with a cotton swab to initiate bleeding so an exact area of pathology can be identified and then cauterized (see Fig. 64–32B). If no bleeding source is found and the bleeding has ceased, pack the nose only if the epistaxis is recurrent. Wait 15 to 20 minutes before deciding on lack of further intervention. If no anterior source is found and bleeding continues down the posterior pharynx, assume a posterior source and pack the nose with an anterior and posterior pack.

Cautery

After an anterior source of bleeding is identified, cautery may be used to obtain hemostasis (Fig. 64–33). Silver nitrate sticks may be used to cauterize but *will not work on an actively bleeding source; hemostasis* must be achieved first. Silver nitrate works well for a small, circumscribed area of bleeding (see Fig. 64–32C). To apply, hold the tip of the silver nitrate stick against the site for 4 to 5 seconds. Apply again if necessary. Wipe away any excess silver nitrate to prevent inadvertent cautery of other areas of the nose. If bleeding restarts, the initial cautery was insufficient and should be applied again. The cauterized area immediately turns white/gray. Electrocautery works in the same manner, but will penetrate more quickly than silver nitrate. In either cautery technique, be careful not to cause septal perforation with overaggressive or repeated cautery. If cautery has not been successful after two attempts, use another technique. Multiple cautery attempts can significantly injure the nasal septum, and bilateral cautery should not be performed. If this is the initial bleed and hemostasis is achieved, no packing is necessary. If this is a recurrent bleed within 72 hours of another, or if cautery does not provide hemostasis, pack the anterior cavity. If hemostasis is accomplished, apply petroleum jelly or antibiotic ointment to the area to prevent desiccation. Loughran and coworkers[40]

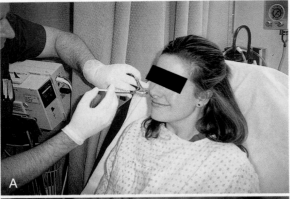

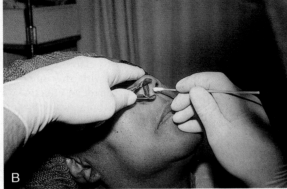

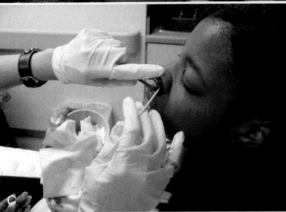

Figure 64–32 *A,* If an arterial bleeding site is found in the nasal septum, both hemostasis and anesthesia for cautery can be accomplished by injecting the mucosa at the base of the bleeder with a small amount of lidocaine with epinephrine via a tuberculin or insulin syringe. This procedure best follows an initial application of topical anesthesia. *It is impossible to cauterize an actively bleeding vessel. B,* If no bleeding site is identified on the septum, lightly brush the entire septum with a cotton swab *under direct vision* to stimulate the bleeding site so it can be directly identified and subsequently cauterized. *C,* The most common way to cauterize a small bleeding site on the anterior septum is with a silver nitrate stick. This burns, causes the patient to sneeze, and is only effective for small sites, not those that are actively bleeding. Apply for 3–4 sec to an area that *is not vigorously bleeding. Do not blindly cauterize.* Treat an identified bleeding site only under direct vision. The area immediately turns gray/white.

found antimicrobial ointment better than petroleum jelly at preventing bleeding. Do not administer aspirin or nonsteroidal anti-inflammatory drugs for 4 days after epistaxis. If bleeding recurs at home, instruct the patient to pinch the nostrils closed for 20 minutes. Instruct the patient to return to the ED if this maneuver is unsuccessful or the bleeding is profuse.

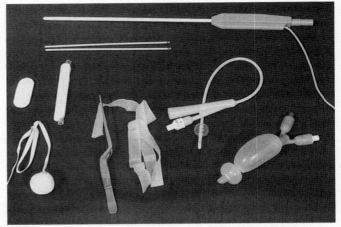

Figure 64–33 **Equipment used for treatment of epistaxis.** *Top,* Electrocautery device and silver nitrate sticks. *Left to right, bottom row,* Merocel nasal tampon, posterior packing ball, Merocel nasal tampon with catheter included (Doyle Pack), anterior packing gauze with bayonet forceps, Foley catheter, Epistat dual-balloon catheter.

Anterior Nasal Packing

Anterior packing achieves hemostasis, prevents desiccation, and protects the area from trauma. However, improperly placed packing may further abrade the area, dislodge prematurely, or migrate into the posterior pharynx. Anterior packing must be placed with adequate analgesia, proper visualization, and deliberate movements. Coating any packing material with antibiotic ointment (if not contraindicated by the manufacturer) aids in its placement and theoretically prevents infection and toxic shock syndrome secondary to nasal packing. *Areas that continue to ooze after cautery are often treated with an anterior pack.*

Traditional petrolatum gauze has been largely supplanted by easier-to-use commercial devices. When used, packing is applied in an "accordion" fashion so that each layer extends the entire length of the nasal cavity. Place the speculum properly to allow visualization of the floor of the nasal cavity. Lay a strip of petroleum gauze 1.2-cm across the nasal floor, with the starting end of the gauze at the naris (Fig. 64–34). Gently pack the gauze strip into the floor of the nose. Measure the gauze to twice the length of the nasal cavity. Grasp the gauze at the midpoint and insert this point all the way back to the posterior aspect of the nasal cavity. Attempt to place this layer of gauze without movement of the underlying layer. Continue this pattern, replacing the speculum after each layer, until the cavity is filled.

Compared with gauze packing, numerous compression devices are easier to place, better tolerated, and very successful. Preformed nasal packing products are convenient alternatives to anterior nasal packing (Figs. 64–35 and 64–36; see also Fig. 64–33). The Merocel packing consists of compressed polyvinyl acetate with or without a drawstring that expands on contact with fluid. The pack can be trimmed with scissors or a scalpel before insertion. The Merocel Doyle nasal pack has an airway tube in the center of the compressed material and is a more anatomic shape. Each are available in various sizes, but usually an 8- × 1.5- × 2-cm standard Merocel or 8- × 1.5- × 3-cm Doyle will suffice. The Rapid Rhino Stat Pac (ArthroCare Corporation, Austin, TX; see Fig. 64–35*C*) is a high-volume, low-pressure balloon device with an open lumen air passage, a pilot cuff to check pressure, and a specialized Gel-Knit (carboxymethyl cellulose) covering designed to

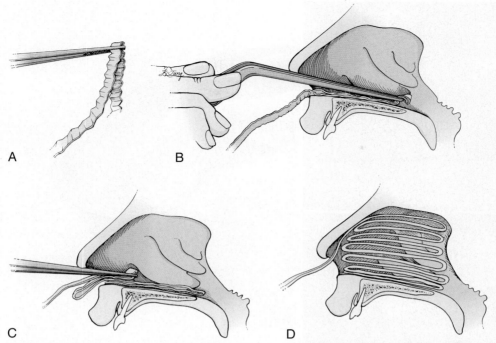

Figure 64–34 The key to placement of an anterior nasal pack that will control epistaxis adequately and stay in place is to lay the packing into the nasal cavity in an "accordion" manner, so that part of each layer of packing lies anteriorly, preventing the gauze from falling posteriorly into the nasopharynx. *A,* Grasp the first layer of 0.25-inch Vaseline gauze strip approximately 2–3 cm from its end. *B,* Then place the first layer on the floor of the nose through the nasal speculum (not pictured). Then withdraw the bayonet forceps and nasal speculum. *C,* Reintroduce the nasal speculum on top of the first layer of packing, and place a second layer in an identical manner. After several layers have been placed, it is often useful to reintroduce the bayonet forceps to push the previously placed packing down onto the floor of the nose, making it tighter and more secure. *D,* A complete anterior nasal pack can tamponade a bleeding point anywhere in the anterior nasal cavity and will stay in place until the clinician or patient removes it.

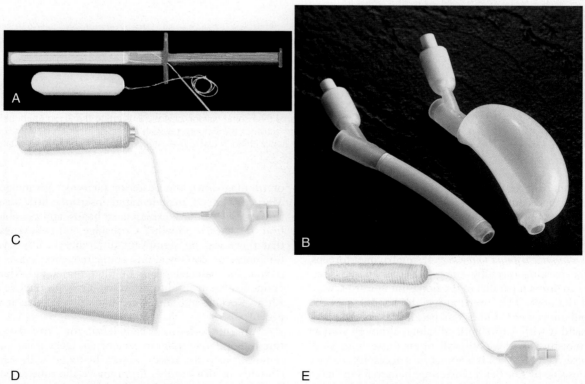

Figure 64–35 **Commerical nasal packings are commonly used in place of the traditional gauze packing.** *A,* Rhino Rocket (manufactured by Shippert Medical, Centennial, CO). *B,* Epi-Stop Balloon Catheter (available from Shippert Medical, Centennial, CO). *C,* Rapid Rhino (ArthroCare Corporation, Austin, TX). *D,* Rapid-Pac (ArthroCare Corporation, Austin, TX). *E,* Rapid Rhino Dual Nasal Pack (ArthroCare Corporation, Austin, TX).

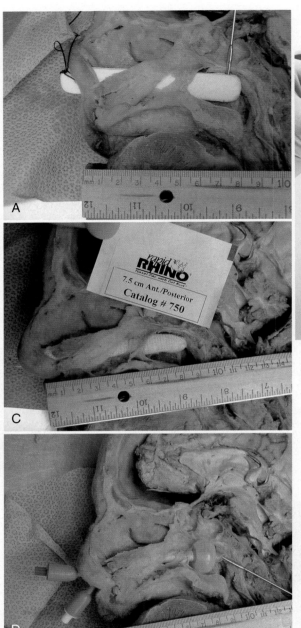

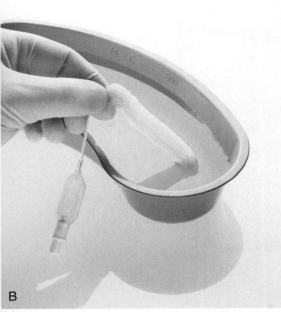

Figure 64–36 **Various packs for epistaxis in a cadaver model.** *A,* The posterior Merocel sponge, not inflated, will stop most nosebleeds and is more comfortable than some balloon devices. *B,* Wetting the Rapid Rhino before placement activates the slippery covering for easier insertion. *C,* Anterior/posterior Rapid Rhino in place. *D,* Posterior pack with the balloon inflated.

promote platelet aggregation. Numerous variations for anterior, posterior, and combination packs are available.

The easily applied nasal tampon is a reasonable first choice for most anterior bleeds. Lubricate the tampon generously with antibiotic ointment and *trim the length and width carefully to minimize trauma to the nose.* Using bayonet forceps, advance the packing carefully along the floor of the nose. Remember to direct it parallel to the floor, not upward toward the top of the nose. The insertion may be painful, so use a single rapid movement. Once the packing is in the nasal cavity, expand it with 5 to 10 mL of saline, although contact with the moisture of the nose will often cause it to swell spontaneously (Fig. 64–37). It is sometimes necessary to place two tampons side by side before inserting them to fill the nasal cavity and provide better pressure on the areas of bleeding.[38,41,42] Observe for 10 minutes after anterior packing to identify continued bleeding either anteriorly from the naris or running down the posterior pharynx. Advantages to the Merocel tampon include rapid insertion, little discomfort, ease of use even in inexperienced hands, and possible inhibition of bacterial growth.[43] Corbridge and colleagues[41] found that there was no significant difference in efficacy, patient tolerance, or complications compared with gauze packing. Singer and associates[44] found that the Rapid Rhino nasal tampon is less painful to insert and easier to remove than the Rhino Rocket, and both were similarly effective at stopping nosebleeds.

Anterior packs are usually left in for 2 to 5 days. Premature removal may result in rebleeding. During use and before removal, keep the nasal tampon hydrated with saline. If it contains an airway tube, first remove the tube, then irrigate the space once occupied by the tube.

Complications. Any packing in the anterior nasal cavity may obstruct drainage of the paranasal sinuses or block the

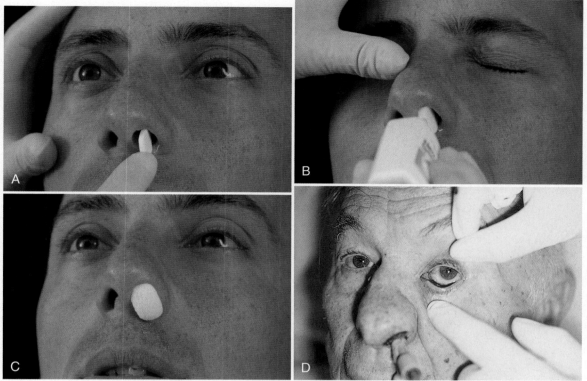

Figure 64–37 A–C, An expanding Merocel tampon is ideal for minor anterior bleeds. The dehydrated pack is *trimmed to fit the nose and generously lubricated with antibiotic ointment.* Apply a vasoconstrictor spray. Use a swift single motion (may be painful) to insert the pack *to its full length.* The pack expands when hydrated with saline. The patient continues to keep the pack moist at home and it is again well hydrated just before removal. D, After packing, blood coming from a nosebleed exiting via the nasolacrimal duct gives the appearance that the eye is bleeding. Although benign, it can be alarming to the patient.

1205

nasolacrimal ducts. Occasionally, blood will exit the duct and be noted in the eye (see Fig. 64–37D). A pack or device may stimulate mucus production and act as an impetus for infection. Oral antibiotics (e.g., cephalexin, amoxicillin, or trimethoprim/sulfamethoxazole) may be prescribed with any packing in the nose after emergency treatment because of the minimal risk of sinusitis and toxic shock syndrome. The necessity of antibiotics for short-term anterior packing is unproved. Decongestants are also prescribed to decrease secretions. Practices vary and no common standards exist. Hollis[43] reported massive pneumocephalus after Merocel nasal tampon insertion in an elderly woman, presumably from fracture of the ethmoid plate. There have been case reports of ethmoid fracture after anterior nasal gauze packing and with the use of an intranasal balloon. Patients with anterior packs are usually discharged with follow-up as outpatients in 3 to 4 days. Minor oozing of blood can be expected.

Posterior Nasal Packing

If no bleeding source is found anteriorly and the patient continues to hemorrhage down the posterior pharynx, the patient most likely has a posterior source of epistaxis. Posterior epistaxis may respond to topical vasoconstrictors. However, anterior nasal packing will not provide hemostasis for a posterior bleed because it will not cover the source of bleeding. A posterior pack directly compresses the sphenopalatine artery and prevents the passage of blood or anterior packing into the nasopharynx.

The posterior nasal gauze pack is the classic method of treating posterior epistaxis. However, because balloon devices are easier to use and less distressing to the patient, formal posterior nasal packing is less commonly used. To place a formal traditional posterior nasal gauze pack, anesthetize the patient's nares and posterior pharynx with topical anesthetic. Prepare a roll of gauze with two silk ties (2-0) secured around the middle and extending in opposite directions. One set of ends will be used to place the posterior pack and the second will remain extruding from the oral cavity to remove the pack. Place a No. 10 red rubber catheter through the bleeding nostril (Fig. 64–38). When it is seen in the posterior pharynx, grasp it with forceps, and guide it out of the mouth. Attach it to one set of ends of the silk ties secured to the gauze pack. Retract the red rubber catheter, thus carrying the No. 2 silk tie through the nasopharynx and out of the nose. Grasp the suture and pull the pack into the nasopharynx. Guide the pack swiftly into the oral cavity and nasopharynx with the other hand. Attach the silk tie that remains in the oropharynx to the patient's cheek to aid in removal or rescue of the posterior pack. Use the silk ties exiting the nostril to maintain the position of the posterior pack. Pack the anterior passage as described for anterior epistaxis. Secure the silk ties over a gauze pad or dental roll. Admit patients with traditional posterior packing to the hospital. Administering humidified air or oxygen makes this pack more comfortable.

Inflatable Balloon Packs. Inflatable balloons come in two varieties. The Foley catheter is often used as a posterior pack because of its availability, ease of use, and successful tamponading effect.[45] Insert a 12-French Foley catheter through the bleeding naris into the posterior pharynx (Fig. 64–39). Inflate the balloon halfway with about 5 to 7 mL of

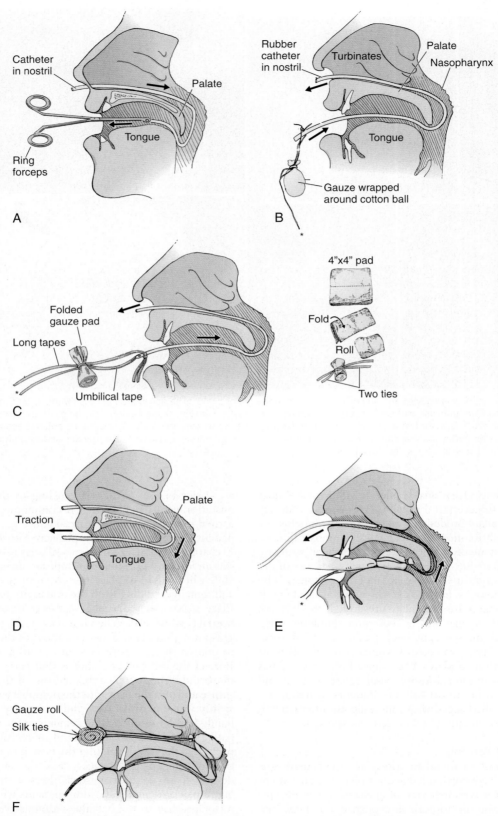

Figure 64–38   Traditional posterior nasal pack. *A,* After applying topical anesthesia, pass a red rubber catheter through the nose and carefully grasp it in the oropharynx with ringed forceps and bring it out through the mouth. *B, upper right,* Make a posterior nasal pack by wrapping a cotton ball in a 4 × 4-inch gauze pad and tying two long silk sutures or umbilical tapes around the neck of the pack. Leave one tie long so that it can be taped to the cheek until needed for removal of the pack. *C, center,* Alternatively, fold a gauze pad and roll it into a cylinder and tie it with two strings. Use two of the long strings to tie the pack to the tip of the catheter and use the other two to remove the pack. *D,* As an option, use a second catheter, which has been passed through the nonbleeding side and brought out the mouth, to retract the palate forward to aid in the placement of the pack (not shown). *E,* Remove the optional "retraction" catheter after the pack is in the proper position. Digitally guide the pack into the nasopharynx. *F,* Use a gauze roll to secure the pack to the nose and tape the rescue ties to the cheek.

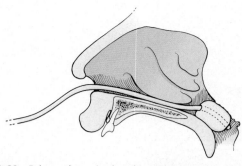

Figure 64–39 Foley catheter is placed into the nasopharynx, inflated with water, and retracted into position. The distal tip of the catheter has been cut off. Then, place an anterior pack (not shown) around the catheter. Protect the ala and columella with gauze padding, and apply a plastic umbilical clamp or nasogastric clamp to the catheter to maintain slight tension on the balloon.

normal saline or water. Slowly pull the Foley into the posterior nasopharynx and secure it against the posterior aspect of the middle turbinate. Finish inflating the balloon with another 5 to 7 mL of normal saline or water. If there is pain or inferior displacement of the soft palate, deflate the balloon until the pain resolves. Ensure proper placement before completely inflating the balloon because the balloon will remain too posterior in the nasopharynx and fail to achieve hemostasis.[46] While maintaining constant gentle anterior tension on the Foley catheter, place an anterior nasal packing using layered petroleum gauze. Pack the opposite nasal cavity to counteract septal deviation. Finally, place a short section of plastic tubing over the catheter and secure it with a nasogastric tube clamp or umbilical clamp. Be careful not to exert undue pressure on the nasal alar because this may cause necrosis.

The second type of inflatable balloon pack is the premade dual-balloon tamponading system. These devices have been a significant advance in the treatment of epistaxis. Several balloon devices are available (Goitschach Nasostat [Sparta Surgical Corp, Hayward, CA], Xomed Epistat [Xomed Inc, Jacksonville, FL], and Epi-Max Balloon Catheter [Shippert Medical, Centennial, CO]). The dual-balloon pack has a posterior balloon that inflates with about 10 mL of air and an anterior balloon that inflates with about 30 mL of air (Fig. 64–40; see also Fig. 64–36D). Each device may vary slightly (Fig. 64–41). After appropriately anesthetizing the naris, place the lubricated pack along the floor of the affected naris as far back as possible. Inflate the posterior balloon about halfway with air and, then, with traction, pull the balloon into place up against the posterior aspect of the middle turbinate. Complete the inflation of the posterior balloon with air. Some clinicians prefer to inflate all balloons with saline instead of air because air may deflate slowly. *Inflate slowly, and stop if pain is felt. This is usually an uncomfortable sensation to the patient.* If the patient complains of pain or if the posterior soft palate deviates downward, deflate the balloon until the symptoms are relieved. Maintain the position of the balloon and inflate the anterior balloon with up to 30 mL of air. Again, halt inflation if the patient experiences increasing pain or deviation of the nasal septum. Some authors suggest packing the opposite naris to prevent this lateral deviation. Place a small piece of gauze between the nose and the external catheter hub to decrease skin irritation.

Patients with bleeding easily controlled with commercial packing can usually be discharged with 1- to 3-day outpatient follow-up unless other conditions exist. Elderly patients

and those with chronic obstructive pulmonary disease may require admission. Minor oozing may be expected for a few days.

Other Techniques. ENT consultation may be required for posterior nosebleeds that do not respond to the posterior packing techniques. Other treatment options include ligation or embolization of the internal maxillary artery and posterior endoscopic cautery.

Complications. Care of posterior nasal packing is of some concern. Posterior nasal packing is uncomfortable and often painful. These bleeds are more complicated than simple anterior septal bleeds. Complications associated with posterior packing include infection, dysphagia, eustachian tube dysfunction, tissue necrosis, and dislodgment. Other serious complications rarely associated with posterior packing are hypoxia, hypercarbia, aspiration, hypertension, bradycardia, arrhythmias, myocardial infarction, and death.[47] For these reasons, most patients with a posterior pack, especially the elderly and those with pulmonary and cardiovascular diseases, should be admitted to the hospital for sedation and monitoring. This recommendation was common for formal posterior packs, but the ease and safety of the balloon devices now allow select patients to be treated as outpatients despite the presence of posterior packing. Rebleeding may also be seen with early pack removal; one series found pack removal within 48 hours increased the risk of rebleeding.[48] Most posterior packs are left in place for 72 to 96 hours.

Infection risk with posterior packing includes toxic shock syndrome, nasopharyngitis, and sinusitis. The packing blocks the sinus ostia, preventing proper drainage of the sinuses. In addition to coating the packing with antibiotic ointment, broad-spectrum antibiotics should be administered. Dysphagia due to the packing can lead to poor oral intake, and intravenous fluid hydration may be required.

A significant decrease in the arterial partial pressure of oxygen (Pa_{O_2}; 7.5–11 torr) and an increase in the arterial partial pressure of carbon dioxide (Pa_{CO_2}; 7–13 torr) are seen in patients with nasal packing who are treated with sedation.[49] A posterior pack will cause vagal stimulation, resulting in varying degrees of bradycardia and bronchoconstriction. This physiologic adaptation may be of concern in patients with underlying lung or heart disease. With the risk of hypercarbia and hypoxia, closely monitor patients with lung disease with posterior nasal packs in an intensive care setting.

Tissue necrosis of the nasal ala, nasal mucosa, and soft palate has been described secondary to improper placement or padding. Protect the skin with gauze placed under the device to reduce skin maceration. The risk of necrosis increases with the duration of the packing, so all packing should be removed in 3 to 5 days. Bleeding from the nasolacrimal duct is a common benign problem with nasal packing.

If the posterior pack becomes dislodged, it will fall into the oropharynx, risking asphyxiation, vomiting, and aspiration. The patient and nursing personnel need to be familiar with the technique for removing the pack. To accomplish this, cut the anterior sutures that exit the naris from the gauze roll if they have not already broken. Grasp the sutures exiting the mouth and guide the packing out of the nasopharynx. It may be necessary to extract the packing with forceps or digits.

Toxic shock syndrome has been rarely described with nasal packing.[42,50] The syndrome is caused by a toxin released by *S. aureus* infection of the packing. Sudden onset of vomiting and diarrhea with high fever, as well as development of

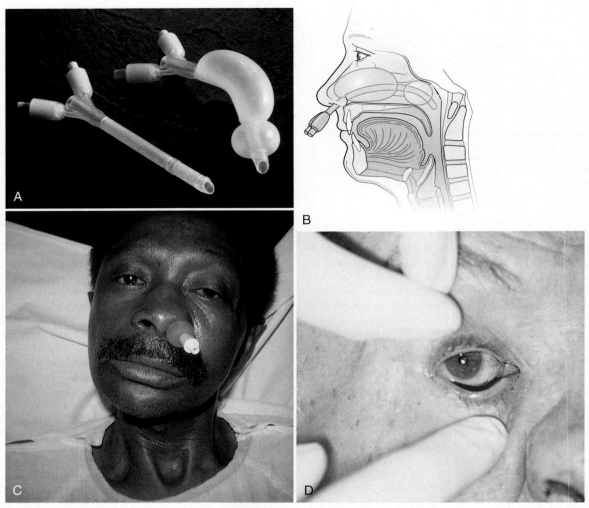

Figure 64–40 *A,* Epi-Max Balloon Catheter (available from Shippert Medical, Centennial, CO). The balloon tamponade device serves as both an anterior and a posterior pack. It is easily inserted and is often successful for the temporary control of posterior epistaxis in the emergency department (ED). Such devices rarely fail for the initial control of bleeding in the ED. *B,* The inflated Epi-max. *C,* This patient had bleeding controlled with a balloon catheter and was treated as an outpatient. If the balloon pack is used for more than a few days, protect the nasal opening with a piece of gauze because skin breakdown is possible. *D,* Although alarming to the patient, blood in the eye from backbleeding via the lacrimal duct from a balloon pack is benign.

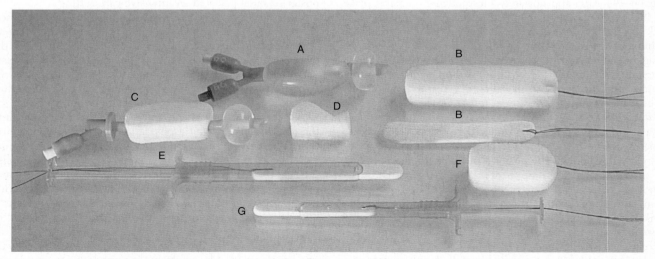

Figure 64–41 Xomed Rhinology Products. *A,* Xomed Epistat nasal catheter. *B,* Pope Flex-Pak nasal packing (shown expanded and compressed). *C,* Xomed Epistat II nasal catheter. *D,* Staxi-Stat pack without drawstring. *E,* Large Fast-Pak nasal pack with applicator. *F,* Weimert epistaxis packing. *G,* Small Fast-Pak nasal pack with applicator.

an erythrodermic rash, heralds the onset of the disease. Untreated, the disease can advance into shock and multisystem organ dysfunction. Therefore, in addition to coating the gauze with antibiotics to decrease the local bacterial concentration, give broad-spectrum antibiotics to any patient with nasal packing. No single antibiotic has been traditionally recommended, but a cephalosporin (such as cephalothin), ampicillin/sulbactam (Unasyn) or ampicillin/clavulanate (Augmentin) are all reasonable. If the patient develops signs of toxic shock syndrome, promptly remove the packing and admit to the hospital for fluid hydration and intravenous nafcillin or vancomycin therapy.

Septal Hematoma

Trauma to the anterior portion of the nasal septum may cause a hematoma to form. A buckling stress tears the submucosal blood vessels. If the mucosa remains intact, the blood will accumulate between the mucoperichondrium and the septal cartilage (Fig. 64–42A). Stagnant blood is an excellent medium for bacterial growth and the formation of an abscess. Common bacteria include *S. aureus*, *Streptococcus pneumoniae*, and group A β-hemoltyic streptococcus. Other complications of an untreated hematoma include septal perforation and cartilage destruction, with resultant saddle-nose deformity. Septal hematomas may present immediately after the trauma or, more commonly, in the first 24 to 72 hours after the injury.[51] The hematoma can cause significant destruction of the nasal cartilage, resulting in a cosmetic deformity.

Most common symptoms of a septal hematoma are nasal obstruction, pain, rhinorrhea, and fever. Most patients will complain of inability to breathe through the affected side, but the absence of nasal obstruction does not rule out a septal hematoma. It is usually possible to diagnose a septal hematoma by inspecting the nasal septum with a speculum for swelling, pain, and a fluctuant area. The presence of septal asymmetry with a bluish or reddish hue of the mucosa is suggestive of a septal hematoma. Direct palpation may be necessary, because newly formed hematomas may not yet be ecchymotic. Inspect both sides, because bilateral hematomas are possible. The best way to palpate for a septal hematoma is to insert the gloved small fingers in each side of the nose and palpate the entire septum, feeling for swelling, fluctuance, or widening of the septal space (Fig. 64–43).

Drainage

Treatment of a septal hematoma consists of evacuation of the clot with subsequent reapproximation of the perichondrium to the cartilage. To drain the hematoma, incise the mucosa horizontally over the hematoma after adequate anesthesia is achieved (see Fig. 64–42B–D). Suction out all of the clot and then irrigate with normal saline. Excise a small amount of mucosa to prevent premature closure of the incision and place a section of a sterile rubber band to act as a drain. Pack the nostril, as in anterior epistaxis, to reapproximate the perichondrium to the cartilage.

Give the patient broad-spectrum antibiotic therapy. Inspect the septum daily for signs of infection, recurrent hematoma, or necrosis. Evacuate recurrent hematomas. When there is no further hematoma formation for a 24-hour period, remove the drain. Pack the affected naris for 1 more day to complete the apposition of the perichondrium to cartilage where the drain had been. If there is any evidence of infection, admit for intravenous antibiotics and surgical débridement.

Nasal Fracture

Nasal fracture is the most common facial fracture. Nasal fractures present with a broad range of symptoms including mild swelling, epistaxis, or periorbital ecchymosis with obvious deformity. As with any trauma to the head, evaluate for coexistent intracranial injury or neck injury. In the evaluation of nasal trauma, rule out the existence of a septal hematoma or cerebrospinal fluid rhinorrhea. In most cases, swelling and soft tissue deformity prevent adequate evaluation, treatment, or both. To evaluate a patient with a suspected nasal fracture, include a thorough history, external nasal examination, and internal nasal examination using a nasal speculum with or

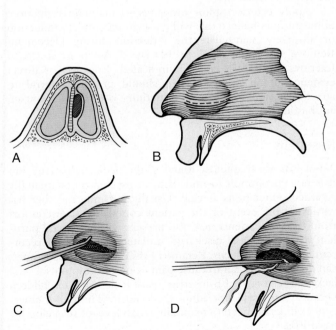

Figure 64–42 *A*, A small left-sided septal hematoma. *B*, After application of appropriate topical anesthesia, supplemented with local infiltration, if necessary, make a horizontal incision through the mucosa and the perichondrium covering the hematoma. *C*, Use a small cup forceps or scissors to remove enough mucosa to prevent premature closure of the wound and reaccumulation of hematoma. *D*, Then place a sterile rubber band as a drain, and pack the naris.

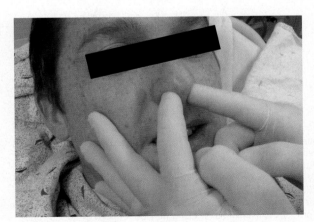

Figure 64–43 If visual inspection of the nose with a speculum does not rule out a septal hematoma, the clinician's gloved fingers, passed posteriorly along both sides of the septum, may feel bulging or fluctuance. The normal septum is thin and smooth.

without the use of a rigid nasal endoscope. Nasal radiographs are not routinely needed because they will not alter the course of treatment or injury.[52,53] Ask the patient to apply ice to the area and keep the head elevated to reduce soft tissue swelling. Refer the patient to an otolaryngologist or plastic surgeon for reexamination and definitive treatment in 3 to 5 days. Stress the importance of reevaluation within 10 days so that the bones do not set in a malaligned state.

Nasal Fracture Reduction

Most fractures, and patients with significant soft tissue swelling, should be seen in follow-up for definitive evaluation and possible fracture reduction. Complicated fractures and septal injuries are usually referred for follow-up (Fig. 64–44). Simple fractures with minimal local swelling can be treated with

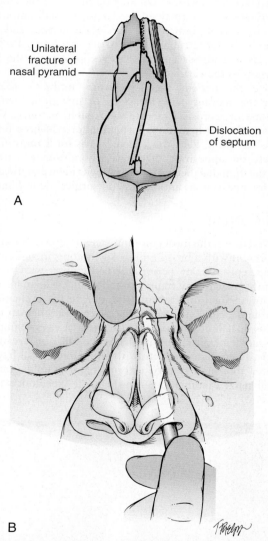

Unilateral fracture of nasal pyramid

Dislocation of septum

A

B

Figure 64–44 Nondisplaced and minimally displaced nasal fractures often do not require manipulation, but the true extent of the deformity is difficult to appreciate initially. *A,* Note that the septum may also require subsequent intervention. Reduction of a depressed and dislocated nasal bone fracture is usually performed in 3–7 days, after swelling has subsided and the true deformity is obvious. *B,* Minor deformities with minimal swelling may be reduced in the ED, and mitigate further therapy. Accomplish this reduction in two steps, after applying anesthesia, by first elevating the depressed nasal bone as illustrated and then manually displacing the pyramid to the midline. Use the handle of a scalpel if an elevator is unavailable.

closed reduction. Some patients prefer immediate correction, are not concerned with aesthetics, or are unable to comply with follow-up, so ED intervention may be an option. To minimize potential litigation, obtain written consent and take pre-reduction and post-reduction photographs. Inform the patient that the outcome is not guaranteed, because impacted fractures may not reduce and greenstick fractures may deform again after reduction. Acute swelling may obscure the extent of the injury.

If minor manipulation is reasonable, anesthetize the mucosa as described earlier. For infiltrative anesthesia, inject lidocaine either deep to the nasal fracture by entering intranasally or externally into the fracture site for a hematoma block. The external approach may be quite uncomfortable for the patient. In the external technique, inject bilaterally at the caudal edge of the nasal bone, midway between the nasal bridge and the maxilla. Bilateral infraorbital blocks may also be used. Debate exists in the literature as to which method provides adequate anesthesia with minimal patient discomfort.[53,54] Intravenous sedation and analgesia may be necessary.

Using the dominant hand, advance Asch forceps, Walsham forceps, or a scalpel handle into the naris with the dominant hand (see Fig. 64–44*B*). Apply pressure in an anterosuperior direction at a right angle to the ridge of the nasal bone. Use the other hand to manipulate the nasal fracture in an anteroinferior direction. Maintain firm, constant pressure until the bone shifts back into its original position. Alternatively, a Boies elevator may be used to lessen the risk of nasal mucosa damage. Be careful not to perforate the cribiform plate when using these surgical instruments. After the maneuver, assess the reduction for malalignment or subsequent displacement secondary to a greenstick fracture. If either occurs, refer the patient to an otolaryngologist to see whether open reduction is necessary.

Apply exterior splint dressings to maintain reduction. Some authors believe this will mask an incomplete reduction or adversely manipulate the reduction during placement. Remove the splint in 7 to 14 days.[55] As in most closed fractures, antibiotics are not indicated. Epistaxis or direct evidence of an open fracture should prompt referral to an otolaryngologist and initiation of broad-spectrum antibiotics.

Nasal FBs

Nasal FBs are frequently found in the pediatric patient, but it is not uncommon to find them in psychiatric or mentally retarded populations as well. Usually, a family member has witnessed the event or the patient complains of discomfort from the FB. Patients may also present with unilateral purulent or bloody nasal discharge, unilateral sinusitis, or recurrent unilateral epistaxis. Retained FBs, especially plastic ones, can initially fail to cause pain or other symptoms.[56] The lack of a history of FB insertion is of little value in children because many will not admit to doing it. Therefore, emergency clinicians need to maintain a high level of suspicion for nasal FBs.

Types of nasal FBs vary widely and include food (e.g., meat, nuts, beans), rubber erasers, paper wads, pebbles, marbles, sponges, beads, jewelry, hardware (e.g., nuts, screws), and even certain living larvae or worms.[56] Alkaline button batteries pose a unique problem because they may cause significant nasal injury within hours to days.[57-59] They are composed of heavy metals like mercury, zinc, silver, nickel, cadmium, and lithium. Injuries can occur including mucosal burns, ulcerations, liquefaction necrosis, septal perforation, synechiae, and stenosis of the nasal cavity.[56-58] It is imperative to remove these batteries promptly before tissue damage occurs from leakage of battery contents, electrical currents, or direct pressure. A relatively new and interesting nasal FB is the magnetic nose ring. These are small, commercially available earth magnets usually worn on either side of the alar cartilage, giving the appearance of a pierced nasal stud. The magnets can be displaced and become polarized across the nasal septum. The magnetic attraction can be quite strong and can lead to pressure necrosis of the nasal mucosa and possibly septal perforation. This attraction can also make removal difficult as well as painful for the patient.[59,60]

Many nasal FBs come to rest on the floor of the anterior or middle third of the nose. Metallic or calcified objects may show up on x-ray, but physical examination remains the most reliable means for diagnosis. Maxillary, ethmoid, or sphenoid sinusitis may also accompany FB retention. Plain radiographs or facial CT scanning may be of value in detecting sinusitis, although these studies are usually not necessary in the acutely retained object.

Failure to remove a nasal FB will necessitate ENT consultation and may result in admission for removal under anesthesia; therefore, it behooves emergency clinicians to be skilled in this procedure. Admission incurs increased cost, inherent procedural risks, and psychological stressors for parents and patients. As with the removal of auricular FBs, the removal of nasal FBs can be both frustrating and time-consuming.

Nasal FB Removal

A cooperative patient is essential; therefore, young children often require procedural sedation or general anesthesia for more posterior FBs. Whereas procedural sedation may aid in removal and preclude the need for admission and general anesthesia, this method will increase the risk of aspiration and must be considered with use of agents that blunt protective airway reflexes. Before attempting removal, anesthetize and vasoconstrict the affected naris, as previously described. Obtain assistance to stabilize the patient's head, and immobilize a younger patient as necessary. Place a more cooperative patient in the sniffing position and use a head lamp for proper illumination. Several of the techniques previously mentioned for EAC FB removal, including the use of cyanoacrylate glue, can also be used in the management of a nasal FB.

Use alligator forceps or bayonet forceps to retrieve more anteriorly lodged FBs that have edges amenable to grasping. For harder or larger objects, carefully pass wire loops, right-angle hooks, or even a properly bent paper clip beyond the object and rotate, allowing it to be pulled from the naris (see Fig. 64–20). Direct mucosal trauma and epistaxis may occur with any of these methods. For a nasal FB with smooth, round edges that are difficult to grasp or get behind, attempt to extract it with a suction-tip catheter in a manner similar to that described earlier for EAC FBs. The Hognose catheter described earlier also works well for nasal FBs. Local vasoconstriction and anesthesia is helpful, and 2% lidocaine with epinephrine (local anesthetic) may be used (Fig. 64–45A).

For an object that cannot be removed with anterior instrumentation, try to remove it with a balloon catheter. A Fogarty catheter can be highly effective in removing a nasal FB (see Fig. 64–45B and C). A No. 4 or 5 vascular Fogarty catheter, a 12-French Foley catheter, and a No. 6 biliary Fogarty catheter are all described in the literature for this use. A biliary catheter is reportedly less apt to rupture. Place the patient in the supine position and apply a vasoconstrictor and anesthetic to the nasal mucosa. With a 5-mL syringe attached and the catheter lubricated with lidocaine gel, pass the tip

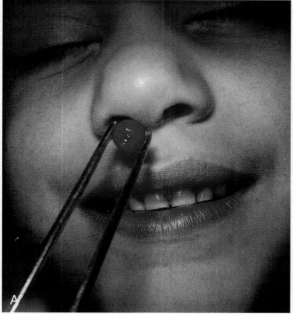
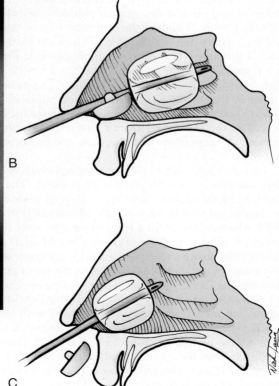
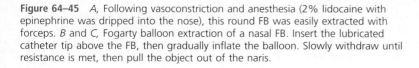

Figure 64–45 *A*, Following vasoconstriction and anesthesia (2% lidocaine with epinephrine was dripped into the nose), this round FB was easily extracted with forceps. *B* and *C*, Fogarty balloon extraction of a nasal FB. Insert the lubricated catheter tip above the FB, then gradually inflate the balloon. Slowly withdraw until resistance is met, then pull the object out of the naris.

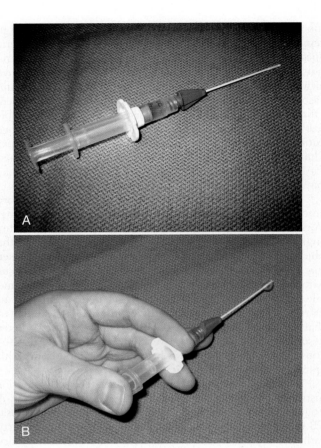

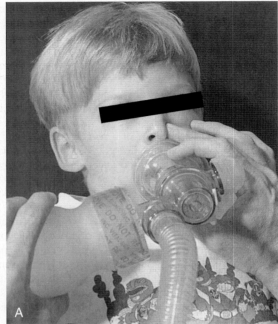

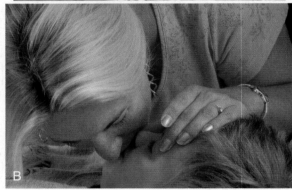

Figure 64–46 The Katz Extractor (InHealth Technologies, Carpinteria, CA) for otorhinonology FB removal. *A,* The device out of package. *B,* The device with the balloon inflated.

Figure 64–47 *A,* Bag-valve-mask technique to blow an FB out of the naris. Ensure that the face mask forms a tight seal around the patient's mouth and that the unaffected nostril is completely occluded. Attempt to firmly compress the bag as the patient exhales (an assistant is helpful to hold the mask snugly and to occlude the other nostril). This technique works best with objects that completely occlude the nostril. *B,* To blow out an FB in the nose, have the parent blow in the mouth while occluding the unaffected side with the thumb.

above the object and into the nasopharynx. Inflate the balloon with air or water (~2 mL in small children and 3 mL in older children) and control the syringe plunger and balloon size with the thumb. Withdraw the catheter until resistance is felt, and then slowly pull out the object. The Katz Extractor otorhino FB remover (InHealth Technologies, CA; Fig. 64–46) is a disposable, single unit, composed of a flexible catheter with balloon tip attached to a syringe. The procedure is similar to that of the Fogarty catheter. Complications mentioned in the literature include mild post-traumatic bleeding, as well as the theoretical risk of airway obstruction by the balloon or aspiration from further displacement of the object.

Another approach to the posteriorly placed nasal FB is to blow the object out with positive air pressure. The simplest way is to ask the child to blow her or his nose while occluding the unaffected nostril. This is really effective only in the older child. Alternatively, place a bag-valve mask[61] over the child's mouth to provide positive pressure (Fig. 64–47*A*). Occlude the opposite nostril and apply the Sellick maneuver to prevent air passage into the esophagus. This technique often requires restraint and can also be threatening to a young child.

Another technique is performed by having the child lie supine and occluding the unaffected nostril with the thumb (see Fig. 64–47*B*).[62,63] Next, as in mouth-to-mouth resuscitation, ask the mother or father to blow a short, sharp puff of air briskly into the mouth, producing an outward pressure behind the object. This either moves the object within grasping reach or pops it completely out of the naris. This method

is called "a parent's kiss." To gain the child's cooperation, tell him or her that the parent is going to "give them a big kiss." The parent is asked to make a firm seal with her or his mouth over the child's open mouth and then to give a short, sharp puff of air into the child's mouth. The opposite nostril is occluded throughout the procedure. If it fails, the technique can be repeated. A study of the parent's kiss by Botma and coworkers[64] found a success rate of 79%, and all parents thought the technique was acceptable and preferable to instrumentation or restraint. Although theoretical complications include barotrauma to the TM or other complications seen with positive-pressure ventilation (pneumothorax, mediastinal emphysema), no reported complications have been published in regard to these positive-pressure techniques.

Another similar technique may be successful.[65] After a nasal decongestant is instilled in the affected side, place a ¼- or ⅛-inch section of rubber or soft vinyl tubing (6–10 inches) into or over the contralateral nostril, holding the tubing in

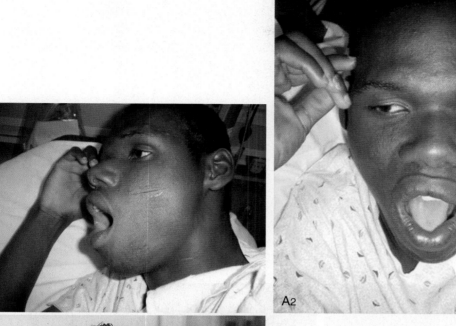

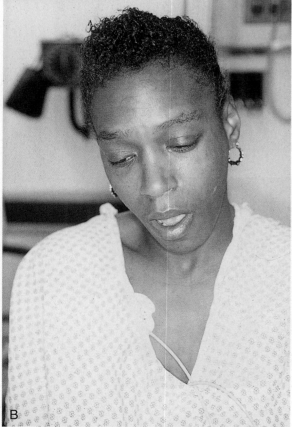

Figure 64–48 *A, 1* and *2,* This patient yawned and then could not close the mouth. This was a recurrent bilateral mandible dislocation. *B,* This patient was suspected of having a dystonic reaction because she could not speak and the mandible was misaligned. It was a unilateral mandible dislocation. *C,* Reduction of the temporomandibular joint (TMJ) dislocation. *Appropriate procedural sedation is the key to success.* The TMJ is shown in both normal and dislocated positions. *1,* Closed position, with the mandibular condyle resting in the mandibular fossa behind the articular eminence. *2,* In the maximally open position, the condyle is just under and slightly behind the eminence. *3,* In the dislocated position, the condyle moves forward and upward slightly above the eminence; muscle spasm then occurs. *4,* To reduce dislocation, place the thumbs intraorally and lateral to the lower molars, apply downward pressure to the lower molar ridge area near the jaw angle in a downward and backward direction. *5,* When the condyle has cleared the articular eminence, muscle contraction will return the jaw to a normal closed position. *D, 1* and *2,* To reduce a dislocated mandible, use sedation generously. Local injection of the TMJ joint with lidocaine is another option. The patient sits on a low chair with the back straight. Face the patient, wrap/protect the thumbs with gauze and place them in the mouth on the back molars, and push down and back. A rocking motion may help. *Inset, E,* The patient in Figure *A* after the dislocation is reduced. *(B, From Amsterdam JT: Oral medicine. In Marx JA, Hockberger RS, Walls RM [eds]: Rosen's Emergency Medicine: Concepts and Clinical Practices, 6th ed. Philadelphia, Elsevier Mosby, 2006, p 1041.)*

Continued

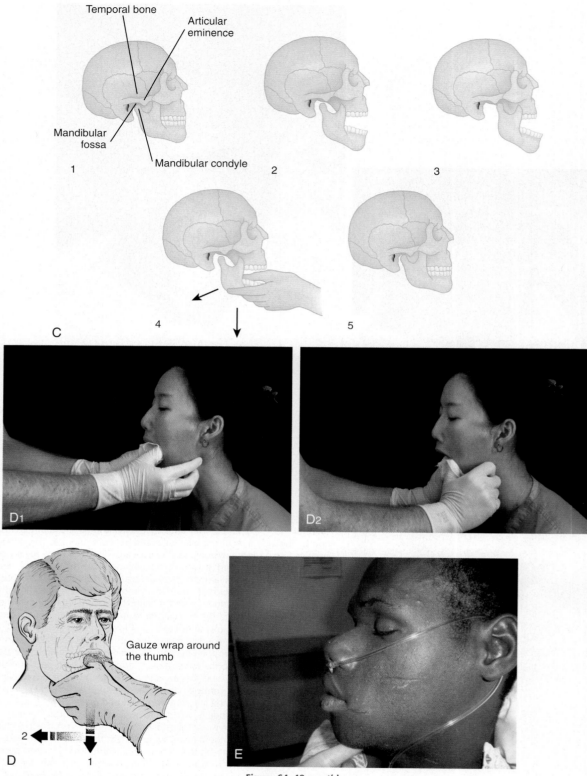

Temporal bone

Articular eminence

Mandibular fossa

Mandibular condyle

C

1

2

3

4

5

D1

D2

Gauze wrap around the thumb

D

2

1

E

Figure 64–48, cont'd

place with the fingers of one hand. Place the free hand gently over the child's mouth, take a good-sized breath, and blow forcefully through the tubing. This step may be repeated up to four times.

MANDIBLE

Mandible Dislocation

Mandibular dislocation is more properly known as *temporomandibular joint (TMJ) dislocation*. It is actually the mandibular condyles that dislocate. It may result from trauma, but more commonly follows extreme opening of the mouth such as may occur in eating, laughing, or yawning. It may also be seen in dystonic reactions to medications or confused with this reaction. Patients with a previous history of TMJ dislocation are more prone to repeat dislocations. The condition can be unilateral or bilateral (Fig. 64–48).

TMJ dislocation occurs when the mandibular condyle(s) moves anteriorly along the articular eminence and become(s) locked in the anterosuperior aspect of the eminence. Spasm of the masseter, internal pterygoid, and temporalis muscles occurs in an attempt to close the mandible. Trismus then results and the condyle cannot return to its normal position. Predisposing factors include anatomic disharmony between the mandibular fossa and the articular eminence and weakness of the capsule and the temporomandibular ligaments.

The diagnosis is usually straightforward, but can be misinterpreted as an acute dystonic reaction. Patients *cannot close the mouth*, and speech is affected. Pain varies, and patients are often very anxious. In unilateral dislocation, the jaw will deviate to the opposite side. More commonly, bilateral dislocation occurs. In traumatic dislocation, radiographic evaluation should be performed to exclude a fracture. A mandibular series, Panorex, or TMJ radiographs are acceptable.

Reduction of a TMJ dislocation is fairly straightforward. Procedural sedation is usually required. Occasionally, injection of lidocaine locally at the TMJ areas is helpful. Face the patient or reach from behind and grasp the mandible with both hands. Rest the *wrapped/protected thumbs* inside the mouth on the posterior molars, and wrap the fingers around the outside of the jaw. Apply downward pressure on the mandible to free the condyles from the eminence; often, a rocking motion helps. Then, guide the mandible posteriorly and superiorly back into the temporal fossa (see Fig. 64–48C).

When discharged, the patient is advised to avoid extreme mouth opening and to have a soft diet for 1 week. Warm compresses, nonsteroidal anti-inflammatory agents, and muscle relaxants may be helpful. The patient may be referred to an ENT or oral and maxillofacial surgeon for further care. Patients with chronic dislocation may require surgical fixation.

Uvulitis/Angioedema of the Uvula

Most cases of acute angioedema of the uvula (uvula hydrops), also known as Quincke's disease, are spontaneous and no cause can be found. The affected patient wakes up with a lump in the throat, or a fullness when swallowing, looks in the mirror, and sees an enlarged uvula (Fig. 64–49). It appears as an edematous, pale, and watery filled structure. This is nonpainful. Most patients are young and otherwise healthy.

Although most of the time, the cause remains unidentified, there are numerous known precipitants, including mari-

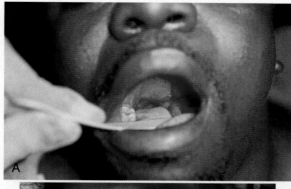

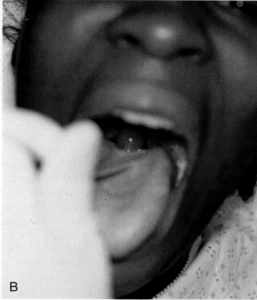

Figure 64–49 *A,* Very elongated uvula secondary to idiopathic angioedema, measuring about 3 cm and reaching past the mid-tongue. *B,* Globular shaped enlarged uvula caused the sensation of a lump in the throat. Both cases were treated as outpatients with antihistamines and prednisone, following 2 doses of subcutaneous epinephrine (0.3 mg) in the ED. Both resolved over 48 hours without sequelae.

juana and cocaine (crack) smoking, trauma to the uvula by endotracheal tubes or suction catheters during general anesthesia, and sticking the finger down the throat to induce vomiting. This is not to be confused with hereditary angioedema (hereditary angioneurotic edema) due to C1 esterase inhibitor deficiency, a recurrent and potentially fatal condition. Uvulitis may rarely be caused by bacterial infection, particularly *H. influenzae* B, and can coexist with epiglottitis. Angiotensin-converting enzyme inhibitor use does not seem related, but nonspecific allergic reactions (food, environmental) have been postulated. This condition, although annoying, is usually benign and self-limited and resolves in 24 to 48 hours. Airway compromise is a theoretical concern, but rarely occurs. Evaluating and maintaining the airway is the most important concern in uvulitis. The enlarging uvula can cause upper airway obstruction, particularly in children.

There are no controlled studies evaluating therapy, but numerous antiangioedema interventions have been used. Treatment includes topical epinephrine (applied with a cotton swab), subcutaneous epinephrine, intravenous H_1 and H_2 histamine blockers, and parenteral or oral corticosteroids.[66,67]

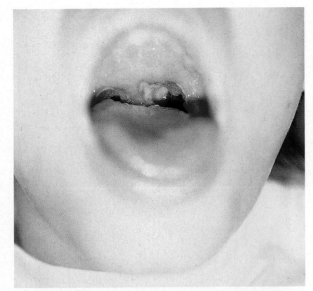

Figure 64–50 Typical appearance of the oral cavity 5–7 days post bilateral tonsillectomy. This is a common time for bleeding.

Inhalation of nebulized vasoconstrictors (such a epinephrine or racemic epinephrine) is an attractive, yet unproven, intervention. For severe cases, otolaryngology consultation is warranted, and invasive techniques, such as needle decompression (scoring the uvula with a needle to drain fluid is described) and uvulectomy, may be necessary. In an acute airway emergency, when intubation is not possible, the base of the uvula can be clamped with a hemostat and the distal portion amputated.

Post-Tonsillectomy Bleeding

Hemorrhage is the most serious complication of adenotonsillectomy with reported rates from 0.5 to 10% depending upon the technique (Fig. 64–50).[68] Bleeding is categorized as intraoperative, primary (within 24 hr) and secondary (between 24 hr and 10 days). Bleeding is serious at all times and must be evaluated and quickly controlled if active. The most common time for delayed bleeding to present to the ED is between the 5th and the 7th postoperative days. Some bleeding is minor, but sudden hemorrhage may be fatal if not managed appropriately. If active bleeding is confirmed by physical examination, consult otolaryngology. The severely bleeding patient should be taken to the operating room immediately for hemostasis. Until the surgeon arrives, apply pressure directly to the bleeding area with a sponge on a long clamp. The sponge may be dipped in epinephrine or thrombin powder if available. Theoretically, the bleeding area can be infiltrated with lidocaine with epinephrine local anesthetic.

If the patient presents to the ED complaining of post-tonsillectomy bleeding, but there is no active bleeding on examination and a blood clot is present, do not remove the clot. Definitive treatment and disposition are best made by the surgeon. Admission for observation is prudent. Obtain laboratory studies for a coagulation profile and a complete blood count.

 REFERENCES CAN BE FOUND ON **EXPERT CONSULT**

CHAPTER 65

Emergency Dental Procedures

Kip Benko

Complaints pertaining to the teeth and the supporting maxillofacial structures are common, and patients frequently present to the emergency department (ED) for evaluation. Complaints may range in scope from a simple chipped tooth to an odontogenic deep space infection or a maxillofacial injury. Treating these patients can be challenging and frustrating for busy emergency clinicians. Many emergency clinicians do not receive specific training in dental emergencies during their training, yet it is important for them to be able to recognize and treat a wide range of dental problems. Some dental emergencies can lead to morbidities such as tooth loss, pain, infection, and craniofacial abnormality whereas others can lead to life-threatening airway compromise.

Management of specific dental emergencies requires a thorough understanding of adult and pediatric dentition. The relevant anatomy of both populations is outlined. The techniques described for management of the various traumatic and infectious problems are, in most cases, temporizing until definitive dental or oral/maxillofacial surgery referral can be obtained. Those conditions requiring emergent consultation are discussed. Topical, local, and regional anesthesia are of particular importance and utility in the management of odontogenic emergencies; the clinician should be very familiar with these techniques.

Although this chapter describes the diagnosis and treatment of dental injuries that may confront the emergency clinician, no standard of care mandates that complex dental problems (e.g., replacement of avulsed teeth, infection drainage) be definitively handled in the ED setting. Advances in ED equipment and clinician training, however, are gradually raising the existing standard of care such that the initial stabilization of fractured, subluxed, luxated, and avulsed teeth is now within the realm of the emergency clinician. It is appropriate to refer all significant dental pathology to a dentist or oral surgeon.

TEETH

The adult dentition normally consists of 32 teeth, comprising four types: 8 incisors, 4 canines, 8 premolars, and 12 molars. From the midline to the back of the mouth, there is a central incisor, a lateral incisor, a canine, two premolars (bicuspids), and three molars, the last of which is the wisdom tooth (Fig. 65–1). The 20 primary or deciduous (baby) teeth comprise 8 incisors, 4 canines, and 8 molars. From the midline to the back of the mouth, there is a central incisor, a lateral incisor, a canine, and two molars (Fig. 65–2). *Agenesis*, or the lack of proper formation of a tooth or teeth, is not uncommon, especially in the maxilla. Likewise, *supernumerary*, or extra, teeth also occur. The adult teeth are numbered from 1 to 32, with the 1st tooth being the right upper third molar and the 16th tooth being the left upper third molar. The left lower third

molar is 17th, and the 32nd tooth is the right lower third molar. Numerous classification and numbering systems of the teeth exist; however, it is probably best for clinicians to simply describe the location and type of tooth in question (e.g., upper left second premolar, lower right canine). This removes any question when discussing a case with a consultant.

A tooth consists of the central pulp, the dentin, and the enamel (Fig. 65–3). The *pulp* contains the neurovascular supply of the tooth, which is responsible for carrying nutrients to the *dentin*, a microporous substance that consists of a system of microtubules. The dentin makes up the majority of the tooth and cushions the tooth during mastication. The *enamel* is the white, visible portion of the tooth and the hardest part of the body. The tooth may also be described in terms of the crown (coronal portion) or the root. The *crown* is that portion covered in enamel; the *root* is the part that serves to anchor the tooth in the alveolar bone.

The following descriptive terminology is used for the different anatomic surfaces of the tooth. These terms are useful when describing the specific tooth injury to a consultant or colleague:

- *Facial*: That part of the tooth that faces the opening of the mouth. This is the part that you see when somebody smiles. This is a general term applicable to all teeth.
- *Labial*: The facial surface of the incisors and canines.
- *Buccal*: The facial surface of the premolars and molars.
- *Oral*: That part of the tooth that faces the tongue or the palate. This is a general term applicable to all teeth.
- *Lingual*: Toward the tongue; the oral surface of the mandibular and maxillary teeth.
- *Palatal*: Toward the palate; the oral surface of the maxillary teeth.
- *Approximal/interproximal*: The contacting surfaces between two adjacent teeth.
- *Mesial*: The interproximal surface facing anteriorly or closest to the midline.
- *Distal*: The interproximal surface facing posteriorly or away from the midline.
- *Occlusal*: Biting or chewing surface of the premolars and molars.
- *Incisal*: Biting or chewing surface of the incisors and canines.
- *Apical*: Toward the tip of the root of the tooth.
- *Coronal*: Toward the crown or the biting surface of the tooth.

THE PERIODONTIUM

The *periodontium*, also known as the attachment apparatus, consists of two major subunits and is necessary for maintaining the integrity of the normal dentoalveolar unit.

The *gingival subunit* consists of the junctional epithelium and the gingival tissue. The gingival tissue is keratinized, stratified, squamous epithelium; it can be divided into the free gingival margin and the attached gingiva. The free gingiva is the cuff of tissue formed around the neck of the tooth. The gingival sulcus is that space between the free gingiva and the tooth. It is rarely greater than 2 to 3 mm in depth in normal healthy dentition. The attached gingiva is the portion of gingiva attached to the alveolar bone and extends apically (away from the tooth) to the mucogingival junction (or the mucobuccal fold). At this point, the tissue, loose and nonkeratinized, is called the alveolar mucosa (or buccal mucosa).

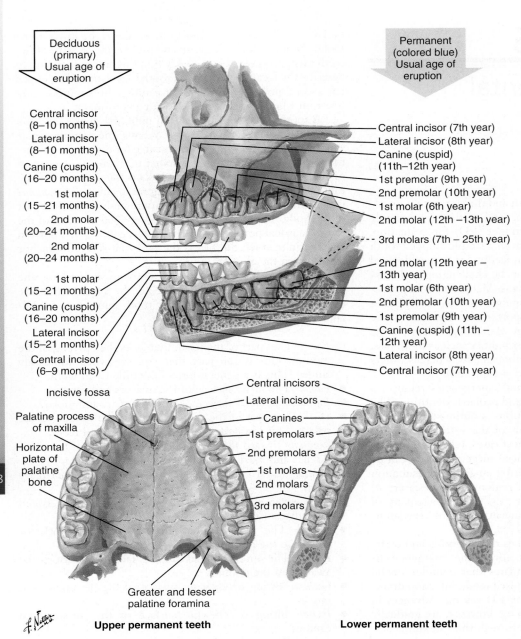

Deciduous (primary) Usual age of eruption

Central incisor (8–10 months)
Lateral incisor (8–10 months)
Canine (cuspid) (16–20 months)
1st molar (15–21 months)
2nd molar (20–24 months)
2nd molar (20–24 months)
1st molar (15–21 months)
Canine (cuspid) (16–20 months)
Lateral incisor (15–21 months)
Central incisor (6–9 months)

Permanent (colored blue) Usual age of eruption

Central incisor (7th year)
Lateral incisor (8th year)
Canine (cuspid) (11th–12th year)
1st premolar (9th year)
2nd premolar (10th year)
1st molar (6th year)
2nd molar (12th –13th year)
3rd molars (7th – 25th year)
2nd molar (12th year – 13th year)
1st molar (6th year)
2nd premolar (10th year)
1st premolar (9th year)
Canine (cuspid) (11th – 12th year)
Lateral incisor (8th year)
Central incisor (7th year)

Incisive fossa
Palatine process of maxilla
Horizontal plate of palatine bone

Central incisors
Lateral incisors
Canines
1st premolars
2nd premolars
1st molars
2nd molars
3rd molars

Greater and lesser palatine foramina

Upper permanent teeth   **Lower permanent teeth**

Figure 65–1 Anatomy of the teeth, primary and permanent. Note: an avulsed primary tooth need not be reimplanted if it is traumatically lost. *(Netter illustrations used with permission of Elsevier Inc. All rights reserved.)*

The *periodontal subunit* includes the periodontal ligament, alveolar bone, and the cementum of the root of the tooth. The periodontal ligament consists of collagen that extends from the alveolar bone to the root of the tooth. One end of the periodontal ligament inserts into the alveolar bone, the other end into the cementum.

The gingival subunit is primarily responsible for maintaining the integrity of the periodontal subunit. Certain disease states such as gingivitis weaken the attachment apparatus and can result in tooth loss.

ACUTE TOOTHACHE IN THE ED

Patients with an acute toothache often come to the ED for dental evaluation and symptomatic relief. Although multiple problems can initially cause pain in the area of the teeth, the etiology is usually dental decay or a cracked tooth (Fig. 65–4). Referral to a dentist is the logical definitive course of action, but pain relief can be initiated in the ED. Dental pain is,

however, also a common complaint in drug seekers. Nonsteroidal anti-inflammatory drugs (NSAIDs), acetaminophen, narcotics, and local nerve blocks provide pain relief, depending on the scenario. Hile and Linklater[1] recently reported significant pain relief for a fractured tooth by applying 2-octyl cyanoacrylate tissue adhesive (Dermabond, Ethicon Products) directly to the tooth. This intervention is currently anecdotal but may also provide temporary pain relief for patients with open decay when air and temperature exacerbate pain. Dry the tooth thoroughly with gauze, and generously apply a few layers of the product to the affected area. This intervention lasts for a few days only but should not interfere with subsequent dental intervention. Note that the use of skin adhesives has not been approved for intraoral use; and these tend to break down quickly in the oral cavity.

Pain in a tooth when exposed to hot liquids usually indicates a dental abscess. Sensitivity to cold can signify simple sensitivity or gum recession but can also indicate decay. Pain while biting down can indicate a fractured tooth or decay.

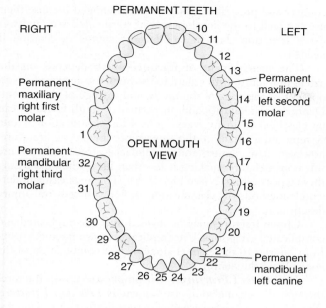

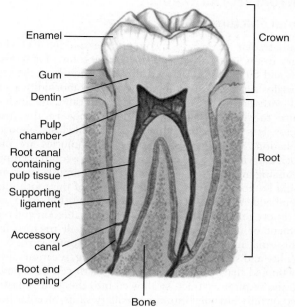

Figure 65–3 The dental anatomic unit.

Figure 65–2 **Identification of teeth, adult and child.** Each tooth has a number assigned to it. By age 14 years, all primary teeth should normally be lost. Do not reimplant an avulsed primary tooth; rather, refer to a dentist to prevent future misalignment of permanent teeth.

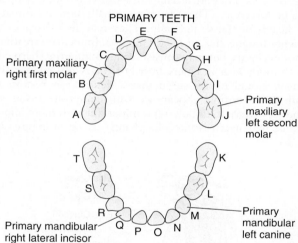

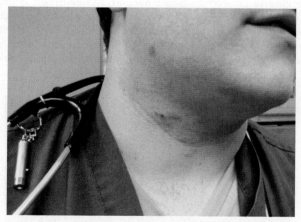

Figure 65–4 This physician had severe pain in the jaw thought to be related to a dental problem. Two days after the onset of pain the rash of herpes zoster appeared, the cause of the pain.

Many fillings can leak and cause pain, and microcracks can occur and not be readily apparent to the nondentist. One cause of microcracks, or even a totally fractured tooth, is constant trauma from metal balls implanted with tongue piercing.

For years, clove oil (contains eugenol) has been a popular and reasonably effective short-term home remedy for an acute toothache or inflamed gingiva. For a cavity or gum pain, saturate a piece of cotton in clove oil and place the cotton directly in the cavity or along the gum. This will provide relief for a few hours. Clove oil should not be used for more than a few applications owing to irritation and possible nerve damage. A paste made of water and activated charcoal has also been suggested.

Acute dental pain may also be referred pain, so a complete evaluation should be conducted if the area appears normal. For example, acute sinusitis can cause tooth pain, and vice versa. Obvious dental infection should be treated with antibiotics (e.g., penicillin, clindamycin, erythromycin) while awaiting dental evaluation. Chronic acetaminophen overdose is a known complication of overaggressive use of analgesics by patients unable to obtain dental care for acute toothache.[2] Unfortunately, many patients have irreversible pulpitis by the time they seek emergency care.[3]

Antibiotics provide no benefit for pain from a simple toothache, dental cavity, or pulpitis, although some clinicians prescribe them because follow-up dental care may be delayed or difficult to obtain.[4]

Individual teeth (except posterior molars) can be temporarily anesthetized with total pain relief by simply giving a periapical injection of a local anesthetic. Recently, articaine (septocaine) has been used for this purpose. It is fast acting and penetrates well. Many dentists have replaced lidocaine with articaine for local tooth anesthesia. Note, however, that *this anesthetic is not used for nerve blocks, only local injection, because persistent paresthesias have been associated with nerve blocks.*

DENTOALVEOLAR TRAUMA

Dental Fractures

Dentoalveolar trauma is a common reason for ED visits. Injury to the maxillary central incisors accounts for between 70% and 80% of all fractured teeth.[5–7] Trauma to the teeth is usually not life-threatening; however, the morbidity associated with dental fractures can be significant and includes failure to complete eruption, color change of the tooth, abscess, loss of space in the dental arch, ankylosis, abnormal exfoliation, and root resorption. Dental injuries are often associated with intraoral lacerations. When a tooth is chipped or missing and there is a concomitant intraoral laceration, it should be noted that the missing portion of the tooth might be embedded in the depths of the laceration (Fig. 65–5).

Some general principles apply to the evaluation and management of dental trauma. First, identify all fracture fragments and mobile teeth. Percuss each tooth surface for mobility and sensitivity. If a tooth is missing, it cannot always be assumed that it has been avulsed. Teeth can be aspirated into the respiratory tract, swallowed into the gastrointestinal tract, or fully intruded into the maxillary sinus, alveolar bone, or nasal cavity. Take radiographs if there is any suspicion of aspiration of tooth fragments or intrusion of fragments into the gingiva or alveolar bone. Second, the dentition is much more easily manipulated if the patient is not in significant discomfort. Tooth infiltration and common dental blocks should be part of the emergency clinician's armamentarium. Third, topical tooth remedies and analgesics, both over-the-counter and prescribed, should be discouraged because their use can lead to the development of sterile abscesses and soft tissue irritation. Fourth, administer tetanus vaccination if needed.

The management of fractured teeth depends on the extent of fracture with regard to the pulp, the degree of development of the apex of the tooth, and the age of the patient. Dentoalveolar injuries and, in particular, tooth fractures can be classified in many ways.[8] The Ellis classification is one system often cited in the emergency medicine literature; however, many dentists and maxillofacial surgeons do not use this nomenclature, making it less than ideal when discussing these types of injuries (see Fig. 65–5).[6] The most easily understood method of classification is one based on injury description.

Crown fractures may be divided into uncomplicated and complicated categories. Uncomplicated crown fractures result from injuries to the enamel alone or to a combination of the enamel and the dentin.

Ellis Class I Fractures. Uncomplicated crown fractures through the enamel only are known as *Ellis class I fractures* (Fig. 65–6A). They are usually not sensitive to either temperature or forced air. These fractures usually pose no threat to the health of the dental pulp. They may feel sharp to the patient's tongue, lips, or buccal mucosa. Immediate treatment is not necessary but may consist of smoothing the sharp edge of the tooth with an emery board or rotary disk sander. The patient should be reassured that a dentist can restore the tooth to its normal appearance with composite resins and bonding materials. Follow-up is important with these injuries because pulp necrosis and color change can occur in rare cases (<1%).[6,9,10]

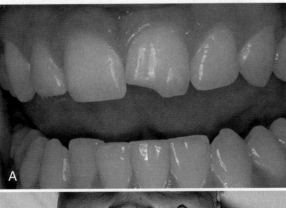

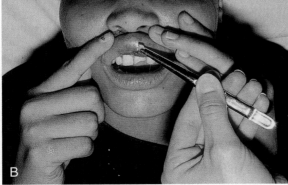

Figure 65–5 *A*, A chipped front tooth after a punch to the mouth can result in a piece of tooth being aspirated or imbedded in the laceration. *B*, When this lip laceration was explored, a piece of tooth was found embedded within the laceration. If this foreign body is not removed, an infection is certain a few days later. Note the obvious chipped upper tooth, the source of the piece found in the upper lip laceration.

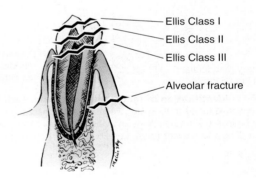

Ellis Class I
Ellis Class II
Ellis Class III

Alveolar fracture

A

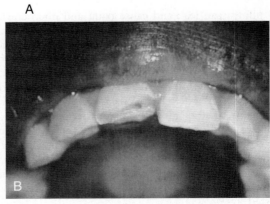

Figure 65–6 *A*, The Ellis classification for fractured alveolar teeth. The easiest method to classify fractured teeth is by description (e.g., fracture through the dentin of the first upper right molar). *B*, A fracture through the dentin puts this tooth at high risk for serious problems. This requires a dental radiograph for definitive diagnosis.

Ellis Class II Fractures. Uncomplicated fractures through the enamel and dentin are called *Ellis class II fractures.* Fractures that extend into the dentin are at higher risk of pulp necrosis and, therefore, need more aggressive treatment by the emergency clinician (see Fig. 65–6). The risk of pulp necrosis in these patients is less than 10%, but this increases as treatment time extends beyond 24 hours.[6] These patients often complain of sensitivity to heat, cold, or forced air. The physical examination reveals the yellow tint of the dentin in contrast to the white hue of the enamel. Fractures closer to the pulp cavity will reveal a pink tinge to the dentin. The tooth is usually sensitive to percussion with a tongue blade. The porous nature of the dentin allows passage of bacteria from the oral cavity to the pulp that may result in inflammation and infection of the pulp chamber. This is more likely to occur after 24 hours of dentin exposure but occurs sooner if the fracture site is closer to the pulp. Likewise, patients younger than 12 years have a pulp-to-dentin ratio larger than that in the mature adult and are at increased risk for pulp contamination. For this reason, younger patients should be treated aggressively and should be seen by their dentist within 24 hours[10,11] (see Fig. 65–6*B*).

The goal of treating dentin fractures is twofold: to cover the exposed dentin, thus preventing secondary contamination or infection, and to provide pain relief. After the tooth is covered, the dentist, using modern composites, can often rebuild the tooth directly over the calcium hydroxide (CaOH) cap that was placed in the ED. Perform a supraperiosteal infiltration or a regional tooth block before any tooth manipulation. This will make the application of the dressing easier because the tooth will become painless. Dressings that may be applied to the surface of the tooth include CaOH, zinc oxide, and glass ionomer composites. Some literature suggests that glass ionomers may be superior to other coverings; however, the difference is probably slight and the increased cost of the glass ionomers is not justified for routine ED use at this time.[5,12] Certain composites may be cured with a bonding light. This is routinely done in the dentist's office and is beyond the scope of most emergency practice. Bone wax and skin glues such as the cyanoacrylates are not recommended as dressings. Most dressings come as a base and a catalyst, which require mixing. This is easily accomplished with a dental spatula and a mixing pad, obtainable from any dental supply house. A commonly used ED dressing is Dycal (calcium hydroxide). Mix the catalyst and the base in equal portions, and place a small amount on the exposed area with an applicator such as a dental spatula or another appropriate instrument (Figs. 65–7 and 65–8).

Dry the tooth surface before application to ensure adherence of the CaOH. Have the patient bite into gauze pads to accomplish this. Dycal will dry within minutes after being exposed to the moist environment of the mouth. Although placing dental foil over the CaOH dressing is recommended, it is not usually necessary if the patient plans to follow up with a dentist within 24 to 36 hours. To prevent dislodging the dressing, instruct the patient to eat only soft foods until seen by a dentist. Begin antibiotic treatment with penicillin or clindamycin until definitive dental treatment can be obtained.[13]

Many patients who sustain a fracture through the dentin will require a root canal or other definitive endodontic treatment. The timely application of an appropriate dressing in the ED, however, may prevent contamination of the pulp and make root canal therapy unnecessary. As with any trauma to

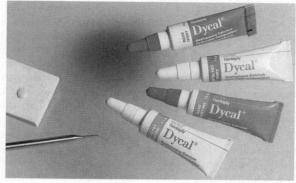

Figure 65–7 Calcium hydroxide paste (Dycal) is one acceptable material to cover dentin or pulp fractures. Mix the calcium hydroxide paste with a spatula on a mixing pad.

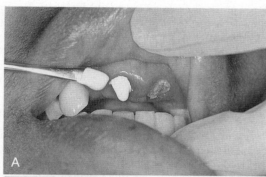
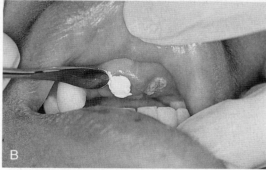

Figure 65–8 Application of the periodontal calcium hydroxide paste to the fractured surface of the tooth. The paste hardens quickly in the moist environment of the mouth.

the anterior teeth, explain to the patient that disruption of the neurovascular supply is possible and that long-term complications such as pulp necrosis, color change, and resorption of the root might occur.

Ellis Class III Fractures. Complicated fractures involving the pulp are also known as *Ellis class III fractures.* Complicated fractures of the crown that extend into the pulp of the tooth are true dental emergencies. These fractures result in pulp necrosis in 10% to 30% of cases even with appropriate treatment.[6] They may be distinguished from fractures of the dentin by the pink color of the pulp. Wipe the fractured surface of the tooth with gauze and observe for frank bleeding or a pink blush, which indicates exposure of the pulp. Fractures through the pulp are often excruciatingly painful, but occasionally, there is a lack of sensitivity secondary to a disruption of the neurovascular supply of the tooth.

Immediate management includes referral to a dentist, oral surgeon, or endodontist. The patient often requires a pulpectomy (complete removal of the pulp) or, in the case of primary teeth, a pulpotomy (partial removal of the pulp) as definitive treatment.[5,9] The longer the pulp is exposed, the greater the likelihood of contamination and abscess formation. If a dentist cannot see the patient immediately, attempt to relieve the pain and cover the exposed pulp. If significant pain is present, perform a dental block. Subsequently, cover the tooth with one of the dressings described earlier. Sometimes, bleeding is brisk. Control this by applying a dressing. Ask the patient to bite onto a gauze pad that has been soaked with a topical anesthetic containing a vasoconstrictor such as epinephrine. Alternatively, inject a small amount of the anesthetic/vasoconstrictor into the pulp to control bleeding. After the covering is applied, instruct the patient to follow up as soon as possible with a dentist. Antibiotics with coverage directed at oral flora (e.g., penicillin, clindamycin) should be considered and only soft foods should be eaten. Removal of the pulp with specialized instruments by the emergency clinician is not recommended, although some authors have advocated this in the past. This procedure is the realm of the dental professional and is likely to result in complications if not done properly.

Luxation, Subluxation, Intrusion, and Avulsion

Luxation and Subluxation. *Subluxation* refers to teeth that are mobile but not displaced. *Luxation* refers to teeth that are displaced, either partially or completely, from their sockets. Luxation injuries are divided into four types (Fig. 65–9):

1. *Extrusive luxation* is an injury in which the tooth is forced partially out of the socket in an axial direction (see Fig. 65–9A).
2. *Intrusive luxation*, or intrusion, occurs when the tooth is forced apically. It may be accompanied by crushing or fracture of the tooth apex (see Fig. 65–9B).
3. *Lateral luxation* occurs when the tooth is displaced either facially, lingually, mesially, or distally (see Fig. 65–9C). This injury is often associated with injuries to the alveolar wall.
4. *Complete luxation*, also known as complete avulsion, results in loss of the entire tooth from the socket.

Even minor trauma to the oral cavity requires meticulous examination for loose or missing teeth. Examine each tooth for mobility by using a back-and-forth motion on each side of the tooth surface with either the fingertips or two tongue blades. Any blood in the gingival crevice (area where the gingiva touches the tooth) suggests a traumatized tooth.

Teeth that are minimally mobile and are not displaced do very well with only conservative treatment. The tooth will tighten up in the socket if not retraumatized. Instruct patients to eat only a soft diet for 1 to 2 weeks and follow up with their dentist as soon as possible. Note that a seemingly lost (avulsed) tooth may actually be deeply intruded into the soft tissue (Fig. 65–10).

Grossly mobile teeth require some form of stabilization as soon as possible. It is important to note that in certain patients with poor gingival health, luxated teeth may not be salvageable owing to disease of the attachment apparatus. Fixation is best performed by the dental specialist with enamel bonding materials or wire ligation. Although many different

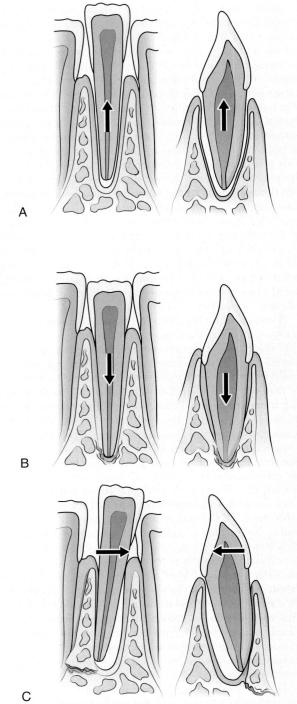

Figure 65–9 Tooth trauma classification. *A,* Extrusive luxation occurs when the tooth is forced partially out of the socket in an axial direction. *B,* Intrusive luxation of a tooth compresses the periodontal ligament and vascular supply of the pulp. It may even crush the apical bone. *C,* Lateral luxation occurs when the tooth is displaced in a lingual, a mesial, a distal, or a facial direction. Fractures of the alveolus frequently accompany lateral luxation injuries. *(A–C, Adapted from King R: Orofacial infections. In Oral-Facial Emergencies—Diagnosis and Management, 1st ed. Portland, OR, JBK Publishing, 1994.)*

"home remedies" exist for splinting loosened teeth in the ED, be aware of the concern for aspiration of teeth if the splint fails. Avoid the use of nonapproved medications in the mouth. Splinting techniques are suitable for the emergency clinician to perform as temporizing measures until definitive care can

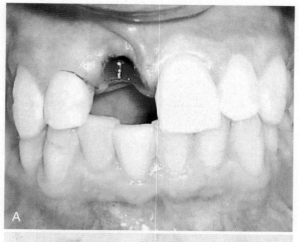

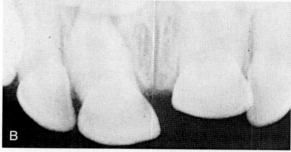

Figure 65–10 **Intruded tooth secondary to trauma.** *A,* On superficial examination, it appears that the tooth was simply knocked out. This missing tooth could be simply lost, fully intruded, or aspirated or swallowed. *B,* In some cases a dental radiograph or computed tomography scan is necessary to determine intrusion or avulsion. Intruded teeth create the potential for infection or cosmetic deformities. Intrusion of an upper tooth into the maxillary sinus can cause recurrent sinusitis. Teeth can also intrude into the nasal cavity and cause infection or bleeding, or they can be aspirated into the airway. The incisors are the teeth most commonly intruded.

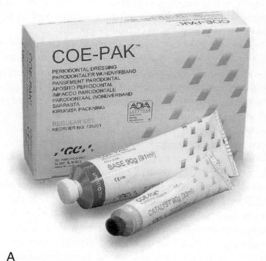

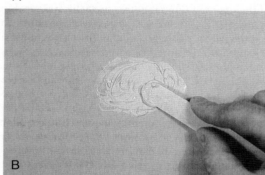

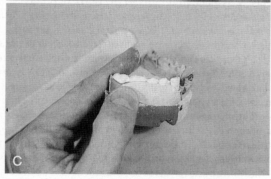

Figure 65–11 **Temporary stabilization of loose teeth.** *A,* Coe-Pax periodontal dressing. *B,* Squeeze out equal-sized ribbons of the periodontal paste. Mix the base and catalyst together with a tongue blade. *C,* Using moistened gloves, apply the paste to the dry enamel and gingiva.

be arranged. One simple technique for emergency use is to apply periodontal paste, commercially available as Coe-pak (Fig. 65–11). Coe-pak consists of a base and a catalyst that, when mixed, form a moderately sticky claylike dressing, which becomes firm after application. It is applied over the enamel and gingiva as well as the adjacent teeth to splint the subluxed tooth into place. Although the splint performs best if placed on the facial and buccal surfaces of the teeth, it is usually sufficient to apply the paste only to the front (facial) surface of the teeth. Make sure that the gingiva and enamel are completely dry. Lubricate your gloves with water or lubricating jelly before applying the dressing. Apply the dressing into the grooves between the teeth as well as to the adjacent teeth. Remind the patient to eat a soft diet until seen in follow up within 24 hours. Coe-pak is fairly simple for the dentist to remove during formal restoration.

Teeth that are luxated in either the horizontal or the axial plane or are slightly extruded can also be splinted with the techniques described earlier. It is important that the loosened tooth is in perfect alignment when the final adjustments are made at the dentist's office. However, the alignment does not need to be precise when the tooth is splinted in the ED. The important point is that the tooth is splinted adequately and follow up is ensured.

Intrusion and Avulsion. Intruded teeth are those that have been forced apically into the alveolar bone. This often results in disruption of the attachment apparatus or fracture of the supporting alveolar bone, especially in permanent teeth with mature roots.[11,14] These teeth are usually immobile and do not require stabilization in the ED. Intruded teeth often require endodontic treatment because of pulp necrosis. It is important to consider the possibility of an intruded tooth anytime there is a space in the dentition (see Fig. 65–10). Undiagnosed intrusion of the teeth can lead to infection and craniofacial abnormalities. Obtain x-rays anytime there is uncertainty as to whether a tooth is intruded or simply avulsed. Intruded teeth are best managed by the dentist or dental specialist; referral should take place within 24 hours. Permanent teeth often require repositioning and immobilization, but primary teeth are usually given a trial period to erupt on their own before any intervention is taken.

Primary teeth are not replaced after avulsion because they can fuse to the alveolar bone and potentially cause craniofacial abnormalities or infection. Reimplanted primary teeth may also interfere with the eruption of the secondary teeth. The parents of these patients need to be reassured that a prosthetic replacement for the avulsed teeth can easily be made and worn until the permanent teeth erupt. See Figures 65–1 and 65–2 as a guide to identifying permanent versus primary teeth.

Avulsed permanent teeth are those that have been completely removed from their ligamentous attachments. These are true dental emergencies. *The majority of patients presenting to the ED with an avulsed tooth will lose that tooth*, so patient and physician expectations should not be overly optimistic. Under ideal circumstances, such as presentation to a dentist's office with a properly stored tooth avulsed less than 60 minutes, this situation may result in a successful reimplantation 80% to 90% of the time but often requires specialized procedures and endodontics (root canal). Emergency clinicians are not expected to save an avulsed tooth, but prompt action may give that replanted tooth some chance for survival.

The first consideration in treating dental avulsions is to ask, "Where is the tooth?" Missing teeth may have been intruded, fractured, aspirated, swallowed, or embedded into the soft tissues of the oral mucosa (see Fig. 65–10). Therefore, x-rays should be considered anytime an avulsed tooth cannot be located. Management of the avulsed tooth in the ED depends on a number of factors, including the age of the patient, the amount of time that has elapsed since the tooth was avulsed, associated trauma to the oral cavity such as alveolar ridge fractures, and the overall health of the periodontium.[14] Time is the other important consideration when deciding whether to replace an avulsed tooth. In general, the longer the tooth is out of the socket, the higher the incidence of periodontal ligament necrosis and subsequent failure of reimplantation. The periodontal ligament cells generally die within 60 minutes outside of the oral cavity if they are not placed in appropriate transport media.[15] A significant amount of research has been conducted on different media used to keep the cells of the periodontal ligament alive. Various transport media have been studied including milk, Hank's Balanced Salt Solution, Save-A-Tooth, saliva, cell culture media, and water. Although certain cell culture media have been developed to stimulate the periodontal ligament cells to proliferate and remain viable, milk and the commercially available Save-A-Tooth and EMT Toothsaver are the best and easiest for both prehospital care and ED storage (Fig. 65–12).[15,16] Milk will preserve the periodontal ligament for 4 to 8 hours; the commercial products will preserve the ligament for 12 to 24 hours. However, reimplantation should take place at the earliest possible opportunity after the socket has been adequately prepared. The key is to get the tooth into the transport media immediately because even 10 minutes outside of some type of storage media can cause desiccation and death of the periodontal ligament cells. Use saliva at the scene if milk, EMT Toothsaver, or Save-A-Tooth is not available. The patient should reimplant the tooth in the prehospital setting, if possible. The principles cited here should be followed when providing instructions to prehospital providers or to a patient who calls for advice. It is always preferable to refer such patients directly to a dentist, rather than the ED, if this is practical. Ask them to:

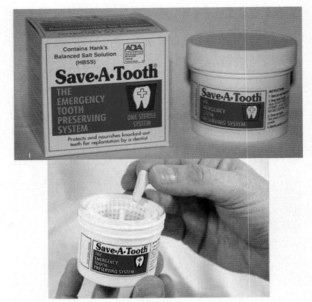

Figure 65–12 Using the "Save A Tooth" system, an avulsed *permanent* tooth is placed into the container and closed. *Avulsed primary teeth are not replanted*. The preservative will increase the life span of traumatized periodontal ligament cells. Unpreserved teeth replanted after 60 min rarely survive; those that do require root canal procedures and close follow-up. This system prolongs the time to successful reimplantation, but does not ensure success.

- Determine whether this is a permanent tooth: By 14 years of age, all primary teeth should have been lost.
- Handle the tooth by the crown only, because handling the tooth by the root can damage the alveolar ligament.
- Do not replace the tooth if it is fractured or if there is significant maxillofacial trauma such as an alveolar ridge fracture.
- If the tooth can be replaced in the prehospital setting, gently *rinse off* the root first to remove any debris. Do not wipe off the root because this removes the periodontal ligament.
- If the tooth cannot be reimplanted successfully in the field, place it in a transport media as described earlier. Do not transport the tooth in the oral cavity such as the cheek because it can be aspirated. This location is also not ideal for keeping the periodontal ligament alive because of the bacterial flora and low osmolality of the saliva.
- Once the patient arrives in the ED, confirm proper placement and alignment. It is not important that the tooth is in perfect position, because the dentist can make final adjustments. Splinting the repositioned tooth with periodontal paste or composite as outlined earlier may be necessary if mobility is present.

Should reimplantation not be successful in the prehospital setting, it must be done in the ED using the following guidelines:

- Store the tooth in appropriate media if reimplantation is delayed for any reason.
- Perform a supraperiosteal dental infiltration before manipulating or replacing teeth to make the procedure more comfortable for the patient and easier to perform.

- Check the oral cavity for trauma. If an alveolar ridge fracture is present or the socket is significantly damaged, do not reimplant the tooth.
- Gently suction the socket first with a Frasier suction tip to remove any accumulated clot. Be careful not to damage the walls of the socket because this can further damage periodontal ligament fibers. Irrigate gently after suctioning. If the clot is not removed, reimplantation and realignment will be difficult. Rinse off any debris on the tooth with saline but do not scrub it. Implant the tooth into the socket using firm, but gentle, pressure. Remember to handle the tooth only by the crown.
- Ask the patient to bite down gently on gauze to help align the tooth. The tooth may require splinting after replacement. If significant mobility is present such that temporizing splints are not adequate, consult the dentist to see whether wiring or arch bars are necessary.
- Update tetanus as necessary.
- Prescribe a liquid diet until the patient is seen in follow up.

Antibiotics are controversial in the treatment of fractured and avulsed teeth. Although the American Association of Endodontics does not recommend the routine use of antibiotics for fractures or avulsions, other authors recommend the use of antibiotics that cover mouth flora (e.g., penicillin, clindamycin) to decrease the inflammatory resorption of the root.[6,17] It is probably reasonable to use antibiotics if the root or socket is heavily soiled; otherwise, treatment should be tailored to the individual patient and discussed with the consultant.

Ideally, but rarely possible in real life, the patient is immediately referred to a dentist, and the reimplanted tooth held in place by biting on gauze. The tooth may be temporarily held into place with Coe-Pax (see Fig. 65–11) or the technique described in Figure 65–13.

Prognosis. The prognosis of a reimplanted tooth depends on many things. As discussed earlier, the time to reimplantation is critical. Likewise, the age of the patient, the stage of development of the root (younger is better), and the overall health of the gingiva are also very important. An individual with gingival disease is more likely to have an unsuccessful reimplantation.

The goal in any tooth avulsion or fracture is to keep the native tooth if at all possible. A tooth that has been avulsed and reimplanted usually loses the majority of its neurovascular supply and undergoes pulp necrosis. However, if the periodontal ligament remains intact, there is a greater chance of a functional tooth. It is important that the patient be aware that some root resorption is always going to occur after reimplantation and loss of the tooth might occur.

Alveolar Bone Fractures

Trauma involving the anterior teeth may be associated with fractures of the alveolus, which is the tooth-bearing portion of the maxilla or mandible. Alveolus or alveolar ridge fractures often occur in multitooth segments and will vary in the number of teeth involved, the amount of displacement, and the mobility of the affected segment. The patient usually complains of pain as well as malocclusion. The diagnosis is usually clinically apparent and is notable for a section of teeth that are misaligned and variable in mobility. Avulsed teeth, fractured teeth, or displaced teeth may be present within the

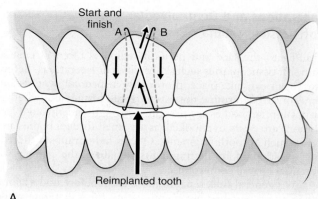
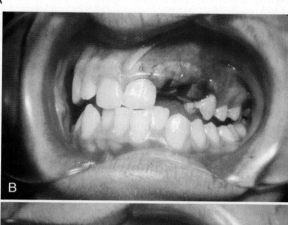
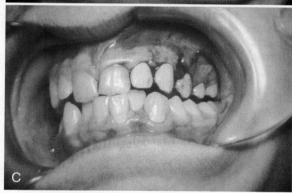

Figure 65–13 **Temporary suturing to hold a replanted tooth in place.** *A,* Use a silk suture. Start by puncturing the gingival at the border of the replaced tooth (*A*). Bring the suture behind the tooth, then cross over the front of the tooth to the other side. Penetrate the gingiva (*B*), go behind the tooth, cross over the front again, and tie the suture (*A*). *B* and *C,* Multiple teeth can be reimplanted.

alveolar segment itself. Dental bite-wing x-rays confirm the diagnosis. In the ED, Panorex or facial films may show the fracture line just apical to the root of the involved teeth; however, these films are often inconclusive or normal.

Treatment of alveolar ridge fractures involves rigid splinting after repositioning of the involved segment. This is usually beyond the scope of the emergency clinician, and urgent consultation with an oral surgeon or dentist is necessary. The role of the emergency clinician is to identify the injury as well as any avulsed or fractured teeth and preserve as much of the alveolar bone and surrounding mucosa as possible. Alveolar bone that is lost, débrided, or missing is difficult for the specialist to restore properly.[12]

Lacerations and Dentoalveolar Soft Tissue Trauma

Trauma to the face and perioral region is often associated with soft tissue injuries such as abrasions or lacerations. Before any repair can take place, thoroughly inspect all wounds and abrasions to determine the extent of the wound and whether or not foreign bodies are present. Through-and-through lacerations are easily overlooked, as are small foreign bodies and debris such as tooth fragments. Obtain radiographs if there is any question of tooth fragments. Evaluate the patient for potential airway compromise.

As a general rule, repair injured teeth before undertaking soft tissue repair because manipulating the soft tissue while repairing teeth may damage sutures already in place in the soft tissues. Begin repairing in the perioral region with standard wound care. After appropriate local or regional anesthesia, débride devitalized, crushed, or macerated tissue. Irrigate profusely. The role of antibiotics in mucosal trauma has not been definitively established, and there is no definitive standard of care. Several studies suggest a minimal benefit; however, this remains to be completely proved.[18] A reasonable guideline to follow is to use antibiotics if a significant amount of devitalized or crushed tissue is present or if the wound is through-and-through. Coverage of oral flora (e.g., penicillin, clindamycin) is fine for mouth lacerations, and additional skin coverage (e.g., clindamycin, dicloxacillin) should be considered for through-and-through lacerations. Dentoalveolar trauma may present the emergency clinician with several different situations that should generally be approached as follows.

Buccal Mucosa. Most small lacerations and abrasions of the buccal mucosa heal quickly and rapidly without repair, but large lacerations (>1–2 cm) should be repaired. Use any absorbable suture such as chromic gut or Vicryl in the mouth, but place the sutures so that the knots are buried. Silk is an alternative, but has a higher reactivity and is nonabsorbable. Avoid using nylon because it is sharp and irritating to the tissues.

Through-and-through lacerations of the oral cavity present a special situation. Evaluate for damage to the salivary ducts (Wharton's duct and Stensen's duct) and to the facial nerve. If they are intact, proceed with repair. Guidelines for closure are controversial, but generally, larger lacerations (>1–2 cm) should be closed. Close the mucosa with absorbable sutures as noted earlier, and close the skin aesthetically with 6-0 nylon, Prolene, or a rapidly absorbable suture. Close the mucosa first so as not to disturb the skin repair. If the mucosal wound is small or is a puncture wound, it is reasonable to close only the skin layer. Refer very large, gaping, or complicated lacerations to an oral surgeon.

Recheck large or through-and-through lacerations of the oral cavity in 2 to 3 days. Remove nonabsorbable sutures in 7 to 10 days. Advise the patient to rinse four to six times a day with saline. Prescribe a soft diet. Apply a topical skin antibiotic for 24 to 48 hours.

Gingiva. Small lacerations of the hard gingiva overlying the maxillary or mandibular alveolus usually heal uneventfully without repair. If the laceration is large, if there is a flap present, or if bone is exposed, approximate the gingiva with a 4-0 or 5-0 Vicryl or Dexon suture. As earlier, silk is another option. It is difficult to suture gingiva because there is little supporting soft tissue underneath. A helpful technique is to wrap the suture around the teeth circumferentially and use

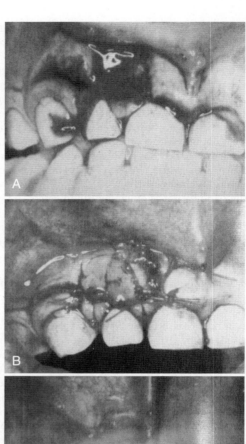

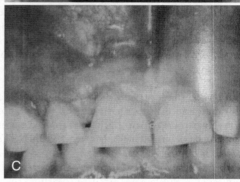

Figure 65–14 *A,* Gingival lacerations sometimes leave little tissue for approximation. *B,* The teeth can be used as anchors for sutures and help approximate the lacerated tissue. *C,* Gingival lacerations usually heal rapidly.

the teeth as anchors (Fig. 65–14). Large lacerations should be repaired to approximate the gingiva and cover the base of the teeth (Fig. 65–15).

Frenulum. The maxillary frenulum rarely requires sutures for simple lacerations. If the laceration is extensive or extends significantly into the surrounding mucosa or gingiva, approximate it with chromic Vicryl or Dexon suture. These wounds are often significantly painful. Prescribe analgesic medications even if the wound does not require suturing. The lingual frenulum is very vascular in nature and often will need a suture or two to control hemostasis. Use a local anesthetic with a vasoconstrictor to aid in hemostasis while the wound is repaired.

The Tongue. Tongue lacerations are challenging. Although they may be tempting to suture, most large lacerations of the body of the tongue, such as those that occur from a seizure, will heal well without suturing. Tongue lacerations that have the wound edges approximated do not need to be sutured. Repair larger lacerations that gape because the cleft left by the wound will epithelialize and leave a grooved or bifid or lateral flap appearance. Approximate wounds that are

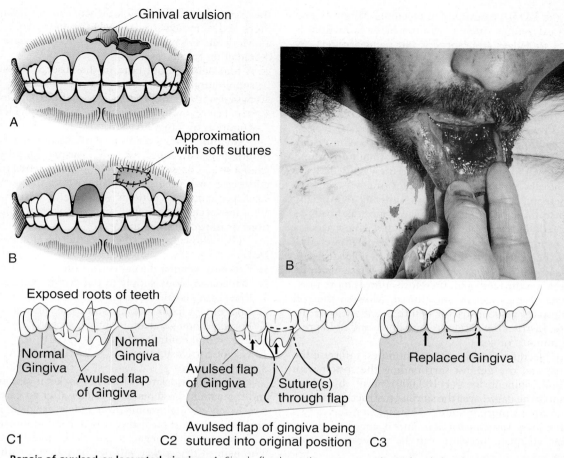

Figure 65–15 Repair of avulsed or lacerated gingiva. *A*, Simple flap lacerations are approximated and closed with interrupted soft sutures, such as Dexon or Vicryl. *B*, Large gingival avulsions should be approximated to an anatomic position with interrupted sutures. *C1*, The exposed roots of the teeth should be covered. The thin and friable avulsed gingiva cannot be sutured to the remaining gingiva or submucosal tissue. *C2*, The suture begins on the outer surface of the avulsed flap and is passed behind an anchoring tooth, like dental floss. The underside of the avulsed segment is then entered by the suture needle so the needle exits on the gingival surface. *C3*, Sutures pull the gingival to an anatomic position to cover the roots of the teeth and are tied on the outer surface. Sutures are removed in 5–7 days (see also Fig. 65–14).

bleeding profusely, are flap-shaped, involve muscle, or are on the edge of the tongue. Small avulsions (divits) or those in the center of the tongue usually heal without intervention.

Explain the procedure in detail to the patient before repairing these wounds. Ask an assistant to secure the tongue by holding it with gauze. If the tongue cannot be secured in this manner, apply a towel clip to the end of the anesthetized tongue. Children with tongue lacerations that need repair usually require sedation or repair by a specialist in the surgical suite, but many of these lacerations are small and heal uneventfully on their own.

Begin the repair with either a local infiltration of anesthetic or a lingual block. To promote hemostatis, infiltrate locally with lidocaine with epinephrine. Use absorbable sutures such as 4-0 chromic, Vicryl, or Dexon. Silk can be used, but it must be removed in 7 to 10 days. Do not use nylon because it is very irritating to the surrounding tissues. For a laceration extending through muscle, close with one deep stitch penetrating both the mucosa and the muscle. When possible, bury the knots of absorbable sutures because they will often work their way loose. Full-thickness lacerations can be closed in a number of ways. Place a suture through all three layers or close the top mucosa and muscle together and do the same thing on the underside of the tongue. Bleeding from large lacerations is almost always controlled with primary

repair. In some instances, hemostasis can be achieved without the use of sutures with the use of Gelfoam impregnated with topical thrombin (see Fig. 65–15).

ORAL HEMORRHAGE

Bleeding from the oral cavity is not unusual and is most commonly associated with dental procedures. It is important to ascertain whether any recent dental work has been performed and what was done. Spontaneous bleeding of the gingiva or oral cavity not associated with dental manipulation or trauma is suggestive of advanced periodontal disease or an underlying systemic process. Ask the patient about other medical conditions that predispose to bleeding (e.g., liver disease, platelet abnormalities) as well as historical factors that may suggest a bleeding abnormality or clotting factor deficiency. Find out whether the patient is taking aspirin or other anticoagulants. Consider laboratory testing if there is a significant concern for a pathologic coagulopathy, but not routinely in the patient presenting after dental manipulation.

Control gingival bleeding after scaling or minor dental procedures with direct pressure and saline/hydrogen peroxide rinses. Bleeding persisting from the gingival areas despite pressure and rinses raises suspicion for a bleeding abnormality. A much more common cause of oral hemorrhage that presents to the ED is postextraction bleeding. Minor oozing from dental extractions, such as wisdom teeth extraction, is normal for 2 to 4 days after surgery, but many patients get concerned when bleeding persists, despite warnings from the oral surgeon. These patients usually present when their dentist cannot be contacted and after futile attempts to stop the bleeding at home. The emergency clinician has a number of options to obtain hemostasis from postextraction bleeding.

Direct Pressure. Although the patient may have been using this technique at home, a few simple procedures may make it more effective. Remove excessive clot built up around the oozing site with a suction catheter and then gently irrigate the area. The clot that is inside the socket (if any is present) should be left intact. Often, this clot is missing or partially missing. Once the clot is removed, place gauze as firmly as possible directly onto the bleeding site. This is best accomplished by using dental roll gauze (see "Dental Materials," later in this chapter). Insert it directly over the bleeding site and then cover with 2 × 2 gauze. Dental roll gauze fits more precisely between the teeth and, therefore, affords more pressure; however, 2 × 2s can be substituted. Moisten the roll gauze with topical vasoconstrictor before placing it over the bleeding site. Instruct the patient to bite down and hold pressure for 15 minutes or so.

If active bleeding persists after 15 minutes, infiltrate the bleeding area and the gingiva surrounding the socket with lidocaine and epinephrine (1:100,000) until blanching occurs. Reapply the gauze over the site and instruct the patient to bite down for 15 more minutes. The injection serves two purposes: It causes vasoconstriction, and it anesthetizes the area so that adequate pressure can be generated during biting.

If bleeding persists, insert a coagulation sponge, such as Gelfoam, into the socket and then loosely close the gingiva surrounding the socket with a 3-0 absorbable figure-of-eight suture. Instruct the patient to bite down on gauze placed over the sutures. Soaking Gelfoam with topical thrombin before placement is a good way to halt minor persistent bleeding (see Fig. 65–19). A new agent showing great promise for oral hemorrhage is the chitosan dental bandage (Hemcon), which is designed specifically for postextraction and oral bleeding. The shrimp-based bandage forms a sticky matrix when it contacts blood and it quickly forms a seal that stops bleeding. If these measures fail to control the bleeding, consult a specialist. It is also reasonable to check blood counts and coagulation profiles at this time.

Patients whose bleeding is controlled can be discharged and instructed not to take anything by mouth for 4 hours and then only liquids and soft foods. Remove silk sutures in 7 days.

ALVEOLAR OSTEITIS (DRY SOCKET)

The pain associated with an extracted tooth is significant but usually manageable with current pharmacologic modalities. The pain associated with dry socket, however, can be very severe and often requires more definitive treatment. Alveolar osteitis, or dry socket, is a localized inflammation that occurs when the alveolar bone becomes inflamed. This condition usually occurs when the clot that is normally present in the socket after a tooth extraction becomes dislodged or dissolves. It is most common in the 2- to 4-day period after a tooth extraction. The examination is essentially unremarkable with the exception of a missing clot where the tooth was extracted. Signs and symptoms of dry socket include

1. Moderate to severe pain localized to the area or frequently radiating to the ear.
2. A foul odor or foul taste in the absence of purulence or suppuration.
3. Symptoms that occur 3 to 5 days after tooth extraction.
4. Absence of swelling or purulence or lymphadenitis.
5. Duration of 5 to 40 days.

Anything that increases negative intraoral pressure in the mouth (e.g., smoking, excessive rinsing, spitting, drinking from a straw), as well as hormone replacement and periodontal disease, will predispose a patient to a dry socket. Only a small percentage of patients will develop a dry socket (2%–5%); however, this number increases with traumatic extractions or impacted third molars.[13,19]

The following contribute to the development of a dry socket:

1. Excessive trauma during extraction.
2. Inadequate blood supply to the extraction site.
3. Preexisting localized infection.
4. Loss of clot from sucking, straw use, rinsing or smoking.
5. Foreign bodies remaining in the socket.
6. Use of oral contraceptives.
7. Use of corticosteroids.
8. Pericoronitis.

The pain associated with a dry socket is extremely severe, and if a patient presents several days after an extraction with a relatively normal examination and severe pain, it is likely a dry socket. It must be distinguished from osteomyelitis, which is characterized by fever, leukocytosis, malaise, and nausea. The pain of dry socket will not be relieved with traditional pain medications, but a dental block usually provides instant relief. Once the block is performed, the alveolar osteitis can be treated. Irrigate the socket and gently suction to remove any accumulated debris. Next, fill the socket to prevent recurrence of pain and allow healing to begin. A variety of materials are suitable to fill the socket again.

Gauze (¼ inch) impregnated with eugenol (oil of cloves) or a local anesthetic may be used. Replace the gauze in 24 to 36 hours because it tends to dry out and loosen. The patient should be seen by a dentist the next day if at all possible. The socket may also be packed with a slurry of Gelfoam and eugenol. The Gelfoam acts as a matrix to hold the eugenol in the socket. Commercial products, such as Dry Socket Paster or Dressol-X (Fig. 65–16) can also be applied by itself into

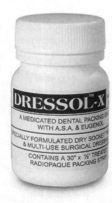

Figure 65–16 Dry socket packing (Dressol-X) with eugenol.

the socket or mixed with Gelfoam and placed into the socket. Dry Socket Paste is a very sticky thick paste containing eugenol. It may stay in place longer than gauze and does not dry out. Whichever packing material is used for a dry socket, one or more packings might be necessary before healing is complete.

Although antibiotics may be given to prevent alveolar osteitis, they are not usually necessary once the socket has been packed and should be prescribed at the discretion of the patient's oral surgeon or dentist.[11-13] NSAIDs should also be prescribed because they seem to work better than narcotics for dry socket.[20]

DENTOALVEOLAR INFECTIONS

Infections of the oral cavity run the spectrum from minor, easily managed abscesses to severe, life-threatening, deep space infections that require airway management and operative drainage. Although dental infections of all severity present to the ED, the most common are those related to pulp disease. Others are associated with the attachment structures of the teeth such as the gingiva, periodontal ligament, and the alveolar bone. These infections are often chronic conditions, but they can progress to the point where periodontal abscesses form and emergency treatment is required.

Emergency clinicians will be called on to drain abscesses of dental origin that do not extend into the deep spaces and that have well-defined boundaries easily accessible by intraoral or external drainage.

Disease of the Pulp

Disease of the pulp can occur from trauma, operations, or other unknown causes, but the most frequent cause is invasion of microorganisms after carious destruction of the enamel. As the enamel is destroyed, caries development progresses more rapidly through the dentin and into the pulp chamber, causing an inflammatory response, referred to as *pulpitis*. If the path of carious destruction through the tooth is adequate for drainage of the developing inflammation, the patient may be asymptomatic for a long time. If drainage is blocked, however, the process progresses forward to rapidly involve the entire pulp cavity and the periapical space. The tooth is usually exquisitely tender at this point. Abscesses in the periapical region are usually picked up on dental x-rays and less commonly on a Panorex. However, unless extension through the cortex exists, it is not important for the emergency clinician to make the distinction between pulpitis and a periapical abscess. Examination often reveals gross decay of one or many teeth and percussion tenderness of the abscessed tooth. A periapical abscess will follow the path of least tissue resistance if not treated. This may be through the alveolar bone and gingiva and into the mouth or into the deep structures of the neck. If the infection has progressed apically through the alveolar bone and localized swelling and tenderness exists, incision and drainage should be performed (discussed subsequently).

In the ED setting, it is uncertain whether a periapical abscess or simple pulpitis exists. Dental x-rays are usually not available. In the absence of trauma or recent instrumentation, it is prudent to begin antibiotic coverage for the typical oral flora. Penicillin and clindamycin are good choices. Analgesia should be provided as well. In most cases, perform supraperiosteal infiltration (tooth block) using a long-acting anesthetic

because this not only provides immediate and long-lasting relief but also decreases the requirement for narcotic analgesics once the anesthetic effect has dissipated. Do not perform a supraperiosteal injection if the abscess has extended through the gingival tissue and is present near the injection site. In this case, perform a regional block away from the infected tissue.

Disease of the Periodontium

Periodontal disease is also very common and affects practically all adults to some degree. *Periodontal disease* refers to infection of the attachment apparatus of the teeth: the gingiva, the periodontal ligament, and the alveolar bone. Unlike pulpal disease, periodontal disease is not usually symptomatic and, therefore, is rarely a primary reason to come to the ED. *Gingivitis* is an inflammation of the gingiva caused by bacterial plaque. In advanced disease, the gingiva becomes red and inflamed and tends to bleed easily. With chronic periodontal disease, an abscess can form when organisms become trapped in the periodontal pocket. The purulent material usually escapes through the gingival sulcus; however, it occasionally invades the supporting tissues, the alveolar bone, and the periodontal ligament (periodontitis). Periodontal abscesses that are not draining spontaneously through the sulcus can be drained in the ED. Saline rinses are encouraged to promote drainage. Antibiotics should be reserved for severe cases or for abscesses that cannot be drained. If it is uncertain whether the abscess is from the pulp or the periodontium, prescribe antibiotics even if the abscess is drained.[13,19]

Pericoronitis is a localized inflammation that occurs when gingiva overlying erupting teeth becomes traumatized and inflamed. Third molars are especially susceptible; however, any tooth can be affected. The gingiva overlying the crown may entrap bacteria and debris. Subsequent infection may develop. Typical signs of inflammation and infection may develop including erythema, edema, pus, and foul breath. Examination of the overlying gingiva with a tongue blade or finger will elicit tenderness and may produce drainage from the infection underlying the tissue flap. Pain may be moderate to severe and referral to the ear region is common. The localized infection occasionally spreads to deeper spaces such as the pterygomandibular or submasseteric spaces. Clinically, patients with significant spread of their pericoronal infection will present with trismus secondary to irritation of the masseter and pterygoid muscles.

ED treatment of pericoronitis is directed at detecting regional spread to the deeper spaces. Trismus or other systemic signs of advanced infection require intravenous antibiotics and urgent consultation for drainage procedures that usually require extraction of the offending tooth. If pericoronal infection is localized, local or nerve block anesthesia is followed by removal of submucosal debris. Saline rinses and oral antibiotics are prescribed with dental follow-up in 24 to 48 hours.

Drainage of Dentoalveolar Infections

The important determination for the emergency clinician to make is whether or not the odontogenic infection is localized, confined, and easily accessible or whether it is complex and involves several potential spaces. Likewise, determine whether the patient appears toxic, has trismus, or exhibits any signs of airway compromise. Patients not meeting these criteria

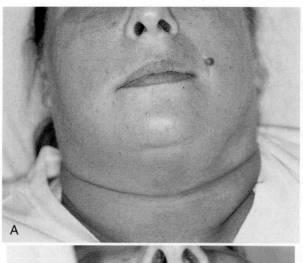

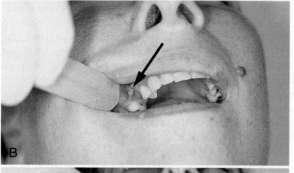

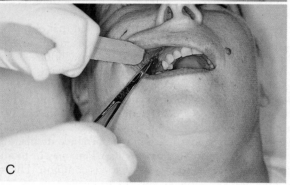

Figure 65–17 *A,* This patient presented with facial swelling up to the right eye. She stated that her sinusitis had returned. She had minor tooth pain but mostly complained of an ache in the face. X-rays revealed maxillary sinusitis with an air-fluid level. *B,* Intraoral examination revealed a pea-sized pointing abscess at the base of an upper tooth, the cause of sinusitis. After local anesthesia was applied, a No. 11 blade punctured the abscess, with drainage of copious pus. *C,* A hemostat was inserted into the abscess cavity and spread open, yielding more pus. Intravenous antibiotics (clindamycin) followed by oral antibiotics were given, and the patient saw her dentist the next day. She recovered fully.

require specialist referral. Dental infections are not always obvious and can be mistaken for sinusitis, or vice versa (Figs. 65–17 and 65–18).

Several anesthetic techniques can make the drainage process more comfortable. Nerve blocks and local injections work best. Benzocaine 20% gel or a combination of lidocaine/prilocaine/tetracaine generally provides good topical anesthesia before injection. Application of these to the dry mucosa before injection of the local anesthetic decreases the pain of injection. After applying the topical anesthetic, slowly infiltrate local anesthetic with a vasoconstrictor until the tissue

blanches. Either a short-acting anesthetic (2% lidocaine) or a longer-acting anesthetic (0.5% bupivacaine) may be used depending on the clinical circumstances. Regional or dental blocks may be performed instead of local infiltration if needle placement would track already infected tissues into healthy areas. Otherwise, consider local infiltration over the site of the abscess. Instruments necessary for drainage of dentoalveolar abscesses are those usually found on a standard incision and drainage tray and include hemostats, scalpel (No. 15 or 11), packing material ($\frac{1}{4}$-inch gauze), and a fenestrated Penrose drain.

Intraoral Technique

Intraoral abscesses do not routinely require any antiseptic mucosa preparation prior to drainage. After anesthetizing the region, make a small incision (0.5–1.0 cm) over the area of fluctuance, keeping the point of the blade toward the alveolar bone. Use a hemostat to bluntly dissect the abscess and break up any loculations. Cultures are not necessary unless the patient is immunocompromised. Irrigate the wound profusely with normal saline. If the wound is large enough to place a drain or gauze inside, tack one end to the mucosa with a silk suture to prevent aspiration. Advise the patient to perform salt water rinses hourly and arrange follow-up in 24 to 48 hours with the dentist or oral surgeon to remove the drain and provide continued management. Because the source of the abscess is not always known to the emergency clinician, prescribe antibiotics.

Extraoral Technique

Most simple dental infections can be drained intraorally, but occasionally, an abscess spreads to the face and requires drainage through the skin. It is important to realize that most dental infections should be drained through the mouth, if possible, because any extraoral drainage will cause some scarring. Abscesses on the face, which should be drained in the ED, are usually very localized and fluctuant and have not spread to any of the deep spaces of the head or neck. It is also important never to make any incisions on the face in direct proximity to important structures such as the facial nerve or the parotid gland and duct.

Prepare the patient for incision and drainage with a skin scrub and povidone-iodine (Betadine) preparation. Drape the face and infiltrate the skin with a local anesthetic containing a vasoconstrictor (1% or 2% lidocaine with epinephrine). Make any incision on healthy skin slightly below the area of fluctuance following the dynamic skin tension lines. After making the incision, use blunt dissection in the fluctuant area until adequate drainage is achieved. Irrigate the abscess cavity profusely. Place a drain or packing in the abscess cavity, being careful not to pack it too tightly but just enough to keep the incision open and draining. Unlike intraoral drainage, suturing the drain in place is not necessary. Instruct the patient to take antibiotics and follow up with the oral surgeon in 24 to 48 hours for packing change and definitive management.

Remember that not all infections about the mouth are the result of a simple dental infection. Osteomyelitis of the mandible, various tumors, and other exotic diseases can present as a dental infection.

Deep Space Infections of the Head and Neck

It is not unusual for odontogenic infections to spread into the various potential spaces of the face and neck. Presenting signs

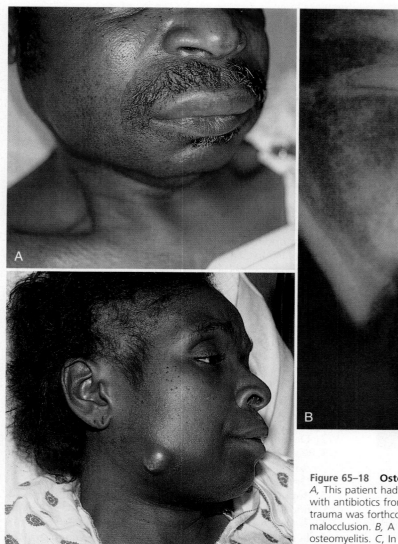

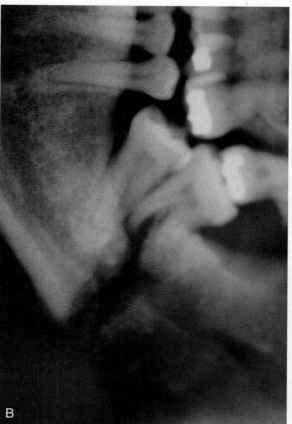

Figure 65–18   Osteomyelitis presenting as a dental infection.
A, This patient had a chronic toothache for months, and got minimally better with antibiotics from numerous emergency departments (EDs). No history of trauma was forthcoming. There was diffuse soft tissue swelling with malocclusion. *B,* A Panorex x-ray revealed nonunion of a fractured mandible with osteomyelitis. *C,* In this case a fractured mandible with osteomyelitis produced an obvious abscess. She had been treated for a presumed dental abscess many times in the past and got temporary relief.

and symptoms consist of fever, chills, pain, difficulty with speech or swallowing, and trismus. Although infections of certain teeth usually spread to particular contiguous spaces, the rapid spread of these infections often makes localizing the exact space difficult. Any space including the buccal, temporal, submasseteric, sublingual, submandibular, parapharyngeal, and others may be involved (Figs. 65–19 to 65–21).

Maxillary extension of periapical abscesses can spread into the infraorbital space and, subsequently, to the cavernous sinus through the ophthalmic veins, resulting in cavernous sinus thrombosis. Cavernous sinus involvement is associated with periorbital cellulitis as well as meningeal signs or a decreased level of consciousness. Periapical infections of the anterior mandibular teeth often spread to the buccinator space or the sublingual space, whereas those of the mandibular molars spread into the submandibular space.

The submandibular space connects with the sublingual space. Infection involving both of these spaces is known as *Ludwig's angina,* which can be life-threatening (Fig. 65–22). The source is usually a decayed lower tooth, with the tooth itself being relatively asymptomatic. Initially, this infection can be subtle, but it can rapidly progress. As infection pro-

gresses, the submandibular, submental, and sublingual spaces all become edematous and there may be elevation of the tongue and the soft tissues of the mouth. This is not a simple abscess that can be readily drained. Intervention includes intravenous antibiotics and oral surgery consultation. Established cases of Ludwig's angina cases are admitted to the hospital and often receive multiple drains. Minor early cases can be treated and observed for 6 to 8 hours in the ED with close follow up if the infection is deemed benign. The soft tissues of the posterior pharynx can also become involved. Securing the airway becomes of paramount importance. The suprahyoid region of the neck appears tense and indurated, and landmarks may be obscured. A computed tomography (CT) scan can further delineate Ludwig's angina if the diagnosis is in doubt.

The management of complicated odontogenic head and neck infections centers on airway management, surgical drainage, and antibiotics. If there is uncertainty as to whether the deep spaces are involved, obtain a CT scan to delineate the extension of the infectious process. Perform airway interventions early if there is any question of compromise, and consider tracheostomy. Consult an oral maxillofacial surgeon

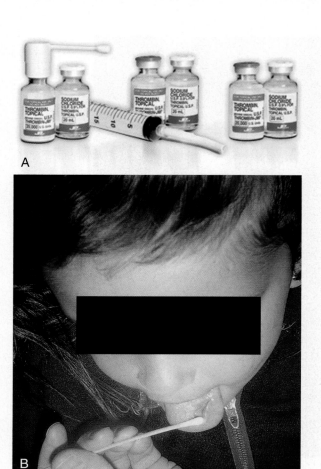

Figure 65–19 *A,* For persistent bleeding of a tongue, mucosa, or dental extraction site, topical thrombin can be used (Thrombin-JM, King Pharmaceuticals). Topical thrombin is available as a spray pump, to be applied with a syringe, or as a reconstituted powder to saturate absorbable Gelfoam. *B,* A tongue laceration like this will heal well without sutures once bleeding is controlled. Topical thrombin may be an option if hemostasis is problematic, such as for a patient taking warfarin.

because drainage and removal of necrotic tissue might be necessary. Administer antibiotics to slow down the spread of the infection and decrease hematogenous dissemination. The bacteria involved are typically a streptococcus/staphylococcus combination but a mixed aerobic and anaerobic infection is also possible. There has been an emergence of β-lactamase–producing organisms in upward of 40% of isolates from odontogenic neck abscesses.[19] Antimicrobials of choice in complicated odontogenic infections are usually the penicillins. The expanded-spectrum penicillins (ampicillin/sulbactam, ticarcillin/clavulanic acid, piperacillin/tazobactam) are effective against β-lactamase–producing bacteria and also cover the anaerobe *Bacteroides fragilis*. Clindamycin is an effective choice in patients who are allergic to penicillin. It should be used in combination with a cephalosporin, such as cefotetan or cefoxitin, in order to cover recently emerging resistant organisms. It is important to realize that in many of these infections, antibiotics are adjunctive therapy and not a substitute for surgical intervention.

DENTAL MATERIALS

As a general rule, EDs should have a well-stocked supply of basic dental materials. Many commercially available products can be used interchangeably with many of the items listed here. These can often be kept with the ear, nose, and throat cart or in another appropriate location. The following is a basic list:

1. Packing gauze.
2. Dental roll gauze.
3. Calcium hydroxide paste, glass ionomer cement, or zinc oxide cement.
4. Dry Socket Paste or eugenol.
5. Topical anesthetic gel (20% benzocaine or 5% lidocaine).
6. Topical bactericidal intraoral solution (Ora-5).
7. Periodontal paste (Coe-pak) or self-cure composite.
8. Articaine (septocaine) cartridges with epinephrine.
9. Save-A-Tooth Tooth Preservation System, EMT Toothsaver or fresh milk.
10. Zinc oxide/eugenol temporary cement (Temrex).

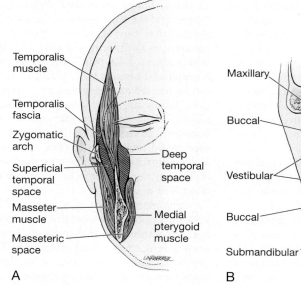

Figure 65–20 *A,* Location of temporal space abscesses. *B,* Route of infection into the buccal space, vestibular spaces, submandibular space, sublingual space, and palatal space. *(From Eisele D, McQuone S [eds]: Emergencies of the Head and Neck, 1st ed. St. Louis, Mosby, 2000.)*

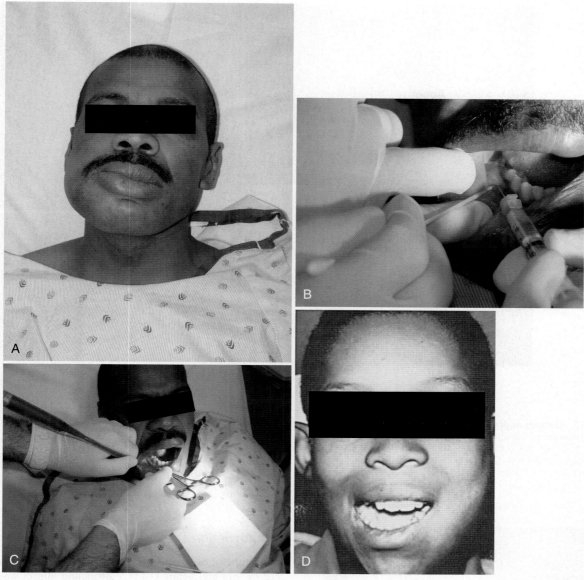

Figure 65–21 *A,* Advanced dental infection with characteristic facial swelling, likely involving the masseter space. *B,* Local anesthesia (lidocaine with epinephrine) is injected with a 27-gauge needle into an area of obvious fluctuance (shown by probe). A mandibular nerve block is an alternative to local injection. *C,* After the site is punctured with a No. 11 blade, a hemostat is inserted into the cavity and spread. Copious pus is drained with a suction catheter. Initial intravenous antibiotics (clindamycin) and outpatient follow-up on oral antibiotics yielded good results. The offending tooth was extracted when the infection was controlled. *D,* Advanced infection of the masseter space causes trismus.

11. Ringed injection syringe.
12. Stainless steel spatula and mixing pads.
13. Oral surgery tray with arch bars and ligature wires.
14. Tongue blades and cotton-tipped applicators.
15. Gelfoam, Hemcom, Surgicel, or topical thrombin.

Regional dental supply houses are good sources for these items. The Dental Box is a commercially available kit that contains many of these items and is designed for ED use. It is available at Thedentalbox.com.

INTRAORAL PIERCING

Dating back to antiquity, body piercing has been practiced in many countries and cultures as part of ceremonial and religious rites. In recent years, body and intraoral piercing has gained tremendous popularity throughout the world as a means of self-expression. In the ED, clinicians may see patients with piercings of the lips, tongue and even uvula. Complications of oral piercing on the gums and teeth include pain, infection, bleeding, increased salivary flow, difficulty swallowing, gingival recession, gingival trauma, and chipped or fractured teeth. Repeated trauma from a metal tongue ball can be quite detrimental to teeth, causing microfractures and a sudden shattered tooth (Fig. 65–23). One study of 400 consecutive patients at a military dental office, found 20% of their patients had at least one type of oral piercing, with the tongue being the most common location.[21] Of these patients, 14% had fractured teeth and 27% had recession of the gums. Another study assessed the impact of time and found that tooth chipping was found on molars and premolars in 47% of patients who had a tongue piercing for longer than 4 years.[22]

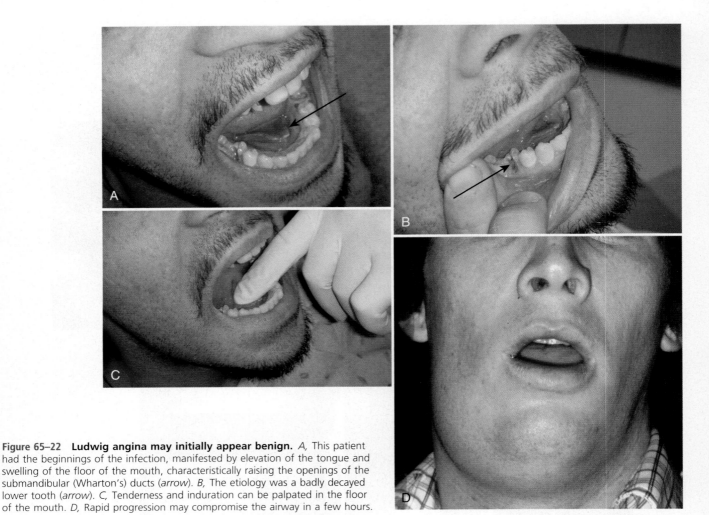

Figure 65–22   Ludwig angina may initially appear benign. *A,* This patient had the beginnings of the infection, manifested by elevation of the tongue and swelling of the floor of the mouth, characteristically raising the openings of the submandibular (Wharton's) ducts (*arrow*). *B,* The etiology was a badly decayed lower tooth (*arrow*). *C,* Tenderness and induration can be palpated in the floor of the mouth. *D,* Rapid progression may compromise the airway in a few hours.

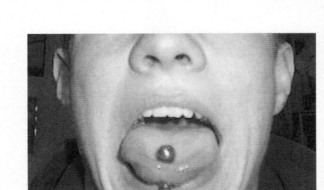

Figure 65–23   Tongue and lip piercing can cause dental and gingival problems. A metal tongue ball and other intraoral piercings can have significant detrimental effects on teeth and gums. This tongue ball can cause microfractures, leading to a suddenly shattered tooth. The longer the post, the greater the tooth damage.

Acknowledgments

The contributions of Robert H. Benko, DDS, to this material are greatly appreciated. The editors and author also wish to acknowledge the contributions of James T. Amsterdam to this chapter in previous editions. The editors would like to thank Michael B. Pavel, DMD, for his review of this manuscript.

REFERENCES CAN BE FOUND ON **EXPERT CONSULT**

CHAPTER **66**

Procedures Pertaining to Hypothermia and Hyperthermia

Heather M. Prendergast and
Timothy B. Erickson

PROCEDURE PERTAINING TO HYPOTHERMIA

With an increase in outdoor activities, changing weather patterns, and the growing epidemic of homelessness in our country, issues pertaining to hypothermia remain in the forefront. Hypothermia not only is a common diagnosis in rural areas but also has become more commonplace in urban centers across the nation secondary to inadequate housing or lack of preparation for cold weather changes.[1] It is also important to note that numerous accidental hypothermia cases are reported every year in areas typically considered warm weather locales such as Florida, Texas, California, and Alabama.[2,3] Every year, many recreational and elite athletes participate in outdoor sporting events. The higher the environmental stress, the greater the potential for performance failure and development of hypothermia.[4] High-altitude expeditions on Mt. Everest in 1996, Mt. Denali in 2003, and most recently, Mt. Hood in 2006, are reminders that even well-protected, acclimitized individuals can sucomb to cold-related fatalities. Optimal treatment for hypothermia remains controversial; however, it is a well-accepted practice that resuscitation of these individuals is carried out for extended periods of time. The medical literature contains numerous anecdotal reports of profoundly hypothermic individuals who are successfully resuscitated and are neurologically intact at the time of discharge.[5-8] Despite these spectacular reports of survival, both morbidity and mortality from hypothermia are common. Between 1972 and 2002, 16,555 deaths were attributed to hypothermia, approximately 689 deaths per year in the United States.[9] Between 1999 and 2002 alone, 4607 death certificates in the United States had hypothermia-related diagnoses listed as the underlying cause of death.[10] The actual number of patients presenting to emergency departments (EDs) with hypothermia is unknown. Poverty, homelessness, alcoholism, and psychiatric illnesses are commonly associated conditions. This chapter critically reviews approaches and procedures appropriate to the management of several categories of hypothermic patients. The recommendations combine treatment efficacy with safety. Before describing procedures and making recommendations, essential terms are defined and the pathophysiology of hypothermia is briefly reviewed.

Definitions

Accidental hypothermia (AH) has been defined as an unintentional decrease in the core (vital organ) temperature below 35°C (<95°F).[5] Victims of hypothermia can be separated into the following categories: *mild hypothermia*, 35°C to 32°C (95.0°F–90.0°F); *moderate hypothermia*, less than 32°C to 30°C (<90.0°F–86.0°F); and *severe hypothermia*, less than 30°C (<86.0°F). Other factors that may be useful in separating groups of patients with AH include the presence of underlying illness,[1,11-14] altered neurologic state on arrival, hypotension, and the need for prehospital cardiopulmonary resuscitation (CPR). A hypothermia outcome score has been developed that incorporates some of these factors and may permit comparison of outcomes for patient groups treated with different modalities.[15]

Risk factors for the development of AH include burn injuries, extremes of age, ethanol intoxication, dehydration, major psychiatric illness, trauma, use of intoxicants, significant blood loss, sleep deprivation, malnutrition, and concomitant medical illnesses.[16,17] Risk factors for development of indoor hypothermia include advanced age, coexisting medical conditions, being alone at the time of illness, being found on the floor, and abnormal temperature perception or regulation.[13] Unlike healthy exposed outdoor enthusiasts, such as skiers or mountaineers, hypothermia in urban populations is most often associated with conditions that impair either thermoregulation or the ability to seek shelter. In the majority of studies of urban hypothermia, death has been attributed to the severity of the underlying disease such as infection.[1]

Because signs and symptoms may be vague and nonspecific, mild to moderate hypothermia may easily be overlooked in the ED. A common error is failure to routinely obtain an accurate core temperature on all patients at risk. Often, the diagnosis is delayed because of false reliance on standard oral temperatures. Presenting symptoms such as confusion in the elderly and combativeness in the intoxicated patient might not initially be recognized as symptoms of hypothermia. *Hypothermic patients frequently will not feel cold or shiver.* This is particularly true in the elderly populations who have impaired thermoregulatory responses because of their advanced age.[18-20] Paradoxical undressing, a cold-induced psychiatric dysfunction, has been described in confused patients who develop the sensation of heat at lowered body temperatures as a result of constricted blood vessels near the body surface, which suddenly dilate. In many cases, these patients are mislabeled as psychotic, leading to further delays in appropriate treatment.[21]

Core Temperature Measurement

Because of the nonspecific nature of symptoms of hypothermia, an accurate temperature assessment is a necessity in any clinical setting in which the diagnosis may be suspected. It is of paramount importance not only for confirmation of the diagnosis but also for guidance in further diagnostic and therapeutic decisions. Any thermometer that does not record temperatures in the hypothermic range is *inappropriate* for evaluating significant hypothermia. Standard glass/mercury thermometers generally cannot record temperatures of less than 34°C (<93.2°F), although some models are available to record temperatures as low as 24°C (75.2°F) (Dynamed, Inc., Carlsbad, CA). An electronic probe and accompanying calibrated thermometer is recommended when monitoring this vital sign. Examples of thermometers with accompanying accuracy at various temperature ranges are shown in Figure 66–1A and B.

Core temperature is traditionally estimated with a rectal probe. The rectal temperature, however, often lags behind the core temperature because of large gradients within the body.[19] Esophageal probes may be used, although they may be affected by warm humidified air therapy, commonly used in severe hypothermia. Other possible sites for temperature measurement include the tympanic membrane, nasopharyngeal passage, and urinary bladder.[1,22,23] Fresh urine temperature can closely approximate core temperature.[24] "Deep forehead" temperatures measured with a Coretemp thermometer (Teramo, Tokyo, Japan) have also demonstrated excellent accuracy and approximation of core temperatures.[25] For continuous-monitoring purposes, rectal or bladder probes are preferred. Infrared tympanic temperatures have demonstrated excellent correlation with core temperatures. Studies show that, although easier to use and faster, infrared tympanic temperatures can be inaccurate at extremes of temperature by underestimating higher temperatures and overestimating lower temperatures.[26] When a rectal probe is used, it should be inserted at least 15 cm beyond the anal sphincter and its

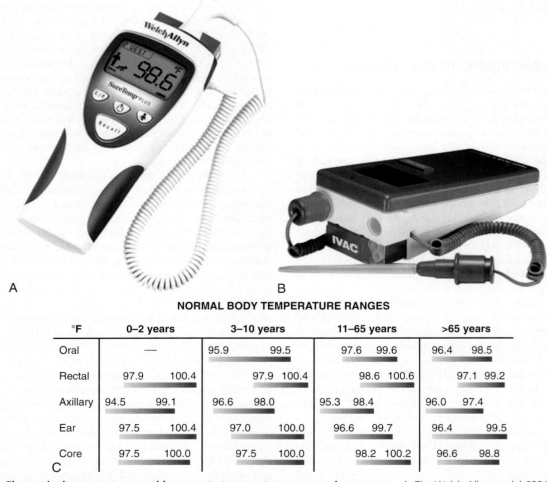

NORMAL BODY TEMPERATURE RANGES

°F	0–2 years		3–10 years		11–65 years		>65 years	
Oral	—		95.9	99.5	97.6	99.6	96.4	98.5
Rectal	97.9	100.4	97.9	100.4	98.6	100.6	97.1	99.2
Axillary	94.5	99.1	96.6	98.0	95.3	98.4	96.0	97.4
Ear	97.5	100.4	97.0	100.0	96.6	99.7	96.4	99.5
Core	97.5	100.0	97.5	100.0	98.2	100.2	96.6	98.8

Figure 66–1 Electronic thermometers provide accurate temperatures over various ranges. *A,* The Welch Allyn model 692/690 SureTemp Plus (oral, axillary, rectal) is accurate from 80°F–110°F. Note the various ranges for normal temperatures from various sites by age. *It is generally accepted that a rectal temperature greater than 100.3 represents a fever, and oral readings can be misleading. B,* The IVAC electronic thermometer is also commonly used in the emergency department (ED; accuracy 88°F–108°F). For severe hypothermia or hyperthermia, it is important to know the accuracy of the thermometer being used. *C,* Graph demonstrates variations in normal body temperature by site and age. (A and B, *Images courtesy of WelchAllyn, Inc.*)

position frequently verified.[6] One should remember that temperature gradients exist in the human body and consistency of monitoring at one or more sites is mandatory. A chart and formula that convert centigrade to Fahrenheit temperatures will assist the clinician in assessing the severity of hypothermia (see Fig. 66–1C).

Pathophysiology

AH results from the failure of the body's thermoregulatory responses to generate enough heat to compensate for heat losses. These thermoregulatory responses include shivering, tachycardia, tachypnea, increased gluconeogenesis, peripheral vasoconstriction, and shunting of blood to central organs.[27] As the core temperature drops despite these compensatory mechanisms, the patient becomes poikilothermic and cools to the ambient temperature.

Four methods of heat loss affect the body: radiation, conduction, convection, and evaporation. *Radiation* involves the transfer of heat from a warmer body to a cooler environment and accounts for approximately 60% of heat loss in a normothermic individual. *Conduction* refers to heat loss from direct contact with a cooler surface. These losses are most profound with immersion hypothermia. *Convection* occurs when cool air currents pass by the body and accounts for 15% of heat loss, especially with a wind chill factor. *Evaporation* refers to significant heat loss through sweating and insensible water losses.[19,27] In hypothermia, the enzymatic rate of metabolism itself decreases two to three times with each 10°C (18°F) drop and cerebral blood flow decreases 6% to 7% per 1°C (1.8°F) drop. Signs and symptoms of hypothermia vary according to the core temperature. The overall functioning of all organ systems is impaired by the cold.[28] The greatest effects, however, are seen with the cardiovascular, neurologic, and respiratory systems (Table 66–1). As the core body temperature drops below 33°C (<91.4°F), the patient becomes confused and ataxic.[29] The initiation of involuntary motor activity (shivering) prevents the reduction in core temperature.[30] Shivering thermogenesis in skeletal muscle operates on acute cold stress. In the malnourished patient, the mechanism may be rendered ineffective secondary to reduced muscle mass.[31] Shivering stops at about 32°C (89.6°F); however, shivering artifact on an electrocardiogram has been associated with increased survival in severe hypothermia.[32] Atrial fibrillation occurs frequently as the temperature continues to drop

and the patient loses consciousness. A J-wave in the electrocardiogram often appears before ventricular fibrillation (Fig. 66–2).[33,34] Although classically considered pathognomonic for hypothermia, the J- or "Osborne" wave has no prognostic or predictive value in cases of hypothermia. Studies found that Osborne waves occurred in 36% of AH survivors and in 38% of nonsurvivors.[32,35] Ventricular fibrillation may occur below 29°C (<84.2°F) and becomes common as the core drops to 25°C (77°F).[36] The electroencephalogram flattens at 19°C to 20°C (66.2°F–68°F).[37] Asystole commonly occurs at 18°C (64.4°F) but has been seen at higher temperatures. Initial core temperature does not necessarily correlate with vital outcome.[38] The lowest recorded temperature for a survivor of AH is 9.0°C (43.7°F).[27]

Initial Evaluation and Stabilization of the Hypothermic Patient

The treatment of hypothermia can be divided into prehospital care and ED management.

Prehospital Care

In the prehospital setting, focus primarily on removing the patient from the current environment to prevent further decreases in core temperature. Studies have shown that oral temperatures are sufficiently accurate for field use.[39] In addition, infrared tympanic thermometers may not be reliable in the prehospital setting.[40] Handle these patients with special care and anticipate the presence of an irritable myocardium, because aggressive measures can inadvertently trigger cardiac dysrhythmias. In addition, hypovolemia and a large temperature gradient between the periphery and the core often exist in the hypothermic patient.[6] Avoid aggressive field management and prolonged transport times.[41,42] After removing the patient's wet clothing, wrap the patient in dry blankets or sleeping bags. "Field rewarming" is a misnomer, because adding significant heat to a hypothermic patient in the field is extremely difficult. Studies have shown that for mild hypothermia, resistive heating (e.g., warming blankets) can be safely used in the prehospital setting. Resistive heating augments thermal comfort, increases core temperature by approximately 0.8°C/hr (33.4°F/hr), and reduces patient pain and anxiety during transport.[39] In one study, resistive heating more than doubled the rewarming rate compared with passive

TABLE 66–1 Signs and Symptoms of Hypothermia

Core Temperature (°C)	Cardiovascular System	Respiratory System	Central Nervous System
34–35	Tachycardia Increased afterload Increased systemic blood pressure	Tachypnea Increased minute ventilation	Lethargy Mild confusion Loss of fine motor coordination
30–34	Progressive bradycardia Decreased cardiac output Hypotension Lengthening of cardiac conduction Atrial/ventricular dysrhythmias	Increased bronchial secretions Diminished gag reflex Depressed cough response	Delirium Slowed reflexes Muscle rigidity Abnormal EEG
<30	Spontaneous ventricular fibrillation Osborne waves at 25°C	Respiratory rate decreased to 5 breaths/min	Aflexia Coma Fixed pupils Rigidity EEG silent at 19°C

EEG, electroencephalogram.

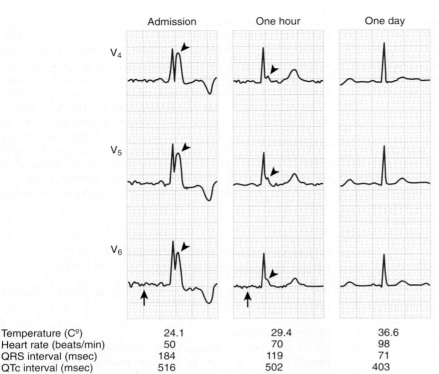

	Admission	One hour	One day
Temperature (C°)	24.1	29.4	36.6
Heart rate (beats/min)	50	70	98
QRS interval (msec)	184	119	71
QTc interval (msec)	516	502	403

Figure 66–2 In severe hypothermia, the electrocardiogram (ECG) exhibits marked elevation of the J deflection, so-called Osborne waves. The height of the J-wave is proportional to the degree of hypothermia, and this finding is usually most marked in the mid-precordial leads. The ECG is of a patient with sinus bradycardia, but approximately half of patients with a temperature below 32°C (89.6°F) develop slow atrial fibrillation, a rhythm that usually converts spontaneously with rewarming. *(Adapted from Krantz MJ, Lowery CM: Giant Osborne waves in hypothermia. N Engl J Med 352:184, 2005. Used with permission.)*

insulation and did not produce an afterdrop.[43] With longer transport times, utilize active rewarming methods limited to heated inhalation and truncal heat application. Place insulated hot water bottles near the patient's axilla or groin. The Res-Q-Air device (CF Electronics, Inc., Commack, NY) is lightweight and portable and delivers heated humidified air or oxygen at temperatures ranging from 42°C to 44°C (107.6°F–111.2°F) and down to ambient conditions of –20°C (–4°F). In more remote settings, another option is to use a modified forced-air warming sytem in the field. The Portable Rigid Forced-Air Cover is heated with a Bair Hugger heater/blower (Augustine Medical, Inc., Eden Prairie, MN). It covers the patient's trunk and thighs and can adapt to various transport vehicle power sources.[6]

Immobilize patients with potential traumatic injuries to the spine or extremities before transport. Pay continuous attention to airway maintenance. Initiate fluid resuscitation with intravenous (IV) crystalloid, preferably 5% dextrose in normal saline (D₅NS). Alternatively, give oral warm glucose-containing drinks to a patient who is awake and alert. Most hypothermic patients are dehydrated because fluid intake is reduced and cold causes a diuresis. Avoid using lactated Ringer's solution because theoretically it can decrease metabolism of lactate by cold-induced hepatic dysfunction. If possible, use warmed IV fluids because they are generally well tolerated.[44,45] If available, use a flameless heater, which is currently being used by military medical units, and provides easy and expedient means of warming fluids in the prehospital setting.[46]

Intubate unresponsive patients but recognize that there is no universal agreement on when to intubate a hypothermic patient who has detectable vital signs. Pulse oximetry is usually not helpful because vasoconstriction limits blood flow to the periphery and readings may be inaccurate or not possible. Some authors suggest that pulseless victims with core temperatures below 32°C (<89.6°F) should be transported with continuous CPR.[44] Other authors believe that it is unneces-sary to perform CPR on a patient who has any perfusing cardiac rhythm because it may precipitate ventricular fibrillation.[47] At this juncture, there is no universally accepted standard for intubation or CPR in hypothermic patients with detectable vital signs.[48]

Definitive prehospital determination of cardiac activity requires a cardiac monitor. Cardiac arrest is a common misdiagnosis because peripheral pulses are difficult to palpate when extreme bradycardia is present along with peripheral vasoconstriction. Some authors report that asystole is a more common presenting rhythm than is ventricular fibrillation. In the field, differentiating ventricular fibrillation from asystole may be impractical.

Transport cold, stiff, cyanotic patients with fixed and dilated pupils because the treatment dictim for prehospital personnel remains, "No one is dead until warm and dead." A succinct summary of prehospital care of the hypothermic patient is rescue, examine, insulate, and transport.[6]

ED Management

Treatment priorities in the ED setting are to prevent further decreases in core body temperature; establish a steady, safe rewarming rate; maintain the stability of the cardiopulmonary system; and provide sufficient physiologic support. Adjust the rate of rewarming and the techniques used based on the degree of hypothermia and the severity of the patient's clinical condition (Table 66–2). Anticipate and prevent complications.

In the pulseless, apneic patient, initiate CPR and continue until the core temperature is above 34°C (>93.2°F). Profound hypothermia results in coma, hyporeflexia, fixed and dilated pupils, severe bradycardia, and often unobtainable blood pressure. In severe hypothermia, a pulse might not be palpable and blood pressure measurement might require the use of a Doppler device. If available, use ultrasound to detect the presence of cardiac wall motion. Follow the heart rate and rhythm with electrocardiographic monitoring. In patients who have anything more than minimal impairment, use arterial blood gas analysis frequently to determine oxygenation, ventilation, and acid-base status. If feasible, establish large-bore IV lines. Avoid central lines if possible because their insertion may exacerbate myocardial irritation. Give maintenance intravenous fluids. Warm all IV fluids to 40°C to 42°C (104°F–107.6°F) but be aware that the usual volumes administered will not contribute significant calories of heat. Furthermore, with long standard IV tubing, the heated IV fluids may actually cool to room temperature before entering the patient's IV site.

With a mild to moderate reduction in core temperature, the level of mentation correlates with the severity of the AH, associated illnesses, or both. Noteworthy exceptions are alcoholics and diabetics who can present in comas at higher core temperatures because of concomitant hypoglycemia. Perform bedside glucose measurements in these patients on their arrival in the ED. A high correlation exists between alcohol consumption and development of hypothermia, especially in colder climates.[1] A review of 68 cases of hypothermic deaths in Jefferson County, Alabama, found that a significant number of cases involved middle-aged men who had consumed alcohol.[3] In the 22 cases of AH reviewed by Fitzgerald,[49] all

but 2 patients were alcoholics. The serum glucose level was less than 50 mg/dL in 41% (9 patients). This study noted glycosuria in 2 patients, even when low serum glucose values were evident, and described a renal tubular glycosuria in AH. Such glycosuria may worsen or cause hypoglycemia; *hence, glycosuria in AH is no guarantee of an adequate serum glucose concentration*. This supports the routine use of supplemental IV glucose unless a normal serum glucose value can be quickly ensured. Also, consider IV thiamine (100 mg) and a trial dose of 0.4 to 2 mg IV naloxone (Narcan) in the comatose patient. Although failure to rewarm spontaneously has been noted in victims with hypothyroidism and other endocrine deficiencies, reserve the use of thyroid hormones and corticosteroids for those patients with suspected thyroid and adrenal insufficiency, respectively.

The thermoregulatory vasoconstriction caused by hypothermia significantly decreases the subcutaneous oxygen tension.[19] A good correlation exists between the incidence of wound infections and the subcutaneous oxygen tension. As core temperatures decrease from 41°C to 26°C (105.8°F–78.8°F), neutrophil function is significantly impaired.[19] Conversely, in animal models, hypothermia appears to decrease leukocyte sequestration within brain parenchyma, offering some resistance to meningitis.[50] Although antibiotics are not routinely indicated in uncomplicated mild hypothermia, some authors advocate the routine empirical initiation of broad-spectrum antibiotic therapy on admission of severely hypothermic patients. In this setting, detection and treatment of the underlying cause, such as infection, may be more critical than treatment of the hypothermia.[1]

Management Guidelines

Hypothermia affects virtually every organ system owing to the generalized slowing of the body. Management goals depend on the severity of hypothermia, but in all cases, the primary goal is to increase the core temperature and prevent further losses. In the patient with mild hypothermia, a conservative approach to rewarming is generally advocated. Overly aggressive methods may be more harmful to the patient by causing a worsening hypotension, a paradoxical decrease in core temperature, and cardiac dysrhythmias. Other complications may include bleeding[19] and infection of surgical incisions. The optimal rewarming rate remains unclear and varies with each case. Standard rewarming rates are a 0.5°C/hr to 2.0°C/hr (0.9°F/hr–3.6°F/hr) rise in temperature *in the otherwise stable patient* (Table 66–3). Carefully consider and individualize invasive therapy to the severity of the hypothermia and the condition of the patient. Avoid *overtreating and overutilizing invasive techniques in an otherwise stable hypothermic patient*. In patients with severe underlying problems such as hypoglycemia, hyperglycemia, sepsis,

TABLE 66–2 Rewarming Techniques

Core Temperature (°C)	Method and Techniques
>32	**PER** • Dry blankets, clothing • Heated intravenous solutions (43°C) D$_5$NS • Warm fluids if fully alert
≤32	**AER** • Heated blankets, heating pads, warm air convection • Radiant heat sources • Alcohol-circulating blankets **ACR** • Peritoneal dialysis • Bladder, gastric, or colonic lavage with warm fluids (43°C) • Heated intravenous fluids • Heated humidified oxygen • Thoracic cavity lavage (43°C) • Extracorporeal blood rewarming • Hemodialysis • Ultrasonic and low-frequency microwave diathermy • Arteriovenous anastomoses rewarming

ACR, active core rewarming; AER, active external rewarming; PER, passive external rewarming.

TABLE 66–3 Warming Rates (°C/hr)

	Passive External	Active External	Inhalation of Warm Air	Peritoneal Lavage	Bladder Lavage
1st hr	1.4	1.5	1.5	1.5	1.3
2nd hr	1.4	2.4	2.0	2.5	1.7
3rd hr	1.8	2.0	1.9	3.2	1.8

Note: Thoracic lavage had a median rewarming rate of 2.95°C/hr (see Plaisier BR: Thoracic lavage in accidental hypothermia with cardiac arrest—Report of a case and review of the literature. Resuscitation 66:99, 2005).
From Danzl D, Pozos RS: Multicenter hypothermia study. Ann Emerg Med 16:1042, 1987.

adrenal crisis, drug overdose, or hypothyroidism, treat these conditions appropriately in addition to treating the hypothermia because long-term outcome may depend more on treatment of the underlying illness than on treating the hypothermia.[1,51]

Passive External Rewarming

The cornerstone of effectiveness for this method relies on the body's ability to restore normal body temperature through its own mechanisms for heat production. Stop further heat loss through insulation and environmental manipulation. Give warm fluids containing glucose to the patient who is fully alert. For patients with mild AH, remove wet clothing and then provide *passive external rewarming* with blankets. The technique is simple; however, the patient must be capable of generating enough body heat for this method to be successful. Give warmed IV fluids to counteract the cold-induced diuresis. Internal heat generation is required for rewarming, and this effect will be relatively slow. In the otherwise stable patient, aggressive intervention with drugs and invasive monitoring might be more harmful than beneficial. Patients who cannot shiver, those who are hypotensive, or those who are intoxicated or malnourished may not have this capability. Survival rates using passive external rewarming have ranged from 55% to 100%.[52-54]

For patients in the moderate or severe category of hypothermia, a more aggressive approach may be warranted. The options available are active external rewarming and active core rewarming. Active core rewarming techniques can be further divided into less invasive and more invasive techniques. Generally, the aggressiveness of therapy depends more on the patient's underlying health, hemodynamic status, and response to initial therapy than on the initial temperature.

Active External Rewarming

The application of heat to the skin of the hypothermic patient has been termed *active external rewarming*.

Indications. Although there is some suggestion that active external rewarming of profoundly hypothermic patients by immersion may be associated with an increase in mortality over other treatments,[15,55] more recent studies suggest that this technique is highly effective for mild hypothermia.[29,56] Use it selectively and limit it to the trunk. Other forms of active external rewarming are increasingly used in the ED as adjunctive care of moderately hypothermic, otherwise healthy individuals. Vasoconstriction limits the ability to increase core temperature using techniques that primarily warm the skin.[57]

Active external rewarming is most beneficial in cases in which heat supplied by the external source is greater than the loss of rewarming heat incurred by the cessation of shivering. In more remote wilderness settings where more aggressive warming techniques are precluded owing to lack of equipment or personnel, active external rewarming with body-to-body contact may be the only option available to the rescuer. However, the rewarming contribution of body-to-body contact appears limited.[58]

Equipment. Traditionally, immersion therapy has used a heated (40°C–42°C [104.0°F–107.6°F]) water tank of the type present in most burn units. Generally, immerse the hypothermic patient entirely except for the extremities and head; however, immersion of the extremities may hasten rewarming.[59-61] A major drawback is the inability to closely monitor the patient undergoing immersion. Alternatively, use a warm water–filled heat exchange blanket (e.g., Blanketrol, Cincinnati Sub-Zero Products, Cincinnati, OH) for conduction warming. Intraoperative studies have demonstrated excellent results.[60] A forced–warm air convection system (Bair Hugger, Augustine Medical, Eden Prairie, MN; Snuggle Warm Convective Warming System, Sins Level 1, Inc., Rockland, MA) has been used for postsurgical rewarming.[60,62] This approach also has been used successfully for ED-based AH therapy. Warm air convection rewarming permits continued monitoring in the ED and is better tolerated than immersion owing to the less rapid development of vasodilatation in peripheral tissues.

Technique. Because profound fluid shifts can occur with conduction warming, give the patient supplemental IV fluid warmed to 40°C (104.0°F; Hotline Fluid Warmer, Sims Level 1, Inc., Rockland, MA), and at a rate sufficient to generate a urinary output of 0.5 to 1.0 mL/kg/hr. Give an initial fluid bolus of 500 mL of D_5NS. Note that blood pressure is not an accurate way to gauge fluid resuscitation because serious hypothermia is always accompanied by "physiologic" hypotension. Because patients requiring mechanical ventilation have rarely been subjected to tank immersion, it cannot be recommended for hypothermic patients who require intubation. Rewarming rates ranging from 0.9°C to 8.8°C (1.6°F–15.8°F) per hour have been reported with immersion therapy.[6,63]

A heat exchange blanket allows the patient to receive other treatments that may be difficult or impossible to carry out in a tub, such as defibrillation, CPR, or more invasive warming techniques. Place the heating blanket and overlying cloth sheet underneath the patient. Set the blanket temperature at 40°C to 42°C (104.0°F–107.6°F), and initiate the measures described under "Passive Rewarming Techniques." Forced-air rewarming (convection) uses a blanket cradle to create an environment through which heated air is blown. Access to the patient is quite good with this system because the overlying blankets can be raised temporarily to evaluate the patient or perform procedures. Experience with mild immersion-induced hypothermia in volunteers suggests that the forced-air technique warms at a rate comparable with that of vigorous shivering, but with less metabolic stress and less afterdrop.[64]

Arteriovenous Anastomoses Rewarming. Arteriovenous anastomoses rewarming (AVR) involves the immersion of the distal extremities (hands, forearms, feet, and lower legs). Advantages include rapid rewarming rates. A study in healthy volunteers using AVR immersion in temperatures of 45°C and 42°C (113.0°F–107.6°F), respectively, demonstrated rewarming rates of 9.9°C/hr (±3.2°C/hr) for the former and rewarming rates of 6.1°C/hr (±1.2°C/hr) (43.0°F ± 34.2°F/hr) for the latter.[65] There was also a decrease in postcooling afterdrop. AVR is well tolerated by patients because of the rapid rise in core temperature and the shortened period of shivering.[59,66]

Complications. There is concern that surface warming with accompanying vasodilatation may produce a relative hypovolemia in the hypothermic patient. Other complications described with the active external rewarming method include core temperature afterdrop and rewarming acidosis. In *core temperature afterdrop*, colder peripheral blood is transported to the warmer core organs, further reducing the core temperature. In *rewarming acidosis*, colder blood and lactic acid return to the core organs, worsening the acidosis. To limit these complications in moderate hypothermia, some authors advocate using active external warming only after active internal techniques have been initiated.[27]

Importantly, CPR and other advanced cardiac therapy and monitoring are impossible with immersion rewarming. Until studied further, active external rewarming should be considered only in a clinically monitored setting for mildly hypothermic patients who can protect their airways. When using a heating device, also monitor the potential for burns to the areas in greatest contact with the heating source.

Active Core Rewarming

There is evidence that active core rewarming may decrease mortality from severe hypothermia exposure compared with other techniques. In the face of circulatory failure, often the best chance of survival is treatment with extracorporeal circulation (ECC) and warming of the blood.[67] Several methods have been described, including the use of warm humidified air through an endotracheal tube or mask, peritoneal lavage, gastric or bladder lavage with warm fluid, thoracic tube lavage, cardiopulmonary bypass, AVR, peripheral vascular extracorporeal warming, hemodialysis, and thoracotomy with mediastinal lavage. These techniques transfer heat actively to the body core, achieving varying rewarming rates. The specific techniques as well as some of the advantages and disadvantages for each procedure follow.

Emergency Warming of Saline in a Microwave.

Under ideal circumstances, keep saline in a standard warming device. When large amounts of saline are required for such procedures as peritoneal lavage, warm 1-L saline bags rapidly in a standard microwave oven.[68] Although devices will vary, a 650-W microwave has been demonstrated to warm 1 L of room temperature non–dextrose-containing saline from 21.1°C to 38.3°C (70°F–101°F) in 120 seconds on the high setting. At midcycle (i.e., after 60 sec), interrupt with agitation, and repeat agitation at end-cycle before infusion.

Inhalation of Heated Humidified Oxygen or Air.

The use of warm humidified oxygen to treat hypothermia has been well established. Average rates of rewarming of 1°C/hr (33.8°F/hr) via mask and 1.5°C/hr to 2.0°C/hr (34.7°F/hr–35.6°F/hr) via endotracheal tube with heated aerosol at 40°C (104.0°F) can be obtained.[6,29] Faster rewarming rates may be accomplished using a maximum safe aerosol temperature of 45°C (113°F). Core rewarming with this technique occurs through the following mechanisms. The warmed alveolar blood returns to the heart, thereby warming the myocardium. The warmed humidified air delivered to the alveoli also warms contiguous structures in the mediastinum by conduction. Finally, warming the inhaled air or oxygen eliminates a major source of heat loss.

Indications and Contraindications. The use of heated humidified air or oxygen is a simple technique that *should be used routinely*, either by itself or in combination with other methods, in all patients with hypothermia, regardless of severity. If the correct equipment is available, it can be used in the field as well as the hospital.[41,42] However, one must address the risk of burns during inhalation of warm air in the field environment.[69] Mouth-to-tube ventilation in the intubated hypothermic prehospital patient has the theoretical advantage of providing warm humidified air without special equipment. The ventilating rescuer can inhale oxygen before expiring into the patient's endotracheal tube to provide air with increased oxygen content. There are no contraindications for or reported complications from the use of warm humidified air for hypothermia, and there is no afterdrop.[70]

Technique. Use a heated cascade nebulizer with a mask for patients with spontaneous respirations. Use a volume ventilator for intubated patients. Monitor the inspired air to maintain a temperature of approximately 45°C (~113.0°F).[71] Temperatures higher than 50°C (122°F) may burn the mucosa, and temperatures lower than 45°C (<113°F) do not deliver maximum heat. Humidify the air or oxygen and note that the heater module may need modification because many units have feedback mechanisms that shut off at a given temperature. As a practical issue, it may be difficult to deliver oxygen at the recommended temperature because of equipment limitations. In many cases the air temperature is only 30°C (86°F).

Summary. Inhalation of warm humidified air or oxygen causes gradual core rewarming and should be the mainstay of rewarming therapy. Studies have suggested that the rewarming rate of inhalation therapy is inferior to that of peritoneal lavage, thoracic lavage, and bath rewarming.[6] However, because inhalation therapy can be combined with any and all other methods of rewarming and because it is relatively noninvasive and inexpensive, consider it as the initial treatment of choice for hypothermic patients.

Peritoneal Dialysis (Lavage).

Peritoneal dialysis (lavage) is an attractive treatment for severe hypothermia because it is available in most hospitals and does not require any unusual equipment or training. Rewarming rates of 2°C to 3°C (3.6°F–5.4°F) per hour, depending on the dialysis rate, can be achieved without sophisticated equipment that may delay therapy or require transfer of the patient to a tertiary care facility.[72] This technique can also be used to help correct electrolyte imbalances.

Peritoneal dialysis rewarming was first used successfully in a patient in ventricular fibrillation with a temperature of 21°C (69.8°F).[73] Since that time, there have been reports of successful rewarming with peritoneal lavage in stable, severely hypothermic patients and unstable hypothermic patients in cardiac arrest.[74,75] Peritoneal lavage works through heat transfer from lavage fluid to the peritoneal cavity. The peritoneal great vessels and abdominal organs provide a large surface area for heat exchange. The use of warmed peritoneal lavage fluid is an effective approach to rewarming.[76] There have been reports of success in the literature using rapid high-volume peritoneal lavage in pediatric patients. The technique involves use of an infra-umbilical "mini-laparotomy" incision followed by placement of a large silicone peritoneal dialysis catheter. The catheter is connected to a rapid infusion device with the delivery of 1 L of warmed normal saline every 90 seconds.[76]

Indications and Contraindications. Peritoneal dialysis is appropriate therapy in a severely hypothermic patient. In practice, however, it is often omitted if other measures appear to be successful. There are no universally agreed on criteria for performing peritoneal lavage in hypothermic patients who have detectable vital signs. Although theoretically less effective than other techniques that directly warm the thorax in the setting of cardiac arrest, it has been used successfully in that situation. It is theoretically useful in hypothermic patients who have overdosed with a dialyzable toxin. Other less invasive methods, such as gastric or bladder lavage or warm nebulized air or oxygen inhalation, may be preferred in stable patients with temperatures higher than 26°C to 28°C (>78.7°F–82.4°F). Peritoneal dialysis should not be performed on patients with previous abdominal surgery. It should be used with extreme caution in patients with a coagulopathy after the risks and benefits have been considered.

Equipment. We recommend using the Seldinger technique with a commercially available disposable kit (e.g., Arrow Peritoneal Lavage Kit, product no. AK-09000, Arrow International, Inc., Reading, PA) because of the ease of performance and minimal morbidity associated with this procedure.

Technique. In the noncritical patient, obtain a coagulation profile before the procedure, but in life-threatening situations, initiate the procedure immediately before laboratory studies. Place the patient in the supine position with a Foley catheter and nasogastric tube in place. After infiltrating with lidocaine, make an infraumbilical stab incision with a No. 11 blade scalpel, and place an 18-gauge needle into the peritoneal cavity directed toward the pelvis at a 45°. Insert a standard flexible J-wire through the needle, and then remove the needle. Pass the 8-French dialysis catheter over the wire with a twisting motion, and then remove the wire.

Lavage rates of 4 to 12 L/hr can be achieved with two catheters. Warm the fluid with a standard blood warmer to 40°C to 45°C (104.0°F–113.0°F). Use a standard 1.5% dextrose dialysate solution. Add potassium (4 mmol/L) if the patient becomes hypokalemic. Saline has also been used successfully. The rate should be at least 6 L/hr and preferably 10 L/hr.[75]

Complications. The Seldinger method has a complication rate of less than 1%.[77] A "mini-lap" using direct dissection may also be used but might have a higher complication rate.[77] Further discussion of potential complications is provided in Chapter 43, Peritoneal Procedures.

Summary. Peritoneal dialysis is a useful method because it uses readily available fluid and can be done with a self-contained disposable kit.[78] If a hospital also treats trauma victims, the same lavage kit can be used for evaluation of abdominal trauma. If this technique is combined with warm nebulized inhalation, warming rates of 4°C/hr (7.2°F/hr) can be achieved.[79] Peritoneal lavage rewarms the liver and restores its synthetic and metabolic properties.[80]

Gastrointestinal and Bladder Rewarming. Gastric or bladder irrigation offers some of the same advantages as peritoneal dialysis without invading the peritoneal cavity. Heat is delivered to structures in close proximity to the core. In the Multicenter Hypothermia Study, gastric/bladder/colon lavage had a 1st-hour rewarming rate of 1.0°C to 1.5°C/hr (33.8°F/hr–34.7°F/hr) and a 2nd-hour rewarming rate of 1.5°C/hr to 2.0°C/hr (34.7°F/hr–35.6°F/hr) for severe hypothermia.[78,81] In a multifactorial analysis of the Multicenter Hypothermia Study, there was a trend toward improved survival in patients on whom this method was used.[15]

Although the amount of heat delivered with gastric lavage appears less than that delivered with peritoneal dialysis, it is somewhat easier to use and less invasive. When combined with other methods, gastric or bladder lavage provides significant warming.[78,79] Serum electrolyte levels should be monitored if large volumes of tap water are used, because dilutional electrolyte disturbances may occur. Children and geriatric patients might be more susceptible to electrolyte changes with tap water irrigation.[82]

Indications and Contraindications. Warmed gastric or bladder lavage may be used as adjunctive therapy in moderate or severe hypothermia. It can be combined with other warming techniques when rapid rewarming is needed. Patients who are obtunded and lack protective airway reflexes should have endotracheal intubation before gastric lavage to prevent aspiration of gastric contents. Refer to the appropriate chapters concerning nasogastric tube placement (see Chapter 40, Nasogastric and Feeding Tube Placement), gastric lavage (see Chapter 42, Decontamination of the Poisoned Patient), and urethral catheterization for specific contraindications to these procedures.

Equipment. Use a large-diameter 32- to 40-French lavage tube with normal saline solution warmed to 40°C to 45°C (104.0°F–113.0°F; in a microwave or blood warmer with verification of temperature before use). Although smaller tubes are easily passed nasally, use oral placement of the large lavage tubes. A modified Sengstaken tube with gastric and esophageal balloons may also be used.

Technique. Instill 200- to 300-mL aliquots of fluid into the stomach before removal by gravity drainage. For bladder irrigation, the optimal volume is not known but avoid bladder distention (100- to 200-mL aliquots should be sufficient). The amount of time that the irrigant should be left before removal is not known, but rapid exchanges with a dwell time of 1 to 2 minutes is suggested.

Complications. Lavage complications include trauma to the nasal turbinates (especially if a large tube is passed nasally), gastric and esophageal perforation, dilutional hyponatremia, inadvertent placement of the tube in the lungs, and pulmonary aspiration. All of these can be minimized by careful, proper technique. Fluid overload or electrolyte disturbances when using tap water are potential complications in pediatric and geriatric patients.

Summary. Gastrointestinal and bladder lavage with heated fluids is easily performed using equipment and solutions available in any hospital. However, the stomach, colon, and bladder are poor sites for body cavity lavage because the surface area for heat exchange is small.[80] Because of its ease and availability, it can be started early in the resuscitation and combined with any other rewarming method to significantly add heat,[64] although the specific effect on morbidity and mortality is not known.

Thoracic Cavity Lavage. Thoracic cavity lavage can be performed either *closed*, through chest tubes placed in the one hemithorax,[83,84] or *open*, after resuscitative thoracotomy.[85] The former approach offers the advantages of being less invasive and an effective form of treatment in hospitals not equipped for cardiopulmonary bypass.[84] Furthermore, closed-chest CPR can be continued while this technique is used. The open thorax approach offers the theoretical advantage of direct heart warming and the option of open-chest cardiac massage. Rapid warming rates of 6°C to 7°C (42.8°F–44.6°F) in 20 minutes have been described.[83,84] Pleural irrigation results in cardiac rewarming and might be the method of choice, particularly if an arrythmia is present.[80]

Indications and Contraindications. Thoracic cavity lavage should be considered for patients requiring rapid core rewarming in the setting of cardiac arrest or inadequate perfusion (e.g., shock, during CPR) when cardiac bypass is not available. Open thoracic lavage should be considered in those patients who will receive open chest massage or thoracotomy for other reasons (e.g., hypothermic arrest with penetrating trauma). Thoracic lavage is not necessary for patients with mild or moderate hypothermia who can be rewarmed by other, less invasive methods. Avoid the technique in the patient with a coagulopathy unless needed as a life-saving measure.

Closed Thoracic Lavage. An alternative that is more practical for the ED is pleural rewarming repeatedly using warmed saline intermittently placed then withdrawn through a chest tube. Place two large-bore thoracostomy tubes (e.g., 36- to 38-Fr in 70-kg adults) in one hemithorax. Infuse one chest tube with 3-L bags of heated normal saline (40°C–41°C [104°F–105.8°F]) using a high-flow fluid infuser (e.g., Level-1 Fluid Warmer, Technologies, Inc., Marshfield, MA). Collect the effluent with an autotransfusion thoracostomy drainage set (e.g., Pleur-evac, Deknatel A-5000-ATS, Fall River, MA). Empty the removable reservoir as needed. Alternatively, use a single chest tube system with a Y-connector arrangement similar to that used for gastric lavage. Place aliquots of 200 to 300 mL with a 2-minute dwell time followed by suction drainage (at 20 cm H_2O).

Provide closed chest massage until adequate spontaneous perfusion occurs. Administer closed chest defibrillation if the patient is warmed to 30°C (86°F) and has persistent ventricular fibrillation. Continue thoracic lavage until the patient's temperature approaches 35°C (95°F).

Open Thoracic Lavage. Perform a left thoracotomy and pour saline warmed to 40°C to 41°C (104.0°F–105.8°F) continuously into the thoracic cavity, bathing the heart while an assistant suctions the excess fluid from the lateral edge of the thoracotomy. Alternatively, add fluid to the thorax and mediastinum intermittently and suction after several minutes. Follow this with more warm saline and repeat. This technique also allows for direct myocardial temperature monitoring. Perform direct cardiac massage until adequate spontaneous perfusion occurs. Perform direct cardiac defibrillation in a patient warmed to 30°C (86°F) with persistent ventricular fibrillation. When defibrillation is successful, continue direct myocardial warming until the patient's temperature approaches 35°C (95°F). If defibrillation is unsuccessful at a core temperature of 30°C (86°F), continue warming while oxygenation, perfusion, and other physiologic parameters are optimized before further defibrillation attempts.

Summary. Thoracic lavage is an effective form of active core rewarming usually reserved for hypothermic arrest patients.[84-86] Thoracic lavage may be considered when vital signs are inadequate or unstable enough to severely limit perfusion. However, precise indications are not clarified beyond the patient in cardiac arrest.

Cardiac Bypass. The use of cardiac bypass or an extracorporeal shunt through either the femoral artery–femoral vein or the aorta-caval procedure can result in rapid rewarming but requires surgical expertise, availability of appropriate equipment, and technical support.[5,11,47] This procedure has not been compared with other rewarming methods in a controlled fashion, and few centers have this modality available in a timeframe that would affect survival rates. Its main advantages appear to be the rapid rate of warming it produces and optimal patient oxygenation and perfusion. Femoral flow rates of 2 to 3 L/min with the warmer set at 38°C to 40°C (100.4°F–104°F) will raise the core temperature 1°C to 2°C (33.8°F–35.6°F) every 3 to 5 minutes.[6] Drawbacks include potential delays in assembling the appropriate team and equipment, delays owing to the time necessary to complete the operation, complications from the operation, the expense of the procedure and bypass equipment, and the potential for infection. Its use in extreme situations that may include cardiac arrest should be based on individual characteristics of the patient, clinician team, and hospital resources. If readily available, it should be strongly considered in hypothermic patients with asystole or ventricular fibrillation.[38] If oxygenation is not a consideration, venovenous rewarming with an extracorporeal venovenous rewarmer can achieve rapid rewarming rates

(2°C/hr–3°C/hr [3.6°F/hr–5.4°F/hr]), although they are slower than cardiopulmonary bypass.[66] Such a device is relatively easy to use, uses readily available technology, and probably does not require heparin. However, it needs to be assembled before patients present with hypothermia.[22] In severely hypothermic patients, extracorporeal rewarming using venovenous hemofiltration has also been successfully described.[65,66] Compared with adults, children, especially smaller ones, require special consideration with regards to IV cannulation because drainage can be inadequate using femoral-femoral cannulation. In smaller hypothermic children, some sources recommend a more aggressive emergent median sternotomy for cardiopulmoary bypass.[87]

Cardiopulmonary bypass is indicated in the following situations: (1) cardiac arrest or hemodynamic instability with a temperature less than 32°C (<89.6°F) (2) no response to less invasive techniques, (3) completely frozen extremities, or (4) rhabdomyolysis with severe hyperkalemia.[2] A 47% long-term survival rate was obtained in a Swiss study of 32 young, otherwise healthy individuals including mountain climbers, hikers, and victims of suicide attempts. Cardiopulmonary bypass is unlikely to confer similar benefit in older, poorly conditioned populations with underlying chronic diseases.[88]

Hemodialysis. Hemodialysis was first described in the management of AH in 1965.[89] It is a rapid and efficient modality of rapid internal rewarming for moderate to severe AH, but it is uncommonly used in clinical practice. One study reported that 26 patients with AH combined with circulatory arrest or severe circulatory failure were rewarmed to normothermia by the use of ECC.[90] Core rewarming by hemodialysis has been achieved after placement of a dialysis catheter or with the use of an existing shunt. Some of the potential advantages and drawbacks of cardiac bypass also apply to this procedure, although slower warming rates have been reported. A range from 0.6°C/hr (33.1°F/hr) to rates as high as 4.5°C/hr (40.1°F/hr) have been achieved with fluid warmed to 40°C (104.0°F).[89] For patients who have ingested a dialyzable toxin (such as barbiturates and toxic alcohols), hemodialysis can be used to both remove the toxin and rewarm the blood. In such cases, its use may be appropriate.

Experimental Techniques. Ultrasonic, radiowave, and low-frequency microwave diathermy rewarming appears to be a rapid, safe, noninvasive technique with promise in animal studies.[62,91] Frequencies of 13.6 MHz to 40.7 MHz are typically used. However, the technique seems less effective than immersion therapy and equivalent to passive rewarming techniques in a volunteer study.[91,92] Total liquid ventilation is currently being studied in animals as a method to rapidly rewarm the core using warmed oxygenated perflurocarbon. Benefits include shorter rewarming times when compared with warm humidified oxygen (1.98 ± 0.5 hr vs. 8.61 ± 1.6 hr; P <.0001), no afterdrop phenomenon, and no increase in lactate dehydrogenase and aspartate aminotransferase.[70]

Very hot IV fluids (65°C [149°F]) have been used in animals with little vascular damage or hemolysis. Trials in humans undergoing burn débridement have been very successful in preventing hypothermia during operative procedures. Patients had saline heated to 60°C (140°F) using modified fluid warmers infused through central venous access. Patients had no evidence of intravascular hemolysis or coagulopathy after infusions.[93] The role of hot IV fluids in the management of AH is currently undefined.

Special Situations

Cardiac Arrest

Cardiac arrest from AH requires immediate treatment for the best chance of a successful outcome. Rapid rewarming and restoration of cardiac rhythm are essential for patients in cardiopulmonary arrest and can best be achieved by a combination of passive and multiple active core rewarming techniques. Because there are numerous cases of survival from hypothermic cardiac arrest with prolonged external cardiac compression,[5,38,94] thoracotomy is not mandatory. Thoracotomy does offer some theoretical advantages, such as increased cardiac output with open chest massage,[85] direct observation of cardiac activity, and direct warming of cardiac tissue with thoracic cavity lavage of warm fluid. Cardiopulmonary bypass is an effective technique for rapid rewarming. Blunt trauma and head trauma victims were previously not ideal candidates for cardiac bypass because of the anticoagulation requirement; however, some authors have advocated this technique using heparin-bonded tubing even in the setting of known traumatic injury.[5] A review of outcome from hypothermic cardiac arrest from one institution found that the average time from thoractomy to development of a perfusing rhythm was 38 minutes (range, 10–90 min).[5] The optimal rate of cardiac compression in hypothermia is not known, but because of decreased oxygen consumption of vital organs, the rate required in hypothermic cardiac arrest is less than that recommended in normothermic cardiac arrest. Cardiac compressions should be initiated at half the normal rate in profoundly hypothermic patients. Guidelines developed by the American Heart Association and the Wilderness Medical Society recommend that CPR should be initiated in accidental hypothermia unless any of the following conditions exist: a "do not resuscitate" (DNR) status is documented and verified, obvious lethal injuries are present, chest wall depression is impossible, any signs of life are present, or rescuers are endangered by evacuation delays and altered triage conditions.[6]

The duration of CPR depends on the time required to raise the core temperature to a level at which defibrillation should be successful (i.e., >30°C [>86°F]). Previously, it was recommended that patients should not receive a set of three countershocks until a core temperature above 30°C (>86°F) can be reached. However, there have been reports of successful defibrillation in patients with profound hypothermia with core temperatures of 25.6°C (78.1°F).[81] The decision to terminate resuscitative efforts remains a clinical one. However, there are certain poor prognostic factors. Certainly, survival is unlikely in patients who persist in asystole or go from ventricular fibrillation to asystole as they are warmed past 32°C (>89.6°F). Prognostic markers for patients with severe hypothermia and cardiac arrest have been proposed as contraindications to ED thoractomy and/or cardiac bypass by some authors.[5] These markers include elevated potassium levels above 10 mmol/L (mEq/L) and pH levels below 6.5. Nonetheless, there are survival reports for patients with higher potassium levels and a pH as low as 6.29.[87] Therefore, the decision to continue resuscitative efforts should not be based solely on specific laboratory values or presenting core temperature.

Isolated reports of survival with prolonged CPR in hypothermic patients make extended efforts to resuscitate such patients reasonable. Children may be the best candidates for heroic measures.[47] Under ideal conditions, hypothermic cardiac arrest patients may reasonably be admitted to an intensive care unit for a 4- to 5-hour trial of rewarming with CPR in progress. Manual CPR should be replaced by mechanical methods if equipment is available. The oxygen-powered "thumper" has been successful during prolonged hypothermic resuscitations. Absence of responsiveness to treatment in conjunction with a highly elevated potassium level is an indication for termination of resuscitative efforts.

Airway Management

Maintain a secure functioning airway for the hypothermic patient, just as in any critically ill patient. In mild hypothermia, deliver heated humidified oxygen by a face mask. Recognize that the hypothermic patient can be combative and uncooperative and may require arm restraints if a mask is used. Intubate the patient with decreased sensorium who cannot reliably maintain her or his airway or the hypothermic patient who may be hypoxic. Endotracheal intubation may be performed safely without the added risk of ventricular dysrhythmias.[14] The technique for endotracheal intubation depends on the specific presenting circumstances and the expertise of the operator. Once an endotracheal tube has been placed and secured, use it to provide warm humidified oxygen. There is no evidence that tracheal intubation is detrimental in the severely hypothermic patient, and it should be considered if indicated for ventilation, oxygenation, or airway protection.

Acid-Base Disturbances

Acid-base disturbances are variable and can lead to metabolic acidosis from carbon dioxide retention and lactic acidosis or metabolic alkalosis resulting from decreased carbon dioxide production or hyperventilation. The interpretation of arterial blood gases in the hypothermic patient has been the cause of some confusion. Previously, it was suggested that all blood gases be corrected for temperature with correlation factors. With a decrease in temperature of 1°C (33.8°F), the pH rises 0.015, the carbon dioxide pressure (Pco_2) drops by 4.4%, and the oxygen pressure (Po_2) drops 7.2% compared with values that would be obtained on blood analyzed under normal conditions. Despite the conversion guide, optimal or normal values in hypothermia have not been well documented.[29] Other recent literature supports the use of uncorrected arterial blood gases to guide therapy with bicarbonate or hyperventilation.[27] This approach appears appropriate to support optimal enzymatic function. A gradual correction of acid-base imbalance will allow for the increased efficiency of the bicarbonate buffering system as the body warms. Arterial pH did not correlate with patient death in the Multicenter Hypothermia Study[79] and should not be used as a prognostic guide to resuscitation.

Coagulopathies

Abnormal clotting frequently occurs in hypothermia, probably because cold inhibits the enzymatic coagulation cascade.[95,96] Hypothermia-induced coagulopathy does not result from excessive clot lysis, but rather from impaired clot formation.[15,19] Platelet function is also impaired during hypothermia because the production of thromboxane B_2 is inhibited. Hypothermia-induced platelet aggregation with or without neutrophil involvement has been associated with neurologic dysfunction in patients undergoing surgical procedures.[11] Hypercoagulability with risks of thromboembolism may also occur, but the main importance of cold-induced coagulopathy is in patients with coincidental trauma. Such victims often have bleeding that is difficult to control. Replace appropriate clotting factors and use warm blood to limit further blood loss and worsening of hypothermia.

Trauma and Hypothermia

Mortality is increased in trauma patients with temperatures below 32°C (<89.6°F). It is not clear whether this increased mortality is actually a result of hypothermia or whether hypothermia is merely an indicator of severe injury and response to a massive transfusion of cold fluid.[19,97] Patients with severe trauma are prone to hypothermia because their injuries often expose them to environmental heat loss. Concurrent alcohol intoxication may add to the heat loss owing to the vasodilatory effects on cutaneous vasculature and prolonged cold exposure secondary to altered mental status. Severe injury victims also lose heat because of exposure during resuscitation and rapid administration of cold fluids.

It is unknown to what degree correcting the hypothermia improves outcome. Nevertheless, devices to rapidly infuse warm fluids such as the Level 1 fluid warmer (Level 1 Technologies, Rockland, MA) and the Thermostat 900 (Arrow International, Reading, PA) are frequently used to warm large-volume fluid transfusions. These devices seem reasonable to prevent the hypothermia associated with massive transfusions (see Chapter 23, Venous Cutdown). Their use in hypothermia not associated with severe trauma is limited by the relatively low fluid requirements of environmental exposure. Another Thermostat device (Aquarius Medical Corp., Phoenix, AZ) is used to accelerate recovery from hypothermia by mechanically distending blood vessels in the hand, thereby increasing transfer of exogenous heat to the body core. One article found that this particular rewarming device was not very effective in accelerating rewarming in hypothermic surgical patients after general anethesia.[98]

Pharmacotherapy and Monitoring

Hypothermia alters the pharmacodynamics of various drugs. It markedly alters drug kinetics, but not enough is known about this phenomenon to define specific therapeutic guidelines. Administer drugs with caution to the hypothermic patient (Table 66–4). Because of the negative effects of hypothermia on both hepatic and renal metabolism, toxic levels of medications can accumulate rapidly after repeated use. Avoid certain drugs, such as digitalis. Sinus bradycardia and most atrial arrhythmias do not require pharmacologic treatment because most resolve with rewarming. Transient ventricular dysrhythmias also do not require treatment. For those patients requiring medication for ventricular dysrhythmias, bretylium is the preferred agent, although lidocaine, magnesium, pro-

pranolol, and amiodarone have been used.[27] For severe acidosis (pH < 7.1), IV sodium bicarbonate can be used with extreme caution. Vasopressors should be used with caution, perhaps in much smaller doses than usual, because of the arrhythmogenic potential and the delayed metabolism. A review of intensive care unit admissions for hypothermic patients found that treatment with vasoactive drugs was an independent risk factor for mortality, but this phenomenon remains poorly understood.[38] In animal studies, use of epinephrine impaired myocardial efficiency in cases of moderate hypothermia.[99] There also was no advantage to repeated doses of epinephrine or high-dose epinephrine in the hypothermic cardiac arrest animal models.[100] The use of inamrinone (formerly known as amrinone) has been investigated in cases of deliberate mild hypothermia. Initial results indicate that amrinone accelerates the cooling rate of core temperature, potentially limiting the usefulness in management of AH.[101]

Administer IV fluids slowly to prevent fluid overload as a result of the decreased cardiac output. In addition, start fluids early because most hypothermic patients have intravascular volume depletion. D5NS has been advocated as the ideal initial resuscitation fluid.[56,58,63] Avoid potassium until electrolytes are measured and normal renal function is confirmed. Check serum levels of creatine phosphokinase in hypothermic patients that may indicate rhabdomyolysis. If elevated, carefully monitor renal function. Replace fluids aggressively because this may help to prevent the development of renal failure. In severely hypothermic patients, place a Swan-Ganz catheter and closely monitor urinary output to assist in the fluid management. The risks of precipitating ventricular fibrillation should be weighed against the potential benefits of the Swan-Ganz catheter.

Finally, it should be emphasized that hypothermic patients exhibit a "physiologic" (and probably somewhat protective) hypotension, hypoventilation, depressed mental status, and bradycardia, the extent of which depends on the core temperature. This observation prohibits precise recommendation on the indications and use of medications, intubation, CPR, and other resuscitative interventions that are better defined in the normothermic patient. Hypothermic patients who present with a blood pressure, respiratory rate, or mental status that would prognosticate certain morbidity in normothermic patients may recover with minimal intervention to their normal prehypothermic state. Avoid aggressive therapies or medications aimed at providing the hypothermic patient with vital signs that would be desirable in the normothermic patient but which may be supraphysiologic in the hypothermic patient.

Frostbite

Hypothermic patients frequently suffer other forms of cold-related injuries in addition to their systemic hypothermia. The mildest form of frostbite is termed *frostnip*, a condition that involves only the skin, sparing the subcutaneous tissues. The skin is blanched and numb, but the injury is immediately reversible with no permanent sequelae if the area is quickly rewarmed. Rewarm rapidly in a water bath at 40°C to 42°C (104.0°F–107.6°F). Frostnip occurs most frequently on the distal extremities, the nose, and the ears. Nonfreezing temperatures also produce *trenchfoot*, an intermediate step in the progression to true frostbite. Trenchfoot is the result of prolonged immersion. Rewarm patients and apply dry dressings.[102,103]

TABLE 66–4 Commonly Used Medications in Hypothermia

Clinical Situation	Medication	Dosage
Hypoglycemia	D50W	1 mg/kg IV
Alcoholic/malnourished	Thiamine	100 mg IV
Altered mental status	Naloxone	0.4–2 mg IV
Ventricular fibrillation	Bretylium*	5 mg/kg IV
	Magnesium sulfate	100 mg/kg IV

*The role of more available antidysrhythmics such as amiodarone in hypothermia remains to be determined.

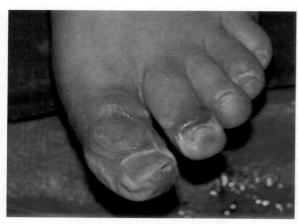

Figure 66–3 Example of frostbite.

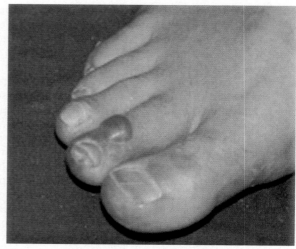

Figure 66–4 Example of frostbite.

In frostbite, the body parts most susceptible are those farthest away from the body's core: the hands, feet, earlobes, and nose. Exposure of the fingers to severe cold leads to cold-induced vasodilatation.[104,105] Apical structures rich with AVRs can shunt blood flow away from tissues. Freezing of the corneas has been reported to occur in individuals who keep their eyes open in high–wind chill situations without protective goggles (e.g., snowmobilers and skiiers).[92]

The pathophysiology of frostbite includes three pathways of tissue freezing: (1) through the extracellular formation of ice crystals, (2) hypoxia as a result of cold-induced local vasoconstriction, and (3) the release of inflammatory mediators. These pathways can and often do occur simultaneously, intensifying tissue damage. At the early stages of frostbite, the "hunting reaction" is observed whereby the body alternates between periods of vasoconstriction and periods of vasodilatation. As the temperature continues to decrease, the reaction stops and vasoconstriction persists.[36,102] Cold also increases blood viscosity, promotes vasospasm, and precipitates microthrombus formation. The release of the inflammatory mediators prostaglandin F_2 and thromboxane A_2 that are found in blister fluid cause further vasoconstriction leading to cell death. The release of these mediators peaks during rewarming, and cycles of recurrent freezing and rewarming only increase their tissue levels. Rewarming must be avoided until refreezing can be prevented.

The clinical signs and symptoms of frostbite vary according to the degree of injury. Although useful clinically, the degree classification does not predict the extent of further tissue damage.[29,87,95] The appearance of the affected extremity will depend on the extent of the frostbite. In superficial frostbite, the affected extremity appears pale, waxy, and numb; has poor capillary refill; and is very painful on rewarming. In deeper frostbite, the affected extremity is hard, solid, and blanched. Hemorrhagic blisters may be present (Figs. 66–3 and 66–4). Initially, there is no pain or feeling in the frostbitten extremity. After rewarming, the affected area develops severe edema and blistering, eventually exhibiting dry gangrene and mummification, leading to tissue sloughing.

Favorable prognostic signs for frostbite include intact sensation, normal color, warm tissues, early appearance of clear blisters, and edema. Early intervention is citical in terms of ultimate outcome. Delay in seeking medical care for more than 24 hours is associated with an 85% likelihood that surgical intervention will be required. Patients who present within the first 24 hours require surgery in less than 30% of cases.[2,103] The predictive value of the initial physical examination is limited; however, the presence of nonblanching cyanosis, hemorrhagic blisters, and impaired sensation appear to indicates a poor prognosis.[2]

Based on early bone scans and retrospective studies, researchers from France proposed a new classification for predicting frostbite outcomes on day 0.[106] Four degrees of severity are defined. With *first degree*, there is complete recovery. *Second degree* often leads to soft tissue amputation. With *third degree*, there is the need for bone amputation, and with *fourth degree*, there are systemic effects.[106]

Rapid rewarming is the treatment of choice for frostbite.[102] The aim is to limit the length of time the tissue remains in the frozen state. The most practical way to rewarm an extremity is to totally immerse the area in warm water at 40°C to 42°C (104.0°F–107.6°F) for 15 to 30 minutes. Carefully protect the affected area to ensure that the tissue is not additionally injured through contact with the sides or rim of the container. After thawing, meticulously protect the area from injury. Elevate the extremity and place cotton or gauze between the toes/fingers to limit maceration. Débride white or clear blisters. Leave hemorrhagic or dark blisters intact because disruption may cause damage to the vascular supply and viable tissue.

Use topical aloe vera (a thromboxane inhibitor) and systemic antiprostaglandins (such as ibuprofen) because they may be helpful. The use of semiocclusive dressings has shown promising results for management of deep frostbite injuries of the fingertips.[107] Provide tetanus prophylaxis. Adjuvant therapies involving the use of heparin or low-molecular-weight heparin, warfarin, vasodilators, corticosteroids, or immediate surgical sympathectomy have failed to improve outcomes.

Mixed success has been achieved with the use of hyperbaric oxygen and thrombolytics.[108] In a small study of frostbite victims, Twomey and coworkers[109] suggested the following treatment algorithm for severe frostbite: (1) rapid rewarming, (2) clinical appearance assessment, (3) early-phase ^{99m}Tc scintiscan to assess distal circulation, (4) IV tissue-type plasminogen activator (tPA; if no contraindications) for patients with digits or limbs showing no flow, (5) tPA at 0.15 mg·kg⁻¹ IV bolus followed by 0.15 mg·kg⁻¹·hr⁻¹ to maximum dose of

100 mg over 4 to 6 hours, (6) therapeutic heparin for 3 to 5 days, (7) warfarin to International Normalized Ration (INR) two times control for 4 weeks, (8) pain management as needed, (9) ibuprofen 400 to 600 mg orally four times daily, (10) light dressings with topical antimicrobials, and (11) no ambulation on frostbitten feet.[109] Bruen and colleagues,[110] in a small retrospective study, likewise reported that tPA within 24 hours of frostbite injury improved tissue perfusion and reduced amputations. The protocol included tPA administered at an initial rate of 0.5 to 1.0 mg/hr into the extremity via the femoral or brachial arterial catheter sheath. Heparin was also administered at 500 U/hr into the intra-arterial catheter.[110] Thrombolytic therapy for frostbite is encouraging, but the exact parameters for use are still being investigated.

Agents that can inhibit the formation of free radicals are also promising. These agents include superoxide dismutase, prostaglandin E_1 analogues, and drugs containing antiplatelet activity such as pentoxifylline.[36,102] The use of antibiotics is controversial, although some authors advocate agents with staphylococcus/streptococcus coverage (e.g., cephalosporins, pencillins). Avoid débridement of tissue in the ED. Give analgesics (IV opioids) as needed.

Cold Water Immersion/Submersion

One of the leading causes of hypothermia remains cold water immersion/submersion.[111] In one retrospective review of AH cases in a 3-year period, submersion hypothermia accounted for the greatest number of cases.[112] Unlike in cases of AH secondary to cold exposure, risk factors (both internal and external) are harder to identify secondary to the high mortality from drowning.[95] Studies have shown that at cold water temperatures (8°C [46.4°F]), core cooling occurs at slower rates in persons with increased body mass and subcutaneous fat and at faster rates when there is increased voluntary activity (e.g., treading water). Risk factors for submersion hypothermia include impaired performance and initial cardiorespiratory response to immersion. A study in healthy volunteers found that swimming efficiency and length of stroke decreased while rate of stroke and swim angle increased as the water temperature dropped.[113]

The body's response to cold water immersion (head-out) has been previously described as occurring in three phases.[62] The initial phase involves the "cold-shock response," which typically occurs within the first 4 to 6 minutes. Signs include peripheral vasoconstriction, gasp reflex, hyperventilation, and tachycardia. At this stage, there is a higher incidence of sudden death resulting from hypocapnia, inability to breath-hold, and increased cardiac output.[62] After the initial cold-shock response, the body undergoes profound cooling of the peripheral tissues. The peripheral cooling tends to be the greatest in the hands, leading to incoordination and grasping difficulties.[62] In prolonged immersion in cold water, heat is lost from the body quicker than it is produced, thus predisposing to hypothermia.[114]

In cases of cold water submersion, researchers found that rapid cooling is protective against neurologic impairment and increases chances of survival. There are numerous reports in the literature of survival after cold water submersion in children, but very few reports in adults. There are reports of survival after up to 66 minutes of cold water submersion.[115] Survival was reported in an elderly male after 22 minutes of submersion.[116] Overall, children tend to have a better prognosis because of the presence of the mammalian dive reflex

and a greater body surface area–to–mass ratio that allows for more rapid cooling. A recent case reported a 2-year-old boy who suffered from severe hypothermia after falling into ice water.[7] On discovery, cardiac arrest and asystole were present and the first measured temperature was 23.8°C (74.8°F). The patient was rewarmed by ECC with cardiopulmonary bypass and was discharged 9 days later without any sequela. Orlowski[117] identified five poor prognostic factors for near-drowning in pediatric patients: (1) maximum submersion time longer than 5 minutes, (2) comatose on arrival to ED, (3) arterial blood gas pH less than 7.10, (4) age younger than 3 years, and (5) resuscitation not attempted for at least 10 minutes after rescue. Adults tend to have higher mortality rates because of the following: (1) the lack of the mammalian dive reflex and (2) slower rates of temperature cooling secondary to lower body surface area–to–mass ratios in adults as compared with children. Recent reports of hypothermia and drowning in commercial fishing deaths in Alaska noted a strong protective association with the use of personal floatation devices, particularly immersion suits, in surviving cold water–related events in adults.[118]

Various mechanisms for brain and body cooling during submersion hypothermia have been described including the mammalian dive reflex, cold-induced changes in neurotransmitter release, and water ventilation.[119] The mammalian dive reflex prevents or delays aspiration or ventilation until the body has cooled to a point at which hypothermia protection occurs. Much attention has focused on the theory of water ventilation as a key component of accelerated brain cooling. Animal studies comparing immersed (head-out) and submersed dogs found that cooling rates were faster in the submersed dogs than in the immersed dogs. The submersed dogs cooled by convective heat exchange in the lungs, whereas the immersed dogs cooled by surface conduction only. Laboratory data obtained after the submersion indicated that there was indeed ventilation exchange in the water.[115] The body also undergoes a relative bradycardia as another protective measure. Bradycardia is inversely proportional to the water temperature with heart rates reaching 18 beats/min in 10°C (50°F) water.[119] Many authors advocate therapies aimed at symptoms resulting from near-drowning rather than severe hypothermia because, in fatal cases of submersion, death occurs too rapidly for hypothermia to be a significant contributor. Complications of near-drowning include pneumonia, lung edema, hemorrhagic pancreatitis, and skin edema.[95]

Conclusion

Mortality rates from AH are decreasing owing to increased recognition and advanced therapy. Caution should be used when extrapolating published data obtained in adults to children.[52] With the exception of severe hypothermia, the prognosis mostly correlates with the presence or absence of underlying disease states. Studies have shown that the prognosis is excellent in patients in whom no hypoxic event precedes hypothermia and no serious underlying disease states exist. Previously healthy individuals usually have a full recovery with mortality rates less than 5%, whereas patients with coexisting medical illnesses have reported mortality rates of greater than 50%.[51]

As a general guideline, take a conservative approach to rewarming the stable hypothermic patient, with avoidance of overtreatment and the selective and careful use of invasive monitoring. Evaluate the patient's "physiologic" hypotension, hypoventilation, and bradycardia with regard to that expected for the core temperature.

Because death is related more to underlying illnesses than to hypothermia, some recent sources do not believe invasive rewarming modalities are useful for the poikilothermic patient with severe underlying disease.[1]

In moderate hypothermia, underlying problems should be sought, passive rewarming and basic support started, and less invasive core rewarming begun. This approach should include mask ventilation with warm humidified air or oxygen in the conscious patient and intubation and ventilation in the unconscious patient. In selected patients, gastric or peritoneal lavage with warm fluid may be considered. For severely hypothermic, *unstable* patients, cardiac bypass and thoracic lavage may offer additional benefits, including rapid warming rates and direct heart warming. The benefits should be weighed against the institutional capabilities, time, expense, and the danger of complications that these procedures entail.

PROCEDURES PERTAINING TO HYPERTHERMIA

Human epidemics of heat-related illness have been well documented historically.[120,121] A Roman army was decimated by heat in 24 bc, and King Edward's heavily armored crusaders were defeated by "heat and fever" during the final battle of the Holy Land. In Peking, 11,000 residents died during a heat wave in 1743. More than 1000 heat-related deaths occurred during a pilgrimage to Mecca in the early 1960s. Recent years have witnessed a considerable number of deaths due to hyperthermia and heat-related illnesses within the United States and worldwide.[122] In the United States from 1999 to 2003, a total of 3442 deaths were attributed to extreme heat exposure. During the heat wave of 2003, France reported 15,000 excess deaths due to the heat wave.[123,124]

In contrast, malignant hyperthermia (MH) and neuroleptic malignant syndrome (NMS) have been recognized and described only since the 1960s.[125,126] These conditions are largely iatrogenic and are most commonly triggered by modern pharmacologic therapy. In addition, the incidence of hyperthermic conditions induced by psychostimulant drugs of abuse, such as cocaine and amphetamine derivatives, is also on the rise.[127]

As with hypothermia, it is important to use the proper thermometer capable of detecting a wide range of body temperatures. Heatstroke remains a common clinical problem with significant morbidity and mortality. Every year, approximately hundreds of people die from heat-related illnesses. As the weather patterns continue to change with a trend toward more hot and humid summers, the number of individuals adversely affected by the heat continues to rise. A variety of cooling techniques have been advocated since World War II. Although some cooling techniques have been compared in controlled human and animal models of heatstroke, our practice decisions are not based solely on the theoretical rate of cooling. Other important factors include the ease of use, rapidity of initiation, and safety.

Before considering the various cooling techniques, it is essential that the underlying disorders of hyperthermia are clearly understood. Heat illness represents a broad spectrum of disease ranging from mild heat exhaustion, which is primarily a volume loss disorder, to severe heatstroke resulting in thermal-related end-organ damage. The latter includes disorders such as MH and NMS. Treatment of this spectrum

of disease requires a discriminating approach, including supportive care only for heat exhaustion and rapid cooling for heatstroke. MH requires specific pharmacologic therapy (e.g., dantrolene) in addition to cooling measures. A brief discussion of hyperthermic disorders is therefore necessary before describing cooling techniques.

Normal Thermoregulation

Body temperature typically follows a diurnal pattern, increasing from about 36°C (96.8°F) in the early morning to 37.5°C (99.5°F) in the late afternoon, and reflects the balance between heat production and heat dissipation.[128,129] Heat is produced as a byproduct of metabolic processes and when ambient temperatures exceed the body temperature. Body temperature increases when the rate of heat production exceeds the rate of heat dissipation. The brain's thermal center is located in the preoptic nucleus of the anterior hypothalamus. In response to rising core temperature, this thermal center activates efferent fibers of the autonomic nervous system to produce vasodilatation and increase the rate of sweating. Vasodilatation dissipates heat by convection, and sweat dissipates heat by evaporation.

Hyperthermia occurs when thermoregulatory mechanisms are overwhelmed by excessive metabolic production of heat, excessive environmental heat, or impaired heat dissipation. Fever, conversely, occurs when the hypothalamic set point is increased by the action of circulating pyrogenic cytokines, causing peripheral mechanisms to conserve and generate heat until the body temperature rises to the elevated set point. Hyperthermia and fever cannot be differentiated clinically on the basis of the magnitude of temperature or on the pattern of its changes.[130-132]

Types of Hyperthermia

Mild Heat Illness

Heat cramps and heat exhaustion are induced by a hot environment.[133-135] The body's heat dissipation mechanisms generally are able to keep up with heat production and absorption in these disorders. Symptoms are largely due to the mechanisms used by the body to dissipate heat, and body temperatures remain at or near normal. Rapid cooling techniques are *not* required, and supportive care and hydration in a cool environment are usually adequate therapy.

Heat cramps are intensely painful but generally benign, involuntary skeletal muscle spasms (most often in the calves, hamstring, or quadriceps muscles). The pain may also be in the arms and back. The cramps may be severe and prolonged but fortunately only rarely lead to rhabdomyolysis. Heat cramps occur after strenuous exercise or heavy labor in a hot environment. Heat cramps were previously felt to be the result of dehydration associated with significant sodium chloride losses, but some clinical observations have proved that heat cramps can occur at rest or during exercise under any environmental conditions.[136] The most recent theory is that heat cramps may be the result of alterations in the spinal neural reflex activity and triggered by fatigue in susceptible individuals. There are no controlled clinical trials evaluating the efficacy of electrolyte replacement, quinine, or other medications.[136] Rest in a cool environment and vigorous oral fluid replacement with isotonic solutions are usually adequate therapy, but in some cases, IV saline is required. A common mistake is to rely on thirst to indicate dehydration. The pain of severe cramping may be resistant to narcotics in the absence of adequate fluid replacement.

Heat exhaustion, commonly referred to as heat syncope, is a poorly defined syndrome with nonspecific symptoms that *occur after heat exposure*. Malaise, flulike symptoms, orthostasis, dehydration, nausea, headache, and collapse may all occur. Heat exhaustion is considered to be the result of dehydration-induced heat retention that is not severe enough to cause heatstroke.[137] Compared with the more severe heat disorders, mental status is normal and body temperature is normal or mildly elevated in heat exhaustion. There does not appear to be any thermoregulatory failure in heat exhaustion. Rehydration, rest, and supportive care in a cool environment are adequate therapy for heat exhaustion.[133] One theory of the etiology of heat exhaustion is that there is a precipitous fall in central rather than circulating blood volume following cessation of exercise that results in postural hypotension. Some authors advocate cooling and placing the patient either in the supine position with the legs elevated or seated with the head between the knees to decrease skin blood flow and increase venous blood flow to the heart.[136,137] Recovery is usually evident within a few minutes to hours. Occasionally, heat exhaustion is accompanied by heat cramps, presenting a confusing scenario if the diagnosis is not suspected. Rapid cooling techniques are not usually required, but patients should be observed for progression to heatstroke because heat exhaustion and heatstroke are a continuum of one disease process.[138]

Heatstroke

When the body's normal heat dissipation mechanisms are overwhelmed, core temperature elevation and heatstroke rapidly develop. Heatstroke is a state of thermoregulatory failure.[29,128,131,139] Two forms of heatstroke are described in the literature. *Classic (nonexertional) heatstroke* usually occurs during summer heat waves. Poor, urban elderly, infants, and persons with impaired mobility are at greatest risk.[134,137,140] Dehydration, lack of air conditioning, obesity, neurologic disorders, hyperthyroidism, cardiovascular disease, impaired mentation, and medications that interfere with heat dissipation (e.g., phenothiazines, diuretics, and anticholinergics) predispose this population to heatstroke. *Exertional heatstroke*, a consequence of strenuous physical activity, usually afflicts a younger segment of the population. Highly motivated, poorly acclimatized, or unconditioned athletes and military recruits are common victims, as are individuals who perform heavy physical labor in hot, humid conditions (Fig. 66–5).[141] In exertional heatstroke, the risk appears to be greatest in those individuals performing high-intensity exercise for relatively short durations.[136] A retrospective review of long-distance cyclists participating in the California AIDS (acquired immunodeficiency disease) Ride found that as the number of chronic medical illnesses increased, so did the risk of developing an exertional heat-related illness. Human immunodeficiency virus seropositivity alone was not associated with an increased risk of exertional heat-related illness.[142]

The degree of hyperthermia necessary to produce heatstroke in humans is unknown. In tissue culture cells, thermal injury is observed in the range of 40°C to 45°C (104°F–113°F). Studies of hyperthermia in cancer therapy reveal that tissue sensitivity to heat is increased by relative hypoxia, ischemia, and acidosis.[143]

The key clinical findings in the diagnosis of heatstroke are (1) a history of heat stress or exposure, (2) a rectal tem-

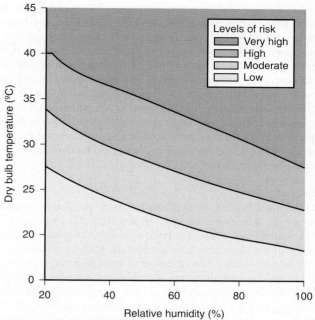

Figure 66–5 Risk of heat exhaustion or heatstroke during intense work in the heat. (Adjusted to the ACSM Position Stand: the prevention of thermal injuries during distance running[2]). *(Adapted from Keystone JS, Freeman DO, Kozarsky PE (eds): Heat illness. In Travel Medicine, 2nd ed. Copyright © 2008 by Mosby, an Imprint of Elsevier. All rights reserved.)*

perature greater than 40°C (>104°F), and (3) central nervous system (CNS) dysfunction (altered mental status, disorientation, stupor, seizures, or coma). The cerebellum is very sensitive to heat, and ataxia may be an early clue. Although anhydrosis is described as a classic sign of heatstroke, investigations demonstrate that cessation of sweating may be a late finding. Failure to consider the diagnosis of heatstroke in a diaphoretic patient with mental status changes could prove disastrous.[137]

The sequelae of heatstroke are caused by thermal damage to multiple organ systems.[128] After a hyperthermic event, tissue injury continues.[144] Delirium, seizures, and coma can result from direct effects of heat on the CNS. Autopsies show profound brain edema after hyperthermic insults. Researchers suggest that in cases of instant death, brain edema due to the increased permeability of the blood-brain barrier causes raised intracranial pressure, papilledema, followed by vascular infarction and brain herniation.[145] Cardiovascular collapse results from dehydration, maximal cutaneous vasodilatation, and direct heat-induced myocardial depression. Coagulopathies and liver dysfunction (elevated levels of bilirubin and transaminases) occur as consequences of thermal breakdown and consumption of serum proteins, as well as direct heat damage to hepatic cells. Children often demonstrate diarrhea. Renal failure can result from myoglobinuria (related to rhabdomyolysis) and acute tubular necrosis.[29,140] Animal studies in rats after hyperthermic events demonstrate significant gastrointestinal changes. In rats successfully cooled to normothermia, delayed secondary deterioration occurs with massive gastrointestinal bleeding.[146] Metabolic acidosis is the primary acid-base alteration observed in heatstroke, with the prevalence increasing with the degree of hyperthermia.[147]

The treatment of these sequelae in acute heatstroke does not differ from that in other heat-related disorders, with the sole exception that rapid cooling is necessary to prevent further damage and reverse heat stress. The more rapidly the rectal temperature is reduced to 38°C (100.4°F), the better the prognosis.[29,134,148] The human body tolerates hyperthermia poorly. Unlike patients with hypothermia, in whom slow, gentle rewarming and supportive care often result in a favorable outcome, victims of severe heatstroke must be aggressively treated with measures designed to rapidly lower the core temperature. Studies investigating precooling techniques to avoid heatstroke have been relatively unsuccessful in attenuating increases in core body temperature and are not recommended.[149] In contrast, whole body precooling increases overall exercise endurance.[150]

MH

MH is a pharmacogenetic disease, which predisposes to the trigger of a life-threatening, hypermetabolic syndrome.[151] MH results from a rare inherited autosomal dominant abnormality of the skeletal muscle membrane with an incidence of 1:50,000 in adults.[126] In response to certain stresses or drugs (Table 66-5), patients with this disorder sustain a massive efflux of calcium from skeletal muscle sarcoplasmic reticulum, resulting in contraction of the sarcomeres; skeletal muscle rigidity; increased skeletal muscle metabolism, elevated serum creatine kinase levels, and heat production; and finally, systemic hyperthermia.[152,153] Hyperthermia is a late development occurring after rigidity has been present for some time and the body's normal heat dissipation mechanisms are overwhelmed. The earliest signs of MH are increased carbon dioxide production, muscle rigidity, and tachycardia.[152,154] Cardiac output and cutaneous blood flow also increase to maximize heat loss. MH is diagnosed based on the clinical triad of (1) exposure to an agent or stress known to trigger the condition, (2) skeletal muscle rigidity, and (3) hyperthermia.

MH is usually encountered in the operating room while patients are undergoing general anesthesia, particularly with halogenated inhalation agents and depolarizing muscle relaxants. Heat production in the anesthetized patient can be profound with as much as a fivefold increase in oxygen consumption.[151] However, cases of MH may be encountered anywhere general anesthetics or neuromuscular blocking agents are used.[155]

As with heatstroke, treatment of MH requires rapid cooling and supportive care for the sequelae described previously. Unlike heatstroke, MH requires specific pharmacologic therapy to stop excess heat production by skeletal muscle. Dantrolene sodium induces muscle relaxation in MH by blocking calcium release from muscle cell sarcoplasmic reticulum.[152,154] In all cases of MH, the inciting stimulus (see Table 66-4) should be discontinued immediately and dantrolene therapy administered (3 mg/kg IV every 10 min for three doses) until the episode resolves.[156] Procainamide has been used successfully when dantrolene is unavailable.[156]

It has been suggested that dantrolene administration speeds cooling of heatstroke victims by reducing skeletal muscle heat production.[157] However, a randomized, controlled trial of the use of dantrolene in heat stroke found no difference between the treatment and the placebo groups in terms of cooling time, complications, or length of stay.[158] In 2005, a meta-analysis concluded that there was no role for dantrolene use in management of heat stroke.[159] Currently, dantrolene administration is best reserved for patients with clinical muscle rigidity or suspected MH. Routine use of this drug in heatstroke patients is not recommended.[160] New and promising treatments for MH are being investigated. Researchers have discovered mutations in the gene coding for the ryanodine receptor calcium release channel (RyRI) in families with MH, which may be the functional basis for MH. Some studies have examined the effects of MH mutations on the sensitivity of the RyRI to drugs and endogenous channel effectors including Ca^{2+} and calmodulin.[151,161]

NMS

First described in the late 1960s, NMS is characterized by hyperthermia, muscle rigidity, altered level of consciousness, and autonomic instability.[125] Mortality from NMS is estimated at 20% of patients who develop the condition.[162,163] This idiosyncratic disorder follows the therapeutic use of neuroleptic drugs, including phenothiazines, butyrophenones, thioxanthenes, lithium, and tricyclic antidepressants. The reaction is triggered by blockade of dopaminergic receptors, resulting in spasticity of skeletal muscle, which generates excessive heat and impairs hypothalamic thermoregulation and heat dissipation.[164] Muscle rigidity, described as "lead-pipe" rigidity in its most severe form,[165] can manifest as oculogyric crisis, dyskinesia, akinesia, dysphagia, dysarthria, or opisthotonos. NMS occurs in 0.2% of patients who receive neuroleptic agents either chronically or acutely. Haloperidol and depot fluphenazine appear to be the most common offending agents.[163] Temperatures can exceed 42°C (107.6°F). Initial agitation often progresses to stupor and coma. Catatonia and mutism may also be present. Autonomic instability is manifested as tachycardia, labile blood pressures, sweating, and incontinence. Ventilations are impaired by chest wall rigidity.

This syndrome is more likely to occur at the initiation of or after an increase in neuroleptic dosage. Researchers suggest that NMS typically occurs over several days (average in patients taking neuroleptic agents). It may also occur if antiparkinsonian drugs are suddenly discontinued.[162,166] NMS resembles MH but usually lasts longer (5–10 days) after the inciting drug is discontinued. The syndrome may be misinterpreted as a worsening of the underlying psychiatric disorder, drug intoxication (e.g., cocaine and amphetamines), a severe dystonic reaction, tetanus, or a variety of CNS infections. In addition to agents with increased dopaminergic blocking activity, other risk factors for NMS include dehydration, prior history of dystonia, catatonia, agitation, and iron

TABLE 66-5 Triggers for Malignant Hyperthermia

Drugs	Conditions
Halothane	Heat stress
Methoxyflurane	Vigorous exercise
Enflurane	Emotional stress
Diethyl ether	
Cyclopropane	
Succinylcholine	
Tubocurarine	
Lidocaine	
Mepivacaine	
Isoflurane	
Ketamine	
Trichloroethylene	
Chloroform	
Gallamine	
Nitrous oxide	

deficiency.[156] The mortality rate is high, and respiratory failure, renal failure, cardiovascular collapse, or thromboembolic disease usually cause death.[167]

Treatment of severe NMS (i.e., hypotension, hyperthermia, marked rigidity) closely follows that of MH, except that therapy must be maintained for several days until symptoms resolve. Therapy of NMS involves discontinuation of the triggering agent, rapid cooling, benzodiazepines, a combination of a central dopamine agonist, bromocriptine or L-dopa, and dantrolene as well as supportive treatment for ensuing organ failure.[166] Although the effects are not immediate, pharmaceutical therapy is directed at overriding the dopaminergic blockade caused by offending neuroleptic agents or dopamine depletion resulting from the cessation of antiparkinsonian medications. There are reports of successful treatment of NMS using subcutaneous apomorphine monotherapy.[168] As with MH, dantrolene (2–3 mg/kg) can be given to treat NMS-induced muscle rigidity.[167] The beneficial response stems not only from the effects at the sarcoplasmic reticulum of skeletal muscles but also from central dopamine metabolism of calcium in the CNS. In addition, bromocriptine, a central dopamine agonist, is reported to be efficacious in NMS therapy at doses of 2.5 to 10 mg three times a day.[164] Although both of these agents have been noted to reduce the duration of hyperthermia, there have been mixed results of success using bromocriptine and dantrolene.[157,164]

A more recently described disorder often confused with NMS is the *serotonin syndrome*.[166] This syndrome involves the newer antidepressants (fluoxetine, paroxetine, citalopram, fluvoxamine, venlafaxine, and sertraline),[156,169] which are selective serotonin reuptake inhibitors (SSRIs). These drugs can adversely react with other stronger serotonin receptor agents such as monoamine oxidase inhibitors (MAOIs) and nonselective serotonin reuptake inhibitors (clomipramine and tricyclic antidepressants) to induce a clinical presentation similar to that of NMS, only milder. Serotonin syndrome classically occurs when two or more drugs that interfere with serotonin metabolism act synergistically on the $5-HT_{1A}$ receptor, leading to overstimulation.[156,169] Drugs that act at any of the other serotonin receptors are not likely to produce the syndrome.[156,169] The range of symptoms varies from mild gastrointestinal upset, insomnia, and agitation to the most severe symptoms that include muscle spasms, seizures, ataxia, rhabdomyolysis, and autonomic instability. Treatment is primarily supportive in milder cases and consists of prompt recognition and withdrawal of the offending agent. Most cases resolve spontaneously within 24 hours. For the more severe cases, aggressive intensive care unit management is warranted to prevent renal failure and death. The drug cyproheptadine (Periactin) has shown promise in managing the agitation often seen with severe cases.[156,169] Cyproheptadine is an antihistamine with antiserotonergic properties. There has been limited success using benzodiazepines and β-blockers in these patients to treat agitation;[156] however, in cases in which serotonin syndrome and NMS cannot be differentiated, benzodiazepines represent the safest therapeutic option.[166] Further study among newer antipsychotic drugs, such as ziprasidone, a powerful $5-HT_{1A}$–receptor blocker, may delineate other possible benefits.[169]

Hyperthermia and Psychostimulant Overdose

As mentioned previously, the recognized incidence of hyperthermia induced by sympathomimetic psychostimulant drugs of abuse is on the rise. The offending agents most commonly described are cocaine, phencyclidine, amphetamine, and the amphetamine derivatives such as 3,4-methylenedioxymethamphetamine (MDMA) ("ecstasy") and 3,4-methylenedioxyethamphetamine (MDEA) ("Eve").[170,171] A number of studies have looked specifically at the club drug MDMA-ecstasy and its impairment of heat dissipation.[127] Animal studies in rats suggest that MDMA-induced hyperthermia results not from MDMA-induced 5-HT release, but from an increased release of dopamine acting at D1 receptors, suggesting a future role for use of dopamine antagonists in clinical treatment.[172]

Hyperthermia is a common feature of these potentially severe to lethal poisonings with sympathomimetic psychostimulant drugs and may be the primary cause of fatality in many cases.[170,173] Because of the nonlinear pharmokinetics of MDMA and γ-hydroxybutyrate (GHB), it is difficult to estimate a dose-response relationship.[170,173] Some have applied a pathophysiologic model of exertional heatstroke or NMS to profound cocaine intoxication.[174,175] In addition to profound hyperthermia (>42°C [>107.6°F]), acute rhabdomyolysis, disseminated intravascular coagulation, psychiatric and cognitive sequelae, renal failure, coma, seizures, and death have been described in these patients.[170-172,174-176] As demonstrated by Roberts and associates,[177] even a patient with a core temperature of 45.5°C (114°F) owing to acute cocaine intoxication may survive with aggressive cooling methods. Treatment requires prompt recognition, maintenance of adequate hydration, rapid cooling, as outlined later, and the aggressive use of sedative and/or paralyzing agents to control agitation. Importantly, the longer that psychostimulant-overdosed patients remain hyperthermic, the higher their morbidity and mortality rates. Agitation and seizures must be chemically controlled, because they lead to continued generation of heat and muscle injury. Therefore, liberal doses of benzodiazepines are recommended.[173] Some have advocated the use of bromocriptine[178] and dantrolene[173] as for MH and NMS, but their efficacy in the setting of drug-associated hyperthermia remains controversial.[179]

Hemorrhagic Shock and Encephalopathy Syndrome

The condition of hemorrhagic shock and encephalopathy syndrome in children (mainly infants, but some older children) resembles heatstroke in adults. The full-blown syndrome includes hyperthermia, coagulopathy, encephalopathy, and renal and hepatic dysfunction.[180] Although there may be an association with concurrent viral illness, the condition generally follows a temperature elevation, which may be triggered by the "bundling" of a child with a low-grade fever. Therapy is largely supportive and includes volume replacement and rapid cooling of the hyperthermic child while sources of bacterial infection are sought and treated.

Cooling Techniques

General Considerations

Heatstroke mortality is proportional to the magnitude and duration of thermal stress measured in degree-minutes.[181] *Delay in cooling may represent the single most important factor leading to death or residual disability in those who survive.*[29,133] In addition, advanced age and underlying disease states are significant contributing factors.[124,128,134,135]

Many exertional heatstroke victims are volume depleted and may present with hypotension. As a result, initial stabilization with cooled (room temperature) IV fluids and correction of electrolyte abnormalities are valuable in the hypotensive patient. Traditional sources recommend a rate of 1200 mL over the first 4 hours;[182,183] whereas others advise a 2-L bolus over the 1st hour, with an additional 1 L/hr for the following 3 hours.[183] Seraj and coworkers[184] challenged this more aggressive recommendation. In their study of pilgrims who suffered heatstroke, 65% had a normal or above normal central venous pressure (CVP) measurement on arrival. These authors found that an average of 1 L of saline was sufficient to normalize the CVP during the cooling period in their patients, who had a mean age of 55 years (range, 31–80 yr). Hence, in older patients, fluid resuscitation should be monitored carefully to avoid pulmonary edema. Regarding antipyretics, *there is no indication for either salicylates or acetaminophen in the setting of heatstroke* because their efficacy depends on a normally functioning hypothalamus. In addition, overzealous use of acetaminophen could potentiate hepatic damage, and salicylates may promote bleeding tendencies.[185] A study comparing acetaminophen and physical cooling methods found that in patients treated with antipyretics only, the mean body temperature increased by 0.2°C (32.4°F) on average.[186]

Given that rapid cooling is accepted as the cornerstone of effective heatstroke therapy, the clinician must choose which cooling technique to use. Studies in animal models are based on the assumption that the fastest cooling technique is the best. In clinical patient care, other factors will also influence the choice of technique. Patient access, monitoring, safety, ease of use, and availability are all considerations, in addition to speed of cooling. A technique that may not be the most rapid but allows easy patient access and is readily available may be preferable to more cumbersome (albeit more rapid, once established) cooling techniques in some clinical settings.

The cooling rates achieved in various human and animal studies of heatstroke are summarized in Table 66–6. The advantages and disadvantages of various cooling techniques are outlined in Table 66–7.

In addition to the cooling procedures outlined later, *it is imperative that the clinician institute the judicious use of sedation and/or muscle paralysis, to control agitation, suppress shivering, reduce energy expenditures, and make the patient receptive to sometimes unpleasant therapies.*[29,137] In general, IV benzodiazepines are the easiest and safest first-line drugs used for sedation.

Indications for Rapid Cooling

Rapid cooling should be instituted as soon as the diagnosis of heatstroke (rectal temperature >40°C [104°F], altered mental status, history of heat stress or exposure) is made. Rapid cooling is also indicated for the treatment of MH and NMS but should be instituted concurrently with discontinuation of the triggering agent or drug and administration of dantrolene. Because studies show that the degree of organ damage correlates with the degree and duration of temperature elevation above 40°C (>104°F), a reasonable clinical goal is to reduce the temperature to below 40°C (<104°F) within 30 minutes to an hour after the start of therapy.[29,128,131,159]

Contraindications for Rapid Cooling

Rapid cooling, per se, is never contraindicated in the presence of heatstroke. Immersion cooling is relatively contraindicated when cardiac monitoring of an unstable patient is required or when limited personnel make constant patient supervision impossible. Iced gastric lavage is contraindicated in patients with depressed airway reflexes unless the airway is protected by endotracheal intubation. Gastric lavage is also contraindi-

TABLE 66–6 Cooling Rates Achieved with Various Cooling Techniques

Technique	Reference	Model	Rate (°C/min)
Evaporative	Poulton & Walker, 1987*	Human	0.10
	Weiner & Khogali, 1980[188]	Human	0.31
	Kielblock et al, 1986[192]	Human	0.09
	Wyndham et al, 1959[187]	Human	0.07
	Daily & Harrison, 1948[†]	Rat	0.93
Immersion (ice water)	Armstrong et al, 1996[‡]	Human	0.20
	Weiner & Khogali, 1980[188]	Human	0.11
	Wyndham et al, 1959[187]	Human	0.14
	Magazanik et al, 1980[200]	Dog	0.27
	Daily & Harrison, 1948[†]	Rat	1.86
	Costrini, 1990[195]	Human	0.15
Selective immersion	Clapp et al, 2001[§]	Human	
	Torso immersion		0.16
	Hand/foot immersion		0.11
Ice packing (whole body)	Kielblock et al, 1986[192]	Human	0.034
Strategic ice packs (towels)	Armstrong et al, 1996[‡]	Human	0.11
	Kielblock et al, 1986[192]	Human	0.028
Evaporative strategic ice packs	Kielblock et al, 1986[192]	Human	0.036
Cold gastric lavage	Syverud et al, 1985[209]	Dog	0.15
	White et al, 1987[208]	Dog	0.06
Cold peritoneal lavage	Horowitz et al, 1989[211]	Human	0.11
	Bynum et al, 1978[ǁ]	Dog	0.56
	White, 1993[193]	Dog	0.14
Cyclic lung lavage	Harris et al, 2001[216]	Dog	0.5

*Poulton TJ, Walker RA: Helicopter cooling of heat stroke victims. Aviat Space Environ Med 58:358, 1987.
[†]Daily WM, Harrison TR: A study of the mechanism and treatment of experimental heat pyrexia. Am J Med Sci 215:42, 1948.
[‡]Armstrong LE, Crago AE, Adams R, et al: Whole body cooling of hyperthermic runners: comparison of two field therapies. Am J Emerg Med 14:355, 1996.
[§]Clapp AJ, Bishop PA, Muir I, et al: Rapid cooling techniques in joggers experiencing heat strain. J Sci Med Sport 4:160, 2001.
[ǁ]Bynum GD, Pandolf KB, Schuette WH, et al: Induced hyperthermia in sedated humans and the concept of critical thermal maximum. Am J Physiol 235:625, 1978.

TABLE 66–7 Advantages and Disadvantages of Various Cooling Techniques

Technique	Advantages	Disadvantages
Evaporative	Simple, readily available Noninvasive Easy monitoring and patient access Relatively fast	Constant moistening of skin required
Immersion	Noninvasive Relatively fast Low mortality rates	Cumbersome Patient access and monitoring difficult Shivering Poorly tolerated by conscious patients
Ice packing	Noninvasive Readily available	Shivering Poorly tolerated by conscious patients
Strategic ice packs	Noninvasive Readily available Can be combined with other techniques	Relatively slower cooling Shivering Poorly tolerated by conscious patients
Cold gastric lavage	Can be combined with other techniques	Relatively slower cooling Invasive Requires airway control Human experience limited
Cold peritoneal lavage	Rapid cooling	Invasive Human experience limited

cated by conditions that preclude placement of an orogastric or nasogastric tube. Cold peritoneal lavage is relatively contraindicated when multiple previous abdominal surgeries make placement of a lavage catheter risky owing to potential bowel perforation.

Evaporative Cooling

Evaporating water is thermodynamically a much more effective cooling medium than melting ice, given an appropriate water-vapor gradient. Evaporating 1 g of water requires 540 kcal. Melting 1 g of ice requires only 80 kcal. In theory, therefore, evaporative cooling should be approximately seven times more efficient than ice packing. In practice, evaporative cooling is more efficient.[148] In separate human studies, Wyndham and colleagues[187] and Weiner and Khogali[188] found evaporative cooling rates were substantially greater than water immersion at 14.4°C (57.9°F).[148] Studies in primate models demonstrated faster cooling rates using evaporative cooling as an adjunct to ice bag placement.[146] Methods using convection and evaporation were more effective than those involving conduction for the treatment of hyperthermia. In clinical practice, ice water immersion or ice packing causes heat loss by conduction as well as by heat consumption by the phase change of melting ice. In healthy volunteers, evaporative cooling techniques (e.g., facial fanning) were associated with decreased thermal sensation and improved thermal comfort.[189]

Despite the continued enthusiasm of some clinicians for ice water immersion, *evaporative cooling is the fastest noninvasive cooling technique in human studies.*[129,189] To maximize evaporative cooling rates, several factors must be optimized. Airflow

rates must be high (large fans are required). The air must be warm (but *not* humid), because evaporation is decreased at lower temperatures. The entire body surface must be exposed to airflow and continuously moistened with water (ideally the patient is suspended in a mesh sling to expose the back to airflow and moisture). Finally, the temperature of the water used to moisten the skin must be tepid (15°C [59°F]). Warm forced air is essential for effective evaporation and crucial to maintaining good peripheral perfusion and preventing shivering by warming the skin.[148] If the water is ice cold, evaporation will be slowed. Conversely, if it is hot, conductive heat gain may occur. Studies conducted in heat-stressed laying hens demonstrated superior cooling rates with ventral cooling regimes over dorsal cooling.[190]

Weiner and Khogali[188] constructed a sophisticated "body cooling unit" (BCU) to maximize evaporative cooling. Patients in the BCU are suspended in a mesh net. High airflow rates (30 m/min) at temperatures of 45°C (113°F) are maintained both anterior and posterior to the mesh net. Atomized water at 15°C (59°F) is continuously sprayed on all body surfaces. For EDs without access to a "body cooling unit," temporary units can be set up using shower sprays and fans, providing the ambient temperature in the ED is relatively cool.[191] An alternative less expensive, portable device developed at King Saud University involves covering the patient with a gauze sheet soaked in water at 20°C (68°F), while two fans direct the room air over the patient.[148] Cooling rates obtained with this device (0.087°C/min [32.2°F/min]) were nearly double the cooling rates achieved with the original BCU developed by Weiner and Khogali.[188]

The realities of clinical practice make these conditions hard to reproduce. Half the body surface (the back) will usually be unavailable for evaporative cooling. Airflow rates and temperatures are usually limited by the ambient temperature in the treatment facility and by the size and power of the fan available. These realities are reflected in the slower cooling rates achieved with evaporative cooling in a clinical setting.

Procedure. For evaporative cooling, undress the patient completely. Position a fan at the foot of the bed or stretcher and as close to the patient as possible. Then sponge or mist the patient's skin with tepid water (15°C [59°F]). Spray water continuously over the skin to create a warm microclimate around the skin and to promote water evaporation.[148] A single care provider can continue the technique and monitor the patient once cooling has been initiated. It is important to keep as much of the body surface area as moist as possible and exposed to airflow. Do not cover with sheets or clothing because this will impede skin evaporation and cooling. Studies of evaporative cooling in heatstroke patients show cooling rates of 0.046°C/min to 0.34°C/min (32.1°F/min–32.6°F/min).[174,192,193]

Complications. Complications of evaporative cooling are rare and more often a result of the underlying disorder than the cooling technique. Wet skin may interfere with electrocardiogram monitoring, but this can usually be avoided by using electrodes on the patient's back. Shivering occurs infrequently with this technique when compared with other cooling methods, because the water is relatively lukewarm.[148] Because the rectal temperature lags behind the core (esophageal) temperature, evaporative cooling should be discontinued when the rectal temperature reaches 39°C (102.2°F). In cases of mild hyperthermia, tympanic temperatures also accurately reflect core temperatures and can be useful in this setting.[194] Continued cooling beyond this temperature may lead to subsequent "overshoot hypothermia" due to continued core temperature drop after active evaporative cooling is discontinued. Shivering indicates that the core temperature has decreased to 37°C (89.6°F) or below.[136]

Immersion Cooling

It would seem obvious that the fastest way to cool a heatstroke patient would be immersion in ice water. In a case series of exertional heatstroke patients, iced water immersion cooled patients to less than 39°C (<102.2°F) within 19.2 minutes.[159] Some contemporary sources recommend ice water immersion as the cooling technique of choice for heatstroke.[148,181,191,195] Plattner and associates[196] demonstrated cooling rates with ice water immersion that were six times faster than rates seen with forced air or circulating water.

Costrini[195] reported no fatalities in 252 consecutive young marine recruits with exertional heatstroke who were treated with ice water immersion within 20 minutes of diagnosis. He regarded ice water immersion as superior in reducing mortality rates when compared with other conventional methods described in the literature.

In clinical trials, cold water immersion remains the second fastest noninvasive cooling technique available (see Table 66–5). Cold water immersion takes advantage of the high conductance properties of water, which is 25 times that of air.[159] In situations in which an adequate evaporative cooling system is not available, immersion may be the cooling technique of choice. Several factors are important in maximizing the rate of immersion cooling. Conductive heat loss depends on cutaneous blood flow to maintain a heat gradient from skin to water. Theoretically, contact with ice water causes skin and subcutaneous vasoconstriction, blocking heat exchange and turning these structures into insulators.[197] Intense cutaneous vasoconstriction will impede conductive heat loss. Mekjavic and coworkers[198] reported that motion sickness actually potentiates core cooling during immersion by attenuating the vasoconstrictor response to skin and core cooling, thereby augmenting heat loss and the magnitude of the decrease in deep body temperature. Careful monitoring is required because this may predispose patients to hypothermia.

Researchers have suggested that the use of ice water immersion may be superior to cold water immersion because of establishment of a steeper thermal gradient between the skin and the environment.[159,197] A study comparing the cooling capacity of ice water immersion (5.2°C [41.4°F]), tepid water immersion (14°C [57.2°F]), and passive cooling in experienced distance runners with body temperatures of 39.3°C to 39.6°C (102.7°F–103.3°F) found comparable cooling rates with ice water or cold water immersion. Both techniques were superior to passive cooling techniques.[199] The optimal water temperature for cooling human heatstroke patients has not been defined. However, aggressive skin cooling may stimulate shivering and peripheral vasoconstriction, thus hindering cooling efficacy. Thus, investigators suggest the inclusion of skin massage as a crucial component of immersion cooling techniques.[148]

Regardless of the water temperature, it is clear that increasing surface area increases conductive heat loss. Maximizing the body surface area in contact with the water will increase cooling rates with immersion cooling. In clinical practice, this means that complete immersion of the trunk and extremities will cool the patient faster than partial immersion of the trunk (back only) with the extremities extended out of the bath.

Procedure. For immersion cooling, undress the patient completely and transfer to a tub of water of a depth sufficient to cover the torso and extremities. Various water containers may be used. A regular bathtub can be used. Most clinical reports describe tubs that can be moved to the emergency treatment area when needed. A child's plastic wading pool and a decontamination tub or stretcher with waterproof sides and drainage capability are examples of the latter approach. Support the patient's head out of the tub at all times. In situations in which tubs are unavailable, place patients on water-impermeable sheets and in a sling apparatus while ice and water are poured into the sling.[191] Securely attach temperature and electrocardiogram leads to the patient if monitoring is to be continued during immersion. Remove the patient from the bath when the rectal temperature reaches 39°C (102.2°F), because core temperature will continue to drop for a short period even after the patient is removed. If available, use an electronic temperature monitor with a long flexible rectal probe for continuous temperature monitoring during immersion. Studies show cooling rates with ice water immersion (1°C–5°C [33.8°F–41.0°F]) in heatstroke patients of 0.15°C/min to 0.23°C/min (32.3°F/min–32.4°F/min).[197,199]

Complications. The common complications of immersion cooling are patient shivering, cutaneous vasoconstriction, patient discomfort, and the loss of monitoring capability. Shivering generates considerable heat through muscle metabolism. Cutaneous vasoconstriction impedes conductive heat loss. If significant shivering does occur, it can be reduced with benzodiazepine agents such as diazepam. Although the use of phenothiazines such as chlorpromazine has been advocated for shivering in the past, their use is currently discouraged because administration of these agents also may impair heat loss by their anticholinergic effects on sweat glands, contribute to hypotension via α-adrenergic blockade, lower the seizure threshold, and cause dystonic reactions. In addition, they possess central dopamine-blocking effects that may exacerbate symptoms of NMS.[164] Benzodiazepines are also valuable if the patient is hyperthermic secondary to sympathomimetic agents such as cocaine. Magazanik and colleagues[200] also suggested that warmer water temperatures (15°C [59°F]) minimize shivering and increase cutaneous blood flow, thereby increasing cooling rates. DeWitte and Sessler[201] reported that shivering occurs only as the body's final defense after maximal arteriovenous shunt vasoconstriction and behavior modifications have proved to be insufficient in maintaining core temperature. Shivering typically occurs after temperatures fall below 37°C (<98.6°F).[136] Patient monitoring is a problem under water. Electrodes can be used on the nonimmersed upper shoulders. Electrocardiogram artifact often becomes a major problem during vigorous shivering. Immersion cooling is not recommended for patients with unstable cardiac rhythms or those who are at risk for developing these rhythms. A significant change in cardiac rhythm might go undetected during the labor-intensive process of immersion cooling.

Patient access for resuscitative procedures is also a major problem with this technique. Should the patient develop ventricular fibrillation, he or she must be removed from the bath and dried before defibrillation. Invasive and diagnostic procedures (e.g., IV access and radiography) cannot be performed during the cooling period. Care must be taken to avoid displacement of IV lines during placement in and removal from the bath.

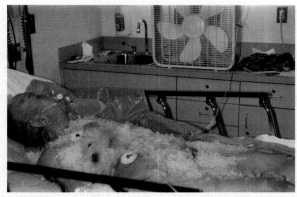

Figure 66–6 It is essential to rapidly lower the core temperature of a severely hyperthermic patient by instituting cooling techniques as soon as possible. Evaporative cooling (see text) is usually quite effective and technically easy. Note the fan for additional cooling. Many such patients require sedation, paralysis, and mechanical ventilation. An alternative aggressive method shown here, in a patient with a rectal temperature at 110°F, is to literally pack the patient in ice. She did not survive.

As body temperature drops, mental status will improve in many heatstroke victims. When awake, most people find ice water immersion difficult to tolerate. IV sedation may be required. Finally, this technique is labor intensive. Several caregivers must be present throughout the process. The patient's head must be maintained out of the bath. If massage is used, one or more individuals will need to immerse their own hands in water to continuously massage the patient. Medications should be given intravenously, and constant attention to temperature and electrocardiogram monitors is also necessary. This cooling technique should be used only if adequate personnel are available.

Whole Body Ice Packing

Packing the heatstroke victim in ice may enhance conductive heat loss without the attendant logistical problems caused by water immersion (Figs. 66–6 and 66–7). Constant attendance, as required for skin moistening with evaporative cooling and as described for immersion cooling, may not be necessary with ice packing. Kielblock and associates[192] demonstrated in a human study of mild, exercise-induced hyperthermia that whole body ice packing cooled just as fast as evaporative cooling (see Table 66–5).

Procedure. For whole body ice packing, undress the patient completely and then cover the extremities and torso with crushed ice. A fan blown over the patient may increase cooling. As with any cooling technique, monitor the temperature constantly using an electric thermometer and a long, flexible rectal probe. A large supply of crushed ice will be needed whenever this technique is used. Logistically, ice packing may be problematic. Whole body ice packing can usually be performed on the ED stretcher without additional equipment. Ideally, the patient is placed in a container that facilitates ice contact with the skin and prevents water from dripping onto the floor. A body bag makes an ideal device. Iced cooling may also be accomplished by placing the patient in a child's lightweight plastic pool, available in toy stores. Lacking this equipment, plastic cloths or trash bags may be placed under the patient with the edges curled up to form a slinglike apparatus. As with immersion cooling, electrocardiogram monitoring can potentially be difficult owing to shivering artifact and displacement of electrodes. If the patient is

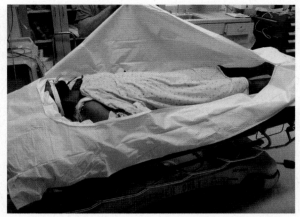

Figure 66–7 A body bag or plastic sheets may keep water from flooding the floor when packing the patient in ice.

alert and cannot tolerate the ice packing, give IV sedation or restraint. Treat excessive shivering with benzodiazepines if needed. Once the rectal temperature reaches 39°C (102.2°F), remove the ice and dry the patient off. Studies show cooling rates with whole body ice packing in heatstroke patients of 0.34°C/min (32.6°F/min).[148]

Strategic Ice Packs

Noakes[202] suggested that selective placement of ice packs over areas of the body where large blood vessels run close to the skin may be an effective cooling technique. Cooling in these areas occurs despite cutaneous vasoconstriction, owing to direct conductive heat loss from the blood within the vessel, across the vessel wall, subcutaneous tissue, and skin to the ice. The most common areas used for strategic ice packing are the anterior neck (carotid and jugular vessels), the axilla (axillary artery and vein), and the groin (femoral vessels). There have been numerous reports of successful cooling using ice packs as primary or adjunctive therapy[191,202] (see Table 66–5). In addition, application of ice packs, although easier to perform than immersion or total body ice packing, limits the conductive cooling offered by the latter two procedures.[203] However, a study in pigtail monkeys demonstrated that a combination of strategic ice packs with evaporative cooling resulted in faster cooling than either technique alone, although the relative increase achieved by adding ice packs to evaporative cooling was small.[204]

In unconscious patients or in awake patients who can tolerate ice packs without excessive shivering, this technique could be added to evaporative cooling. Kielblock and associates[192] found that the combination of strategic ice packs with evaporative cooling yielded higher cooling rates than either method individually (0.036°C/min vs. 0.027°C/min and 0.034°C/min). However, the clinical value of strategic ice packs alone or in combination with other techniques remains to be determined. Anecdotally, during the Chicago heat wave of 1995, the majority of heatstroke patients who presented to EDs survived after being effectively cooled using the evaporation method accompanied by strategic placement of ice packs.

Procedure. Place large plastic bags filled with crushed ice or an ice water mixture in both axillae and over both femoral triangles. If the neck is used, place the packs laterally so as to not compress the trachea or apply excessive weight over the carotid arteries. Do not pack the neck if the patient has carotid bruits or a history of cerebrovascular disease.

Some sources advocate rubbing the body surface briskly with plastic bags containing ice after the body has been wet down with water. This is effective, provided it is combined with evaporation therapy.[181] Studies show ranges of cooling rates with strategic ice packs in heatstroke patients of 0.028°C/min to 0.087°C/min (32.0°F/min–32.2°F/min).[192]

Complications. Complications of strategic ice packing are limited to shivering and patient discomfort, as described previously for whole body ice packing. The ice packs are removed when the rectal temperature reaches 39°C (102.2°F) to avoid excessive core temperature drop.

External versus Core Cooling

All of the external cooling techniques described previously are noninvasive and use heat loss by evaporation or conduction across the skin as the primary cooling mechanism. With each of these techniques, dropping of the central temperature will continue even after the technique is discontinued and the skin is dried. This is due to a delay in the establishment of an equilibrium between the cold skin and the core. The amount of "core afterdrop" can exceed 2°C (>35.6°F).[196,205] For this reason, cooling is discontinued when the core temperature reaches 39°C (102.2°F).

Because the sites of significant cell damage with heatstroke are centrally located (e.g., liver, kidney, heart), central cooling techniques theoretically are preferable to external techniques. Core cooling techniques studied in both animal and human models include iced gastric lavage, intravascular cooling, bladder lavage, and peritoneal lavage.[193,196,205,206] Central venous cooling is effective in rapidly decreasing core temperatures.[207] Studies conducted in healthy volunteers demonstrated that reductions of core temperatures varied according to the temperature of the infused fluid. Subjects receiving 30-minute infusions of fluid at 4°C (39.2°F) experienced decreases in core temperatures of 2.5°C ± 0.4°C (36.5°F ± 32.7°F). Subjects receiving 30-minute infusions of fluid at 20°C (68°F) experienced decreases of 1.4°C (±0.2°C [34.5°F ± 32.4°F]).[207] Clinical trials investigating this method showed that cooling via the respiratory tract had no significant impact on temperature changes when used exclusively; however, it did demonstrate effectiveness as an adjunctive measure to other external cooling techniques.[194] Cool air (10°C [50°F]) was administered via a hood or mask. Cooling via the respiratory tract has been studied in animals but not investigated clinically.[194] Central cooling techniques are necessarily more invasive than external techniques and, therefore, have the potential for more significant complications.

Cold Gastric Lavage

The stomach lies in close proximity to the liver, great vessels, kidneys, and heart. The gastric mucosa is not subject to the intense vasoconstriction observed on skin exposure to ice water.[208] For these reasons, lavage of the stomach might be expected to be an effective central cooling method. Studies of cold gastric lavage in a canine model produced cooling rates five times greater than controls exposed to ambient air at room temperature (0.15°C/min vs. 0.03°C/min).[209] In one human trial, ice water lavage at a rate of 500 mL every 10 minutes was associated with increased abdominal cramping and diarrhea.[196,205] Human heatstroke victims have been successfully cooled with gastric lavage, but only in combination with external techniques. Cold gastric lavage seems best suited for use in patients with severe hyperthermia who are cooled at a slow rate with external techniques alone. The presence

of an endotracheal tube and the passage of a large-bore gastric tube make rapid lavage without aspiration possible. This technique should be reserved for a patient whose airway is protected by endotracheal intubation and who does not have a contraindication to gastric tube placement.

Procedure. For cold gastric lavage, instill 10 mL/kg of iced tap water into the stomach as rapidly as possible (usually over 30–60 sec). After a 30- to 60-second dwell time, remove the water by suction or gravity.[193] Cooling, theoretically, will be faster if a high temperature gradient is maintained in the stomach. A faster lavage rate can be maintained if suction is used to withdraw instilled fluid. A large container of ice-temperature water maintained 1 to 1.5 m above the patient's body will facilitate instillation of fluid. Connect this container directly to the lavage tubing and ideally allow passage of water but not ice, which may occlude the tube. Because large volumes of water are needed, it is helpful if additional ice can be added to the container without interrupting the lavage. A large syringe can be used as an alternative to gravity instillation, but this is usually slower.

A simple system that accomplishes this procedure can be devised from readily available equipment in most EDs. Use a standard lavage setup (for use in drug overdoses) and a large-bore gastric tube. Cut the lavage bag open at the top to allow water and ice to be added. Suspend this above the patient's body and connect it to the orogastric tube by Y tubing with clamps. Connect the other arm of the Y tubing to suction. Using the clamps, intermittently instill ice water by gravity and withdraw it by suction.

Complications. A major potential complication of cold gastric lavage is pulmonary aspiration. The use of a cuffed endotracheal tube minimizes the incidence of this complication. Owing to the large volume of water used and the frequent depression of airway reflexes seen with severe heatstroke, this technique should rarely be used in a patient who is not endotracheally intubated.

If tap water is used, water intoxication, hyponatremia, and other electrolyte disturbances are *potential* complications, particularly in the pediatric or geriatric patients. Water is absorbed from the stomach and, with large-volume lavage, may pass the pylorus into the small intestine. In canine studies, large-volume gastric lavage with tap water did not cause electrolyte abnormalities.[209] The actual incidence of these potential complications in human heatstroke has not been determined. The use of normal saline instead of tap water would eliminate this potential problem.

Theoretically, the passage of cold water through the esophagus, located directly behind the heart, has the potential to induce cardiac dysrhythmias. Dysrhythmias have not been observed in canine studies or in case reports of human heatstroke victims cooled with this technique.[208,209]

Cold Peritoneal Lavage

The surface area and blood flow of the peritoneum greatly exceed those of the stomach. Peritoneal lavage is, therefore, expected to exchange heat much faster than is possible with gastric lavage. Peritoneal lavage demonstrates some of the fastest cooling rates ever reported in large animal or human studies (see Table 66–5). A case report of cold peritoneal lavage cooling for hyperthermia after ecstasy ingestion demonstrated rapid cooling.[210] As with gastric lavage, this central cooling technique offers the advantage of directly cooling the core organs that are most susceptible to thermal damage. Unlike with gastric lavage, endotracheal intubation is not required. Peritoneal lavage is used extensively to treat hyperthermia under various conditions and typically decreases core temperatures 5°C/hr to 10°C/hr (41°F/hr–50°F/hr).[196,205,206,210]

Peritoneal lavage is a more invasive cooling technique. Because heat exchange is more efficient across the peritoneum, smaller volumes of fluid can be used. Surgical placement of the lavage catheter is necessary. This cooling technique is relatively contraindicated by conditions that preclude placement of a lavage catheter (e.g., multiple abdominal surgical scars).

Peritoneal lavage is the most rapid central cooling technique. It can theoretically be combined with other techniques to speed cooling of the heatstroke patient with refractory hyperthermia. Being the most invasive cooling technique, it requires time, proper equipment, and surgical expertise to institute. Its use is probably best suited to situations in which heatstroke patients are not responding to external cooling and adequate equipment and personnel are readily available.

Procedure. To institute peritoneal lavage cooling, immerse 2 to 8 L of sterile saline in an ice water bath to cool while the catheter is being placed. Place a standard peritoneal lavage catheter (as for diagnostic use in trauma patients) using any of the techniques described in Chapter 43, Peritoneal Procedures. Standard contraindications apply. Use of a larger peritoneal dialysis catheter may speed fluid instillation and withdrawal. Actual lavage volumes and rates have not been established. One approach is to instill and withdraw 500 to 1000 mL every 10 minutes until adequate cooling is achieved. Rectal temperature may be falsely low during the lavage owing to the presence of cold water about the rectum at the level of the rectal temperature probe.[193,211] It may be preferable to monitor temperature by the tympanic membrane or esophagus when using this technique. Stop the lavage when core temperature reaches 39°C (102.2°F) to avoid excessive core temperature afterdrop.

Complications. The potential complications of peritoneal lavage cooling are primarily related to placement of the catheter and include bowel or bladder perforation and placement into the rectus sheath rather than the peritoneum.

Other Cooling Techniques

"Rewarming" techniques are used to minimize ongoing heat loss via the respiratory tract in hypothermic patients.[63] Although high-frequency jet ventilation (HFJV) causes core cooling in critically ill patients,[212] efforts to use the respiratory tract to cool heatstroke victims have been unsuccessful. In a canine model of heatstroke, the use of HFJV was shown to be a relatively ineffective cooling technique.[213] Heat loss by convection (air transfer) is relatively inefficient compared with the conductive heat loss mechanism used by other cooling techniques. The use of dry, hot air to maximize evaporative heat loss from the lungs might cause respiratory complications.[212]

In human trials, ice water lavage of the bladder (300 ml iced Ringer's solution every 10 min) provided only minimal cooling with rates of 0.8°C/hr (±0.3°C/hr [33.4°F/hr ± 32.5°F/hr]).[205] Iced water lavage of the rectum would theoretically provide faster cooling rates secondary to the increased surface area and better perfusion; however, it has not been investigated in human trials.[196]

Hemodialysis or partial cardiopulmonary bypass could theoretically be used to cool heatstroke patients. Prior to the availability of dantrolene in 1979, partial cardiopulmonary bypass was one of the treatments for MH.[214] Drawbacks could potentially include technical expertise as well as preparation time for the procedure. A recent case report described successfully treating a heatstroke patient with multiple organ failure refractory to conventional cooling techniques with cold hemodialysis initially 30°C (86°F) and later at 35°C (95°F), followed by continuous hemodiafiltration with cold dialysate (35°C [95°F]) at a high flow rate of 18,000 mL/hr. Within 3 hours of starting this particular technique, the patient's body temperature was below 38°C (<100.4°F).[215]

Cyclic lung lavage using cold perflurochemical lung lavage in animal models is currently under investigation. Benefits include rapid cooling rates of 0.5°C/min (32.9°F/min) and minimally invasive in the already mechanically ventilated subject.[216,217]

Intravascular cooling catheters have demonstrated efficiency as up-and-coming cooling devices. Intravascular cooling catheters circulate temperature-controlled sterile saline placed in the bladder or inferior vena cava. Although these devices have not been used in heatstroke patients, studies have found the cooling catheters to be very effective in neurologic conditions in both human and animal models.[218,219] Another promising cooling technique involves the use of a hypothermic retrograde jugular vein flush (HRJVF) for heatstroke. HRJVF has been studied only in animal models thus far. This technique involves infusion of 4°C (39.2°F) isotonic sodium chloride solution through the external jugular vein (1.7 mL/100g of body weight over 5 min). Use of HRJVF was found to increase survival rates during heatstroke by attenuating cerebral oxidative stress, tissue ischemia/injury, systemic inflammation, and activated coagulation.[220]

In addition to physical cooling techniques, pharmacologic agents have demonstrated merit as adjunctive agents in the management of hyperthermia. There are anecdotal reports of enhanced temperature reduction using IV ketoralac. Cienki and colleagues[221] demonstrated enhanced temperature decreases using ketorolac 30 mg intravenously. All patients received standard treatment for hyperthermia (e.g., ice packs, iced lavage, circulating air). Patients were randomized to receive ketorolac versus saline. In the group receiving ketorolac, the average rectal temperature after 90 minutes was two times lower than those receiving placebo saline (3.7°C vs. 1.6°C [38.7°F vs. 34.9°F]).

Conclusion

Rapid cooling is the key step in the emergency management of heatstroke patients. Survival approaches 90% when elevated temperatures are lowered in a timely fashion.[135,140,181] The highest documented temperature in the medical literature with survival is 48.8°C (115°F). In this case, the patient was rapidly cooled and recovered without neurologic sequelae.[222] Evaporative cooling appears to be the technique of choice. It combines the advantages of simplicity and noninvasiveness with the most rapid cooling rates achieved with any external technique. It is also logistically easier to institute, maintain, and monitor evaporative cooling than any other cooling technique. If a patient is not cooling rapidly with evaporative cooling, other techniques can be added. Strategic ice packs can be used. If the patient is endotracheally intubated, gastric lavage can be instituted. If facilities and personnel are available, peritoneal lavage cooling can be used as a rapid central cooling technique. If muscle rigidity is present or MH is suspected, dantrolene sodium should be administered. In addition, the clinician should have a heightened index of suspicion for NMS and sympathomimetic drug toxicity. Regardless of the cause, a reasonable clinical goal is to reduce the rectal temperature to 40°C (104°F) or below within 30 minutes of instituting therapy.[191]

Immersion cooling is best limited to centers with the proper equipment and skilled medical personnel experienced in managing hyperthermic patients. This method may also be effective in conditions in which electric power for evaporative cooling is unavailable (e.g., in wilderness settings where bodies of cool water are available nearby and the victim is far from more sophisticated medical care). Central venous cooling with iced saline is a promising cooling technique for rapid cooling for severe hyperthermia. Other cooling techniques require further study before a clear recommendation as to their efficacy can be made.

Acknowledgments

The authors wish to acknowledge and thank Dwight E. Helmrich, Scott A. Syverud, David Doezema, and David P. Sklar for their contributions and authorship in previous editions.

 REFERENCES CAN BE FOUND ON EXPERT CONSULT

CHAPTER 67

Ultrasound-Guided Procedures

Sarah A. Stahmer and
Lisa Mackowiak Filippone

Sonographic guidance for invasive procedures is a logical addition to the practice of emergency medicine. Bedside sonography allows visualization of subcutaneous structures (e.g., blood vessels, bones, and muscle) and deep tissue spaces. The ability to "see" beneath the skin increases the chances of successfully performing a wide range of invasive procedures and minimizes potential complications. This chapter is not meant to be a comprehensive description of the ultrasound (US) examination, nor should it be viewed as a tutorial for emergency clinicians unskilled in the use of US. It is assumed that the emergency clinician using US has had some formal training in the performance and interpretation of directed bedside US. This chapter describes those procedures within the scope of practice of emergency clinicians for which there is a role for bedside US. The procedures described here are covered in detail elsewhere in the text; this chapter focuses primarily on the role of US. At the current time, most emergency clinicians do not have significant training or expertise in ultrasonography. Whereas emergency department (ED) US is quite acceptable and strongly supported, it is not yet standard that all clinicians use this technique at the bedside.

PHYSICS

US images are created by high-frequency sound waves, which are generated and interpreted by a transducer and then converted electronically to form an image on a screen. The transducer is a probe that contains crystals that change shape and vibrate when an electrical current is applied, creating sound waves. This is referred to as the *piezoelectric effect*. The crystals emit sound for a brief moment, and then wait for the returning echo reflected from the structures in the plane of the sound beam. When the echo is received, the crystals vibrate, generating an electrical voltage proportional to the strength of the returning echo. This is then converted electronically into an image on the viewing screen.

Sound waves are reflected back to the transducer from tissue interfaces that have different acoustic impedances (the density of the tissue times the speed of sound in tissue). Tissues of higher density, such as bone, that interface with lower-density substances, such as muscle or fluid, will reflect nearly all the sound waves and appear on the monitor as brightly echogenic (white) structures. Fluid transmits nearly all the sound waves and will appear black or anechoic. Tissues will vary in their echogenicity or brightness based on their density, compliance, and adjacent structures (Fig. 67–1).

The purpose of using US during a procedure is to allow the clinician to "see" the area of interest below the skin's surface. The area on the body surface that will provide the best images is referred to as the *acoustic window*. Some general principles help determine the suitability of an area as an acoustic window. Sound waves travel best through structures composed of closely packed molecules. Air, because the molecules are widely spaced, is a very poor conductor of sound. Therefore, structures that contain air, such as the lungs and bowel, cannot be imaged with US. In addition, structures that lie beneath an air-filled structure (such as the aorta, which lies beneath loops of small bowel) may not be clearly visualized. In contrast, fluids have tightly packed molecules and conduct sound well. Fluid-filled structures are readily visualized with US because the fluid-tissue interface is highly reflective, creating a clear image. Fluid-filled structures also serve as excellent acoustic windows to structures that lie beneath them. Therefore, procedures involving entry into a fluid-filled space are best suited to sonographic guidance. Where appropriate, the optimal acoustic window is described for each of the procedures discussed in this chapter.

INDICATIONS AND CONTRAINDICATIONS

US may be used to guide cannulation of vessels, aspirate fluid collections within cavities (e.g., pericardium, pleura, peritoneum, bladder, or joints), identify purulent fluid collections for drainage, and locate soft tissue foreign bodies (FBs). US may be used to mark the site for skin puncture or provide continuous real-time visualization throughout the procedure. The real and potential applications for bedside sonography continue to expand as technology improves and clinical expertise in the hands of emergency clinicians grows. It is truly an extension of the examining clinician's eyes and hands and may be used to visualize any portion of the anatomy that is amenable to sonographic imaging. US is especially helpful in answering clinical questions regarding depth, size, and nature of subcutaneous masses or collections and determination of the presence of fluid within body cavities.

Lack of training and experience in the use of US technology and image interpretation is the only absolute contraindication for using US to guide procedures in the ED. There are no other absolute contraindications for its use. For the remainder of this chapter, it is assumed that the clinician performing an US-guided procedure has appropriate training and experience. To avoid redundancy, we will not restate this point. That is, lack of sonographic training and/or experience is a contraindication for incorporating bedside sonography with any procedure.

EQUIPMENT

The crystals determine transducer frequencies. Those used most commonly for medical diagnostic imaging range from 2 MHz to 10 MHz. Higher-frequency sound waves allow for better resolution and sharper images, but are unable to penetrate deeper tissues. Lower-frequency sound waves are able to better penetrate deeper structures and tissue spaces, but produce lower-resolution images. As a result, higher-frequency probes are used when high-resolution images of fairly superficial structures, such as veins and subcutaneous tissues, are needed. High-frequency probes are also recommended for use in children and very thin adults. Lower-frequency probes are used for viewing deeper structures, such as the heart or the aorta, and larger patients, in whom lower-resolution images are adequate. As a general rule, use the highest possible frequency probe that can image the desired structure or space because it will provide superior resolution.

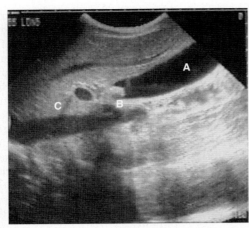

Figure 67–1 **Longitudinal image of the gallbladder demonstrates variability in tissue echogenicity.** *A,* The anechoic appearance of fluid. Water, plasma, nonclotted blood, and urine will have the same appearance. *B,* The highly reflective appearance of a calcified stone in the gallbladder. Foreign bodies, needles, and bone will have a similar brightly echogenic appearance. *C,* The relatively hypoechoic appearance of tissue. Clotted blood, particulate material within fluid (lipid or purulent material) will appear the same, with echogenicity intermediate to that of bone and fluid.

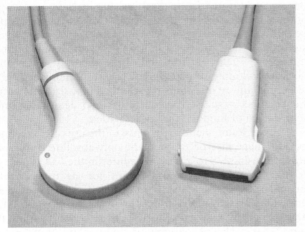

Figure 67–2 The curvilinear array probe is used for lower-frequency (2–5 MHz) scanning of abdominal and thoracic structures. The linear array probe is used for high-frequency (6–10 MHz) scanning of superficial tissues, vessels, subcutaneous masses, and foreign bodies.

Transducers vary also in the array of their piezoelectric elements, or crystals. The nature of the array will affect the overall field of imaging. The transducer array with the widest range of applications for emergency sonography is the curvilinear array, which has a narrow near-field and pie-shaped window, allowing for a small acoustic window and large imaging area. This is ideal for imaging between ribs and curved surfaces. The linear array is used for high-frequency scanning of superficial tissues and is ideal for imaging vessels, subcutaneous masses, and fluid collections (Fig. 67–2). With the increasing use of sonography for intravenous line placement, other probes, such as the "hockey-stick"–shaped probe are becoming more popular. The hockey-stick probe has a small footprint and high frequency that are ideal for locating vessels for intravenous line placement (Fig. 67–3).

Several needle guidance systems are available, which have a metal or plastic device attached to the probe through which

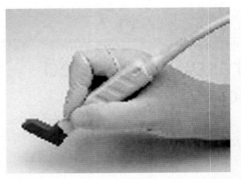

Figure 67–3 The linear array "hockey-stick" probe is used for very high frequency (6–13 MHz) scanning of superficial vessels and superficial tissues. *(Courtesy of SonoSite, Inc., Bothel, WA.)*

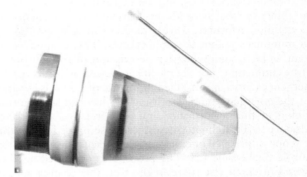

Figure 67–4 An ultrasound needle guide is ideally used to guide needle placement into deep or small structures. *(Courtesy of Dymax Corp, a subsidiary of Bard Access Systems, Salt Lake City, UT.)*

the needle passes (Fig. 67–4). Although these systems are designed to improve the accuracy of needle insertion, the path of the needle is determined by the probe angle, which can be altered by even subtle hand movements. Needle guidance systems are most useful when the target organ is deep or small in size and are usually not necessary for the majority of ED procedures.

GENERAL APPROACH

Most procedures facilitated by the use of bedside US require the use of two hands. Therefore, the clinician must make a decision whether to have an assistant hold the probe, perform the procedure with one hand while holding the probe in the other (freehand), or use the US probe to simply mark the point of entry before the procedure (blind approach). When the actual procedure requires two hands, it is best to have an assistant hold the probe. This is particularly important when one needs to visualize needle entry into a space or vessel. The freehand approach requires the operator to hold the probe in one hand while performing the procedure with the other. This is best suited for procedures that require only one hand, such as needle aspiration of large joint spaces or abscesses.

The blind approach is best used for large collections of fluid such as ascites or large pleural effusions. Identify the optimal site before the start of the procedure and mark the area with a sterile pen. The depth of the collection is noted by referring to the depth markers to the right of the imaging screen, which indicate the distance from the skin surface to the most anterior margin of the collection or vessel. Depending on the area of interest, it may be necessary to note the patient's position and phase of respiration when identifying the point of entry. This is especially important when attempting thoracentesis (phase of respiration) or paracentesis (patient positioning).

Catheters, wires, and needles appear as brightly reflective structures within the fluid-filled anechoic space. Keep the needle perpendicular to the plane of the US beam to maximize the chance of visualizing the needle. Other methods that have been reported to improve needle visualization include placing the focal zone in the near field and bobbing the needle. The latter requires an in-and-out jiggling movement that moves the needle within the sonographic window.[1]

When the probe is left in place during the procedure, cover it with a sterile rubber sheath. Commercially available probe covers are preferred because they incorporate part of the cord and are shaped to accommodate the probe, reducing the likelihood of air bubbles becoming trapped and interfering with image interpretation. If a commercial probe cover is not available, use a sterile glove to cover the probe and wrap a standard sterile drape around the cord. Alternatively, use a transparent sterile drape to cover the area being examined. Place a layer of acoustic gel between the probe and the sterile cover or drape and a second layer between the skin surface and the probe cover or drape. Remember that air bubbles may interfere with sound transmission and must be removed before the procedure.

COMPLICATIONS

Clinical errors directly related to the use of bedside US usually result from incorrect use of the technology or misinterpretation of sonographic images. Technologic errors may occur when the wrong probe is used. For example, procedures requiring high resolution (central vein cannulation or FB detection) should be guided with a high-frequency probe. Lower-frequency probes may not adequately delineate the desired structures and, hence, lead to error. Imaging of the heart often requires a probe with a small "footprint" that will allow for imaging between the ribs; a larger-footprint probe will include rib shadows that may affect the quality of the examination. Inadequate amounts of gel and air bubbles in the probe cover can create artifacts that adversely affect the technical quality of the images. Finally, the sonographer must be familiar with the various settings on the machine that determine image quality. For example, inappropriate gain settings are common sources of error and image misinterpretation; too much gain may give the appearance of echogenic shadows within spaces that may be interpreted as tissue or clot.

Problems with interpretation usually arise when the clinician is attempting to interpret an image that is suboptimal owing to poor patient preparation or positioning, when there are air-filled structures between the probe and the structure of interest, or when there is a lack of appreciation of sonographic artifacts. Emergency clinicians are often required to perform procedures under suboptimal conditions, and the same is true for sonography. Bedside sonography is often performed simultaneously with other procedures on a patient who may be unable or unwilling to fully cooperate. The patient may be receiving active chest compressions or be profoundly hypotensive, leaving vessels flaccid with poor flow. There may be subcutaneous air or significant soft tissue swelling between the probe and the object of interest, and veins may be filled with clot or scar from previous central lines. For this reason, the clinician using sonography must adhere to a few important principles. First, do not attempt to interpret a sonographic image that does not clearly depict the structure or organ of interest. Second, interpret the sonographic image in the context of the clinical picture—what you see must make sense to what is happening clinically. Finally, if you are not sure what you are seeing, obtain an alternative imaging study or expert assistance.

PERIPHERAL VENOUS LINE PLACEMENT

Obtaining vascular access is central to the care of many patients in the ED. Although the majority of patients have peripheral venous catheters placed without the aid of US, in selected groups US guidance may be helpful. These include patients with a history of intravenous drug use, obese patients, and those who have required multiple previous peripheral venous lines. In addition, any patient who has failed the standard blind approach may benefit from an attempt at peripheral vein cannulation utilizing US guidance.

Background

Common sites for peripheral venous cannulation include the metacarpal and dorsal veins in the hand, the basilic and cephalic veins in the forearm, and the median cubital and brachial veins in the antecubital fossa. With the exception of the metacarpal and dorsal veins on the dorsum of the hand, the other vessels are easily identified with US. In addition, less commonly used vessels such as the proximal cephalic and basilic veins in the upper arm may be identified and accessed with the aide of US.

Studies have demonstrated the superiority of sonographic guidance over traditional approaches for peripheral vein cannulation.[2,3] Costantino and coworkers[3] demonstrated a 97% success rate in placing a peripheral venous catheter in difficult intravenous access patients compared with a 33% success rate in the traditional placement group. They also demonstrated a shorter time to cannulation, fewer percutaneous punctures, and greater patient satisfaction with US guidance.

Indications and Contraindications

Sonographic guidance should be considered in those patients that require peripheral venous cannulation but in whom there are no visible or palpable upper extremity veins. In addition, sonography should be tried in any patient who has undergone a number of failed attempts using the standard approach. US may be considered first line in those patients who have a high likelihood for failure via the traditional method (e.g., intravenous drug users, obese patients, patients who have had multiple previous peripheral venous catheters).

Equipment

A high-frequency probe (≥ 7.5 MHz) is required for identifying superficially located peripheral veins in the upper extremity. A probe with a small footprint is particularly helpful, because there is less hardware on the patient during catheterization (see Fig. 67–3). If a linear probe is not available, any high-frequency probe, such as the endovaginal probe, can be used. A needle guide may be helpful for deep or small veins, but may make coordinating imaging and access more difficult for less experienced sonographers (see Fig. 67–4). Unlike central line placement, peripheral vein cannulation does not

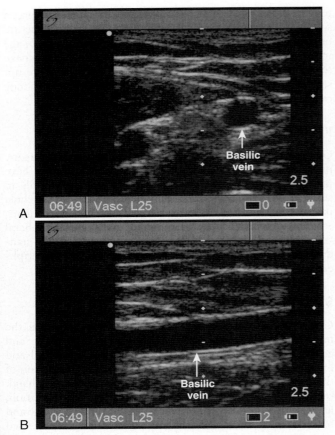

Figure 67–5 Sonographic images of the basilic vein in the upper extremity in transverse (*A*) and longitudinal (*B*) views. (*A and B, Courtesy of SonoSite, Inc., Bothel, WA.*)

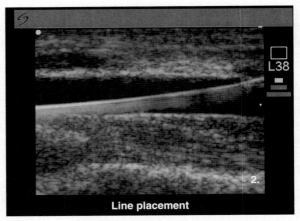

Figure 67–6 Sonographic image of a needle within the basilic vein. The basilic vein is imaged in a longitudinal orientation. (*Courtesy of SonoSite, Inc., Bothel, WA.*)

require sterile technique; however, a sterile probe cover and sterile acoustic gel are preferred. A sterile glove can be used to cover the probe, but a sterile sheath specifically designed for the US probe is better (see "General Approach," earlier).

For superficial vessels, use a standard intravenous catheter. However, for deeper vessels, a longer and stiffer catheter, such as those used for arterial lines, will help reduce the likelihood of kinking and are less easily dislodged.

Image Interpretation

The basilic vein in the distal upper extremity courses along the posterior ulnar aspect of the forearm. The cephalic vein is located along the radial aspect of the forearm. With the US placed perpendicular to the long axis of the vessel, the veins appear round and anechoic (black) on the monitor (Fig. 67–5*A*). They are superficial in location (close to the top of the screen), thin walled, and easily compressible. These veins can also be located more proximally in the arm, but will be deeper in this location.

With the probe placed perpendicular to the long axis of the arm in the antecubital fossa, the median cubital vein is located superficially and lateral to the brachial vessels. The brachial artery and vein can be distinguished from one another with the aid of color-flow or Doppler. The artery will demonstrate pulsatile flow, whereas the vein will demonstrate a steady snowstorm-like flow. Also, compression of the forearm will augment flow in the vein.

Peripheral vessels can also be viewed from the longitudinal approach (see Fig. 67–5*B*). In this view, the length of vein can be visualized to ensure patency and the needle can often be seen directly entering the vein (Fig. 67–6). The drawback to this approach is that small-caliber vessels may be difficult to keep aligned within the sonographic window, and it may be difficult to keep the adjacent artery in view.

Procedure and Technique

The procedure is the same regardless of the peripheral vein chosen. Two persons are usually required: one to perform the US while the other obtains vascular access. With experience, one person may perform the entire procedure. To begin, place a tourniquet around the extremity proximal to the desired cannulation site and prepare the probe with a sterile cover and sterile acoustic gel as described earlier (see "General Approach"). Then place the probe over the vessel to be cannulated. The probe may be oriented either parallel (longitudinal approach) or perpendicular (transverse approach) to the vessel of interest; however, the authors recommend perpendicular orientation for ease of image acquisition and maintenance (Fig. 67–7).

Once located, center the vessel on the screen and have an assistant puncture the skin using the middle of the probe as a guide. Advance the needle toward the vessel, which will first indent and then collapse as the needle contacts and applies pressure to the vessel wall. Once the catheter enters the lumen, the vessel will resume its normal diameter and the catheter may be seen as a brightly echogenic dot within the vessel. Blood return and easy flushing with saline (after tourniquet removal) further verifies correct catheter placement. If there is any doubt regarding proper catheter location, rapidly administer 5 to 10 mL of sterile saline into the catheter, which will cause the vessel to enlarge on the US monitor. Alternatively, if colorflow or Doppler is available, a sudden increase in signal is observed within the vessel with proper placement.

Complications

Complications of peripheral vein cannulation include phlebitis, infiltration, infection, arterial or nerve injury, air embolism, thrombosis, hematoma, and line failure; these are

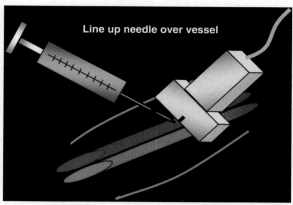

Figure 67–7 Schematic representation of ultrasound-guided peripheral venous cannulation. To image the antecubital vessels, place a high-frequency linear probe lightly over the arm in the transverse plane. Too much pressure will collapse the veins, even after a tourniquet is applied. The artery will appear as a small, noncompressible vessel with pulsatile flow if color-flow Doppler is used. The adjacent vein will be thin walled, collapse under pressure, and have augmented flow when the distal forearm is squeezed.

discussed in Chapter 21, Peripheral Venous Access. Some of these, such as injury to adjacent structures or hematoma formation, may occur less often with US guidance.

Using US to locate and cannulate deeper vessels may produce a higher incidence of subsequent line failure owing to kinking of the catheter and/or dislodgment of the catheter with extravasation of infusate into the surrounding tissues. Using longer, more rigid catheters when cannulating deeper vessels can reduce the incidence of these complications. Immobilizing the patient's arm may also be beneficial.

Complications may also arise from image misinterpretation. Arteries may be confused with veins if care is not taken to ensure that the vessel being cannulated collapses under light pressure or, if available, use of color-flow or Doppler demonstrates the typical steady snowstorm-like blood flow seen with veins (as opposed to the pulsatile flow of an artery). In the forearm, veins may be in close relation to tendons, which may be confused with vessels. Keeping the probe perpendicular to the desired vessel may remove this artifact.

CENTRAL VENOUS LINE PLACEMENT

Central vein cannulation is a frequently performed procedure in the ED. Bedside US has been shown to improve the chance of successful central vein cannulation and to reduce the number of complications and attempts, particularly in difficult subjects such as obese patients, those with failed prior attempts at blind cannulation, and those with prior central lines. As a result, US guidance for central vein cannulation has been recommended by the U.S. Department of Health and Human Services. In a report prepared in 2001 by the Agency for Healthcare Research and Quality, US guidance for central vein cannulation was listed as one of its 11 most highly rated safety practices.[4]

Because of their location, the internal jugular and femoral veins are easy to locate and visualize using US. The subclavian vein is more difficult to visualize sonographically secondary to the presence of the clavicle, but with practice, US can be used to facilitate subclavian vein cannulation. The use of US guidance for cannulation of each vessel is discussed later.

Background

Sonographic guidance (using two-dimensional echo) of internal jugular vein cannulation was first described in 1986;[5] since then, the benefits of US guidance have been well documented.[6,7] The largest prospective trial to date compared 302 US-assisted internal jugular vein cannulations with 302 attempts using the standard landmark-guided technique. The authors of this study demonstrated that use of US was associated with a higher success rate (100% vs. 88.1%), fewer attempts, a shorter mean time to cannulation, and a lower incidence of carotid puncture, brachial plexus injury, and hematoma formation.[6] Similar results have been demonstrated in several ED studies comparing US-guided internal jugular vein catheterization with the standard landmark technique.[7,8] In addition, Milling and colleagues[9] found that using US to simply mark the location of the internal jugular vein (and then cannulate the vessel using standard technique) was associated with higher first-attempt success rates (50% vs. 23%) and greater overall success rates (82% vs. 64%) compared with using landmarks alone.

The benefits of using US for internal jugular vein cannulation have also been demonstrated in children.[10,11] This is no surprise because children's vessels are smaller, cooperation unpredictable, and tensions often high when performed under emergent conditions. In a study of infants younger than 12 months undergoing preoperative central line placement, cannulation of the internal jugular vein was successful in 100% of infants using US guidance ($n = 43$) vs. 77% in infants using the standard landmark-guided technique ($n = 52$).[10] The time for cannulation was also significantly reduced (3.3 min vs. 10 min) and incidence of carotid punctures lower (0% vs. 25%) in the US group.[10]

Few studies have specifically evaluated the use of US for femoral vein access, but because these vessels are readily visualized on US, the advantages seen with cannulation of the internal jugular vein are likely to be found with this procedure as well. In 1997, Kwon and associates[12] demonstrated greater success (100%) in cannulating the femoral vein using US guidance than with the standard landmark-guided technique (89%) in patients requiring central venous access for hemodialysis. Complication rates were also lower in the US-guided group.[12] In another study, Hilty and coworkers[13] compared success and complication rates of US-guided femoral line placement with that of the standard landmark-guided approach in ED patients during cardiopulmonary resuscitation (CPR). The success rate using US was 90% versus 65% in the control group. There were no arterial punctures in the US group; however, the femoral artery was punctured in 20% of blind attempts.

Data are also very limited regarding the impact of sonographic guidance on the efficacy and safety of subclavian vein cannulation, but available data indicate that compared with the landmark technique, US guidance increases the probability of successful catheter placement, reduces the number of complications encountered, and decreases the need for multiple attempts.[14,15] In one of the few studies comparing US guidance with the standard landmark technique for subclavian vein cannulation, Gualtieri and colleagues[15] found that patients in the US group had a higher success rate (92% vs. 44%), fewer complications (1 complication in 25 attempts vs. 11 complications in 27 attempts), and fewer attempts (1.4 vs. 2.5).

Equipment

A high frequency (7.5- to 10-MHz) linear probe is highly recommended for imaging the relatively superficial internal jugular, subclavian, and femoral veins. A needle guide may be helpful for deep or small veins, but as mentioned earlier, it may make coordinating imaging and access more difficult for less experienced sonographers (see Fig. 67–4). If a linear probe is not available, any high-frequency probe, such as the endovaginal probe, can be used. A sterile probe cover (or glove) as well as sterile conductive medium is required. A sterile marking pen can be used to mark the location of the vein if the US probe is removed before puncture (see later).

Indications and Contraindications

If sonographic equipment is readily available, the ED clinician should have a very low threshold for using it to guide central venous cannulation. It is especially helpful when access is required on a patient with distorted anatomy, obesity, history of multiple prior central lines, coagulopathy, or hypotension and when blind attempts have been unsuccessful. The benefits include localization of the vein and adjacent artery and assessment of venous patency through ease of compression and demonstration of free flow (if Doppler is available). US can also identify the optimal vessel for cannulation (larger is always better) and the relationship between the vein and the adjacent artery.

There are no reported contraindications specific to sonographic guidance for central venous cannulation.

Procedure

Whereas there are slight variations in the techniques used for accessing different central veins (see later), two persons are usually required; one to perform the US while the other obtains vascular access. Preparation of the probe is the same regardless of which vessel is being cannulated and includes use of a sterile probe cover and sterile acoustic gel (see "General Approach"). Antiseptic skin preparation and draping are also similar for each site.

Internal Jugular Vein

Image Interpretation. The internal jugular vein and carotid artery will appear as relatively superficial structures on the monitor. When viewed in the transverse plane, the internal jugular vein is a thin-walled, circular, anechoic structure anterior and lateral to the carotid artery (Fig. 67–8). However, some variability in the relationship between the two vessels exists.[9,16,17] In a small percentage of patients, the internal jugular vein may be found medially (overlying the carotid artery), laterally or may not be visualized at all (presumably because of thrombosis).[9,16] Turning the patient's head will also alter the relationship between the vein and the artery, usually moving the vein medially over the artery.

When patent, the internal jugular vein will increase in size with inspiration and Valsalva maneuvers. Having the patient blow on her or his thumb is often helpful in creating a sustained Valsalva maneuver that will readily identify a patent internal jugular vein. Light pressure applied with the probe directly over the vessels will easily compress the internal jugular vein and only one anechoic circular structure, the carotid artery, will be seen on the monitor. Once pressure is released, the lumen of the internal jugular vein will reappear. Because of its superficial location and compressibility, the external jugular vein is usually flattened by placement of the probe on the neck and, therefore, is not seen on the monitor.

Technique. To access the internal jugular vein, place the patient in the supine position with the head turned slightly to the side opposite the vein being cannulated. Prepare and drape the lateral aspect of the neck in the usual fashion and prepare the probe as described earlier (see "General Approach").

Place the US probe parallel and superior to the clavicle over the groove made by the two heads of the sternocleidomastoid muscle (Fig. 67–9). The beam of the US probe should intersect the carotid artery and the internal jugular vein in a transverse or cross-sectional plane. At this level, the internal jugular vein is usually anterior and lateral to the carotid artery. Additional maneuvers that can help differentiate the internal jugular vein from the carotid artery are described earlier (see "Image Interpretation") and include having the patient "blow on his or her thumb" (this creates a sustained Valsalva maneuver) and applying gentle pressure to the vein (this will cause the vein to collapse, leaving only the carotid artery visible on the monitor). Use of color-flow or Doppler can also readily distinguish vein from artery. Pulsatile flow within the carotid appears quite different from lower-amplitude, phasic venous flow that augments with Valsalva maneuvers. Once the internal jugular vein is visualized, center it on the monitor screen, using the center of the probe as a guide for needle puncture.

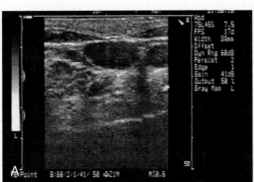 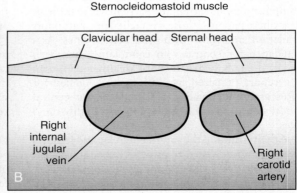

Figure 67–8 The internal jugular vein and carotid artery. *A,* Sonographic image. *B,* Schematic representation. The beam of the ultrasound should intersect the carotid artery and the internal jugular vein in a transverse or cross-sectional plane. The internal jugular vein is easily identified by its compressibility and response to Valsalva maneuvers (i.e., it increases in diameter).

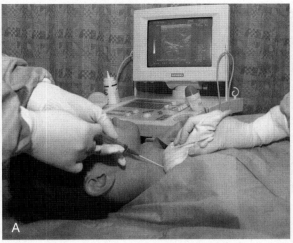

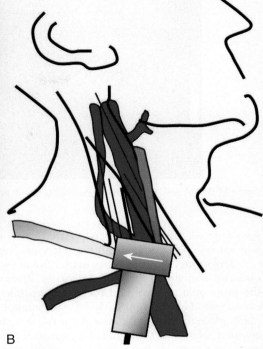

Figure 67–9 Imaging window for the internal jugular vein and carotid artery.
A, Cover the ultrasound probe with acoustic gel and then a sterile cover or glove. Place an additional layer of sterile gel over the cover. Then place the probe parallel and superior to the clavicle over the groove made by the two heads of the sternocleidomastoid muscle. Point the probe toward the patient's right. Take care not to apply undue pressure on the probe to avoid compression of the easily collapsible internal jugular vein. Asking the patients to "blow on their thumb," or Valsalva, will increase the luminal diameter of the vein. *B,* Schematic representation of probe placement and vessel location. *(A, Lydia F. Roberts, Photographer.)*

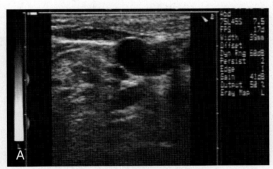

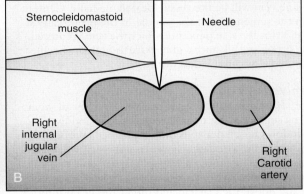

Figure 67–10 *A* and *B,* Once the vein is positioned directly under the probe, attempt needle aspiration. If the site of skin puncture is correct, the needle will indent the vein and the vein will appear to collapse as it is entered.

The needle will first indent the vein and then the vein will appear to collapse on the monitor just before it is entered (Fig. 67–10). Advance the needle slightly further and the vein will reexpand once it has been entered. The needle may be seen on the monitor as a brightly echogenic dot in the lumen of the vessel (Fig. 67–11). Once venous blood is aspirated, remove the US probe. Then thread a guidewire through the needle and place the catheter.

An alternative method, requiring only one operator, is to use the US to locate the underlying vein and then mark its location with a sterile pen. The internal jugular vein is usually a very superficial structure between the two heads of the sternocleidomastoid muscle and easily accessed once its location and patency are confirmed with US. Take care not to readjust the position of the patient's head at this time. Rotating the head further away from the vessel being cannulated will usually cause the vein to move medially over the carotid and increase the risk of inadvertent puncture of the artery.

Remove the probe after the vein has been located and perform needle puncture.

Femoral Vein

Image Interpretation. The femoral artery and vein also appear as superficial anechoic circular structures when viewed in the transverse plane. The vein is located medially and the artery is located laterally. As the probe is moved toward the patient's head, this relationship changes, with the vein eventually lying behind the artery. Other sonographic findings helpful in distinguishing the femoral vein are that it is easily compressed and will increase in size when the thigh is squeezed. The artery is not readily compressed and can be seen to pulsate. One exception to this may be in patients who are undergoing CPR in whom pulsations will be seen primarily in the femoral vein and not the artery. Coletti and associates[18] described the presence of femoral pulses in canines when CPR was in progress and the proximal femoral artery

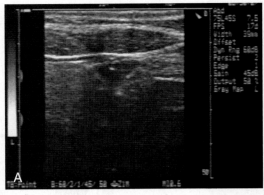
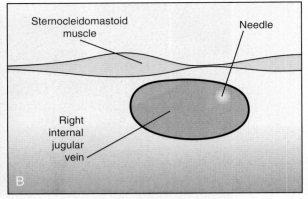

Figure 67–11 *A* and *B*, The needle may be visualized within the vessel lumen and will appear as a brightly echogenic structure.

1266

was clamped. These pulses disappeared when the proximal femoral vein was clamped and the artery unclamped.

Technique. Place the patient supine with the leg extended and slightly rotated externally. Prepare and drape the groin area as usual and prepare the probe as described earlier (see "General Approach"). If the patient has a palpable pulse, place the US probe over the pulse in a transverse orientation inferior to the inguinal ligament. If the patient does not have a palpable pulse, place the probe midway between an imaginary line drawn from the anterior superior iliac spine to the ipsilateral pubic tubercle just inferior to the inguinal ligament. The vein will be the vessel located medially. Center the vein on the screen so that the middle of the probe can be used as a guide for the skin puncture. Once the vein is entered, remove the probe and advance a guidewire though the needle. Perform subsequent cannulation of the vein.

Subclavian Vein

Image Interpretation. Visualize the subclavian vein using either a supraclaviclar or an infraclavicular window. The imaging window chosen depends on the planned approach to cannulating the vein. The supraclavicular approach will allow visualization of the juncture of the subclavian vein and the internal jugular vein. To obtain this view, place the probe parallel to and above the clavicle and direct the beam inferiorly. The internal jugular vein should be readily seen and then followed down to where it joins the subclavian vein.

Obtain the infraclavicular imaging window by placing the probe parallel to and below the most lateral aspect of the clavicle (Fig. 67–12*A*). The subclavian vein usually lies above the artery in this plane and can be identified by its thin wall and change in diameter in response to breathing and Valsalva maneuver. It will also be compressed with application of gently pressure from the probe. If color-flow or Doppler is available, venous flow will appear as a steady hum in contrast to the pulsatile arterial flow (see Fig. 67–12*B*).

Technique. Prepare and drape the skin and sheath the probe using sterile technique as described earlier (see "General Approach"). Place the probe just inferior to the most lateral aspect of the clavicle (infraclavicular approach). The plane of the US beam should lie parallel to the clavicle, catching the subclavian vein and artery in the transverse plane (see Fig. 67–12). To ensure the presence of normal anatomy up to the point of needle insertion, image the vein along its length for an additional 2 to 3 cm by moving the probe medially beneath the clavicle. The subclavian vein may also be viewed from the

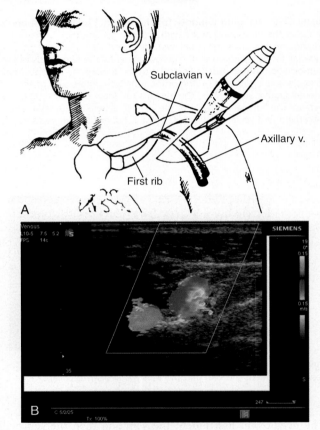

Figure 67–12 The infraclavicular imaging window. *A,* Schematic view demonstrates placement of a high-frequency probe transversely just below the distal clavicle. *B,* Sonographic appearance using color-flow enhancement. Note that the artery appears as a small, red, noncompressible vessel with pulsatile flow, whereas the adjacent vein appears as a blue, thin-walled vessel that readily collapses under pressure.

supraclavicular window, with the sonographic beam angled inferiorly and the vein seen in the longitudinal plane. Puncture the skin and advance the needle. Needle entry is best seen using the supraclavicular window and the longitudinal plane to image the vessel. However, because of its location under the clavicle, it may be difficult to visualize the needle entering the subclavian vein. Evidence that the needle is in close prox-

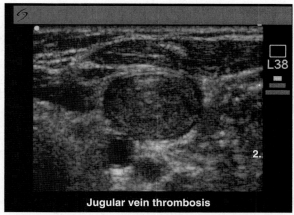

Figure 67–13 **Sonographic image of a thrombus within the internal jugular vein.** Thrombus is identified by the presence of echogenic material within the vessel lumen. The vessel will be noncompressible, and no flow (or only a trickle around the clot) will be observed. *(Courtesy of SonoSite, Inc., Bothel, WA.)*

imity to the vein includes indentation and collapse of the vein as it is entered and rapid rebound once cannulated.

Complications. Complications of internal jugular, femoral, and subclavian line placement are discussed elsewhere. Complications unique to using US are rare and usually due to poor technique or misinterpretation of the images obtained. One commonly encountered problem is the patient with proximate clot or stricture in the vein from prior central lines. In these patients, the vein will be seen and readily accessed, yet there will be little to no flow. A clue to this problem is a vein that does not easily compress. On occasion, the clot can be visualized directly with US (Fig. 67–13). When in doubt, comparison with the opposite side may be helpful. In addition, the use of color-flow or Doppler US can also be very helpful in identifying vessels with proximate obstruction by demonstrating reduced or absent flow in the occluded vessel.

PERICARDIOCENTESIS

The role of bedside sonography in the management of patients with suspected pericardial effusion is to establish the diagnosis and visualize placement of a drainage catheter within the pericardial sac. The diagnosis of a clinically significant pericardial effusion is readily determined by bedside sonography and is far superior to physical examination alone. Sonography is the study of choice for identifying pericardial effusions, and the availability of bedside US has the potential to shorten time to diagnosis of patients with clinically significant effusions.[19-22] For the subset of patients who are hemodynamically compromised by their effusion, pericardiocentesis performed under sonographic guidance is a safe and effective alternative to blind aspiration.

Background

Aspiration of the pericardial sac by emergency clinicians is usually a last-ditch effort to resuscitate patients with pulseless electrical activity and is often unsuccessful. This is because the diagnosis is usually considered only after the patient has become unstable and pericardiocentesis is performed late in the resuscitation effort. Several studies have shown that,

although large pericardial effusions are a rare cause of hemodynamic instability in the ED, a low threshold for performing bedside US may increase detection of effusions before they become hemodynamically significant.[19-21]

The traditional approach to the patient with a suspected clinically significant effusion has been to blindly access the pericardial sac using the subxiphoid approach. This technique is associated with a variety of complications including puncture of the liver, lungs, myocardium, and epicardial vessels[22] (see Chapter 16, Pericardiocentesis). In hemodynamically stable patients, a surgical window is usually performed in order to avoid the complications of blind aspiration. Over the past decade, there has been increased enthusiasm for echocardiographically guided pericardiocentesis. The techniques first described in 1998 are applicable to the ED setting and can be used for management of patients with hemodynamically significant pericardial effusions.[22]

Indications and Contraindications

Patients presenting with acute and subacute cardiac tamponade usually do not display the classic triad of hypotension, neck vein distention, and muffled heart tones. Waiting for their appearance to order a confirmatory test will often delay diagnosis and possibly jeopardize the safety of the patient. Image the heart whenever a clinically significant pericardial effusion is suspected. Scenarios warranting consideration of a pericardial effusion include a patient with hypotension of unclear etiology, particularly those patients with known malignancies, recent myocardial infarction, end-stage renal disease, and victims of trauma, both blunt and penetrating.[20,21] Early demonstration of a large pericardial effusion will guide further work-up, support early consultation from either cardiology or cardiothoracic surgery, and facilitate therapeutic drainage for those patients who remain hypotensive in spite of fluid resuscitation. For patients in extremis, the clinician most clinically experienced in both sonography and aspiration of the pericardial sac should perform pericardiocentesis without delay. For patients with large effusions who are relatively stable, management options are greater and may include a pericardial window. Consultation with either cardiology or cardiothoracic surgery is advised before performing aspiration of stable patients.

Equipment

The optimal probe frequency is 2 to 4 MHz. It should have a small enough footprint to allow for imaging between the rib spaces, particularly if the parasternal windows are used. For the subxiphoid view, the standard 2- to 3.5-MHz curvilinear probe will provide excellent images.

Acoustic Windows

The cardiac examination is dynamic and the sonographer must identify the acoustic window that provides those images that best demonstrate the effusion or cardiac chamber(s) of interest. It is important for the sonographer to develop expertise in using a variety of imaging windows to obtain the necessary clinical information. Although it is beyond the scope of this chapter to describe all of the possible cardiac imaging windows, the two most useful and commonly used views, the subxiphoid and parasternal, are described.

Subxiphoid View

The subxiphoid cardiac window provides the most comprehensive information for a single view when screening for pericardial effusions. It will readily identify a circumferential pericardial effusion and allow assessment of overall cardiac wall motion. To obtain the subxiphoid view, place the probe transversely at the left costal margin at the level of the xiphoid process with the beam aimed at the left shoulder (Fig. 67–14). The transverse plane is ideal for identification of the effusion. Adjust the angle and rotate the probe to obtain the appropriate views. The structures closest to the probe will appear at the top of the display and include the liver, diaphragm, pericardial space, and right ventricle (Fig. 67–15).

For guiding needle placement, some clinicians prefer using the subxiphoid view in the longitudinal plane because it helps avoid puncturing the liver (Fig. 67–16). In reality, any imaging window that demonstrates the effusion and identifies a "best path" for aspiration may be used. Often, this is a hybrid view that identifies a needle path where the effusion is closest to the probe (chest wall) and farthest from the liver, lungs, and heart. This is typically over the anterior chest wall or apex of the heart (Fig. 67–17).

Parasternal View

The next most useful view is the parasternal long-axis view. To obtain this view, place the transducer in the left parasternal area between the second and the fourth intercostal spaces. The plane of the beam should be parallel to a line drawn from the right shoulder to the left hip with the marker pointing to the right shoulder (reverse if the image is not set for cardiac views) (Fig. 67–18). The parasternal view provides excellent images of the left atrium, mitral valve, left ventricle, aortic valve, and proximal ascending aorta. It is also the best view to identify small dependent collections within the pericardial sac (Fig. 67–19).

Image Interpretation

The normal pericardium will appear as a single, brightly echogenic stripe adjacent to the myocardium. Fluid within the pericardial space will collect between the visceral and the parietal pericardium and will appear as a large, nonbeating anechoic area adjacent to the ventricular myocardium (Fig. 67–20). A small amount of fluid in the dependent portion of the pericardial sac is normal. The sonographic appearance of the clinically significant effusion is distinct. The sonogram

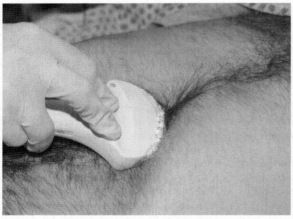

Figure 67–14 To obtain a subxiphoid view of the heart and pericardium, place the probe beneath the xiphoid process with the probe marker pointing to the patient's right. Angle the probe upward and slightly to the left. (*Lydia F. Roberts, Photographer.*)

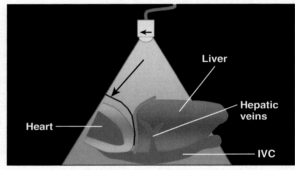

Figure 67–16 **Schematic diagram of the subxiphoid imaging window in the longitudinal plane.** Some clinicians prefer the longitudinal plane for aspirating a pericardial effusion, because it helps avoid puncturing the liver (*arrow*).

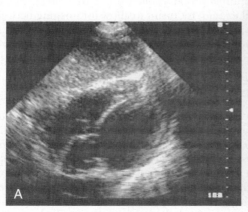
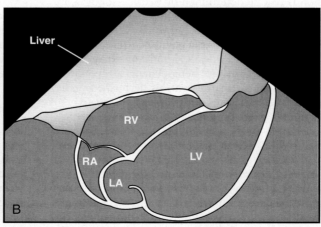

Figure 67–15 *A,* Sonographic appearance of a normal heart and pericardium obtained through the subxiphoid window in the transverse plane. The right ventricle will be the most anterior cardiac structure, bordered superiorly by the pericardium and diaphragm. *B,* Schematic representation. LA, left atrium; LV, left ventricle; RA, right atrium; RV, right ventricle.

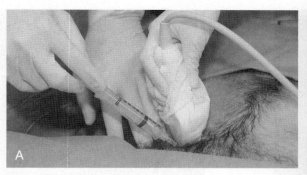

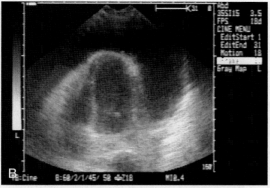

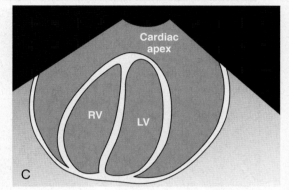

Figure 67–17 Photograph (*A*), sonographic image (*B*), and schematic representation (*C*) demonstrate the sonographic window that places the largest area of accumulated fluid nearest the probe (*top of screen*). There should be no vital structures between the probe and the pericardial space when the aspirating needle/catheter is placed over the superior border of the rib closest to the anechoic area. LV, left ventricle; RV, right ventricle. (*Lydia F. Roberts, Photographer.*)

1269

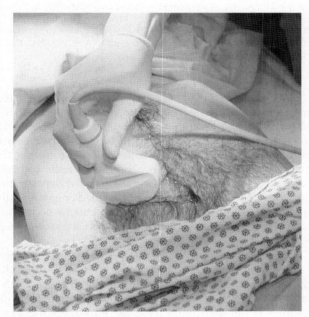

Figure 67–18 To obtain a parasternal view of the heart, place the probe adjacent to the left sternal border in the left second or third intercostal space. The patient's head is at the lower edge of the photograph. (*Lydia F. Roberts, Photographer.*)

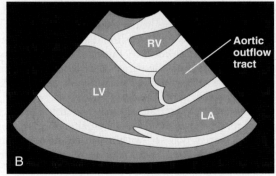

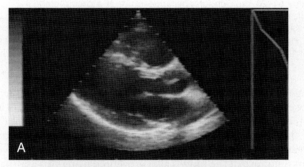

Figure 67–19 *A*, Sonographic appearance of a normal heart and pericardium obtained through the parasternal long-axis window. This view is an excellent imaging window for posterior effusions. *B*, Schematic representation. LA, left atrium; LV, left ventricle; RA, right atrium.

will reveal a hyperkinetic heart within a circumferential pericardial effusion, with diastolic collapse of the right-sided chambers. This reflects pressures within the pericardial space that are greater than the right ventricular filling pressure during diastole. The inferior vena cava will be dilated and not show respiratory variation or collapse when the patient is asked to "sniff."

Procedure and Technique

Tsang and coworkers[22] described the technique for US-guided pericardiocentesis in 1998. The ideal site of skin puncture is where the largest area of fluid accumulation is closest to the skin surface. On US, this is demonstrated by visualizing a

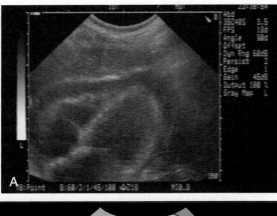

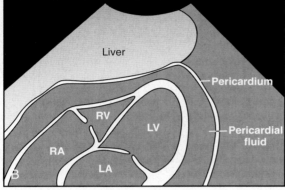

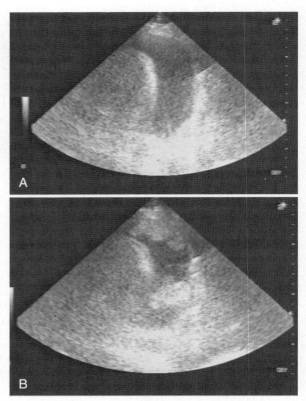

Figure 67–20 *A,* Sonographic appearance of a circumferential pericardial effusion obtained through the subxiphoid window. The effusion is seen as an anechoic stripe surrounding the heart. *B,* Schematic representation. LA, left atrium; LV, left ventricle; RA, right atrium; RV, right ventricle.

Figure 67–21 *A,* This image reveals a large pericardial effusion that is viewed from the subxiphoid window. The aspirating catheter can be seen within the effusion. *B,* Inject agitated saline through the catheter to confirm placement; and it can be seen as echogenic clouds within the pericardial sac that rapidly dissipate.

large anechoic area at the top of the screen (the body area closest to the probe) and usually corresponds to either the left anterior chest wall or, less often, the subcostal region (see Fig. 67–17). The anterior chest approach is usually preferred because it reduces the chances of injuring the liver. Inadvertent puncture of the lung is also prevented using this approach because air in the lung will not conduct sound waves and will prevent visualization of the heart when located immediately beneath the probe. The clinician should avoid choosing a site that might puncture either the internal mammary artery, which lies 3 to 5 cm from the parasternal border, or the neurovascular bundle located at the inferior rib border. Mark the best site with a sterile pen.

Confirm the needle trajectory and depth before skin puncture. Repositioning the patient will alter the position of the heart and pericardial sac within the chest and requires reassessment. Prepare the skin antiseptically (see Chapter 16, Pericardiocentesis) and place a sterile cover over the probe as described previously (see "General Approach"). If time permits, anesthetize the selected area with 1% to 2% lidocaine, using the superior border of the adjacent rib as a landmark. The needle should ideally have an over-the-needle sheath that allows the needle to be withdrawn after the pericardial space is entered. This helps avoid injury to the heart and other vital structures. A 16- to 18-gauge needle that is 5 to 8 cm in length is ideal. Attach a saline-filled syringe to the needle, and apply gentle aspiration while the needle is advanced. The US probe can remain on the chest wall immediately adjacent to the aspiration site or be removed after the fluid is localized.

Once the pericardial space is entered, inject agitated saline to confirm needle placement, particularly if the pericardial fluid is grossly bloody or there is any question concerning needle position. Prepare saline echo contrast medium by using two 5-mL syringes, one with saline and the other air, connected via a three-way stopcock to the needle catheter sheath. Saline in one syringe is rapidly injected between the syringes and then injected into the sheath. Sonographically monitor the entrance of the agitated saline into the pericardial space; it will appear as a brightly echogenic stream (Fig. 67–21).

After confirming needle placement, pass a wire through the sheath and place a dilator (6- to 8-Fr Cordis) over the wire. Remove the dilator and place an introducer sheath–dilator (6- to 8-Fr Cordis) over the wire. Then remove both the wire and the sheath and leave the introducer sheath in place. Insert the pigtail angiocatheter through the introducer sheath and aspirate fluid to confirm placement.[22]

Complications

The potential complications associated with US-guided pericardiocentesis are the same as those with blinded aspiration. The use of US will help minimize the risk of many of these complications, especially inadvertent puncture of the myocardium, epicardial vessels, and liver.[19,22] Additional complications uniquely associated with US are due to misinterpretation of the sonographic image. For example, epicardial fat pads are common in obese patients and can be misinterpreted as clot or fluid within the pericardial space.[19] Although they have a similar echogenicity, a number of important findings can aid in differentiating an epicardial fat pad from clot or fluid in the pericardial space.

First, the epicardial fat pad is an anterior structure. Clot in the anterior pericardial space suggests that the effusion is circumferential and, therefore, should also be seen in the dependent portion of the pericardial space. This is best demonstrated using the parasternal long-axis view. Alternatively, align the probe longitudinally so that the inferior vena cava is visualized as it enters the right atrium. The right side of the heart can be seen adjacent to the diaphragm, and blood or fluid within the pericardial sac can be readily identified (as long as it is not loculated).[19]

Second, the inferior vena cava should collapse when the patient sniffs; collapse of less than 50% indicates that there is increased intrathoracic pressure and possibly tamponade. Third, blood clotting is a dynamic process, with clots continuously forming and being broken down. If blood is present within the pericardial sac, careful examination may reveal amorphic clot (of medium echogenicity) within an anechoic (black) pericardial space. In the acutely ill patient, such as one with penetrating cardiac injury or myocardial rupture, clot is rarely present. Finally, and most importantly, an anterior fat pad should not cause collapse of the right ventricular free wall. If after careful examination doubt still exists as to the presence of an effusion, hemodynamically stable patients should have a formal echocardiogram or computed tomography (CT) scan performed.

Also remember that fluid within the pericardial space is not always pathologic. A small (<0.5- to 0.9-cm) effusion may not be clinically significant, and the sonographer should exercise caution in over-reading an effusion, particularly when the patient is hemodynamically stable. The patient who is hemodynamically compromised by a pericardial effusion should have a sizable effusion (the size can vary) with diastolic collapse of the right ventricular free wall, septal bulging, and dilatation of the hepatic veins and inferior vena cava. The heart is usually beating rapidly with hyperkinetic wall motion and may appear to swing to and fro within the pericardial sac.

TRANSVENOUS PACEMAKER INSERTION

Transvenous cardiac pacing can be life saving in patients with symptomatic bradycardia or heart block. Optimal conditions for placement of a transvenous pacemaker (TVPM) are the presence of forward flow to float the catheter into the right ventricle and fluoroscopy to guide placement. Unfortunately, ED patients who require emergent pacing are usually hemodynamically compromised by their rhythm and have poor forward flow. In the absence of flow, pacing wires may fail to pass through the tricuspid valve, coil in the right atrium, or fail to make contact with the right ventricular wall. Bedside sonography can readily demonstrate the passage of the pacing wire into the right ventricle, confirm contact with the right ventricular myocardium, and verify successful capture of the ventricle.

Background

Success rates for blind TVPM insertion with capture of the heart are highly variable, ranging from 10% to 90%.[23-25] Reasons for failure are often difficult to determine without adjunctive imaging, but malposition of the pacemaker wire is likely to play a role. US can not only readily demonstrate the passage of the pacing wire into the right ventricle but also confirm contact with the myocardium. Bedside sonography has been shown to be extremely helpful in guiding pacemaker wire placement and demonstrating capture in patients with hemodynamically significant bradyarrhythmias.[24,25] In addition, US can detect complications of blind pacemaker placement, including malposition of pacemaker wires and intraventricular septal perforation.[23]

Indications and Contraindications

Patients with symptomatic bradycardia or heart block for whom the placement of a TVPM is clinically indicated are excellent candidates for US-guided pacemaker wire placement. Although there are no absolute contraindications, the presence of obesity or hyperinflated lungs (e.g., patients with chronic obstructive pulmonary disease) may interfere with visualization of the heart and pacing wire.

Equipment

Use a 2- to 3.5-MHz probe to optimally visualize the right ventricle.

Acoustic Window

The subxiphoid view is usually the best imaging window for placing a TVPM because it provides excellent views of the four cardiac chambers, pericardial space, and overall cardiac wall motion. To obtain the subxiphoid view, place the probe at the left costal margin at the level of the xiphoid process with the beam aimed at the left shoulder (see Fig. 67–14).

Image Interpretation

Using the subxiphoid window, the structures closest to the probe will appear at the top of the display and include the liver, diaphragm, pericardial space, and right ventricle (see Fig. 67–15). Pacing catheter wires are highly reflective of sound waves and appear as bright linear echoes within the heart (Fig. 67–22).

Procedure and Technique

Once central venous access has been obtained (usually in the right internal jugular vein for TVPM insertion), place the probe at the left costal margin at the level of the xiphoid process with the beam aimed at the left shoulder. The pacing wire appears as a bright linear echo and can be tracked as it passes into the right ventricle and is placed in the right ventricular apex (see Fig. 67–22). Myocardial capture is readily demonstrated sonographically as rhythmic contractions of the heart at a rate determined by the pacemaker settings.

Complications

No complications specific to the use of US have been reported, although experience to date is limited.

THORACENTESIS

Clinicians typically have localized fluid within the pleural space by percussing the patient's chest and listening for

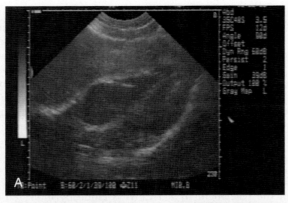

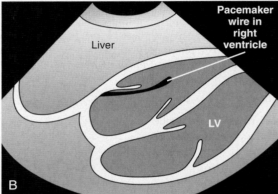

Figure 67–22 **Pacing wire within the right ventricle.** *A,* Sonographic image. *B,* Schematic representation. The right ventricle is seen through the subxiphoid window, which provides excellent views of the heart without interfering with pacemaker line placement. The pacemaker wire is seen as a brightly echogenic structure within the right ventricle. LV, left ventricle.

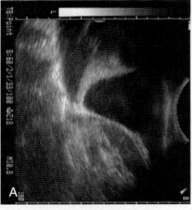

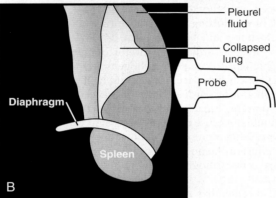

Figure 67–23 Sonographic appearance (*A*) and schematic representation (*B*) of a pleural effusion. Fluid will appear as an anechoic area over the brightly echogenic diaphragm. The collapsed lung can usually be seen as a wedge-shaped echogenic structure moving with respirations within the fluid. Note that the sonographic image has been rotated 90° clockwise to match the schematic drawing.

dullness. This can be unreliable and inexact, particularly in obese or very muscular patients. US is an excellent tool for identification and aspiration of pleural effusions, and can detect even small amounts of fluid within the pleural space. It has been shown to be at least comparable, and in some studies superior, to chest radiography in the detection of pleural fluid.[26–30] US offers several advantages in the ED management of pleural effusions. The examination is rapid, it can be performed at the bedside with suboptimal patient positioning, and percutaneous insertion of the needle is not blind. This reduces the risk of inadvertent puncture of a vessel, a lung, or subdiaphragmatic organs.

Background

The use of US to identify the presence of pleural fluid and guide aspiration is not new, and has become routine for many pulmonary and critical care practitioners managing pleural effusions. Prior to the use of US, complications associated with blind thoracentesis included pneumothorax, dry aspiration, inadvertent liver or splenic lacerations, and subcutaneous hematoma. These complications are significantly reduced when performed under sonographic guidance.[30,31] In addition, US can readily distinguish between tissue masses and fluid in patients with chest radiographs that show a "white lung" or opacifications that do not layer freely.

Indications and Contraindications

Any patient with a suspected pleural effusion is a potential candidate for sonographic imaging. Patients who are at greater risk for complications such as those with small effusions, underlying malignancies, or for whom there are concerns regarding whether the fluid is free flowing are ideal candidates. There are no absolute contraindications to the use of US. However, the study may be limited when there is subcutaneous emphysema or morbid obesity.

Equipment

A 3.5- to 5.0-MHz probe can readily identify most pleural effusions.

Image Interpretation

In the normal chest, the interface between the air-filled lung and the visceral pleura is highly reflective and blocks further transmission of sound waves into the chest. The image on the screen will appear as a uniform pattern of bright echoes, which are due to reverberation artifacts. Free fluid within the pleural space will appear as an anechoic area bounded inferoposteriorly by the brightly echogenic diaphragm (Fig. 67–23). The atelectatic lung will appear to flap within the pleural fluid

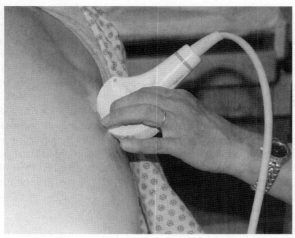

Figure 67–24 Probe positioning for identification of a pleural effusion. Place the probe longitudinally over the lateral or posterior chest wall on the side of the suspected effusion. Move the probe inferiorly to identify the kidney, liver or spleen, and diaphragm. *(Lydia F. Roberts, Photographer.)*

with respiratory efforts. Echogenic material within the pleural fluid may indicate clotted blood or pus depending on the underlying etiology. Effusions due to chronic inflammatory conditions or malignancy may be loculated or contain septations.[31,32]

Procedure and Technique

All patients should have a chest radiograph before starting the procedure, which will demonstrate the presence and general location (e.g., left or right pleural space) of the fluid. The optimal position for thoracentesis is to have the patient sit upright with her or his arms resting on a bedside table. This will allow fluid to collect in a dependent position. Position the probe on the chest wall at the midaxillary line, above either the spleen or the liver (Fig. 67–24). The lung should be seen moving freely within the fluid as the patient breathes. The diaphragm must be visualized to avoid puncture of the liver or spleen. Accomplished by first locating the kidney, which is usually readily identified. Move the probe superiorly to identify the diaphragm. The pleural fluid will be seen above the diaphragm (see Fig. 67–23). For large effusions, advance the thoracentesis needle over the rib that is immediately adjacent to the fluid. If the fluid pocket is small, perform the aspiration under directed sonographic guidance by covering the transducer with a sterile cover (see "General Approach") and puncturing the chest wall directly alongside the transducer.

Complications

Although rare, complications directly related to use of US may occur owing to misinterpretation of the images or failure to identify free-flowing fluid within the pleural space. Echogenic material within the pleural fluid can suggest the presence of clot, pus, tumor, and even bowel depending on the sonographic appearance. Clot will appear as globules that typically migrate to the most dependent area of the effusions and may appear to wave within the fluid as the patient breathes. Pus will layer in the most dependent area and appears as an echogenic base upon which the fluid rests. Solid masses adhere

to the pleura, do not move with respirations, and do not sink to the most dependent region. Bowel has a distinct sonographic appearance, a brightly echogenic border (seen in cross-section) surrounding a hypoechoic internal lumen, and can be readily identified when peristalsis is observed.

Fluid contained within cysts, masses, or loculations can be confused with free fluid in the pleural space. The best way to differentiate the two is to visualize the borders of the fluid. Fluid located in the pleural space is bounded by pleural creases and reflections, giving it sharply angled edges. In contrast, fluid contained within a cyst, mass, or loculation will have rounded borders. If there is any doubt as to the location or free movement of the fluid, obtain a CT scan of the chest to clarify the anatomy.

PARACENTESIS

US is a very sensitive tool for identification of fluid within the peritoneal cavity and has virtually replaced diagnostic peritoneal lavage in patients with traumatic injuries and suspected hemoperitoneum.[33] In such patients, demonstration of free fluid is presumed to be blood and most patients will subsequently undergo exploratory laparotomy or CT scanning. Patients requiring paracentesis in the ED usually have atraumatic peritoneal fluid collections. The benefits of paracentesis for these individuals include diagnosis of spontaneous bacterial peritonitis, differentiation of transudative from exudative effusions, and therapeutic aspirations for patients with large amounts of ascitic fluid.

Background

US is the diagnostic study of choice for demonstration of intraperitoneal fluid. The primary use in the ED is for identification of patients with intraperitoneal blood secondary to both blunt and penetrating trauma.[33–37] Demonstration of free fluid in these patients usually leads to exploratory laparotomy or CT scanning to further delineate the extent of intra-abdominal injury and rarely results in paracentesis. Patients requiring paracentesis in the ED are generally those with nontraumatic fluid collections requiring either a diagnostic or a therapeutic tap. Many of these patients have end-stage liver disease or underlying malignancy.

Although relatively rare, intraperitoneal hemorrhage, abdominal wall hematomas, and bowel perforation are reported complications of blind paracentesis. US can minimize these risks by identifying the largest pocket of readily accessible fluid. In addition, US will identify the presence of other abnormalities mistakenly thought to be ascitic fluid (e.g., cystic mass, ventral hernia) and has been shown to significantly increase the success rates of paracentesis in the ED.[38]

Indications and Contraindications

Specific indications for sonographic imaging include obese patients and those with prior abdominal surgeries, small fluid collections, failed blind aspirations, and no prior history of ascites. US is the study of choice to determine the presence of intraperitoneal fluid, estimate the size of the collection, and identify the best site for aspiration. Ascitic fluid in patients with prior abdominal surgeries may be loculated, and US can identify areas of free-flowing fluid. There are no specific contraindications to the use of US.

Equipment

A 3.5- to 5.0-MHz probe can readily identify free fluid within the peritoneal cavity.

Image Interpretation

Free fluid will appear as an anechoic, black, sharp-edged collection in the most dependent portion of the peritoneal cavity. In contrast to the usual snowstorm appearance created by the air-filled loops of bowel, large amounts of fluid will appear to fill the peritoneal cavity and floating loops of bowel can be clearly seen outlined by the fluid (Fig. 67–25). Blood clots, if present, will layer or appear as fronds floating within the fluid. Structures within the peritoneal cavity, particularly bowel and bladder, are easily identified and avoided during needle aspiration.

Procedure and Technique

Image the patient in either the supine or reverse Trendelenburg position to allow flow of smaller amounts of fluid into the pelvis. Clean and drape the abdominal wall and prepare the probe as described earlier (see "General Approach"). A

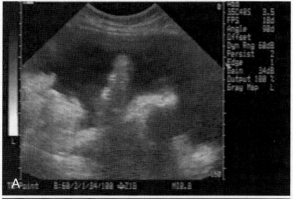

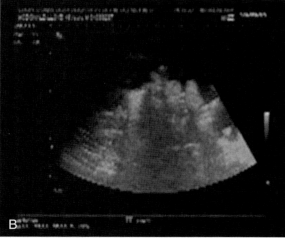

Figure 67–25 *A,* Sonographic appearance of peritoneal free fluid. Fluid will appear as a large anechoic area with loops of bowel floating freely. The optimal area for needle insertion is where there is a large pocket of fluid just under the skin surface, closest to the probe. *B,* In this view, the aspirating needle can be seen as a brightly echogenic dot within the ascitic fluid.

full bladder can be confused with an intraperitoneal fluid collection; it should be emptied before the procedure. Identify the liver, spleen, bladder, and loops of bowel to avoid inadvertent puncture. For the best result, locate the largest pocket of free fluid. This is usually found in the lower quadrant of the abdomen and will appear as a black, anechoic area.

When performing the procedure alone, identify a site directly over the area of the largest fluid collection and mark it with a sterile marking pen. Then perform paracentesis, carefully avoiding the bladder and inferior epigastric arteries. Alternatively, if an assistant is available, keep the US probe on the abdominal wall and visualize needle entry into the fluid collection on the monitor.

Complications

Complications directly related to the use of US are rare and likely to be due to misinterpretation of the images. A full bladder or large cystic masses within the abdomen (e.g., ovarian) may be confused with intraperitoneal fluid. To avoid this confusion, remember that ascitic fluid will have an irregular appearance superiorly owing to bowel indentation, whereas fluid in the bladder or in a cyst will have a smooth curved surface all the way around. In addition, free intraperitoneal fluid will collect dependently and will have a sharp-edged appearance when bounded by peritoneal reflections. In contrast, fluid contained in the bladder or cyst will have rounded edges.

JOINT ASPIRATION

Joint pain is a common complaint in the ED, and identification of fluid within the joint space has important implications for both diagnosis and treatment. For the patient presenting with a warm, swollen joint, it is often difficult to differentiate cellulitis, soft tissue abscess, or septic/inflammatory arthritis by physical examination alone. US has been widely used by rheumatologists as an adjunct to their clinical examination to define joint and synovial pathology and monitor response to treatment.[39,40] In the hands of the emergency clinician, it can aid in identification of clinically significant fluid within the joint, determine extra-articular sources of pain, and guide aspiration of joint spaces.

Background

US can demonstrate the presence of intra-articular fluid in any joint space that has a sonographic "window," in particular the hip, shoulder, knee, ankle, and wrist.[41-45] Although some joints, such as the knee, are readily aspirated using the blind approach, other joints are often difficult to aspirate successfully and might require multiple attempts. US will not only confirm the presence of fluid, which in itself is of clinical value, but can also identify the optimal site for joint aspiration.

Additional benefits to sonographic imaging of the joints include characterization of the joint fluid and identification of extra-articular sources of pain. When no fluid is seen within the joint space and the patient has pain and/or swelling, it can be assumed that the source of discomfort is outside the joint space (e.g., involving skin, tendon, bone, ligament, or extra-articular bursa). In experienced hands, US can also diagnose disease of the periarticular tissues.[41]

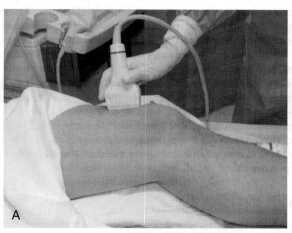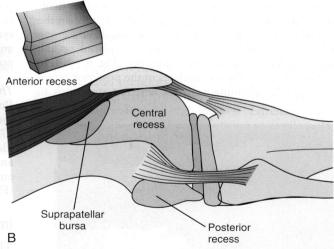

Figure 67–26 *A,* Probe positioning for sonographic imaging of the suprapatella bursa. Place the probe in the longitudinal position superior to the patella. After identifying fluid within the bursa, rotate the probe transversely to identify the medial and lateral extent of the fluid. *B,* Schematic representation. *(A, Lydia F. Roberts, Photographer.)*

Indications and Contraindications

Sonographic examination of the joint is indicated whenever identification of fluid within the joint space is clinically relevant. This includes patients presenting with acute joint pain due to trauma and those with suspected inflammatory or infectious arthritis and nontraumatic hemarthrosis, particularly associated with coagulopathic states. There are no reported contraindications to the use of US.

Equipment

The most commonly utilized probe for assessment of the joint space is a high-frequency linear array probe (7.5–10 MHz).

Acoustic Windows

A detailed discussion of the sonographic anatomy of all joints is beyond the scope of this section. The knee, shoulder, and ankle are most often involved in traumatic and inflammatory conditions, and the sonographic windows for these joints are discussed.

The Knee

Knee effusions are often difficult to reliably identify on physical examination alone, particularly when the patient is obese or severe pain limits the examination. Flex the knee (~20°) and place a roll behind the popliteal fossa. Begin the anterior views of the knee with a longitudinal scan above the patella, which is the bony landmark for imaging the suprapatellar bursa.[41,43] The suprapatellar bursa communicates with the knee joint, extending approximately 6 cm above the patella just deep to the quadriceps tendon (Fig. 67–26). Then view the medial and lateral recesses of the knee (extensions of the suprapatellar bursa) in longitudinal and transverse orientation. In a normal joint, the bursa is a thin hypoechoic line no more than 2 mm thick. Fluid within the bursa will appear as an anechoic stripe beneath the quadriceps tendon[41,44] (Fig. 67–27). Extra-articular fluid commonly located in the prepatellar bursa can also be readily identified as a fluid collection anterior to the patella.

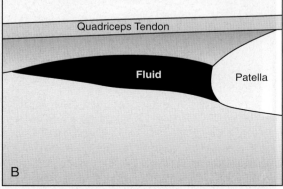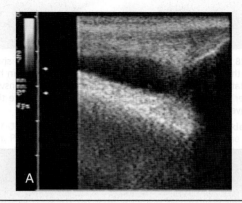

Figure 67–27   Sonographic appearance of a suprapatellar effusion. *A,* Fluid will appear as an anechoic area superior to the patella and beneath the quadriceps tendon. *B,* Schematic representation.

The Shoulder

The shoulder joint can be imaged using anterior or posterior windows. The anterior window is the easier of the two approaches to acquire and consists of longitudinal and transverse scans of the long head of the biceps tendon (Fig. 67–28). To image through the anterior window, place the patient in the sitting position with the elbow adducted and the hand on the affected side positioned palm-up. The biceps tendon has a synovial sheath, an extracapsular extension of the joint

BLADDER ASPIRATION

Needle aspiration of the bladder may be required when a patient, usually an infant, is unable to provide a sterile urine specimen. The bladder is a superficial structure that is readily identified with US. The role of US is to localize the bladder, demonstrate that the bladder is full, and guide needle aspiration.[57,58] A secondary role of bladder sonography is to assess bladder volume, which may be particularly helpful when the patient is unable to provide a spontaneous urine sample and the differential diagnosis includes dehydration versus bladder outlet obstruction.[59]

Background

The approach to blind suprapubic bladder aspiration requires localization of the bladder by percussion and palpitation. Although relatively straightforward in most children and adults, it may be difficult in infants in whom the bladder is an intra-abdominal organ and in children who are agitated or volume depleted or have abdominal distention. US can help locate the bladder, estimate bladder volumes, and guide suprapubic aspiration.[57–59] Studies have shown that US guidance increases the likelihood of successful bladder aspiration. In a study of 140 male infants younger than 2 years, Ozkan and associates[58] demonstrated a 90% success rate in the US-guided group compared with 64% (P < .05) in the blind aspiration group. In addition, the US group required fewer attempts. A similar study evaluated the impact of bedside US on bladder aspiration in 59 infants.[60] Aspiration was successful on the first attempt in 26 of 28 patients (93%) with US guidance, but in only 13 of 21 patients (62%) undergoing blind aspiration.[60] The authors of these studies found that complications were rare in both the experimental and the control groups.

Indications and Contraindications

US-guided aspiration is indicated in the infant, child, or adult for whom blind aspiration is unsuccessful or in whom localization of the bladder may be difficult owing to dehydration or abdominal distention. In the child who is agitated, clear localization of the bladder may facilitate the speed and success of the procedure. Adult patients with prior abdominal surgery or irradiation may have adhesions of the bowel to the bladder and may also benefit from sonographic guidance. US can also be used to guide placement of a cystostomy tubes in adults. There are no contraindications specific to the use of US.

Equipment

A 5-MHz curvilinear probe is usually adequate for pediatric patients. A lower-frequency (i.e., 3.5-MHz) probe should be used for adults.

Image Interpretation

The bladder should be full for best results. Place the probe just above the pubic symphysis and image the bladder in both the longitudinal and the transverse planes. The bladder will appear as an anechoic structure immediately beneath the skin surface, with a characteristic rhomboid appearance on transverse view (Fig. 67–35).

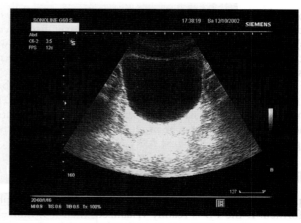

Figure 67–35 Sonographic appearance of the bladder in transverse view. The bladder will appear as an anechoic structure immediately beneath the skin surface, with a characteristic rhomboid appearance on transverse view.

Procedure and Technique

Prepare and position the patient and ready the probe with a sterile cover and acoustic gel as described previously (see "General Approach"). Puncture the skin immediately above the portion of the bladder closest to the skin surface (at the top of the imaging screen). Either mark the site with a sterile pen before skin puncture or leave the probe to guide aspiration.

Complications

Complications of bladder aspiration include viscous perforation, microhematuria, and unsuccessful aspiration. Complications directly related to the use of US are rare, but might occur if aspiration is attempted and the bladder is not full or if there is free fluid in the peritoneal cavity that is mistaken for urine in the bladder. The outlines of the bladder wall may be difficult to identify when there is peritoneal fluid, particularly if the fluid is loculated. In general, bladder fluid has a curved outline, whereas fluid within the peritoneal cavity will be indented by loops of free-floating bowel.

FLUID COLLECTIONS AND CUTANEOUS ABSCESSES

US is a very useful adjunct for identification of subcutaneous masses. It can readily differentiate solid from fluid-filled masses, estimate the size and depth of the fluid collection, and demonstrate the presence of septations or FBs.[51,61] US is particularly helpful when confronted by a patient with a mass in whom aspiration is "limited" or unsuccessful,[62] by the substance-abusing patient with an antecubital "mass" that may be an abscess or fistula, or by a restless child with a suspected peritonsillar abscess. US can also provide critical information regarding the extent of the collection and its proximity to important structures such as blood vessels and vital organs.

Background

US is an important adjunct to the clinical assessment of soft tissue collections, which include subcutaneous abscesses, hematomas, and solid tumors. It can identify the presence of

FBs that might serve as a nidus for infection and the location of adjacent structures that should be avoided during attempted drainage.

Indications and Contraindications

Image any subcutaneous mass when demonstration of a fluid collection is of clinical significance. It is particularly important when the collection is near vital structures, the extent of the collection is difficult to assess owing to location or body habitus, and prior attempts at aspiration have been unsuccessful. There are no contraindications to the use of US for this purpose.

Equipment

The depth and size of the collection will determine optimal probe selection. The vast majority of percutaneous aspirations and/or drainages are performed on relatively superficial "masses," which are best seen with higher-frequency (e.g., 7.0- to 10.0-MHz) linear probes, whereas large or deep collections are better imaged with lower-frequency (e.g., 3.5- to 5.0-MHz) probes.

Acoustic Window

In most cases, place the probe directly over the mass or fluid collection being evaluated. Image in both the longitudinal and the transverse planes to demonstrate the full depth and extent of the fluid collection or mass.

A water bath can be a useful adjunct to imaging areas that are exquisitely painful to touch, are very superficial, or have an uneven imaging surface. When imaging underwater, the probe does not have to touch the patient, hence reducing pain and eliminating contact issues encountered with uneven surfaces. In addition, very superficial structures can often be visualized more clearly owing to the acoustic window provided by the surrounding water bath.[63,64]

To use this acoustic window, place the extremity under water and hold the probe close to the skin surface. The distance between the probe and the skin surface is usually less than 1 cm and can be adjusted to optimize image quality.

Image Interpretation

In the early stages of abscess formation, the affected tissue will contain an increased amount of fluid, which will appear as horizontal bands of hypoechoic or anechoic areas.[61] As the abscess forms, the central area liquefies and the surrounding tissue forms a wall of scar tissue. Sonographically, an abscess appears as a discrete anechoic area often surrounded by a brightly reflective wall (Fig. 67–36). The fluid will usually be black, but will often contain scattered echoes representing purulent material or necrotic debris. The fluid may contain septations, which appear as echogenic walls traversing the fluid cavity.

Procedure and Technique

Identify surrounding structures, particularly blood vessels, before aspiration or incision and drainage. The use of Doppler (either color-flow or power) to demonstrate absence of flow within the collection can add an additional measure of safety (but is not required). Determine the depth of the collection

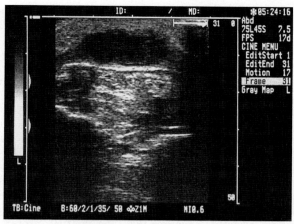

Figure 67–36 **Sonographic appearance of a subcutaneous fluid collection.** An abscess appears as a discrete anechoic area that may be surrounded by a brightly reflective wall. The fluid will be anechoic, but will often contain scattered echoes representing purulent material or necrotic debris. The fluid may also contain septations, which appear as echogenic walls traversing the fluid cavity.

by using the depth markers on the right side of the monitor screen.

When aspirating a soft tissue mass, mark the puncture site with a sterile pen and perform the aspiration blindly. Alternatively, have an assistant hold the sterilely prepared probe over the mass during the aspiration attempt. The needle will appear as a brightly echogenic structure entering the fluid-filled cavity. When performing abscess incision and drainage, mark the incision site with a pen and remove the probe from the skin. Then perform incision and drainage.

Complications

Although image interpretation is usually straightforward, complications may occur owing to misinterpretation of like images. Cellulitic areas will have a heterogeneous, layered appearance (alternating bands of anechoic and echogenic layers) that may be mistaken for a discrete fluid collection. In contrast, the majority of abscesses will not appear as a simple anechoic collection. This is due to the presence of pus and/or sebaceous material within the abscess cavity, which create echogenic shadows. When in doubt, look for the brightly echogenic capsule that outlines the borders of an abscess cavity.

Blood vessels, when imaged in the transverse plane, can appear as a cystic fluid collection, undermining the importance of imaging the collection in both the longitudinal and the transverse planes and, if available, the liberal use of color-flow or Doppler. This is especially important when the differential diagnosis includes a vascular aneurysm. Also remember that fluid collections do not always indicate an abscess and may be Baker's cysts, bursae, or hematomas. Always exercise clinical judgment during image interpretation.

PERITONSILLAR ABSCESS

The diagnosis of peritonsillar abscess is usually based on clinical findings, and both the diagnosis and the treatment depend on needle aspiration of purulent material. Intraoral US can be a very useful adjunct in identifying a fluid collection and guiding aspiration.

Background

Emergency clinicians and otolaryngologists have used intra-oral US to improve the diagnosis and management of peritonsillar abscesses.[65,66] When blind aspiration of a suspected peritonsillar abscess is unsuccessful, it is often not clear whether this is due to poor technique or a lack of fluid. Indeed, distinguishing peritonsillar abscess from cellulitis is difficult, and patients without fluid may be subjected to repeated unsuccessful attempts at aspiration. US can be used to identify the presence of peritonsillar fluid collections, determine the depth and size of the collection, and locate important adjacent structures (e.g., the internal carotid). A small case series of patients with suspected peritonsillar abscess showed that emergency clinicians were able to diagnose 100% of all true abscesses.[66]

Indications and Contraindications

US is extremely helpful in managing patients in whom the diagnosis of peritonsillar abscess is not clear, such as those with bilateral findings or early abscess formation. Early in the course of infection, there may be trismus and distortion of peritonsillar anatomy without frank bulging, uvular deviation, restricted palatal movement, and/or voice alteration. Patients who have undergone repeated attempts at aspiration without success are also ideal candidates to determine if there is truly a fluid collection. Finally, those patients for whom aspiration is expected to be difficult owing to inability to open their mouths or fully cooperate with the procedure will often benefit from identifying the exact location of the abscess. There are no specific contraindications to using US to manage peritonsillar abscesses.

Equipment

A dedicated intraoral probe is the optimal tool to use for this procedure, but is often unavailable in the ED. The high-frequency intracavitary probe is a reasonable alternative.

Image Interpretation

A peritonsillar abscess will appear as a heterogeneous collection usually bounded by a brightly echogenic capsule surrounding a relatively hypoechoic center. Estimate the size and depth of the collection from the image by measuring the distance from the skin surface/probe interface to the center of the collection (Fig. 67–37).

Procedure and Technique

If an intracavitary probe is used, cover it with a layer of gel and a probe cover. With the patient sitting up, insert the probe into the mouth and direct it to the side of the suspected abscess. It is often helpful to ask the patient to insert the probe

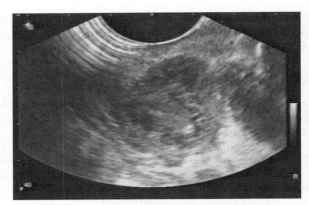

Figure 67–37 **Sonographic image of a peritonsillar abscess.** The abscess is seen as a discrete collection of hypoechoic material surrounded by an echogenic capsule.

himself or herself, which relieves anxiety and the chance of gagging.

Once a fluid collection is identified, determine the size and depth of the collection and choose the appropriate needle length. The probe is usually removed before aspiration because of the patient's limited ability to fully open her or his mouth. Once the fluid collection is identified, proceed with aspiration.

Complications

Complications directly due to the use of US are rare and usually due to misinterpretation of the sonographic images, which were discussed in the previous section.

SUMMARY

US has become a valuable adjunct to the performance of a wide range of procedures in the ED. The principles and approaches described in this chapter can be applied to most procedures involving percutaneous cannulation or aspiration of a fluid-filled body cavity. The role of US includes identifying and then localizing (e.g., size and depth) the structure of interest; delineating the surrounding anatomy and identifying the presence of anatomic variants or other pathologic conditions; and guiding the placement of needles, catheters, and wires. The primary goal of US is to improve the safety and efficiency of the procedure.

Although sonography is now within the scope of practice of emergency clinicians, the individual practitioner must take care to understand the limitations of the sonographic examination and obtain appropriate training before using it to guide clinical practice. In addition, use nonemergency clinician-sonographers to provide sonographic guidance for procedures when no skilled sonographer is in the ED or when concerns exist with the examination performance or interpretation.

 REFERENCES CAN BE FOUND ON EXPERT CONSULT

CHAPTER 68

Bedside Laboratory and Microbiologic Procedures

Anthony J. Dean and David C. Lee

ASSESSMENT OF URINE

Obtaining a Urine Specimen

Several methods are available for obtaining a urine specimen. These can be listed in order of increasingly precise collection techniques, which tend to come at the cost of increasing difficulty and/or patient discomfort:

1. *Random voided*: Any specimen provided by the patient.
2. *Midstream voided*: No skin preparation; container placed in urinary stream 2 to 3 seconds after the initiation of micturition.
3. *Clean catch*: Same as item 1, with antiseptic cleansing of the urethral area. In males, retract the prepuce (the labia in females) and cleanse the meatus in an anterior to posterior direction using three swabs soaked in povidone-iodine (or some other antiseptic solution). For female patients who are physically capable, ideally have the patient sit astride a toilet, facing backward. This helps to separate the labia and position the cup for specimen collection.
4. *Midstream clean catch (MSCC)*: Cleanse as in item 3, with midstream collection as in item 2.
5. *Catheterized*: Obtained from a newly placed catheter.
6. *Suprapubic aspiration (SPA)*: see Chapter 55, Urologic Procedures.

The low levels of bacteriuria induced in 2% to 8% of patients after straight catheterization are generally below the threshold that defines the presence of urinary tract infection (UTI). Catheterization does cause minor local injury, as reflected by low-level hematuria in 15% of patients.[1] Some clinicians continue to advocate SPA for neonates when accurate diagnosis is essential and the risk of infection must be minimized. Both SPA (see Chapter 55, Urologic Procedures) and catheterization have an approximately 25% "failure rate" owing to an empty bladder.[2] This problem, as well as associated complications, can be avoided by a bedside ultrasound performed before the procedure.[2,3] SPA may spuriously lower leukocyte or bacterial colony counts owing to the necessity of filling the bladder before the procedure is performed. A study in infants demonstrated the discomfort of SPA to be greater than that of catheterization,[4] although perhaps surprisingly, older men who underwent both catheterization and SPA strongly preferred the latter.

Recommendations for Urine Collection

Since the mid-1950s, each technique has had its proponents and opponents. In choosing a method for obtaining a urine specimen, the disease under consideration influences both the choice of specimen collection method and the interpretation of the results. For the purposes of this discussion, the diagnostic categories can broadly be divided into infectious and noninfectious. With the exception of testing for blood, most of the noninfectious tests (e.g., ketones, glucose, bilirubin, protein) are not affected by collection method. Because detection of infection is the most common purpose of urine testing in emergency practice, this is considered first.

UTIs are either symptomatic or asymptomatic. The group to which a patient belongs is the first step in determining the collection method (Fig. 68–1). This is because in *symptomatic* UTI, extremely low levels of bacteriuria (10^2 colony-forming units [CFU]/mL) and pyuria are of clinical significance.[5] This fact has been obscured by studies on *asymptomatic* patients showing that the threshold for "significant bacteriuria" is 10^5 CFU/mL or greater. Another misconception is that a contaminated specimen is signaled by isolation of multiple pathogens. In fact, up to 50% of symptomatic women may have polymicrobial infections.[5] Although several studies have failed to demonstrate a statistical difference in contamination rates with less stringent urine collection techniques, most studies show trends in favor of more meticulous and/or invasive collection methods.[6] These methods are likely to provide more reliable information in the *symptomatic* group in whom the margin of error for the test is narrower.

At first glance, the issue of whether a patient is "symptomatic" might appear trivial, but the clinical practice of checking for UTI in most patients with any kind of abdominal pain has important implications. Studies of urine collection and testing in "symptomatic" patients focus on the classic signs and symptoms of UTI (e.g., urgency, frequency, dysuria, flank pain, costovertebral angle tenderness) and do not include patients with nonspecific abdominal pain. Whether undifferentiated abdominal pain or fever constitute "symptoms" of UTI has never been studied, and how to apply the results of studies done on patients with classic symptoms to those with nonspecific symptoms is unclear.[7] Certainly, patients with classic symptoms need the most careful urine collection method practicable because they have the most riding on the outcome of the test, whether it be positive or negative. To this group of patients might be added those with systemic signs of infection (e.g., fever and chills) who are unable to accurately report on symptoms[7] and patients in whom failure to diagnose asymptomatic bacteriuria would be potentially dangerous (e.g., the immunocompromised, neonates and infants, pregnant patients, diabetics) or for whom urine cultures are going to be necessary because of a history of relapsing, recurrent, complicated, or childhood UTI.[7]

In cooperative, motivated males and females with symptoms of uncomplicated lower UTI or pyelonephritis who are capable of diligently performing the necessary maneuvers, an MSCC specimen is as accurate as a catheterized specimen, especially when the possibility of urethral and/or prostatic trauma and patient discomfort are considered. In patients unable to provide an MSCC specimen, a catheterized specimen is usually warranted.

If no symptoms of UTI are present, the urine examination can be considered as a "screening" test. In the asymptomatic patient, routine screening for bacteriuria is unwarranted in all but two clinical situations: pregnant women and all patients for whom urologic surgery has been scheduled.[8] If only a urine culture is to be performed, some would argue that any spontaneously voided specimen would suffice, because the diagnosis of asymptomatic bacteriuria depends on 10^5 CFU or greater of a single pathogen per milliliter of

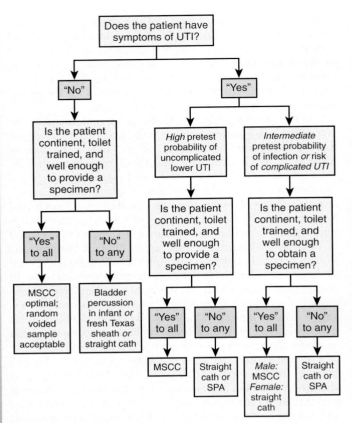

Figure 68–1 Algorithm for deciding method of obtaining urine specimen for evaluation of possible urinary tract infection. MSCC, midstream clean catch; SPA, suprapubic aspiration; UTI, urinary tract infection.

urine, and with such criteria, contaminants are usually easily identified.[6] However, performing cultures in all such patients is prohibitively costly, so that dipstick and/or urinalysis (UA) is commonly used for screening. With these tests, contamination by bacteria, leukocytes, or erythrocytes can still cause diagnostic confusion. Thus, the advantages of a less contaminated specimen are worth the minimal extra effort of asking the patient to provide an MSCC sample. The approach presented in Figure 68–1 covers the vast majority of situations. A few circumstances and techniques deserve special mention.

Bladder Percussion and the Midstream Specimen in Infant Males

The emergency clinician is familiar with how frequently a urine stream is generated in infants who are confronted by the alarming emergency department (ED) environment and a cold stethoscope. Rather than wasting a potentially perfect MSCC specimen on a laboratory coat, with an ensuing delay in obtaining urine, the clinician can exploit the situation by approaching an infant with an open sterile urine container in hand in case of spontaneous micturition. The process is facilitated with the application of cold povidone-iodine to the genitalia. Such an approach has been shown to generate a urine sample in a median time of 10 minutes.[9] This is less than the typical time needed for straight catheterization or SPA, especially because it can be performed concomitant with the history and physical examination and it circumvents an invasive procedure. If the urine specimen is not immediately

forthcoming, instruct a parent to catch the specimen in the sterile container, freeing up ED staff for other tasks.

Two techniques to actively induce voiding in infants have been described. The first, which is useful in newborns, exploits the Perez reflex.[10] After cleansing the genitalia, hold the infant in one hand while the paraspinal muscles are stroked, cephalad to caudad. This causes extension of the back and flexion of the hips and induces micturition in less than 5 minutes in the majority of cases.[10] The second technique is known as "bladder tapping." After urethral cleansing, if there is still no urine, tap two fingers on the suprapubic area at a rate of approximately once per second for a full minute, followed by a minute's rest. Then repeat the cycle until urine is produced. The mean time before the production of urine is about 5 minutes. This technique, although not practicable for the staff in a busy ED, can provide an infant's parents with a task that invests them in the clinical process.

Bag Collection in Non–Toilet-Trained Children

The incidence of unsuspected UTI in the febrile neonate or infant is about 5%.[11] Because a true UTI in an infant or child requires a subsequent evaluation for urinary tract pathology and the disease may produce significant morbidity (e.g., hypertension, renal disease), one must be certain of the presence or absence of infection in this subgroup. Numerous studies have demonstrated the disutility of urine specimens obtained *for culture* from a collection bag stuck to an infant's perineum.[10,12,13] However, bag specimens may be more sensitive than catheter specimens when used for UA and/or microscopy to identify infection in children at low or moderate risk of UTI.[14] Thus, in this group, the current recommendation is screening UA and/or microscopy of a bag specimen.[15,16] If this is negative, UTI is ruled out; if positive (leukocyte esterase [LE] or nitrites or >5 white blood cells [WBCs]/high-power field [HPF] on spun urine or bacteria on unspun Gram stain specimen), follow it with catheterization and culture, with treatment usually pending culture results.[12,15,16] If a urine specimen is needed solely for chemical analysis (e.g., glucose, ketones, specific gravity), a bag specimen will suffice.

Urine Specimens from Patients with Chronic Urinary Drainage Systems

All urinary catheters quickly become colonized with bacteria; it simply cannot be prevented. Therefore, urine obtained from any part of a chronic urinary drainage system is highly inaccurate for bacteriologic purposes and will demonstrate infection. If UTI is suspected, insert a new catheter and subsequently obtain fresh bladder urine specimens.[17] A small study advocating replacement of a chronically applied "Texas sheath" catheter with a fresh one was performed on subjects who did not have symptoms of UTI. Such a method might be sufficiently accurate for screening of asymptomatic patients, but use a Foley catheter to obtain urine from patients with sheath catheters who have signs or symptoms of acute UTI.

Urine Dipstick

Urine dipstick tests are available to test for 10 separate parameters. The unassuming appearance and commonplace use of the urine dipstick might lead one to mistakenly underestimate its technical sophistication. Because each colored square on a urine dipstick involves a complex assay, it is essential to *meticulously follow the manufacturer's instructions for storage and use.*[18] If the top of the container is off, the dipsticks quickly lose accuracy. Even with optimal storage and testing conditions, the false-negative and false-positive rates of these tests are problematic. In addition, most of the tests are susceptible to interference from a variety of substances (Table 68–1).

Method

Urine specimens should be tested as soon as possible after they are collected. If urine has been standing, it should be stirred or shaken well, because cells rapidly sink in a container. Completely immerse the test strip for 1 second or less. Draw the edge of the strip along the rim of the specimen container; it can also be lightly tapped to remove excess urine,

thus avoiding mixing of the reagents between different test patches. Hold the strip horizontally or place it on a clean gauze pad until the recommended time has elapsed. Most strips are designed so that all of the tests can be read together after 1 to 2 minutes. The proper method of using the dipstick is demonstrated in Figure 68–2.

Interpretation

Glucose. The urine glucose test is normally negative. Urine glucose testing has limited usefulness in quantitative testing because the serum glucose level at which spillage occurs varies (although in most patients it starts at between

TABLE 68–1 Overview of Urine Dipstick Tests

Test	Sources of Error and Artifact	Comments
Glucose	**False positive** with peroxide and hypochlorite, ketonuria, levodopa, dipstick exposed to air. **False negative** with ascorbate, ketones, uric acid, and high specific gravity.	Hypothermia may cause glycosuria despite systemic *hypoglycemia.*
Ketones	**False positive** with ascorbate, acidic urine, high specific gravity, levodopa, valproate, pyridium, *N*-acetyl cysteine, high-protein diet, phenylketones, phthalein compounds.	Very susceptible to deterioration with humidity and delay in analysis, causing false negative.
Nitrites	**False positive** with pyridium, contamination, dipstick exposed to air. **False negative** with high specific gravity, ascorbate, high urobilinogen, low urine pH, and urine standing in specimen cup > 2 hr.	75% false negative rate when exposed to air for 15 days. Negative in the presence of reductase-negative bacteria.
Protein Not clinically significant unless ≥ 3+, detects mainly albumin	**False positive** with pH > 7, and chlorhexidine, some iodinated contrast material. **False negative** with low pH, very dilute urine.	Only reliable for albumin (glomerular proteinuria). Negative if primary protein is not albumin, such as Bence-Jones protein
Blood Test depends on peroxidase activity of RBCs, a very sensitive test positive with 1–2 RBCs/HPF.	**False positive** with myoglobinuria, semen in urine, povidone-iodine, certain (peroxidase-producing) bacteria, hypochlorite, menstrual blood, highly alkaline. **False negative** with high specific gravity, pH < 5, heavy proteinuria, and high concentrations of urinary nitrites, ascorbate (vitamin C), or captopril, dipstick exposed to air.	Positive test with speckles or dots implies nonhemolyzed blood. Positive test with diffuse pattern implies hemolyzed RBC or myoglobin. Severe exercise causes false position owing to myoglobinuria.
Bilirubin	**False positive** with iodine, stool contamination, chlorpromazine, mefenamic acid. **False negative** after prolonged standing.	Hard to read with agents causing marked urine discoloration.
Urobilinogen	**False positive** with pyridium, gantrisin, sulfonamides, porphyrin, methyldopa, procaine, aminosalicylic acid, 5-hydroxyindolacetic acid. **False negative** with gantrisin and pyridium.	Use fresh specimen: rapidly broken down by light and in acid urine.
Leukocyte esterase	**False positive** with vaginal contamination, oxidizing agents, eosinophils in the urine, *Trichomonas.* **False negative** with high glucose, ketones, protein (especially albumin), pH, specific gravity, cephalexin, tetracycline, oxalates, ascorbic acid, neutropenia.	Commonly positive with vaginal secretion contamination. Sterile pyuria seen with tuberculosis, nephrolithiasis, interstitial nephritis.
pH	Urea-splitting bacteria elevate pH. Runoff from protein strip can falsely lower pH.	Use fresh specimen: standing raises pH by loss of CO_2
SG Most accurate analysis requires osmometer	Overestimates SG with low pH, ketoacidosis, and protein. Underestimates SG owing to glucose, urea, or with pH > 7. Elevated with use of dextran, IV contrast, proteinuria.	Not reliable at SG. > 1.025.

HPF, high-power field; RBCs, red blood cells; SG, specific gravity.

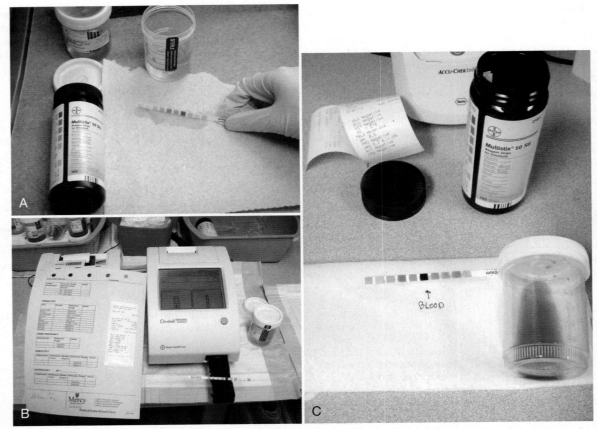

Figure 68–2 *A,* Totally immerse the dipstick in urine for a few seconds and place it on its side on a paper towel to allow drainage of urine, limiting cross-contamination of the individual testing squares. Note that the bottle of test strips should be closed immediately because prolonged exposure to air will produce false results. *B,* Formal reading of the test strip is accomplished electronically rather than only by the naked eye, for quality assurance and a permanent record. *C,* Myoglobinuria: strongly positive for blood on dipstick, with no red blood cells (RBCs) on microscopy.

180 and 200 mg/dL).[19] Changes in urine glucose lag behind changes in blood glucose by approximately half the interval between voids. Glycosuria in the absence of hyperglycemia suggests renal tubular dysfunction. Glycosuria may occur in hypothermic patients in the absence of hyperglycemia and may mask true hypoglycemia in hypothermic patients.

Ketones. Ketones are found in the urine during starvation, inadequate carbohydrate intake, diabetic ketoacidosis (DKA) and alcoholic ketoacidosis, isopropyl alcohol poisoning, or glycogen storage disease. Urine testing for ketones is not sensitive to all forms of ketonemia or ketonuria, and the absence of a positive ketone test by dipstick should not categorically dismiss a significant ketotic state. Tests for urine ketones are 5 to 10 times as sensitive to acetoacetate as to acetone. Similar to the serum "acetone test," dipsticks do not detect β-hydroxybutyrate, which makes up 80% to 95% of the three "ketone bodies" and is the predominant form in the setting of ketoacidosis. However, urine ketone testing is significantly *more* sensitive than serum ketone testing. Indeed, there is generally no need to obtain "serum acetones" to diagnose or manage DKA when urine ketone monitoring is coupled with blood gas and anion gap analyses.

LE. This portion of the dipstick test is designed to detect enzymes from the azurophilic granules in neutrophils. Normally, the test is negative. Studies report a wide and clinically important range of thresholds for dipstick testing sensitivity, from 10 to 100 WBCs/µL urine. Studies suggest that the test is between 50% and 96% sensitive in detecting infection. The specificity for presence of WBCs is between 91% and 99%. The most common cause of a false-positive LE test is vaginal contamination.

Nitrites. Normally, urine does not contain nitrites. Nitrites are specific (~95%), but not sensitive (~45%) indicators of UTI.[20] Urinary nitrates are converted to nitrites most strongly by enteric coliform bacteria, explaining the nitrite test's 90% sensitivity in detecting UTI caused by *Escherichia coli.* *Enterococcus*, a moderately frequent urinary pathogen, *Pseudomonas* species, and *Acinetobacter* do not convert nitrates to nitrites and, therefore, are not detected by this test. False-negative results also occur because of lack of dietary nitrate, frequent voiding, and/or diuresis. Early-morning voided specimens are ideal (allowing time for conversion of nitrate to nitrite), but rarely available in the ED; if possible, a specimen obtained longer than 4 hours after the last voiding is preferred.

Protein. Proteins with molecular weight below 50,000 to 60,000 Daltons can pass through the glomerulus to be reabsorbed in the proximal tubule. Normal protein passage in the urine is less than 150 mg/24 hr, or approximately 10 mg/dL of urine. About 10% to 33% of urinary protein is albumin, 33% is Tamm-Horsfall glycoprotein (secreted by renal tubular cells), and the balance is made up of a variety of immunoglobulins and other proteins. Proteinuria is a finding noted in about 5% of routine urine screens in men. This may represent a normal variant, because 3% to 5% of healthy adults have postural proteinuria (proteinuria when standing, but not when recumbent).[19] The dipstick detects negatively charged proteins more strongly than positively charged ones; it is therefore most sensitive to albumin. A study of ED patients with severe acute hypertension identified renal dysfunction (defined as an elevated serum creatinine) with 100% sensitivity using urine dipstick detection of 1+ proteinuria or hematuria. The urine dipstick test is positive for protein with pyuria of more than 6 WBCs/HPF. This is a false-positive finding for protein but is useful when the urine dipstick is being used to screen for a UTI, because the threshold for LE is often much higher. Hematuria only slightly elevates urine protein levels.

In assessing a patient with proteinuria, it is helpful to divide the list of causes into those that are and those that are not associated with hematuria. These are listed in Table 68–2. Elevated urinary protein is more commonly due to renal than systemic causes. The source is either glomerular, with passage of normally unfiltered proteins, or tubular, with failure to reabsorb physiologically filtered, low-molecular-weight globulins. The former condition causes albuminuria. Renal tubular proteinuria is characterized by low levels of urinary albumin and therefore more likely to be missed.

"Blood." The blood section of the urine dipstick is positive if exposed to red blood cells (RBCs), hemoglobin (Hb), or myoglobin. Urine in healthy volunteers contains fewer than 7 RBCs/μL. Studies have shown that the urine dipstick is very sensitive to 10 RBCs/μL. Hence, false-negative results are confined to clinically insignificant hematuria.[21] The dipstick pad should be inspected for discrete positive "dots," indicative of nonhemolyzed RBCs. Moderate intravascular hemolysis does not cause hemoglobinuria because the Hb is tightly bound to haptoglobin and therefore not filtered (see Fig. 68–2*C*). Massive intravascular hemolysis gives rise to free plasma Hb with a molecular weight of 32,000 Daltons, which easily passes through the glomerulus. Myoglobin has a molecular weight of 17,000 Daltons, also allowing easy glomerular passage. Guidelines for distinguishing hematuria, hemoglobinuria, and myoglobinuria are outlined in Table 68–3. In asymptomatic men older than 50 years, significant disease can be signaled by intermittent hematuria, mandating follow-up of patients with this incidental finding.

Dipsticks are vitiated by humidity and air, which cause false-negative results after improper storage. Because RBCs may lyse rapidly, delays in performing the UA may misleadingly suggest myoglobinuria or hemoglobinuria. Microscopy or dipstick testing of a *freshly* obtained specimen can clarify this issue. Conversely, high specific gravity or low pH can inhibit lysis of erythrocytes, which is necessary for the dipstick chemical reaction to occur, thus causing false-negative results.

A study reproducing clinical conditions has demonstrated that povidone-iodine does not cause false-positive results on dipstick. Iatrogenically caused trace positive results may occur after catheterization in 15% of cases, but at such low levels that they should not be a source of confusion with emergency urologic conditions.[1]

TABLE 68–2 Some Causes of Proteinuria with and without Hematuria

Proteinuria usually with Hematuria	Proteinuria usually without Hematuria
(Usually indicates glomerular disease. Most etiologies in early stages can present without hematuria.)	(Usually indicates tubular/interstitial disease, or high serum levels causing "overflow." In advanced disease, can develop hematuria.)
Infectious Diseases	**Systemic Conditions**
Post-streptococcal GN, pneumococcal pneumonia, ABE, meningococcemia, secondary syphilis, hepatitis B, severe viral infections, malaria, toxoplasmosis, Guillain-Barré	Physiologic: postexercise, postural (with standing) Pathologic: fever, shock states, severe hypovolemia, dehydration, CHF Diabetes Amyloidosis Sarcoidosis "Overflow states": multiple myeloma, lymphoma, leukemia, rhabdomyolysis Renovascular hypertension
Multisystem Diseases	
Vasculitides: Henoch-Schönlein purpura, PAN, Wegener's granulomatosis, Kawasaki disease, etc. Connective tissue diseases (SLE, RA, scleroderma) Neoplasia Rhabdomyolysis (artifactual hematuria) Goodpasture's syndrome Cryoglobulinemias Toxemia of pregnancy Serum sickness	**Medications, Drugs, and Toxins** NSAIDs, gold, penicillamine, probenicid, captopril, lithium, cyclosporin Heroin Heavy-metal nephropathy: lead, mercury, or cadmium
Primary Glomerular Diseases	**Renal Diseases** Chronic pyelonephritis Interstitial nephritis Fanconi's syndrome

ABE, acute bacterial endocarditis; CHF, congestive heart failure; GN, glomerular nephritis; NSAIDs, nonsteroidal anti-inflammatory drugs; PA, polyarteritis nodosa; RA, rheumatoid arthritis; SLE, systemic lupus erythematosus.

TABLE 68–3 Aids in Distinguishing Hematuria, Intravascular Hemolysis, and Myoglobinuria.

	Hematuria	Myoglobinuria	Intravascular hemolysis
Serum findings	Color: clear.	Color: clear. Haptoglobin: normal.	Color: pink Haptoglobin: low.
Urine appearance	Color: Clear to brown, clears with centrifugation.	Color: clear to red/brown; no clearing with centrifugation.	Color: clear to brown; no clearing with centrifugation.
Urine microscopy	RBCs, RBC casts, and protein: imply glomerular source. No RBC casts, tubular cells, small protein: nephron source. Just RBC: source distal to nephron. (e.g., ureterolithiasis)	Possible occasional RBCs and tubular cells secondary to rhabdomyolysis-induced renal damage.	Usually unremarkable.

RBCs, red blood cells.

Urine Bilirubin. Urine bilirubin represents the filtered, soluble, conjugated form of bilirubin. Unconjugated bilirubin is protein-bound and does not pass through the glomerulus. Bilirubinuria is therefore due to intrahepatic or extrahepatic cholestasis. Bilirubinuria will be detected significantly earlier than clinical jaundice. Urinary bilirubin excretion is enhanced by alkalosis. Test a fresh sample of urine, because bilirubin glucuronide is hydrolyzed when exposed to light. Ascorbic acid and high levels of urinary nitrites decrease the sensitivity of the test to bilirubin.

Urobilinogen. In a healthy person, conjugated bilirubin is excreted in bile. In the colon, it is broken down into a number of compounds, which includes urobilinogen. Most of these compounds are excreted in the stool, giving the characteristic color. A small amount of urobilinogen is absorbed from the colon, and if it is not taken up on the first pass through the liver, it enters the circulation. Ultimately, some of this urobilinogen may enter the urine, so that it is normal to have zero to moderate levels of urinary urobilinogen on dipstick testing. Most diseases causing hepatocyte dysfunction (e.g., hepatitis, cirrhosis, passive liver congestion) increase urinary urobilinogen excretion by impairing hepatic uptake of urobilinogen. It is rarely helpful as a qualitative test with a wide range of normal values, but it can have diagnostic significance in evaluating a patient with jaundice (Table 68–4).

pH. Average daily excretion of 50 to 100 mmol of H^+ in the urine gives rise to a typical urine pH of around 6 with a range from 4.5 to 8. Dietary protein lowers urinary pH, whereas fruit (especially citrus) and vegetables tend to raise it. The significance of pH testing is in the assessment of normal renal function. In most states of alkalosis and acidosis, the healthy kidneys maintain homeostasis by conserving or excreting H^+. Failure to do so suggests renal disease, especially renal tubular acidoses. An exception is the "paradoxical aciduria" of hypokalemic alkalosis secondary to volume contraction, hypercorticism, or diuretics, in which the highest priority of the renal tubule is to conserve sodium. pH is elevated by the action of urea-splitting bacteria, especially *Proteus* species. This can occur with "stasis" of urine, either in the bladder or in specimen cups. A persistently alkaline urine is seen in patients with struvite (triple phosphate) urolithiasis.

Specific Gravity. The dipstick tests for urine-specific gravity assays for the primary urinary cations sodium and potassium. True specific gravity, which is also dependent on anions, albumin, proteins, urea, and glucose, is therefore not measured. Artifactually low specific gravity readings are obtained in alkaline urine. Acid urine and albumin falsely elevate the specific gravity reading. Some investigators believe that these strips on the dipstick test are of marginal clinical utility. Other clinical indicators of a patient's hydration status are probably more reliable. If necessary, use a refractive-specific gravitometer or a hygrometer.

Microscopic UA

Microscopic UA is performed to identify cells, bacteria, and other microbes as well as formed elements such as casts and crystals (Fig. 68–3). The following discussion focuses on the findings of significance in diagnosing UTI: WBCs, bacteria, and WBC casts. The presence of WBCs with bacteria distinguishes infection from colonization (bacteriuria without pyuria). Some authorities state that significant infection without pyuria occurs in less than 5% of cases, making pyuria a sensitive marker of infection.[22,23] Other studies do not support reliance on pyuria as an indicator of infection. The presence of WBC casts distinguishes pyelonephritis ("upper UTI") from cystitis ("lower UTI").

Perform microscopic UA using one of five methods. Traditionally, the most common technique has been the examination of unstained centrifuged urine. It has the advantage of concentrating formed elements that might otherwise be missed. The disadvantage is that the presence and quantity of elements in a specimen will vary depending on many uncontrolled factors: the volume of the specimen, the time and speed of centrifugation, the fragility of the formed elements, the volume of the "drop" in which the pellet is resuspended, and the size of the microscope's "high-power field."[8,24]

1. **Examination of unspun urine in a hemocytometer counting chamber.** The hemocytometer is a precisely milled slide etched with measured squares, allowing for the exact enumeration of cells in each square. Because the distance between the etched surface and the coverslip is exactly known, it is possible to determine the number of cells per unit volume of specimen. Enough fresh unspun urine is placed on the slide to fully cover the counting area, and the cells are counted. There should usually be fewer than 1 WBC/μL, although more than 10 WBCs/μL and more than 5 RBCs/μL are unequivocally abnormal. The threshold for diagnosing UTI is usually set at 8 WBCs/μL or greater.[13,24,25] Bacteria do not sink to the surface of the hemocytometer, so that counting them through the many focal planes of the chamber is not possible, although methods to estimate the bacterial count per unit volume have been described.

   The hemocytometer is accurate, fast (time need not be spent in staining or centrifugation), and relatively easy to master. Its major drawbacks are cost (around $150 for the slide and coverslip) and fragility (easily destroyed if dropped). These characteristics are problematic given conditions and resources in many EDs, although some advocate their use. Formed elements other than WBCs and RBCs (e.g., casts) occur in such low concentrations that they are encountered only by chance in the hemocytometer, and microscopy of spun urine is needed for their identification.

TABLE 68–4 Relationship between Urinary Bilirubin, Urobilinogen, and Stool Color in the Jaundiced Patient

	Healthy Normal	Complete Biliary Obstruction	Intravascular Hemolysis	Hepatocellular Disease
Urinary bilirubin	None	Elevated	None	Elevated
Urinary urobilinogen	None or present	None	Present, sometimes large	Normal early Increased late
Stool color	Normal	Acholic	Normal	Normal

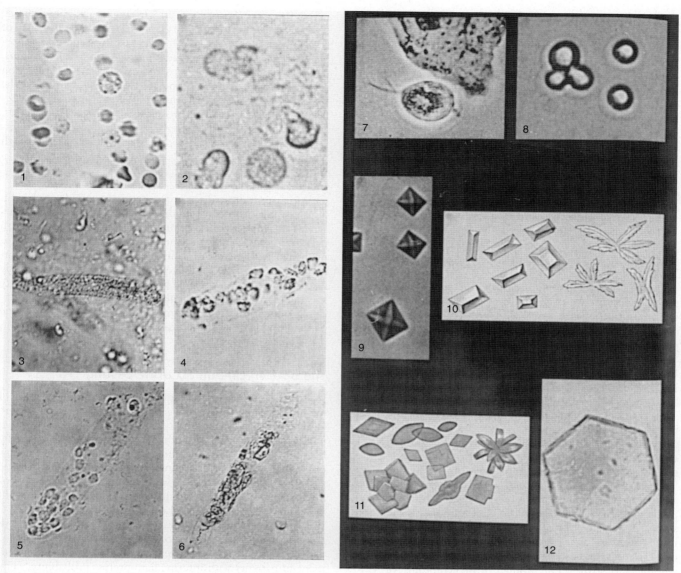

Figure 68–3 *1,* RBCs and white blood cells (WBCs). *2,* WBCs with bacteria in an infected urine specimen. *3,* Fine granular cast. *4,* WBC cast (seen in intrinsic renal diseases such as pyelonephritis and glomerulonephritis; note the discernible nuclei and cell boundaries). *5,* RBC cast (the distinct and uniformly spherical shape of the erythrocyte is visible). *6,* Epithelial cast (present in tubular disease). *7, Trichomonas vaginalis. 8,* Budding yeast forms. *9,* Calcium oxalate crystals. *10,* Phosphate crystals. *11,* Urate crystals. *12,* Cystine crystal (indicative of cystinuria). *(1, 3–9, and 12, From Urine under the Microscope. Montclair, NJ, ROCOM Press, 1975; 2, from Birch DF, et al: A Color Atlas of Urine Microscopy. Chapman & Hall, 1994; 10 and 11, from Netter FH, Shapter RK, Yonkman FF [eds]: The Ciba Collection of Medical Illustration. 6:80, 1973.)*

2. **Examination of unspun, unstained urine placed on a regular microscope slide** is a qualitative method sometimes used in the diagnosis of UTI. Using 1 organism/HPF as a positive result, the sensitivity and specificity in detecting 10^5 CFU/mL are between 60% and 90%. This method only identifies 1 WBC/HPF with the highly pyuric state of 250 WBCs/μL,[25] leading some to advocate the use of more than 1 WBC/low-power field as a criterion for infection.

3. **Examination of unstained, centrifuged urine** is performed by centrifuging 10 mL of urine at approximately 450 g (1000–4000 revolutions per minute [rpm]) for 3 to 5 minutes. Pour off roughly 9 mL of supernatant , and resuspend the pellet in the remaining fluid. Place this suspension on a slide with a coverslip and examine it. The larger formed elements, especially casts, tend to migrate to the edge of the coverslip, and they can be seen with low

magnification. One or two casts, depending on the clinical context, may be normal; more are not. The morphology of the more commonly encountered formed elements of urine sediment is shown in Figure 68–2. The significance of each is beyond the scope of this text, but this information can be found in a standard textbook of clinical laboratory procedures and diagnostic testing.[19] When examining centrifuged urine, more than 5 WBCs/HPF seen in the middle of the coverslip has traditionally been taken as indicative of abnormal pyuria. Most authors have estimated that 10 WBCs/μL are equivalent to approximately 1 WBC/HPF; thus, this oft-cited threshold for diagnosing UTI is actually equivalent to 50 WBCs/μL.[24,25]

Because the "gold standard" for diagnosis of UTI is 8 WBCs/μL or greater, many infections will escape detection using this method. Various numbers of bacteria per high-power field have been used as criteria for the diagnosis of UTI. A threshold of 10 to 20 organisms/HPF has been recommended to rule out bacteriuria at the 10^5 CFU/mL level. This threshold does not exclude infection in symptomatic patients.

4. **Examination of Gram-stained, uncentrifuged urine** is also a semiquantitative measurement. It is estimated that 1 bacterium/HPF is equivalent to 10^5 CFU/mL in bacterial culture.[19]

5. **Gram stain of centrifuged urine** is probably the optimal technique, short of culture, in the assessment of bacteriuria. It is more than 95% sensitive and more than 60% specific to 10^4 CFU/mL—a concentration of bacteriuria an order of magnitude lower than the previously described methods. Detection of 1 organism/oil-immersion field constitutes a positive result. Specificity is increased to 95% if 5 organisms/HPF are seen.

Summary of Tests Used in the Diagnosis of UTI

The three tests commonly used to evaluate a patient for the presence or absence of UTI are urine dipstick, microscopic UA, and urine culture. Each represents an increasing degree of expense, delay, and resources. A brief discussion of their relative strengths and weaknesses ensues.

Urine Dipstick

Dipstick testing of urine is faster than microscopic UA; is less labor-intensive, thus cheaper; and circumvents multiple sources of potential and proven error.[26] Is it sufficiently accurate to replace it? Using *either* LE *or* nitrites to indicate infection, the dipstick is still only 50% to 90% sensitive to culture-proven infection. This is clearly not adequate to rule out infection in symptomatic patients (in whom the prevalence of disease is high) but may be acceptable in asymptomatic patients in whom the test has a serviceably high negative predictive value of 95% to 99%.[26] In symptomatic men, sensitivity is enhanced by taking a positive result in *any one* (or more) of *either* LE *or* nitrites *or* protein *or* blood as indication of a UTI and can be augmented by allowing extra time before reading the strip.[27] For women with symptoms of UTI, empirical treatment is recommended because no test can rule out infection. A negative dipstick test in a patient with high pretest probability of UTI should prompt a search for an alternative source of the patient's symptoms. Clearly, maneuvers to enhance the dipstick's sensitivity diminish specificity, which may be as low as 26%,[7] leading some to advocate microscopic UA for all urines abnormal by dipstick. However, this probably adds little to a carefully performed dipstick test. Read the dipstick by electronic methods rather than only the naked eye, for quality assurance and to produce a permanent record (see Fig. 68–2B).

Microscopic UA

If the urine dipstick has such poor specificity when it is used as a test with adequate sensitivity, should it be discarded altogether and microscopic UA relied upon instead? Apart from the hemocytometer, the most reliable method for identifying significant bacteriuria is oil-immersion microscopy of Gram-stained, centrifuged urine. Despite this, the practice in most hospital laboratories is to examine the resuspended pellet of unstained, centrifuged urine. The problems with this method have been discussed. In various studies, a range between 1 and 10 organisms/HPF or 5 WBCs/HPF has been considered a "positive" test (as the threshold number rises, so does specific-

ity, at the price of sensitivity).[28] In aggregate, the accuracy of microscopy in the diagnosis of UTI is similar to that of the dipstick alone, with 22% false-positive, and 23% false-negative rates when compared with those of culture.[29] Thus, microscopic UA, like the dipstick, cannot rule out infection in symptomatic patients. The specificity of pyuria will be improved when viewed as a marker of all genitourinary infections including urethritis, prostatitis, epididymitis, vaginitis, and cervicitis. Always entertain these diagnoses in patients with urinary symptoms, especially if the urine is sterile with pyuria.

Urine Culture

Cultures are indicated for any potentially complicated UTI. This includes those in children; men; women with recurrences or relapses; the immunocompromised; patients with urinary tract pathology, including stones and possible pyelonephritis; and pregnant patients. They are usually recommended around the 16th week of gestation. As previously discussed, every effort should be made to obtain a high-quality specimen owing to the difficulty of distinguishing contamination from significant low-count bacteriuria in symptomatic patients and in view of the expense of cultures and treatment, if the culture is positive.

The Bottom Line on ED Urine Testing

It is well established that female patients with symptoms of uncomplicated lower UTI can be treated without culture because the prevalence of disease is 50% or more in women with classic urinary symptoms.[8,20] Treatment is generally benign, and 95% of urine cultures that are positive will grow out a limited number of organisms with predictable antibiotic susceptibilities.[8] Some authors recommend dipstick and/or microscopic UA in this group because a negative test might prompt more careful consideration of alternative diagnoses.[8,20] If none is found, treat such patients empirically with trimethoprim-sulfamethoxazole.

Urine testing is more likely to influence clinical management in patients with intermediate pretest probability.[7] The urine microscopy can also help in distinguishing pyelonephritis (WBC casts), vaginitis (absence of pyuria or hematuria on catheterized specimen), and urethritis (pyuria, rarely hematuria) from cystitis (pyuria and often hematuria).[8] In the ED, the ease of obtaining a dipstick argues for its use without UA because it is equally sensitive, unless formed elements such as casts, crystals, *Trichomonas*, or other parasites are suspected. In patients with pyelonephritis, urine cultures are probably warranted because they alter therapy in about 5% of cases.[30] In most asymptomatic patients, a negative dipstick or UA has sufficient negative predictive value to rule out disease unless the patient is pregnant or getting urologic surgery. Special clinical considerations in some patients (e.g., the immunocompromised, diabetic females at high risk for UTI) might mandate adjustments of this approach. Cultures are recommended for febrile infants younger than 2 months and for children who appear sick or have high pretest probability of infection.[12,31]

TESTING FOR PREGNANCY

Pregnancy tests are based on the detection of β-human chorionic gonadotropin (β-hCG) in serum or urine. β-hCG is secreted by trophoblastic cells of the placenta starting from the time of implantation of the blastocyst. Qualitative serum tests and the urine test detect β-hCG levels of between 15 and 25 mIU/mL. The concentration of β-hCG is usually lower in urine than in serum, which accounts for the slight advantage of serum tests in detection of early pregnancy. Optimal urine pregnancy tests are obtained on first-voided concentrated morning specimens. Home urine pregnancy test kits detect levels of β-hCG of about 50 mIU/mL in the urine.

If fertilization has occurred, β-hCG levels of 5 to 8 mIU/mL (the threshold of the quantitative serum test) correspond to the 9th to 11th day after ovulation (23–25 days after the 1st day of the last normal menstrual period). In a viable intrauterine pregnancy, the β-hCG level doubles approximately every 2 days during the first 4 weeks of gestation, reaching a serum level of greater than 25 mIU/mL, detectable by virtually all pregnancy tests on the 1st day of the missed menstrual period. The doubling rate declines to every 3rd day thereafter. The quantitative β-hCG (Q β-hCG) reaches a peak of between 100,000 and 200,000 mIU/mL between the 10th to the 14th gestational weeks and declines to 10,000 to 20,000 mIU/mL for the rest of the pregnancy (Table 68–5). There is a wide range of β-hCG levels among different women at the same stage of gestation, making definite clinical determinations on the basis of a single quantitative test impossible.[32] False-positive tests have been described in association with molar pregnancy, choriocarcinoma, teratoma, occasional malignancies outside the genitourinary tract, and very high levels of proteinuria. There is one report of a positive urine hCG (but normal serum hCG) associated with tubo-ovarian abscess.

Although a previous Q β-hCG level is rarely available to the emergency clinician, doubling rates are an important part of the assessment of a healthy first-trimester pregnancy. Fetal nonviability, ectopic pregnancy, and intrauterine demise are signaled by abnormalities in the predicted rise in Q β-hCG.[33] A serum Q β-hCG level that does not increase by 66% every 48 hours has a 75% chance of being due to a nonviable pregnancy. The β-hCG levels in a healthy intrauterine pregnancy (IUP) and associated sonographic findings are listed in Table 68–5.

The rate of decline of Q β-hCG after gestation varies depending on the reason for the conclusion of the pregnancy. After a term delivery, β-hCG falls to zero in 2 weeks. After surgery for an ectopic pregnancy, the range is 1 to 31 days, with a median of 8.5 days; after a first-trimester spontaneous abortion, the range is 9 to 35 days (median, 19 days); and after first-trimester elective abortion, the range is 16 to 60 days (median, 30 days).[19]

The association between β-hCG levels and gestational dates has led to the concept of the "discriminatory zone." In a normal pregnancy with a Q β-hCG level of 1500 mIU/mL, at least a double decidual sac should be sonographically identifiable by transvaginal ultrasound. The discriminatory threshold for identifying this sign by transabdominal ultrasound is considered to be 6500 mIU/mL. If these ultrasound findings are absent at these thresholds, the pregnancy is almost certainly abnormal, with a significant possibility of ectopic. However, the converse—that there is no point in trying to exclude ectopic if the Q β-hCG is less than 1000 mIU/mL—is *not* true. This is because (1) the discriminatory zone does not preclude the possibility of identifying a double decidual sac (or more definitive features of an IUP such as a yolk sac) before the Q β-hCG reaches 1500 mIU/mL and (2) ectopic masses are frequently identified in the adnexa with Q β-hCGs of less than 1000 mIU/mL. Ectopic gestational sacs have a variety of pathologic characteristics and implantation sites, leading them to generate highly variable Q β-hCG levels. One percent of ectopic pregnancies having a Q β-hCG of less than 10 mIU/mL and approximately one third of ectopics are diagnosed in patients presenting with a Q β-hCG less than 1000.[34,35] Even if no definitive diagnosis can be made, the clinician should be aware that pregnant ED patients with pelvic complaints and a β-hCG level of 1000 mIU/mL or less have a fourfold *increased* risk of ectopic pregnancy compared with those with the same symptoms and a β-hCG level of 1000 mIU/mL or greater.[36]

For this reason, the "discriminatory zone" provides a basis for *interpreting* the ultrasound, but not a basis for *deciding whether or not to get* the ultrasound.[34,36,37] Although the percentage of patients below the "discriminatory zone" who will receive a definitive diagnosis by ultrasound is much lower than that among those above it (25% vs. 90%), even a 25% diagnosis rate would seem to merit pursuit in a potentially lethal disease; especially because follow up for patients whose evaluation is "indeterminate" on their ED visit is time-consuming and resource-intensive.[35]

TABLE 68–5 Relationship between Gestational Age, Quantitative β-Human Chorionic Gonadotropin Levels, and Ultrasound Findings

Time Elapsed from 1st Day of Last Normal Menstrual Period	Quantitative β-HCG Level (mIU/mL) Using the IRP	Ultrasound Findings
<28 days	5–50	
4–5 wk	50–500	From about 4.5 wk and Q β-HCG 1000–1500. EVU can show signs of IUP
5–6 wk	100–10,000	Definitely abnormal if no DDS seen by TVU with Q β-hCG > 2000 or by TAU with Q β-hCG > 6500 Abnormal if no YS with MSD > 10 mm
6–7 wk	1000–30,000	FP, cardiac activity 5.5–7 wk, Qβ-hCG > 10,000 Abnormal if no FP with MSD > 18 mm
7–8 w	3500–115,000	
8–14 wk	12,000–270,000	
>10 wk	270,000–15,000	

DDS, double decidual sac; EVU, endovaginal ultrasound; FP, fetal pole; IRP, international reference preparation; IUP, intrauterine pregnancy; MSD, mean sac diameter; Q β-hCG , quantitative β-human chorionic gonadotropin; TAU, transabdominal ultrasound; TVU, transvaginal ultrasound; YS, yolk sac.

BLOOD CULTURES IN THE ED

Indications

Blood cultures are indicated when there are clinical findings suggestive of an otherwise unidentifiable bacteremic state (Table 68–6). Twenty-five percent of patients with documented bacteremia have periods without fever. In the elderly, the proportion is even higher, with 50% of bacteremic patients over 65 having a temperature between 97.1°F (36.2°C) and 100.9°F (38.3°C); and at least 13% with no documented temperature greater than 99.1°F (37.3°C) at any time.[38] In the elderly, increasing age, vomiting, altered mental status, urinary incontinence, presence of a Foley catheter, or greater than 6% band forms is predictive of positive blood cultures. The subjective impression of "having fever" in adults is not a reliable indicator of the presence of fever, although the subjective impression of "no fever" is much more likely to be accurate. Prediction models to optimize the utilization of this costly test have been explored, but are cumbersome, add little to educated clinical judgment, and lack widespread validation or acceptance.[39] Many studies have shown that blood cultures in patients with uncomplicated pneumonia or pyelonephritis are of very limited clinical value.[30,40–42]

In children, the traditional teaching that blood cultures are indicated for all patients younger than 2 years with fever greater than 38.6°C (>101.5°F) and without obvious source is being modified by the widespread availability and use of pneumococcal conjugate (PC) and *Haemophilus influenzae* type B (HIB) vaccines.[43–45] In the post-PC and -HIB vaccines era, the incidence of occult bacteremia in otherwise well-appearing febrile children is probably under 1%, making the false positive rate at least four times as high.[44,45] It therefore seems reasonable to withhold blood cultures and empirical antibiotic coverage in otherwise well-appearing febrile children with reliable parents. The risk of bacteremia in a child is positively correlated with the degree of fever, WBC count, and rapidity of onset of illness. It is inversely proportional to the patient's age. In infants younger than 2 months with temperatures higher than 38°C (>100.5°F), some authorities would recommend blood cultures regardless of the presence or absence of a source, although this approach is subject to modification by experienced clinicians based on the patient's age and clinical setting. A child with a normal temperature in the ED and a history from the parents of tactile fever needs to be approached in the same way as a patient with fever documented on physical examination for several reasons. First, bacteremic children, like adults, have intermittent fever, with up to 50% afebrile rates in children with demonstrated bacteremia. Second, parents' tactile impression of fever has been shown to be reliable.

The Controversy Regarding "Outpatient Blood Cultures"

There is a longstanding debate regarding the utility of outpatient blood cultures (i.e., blood cultures on patients who are discharged from the ED pending results). Arguments for and against outpatient blood cultures are summarized in Table 68–7. The data on the subject are still inconclusive. Opponents cite medicolegal issues, problems with follow-up, high contamination rates, low rates of positive cultures, and even lower rates of frequency of patients in whom therapy is changed because of culture results. Proponents also cite medicolegal concerns, positive rates similar to those seen with inpatient blood cultures, cost savings, and the benefit of diagnosing significant, yet subtle, bacteremic states (such as endocarditis).[46,47] They also point out that the high false-positive rates seen in many ED series should be an indictment of poor technique, not of the test itself.

On the basis of current data, it would seem to be fiscally extravagant to admit all patients in whom a bacteremic state is possible and injudicious to deny blood cultures solely on the basis of a patient not appearing "toxic enough" to warrant admission. With mounting societal and economic pressures to avoid hospital admissions whenever possible, it would seem that outpatient blood cultures, with due attention to collection technique, patient selection, and diligent follow-up, will continue to be a necessary component of ED practice.

Technique for Obtaining Blood Cultures

Studies have demonstrated sources of contamination at every stage of the process of obtaining and processing blood cultures. In addition to obvious sources of contamination from the patient's and the phlebotomist's skin, antiseptic agents[48] and gloves have been implicated. Some authorities have argued that the primary source of contamination is in the laboratory processing of specimens.[49] However, the consensus

---

TABLE 68–6 Summary of Indications for Obtaining Blood Cultures

Patients with Fever and Any of the Following

Unexplained alterations in mental status, functional status, or autonomic status in a previously healthy patient between the ages of 5 and 65, or

No source, if <2 yr of age, >65 yr, or immunocompromised, or Age < 2 mo

Patients with or without Fever and Any of the Following

Rigors,

Toxic or "septic" appearance (e.g., unexplained hypotension, altered mental status, shock),

Suspicion of infectious endocarditis, or

Serious focal infections (e.g., meningitis, septic arthritis, osteomyelitis)

TABLE 68–7 Summary of Arguments for and against the Performance of Outpatient Blood Cultures

Arguments *against* Outpatient Blood Cultures

Low true-positive rates.

True positives are rarely clinically significant.

High false-positive rates are expensive and time-consuming for both patient and health care system.

Difficulty of emergency department follow-up makes positive blood culture results a medicolegal liability.

Arguments *for* Outpatient Blood Cultures

Permits outpatient evaluation/management in patients with low probability of disease (especially infectious endocarditis).

Financial, psychological, and nosocomial cost savings for patients who are spared admission.

Financial and nosocomial cost savings for society by avoidance of hospital admissions.

Allows initiation of antibiotics without irrevocable loss of opportunity for blood cultures.

is that the most common source of contamination is the process of phlebotomy and inoculation of blood culture bottles. Obviously, this is the single step over which emergency clinicians have control, either directly or via protocols of technique for blood culture phlebotomy. Contamination rates are typically between 1.5% and 3%,[43,50] although many ED series show much higher rates than this.

A high degree of sensitivity is required of blood cultures. Many significant bacteremic illnesses have been documented with as little as 1 CFU/10 mL of blood.[51] Human skin has a bacterial concentration between 10^3 and 10^6 CFU/mL, on the forearm and groin, respectively.[52] Designed to detect vanishingly low concentrations of bacteria, the test is clearly susceptible to false-positive results (impaired specificity) when blood must necessarily be obtained by passing a needle through the skin. Eighty percent of the skin flora is transient, superficial, and removable; 20% inhabit the sebaceous ducts and hair follicles and are not removable without destroying the skin.[52] The former group are predominantly gram-positive and gram-negative aerobes and are the target of skin disinfectants.

The primary agents for skin disinfection are iodine compounds, alcohols, chlorhexidine, and hexachlorophene. Iodine solution remains a gold standard, killing bacteria, fungi, protozoa, and viruses, but has been replaced in many institutions owing to concerns about skin burns and allergic reactions. Reports of the former were probably due to the use of 7% solution. The risk of a burn or an allergic reaction is thought to be negligible with the currently available 2% preparation. The most effective cleansing agent is tincture of iodine, which is a mixture of 2% iodine solution and 70% alcohol. Povidone-iodine 10% solution (Betadine) has a much lower free iodine concentration than iodine solution and is therefore less potent. Iodine is superior to hexachlorophene and chlorhexidine in killing gram-negative bacteria. Iodine, like other antiseptic agents, is inhibited by the presence of organic matter, emphasizing the need for thorough skin cleansing before the application of any skin disinfectant.

Ethyl or isopropyl alcohol should be used in 60% to 80% solution. Alcohol preparation pads, which generally contain 70% isopropanol, have solved traditional concerns regarding evaporation of alcohol from cotton balls stored in jars. Alcohol is a less powerful germicide than iodine in vitro and kills only 90% of surface bacteria after a full 2 minutes with reapplication to prevent drying. Alcohol foam applicators can avoid premature drying. Alcohol is inactive against fungi, spores, and viruses; however, in vivo studies of blood culture contamination rates have shown it to compare favorably with iodine. Because iodine solution is often not available and iodophor solutions are less potent, alcohol still has an important place in skin antisepsis. In addition, alcohol is an excellent solvent, so that alcohol pads are a good tool for skin preparation before the application of iodine compounds.

Chlorhexidine (Hibiclens) and hexachlorophene (pHisoHex) are antiseptics that are more effective against gram-positive than gram-negative bacteria. Both agents have intradermal absorption, which causes prolonged antimicrobial activity and is the basis of their popularity as surgical scrub and operative site preparations. This also makes them preferable agents where indwelling lines, especially central lines, are being placed. For routine blood culture phlebotomy, they are not as effective as alcohol and iodine combinations, although they are superior to povidone-iodine solution. Most studies show chlorhexidine to be more potent than hexachlorophene, and

TABLE 68–8 Skin Preparation and Technique for Drawing Blood Cultures

Cleanse the skin with alcohol swabs three times, or until swabs appear entirely free of surface dirt.
Allow to dry.
Apply 10% povidone-iodine, or (preferably) 2% iodine solution, or (ideally) 2% tincture of iodine in 70% alcohol, three times, in centrifugal circles from anticipated site of venipuncture.
After third swab, allow to dry for at least 60 sec.
During this period:
  Remove covers and sterilize rubber stoppers of blood culture bottles with iodine and/or alcohol.
  Lay out sterile gloves.
  Use paper glove wrapper as a sterile field for the needle and syringe (not necessary if using a Vacutainer system).
Wipe off dry iodine at venipuncture site with alcohol. Substitute chlorhexidine if placing an indwelling catheter.
Obtain at least 20 mL of blood to place in two bottles.
  If short, use at least 10 mL for **aerobic** bottle.
  If >20 mL, use additional **aerobic** bottles. No more than 10 mL blood/bottle.
Inoculate bottles without changing needles between bottles.
However many bottles are filled, this is **one** "set" of blood cultures.
Do not fill second set of bottles from this site.

it has not been associated with induction of seizures in infants.

Table 68–8 presents a skin preparation protocol addressing. Optimal results seem to be obtained by alcohol-iodine mixtures.[52] The most important concept in skin disinfection is that bacteria do not die at the instant of contact with disinfectant agents. Iodine (2%), which is twice as potent as 10% povidone-iodine, requires at least 90 seconds in contact with the skin to kill 90% of surface bacteria. In many ED patients, it will be necessary to use alcohol preparation pads to remove gross dirt and debris from phlebotomy sites before initiating the steps of the formal skin preparation.

Special Considerations in Obtaining Blood Cultures

"Changing the Needle" after Phlebotomy

In considering this issue, it is important to emphasize the distinction between *needle changing* and *needle recapping*. The latter is a well-established risk to health care workers. It contravenes standard recommendations for universal precautions and *should not be performed*. Needle replacement using the standard needle removal device on "sharps" containers is an unquantified risk, but clearly much less dangerous than recapping.

Based on little scientific data, it was long considered essential to change the phlebotomy needle before inoculating blood culture bottles. With increasing awareness of the risks of needle-stick injuries, this practice has come under scrutiny. Studies generally show trends toward lower contamination rates with needle change, without reaching statistical significance.[53,54] Thus, not changing needles before blood culture bottle inoculation is acceptable practice for obtaining routine blood cultures. In situations in which the results of blood cultures are of paramount importance (e.g., suspected infectious endocarditis, in which empirical antibiotics are to be started immediately), needles can be changed before inoculation of culture bottles (without recapping).

Special Access Sites

Most studies show that newly placed intravenous (IV) catheters are an acceptable source of blood culture specimens, providing that the usual measures are taken in skin preparation.[50,55] Chronically placed lines either trend toward or show statistically significant increased contamination rates.[56] An exception can be made for carefully tended central venous access ports in cancer patients, which may have increased sensitivity in identifying bacteremia, possibly owing to the fact that the catheters themselves are often a source of bacteremia in those patients.[57]

Heel Stick in Neonates

This technique resulted in recovery rates of bacteria equivalent to phlebotomy in two studies.[58] Because approximately 25% of bacteremic infants have less than 5 CFU/mL of blood, this proportion (25%) will be missed if 0.2 mL or less is obtained for culture. For this reason, heel stick should be considered as a source of last resort for blood culture.

Intraosseous Specimens

This technique may also be used when phlebotomy is impossible.

Timing of Blood Cultures

In most circumstances, the timing of blood cultures is moot in the ED. Patients are sick enough to warrant the initiation of empirical antibiotics, or are well enough for discharge, so that two or more sets need to be drawn immediately. The situation in which the timing of blood cultures might become a consideration is in a patient requiring admission but in whom the diagnosis of bacteremia is in doubt so that empirical antibiotic therapy is withheld. Contrary to time-honored beliefs, the true positive blood cultures are more likely if drawn in the 12 hours *before* a fever spike. Furthermore, excepting infectious endocarditis, most clinically significant bacteremia is thought to be intermittent, so that multiple sets of cultures obtained at one time would heighten the risk of missing the period of bacteremia. Therefore, for patients admitted to the hospital with the tentative diagnosis of sepsis, it is theoretically advantageous to draw the three sets of blood cultures over the first 12 to 24 hours of admission. If immediate administration of antibiotics is indicated, the two or three sets of cultures should be obtained before initiation of antibiotic therapy.

Blood Culture Volumes

Volumes in Adults

A large number of studies almost uniformly demonstrate that the sensitivity of blood cultures is directly related to the volume of blood cultured.[59-61] In a representative study, Ilstrup and Washington[62] showed that 20 mL and 30 mL of blood yielded, respectively, 38% and 62% more true-positive results than 10 mL. Mermel and Maki[60] showed that each additional milliliter of blood yields an average of 3% more true-positive results. This finding is also consistent with the fact that 40% of adults with bacteremia have fewer than 1 CFU/mL of blood and that 20% have fewer than 1 CFU/10 mL.[51] Alternatively expressed, if 10 mL of blood is obtained for culture,

20% of patients with continuous bacteremia will be missed. Because most bacteremia is intermittent, and because endogenous factors in blood will cause some inhibition of bacterial growth even with modern lysis- and filtration-centrifugation techniques, the false-negative rate in clinical practice will always be significantly higher. On purely mathematical grounds, 10 mL per set of blood cultures is a bare minimum for culture. In adults, most authorities recommend at least 30 mL of blood per culture site/set.[63] To ensure dilution of the blood's antibacterial properties (e.g., immunoglobulins, complement, WBCs), place blood in a concentration less than 10% (i.e., not > 1 part of blood/10 parts of medium). Thus, if 30 mL of blood is obtained from one site, it should be equally divided into three of the usual 100-mL broth bottles.

Volumes in Children

A blood volume of 30 mL from a 70-kg adult is equivalent to 0.5 mL of blood in a 3.5-kg neonate. Fortunately (for the utility of the blood culture), it has been shown that levels of bacteremia are typically 10-fold higher in neonates than in adults and that the sicker the child, the greater the likelihood of a high level of bacteremia. As the immune system matures during infancy, levels of bacteremia might be expected to fall toward those seen in adults, so that small culture volumes are at increased risk of false-negative results, as is the case in adults.[55,64] As a rule of thumb, a similar volume of blood with respect to body mass should be drawn in children as would be drawn in adults: approximately 1 mL/2.5 kg, or *4 mL blood/ 10 kg body mass.*[65]

How Many Sets of Blood Cultures Are Needed?

A set of blood cultures is the sample obtained from a single site. A 1-mL specimen from a neonate placed in an aerobic bottle and a 30-mL specimen from an adult divided between fungal, aerobic, and anaerobic bottles are both considered a *single set* of blood cultures. Two or more sets of blood cultures make up a *series*. The information derived from the blood culture sets is pooled in such a way as to make both the sensitivity and the specificity of the series greater than that of the component sets. Sensitivity is enhanced because even with continuous bacteremia, an individual set is usually only 80% sensitive. Specificity is improved by determining whether pathogens that are also frequently contaminants are found in more than one set of the series.

Whereas this conceptual process is applied to all blood culture series, the focus of inquiry varies depending on the infectious process being ruled in or out. For example, in an elderly patient with sepsis and a chronic indwelling Foley, it is extremely unlikely that the causative organism is a typical skin contaminant. The usual causes of "false-positive" blood cultures will therefore be easily recognized, thus lowering the false-positive rate for the series and making for a test with intrinsically higher specificity. At the same time, with typical pathogens in this clinical context being nonfastidious organisms, sensitivity is typically around 99% with two sets of 20 mL blood/set. Conversely, in a patient with a prosthetic heart valve, fever, and signs of septic emboli, many likely pathogens are also skin contaminants, lowering the specificity of each individual blood culture set. Thus, at least two sets of cultures must be *positive* with such organisms before the overall test (i.e., the *series*) is considered positive. At the same time, this clinical picture makes the pretest probability of

TABLE 68–9 Numbers of Blood Culture Sets to Be Obtained in Various Clinical Situations in Adults

Number of Sets (Minimum)	Clinical Context
Two sets	Etiology is likely to be easily distinguished from contaminants, and pretest probability of bacteremia is low to moderate.
Three sets	Skin contaminants are possible causes of infectious process, pretest probability of bacteremia is high, or infectious endocarditis is a consideration, but with low to moderate pretest probability.
Four sets	Infectious endocarditis AND either moderate to high pretest probability or the patient has recently been on antibiotics.

TABLE 68–10 Blood Culture Types to Be Used in Various Clinical Settings

Clinical Situation	Bottles to Be Obtained
Children <12 yr	Aerobic bottles only unless patient has peritonitis or fasciitis (in which case, draw standard aerobic and anaerobic cultures).
Adults and children >12 yr	Anaerobic infection unlikely, immunocompetent patient: aerobic bottles only. Anaerobic infection unlikely, immunocompromised patient: aerobic bottle, one bottle for fungal culture (usually effective in aerobic bottles: consult laboratory for guidance). Possibility of anaerobic infection: one aerobic and one anaerobic bottle per set.

TABLE 68–11 Clinical Settings at Higher Risk for Anaerobic Bacteremia

Infectious Foci

Abdominal/pelvic infections
Soft tissue or wound infections (e.g., myofasciitis)
Sepsis with decubitus ulcers or necrotic tissue
Aspiration pneumonia
Odontogenic head and neck infections

Predisposing Clinical Features

Malignancy
Immunosuppressive medications
Recent abdominal or pelvic surgery
Diabetes

disease very high (diminishing the negative predictive value of a negative set), so that an extremely sensitive overall test (i.e., series) will be needed to adequately rule out disease. Thus, in this setting, most authorities would recommend four sets of blood cultures, with good volumes in each. Except in infants, single sets of blood cultures are of insufficient sensitivity or specificity to be of any utility and should not be drawn. Recommended numbers of sets of blood cultures as they relate to the pretest probability of disease as well as causative organism are summarized in Table 68–9.

Aerobic versus Anaerobic (vs. Other) Bottles

Anaerobic infections tend to occur in poorly perfused tissues or locations, frequently evolving into abscesses, which further isolate them from the bloodstream, decreasing the likelihood of bacteremia and detection by blood cultures. For these reasons, it is not surprising that anaerobic isolates account for 0.5% to 12% of positive blood cultures. Thus, with a typical true-positive blood culture rate of about 5%, and with 5% or less of positive blood cultures being anaerobic, more than 400 patients need to have complete series of blood cultures drawn to detect one case of anaerobic bacteremia.[66,67] If, as is often reported, more than 50% of anaerobic infections are clinically evident before the culture, 800 or more blood culture series need to be drawn to generate a single anaerobic result that would alter clinical management. Anaerobic cultures might also have the unintended consequence of compromising the sensitivity of aerobic cultures in situations in which less than the ideal 20 mL of blood is drawn for a blood culture set.[60] The use of blood culture specimens in anaerobic bottles will also diminish the likelihood of identifying fungal infections, which are increasingly common, especially in immunocompromised patients.

In addition to these pathophysiologic considerations, there was a widely reported decrease in the positive anaerobic blood culture rate in the 1980s and 1990s, although some authors have recently suggested a resurgence of anaerobic bacteremia rates.[67] At the current time, the arguments for a selective use of anaerobic blood cultures are compelling, especially if working in an institution where there is a low rate of anaerobic bacteremia. Based on review of several articles on this topic, Table 68–10 suggests a possible approach to the allocation of blood specimens to various blood culture media after phlebotomy. Clinical features that place a patient at high risk of anaerobic bacteremia are listed in Table 68–11.

Identifying Contaminants

The emergency clinician may receive calls from the laboratory about results of positive blood cultures obtained on previous shifts. These may be "true positives," due to true contamination, or caused by the intermittent bacteremia that occurs in normal, healthy people. This situation has been complicated by increasingly common identification of *Staphylococcus epidermidis* and *Streptococcus viridans* and fungi as real pathogens in blood culture series.[57] The expense of false-positive blood cultures has been estimated at $900 per episode for discharged patients, and more than $5,000 per episode for inpatients. These costs emphasize the importance of good technique in obtaining blood cultures.[68] Distinguishing contaminants from clinically significant bacteremia is based both on microbiologic information and the patient's clinical condition. Features of false-positive blood culture results are listed in Table 68–12. Notwithstanding these guidelines, it would probably be prudent to contact discharged patients with positive blood cultures even when contamination is suspected on

TABLE 68–12 Features Suggestive of Contaminant ("False-Positive") Blood Culture Results

Coagulase-negative staphylococci (*Staphylococcus epidermidis*) or *S. viridans* in a single bottle in patients not suspected of infectious endocarditis and without chronic indwelling intravenous access catheters are usually contaminants.

Corynebacteria (previously known as "diphtheroids"), *Propionobacterium acne*, and bacillus species are usually contaminants, but can be pathogenic in the immunocompromised.

Multiple organisms in a series suggest contamination.

Species that grow out after prolonged culture have a higher likelihood of being contaminants. Conversely, early-growing bacteria have a much higher likelihood of being pathogens.

The patient's symptoms have resolved or are inconsistent with sepsis (beware with infectious endocarditis, which can have an indolent course).

A primary source (e.g., sputum or urine) has a different pathogen isolated.

a microbiologic basis, to ensure that their condition is improving.

Fungal Cultures

Generally, fungi are difficult to isolate in blood cultures, and it may take 4 to 6 weeks to obtain a positive yield. If a fungemia is suspected, it is best to discuss culture media and technique with the laboratory before cultures are taken. Cultures of bone marrow are occasionally positive in deep mycoses when blood cultures are negative.

BEDSIDE TESTS FOR GASTROINTESTINAL HEMORRHAGE

Detection of Blood in the Stool

Bedside fecal blood tests make use of the peroxidase-like activity of Hb. The test card is impregnated with a compound that exhibits a blue color reaction when oxidized. The original test used guaiac, but current tests use more sensitive and more reliable dyes. The addition of hydrogen peroxide developer solution will oxidize the dye in the presence of a peroxidase (e.g., Hb).

Testing for occult blood in the stool is associated with false-positive and false-negative results, but in its primary role in emergency medical practice, the test is usually reliable in detecting significant acute gastrointestinal (GI) hemorrhage. Low pH, heat, dry stools, reducing substances (e.g., ascorbate), and antacids can cause false-negative findings.[69,70] Slow bleeding in the upper GI tract in which heme can be converted (denatured) to porphyrin during transit through the gut might not be identified by stool testing. *False-positive results* have been attributed to the ingestion of partly cooked or large quantities of meat (dietary sources of myoglobin and Hb) and peroxidase-rich food.[70] Most vegetables contain peroxidase, including (in decreasing order) broccoli, turnips, cantaloupe, red radishes, horseradish, cauliflower, parsnips, Jerusalem artichokes, bean sprouts, beans, lemon rind, mushrooms, parsley, and zucchini. However, a simple in vivo study convincingly called into question the possibility of peroxidase's passing through the stomach without being denatured.[71] False-positive tests can also be caused by the presence of

povidone-iodine solution in concentrations less than 0.1% (a 1% dilution of the 10% solutions commonly available at the bedside), but are uncommon. *A positive test should be considered evidence of the presence of blood until proved otherwise.* Routine iron supplementation does cause black stool but does *not* a cause a positive Hemoccult test result, despite early in vitro studies to the contrary that are still frequently cited.[72,73]

Normal GI blood loss is limited to less than 2.5 mL/day, which translates to less than 2 mg Hb/g of stool (0.2% by weight). The sensitivity of the Hemoccult test varies both with the concentration of Hb present in the stool and the extent to which Hb is exposed to the proteolytic effects of the digestive tract. The Hemoccult test is 37% sensitive to stool containing 2.5 mg Hb/g of stool, but 95% sensitive when the concentration is 20 mg Hb/g of stool, indicating that low to moderate levels of blood may be missed.[19] The test is much more likely to detect lower GI hemorrhage than an identical rate of upper GI bleeding owing to the 100-fold diminution of peroxidase activity of blood during transition through the GI tract. Impaired detection of Hb may also occur as a result of dilution due to diarrheal illness.[19] In the event of a trace positive Hemoccult test that is not the source of an emergent illness, notification of the patient and advice regarding further outpatient evaluation should not be overlooked.[74]

Method

Smear the stool specimen onto the reagent area on the card and add a drop of developer (Fig. 68–4). Because the reaction must occur in an aqueous medium, add a drop of water to very dry specimens and allow them to moisten before addition of developer. Adding water will increase the false-positive rate, however.[70] Formation of a blue color on the paper anywhere around or under the specimen within 60 seconds should be considered a positive result. Allow the stool to penetrate (fix) on the card for 2 to 3 minutes, then read the test within 60 seconds. Always use the control areas for comparison and accuracy.

Testing for Gastric Blood

Heme tests designed for use on stool specimens can be unreliable when applied to gastric juices, with increasing inaccuracies reported as pH decreases.[75] Thus, whereas a positive test of gastric contents using a fecal Hemoccult card is likely to be accurate, a negative test with the fecal Hemoccult card does not rule out the presence of blood. The Gastroccult card uses a modified guaiac developer containing buffers to neutralize gastric acid, thereby facilitating accurate Hb detection. The test works on the same basis as the fecal guaiac test using the properties of Hb as a peroxidase. In product testing, the Gastroccult card was 100% sensitive in detecting specimens of 500 or greater parts per million of blood by volume, equivalent to 0.05%, or 0.25 mL of blood in 500 mL of gastric contents.

Method

Apply a drop of gastric aspirate to the test area. Apply two drops of developer to the sample. Look for formation of a blue dye within 1 minute. Do *not* use fecal blood test developer. In a specimen that is already a bilious green, the test is considered positive only if new *blue* color is formed. The Gastroccult card also contains a pH-testing strip located close to the occult blood testing area, which might be useful in testing emesis after an acid or alkali ingestion. Inaccurate

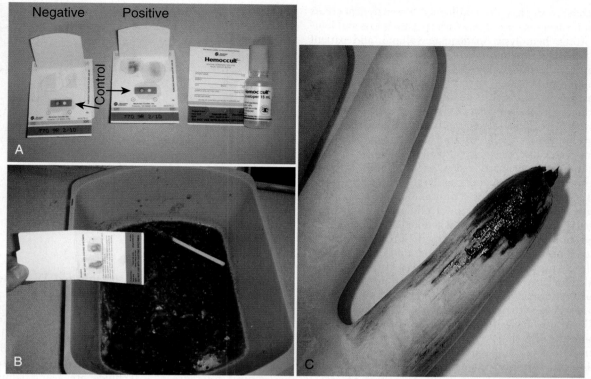

Figure 68–4 *A,* Hemoccult testing (see text): Test cards contain guaiac resin; the developer contains hydrogen peroxide (5%) and ethyl alcohol (75%). The test is based on the oxidation of guaiac by peroxide in the presence of hemoglobin catalyst, to produce a blue-colored quinolone compound. *Caveats of testing:* Two areas of stool can be tested; use the positive and negative controls; allow specimen to dry (fix) for 2 mins, read within 60 sec; *any blue color is a positive test. Positive test:* Any source of gastrointestinal bleeding, from lesion or drug-induced (aspirin, warfarin, heparin, nonsteroidal anti-inflammatory drugs [NSAIDs]). Acetaminophen use does not alter results. *Note:* Do not consider iron supplements as a cause of a false-positive test. *False negative test:* Large doses of antioxidants, such as vitamin C (pills, citric juices), can cause a false-negative test. *B,* Although Hemoccult will also detect gastric blood, use the Gastroccult card/developer to test gastric contents for blood. *C,* Iron causes a black stool, but not a reaction on the Hemoccult test. Do not attribute a positive test for blood in the stool to iron therapy.

results might be anticipated in the presence of the same confounding substances identified for the Hemoccult test: meats, peroxidase-rich foods, and reducing substances such as ascorbic acid. The accuracy of Gastroccult should not be affected by the presence of cimetidine or sucralfate.

PRINCIPLES AND PITFALLS IN PHLEBOTOMY FOR BLOOD TESTING

A number of blood tests are ordered as a part of emergency practice, but by far the most common are the complete blood count (CBC) and serum chemistries. Many medications, substances, and diseases have been identified as causes of hematologic abnormalities besides the familiar categories of infectious, inflammatory, stress-related, neoplastic, and hematopoetic processes. These include antibiotics (especially sulfonamides), antineoplastic and therapeutic drugs, immunosuppressives, and toxins (mercury and black widow spider envenomation causing leukocytosis, and arsenicals causing leucopenia). In addition, some substances and disease processes cause purely artifactual errors by interfering with the equipment and/or procedures used to perform the test. Examples include in vivo and in vitro hemolysis, cellular clumping, and markedly elevated platelet, leukocyte, or triglyceride levels, all of which can perturb the proper functioning of machinery used to perform blood assays. Because the less common causes—both pathophysiological and artifactual—of

TABLE 68–13 Artifactual Causes of False Values of the Complete Blood Count*

	Artifactual Increase	Artifactual Decrease
White blood count	Nucleated RBCs (such as sickle cell disease)	Multiple myeloma and other monoclonal gammopathies
Hemoglobin and hematocrit	Severe leukocytosis (>30,000), hyperlipemic serum, giant platelets, cryoproteins	Microcytic anemia, in vitro hemolysis

*Improper collection techniques are the most common cause of errors in all categories.
RBCs, red blood cells.

laboratory abnormalities are legion, it is necessary for most clinicians, when encountering a confirmed laboratory abnormality, to resort to standard reference texts and/or on-line sources to review potential causes or sources of error. Some of the analytical causes of false laboratory values in the CBC are listed in Table 68–13.

However, before checking for obscure or uncommon causes of laboratory abnormalities, bear in mind that the most common source of error (by far) in laboratory blood tests is in the "preanalytical phase."[76-79] This is the part of the laboratory process that actively involves the practicing clinician and over which he or she has direct influence. Preanalytical errors have been broken into problems with specimen loss and handling, clotting, hemolysis, inadequate volume, and patient identity.[78] In one series, more than 90% of these errors related to specimen collection.[80] These key components and their most common pitfalls are

1. **Preparation of the site**. The importance of aseptic technique in the preparation of a site for blood culture has been discussed. For hematologic and serum analysis, allow enough time for drying of the alcohol, because trace amounts can cause hemolysis. Povidone-iodine can cause errors in several chemistry assays, so if it is used, it should be cleaned off with alcohol, as described under "Techniques for Obtaining Blood Cultures."

2. **Venous occlusion**. Both intracellular and chemical changes start occurring in blood as soon as a tourniquet is applied, not, as is often thought, only after it has passed through a needle into a specimen container. Serum potassium levels may increase by 6% in a vessel that has been occluded for only 3 minutes.[77] Prepare venous access sites, if visually identifiable, before placing a tourniquet; after which, proceed with phlebotomy and sample acquisition as rapidly as possible, ideally within 30 seconds.[81] Avoid pumping the fist, if possible, because it increases serum concentrations of potassium, lactate, and phosphate.[77]

3. **Routine phlebotomy**. Smaller-gauge needles and higher suction pressures are associated with hemolysis. Overexuberant application of suction to a syringe is doubly counterproductive because, in addition to causing hemolysis, it is likely to occlude the needle with the vein wall, thus increasing the likelihood of unsuccessful phlebotomy as well as iatrogenic injury to the patient. Clinicians should remember that, counterintuitively, when applying negative or positive pressure to a syringe, a given amount of force on the plunger causes *higher* pressure within the chamber of a *smaller*-diameter syringe (pressure is proportional to $1/radius^2$). Blood drawn into either a standard Vacutainer or a syringe via a butterfly and tubing causes similar hemolysis rates.[81] If a phlebotomy site is tenuous, obtain specimens in order of clinical priority, but in most cases, fill the tubes in the following order to avoid cross-contamination of chemicals: blood cultures, red, blue, speckled-red, green, lavender, gray.[77]

4. **Phlebotomy through a freshly placed IV catheter**. Routine phlebotomy typically causes a hemolysis rate of less than 2%.[82] Reported hemolysis rates in ED patients are often 7% to 15%.[83–85] This might be due to any or all of the reasons considered here, but one contributing factor is probably the number of blood specimens drawn in the ED through a catheter being placed for therapeutic use. Several studies have shown that this arrangement significantly increases rates.[83,85,86] The popularity of this technique in emergency care is most probably owing to limitations of personnel and temporal resources and the attempt to enhance patient comfort by avoiding an extra needle stick. Because tourniquet times are probably longer in catheter placement than in simple phlebotomy, this likely contributes to hemolysis, although this has never been experimentally verified. Perceived ease of blood aspiration, larger-bore catheters, and small aliquots drawn through the catheter have been associated with lower rates of hemolysis.[84,86] Laboratory results of specimens obtained in this manner are accurate within clinically acceptable margins of error.

TABLE 68–14 Laboratory Values That Are Accurate When Venous Blood Is Obtained from an Indwelling Intravenous Catheter or Saline Lock, Carefully following the Procedure Outlined in Text

Hemoglobin
Hematocrit
Sodium
Potassium
Bicarbonate
Chloride
Glucose
Creatine phosphokinase
Troponin I

5. **Phlebotomy through an established IV catheter**. An established IV line appears to be a reliable source of blood for analysis, although success rates are lower and hemolysis rates higher than for phlebotomy from a fresh site. Table 68–14 lists common blood tests that are accurate by analysis of blood from an established IV site.[87,88] As with the use of a freshly placed catheter, results are accurate within clinical tolerances.[89,90] If fluids are being administered through the catheter, turn it off for at least 3 minutes *before* applying a tourniquet for phlebotomy. A typical 18-gauge 30-mm-long plastic IV catheter without a heparin well has a volume of 0.07 mL. The heparin well adds a volume of 0.05 mL to make a combined volume of 0.12 mL. Thus, using a syringe directly attached to the heparin well (IV tubing detached), just 1 mL of aspirated fluid should have replaced the entire volume of the heparin well at least six times. Most studies have discarded at least three times that volume. Some have suggested a "push-pull" technique (aspirating a small volume into the syringe and reinjecting before drawing a final 3 mL for discarding) in order to minimize the likelihood of small sequestered pockets of IV fluid in the heparin well.[91] The use of the standard distal port of the IV tubing (usually 25 cm from the end) is not recommended. The IV tubing has a volume (combined with the heparin well and catheter) of about 1.6 mL, making it necessary to discard large volumes of blood, in addition to the risk of contamination from IV fluids entrained in the specimen from the main IV line during aspiration through the port

6. **Disposition of the specimen after phlebotomy**. If blood has been drawn into a syringe, promptly decant it into the appropriate containers for the laboratory. If it has already started to clot, do not force it, because this would cause hemolysis of the specimen. Because cells and platelets are fragile, specimens requiring agitation (all except red- and speckled-red–top tubes) should be *rocked gently, not shaken*. If specimens are sent to the laboratory in pneumatic tubes, surround them with shock-absorbing material. Artifactual increase of measured HCO_3 occurs fairly rapidly at room temperature.[89] Progressive hemolysis of blood occurs with prolonged standing, and it is likely that specimens are of little utility after more than 2 to 3 hours of typical ED storage conditions, although one study showed that unrefrigerated *nonagitated* samples were reliable for up to 8 hours.[92]

DIAGNOSTIC AND THERAPEUTIC TOXICOLOGIC BEDSIDE PROCEDURES

The management of patients who present with an altered mental status can be challenging, especially if the clinician suspects a drug overdose or poisoning. These patients often present with no available history or an inaccurate history. Clinicians must rely heavily on physical examination findings and other sources of information to diagnose or confirm their clinical suspicions of poisoning or overdose. The hospital toxicology laboratory can be valuable in select cases. Limited screening tests for commonly ingested drugs are available, and ascertaining levels of specific drugs (e.g., acetaminophen, lithium, digoxin, phenytoin) can help guide management. However, hospital laboratories are not equipped to perform timely analytical procedures for the thousands of possible drugs or toxins. In fact, drugs-of-abuse screening panels that most hospitals employ have been shown to rarely influence medical management of adult ED patients. Conversely, these drug screens in select pediatric patients may have more of an impact on medical management.

Diagnostic bedside testing for specific poisons or toxins has the advantage of being cost-effective and timely. When applied appropriately, certain bedside tests provide immediate information to the clinician and can significantly influence medical management in a timely manner. Unfortunately, with the establishment of Clinical Laboratory Improvement Amendments of 1988 (CLIA), bedside laboratory testing has undergone stricter oversight. This federal regulation has jurisdiction on any laboratory tests performed on humans and has added a layer of complexity to bedside testing. Tests that are not performed on humans, such as the Meixner test or mothball testing, are not covered by the CLIA act. This section discusses bedside diagnostic and therapeutic toxicologic procedures.

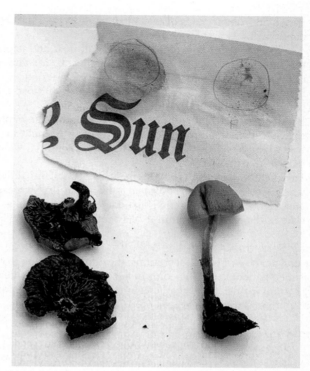

Figure 68–5 The Meixner test is a crude assay for amatoxins. Place portions of the unknown dried mushroom on low-grade newsprint and add 10-N hydrochloric acid. The dried-up mushroom (*left*) is *Galerina marginata*, which yields a blue reaction (positive = probably deadly poisonous); the little brown mushroom (*right*) does not (negative = toxicity uncertain). This test is the only one readily available but has varying accuracy and depends on the paper being used (regular newsprint is shown here). (*Courtesy of Kathie T. Hodge and Kent Loeffler [photographer], Cornell University. http://blog.mycology.cornell.edu*)

1299

Noninvasive Diagnostic Procedures

Amatoxin: Meixner Test

The ingestion of several types of mushrooms (e.g., *Amanita phalloides*) can be fatal. The most poisonous of these mushrooms contain amatoxins. Patients who have ingested amatoxins often complain of GI symptoms consisting of nausea, vomiting, diarrhea, and abdominal cramping beginning 6 to 8 hours after ingestion. They often bring in specimens of the mushrooms chopped, crushed, cooked, or mixed with stool or gastric contents. Standard hospital laboratories cannot confirm or exclude the diagnosis of amatoxin poisoning; therefore, treatment decisions are made on clinical grounds.

A simple colorimetric test for detecting amatoxins (Meixner test) has been developed that can be used on gastric contents, stool, or actual mushroom samples. The basis of this test is the acid-catalyzed color reaction of amatoxins with lignin, a complex organic compound found in wood pulp (Fig. 68–5). Cheaper grades of paper (e.g., newsprint or the whiter pages of a telephone book) contain high amounts of lignin. Although there have been no extensive reports of in vivo studies, in vitro tests have shown this method to be somewhat sensitive and relatively specific for amatoxins, but it should be considered an *adjunctive test only*. Psilocybin-containing mushrooms can cause false-positive results for amatoxin.[93]

The procedure for the qualitative detection of amatoxin consists of squeezing a drop of liquid from a fresh mushroom sample or squashing a piece of fresh mushroom onto a piece of newspaper. If stool or gastric samples are the only available specimens, mix the sample with reagent-grade methanol (99.8%) to extract the amatoxin. If the samples are mixed with methanol, centrifuge and filter them. Then place a drop of the liquid extract on newspaper. Gently air-dry all specimens at room temperature and avoid direct sunlight. Add two to three drops of concentrated hydrochloric acid (37%) to the dried specimen. Use an adjacent area for a control. High amounts of amatoxin in the dried samples exhibit a blue color in 1 to 2 minutes. Small amounts of amatoxin show a blue color in the sampled area in 10 to 20 minutes. This procedure has *not* been proved effective using other bodily secretions, such as blood or urine.[93]

Mothball Identification

At present, commercial mothballs are composed of either nontoxic paradichlorobenzene or possibly toxic naphthalene. Naphthalene can cause a hemolytic reaction in neonates and patients with glucose-6-phosphate dehydrogenase (G6PD) deficiency.[94] In the past, mothballs have also been produced from camphor, which can cause central nervous system depression and seizures. Fortunately, camphor mothballs are no longer commercially available, although they may still exist in older households. A rapid differentiation between these groups of mothballs can expedite patient management and disposition. Several bedside tests have been reported to facilitate this.

1. Paradichlorobenzene is heavier than naphthalene. In turn, naphthalene is heavier than camphor.

   In lukewarm tap water, camphor will float and naphthalene and paradichlorobenzene will sink. In a solution of 3 tbsp. of table salt thoroughly dissolved in 4 ounces of lukewarm water, camphor, and naphthalene will float and paradichlorobenzene will sink.

2. Paradichlorobenzene has a lower melting point than naphthalene. Paradichlorobenzene mothballs will melt in a water bath at 53°C, whereas naphthalene requires a water bath hotter than 80°C.

3. Paradichlorobenzene is described as "wet and oily," whereas naphthalene is described as having a "dry" appearance. Paradichlorobenzene is familiar to many people as a cake of disinfectant used in urinals and diaper pails.

Body Secretion Analysis

Careful analysis of bodily secretions, the odor emanating from poisoned patients, and the color of their urine can help identify certain toxins. Some characteristic smells and urine colors are noted in Tables 68–15 and 68–16.

Bedside Toxicologic Tests on Urine

Ethylene Glycol. Evaluation of the urine of patients who may have ingested ethylene glycol can be helpful. Urine should be tested for fluorescence (an additive in many commercial antifreeze products) under an ultraviolet light and the presence of calcium oxalate crystals (a metabolic byproduct of ethylene glycol metabolism).

Microscopic inspection of urine for the presence of *calcium oxalate crystals* (either envelope-shaped calcium dihydrate or needle-shaped calcium monohydrate) indicates high oxalate levels in the serum (Fig. 68–6; see also Fig. 68–3). Calcium monohydrate crystals can be easily confused with sodium urate crystals; therefore, the presence of the dihydrate crystal tends to be more specific for ethylene glycol ingestion. The lack of these crystals does not rule out significant ethylene glycol ingestion because the excretion of these may occur late in the ingestion (>6 hr) and occasionally does not occur at all.[95,96]

Visual inspection of urine under a Wood's lamp or ultraviolet light to ascertain *fluorescence* may also be helpful in the diagnosis of ethylene glycol exposure. Antifreeze is the most common source of ingested ethylene glycol. Fluorescein, the actual fluorescing material, is often placed in commercially available antifreeze to enable mechanics to detect radiator leaks with a Wood's lamp or other ultraviolet light source. Fluorescein is a nontoxic inert vegetable dye that is eliminated unchanged in the urine. Therefore, high levels of fluorescein in urine suggest significant ethylene glycol ingestion. However, a lack of fluorescein does not rule out a significant exposure, because *not all antifreezes contain fluorescein or high concentrations of fluorescein in relation to ethylene glycol.* False-positive findings can occur if certain plastic urine containers are used.[97]

To perform this procedure, place the test urine sample and control samples into separate glass test tubes. Inspect for fluorescence under a Wood's lamp in a dark room. Always perform this test using controls that include urine that does not contain fluorescein and urine that does contain fluorescein. The use of controls may increase sensitivity and specificity from 49% and 75% to a sensitivity and specificity of

TABLE 68–15 Diagnostic Odors

Characteristic Odor	Responsible Drug or Toxin
Acetone (sweet, fruity; pearlike)	Lacquer, ethanol, isopropyl alcohol, chloroform, diabetic ketoacidosis, alcoholic ketoacidosis, trichloroethane, paraldehyde, chloral hydrate, methylbromide, *Pseudomonas* infections
Alcohols	Ethanol, (congeners) isopropyl alcohol
Ammonia-like	Uremia
Automobile exhaust	Carbon monoxide (odorless, but associated with exhaust)
Beer (stale)	Scrofula
Bitter almond	Cyanide
Carrots	Cicutoxin (or water hemlock)
Coal gas (stove gas)	Carbon monoxide (odorless, but associated with coal gas)
Disinfectants	Phenol, creosote
Eggs (rotten)	Hydrogen sulfide, carbon disulfide, mercaptans, disulfiram, *N*-acetylcysteine
Feculent	Intestinal obstruction
Fish or raw liver (musty)	Hepatic failure, zinc phosphide, hypermethioninemia, trimethylaminuria
Fruitlike	Nitrites (e.g., amyl, butyl), ethanol (congeners), isopropyl alcohol
Garlic	Phosphorus, tellurium, arsenic, parathion, malathion, selenium, dimethyl sulfoxide (DMSO), thallium
Halitosis	Acute illness, poor oral hygiene
Hay	Phosgene
Mothballs	Naphthalene, *p*-dichlorobenzene, camphor
Peanuts	*N*-3-pyridyl-methyl-*N*-*p*-nitrophenyl urea (Vacor)
Pepper-like	*O*-chlorobenzylidene malonitrile
Putrid	Anaerobic infections, esophageal diverticulum, lung abscess, scurvy
Rope (burned)	Marijuana, opium
Shoe polish	Nitrobenzene
Sweating feet	Isovaleric acid acidemia
Tobacco	Nicotine
Vinegar	Acetic acid
Vinyl-like	Ethchlorvynol (Placidyl)
Violets	Turpentine (metabolites excreted in urine)
Wintergreen	Methyl salicylate

From Chiang WK: Otolaryngologic principles. In Goldfrank LR, Flomenbaum NE, Lewin NA, et al (eds): Goldfrank's Toxicologic Emergencies, 5th ed. East Norwalk, CT, Appleton & Lange, 1994, p 374.

TABLE 68–16 Drugs That Color Urine Yellow

Yellow
   Quinacrine (Atabrine) in acid urine
   Riboflavin (large doses)
Yellow-green
   Methylene blue, see Blue
Yellow-orange
   Fluorescein sodium
Yellow-pink
   Cascara* in alkaline urine, see Yellow-brown, Brown, Black
   Senna* in alkaline urine, see Yellow-brown, Brown
Yellow-brown
   Cascara* in acid urine, see Yellow-pink, Brown, Black
   Nitrofurantoin* (Furadantin and others), see Brown
Orange
   Phenazopyridine* (Pyridium), see Red
Orange-red
   Rifampin (Rifadin, Rifamycin, Rimactane)
Pink
   Phenothiazines,* see Red, Red-brown
   Phenytoin* (Dilantin), see Red, Red-brown
Red
   Anthraquinone in alkaline urine
   Deferoxamine (Desferal)
   Methydopa (Aldomet), see Brown, Black
   Phenazopyridine* (Pyridium), see Orange

   Phenothiazines,* see Pink, Red-brown
   Phenytoin* (Dilantin), see Pink, Red-brown

Red-purple
   Phenacetin,* see Brown
Red-brown
   Phenothiazines,* see Pink, Red
   Phenytoin* (Dilantin), see Pink, Red
Brown
   Cascara* in alkaline urine, see Yellow-brown, Yellow-pink, Black
   Levodopa (Dopar)
   Methocarbamol* (Robaxin), see Green, Black
   Metronidazole (Flagyl)
   Methyldopa* (Aldomet), see Red, Black
   Nitrofurantoin* (Funadantin and others), see Yellow-brown
   Phenacetin,* see Red-purple
   Quinine,* see Black
   Senna* in alkaline urine on standing, see Yellow-brown, Yellow-pink
Blue
   Methylene blue,* see Green
   Triamterene (Dyrenium), fluorescent
Blue-green
   Amitryptyline (Elavil, Endep)
Green
   Indomethacin (Indiocin) from liver damage
   Methocarbamol* (Robaxin), see Brown-black
Black
   Cascara* in alkaline urine on standing, see Yellow-brown, Yellow-pink, Brown
   Iron sorbitex* (Jectofer), see Brown
   Methocarbamol* (Robaxin), see Brown, Green
   Methyldopa (Aldomet), see Red, Brown
   Quinine,* see Brown

*Drug imparts more than one color to urine and is listed under each color it adds.
From Thoman M: Physicians' primer on the toxicology of adolescent drug use. Vet Hum Toxicol 31:384, 1989.

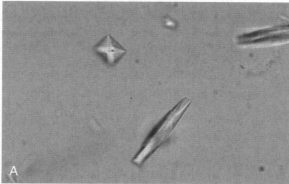
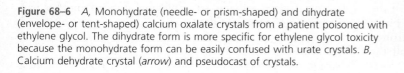
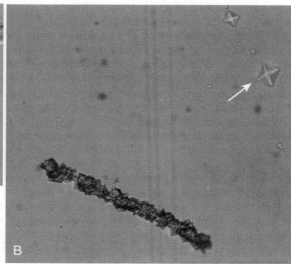

Figure 68–6 *A,* Monohydrate (needle- or prism-shaped) and dihydrate (envelope- or tent-shaped) calcium oxalate crystals from a patient poisoned with ethylene glycol. The dihydrate form is more specific for ethylene glycol toxicity because the monohydrate form can be easily confused with urate crystals. *B,* Calcium dehydrate crystal (*arrow*) and pseudocast of crystals.

100%.[98] Fluorescein is readily available because fluorescein-containing strips are commonly used in ophthalmologic procedures (see Chapter 63, Ophthalmologic Procedures).

Salicylates. Several bedside tests have been developed to qualitatively detect salicylates in urine. These include 10% ferric chloride solution, Trinder's solution, or Phenistix reagent strips. All of these are rapid, inexpensive, sensitive tests that give a qualitative rather than a quantitative result.

Ferric chloride and Trinder's solution both have sensitivities of 100% with serum salicylate levels of 5 mg/dL. False

positives can occur with both tests. Acetoacetic acid, acetone, and phenylpyruvic acid will cause false-positive results. Thus, this test may be falsely positive in patients with diabetic, alcoholic, or starvation ketoacidosis. Phenol-containing drugs such as diflunisal, sulfasalazine, and salicylamide may also produce false positives. Any positive result requires a confirmatory quantitative serum salicylate assay.[99]

The *ferric chloride test* is a commonly used rapid, qualitative, urinary screening procedure. To perform this test, add several drops of 10% ferric chloride to 1 or 2 mL of urine

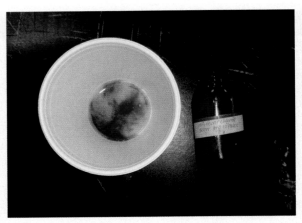

Figure 68–7 Adding ferric chloride (10%) to a few milliliters of urine immediately turns a deep purple color in the presence of small quantities of aspirin. Beware of other color changes, such as gray or brown, that are not a *positive test*. This test is also positive in ketoacidotic states, such as diabetic ketoacidosis.

that has been collected in a test tube. The immediate appearance of a bluish-purple color signifies that salicylates are present in urine (Fig. 68–7). This test is very sensitive, and as few as 1 aspirin taken within 12 to 24 hours will give a positive result. It will require 60 to 120 minutes from time of ingestion for this reaction to become positive in patients with normal renal function; so early test results may be misleading.

The *Trinder test* uses a mixture of mercuric chloride and ferric nitrate in deionized water. To perform this test, mix 1 mL of urine with 1 mL of Trinder's solution. A violet or purple color signifies the presence of salicylates. Acetoacetic acid and high levels of phenothiazines may give false-positive results.

Phenistix reagent strips were originally developed to detect phenylketonuria. However, Phenistix strips also turn brown in presence of salicylates. False-positive findings for salicylates can occur if phenothiazines are present.

Bedside Toxicologic Tests on Oral Secretions and Breath: Ethyl Alcohol

Several bedside devices have been developed to measure alcohol concentrations in bodily fluids. Measurements of alcohol concentration in expired air or saliva have been shown to correlate well with blood alcohol concentrations in the appropriate settings.

Breath alcohol analyzers have been developed since the 1950s and are currently used in law enforcement. These devices typically use an infrared spectral analysis to determine the concentration of alcohol in expired air. Almost all the alcohol found in expired air at the level of the mouth is secondary to alcohol diffused from the bronchial system rather than the alveolar system.[100] Minor alterations in breathing patterns can cause large variations in readings. Thus, uncooperative patients who do not exhale properly will cause an inaccurate reading. Other causes of inaccurate readings include the recent use of alcohol-containing products such as ingestion of alcohol-containing products, belching or vomiting, use of inhalers, poor technique, or restrictive pulmonary pathology.

Alcohol concentrations in saliva have been shown to correlate to serum concentrations. Bedside measurement

of salivary alcohol concentrations can also be obtained using a dipstick-like device. These devices use an enzymatic reaction involving alcohol dehydrogenase to measure alcohol concentrations.[101] Patients who are dehydrated (a common occurrence in alcohol-intoxicated patients) are often unable to provide adequate saliva samples, and inaccurate readings have occurred in patients with high blood alcohol concentrations.[102,103]

Bedside Toxicologic Tests on Blood: Methemoglobinemia

Patients with methemoglobinemia will often have a normal partial pressure of oxygen (Po_2) on routine arterial blood gas analysis, a normal *calculated* Hb saturation, a *nondiagnostic pulse oximeter reading*, and a cyanosis that does not clear with O_2 administration. Newer models of co-oximeters are able to reliably measure methemoglobin levels. Bedside visual inspection of venous or arterial blood may be helpful in the diagnosis of methemoglobinemia. Methemoglobinemia occurs when normal Hb is exposed to an oxidant stress (Fe^{2+} converted to Fe^{3+}). If the erythrocytes are not able to handle such stress, such as in the presence of G6PD deficiency, Hb remains in an oxidized state (methemoglobin), causing a color change in the molecule.

To evaluate for methemoglobinemia, place a drop of sample blood on a white background (a white coffee filter is appropriate) in a well-lit environment. Next to this, place a drop of normal blood as a comparison control sample. Blood with methemoglobinemia appears "darker" or "chocolate-brown."[104] This method relies on the ability of the examiner to distinguish color changes and therefore may have a degree of interobserver variance. Methemoglobin levels of less than 10% may only slightly alter the color of blood and thereby cause a false-negative finding. Methemoglobin levels of between 12% and 14% may cause a false-negative reading 50% of the time. Methemoglobin levels greater than 15% are reported to cause a cyanotic appearance in patients. With levels of 35% or greater, the identification of methemoglobinemia by visual inspection of the color of blood is quite accurate.[104] At this level, almost all patients are obviously cyanotic and symptomatic.

Invasive Diagnostic Procedures

Several invasive diagnostic bedside procedures can be useful in the assessment of possible drug overdoses. The basic premise of these procedures is that patients who have been exposed to a certain drug or poison will respond in a particular fashion if given a diagnostic challenge dose of another particular drug or true antidote.

Naloxone

Naloxone hydrochloride (Narcan) is a μ-opioid receptor antagonist. A diagnostic challenge of IV naloxone has been recommended for all patients with central nervous system depression.[105] Certain clinical findings such as miosis, decreased respiratory rate, and evidence of illicit drug use can predict many patients who will respond to a challenge dose of naloxone.[106] If a patient's mental status improves significantly after a dose of naloxone, the patient should be considered to have been exposed to an opioid substance. This is true even if a laboratory drug screen is negative for opioids. Furthermore, many of the synthetic opiates, such as fentanyl, propoxyphene, meperidine, methadone, and pentazocine, may not be detected by the routinely used immunoassay drug screen. Although cases have been reported of patients with nonopioid overdoses (such as alcohol or phencyclidine) responding to naloxone, these single observations have not been confirmed in controlled animal or human studies.

The traditional challenge dose of naloxone in an adult or child is 2 mg every 2 minutes intravenously until a response is achieved or 10 mg is given.[107] Some clinicians prefer to use much smaller doses (0.1–0.2 mg) and titrate to effect. This may partially reverse opioid overdose–related symptoms and confirm the diagnosis without precipitating the opioid withdrawal syndrome seen in patients with opioid dependency. Most patients with an opioid overdose will exhibit some response to 1 to 4 mg of naloxone, but some massive overdoses might require larger amounts. A patient who does not respond at all to 10 mg of naloxone probably does not have a pure opioid overdose. High doses of naloxone may be needed to reverse many synthetic opiates, such as propoxyphene and methadone. Lower doses can be given (0.4–0.8 mg in adults or 0.01 mg/kg in children) to reverse known opioid-induced respiratory depression without reversing analgesia. Because naloxone has a half-life between 30 and 60 minutes, a continuous drip of naloxone can be used to avoid re-sedation. A reasonable choice is to use two thirds of the initial bolus dose that achieved the desired reversal effect as the hourly IV dose. For example, a patient who satisfactorily responded to 1.5 mg of naloxone might receive a naloxone solution of 10 mg of naloxone in 500 mL of normal saline at a rate of 1 mg (50 mL) per hour intravenously. Nalmefene, a long-acting opioid receptor antagonist that has a terminal half-life of roughly 11 hours, can also be given to patients with suspected overdoses. Theoretically, a single dose of nalmefene will be effective longer than the effects of heroin or most abused opiate substances. The initial recommended dose is 1.0 to 1.5 mg intravenously.

Naloxone and nalmefene have minimal significant side effects, but they can precipitate withdrawal in patients addicted to opioids. Unlike alcohol withdrawal, naloxone-induced opioid withdrawal in adults is short-lived and is usually not life threatening. Withdrawal can be avoided if lower initial doses of naloxone or nalmefene are given and then are slowly titrated upward to the desired effect.

Re-sedation may occur if the ingested drug (e.g., methadone, oxycontin, morphine sulfate [MS Contin]) has a *clinical effect* longer than that of naloxone. Calculated drug half-lives have minimal clinical validity. If no narcotic effect is evident in 60 to 120 minutes after standard doses of naloxone (common with heroin, for example), no clinically significant re-sedation is expected. Larger naloxone doses may prolong the expected antidote effect of naloxone, and longer observation is required. All timing and dose recommendations are guidelines, and all clinical decisions with regard to re-sedation should be individualized.

Flumazenil

Flumazenil (Romazicon) is a competitive benzodiazepine receptor antagonist that has the ability to reverse the central nervous system depression caused by all currently commercially available benzodiazepines. Its routine use in the setting of possible benzodiazepine overdose is controversial but is supported as a diagnostic and therapeutic agent in selected cases. Unlike naloxone, flumazenil can have significant side effects, but only in certain subsets of patients,[106] and its downsides are likely exaggerated in many texts. Complications

include precipitating seizures or a withdrawal syndrome in benzodiazepine-dependent patients. To minimize the chance of seizures, flumazenil should be avoided in known benzodiazepines-dependent patients and those who may have ingested epileptogenic drugs (e.g., cyclic antidepressants, cocaine, theophylline, lithium, carbamazepine, or isoniazid).

In suspected benzodiazepine overdoses in which patients present with obtundation and have no history of seizures or suspicion of involvement of epileptogenic agents, flumazenil can be administered intravenously at a dose of 0.2 to 0.5 mg/min. Most benzodiazepine-overdosed patients show mental status improvement with 1 mg of flumazenil and almost all respond to 3 to 5 mg. Small, escalating doses given slowly (maximally, 0.5 mg/min) have been recommended. Larger doses can be given at one time as a bolus, although this increases such side effects as anxiety, agitation, and emotional lability; it also increases the chances of precipitating withdrawal in benzodiazepine-dependent patients. Fortunately, seizures that occur after flumazenil use are usually transient and can usually be controlled with additional benzodiazepines. In rare cases, higher doses of benzodiazepines, barbiturates, and phenytoin might be required.

If a patient responds to flumazenil with an improvement in depressed mental status, this suggests only that the patient is under the influence of a benzodiazepine. Flumazenil can partially reverse the effects of many of the newer nonbenzodiazepine sleeping agents that affect the γ-aminobutyric acid (GABA) pathway, such as zolpidem, zoplicone, and eszopiclone. Flumazenil can improve the mental status in patients with hepatic encephalopathy.[108–110] It does not have any significant effect on alcohol, barbiturates, and other nonbenzodiazepine sedative-hypnotics.

Re-sedation is possible if the ingested drug has a *clinical duration* longer than that of flumazenil. Calculated drug half-lives have minimal clinical validity. If no re-sedation has occurred 60 to 90 minutes after standard doses of flumazenil, clinically significant re-sedation is not expected. If higher flumazenil doses have been used, additional observation may be warranted. All timing and dose recommendations are guidelines, and all clinical decisions with regard to re-sedation should be individualized.

Physostigmine

Physostigmine is an acetylcholinesterase inhibitor that can penetrate into the central nervous system and thus can reverse both the central and the peripheral effects of anticholinergic agents. In the majority of patients with anticholinergic toxicity, no laboratory tests are available to rapidly confirm the diagnosis, and testing for specific drugs is limited or unavailable. A clinical picture that may consist of mydriasis, dry and flushed skin, dry mucous membranes, urinary incontinence, absent bowel sounds, tachycardia, hyperthermia, hallucinations, agitation, and seizures suggests an anticholinergic syndrome. In some cases (low-dose antihistamines and others), only a central nervous system syndrome exists, characterized by hallucinations, agitation, and confusion. A rapid and dramatic response to physostigmine often confirms a diagnosis of anticholinergic toxicity. In these patients, physostigmine often decreases the degree of agitation and confusion.[111–113] The use of physostigmine as a diagnostic challenge can be helpful in select situations, but similar to flumazenil, the routine use of physostigmine as a diagnostic bedside challenge in all obtunded patients, especially in those without anticholinergic findings, should be discouraged. In some cases, the agitation produced by potent anticholinergics, such as scopolamine, is totally resistant to benzodiazepines, and the judicious use of physostigmine is warranted to avoid excessive sedation or chemical paralysis/ventilation. Physostigmine has recently been used to reverse a curious anticholinergic syndrome precipitated by propofol sedation.

As a diagnostic challenge or therapeutic intervention, physostigmine can be administered intravenously under constant cardiac monitoring at a dose of 1 to 2 mg in adults and 0.02 mg/kg in children, over 3 to 5 minutes. It will take 2 to 4 minutes for the central nervous system effect to be apparent. *Some clinicians empirically pretreat with a benzodiazepine to prevent seizures.* Because the half-life of physostigmine is 30 to 60 minutes, a repeat dose of 0.5 to 2 mg can also be given as clinically indicated.

Similar to flumazenil, physostigmine has been reported to interact detrimentally with cyclic antidepressants, often causing life-threatening dysrhythmias. Physostigmine also can cause an excess of acetylcholine and a resultant cholinergic crisis. This syndrome includes salivation, lacrimation, urination, defecation, bradycardia, bronchorrhea, and seizures. For this reason, 1 mg of atropine, intravenously, should be readily available to reverse potential cholinergic excess when using physostigmine.

Deferoxamine

Deferoxamine is an organic compound derived from the bacterium *Streptomyces pilosus* and can chelate iron. It can be used as a therapy or as a diagnostic challenge in patients with iron overdoses. Patients who have unstable vital signs or significant GI or central nervous system symptoms usually require therapeutic doses of deferoxamine. *Asymptomatic* patients with a history of iron overdose usually require supportive care only. Patients with persistent but mild symptoms, such as vomiting and diarrhea, may be given a diagnostic challenge dose of deferoxamine. A diagnostic challenge is preferential over ancillary laboratory testing because tests such as iron levels and total iron-binding capacity in the setting of iron overdose can be inaccurate, misleading, and time-consuming.[114]

A diagnostic challenge dose of deferoxamine is administered intramuscularly or intravenously over 45 minutes at doses of 40 to 90 mg/kg up to a maximum of 1 g in children and 2 g in adults. Deferoxamine can also be administered intravenously as a constant infusion of 15 mg/kg/hr. A positive result occurs when chelated iron in the form of ferrioxamine appears in the urine. This usually causes the urine to turn a reddish orange or "vin rose" color in 2 to 3 hours after initiation of treatment. The color change is qualitative only and has no prognostic significance. Color change caused by ferrioxamine is pH- and concentration-dependent, and false-negative test results occur.

Chronically administered deferoxamine has been reported to have multiple adverse effects, such as adult respiratory distress syndrome (ARDS), visual defects, and enhancement of *Yersinia enterocolitica* infections. In the setting of the single-challenge dose, flushing, erythema, tachycardia, urticaria, and hypotension caused by rapid administration of deferoxamine are the most serious side effects.

Invasive Therapeutic Procedures

The indications and rationale for use of certain therapeutic procedures in toxicology are often misunderstood.

TABLE 68–17 Drugs That Have Increased Elimination with Urinary Alkalinization

Chlorpropamide
2,4-Dichlorophenoxyacetic acid
Formate
Methotrexate
Phenobarbital
Salicylates

Alkalinization of Urine and Blood

Alkalinization of urine consists of manipulating the pH of urine to enhance excretion of certain drugs (Table 68–17). Weak acids remain in ionic form in a basic milieu. The ionic form often prevents reabsorption of that drug in the proximal tubule, and urinary alkalinization can therefore promote elimination in the urine. For certain drugs, this can play a significant role in their elimination. For example, salicylate elimination increases proportionately to the urinary flow rate, but it increases *exponentially* with increases in the urinary pH. The increased serum clearance attributed to alkalinization does not correlate well with outcome or length of hospitalization.

Recommendations differ on the actual method or formula to achieve urinary alkalinization. No body of literature exists that supports one method of urinary alkalinization over another. In general, this procedure should be titrated to the patient's fluid and acid-base status to achieve a urinary pH of 7.5 to 8.0. One method uses a constant infusion of a relatively isotonic solution consisting of 3 ampules of sodium bicarbonate (44 mmol/ampule) added to 1 L of 5% dextrose in water (D_5W). Another formula is to begin with a bolus of 2 ampules of IV sodium bicarbonate, or 1 to 2 mmol/kg of body weight. The bolus is followed with a constant infusion of 3 ampules of sodium bicarbonate in 1 L of D_5W solution with 20 to 40 mmol of potassium infused at 100 to 300 mL/hr. These formulas assume that the patient has a normal renal function. Repetitive boluses of sodium bicarbonate ampules also can be used, but this may increase the chances of hypernatremia, hypokalemia, relative hypocalcemia, fluid overload, and alkalemia. All of these are potential adverse effects of aggressive urinary alkalinization. The actual amount of fluids and bicarbonate administered requires titration to the patient's clinical condition, and careful monitoring of electrolyte, pH, and fluid status is encouraged.

Urinary alkalinization can sometimes be difficult to achieve or maintain. Hypovolemia is probably the leading cause of an inability to achieve alkaline urine. Other theoretical causes are hypokalemia, hypomagnesemia, and hypochloremia. Several authors have suggested that in patients with severe salicylate poisoning, urinary alkalinization may be difficult, if not impossible, to achieve.[115] Some will empirically add potassium and magnesium to the diuresis fluid.

Ethanol Infusion

Fomepizole (4-methylpyrazole) has been approved by the U. S. Food and Drug Administration for the treatment of ethylene glycol poisonings. It has also been used successfully in treating methanol poisonings.[116,117] Compared with the traditional treatment of toxic alcohol poisoning, namely ethanol, fomepizole has the advantages of ease of use, lower side effects

TABLE 68–18 Ethanol in Methanol or Ethylene Glycol Poisoning*

Intravenous Ethanol: Loading Dose (using a 10% ethanol solution)[a] (A 10% volume/volume concentration yields approximately 100 mg/mL)

	Volume of Loading Dose (given over 1–2 hr as tolerated)[a]					
	10 kg	15 kg	30 kg	50 kg	70 kg	100 kg
Loading dose of 1000 mg/kg of 10% ethanol (infused over 1–2 hr as tolerated); *assumes a zero ethanol level to start* Aim is to produce a serum ethanol level of 100–150 mg/dL	100 mL	150 mL	300 mL	500 mL	700 mL	1000 mL

Oral Ethanol: Loading Dose (A 20% volume/volume concentration yields approximately 200 mg/mL)

	Volume of Loading Dose					
	10 kg	15 kg	30 kg	50 kg	70 kg	100 kg
Loading dose of 1000 mg/kg of 20% ethanol,[b] diluted in juice; may be administered orally or via nasogastric tube; *assumes a zero ethanol level to start* Aim is to produce a serum ethanol level of 100–150 mg/dL	50 mL	75 mL	150 mL	250 mL	350 mL	500 mL

Intravenous Ethanol: Maintenance Dose (using a 10% ethanol solution)[c] (A 10% volume/volume concentration yields approximately 100 mg/mL. Infusion to be started immediately following the loading dose. Aim is to maintain serum ethanol level of 100–150 mg/dL[†])

	Infusion Rate (mL/hr for various weights)[c]					
	10 kg	15 kg	30 kg	50 kg	70 kg	100 kg
Normal Maintenance Range (mg/kg/hr)						
80	8	12	24	40	56	80
110	11	16	33	55	77	110
130	13	19	39	65	91	130
Approximate Maintenance Dose for Chronic Alcoholic						
150[‡]	15	22	45	75	105	150
Range Required during Hemodialysis						
250[‡]	25	38	75	125	175	250
300[‡]	30	45	90	150	210	300
350[‡]	35	53	105	175	245	350

Oral Ethanol: Maintenance Dose (A 20% volume/volume concentration yields approximately 200 mg/mL; infusion to be given each hour immediately following a loading dose; aim is to maintain seum ethanol level of 100–150 mg/dL;[†] each dose may be diluted in juice and given orally or via nasogastric tube)

	Infusion Rate (mL/hr[§] for various weights[¶])					
	10 kg	15 kg	30 kg	50 kg	70 kg	100 kg
Normal maintenance Range (mg/kg/hr)						
80	4	6	12	20	28	40
110	6	8	17	27	39	55
130	7	10	20	33	46	66
Approximate Range for Chronic Alcoholic or for Patient Receiving Continuous Oral Activated Charcoal						
150	8	11	22	38	53	75
Range Required during Hemodialysis						
250	13	19	38	63	88	125
300	15	23	46	75	105	150
350	18	26	52	88	123	175

[a]If a 5% ethanol solution is used, *double* the volume of the loading dose.
[b]Equivalent to a 40-proof solution.
[c]If a 5% ethanol solution is used, *double* the volume rate; monitor closely for potential volume overload.
*Note: *Concentrations > 10% are not recommended for IV administration. Concentrations > 30% are not recommended for oral administration.* The dose schedule is based on the premise that the patient initially has a *zero* ethanol level. The aim of therapy is to maintain a serum ethanol level of 100–150 mg/dL, but constant monitoring of the ethanol level is required because of wide variations in endogenous metabolic capacity. Ethanol is removed by dialysis, and the infusion rate of ethanol must be increased during dialysis. Prolonged ethanol administration may lead to *hypoglycemia*. Note: 10% ethanol for infusion may be difficult to find in the hospital pharmacy. To formulate 10% ethanol for infusion (1) remove 50 mL from a 1-L bottle of 5% ethanol/D_5W and replace it with 50 mL of 100% ethanol, or (2) remove 100 mL from a 1-L bottle of D_5W and replace it with 100 mL of 100% ethanol.
[†]Serum ethanol levels should be monitored closely.
[‡]At higher infusion rates, it may be necessary to administer by volume rather than by mL/hr.
[§]For a 30% concentration, divide the amount by 1.5.
[¶]Rounded off to nearest milliliter.

(specifically hypoglycemia), and ability to maintain therapeutic levels.[116,118] Fomepizole is considered the antidote of choice; however, owing to the cost and the logistics of stocking this antidote, many hospitals might not have this drug readily available.

Ethanol can be used as a therapeutic intervention in patients with methanol or ethylene glycol poisoning owing to ethanol's much greater affinity for alcohol dehydrogenases. These enzymes metabolize methanol and ethylene glycol to toxic byproducts. However, with serum ethanol levels of 100 mg/dL, minimal amounts of ethylene glycol or methanol are metabolized by alcohol dehydrogenases.[116,118] Ethanol infusions are not useful in the treatment of isopropyl alcohol poisoning.

Ethanol can be administered orally or intravenously (Table 68–18). IV ethanol has the advantages of obtaining therapeutic levels rapidly, ensuring complete absorption, limiting chances of aspiration, and avoiding gastritis. A 5% concentration of ethanol, which can be given in a peripheral vein, requires the use of large fluid volumes. In a 70-kg patient, a loading dose requires 1.4 L of 5% solution, with a maintenance dose of 700 mL/hr. If IV ethanol is given, maintain careful attention to cardiopulmonary status. In contrast, oral loading can be achieved using much lower volumes. However, oral loading can be difficult in the uncooperative or unconscious patient or if vomiting or GI hemorrhage is present. A therapeutic level is reached more slowly with oral loading.

Ethanol metabolism can vary widely, and ethanol is dialyzable. Therefore, it may be difficult to maintain appropriate ethanol levels during dialysis therapy of ethylene glycol or methanol. Frequent measurements of ethanol should be obtained and the infusion adjusted accordingly. When patients are given ethanol infusions, central nervous system depression, hypothermia, hypotension, hypoglycemia, and phlebitis are common adverse effects, especially in children. Serial levels of ethanol and glucose should be obtained.

 REFERENCES CAN BE FOUND ON **EXPERT CONSULT**

CHAPTER 69

Standard Precautions and Infectious Exposure Management

Peter Erik Sokolove

Body fluid contamination of health care workers is a frequent occurrence in the emergency department (ED). In a prospective study of ED health care workers, skin and clothing contamination with body fluids occurred in 1 of 35 patient visits.[1] These fluids may contain various transmissible infectious diseases, as the prevalence of human immunodeficiency virus (HIV) infection, hepatitis, and other communicable diseases can be high in certain ED patient populations.[2-5] For example, investigators from an inner-city ED reported a patient seroprevalence of 6% for HIV infection, 18% for hepatitis C virus (HCV), and 5% for hepatitis B surface antigen (HBsAg).[6] One in four patients tested positive for at least one of these diseases. Patient characteristics were found to be poor predictors for hepatitis positivity, making it more difficult to identify which patients pose a risk to health care workers.

Unfortunately, compliance with standard precautions, formerly known as universal precautions, is far from universal.[7-9] Baraff and Talan[7] reported poor compliance, even in the setting of treating critical trauma patients. Compliance rates were 75% for gloves, 27% for gowns, 19% for eyewear, and only 2% for masks. Despite health care workers having recently received education about standard precautions, Hammond and coworkers[8] also reported low compliance rates during invasive procedures and with high-risk patients. Compliance improved when equipment was organized and placed in trauma resuscitation rooms. In 1985, this combination of high-risk illness with low compliance barrier use prompted the Centers for Disease Control and Prevention (CDC) to recommend guidelines for the protection of health care workers.[10] In 1991, these recommendations were enacted into law by mandate of the Occupational Safety and Health Administration (OSHA).[11]

The primary focus of the CDC guidelines is to reduce mucocutaneous body fluid exposures by encouraging hand washing and barrier protection. However, these measures do little to protect from percutaneous exposures, which are the most efficient exposures in the transmission of hepatitis and HIV.[12,13] The current strategy for risk reduction in the ED includes immunization against hepatitis B virus (HBV), use of standard precautions (including re-engineered safety products), and prompt initiation of postexposure prophylaxis (PEP) when appropriate.

STANDARD PRECAUTIONS GUIDELINES

Appropriate precautions for all patient contact must be viewed as a consistent practice or "way of life" in the ED. The following guidelines, based upon the CDC recommendations, should be used when there is any possibility of body fluid contact:

Barrier Precautions

1. Use gloves for any patient contact with the risk of body fluid exposure. Both cutaneous and percutaneous exposures can be reduced by the use of gloves. In an animal model, Mast and colleagues[14] reported a 46% to 86% reduction in the volume of blood transferred via needle-stick injury when the needle first punctured a glove. Fisher and associates[15] compared the biomechanical performance of powder-free, latex, and nitrile examination gloves. The nitrile examination gloves exhibited greater puncture resistance, despite being thinner than the latex examination gloves.
2. Wear mask and protective eyewear when exposure to body fluid aerosols is possible (e.g., wound irrigation, traumatic chest wound).
3. Wear gown and shoe covers when there is the risk of large splash volumes of body fluids (e.g., chest tube, thoracotomy).

Sharps Precautions

Most importantly, this means no recapping, bending, or breaking of needles. If needle recapping is deemed necessary, use a single-handed technique (Fig. 69–1). A safer alternative is to immediately dispose of the needle into an approved sharps container without recapping. In an observational study of ED employees, the rate of needle recapping was 34%; most practitioners used a two-handed technique.[16] Various re-engineered products are available for use in the ED, including retracting scalpels, auto-capping needles, and needle-less intravenous systems. Using such devices decreases percutaneous injury rates among health care workers.[17] A survey of infection control professionals at Iowa and Virginia hospitals found that implementation of such devices was the most common action taken to decrease percutaneous injuries.[18]

Respiratory Precautions

During contact with patients with suspected or confirmed pulmonary tuberculosis (TB), wear a National Institute of Safety and Health (NIOSH)–approved N-95 particulate respirator. These masks are designed to efficiently filter 1- to 5-μm particles, and are less costly and more comfortable than high-efficiency particulate air (HEPA)–filtered masks. In addition, place such patients in a respiratory isolation room with negative pressure, high circulation (optimally at least 12 air changes/hr), and external exhaust. While in the ED, avoid procedures resulting in increased release of infectious droplets, such as sputum induction. Make sure that all potentially infectious patients wear a surgical-type mask themselves, especially during transportation outside of the respiratory isolation room (e.g., to radiology).[19]

Hand Washing. Immediately wash any skin surface coming into contact with body fluids with soap and water.

Annual Education. Make sure that all workers receive a mandatory annual review of infection control and safe practices.

OCCUPATIONAL DISEASE EXPOSURE

Occupationally acquired infections cause considerable morbidity and mortality among health care workers despite OSHA requirements for precautions. Given the often-occult presen-

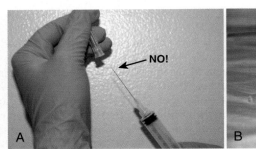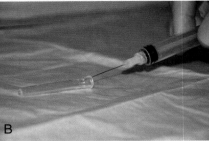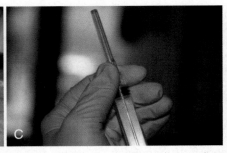

Figure 69–1 *A,* Recapping a needle by holding the cap in the hand is the most common way to sustain a needle puncture. *B,* It is best to discard the needle/syringe without recapping, but an alternative is to partially recap **without** holding the needle cap. *C,* Make sure that at least 80% of the needle is covered before completing the recapping with the second hand (by holding the base of the needle cap).

TABLE 69–1 Recommendations for Hepatitis B Prophylaxis after Percutaneous or Permucosal Exposure

Exposed Person	Source		
	HBsAg-Positive	**HBsAg-Negative**	**Source Unknown or Not Available**
Unvaccinated	HBIG × 1* and HB vaccine series	Initiate HB vaccine series	Initiate HB vaccine series
Vaccinated			
Known responder	No treatment	No treatment	No treatment
Known nonresponder	HBIG × 2 or HBIG × 1 and initiate revaccination[†]	No treatment	If known high-risk source, treat as if source were HBsAg-positive
Response unknown	Test exposed person for anti-HBs 1. If adequate,[‡] no treatment 2. If inadequate, HBIG × 1 plus vaccine booster	No treatment	Test exposed person for anti-HBs 1. If adequate, no treatment 2. If inadequate, HB vaccine booster and recheck titer in 1–2 mo

*HBIG dose = 0.06 mL/kg IM.
[†]The option of giving one dose of HBIG and reinitiating the vaccine series is preferred for nonresponders who have not completed a second three-dose vaccine series.
    For persons who previously completed a second vaccine series but failed to respond, two doses of HBIG are preferred.
[‡]Adequate anti-HBs = 10 mIU/mL.
HB, hepatitis B; HBIG, hepatitis B immunoglobulin; HBsAg, hepatitis B surface antigen.
Adapted from Updated U.S. public health service guidelines for the management of occupational exposures to HBV, HCV, and HIV and recommendations for postexposure prophylaxis. MMWR Recomm Rep 50:1, 2001.

tation of disease in the ED patient population, emergency health care workers are at high risk for significant exposure from many pathogens. Owing to the high prevalence of particular diseases among ED patients and specific concerns for pathogens associated with high morbidity and mortality, this chapter focuses on HIV, HBV, HCV, and TB.

HBV

HBV Transmission
HBV is a well-recognized occupational risk for health care providers; multiple studies have documented the high prevalence of hepatitis among ED patients.[6,20,21] Despite the attention focused on transmission of HIV, the infectivity of HBV is significantly higher because of the virulence of the organism and relatively small inoculum required for disease transmission.[22] Percutaneous injuries are among the most efficient modes of HBV transmission, but many infected health care workers do not recall a specific injury.[23,24] Many body fluids other than blood contain HBsAg, but the levels of infectious HBV particles in blood-free body fluids are 100 to 1000 times lower than blood itself. Because of implementation of the CDC's standard precautions, along with the OSHA regulations for barrier protection and pre-exposure vaccination, the incidence of HBV transmission has sharply declined.[25]

To understand the risk of HBV transmission resulting from occupational exposure, familiarize yourself with a few key serologic markers for HBV. HBsAg is a marker of active

infection in the source patient. From a practical standpoint, HBV can be transmitted when HBsAg is present, and it is generally not transmissible when this marker is absent. Hepatitis B surface antibody (HBsAb) is a protective antibody against HBV. In vaccinating health care workers, the goal is to stimulate the immune system to produce a sufficient quantity of this antibody. Hepatitis Be antigen (HBeAg) can be found in the bloodstream of HBV-infected individuals during times of peak virus replication. When a source is positive for HBeAg, her or his bloodstream contains a much larger number of infectious HBV particles. If a nonimmune individual sustains a needle stick from an HBsAg-positive patient, the risk of HBV transmission depends on the HBeAg status of the source.[26] The risk of clinical hepatitis is approximately 2% (range, 1%–6%) if HBeAg is absent, compared with a risk of 22% to 31% if HBeAg is present.[27]

HBV Postexposure Management
PEP following exposure to an HBsAg-positive source may require hepatitis B vaccine, hepatitis B immunoglobulin (HBIG), both, or neither (Table 69–1). This depends on the vaccination and antibody response status of the exposed health care worker. HBIG is derived from pooled human plasma and provides passive immunization for nonimmune exposed individuals. This preparation is very safe and not known to transmit disease.[25,27] When HBIG is used for PEP, give it ideally within 24 hours after exposure and note that it is of questionable value beyond 7 days.[28] Hepatitis B vaccine may also be

given for PEP. Provide routine vaccination against hepatitis B for all health care workers who have any chance of exposure to infectious body fluids. Adverse reactions to the hepatitis B vaccine are generally quite mild, and it is even safe to give during pregnancy. For primary immunization, give an initial intramuscular (IM) injection, followed by subsequent IM vaccinations at 1 and 6 months. Check antibody levels (HBsAb) at 4 to 6 weeks after the series is completed to confirm that the desired titer of at least 10 mIU/mL has been attained. Vaccinated individuals who achieve this antibody level are referred to as "responders" and are believed to be immune for life. Although about 25% to 50% of vaccine responders demonstrate a decline in HBsAb levels to below 10 mIU/mL within 5 to 7 years, these individuals are still protected against clinical disease. This results from a robust immune system memory or anamnestic response.[29] PEP with these agents is not contraindicated during pregnancy or lactation. Health care workers who have previously been infected with HBV are immune to re-infection, so PEP is not indicated in such individuals.

HCV

HCV Transmission
Approximately 1.6% of Americans (4.1 million) are infected with HCV,[30] and many of these individuals are unaware that they are infected. Percutaneous transmission is the most efficient route. The incidence of seroconversion after an HCV-positive needle stick is about 1.8% (estimates range from 0% to 7%).[27] HCV is often acquired from injection drug use. It was once commonly transmitted by blood transfusion but is fortunately rare now with modern screening. Although HCV can be transmitted sexually, this a minor route. Mucous membrane transmission of HCV is possible but much less common. It is useful to remember that the risk of HCV transmission after a needle stick is similar to that of HBV transmission when the source is HbeAg-negative. When seroconversion does occur, 80% of patients will demonstrate antibodies at 15 weeks and 97% at 6 months after exposure. Although the clinical course of HCV is often asymptomatic or mild, approximately 85% of patients will develop chronic hepatitis, 10% to 20% cirrhosis, and 1% to 5% hepatocellular carcinoma.[31-33]

HCV Postexposure Management
Unfortunately, PEP for HCV exposure is currently not available. HCV exhibits a high degree of genetic heterogeneity and a very rapid mutation rate, making the development of a vaccine extremely difficult. The use of postexposure immune globulin is probably not helpful, and there are currently no published clinical trials of agents such as interferon or ribavirin for HCV PEP.[27]

HIV

HIV Transmission
According to the CDC, through June 2000, 56 cases of occupational HIV transmission to health care workers occurred in the United States. In addition, another 138 health care workers demonstrated HIV seroconversion, which may have been occupationally related.[34] The risk of contracting HIV from working in the ED depends on the prevalence of HIV in the local patient population. One study reported an annual HIV seroconversion risk of 1 in 3800 for high-prevalence EDs and 1 in 55,000 for low-prevalence EDs.[13] Wears and coworkers[35] estimated the cumulative career risk of contracting HIV from occupational exposure in a high-prevalence ED to be as high as 1.4%. The overall risk of HIV seroconversion is about 1 in 300 (0.3%) after needle stick and less than 1 in 1000 for mucous membrane exposures. Cardo and colleagues[36] demonstrated that the risk for HIV seroconversion after needle stick injuries is not uniform. Seroconversion was found to be more likely for deep injuries (odds ratio [OR] = 15), if blood was visible on the device (OR = 6.2), if the needle had been used in a source patient's artery or vein (OR = 4.3), or if the source patient suffered from terminal acquired immunodeficiency syndrome (AIDS; OR = 5.6). It is essential to gather information regarding the nature of the injury to "risk stratify" the exposure.

When seroconversion occurs, HIV antibodies can be detected as early as 3 weeks after exposure and are almost always present by 6 months. Seroconversion at 6 to 12 months is rare, but has been reported with HIV and HCV virus co-infection. Thus, follow-up HIV testing is recommended for 12 months for health care workers who become infected with HCV from a dual exposure to both HCV and HIV.[37] Acute retroviral syndrome is a clinical manifestation of HIV seroconversion that occurs in approximately 80% of newly infected individuals at a median of 25 days after exposure. The presentation of acute retroviral syndrome is similar to that of mononucleosis, with fever, lymphadenopathy, and rash.

HIV Postexposure Management[27]
Evidence Supporting PEP. In 1998, the U.S. Public Health Service recommended using PEP for selected HIV exposures.[32,33] These recommendations were based on a number of animal and human studies suggesting that PEP might be effective. Although animal studies are mixed in both methodology and outcomes, PEP with various agents has successfully prevented HIV infection. In human studies, the use of antiretroviral agents during pregnancy decreased perinatal HIV transmission by 67%.[38] In addition, when children born to HIV-positive mothers were given HIV PEP within 48 hours of birth, HIV transmission was also decreased.[39] Although perinatal exposures are different than occupational needle sticks, this evidence supports the concept of a "window of opportunity" during which PEP may prevent HIV transmission to an exposed individual. The most important human study of the efficacy of PEP is a CDC-sponsored case-control study undertaken in the United States, France, the United Kingdom, and Italy.[36] This investigation compared 33 health care workers who seroconverted after HIV exposure with 665 control health care workers who did not seroconvert after HIV exposure. About 90% of patients in this study were exposed via hollow-bore needles. When postexposure zidovudine (azidothymidine [AZT]) was used, the risk for HIV infection was reduced by 81% (95% confidence interval, 48%–94%). Although the study methodology is limited by its retrospective design and the potential for recall bias, these results strongly support the efficacy of AZT for PEP. Currently, there are no published randomized, controlled human trials of agents for HIV PEP. Given the results of the CDC case-control study, it is highly unlikely that such trials will ever be conducted or published, because the use of a control group is now considered unethical.

Selecting Patients for PEP. In both 2001 and 2005, the U.S. Public Health Service published updated recommendations regarding the use of HIV PEP.[27,37] In general, the decision to use PEP depends on the type of exposure and the source's HIV status. The first step in determining whether PEP is indicated is to assess the exposure severity. Percutaneous exposures can be categorized as "less severe" or "more severe." A less severe exposure involves a solid needle, a superficial injury, and no visible blood on the device. All other percutaneous injuries are categorized as more severe. Exposure to mucus membranes and nonintact skin are categorized as either "small volume" (a few drops of blood) or "large volume" (a major blood splash). There are no reported cases of HIV seroconversion after blood exposure to intact skin.

After assessing the exposure severity, determine the potential infectivity of the source. Consider PEP only for blood and body fluid exposures from a source known or likely to be HIV-positive. Exposures from an HIV-negative source do not require PEP. Do not test sharp instruments for HIV because this is not reliable or recommended. Categorize HIV-positive source patients as either "lower risk" (class 1) or "higher risk" (class 2). Class 1 patients have asymptomatic HIV infection and a low viral load (<1500 RNA copies/mL). Higher-risk patients include those with symptomatic HIV, AIDS, acute seroconversion, or a high viral load. Once exposure severity and source HIV status are determined, use Tables 69–2 and 69–3 to guide the proper PEP regimen. For skin and mucous membrane exposures, choose a PEP regimen from three general categories. For small-volume exposures from an HIV class 1 source, consider using the basic regimen (two drugs). If either the exposure is of large volume or the source is HIV class 2, then recommend the basic regimen. In cases in which there is both a large-volume exposure and an HIV class 2 source, recommend the expanded regimen (at least three drugs). For most percutaneous exposures, recommend the expanded regimen. However, for less severe percutaneous exposures from an HIV class 1 source, recommend the basic regimen.

A number of special circumstances may arise when determining the need for HIV PEP. When a source is known but his or her HIV status is pending, decide about the use of PEP on a case-by-case basis. When the source is high-risk, initiate PEP and then stop or modify it later once the HIV status is determined. When a source can be identified but his or her HIV status is unknown and will not become available, PEP is generally not recommended. However, if the source has HIV risk factors, consider using the basic two-drug regimens. Sometimes, an exposure will occur in which the source is completely unknown. Although PEP is generally not recommended for such exposures, the basic regimen should be considered if the exposure occurred in an HIV-likely setting (e.g., exposure to a discarded needle on an AIDS ward).

Choice of PEP Medications. When HIV PEP is administered, a minimum of two drugs is recommended. Although there is no direct evidence that combination PEP regimens are beneficial, concerns about antiretroviral resistance and the synergistic effects of antiviral medications when treating patients with AIDS supports such an approach. As discussed earlier, the U.S. Public Health Service recommends using a basic (two-drug) PEP regimen for lower-risk HIV exposures and an expanded (at least three-drug) PEP regimen for higher-risk exposures. The basic PEP regimen consists of either two nucleoside reverse transcriptase inhibitors or a nucleoside reverse transcriptase inhibitor plus a non-nucleoside reverse transcriptase inhibitor. The traditional regimen is AZT plus lamivudine (3TC). Alternative basic regimens include AZT plus emtricitabine (FTC), 3TC plus tenofovir (TDF) or TDF plus FTC. When using the expanded PEP regimen, add a protease inhibitor to the basic regimen. In the currently preferred expanded regimen, the combination medication lopinavir/ritonavir is added to the basic regimen. A number of second-line and alternative agents may be chosen for HIV PEP. Expert consultation is recommended, especially if antiretroviral resistance is suspected. An important resource for

TABLE 69–2 Recommended HIV Postexposure Prophylaxis for Percutaneous Injuries

Exposure Type	Infection Status of Source		Source of Unknown HIV Status[†]	Unknown Source[‡]	HIV-Negative
	HIV-Positive Class 1*	HIV-Positive Class 2*			
Less severe[§]	Recommend basic two-drug PEP	Recommend expanded ≥ three-drug PEP	Generally, no PEP warranted; however, consider basic two-drug PEP[‖] for source with HIV risk factors[¶]	Generally, no PEP warranted; however, consider basic two-drug PEP[‖] in settings where exposure to HIV-infected persons is likely	No PEP warranted
More severe**	Recommend expanded three-drug PEP	Recommend expanded ≥ three-drug PEP	Generally, no PEP warranted; however, consider basic two-drug PEP[‖] for source with HIV risk factors[¶]	Generally, no PEP warranted; however, consider basic two-drug PEP[‖] in settings where exposure to HIV-infected persons is likely	No PEP warranted

*HIV-positive, class 1—asymptomatic HIV infection or known low viral load (e.g., <1500 RNA copies/mL). HIV-positive, class 2—symptomatic HIV infection, AIDS, acute seroconversion, or known high viral load. If drug resistance is a concern, obtain expert consultation. Initiation of PEP should not be delayed pending expert consultation, and because expert consultation alone cannot substitute for face-to-face counseling, resources should be available to provide immediate evaluation and follow-up care for all exposures.
[†]Source of unknown HIV status (e.g., deceased source person with no samples available for HIV testing).
[‡]Unknown source (e.g., a needle from a sharps disposal container).
[§]Less severe (e.g., solid needle or superficial injury).
[‖]The designation "consider PEP" indicates that PEP is optional and should be based on an individualized discussion between the exposed person and the treating clinician regarding the risks versus benefits for PEP.
[¶]If PEP is offered and administered and the source is later determined to be HIV-negative, PEP should be discontinued.
**More severe (e.g., large-bore hollow needle, deep puncture, visible blood on device, or needle used in patient's artery or vein).
AIDS, acquired immunodeficiency syndrome; HIV, human immunodeficiency virus; PEP, postexposure prophylaxis.
Adapted from Updated U.S. Public Health Service Guidelines for the Management of Occupational Exposures to HIV and Recommendations for Postexposure Prophylaxis. MMWR Recomm Rep 54(RR-9):3, 2005.

TABLE 69–3 Recommended HIV Postexposure Prophylaxis for Mucous Membrane Exposures and Nonintact Skin* Exposures

| Exposure Type | Infection Status of Source | | Source of Unknown HIV Status[‡] | Unknown Source[§] | HIV-Negative |
	HIV-Positive Class 1[†]	HIV-Positive Class 2[†]			
Small volume[‖]	Consider basic two-drug PEP[¶]	Recommend basic three-drug PEP	Generally, no PEP warranted; however, consider basic two-drug PEP[¶] for source with HIV risk factors**	Generally, no PEP warranted; however, consider basic two-drug PEP[¶] in settings where exposure to HIV-infected persons is likely	No PEP warranted
Large volume	Recommend basic three-drug PEP	Recommend expanded three-drug PEP	Generally, no PEP warranted; however, consider basic two-drug PEP[¶] for source with HIV risk factors**	Generally, no PEP warranted; however, consider basic two-drug PEP[¶] in settings where exposure to HIV-infected persons is likely	No PEP warranted

*For skin exposures, follow-up is indicated only if there is evidence of compromised skin integrity (e.g., dermatitis, abrasion, or open wound).

[†]HIV-positive, class 1—asymptomatic HIV infection or known low viral load (e.g., <1500 RNA copies/mL). HIV-positive, class 2—symptomatic HIV infection, AIDS, acute seroconversion, or known high viral load. If drug resistance is a concern, obtain expert consultation. Initiation of PEP should not be delayed pending expert consultation, and because expert consultation alone cannot substitute for face-to-face counseling, resources should be available to provide immediate evaluation and follow-up care for all exposures.

[‡]Source of unknown HIV status (e.g., deceased source person with no samples available for HIV testing). Unknown source (e.g., splash from inappropriately disposed blood).

[§]Large volume (e.g., major blood splash).

[‖]Small volume (e.g., a few drops).

[¶]The designation "consider PEP" indicates that PEP is optional and should be based on an individualized discussion between the exposed person and the treating clinician regarding the risks versus benefits for PEP.

**If PEP is offered and administered and the source is later determined to be HIV-negative, PEP should be discontinued.

HIV, human immunodeficiency virus; PEP, postexposure prophylaxis.

Adapted from Updated U.S. Public Health Service Guidelines for the Management of Occupational Exposures to HIV and Recommendations for Postexposure Prophylaxis. MMWR Recomm Rep 54(RR-9):3, 2005.

emergency clinicians is the National Clinicians' Postexposure Prophylaxis Hotline at UCSF/San Francisco General Hospital. Expert consultation can be obtained by calling 888-448-4911.

PEP Timing, Duration, and Side Effects. HIV exposure should be considered a true emergency. Administer PEP as soon as possible after exposure, ideally within 1 hour. Animal studies indicate that the efficacy of PEP diminishes with delayed initiation.[40] HIV PEP regimens consist of a 4-week course of therapy. In the ED, patients can be prescribed the first 3 days of medications, as long as outpatient follow-up is arranged. Side effects are experienced by about 50% of health care workers taking PEP, causing approximately 33% of health care workers to discontinue therapy prematurely.[41] Depending on the choice of PEP medications, patients should also be prescribed antiemetics and antidiarrheal agents when PEP is initiated.

TB

TB Transmission

During the mid-1980s, the United States experienced a resurgence in TB, especially among HIV-positive patients. Although the incidence of TB cases in the United States has since declined, almost 14,000 cases were reported in 2006.[42] Thus, TB continues to pose a serious risk to both public health and health care workers. TB is transmitted by infectious droplets 1 to 5 μm in size. Primary infection occurs when one to three organisms are inhaled into the alveoli, where they begin to replicate. Host defenses usually stop infection within 2 to 10 weeks, and the patient enters the latent period. During this time, patients are asymptomatic and not contagious. Reactivation occurs when cell-mediated immunity wanes, and patients are again contagious. This can

be due to advancing age, HIV infection, steroid use, malignancy, malnutrition, or other causes of immune suppression. The lifetime risk of reactivation is 5% to 10%, with about half of this risk occurring in the first few years after primary infection. Patients with increased infectivity include those with pulmonary or laryngeal TB, an active cough, positive sputum smears for acid-fast bacilli, cavitation on chest radiographs, and those on inadequate therapy. Overall, children are less contagious than adults, but can still transmit the disease. Extrapulmonary TB is contagious only in the cases of an open skin lesion or oral cavity involvement.[19]

Depending on the patient population and geographic location, ED personnel can be at high risk for occupational TB infection. In a 1993 study at a county hospital in Los Angeles, it was reported that 31% of ED workers became purified protein derivative (PPD)–positive during employment, including 20% of attendings, 32% of nurses, and 33% of residents.[43] PPD conversion risk was found to be 6% after 1 year of ED employment, 14% after 2 years, and 27% after 4 years. EDs typically care for higher-risk patients—those who are homeless, foreign-born, recently incarcerated, or chronically debilitated. Overcrowding can lead to extended waiting periods and delays in admissions. The clinical presentation of TB in ED patients is often atypical, which can lead to delayed diagnosis.[44,45] This is especially true for HIV-infected patients, in whom symptoms may mimic *Pneumocystis jiroveci* pneumonia, skin tests are often negative, chest radiographs are commonly atypical, and sputum tests may be less sensitive.[46-52] In one study of ED patients with TB, the mean time from ED registration to respiratory isolation was 6.5 hours, and 46% of patients were first isolated on the hospital ward.[53]

Preventing TB exposure requires a multifaceted approach.[19] Proper ED ventilation plays a key role; inadequate ventilation has been a contributing factor in many nosocomial outbreaks. Ideally, install single-pass airflow from waiting rooms to the outside. Within the ED, make sure that air flows from clean areas to less clean areas, not vice versa. If patients with TB are seen frequently, provide at least one true respiratory isolation room in the ED. Make sure that such rooms have at least 12 air changes/hr and that they are "negative-pressure" rooms in which air flows into the room from other ED areas. Other engineering approaches to TB infection control include using HEPA filters and upper room ultraviolet light irradiation.

Familiarize all ED personnel with the appropriate use of respiratory protection against TB. Provide surgical masks (e.g., string-tie masks) for source control. Place these masks on potentially contagious patients to decrease the passage of infectious droplets into the air. Because air can leak around such masks, they are not optimal for health care worker protection. In late 1995, NIOSH certified a new class of masks known as N-95 particulate respirators.[54] These filter 1-μm-size particles with at least 95% efficiency and are generally the preferred mask for health care workers. In some circumstances, such as when patients are undergoing cough-inducing or aerosol-generating procedures, health care workers need better protection. Thus, N-95 masks are usually the appropriate choice for ED use, but these masks should be thought of as the minimum required level of respiratory protection against TB.[19]

Initiate early respiratory isolation of patients with suspected pulmonary TB as soon as possible in the ED, ideally at triage. Screening protocols at triage can detect patients with more classic presentations of TB, but unfortunately, reported protocols are only moderately sensitive and somewhat cumbersome.[44,45] Consider immediate respiratory isolation for patients with high-risk chief complaints, such as HIV-positive patients with cough, those with hemoptysis, or patients with a history of TB presenting with cough or fever. The best guideline is to initiate respiratory isolation as soon as TB is considered to be a possible diagnosis. Place masks on such patients before obtaining chest radiographs.

TB Postexposure Management

If health care workers are exposed to patients with active pulmonary TB, refer them to either employee health care or their primary care clinician for follow-up testing and treatment. To establish a health care worker's baseline PPD status, perform skin testing within days after exposure. If the baseline test is negative, perform a follow-up skin test 8 to 10 weeks later to determine whether PPD conversion has occurred. A positive baseline test ($\geq$10-mm induration) indicates previous exposure or infection. A positive test has 5-mm induration after a negative baseline test, or an increase of at least 10-mm induration after a baseline test of 1-mm to 9-mm induration. Health care workers who convert their PPD to positive after an exposure should undergo chest radiography to screen for active pulmonary TB.[19] If active disease is present, initiate treatment with at least four antituberculous medications. In PPD converters who do not have active disease, consider chemoprophylaxis. When deciding whether or not to initiate chemoprophylaxis, balance the potential benefit of TB prevention with the risk of medication-associated hepatitis. In general, give chemoprophylaxis in the case of a recent ($\leq$2 yr) PPD conversion, a known TB contact, a patient who is medically predisposed to TB, HIV-infected, intravenous drug user, or younger than 35 years. For occupationally exposed health care workers who are PPD converters, give chemoprophylaxis, regardless of age. The preferred regimen for HIV-negative persons is daily isoniazid (INH) for 9 months, although acceptable alternative regimens can be considered.[55] Some health care workers may become exposed to strains of TB that are resistant to INH. In 2005, there were 124 reported cases of multidrug-resistant TB (MDR-TB) in the United States, mostly among foreign-born persons.[42] For exposures to MDR-TB, consult an expert when selecting an individualized chemoprophylaxis regimen. Baseline and serial liver function testing is not necessary for chemoprophylaxis administration in most cases, but monitor closely for clinical symptoms suggestive of hepatotoxicity.

Acknowledgment

The editors and author wish to acknowledge the contributions of Kevin Rodgers and Aaron Bair to this chapter in previous editions.

 REFERENCES CAN BE FOUND ON EXPERT CONSULT

CHAPTER 70

Educational Aspects of Emergency Department Procedures

Catherine B. Custalow and Amita Sudhir

Learning to perform emergency department (ED) procedures is a complex and highly individualized educational process. Many of these procedures, particularly those that are rare, are difficult to learn, but emergency clinicians can become proficient in their performance when provided with adequate training and sufficient practice.

BASIC PROCEDURAL SKILL TRAINING

Interns, residents, and medical students love to do procedures. This willing attitude opens the door to learning, but teaching complex procedural skills is still a challenging task. To be successful, begin by understanding the procedure yourself. Familiarize yourself with the procedure. Develop a working understanding of its indications, contraindications, necessary equipment, procedural steps, complications, and critical actions. Teach procedures in a consistent and organized manner. Appreciate that it is challenging to teach adult learners a complicated psychomotor skill. Finally, respect and adapt your teaching method to each individual's learning style.

Formal Education

Chapman[1] described a set of eight steps to use as a framework for procedural learning; these are shown in Table 70–1. These steps incorporate the different stages of learning and are important to understand when teaching a procedural skill. To introduce a new procedure, provide a variety of instructional materials such as lectures (Fig. 70–1), small group sessions (Fig. 70–2), computerized instructional materials, procedural texts, and atlases.

Bedside Teaching

Procedural training at the bedside is an important part of learning a new skill in the ED. As discussed previously, make sure that the learner has gone through formal training in the procedure before attempting it on a human patient. Select and provide an appropriate clinical setting (Fig. 70–3A) with adequate time to explain the procedure in detail. Review the procedure beforehand with the learner. Discuss the indications, contraindications, equipment, procedural steps, critical actions, and complications (see Fig. 70–3B). Provide this review either outside the patient's room or at the bedside, depending on the patient and the clinical scenario. Observe the learner as she or he performs the procedure and provide guidance and assistance when needed. After the procedure, examine the patient and assess the adequacy of the procedure (see Fig. 70–3C). Finally, discuss problems that occurred

during the procedure, offer suggestions for improvement, and provide a review of postprocedural care.

Long-Term Procedural Skill Retention

When teaching procedures, aim for long-term retention because decay of procedural skills is natural over time. As mentioned, skill retention depends, in part, on the adequacy of the initial educational experience.[2] Information is lost from short-term memory through decay and interference, but fortunately, once committed to long-term memory, it is virtually permanent.[3,4] This is analogous to certain learned skills that are retained indefinitely, such as riding a bicycle. These skills are never forgotten owing to a process called overlearning. Allowing students to practice and execute movements actively during learning results in better recall than when they learn from a passive demonstration.[5,6] How long the effect of procedural training will last for each individual is unknown. For most ED procedures, which are rarely overlearned, practice is required in order to maintain those skills.[1] Kovacs and colleagues[7] demonstrated that airway management skills decline early after initial training but performance may be maintained effectively with independent practice and periodic feedback. In summary, continued practice is essential in order to maintain speed and accuracy, particularly for resuscitative and rare procedures.

PROCEDURAL TRAINING DURING EMERGENCIES

Procedural training in the ED is often complicated by the exigent circumstances under which emergency procedures are performed. Procedures must be performed rapidly and competently in order to be life saving. The adage "see one, do one, teach one" is particularly unconscionable in the ED.[8] When a patient arrives with a life-threatening condition that mandates emergent intervention, let the most experienced member of the resuscitation team perform the procedure as quickly and as competently as possible in order to save a life.[9,10] In this setting, the teacher lacks the time and the circumstances necessary to explain the rationale and details of life-saving surgical procedures to residents in training.[11,12] Hedges[13] wrote that in the case of an unfavorable teaching scenario, it is better for the educator to teach while he or she does the procedure. Although this may be less satisfying for the learner, there are still many things to be learned from observing the patient-clinician interaction, procedural setup, critical actions, and postprocedural care.

PROCEDURAL TRAINING FOR UNCOMMON PROCEDURES

The opportunity for learners to practice certain critical resuscitative procedures on human patients in the ED may be limited because they are performed so infrequently. Residents, therefore, have limited opportunity to acquire procedural competency and speed in these rare procedures.

The rate of performance of certain resuscitative procedures in recent years has declined owing to a number of factors. Critical analyses of patient outcomes after ED thoracotomy have identified key predictors of successful outcome, most notably penetrating trauma to the chest, which have also virtually eliminated performing this procedure in victims of blunt trauma.[14,15] With clinicians now using a more selective

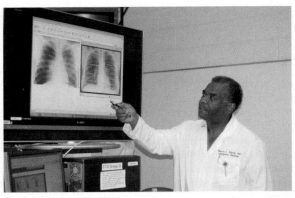

Figure 70–1 Formal lecture to teach a new procedure.

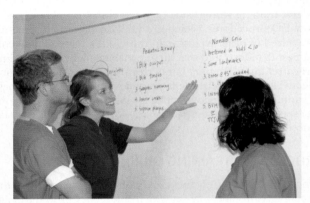

Figure 70–2 Small group review for free discussion between teacher and fellow students.

TABLE 70–1 Eight Steps of Procedural Skill Learning

1. Identify an acceptable skill level.
2. Identify when to perform the procedure.
3. Select the instruments and equipment needed to perform the procedure.
4. Identify the critical steps of the procedure.
5. Memorize the sequential order of the steps.
6. Develop a mental image of performing the procedure.
7. Practice procedural movements with feedback.
8. Assess procedural competence.

---

approach for thoracotomy, procedural competency is more difficult to obtain in the ED setting. Chang and associates[16] reported a significant decline in the rate of cricothyroidotomies performed on trauma patients following the beginning of a new emergency medicine (EM) residency-training program. They attributed this to several possible causes, including the widespread application of rapid-sequence intubation techniques, the presence of supervisory EM faculty 24 hours a day, and the diminished concern regarding orotracheal intubation of patients whose cervical spines have not been radiographically cleared. There is also competition for procedures between EM residents and residents from other specialties such as surgery.[17] In fact, a 1995 survey completed by program directors of EM residencies found that, overall, emergency clinicians perform only 50% of 10 index proce-

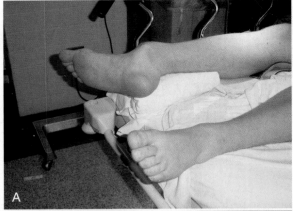

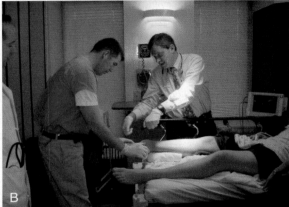

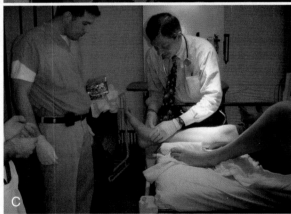

Figure 70–3 Procedural training at the bedside is an important part of learning a new skill. *A,* This ankle dislocation requires prompt relocation in the emergency department (ED). *B,* The instructor first reviews the procedure with the trainee, including indications, contraindications, procedural steps, and complications. The trainee then performs the reduction while the instructor observes and provides guidance during the procedure. *C,* After the procedure, the instructor examines the patient and assesses the adequacy of reduction.

dures in the ED whereas residents from other specialties perform the remainder.[18] Finally, how often residents have the opportunity to perform surgical procedures is often determined by chance.[5,19]

One study found that a significant number of residents perform fewer than five each of certain critical resuscitative procedures during their training.[20] This confirms the findings of earlier published reports that certain emergency procedures, particularly venous cutdown, thoracotomy, and cricothyroidotomy, are performed infrequently.[21,22]

ASSESSING PROCEDURAL COMPETENCY

Developing the skills necessary to perform a procedure independently is different for everyone, and successful learning depends on both the quality of each procedural experience and the number of procedures performed.[20] If procedures have been taught or practiced incorrectly, experience is not a useful predictor of procedural competency. When a learner performs a manual skill incorrectly, even once, it is much more difficult to relearn the correct technique.[23] If procedures are learned incorrectly without the benefit of guidance and remediation, the learner becomes the instructor and then passes mistakes on to other learners through the teaching process.[24] To avoid this, particularly in the beginning, observe learners closely and correct them as they perform the procedure. In the words of Red Auerbach, the legendary coach of the Boston Celtics, "Practice does not make perfect; perfect practice makes perfect."[23]

With so few of these rare procedures being done, and if there are no training alternatives provided, it is unlikely that EM residents will have achieved procedural competency for some procedures during their training.[16,25] The actual number of procedures necessary to ensure competency is unknown. A study by Chapman and colleagues failed to show a significant correlation between the clinician's previous procedural experience and actual thoracotomy performance as assessed by written, computerized, or animal models. Similarly, knowledge of thoracotomy content and procedural steps did not predict procedural competency.[26] Typically, the number of procedures previously performed is taken as predictive of procedural competency; however, these findings suggest that procedural competency cannot be predicted by numbers. Despite these findings, many hospitals use the number of procedures previously performed as a criterion for hospital credentialing and for granting the privilege to perform procedures independently.[24] Some surgical residencies have adopted competency-based education and report success using fresh cadavers as models to achieve rapid improvement in surgical skills.[27]

The learning curve is steep for certain procedures. In a report by Konrad and coworkers,[28] initial intubation success rates for anesthesia residents in the operating room may be as low as 50% with their first 10 patients, and the curve does not rise to 90% until a mean of 57 attempts.

Regardless of the reasons, when procedures are performed infrequently, competency becomes an issue and complications may be prevalent. Cricothyroidotomy is an example of an uncommon procedure, and published reports of complication rates vary widely.[29–32] However, despite a high incidence of complications, successful cricothyroidotomy is an essential skill because the alternative is failing to establish an airway, which in most cases results in certain death.[33]

Chapman[25] is an advocate of establishing procedural competency expectations for emergency procedures and resuscitations to ensure the competency of EM graduates. Currently no competency criteria are set by the American Board of Emergency Medicine (ABEM) for emergency procedures and resuscitations, and the minimum number of procedures has not been established. ABEM has, likewise, not established a mechanism for testing procedural competency and must rely on residencies to provide the necessary training, evaluation, and assurance of competency.[34] Braen and Munger[34] described early efforts of ABEM to evaluate procedural skills, but these were not implemented, primarily owing to a lack of reliable equipment and resources to examine large pools of candidates in a high-stakes national examination. To standardize testing, there must be an assurance that examiners will be able to reliably evaluate candidates. Bullock and colleagues[35] demonstrated good inter-rater reliability by both expert and nonexpert observers when they were given structured checklists to assess procedural skills. Custalow and associates[36] likewise observed excellent inter-rater reliability among expert reviewers for the evaluation of critical step performance of saphenous vein cutdown, thoracotomy, and cricothyroidotomy. Ideally, a national procedural competency examination might incorporate animal, cadaver, and virtual reality simulation laboratories to evaluate candidates.[25]

EDUCATIONAL ALTERNATIVES FOR PRACTICING PROCEDURES

To ensure residents' procedural competency upon completion of residency training and with limited available clinical experience, explore alternative methods for training. Many educational methods are in use. Unfortunately, many alternatives to clinical experience have substantial limitations and few have been tested for their efficacy and applicability to the performance of procedures on human patients. The following is a description of the currently available educational techniques. As mentioned earlier, it is ideal to introduce the procedure via formal review before the learner practices the skill using one of the following procedural models. This may include listening to lectures, watching videotapes, using computerized instructional materials, and reading and reviewing procedural texts and atlases.

Volunteers

Human volunteers (paid or unpaid) are commonly used for teaching procedures. Use a human volunteer to practice noninvasive procedures such as casting and splinting, and consider using a volunteer for certain minimally invasive procedures such as intravenous catheter or nasogastric tube insertion. Volunteers are clearly not appropriate for most invasive procedures.

Living Patients in Operating Rooms

Provide opportunities for residents to practice endotracheal intubations during anesthesia rotations in the controlled setting of the operating room. Be aware that if there is also an anesthesia residency–training program at the hospital, residents may compete for these cases.

Mannequins

Use mannequins, such as the popular "Resusci-Annie," to teach procedures when available (Fig. 70–4). Models are available for virtually any procedure including cardiopulmonary resuscitation, peripheral venipuncture, arterial puncture, intraosseous infusion, umbilical vessel catheterization, central line catheterization, lumbar puncture, endotracheal intubation, needle thoracostomy, urinary catheter placement, suturing, and emergency childbirth. Stratton and coworkers[37] found that paramedics who train in endotracheal intubation using a mannequin-only teaching program achieve equal success rates in field intubations compared with those receiv-

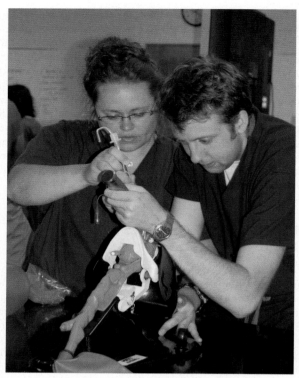

Figure 70–4 Mannequins are available to teach many procedures, including endotracheal intubation.

ing additional training on human cadavers. Mannequins can serve as useful adjuncts for teaching procedures but are limited by the lack of certain physical properties of living tissue, including hemorrhage, a beating heart, and breathing lungs. Most mannequins are designed for durability and not for realistic simulation. They are very different from the human patient in whom pliable structures (such as the tongue and epiglottis) bend easily and move with the instruments.[38]

Video Imaging

Videotaping may be used to teach a procedure and also to review the procedure once it has been completed. The Airway Cam Direct Laryngoscopy Video System includes a miniature video camera that is worn by the trainee, thus allowing a supervisor to assist. The advantage is that the instructor provides real-time feedback to trainees. Recording the trainee's performance allows for review at a later time.[39] In a study of initial success rates of paramedic trainees in an operating room setting, Levitan and colleagues[40] observed a mean improvement in intubation success rates of 41% after paramedics watched a 26-minute instructional videotape recorded using this video camera system.

In another study, after watching a 30-minute videotape demonstration of thoracotomy, medical students were able to perform this emergent procedure on dog and pig models with surprising accuracy. The presentation of complicated anatomy to novices appears to be an important prerequisite to performing procedures accurately.[1,24]

Medical Simulators

We are now well into the information age, and medical simulation is taking an increasingly important role in medical education. An invaluable teaching tool, medical simulation can be used to improve a learner's competence and confidence, expose a learner to rare, but potentially life-saving procedures, and decrease the rate of procedural errors. With a simulator, the learner has the opportunity to practice every procedure that she or he needs to know under a variety of different conditions. The educator can vary the difficulty of the situation based on the level of training of the learner. Complications can be simulated and the learner has the opportunity to learn how to avoid them or deal with the consequences should they arise. Debriefing is an important part of the simulator educational method.

Different types of simulators are available. Part-task simulators, such as intravenous arms or chest tube mannequins, are designed to teach specific procedural skills. Full-scale simulation is designed to mimic a real-life medical scenario, including the procedures, decision-making skills, and possible permutations that may occur.[41] Full-scale simulation requires a high-fidelity mannequin, a team leader/instructor, a script, a scenario, and a debriefing. The instructor's responsibility is to create an environment that resembles reality as closely as possible.[42] Whereas the script is standardized, the software and mannequin can take into account the unpredictable actions of participants. If this is not possible, the team leader may redirect participants to take an action that will result in a predetermined response. The debriefing process is also an important learning opportunity in which mistakes can be discussed and alternate courses of action can be explored.

In a review of simulation technology, Reznek and associates[42] wrote that to be an effective teaching tool, a simulator must provide both educationally sound and realistic feedback to a user's questions, decisions, and actions. Force and tactile feedback have proved to be the most difficult parts of the virtual environment to simulate. Modern human patient simulators have been developed, or are currently under development, for endotracheal intubation, chest compression, electrical cardioversion, cricothyroidotomy, chest tube insertion, pericardiocentesis, diagnostic peritoneal lavage, emergency thoracotomy, lumbar puncture, skin suturing, insertion of peripheral venous/arterial catheters, insertion of central venous lines, and virtually any procedure (Fig. 70–5).[42] Many studies have demonstrated the efficacy and applicability of simulation education.[43-45]

Cadaver Laboratories

Use fresh cadavers to teach procedures when available. To clarify, these are the bodies of individuals who have given consent for their bodies to be used for teaching. The advantage of using a fresh cadaver is that it more clearly resembles the tissue properties and pliability of a live human. The disadvantages are cost, limited availability, and potential risk for transmission of disease.[11]

Use preserved cadavers if these are more readily available at your institution. A cadaver laboratory offers the advantage of a standardized reproducible laboratory experience under the guidance of an instructor and with no risk to the patient.[46] Disadvantages of preserved cadavers are that they do not bleed and they suffer from tissue adherence owing to the preservation process, so although excellent for learning the anatomy of procedures, they may not completely simulate the in vivo experience.[47]

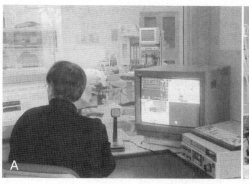
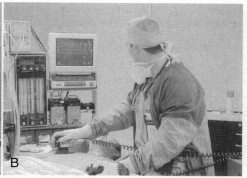

Figure 70–5 **Human patient medical simulator.** *A,* In the control room, the educator is able to create and monitor clinical scenarios. *B,* The trainee performs electrical cardioversion on a human patient simulator and receives feedback from his or her actions by watching the monitor (successful conversion of ventricular tachycardia to sinus rhythm).

Newly Deceased Patients

Newly deceased patients—those who have not expressly given consent for the use of their bodies—have also been used to practice procedures. A survey of program directors of EM and critical care training programs found that 63% of EM programs allow procedures to be performed on newly dead patients.[48]

Performing invasive procedures on the newly dead may be limited by certain debated ethical concerns.[48–55] Whether consent should be obtained before performing procedures on the newly dead is a question that has been discussed extensively in the literature. Advocates of practicing procedures without consent believe that the dead have no claim to autonomy and that this is a function of personhood. Iserson[51] stated that consent for procedures on the newly dead is, therefore, an inappropriate extension of patient autonomy. In addition, given the absence of suitable alternative training models, it is in society's best interest to have adequate numbers of medical care providers who are experienced in life-saving procedures. Finally, families are often less altruistic on behalf of their relatives than the individual would be, and requesting permission from relatives may supersede the individual's own wishes and create excessive emotional barriers between the provider and a distraught family.[51]

Those who advocate obtaining consent claim that practicing procedures on the newly dead without consent is unlawful and unethical. Goldblatt[50] wrote that proxy consent by a family member is required when patients cannot give consent themselves and that the next of kin have "quasi-property rights" for the body of a dead family member. He suggested that by framing a request to the family, such as, "What would the deceased have wanted?," the protective instincts of the next of kin may be decreased and permission granted.

In a survey involving theoretical clinical scenarios, people responded that they would agree to after-death procedures on themselves in 75% of cases and on their relatives in 70% of cases. However, without prior consent, they would allow such procedures only 40% of the time on themselves and only 50% on their family members.[53] In actual clinical practice, consent given by family members has traditionally been lower. Families gave consent for retrograde wire intubation of newly deceased adults in 59% of cases,[54] and for cricothyroidotomy of newly deceased adults in 39% of cases.[55]

Isolated Animal Tissues

Use isolated animal tissues such as pig's feet to teach basic wound closure techniques (Fig. 70–6).[56] Isolated sheep or pig tracheas are useful to practice the technique of cricothyroid-

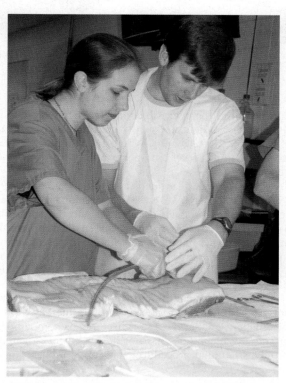

Figure 70–6 Isolated pig's chest wall is a useful model to teach tube thoracostomy.

otomy but lack the external anatomy of the cricothyroid membrane in situ. Others have experimented with the use of chicken or turkey bones to teach the technique of intraosseous line placement.

Live Animal Laboratories

Live animal laboratories provide for a realistic, stimulating teaching environment that imparts a level of understanding vastly different from other educational methods.[57] Although no alternative to performing procedures on a human patient is completely suitable, animal laboratories can provide a reasonable training alternative in which procedures may be performed with close supervision and under controlled conditions (Fig. 70–7).[10] Animal laboratories offer the advantages associated with performing procedures on living, bleeding tissues. Many feel that there is no substitute for this experience and that these learning experiences cannot be duplicated by simulations.[57] Students experience a feeling of responsibility and receive immediate feedback for their actions.[58] Moreover,

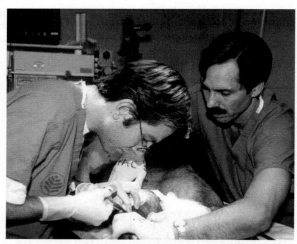

Figure 70–7 In the live animal laboratory, an instructor assists while the trainee performs a venous cutdown.

animal laboratories may instill confidence in performing procedures on real patients. A survey of clinicians participating in a swine procedure laboratory reported a significant change in their comfort level in performing six resuscitative procedures.[59]

A survey of American medical colleges found that 92 of 126 medical schools (73%) use live animal laboratories at some point in their regular curriculum.[56] In this study, more than half of the schools without animal laboratories cited increasing expense of animals and equipment as the primary reason for not continuing them. Only two schools noted pressure from animal rights activists or student complaints as significant issues in discontinuing animal laboratories.[56]

The time, space, and money required to provide animal laboratory training for residents are considerable, yet the effectiveness of animal laboratory training as compared with other training techniques has not been well investigated. In one study, an animal procedure laboratory emphasizing skill repetition improved tube thoracostomy procedural skills and speed, and these skills were retained on retesting of subjects 18 days later. However, all participants in this study received animal laboratory training, and there was no comparison with subjects receiving instruction using conventional training techniques.[9] A 2002 study by Custalow and associates[36] compared residents who had received animal laboratory training with those without animal laboratory training and found significant long-term improvements in procedural competency and speed in the performance of resuscitative procedures in those who received animal laboratory training.

One disadvantage of using animals for medical training, however, is the considerable cost involved. Furthermore, many question whether an animal model provides the best available simulation of the performance of procedures in humans. Finally, debate continues on the appropriate balance between animal rights and the benefits of using animals for medical training and research.[6,9,60,61]

CONCLUSION

Numerous educational alternatives are available for teaching ED procedures, each with advantages and disadvantages. Optimally, residencies will have the space and resources to use a combination of training techniques to ensure competent performance of procedures by EM graduates. Educators may then find new ways to teach time-proven techniques, refine these techniques, or even develop new ones such as the Brofeldt four-step cricothyroidotomy.[62,63] Many questions remain unanswered regarding the best educational methods, but EM has the foundation for building a comprehensive instructional system to ensure the competency of trainees and maintenance of procedural skills throughout life. With repetition and reinforcement, these skills may then be committed to long-term memory for retrieval when they are most needed in the ED.

 REFERENCES CAN BE FOUND ON **EXPERT CONSULT**

CHAPTER **71**

Physical and Chemical Restraint

Charles J. Fasano and Gregory Schneider

Emergency clinicians are often faced with the challenge of caring for agitated, combative, and violent patients who are a danger to themselves and medical and prehospital personnel.[1,2] Psychiatric illness, acute intoxication or withdrawal, delirium, medical illness, uncontrolled rage, and rarely, central nervous system trauma and infection are frequent causes of agitated or violent behavior in the emergency department (ED).[2] The term *excited delirium*, a condition described as an individual totally out of control, unable to be reasoned with or talked down, and possessing great feats of strength is somewhat vague and ill defined; but it is well known to any police officer, paramedic, or emergency clinician (Fig. 71–1).

Patients who abuse alcohol, sympathomimetic agents such as cocaine or methamphetamines, or hallucinogenic drugs such as phencyclidine (PCP) are the subset of individuals who most commonly present with severe uncontrolled agitation. Alcohol withdrawal may progress to delirium tremens, a condition typified by excessive agitation. Schizophrenia, schizoaffective disorder, and the manic phase of bipolar disorder can all lead to an impaired perception of reality. Patients with these disorders often develop paranoid delusions, hallucinations, and hostile moods that can easily lead to severe agitation.

Any medical condition that leads to brain dysfunction may also result in agitated, combative, or frankly violent behavior (Table 71–1). Well-documented examples include hypoglycemia, hypoxia, medication intoxication, encephalitis, meningitis, intracranial hemorrhage, thyrotoxicosis, traumatic brain injury, febrile illnesses in the elderly, and dementia.[3]

The need to prevent these patients from harming themselves and those around them and to perform monitoring and diagnostic testing and institute timely treatment often necessitates physical and chemical restraint.

During the late 1980s and early 1990s, reports of restraint-associated deaths in psychiatric and extended care facilities[4] led lawmakers to pass legislation that established regulations for restraint use.[5] Since then, the Joint Commission for Accreditation of Healthcare Organizations (JCAHO) and the Center for Medicare and Medicaid Services (CMS) have created standards governing the use of restraints in a variety of health care settings, including acute care hospitals and the EDs they operate.[6,7] These standards allow the use of restraints for limited periods of time, and only after a physician or licensed practitioner has evaluated the patient and determined that less restrictive interventions have been ineffective and physical restraint is needed to improve the patient's well-being. The standards also include requirements for written policies and procedures governing restraint use (Table 71–2), which must address indications, staff training and education, patient assessment and re-evaluations, appropriate documentation, and patient-focused issues such as maintaining dignity and respect. Hospitals and extended care facilities are required

by law to report any death or adverse event related to restraint use.[7]

Some authors advocate for "restraint-free" environments in nursing homes, extended care facilities, and acute care hospitals.[8,9] Although this concept is laudable, mandating a restraint-free ED is impractical and potentially dangerous. Emergency clinicians need to be vigilant regarding the potential risks inherent to patient restraint but should not be deterred from using both physical and chemical restraint in appropriate patients who are a danger to themselves, fellow patients, or ED staff. Indeed, the American College of Emergency Physicians, in a 2001 Policy Statement,[10] supports the careful and appropriate use of patient restraints or seclusion.

MEDICOLEGAL CONCERNS

Emergency clinicians need to be cognizant of the potential legal ramifications stemming from physically restraining patients. Such patients are often young and previously medically well, and a death is usually highly charged with social and racial issues, police brutality complaints, and charges of clinician indifference. The risk of litigation can be mitigated by strict adherence to written institutional and/or departmental policies regarding the use of restraints and medications. Emphasis should be placed on a timely and comprehensive prerestraint assessment, regular patient re-evaluations, limitations on the time spent in restraints, and detailed documentation in the ED record. Furthermore, clinicians need to recognize that competent patients do have the legal right to refuse medical treatment even if the result of their refusal is death or serious bodily harm. Coercive measures, including physical restraints or the threat of physical restraints, should not be used simply because a competent patient refuses treatment or as retaliation for perceived disruptive behavior.[11] *Nonetheless, emergency clinicians should not be deterred from using both physical and chemical restraints in appropriate patients who are determined to be a danger to themselves or others.* If any uncertainty surrounds the appropriateness of restraining a particular patient, early psychiatric consultation and discussion with hospital administration and legal counsel are advised, but rarely available in practical terms.

PATIENT ASSESSMENT

A complete and thorough assessment is mandatory for all patients requiring physical or chemical restraint in the ED. Emergency clinicians must avoid ascribing agitated or abusive behavior to drug or alcohol intoxication or underlying psychiatric disease before considering the potentially more serious or life-threatening diagnoses (see Table 71–1).

Every attempt should be made to obtain a detailed history surrounding the patient's presentation, as well as her or his past medical and psychiatric histories, including medications, drug and alcohol use, and prior similar events. In reality, *such information is rarely available or accurate, leaving clinical judgment of the treating clinician the only alternative*. If time permits, an unusual luxury, the clinician may question emergency medical service providers and/or contact family members to elucidate the circumstances before ED arrival and obtain information about previous abnormal or violent behavior. Five groups of patients have been identified as being at risk for the presence of an underlying medical problem: the elderly, those with a history of substance abuse, patients without a prior psychiatric disorder, those with preexisting or

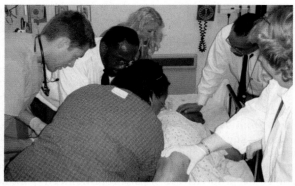

Figure 71–1 The first action when dealing with excited delirium is to physically restrain the patient, gain control, then consider chemical restraint.

new medical complaints, and individuals from lower socioeconomic groups.[12,13] Of these, patients presenting with new psychiatric symptoms are especially worrisome and require careful evaluation for underlying medical illness.[14]

Physical examination should be aimed at identifying organic causes of the patient's behavior such as trauma, infection, and metabolic derangements. Temperature measurements may have to wait until the patient calms down or has been restrained, but should not be overlooked, because an elevated temperature may be the only clue to the presence of an underlying infection such as meningitis or encephalitis or a toxidrome such as sympathomimetic or anticholinergic poisoning. Signs of head trauma in patients who appear intoxicated warrant investigations to rule out traumatic brain injury.

Rapid beside serum glucose determination should be part of any patient presenting with agitated or combative behavior. Additional studies are based on the results of the history and physical examination and may include both radiologic and laboratory testing.

Once a patient has been restrained, frequent periodic re-evaluation is paramount to the patient's safety and is required by the JCAHO (see Table 71–2).[15] Re-evaluations should include a careful appraisal of the patient's vital signs and neurologic condition including mental status, cardiorespiratory system, and extremity perfusion (Table 71–3). Remove physical restraints as soon as the patient's condition has changed sufficiently so as not be a threat to herself or himself or others.

DE-ESCALATION TECHNIQUES

Although many patients cannot be reasoned with, several de-escalation techniques have been shown to help quell agitated and violent patients.[1] A simple, yet effective, practice is to verbally engage the patient and ask him or her "how can we help you?" This display of empathy on the part of the treating clinician and staff will often calm the patient. Similarly, offering something to eat or drink will often soothe an agitated patient. Along with these displays of caring and empathy, it is important to communicate to the patient that violent behavior will not be tolerated and will be dealt with quickly and firmly.[1] If the patient continues to demonstrate agitated or violent behavior, enlisting the aid of a family member or a specially trained individual, such as a social worker, psychiatric counselor, or member of the clergy, may also be beneficial.

TABLE 71–1 Conditions That May Cause Agitated and Violent Behavior

Endocrine

- Hypoglycemia
- Hyperglycemia
- Thyrotoxicosis/thyroid storm
- Myxedema

Infectious

- Meningitis
- Encephalitis
- Sepsis
- Urinary tract infection

Metabolic

- Hypoxia
- Hypercarbia
- Hyponatremia
- Hypernatremia

Toxicologic

- Acute alcohol intoxication
- Sympathomimetic intoxication
- Anticholinergic intoxication
- Delirium tremens
- Alcohol withdrawal
- Benzodiazepine withdrawal
- Narcotic withdrawal

Traumatic

- Intracranial hemorrhage
- Diffuse axonal injury
- Hypoxia
- Low flow states due to systemic hemorrhage

Neurologic

- Status epilepticus
- Postictal states
- Acute delirium
- Subarachnoid hemorrhage
- Cerebral vascular accident

TABLE 71–2 Joint Commission for Accreditation of Healthcare Organization Requirements for Patient Restraint Protocols and Documentation

Restraint Protocols Should Include

- Guidelines for assessing the patient
- Criteria for applying restraint
- Criteria for monitoring the patient and reassessing the need for restraint
  - Monitoring at least every 2 hr or sooner based on patient needs
- Criteria for terminating restraint

Documentation Should Include

- Relevant orders for use
- Results of patient monitoring
- Reassessment
- Significant changes in the patient's condition

TABLE 71–3 Recommended Areas to Assess during Re-evaluation of Restrained Patients

Neurologic Status

- Level of alertness
- Degree of agitation
- Pupillary examination
- Motor examination
- Sensory examination

Vascular Status

- Capillary refill
- Distal pulses

Vital Signs

- Blood pressure
- Heart rate
- Respiratory rate
- Oxygen saturation
- Temperature

Patient Comfort

- Skin under and around the restraints
- Hydration
- Personal hygiene
- Toileting needs

Assessment for Restraint Removal

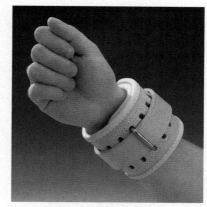

Figure 71–2 Leather extremity restraint. *(Courtesy of Posey Company, Inc., Arcadia, CA.)*

Physical Restraint

Research in the area of ED restraints is limited. In one prospective study of restraint-associated complications in 298 ED patients, minor complications were seen in only 7% of patients, and there were no serious complications or deaths.[22] The author of this study concluded that dangers of ED patient restraint promulgated by professional organizations and health care regulators may be overstated.[22] This study appears to support the safe use of restraints by emergency clinicians, who by virtue of their training and experience are experts in recognizing signs of deterioration and skilled in airway management and resuscitation.

Although the actual prevalence of patient restraint in EDs is unknown, it has been estimated that 25% of teaching hospitals physically restrain at least one person per day.[2]

Restraint Devices

Limb Holders (Restraints). Restraining a patient's extremities is the primary method of physical restraint used in the ED. Limb restraints are constructed from a variety of materials including leather, synthetic leather, cotton, and single-use foam material. These materials provide restraints that differ in strength, ease of removal, and cleaning.

Hard leather and synthetic leather limb holders are virtually impossible to break or tear but are difficult to sterilize if they become soiled with blood or bodily fluids (Fig. 71–2). They are more rigid than soft restraints, also making them somewhat more difficult and time consuming to apply. More importantly, most leather limb holders require a key to unlock and, as a result, might take longer to remove after an adverse event such as vomiting or respiratory arrest. Leather limb holders are generally used to restrain combative and violent patients, in whom the need for indestructible secure restraints outweighs the more time-consuming application and removal process.

Soft limb restraints are usually made from cotton and/or foam materials (Fig. 71–3). They are single-use devices, which obviates the need for cleaning and sterilization. Soft limb restraints are less rigid than leather limb restraints, making them easier to apply. In addition, because they are fastened without the use of a key, soft limb restraints are more easily removed. Soft restraints are typically used for agitated and less combative patients because they are not as secure as leather limb holders.

Belts/Fifth-Point Restraint. A fifth-point restraint is a belt apparatus used to supplement the use of four limb

If these conservative measures fail, summon hospital security to ensure the safety of the patient and staff. In these situations, security staff should not rush to the patient's bedside, but should instead gather outside the door or close by, remaining within eye contact of the patient's room. *A strong show of force* may calm a potentially violent patient without the need for restraints.

TYPES OF PATIENT RESTRAINT

Seclusion

The utility of seclusion in psychiatric evaluation units and inpatient hospital wards is well documented in both adult and pediatric populations.[16–19] In the mid-1980s, seclusion was commonly used to calm combative and violent ED patients, but its popularity has declined since then.[2,20] Reasons for this decline are unclear, but probably include lack of adequate space and concerns regarding the provision of medical care and compliance with regulatory agencies.[20] Nevertheless, at institutions with adequate physical space and well-designed policies and procedures, experience has shown that seclusion is an effective, although underutilized, ED practice for selected patients.[20,21]

Seclusion is often used in conjunction with chemical and/or physical restraints.[20] Place agitated and violent patients in seclusion on dedicated hospital stretchers or beds secured in place to prevent injury. The seclusion room should be located near ED staff and allow for constant patient observation. Reassess patients placed in seclusion at regular frequent intervals, similar to restrained patients (see Table 71–3).

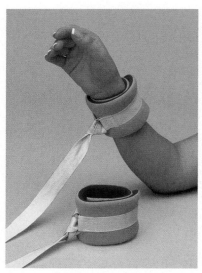

Figure 71–3 Cotton extremity restraint. *(Courtesy of Posey Company, Inc., Arcadia, CA.)*

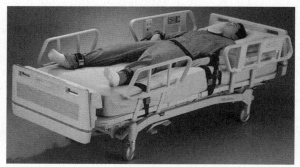

Figure 71–4 Fifth-point restraint. *(Courtesy of Posey Company, Inc., Arcadia, CA.)*

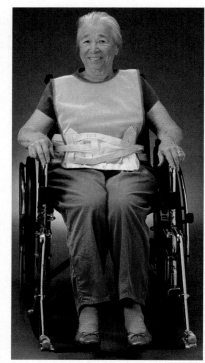

Figure 71–5 Restraint vest. *(Courtesy of Posey Company, Inc., Arcadia, CA.)*

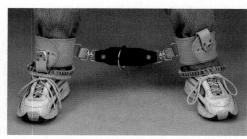

Figure 71–6 Hobble leg restraint. *(Courtesy of Posey Company, Inc., Arcadia, CA.)*

restraints by holding down the thighs, chest, or pelvis (Fig. 71–4). A fifth-point restraint is used for patients who continue to be at risk for harming themselves, despite adequate limb restraints, and for those whose continued combative behavior interferes with diagnostic or therapeutic interventions. Patients restrained across the thighs, chest, or pelvis require close monitoring for adverse events, especially vomiting, because they may not be able to sit up or turn onto their side. Place the side rails of the stretcher in the upright position at all times and place the belt snugly enough to prevent the patient from slipping under the device, increasing the risk of accidental suffocation. Fifth-point restraints are usually made out of synthetic material and are available with both quick-release and key-release locks.

Jackets and Vests. Jackets and vests are generally used on inpatient wards and extended care facilities for the prevention of falls; they have little utility in the ED (Fig. 71–5). Moreover, these products have been implicated in a number of restraint-associated deaths secondary to choking and suffocation, prompting recommendations from the American Geriatric Society to abandon their use.[9] We do not recommend the use of restraint jackets and vests in the ED.

Hobble Leg Restraints. Hobble leg restraints limit movement by securing the patient's ankles with connecting locking cuffs (Fig. 71–6). Hobble leg restraints are commonly used by law enforcement agencies because they impede running and kicking, making them an effective method to transport potentially violent patients and those who pose a flight risk. Hobble leg restraints are seldom used in the ED, but their use by law enforcement agencies and prison authorities means that most emergency clinicians will encounter patients placed in these devices. The combination of prone positioning, hobble leg restraints, and binding a patient's hands behind her or his back, commonly referred to as a *hog tie*, was a common method for restraining prisoners and violent psychiatric patients (Fig. 71–7). However, this practice is no longer widely used (see "Positional Asphyxia," later).

Indications

Limb restraints are indicated to prevent agitated, combative, or violent patients from harming themselves or others. Often, the use of restraints can be delayed while verbal de-escalation techniques are attempted (see "De-Escalation Techniques," earlier). However, if a patent is deemed an immediate threat to himself or herself or others, restrain him or her without delay. Patients with altered mental status often require limb restraints so that important diagnostic tests can be performed and/or appropriate treatment rendered. Limb restraints are

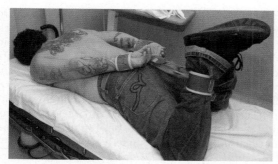

Figure 71–7 The "hog-tie" method of restraint. The combination of prone positioning, hobble leg restraints, and binding a patient's hand behind his or her back, is commonly referred to as a *hog tie*. Although this was a common method for restraining prisoners and violent psychiatric patients in past, the hog tie is no longer recommended. The exact physiologic and metabolic derangements from this position by itself is likely minimal, but the practice is strongly discouraged.

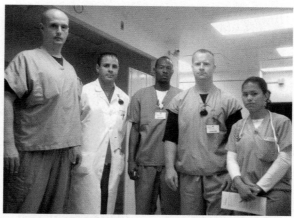

Figure 71–8 Show of force. A minimum of five well-trained individuals should be available to restrain a patient. This show of force may help discourage the patient from resisting and is an important part of the restraint process.

also used to prevent patients from removing or interfering with potentially life-saving devices, such as endotracheal tubes and indwelling intravenous lines and catheters.

The addition of a fifth-point restraint is indicated in patients who continue to be at risk for harming themselves, despite adequate limb restraints, and for those patients whose continued combative behavior interferes with diagnostic or therapeutic interventions. In general, the ED use of restraining vests and jackets and hobble leg restraints is not recommended.

Contraindications

In the appropriate situations, physical restraint may be delayed in favor of an attempt at verbal de-escalation. Do not place limb restraints on extremities with fractures, open wounds, or acute skin and soft tissue infections and use them cautiously in patients with uncertain or unreliable extremity perfusion, such as those with peripheral vascular disease or previous arterial injury or surgery.

Avoid fifth-point restraint of the abdomen and pelvis region in patients with pelvic fractures, suprapubic tubes, ostomies, and percutaneous feeding tubes. In addition, it is important to note that patients with underlying pulmonary or cardiac disease may not tolerate restraint of their thorax.

Procedure

A minimum of five people, all of whom have had training in restraint technique and patient safety, should be available to restrain a patient (Fig. 71–8). This show of force may help discourage the patient from resisting and is an important part of the restraint process. The individuals making up the restraint team may include clinicians, nurses, technicians, and police or hospital security. When possible, undress the patients and place them in a hospital gown before restraining them. When this is not practical, the patient can still be restrained, but should be promptly searched and all potentially harmful possessions, such as guns, knives, razors, combs, matches, and lighters, taken for safekeeping.

Always restrain patients in the supine, rather than the prone, position. Assign one person to each limb, which they hold firmly against the stretcher by applying direct pressure proximal to the elbows and knees. The fifth member of the team places restraints around the wrists and ankles (Fig. 71–9). Control above the elbow and knees reduces the risk of

injury to these joints and concentrates force closer to the patient's center of gravity. Such patients rarely perceive pain, so the practice of manipulating or twisting the patient's digits, nose, or ears should be avoided because it is generally useless and might further escalate the patient's combative and violent behavior.

Apply the limb holders snugly enough to control movement and prevent escape, but not so tight as to cause pain or impair circulation. If necessary, place a fifth-point restraint across the patient's thighs, pelvic, or chest to further limit motion. A surgical mask may be temporarily placed over the patient's mouth to prevent her or him from spitting at members of the restraint team or ED staff.

Once the patient has been safely restrained, frequent re-evaluation in accordance with your institution's policies and procedures is the key to preventing complications (see Table 71–3). If leather restraints are used, have a restraint key readily available in the event that the restraints need to be removed urgently. Restraints should have well-defined time limits and should be removed as soon as the patient's condition has changed sufficiently that he or she is no longer a threat to himself or herself or others.

Complications

Increased Agitation. For some patients, being placed in physical restraints is so emotionally disturbing that it actually increases agitation and combative behavior. Patients who continue to struggle despite restraints are at risk for a number of potentially serious adverse events including skin damage, ischemia, metabolic acidosis, and even death (see "Other Complications," later). In these patients, the addition of chemical sedation is highly recommended (see "Chemical Restraint," later). In contrast, the use of extremity restraints alone is often effective in the alcohol-intoxicated patient because the natural progression of alcohol intoxication is sedation and sleep. Intoxicated patients may benefit from a brief period of observation before a decision is made to administer chemical sedation. Most of these patients will fall asleep, obviating the need for sedation and the accompanying risks.

Local Skin Complications. Restraints may cause skin irritation or breakdown. Risk factors include restraints that have been placed too tightly and those that have been left on for prolonged periods of time. Leather restraints are more

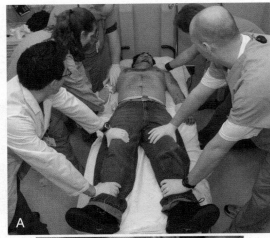

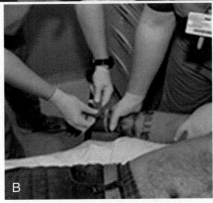

Figure 71–9 Technique to restrain a violent patient. *A,* Patients should always be restrained in the supine position. One person is assigned to each limb, which they hold firmly against the stretcher by applying direct pressure proximal to the elbows and knees. *B,* The fifth member of the team places restraints around the wrists and ankles. The limb holders should be applied snug enough to control movement and prevent escape, but not so tight as to cause pain or impair circulation. If necessary, a fifth-point restraint may be placed across the patient's thighs, pelvis, or chest to further limit motion.

likely than soft restraints to cause skin damage. This is particularly true in patients who continue to struggle despite being placed in restraints. Using soft restraints whenever possible, avoiding overly tight restraints, limiting restraint time, and reevaluating frequently (see Table 71–3) will help prevent skin complications. In addition, the judicious use of chemical restraint will help avoid skin damage in patients who continue to struggle. It is also important not to ignore a patient's complaints of restraint pain without first evaluating the possibility of an adverse event.

Vascular Compromise. Restraints have the potential to impede blood flow to the hands and feet. In extreme cases, this could result in ischemia of the distal extremity. Ischemia is more likely to occur in patients whose restraints are placed too tightly and in those who develop swelling from an occult injury. Struggling against the restraints may further increase this risk. A thorough search for occult injuries, attention to proper fit, and limiting restraint time will help avoid ischemia. Frequent assessment of pulses, capillary refill, skin color and temperature, and motor and sensory function are also extremely important. As mentioned previously, it is also important not to ignore a restrained patient's complaints regarding extremity pain without first evaluating the possibility of ischemia.

Respiratory Compromise. Restraints may impair respiratory mechanics in some patients. This is more likely to occur in patients restrained in the prone or hog-tie positions and those with underlying pulmonary disease.[23–27] Patients with chronic obstructive pulmonary disease (COPD) may not tolerate a fifth-point restraint across the chest. Respiratory complications can be avoided by not restraining patients in the prone or *hog-tie* positions. In addition, the use of adequate chemical sedation may negate the need to use a supplemental restraint belt in patients with underlying COPD.

Positional Asphyxia. *Positional asphyxia*, a severe respiratory complication attributed to restraint use, is unexpected death due to asphyxia theoretically solely related to patient positioning. The specifics of respiratory embarrassment secondary to restraint are vague and unproved, and volunteer subjects do not seem to experience severe pulmonary compromise from restraint. *Although often implicated, the exact contribution of restraint to sudden death is unclear.* Obesity, underlying cardiac and pulmonary disease, prone positioning, and concurrent stimulant use are thought to be contributing factors.[23,25,27–30] The hog-tie position places patients at theoretical risk for positional asphyxia and therefore should not be used in the ED.[23–26,29,31–33] Restraining patients in the supine position and frequently re-evaluating will help prevent positional asphyxia. Extremely close monitoring of respiratory status is indicated in patients with obesity and COPD and those using cocaine or other stimulant drugs.

Cocaine-Associated Agitated Delirium. *Cocaine-associated agitated delirium* is a syndrome of hyperthermia with delirium and severe agitation that can progress to respiratory arrest and death.[25,27,30,31,34] Restrained patients appear to be at particularly high risk for this syndrome. The syndrome was first described in 1985, but the incidence increased significantly in the 1990s owing to the popularity of crack cocaine.[31,32]

The pathophysiology of cocaine-associated agitated delirium is a complex process involving down-regulation of dopamine receptors with subsequent dopamine excess during times of cocaine binges.[31,35–37] When patients with cocaine-associated agitated delirium are restrained, especially in the prone position, interference with normal respiratory mechanics increases the likelihood of hypoventilation, hypercarbia, and hypoxemia, ultimately leading to asphyxia and death. It has also been suggested that stress caused by the restraining process increases the risk of fatal cardiac arrhythmias due to catecholamine surge in an already cocaine-sensitized myocardium.[31] Chronic stimulant use leads to adrenergic-induced cardiomyopathy, often clinically silent until the individual is severely stressed. The potential for malignant arrhythmias is unknown, but this pathophysiology has been implicated in some cases of sudden death in restraint.

Metabolic Acidosis. In patients who have been restrained, continued agitation and struggling can lead to severe metabolic acidosis.[34] The pH is often less than 7.0. The etiology of this acidosis is unclear, but probably involves the production of lactic acid from physical exertion compounded by sympathetic-induced vasoconstriction. Such vasoconstriction may result from agitation or cocaine (and other stimulant) use and is believed to enhance exercise-induced lactic acidosis by impeding lactate clearance by the liver.[38,39] In some patients, the buildup of lactate is further increased by the presence of psychosis and delirium, which may alter pain sensation, allowing exertion far beyond normal physiologic limits.[34] In addition, some restraint positions (e.g., prone, hog tie) may not allow adequate respiratory compensation, resulting in further enhancement of the acidosis. The common scenario is an out-of-hospital cardiac arrest, in which the severely agitated individual suddenly stops struggling and experiences a bradycardic/asystolic death that is not immediately recognized. Such patients may have been subdued by force, Tasered, or maced/pepper-sprayed, leading to unproven speculation that these interventions may have been culpable.

Regardless of the etiology, profound metabolic acidosis has been associated with cardiovascular collapse and sudden and unexpected death in restrained patients.[34] Patients who remain combative despite restraints, especially those who have used cocaine or other sympathomimetic agents, are at particularly high risk for death.[34] Clues to the presence of a metabolic acidosis include severe agitation, abnormal vital signs (e.g., persistent tachycardia, tachypnea, and hyperpyrexia), and decreased or concentrated urine output despite adequate intravenous fluid administration. Laboratory testing, including arterial blood gas analysis, serum electrolytes, and serum creatine phosphokinase are recommended in patients with signs and symptoms suggestive of metabolic acidosis and in those with a suspicion of a potentially lethal co-ingestion (e.g., salicylates and toxic alcohols).

Restrained patients with severe metabolic acidosis should receive aggressive saline hydration and sedation with benzodiazepines to counter sympathetic hyperactivity.[34] The utility of sodium bicarbonate is unknown but is probably best reserved for patients with pH below 7.0. However, once cardiac arrest has occurred, resuscitative efforts are usually futile.

Chemical Restraint

Chemical restraint is the use of medication to induce tranquility, quell dangerous behavior, limit pathophysiologic derangements, and permit a more thorough evaluation of a patient's underlying condition. The term "chemical restraint" carries with it a negative connotation to many practitioners. Others have used the term *rapid tranquilization*, which seems more descriptive and less pejorative.

The CMS states a chemical restraint is "a medication used to control behavior or to restrict the patient's freedom of movement and is not a standard treatment for the patient's medical or psychiatric condition."[7] The JCAHO defines chemical restraint as "the inappropriate use of a sedating psychotropic drug to manage or control behavior."[15] These definitions lack perspective on the use of chemical restraint in the ED where these medications are typically employed after all other measures fail and the health and safety of the patient and/or staff are threatened. *Such statements do not reflect standard care in the ED, and should not be interpreted as prohibition of the appropriate short-term use of chemical restraint.*

The pathogenesis of agitation is poorly understood, but is thought to arise from increases in dopamine and noradrenalin with concomitant decreases in γ-aminobutyric acid (GABA). Prior to the development of antipsychotic medications, pharmacologic management of agitation included barbiturates, insulin coma therapy, bromides, and various anesthetic agents. These treatments had a number of undesirable side effects and, in some cases, resulted in death.[3] The discovery of antipsychotic medications revolutionized the treatment of acute agitation. Not only did tranquilization become safer, but many of these new agents had the added benefit of treating underlying psychotic states.[3] The develop-

ment of benzodiazepines added another medication to the arsenal. These agents, because of their solid safety profile, have virtually replaced barbiturates in the treatment of acute agitation. Recently, intramuscular preparations of "atypical antipsychotic" medications such as olanzapine and ziprasidone have provided additional treatment options for rapid tranquilization.[64,66]

The emergency clinician is often faced with an uncontrollable individual with an undifferentiated etiology for the delirium and one who has been resistant to reason and physical restraint. Such an individual must be quickly controlled in the ED, and this equates to the use of chemical restraint. The ideal drug for chemical restraint should have multiple routes of administration (i.e., intramuscular, intravenous, transmucosal), a rapid onset of action, and negligible hemodynamic effects, should be familiar to the clinician, should possess a good safety record with minimal side effects. No one medication fits this profile for every patient, but with proper patient assessment and careful drug selection, most ED patients can be rapidly and safely sedated. In the ED setting in which rapid tranquilization is usually the goal, medications should be administered intramuscularly (IM) or intravenously (IV); other routes may be used when parenteral administration is not practical or feasible. The remainder of this chapter discusses the safety, efficacy, side effect profile, and recommended dosages for the medications most commonly used for chemical restraint. Recommendations for the drug selection are also discussed (Table 71–4).

Indications

Chemical restraint is used to prevent injury to the patient and others, attenuate psychosis, decrease the time spent in physical restraints, and calm the patient enough to permit a medical history and physical examination and perform diagnostic tests and procedures.

Contraindications and Adverse Effects

Absolute and relative contraindications and adverse effects vary by agent and are discussed separately for each agent.

Neuroleptic Agents

The antipsychotic effects of neuroleptic agents usually do not occur for 7 to 10 days, but the onset of sedation is rapid, making them useful in the acutely agitated patient. Potent neuroleptic agents such as haloperidol and droperidol are preferred because they lack tolerance with repeated use, have a low addiction potential, and possess a high therapeutic index (see Table 71–4). *Despite recent concerns about unapproved intravenous administration and QT prolongation, these agents have been used safely and effectively for years in the ED patient with undifferentiated agitated delirium.* Low-potency neuroleptics such as chlorpromazine are less desirable owing to a higher incidence of hypotension, seizures, and anticholinergic effects.[40]

Contraindications. Haloperidol and droperidol are contraindicated in patients with thyrotoxicosis (neurotoxicity may develop), Parkinson disease, or severe hepatic disease. These drugs can lower the seizure threshold, so they should be used with caution or not at all in patients with a history of seizures or trauma patients who may be at risk for seizures. Nevertheless, droperidol has been used safely in patients with a seizure disorder.[41] In addition, like all neuroleptic agents, haloperidol and droperidol can cause QT prolongation, so they should be used with caution in patients at risk for QT prolongation and torsades de pointes (Table 71–5). Droperi-

TABLE 71–4 Drugs Used for Chemical Restraint in the Emergency Department

Agent	Dosage	Onset/Duration of Action	Indications	Contraindications	Adverse Events	Comments*
Haloperidol	Adults: 5 mg IM/IV Children: 6–12 yr: 12.5 mg >12 yr: 2.5–5 mg	Onset: 30–45 min Duration: 4–24 hr	All forms of agitation	Patients with a history of QT prolongation, thyrotoxicosis, Parkinson disease, and severe hepatic disease	Extrapyramidal symptoms: QTc prolongation, neuroleptic malignant syndrome, hypotension, cholinergic blockade	Can be given alone or in combination with a benzodiazepine; may lower the seizure threshold
Droperidol	Adults: 5 mg IM/IV Children: 0.03–0.07 mg/kg (maximum, 2.5 mg)	Onset: 3–10 min Duration: 2–12 hr	All forms of agitation	Patients with a history of QT prolongation, thyrotoxicosis, Parkinson disease, severe hepatic disease, and intoxication with LSD	Extrapyramidal symptoms, QTc prolongation, neuroleptic malignant syndrome, hypotension, cholinergic blockade	Black box warning regarding QT prolongation and serious arrhythmias; rapid onset IM; use with caution in children
Lorazepam	Adults: 2–4 mg IM/IV Children: 0.05–0.1 mg/kg	Onset: IV: 15–20 min IM: 30–45 min Duration: 8–10 hr	All forms of agitation	Patients with respiratory depression and pregnant women	Respiratory depression, ataxia, hypotension	First-line therapy for children; use with caution in patients with alcohol intoxication owing to the risk of respiratory depression
Midazolam	Adults: 5 mg IM/IV Children: 0.1–0.2 mg/kg	Onset: IV: 3 min IM: 5 min Duration: 30–120 min	All forms of agitation	Patients with respiratory depression and pregnant women	Respiratory depression, ataxia, hypotension	First line therapy for children; rapid IM onset; use with caution in patients with alcohol intoxication owing to the risk of respiratory depression
Ziprasidone	Adults: 10–20 mg IM Children: Not indicated	Onset: 15–30 min Duration: 4 hr	Psychoses, intoxications	Patients with dementia	QT prolongation, somnolence, EPS	Lower incidence of EPS compared with haloperidol and droperidol; black box warning regarding use in elderly patients with dementia
Olanzapine	Adults: 10 mg IM Children: Not indicated	Onset: 15–30 min Duration: 2–24 hr	Psychiatric illness	Patients with dementia	Somnolence, EPS	Lower incidence of EPS compared with haloperidol and droperidol; black box warning regarding use in elderly patients with dementia

*Many of the caveats concerning the safety and efficacy of long-term use cannot be equated to short-term ED use. These medications are currently often used with safety and efficacy for short-term sedation in clinical ED practice.

EPS, extrapyramidal symptoms; LSD, lysergic acid diethylamide.

dol has also been associated with serotonin syndrome in patients taking lysergic acid diethylamide (LSD) and should be avoided in these patients.[40]

Adverse Effects. Adverse effects common to all neuroleptic agents include extrapyramidal symptoms (EPS), QTc prolongation, neuroleptic malignant syndrome (NMS), hypotension, and cholinergic blockade (see Table 71–4).

EPS include akathisia (restlessness), dystonia (muscular spasms of neck, eyes [oculogyric crisis], tongue, or jaw), drug-induced parkinsonism (muscle stiffness, shuffling gait, drooling, tremor), and tardive dyskinesia. These effects are due to the drugs' antidopaminergic action and, although bothersome, are seldom if ever life threatening. Anticholinergic agents such as diphenhydramine (25–50 mg orally [PO], IM, or IV) and benztropine (1–2 mg IM/IV) are very effective in preventing or minimizing EPS.

A potentially deadly, but exceeding rare, effect of neuroleptic drug use is prolongation of the QTc interval, leading

TABLE 71–5 Risk Factors for QTc Prolongation and Torsade de Pointes

Nonpharmacologic

- Congenital long QT syndromes
- Cardiac disorders (ventricular hypertrophy, heart failure, bradycardia)
- Electrolyte imbalance (especially hypokalemia)
- Overdose of antipsychotic drug
- Female sex
- Restraint use and psychological stress
- Substance abuse
- Miscellaneous factors
- Elderly patients
- Renal and hepatic impairment

Pharmacologic

Pharmacokinetic Factors

- Inhibition of specific cytochrome P-450 enzymes
- Competition for specific cytochrome P-450 enzymes

Pharmacodynamic Factors

- Independent QTc prolongation

TABLE 71–6 U.S. Food and Drug Administration "Black Box" Warning for Droperidol*

Cases of QT prolongation and/or torsades de pointes have been reported in patients receiving INAPSINE at doses at or below recommended doses. Some cases have occurred in patients with no known risk factors for QT prolongation and some cases have been fatal.

Due to its potential for serious proarrhythmic effects and death, INAPSINE should be reserved for use in the treatment of patients who fail to show an acceptable response to other adequate treatments, either because of insufficient effectiveness or the inability to achieve an effective dose due to intolerable adverse effects from those drugs (see package insert Warnings, Adverse Reactions, Contraindications, and Precautions).

Cases of QT prolongation and serious arrhythmias (e.g., torsades de pointes) have been reported in patients treated with INAPSINE. Based on these reports, all patients should undergo a 12-lead ECG prior to administration of INAPSINE to determine if a prolonged QT interval (i.e., QTc greater than 440 msec for males or 450 msec for females) is present. If there is a prolonged QT interval, INAPSINE should <u>NOT</u> be administered. For patients in whom the potential benefit of INAPSINE treatment is felt to outweigh the risks of potentially serious arrhythmias, ECG monitoring should be performed prior to treatment and continued for 2–3 hours after completing treatment to monitor for arrhythmias.

INAPSINE is contraindicated in patients with known or suspected QT prolongation, including patients with congenital long QT syndrome.

INAPSINE should be administered with extreme caution to patients who may be at risk for development of prolonged QT syndrome (e.g., congestive heart failure, bradycardia, use of a diuretic, cardiac hypertrophy, hypokalemia, hypomagnesemia, or administration of other drugs known to increase the QT interval). Other risk factors may include age over 65 years, alcohol abuse, and use of agents such as benzodiazepines, volatile anesthetics, and IV opiates. Droperidol should be initiated at a low dose and adjusted upward, with caution, as needed to achieve the desired effect.

*The relevance of these observations and recommendations for short-term use of such agents in the ED is unknown, and long-term or high dose use are not necessarily applicable to ED care. Droperidol is currently often used with safety and efficacy for short-term sedation in clinical ED practice.
ECG, electrocardiogram.

1327

to torsades de pointes, a polymorphic ventricular arrhythmia that can progress to ventricular fibrillation and sudden death.[3] Droperidol has been the most publicized agent associated with QTc prolongation and is currently the only neuroleptic agent that has been tagged with a "black box warning" (Table 71–6) regarding its propensity to cause QTc prolongation and sudden death.[42] In addition, a number of case reports and small case series document QTc prolongation and torsades de pointes after administration of haldol.[43] Ziprasidone has been shown to prolong the QTc interval more than all antipsychotic agents except thioridazine, but to date, it has not been associated with any cases of torsades de pointes.[43] Risk factors for QTc prolongation and torsades de pointes are listed in Table 71–5.

Symptoms of NMS include rigidity, hypertension, hyperthermia, and altered mental status. Treatment includes administration of dantrolene, cooling measures, sedation with benzodiazepines, and in severe cases, neuromuscular paralysis and endotracheal intubation.[40]

Hypotension is usually orthostatic in nature and tends to be more pronounced when the drugs are given IV. In general, haloperidol and droperidol have a lower incidence of hypotension than lower-potency neuroleptic agents. Likewise, the anticholinergic effects (e.g., confusion, dry mouth, blurred vision, urinary retention) of haloperidol and droperidol are much less severe than the lower-potency agents.

Haloperidol. Haloperidol (Haldol) is a neuroleptic and a butyrophenone (see Table 71–4). It is categorized as a high-potency neuroleptic due to its strong antidopaminergic activity. The antidopaminergic activity is responsible for both its intended effects against delusions, hallucinations, and psychomotor agitation and its unintended parkinsonian symptoms. Haloperidol has been evaluated in a large number of clinical trials alone and in combination with benzodiazepines.[44–49] *These studies demonstrate that intramuscular haloperidol is both safe and effective in the treatment of agitation caused by virtually any etiology.* Haloperidol is universally used IV, despite lack of U.S. Food and Drug Administration (FDA) approval, in the

ED for undifferentiated agitated delirium. It is usually combined with benzodiazepines.

Dosage and Administration. Haloperidol can be administered PO, IV, and IM and has a low incidence of oversedation regardless of which route is chosen.[3] The recommended dosage for rapid tranquilization in agitated patients is 5 mg IM or IV or 5 to 10 mg PO. In elderly patients, the dose should be halved. In children aged 6 to 12 years, the dosage is 1 to 3 mg IM every 4 to 8 hours with a maximum of 0.15 mg/kg/day. Children older than 12 years can receive the adult dosage. Although it is common practice, the use of intravenous haloperidol is not FDA approved. *Years of clinical experience with IV haloperidol, however, attest to its safety in standard doses required for the short-term control of agitated delirium.* IM, haloperidol has a peak clinical effect within 30 to 45 minutes and may last up to 24 hours when given for acute agitation. When given PO, its bioavailability is 60% and the onset of action is 30 to 60 minutes. Haloperidol is metabolized by the liver and excreted by the kidneys[50] (see Table 71–4).

Droperidol. Droperidol, an analogue of haloperidol, is a high-potency butyrophenone with rapid tranquilizing effects. Like haloperidol, droperidol possesses significant antidopaminergic activity (see Table 71–4). Droperidol was initially FDA approved in 1970 as an antiemetic and antipsychotic agent. Soon after, psychiatric EDs found it useful for chemical restraint.[51] Many physicians prefer droperidol to haloperidol owing to its more rapid onset and shorter duration of action.

Droperidol's use as a chemical restraint increased in popularity until 2001 when the FDA issued a "black box" warning, stating that it had the potential to cause fatal dysrhythmias (see Table 71–6).[52] This prompted many hospitals and pharmacies to restrict or prohibit its use. The black box warning sparked harsh reaction from anesthesiologists who used droperidol frequently for treating postoperative nausea[53] and emergency clinicians and psychiatrists who used it for rapid tranquilization with excellent results.[51,54] Indeed, two large retrospective studies encompassing over 15,000 patients failed to demonstrate increased morbidity or mortality with droperidol use for the treatment of acute agitation.[41,51] This controversy prompted an independent review of the data submitted to the FDA that led to the black box warning. The authors of this review found a number of anomalies and duplicate reports. *They concluded that droperidol is a safe drug when used at the recommended dosage (i.e., 5–10 mg).*[54] Despite the apparent lack of evidence behind the black box warning, the use of droperidol has declined dramatically.[55]

Studies comparing a variety of agents for rapid tranquilization found that droperidol provides more rapid and effective control than lorazepam,[56] haloperidol,[44] midazolam,[57,58] and ziprazidone.[57] In addition, droperidol has proved safe in patients with head injuries, alcohol and cocaine intoxication, and seizure disorders.[41]

Dosage and Administration. The initial dosage used for sedation is 5 mg IM or IV. There is no oral formulation. The onset of action is 3 to 10 minutes with a peak clinical effect at 30 minutes. The elimination half-life is 2 to 4 hours, but droperidol's sedative effects may last up to 12 hours[59] (see Table 71–4).

Benzodiazepines

All benzodiazepines enhance GABA neurotransmission, resulting in anxiolysis, sedation, hypnosis, and muscle relaxation. This combination makes them an excellent choice for tranquilization of agitated patients. The differences in clinical effects (e.g., onset, duration, adverse effects) are primarily related to dosage, route of administration, and pharmacokinetics. Benzodiazepines can be used alone or in combination with an antipsychotic agent. Lorazepam and midazolam are the benzodiazepines most commonly used for chemical restraint. This is likely due to their rapid and predictable absorption when given IV or IM and a long history of safe and successful ED use. Unlike the neuroleptics, benzodiazepines do not treat underlying psychiatric disorders, even when used long term. There is some support for the preferred use of intravenous diazepam because the effects and toxicity are evident sooner than other benzodiazepines, usually within 5 minutes.

Contraindications. There are few contraindications to the use of benzodiazepines as a chemical restraint. Because of the possibility of respiratory depression, use benzodiazepines with caution in patients in respiratory distress (see Table 71–4). Respiratory depression is, however, very unlikely in most patients suffering from agitated delirium, and large doses of all benzodiazepines have been safely used.

Adverse Effects. Benzodiazepines may cause respiratory depression, hypotension, oversedation, and ataxia. However, when given in the typical dose to treat agitation, these events are rare, making benzodiazepines the drugs of choice in most circumstances.

Respiratory depression is the most worrisome complication associated with benzodiazepine use. The severity of respiratory compromise is dose-dependent and greatly enhanced in the presence of ethanol or other depressive drugs, especially barbiturates.[60,61] Therefore, use benzodiazepines cautiously when treating agitated patients who have consumed alcohol or taken opiates or barbiturates. The risk of respiratory depression is also greater in the elderly and in those with COPD, but not in the doses typically used in the ED.

Hypotension is usually mild and clinically insignificant. However, benzodiazepines may cause a considerable drop in blood pressure in patients with moderate or severe dehydration or occult blood loss. Although exceedingly rare, paradoxical disinhibition may occur, especially in patients with developmental delay, organic brain syndromes, and dementia.[3] Benzodiazepines are not associated with EPS (see Table 71–4).

The best benzodiazepine to use is the one that is most familiar to the clinician. All are given in titrated amounts, preferably IV. Propylene glycol, the preservative in benzodiazepines, can elevate the osmolal gap and rarely cause metabolic acidosis when gargantuan doses are used. For some reason, patients resistant to one benzodiazepine may be sensitive to another, so changing the drug may be preferable to switching to another class.

Lorazepam. Lorazepam (Ativan) is the benzodiazepine most frequently used to treat agitation. It enjoys popularity as part of the well-established "five and two" treatment regimen, consisting of intramuscular haloperidol, 5 mg, and lorazepam, 2 mg.[62] In a number of clinical trials, lorazepam was shown to be an effective drug for rapid chemical restraint.[45,48,49,56] In these studies, lorazepam had no extrapyramidal effects and was better tolerated than neuroleptics. However, when compared with haloperidol, droperidol, midazolam, and a combination of haloperidol and lorazepam, the onset of sedation after an intramuscular dose of lorazepam is more protracted (see Table 71–4).[45,48,49,56]

Dosage and Administration. When used alone, lorazepam is usually given in 2- to 4-mg doses and can be administered PO, sublingually, IM, IV, or rectally (see Table 71–4). No maximum dose has been established. Following an intramuscular injection of lorazepam, adequate sedation is usually achieved in 30 to 45 minutes.[56] When given IV, tranquilization occurs in 15 to 20 minutes.[48,49] The elimination half-life is 12 to 15 hours, which produces a duration of effect of 8 to 10 hours. This makes lorazepam a better choice when long-term sedation is the goal. Lorazepam is rapidly conjugated to an inactive glucuronide. This does not require involvement of the cytochrome P-450 system, so lorazepam has few drug-drug interactions. The intravenous or intramuscular preparation of lorazepam must be refrigerated, thus potentially limiting its use in underdeveloped countries and in the prehospital setting.[3]

Midazolam. Midazolam (Versed) is another benzodiazepine shown to be effective for rapid tranquilization.[47,48,57,58] It differs from other benzodiazepines by virtue of its more rapid onset and shorter duration of action. Midazolam is the benzodiazepine of choice when rapid, short-term sedation is desired, whereas lorazepam is used for patients who require a longer period of restraint (see Table 71–4).

Midazolam compares favorably with haloperidol, loraze-pam, droperidol, and ziprazidone for treatment of agitation in the ED.[47,48,58] It was found to have a more rapid onset of sedation than the other drugs except droperidol, which had a similar time of onset (5–10 min). The studies also noted that midazolam, as expected, had a shorter duration of effect than the other medications. This may be advantageous in certain circumstances and undesirable in others.

Dosage and Administration. The initial dosage for an agitated adult is 5 mg IV or IM, which may be repeated at 5- to 10-minute intervals. No maximum dose has been estab-lished. Owing to first-pass metabolism, only 40% to 50% of a PO-administered dose reaches the systemic circulation, therefore twice the parenteral dose (i.e., 10 mg) should be given. It may be given nasally in oral dosing regimens. The onset of sedation occurs approximately 3 minutes after an intravenous dose, 5 minutes after an intramuscular injection, and 15 minutes after oral, nasal, or rectal administration (see Table 71–4). Midazolam is hydroxylated by the cytochrome P-450 system to its primary metabolite, α-hydroxy-mid-azolam, which undergoes glucuronide conjugation before being excreted in the urine. The duration of action is between 30 and 120 minutes and does not vary significantly by route of administration[48,63] (see Table 71–4).

Diazepam. Diazepam (Valium) has a long positive safety record for the treatment of agitated delirium, especially delir-ium tremens/alcohol withdrawal. The standard dose is 5 to 10 mg IV every 5 to 10 minutes. No maximum dose has been established and doses of 500 to 2000 mg have been safely used. Intramuscular diazepam should not be used. In about 5 to 6 minutes, the maximum effect and maximum respiratory depression of diazepam have been reached, allowing for addi-tional titrated doses.

Atypical Antipsychotic Agents

Atypical antipsychotic agents have a high affinity for 5-HT (serotonin) receptors, and less affinity for D_1 and D_2 recep-tors. As a result, they have a lower incidence of EPS than haldol and droperidol.[64] Previously, medications in this class were available only in an oral formulation, limiting their use in the management of acute agitation. Recently, intramuscu-lar formulations of ziprasidone (Geodon) and olanzapine (Zyprexa) have been developed. The combination of intra-muscular formulation and low incidence of EPS make these newer agents an attractive option for rapid tranquilization in the undifferentiated patient in the ED.

Contraindications. In 2005, a meta-analysis of placebo-controlled trials demonstrated an increased risk of death asso-ciated with atypical antipsychotic agents used to treat *elderly patients with dementia-related psychosis.*[65] This report led the FDA to issue a black box warning regarding the use of atypical antipsychotics for "behavioral disorders" in elderly patients with dementia (Table 71–7).[42] *Such warnings have not been translated into the prohibition of such agents for short-term use in the ED.* The FDA has also advised caution with ziprasidone owing to its tendency to prolong the QTc interval, especially when used in patients taking other drugs or with medical conditions that increase the risk of QTc prolongation (see Table 71–6).[65] However, the QTc interval may not be avail-able when the use of these drugs is indicated. Ziprasidone prolongs the QTc interval more frequently than haloperidol, droperidol, and olanzapine,[3] but the degree of prolongation

is generally considered minor. To date, there have been no clinical reports of adverse events due to QTc prolongation with the short-term ED use of atypical antipsychotic agents. Experience with these agents in the undifferentiated acutely delirious patient in the ED is limited, but their use is increas-ing, and initial reports are supportive but not yet definitive.

Adverse Effects. Atypical antipsychotic agents may cause somnolence, EPS (although EPS occur less often than with haldol and droperidol), QTc prolongation, and less often, anticholineric symptoms and muscle weakness.

Ziprasidone. Ziprasidone (Geodon) is a benzylisothia-zolylpiperazine antipsychotic agent whose mechanism of action remains unknown. It was the first atypical antipsychotic agent available in a fast-acting intramuscular preparation and is the only intramuscular atypical antipsychotic agent that has been studied for undifferentiated agitation in the ED. In a double-blind, randomized study, Martel and coworkers[57] noted that ziprasidone was as effective as midazolam and droperidol in controlling acute agitation. Patients receiving ziprasidone and droperidol took longer to be sedated (30 min, compared with 15 min for midazolam), but were more deeply sedated at 60 and 120 minutes.[57] In a prospective, open-label study, ED patients receiving ziprasidone had progressive improvement in anxiety, hostility, and uncooperativeness starting at 15 minutes and continuing through the 90-minute study period.[66] In an observational study of agitated psychiat-ric ED patients with nonspecific psychosis, alcohol intoxica-

---

TABLE 71–7 U.S. Food and Drug Administration "Black Box" Warning for Use of Atypical (Second-Generation) Antipsychotic Medications in Elderly Patients with Dementia*

The Food and Drug Administration has determined that the treatment of behavioral disorders in elderly patients with dementia with atypical (second-generation) antipsychotic medications is associated with increased mortality. Of a total of seventeen placebo-controlled trials performed with olanzapine (Zyprexa), aripiprazole (Abilify), risperidone (Risperdal), or quetiapine (Seroquel) in elderly demented patients with behavioral disorders, fifteen showed numerical increases in mortality in the drug-treated group compared to the placebo-treated patients. These studies enrolled a total of 5106 patients, and several analyses have demonstrated an approximately 1.6–1.7 fold increase in mortality in these studies. Examination of the specific causes of these deaths revealed that most were either due to heart-related events (e.g., heart failure, sudden death) or infections (mostly pneumonia).

The atypical antipsychotics fall into three drug classes based on their chemical structure. Because the increase in mortality was seen with atypical antipsychotic medications in all three chemical classes, the Agency has concluded that the effect is probably related to the common pharmacologic effects of all atypical antipsychotic medications, including those that have not been systematically studied in the dementia population. In addition to the drugs that were studied, the atypical antipsychotic medications include clozapine (Clozaril) and ziprasidone (Geodon). All of the atypical antipsychotics are approved for the treatment of schizophrenia. None, however, is approved for the treatment of behavioral disorders in patients with dementia.

*The relevance of these observations and recommendations for the short-term use of such agents in the ED is unknown. Such cautions and concerns extrapolated from long-term retrospective data are not necessarily applicable to their short-term use in the ED. These medications are currently often used with safety and efficacy for short-term sedation in clinical ED practice.

tion, or substance-induced psychosis, 20 mg of intramuscular ziprasidone was effective in tranquilizing patients as early as 15 minutes.[67]

Dosage and Administration. The recommended dosage of ziprasidone is 10 mg IM, which can be repeated at 2 hours, or 20 mg IM, which may be repeated at 4 hours. The drug reaches peak plasma concentrations in 30 to 45 minutes and has an elimination half-life of 2 to 4 hours. Following an intramuscular injection, sedation usually begins within 15 to 30 minutes and peaks at around 2 hours. The clinical effects usually last at least 4 hours.[68]

Olanzapine. Olanzapine (Zyprexa) is a second-generation thienobenzodiazepine antipsychotic agent that is thought to exert its effects through antagonism of both dopamine and serotonin type 2 receptors. Olanzapine has recently been approved by the FDA in an intramuscular formulation for the treatment of agitation in acutely psychotic patients. Intramuscular olanzapine has been shown to be comparable with haloperidol or lorazepam monotherapy in managing acute agitation associated with schizophrenia and dementia[46,69,70] and superior to lorazepam monotherapy in the management of agitation associated with bipolar disorder.[71] To date, there have been no clinical trials using intramuscular olanzapine in undifferentiated agitation in the ED.

Dosage and Administration. The recommended dosage for treatment of acute agitation is 10 mg IM. Additional doses may be considered 2 to 4 hours after the preceding dose with a maximum recommended dose of 30 mg/day. Olanzapine reaches peak plasma concentrations in 15 to 45 minutes and has an elimination half-life of 21 to 54 hours. The onset of sedation usually begins 15 to 30 minutes after an intramuscular injection and typically lasts at least 2 hours. In some patients, the clinical effects have lasted as long as 24 hours. The drug is metabolized via direct glucuronidation and cytochrome P-450–mediated oxidation.[72]

Ketamine. Ketamine is a widely used anesthetic. It has been used safely throughout the world for major surgery and with minimal monitoring.[73] Many clinicians are familiar with ketamine as a safe and rapidly effective dissociative anesthetic for children undergoing painful procedures in the ED, where it has become standard practice. Ketamine has no significant adverse effects on blood pressure or respirations. A ketamine-related catecholamine release supports blood pressure and promotes bronchodilatation. Minor hypertension and tachycardia may be seen. Commonly raised as a caution, there is no proven issue with ketamine causing harmful increased intracranial pressure.[74] Possible side effects of ketamine include salivation, vomiting, laryngospasm, or the emergence phenomenon consisting of short-lived bizarre thoughts and hallucinations. The co-administration of atropine or glycopyrrolate can dry secretions, and benzodiazepines may quell the emergence issues; but neither has been routinely given as adjuncts for ketamine anesthesia in the ED.

Although ketamine is not commonly used to control agitated and delirious patients, its pharmacologic profile lends itself to this use, and case reports support such a role.[75-77] Melamed and colleagues[75] reported the successful use of ketamine for the prehospital management and transport of combative trauma patients. Other case reports describe ketamine to chemically control an acutely agitated cocaine-intoxicated patient[76] and for an agitated patient bent on suicide.[77]

The dose of ketamine to produce profound dissociation is 1 to 1.5 mg/kg IV, or 4 to 5 mg/kg IM, with the intramuscular route lending itself to ED use when intravenous access

is problematic. Both routes are effective within 30 seconds (IV) to 2 to 5 minutes (IM). At the current time, the exact role of ketamine for the chemical control of the acutely agitated and delirious patient in the ED has not been clarified.

Choosing the Best Agent

The Undifferentiated Patient. The most common scenario is a patient brought to the ED with acute agitated delirium with little or no history, who must be expeditiously controlled for medical evaluation and monitoring. The safest agent has traditionally been an intravenous benzodiazepine, often with judicious doses of haloperidol. Newer atypical antipsychotics are gaining favor, but their track record is short. *Large doses of benzodiazepines seem to be the most prudent choice in such circumstances because of familiarity to clinicians and the drugs' safety record and safety profile.* There is little concern for respiratory or cardiovascular depression with the prudent use of carefully titrated intravenous benzodiazepines in the monitored setting.

Agitation Due to Alcohol and Drugs of Abuse. For patients who are obviously intoxicated with alcohol or other sedative agents, haloperidol, droperidol, or ziprasidone will provide rapid, safe, and effective tranquilization.[41,51,57] Benzodiazepines should be administered with caution to alcohol-intoxicated patients and those taking sedative agents owing to the possibility of respiratory depression.[60,61] In contrast, benzodiazepines are the *drugs of choice* in patients who are agitated due to *alcohol withdrawal.* Large doses may be required, and the safety profile is wide. Patients who are agitated owing to sympathomimetic agents such as cocaine, methamphetamines, hallucinogens such as PCP or LSD may be safely treated with large doses of benzodiazepines or butyrophenones or a combination of the two.[41,45,56] Droperidol has been associated with serotonin syndrome in patients taking LSD, and should be avoided in these patients.[40]

Agitation Due to Medical Illness. In patients who are agitated due to medical illness, treatment should be aimed at correcting the underlying pathology. If rapid tranquilization is required, typical antipsychotics or benzodiazepines should be used as first-line therapy. If the patient is frail or elderly or has known renal impairment, consider using smaller doses of a single agent.

Agitation Due to an Underlying Psychiatric Disorder. Patients with an established psychiatric history and agitation attributed to schizophrenia, schizoaffective disorder, or the manic phase of bipolar disorder may be treated with typical antipsychotic agents, atypical antipsychotic agents, or benzodiazepines. However, a growing body of evidence seems to support the use of atypical antipsychotic agents in this patient population.[46,57,66,67,69,70,76] Moreover, ziprasidone has been shown to be safe in patients with undifferentiated agitation, substance-induced psychosis, and alcohol intoxication, common findings in acutely agitated ED patients.

Agitation in Children. Owing to years of experience and a proven safety record, benzodiazepines are considered first-line therapy for the management of agitation in children. The intramuscular dose of lorazepam is 0.05 to 0.1 mg/kg and the intramuscular dose of midazolam is 0.1 to 0.2 mg/kg (see Table 71–4). Neuroleptic agents have also been used to manage agitation in children. The dose of intramuscular haloperidol is 0.025 to 0.075 mg/kg, with a maximum dose of 2.5 mg. Children older than 12 years can receive the adult dose, usually 2.5 to 5.0 mg (see Table 71–4). Although droperidol is a highly effective drug for rapid tranquilization in adults, there is a paucity of literature supporting its use in children. The pediatric dose of droperidol is 0.03 to 0.07 mg/kg with a maximum initial dose of 2.5 mg[40] (see Table 71–4). Combination therapy is generally not recommended for children.[62]

Agitation in Pregnancy. Psychotropic medications should be used during pregnancy only when the potential risk to the fetus from exposure is outweighed by the risk of the untreated maternal disorder.[78] Based on years of accumulated clinical experience, but very little scientific data, conventional antipsychotic agents such as haldol and droperidol are recommended to control agitation in pregnant women.[79] Benzodiazepine are also commonly used short term.

Agitation in the Elderly. Patients 65 years of age or older are particularly susceptible to adverse drug reactions owing to coexisting medical illness, use of multiple prescription medications (which increase the risk of drug-drug interactions), and age-associated changes in pharmacokinetics and pharmacodynamics. Research suggests that conventional antipsychotic medications such as haloperidol and droperidol are safe and effective for both psychotic symptoms and nonpsychotic agitated behavior.[80] Low doses (e.g., half the usual dose) of benzodiazepines can also be used, but require close observation for respiratory depression. Atypical antipsychotic agents should be avoided in this population owing to the risk of death associated with dementia-related psychosis.[65]

Conducted Electrical Weapons

Conducted electrical weapons (Tasers, stun guns) are used by law enforcement agencies throughout the world. These non-lethal weapons use a temporary high-voltage low-current electrical discharge to overcome the body's muscle-triggering mechanisms, resulting in widespread uncontrollable muscle contractions that incapacitate the victim. The current is delivered by direct contact with a handheld device (i.e., electric shock prods) or via a small dartlike electrode fired from a gun using small gas charges (e.g., Taser) similar to some air rifle propellants. There are also electrical weapons that cause intense pain without incapacitating the target, so-called *drive stun devices*. Law enforcement and correctional personnel typically use drive stun devices as a pain compliance technique.

Despite claims of lethality in the lay press, there are no documented immediate deaths directly caused by a Taser discharge in humans. Volunteer studies and animal models fail to provoke cardiac arrest or significant cardiorespiratory or metabolic derangements after standard electrical discharges. Although considered safe by limited scientific studies, conducted electrical weapons have been temporally linked to a number of fatalities.[81] The majority of these cases also involved drug overdoses (e.g., cocaine, methamphetamines) and/or the use of additional excessive physical force.[82] Efforts to define the actual cause of death in forensic investigations of individuals dying unexpectedly after having been shocked while in police custody, or during efforts to subdue or incapacitate, fail to show definitive causation. The role of severe sympathomimetic/drug intoxication or underlying cardiac pathology (such as clandestine catecholamine-induced cardiomyopathy) obscure the exact etiologic contribution of these electrical devices to deaths occurring in police custody. For a complete discussion of this topic, the reader is referred to the excellent text by Kroll MW and Ho JD: TASER® Conducted Electrical Weapons: Physiology, Pathology, and Law. New York: Springer Science, 2009. Because darts often penetrate the skin and must be removed, the remainder of this section focuses on the procedure for removing embedded Taser electrodes.

Taser Electronic Control Devices

Taser is an acronym for "Thomas A. Swift's Electric Rifle" and has been in existence since the early 1990s (Fig. 71–10). More than 11,000 law enforcement, correctional, and military agencies in 44 countries deploy Taser devices and many municipalities in the United States allow civilians to purchase and carry these weapons for personal protection.[83] Taser uses compressed nitrogen to propel two electrode-tipped barbs that are attached to the device by two thin wires. The barbs are similar in size to a No. 8 fishhook measuring 4 mm in length (Fig. 71–11). The barbs may attach to clothing and fail to penetrate the skin, or they may become embedded in the skin and must be removed.

Removal Techniques. Barbs embedded in soft tissues can be easily removed with direct pressure. Place one hand on the skin surrounding the barb to hold the skin taught and use the other hand to apply direct pressure to the barb[83,84] (Fig. 71–12). If the patient cannot tolerate the procedure, inject a small amount of local anesthetic near the barb and use a No. 11 scalpel to cut down through the soft tissue to the tip of the barb.[83] Owing to the small size and linear shape of the barb, there is no need to advance the barb through the skin to remove the tip as is commonly performed during the removal of fishhooks.[84] After removal, clean and dress the wound (see Chapter 35, Methods of Wound Closure), but do not suture it. Analgesics (e.g., nonsteroidal anti-inflammatory drugs, acetaminophen) may be administered.

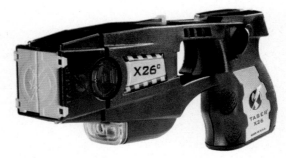

Figure 71–10 TASER electrical control device.

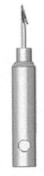

Figure 71–11 TASER electrode-tipped barb.

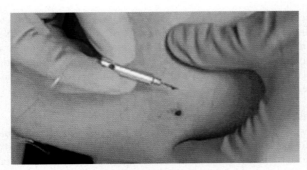

Figure 71–12 **Removal of an electrode-tipped barb.** Barbs embedded in soft tissues can be easily removed with direct pressure. Place one hand on the skin surrounding the barb to hold the skin taught and use the other hand to apply direct pressure to the barb.

After removing the barb, provide standard wound care. Advise the patient to watch for signs of infection; a 48-hour wound check may be prudent in contaminated wounds, when the barb was difficult to remove, and if there is a concern for a retained foreign body. Significant infection after barb removal is rare, and prophylactic antibiotics are unnecessary. Following removal of a TASER dart, the disposition of the patient is based on the individual real time scenario, and long-term ED observation is not required.

Complications. Owing to the small size of the barb, the risk of significant injury to the heart, lungs, or bowel from a TASER device is small. a theoretical risk of injury to vascular structures and genitalia exists, although there have been no reported cases in the literature. There have been case reports of serious intraocular and intracranial injuries resulting from a TASER barb, but these are rare.[85-87] A barb embedded in a vascular structure can probably be removed with manual traction followed by direct pressure on the wound because the size of the barb is similar to devices used to obtain central venous access.[84] Consultation with a vascular surgeon may be required in complicated cases. Severe muscle contraction from the electrical discharge has been implicated as a cause of acute thoracic compression fractures.[88]

 REFERENCES CAN BE FOUND ON EXPERT CONSULT

Commonly Used Formulas and Calculations

Brent E. Ruoff and Eric D. Katz

WEIGHT CONVERSION FROM POUNDS TO KILOGRAMS

Patients frequently express body weight in pounds, but many medical calculations require conversion to kilograms. The formulas for conversion between these two units are

$$1 \text{ kg} = 2.2 \text{ lb}$$

Example: A dehydrated child requires intravenous (IV) fluid. The clinician plans to infuse a fluid bolus of 20 mL/kg. The patient's mother states that the child weighs 35 lb. The fluid bolus is:

$$16 \text{ kg} \times 20 \text{ mL} = 320 \text{ mL}$$

TEMPERATURE CONVERSIONS FROM CELSIUS TO FAHRENHEIT

Fahrenheit (F) and Celsius (C) are the temperature units most commonly used. Table A–1 lists approximate F/C equivalents. The formulas for conversion between units are as follows:

$$°F = (°C \times 1.8) + 32$$

$$°C = (°F - 32) \times 1.8$$

Example: A mother reports her child's temperature is 104 °F. To convert to °C:

$$°C = (104°F - 32) \times 1.8 = 40°C$$

Example: A child's temperature in the emergency department (ED) is 39.6°C. His mother wants to know what the temperature is in °F. To convert to °F:

$$°F = (39.6°C \times 1.8) + 32 = 103.3°F$$

CALCULATION OF THE MEAN ARTERIAL PRESSURE

Calculation of the mean arterial pressure (MAP) provides a weighted average of the systolic blood pressure (SBP) and the diastolic blood pressure (DBP). It is a determination of tissue perfusion pressure and is normally 70 to 100 mm Hg in adults. To determine the MAP:

$$MAP = [SBP + (2 \times DBP)]/3$$

Example: An elderly, hypertensive patient is diagnosed with an acute hemorrhagic stroke. The neurologist recommends lowering the MAP to less than 130 mm Hg. The patient's current blood pressure is 210/120. To calculate the current MAP:

$$MAP = [210 + (2 \times 120)]/3 = 150 \text{ mm Hg}$$

QT AND QTC INTERVALS

The QT interval on the electrocardiogram (ECG) represents the period of ventricular electrical activity from activation to repolarization. The most important determinant of the QT interval is the heart rate. As the heart rate increases, the QT interval shortens. To calculate the rate-corrected QT interval (QTc), divide the QT interval by the square root of the R-R interval (the interval between the R on two consecutive QRS complexes). The R-R interval is calculated as 60 divided by the heart rate (in beats per minute [bpm]). The interval is represented in seconds or milliseconds:

$$QTc = QT/\sqrt{(R\text{-}R)}$$

QTc is normally less than 0.46 sec for men and 0.44 sec for women.

Table A–2 shows the normal range of the QT interval for adults.

Example: A 21-year-old man ingested a large quantity of amitriptyline (tricyclic antidepressant) tablets. His ECG reveals a QT interval of 0.37 sec and a heart rate of 120 bpm. The QTc is calculated as

$$R\text{-}R \text{ interval: } 60/120 = 0.50$$

$$QTc = 0.37/\sqrt{0.5} = 0.53 \text{ sec} = 520 \text{ msec}$$

The patient's QTc is significantly prolonged for his heart rate and indicates significant cardiac effects from a tricyclic antidepressant overdose.

Causes of prolonged QT interval are shown in Table A–3.

PREDICTED PEAK EXPIRATORY FLOW RATE

The peak expiratory flow rate (PEFR), measured in liters per minute (L/min), is a useful means of assessing airway obstruction. It is measured by having a patient exhale maximally through a peak flow meter. Normal values range from 350 to 600 L/min. A patient's prognosis in asthma exacerbations can be followed by comparing the initial and post-treatment PEFR. Patients with an initial PEFR of less than 20% predicted or with a subsequent value of less than 60% predicted after initial therapy may require further evaluation, treatment,

TABLE A–1 Approximate Fahrenheit and Celsius Equivalents

°C	°F
30	86
32	89.6
34	93.2
35	95
35.5	95.9
36	96.8
36.5	97.7
37	98.6
37.5	99.5
38	100.4
38.5	101.3
39	102.2
39.5	103.1
40	104
40.5	104.9
41	105.8

TABLE A–2 Normal Range of QT Interval for Adults

Heart Rate (bpm)	Normal QT Range (sec)
40	0.42–0.53
50	0.37–0.48
60	0.34–0.44
70	0.31–0.41
80	0.29–0.38
90	0.28–0.36
100	0.27–0.34
110	0.25–0.32
120	0.24–0.31
130	0.23–0.30
140	0.22–0.29
150	0.21–0.28

TABLE A–3 Conditions/Medications That May Cause QT Prolongation and/or Induce Torsades de Pointes

Conditions That May Cause QT Prolongation

Metabolic Abnormalities
- Hypokalemia
- Hypocalcemia
- Hypomagnesemia

Bradyarrhythmias
- Complete atrioventricular block
- Any bradyarrhythmia, even transient

Starvation
- Anorexia nervosa
- "Liquid protein" diets
- Gastroplasty and ileojejunal bypass
- Celiac disease

Nervous System Injury
- Subarachnoid hemorrhage
- Thalamic hematoma
- Right neck dissection or hematoma
- Pheochromocytoma

Medications That Can Prolong the QT Interval and/or Induce Torsades de Pointes

Antipsychotics
- Chlorpromazine*
- Haloperidol—QT, TdP
- Mesoridazine—QT, TdP
- Pimozide—QT, cases
- Quetiapine—QT
- Risperidone—QT
- Thioridazine—QT, TdP
- Ziprasidone—QT

Antiarrhythmics
- Amiodarone—QT, TdP
- Disopyramide—QT, TdP
- Dofetilide—QT, TdP
- Flecainide[†]—QT, TdP
- Ibutilide—QT, TdP
- Procainamide—QT, TdP
- Quinidine—QT, TdP
- Sotalol—QT, TdP

Antidepressants
- Amitripyline[‡]–cases
- Desipramine[‡]–cases
- Doxepin[‡]–cases
- Fluoxetine—QT, TdP
- Imipramine[‡]–cases
- Paroxetine—TdP
- Sertraline[†]—QT, TdP
- Venlafaxine—QT

Anticancer
- Arsenic Trioxide—QT, TdP, cases
- Tamoxifen—QT

Miscellaneous Cardiac
- Bepridil—QT, TdP
- Isradipine—QT
- Moexipril/hetz—QT
- Nicardipine—QT

GI stimulant
- Cisapride—QT, TdP

Antibiotics
- Clarithromycin–cases
- Erythromycin—QT, TdP
- Gatifloxacin—QT
- Levofloxacin—TdP
- Moxifloxacin—QT
- Sparfloxacin—QT, TdP

Antimigraine
- Naratriptan—QT
- Sumatriptan—QT
- Zolmitriptan—QT

Miscellaneous
- Dolasetron—QT Droperidol—QT, TdP, cases
- Fascarnet—QT
- Felbamate—TdP
- Fosphenytoin—QT
- Halofantrine—QT, TdP
- Indapamide—QT, cases
- Levomethadyl—QT
- Methadone
- Octreotide—QT
- Pentamidine—QT, TdP
- Salmeterol—QT
- Tacrolimus–cases
- Tizanidine—QT

*Nonspecific QT changes.

†Association not clear.

‡Tricyclic antidepressants used alone or in combination with drugs that prolong the QT interval may predispose patients to cardiac arrythmias.

QT, Prolongation is mentioned in the u.s. Food and Drug Administration (FDA)–approved labeling as a known action of the drug.

TdP, The FDA-approved labeling includes mention of cases or a risk of torsades de pointes.

Cases, There are case reports of TdP in the medical literature.

Reference: Drugs that prolong the Q-T interval and/or induce torsades de pointes. Available at http://www.torsades.org (ccessed September 12, 2000).

From Viskin S: Long QT syndromes and torsade de pointes. Lancet 354:1625, 1999.

or both. Many patients monitor PEFR on themselves and are able to state a personal best, which is the preferred standard for that individual. Other patients may be monitored using an estimated PEFR. PEFR is primarily based on a patient's gender, age, and height. Whereas graphs and tables are available to provide values across a range of ages and heights, PEFR can also be approximated using the following formulas:

$$\text{Adults: PEFR} = 13 \times (\text{height [inches]} - 40) + 110$$

$$\text{Children/adolescents: Female: PEFR} = \text{Height (m)} \times 5.5 - \text{Age (yr)} \times 0.03 - 1.11$$

$$\text{Male: PEFR} = \text{Height (m)} \times 6.14 - \text{Age (yr)} \times 0.043 + 0.15$$

ENDOTRACHEAL INTUBATION AND MECHANICAL VENTILATION

Patients with respiratory failure may require endotracheal intubation and mechanical ventilation in the ED. The following are guidelines for choosing the endotracheal tube (ETT) size and for calculating the initial ventilator settings.

Selecting the ETT

Adults: Select the largest diameter ETT that can be tolerated for adults. A size 7.5-mm cuffed ETT is well tolerated by most adult female patients. A size 8.0-mm cuffed ETT is well tolerated by most adult male patients.

Pediatrics: An uncuffed ETT should be used for children under the age of 8 years. A number of techniques are available for estimating the appropriate ETT size in children. The formula most commonly used is

$$\text{ETT size (mm)} = (\text{Age [yr]} + 16)/4$$

To estimate the depth of insertion for a child older than 2 years:

$$\text{Depth of insertion} = 3 \times \text{internal diameter of the ETT}$$

Determining Initial Ventilator Settings

The recommended initial ventilator settings follow. Adjustments in these ventilator settings may be made according to the patient's clinical situation:

Tidal volume (TV) = 6–12 mL/kg*
Rate = 10–12 breaths/min for adults, 16–20 breaths/min for children and 20–30 breaths/min for infants
FI_{O_2} = 50%–100% initially; reduce the FiO_2 as quickly as possible to avoid oxygen toxicity to the lungs
I:E ratio = 1:2. To allow complete exhalation, the inspiratory-to-expiratory ratio should be at least 1:2.

Example: A 6-year-old female with asthma has respiratory distress and altered mental status, requiring ETT intubation. Her weight is 20 kg. To prepare for intubation and mechanical ventilation:
ETT size (mm): (6 + 16)/4 = 5.5 ETT (uncuffed)
Depth of insertion: 3 × 5.5 = 16.5 cm
TV = 12 mL/kg × 20 kg = 240 mL
Respiratory rate = 16 breaths/min
FI_{O_2} = 100%
I:E ratio = 1:2

*Adjust tidal volume to limit inflation pressures to 30 cm H_2O or less.

RENAL FUNCTION

Creatinine clearance (Cr_{Cl}) is best calculated using a collection of urine over a 24-hour period. However, if the patient's Cr_{Cl} is in steady state (i.e., without recent change), it is possible to estimate Cr_{Cl} by using a formula that incorporates serum creatinine, weight, age, and gender:

$$Cr_{Cl} \text{ (men)} = [(140 - \text{age [yr]}) \times (\text{lean body weight [kg]})]/ [72 \times \text{serum creatinine (mg/dL)}]$$

$$Cr_{Cl} \text{ (women)} = 0.85 \times [(140 - \text{age \{yr\}}) \times (\text{lean body weight [kg]})]/[72 \times \text{serum creatinine (mg/dL)}]$$

Normal values: 74–160 mL/min
Mild renal impairment: 40–60 mL/min
Moderate renal impairment: 10–40 mL/min
Severe renal impairment: <15 mL/min (= indication for renal dialysis)

Example: A 64-year-old woman has upper abdominal tenderness. A computed tomography (CT) scan is planned, but the radiologist is concerned about the risk of IV contrast. The patient's serum creatinine is 1.8 mg/dL and she weighs 75 kg. To calculate her Cr_{Cl}:

$$Cr_{Cl} \text{ (women)} = 0.85 \times [(140 - 64)/(75 \text{ kg} \times 72)] = 37.4 \text{ mL/min}$$

The patient has moderate renal impairment.

ACID-BASE, FLUID, AND ELECTROLYTE BALANCE

The anion gap (AG) is an estimate of the amount of negatively charged (unmeasured) ions in the serum that are not bicarbonate (HCO_3^-) and chloride (Cl^-). The AG is calculated by subtracting the sum of HCO_3^- and Cl^- values from the sodium (Na^+), which is the major positive charge in the serum. Potassium (K^+) is not used in the calculation because most of the body's potassium is intracellular and there is a relatively small amount of K^+ in the serum. An elevated AG usually means that there is some unmeasured anion, toxin, or organic acid in the blood. The AG is normally 8 to 12 mmol/L:

$$AG = Na - (Cl^- + HCO_3^-) = 8\text{–}12 \text{ mmol/L}$$

An increase in the AG is usually associated with acidosis, referred to as an *anion gap acidosis*. Table A–4 lists many substances that can cause an anion gap acidosis.

Example: A suicidal young male drank an unknown amount of antifreeze. His electrolyte levels are Na^+ 144, K^+ 3.1, Cl^- 108, and HCO_3^- 14. The AG is calculated as follows:

$$AG = [144 - (108 + 14)] = 22 \text{ mmol/L}$$

The AG is abnormally elevated, presumably owing to ethylene glycol ingestion.

Calculating the Osmolal Gap

Serum osmolality can be measured in the laboratory by freezing point depression. The measured serum osmolality is normally higher than the calculated osmolality and the difference is termed the *osmolal gap* (OG). The OG is normally 5 to 10 mOsm/kg. If there is a higher gap, the osmols unaccounted for may represent methanol, ethylene glycol, isopropyl alcohol, or other solutes (Table A–5). To calculate serum osmolality (Osm_{calc}) and the OG:

TABLE A–4 Substances Associated with High Anion Gap*

Aspirin
Methanol, metformin
Uremia
Diabetic ketoacidosis
Paraldehyde, phenformin
Isoniazid, iron
Lactate (multiple causes)
Ethylene glycol
Carbon monoxide, cyanide
Alcoholic ketoacidosis
Toluene

*Follows the mnemonic A MUDPILE CAT.

TABLE A–5 The Effect of Some Solutes on Serum Osmolality

Each mg/dL Of	Increases Serum mOsm/kg By	For Each Serum mOsm/kg Increase Due To	The Corresponding mg/dL Change Is (= mol wt/10)
Methanol	0.31	Methanol	3.2
Ethanol	0.22	Ethanol	4.6
Acetone	0.17	Acetone	5.8
Isopropyl alcohol	0.17	Isopropyl alcohol	6.0
Ethylene glycol	0.16	Ethylene glycol	6.2
Glycerol	0.11	Glycerol	9.2
Mannitol	0.05	Mannitol	18.2

Adapted from Kullig K, Duffy JP, Linden CH, et al: Toxic effects of methanol, ethylene glycol and isopropyl alcohol. Top Emerg Med 6(2):16, 1984.

$$Osm_{calc} = 2 \times Na^+ + [BUN(mg/dL)/2.8] + [glucose(mg/dL)/18]$$
$$= normally\ 280\text{–}295$$

$$OG = Osm_{meas} - Osm_{calc}$$

where BUN indicates blood urea nitrogen.

Table A–5 shows the effect of some solutes on serum osmolality. In general, the increase in osmolality caused by a solute can be calculated by dividing its serum concentration by the tabulated value.

Example: An intoxicated patient has serum chemistry results as follows: Na^+ 142, K^+ 4.5, Cl^- 100, HCO_3^- 22, glucose 90, BUN 14. His ethanol level is 240 and his measured serum osmolality is 348. To calculate his serum osmolality:

$$Osm_{calc} = 2 \times 142 + (14/2.8) + (90/18) = 294$$

To evaluate for the effect of ethanol, refer to Table A–5, adding the alcohol level divided by 4.6:

$$240/4.6 = 52$$

$$Osm_{calc} = 294 + 52 = 346$$

Finally, calculate the OG:

$$OG = Osm_{meas} - Osm_{calc} = 348 - 346 = 2$$

HYPONATREMIA

Factitious hyponatremia may be due to hyperglycemia. In this hyperosmolal state, glucose tends to stay in the extracellular fluid, drawing water out of the cells and into the extracellular fluid. Serum sodium is decreased by about 1.6 mmol/L for each 100 mg/dL of excess glucose. To calculate the corrected sodium:

$$Corrected\ Na^+\ (mmol/L) = Measured\ Na^+\ (mmol/L) + [1.6 \times (measured\ glucose\ [mg/dL] - 100)/100]$$

Many laboratories automatically make this adjustment, so it is important to check with your laboratory to determine the necessity of this correction.

Example: An obtunded elderly man appears dehydrated. His sodium level is 126 mmol/L and his glucose is 1000 mg/dL.

$$Corrected\ Na^+ = 126\ mmol/L\ [1.6 \times (1000 - 100)/100]$$
$$= 126 + 14.4 = 140.4\ mmol/L$$

His corrected Na^+ suggests that he has factitious hyponatremia due to hyperglycemia.

HYPERNATREMIA

Elevation of serum sodium concentration is proportionate to free water deficit when volume is depleted. Because 60% of the adult body is water, total body free water deficit is calculated using measured Na^+, desired Na^+, and body weight in kilograms. To calculate the free water deficit:

$$Ideal\ total\ body\ water\ (TBW) = 60\% \times weight\ (kg)$$

$$Current\ TBW = (desired\ serum\ Na^+ - measured\ Na^+) \times ideal\ TBW/measured\ Na^+$$

where desired Na^+ is assumed to be 140 mmol/L.

$$Free\ water\ deficit = ideal\ TBW - current\ TBW$$

Example: An elderly man is brought to the ED in a coma. He has signs of severe dehydration. His ideal body weight is 70 kg. His serum Na^+ is 165 mmol/L. To determine his free water deficit:

$$Ideal\ TBW = 0.6 \times 70\ kg = 42\ L$$

$$Free\ water\ deficit = (165 - 140) \times 42\ L/140\ mmol/L = 7.5\ L$$

Fluid correction for hypernatremia should take place over 48 to 72 hours to avoid the potential for cerebral edema.

The following formula may be used to calculate the Na^+ deficit in hyponatremia:

$$Na^+\ deficit = 60\% \times weight\ (kg) \times (desired\ Na^+ - measured\ Na^+)$$

Symptoms related to hyponatremia are variable and the severity of symptoms should guide therapy. Sodium replacement is most commonly given as isotonic saline, which contains 154 mmol of Na^+/L. Patients who are severely symptomatic may require 3% saline solution that contains 513 mmol of Na^+/L. The volume of solution needed to replace the Na^+ deficit (in millimoles) can be calculated using the concentrations in the saline solutions listed earlier.

Example: A young man is seizing on arrival to the ED. He is known to have schizophrenia and compulsive water drinking. His Na^+ is 116 mmol/L. He weighs 65 kg. To determine his sodium deficit:

$$Na^+ \text{ deficit} = 0.6 \times 65 \text{ kg} \times (140 - 116) = 936 \text{ mmol of } Na^+$$

This amount of Na^+ deficit can be administered as approximately 6 L of isotonic saline or 1.8 L of hypertonic saline. Na^+ should be replaced very slowly to avoid the possibility of inducing central pontine myelinolysis (CPM), which results from overaggressive correction of sodium.

POTASSIUM

Serum potassium (K^+) levels change with the acid-base status. In acidemic states, K^+ moves out of cells as H^+ moves in, thus raising serum K^+ levels. In alkalemic states, K^+ moves into cells as H^+ moves out, thus lowering serum K^+ levels. The change in K^+ varies inversely with pH at the following rate:
Serum K^+ concentration increases 0.6 mmol/L for each 0.1 unit decrease in pH.
Serum K^+ concentration decreases 0.6 mmol/L for each 0.1 unit increase in pH.

Approximately 50% of serum calcium is bound to serum proteins (primarily albumin), 40% is in the free ionized state (the physiologically active form), and 10% is mixed with serum anions (phosphate, bicarbonate, citrate, and lactate). For this reason, serum calcium is lowered about 0.8 mg/dL for every decrease in albumin of 1 g/dL. To correct for decreased albumin (at levels < 4 g/dL), the following formula can be used:

$$\text{Corrected } Ca^{2+} \text{ (mg/dL)} = \text{serum } Ca^{2+} \text{ (mg/dL)} + (0.8 \times [4.0 - \text{serum albumin } \{g/dL\}])$$

Example: A malnourished man has a serum calcium level of 7.5 mg/dL and a serum albumin level of 2 g/dL. To calculate his corrected calcium level:

$$\text{Corrected } Ca^{2+} \text{ (mg/dL)} = 7.5 \text{ mg/dL} + [0.8 \times (4.0 - 2.0 \text{ g/dL})] = 9.1$$

MAINTENANCE IV FLUID RATE

To calculate maintenance IV fluids for a pediatric patient, use the following formula:
4 mL/kg/hr for the first 10 kg, plus
2 mL/kg/hr for the second 10 kg, plus
1 mL/kg/hr for each further kg

Example: A 5-year-old boy weighs 19 kg and requires maintenance IV fluids. To calculate his IV fluid rate:

4 mL/kg/hr for the first 10 kg: $4 \times 10 \text{ kg} = 40 \text{ ml/hr}$, plus

2 mL/kg/hr for the second 10 kg: $2 \times 9 \text{ kg} = 18 \text{ ml/hr}$

$$40 \text{ kg/hr} + 18 \text{ kg/hr} = 58 \text{ ml/hr}$$

BURN PATIENT FLUID RESUSCITATION

Various formulas for IV fluid resuscitation in burns have been recommended. The Parkland formula is commonly used, and is calculated as follows:

$$\text{Replacement fluid} = 4 \text{ mL} \times (\text{weight [kg]}) \times (\% \text{ body surface area [BSA] burned}).$$

Count only second- and third-degree burns in calculating BSA.

The total volume should be given in the first 24 hours with half the fluid given in the first 8 hours and the remaining half given in the next 16 hours. Clinical parameters including urine output, vital signs, and central venous pressure or pulmonary capillary wedge pressure should be monitored carefully to assess the adequacy of resuscitation.

Example: A 65-kg woman has second- and third-degree burns covering 35% of her body. To determine her anticipated 24-hour fluid resuscitation needs:

$$\text{Replacement fluid (L)} = 4 \text{ mL} \times 65 \times 0.35 = 9100 \text{ mL}$$

Half is given in the first 8 hours: 9100/2 = 4550 mL.

$$4550 \text{ mL/8 hr} = 569 \text{ mL/hr for the first 8 hr}$$

Half is given in the second 8 hours = 284 mL.
Do not forget to add maintenance fluid rates to the results of the Parkland formula.

ARTERIAL BLOOD GAS ANALYSIS

The alveolar-arterial oxygen gradient (A-a gradient) is the difference between the partial pressure of oxygen in the alveolar air (PA_{O_2}) and the arterial blood (Pao_2). It is used primarily to differentiate between hypoxia due to hypoventilation (in which the A-a gradient is normal) and hypoxia due to ventilation-perfusion mismatch (in which the A-a gradient is abnormal). In conditions in which there is abnormal oxygen exchange between the alveoli and the arterial blood, the A-a gradient will be increased.

The partial pressure of oxygen in the alveolar air (PA_{O_2}) cannot be directly sampled and is therefore calculated from the alveolar air equation. Because it is difficult to determine the actual amount of oxygen delivered to the alveoli when the patient is breathing supplemental oxygen, the equation is most accurate when the patient is breathing room air.
$PA_{O_2} = [FI_{O_2} \times (\text{barometric pressure} - PH_2O)] - Pco_2/RQ$
PA_{O_2} = partial pressure of oxygen in the alveolar air
FI_{O_2} = fraction of the inspired air that is oxygen (21% for room air)
Barometric pressure (at sea level) = 760 mm Hg
PH_2O = 47 mm Hg (partial pressure of water vapor at 37°C and sea level)
Pco_2 as measured by arterial blood gas (ABG) analysis
RQ = 0.8 (respiratory quotient, the ratio of CO_2 produced per unit of oxygen consumed)

To simplify the equation assuming sea level barometric pressure and room air:

$$PA_{O_2} = [0.21 \times (760 - 47)] - (Pco_2/0.8)$$

$$PA_{O_2} = 150 - (Pco_2/0.8)$$

To determine the A-a gradient, the partial pressure of oxygen in the arterial blood (Pao_2) (as determined by the ABG) is subtracted from the calculated partial pressure of oxygen in the alveolar air (PA_{O_2}):

$$\text{A-a gradient: } PA_{O_2} - Pao_2 = [150 - (Pco_2/0.8)] - Pao_2$$

The normal A-a gradient is less than 10 mm Hg in a young person; however, because alveolar oxygen diffusion decreases with age, an increase in the A-a gradient is expected with age. To estimate this change, use the following formula:

$$\text{Age-corrected A-a gradient} = 10 + (\text{age}/10)$$

Example: A 60-year-old man is found confused at home. He is tachypneic and diaphoretic. Oxygen saturation is 92% by pulse oximetry. A room air ABG showed pH = 7.48, Pco_2 = 27, Po_2 = 72. To calculate the A-a gradient:

$$\text{A-a gradient:} (150 - 27/0.8) - 72 = 116 - 72 = 44 \text{ mm Hg}$$

$$\text{Age adjusted A-a gradient:} 10 + 60/10 = 16$$

The A-a gradient is abnormally elevated beyond the adjustment for age, suggesting a ventilation-perfusion ($\dot{V}/\dot{Q}$) mismatch.

ACID-BASE BALANCE

Using the combination of an ABG sample and serum electrolyte levels, a patient's acid-base status can be evaluated. The following basic steps are required.

Knowledge of normal values:
Normal serum pH = 7.40
Normal Pco_2 = 40 mm Hg

First, determine the pH status. Acid-base changes are either metabolic or respiratory. Simple disturbances are categorized by examining the pH and the Pco_2 and HCO_3^- (Table A–6). If the pH is less than normal (<7.35), the patient is acidemic. If the pH is above normal (>7.45), the patient is alkalemic. If the patient is acidemic and the Pco_2 is elevated (>45 mm Hg) as a primary disorder, then respiratory acidosis is present. If the patient is alkalemic and the Pco_2 is decreased (<35 mm Hg) as a primary disorder, then respiratory alkalosis is present. If the patient is acidemic and the arterial HCO_3^- level is less than normal (<22 mm Hg) as a primary disorder, then a metabolic acidosis is present. If the patient is alkalemic and the HCO_3^- level is greater than normal (>26 mm Hg) as a primary disorder, then a metabolic alkalosis is present.

Acid-base homeostasis is normally maintained because a change in pH will normally trigger a compensatory change to minimize the pH change, although the compensation is never complete. The degree and timing of compensation are determined by the primary disturbance itself and by individual physiology. Respiratory compensation for metabolic disorders is rapid and occurs by adjusting the Pco_2. Full metabolic compensation for a respiratory disturbance requires renal adjustment of HCO_3^- and takes 3 to 5 days. The predicted compensatory responses for the primary disturbances are shown in Table A–6. It is important to remember that physiologic compensatory mechanisms may themselves be compromised or overwhelmed by the acid-base disorder (Fig. A–1).

Example 1: A 58-year-old woman has had profuse diarrhea for 1 week. Initial laboratory data include the following:
Sodium, 133 mmol/L
Potassium, 2.8 mmol/L
pH, 7.26
Chloride, 118 mmol/L
Pco_2, 13 mm Hg
HCO_3^-, 5 mmol/L
1. Acidemia is present (pH < 7.40).
2. The primary process is metabolic (HCO_3^- < 22 mmoL, and Pco_2 is not increased).
3. Compensation: In primary metabolic acidemia, the formula that checks for compensation is

$$Pco_2 = 1.3 \times \Delta HCO_3^-$$

$$Pco_2 = 1.3 \times (25 - 5) = 26 \text{ mm Hg}$$

The predicted Pco_2 is $40 - 26 = 14$

The actual Pco_2 is 13 mm Hg

Compensation is normal.

Example 2: A 74-year-old nursing home resident is admitted to the hospital with hypotension (96/70) and fever (39°C). He has had a positive urine culture for *Escherichia coli* and two positive blood cultures with the same organism. The laboratory values are as follows:
Sodium, 138 mmol/L
Potassium, 3.2 mmol/L
Chloride, 105 mmol/L
pH, 7.49
Pco_2, 25 mm Hg
HCO_3^-, 22 mmol/L
1. Alkalemia is present (pH > 7.44).
2. The primary process is respiratory (Pco_2 < 40 mm Hg and the HCO_3^- was not increased).
3. Compensation: The decrease in the Pco_2 is $40 - 25$ or 15 mm Hg. The formula for an expected decrease in HCO_3^- is 2 mmol for every 10 torr decrease in the Pco_2. In this instance, the expected decrease in HCO_3^- for the 15 mm Hg decrease in Pco_2 is 3 mmol/L, which is nearly identical to the actual decrease (i.e., $25 - 22$). Therefore, only acute respiratory alkalemia is present with normal compensation.

WINTER'S FORMULA

In a pure primary metabolic acidosis, the normal body response is a change (decrease) in the Pco_2. The expected compensation can be predicted by Winter's formula:

$$\text{Expected } Pco_2 = 1.5 \times HCO_3 + 8 \pm 2$$

Example: The HCO_3 calculated from an ABG is 10 mEq/L. In a pure metabolic acidosis the expected Pco_2 is:

$$\text{Expected } Pco_2 = 1.5 \times 10 + 8$$

$$\text{Expected } Pco_2 = 23 \text{ mm Hg (range } 21–25 \text{ mm Hg)}$$

TABLE A–6 Acidosis and Compensatory Response

Primary Disturbance	Predicted Compensatory Response
Metabolic acidosis	↓ in Pco_2 = 1.3 ×↓ in HCO_3^-
Metabolic acidosis	↑ in Pco_2 = 0.6 ×↑ in HCO_3^-
Respiratory acidosis	*Acute*: For every Pco_2 ↑ of 10 mm Hg, ↑ by 1 mmol/L
	Chronic: For every Pco_2 ↑ of 10 mm Hg, HCO_3^- ↑ by 4 mmol/L
	Acute: For every Pco_2 ↓ of 10 mm Hg, HCO_3^- ↓ by 2 mmol/L
	Chronic: For every Pco_2 ↓ of 10 mm Hg, HCO_3^- ↓ by 5 mmol/L

Adapted from Rutecki GW, Whittier FC: Acid-base interpretation. Consultant, November 1991, pp 44–59.

ACID-BASE MAP

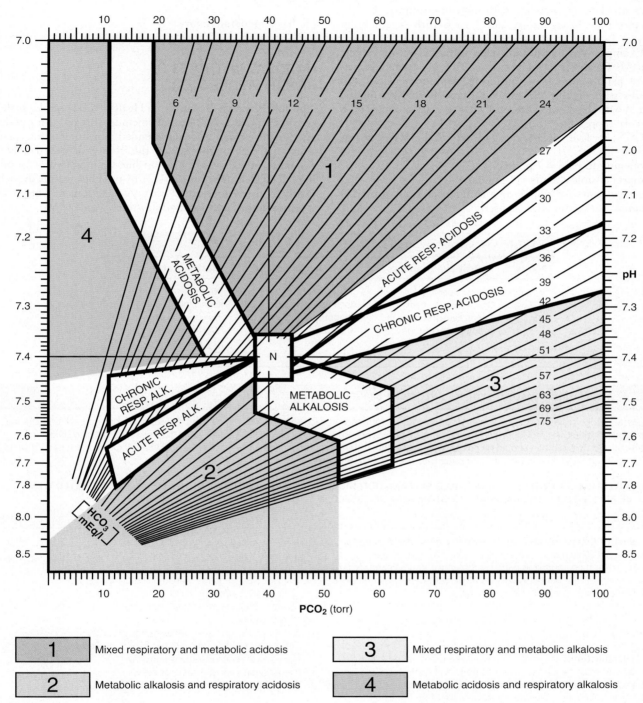

Figure A–1 Acid-base map.

	1	Mixed respiratory and metabolic acidosis		3	Mixed respiratory and metabolic alkalosis
	2	Metabolic alkalosis and respiratory acidosis		4	Metabolic acidosis and respiratory alkalosis

If the measured Pco_2 is higher than the expected Pco_2, a concomitant respiratory acidosis is also present. Normocapnia or hypercapnia in the presence of a severe metabolic acidosis may be a harbinger of impending respiratory failure, and suggest the possible need for mechanical ventilation.

A lower Pco_2 would suggest a concomitant respiratory alkalosis, such as seen in salicylate poisoning.

Another useful tool in estimating the Pco_2 in metabolic acidosis is the recognition that the Pco_2 is approximately equal to the last 2 digits of the pH. In the above example, the expected pH should be 7.23.

GLASGOW COMA SCALE

For head injured patients, the Glasgow Coma Scale (GCS) is a frequently referenced assessment of neurologic function. This is calculated using best result of neurologic testing of eye opening, motor function, and verbal function. Each of the three subscores is determined using verbal and painful stimuli. Point assessments are listed in Table A–7. It is very important to remember to use the best score in each category when assigning points. For example, a person with right-sided motor deficits but otherwise normal function would have a normal GCS because her or his left-sided function is normal. Scores of 13 to 15 correlate with mild brain injury, 9 to 12 with moderate brain injury, and 3 to 8 with severe brain injury.

Example: An intoxicated male suffers a motor vehicle crash (MVC) and is brought to your ED. He opens his eyes only to painful stimuli, is muttering incomprehensibly, and localizes pain on the left and withdraws from pain on the right. What is his GCS score, and what severity of injury does this score represent?

GCS = Eye opening + verbal response + motor response

Eye opening to pain = 2 points

Incomprehensible sounds = 2 points

Localizing pain is 5 points and withdrawal from pain is 4 points. The better score is used.

$$2 + 2 + 5 = 9 \text{ points}$$

He has a moderate injury.

NATIONAL INSTITUTES OF HEALTH STROKE SCORE

The full National Institutes of Health (NIH) stroke scale is shown in Table A–8. The scale includes directions for patient assessment as well as recommended adjustments for special situations that might impair the ability of the patient to respond to the assessor. Free on-line training (with Continuing Medical Education [CME]) to use the scale is available through the American Heart Association at: http://asa.trainingcampus.net/uas/modules/trees/windex.aspx

TABLE A–7 Glasgow Coma Scale Score

Points	Best Eye Response	Best Verbal Response	Best Motor Response
1	No eye opening	No verbal response	No motor response
2	Opens eyes to pain	Incomprehensible	Extension to pain
3	Opens eyes to command	Inappropriate words	Flexion to pain
4	Spontaneous eye opening	Confused	Withdrawal from pain
5		Orientated	Localizes pain
6			Obeys commands

TABLE A-8 National Institutes of Health Stroke Scale

Administer stroke scale items in the order listed. Record performance in each category after each subscale exam. Do not go back and change scores. Follow directions provided for each exam technique. Scores should reflect what the patient does, not what the clinician thinks the patient can do. The clinician should record answers while administering the exam and work quickly. Except where indicated, the patient should not be coached (i.e., repeated requests to patient to make a special effort).

IF ANY ITEM IS LEFT UNTESTED, A DETAILED EXPLANATION MUST BE CLEARLY WRITTEN ON THE FORM. ALL UNTESTED ITEMS WILL BE REVIEWED BY THE MEDICAL MONITOR, AND DISCUSSED WITH THE EXAMINER BY TELEPHONE.

Instructions	Scale Definition	Score
1a. Level of Consciousness: The investigator must choose a response, even if a full evaluation is prevented by such obstacles as an endotracheal tube, language barrier, orotracheal trauma/bandages. A 3 is scored only if the patient makes no movement (other than reflexive posturing) in response to noxious stimulation.	0 = Alert; keenly responsive. 1 = Not alert, but arousable by minor stimulation to obey, answer, or respond. 2 = Not alert, requires repeated stimulation to attend, or is obtunded and requires strong or painful stimulation to make movements (not stereotyped). 3 = Responds only with reflex motor or autonomic effects or totally unresponsive, flaccid, areflexic.	_____
1b. LOC Questions: The patient is asked the month and his/her age. The answer must be correct—there is no partial credit for being close. Aphasic and stuporous patients who do not comprehend the questions will score 2. Patients unable to speak because of endotracheal intubation, orotracheal trauma, severe dysarthria from any cause, language barrier or any other problem not secondary to aphasia are given a 1. It is important that only the initial answer be graded and that the examiner not "help" the patient with verbal or non-verbal cues.	0 = Answers both questions correctly. 1 = Answers one question correctly. 2 = Answers neither question correctly.	_____
1c. LOC Commands: The patient is asked to open and close the eyes and then to grip and release the non-paretic hand. Substitute another one step command if the hands cannot be used. Credit is given if an unequivocal attempt is made but not completed due to weakness. If the patient does not respond to command, the task should be demonstrated to them (pantomime) and score the result (i.e., follows none, one, or two commands). Patients with trauma, amputation, or other physical impediments should be given suitable one-step commands. Only the first attempt is scored.	0 = Performs both tasks correctly 1 = Performs one task correctly 2 = Performs neither task correctly	_____

TABLE A-8 National Institutes of Health Stroke Scale—cont'd

Instructions	Scale Definition	Score
2. Best Gaze: Only horizontal eye movements will be tested. Voluntary or reflexive (oculocephalic) eye movements will be scored but caloric testing is not done. If the patient has a conjugate deviation of the eyes that can be overcome by voluntary or reflexive activity, the score will be 1. If a patient has an isolated peripheral nerve paresis (CN III, IV or VI) score a 1. Gaze is testable in all aphasic patients. Patients with ocular trauma, bandages, pre-existing blindness or other disorder of visual acuity or fields should be tested with reflexive movements and a choice made by the investigator. Establishing eye contact and then moving about the patient from side to side will occasionally clarify the presence of a partial gaze palsy.	0 = Normal 1 = Partial gaze palsy. This score is given when gaze is abnormal in one or both eyes, but where forced deviation or total gaze paresis are not present. 2 = Forced deviation, or total gaze paresis not overcome by the oculocephalic maneuver.	_____
3. Visual: Visual fields (upper and lower quadrants) are tested by confrontation, using finger counting or visual threat as appropriate. Patient must be encouraged, but if they look at the side of the moving fingers appropriately, this can be scored as normal. If there is unilateral blindness or enucleation, visual fields in the remaining eye are scored. Score 1 only if a clear-cut asymmetry, including quadrantanopia, is found. If patient is blind from any cause, score 3. Double simultaneous stimulation is performed at this point. If there is extinction, patient receives a 1 and the results are used to answer question 11.	0 = No visual loss 1 = Partial hemianopia 2 = Complete hemianopia 3 = Bilateral hemianopia (blind including cortical blindness)	_____
4. Facial Palsy: Ask, or use pantomime to encourage, the patient to show teeth or raise eyebrows and close eyes. Score symmetry of grimace in response to noxious stimuli in the poorly responsive or non-comprehending patient. If facial trauma/bandages, orotracheal tube, tape, or other physical barrier obscures the face, these should be removed to the extent possible.	0 = Normal symmetrical movement 1 = Minor paralysis (flattened nasolabial fold, asymmetry on smiling) 2 = Partial paralysis (total or near-total paralysis of lower face) 3 = Complete paralysis of one or both sides (absence of facial movement in the upper and lower face)	_____
5 & 6. Motor Arm and Leg: The limb is placed in the appropriate position: extend the arms (palms down) 90 degrees (if sitting) or 45 degrees (if supine) and the leg 30 degrees (always tested supine). Drift is scored if the arm falls before 10 seconds or the leg before 5 seconds. The aphasic patient is encouraged using urgency in the voice and pantomime but not noxious stimulation. Each limb is tested in turn, beginning with the non-paretic arm. Only in the case of amputation or joint fusion at the shoulder or hip may the score be "9" and the examiner must clearly write the explanation for scoring as a "9."	0 = No drift, limb holds 90 (or 45) degrees for full 10 seconds. 1 = Drift, limb holds 90 (or 45) degrees, but drifts down before full 10 seconds; does not hit bed or other support. 2 = Some effort against gravity, limb cannot get to or maintain (if cued) 90 (or 45) degrees, drifts down to bed, but has some effort against gravity. 3 = No effort against gravity, limb falls. 4 = No movement 9 = Amputation, joint fusion explain: _____ **5a. Left Arm** **5b. Right Arm** 0 = No drift, leg holds 30 degrees position for full 5 seconds. 1 = Drift, leg falls by the end of the 5-second period but does not hit bed. 2 = Some effort against gravity; leg falls to bed by 5 seconds, but has some effort against gravity. 3 = No effort against gravity, leg falls to bed immediately. 4 = No movement 9 = Amputation, joint fusion explain: _____ **6a. Left Leg** **6b. Right Leg**	_____ _____ _____
7. Limb Ataxia: This item is aimed at finding evidence of a unilateral cerebellar lesion. Test with eyes open. In case of visual defect, insure testing is done in intact visual field. The finger-nose-finger and heel-shin tests are performed on both sides, and ataxia is scored only if present out of proportion to weakness. Ataxia is absent in the patient who cannot understand or is paralyzed. Only in the case of amputation or joint fusion may the item be scored "9" and the examiner must clearly write the explanation for not scoring. In case of blindness, test by touching nose from extended arm position.	0 = Absent 1 = Present in one limb 2 = Present in two limbs If present, is ataxia in Right arm 1 = Yes 2 = No 9 = Amputation or joint fusion, explain _____ Left arm 1 = Yes 2 = No 9 = Amputation or joint fusion, explain _____ Right leg 1 = Yes 2 = No 9 = Amputation or joint fusion, explain _____ Left leg 1 = Yes 2 = No 9 = Amputation or joint fusion, explain _____	_____ _____ _____

1341

Continued

TABLE A-8 National Institutes of Health Stroke Scale—cont'd

Instructions	Scale Definition	Score
8. Sensory: Sensation or grimace to pinprick when tested, or withdrawal from noxious stimulus in the obtunded or aphasic patient. Only sensory loss attributed to stroke is scored as abnormal and the examiner should test as many body areas [arms (not hands), legs, trunk, face] as needed to accurately check for hemisensory loss. A score of 2, "severe or total," should only be given when a severe or total loss of sensation can be clearly demonstrated. Stuporous and aphasic patients will therefore probably score 1 or 0. The patient with brainstem stroke who has bilateral loss of sensation is scored 2. If the patient does not respond and is quadriplegic score 2. Patients in coma (item 1a = 3) are arbitrarily given a 2 on this item.	0 = Normal; no sensory loss. 1 = Mild to moderate sensory loss; patient feels pinprick is less sharp or is dull on the affected side; or there is a loss of superficial pain with pinprick but patient is aware he/she is being touched. 2 = Severe to total sensory loss; patient is not aware of being touched in the face, arm, and leg.	_____
9. Best Language: A great deal of information about comprehension will be obtained during the preceding sections of the examination. The patient is asked to describe what is happening in the attached picture, to name the items on the attached naming sheet, and to read from the attached list of sentences. Comprehension is judged from responses here as well as to all of the commands in the preceding general neurological exam. If visual loss interferes with the tests, ask the patient to identify objects placed in the hand, repeat, and produce speech. The intubated patient should be asked to write. The patient in coma (question 1a = 3) will arbitrarily score 3 on this item. The examiner must choose a score in the patient with stupor or limited cooperation but a score of 3 should be used only if the patient is mute and follows no one step commands.	0 = No aphasia, normal 1 = Mild to moderate aphasia; some obvious loss of fluency or facility of comprehension, without significant limitation on ideas expressed or form of expression. Reduction of speech and/or comprehension, however, makes conversation about provided material difficult or impossible. For example, in conversation about provided materials examiner can identify picture or naming card from patient's response. 2 = Severe aphasia; all communication is through fragmentary expression; great need for inference, questioning, and guessing by the listener. Range of information that can be exchanged is limited; listener carries burden of communication. Examiner cannot identify materials provided from patient response. 3 = Mute, global aphasia; no usable speech or auditory comprehension.	_____
10. Dysarthria: If patient is thought to be normal, an adequate sample of speech must be obtained by asking patient to read or repeat words from the attached list. If the patient has severe aphasia, the clarity of articulation of spontaneous speech can be rated. Only if the patient is intubated or has other physical barrier to producing speech, may the item be scored "9," and the examiner must clearly write an explanation for not scoring. Do not tell the patient why he/she is being tested.	0 = Normal 1 = Mild to moderate; patient slurs at least some words and, at worst, can be understood with some difficulty. 2 = Severe; patient's speech is so slurred as to be unintelligible in the absence of or out of proportion to any dysphasia, or is mute/anarthric. 9 = Intubated or other physical barrier, explain _____	_____
11. Extinction and Inattention (formerly Neglect): Sufficient information to identify neglect may be obtained during the prior testing. If the patient has a severe visual loss preventing visual double simultaneous stimulation, and the cutaneous stimuli are normal, the score is normal. If the patient has aphasia but does appear to attend to both sides, the score is normal. The presence of visual spatial neglect or anosagnosia may also be taken as evidence of abnormality. Since the abnormality is scored only if present, the item is never untestable. Additional item, not a part of the NIH Stroke Scale score.	0 = No abnormality. 1 = Visual, tactile, auditory, spatial, or personal inattention or extinction to bilateral simultaneous stimulation in one of the sensory modalities. 2 = Profound hemi-inattention or hemi-inattention to more than one modality. Does not recognize own hand or orients to only one side of space.	_____
A. Distal Motor Function: The patient's hand is held up at the forearm by the examiner and patient is asked to extend his/her fingers as much as possible. If the patient can't or doesn't extend the fingers the examiner places the fingers in full extension and observes for any flexion movement for 5 seconds. The patient's first attempts only are graded. Repetition of the instructions or of the testing is prohibited.	0 = Normal (No flexion after 5 seconds) 1 = At least some extension after 5 seconds, but not fully extended. Any movement of the fingers which is not command is not scored. 2 = No voluntary extension after 5 seconds. Movements of the fingers at another time are not scored. **a. Left Arm** **b. Right Arm**	_____ _____

TABLE A–9 Definitions of Commonly Used Epidemiologic Terms

Prevalence	$= (a + c)/(a + b + c + d)$	= incidence of disease in population tested
Sensitivity	$= a/(a + c)$	= probability of positive test result, disease present
Specificity	$= d/(b + d)$	= probability of negative test result, disease absent
False-negative rate	$= c/(a + c)$	= probability of negative test result, disease present
False-positive rate	$= b/(b + d)$	= probability of positive test result, disease absent
Positive predictive value	$= a/(a + b)$	= probability of disease presence, test positive
Negative predictive value	$= d/(c + d)$	= probability of disease absence, test negative
Overall accuracy	$= (a + d)/(a + b + c + d)$	= probability of a "true" test result

Test Result	Disease State		
	Present	**Absent**	
Positive	a (true positive)	b (false positive)	a + b = all positive tests
Negative	c (false negative)	d (true negative)	c + d = all negative tests
	a + c = all patients with disease	b + d = all patients without disease	a + b + c + d = all patients tested

Modified from Goldman L: Quantitative aspects of clinical reasoning. In Isselbacher KJ, Braunwald E, Wilson JD (eds): Harrison's Principles of Internal Medicine, 13th ed. New York, McGraw-Hill, 1994, p 44.

The scale itself, in unedited format, is listed in Table A–8. Scores range from zero (normal neurologic function) to 34 (maximal injury). Thrombolytic use has been suggested for patients with scores between 8 and 26, who have no contraindications and who can receive the intervention within 3 hours of symptom onset.

Example: A 74-year-old, left-handed woman presents to the ED 90 minutes after the onset of left-sided arm and leg weakness. She has no headache. By 2 hours from symptom onset, she has a normal head CT (read by the neuroradiologist) and does not have contraindications to thrombolytics. Her symptoms have not changed in any way since onset. In consultation with the neurologist, you feel she may be a candidate for thrombolysis and apply the NIH stroke scale. On cognitive testing, you find that she is keenly responsive (0 points), knows her age and the current month (0 points), and can follow two-step commands with the unaffected side (0 points). She has a partial gaze palsy without forced deviation (1 point); partial hemianopsia (1 point); unilateral, complete paralysis of the face (3 points); no drift on the right arm (0 points); no movement of the left arm (4 points); no drift on the right leg (0 points); and some effort of the left leg against gravity, although it falls to the bed within 2 seconds of elevation (2 points). She has no ataxia (0 points). Her sensation to pinprick is decreased, although she is aware of the testing (1 point). She has a mild expressive aphasia but is easily comprehensible (1 point); and some slurring of words, but is still comprehensible (1 point); and no evidence of neglect (0 points). Her total NIH score is 14, and she may receive thrombolytic therapy.

DIAGNOSTIC PROBABILITY

The probability of obtaining a certain test result, in the presence or absence of a particular disease entity, for a given population with a given disease prevalence is presented in Table A–9.

No medical test is totally accurate. The parameters listed in Table A–9, when available, can help guide a clinician's test selection. When this information is not available, it may be difficult to identify random laboratory errors or detection failures. Knowledge of disease prevalence, combined with the sensitivity and specificity of the test, yields the positive (or negative) predictive value of that test. For a given sensitivity and specificity, predictive value is directly proportional to prevalence. Hence, even a test with high sensitivity and specificity may not detect a rare disease. This underscores the importance of pretest clinical evaluation.

Acknowledgment

The editors and authors wish to acknowledge the contributions of M. John Mendelsohn to this Appendix in previous editions.

Note: Page numbers followed by f refer to figures; page numbers followed by t refer to tables; page numbers followed by b refer to boxes.

1353